Imaging of the Musculoskeletal System

Imaging of the Musculoskeletal System

Volume II

Thomas Lee Pope, Jr, MD, FACR

Professor of Radiology and Orthopaedics
Medical University of South Carolina
Charleston, South Carolina

Hans L. Bloem, MD, PhD

Chairman and Professor of Radiology
Leiden University Medical Center
Leiden, The Netherlands

Javier Beltran, MD, FACR

Clinical Professor of Radiology
Mount Sinai School of Medicine
Chairman, Department of Radiology
Maimonides Medical Center
New York, New York
Director of Medical Education
Franklin & Seidelmann, Inc., Subspecialty Radiology
Beachwood, Ohio

William Brian Morrison, MD

Associate Professor of Radiology
Thomas Jefferson University
Director, Division of Musculoskeletal and General Diagnostic Radiology
Thomas Jefferson University Hospital
Philadelphia, Pennsylvania

David John Wilson, MBBS, FRCP, FRCR, MFSEM

Consultant Musculoskeletal Radiologist
Nuffield Orthopaedic Centre
and Oxford Radcliffe Hospital
Senior Clinical Lecturer
University of Oxford
Oxford, United Kingdom

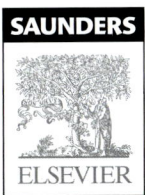

SAUNDERS

ELSEVIER

SAUNDERS
ELSEVIER

1600 John F. Kennedy Blvd.
Ste 1800
Philadelphia, PA 19103-2899

Imaging of the Musculoskeletal System ISBN: 978-1-4160-2963-2

Notice

Knowledge and best practice in this field are constantly changing. As new research and experience broaden our knowledge, changes in practice, treatment and drug therapy may become necessary or appropriate. Readers are advised to check the most current information provided (i) on procedures featured or (ii) by the manufacturer of each product to be administered, to verify the recommended dose or formula, the method and duration of administration, and contraindications. It is the responsibility of the practitioner, relying on their own experience and knowledge of the patient, to make diagnoses, to determine dosages and the best treatment for each individual patient, and to take all appropriate safety precautions. To the fullest extent of the law, neither the Publisher nor the Editors assume any liability for any injury and/or damage to persons or property arising out of or related to any use of the material contained in this book.

The Publisher

Library of Congress Cataloging-in-Publication Data

Imaging of the musculoskeletal system / [edited by] Thomas Lee Pope Jr., [et al.]. 1st ed.
  p. ; cm.
ISBN 978-1-4160-2963-2
  1. Musculoskeletal system—Imaging. I. Pope, Thomas Lee.
  [DNLM: 1. Musculoskeletal Diseases—diagnosis. 2. Diagnostic Imaging—methods.
  3. Musculoskeletal System—injuries. WE 141 I305 2008]
RC925.7.I4356 2008
616.7 0754—dc22   2007000890

Acquisitions Editor: Judith Fletcher
Developmental Editor: Jennifer Shreiner
Publishing Services Manager: Tina Rebane
Project Manager: Norm Stellander
Design Direction: Steve Stave

Printed in China

Last digit is the print number: 9 8 7 6 5 4 3 2 1

Contributors

Faustino Abascal, MD
Radiologist, Department of Radiology, Clínica Mompía, Cantabria, Spain
17 Soft Tissue Injuries of the Hand and Wrist

Judith E. Adams, MBBS, FRCP, FRCR
Professor of Diagnostic Radiology, Imaging Science and Biomedical Engineering, University of Manchester; Honorary Consultant Radiologist, Clinical Radiology, Manchester Royal Infirmary; Central Manchester and Manchester Children's University NHS Trust, Manchester, United Kingdom
75 Osteoporosis

Joong Mo Ahn, MD
Associate Professor, Department of Radiology, University of Iowa, Carver College of Medicine, Iowa City, Iowa
38 Stress Injury

Jorge Albareda, MD
Associate Professor, Faculty of Medicine, University of Zaragoza; Adjunct Medical Specialist in Trauma and Orthopaedic Surgery, Department of Trauma and Orthopaedic Surgery, University Hospital "Lozano Blesa," Zaragoza, Spain
20 Acute Osseous Injury to the Hip and Proximal Femur

Gina M. Allen, BM, DCH, MRCGP, MRCP, FRCR, MFSEM
Consultant, Department of Radiology, University Hospitals, Birmingham, United Kingdom
71 Hemophilia and Related Disorders; 89 The Patient with a Soft Tissue Lump

Arash Anavim, MD
Assistant Clinical Professor and Residency Program Director, Radiological Sciences, University of California, Irvine, Orange, California
CD-8 Discography

Mark W. Anderson, MD
Associate Professor of Radiology and Clinical Orthopaedic Surgery, Department of Radiology, University of Virginia, Charlottesville, Virginia
CD-2 Normal Variants

Suzanne E. Anderson, MD, PD
Honorary Professor, Musculoskeletal Radiology, Department of Diagnostic, Pediatric, and Interventional Radiology, University of Bern, Inselspital, Bern, Switzerland; Associate Professor, Department of Radiology, Royal Melbourne Hospital; Associate Professor, Department of Medicine, University of Melbourne, Melbourne, Australia
40 Complications of Osseous Trauma

Francisco Aparisi, MD, PhD
Associate Professor of Radiology, Department of Fisiotherapy, Universidad Cardenal Herrera; Chief of Musculoskeletal Radiology, Department of Radiology, University Hospital La Fe, Valencia, Spain
18 Pelvis-Hip: Technical Aspects, Normal Anatomy, Common Variants, and Basic Biomechanics; 19 Acute Osseous Injury to the Pelvis and Acetabulum

Pilar Aparisi, MD
Department of Radiology, Hospital de la Ribera, Alzira, Valencia, Spain
19 Acute Osseous Injury to the Pelvis and Acetabulum

Derek R. Armfield, MD, MS
Chairperson, Radiology, Jefferson Regional Medical Center, Pittsburgh, Pennsylvania
108 The Postoperative Hip

Bridget Atkins, MD
Consultant Physician, Bone Infection Unit, Nuffield Orthopaedic Centre NHS Trust, Oxford, United Kingdom
61 Soft Tissue Disease: Cellulitis, Pyomyositis, Abscess, Septic Arthritis

Lisa O. Ballehr, DO
National Orthopedic Imaging Associates, and
Arizona Advanced Imaging Center—Medical
Division, Novato, California

*28 Ankle/Foot: Technical Aspects, Normal Anatomy, Common
Variants, and Basic Biomechanics*

Romulo Baltazar, MD
Resident, Department of Radiology, Maimonides
Medical Center, Brooklyn, New York

87 Drug-Related Bone and Soft Tissue Disorders

Laura W. Bancroft, MD
Associate Professor and Consultant,
Department of Radiology, Mayo Clinic College of
Medicine; Radiologist, Department of Radiology,
St. Luke's Hospital, Jacksonville, Florida

64 Complications of Infection

Michelle S. Barr, MD
Associate Professor of Radiology, Department of Radiology,
University of Virginia, Charlottesville, Virginia

CD-7 Spinal Injections

D. Barron, MD
Consultant Musculoskeletal Radiologist, Department
of Radiology, Leeds Teaching Hospitals Trust, Leeds,
United Kingdom

36 Lower Extremity Injuries in Children (Including Sports Injuries)

Andrea Baur-Melnyk, MD
Associate Professor, Department of Clinical Radiology,
University of Munich, Munich, Germany

91 Myeloma

Francesca Beaman, MD
Director, Musculoskeletal Imaging Section,
Center Radiology, P.C., Washington Hospital Center,
Washington, DC

64 Complications of Infection

Javier Beltran, MD, FACR
Clinical Professor of Radiology,
Mount Sinai School of Medicine, New York, New York;
Chairman, Department of Radiology, Maimonides
Medical Center, Brooklyn, New York; Director of
Medical Education, Virtual Subspecialty Radiology,
Franklin & Seidelmann, Inc., Beachwood, Ohio

*6 Normal Shoulder; 10 Normal Elbow; 12 Soft Tissue Injury to the Elbow;
87 Drug-Related Bone and Soft Tissue Disorders;
CD-A6: Compressive and Entrapment Neuropathies of the
Upper and Lower Extremities*

Luis S. Beltran, MD
Resident, Thomas Jefferson University, Philadelphia,
Pennsylvania

*86 Tuberous Sclerosis; CD-A6 Compressive and Entrapment
Neuropathies of the Upper and Lower Extremities*

Jenny T. Bencardino, MD
Associate Professor of Radiology,
Department of Radiology,
New York University School of Medicine;
Director of Clinical Musculoskeletal MRI,
Hospital for Joint Diseases,
New York, New York

12 Soft-Tissue Injury to the Elbow

Thomas H. Berquist, MD, FACR
Professor of Diagnostic Radiology, Mayo Clinic College
of Medicine, Mayo Clinic Jacksonville, Jacksonville,
Florida

33 Acute Osseous Injury to the Foot

M. Biervliet, MD
Clinical Geneticist, Center of Medical Genetics,
University Hospital Antwerp, Antwerp, Belgium

82 Marfan Syndrome

Donna G. Blankenbaker, MD
Associate Professor, Department of Radiology,
Musculoskeletal Division, University of Wisconsin
School of Medicine and Public Health, Madison,
Wisconsin

4 Cervical Spine Injuries

Hans L. Bloem, MD, PhD
Chairman and Professor of Radiology,
Department of Radiology, Leiden University Medical
Center, Leiden, The Netherlands

*62 Infection in the Appendicular Skeleton (Including Chronic Osteomyelitis);
88 The Patient with a Tumor or Tumor-like Lesion of Bone;
98 Staging Bone and Soft Tissue Tumors; 99 Monitoring Therapy
in Bone and Soft Tissue Tumors*

Marcy B. Bolster, MD
Associate Professor of Medicine, Department of
Internal Medicine, Division of Rheumatology and
Immunology, Medical University of South Carolina,
Charleston, South Carolina

46 Rheumatoid Arthritis

Peyman Borghei, MD
Research Fellow, Diagnostic Radiology,
University of California Irvine Medical Center,
Orange, California

CD-8 Discography

Robert Downey Boutin, MD
Chief, Musculoskeletal Imaging, and Medical Director,
MedTel, Davis, California

41 Muscle Injury and Sequelae

Patrick A. Brouwer, MD, MSc
Interventional Neuroradiologist, Department of
Radiology, Leiden University Medical Center,
Leiden, The Netherlands

CD-10 Percutaneous Intradiscal Therapies

Ángel Bueno, MD
Jefe De Unidad, Diagnóstico por Imagen, Fundación Hospital Alcorcón, Alcorcón, Madrid, Spain
CD-A3: Fractures with Names

Michele Calleja, MD, FRCR
Department of Musculoskeletal Radiology, Nuffield Orthopaedic Centre, Oxford; Department of Radiology, Horton Hospital and Capio Orthopaedic Treatment Centre, Banbury, Oxfordshire, United Kingdom
102 Coalitions

Ana Canga, MD
Radiology Department, Hospital Universitario Marqués de Valdecilla, Santander, Spain
17 Soft Tissue Injuries of the Hand and Wrist

Victor N. Cassar-Pullicino, MD, LRCP, MRCS, DMRD, FRCR, FSEM (UK)
Department of Radiology, The Robert Jones and Agnes Hunt Orthopaedic Hospital, Oswestry, Shropshire, United Kingdom
63 Spinal Infection

Conrado F. A. Cavalcanti, MD
Department of Radiology, University of São Paolo School of Medicine, Hospital das Clinicas – INRAD; Department of Radiology, Hospital Sirio-Libanes, São Paolo, Brazil
42 Complex Regional Pain Syndrome

Luis Cerezal, MD
Chairman, Department of Radiology, Clínica Mompía, Santander, Spain
17 Soft Tissue Injuries of the Hand and Wrist; 32 Soft Tissue Injury to the Ankle: Osteochondral Injury and Impingement

Patrick Chastanet, MD
Service de Radiologie Ostéoarticulaire, Hopital Roger Salengro, Lille, France
CD-4 Percutaneous Biopsy of the Appendicular Skeleton; CD-5 Percutaneous Biopsy of the Spine

Qi Chen, MD
Attending Radiologist, Department of Radiology, Maimonides Medical Center, Brooklyn, New York
6 Normal Shoulder

Yvonne Y. Cheung, MD
Assistant Professor, Department of Radiology, Dartmouth Hitchcock Medical School; Attending Radiologist, Dartmouth Hitchcock Medical Center, Lebanon, New Hampshire
30 Soft Tissue Injury to the Ankle: Ligaments

Aaron Cho
Radiology, Naval Medical Center Portsmouth, Portsmouth, Virginia
CD A2 Orthopedic Devices

Christine B. Chung, MD
Associate Professor of Radiology, University of California School of Medicine, San Diego; Associate Professor of Radiology, Veterans Affairs Medical Center, San Diego, California
107 The Postoperative Elbow, Wrist, and Hand

Claire Coggins, MD
Assistant Professor, Department of Radiology, Virginia Commonwealth University Health System, Richmond, Virginia
56 Ochronosis; 57 Diffuse Idiopathic Skeletal Hyperostosis and Ossification of the Posterior Longitudinal Ligament

Anne Cotten, MD
Professor and Head, Department of Musculoskeletal Radiology, Hopital Roger Salengro, Lille, France
CD-4 Percutaneous Biopsy of the Appendicular Skeleton; CD-5 Percutaneous Biopsy of the Spine

Winnie Courtens, MD
Professor of Genetics, Université Catholique de Louvain, Brussels, Belgium
100 Focal Growth Disturbances

Christian Czerny, MD
Department of Radiology, General Hospital and Medical University of Vienna, Vienna, Austria
21 Internal Derangements of the Hip and Proximal Femur (Including Intra- and Extra-articular Snapping Hip)

Richard H. Daffner, MD, FACR
Professor of Radiologic Sciences, Drexel University College of Medicine, Philadelphia, Pennsylvania; Director, Division of Musculoskeletal Trauma and Emergency Imaging, Diagnostic Radiology, Allegheny General Hospital, Pittsburgh, Pennsylvania
4 Cervical Spine Injuries

A. Mark Davies, MD, FRCR
Consultant Radiologist, Department of Radiology, Royal Orthopaedic Hospital, Birmingham, United Kingdom
90 Primary Bone Tumors; 92 Tumor-like Lesion of Bone

Kirkland W. Davis, MD
Associate Professor, Department of Radiology, University of Wisconsin School of Medicine, Madison, Wisconsin
4 Cervical Spine Injuries; 105 General Principles of Fixation, Fusion, and Joint Replacement

José Luis del Cura, MD, PhD
Associate Professor, Surgery, Radiology and Physical Medicine, Basque Country University, and Department of Radiology, Hospital de Basurto-Basurtoko Ospitalea, Bilbao, Spain
CD-A1: Measurements Most Frequently Used in Orthopedic Imaging

Bradley N. Delman, MD
Assistant Professor, Department of Radiology, The Mount Sinai School of Medicine of New York University, New York, New York
2 Imaging of Facial and Skull Trauma

Michel O. De Maeseneer, MD
Division of Radiologic Sciences, Wake Forest University, Winston-Salem, North Carolina
22 Knee: Technical Aspects, Normal Anatomy, Common Variants, and Basic Biomechanics

Arthur M. De Schepper, MD, PhD
Emeritus Professor, Department of Radiology, University Hospital, Antwerp, Belgium; Emeritus Consultant Professor, Department of Radiology, Leiden University Medical Centre, Leiden, The Netherlands
93 Soft Tissue Tumors; 94 Tumor-like Soft Tissue Lesions

Sachin Dheer, MD
Associate Radiologist, Regional Diagnostic Imaging, LLC; Attending Physician, South Jersey Regional Medical Center, Vineland, New Jersey
58 Gout

Rodrigo Dominguez, MD
Clinical Professor of Radiology, Mount Sinai School of Medicine of New York University, New York, New York; Chief of Pediatric Radiology, Maimonides Medical Center, Brooklyn, New York
78 Pituitary and Thyroid Disorders; 80 Storage Diseases (Mucopolysaccharidoses/Glycogenoses)

Davide Donati, MD
Professor of Orthopaedics, University of Bologna; Director of the Laboratory of Bone Tissue Regeneration, Musculoskeletal Oncology, Istituto Ortopedico Rizzoli, Bologna, Italy
97 Treatment Strategies for Musculoskeletal Tumors and Tumor-like Lesions

A. Bassem Elaini, MD
Clinical Associate, Department of Radiology, Harvard Medical School and Massachusetts General Hospital, Boston, Massachusetts
29 Acute Osseous Injury to the Ankle

Georges Y. El-Khoury, MD
Associate Professor, Department of Radiology, Orthopedics and Rehabilitation, University of Iowa, Carver College of Medicine, Iowa City, Iowa
38 Stress Injury

Chris Fang, MD
Musculoskeletal Radiology Fellow, Department of Radiology, Nuffield Orthopaedic Centre, Oxford, United Kingdom
71 Hemophilia and Related Disorders

J. Farrant, MD
Consultant Radiologist, Department of Clinical Radiology, The Royal Free Hospital, London, United Kingdom
36 Lower Extremity Injuries in Children (Including Sports Injuries)

Laura M. Fayad, MD
Assistant Professor of Radiology and Orthopaedic Surgery, The Russel H. Morgan Department of Radiology and Radiologic Science, The Johns Hopkins University, Baltimore, Maryland
111 Imaging of the Residual Limb after Amputation

Pilar Ferrer, MD
Staff, Radiology Department, Universidad Católica de Valencia, Valencia; Staff, Radiology Department, Hospital Universitario de la Ribera, and Chief of Radiology Services, Radiology Department, Clinica Tecma, Alzira, Spain
18 Pelvis-Hip: Technical Aspects, Normal Anatomy, Common Variants, and Basic Biomechanics

Steven Finden, MD, DDS
Assistant Professor, Department of Radiology, Thomas Jefferson University Hospital, Philadelphia, Pennsylvania
3 Temporomandibular Joint

Donald J. Flemming, MD
Associate Professor, Department of Radiology, Penn State Milton S. Hershey Medical Center, Hershey, Pennsylvania
41 Muscle Injury and Sequelae; 96 Metastatic Disease

Jürgen Freyschmidt, MD
Professor, Consulting Center for Skeletal Radiology, Central Hospital Bremen-Mitte, Bremen, Germany
47 Psoriatic Arthritis and Psoriatic Spondylarthropathy; 50 Progressive Scleroderma

Michael S. Gibson, MD
Assistant Professor of Radiology/Radiological Sciences, F. Edward Hébert School of Medicine, Uniformed Services University of the Health Sciences; Section Chief, Musculoskeletal Radiology, Department of Radiology, National Naval Medical Center, Bethesda, Maryland
77 Amyloidosis; 84 Hypertrophic Osteoarthropathy; 95 Tumoral Calcinosis

Louis A. Gilula, MD
Professor of Radiology, Musculoskeletal Radiology, Washington University School of Medicine, St. Louis, Missouri
13 The Normal Wrist

Angela Gessner Gopez, MD
Assistant Professor of Radiology, Department of Radiology, Jefferson Medical College, Thomas Jefferson University Hospital, Philadelphia, Pennsylvania
CD-A2: Orthopedic Devices

Punita Gupta, MD
Clinical Instructor, Department of Radiology, Mallinckrodt Institute of Radiology, SCOH Radiological, Inc., St. Louis, Missouri
13 The Normal Wrist

Andrew Haims, MD
Associate Professor, Department of Radiology, Yale University School of Medicine, New Haven, Connecticut

15 Internal Derangement of the Wrist

John H. Harris, Jr., MD, DSc
Professor Emeritus, Department of Diagnostic and Interventional Radiology, University of Texas–Houston Medical School, Houston, Texas

1 Introduction and General Principles

Curtis W. Hayes, MD, FACR
Professor of Radiology and Orthopedic Surgery, Department of Radiology, Virginia Commonwealth University School of Medicine, Richmond, Virginia

56 Ochronosis; 57 Diffuse Idiopathic Skeletal Hyperostosis and Ossification of the Posterior Longitudinal Ligament

Tamara Miner Haygood, MD, PhD
Assistant Professor, Department of Diagnostic Radiology, The University of Texas M.D. Anderson Cancer Center, Houston, Texas

39 Radiation Effects in the Musculoskeletal System

Victoria Higueras, MD
Department of Radiology, Hospital de la Ribera, Alzira, Valencia, Spain

19 Acute Osseous Injury to the Pelvis and Acetabulum

Siegfried Hofmann, MD
Associate Professor of Orthopedic Surgery, Head Joint Reconstruction, General and Orthopedic Hospital Stolzalpe, Stolzalpe, Austria

21 Internal Derangement of the Hip and Proximal Femur (Including Intra- and Extra-articular Snapping Hip)

Peter A. Hrehorovich, MD
Attending Radiologist, Radiology Department, Florida Hospital, Sebring, Florida

14 Acute Osseous Injury to the Wrist; 16 Acute Osseous Trauma to the Hand

Ana M. Hualde, MD
Medico Adjunto Especialista en Traumatología y Cirugía Ortopédica, Servicio de Tramatología y Cirugía Ortopédica, Hospital Clínico Universitario "Lozano Blesa," Zaragoza, Spain

20 Acute Osseous Injury to the Hip and Proximal Femur

Wouter C. J. Huysse, MD
Department of Radiology, Gent University, Gent, Belgium

27 Internal Derangement of the Knee: Cartilage and Osteochondral Injuries

Hakan Ilaslan, MD
Assistant Professor, Department of Radiology, Cleveland Clinic Lerner College of Medicine; Staff, Department of Radiology, Cleveland Clinic, Cleveland, Ohio

85 Sarcoidosis

Karsten Jablonka, MD
Department of Pediatric Radiology, University of Giessen, Giessen, Germany; Head of the Department, Pediatric Radiology, Klinikum Bremen-Mitte, Bremen, Germany

47 Psoriatic Arthritis and Psoriatic Spondylarthropathy; 50 Progressive Scleroderma

Bryan T. Jennings, MD
Staff Radiologist, Radiology Associates, P.A., Little Rock, Arkansas

77 Amyloidosis; 95 Tumoral Calcinosis

Ann M. Johnson, MD
Assistant Professor of Clinical Radiology, Department of Radiology, University of Pennsylvania Medical School; Head of Body MRI, Department of Radiology, Children's Hospital of Philadelphia, Philadelphia, Pennsylvania

35 Upper Extremity Injuries in Children (Including Sports Injuries)

Karl Johnson, MD
Consultant Radiologist, Department of Radiology, Birmingham Children's Hospital, Birmingham, United Kingdom

53 Juvenile Idiopathic Arthritis

Apostolos Karantanas, MD
Associate Professor of Radiology, Department of Radiology, University of Crete; Chief, Musculoskeletal Section, Department of Radiology, University Hospital, Heraklion, Greece

73 Thalassemia

David Karasick, MD, FACR
Professor of Radiology, Department of Radiology, Thomas Jefferson University, Philadelphia, Pennsylvania

23 Acute Osseous Injury to the Knee

Theodoros Katsivas, MD
Associate Professor, Department of Medicine, University of California, San Diego, San Diego, California

67 Human Immunodeficiency Virus Infection and Acquired Immunodeficiency syndrome

Eoin C. Kavanagh, MB, BCh, BAO, MRCPI, FFR, RCSI, MSc
Senior Lecturer, Radiological Science, University College of Dublin; Consultant Radiologist and Senior Lecturer, Radiology, Mater Misericordiae Hospital, Dublin, Ireland

74 Myelofibrosis; 108 The Postoperative Hip

Theodore E. Keats, MD
Alumni Professor, Department of Radiology, University of Virginia; Professor of Radiology, Department of Radiology, University of Virginia Health Sciences, Charlottesville, Virginia

CD-2 Normal Variants

Shah H. M. Khan, MBBS, FRCR
Consultant Radiologist, Department of Radiology, Royal Blackburn Hospital, Blackburn, Lancashire, United Kingdom
62 Infection in the Appendicular Skeleton (Including Chronic Osteomyelitis)

Digna R. Kool, MD
Staff Radiologist, Department of Radiology, University Medical Centre Nijmegen, St. Raboud, Nijmegen, The Netherlands
5 Injury to the Thoracic Cage and Thoracolumbar Spine

George Koulouris, MBBS, FRANZCR, M Med
Assistant Professor, Department of Radiology, New York University Medical Center; Assistant Professor, Department of Radiology, Hospital for Joint Diseases, New York, New York
108 The Postoperative Hip

Josef Kramer, MD, PhD, MMSc
Institute for CT and MRI at Schillerpark, Linz, Austria
21 Internal Derangements of the Hip and Proximal Femur (Including Intra- and Extra-articular Snapping Hip)

Herman M. Kroon, MD, PhD
Senior Consultant Radiologist, Department of Radiology, Leiden University Medical Center, Leiden, The Netherlands
88 The Patient with a Tumor or Tumor-Like Lesion of Bone; 98 Staging Bone and Soft Tissue Tumors

Cornelis van Kuijk, MD, PhD
Professor and Chair, Department of Radiology, Vrije Universiteit Amsterdam Medical Center, Amsterdam, The Netherlands
5 Injury to the Thoracic Cage and Thoracolumbar Spine

Susanne W. Y. Lardenoye-Bröker, MD
Department of Radiology, Leiden University Medical Center, Leiden, The Netherlands
37 Skeletal Manifestation of Child Abuse

Hans Peter Ledermann, MD, PD
IMAMED Radiologie Nordwest, Basel, Switzerland
65 Diabetic Pedal Infection

Gerwin M. Lingg, MD
Head, Department of Radiology, Academic Hospital, Johann Gutenberg University, Mainz; Sana Rheumazentrum Rheinland Pfalz, Bad Kreuznach, Germany
49 Ankylosing Spondylitis; 51 Systemic Lupus Erythematosus; 52 Mixed Connective Tissue Disease

Brandon Y. Liu, MD
Department of Radiology, Maimonides Medical Center, Brooklyn, New York
11 Acute Osseous Injury of the Elbow and Forearm

Patrick T. Liu, MD
Assistant Professor of Radiology, Department of Radiology, Mayo Clinic College of Medicine, Scottsdale, Arizona
CD-3 Biopsy: Soft Tissue

Eva Llopis, MD
Department of Radiology, Hospital de la Ribera, Alzira, Valencia, Spain
17 Soft Tissue Injuries of the Hand and Wrist; 18 Pelvis-Hip: Technical Aspects, Normal Anatomy, Common Variants, and Basic Biomechanics; 19 Acute Osseous Injury to the Pelvis and Acetabulum; 20 Acute Osseous Injury to the Hip and Proximal Femur

Calvin T. Ma, MD
Radiology Resident, Department of Radiology, Maimonides Medical Center, Brooklyn, New York
78 Pituitary and Thyroid Disorders; CD-A6: Compressive and Entrapment Neuropathies of the Upper and Lower Extremities

Matthew A. Marcus, MD
Assistant Professor, Department of Diagnostic Imaging, The Warren Alpert Medical School of Brown University, Providence, Rhode Island
35 Upper Extremity Injuries in Children (Including Sports Injuries)

José Martel, MD, PhD
Jefe De Unidad, Diagnóstico por Imagen, Fundación Hospital Alcorcón, Alcorcón, Madrid, Spain
A3: Fractures with Names

Paul Marten, MD
Staff Radiologist, Department of Radiology, University of Pennsylvania, The Children's Hospital of Philadelphia, Philadelphia, Pennsylvania
78 Pituitary and Thyroid Disorders

Manesh Mathew, MD
Attending Physician, Department of Radiology, Maimonides Medical Center, Brooklyn, New York
14 Acute Osseous Injury to the Wrist; 16 Acute Osseous Trauma to the Hand

Iain W. McCall, MD, NIB, ChB, FRCR
Professor, Radiologic Sciences, Keele University, and Honorary Consultant Radiologist, Department of Radiology, University Hospital of North Staffordshire, Stoke on Trent, North Staffordshire; Consultant Radiologist, Department of Radiology, Robert Jones and Agnes Hunt Orthopaedic Hospital, Shropshire, United Kingdom
43 Degenerative Disorders of the Spine

Eugene G. McNally, MB, Bch, BAO (Hon), FRCR, FRCPI
Consultant Musculoskeletal Radiologist, Department of Radiology, Nuffield Orthopaedic Centre; Honorary Senior Lecturer, Nuffield Department of Orthopaedic Surgery, Oxford University, Oxford, United Kingdom
25 Internal Derangement of the Knee: Ligament Injuries

José M. Mellado, MD
Attending Radiologist, Radiology Department, Hospital Reina Sofia, Tudela, Navarra, Spain
19 Acute Osseous Injury to the Pelvis and Acetabulum; 20 Acute Osseous Injury to the Hip and Proximal Femur

Theodore T. Miller, MD, FACR
Assistant Professor of Radiology, Weill Medical College of Cornell University; Attending Radiologist, Department of Radiology and Imaging, Hospital for Special Surgery, New York, New York
6 Normal Shoulder; 10 Normal Elbow; 26 Internal Derangement of the Knee: Tendon Injuries

Douglas N. Mintz, MD
Associate Professor of Clinical Radiology, Weill Medical College of Cornell University; Associate Attending Radiologist, Department of Radiology and Imaging, Hospital for Special Surgery; Associate Attending Radiologist, Department of Radiology, The New York-Presbyterian Hospital, New York, New York
109 The Postoperative Knee

Johnny U. V. Monu, MD
Associate Professor of Radiology and Orthopedics, Department of Imaging Sciences, University of Rochester, Rochester, New York
46 Rheumatoid Arthritis

Sandra L. Moore, MD
Assistant Professor, Department of Radiology, New York University School of Medicine; Attending, Department of Radiology, New York University Medical Center, New York, New York
60 Neuropathic Osteoarthropathy; 67 Human Immunodeficiency Virus Infection and Acquired Immunodeficiency Syndrome

William B. Morrison, MD
Associate Professor, Department of Radiology, Thomas Jefferson University; Director, Division of Musculoskeletal and General Diagnostic Radiology, Thomas Jefferson University Hospital, Philadelphia, Pennsylvania
65 Diabetic Pedal Infection

Timothy J. Mosher, MD
Associate Professor of Radiology and Orthopaedic Surgery, and Vice Chair, Radiology Research, Department of Radiology, Penn State University College of Medicine; Chief, Musculoskeletal Imaging and MRI, Department of Radiology, Penn State Milton S. Hershey Medical Center, Hershey, Pennsylvania
45 Degenerative Disease: Cartilage Anatomy, Physiology, and Advanced Imaging

Michael E. Mulligan, MD
Associate Professor of Radiology, Department of Radiology and Nuclear Medicine, University of Maryland School of Medicine; Chief, Division of Radiology, The J.L. Kernan Hospital, Baltimore, Maryland
96 Metastatic Disease

Mark D. Murphey, MD
Professor of Radiology, Department of Radiology, Walter Reed Army Medical Center, Bethesda, Maryland; Chief, Musculoskeletal Radiology, Department of Radiologic Pathology, Armed Forces Institute of Pathology, Washington, DC
84 Hypertrophic Osteoarthropathy; 95 Tumoral Calcinosis; 96 Metastatic Disease

William A. Murphy, Jr., MD
Professor of Radiology, John S. Dunn, Sr. Distinguished Chair in Diagnostic Imaging, Department of Diagnostic Radiology, The University of Texas M.D. Anderson Cancer Center, Houston, Texas
39 Radiation Effects in the Musculoskeletal System

Daniel B. Nissman, MD, MPH, MSEE
Department of Radiology, Medical University of South Carolina, Charleston, South Carolina
48 Reactive Arthritis

George C. Nomikos, MD
Assistant Professor of Radiology, New York University School of Medicine; Assistant Professor of Radiology, New York University Hospital for Joint Diseases; Assistant Attending, Department of Radiology, Bellevue Hospital Center, New York, New York
8 Shoulder Impingement Syndromes

Willem R. Obermann, MD, PhD
Senior Medical Specialist, Radiological Department, Leiden University Medical Center, Leiden, The Netherlands
CD-6 Tumor Ablation

Philip J. O'Connor, MD, MBChB, BSc, MRCP, FRCR
Department of Radiology, Leeds Teaching Hospitals Trust, Leeds, United Kingdom
36 Lower Extremity Injuries in Children (Including Sports Injuries)

Amaka Offiah, BSc, MBBS, MRCP, FRCR, PhD
Honorary Senior Lecturer, Department of Radiology and Physics, Institute of Child Health; Consultant (Academic), Department of Radiology, Great Ormond Street Hospital for Children, London, United Kingdom
103 Dysplasias

Richard J. Oh, MD
Resident, Department of Radiology, Maimonides Medical Center, Brooklyn, New York
16 Acute Osseous Trauma to the Hand

Imran M. Omar, MD
Instructor, Department of Radiology, Northwestern University Feinberg School of Medicine; Department of Radiology, Northwestern Memorial Hospital; Department of Radiology, Rehabilitation Institute of Chicago, Chicago, Illinois
CD-A5: Classic Signs and Findings in Musculoskeletal Radiology

Oleg Opsha, MD
Radiologist, Diagnostic Radiology, Maimonides Medical Center, Brooklyn, New York
CD-A4: Diseases with Names

Simon Ostlere, FRCR
Radiology, Nuffield Orthopaedic Centre, Oxford, United Kingdom
102 Coalitions

Joshua M. Owen, MS, MD
Radiology Resident, Department of Radiology, Maimonides Medical Center, Brooklyn, New York
16 Acute Osseous Trauma to the Hand

William E. Palmer, MD
Assistant Professor of Radiology, Harvard Medical School; Director, Musculoskeletal Imaging, Massachusetts General Hospital, Boston, Massachusetts
29 Acute Osseous Injury to the Ankle

Mario Padron, MD
Chief, Department of Radiology, Clinica CEMTRO, Madrid, Spain
6 Normal Shoulder

Narayan Babu Paruchuri, MD
Radiology Attending, Doshi Diagnostics, New York, New York
106 Postoperative Imaging of the Shoulder

Mini N. Pathria, MD
Professor of Clinical Radiology, Department of Radiology, University of California, San Diego; Professor of Clinical Radiology, Department of Radiology, University of California, San Diego, Medical Center, San Diego, California
55 Hemochromatosis

Rogerich T. Paylor
Associate, Radiology Associates, P.A., Little Rock, Arkansas
77 Amyloidosis

Christian W. Pfirrmann, MD
Department of Radiology, Orthopedic University Hospital Balgrist, Zurich, Switzerland
21 Internal Derangements of the Hip and Proximal Femur (Including Intra- and Extra-articular Snapping Hip)

Michael Pharoah, DDS, MSc, Dipl Oral Rad, FRCD(C)
Professor and Head of Oral Radiology, Faculty of Dentistry, University of Toronto; Staff Radiologist, Department of Dentistry, Princess Margaret Hospital; Consultant, Department of Diagnostic Imaging, Toronto General Hospital, Toronto, Ontario, Canada
CD-1 Dental Imaging

Marc J. Philippon, MD
Clinical Assistant Professor, University of Pittsburgh Medical Center, Pittsburgh, Pennsylvania; Orthopaedic Surgeon, Steadman Hawkins Clinic, Vail, Colorado
108 The Postoperative Hip

Thomas Lee Pope, Jr, MD, FACR
Professor of Radiology and Orthopedics, Department of Radiology, Medical University of South Carolina, Charleston, South Carolina
48 Reactive Arthritis; 72 Sickle Cell Anemia; CD-2 Normal Variants

Linda J. Probyn, MD, BSc, PT
Lecturer, Medical Imaging, University of Toronto, Toronto, Ontario, Canada
24 Internal Derangement of the Knee: Meniscal Injuries

Mahvash Rafii, MD
Adjunct Professor, Department of Radiology, New York University School of Medicine, New York, New York
8 Shoulder Impingement Syndromes

James J. Rankine, MD, MRCP, MRad, FRCR
Senior Clinical Lecturer, Department of Orthopaedic Surgery, University of Leeds; Consultant Radiologist, Department of Radiology, Leeds General Infirmary, Leeds, United Kingdom
104 Spinal Deformity

Nisha Rao, MD
Radiology Resident, Department of Radiology, Maimonides Medical Center, Brooklyn, New York
14 Acute Osseous Injury to the Wrist

Vijay M. Rao, MD, FACR
Professor and Chair, Department of Radiology, Thomas Jefferson University Hospital, Jefferson Medical College, Philadelphia, Pennsylvania
3 Temporomandibular Joint

Lisa Georgianne Rider, MD
Deputy Chief, Environmental Autoimmunity Group, National Institute of Environmental Health Sciences, National Institutes of Health, Bethesda, Maryland
54 Idiopathic Inflammatory Myopathy

Catherine C. Roberts, MD
Associate Dean, Mayo School of Health Sciences; Associate Professor of Radiology, Mayo Clinic, Phoenix, Arizona
CD-3 Biopsy: Soft Tissue

Lee F. Rogers, MD
Professor, Department of Radiology, University of Arizona Health Services Center; Diagnostic Radiologist, University Medical Center, Tucson, Arizona

58 Gout

Alejandro U. Rolón, MD
Department of Radiology, Universidad de Buenos Aires; Radiologist, Centro de Diagnóstico Dr. E. Rossi, Buenos Aires, Argentina

17 Soft Tissue Injuries of the Hand and Wrist

Zehava Sadka Rosenberg, MD
Professor of Radiology and Orthopedic Surgery, New York University School of Medicine; Attending Radiologist, New York University–Hospital for Joint Diseases, New York, New York

30 Soft Tissue Injury to the Ankle: Ligaments

Lorne Rosenbloom, MDCM, FRCPC
Assistant Professor, Department of Radiology, McGill University; Diagnostic Radiologist, Sir Mortimer B. Davis–Jewish General Hospital, Montreal, Quebec, Canada

2 Imaging of Facial and Skull Trauma

Daniel Rosenthal, MD
Professor, Department of Radiology, Harvard Medical School; Associate Chair, Radiology, Massachusetts General Hospital, Boston, Massachusetts

79 Gaucher Disease

David A. Rubin, MD
Associate Professor of Radiology, Department of Radiology, Washington University School of Medicine; Chief, Musculoskeletal Section, Mallinckrodt Institute of Radiology, Barnes-Jewish Hospital, St. Louis, Missouri

110 The Postoperative Ankle and Foot

Rodrigo A. Salgado, MD
Staff Member, Radiology Department, University Hospital Antwerp, Antwerp, Belgium

94 Tumor-like Soft Tissue Lesions

Barry Schenk, MD
Department of Radiology, Leiden University Medical Center, Leiden, The Netherlands

CD-10 Percutaneous Intradiscal Therapies

Anna Scheurecker, MD
CT/MRT-Institut am Schillerpark, Linz, Austria

21 Internal Derangements of the Hip and Proximal Femur (Including Intra- and Extra-articular Snapping Hip)

Jean Schils, MD
Section Head, Musculoskeletal Radiology and Emergency Imaging, Imaging Institute, Cleveland Clinic, Cleveland, Ohio

76 Hyperparathyroidism, Renal Osteodystrophy, Osteomalacia, and Rickets

Corinna Schorn, MD
Department of Radiology, Sana-Rheumazentrum Rheinland Pfalz, Bad Kreuznach, Germany

49 Ankylosing Spondylitis; 51 Systemic Lupus Erythematosus; 52 Mixed Connective Tissue Disease

Mark E. Schweitzer, MD
Professor of Radiology and Orthopaedic Surgery, Chief of Musculoskeletal Imaging and Chief of Radiology, Department of Radiology, New York University Hospital for Joint Diseases, New York, New York

42 Complex Regional Pain Syndrome

Jon K. Sekiya, MD
Associate Professor, Department of Orthopaedic Surgery, University of Michigan Medical Center, Ann Arbor, Michigan

108 The Postoperative Hip

Maryam Shahabpour, MD
Clinical Professor of Radiology, Department of Radiology, Vrije Universiteit Brussel; Chief of Clinic, Musculoskeletal Imaging, Radiology and Medical Imaging, Universitair Ziekenhuis Brussel, Vrije Universiteit Brussel, Brussels, Belgium

22 Knee; Technical Aspects, Normal Anatomy, Common Variants, and Basic Biomechanics

Steven Shankman, MD
Assistant Professor, Clinical Radiology, Department of Radiology, Mt. Sinai School of Medicine, New York, New York; Vice Chairman and Program Director, Department of Radiology, Maimonides Medical Center, Brooklyn, New York

11 Acute Osseous Injury of the Elbow and Forearm; CD-A4: Diseases with Names

Roger Smith, MD
Consultant Rheumatologist, Nuffield Orthopaedic Centre, Oxford United Kingdom

81 Osteogenesis Imperfecta

Annemie Snoeckx, MD
Department of Radiology, University Hospital Antwerp, Antwerp, Belgium

82 Marfan Syndrome; 100 Focal Growth Disturbances

Travis G. Snyder, MD
Musculoskeletal Fellow, Diagnostic Radiology, Yale University, New Haven, Connecticut

15 Internal Derangement of the Wrist

Peter M. Som, MD
Professor of Radiology, Otolaryngology and Radiation Oncology, Department of Radiology, The Mount Sinai School of Medicine of New York University, New York, New York

2 Imaging of Facial and Skull Trauma

Raphaëlle Souillard, MD
Musculoskeletal Imaging, Université de Médecine, Université Henri Warembourg, Lille, France

CD-4 Percutaneous Biopsy of the Appendicular Skeleton; CD-5 Percutaneous Biopsy of the Spine

Alan Sprigg, MBChB, FRCR, FRCPCH
Senior Clinical Lecturer, Radiodiagnostics, University of Sheffield; Consultant, Paediatric Radiology, Sheffield Children's Hospital, Sheffield, United Kingdom

37 Skeletal Manifestations of Child Abuse

Alison R. I. Spouge, MD, FRCPC
Associate Professor, Department of Diagnostic Radiology, University of Western Ontario; Staff Radiologist, London Health Science Center, University Hospital, London, Ontario, Canada

31 Soft Tissue Injury to the Ankle: Tendons

Lynne S. Steinbach, MD
Professor of Clinical Radiology and Orthopaedic Surgery, Department of Radiology, University of California, San Francisco; Chief, Musculoskeletal Imaging, Department of Radiology, University of California, San Francisco, Medical Center, San Francisco, California

107 The Postoperative Elbow, Wrist, and Hand

Murali Sundaram, MD, FRCR
Professor of Radiology, Lerner College of Medicine, Cleveland Clinic Foundation; Staff, Musculoskeletal Radiology, Cleveland Clinic, Cleveland Clinic Foundation, Cleveland, Ohio

76 Hyperparathyroidism, Renal Osteodystrophy, Osteomalacia, and Rickets; 85 Sarcoidosis

Mihra S. Taljanovic, MD, MA
Associate Professor of Radiology and Orthopaedic Surgery, Department of Radiology, University of Arizona Health Sciences Center, Tucson, Arizona

68 Atypical Mycobacterial Infection

James Teh, BSc, MBBS, MRCP, FRCR
Honorary Senior Clinical Lecturer, Faculty of Medicine, Oxford University; Consultant Musculoskeletal Radiologist, Department of Radiology, Nuffield Orthopaedic Centre, Oxford, United Kingdom

81 Osteogenesis Imperfecta

Jamshid Tehranzadeh, MD
Professor of Radiology and Orthopaedics, Director of Musculoskeletal Radiology, Department of Radiological Sciences, University of California, Irvine Medical Center, Orange, California

CD-8 Discography

Bernhard Johannes Tins, MD, PD
Consultant Radiologist, Department of Radiology, Robert Jones and Agnes Hunt Orthopaedic and District Hospital, Oswestry, Shropshire, United Kingdom

63 Spinal Infection

Dechen W. Tshering, MD, MBBS
Department of Radiology, University of Bern, Inselspital; Department of Diagnostic, Interventional and Pediatric Radiology, University Hospital Bern, Inselspital, Bern, Switzerland

40 Complications of Osseous Trauma

Michael J. Tuite, MD
Professor, Department of Radiology, University of Wisconsin Medical School; Director of Musculoskeletal Radiology, Department of Radiology, University of Wisconsin Hospital, Madison, Wisconsin

9 Glenohumeral Instability

Hilary Umans, MD
Clinical Associate Professor, Department of Radiology and Orthopaedic Surgery, Albert Einstein College of Medicine; Director of Musculoskeletal Radiology, Department of Radiology, Jacobi Medical Center, Bronx, New York

34 Imaging of the Forefoot; 72 Sickle Cell Anemia

Bruno C. Vande Berg, MD
Professor of Radiology, Medical Imaging, Universite Catholique de Louvain; Chief of Department, Medical Imaging, Cliniques Universitaires Saint Luc, Brussels, Belgium

69 General Principles of Magnetic Resonance Imaging of the Bone Marrow; 70 Ischemic Bone Lesions

Filip M. Vanhoenacker, MD, PhD
Lecturer, Faculty of Medicine, University of Antwerp, Wirijk, Belgium; Consultant Radiologist, Department of Radiology, University Hospital Antwerp, Edegem, Belgium

82 Marfan Syndrome; 100 Focal Growth Disturbances

Catharina S. P. van Rijswijk, MD, PhD
Department of Radiology, Leiden University Medical Center, Leiden, The Netherlands

99 Monitoring Therapy in Bone and Soft Tissue Tumors

Koenraad L. Verstraete, MD, PhD
Professor of Radiology, Gent University; Chief, Department of Radiology, Gent University Hospital, Gent, Belgium

27 Internal Derangement of the Knee: Cartilage and Osteochondral Injuries

Iain Watt, FRCP, FRCR
Professor, Department of Radiology, Leiden University
Medical Center, Leiden, The Netherlands
44 Normal Aging; 59 Crystal-Related Arthritis; 83 Paget's Disease

Lawrence M. White, MD, FRCPC
Professor and Head, Division of Musculoskeletal
Imaging, Department of Medical Imaging, University
of Toronto; Staff Radiologist, Head of Division of
Musculoskeletal Imaging, Mount Sinai Hospital and
the University Health Network, Toronto, Ontario,
Canada
24 Internal Derangement of the Knee: Meniscal Injuries

Helen J. Williams, MB, ChB
Honorary Senior Clinical Lecturer, Division of
Reproductive and Child Health—Paediatrics,
University of Birmingham; Consultant Paediatric
Radiologist, Radiology Department, Birmingham
Children's Hospital, Birmingham, United Kingdom
66 Pediatric Infections

Kevin R. Willits, MD, FRCS(C)
Assistant Professor, Department of Surgery, Fowler
Kennedy Sport Medicine Clinic, University of
Western Ontario, London, Ontario, Canada
31 Soft Tissue Injury to the Ankle: Tendons

David John Wilson, MBBS, FRCP, FRCR, MFSEM
Senior Clinical Lecturer, Department of Radiology,
University of Oxford; Consultant Musculoskeletal
Radiologist, Nuffield Orthopaedic Centre, Oxford,
United Kingdom
*61 Soft Tissue Disease: Cellulitis, Pyomyositis, Abscess, Septic Arthritis;
71 Hemophilia and Related Disorders; 101 Developmental
Dysplasia of the Hip; CD-9 Vertebroplasty and Kyphoplasty; CD-11
Ultrasound Procedures*

Emad Yacoub, MD
Resident, Department of Radiology, Maimonides
Medical Center, Brooklyn, New York
10 Normal Elbow

Lawrence Yao, MD
Special Volunteer, Diagnostic Radiology Department,
Clinical Center, National Institutes of Health,
Bethesda, Maryland
54 Idiopathic Inflammatory Myopathy

Joseph S. Yu, MD
Professor of Radiology, Vice-Chair for Education,
Director of Musculoskeletal Imaging, Department of
Radiology, The Ohio State University Medical Center,
Columbus, Ohio
7 Osseous Injuries of the Shoulder Girdle

Natalie Zelenko, MD
Department of Radiology, Maimonides Medical Center,
Brooklyn, New York
87 Drug-Related Bone and Soft Tissue Disorders

Michael B. Zlatkin, MD
Voluntary Professor of Radiology, Miller School of
Medicine, University of Miami, Miami, Florida
106 Postoperative Imaging of the Shoulder

Adam C. Zoga, MD
Assistant Professor of Radiology,
Department of Radiology, Thomas Jefferson University,
Philadelphia, Pennsylvania
23 Acute Osseous Injury to the Knee

Foreword

This magnificent two-volume text on musculoskeletal imaging, designed and edited by internationally acclaimed musculoskeletal radiologists Drs. Pope, Bloem, Beltran, Morrison, and Wilson, differs from conventional textbooks on the subject in several ways. The editors have chosen to expand the concept of the traditional axial and appendicular musculoskeletal system to include imaging of adjacent musculoskeletal anatomic areas such as the skull and face, temporomandibular joints, and mandible and teeth, along with normal variants and postsurgical imaging and complications. Excellent appendices include such topics as orthopedic measurements, orthopedic devices, and entrapment neuropathies of the extremities, which are also unique to this text.

Each chapter, except for the first ("Introduction and General Principles"), follows the identical format. This uniform presentation greatly facilitates information accessibility.

Another unique feature of *Imaging of the Musculoskeletal System* is that the extensive list of authors is a veritable international "who's who" in musculoskeletal radiology. These authors were specifically chosen for their recognized expertise in the subject that each presents.

The organization of the text into parts, subsections, and chapters within each subsection allows the reader rapid access to the specific subject information being sought. Each chapter discusses a single topic (e.g., injuries to a specific anatomic region, a specific disease entity, a group of closely related diseases, or a detailed description of an orthopedic interventional procedure). Thus, the chapter index leads the reader to his or her particular subject of interest. The text material for each chapter is well written, clear, and authoritative and without the tedium of being encyclopedic. Each chapter is supported by a list of suggested readings and of specific, appropriate references. The images are of excellent quality and fulfill their intended purpose. The drawings, all by Dr. Salvador Beltran, are superb and clearly illustrate the intended anatomy and pathology. This is particularly apparent in the appendix "Compressive and Entrapment Neuropathies of the Upper and Lower Extremities."

Imaging of the Musculoskeletal System is equally clinically relevant for musculoskeletal radiologists and non–musculoskeletal radiologists who interpret musculoskeletal images as part of their practice. As a general radiologist, I wish this reference source had been available years ago.

Imaging of the Musculoskeletal System, a classic at its genesis and the definitive work on musculoskeletal imaging, should be in the reading area of every private practicing radiologist who examines musculoskeletal images or performs musculoskeletal interventions.

Imaging of the Musculoskeletal System should also be able to find a home in the library of every academic department of radiology, orthopedic surgery, internal medicine, and emergency medicine.

John H. Harris, Jr. MD, DSc, FACR, FRACR (Hon)
Emeritus Professor of Radiology
University of Texas–Houston Medical School
Houston, Texas

Preface

When I was contacted in early 2005 by Elsevier to assume the editorship of *Imaging of the Musculoskeletal System*, I was excited by the opportunity. One of the most enticing aspects of the proposal was the subspecialty they had chosen as one of their initial offerings in the new *Expert Radiology* series. Elsevier's research had shown that the imaging market needed a comprehensive product that contained a good balance of text and pedagogical features, including tables, figures, and boxed or highlighted information. In order to offer a useful and user-friendly format to the audience, the book was meant to be highly formatted so that the individual writing styles of the authors could be kept as uniform as possible. I was delighted that Elsevier had contacted me and began recruiting coeditors immediately.

Within a week I had the great fortune to recruit three of the other four coeditors of this project: Dr. Javier Beltran, Dr. Hans Bloem, and Dr. Bill Morrison. Each of these experts accepted the invitation with enthusiasm. I must say that they have been a tremendous asset to the project, and it would never have come to fruition without them. In early December 2005 the editorial team met with the Elsevier staff to hammer out a list of contents, the specifics of each chapter template, and potential authors. Each of us then returned home with an enthusiastic endorsement of the book's conceptual framework. In less than six weeks we had contributor commitments for most of the chapters.

Later in the project, Hans Bloem contacted Dr. David Wilson, who kindly agreed to act as our pediatric musculoskeletal radiologist and began working to recruit many world-renowned pediatric radiologists as authors. As you will see, these individuals have ultimately made substantial contributions to the book. Dr. Wilson himself went on to author several adult-oriented chapters in the text as well, contributing greatly to the overall scope and focus of the final product.

So why do the editors believe this book should be read by anyone interested in musculoskeletal diseases? First and foremost, the international authorship of the book provides a global perspective on the field of musculoskeletal imaging. We have assembled 188 experts from 15 different countries to contribute 122 chapters on almost every conceivable aspect of musculoskeletal radiology. As nearly as possible and when relevant, each chapter contains the following section headings: Anatomy, prevalence and epidemiology, biomechanics, pathology, clinical presentation, manifestations of the disease (radiography, computed tomography, MR imaging, ultrasonography, nuclear medicine), and synopsis of treatment options (medical and surgical). The goal is to make the internal flow of the book as even and predictable as possible so that readers will always know where and how to find key information. The text is designed to be succinct and not overwhelming; as you'll see, it has been richly supplemented by some 5500 illustrations of excellent quality from all modalities, tables and diagrams of vivid color, and near-perfect anatomic drawings done by Dr. Salvador Beltran, the extremely talented and gifted brother of one of our editors. The chapters have color boxes for the following: Key Points, Classic Signs, and What the Referring Physician Needs To Know — a key feature designed to help radiologists communicate more effectively with referring physicians. Also included with each textbook is a fully searchable CD, featuring full-text chapters on major procedures in musculoskeletal radiology and extensive appendices presenting a full range of classic signs, instrumentation, fractures, and much more. Finally, the references have, in most cases, been limited to comprehensive up-to-date and extensive reviews on the chapter subject matter. In today's electronic environment, literature searches can be performed with such speed and accuracy that printed bibliographies are no longer essential. We therefore chose not to take up valuable subject space listing thousands of references that could be found easily online.

Perhaps the most exciting element of the project is its inclusion in the new Elsevier initiative entitled *Imaging Consult*, an online diagnosis- and decision-support tool for radiologists that contains content organized by organ system — including musculoskeletal imaging. This book forms the basis for a major component of *Imaging Consult*, which will feature annotated images, high-yield content for quick answers to clinical questions, more extensive references linked to PubMed, patient cases with images focusing on the desired clinical topic, and links within the program to full reference content. Volumes in the *Expert Radiology* series will be a prominent component of *Imaging Consult* over the next few years.

So we have explained why we, the editors, think this reference is unique and why we think it should be read and used by those interested in musculoskeletal imaging. However, you, our readers, are the ultimate judge, jury, and verdict. We hope and trust that you will take a close look at the book and agree with our assessment. By the same token, please let us know of its weaknesses. Writing and editing a major reference work such as this is a human endeavor, and as in all human actions, there is the potential for error. If you find one, let us know. Otherwise read, enjoy, and learn, as this was our primary intent in putting all of this knowledge together in one place!

I must express my sincerest appreciation for the support of all our coeditors, Dr. Hans Bloem of Leiden University in the Netherlands, Dr. Javier Beltran of Maimonides in New York, Dr. Bill Morrison of Thomas Jefferson University in Philadelphia, and Dr. David Wilson in Oxford, England. They have been absolutely fantastic in their dedication to the project, and it would never have been completed if they had not made the effort that they did. To all of our chapter authors, we express our deepest and heartfelt appreciation for their contributions because we know that this book would not have been produced without them. We know that they have spent many hours separated from family and friends and likely many nights and weekends thinking, writing, editing, searching for the best images, and borrowing from colleagues to create their chapters for us. All of them have fulfilled these responsibilities admirably, and we thank them from the bottom of our hearts. We, the editors, would especially like to thank Dr. Jack Harris, who ever so kindly agreed not only to write the first chapter of the book but to compose the Foreword for us at the last minute. Jack, thanks very much for everything. And finally, tremendous credit is due the people at Elsevier behind the scenes, who worked with all of us to coordinate the whole project from start to finish. To Jennifer Shreiner, we give a special thanks. She has been with us for the duration of the project and has been a kind and considerate liaison between the authors and the editors and has performed well above and beyond the call of duty. Also, we would like to thank Judith Fletcher for her leadership as the overall project manager for Elsevier and Norman Stellander for his hard work on the galley proofs. All have been a true pleasure to work with.

Contents

VOLUME II

PART TWO: ARTHROPATHIES AND NEUROLOGIC/MUSCULAR DISORDERS AND CONNECTIVE TISSUE DISEASE

CD Contents

Please see abstracts of these chapters on page 2121.

Arthropathies and Neurologic/ Muscular Disorders and Connective Tissue Disease

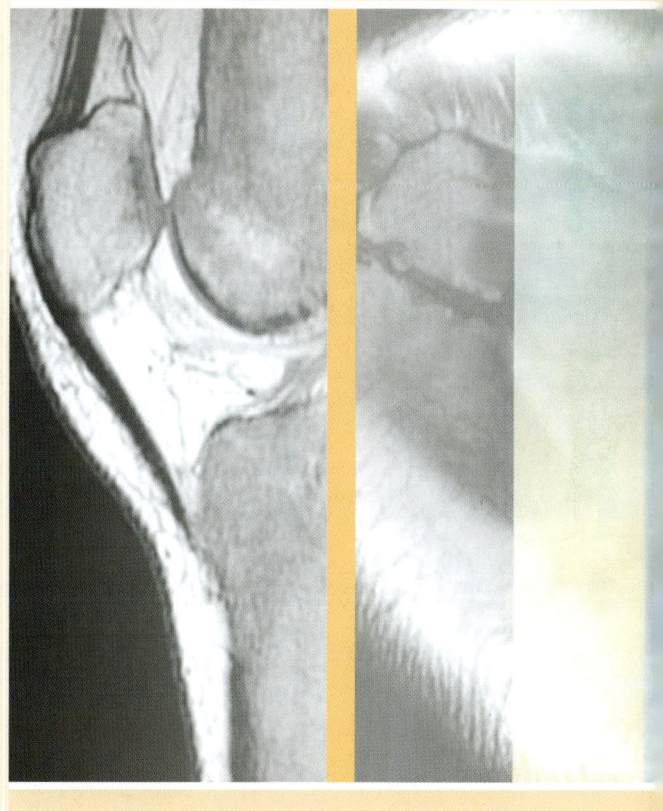

CHAPTER 43

Degenerative Disorders of the Spine

Iain McCall

ETIOLOGY

Degeneration of the spine is universal and involves structural changes in the disc, bone, ligaments, and articular cartilage of the facet joints. Despite the high prevalence of degeneration, the underlying etiology is still only partially understood. There is, however, an interrelationship of the different components of the spine in that changes in one component, such as the disc, will have an effect on another, such as altered biomechanics of the facets. Similarly, alterations in the structure of the vertebral end plate may affect the nutrition of the disc and the viability of the chondrocytes.

Degeneration of the spine is a natural aging process and increases in extent and severity with age. Miller and associates[1] reported an increase in disc degeneration from 16% at age 20 to 98% at age 70 based on microscopic disc degeneration grades of 600 autopsy specimens. Reduction in disc signal intensity on MRI is one of the degenerative findings most highly associated with age.[2] Environmental factors such as heavy physical loading related to occupation have been suggested as a factor, but the evidence is not conclusive and may be influenced by confounding factors including socioeconomic status and lifestyle. Series of studies with monozygotic twins found that heavy physical loading demands at work and leisure explained only a minor portion of the overall variance in lumbar disc degeneration.[3] Driving has also been proposed as a possible etiologic factor, but the current weight of evidence suggests no notable effect of driving on disc degeneration. The only chemical exposure associated with disc degeneration is smoking.

Finally, there is likely to be a genetic influence on degeneration, and initial results suggested a substantial family influence on degenerative findings. A study of both cervical and lumbar spine using MRI showed heritable estimates were very high for both lumbar and cervical spine after adjusting for age, weight, smoking, occupation, and physical activity; and disc bulging and height were the primary contributors to the disc degeneration summary score that relate to the genetic determination.[4] Disc bulging and disc height are the individual features that are the most highly heritable in both cervical and lumbar spine.[4]

PREVALENCE AND EPIDEMIOLOGY

Low back and neck pain are common ailments in developed countries, with an estimated 40% to 70% of adults having suffered low back pain. Low back and neck pain are a major source of disability and loss of working time.

KEY POINTS

- Forty to 70 percent of adults have experienced low back pain, but the prevalence of symptomatic herniated nucleus pulposus is only 1%.
- The prevalence of asymptomatic herniated nucleus pulposus reaches 76% in the adult population.
- There is no correlation between symptoms and imaging features of disc degeneration.
- Incidence of posterior annular tears increases with age; they are common in the asymptomatic population, but it is uncertain whether high signal intensity zones on MRI are more commonly painful.
- The importance of imaging is to demonstrate anatomic features and extent of herniation and its effect on nerve roots.
- Potential disc herniations are, based on morphologic criteria, classified as normal, bulging, protrusion, extrusion, and sequestration.
- Cysts and osteoarthritis of facet joints, including degenerative spondylolisthesis, are diagnosed and classified using well-defined criteria and may be an important cause of low back pain.
- Spinal stenosis is accurately diagnosed using conventional radiographs and especially CT and MRI.

In most cases the pain resolves, but recurrent episodes may occur, ranging from 20% to 44% within 1 year after an episode of acute low back pain, with 80% suffering a recurrence within 10 years. For approximately 5% of the adult population low back pain becomes persistently disabling and chronic. The incidence and prevalence of symptomatic herniated nucleus pulposus are much lower, with 1% of those between 17 and 64 years reporting discomfort from lumbar intervertebral disc herniation and between 0.1% and 0.5% of the population per year within the age range of 20 to 64 having a new clinically manifest herniated nucleus pulposus,[5] with a peak incidence between 38 and 44 years of age.

CLINICAL PRESENTATION

There is no correlation between the presence of symptoms and the imaging features of disc degeneration.

Pain may arise from the structures of the spine—sclerotomal pain—or be due to compression of the nerve roots passing through the spinal canal—dermatomal pain. The sclerotomal pain may be localized to the spinal region or may be referred to adjacent areas or to the limbs. Cervical sclerotomal pain is often referred to the shoulder, and lumbar pain is often referred to the buttocks and thighs, although more distal limb referral may occur. Dermatomal pain may also be present in the region of the spine but will often be present in the limbs in the distribution of the compressed nerve.

The discogenic pain is exacerbated by activity such as bending or lifting and relieved by rest, especially in recumbency. The individual begins the day relatively free of pain.[6] Patients may occasionally find themselves immobilized by pain and spasm. On examination, the erector spinae muscles are tense and movement is limited and there may be a variable degree of tenderness on palpation. Neurologic examination does not identify any objective loss, although straight-leg raising may be limited.

Facet pain may be aggravated by rest, resulting also in sleep disturbances, whereas movement decreases pain.[7,8] Pain and stiffness are present on rising but improve during the day. Symptoms may be exacerbated by extended periods of sitting or standing with the spine in a lordotic position. Examination is unremarkable except that the patient may flex the cervical spine or touch the toes but may be significantly restricted in extension. Deep palpation may reveal tenderness in the region of the affected facet joints and no neurologic deficit.

Discogenic and facet pain may occur together, resulting in a combination or mixture of clinical features sometimes resulting in constant pain[6] and marked restriction of spinal movement in all directions and considerable tenderness.

The pain in nerve root compression by degeneration in the spine is usually in the distribution of the nerve root but may not affect the whole extent of the distribution, and there is overlap between dermatomes. In the cervical spine, compression of the cord may also affect the distribution of the pain; and in the thoracic spine, disc herniations commonly present as back pain that is nonspecific or a myelopathy that includes progressive paraparesis, hyperreflexia, altered sensation and pinprick levels, and, occasionally, urinary problems. Nerve root compression will also lead to motor and sensory changes, and examination includes assessment of motor strength, sensory loss, and deep tendon reflexes in the extremities. Central nuclear herniations may produce severe back pain and bilateral leg pain. Lesions of the peripheral nerve roots must always be distinguished from root irritation by the degenerate spine. Pain from root compression in the upper cervical spine may extend into the occiput.

PATHOPHYSIOLOGY

Anatomy

The spine consists of a column of vertebrae with a vertebral body linked by two pedicles to the lamina, which has two superior and two inferior articular processes and a spinous process. Each vertebra, with the exception of the sacrum and coccyx, is linked as a three-joint complex. The intervertebral disc with associated vertebral cartilage end plates forms the anterior component, whereas the facet joints form the posterior component. The intervertebral disc is made up of two components, the outer being the annulus that surrounds the inner nucleus pulposus. The annulus is divided into outer and inner concentric rings with dense fibrous lamellae containing fibroblasts in the outer ring and less densely packed collagen with chondrocytes and some ground substance in the inner ring. The central nucleus pulposus has an infrastructure of collagen with chondrocytes and a high content of hydrophilic proteoglycans and thus water content. The intervertebral disc and adjacent vertebral end plates form a continuum with the collagen fibers of the disc passing directly into the cartilage of the central part of the vertebral end plate and directly into the bone at the anterior and posterior rims of the vertebra called the enthesis. The collagen from the cartilage is in continuity with the subchondral bone of the vertebra. Because the intervertebral disc is avascular, it obtains most of its nutrients by diffusion through the cartilage end plate from the vascular arcade along the subchondral trabecular bone, with a small component in the outer annulus from vessels around the outer rim of the disc. The transport of water, nutrients, and metabolic waste products to and from the disc is enhanced by pressure, and the nucleus pulposus loses water and metabolic waste products during the day in the upright posture, resulting in reduction in height; while a person is in the recumbent position, water and metabolites reenter the disc, increasing its height.

The facet joints have appositional articular cartilage surfaces and are lined by synovium. The inner capsule is continuous with the ligamentum flavum, and the outer capsule is covered by the ligaments. The alignment of the facets is site dependent, with more horizontal alignment in the cervical spine that facilitates flexion and extension, with some limited potential for rotation and lateral flexion. In the thoracic spine the facets have coronal and more vertical alignment and there is only a limited range of movement. In the lumbar spine the upper facets are aligned vertically in the sagittal plane but become more coronal in the lower lumbar spine.

The motion segments are connected throughout the spine by the anterior and posterior longitudinal ligaments, the ligamentum flavum, and the interspinous ligaments posteriorly. The anterior longitudinal ligament is attached to the anterior vertebral wall and end-plate rim but is not attached to the intervertebral disc. The posterior longitudinal ligament is inserted at the enthesis of each vertebral end plate and is firmly attached to the intervertebral disc by lateral expansions but is not attached to the posterior wall of the vertebral body.

In the lumbar spine the anterior elements of the vertebral column are surrounded by a plexus of nerves derived anteriorly from the sympathetic trunks, laterally from the gray rami communicantes, and posteriorly from the sinu-vertebral nerve. The plexuses supply the anterior longitudinal ligaments, the periosteum of the vertebral body, penetrating branches into the vertebral body, the posterior longitudinal ligament, the ventral aspect of the dural sac, and the outer third of the annulus.

The facet joints are innervated by the medial branches of the dorsal rami and have multisegmental innervation.[9]

The epidural space mainly contains fat and blood vessels, which make up the epidural venous plexus. The anterior epidural veins pass over the discs on either side of the midline. The vertebral bodies are supplied by a central artery that arborizes out to the vertebral end plates, and the veins drain back into a central vein in a similar fashion.

The vertebral/intervertebral disc combination, pedicles, facet joints, and foramina at each level also provide a conduit for the spinal cord and nerve roots. The cord terminates at T12-L1 and becomes the cauda equina. Nerve roots emerge from the dural sac passing under the lamina and out through the foramina.

Pathology

Degeneration is a natural process in the spine, with autopsy studies showing changes of spondylosis in 60% of women and 80% of men by the age of 49 years and in 95% of both by the age of 70.[10] Disc degeneration begins with a gradual loss of hydration of the nucleus with a drop from 90% at birth to about 75% in the third decade. There is a gradual centripetal encroachment of collagen into the nucleus from the annulus, a reduction of chondrocytes, and changes in the proteoglycans of the nucleus. Subsequently, the nucleus becomes solid, nonturgescent, and dry, with a marked increase in collagen content and no discernable differentiation from annulus. In middle age, splits and clefts form parallel with the end plate toward the upper and lower parts of the nucleus; and as aging progresses, they extend to the outer parts of the annulus, where vascular ingrowth may occur.[11] In the annulus, initially fragmentation of fibers, mucinous degeneration, and cracks and cavities occur that may result in tears at the annular rim of the vertebral body, which are commonly present by age 50 years.[12] Concentric circumferential cracks or tears develop between the layers of the collagen in the annulus, and radiating ruptures may also occur radially from the nucleus to the periphery. These radial tears may or may not extend through the outer annular fibers and are also the conduit for nuclear material to pass through the annulus and produce a herniation of

the nucleus pulposus. Such prolapses have been shown to often contain fibrocartilage in both the cervical and lumbar spine. Early degenerative changes of the cartilage end plate include fibrillation, longitudinal fissures, and cleft formation. This may also be enhanced by calcification of the end plates and occlusion of the marrow contact channels that is observed with advancing age.[13] As degeneration progresses, there is extensive loss of cartilage with vascular ingrowth and ossification with islands of residual cartilage. The irregular ossification may be extensive with dense bony sclerosis in the adjoining vertebral bodies and irregularity of the residual vertebral bony end plate.

Osteophyte formation at the peripheral margins of the vertebral bodies is present where there are degenerative changes in the disc. They form initially at the vertebral rim by advancing endochondral ossification of the annulus and increase in size by the formation of subperiosteal new bone. The osteophytic bone is initially coarsely trabeculated or compact but becomes cancellous with marrow cavities continuous with the vertebral body[11] and may vary in size but only rarely becomes united across the disc.

Degeneration may affect a number of motion segments but most commonly involves the mid cervical and lower lumbar spine. In some cases it may begin at a relatively early age and be associated with trauma or overuse. Degeneration may also result in compression of the cord or nerve roots due to herniation of the nucleus pulposus through the annulus, bulging of the annulus, osteoarthritis of the facet joints, or instability of the motion segment secondary to the degenerative changes.

MANIFESTATIONS OF THE DISEASE

Intervertebral Disc Degeneration

Radiography

Radiographs of the spine delineate the vertebra satisfactorily but have significant limitations in demonstrating spinal soft tissue. The demonstration of disc changes is limited to the evaluation of disc height; although the later stages of disc height loss are clearly demonstrated (Fig. 43-1), early disc space loss may be subject to interobserver variation and difficulties of lateral angulation and rotation of the radiographs.[14] Comparison is made to adjacent discs to see early reduction, but it should be noted that disc height normally gradually increases in the lumbar spine between L1 and L4-L5, whereas L5-S1 height is again less. Disc space narrowing may be asymmetric and should be assessed on both anteroposterior and lateral views of the spine. Bony vertebral end-plate irregularity is usually accurately assessed, but sclerosis is a relative feature and varies normally between subjects and may be limited to part of the end plate if there is asymmetric narrowing and particularly if it is related to vertebral osteoporosis. In the thoracic spine, disc space narrowing associated with end-plate irregularity may be seen in conjunction with loss of anterior vertebral height. Although individual disc levels may be affected, if three or more consecutive disc levels are involved, it is referred to as Scheuermann's disease and the presence of these changes in adolescence may result in a degree of kyphosis in severe cases.[15]

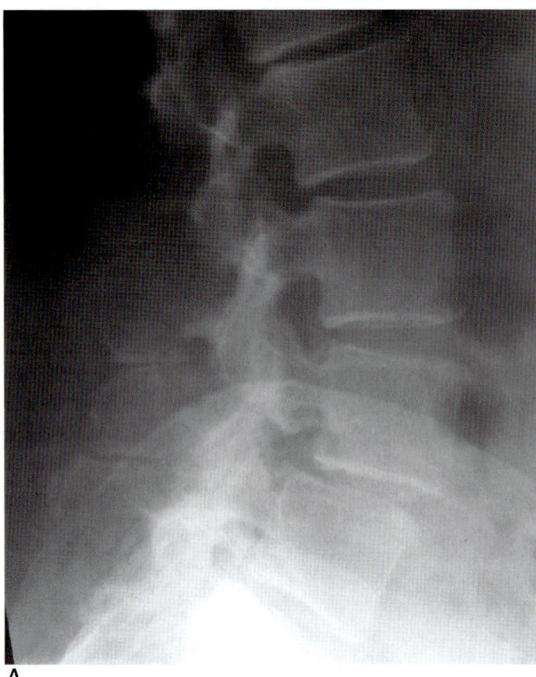

A

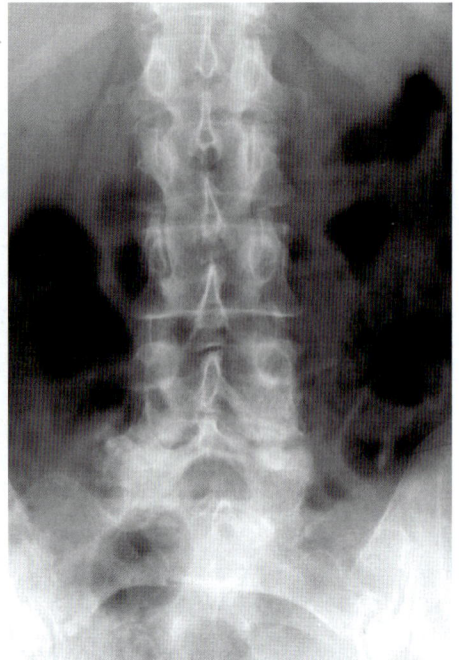

C

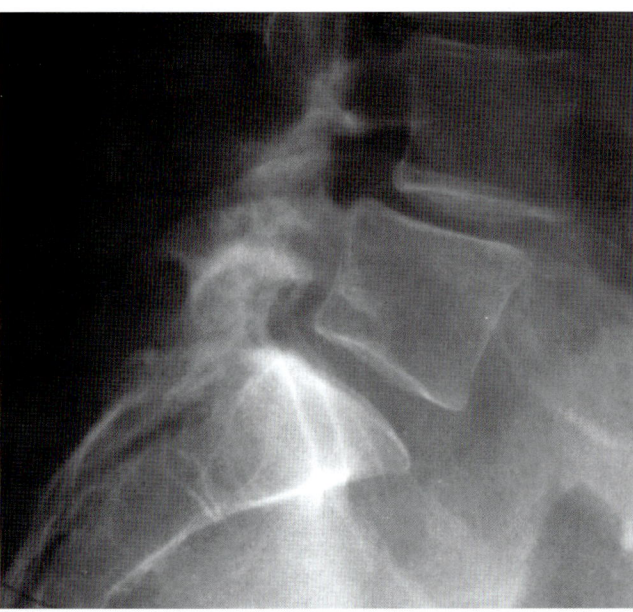

B

■ **FIGURE 43-1** Radiographs of the lumbar spine. Lateral (**A**) and coned lateral (**B**) views demonstrate narrowing of the L4-L5 disc space associated with a forward displacement of L4 on L5 as a degenerative spondylolisthesis due to osteoarthritis of the facet joints. **C,** Anteroposterior radiograph shows sclerosis at the L4-L5 facet joints and a mild lateral curve.

A vacuum phenomenon appearing as low attenuation areas within the disc may be seen that is enhanced by extending the spine. These areas may be limited to the vertebral rim at the insertion of the annulus and may be associated with osteophyte formation. A vacuum phenomenon within the disc substance reflects the cleft formation and is also helpful in excluding infective pathology, which is rare as a cause of disc gas.

The presence of total disc resorption with severe sclerosis of the end plate at only one level in an otherwise normal-looking spine is seen in some younger patients and has been reported as a separate entity.[16]

Multiple disc space narrowing, sclerosis, and osteophyte formation may be present in older subjects in the cervical (Fig. 43-2) and lumbar spine and may be associated with a degenerative scoliosis in the latter, with asymmetric disc space narrowing.

Osteophytes appear as bony projections from the rim of the vertebral body usually slightly below the end plate, less commonly from the end-plate rim. Osteophytes must be differentiated from the flowing ossification of the anterior longitudinal ligament of diffuse idiopathic skeletal hyperostosis (Forestier's disease), which may bridge the whole disc space and involves the anterior surface of the vertebral body.

Lateral radiographs in flexion and extension have also been used to evaluate relative linear and rotational interbody displacement. The normal range of movement has

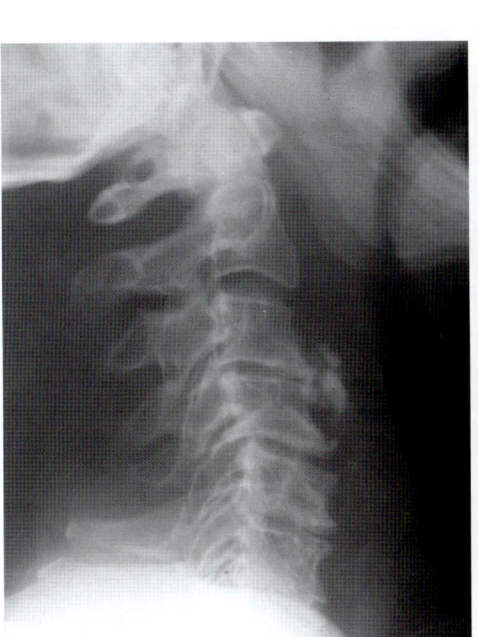
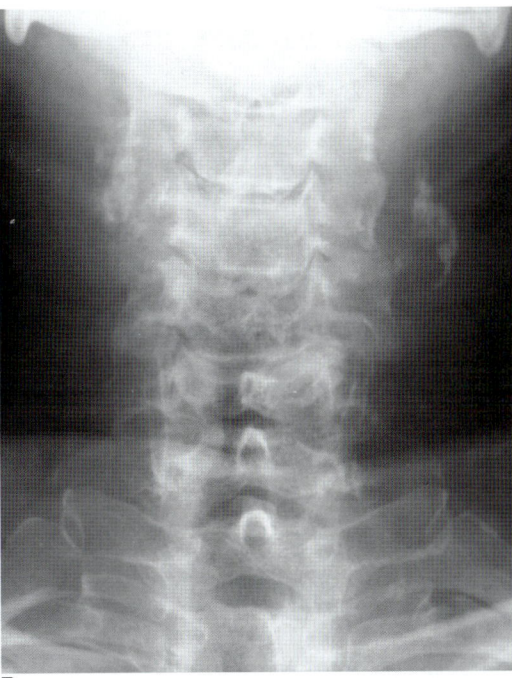

A   B

■ FIGURE 43-2 **A,** Lateral radiograph of the cervical spine demonstrates multiple narrowed disc spaces with anterior osteophyte formation and a retrolisthesis of C4 on C5. Facet joint space narrowing with some sclerosis is present. **B,** Anteroposterior view demonstrates osteoarthritic osteophyte proliferation along the lateral margins of the facet joints and narrowing and sclerosis of the neurocentral joints.

been a subject of dispute. In both the cervical and lumbar spine, translation in the lumbar spine of 4 mm or more was seen in 20% of normal subjects and 10% had 3 mm or more at all levels except L5-S1.[17]

Magnetic Resonance Imaging

The process of intervertebral disc degeneration is best visualized on MRI. The normal nucleus is high signal on the spin-echo, T2-weighted MR sequence, and the surrounding annulus is of low signal. The appearance of the disc on a T2-weighted, spin-echo MR sequence has been graded by Pfirrmann and coworkers (Table 43-1; Fig. 43-3).[18] Grade 1 is described as a "cotton ball" with a uniform high signal throughout the disc and is the appearance in young people. Grade 2 differs only by the presence of a central horizontal low signal cleft and is also considered to be normal. In grade 3 there is a reduction of high signal in the nucleus without loss or with minor loss of disc height representing the early stages of degeneration, and there may be loss of distinction between the nucleus and the annulus. Grade 4 shows some loss of disc height, which can also be appreciated on the plain radiographs, with a generalized loss of signal. Grade 5 represents the end stage with almost complete loss of the disc space.

This grading system has good intraobserver and interobserver correlation and is useful as a descriptive method, although there is no relationship with symptoms. Disc height may be measured on the monitor directly and special techniques may be used, but comparison with an adjacent disc is most commonly utilized. The degenerative process also results in the annulus losing its strength and bulging outward beyond the outline of the vertebral rim. This is a circumferential process, although it may be greater in one area than another, depending on the compressive forces on the disc. In the axial plane, the annulus is seen extending beyond the vertebral body outline uniformly around the whole vertebra; and on sagittal MR images the annulus will be seen to be bulging beyond the vertebra on each section (Fig. 43-4). Cervical discs begin the process of degeneration at a relatively early age with

---

TABLE 43-1 Classification of Disc Degeneration Based on Sagittal T2-Weighted Magnetic Resonance Imaging

Grade	Differentiation*	Signal Intensity†	Disc Height
I	Yes	Homogeneously hyperintense	Normal
II	Yes	Hyperintense with horizontal dark band	Normal
III	Blurred	Slightly decreased, minor irregularities	Slightly decreased
IV	Lost	Moderately decreased, hypointense zones	Moderately decreased
V	Lost	Hypointense, with or without horizontal hyperintense band	Collapsed

*Of nucleus pulposus from annulus.
†Of nucleus pulposus.
Data from Pfirrmann CW, Metzdorf A, Zanetti M, et al. Magnetic resonance classification of lumbar intervertebral disc degeneration. Spine 2001; 26:1873-1878.

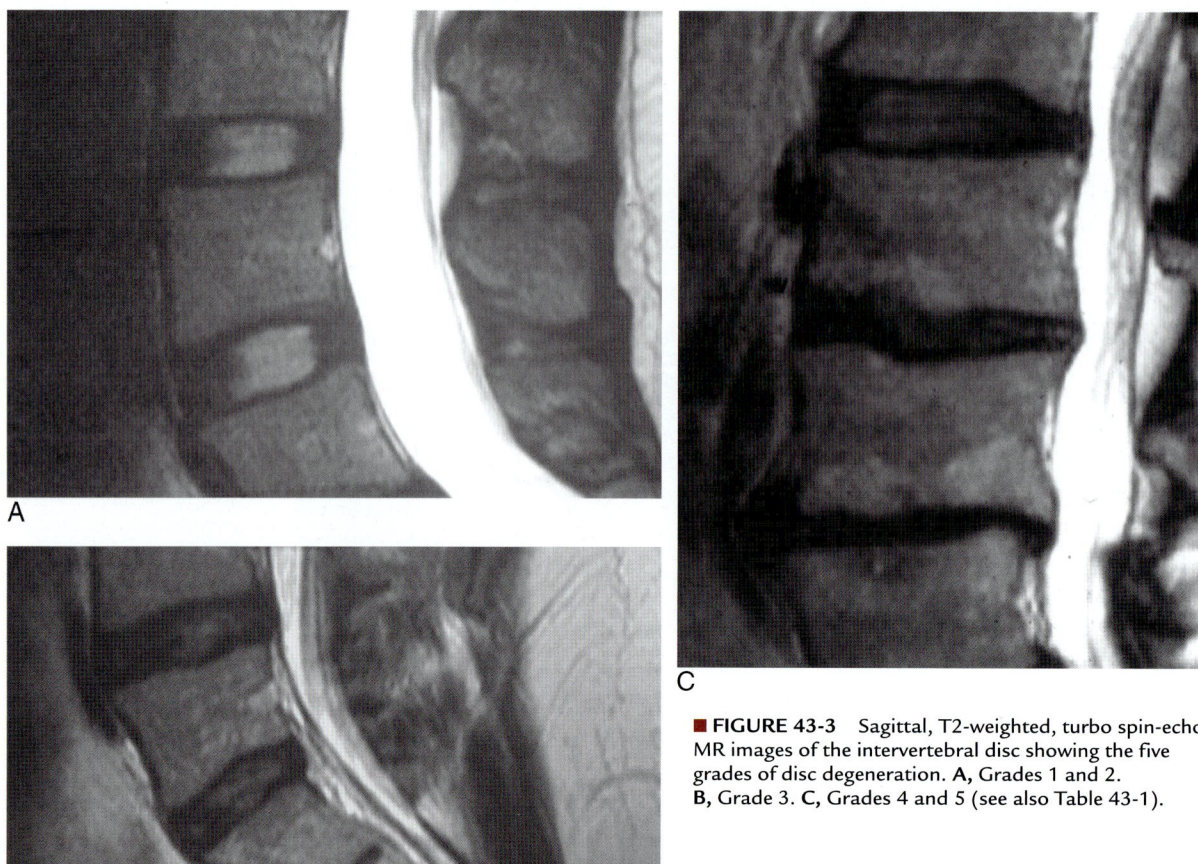

■ **FIGURE 43-3** Sagittal, T2-weighted, turbo spin-echo MR images of the intervertebral disc showing the five grades of disc degeneration. **A,** Grades 1 and 2. **B,** Grade 3. **C,** Grades 4 and 5 (see also Table 43-1).

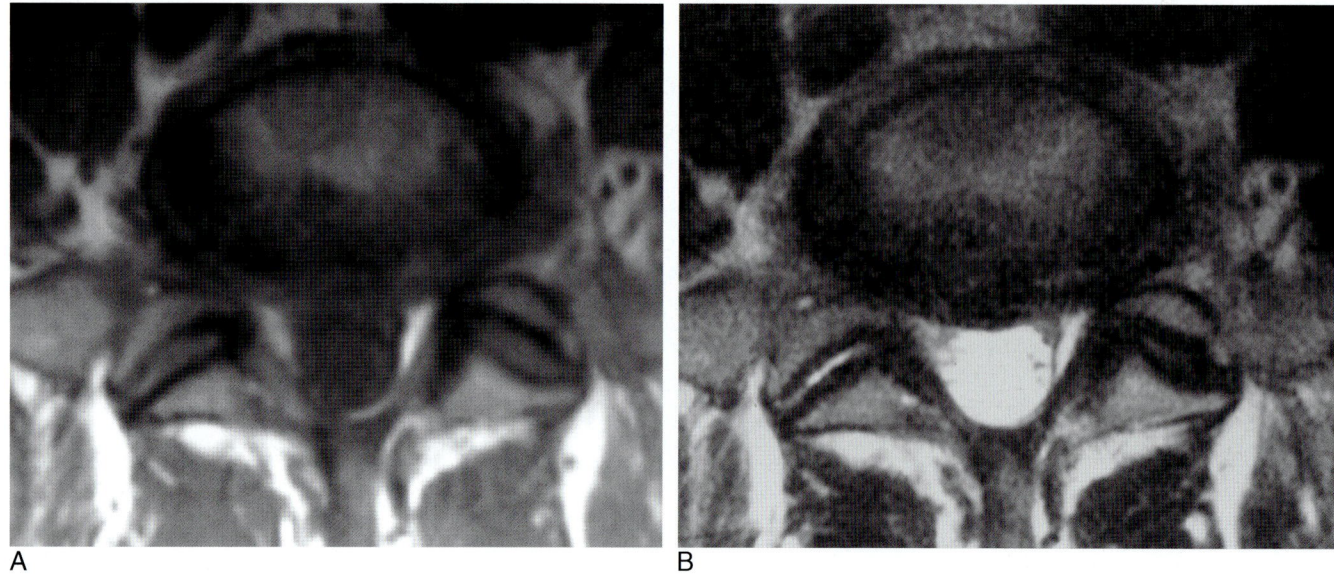

■ **FIGURE 43-4** Disc bulge. Axial T1-weighted (**A**) and T2-weighted (**B**) turbo spin-echo MR images demonstrate the disc extending circumferentially beyond the outline of the vertebral body.

the development of clefts in the posterolateral aspects of the disc from the nucleus into the neurocentral joints.

Focal linear areas of high signal within the degenerated disc occasionally occur that are thought to be due to free water within degenerate clefts, and the presence of gas in the disc may result in low signal on T1- and T2-weighted images. Calcification within the degenerated disc will produce low signal on T1, but occasionally fine calcification may lead to T1 shortening and increased signal intensity.

Discography

Although MRI demonstrates the features of degeneration well, attempts to predict the source of back pain have proven unreliable, especially when more than one disc has degenerated. If accurate delineation of a painful level is required before surgery, an injection of water-soluble contrast agent into the nucleus will confirm the degenerate changes and may provide confirmation of the disc as a source of pain (Fig. 43-5). CT may be performed in conjunction with the injection because this enables internal annular changes to be demonstrated as concentric rings of contrast medium and thus the degree of degeneration to be graded.[19] A good correlation between discographic and MR morphology has been shown, but discograms have identified abnormalities on apparently normal MR images.[20]

Pain production is assessed during and after injection of the contrast agent and is rare if the disc is normal. Symptom provocation from degenerated or injured discs is variable, but in a study of discography in asymptomatic control subjects pain was not produced from abnormal discs,[21] although others have found a higher false-positive rate.[22] The diagnostic accuracy of discography is still unclear because double-blind controlled trials have not been performed.

However, using successful surgical fusion as an end point, an 82% accuracy with an 89% sensitivity has been recorded. The specificity was low at 43%, but abnormal discs with no pain reproduction that were left at surgery did not result in poor results.[23] However, if discography is used only for cases in which all other clinical and diagnostic criteria for the diagnosis of discogenic pain are fulfilled in sequence, the false-positive rate is decreased. Discography is most accurate and useful when the diagnosis of discogenic pain is highly probable.[24]

In the cervical spine there is a greater degree of discordance between MRI and discography owing to posterolateral cleft formation. The accuracy of cervical discography is less clear, and there is an increased potential for infection in the disc after the investigation.

Posterior Annular Tears

Clefts may develop in the annular fibers between the concentric fibers or in a radial pattern, or a combination of the two may occur. This process may be associated with a traumatic episode, particularly in younger patients, but it has been demonstrated with increased frequency with age, as shown in cadaver studies. These clefts are only demonstrated by MRI or discography.

Magnetic Resonance Imaging and Computed Tomographic Discography

The posterior tears can be seen on MR sagittal studies. The disc height is usually maintained on the T1-weighted image and is associated with a small central bulge of the posterior annulus on the midline image and on the axial scan through the disc. On T2-weighted, fast spin-echo MR sequences there is a high signal intensity linear

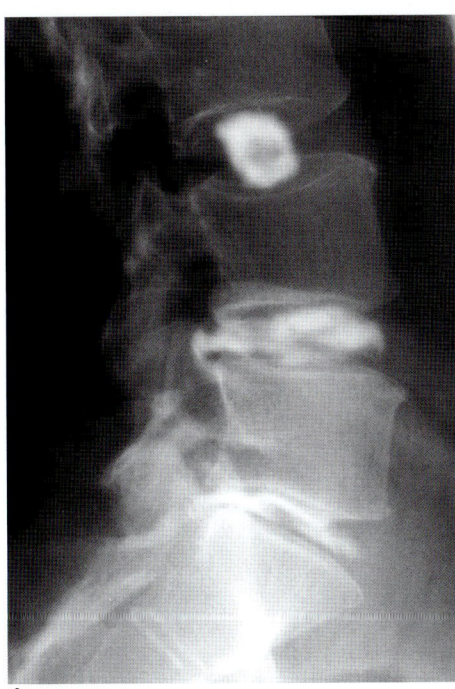

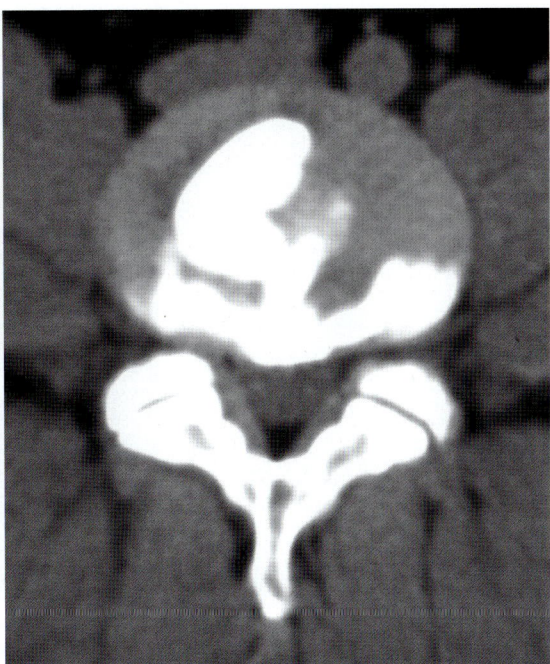

■ **FIGURE 43-5** Disc degeneration. **A,** Three-level discogram shows a normal delineation of the nucleus at L3-L4, degeneration with circumferential posterior annular disruption at L4-L5, and marked degeneration at L5-S1. **B,** CT discography demonstrates that the contrast medium injected into the nucleus has extended through the posterior annular fibers and circumferentially between the fibers.

A

B

track through the low-signal annulus and a small central bulge. In some cases they may be seen as a bright focus within the outer annulus, which is separated from the remainder of the nucleus as a high intensity zone (Fig. 43-6). Posterior annular tears may not be visible on MRI; compared with cadaver anatomic sections, MRI only had a 67% sensitivity.[25] If gadolinium diethylenetriamine pentaacetic acid (Gd-DTPA) is injected, enhancement of the posterior annular cleft may be visualized, and enhancement of the posterior annular tear almost always occurs in the presence of a high intensity zone.

Posterior annular tears are best demonstrated by discography with the injection of contrast medium directly into the nucleus, followed by CT, which will define the pattern of flow in the annulus. The tears with high intensity zones on MRI have been shown on CT discography to represent a combination of radial and concentric tears (see Fig. 43-6), and the significance in relation to symptoms has been the subject of considerable debate. Aprill and Bogduk[26] found that the presence of high intensity zones had a positive predictive value of 86% for a severely disrupted and symptomatic disc. They concluded that a high intensity zone was a sign of painful internal disc disruption. Subsequent investigators looking for correlation between high intensity zones and pain on discography have come to conflicting conclusions. The sign has also been reported to have a high specificity and positive predictive value (95.2% and 88.9%, respectively) for discography-induced pain but was limited by poor sensitivity (26.7%).[27] A high rate of concordance between high intensity zones and painful discography was also reported by other authors.[28] However, other studies have also found no statistical correlation between the presence of high intensity zones and pain response on discography.[29] To further complicate this issue, discographic injection in subjects with high intensity zones provoked significant pain in approximately 70% of subjects whether symptomatic with low back pain or not.[30]

In studies of MRI of the lumbar spine, high intensity zones have been reported to be a common finding (prevalence, 45.5%) in patients with low back and leg pain but a group of patients with particular clinical features was not defined.[31] A high incidence of high intensity zones in asymptomatic volunteers between ages 20 and 50 years (32% and 33% between two observers) has also been reported.[32] A recent study of the natural history of high intensity zones has shown that many stay unchanged, whereas others regress or increase in intensity and that no correlation existed between improvement or exacerbation of high intensity zones and changes in symptoms.[33] On the basis of all available evidence, posterior annular tears increase in incidence with age and are common in the asymptomatic population. They may be a source of pain, but it is uncertain whether high intensity zones are more commonly painful than other posterior annular tears.

Herniation of the Nucleus Pulposus

Radial tears in the posterior annulus enable the nucleus pulposus to pass through the annulus and result in a herniation extending beyond the normal margin of the disc and delineated by the margins of the vertebral body end plate. Such herniations may include annular and endplate material, especially in the cervical spine.

The importance of imaging is to demonstrate the precise anatomic features and extent of the herniation and its effect on the nerve roots. Classification of disc herniations is most commonly based on the morphologic model, with categories of normal disc, bulging disc, protrusion, extru-

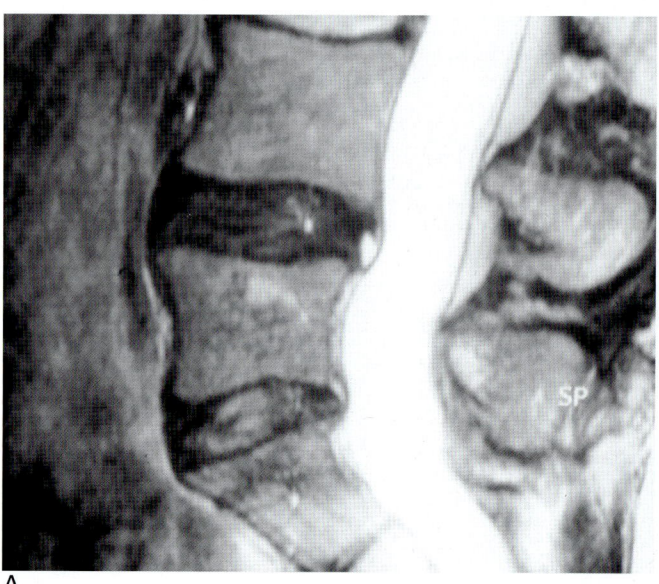
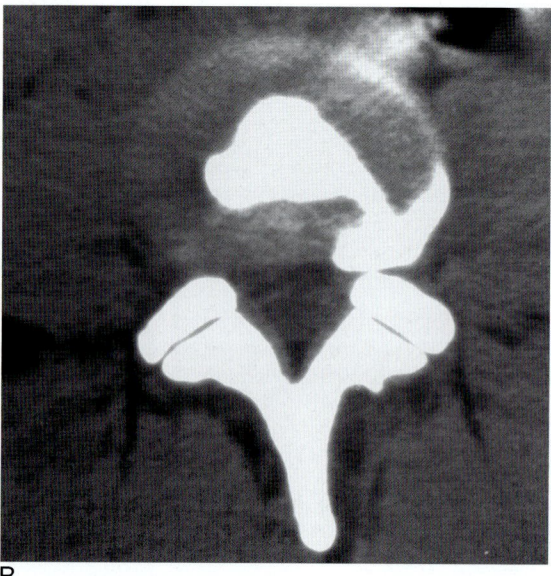

■ **FIGURE 43-6** Posterior annular tear. **A,** Sagittal, T2-weighted, turbo spin-echo MR image demonstrates a high signal zone in the outer fibers of the annulus with no evidence of nuclear material herniating through the posterior annulus. **B,** CT discography demonstrates a radial posterolateral tear through the annulus with a concentric component.

sion, and sequestration. A bulging disc refers to a circumferential symmetric disc extension beyond the disc space. A protrusion indicates focal or asymmetric disc extension beyond the interspace with preservation of the outer annular/posterior longitudinal ligament complex with the base against the parent disc broader than any other diameter of the protrusion and with continuity of nuclear material to the nucleus pulposus. An extrusion is focal with disruption of the outer annular fibers; the base against the parent disc is narrower than any diameter of the extruding material, but continuity with the parent nucleus is maintained. Finally, sequestration indicates complete loss of continuity of the disc material with the parent disc with migration away from the disc in some cases (Table 43-2).[34]

Radiography

Plain radiographs are of little value in the diagnosis of disc herniation and cannot visualize neurologic structures either directly or indirectly. They only provide information on disc height, instability, bony canal size in the cervical spine, and more severe causes of neck pain, such as infection or neoplasm. In the cervical spine, if the herniation is chronic it may be associated with a visible osteophyte, which may be important in surgical planning but does not provide any information about the soft tissue mass. Similarly, in the thoracic and lumbar spine, an old calcified disc herniation may be visible on lateral plain radiographs in chronic cases. Anteroposterior radiographs are useful in the lumbar spine in the presence of transitional vertebra to confirm the level before surgery.

Computed Tomography

Computed tomography can demonstrate a disc herniation in the spinal canal and is an alternative method of investigation in patients in whom MRI is contraindicated.

In the cervical spine there may be streak artifacts from the shoulders, but this is unusual with multislice scanners and can be partially negated by reconstructions. Unenhanced CT does not differentiate the cord from the theca in the cervical and thoracic spine. On CT, the herniated disc material will appear as a focal mass contiguous with the disc, having an attenuation value of 50 to 100 Hounsfield units and encroaching on the spinal canal either centrally or posterolaterally. The low-attenuation epidural fat will be obliterated and the dural sac deformed. The nerve root will be displaced posteriorly and may be compressed against the bony margin of the canal. Fragments that have migrated should be carefully evaluated and not confused with epidural veins, conjoint

nerve roots, and dorsal root ganglia. Large herniations that occupy most of the canal may be misdiagnosed owing to loss of clarity between the disc and dural sac. CT is ideal for demonstrating calcification in the disc material, which has been reported to occur in up to 75% of thoracic disc herniations, and any associated osteophyte formation or end-plate fragments, particularly in the cervical spine.

It is difficult to differentiate between protrusions and extrusions on CT, but disc herniation and nerve root compression in the foramen is visualized and is further improved on multislice CT systems by volume acquisition and reconstructions in the sagittal plane. The reported accuracy of CT in the cervical spine ranges from 72% to 91%, but these studies were performed before multislice CT.[35,36] The accuracy in the lumbar spine has been reported to be between 73% and 83%.[37,38]

In the cervical and thoracic spine the CT examination should be combined with an intrathecal injection of contrast agents, which will increase visualization of the nerve roots and cord, with accuracy reported up to 96%.[35]

Magnetic Resonance Imaging

Magnetic resonance imaging is the imaging modality of choice for evaluating a patient with a suspected disc herniation. Most centers will perform T1- and turbo spin-echo (TSE) T2-weighted sequences in the sagittal and axial planes, although some advocate more limited initial sequences. In the cervical spine a gradient-echo, T2-weighted, axial MR sequence may be preferred. On the T1-weighted, sagittal image the disc is of uniformly intermediate signal with the prolapse extending posteriorly behind the line of the posterior rim of the vertebral body on one or two images. The degree of indentation of the low-signal dural sac is dependent on the position of the herniation and on the thickness of the high-signal epidural fat. On the sagittal T2-weighted, turbo spin-echo sequence the herniated nuclear material will show as increased signal through the low-signal posterior annulus that projects beyond the posterior vertebral line. The relationship of the protrusion to the nerve root is clearly defined, and root deformity and displacement can be identified. The evaluation of this relationship is of major importance and has been graded depending on whether the disc is touching, displacing, or compressing the nerve root.[39]

A *protrusion* will show a low-signal intact line of outer annular fibers and the posterior longitudinal ligament. On the axial T1-weighted studies the localized protrusion can be identified outlined against the low-signal dural sac and high-signal epidural fat (Fig. 43-7). The T2-weighted sequence will demonstrate the nerve roots in and emerging from the dural sac. *Extruded herniations* that have penetrated the outer annular fibers appear as a globular mass of intermediate signal on T1-weighted images with incomplete outer low-signal fibers but with continuity of the herniated material maintained with the nucleus pulposus. The height of the disc of origin is narrower at the base of the herniation than the diameter of the extruding material on the sagittal view, and/or the diameter of the base of the herniated material on the axial view is similar or narrower than the anteroposterior measurement of the herniated material (Fig. 43-8). The extruded disc

TABLE 43-2	Classification of Disc Herniations
Bulging disc	Circumferential symmetric disc extension
Protrusion	Focal/asymmetric disc extension, preserved annulus/PLLC
Extrusion	Focal extension with disruption of annulus/PLLC
Sequestration	Loss of continuity fragment—parent disc

PLLC, posterior longitudinal ligamental complex.

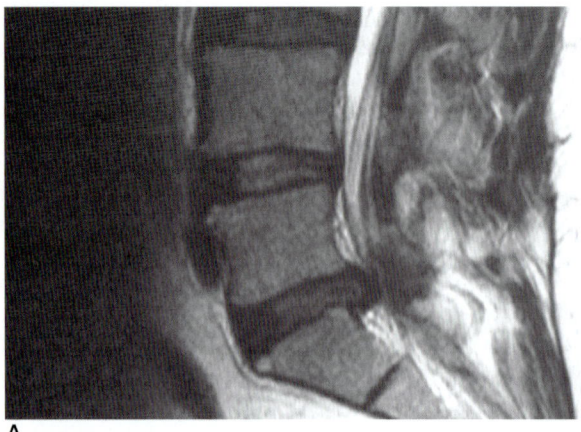

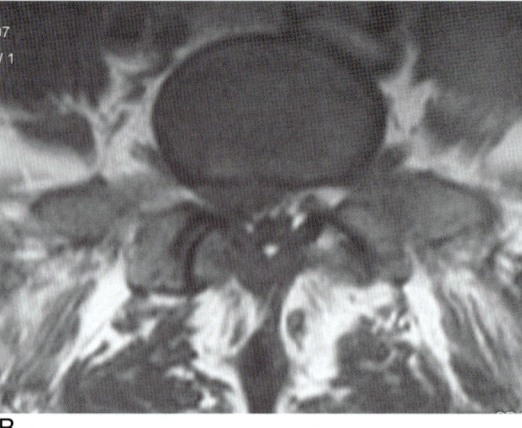

■ **FIGURE 43-7** Disc protrusion. **A,** Sagittal, T2-weighted, turbo spin-echo MR image shows the herniation continuous with the nucleus pulposus, similar width to the disc space, and an intact low signal annular margin. **B,** Axial, T1-weighted MR image shows the base of the herniation is much wider than the height. The right nerve root is compressed, and the surrounding epidural fat is obliterated.

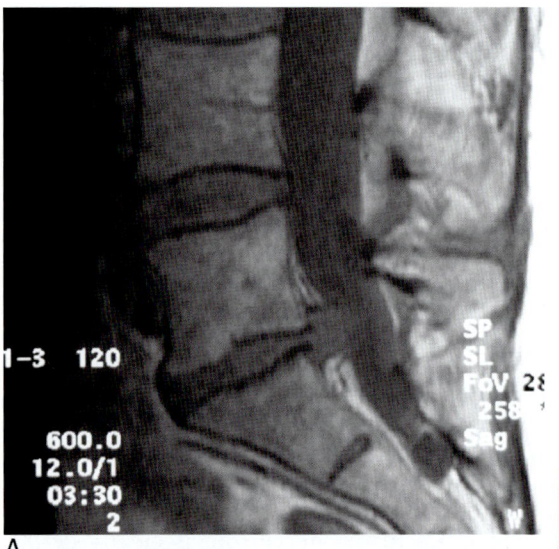

■ **FIGURE 43-8** Disc extrusion. **A,** Sagittal, T1-weighted, turbo spin-echo MR image demonstrates a large L5-S1 herniated nucleus pulposus that has no low signal outline of outer annular fibers. **B,** Sagittal, T2-weighted, turbo spin-echo MR image shows the herniated material remains with increased signal and has not migrated away from the remainder of the disc. **C,** Axial, T2-weighted, turbo spin-echo MR image shows the herniation with a narrow base that is similar to the height of the prolapse. There is grade 3 compression of the right S1 nerve root.

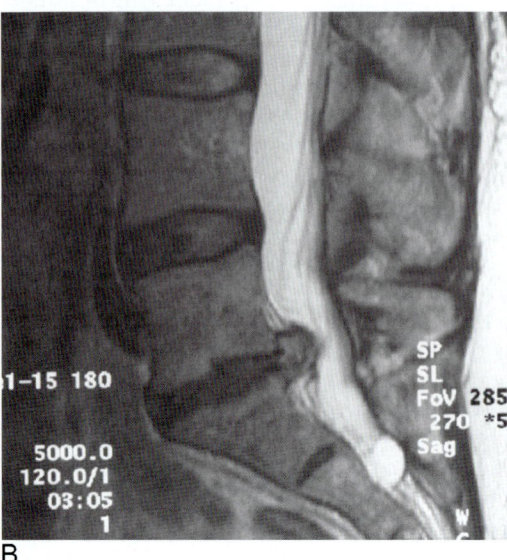

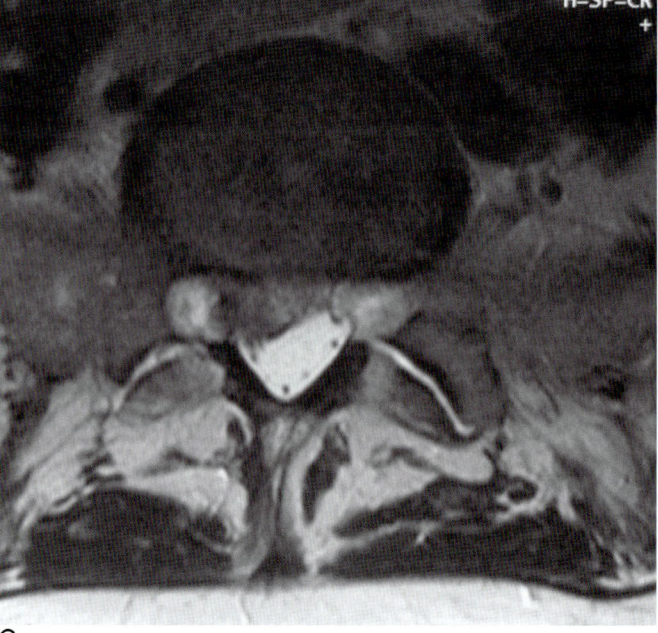

may remain deep to the posterior longitudinal ligament or may penetrate it, but differentiation on MRI has been reported to have a low accuracy.[40] If the nuclear material becomes sequestrated, the continuity with the parent nucleus pulposus is lost and fragments may migrate behind the adjacent vertebra (Fig. 43-9). Careful evaluation of the MRI is required to identify free fragments that have migrated particularly into the nerve root canals.

If the disc herniation is acute, the herniated material is of high signal on T2-weighted images, but persistent herniations become dehydrated and lose signal. Herniations may occur into the foramen in a far-out posterolateral position and may displace the nerve root outside the foramen or compress the root in the foramen (Fig. 43-10).

Paramagnetic contrast agents have not been found to be of great value in the evaluation of uncomplicated disc herniations,[41] although the perception of size and location of the herniation may be significantly changed by the contrast medium enhancement and improved delineation between disc material and nerve root. Contrast medium enhancement may be useful in recurrent herniations and in the postoperative evaluation for differentiating between

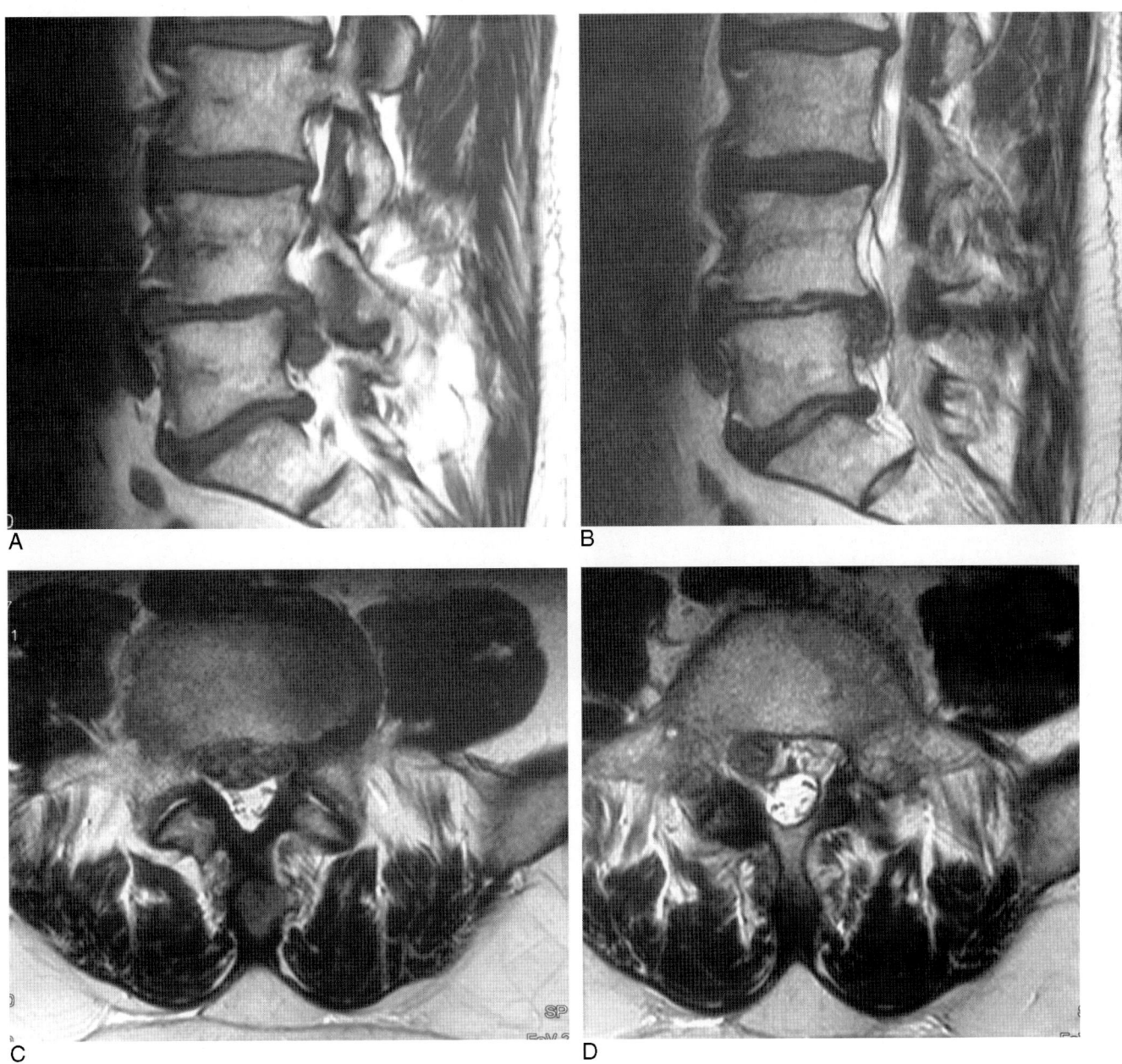

■ **FIGURE 43-9** Disc sequestration. Sagittal T1-weighted (**A**) and T2-weighted (**B**) turbo spin-echo MR images demonstrate a large mass of herniated nucleus pulposus that has migrated away from the disc behind the body. **C** and **D,** Axial T2-weighted turbo spin-echo MR images show the mass of nuclear material behind the vertebral body and migration into the right nerve root canal compressing the nerve root.

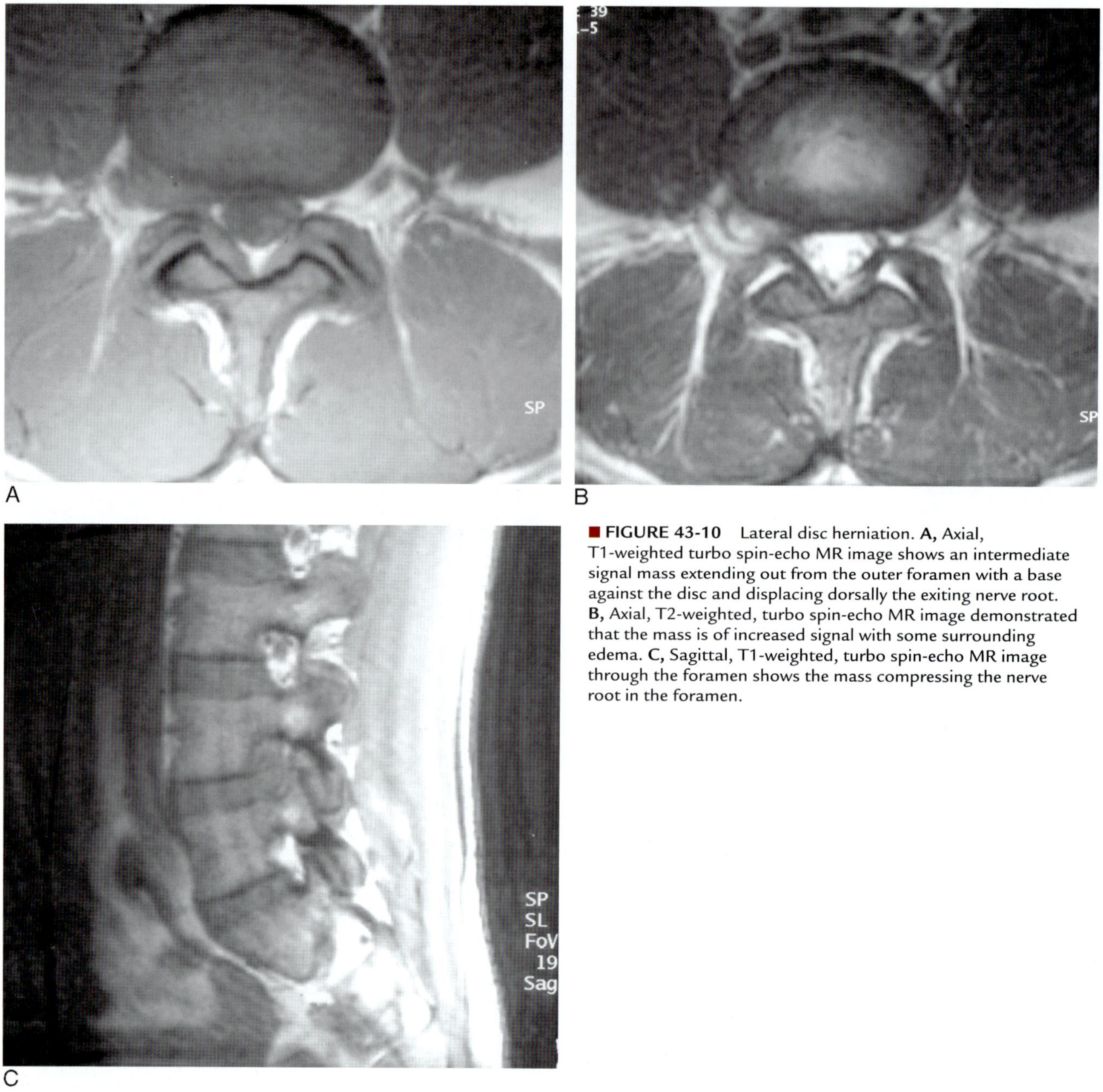

A

B

C

■ FIGURE 43-10 Lateral disc herniation. **A,** Axial, T1-weighted turbo spin-echo MR image shows an intermediate signal mass extending out from the outer foramen with a base against the disc and displacing dorsally the exiting nerve root. **B,** Axial, T2-weighted, turbo spin-echo MR image demonstrated that the mass is of increased signal with some surrounding edema. **C,** Sagittal, T1-weighted, turbo spin-echo MR image through the foramen shows the mass compressing the nerve root in the foramen.

fibrosis and recurrent herniation and between a lateral disc herniation and a nerve sleeve tumor. Enhancement of compressed nerve roots has been demonstrated in a number of series, although the percentage of cases with enhancement has varied between 21% and 68%.[42,43] Tyrrell and colleagues,[44] in a large series of patients, found a statistically significant relationship between nerve root enhancement and the presence of a sequestrated disc, but the sensitivity of nerve root enhancement overall was 23.5%.

Finally, an epidural hematoma associated with a posterior annular tear may result in symptoms indistinguishable from a disc herniation. On MRI the hematoma appears as an extradural mass that is often largest at the level of the midvertebral body, with a tapered indistinct margin at the level of the disc (Fig. 43-11). It may have a high intensity on T1-weighted images and an intermediate signal on T2-weighted images, although the timing of the imaging will affect the signal characteristics and resorption is usually rapid.[45-48]

Vertebral End Plate

Vertebral end-plate changes occurring in conjunction with disc degeneration vary considerably in severity, depending on the degree of disruption of the cartilage end plates and the response of the adjacent subchondral bone.

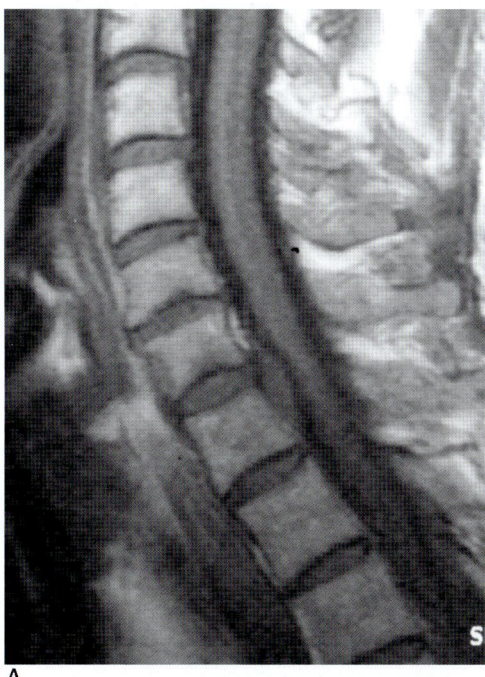
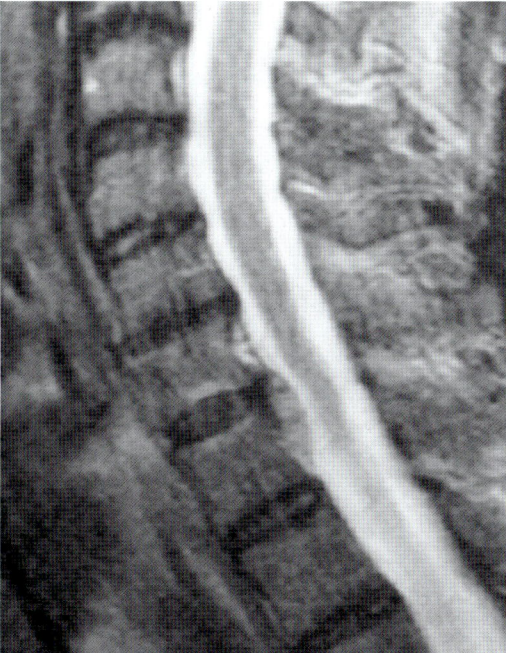

A   B

■ **FIGURE 43-11** Cervical epidural hematoma. Sagittal T1-weighted (**A**) and T2-weighted (**B**) turbo spin-echo MR images show a tapered mass behind the body that is of intermediate signal on the T1-weighted image and of increased signal on the T2-weighted image. Six weeks later there was complete resolution of the hematoma.

Radiography

The most common lesion seen on the lateral radiograph of the thoracic and lumbar spine is the Schmorl node, which appears as a well-defined indentation of the bony end plate just posterior to the midline. More extensive interosseous end-plate herniations may occur, especially anteriorly, and these may result in increased anteroposterior growth of the vertebral bodies with slight wedging. The end plate may be irregular and sclerotic if there is moderate to severe disc degeneration, and in some cases hemispheric sclerosis of the anterior part of the vertebral body may be present. End-plate irregularity and Schmorl's nodes are also a feature of Scheuermann's disease.

Magnetic Resonance Imaging

Schmorl's nodes appear on MRI as indentations of the end plate containing small extensions of high signal intensity in the nucleus within them on T2-weighted sequences. MRI may show a rim of low signal in the vertebral marrow on T1 weighting around the interosseous herniation, with high signal on T2 weighting, suggesting some marrow reaction to the herniation.

Signal intensity changes are also seen in the end plates and adjacent vertebral bodies of both cervical and lumbar vertebrae in association with disc degeneration. These changes tend to fall into three main categories, as described by Modic and coworkers,[49] but mixed features may also be present: type 1 changes have areas of low T1 and high T2 signal and have high signal on the short tau inversion recovery (STIR) sequence (Fig. 43-12) and enhancement after paramagnetic contrast injection and have been shown on histology to relate to an increase in marrow vascularity, with some inflammatory cell infiltration. Type 2 changes are more common and have a high T1-weighted signal and isointense or slightly hyperintense T2 signal, with a low signal on STIR (Fig. 43-13) and no evidence of enhancement. Histologic studies have shown thickened trabeculae and replacement of normal marrow by fat. Type 3 is characterized by low T1- and T2-weighted signals and is associated with sclerosis on radiographs due to marked trabecular thickening. This classification has been shown to be reliable and reproducible. In some patients, type 1 and type 2 changes may occur at different levels in the same patient and a mixture of types 1 and 2 may occur at the same level. Type 1 changes are considered to be the earliest and the most active stage in the process with evolution to type 2,[49] although recent longitudinal studies have demonstrated some type 2 changes converting to type 1.[50]

The symptomatic significance of these changes is still being evaluated with varying result. Type 1 lesions were not reported in a series of asymptomatic subjects, but a recent study has identified all types of end-plate changes in a series of subjects without significant recent back pain. Comparative studies with pain provocation at discography have suggested a close relationship between type 1 changes and back pain reproduction,[51] as well as a high specificity and positive predictive value for the various types of end-plate changes as an indicator of a painful disc at discography.[52,53] In a small longitudinal study, which included six patients with type 1 changes, Modic and colleagues[49] suggested a temporal evolutionary trend of type 1 to type 2. A recent longitudinal study has shown that type 1 end-plate changes are dynamic lesions that either increase in size or convert to type 2; if the type 1 lesion does convert to type 2, it starts to do so within 2 years in most cases. There is also evidence, although not at a statistically significant level, that conversion from type 1 to type 2 is related to an improvement in a patient's symptoms.[54]

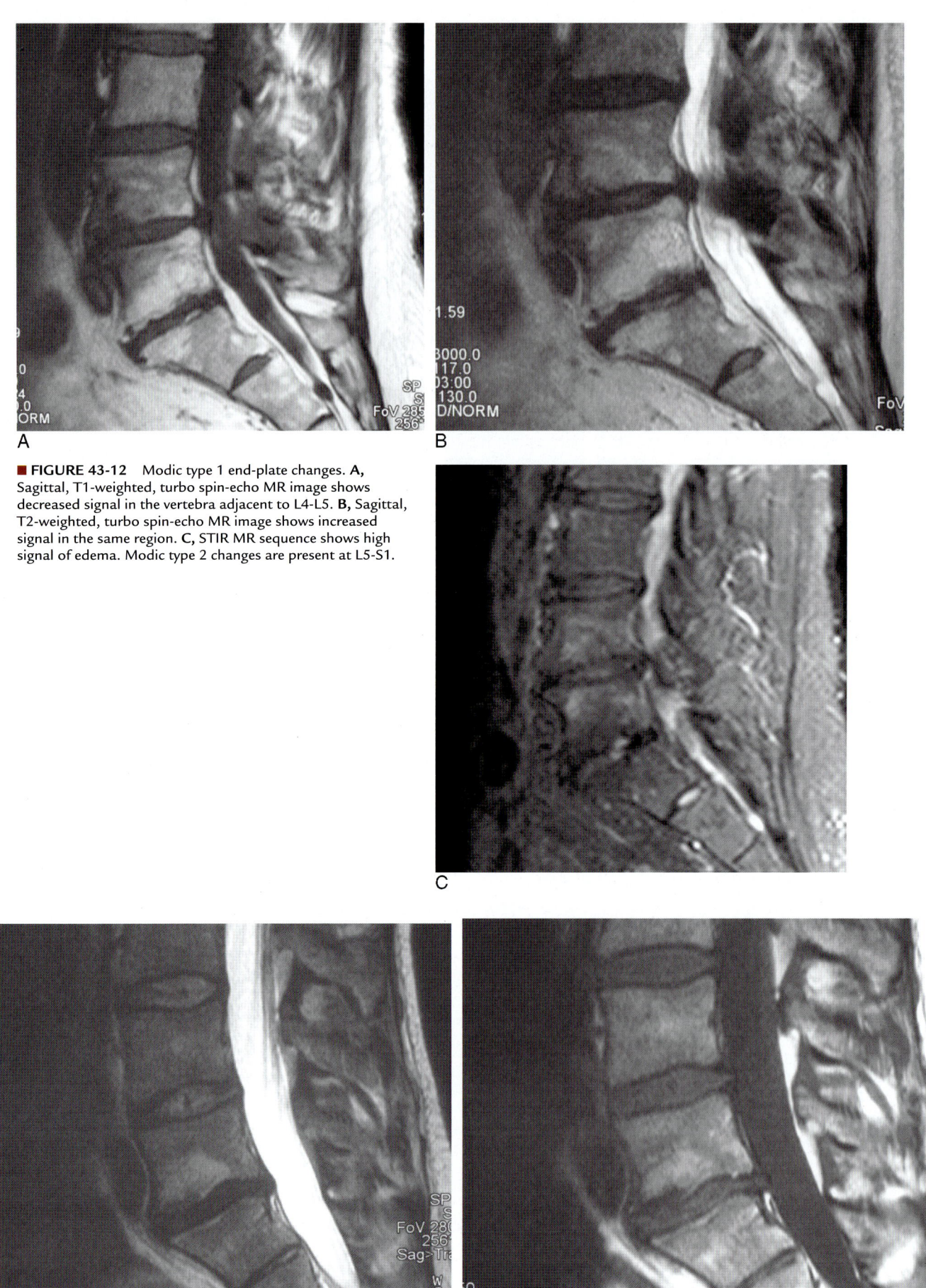

■ **FIGURE 43-12** Modic type 1 end-plate changes. **A,** Sagittal, T1-weighted, turbo spin-echo MR image shows decreased signal in the vertebra adjacent to L4-L5. **B,** Sagittal, T2-weighted, turbo spin-echo MR image shows increased signal in the same region. **C,** STIR MR sequence shows high signal of edema. Modic type 2 changes are present at L5-S1.

■ **FIGURE 43-13** Modic type 2 end-plate changes. T2-weighted (**A**) and T1-weighted (**B**) turbo spin-echo MR images show focal irregularity of the cartilage end plate and subchondral bone with increased signal in the adjacent vertebral bodies on both sequences.

Osteoarthritis of the Facet Joints

Facet joint pain has been described as an ache in the neck or low back and may refer to the shoulder and buttock, respectively. The pain may also refer to both upper and lower limbs, respectively, and in the lower limbs may refer along the back of the leg, sometimes to the ankle. It may be increased in extension and in the case of the lumbar spine may be eased by exercise. In the neck, muscle spasm secondary to facet joint pain may produce a torticollis.

Osteoarthritis of the facet joints is seen as early as 30 years of age and is almost constant after 60 years of age.

Radiography

Radiographic features are present on the lateral and anteroposterior views of the cervical and lumbar spine but are more difficult to appreciate in the thoracic spine owing to the overlying ribs and the alignment of the joints. The initial loss of cartilage thickness is not visualized, but once articular cartilage loss is well established, resultant joint space narrowing will be seen where the joint spaces are parallel to the beam, in particular the lateral cervical projection or the anteroposterior view of the upper lumbar spine. Sclerosis of the subchondral bone and marginal osteophyte formation with hyperostosis results in increased density in the region of the facet and hypertrophy of the apophyseal process, which may be seen projecting laterally on an anteroposterior radiograph, particularly in the cervical spine (see Fig. 43-2) and lower lumbar spine. On the lateral view, remodeling may be seen but subchondral cysts are difficult to appreciate on plain radiographs. Oblique views may show the facet joint spaces more clearly when they are more coronally aligned, as in the lower lumbar spine. The articular process of the facet joints may impinge on the upper surface of the lamina above and below, causing further sclerosis.

Computed Tomography

Computed tomography is considerably superior to radiographs in demonstrating the facet joints in the thoracic and lumbar spine. The horizontal orientation of the joints in the cervical spine requires volume acquisition and multiplanar reconstruction. Although the cartilage is not visualized, the joint space can be accurately evaluated and bony articular surface irregularities, subchondral sclerosis, and subchondral cysts all clearly seen. Osteophyte formation occurs on both dorsal and ventral margins of the joint, resulting in displacement of the capsule and ligaments, and ventral osteophytes may cause compression of adjacent nerve roots. CT appearances of degeneration have been graded in the lumbar spine (Fig. 43-14).[55] Grade 0

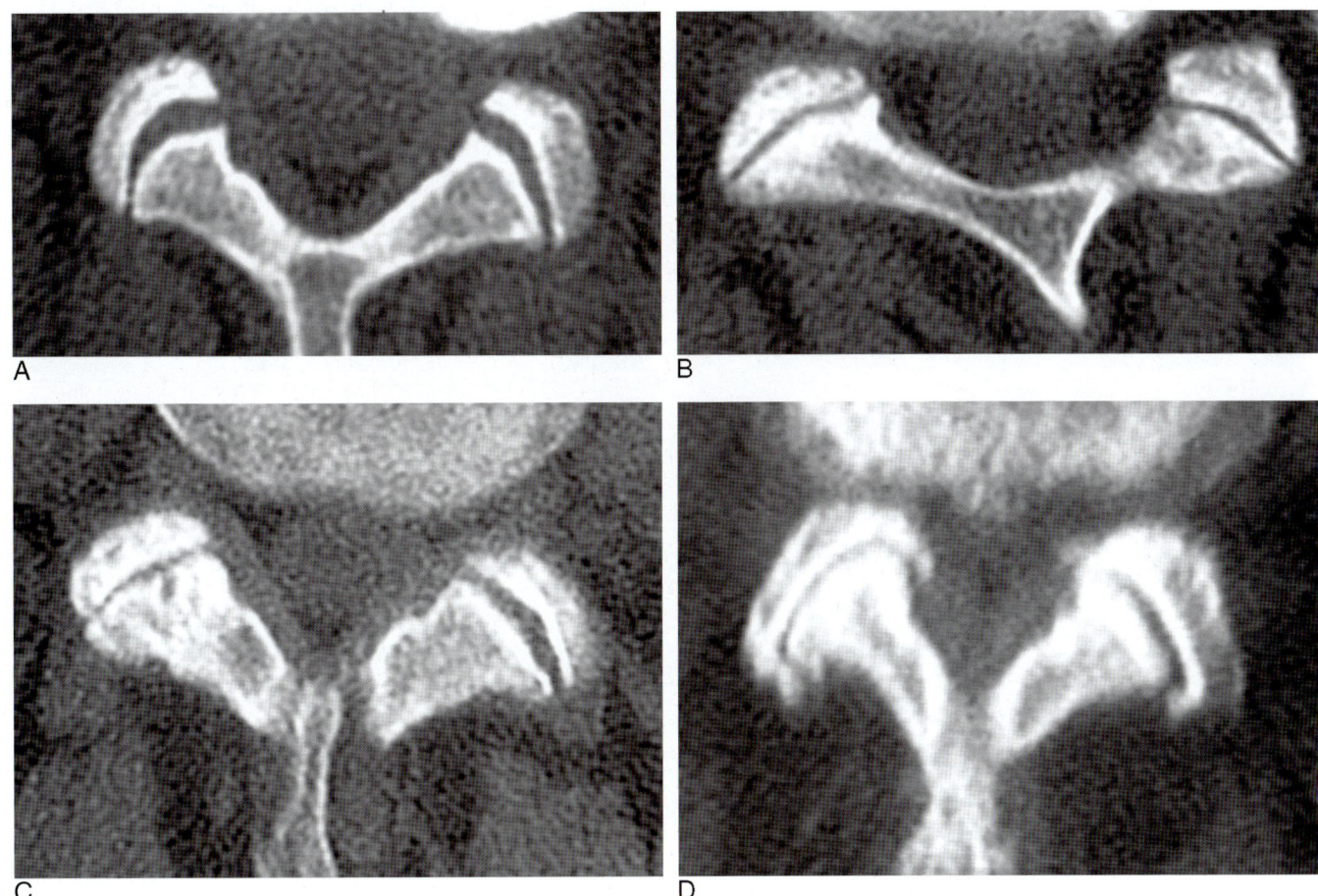

A B C D

■ **FIGURE 43-14**   Facet osteoarthritis. CT of facet joints. **A,** Grade 0: normal joint space and subchondral bone. **B,** Grade 1: both facet joint spaces are narrowed and slightly hypertrophied. **C,** Grade 2: The joint space is narrowed with subchondral sclerosis and small cysts and mild osteophyte formation. **D,** Grade 3: severe degeneration with joint space irregularity, marked osteophyte formation, and bone sclerosis.

is normal with a joint space of 2 to 4 mm. In grade 1, the joint space is reduced to less than 2 mm and/or minor osteophytes and/or hypertrophy of the articular process are present. Grade 2 has narrowing of the joint space with or without any combination of moderate osteophyte formation and articular process hypertrophy, but mild subchondral irregularity is present. Finally, grade 3 has joint space narrowing, severe subarticular bone irregularity, and/or severe osteophytes and/or articular process hypertrophy. When this system of grading was used, interobserver correlation was 0.6 with one grade agreement in 95% to 97%.[55] The severity of CT changes in the lumbar spine does not, however, correlate with the presence of back pain.[56]

Magnetic Resonance Imaging

Magnetic resonance imaging particularly in the axial plane can similarly demonstrate the features of osteoarthritis of the facet satisfactorily but, unlike CT, the articular cartilage is seen as intermediate signal on T1- and proton density–weighted sequences, although the separation of the two surfaces is rarely possible unless an effusion is present. Subchondral line irregularity is not as clearly seen on MRI, but T2-weighted sequences demonstrate effusions and cysts as fluid collections with high signal intensity within the joint or in the subchondral bone, respectively (Fig. 43-15). Osteophytes may also be demonstrated on both T1- and T2-weighted sequences, but bone sclerosis is less easily appreciated. The same grading system can be used for MRI as CT, but the interobserver correlation is lower at 0.41; however, one grade agreement was again 95% to 97%.[55] Both CT and MRI will also demonstrate the ligamentum flavum, which may appear thickened or buckled, and the capsular ligamentum flavum combination is better seen with MRI. Calcification in the ligamentum flavum is difficult to define on MRI, and CT is the imaging method of choice if this feature is of diagnostic importance.

Pain Testing

To precisely relate the symptoms of neck or back capsular pain to the facet joints, image-guided injections of local anesthetic are required. The rationale is to identify whether the patient's neck, back, and/or limb pain

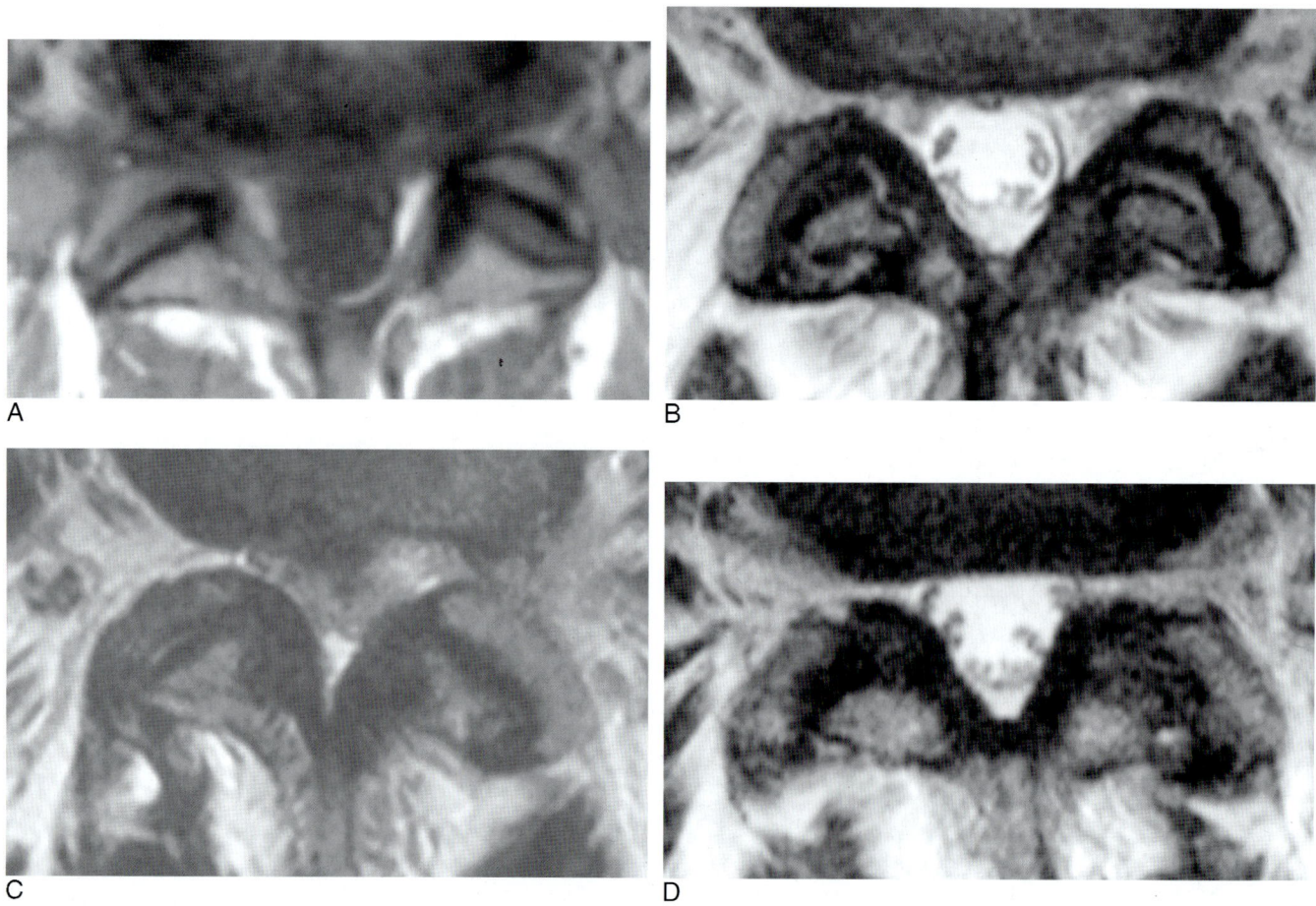

A

B

C

D

■ FIGURE 43-15 Facet osteoarthritis. MRI of facet joints. **A,** Grade 0 normal cartilage thickness is seen with a smooth, low signal, subchondral bone line. **B,** Grade 1: the joint spaces are reduced with slight bony hypertrophy. **C,** Grade 2: joint space loss and mild to moderate osteophyte formation. **D,** Grade 3: there is marked irregularity of the articular surfaces, joint space loss, and marked osteophyte formation.

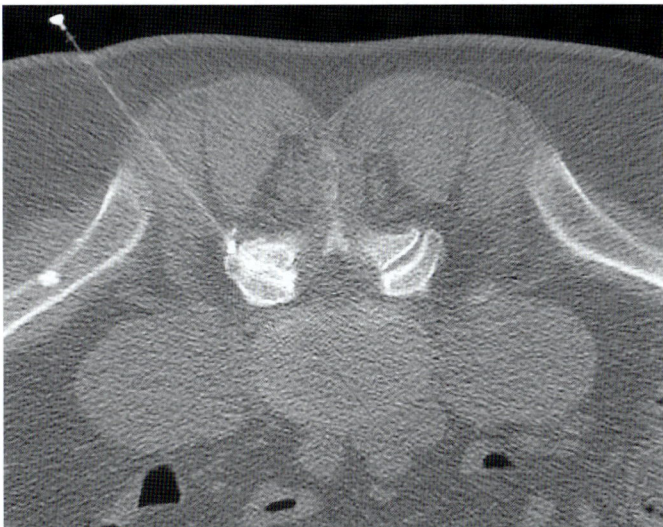

■ **FIGURE 43-16** Facet injection. CT-guided needle is inserted into the posterior capsule of the facet and a very small quantity of contrast agent is injected to check the position, followed by local anesthetic. Corticosteroid may also be injected for therapeutic purposes.

is significantly reduced or removed by the injection of local anesthetic into the facet joint. The needle may be placed in the cervical or lumbar facets using either fluoroscopic or CT guidance (Fig. 43-16). A small quantity of contrast medium may be injected to confirm the intraarticular position, and this is followed by up to 1 mL to avoid rupture or epidural extravasation of a longer-acting local anesthetic. The response to the injection is provided by the patient over the following 2 or 3 hours. A corticosteroid may be added after the local anesthetic as a therapeutic element, but it is not part of the diagnostic test. Studies of the effectiveness of this examination as a diagnostic test have been conflicting, which is compounded by the absence of a clear gold standard. The injections, however, may provide short- or longer-term relief, enabling mobilization and exercise programs to be instituted.

Cysts of the Intervertebral Facet Joints

Juxta-articular cysts of the facet joints of the lumbar spine have been recognized to be more common with the advent of CT and MRI. They may be synovial, arising from the facet joints containing xanthochromic fluid, or ganglion cysts containing gelatinous material and may or may not communicate with the joint. They have an incidence of 0.65% in the lumbar spine and are much less commonly documented in the cervical spine.[57] They more commonly occur in women, with an age range of 16 to 81 years and a mean of 57 years. These patients have low back pain and are often diagnosed only after imaging, but they also present with, or exhibit, radicular symptoms. The majority occur at L4-L5, but other lumbar levels may be affected, and bilateral cysts may occur. Facet osteoarthritis is an almost universal finding, and the incidence of degenerative spondylolisthesis varies between 42% and 65%.

Computed Tomography

The typical appearance is of a rounded juxtafacet mass with relatively low attenuation contents. Calcification may occur within the cyst or in the wall and is well demonstrated by CT (Fig. 43-17). Gas may also be present in the cyst, appearing as low attenuation and sometimes associated with gas in the facet joint. The associated osteoarthritis of the facet joint is well demonstrated on CT, which can also be utilized to guide injections of local anesthetic or corticosteroid into the cyst either directly or via the facet.[58]

Magnetic Resonance Imaging

Facet cysts are usually situated posterolaterally in the spinal canal and proportionally vary in size relative to the surface area of the spinal canal from 20% to 90%, resulting in varying degrees of nerve root and thecal compression. The cysts are best seen on T2-weighted sequences, where they have a discrete low-signal wall less than 3 mm thick. On T1-weighted images the wall may be mildly hyperintense or isointense, with the thecal contents making the cyst difficult to visualize, although the rim does enhance in the majority of cases in which contrast agent was administered. The cyst exhibits a variable pattern, depending on its contents; in the majority, the contents are hyperintense on T2-weighted images and isointense on T1-weighted images (see Fig. 43-17). However, nearly 25% of cysts have been reported to be hyperintense on T1-weighted images and hypointense on T2-weighted images. The mild T1 hyperintensity has been ascribed to a number of factors, including a high protein content or breakdown products of hemorrhage. Uncommonly, cysts may be hypointense or hyperintense on both sequences. Facet cysts must be distinguished from conjoint nerve roots, a sequestrated disc herniation, an intraspinal cyst, or a cystic neurofibroma. The natural history of cysts is variable, with spontaneous regression being seen in some cases. If symptomatic radicular compression is present, injections of corticosteroid may result in regression, but surgery remains the definitive treatment.

Degenerative Spondylolisthesis

The displacement of one vertebra on another is dependent on a biomechanical failure of the support of the posterior elements and may be anterolisthesis or retrolisthesis depending on the direction of stress of the vertebral bodies. Thus, retrolisthesis is more common in the upper lumbar spine, whereas degenerative anterolisthesis is more frequent at L4-L5. The prevalence of anterolisthesis in the lumbar spine increases sharply with age, with approximately 25% of those persons older than age 75 years showing subluxation of 5 mm or more; women may be affected more often than men.[59] Degeneration of the facet joints is the most common cause of spondylolisthesis.

In the cervical spine, the facet joints are horizontally aligned and osteoarthritic changes in the facet joints may lead to a loss of support of the vertebral body by the posterior elements, with forward displacement of the vertebral body. The pathology is that of severe osteoarthritis of the facet joints, with destruction of the articular surfaces, and loss of support of the ligamentum flavum and facet capsule.

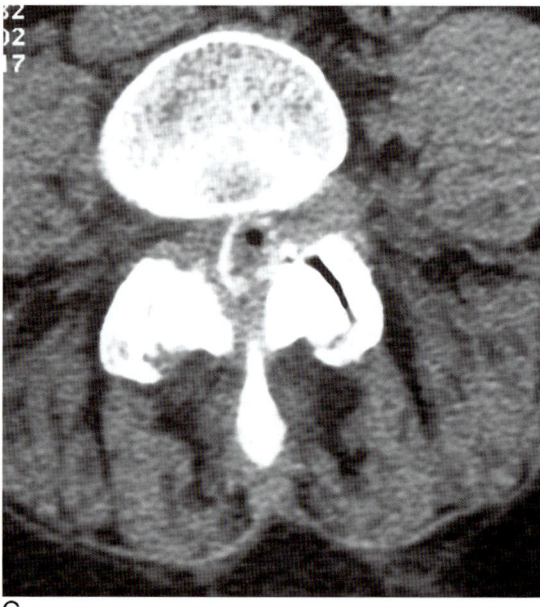

■ **FIGURE 43-17** Facet cyst. **A,** Axial, T2-weighted, turbo spin-echo MR image demonstrates the cyst with the base on the inner aspect of the facet joint. The outer wall of the cyst is of low signal, whereas the contents are of increased signal. The nerve root and dural sac are compressed by the cyst. **B,** Sagittal, T2-weighted, turbo spin-echo MR image shows the cyst occupying the spinal canal. **C,** CT shows extensive calcification with the wall of the cyst and air within the fluid content.

In most cases of degeneration of lumbar spondylolisthesis, the facets are aligned in the sagittal plane. The presence of a marked coronal alignment of the facets tends to reduce the likelihood of a degenerative spondylolisthesis. Disc degeneration may also lead to forward displacement of one vertebral body on another.

The presence of a degenerative spondylolisthesis may be associated with pain, and this may be due to osteoarthritis of the facets, the presence of disc degeneration, or a combination of these causing nerve root ischemia. There is a good correlation between the presence of low back and leg pain and the presence of degenerative spondylolisthesis.[60]

Radiography

The recorded normal range of forward displacement of one lumbar vertebra on another has been wide, with up to 5 mm being quoted as normal, but 3 mm should be used as the upper limit of normal. Recent studies indicate overall incidence of anterolisthesis in women older than the age of 65 as 28.9% and those with retrolisthesis as 14.2%, whereas if 5-mm slip is used as a guide, then the prevalence drops to 14.2% and 3.2%, respectively.[61] Most degenerative spondylolisthesis is at a single level, with 10% at two levels, and rarely exceeds 25% of the adjacent vertebral body. The lateral radiograph will demonstrate the forward displacement of the superior vertebral body with the lamina and spinous process, and the extent of the slip is measured from the posterior rim of the adjacent vertebral end plates (see Fig. 43-1). Disc degeneration is usually present with narrowing of the disc space, and some sclerosis of the vertebral end plate may also be seen. Sclerosis and bone proliferation are often present in the facet joints. On the anteroposterior radiographs the facet joints are usually sagittally aligned, and this can be confirmed on CT, which will also demonstrate the severe facet osteoarthritis that may produce considerable osteophyte formation and ossification of the ligamentum flavum. Dynamic demonstration of the effect on the dural sac by the degenerative spondylolisthesis can be achieved with flexion and extension views in combination with myelography, which shows increased dural sac compression on extension and widening of the dural sac on flexion.

Magnetic Resonance Imaging

The sagittal studies demonstrate the disc degeneration and the distortion of the posterior annulus due to the vertebral displacement, which results in the posterior disc margin being stretched and sometimes bulging into the canal. The axial scans will demonstrate the pseudo-disc appearance of spondylolisthesis, because the slice through the disc will demonstrate the position of the disc in relation to the inferior vertebral body, with an apparent absence of a superior vertebral body, giving the appearance of a disc prolapse. The smooth nature of the disc and its uniform curvature will differentiate this

pseudo-disc appearance of spondylolisthesis from a disc prolapse (Fig. 43-18). The facet joint degeneration is shown by the irregularity of the articular surface, cartilage loss, and proliferation of osteophyte formation.

The combination of forward displacement and disc degeneration and bulging, associated with the reparative changes around the osteoarthritic facets, and thickening or buckling of the ligamentum flavum is a common cause of spinal stenosis. This may be severe, with central canal stenosis causing compression of the nerve roots within the dural sac and narrowing of the subarticular space by the ventral slip of the inferior articular process reducing the entry zone of the nerve root canal. The intervertebral foramen at the involved level assumes a more horizontal configuration, resulting in reduced foraminal height; and in combination with the bulging annulus into the foramen, this results in foraminal stenosis. The degree of stenosis is well demonstrated on MRI, which will also clearly demonstrate, in the sagittal plane, the degree of dural sac compression and the relationship of the disc, the facets, and the ligamentum flavum as to their relative contribution to the degree of stenosis. Dynamic sagittal views in flexion and extension may be helpful in assessing the degree of stenosis.

Spinal Stenosis

Spinal stenosis has been defined as any type of narrowing of the spinal canal causing compression of the content of the canal due to conflict between the available space and its content. The stenosis may involve the central canal, the entry zones of the nerve root canals, or the intervertebral

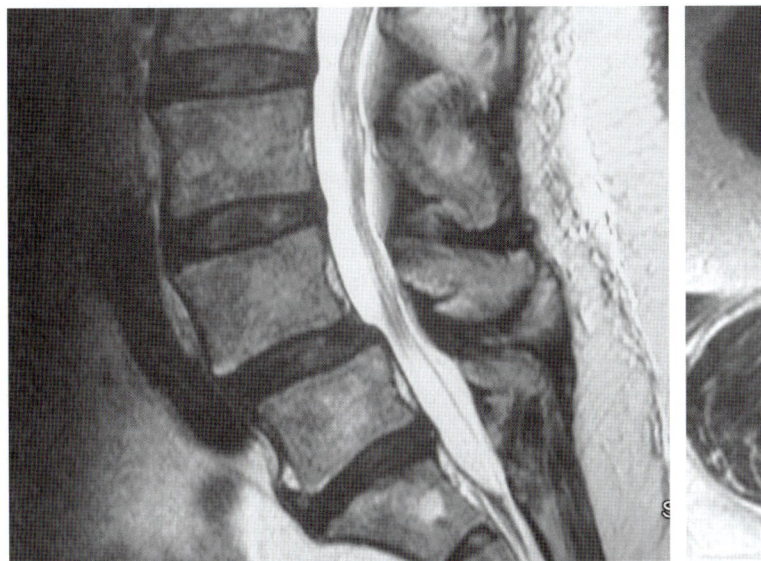
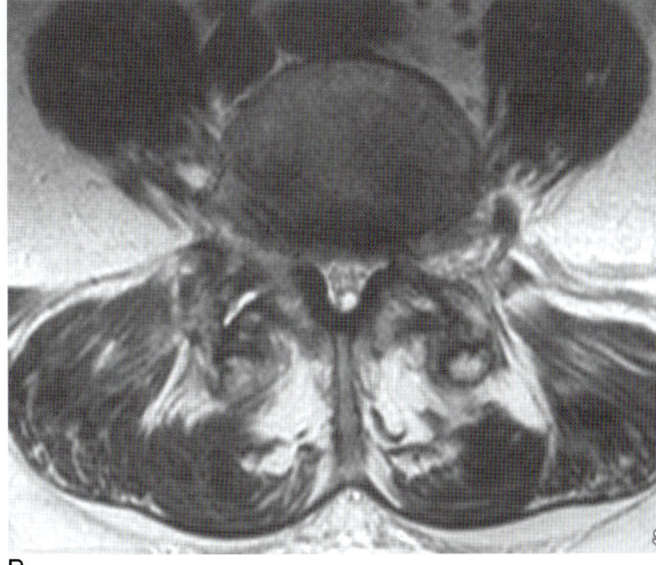

A B

■ **FIGURE 43-18** Degenerative spondylolisthesis. **A,** Sagittal, T2-weighted, turbo spin-echo MR image demonstrates the forward displacement of L4 on L5 with stretching of the posterior annulus and degeneration of the disc. **B,** Axial, T2-weighted, turbo spin-echo MR image shows grade 4 osteoarthritis of the facet joints with the posterior overlap of the annulus producing a mild pseudo-disc appearance.

foramina and, in many cases of degenerative stenosis, a combination of narrowing. Degenerative stenosis particularly involves the cervical and lumbar spine, and underlying developmentally short pedicles and a small spinal canal will increase the likelihood of degenerative stenosis. Degenerative spinal stenosis is due to osteoarthritis of the facet joints with or without hypertrophy, osteophyte formation on the posterior vertebral rim, degenerative bulging of the intervertebral discs, and degenerative changes in the ligamentum flavum. It occurs increasingly with increasing age and presents as long tract or root signs in the cervical spine and root compression in the lumbar spine.

In cervical stenosis with spinal cord myelopathy, the symptoms may be long tract or segmental. Long tract involvement is shown by exaggerated tendon reflexes, the presence of pathologic reflexes, spastic quadriplegia, a spastic type of myelopathy of the hand, glove and stocking sensory loss, and bladder and bowel disturbance, whereas segmental signs are motor deficits affecting that segment.[62] Stenotic impingement of the cervical nerve root usually manifests as occipital, posterior neck, shoulder, or upper extremity radicular symptoms.

Pain radiation to the legs may be unilateral or bilateral and may involve single or multiple nerve root distributions. Claudication is commonly related to the position of the lumbar spine, and the walking distance may vary, with greatest limitation being related to the more severe level of pain. Symptoms fluctuate in severity and increase gradually in most patients over a period of years. Motor and sensory disturbances vary in incidence, with sensory disturbances in the legs being common, weakness being less common, and bowel and bladder disturbances being unusual.

Radiography

In the cervical spine, central canal stenosis is caused by osteophytosis and ligamentous thickening. Quantitative measurements of the width of the cervical spinal canal are frequently performed on radiographs because these measurements are predictive for the presence of spinal canal stenosis. The spinal canal width is calculated as the ratio between the anteroposterior diameter of the spinal canal and the anteroposterior diameter of the vertebral body. In normal volunteers, this ratio is about 1. If the ratio is below 0.8, a developmental spinal canal stenosis may be present.[63] On conventional lateral radiographs the distance between the posterior surface of the vertebral body and the spinolaminar line can be measured. A spinal cord compression may occur if this distance is 10 mm or less. On the other hand, if this distance is 13 mm or more, spinal canal stenosis is unlikely. In the lumbar spine the anteroposterior diameter of the canal is measured from the posterior aspect of the vertebral body to the line joining the upper and lower tips of the articular process, and at L4 the normal mean is 13 mm (range, 10 to 16 mm).[63] On the anteroposterior lumbar films, interpedicular distance has a mean at L4 of 23 mm (range, 19 to 27 mm) but sagittal alignment of the facet joints lying inside the pedicles with a short lamina is particularly prone to spinal stenosis. Plain radiographs are unable to demonstrate the shape of the canal or the size of the dural sac.[64,65]

Computed Tomography

Computed tomography enables the cross-sectional shape and area of the spinal canal to be measured. The combination of the internal canal soft tissue and bony dimensions is of major relevance with regard to the space for the dural sac. In the majority of cases the minimal cross-sectional area in both the cervical and lumbar spine is at the level of the discs and facet joints. In the cervical spine, a cross-sectional area of 60 mm^2 is reported to be predictive of cervical spinal stenosis. CT of the cervical spine will also demonstrate the presence of ossification of the posterior longitudinal ligament (OPLL), which is a major cause of spinal stenosis, particularly in Japan. OPLL is more frequently present in men than in women and typically manifests in the fifth to seventh decades. The diagnosis of OPLL is established by its characteristic appearance on CT as a dense ossified strip of variable thickness that is evident along the posterior margins of the vertebral bodies and the intervertebral disc. OPLL may extend over multiple levels but also can be segmental. In the lumbar spine, the cross-sectional area of the lumbar spinal canal, including the ligamentum flavum, is normally 2.5 cm^2; and less than 1.45 cm^2 would be considered small, but below 0.75 cm^2 impairment of circulatory and nerve function will occur. In the cervical spine, accurate evaluation of the cross-sectional size of the dural sac usually requires intradural administration of a contrast agent; and on CT myelography a measurement below 60 mm^2 would confirm significant stenosis. CT myelography will also enable dynamic evaluation of flexion and extension on the spinal canal to assess the effect on the degree of stenosis of buckling of the ligamentum flavum and disc bulging in extension. It will also assist in the cervical spine in the differentiation of nerve and cord compression between osteophytes and disc bulge or herniation if this is of therapeutic importance or in patients in whom the results of MRI were ambiguous or technically suboptimal. Comparison with MRI has shown only moderately good concordance, with CT myelography tending to upgrade the degree of spinal compromise, neural foraminal encroachment, and cord diameter reduction.[66]

Magnetic Resonance Imaging

Magnetic resonance imaging is the preferred method for evaluating spinal stenosis in both the cervical and lumbar spine, particularly utilizing the T2-weighted sequence as it enables both the bony and soft tissue effect on the dural sac dimensions and cord and nerve roots to be assessed without the use of intrathecal contrast agents. However, in most cases osteophytes and disc bulge or herniation cannot be differentiated, particularly in the cervical spine on MRI and thus are referred to as disc-osteophyte complex by some authorities. The T2-weighted sequences show loss of cerebrospinal fluid in front and behind the cord in the sagittal and axial planes with flattening of the cord. The normal differential of gray and white matter may be lost on the T2-weighted, gradient-echo, axial MR studies. In severe cases of cervical cord compression the cord may have high signal intensity within its substance on the T2-weighted images (Fig. 43-19).

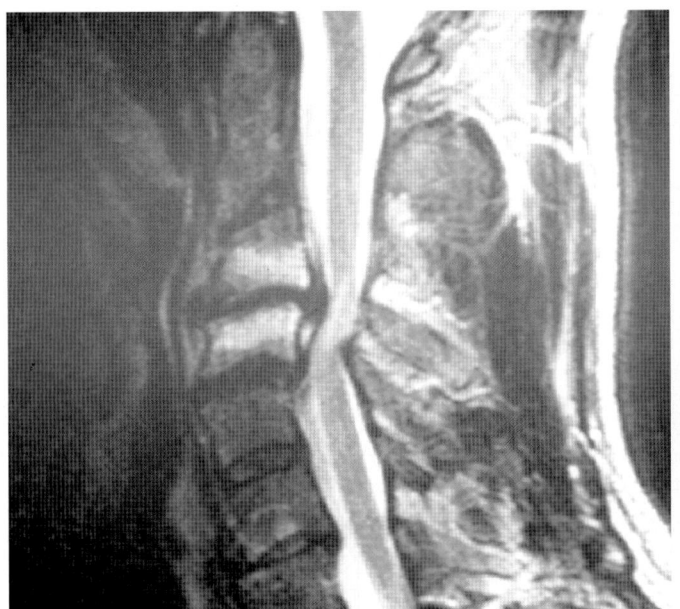

A

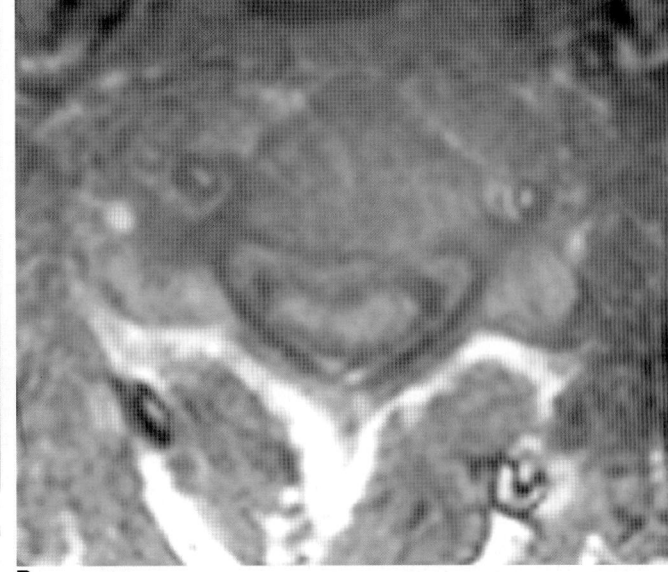

B

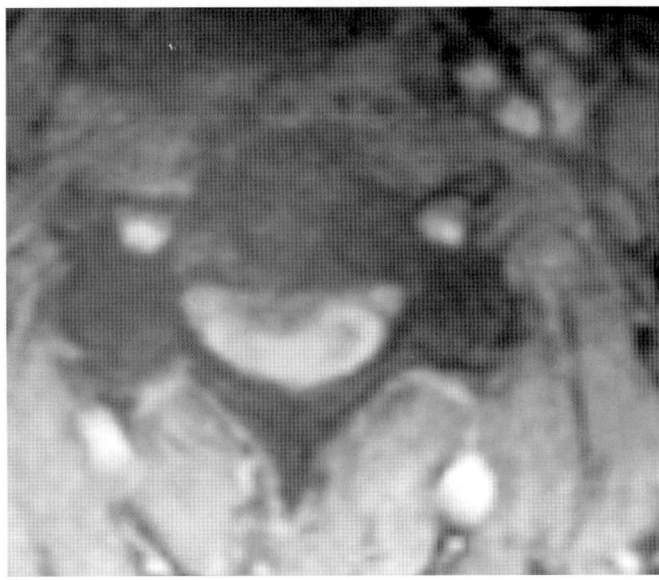

C

■ **FIGURE 43-19** Cervical spondylitic myelopathy. **A,** Sagittal, T2-weighted, turbo spin-echo MR image shows compression of the canal and cord by degenerative retrolisthesis of C3-C4 combined with extruded disc material and indentation posteriorly by the buckled ligamentum flavum. A line of high signal intensity is present in the cord at the site of compression. **B,** Axial, T1-weighted, turbo spin-echo MR image demonstrates the flattened and distorted cord. **C,** Axial, T2-weighted, gradient-echo MR image shows the flattened cord with high signal intensity in the gray and white matter due to myelopathy.

In the lumbar spine, loss of the high signal intensity of the cerebrospinal fluid around the nerve roots on T2-weighted axial images is also valuable for assessing clinically relevant spinal stenosis. In central stenosis, the dural sac is compressed at the disc level anteriorly by the bulging disc and posterolaterally by the osteophytes of the osteoarthritic facets and the buckled ligamentum flavum. Individual nerve roots are not seen on either the axial or sagittal images because they are compressed together (Fig. 43-20). On the axial sequences the nerve roots in the lateral recess can be identified. The lateral recess is bordered posteriorly by the superior articular facet, laterally by the pedicle, and anteriorly by the vertebral body and disc. Lumbar lateral recess stenosis occurs when a hypertrophic superior facet encroaches on the recess, often in combination with a narrowing due to a bulging disc and osteophyte. Foraminal stenosis occurs when a hypertrophic facet, vertebral body osteophyte, or bulging disc narrows the neural foramen and encroaches on the nerve roots. The foramina are assessed on both the sagittal and axial studies because stenosis may be in the anteroposterior direction, craniocaudal, or a combination of both and visualization of the nerve root is the clinically relevant feature. When the epidural fat surrounding the nerve root within the foramen is obliterated on sagittal T1-weighted scans, marked encroachment is present. The nerve root may also be compressed in one plane only.

A systematic review of the accuracy of diagnostic tests for lumbar spinal stenosis concluded that the quality of

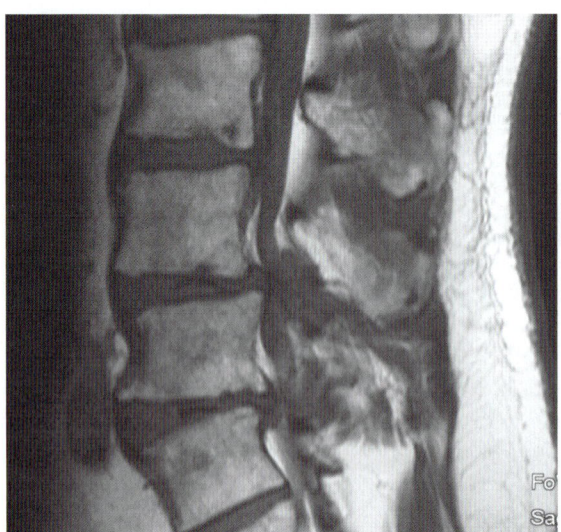

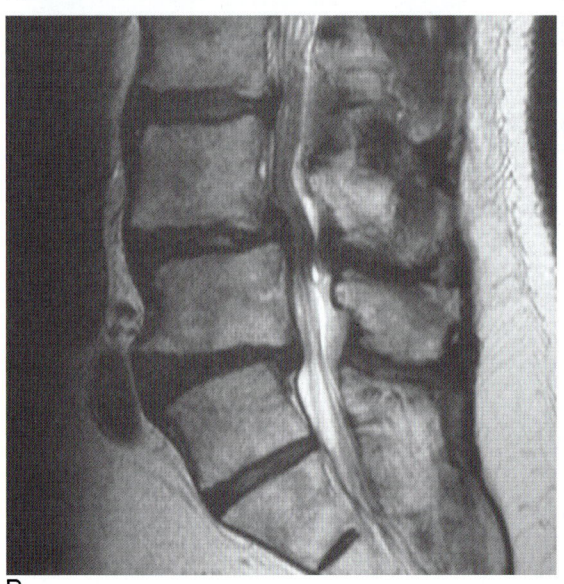

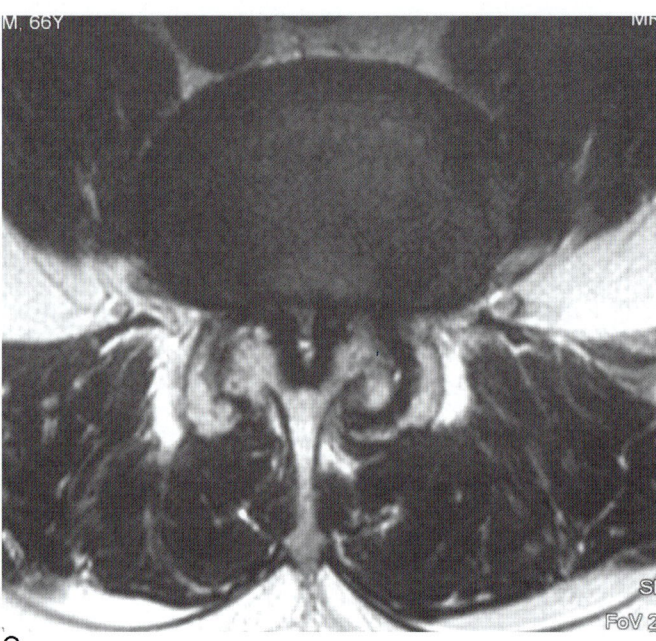

■ **FIGURE 43-20** Lumbar spinal stenosis. **A,** Sagittal, T1-weighted, turbo spin-echo MR image demonstrates marked narrowing of the spinal canal at each disc level. **B,** Sagittal T2-weighted, turbo spin-echo MR image shows the compression of the dural sac at the disc levels due to bulging and facet indentation. **C,** Axial, T2-weighted, turbo spin-echo MR image shows grade 3 degeneration of the facets, shortened pedicles, and severe compression of the dural sac. There is no cerebrospinal fluid remaining around the nerve roots in the dural sac.

the studies' design was insufficient to draw a conclusion on which imaging modality is most accurate.[67]

Foraminal stenosis may occur at more than one level, there may be a discrepancy between the clinical evaluation and the imaging, or the symptoms and signs may be equivocal for chronic nerve root compression. In these circumstances a CT-guided selective nerve root block (Fig. 43-21) with local anesthetic may be helpful in isolating the symptomatic level or confirming the origin of the symptoms. Localized injections of corticosteroids around the nerve root have also been performed.

DIFFERENTIAL DIAGNOSIS

Correlation between Clinical and Imaging Findings

Imaging has been extensively used to demonstrate degenerative changes in the spine in subjects with neck and low back pain, and MRI in particular has become the gold standard in evaluation of spinal pathology. However, there is a lack of correlation between the presence or absence of symptoms and the imaging findings. The advent of MRI, which is noninvasive and enables the different components of the spine and the cord and nerve roots to be imaged, has enabled the detailed evaluation of asymptomatic subjects. A number of studies have now documented a high rate of abnormal imaging findings in the lumbar spine of an asymptomatic subject (Table 43-3).[32,68-72] Only the presence of a disc extrusion and sequestration may represent a clinically significant finding if the symptoms of the patient correspond to the imaging findings. The role of Modic changes is still a subject of debate. Neural compromise, however, is important in the correlation between symptoms and MRI findings. The only substantial morphologic difference between symptomatic patients and asymptomatic volunteers was with the presence of neural compromise (83% vs. 22%), differentiating between asymptomatic subjects and symptomatic disc herniation patients matched according to age, sex, and occupational risk factors.[69]

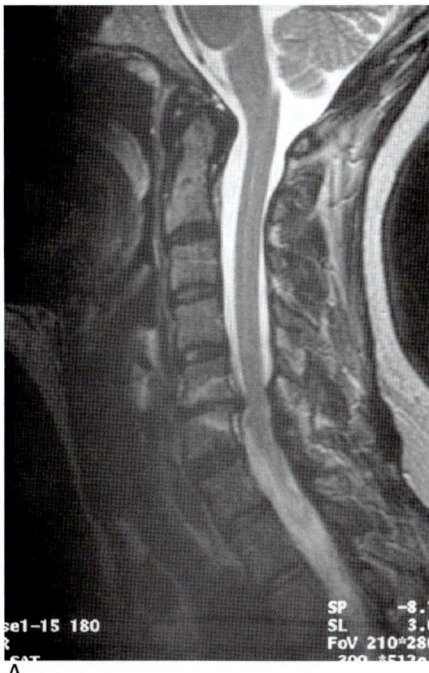

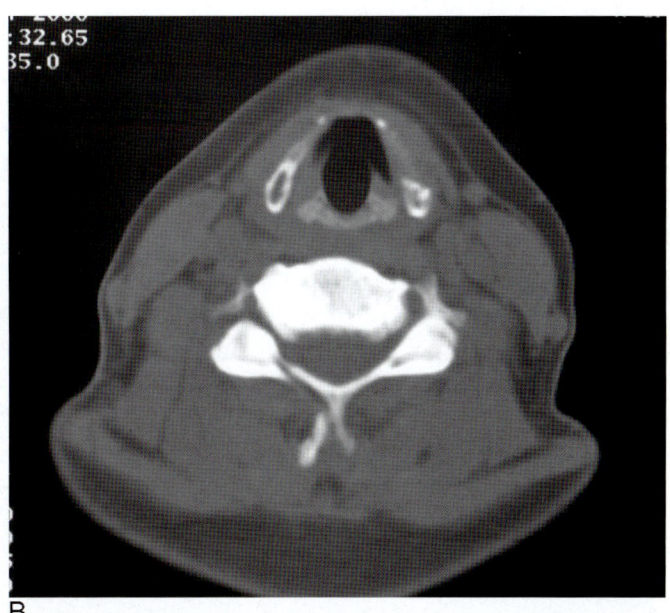

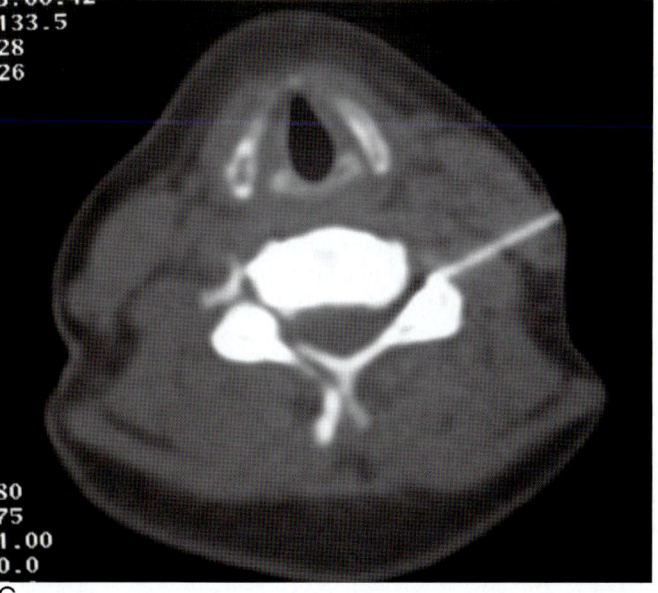

■ **FIGURE 43-21** Nerve root injection. **A,** Sagittal, T2-weighted, turbo spin-echo MR image shows degeneration at the C5-C6 disc with osteophytes and degenerative end-plate changes. **B,** CT demonstrates narrowing of the foramen by osteophyte formation in the neurocentral joints. **C,** CT-guided needle placement posterior to the root and the vertebral artery.

The pathophysiologic mechanisms that cause nerve root symptoms are still not completely understood. Currently, two concepts are discussed: mechanical nerve root compression and nerve root inflammation caused by inflammatory cytokines present in the herniated nucleus pulposus.

SYNOPSIS OF TREATMENT OPTIONS

Disc herniations vary in their natural history, and the majority are treated conservatively. Follow-up studies have indicated that protrusions remained little changed, but larger extrusions and particularly sequestrations may be completely resorbed.[45] These findings are supported by a study of asymptomatic subjects that showed little change in protrusions over an average 5-year period.[46]

A recent report also indicated that the MR appearances of the disc herniation are not of value in planning conservative care.[47] However, if nerve root pain is severe and motor sensory disturbances are present, microdiscectomy may be required. Evidence indicates that surgery provides more rapid relief of symptoms in these cases, but the long-term results between conservative and surgical therapy are similar. If the herniation is large and cauda equina symptoms are present, surgical intervention on an emergency basis is required. The rates of surgical intervention for nerve root compression due to disc herniation vary considerably in different health care systems.

Spinal stenosis is usually initially treated conservatively, but surgical decompression of the cervical or lumbar canal may be required in severe cases. The results of decompression are unpredictable because permanent structural and vascular changes in the nerve roots or cord may have occurred, resulting in a relatively poor outcome.

The treatment of nonradicular neck and low back pain is considerably more controversial, with many different

TABLE 43-3 Prevalence of Disc Abnormalities on Magnetic Resonance Imaging in Asymptomatic Subjects

Study, Year	Age Group No. Subjects	HNP	Bulging Disc	Degenerated Disc	HIZ	Other
Weishaupt, 1998[32]	20-50 yr (mean, 35) n = 60	60%	20%	72%	33%	Nerve root contact or deviation, 26% Nerve root compression, 2%
Stadnik, 1998[68]	17-71 yr (mean, 42) n = 36	33%	81%	72%	56%	
Boos, 1995[69]	20-50 yr (mean, 36) n = 46	76%	51% of discs	85%	14%	No sequestered disc; nerve root contact or deviation, 22%; 64% had disc bulge, protrusion, or extension
Jensen, 1994[70]	20-80 yr (mean, 42) n = 98	28%	52%			
Boden, 1990[71]	< 60 yr, n = 53 > 60 yr, n = 14	22% 36%	54% 79%	46% 93%		
Weinreb, 1989[72]	females, 19-24 yr (mean, 28) n = 86	9%	44%			

HNP, herniated nucleus pulposus; HIZ, high intensity zone.

therapies available, including drugs for pain relief and to treat inflammation, manipulation, physiotherapy, cognitive therapy, and many others. Image-guided local anesthetic injections may provide temporary or longer-term relief and may be repeated. Surgery in the form of spinal fusion is usually reserved for intractable cases and may be performed with or without supplementary metal fixation. The role of disc replacement is still being clinically evaluated, and cellular regeneration of the nucleus pulposus remains at the experimental stage.

What the Referring Physician Needs to Know

■ Are the findings related to normal aging or abnormal?
■ What is the specific nature of the abnormality?
■ What is the location of abnormalities in relation to the nervous system?
■ Can the abnormal findings explain the clinical findings?

SUGGESTED READINGS

Boutin RD, Steinbach LS, Finnessey K. MR imaging of degenerate disease in the cervical spine. Magn Reson Imaging Clin North Am 2000; 8:471-490.
Loredo JD (ed). Imaging of low back pain. Radiol Clin North Am 2000; 36(6).
Loredo JD (ed). Imaging of low back pain. Radiol Clin North Am 2001; 37(1).
Saal JS. General principles of diagnostic testing as related to painful lumbar spine disorders. Spine 2002; 27:2538-2545.

REFERENCES

1. Miller JA, Schmatz C, Schultz AB. Lumbar disc degeneration: correlation with age, sex, and spine level in 600 autopsy specimens. Spine 1988; 13:173-178.
2. Videman T, Nummi P, Battie MC, et al. Digital assessment of MRI for lumbar disc desiccation: a comparison of digital versus subjective assessments and digital intensity profiles versus discogram and macroanatomic findings. Spine 1994; 19:192-198.
3. Batttie MC, Videman T, Gibbons IE, et al. Determinants of lumbar disc degeneration: a study relating life-time exposures and magnetic resonance imaging findings in identical twins. Spine 1995; 20:2901-2612.
4. Sambrook PN, MacGregor AJ, Spector TD. Genetic influences on cervical and lumbar disc degeneration: a magnetic resonance imaging study in twins. Arthritis Rheum 1999; 42:366-372.
5. Kelsey JL, White AA III. Epidemiology and impact of low back pain. Spine 1980; 5:133-142.
6. Coste J, Paolaggi JB, Spira A. Classification of non-specific low back pain: II. Clinical diversity of organic forms. Spine 1992; 17:1038-1042.
7. Mooney V, Robertson J. The facet syndrome. Clin Orthop Relat Res 1976; 115:149-156.

8. Eisenstein SM, Parry CR. The lumbar facet arthrosis syndrome: clinical presentation and articular surface changes. J Bone Joint Surg Br 1987; 69:3-7.

9. Bogduk N. The sources of low back pain. In Jayson M (ed). The Lumbar Spine and Back Pain, 4th ed. Edinburgh, Churchill Livingstone, 1992, p 64.

10. Schmorl G, Junghanns H. The Human Spine in Health and Disease (E. F. Besemann, trans.). New York, Grune & Stratton, 1971.

11. Vernon RB. Aged related and degenerative pathology of intervertebral discs and apophyseal joints. In Jayson M (ed). The Lumbar Spine and Back Pain, 4th ed. Edinburgh, Churchill Livingstone, 1992, pp 21-22.

12. Hilton RC, Ball J. Vertebral rim lesions in the dorsolumbar spine. Ann Rheum Dis 1984; 43:302-307.

13. Roberts S, Urban JP, Evans H, et al. Transport properties of the human cartilage endplate in relation to its composition and calcification. Spine 1996; 21:415-420.

14. Andersson GBJ, Schultz A, Nathan A, et al. Roentgenographic measurement of lumbar intervertebral disc height. Spine 1981; 6:154-158.

15. Sorensen HK. Scheuermann's Kyphosis: Clinical Appearances, Radiography, Aetiology and Prognosis. Copenhagen, Munksgaard, 1964.

16. Venner RM, Crock HV. Clinical studies of isolated disc resorption in the lumbar spine. J Bone Joint Surg Br 1981; 63:491-494.

17. Hayes A, Howard TC, Gruel CR, et al. Roentgenographic evaluation of lumbar spine flexion-extension in asymptomatic individuals. Spine 1989; 14:327-331.

18. Pfirrmann CW, Metzdorf A, Zanetti M, et al. Magnetic resonance classification of lumbar intervertebral disc degeneration. Spine 2001; 26:1873-1878.

19. Sachs B, Vanharanta H, Spivey MA, et al. Dallas discogram description: a new classification of CT discography in low back disorders. Spine 1987; 12:287-294.

20. Osti OL, Fraser RD. MRI and discography of annular tears and intervertebral disc derangement. J Bone Joint Surg Br 1992; 74:431.

21. Walsh TR, Weinstein JN, Spratt KF, et al. Lumbar discography in normal subjects. J Bone Joint Surg Am 1990; 77:1081-1088.

22. Carragee EJ, Tanner CM, Khurana S, et al. The rates of false-positive lumbar discography in selected patients without low back symptoms. Spine 2000; 25:1373-1381.

23. Colhoun E, McCall IW, Williams W, et al. Provocative discography as a guide to planning operations on the spine. J Bone Joint Surg Br 1988; 70:267-271.

24. Saal JS. General principles of diagnostic testing as related to painful lumbar spine disorders. Spine 2002; 27:2538-2545.

25. Yu S, Sether LA, Ho PSP, et al. Tears in the annulus fibrosus: correlation between MR and pathologic findings in cadavers. Am J Neuroradiol 1988; 9:367-370.

26. Aprill C, Bogduk N. High intensity zone: a diagnostic sign of painful lumbar disc on magnetic resonance imaging. Br J Radiol 1992; 65:361-369.

27. Saifuddin A, Braithwaite I, White J, et al. The value of lumbar spine magnetic resonance imaging in the demonstration of annular tears. Spine 1998; 23:453-457.

28. Schellhas K, Pollei S, Gundry C, Heithoff K. Lumbar disc high-intensity zone. Spine 1996; 21:79-86.

29. Ricketson R, Simmons J, Hauser B. The prolapsed intervertebral disc: the high-intensity zone with discography correlation. Spine 1996; 21:2758-2762.

30. Carragee E, Paragioudakis S, Khurana S. Lumbar high-intensity zone and discography in subjects without low back problems. Spine 2000; 25: 2987-2992.

31. Rankine J, Gill K, Hutchinson C, et al. The clinical significance of high-intensity zone on lumbar spine magnetic resonance imaging. Spine 1999; 24:1913-1920.

32. Weishaupt D, Zanetti M, Hodler J, Boos N. MR imaging of the lumbar spine: prevalence of intervertebral disc extrusion and sequestration, nerve root compression, end plate abnormalities and osteoarthritis of the facet joints in asymptomatic volunteers. Radiology 1998; 209:661-666.

33. Mitra D, Cassar-Pullicino VN, McCall IW. Longitudinal study of high intensity zones on MR of lumbar intervertebral discs. Clin Radiol 2004: 59:1002-1008.

34. Milette PC. Classification, diagnostic imaging, and imaging characterization of a lumbar herniated disc. Radiol Clin North Am 2000; 38:1267-1292.

35. Landman JA, Hoffman JC, Braun IF, et al. Value of computed tomographic myelography in the recognition of cervical herniated disc. Am J Neuroradiol 1988; 5:391-394.

36. Jahnke RW, Hart BL. Cervical stenosis, spondylosis and herniated disc disease. Radiol Clin North Am 1991;29:777-793.

37. Modic MT, Masaryk TJ, Boumphrey F, et al. Lumbar herniated disc disease and canal stenosis: prospective evaluation by surface coil MR, CT, and myelography. Am J Neuroradiol 1986; 7:709-717.

38. Jackson RP, Cain JE, Jacobs RR, et al. The neuroradiographic diagnosis of lumbar herniated nucleus pulposus: a comparison of computed tomography (CT), myelography, CT myelography, and magnetic resonance imaging. Spine 1989; 14:1362-1367.

39. Pfirrmann CW, Dora C, Schmid MR, et al. MR image-based grading of lumbar nerve root compromise due to disk herniation: reliability study with surgical correlation. Radiology 2004; 230:583-588.

40. Silverman CS, Lenchik L, Shimkin PM, et al. The value of MR in differentiating subligamentous from supraligamentous lumbar disc herniations. Am J Neuroradiol 1995; 16:571-579.

41. Modic MT, Ross JS, Obuchowski NA, et al. Contrast enhanced MR imaging in acute radiculopathy: a pilot study of the natural history. Radiology 1995; 195:429-435.

42. Toyone T, Takahashi K, Kitahara H, et al. Visualisation of symptomatic nerve roots. J Bone Joint Surg Br 1993; 75:529-533.

43. Jinkins JR. MR of enhancing nerve roots in unoperated lumbar spine. Am J Neuroradiol 1993; 14:193-202.

44. Tyrrell PNMT, Cassar-Pullicino VN, McCall IW. Gadolinium DTPA enhancement of symptomatic nerve roots in MRI of the lumbar spine. Eur Radiol 1998; 8:116-122.

45. Komori H, Shinomiya K, Nakai O, et al. The natural history of herniated nucleus pulposus with radiculopathy. Spine 1996; 21:225-229.

46. Boos N, Semmer N, Elfring A, et al. Natural history of individuals with asymptomatic disc abnormalities in magnetic resonance imaging. Spine 2000; 25:1484-1492.

47. Modic MT, Obuchowski NA, Ross JS, et al. Acute low back pain and radiculopathy: MR imaging findings and their prognostic role and effect on outcome. Radiology 2005; 237:597-604.

48. Gundry CR, Heitoff KB. Epidural haematoma of the lumbar spine: 18 surgically confirmed cases. Radiology 1993; 187:427-431.

49. Modic M, Steinberg P, Ross J, et al. Degenerative disk disease: assessment of changes in vertebral body marrow with MR imaging. Radiology 1988; 166:193-199.

50. Kuisma M, Karppinen J, Niinimaki J, et al. A three year follow-up of lumbar spine endplate (Modic) changes. Spine 2006; 31:1714-1718.

51. McCall IW, Cassar-Pullicino VN, Tyrrell PN. MR vertebral changes and back pain. Abstracts presented at the 25th annual meeting of the International Society for the Study of the Lumbar Spine, Singapore, 1998.

52. Braithwaite I, White J, Saifuddin A, et al. Vertebral end-plate (Modic) changes on lumbar spine MRI: correlation with pain reproduction at lumbar discography. Eur Spine J 1998; 7: 363-368.

53. Weishaupt D, Zanetti M, Hodler J, et al. Painful lumbar disk derangement: relevance of endplate abnormalities at MR imaging. Radiology 2001; 218:420-427.

54. Mitra D, Casssar-Pullicino VN, McCall IW. Longitudinal study of vertebral type-1 endplate changes on MR of the lumbar spine. Eur Radiol 2004; 14:1574-1581.

55. Weishaupt D, Zanetti M, Boos N, Hodler J. MR imaging and CT in osteoarthritis of the lumbar facet joints. Skeletal Radiol 1999; 28:215-219.

56. Schwartzer AC, Wang SC, O'Driscoll D, et al. The ability of computed tomography to identify a painful zygapophyseal joint in patients with chronic low back pain. Spine 1995; 20:907-912.

57. Apostolaki K, Davies AM, Evans NM, Cassar-Pullicino VN. MR imaging of lumbar facet joint synovial cysts. Eur Radiol 2000; 10:615-623.

58. Lim AKP, Higgins SJ, Saifuddin A, Lehovsky J. Symptomatic lumbar synovial cyst: management with direct CT-guided puncture and steroid injection. Clin Radiol 2001; 56:990-993.

59. Rosenberg NJ. Degenerative spondylolisthesis, predisposing factor. J Bone Joint Surg Am 1975; 57:467-474.
60. Magora A, Schwartz A. Relationship between low back pain syndrome and x-ray findings: lysis and olisthesis. Scand J Rehabil Med 1980; 12:47-52.
61. Vogt MT, Rubin D, San Valentin R, et al. Lumbar olisthesis and lower back symptoms in elderly white women. Spine 1998; 23:2640-2647.
62. Yonenobu K: Cervical radiculopathy and myelopathy: when and what can surgery contribute to treatment? Eur Spine J 2000; 9:1-7.
63. Pavlov H, Torg JS, Robie B, Jahre C. Cervical spinal stenosis: determination with vertebral body ratio method. Radiology 1987; 164:771-775.
64. Eisenstein SM. The morphometry and pathological anatomy of the lumbar spine in South African Negros and Caucasoids with specific reference to spinal stenosis. J Bone Joint Surg 1977; 54:173-180.
65. Schonstrom NSR, Bolender NF, Spengler DM. The pathomorphology of spinal stenosis as seen on CT scans of the lumbar spine. Spine 1985; 10:806-812.
66. Shafaie FF, Wippold FJ, Gado M, et al. Comparison of computed tomography myelography and magnetic resonance imaging in the evaluation of cervical spondylotic myelopathy and radiculopathy. Spine 1999; 24:1781-1785.
67. de Graaf I, Prak A, Bierma-Zeinstra S, et al. Diagnosis of spinal stenosis. Spine 2006; 31:1168-1176.
68. Stadnik TW, Lee RR, Coen HL, et al. Annular tears and disk herniation: prevalence and contrast enhancement on MR images in the absence of low back pain or sciatica. Radiology 1998; 206:49-55.
69. Boos N, Rieder R, Schade V, et al. 1995 Volvo Award in clinical sciences. The diagnostic accuracy of magnetic resonance imaging, work perception, and psychosocial factors in identifying symptomatic disc herniations. Spine 1995; 20:2613-2625.
70. Jensen MC, Brant-Zawadzki MN, Obuchowski N, et al. Magnetic resonance imaging of the lumbar spine in people without back pain. N Engl J Med 1994; 331:69-73.
71. Boden SD, Davis DO, Dina TS, et al. Abnormal magnetic-resonance scans of the lumbar spine in asymptomatic subjects: a prospective investigation. J Bone Joint Surg Am 1990; 72:403-408.
72. Weinreb JC, Wolbarsht LB, Cohen JM, et al. Prevalence of lumbosacral intervertebral disk abnormalities on MR images in pregnant and asymptomatic nonpregnant women. Radiology 1989; 170:125-128.

44

Aging

Iain Watt

WHAT IS AGING?

The processes and inevitability of aging are as certain as death and paying taxes! In the past 5 years the population of the world has grown by approximately 1.7% per year. On the other hand, the number of elderly people has increased by 2.7% per year. In the developing world, the number of people older than age 65 years will increase by 200% to 400% in the next 30 years. By 2030 70 million people will be older than the age of 65 in the United States and by 2050 22% of the United States population will be considered elderly.[1]

It is generally agreed that with increasing longevity and health, especially in the developed world, the enlarging graying population will create a significant imbalance in health and welfare provision while, at the same time, the younger, wealth-creating proportion of the population will carry an unsustainable burden to support them. Traditional views about retirement age, the naïve view that older people have reduced expectations about the duration and quality of their lives, and the need for older people to contribute to the gross domestic product are being realized slowly. Already, retirement ages are being moved upward in those countries where they still apply.

Age-related chronic diseases may be expected to increase, especially those with major health care provision needs such as cerebrovascular and cardiovascular diseases, dementia, malignancy, osteoarthritis, and degenerative disc disease. Perhaps more importantly, the healthy but aging population will demand as full and a rewarding standard of health as can be achieved. The understanding, arrest, or even reversal of the processes of aging will become a major research issue in the expectation that a healthy, long-living older population can not only expect a fulfilled life but also, in exchange, contribute to the wealth of society as a whole.

It may be time also to revise an important benchmark in medicine. When studying the effect of age on the musculoskeletal system, an important consideration arises. That is, what is normal? For example, currently, bone density and the diagnosis of osteoporosis is made in comparison to peak bone mass in the young, mature skeleton. Is this reasonable? Can what is seen as normal for a 25-year-old really apply to an 80-year-old? That we grow old and our skeletons continue to remold and adapt is obvious. That the processes involved alter with time is irrefutable. Archaeologists and anthropologists have long used these molding changes to assess the probable age of their clients in funerary and other collections. Hence, thickening of the skull vault, progressive closure of the cranial sutures, deepening of dural venous indentations, and roughening of the articular surfaces of the symphysis pubis are but a few of the signs that are relied upon. Perhaps, rather than consider the majority of older people to be abnormal by young adult standards, it would be more rewarding to ask why some older people have been able to maintain the standards of youth in their old age?

KEY POINTS

- Genotype largely determines the onset and progression of osteoarthritis.
- Age-related hyaline cartilage degeneration starts in the unloaded parts of the joint before migrating to weight-bearing zones.
- Bone remodeling decreases from childhood up to skeletal maturity, but accelerates again over the age of 60 years.
- Decrease of hyaline cartilage thickness and function with advancing age is related to increased joint surface area. The distinction between this normal aging process and similar changes that occur in osteoarthritis is not always clear.
- The decrease of bone marrow perfusion and increase in intraosseous blood volume (venous engorgement) with advancing age may be factors in developing osteoarthritis.
- Because function, morphology, and consistency of all joint components (cartilage, bone, marrow, ligaments, capsule) change with advancing age, intervention aimed at only one joint structure seems conceptually flawed.

MECHANISMS OF AGING

The means by which the human animal grows old are unclear. Obviously environmental issues are important. A life spent in a coal mine or a childhood without adequate nutrition will inevitably prejudice against a long and healthy life span. A number of complex cellular processes are working also toward entropy. One such may be telomere length. Telomeres are repeated sequences of five bases that preserve the integrity of genes during DNA replication. Their function has been likened to preventing the DNA strands from unraveling. The telomere chain length varies in individuals at birth, but every time a cell replicates daughter cells have shorter chains until they are spent. Older people with shorter telomeres are eight times more likely to die from an infectious disease and three times more likely to have a heart attack. On the other hand, it has been suggested that deficient telomere chains may be beneficial by inhibiting further cell replication and thereby be a means of inhibiting malignant transformation. It also has been suggested that an inverse relationship may exist between life span and the number of children borne to an individual.

Widespread endocrine changes occur also in the older human. These include the menopause in women, androgen deficiency in men, subsequent loss of skeletal mass of about 1% per year when older than the age of 50 years, decreased concentration of serum growth hormone, and increased incidence of type 2 diabetes. For example, growth hormone loss is associated with reduced gonadal steroids in serum, increasing body fat, reduced muscle mass, and decreasing bone mass. The inherent substantial physiologic organ reserve of youth becomes lost, together with the impact of increasing other pathologic processes.[2] These include the problems of frailty, vascular disease, and loss of cognitive function.

A third area of recent interest is the understanding of age-related changes in mitochondrial function. The essential function of mitochondria is to burn sugars to produce intracellular energy. However, errors or interruptions in this process can result in the production of excess quantities of highly reactive free radicals that damage both mitochondrial and nuclear DNA. Mitochondrial DNA has 13 genes but lacks the crucial ability of nuclear DNA to repair genome damage, such as that associated with cell replication. Furthermore, as mitochondrial DNA is replaced more frequently than nuclear DNA, uncorrected mutations may contribute to the aging process. Research in a mouse model has shown that animals whose ability has been impaired to proofread accurately copies of mitochondrial DNA show reduced life span and premature onset of aging-related phenotypes such as weight loss, reduced subcutaneous fat, alopecia (hair loss), kyphosis, osteoporosis, anemia, reduced fertility, and heart enlargement.[3]

Whatever processes are involved, it is clear that a familial or genetic tendency occurs with some disorders that are age related. For example, osteoarthritis is known to have strong linkages in first-degree female relatives and data from population studies have suggested that progression of osteoarthritis in probands is strongly associated with progression in their siblings.[4] Similarly, hyaline cartilage defects in the knee have a genetic component related to symptomatic knee pain and bone size.[5]

THE AGING MUSCULOSKELETAL SYSTEM

The individual components of the skeleton are each associated with specific age-related changes, some of which overlap. For convenience, each component will be considered separately. However, the concept that a joint is a whole organ within a whole patient must never be forgotten. Thus, a stumbling old man who fractures his hip is more than just an osteoporotic individual. His variable, weak gait may correlate with depression scores rather than his age, gender, muscle strength, or neurologic features, except in terms of frontal lobe and extrapyramidal function. His cautious gait equates to loss of higher cerebral function. In other words, gait changes in older adults, who may walk in fear of falling, may be an appropriate response to unsteadiness and are likely to be a marker of an underlying cerebral pathologic process and not simply a physiologic or psychological consequence of normal aging.[6]

Within the Joint Organ as a Whole

Age-related hyaline cartilage degenerative changes appear to occur first in unloaded parts of a joint but spread to the more central, weight-bearing zones with increasing age. The argument is that a normal, young joint resembles a ball within a Gothic arch. Initial loading contact is made at the periphery of the joint. With increasing load, both bone and cartilage, being viscoelastic structures, deform and the contact between the joint surfaces increases, distributing the load more evenly. This type of designed incongruent geometry provides for stability, ease of motion, and physiologic loading (Fig. 44-1). Furthermore, and perhaps the most important role, is the normal nutrition of hyaline cartilage. Chondrocytes, that without a blood supply produce all of the crucial components of hyaline cartilage, are dependent solely on circulating synovial fluid for their energy requirements. Thus, the circulation of synovial fluid with oxygen and sugars is facilitated by the pump action of a deformable joint congruence.[7] Aging is associated with a progressive alteration in this crucial joint morphology. Joints become more congruent and deeper and fit more precisely with age (Fig. 44-2).[8] Congruence is achieved by progressive remolding of the articular surfaces as a result of vascular invasion and endochondral ossification of calcified cartilage. In the case of the femoral head, vascular invasion is predominantly superior and gradually declines until the age of about 60 years when a dramatic and persistent increase occurs that continues into old age. Why this should happen is not known, nor why the threshold age should be 60. Other work has shown that a high hip contact stress relates to cartilage degeneration and osteoarthritis. Hip joints that remain

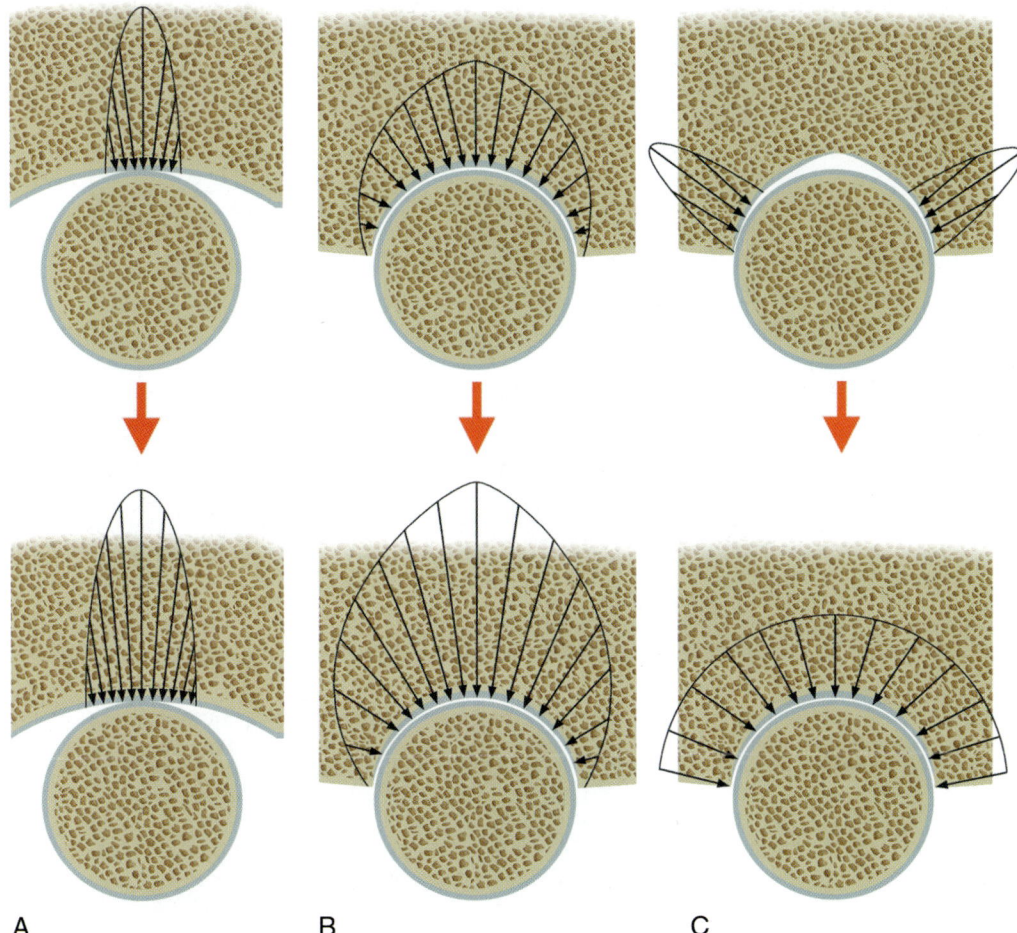

■ **FIGURE 44-1** Diagram of the effect of geometry on the distribution of stress in the loaded joint. Too narrow a contact point causes high focal loading and inherent instability (**A**). Too broad a cup evens out load initially but becomes more focal as it increases. Congruity is total, and synovial fluid circulation is inhibited (**B**). Only in **C**, when the ball fits into the Gothic arch with a narrower diameter of contact, can load become more evenly distributed, stability increase, and synovial fluid be pumped around the joint. *(Reprinted by permission from Teitelbaum SL, Bullough PG: The pathophysiology of bone and joint disease. Am J Pathol 1979; 96:282-354.)*

A   B   C

anatomically normal in older age have a lower estimated peak contact stress (body weight corrected) than those that do not.[9]

Changes are occurring also in hyaline cartilage. Data from both femoral and humeral heads show that the thickness of the calcified zone decreases with age while, at the same time, the number of tidemarks increases, especially in those older than the age of 60. The changes in thickness of calcified cartilage depend on progressive endochondral ossification, resulting in additional subchondral bone and secondary thinning of calcified cartilage. Endochondral ossification occurs continuously throughout life in the calcified zone, but the rate of remodeling is variable, falling progressively from skeletal maturity until the sixth decade when a sudden increase in the number of tidemarks occurs.[10] It is unclear why bone remodeling accelerates with increasing older age. Thus, an intimate interrelationship exists between bone and cartilage remodeling. Not surprisingly, correlations are reported in the knee between increasing patient age, the severity of hyaline cartilage defects and their prevalence, cartilage thinning, and increased bone surface area.[11] How much of this represents age-related, "normal" findings and how distinct it is from what we call osteoarthritis remain unanswered.

Age-Related Changes within Bone

Bone mineral density and total bone mass increase until about the age of 20 years. Both remain stable until about the age of 35 years. The peak bone mass determines the subsequent chance of osteoporosis and is a factor in predicting fracture risk. The determinants of peak bone mass include genetic and environmental factors. Bone mass declines after the age of 35 years at a relatively steady rate throughout the remainder of life. Ovarian failure in women starts around the age of 40 years, and reproductive ovarian function ceases about 15 years later. At the menopause, rapid bone loss occurs with an associated increase in cardiovascular risk. The loss is secondary to reduced estrogen added to the underlying age-related bone loss. Thus, women may lose 5% to 15% of their bone mass in the perimenopausal period, with 80% coming from trabecular bone because it is metabolically more active than cortical bone. At the same time, although serum parathyroid hormone and vitamin D levels remain normal, a rapid increase in bone resorption occurs. The result is a secondary increase in bone formation. However, the net outcome is bone loss, suggesting that the osteoblastic response of aging bone may be hindered. It seems likely that the increased rate of bone loss is attributable, at least

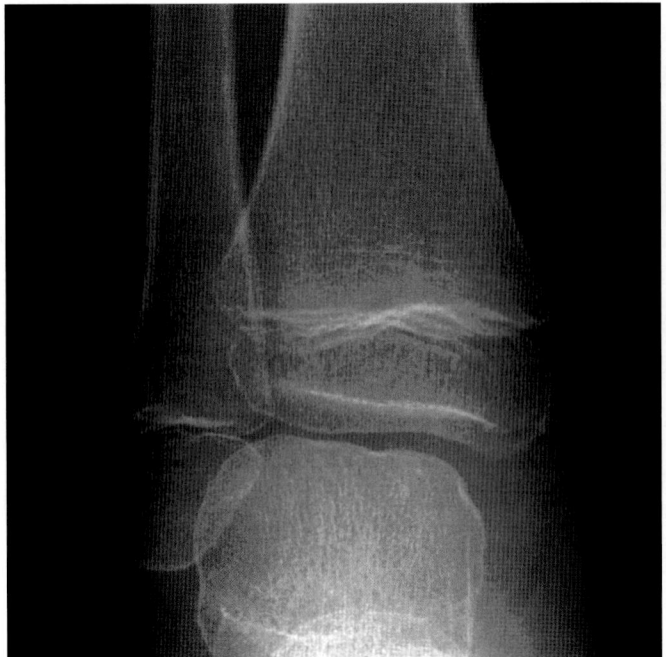

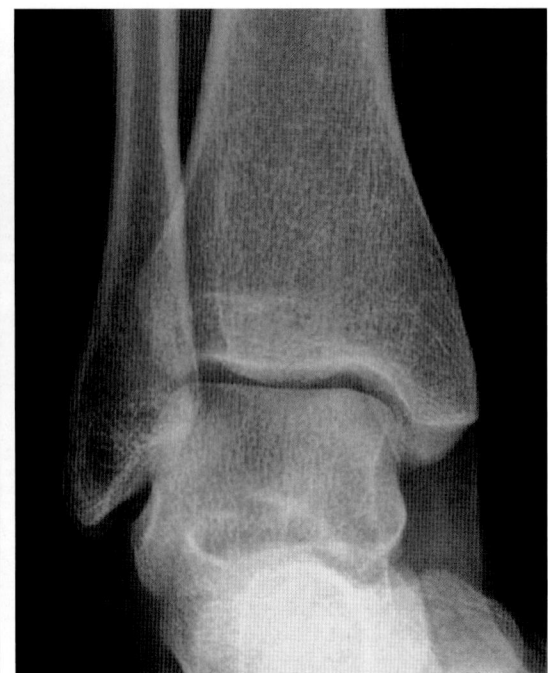

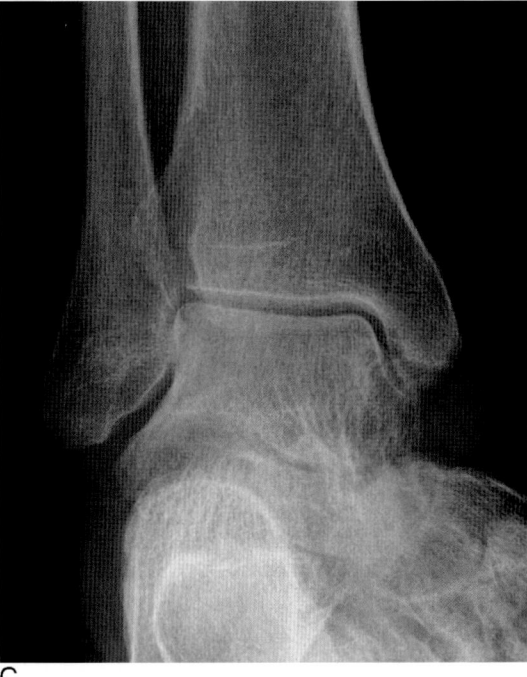

■ FIGURE 44-2 Radiographs of the ankle in a young child
(A), a mature male (B), and an old adult (C) show the obvious
deepening of the ankle mortise and increasing congruity with age.

partly, to the increased number of resorption cycles, in each of which bone resorption is unmatched by bone formation.[2] As the result, one third of women older than the age of 50 have osteoporosis with increased fracture risk. Peak bone mass, and the rate of postmenopausal bone loss, may be related also to ethnicity. A study of Native American women suggested that peak bone mineral density may be higher but the rate of postmenopausal bone loss greater than in white women.[12] Age is associated with

a third factor that enhances bone loss, beyond the effects of normal age-related loss and gonadal failure, and that is pure atrophy. Many older people are incapacitated, even chair- or bed-bound. In these circumstances unloading of the skeleton occurs also, akin to the bone loss of astronauts.

In aging men levels of free and bioavailable testosterone decline. Levels of sex hormone–binding globulin also increase, further reducing available hormone.

An andropause does not seem to exist, but the gradually reducing serum testosterone is associated with reducing blood hemoglobin, lean body mass, and bone mass and perhaps with memory changes. Testosterone replacement may partially reverse these changes but is not a widespread therapy.

Some data suggest that the reduction in bone mineralization is not uniform. Change in distribution of bone density within cancellous bone has been shown to vary with age in the femoral neck. Bone loss is greater, and more variable, in the inferior aspect of the femoral neck and trochanteric region.[13] Does this explain the varus impaction nature of elderly femoral neck fractures? Similarly, tibial plateau fractures are age related and may be a common cause of knee pain in the elderly.[14] Certainly, subchondral insufficiency fractures of the tibial plateaus and many cases of so-called spontaneous osteonecrosis of femur are due to subchondral insufficiency fractures, leading to rapidly progressive osteoarthritis.[15]

Cardiovascular disease is clearly a major age-related factor. However, very little is known about the normal rate of bone blood flow in the aging skeleton and the possible contribution of vascular disease to bone and joint pathology. The rate of vertebral bone marrow perfusion is significantly decreased in subjects older than 50 years. Women demonstrate a higher marrow perfusion rate than men younger than 50 years and a more marked decrease than men older than 50 years.[16] Furthermore, a correlation may exist between perfusion, bone marrow fat content and osteoporosis. It has been shown that the greater the degree of bone loss, the greater the reduction in perfusion, as assessed by MR spectroscopy, and marrow fat content.[17] Another study using positron emission tomography in the femoral head has shown that bone blood flow becomes reduced with age while, at the same time, intraosseous blood volume increases.[18] These data serve to confirm the nearly 40-year-old concept that venous engorgement and slow bone blood flow with a high intraosseous blood volume may be underlying factors in hip osteoarthritis[19] and underpin older decompression strategies for relieving joint pain in the hip and knee.

Age-Related Changes in Hyaline Cartilage

In addition to the hyaline cartilage and subchondral bone changes, articular cartilage undergoes significant intrinsic structural, matrix composition, and mechanical changes with increasing age. These changes are distinct from those of osteoarthritis. Although osteoarthritis is age related, it is not an inevitable consequence of age. In aging, articular surface fibrillation is almost universal and more common in some joints than others. It is asymptomatic and does not necessarily lead to the degeneration and structural failure associated with osteoarthritis. Within the cartilage matrix the size of proteoglycan aggregates decreases significantly with age as aggrecan molecules become shorter and the mean number of aggrecans in each aggregate decreases.[20] It is not known if this is due to deficient synthesis or degradation in the matrix or both. It may be due to reduced func-

tion of aging chondrocytes as shown in culture experiments. Age is also associated with reducing collagen cross-linkages and reduced water concentration secondary to the less hydrophilic negative charge of these older aggrecans. The overall effect is to reduce tensile stiffness and strength, making cartilage more susceptible to injury. Chondrocyte mitotic and synthetic abilities also reduce with age; in particular, chondrocytes exhibit an age-related decline in anabolic response to insulin-like growth factor (IGF-1). IGF-1 appears to have a critical role in stimulating chondrocyte synthetic activity that, in turn, stimulates maintenance and repair of the articular cartilage matrix.[20] How do these changes relate to osteoarthritis, which has a marked age-related incidence? Older cartilage is less able to repair and restore itself, compared with younger individuals. Hence, the risk of developing post-traumatic osteoarthritis after an intra-articular fracture increases threefold to fourfold after the age of 50. However, although older cartilage is less able to repair itself, it does not explain the quite different pathologic process of osteoarthritis per se.

In MRI T2 relaxation times are sensitive to the organization of collagen fibers in hyaline cartilage. Hence, if aging is associated with collagen degeneration, T2 values could be used as a surrogate marker. T2 values are indeed longer in the superficial 40% of cartilage in the 46- to 65-year age group as opposed to 18- to 30-year-old subjects. This suggests that age-related changes in collagen occur near the articular surface,[21] perhaps alongside the fibrillation changes described earlier.

As hyaline cartilage becomes thinner as the result of aging, it also displays a different degree of deformation under load compared with younger subjects. A study of knee cartilage confirmed that patellar cartilage thins significantly in older women (−12%) but not in men (−6%). Femoral cartilage was thinner in both sexes (women, −21%; men, −13%), whereas tibial cartilage showed nonsignificant trends. The striking feature is the reduced ability of cartilage to deform under load at the patella when compared with a younger knee. In other words, older cartilage is less efficient at load shedding.[22] The relationship between load shedding in cartilage and subchondral bone dictates the relative size of the articular surfaces of joints compared with the midshaft cross-sectional area. In the normal long bone, the articular surface area is approximately five times greater than that of the midshaft. Hence, in older subjects with less effective cartilage, it is to be expected that the area of the subarticular bone will increase in compensation. Thus, medial and lateral tibial bone surface area and patellar bone volume increase with age.[11] From these data we must learn that the normal aging joint shows thinner hyaline cartilage and minor marginal spurs that reflect the effects of age and should not be confused with the more progressive and devastating pathology we call osteoarthritis (Fig. 44-3).

Age-Related Changes in Skeletal Muscle

Men have significantly more skeletal muscle than women, both in absolute terms and also in relation to total body mass. These gender differences are greater in the upper than the lower body.[23] Skeletal muscle mass decreases

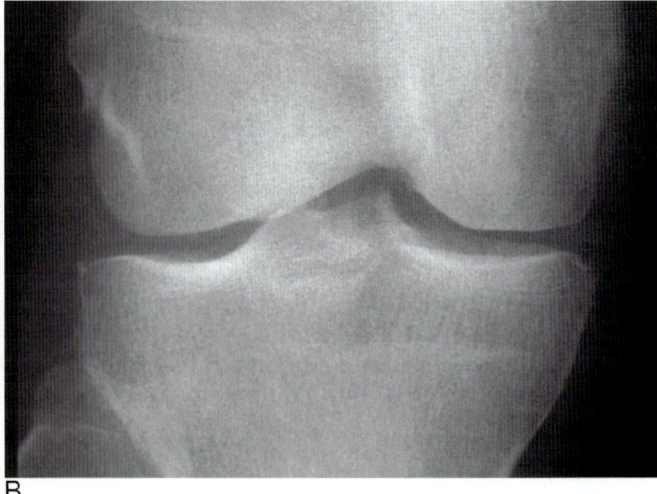

A

B

■ FIGURE 44-3 Two examples of normal, age-related changes in joint architecture. Both the hip (**A**) and the knee (**B**) show modest hyaline cartilage thinning and minor marginal spurs. These features should not be confused with the more destructive process of osteoarthritis.

from the third decade but becomes more noticeable from the fifth decade. Lean body mass decreases steadily with age from the fifth or sixth decades onward. This is due mainly to a loss of lower body muscle mass. At the same time body fat increases until about the age of 65 when it begins to decrease again. To what extent such changes actually cause decreased strength or function or vice versa are unclear. Naturally, the reducing muscle mass has an effect on the activities of normal daily living. For example, it correlates with reduced ability to climb stairs (quadriceps and psoas muscle cross-sectional areas).[24] Furthermore, in the elderly, maximal voluntary contraction torque is reduced owing to incomplete muscle activation. However, prolonged exercise programs (12 months or more) show that muscle bulk and activation can be increased significantly compared with controls.[25] On MRI, features of muscle atrophy and fatty infiltration can be seen in the older patient. More subtle changes include an increase in T2 relaxation time of fast-twitch muscle with age (e.g., the gastrocnemius muscle) due mainly to increased extracellular space reflecting age-related type II fiber atrophy. However, slow-twitch muscle does not show such a change (e.g., the soleus muscle).[26]

Age-Related Changes in Ligaments and Tendons

Age-related changes in tendons have been studied in the rotator cuff and lateral epicondyles at post mortem. They are similar at each site and comprise minor blood vessel wall changes, loss of tenocytes, and patchy calcification. The most frequent finding was glycosaminoglycan

infiltration and fibrocartilaginous transformation. These changes occurred in less than 17% of younger specimens but rise to 40% to 50% in later life.[27] Cystic changes in bone are common around the shoulder in older patients and are held to be evidence of rotator cuff disease. A study of 140 painful shoulders in 136 older patients has clarified this. Of these patients 35% had cystic lesions. The most common site was the bare area around the humeral neck. Lesions here were equally common in patients with or without cuff pathology, whereas cystic lesions at the insertion of either supraspinatus or subscapularis tendons were specific to cuff tears.[28]

Other histologic changes are occurring concurrently in aging ligaments and tendons. In the young anterior cruciate ligament, the diameter of the collagen fibrils that comprise it are highly variable. In adults and older subjects the maximal diameter decreases remarkably and fibril concentration increases considerably. The reduction in diameter and the relative changes in fibril concentration may relate to changes in elastic stiffness in the older ligament. Similar findings are recorded in the Achilles tendon.[29] However, whereas elastic quality may be altered by age, the question arises as to whether the older tendon heals less well after trauma. This is the commonly held wisdom, yet a recent study suggests that, at least in the experimental situation, no reduction occurs in the biomechanics of an older healing tendon.[1]

Enthesis ossification in the form of "osteophytes" occurring at the margins of the intervertebral discs and more florid ossification in the anterior longitudinal ligament, especially in the form usually described as diffuse idiopathic skeletal hyperostosis, are also age related.

However, risk factors for diffuse idiopathic skeletal hyperostosis extend beyond age and include a greater body mass index, as compared with patients with disc degeneration alone. These patients also have higher serum levels of uric acid and a greater likelihood of diabetes mellitus.[30]

The biomechanics of the anterior longitudinal ligament have been studied with regard to bone density, disc degeneration, and tensile stress-strain characteristics. In the young anterior longitudinal ligament, the elastic modulus of the insertion and substance of the ligament was similar. During aging, the elastic modulus of the substance increased twofold, whereas that of the insertion decreased threefold. Thus a fivefold change occurs. At the same time, the strength of the bone-ligament complex decreased by half during aging. The outer portions of the anterior longitudinal ligament consistently had the highest peak tensile strains. Whether this is related to the etiology of diffuse idiopathic skeletal hyperostosis is unknown. Equally of interest is the interrelationship between these findings, disc disease, and bone density. Experiments on preparations with normal discs and high bone density were significantly stronger than in the converse. Older patients with degenerative discs and lower bone density fail mechanically at the ligament insertion regions.[31] Other data support these findings insofar as the mechanical strength of the lumbar posterior spinal ligaments decreases with age owing to a negative correlation between age and tensile strength and is even worse in the presence of facet joint osteoarthritis.[32]

Other Age-Related Changes in the Spine

Apart from morphologic changes directly associated with osteoporosis, changes in the bony shape of vertebrae also occur. The bony neural canal becomes narrower with age in the cervical spine,[33] as it does in the lumbar canal. Although slow bone accretion and narrowing occur per se, they are enhanced by associated degenerative changes.[34] The reduction in area can be demonstrated and quantified using cross-sectional imaging. In addition to axial age-related changes, an MRI study demonstrated a linear age-related decline in anteroposterior height ratio occurs in the thoracic spine (anterior wedging) with increasing vertebral biconcavity. These changes were not corrected for possible osteoporosis, however. At the same time an age-related increase occurs in annular, nuclear, and disc margin abnormalities on MRI data, particularly in the middle and lower thoracic spine. The degree and extent of disc degenerative changes are greater in males.[35]

The intervertebral discs comprise about one third of the total height of the vertebral column. That we shrink with age is self-evident, just as we are shorter in the evening than when we first arise from bed in the morning. These changes are held to be due to hydration loss within the turgid proteoglycan of the nucleus pulposus, reflecting degenerative disease. As in hyaline cartilage, age-related degradation of proteoglycan reduces the hydrophilic ability of the nucleus to maintain turgidity. The elastic, constraining quality of the annulus fibrosus is reduced

also. However, unlike findings in hyaline cartilage, the distinction between aging and degeneration in the spine is not clear.[36] As a person ages the water content of the nucleus pulposus decreases, the turgidity reduces, and gaps and a system of fissures develop, radiating out into the annulus fibrosus. The fissures may fill with vapor to create the vacuum phenomenon typical of degenerative discs as seen on radiographs. The fissures may become filled with liquid also on T2-weighted images. The progressive reduction in water content is associated with signal intensity loss on T2-weighted sequences and reduced disc space height. Careful measurement of signal intensity change has confirmed a significant correlation with age, although signal intensity changes less than 8% by 80 years of age![37] Calcification also may be part of the aging process, occurring most frequently in thoracic discs.

Normal discs exhibit a diurnal variation in T2 values, reflecting water loss associated with weight bearing. This variation disappears after the age of 35 years, which is also thought to be a specific feature of aging.[38] Aging changes occur also in the annulus fibrosus. Typically, this results in a loss of distinction between the annulus and the nucleus, with also the development of annular fissures. The end plates as they degenerate may exhibit fractures, cleft formation, increased vascular permeability, and calcification.

Age-Related Changes in the Whole Joint Organ

It must never be forgotten that a tissue does not exist in isolation in life. A joint is an organ comprising hyaline cartilage, bone, marrow constituents, and ligaments that is surrounded by a capsule and controlled by muscles. From the foregoing it is clear that a number of parallel processes are in operation as we grow old. At present, aging is an inevitable "normal" process. To arrest it requires more than simple protection of chondrocytes, for example. The combination of reducing cognitive function, falling bone density, increasing cartilage deformability, and poor muscle strength will predicate toward falls and injury, perhaps often forgotten or undocumented. For example, they may promote tibial and femoral subchondral fractures, previously thought to be idiopathic necrosis or sudden-onset necrosis of the condyle, and promote sudden and catastrophic joint failure. The combination of disc dehydration, reducing bone mass, and postural control lead to a thoracic kyphosis, increased skeletal loading, and wedge compression fractures. Indeed, bone density does not correlate with the degree of thoracic kyphosis; the severity of disc degeneration does.[39]

At the outset, the question was posed—what is normal for an older person? At what stage do these age-related processes become abnormal? Is it from the moment of conception, or birth, or peak skeletal maturity? Or, would it be more appropriate to dissect out the age-related from the other changes to which we are susceptible so that therapy can be directly more specifically? Our aging populations will demand it!

REFERENCES

1. Dressler MR, Butler DL, Boivin GP. Age-related changes in the biomechanics of healing patellar tendon. J Biomech 2006; 39:2205-2212.
2. Perry MH III. The endocrinology of aging. Clin Biochem 1999; 45:1369-1376.
3. Trifunovic A, Wredenberg A, Falkenberg M, et al. Premature ageing in mice expressing defective mitochondrial DNA polymerase. Nature 2004; 429:417-423.
4. Botha-Scheppers SA, Watt I, Slagboom E, et al. Radiological disease progression over two years is influenced by familial factors in siblings with generalized osteoarthritis. The GARP study. Arthritis Rheum (in press).
5. Ding C, Cicuttini F, Scott F, et al. The genetic contribution and relevance of knee cartilage defects: case-control and sib-pair studies. J Rheumatol 2005; 32:1937-1942.
6. Herman T, Giladi N, Gurevich T, Hausdorff JM. Gait instability and fractal dynamics of older adults with a "cautious" gait: why do certain older adults walk fearfully? Gait Posture 2005; 21:178-185.
7. Bullough PG. The role of joint architecture in the etiology of arthritis. Osteoarthritis Cartilage 2004; 12:S2-S9.
8. Bullough PG. The geometry of diarthrodial joints, its physiologic maintenance, and the possible significance of age-related changes in geometry-to-load distribution and the development of osteoarthritis. Clin Orthop Relat Res 1981; 156:61-66.
9. Mavcic B, Slivnik T, Antolic V, et al. High contact hip stress is related to the development of hip pathology with increasing age. Clin Biomech 2004; 19:939-943.
10. Lane LB, Bullough PG. Age-related changes in the thickness of the calcified zone and the number of tidemarks in adult human articular cartilage. J Bone Joint Surg 1980; 62:372-375.
11. Ding C, Cicuttini F, Scott F, et al. Association between age and knee structural change: a cross sectional MRI based study. Ann Rheum Dis 2005; 64:549-555.
12. Perry HM III, Bernard M, Horowitz M, et al. The effect of aging on bone mineral metabolism and bone mass in Native American women. J Am Geriatr Soc 1998; 46:1418-1422.
13. Lundeen GA, Vajda EG, Bloebaum RD. Age-related cancellous bone loss in the proximal femur of Caucasian females. Osteoporosis Int 2000; 11:505-511.
14. Luria S, Liebergall M, Elishoov O, et al. Osteoporotic tibial plateau fractures: an underestimated cause of knee pain in the elderly. Am J Orthop 2005; 34:186-188.
15. Yamamoto T, Bullough PG. Spontaneous osteonecrosis of the knee: the result of subchondral insufficiency fracture. J Bone Joint Surg 2006; 82:858-866.
16. Chen WT, Shih TT, Chen RC, et al. Vertebral bone marrow perfusion evaluated with dynamic contrast-enhanced MR imaging: significance of aging and sex. Radiology 2001; 220:213-218.
17. Griffith JF, Yeung DKW, Antonio GE, et al. Vertebral bone mineral density, marrow perfusion, and fat content in healthy men and men with osteoporosis: dynamic contrast-enhanced MR imaging and MR spectroscopy. Radiology 2005; 236:945-951.
18. Kubo T, Kimori K, Nakamura F, et al. Blood flow and blood volume in the femoral heads of healthy adults according to age: measurement with positron emission tomography (PET). Ann Nucl Med 2001; 15:231-235.
19. Brookes M, Helal B. Primary osteoarthritis, venous engorgement and osteogenesis. J Bone Joint Surg Br 1968; 50:493-504.
20. Martin JA, Buckwalter JA. Aging, articular cartilage chondrocyte senescence and osteoarthritis. Biogerontology 2002; 3:257-264.
21. Mosher TJ, Liu Yi, Yang QX, et al. Age dependency of cartilage magnetic resonance imaging T2 relaxation times in asymptomatic women. Arthritis Rheum 2004; 50:2820-2828.
22. Hudelmaier M, Glaser C, Hohe J, et al. Age-related changes in the morphology and deformational behavior of knee joint cartilage. Arthritis Rheum 2001; 44:2556-2561.
23. Janssen I, Heymsfield SB, Wang Z, Ross R. Skeletal muscle mass and distribution in 468 men and women aged 18-88 yr. J Appl Physiol 2000; 89:81-88.
24. Masuda K, Kinugasa R, Tanabe K, Kuno SY. Determinants for stair climbing by elderly from muscle morphology. Percept Motor Skills 2002; 94:814-816.
25. Morse CI, Thom JM, Mian OS, et al. Muscle strength, volume and activation following 12-month resistance training in 70-year-old males. Eur J Appl Physiol 2005; 95:197-204.
26. Hatakenaka M, Ueda M, Ishigami K, et al. Effects of aging on muscle T2 relaxation time: difference between fast- and slow-twitch muscles. Invest Radiol 2001; 36:692-698.
27. Chard MD, Cawston TE, Riley GP, et al. Rotator cuff degeneration and lateral epicondylitis: a comparative histological study. Ann Rheum Dis 1994; 53:30-34.
28. Sano A, Itoi E, Konno N, et al. Cystic changes of the humeral head on MR imaging: relation to age and cuff tears. Acta Orthop Scand 1998; 69:397-400.
29. Strocchi R, De Pasquale V, Facchini A, et al. Age-related changes in human anterior cruciate ligament (ACL) collagen fibrils. Ital J Anat Embryol 1996; 101:213-220.
30. Kiss C, Szilagyi M, Paksy A, Poor G. Risk factors for diffuse idiopathic skeletal hyperostosis: a case-controlled study. Rheumatology (Oxford) 2002; 41:27-30.
31. Neumann P, Ekstrom LA, Keller TS, et al. Aging, vertebral density, and disc degeneration alter the tensile stress-strain characteristics of the human anterior longitudinal ligament. J Orthop Res 1994; 12:103-112.
32. Iida T, Abumi K, Kotani Y, Kaneda K. Effects of aging and spinal degeneration on the mechanical properties of lumbar supraspinous and interspinous ligaments. Spine 2002; 2:95-100.
33. Ishikawa M, Matsumoto M, Fujimura Y, et al. Changes of cervical spinal cord and cervical spinal canal with age in asymptomatic subjects. Spinal Cord 2003; 41:159-163.
34. Szpalski M, Gunzburg R. Lumbar spinal stenosis in the elderly: an overview. Eur Spine J 2003; 12(Suppl 2):S170-S175.
35. Goh S, Tan C, Price RI, et al. Influence of age and gender on thoracic vertebral body shape and disc degeneration: an MR investigation of 169 cases. J Anat 2000; 197:647-657.
36. Cassar-Pullicino VN. MRI of the ageing and herniating intervertebral disc. Eur J Radiol 1998; 27:214-228.
37. Sether LA, Yu S, Haughton VM, Fischer ME. Intervertebral disk: normal age-related changes in MR signal intensity. Radiology 1990; 177:385-388.
38. Karakida O, Ueda H, Ueda M, Miyasaka T. Diurnal T2 value changes in the lumbar intervertebral discs. Clin Radiol 2003; 58:389-392.
39. Manns RA, Haddaway MJ, McCall IW, et al. The relative contribution of disc and vertebral morphometry to the angle of kyphosis in asymptomatic subjects. Clin Radiol 1996; 51:258-262.

45

Degenerative Disease: Cartilage Anatomy, Physiology, and Advanced Imaging

Timothy J. Mosher

ETIOLOGY

Degeneration and loss of joint function is a common end point for many arthropathies, the most prevalent of which is osteoarthritis (OA). The American College of Rheumatology defines OA as a heterogeneous group of conditions that leads to joint signs and symptoms that are associated with defective integrity of articular cartilage and associated changes in the underlying bone and at the joint margins.[1] Although OA is a multifactorial disease process, the degeneration and ultimate loss of articular cartilage is a central feature and a significant contributor to clinical symptoms. Despite a high prevalence of this disease, the etiology and pathogenesis of this condition are poorly understood. It is generally accepted that damage to articular cartilage occurs when local biomechanical forces exceed the material properties of cartilage, leading to structural and biochemical changes in the cartilage matrix and alteration in gene expression of the chondrocyte. These biomechanical forces are determined by many variables, including body habitus, intensity and type of physical activity, stiffness of the subchondral bone, joint trauma, as well as alignment of the joint and laxity in the stabilizing tissues. The material properties of cartilage are also influenced by many factors, including senescent changes as a result of normal aging, genetics, diet, exercise, and coexisting systemic diseases or conditions. The complex interplay of these many variables produces an imbalance in cartilage homeostasis in which degradation of the cartilage matrix exceeds synthesis, ultimately progressing to structural loss of tissue.

Although OA involves the entire joint, the primary focus of this chapter is articular cartilage, with particular emphasis on MRI for identification of early cartilage injury.

PREVALENCE AND EPIDEMIOLOGY

Current estimates are that symptoms and disability related to OA afflict more than 20 million Americans. With a rising mean age of the American population and growing incidence of secondary OA in younger individuals it is projected that by the year 2020 OA will afflict more than 60 million Americans.

Age is the primary risk factor for development of both radiographic and clinical OA. In individuals younger than age 45 the prevalence of OA increases slowly in a linear fashion with age. After age 45 the rate of disease prevalence of OA increases exponentially with age, afflicting approximately 50% of people at age 65, increasing to 85% in those individuals 75 years or older.[2]

Obesity has been shown to be a risk factor for knee OA; however, the relative risk for hip OA is less conclusive. Studies have shown weight loss can reduce the risk of OA. Of note, obesity has been shown to increase the risk of OA in non–weight-bearing joints such as the interphalangeal joints of the hand, suggesting that systemic as well as local biomechanical factors may be responsible.

Physical activity, particularly that related to long-term repetitive activities associated with particular occupations, can increase the risk of OA. Hip arthritis is more common in farmers. Hip and spine OA is more prevalent

KEY POINTS

- The primary constituents of articular cartilage are water, type II collagen, and large molecules of aggregating proteoglycans (aggrecan).
- The composition and structure of the cartilage matrix vary with depth of the articular surface as well as with location in the joint.
- Normal cartilage biomechanics relies on a high interstitial tissue pressure that is generated by swelling of hydrated proteoglycans and constraint by the surrounding type II collagen matrix.
- MR T2-weighted images are sensitive to variation in the cartilage matrix as a result of differences in collagen fibril orientation and water content.
- Loss of normal spatial variation in MRI T2-weighted signal intensity is an early finding in cartilage degradation.
- More severe grades of cartilage damage are associated with loss of tissue and surface irregularity.
- Cartilage delamination occurs when cartilage fibrils are cleaved, thereby separating cartilage from subchondral bone. It is characterized by linear high MRI T2-weighted signal at the bone-cartilage interface.
- Underlying bone marrow MRI T2-weighted hyperintensity (bone marrow edema) is an important secondary sign of cartilage injury.

in miners. Unusual repetitive activities may lead to OA in atypical joints. For example, there is an increased frequency of upper extremity OA in pneumatic drill operators. Although a slightly higher incidence of OA is observed in high-performance competitive athletes, this is frequently associated with prior joint trauma, which is strongly associated with secondary OA. Moderate recreational exercise such as running has not been associated with an increased risk of OA.

CLINICAL PRESENTATION

Pain along with loss of joint mobility is a common symptom of OA. Typically, the pain is poorly localized around the joint, increases with activity, and is relieved with rest. The source of pain in OA is not entirely clear but may be associated with the presence of joint effusion, mild synovitis, and changes in subchondral bone marrow. Radiographic features of OA such as joint space narrowing and osteophyte formation correlate poorly with clinimetric measures of pain.

OA may be associated with transient episodes of morning stiffness. With further progression of the disease, loss of joint congruity and development of osteophytes and intra-articular osteochondral bodies can lead to loss of joint function and disability with difficulties in activities of daily living. Complaints of joint instability are common, particularly in knee OA.

Focal chondral or osteochondral lesions may have a clinical presentation that mimics meniscal pathology in the knee or labral pathology in the hip or shoulder. Symptoms consist of nonspecific pain or episodes of locking. With MRI, focal chondral abnormalities are frequently

observed in subjects without joint symptoms and in otherwise healthy volunteers. Because cartilage lacks nociceptive receptors, cartilage injury alone is not responsible for pain but may contribute secondarily to pain through associated changes in subchondral bone marrow or synovium.

PATHOPHYSIOLOGY

Anatomy

Under physiologic conditions articular cartilage is exposed to high compressive and shear forces. For example, it is estimated that during a squatting maneuver, patellar cartilage undergoes compressive loads that are greater than six times body weight, with transient pressures that may be substantially higher.[3] These forces are applied repetitively many times a day throughout the course of a lifetime. What is remarkable is not that cartilage degrades but that it is capable of functioning normally under these conditions throughout a human life span.

The biomaterial properties of articular cartilage are a result of the composition and organization of the extracellular matrix. Cartilage is 65% to 85% water, with water content decreasing slightly with depth from the articular surface. The major solid components of the extracellular matrix are type II collagen, which comprises 10% to 20% of the wet weight of cartilage, and large molecules of aggregating proteoglycans, termed aggrecan, that contribute 5% to 10% wet weight. The content and structure of collagen and proteoglycans in the matrix differ substantially from bone to the articular surface and strongly influence the biomaterial properties of cartilage. The components of type II collagen, tropocollagen molecules, are polymerized into larger collagen fibrils, which in turn are organized into a leaf-like architecture.[4] As illustrated in Figure 45-1, the orientation and alignment of the collagen matrix vary with depth from the articular surface as well as regionally within the joint. Collagen fibrils cross the bone-cartilage interface at the tidemark zone and secure cartilage to the subchondral bone. In the deep layer of cartilage near bone, collagen fibrils have a preferential orientation perpendicular to the bone surface. This is frequently termed the *radial zone*, referring to the radial orientation of the collagen matrix as well as the columnar alignment of chondrocytes observed in this layer. Near the surface the orientation of the collagen matrix curves tangentially in the transitional zone, becoming parallel to the articular surface in the superficial zone. The superficial layer is covered with a distinct layer of dense collagen fibers termed the *lamina splendens*. The tangential and superficial layers of cartilage are relatively thin in regions of the joint habitually exposed to high compressive loads, such as the central portion of the femoral condyle and tibial plateau uncovered by the meniscus. These layers are thicker in regions exposed to less load, such as articular surfaces covered by the meniscus.

Interposed in the meshwork of type II collagen fibrils are large molecules of aggregating proteoglycans consisting of aggrecan (Fig. 45-2). Concentration of proteoglycans also varies within cartilage, with the highest levels found below the articular surface and decreasing in

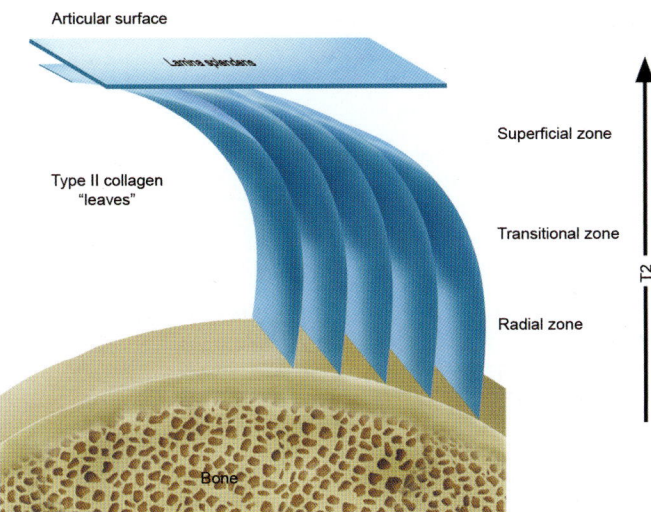

■ FIGURE 45-1 Schematic illustration of type II collagen matrix in cartilage. The primary constituents of the cartilage matrix are water, type II collagen, and aggregating proteoglycans (aggrecan). The structural organization of the collagen matrix varies with depth from the articular surface and influences the T2 relaxation time of cartilage. In the radial zone the collagen matrix is aligned perpendicular to bone. This high degree of orientation or anisotropy provides an efficient mechanism for spin-spin relaxation, leading to short T2 values. Toward the articular surface, the oblique orientation and lower anisotropy in the transitional zone leads to a lengthening of T2, resulting in high signal intensity on T2-weighted images. At the surface, fibrils are aligned parallel to the articular surface. At the articular surface, a distinct surface layer, or lamina splendens, is adherent to the horizontally oriented fibers of the superficial collagen leaves. This layer is generally too thin to resolve with clinical MR images.

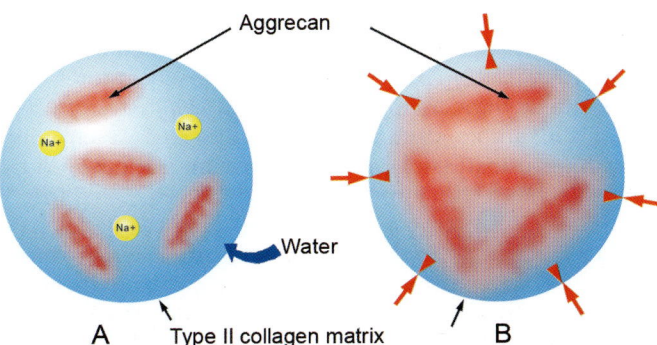

■ FIGURE 45-2 Cartilage swelling pressure. Large molecules of aggregating proteoglycans (aggrecan) are imbedded within the fibrils of the type II collagen matrix. When aggrecan is hydrated, the high density of negative charges draws in sodium and water, causing the aggrecan molecule to swell. Aggrecan swelling is restrained by the surrounding collagen fibrils, resulting in a large interstitial swelling pressure responsible for the compressive stiffness of cartilage. In early cartilage damage, fragmentation of the collagen matrix allows unrestrained swelling of aggrecan and lowers the internal pressure of cartilage. This makes the cartilage more compressible and susceptible to further degeneration.

concentration near bone. The aggrecan molecules consist of a central core fiber of hyaluronic acid. Bound to this fiber are numerous, large, negatively charged glycosaminoglycan molecules consisting of chondroitin sulfate and keratin sulfate. When these molecules are hydrated, the

high density of negative charges on the proteoglycans bind sodium and draw water into cartilage, causing the proteoglycans to swell. Swelling of the proteoglycans is constrained by the surrounding collagen meshwork, producing an interstitial fluid pressure of approximately 9 MPa. This large pressure contributes to the compressive stiffness of cartilage. As such, the balance of aggrecan swelling and an intact collagen matrix is an essential feature for normal cartilage function.

The MRI relaxation properties of articular cartilage and the appearance of cartilage with standard clinical MRI techniques are strongly influenced by the composition and structure of the extracellular matrix. As a result of this sensitivity, MRI has the potential to function as a noninvasive image marker of changes in the extracellular matrix that occur during early cartilage injury that precedes fibrillation and loss of tissue. Because these observations can be made noninvasively in human joints, MRI is a valuable clinical research technique, providing unique information regarding the natural history of OA, human cartilage physiology, and in situ biomechanics.

The influence of cartilage structure and composition on MRI signal intensity is most evident on T2-weighted images. As illustrated in Figure 45-3, the signal intensity of cartilage varies with location in the joint as well as with depth from the articular surface. This is primarily a function of regional and zonal differences of the type II collagen matrix, which influences T2 relaxation of cartilage as well as variation in water content. Within the radial zone the high content and anisotropic orientation of collagen fibrils provide efficient T2 relaxation, leading to low signal intensity on proton-density (PD)– or T2-weighted images. With very high resolution images, the darker radial zone has a striated appearance with alternating fine bands of high and low signal intensity radiating from the bone cartilage interface. In lower-resolution images, individual striations are not resolved and, instead, this layer is characterized by low signal intensity. Closer to the articular surface less fibril anisotropy and oblique orientation of the collagen matrix lead to a gradual increase in T2 relaxation time and thus a relative increase in signal intensity on T2-weighted images. At the articular surface collagen fibers are oriented parallel to the articular surface. The superficial tangential layer and the lamina splendens are approximately 20 μm thick and can be identified on MR microscopy images of excised cartilage specimens as a thin hypointense layer; however, it is too thin to resolve on routine clinical MR images.

The organization and orientation of collagen within the cartilage matrix have a strong influence on the MRI appearance of cartilage. In connective tissues such as tendons, ligaments, and articular cartilage, the highly ordered arrangement of collagen fibers produces residual quadripolar coupling with mobile protons, an efficient mechanism for T2 relaxation. For these tissues with a highly preferred or anisotropic organization of collagen fibrils, T2 relaxation is dependent on the relative orientation of the collagen fibers with the static magnetic field (B0).[5] Tissues containing fibers oriented parallel or perpendicular to B0 have efficient T2 relaxation and low signal intensity on T2-weighted images. However, when fibers are oriented 54 degrees relative to B0, there

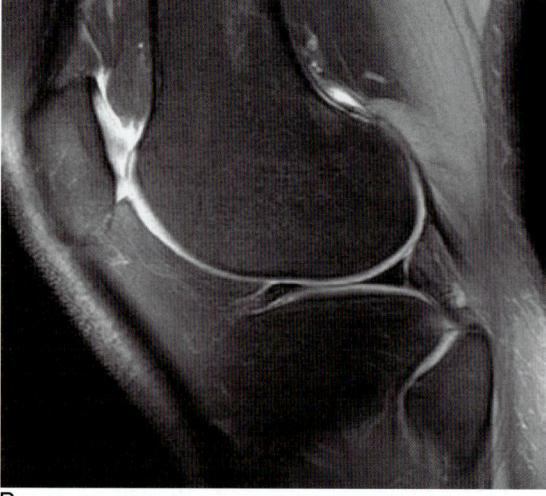

■ **FIGURE 45-3** **A,** Coronal, 3T, fat-suppressed, PD-weighted, TSE MR image of the knee illustrating normal spatial variation in cartilage signal intensity. Areas chronically exposed to high compressive loads such as the uncovered cartilage of the medial compartment (*arrows*) demonstrate a striated hypointense signal intensity of the radial zone, with a thin hyperintense superficial zone. This is a result of the high type II collagen content of the radial zone that has an anisotropic orientation perpendicular to the bone-cartilage interface. The hyperintense superficial zone is thicker in regions of the joint with less compressive load. **B,** Sagittal, 3T, fat-suppressed, PD-weighted, TSE MR image of the knee illustrating uniformly high cartilage signal intensity in the trochlea and posterior femoral condyle. Note the striated appearance of the central load-bearing regions of the femoral condyle and tibial plateau.

is averaging of the residual quadripolar coupling, which minimizes this contribution to T2 relaxation and leads to an increase in signal intensity. Because of this effect, 54 degrees is termed the "magic angle,"[6] derived from the technique of magic angle spinning used to increase the T2 relaxation of crystalline samples in solid-state nuclear magnetic resonance spectroscopy.

The high concentration of collagen in the radial zone also decreases signal intensity through magnetization transfer. As suggested by the name, magnetization transfer is a process in which magnetization from a proton located on collagen is transferred to the mobile proton pool that gives rise to the MR signal.[7] Magnetization transfer effects are most pronounced for techniques that use a large number of radiofrequency pulses such as multislice fast spin-echo (FSE) or turbo spin-echo (TSE) techniques. The rapid application of off-resonance radiofrequency energy quickly saturates protons bound to the collagen molecules but does not saturate the mobile pool in the surrounding water. This saturated magnetization is then transferred either through chemical exchange or exchange of magnetization to nearby water protons in the mobile pool. Type I and II collagen demonstrate substantial magnetization transfer with FSE techniques.[8,9] The effect of magnetization transfer is to decrease signal intensity of tissues rich in collagen on the MR image.[10] For tissues such as cartilage, incidental magnetization transfer reduces signal intensity by 15% to 20% as the number of slices and thus the amount of off-resonance irradiation increases.[11] Because gradient-echo techniques use significantly less radiofrequency energy, there is less incidental magnetization transfer with gradient-echo techniques compared with spin-echo (SE) and FSE techniques. As a result of less magnetization transfer and T2 weighting, cartilage has relatively uniform high signal intensity on T1-weighted fat-suppressed gradient-echo images.

Recognizing the normal heterogeneity of cartilage is important to avoid erroneously interpreting nonuniform signal as disease on T2-weighted images. As discussed previously, the signal intensity of cartilage normally increases toward the surface. In addition to variation in signal intensity with respect to depth from the articular surface, there are differences with respect to location in the joint and relative orientation of cartilage to the applied magnetic field. This variation in signal intensity closely follows variation in histologic and biomechanical properties of cartilage. For example, cartilage consistently exposed to high compressive load such as tibial cartilage not covered by meniscus has a thin superficial layer of high signal intensity, whereas the covered portion of tibial cartilage has a thicker layer of superficial hyperintensity. Goodwin and associates have correlated this regional variation in signal intensity with obliquity of the collagen matrix cleavage planes on freeze-fracture specimens, indicating that the relative orientation of the cartilage matrix to the applied magnetic field is a major factor.[12]

Regional differences in cartilage T2 relaxation are most pronounced in the femoral condyle. This is a result of two processes. First, there are substantial differences in the organization of extracellular matrix and chondrocytes between the central femoral surface and posterior femoral condyles, which are not habitually exposed to high compressive load but experience shear forces during knee flexion. Whereas type II collagen in the central femoral condyle has a high degree of anisotropy, results from electron microscopy and x-ray diffraction studies indicate the collagen matrix in the posterior femoral condyle has less anisotropy and has a fine fibrillar organization. This region of cartilage lacks the regular bands of condensed collagen seen in the central femoral condyle. Second, the oblique orientation of the collagen matrix in this region with respect to the direction of B0 is close to the magic angle of 54 degrees. As a result of differences in organization and orientation of the type II collagen matrix, cartilage in the posterior femoral condyle demonstrates uniformly high signal intensity compared with the layered pattern of signal intensity observed in the central femoral condyle. Although regional variation in the MRI appearance of cartilage has been extensively studied for the knee, similar variation is observed in other joints with MR images of sufficient resolution.[13]

Pathology

Normal cartilage function depends on a balance of aggrecan swelling and constraining forces provided by the collagen meshwork. Investigators in the early 1970s proposed that one of the earliest processes of cartilage degeneration was fragmentation of the collagen matrix. Because damaged collagen no longer constrains the proteoglycans, they swell and draw in more water. The increased water content and loss of interstitial fluid pressure allow water to move more freely through the tissue. As a result, more compressive load is carried by the solid components, leading to structural fatigue. This results in a cascade of events in which damage to the solid matrix increases mobility of water, thereby transferring more of the compressive load onto the matrix and producing further damage. Eventually, this leads to gross loss of cartilage.

Although chondrocytes are capable of producing new proteoglycan, there is limited capacity to repair collagen damage. Most investigators believe damage to the collagen meshwork is irreversible. Several factors can increase susceptibility of cartilage collagen to damage. First, genetic mutations of the type II collagen gene have been implicated in several syndromes associated with premature onset of OA (Fig. 45-4). These are collectively known as type II collagenopathies and include Stickler's syndrome, Kniest's dysplasia, and spondyloepiphyseal dysplasia, along with other conditions. With the relatively large degree of genetic diversity in the type II collagen gene it is likely that inherited factors contribute to the relative risk of OA in the general population. Additional mutations have been identified in genes encoding for other cartilage macromolecules. Second, senescent accumulation of advanced glycation end products in cartilage and cross-linking of collagen fibrils make the collagen matrix more brittle and prone to fracture. Because of the slow turnover of collagen in cartilage, these byproducts accumulate with age. Age also influences chondrocyte metabolism; in particular there appears to be a diminished capacity of older chondrocytes to synthesize proteoglycan. As a result, older cartilage may be more susceptible to damage from fatigue fractures and may have less capacity to replenish aggrecan, thereby predisposing older individuals to development of OA. Third, two families of enzymes are observed to be unregulated in early OA and may contribute to progression of cartilage damage. Matrix metalloproteinases break down collagen, whereas aggrecanases degrade aggrecan. In the healthy state the activity of these degradative enzymes is balanced by that of synthetic enzymes, as well as production of specific enzyme inhibitors. Inflammatory mediators such as interleukin-1 and tumor necrosis factor are increased in OA and tip the balance of enzymatic pathway toward the side of matrix degradation.

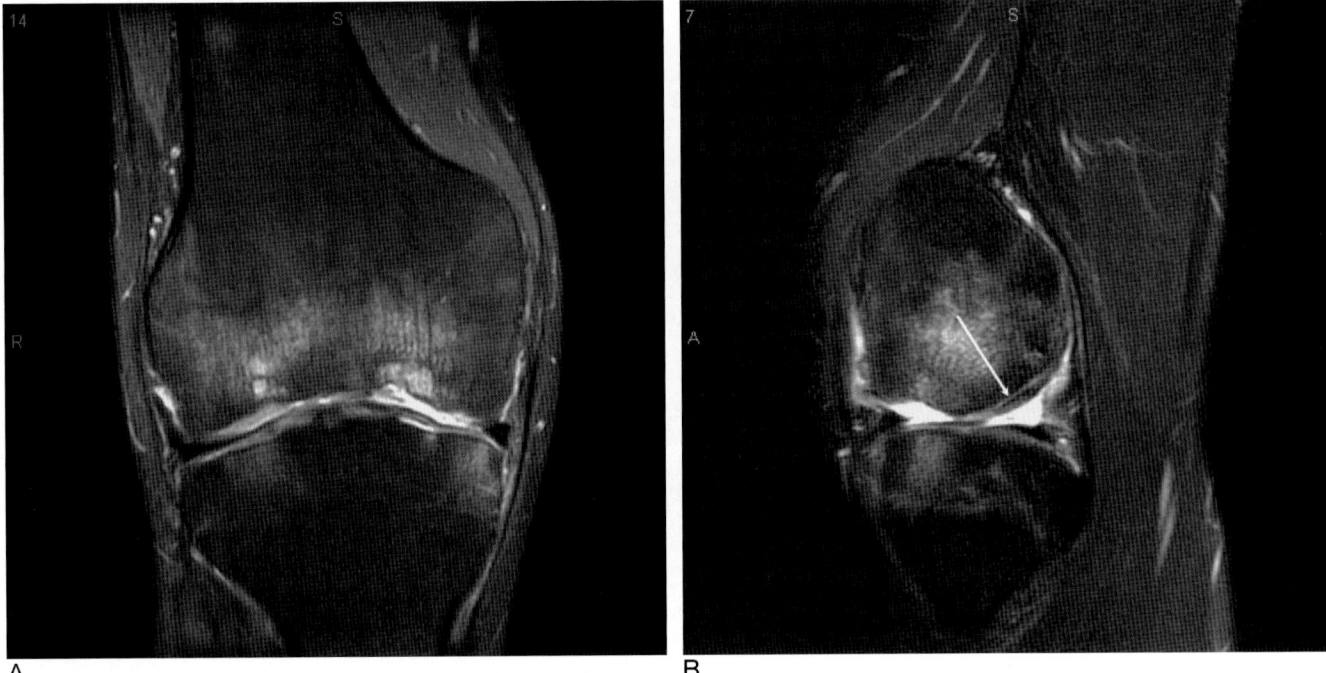

■ **FIGURE 45-4** **A,** Coronal, fat-suppressed, PD-weighted, FSE MR image of a 27-year-old man with Stickler's syndrome, an inherited point mutation of the type II collagen gene. Extensive cartilage loss is present in the medial compartment with associated degenerative changes in the subchondral bone. Although there is normal thickness of cartilage in the lateral compartment, note the loss of spatial variation in signal intensity observed in normal cartilage. **B,** Sagittal, fat-suppressed, T2-weighted MR image of same patient as in **A.** Note the linear hyperintensity at the bone-cartilage interface compatible with cartilage delamination (*arrow*).

BIOMECHANICS

Normal cartilage biomechanics relies on a balance of aggrecan swelling pressure and constraint by the surrounding collagen meshwork. This balance is similar to an automobile tire in which the swelling pressure from the proteoglycans is analogous to the tire pressure from the air and the constraint of the collagen meshwork is like the walls of the tires. Just as driving on tires with low air pressure leads to rapid deterioration of the tire, low interstitial pressure in cartilage leads to deterioration of the matrix. High fluid pressure, along with the high osmolarity, viscosity, and electrostatic forces of the extracellular cartilage matrix restrict the movement of interstitial water and provides compressive stiffness to cartilage. When cartilage is compressed, the energy imparted into the tissue is dissipated by frictional drag forces as water moves through the extracellular matrix. For cartilage to resist compression the movement of water through the extracellular cartilage matrix must be restricted. Under normal conditions, approximately 90% of the load is carried by water, which is the primary reason cartilage is so resilient to repetitive compression.

In addition to compression, cartilage is also exposed to shear stress as one articular surface moves against another. The normal articular surface of cartilage has an extremely low coefficient of friction, allowing the surfaces to move smoothly. Damage to the surface such as fibrillation or focal cartilage defects increases friction at the surface and tensile strain in the extracellular matrix. Shear stiffness in cartilage is a function of tensile strain that develops in the type II collagen matrix. Aggrecan also contributes to shear stiffness by buttressing the collagen fibers and inflating the collagen meshwork.

Mechanical factors influence the susceptibility of cartilage to damage. It is acknowledged that high mechanical load such as impact injuries may exceed the material properties of even healthy tissue, producing fracture fissures through the matrix. However, a certain amount of mechanical loading is necessary for normal cartilage health. Moderate cyclical loading has been shown to increase proteoglycan production in cultured chondrocytes; however, high compressive forces, particularly static forces, have a deleterious effect on cartilage physiology. Increased levels of exercise have been shown to increase proteoglycan levels in cartilage, indicating the tissue has the potential to adapt to changes in demands.[14] In contrast, joint immobilization leads to rapid depletion of proteoglycan and increased susceptibility to cartilage injury.

An emerging theory for the etiology of OA and cartilage degradation is based on a growing body of evidence that indicates cartilage adapts to local biomechanical forces in the joint. In this theory cartilage is conditioned to withstand the local forces applied to it. When local forces are substantially altered, such as after meniscal resection, with abnormal joint alignment, or with increased joint laxity, biomechanical forces are transferred to unconditioned cartilage that exceeds the stress threshold of the tissue, leading to progressive deterioration of tissue.

IMAGING TECHNIQUES

Techniques and Relevant Aspects

Historically, clinical evaluation of articular cartilage has primarily relied on two acquisition techniques: 3D fat-suppressed T1-weighted spoiled-gradient-echo (SGE) and 2D PD-weighted FSE techniques. Each has relative advantages and disadvantages with respect to evaluation of articular cartilage and diagnosis of osteochondral injuries.

Initial MRI investigations of focal cartilage lesions used 3D T1-weighted gradient-echo acquisitions to identify focal defects. This technique provides high-resolution images with excellent differentiation of cartilage and underlying subchondral bone. As demonstrated in Figure 45-5, the major advantage of this technique is high spatial resolution, which is particularly important in evaluation of small joints or curved articular cartilage surfaces such as the talar dome or femoral head, in which thin sections are needed to clearly delineate cartilage interfaces and minimize volume averaging. Using this technique at 1.5 tesla (T), it is possible to obtain images with a 1 to 2 mm section thickness and in-plane resolution of 200 to 350 μm per pixel. For comparison, 2D FSE techniques are generally limited to 3- to 4-mm section thickness and 300- to 500 μm in-plane resolution. Because of high spatial resolution, 3D T1-weighted gradient-echo acquisitions are becoming valuable tools in clinical research applications to quantitatively determine cartilage volume, thickness, and surface area. These tissue measures are being explored as possible end points in assessment of new chondroprotective therapies.[15]

Several disadvantages limit routine clinical application of gradient-echo techniques in larger joints where spatial resolution is less of a premium. A practical limitation of the 3D acquisition is the relatively long imaging times, ranging from 6 to 10 minutes, needed for coverage of large joints such as the knee. Imaging times can be shortened by approximately 30% by using more efficient water excitation techniques rather than chemical shift fat suppression. This is particularly effective at 3 T where greater separation of the fat and water resonances places less stringent demands on frequency-selective excitation pulses. A second limitation of the gradient-echo technique is relatively poor image contrast, particularly at the articular surface. Although the technique produces reliable high-contrast images of cartilage and subchondral bone, contrast at the articular surface can vary depending on protein content or blood degradation products in the synovial fluid. This can lower sensitivity for detection of superficial fibrillation or fissures occurring with cartilage injury. In addition, the T1-weighted technique is relatively insensitive to signal alterations within the cartilage or subchondral bone marrow that can be important indicators of osteochondral injury.

In the knee the T1-weighted, fat-suppressed, gradient-echo technique has a diagnostic accuracy of 65% to 95% for detection of focal cartilage defects. Diagnostic sensitivity has generally been shown to be substantially lower for superficial cartilage lesions confined to the outer 50% of cartilage. The ability to characterize the size of the lesion can be helpful for preoperative planning. In validation studies of focal cartilage defects, MRI has been shown to

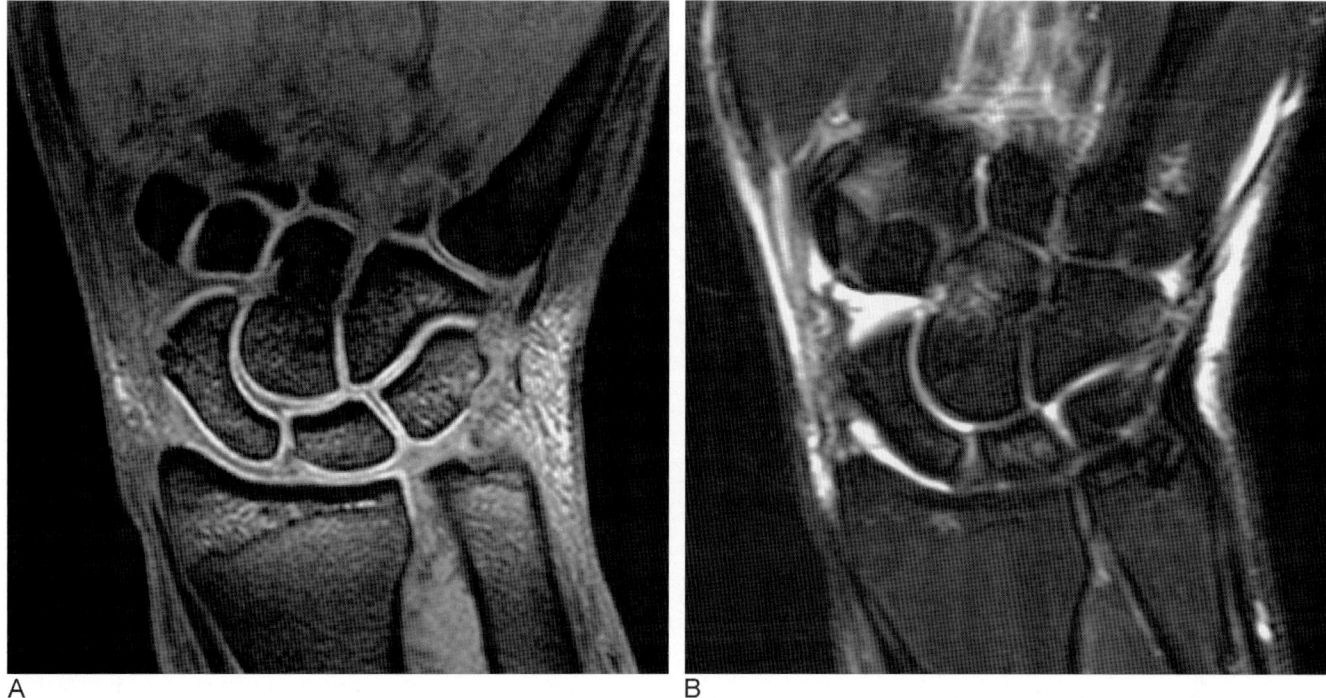

A   B

■ **FIGURE 45-5** **A,** A 3T, 3D, coronal, water-excited, T1-weighted, SGE MR image of a 22-year-old professional hockey player with a nondisplaced fracture of the capitate. This provides high-resolution evaluation of the thin articular cartilage of the wrist but is insensitive to the marrow edema observed in the capitate and lunate on the fat-suppressed T2-weighted TSE image shown in **B**. The 3D, SGE sequence is particularly useful in evaluating thin articular cartilage of small joints such as the wrist and elbow and curved articular surfaces such as the hip and ankle and for providing quantitative assessment of cartilage morphology for research applications.

underestimate the depth of the articular defect. Size of the lesion has been shown to be important in accuracy of MRI. Although MRI is relatively accurate for measuring knee cartilage lesions 5 mm or larger, it has been shown to overestimate size of smaller lesions.

Routine clinical evaluation of articular cartilage, particularly in the knee, relies heavily on PD-weighted FSE images either with or without fat suppression. The primary advantage of this technique is excellent soft tissue contrast with relatively modest image acquisition times of 3 to 4 minutes. As discussed previously, the fat-suppressed, PD-weighted FSE technique demonstrates heterogeneity of the cartilage signal resulting from regional and zonal differences in composition and structure of the extracellular cartilage matrix. This sensitivity to internal cartilage damage is particularly important for identifying injuries of the bone-cartilage tidemark zone that may not be associated with a visible cartilage surface defect but can have long-term consequences for tissue integrity. Also with the addition of chemical shift fat suppression, the technique is sensitive to elevated T2-weighted signal in the subchondral bone marrow that is frequently associated with overlying cartilage injury. The technique also provides clinically useful information regarding other articular tissues, such as menisci and ligaments. The primary disadvantage of the technique is lower spatial resolution compared with 3D acquisitions.

Initial studies by Potter and coworkers report an accuracy of 92% for diagnosis of focal cartilage lesions in the knee using the PD-weighted FSE technique.[16] Similar accuracy has been identified in subsequent studies for full-thickness defects and for partial-thickness defects involving greater than 50% cartilage thickness. As with gradient-echo techniques, sensitivity is generally less than 50% for diagnosis of superficial fibrillation and erosion.

New techniques based on the steady-state free precession gradient-echo sequences and multi-echo T2*-weighted sequences have been proposed for cartilage imaging. These techniques provide high resolution images of cartilage with image contrast similar to that obtained with FSE techniques. Although preliminary results are promising, these techniques are not widely available and have undergone limited validation for routine clinical use.

Controversies

Evaluation of cartilage injury requires high contrast resolution and places a premium on a high signal-to-noise ratio (SNR) of the image. With other acquisition parameters remaining constant, the SNR of the MR image increases with magnetic field strength. Whereas low-field open configuration or dedicated extremity magnets have demonstrated accuracy comparable with 1.5T scanners in diagnosis of meniscal or anterior cruciate ligament tears, accuracy in diagnosis of cartilage injury is substantially lower on low-field scanners. This is particularly true for partial-thickness cartilage lesions. Although clinical experience with 3T in cartilage is limited, preliminary results suggest the higher field strength provides improved contrast resolution and greater diagnostic accuracy in detection of focal defects. For quantitative determination of cartilage morphology, preliminary findings indicate higher spatial resolution images available at 3T improve reproducibility but have not been shown to improve accuracy in defining the size of focal defects.

MANIFESTATIONS OF THE DISEASE

Grade I Lesions

Current MRI grading systems of articular cartilage damage are based on modifications of the Outerbridge classification originally described for surgical grading of patellar lesions.[17] The original Outerbridge surgical classification is based on size of surface fragmentation and fissuring. As shown in Table 45-1, the MRI modification of the Outerbridge classification incorporates the depth of the lesion from the articular surface. Arthroscopic grading of cartilage frequently uses the Noyes classification.[18]

Magnetic Resonance Imaging

In the surgical Outerbridge classification, grade I lesions are identified by a subjective assessment of cartilage softening with an intact articular surface. Because there is no direct MRI finding that corresponds to cartilage softening, this has been modified to reflect MRI signal changes without morphologic changes of the cartilage surface. Early studies found poor correlation between grade I MRI lesions and arthroscopy, as well as low sensitivity in MRI detection of patellar cartilage softening found at arthroscopy. A lack of correlation should not be interpreted as a deficiency in either MRI or arthroscopy. Studies in isolated osteochondral samples indicate the two techniques are evaluating different properties of cartilage damage. In studies on enzymatically treated cartilage specimens, degradation of the type II collagen matrix is correlated with elevation in cartilage T2, whereas removal of proteoglycans has minimal effect. In correlation studies between biomechanical testing and MRI of cartilage specimens it has been shown that while

removal of proteoglycan significantly decreases cartilage stiffness, elevation of T2 with degradation of the collagen matrix does not substantially change cartilage compressibility. In light of these results it is likely that elevation in T2-weighted signal intensity reflects structural changes of the collagen matrix that do not substantially alter the biomechanical qualities of cartilage evaluated at surgery that are primarily related to alterations in cartilage proteoglycans.

Remote areas of T2 hyperintensity are frequently found in patients with more advanced areas of focal cartilage loss. Although the clinical significance of this finding is unknown, small longitudinal studies suggest grade I lesions are common and progress to sites of morphologic damage. The pattern of T2 elevation can reflect the underlying mechanism of cartilage injury. A more diffuse heterogeneous pattern of high T2-weighted signal can be observed after acute trauma, frequently in association with hyperintensity in the adjacent subchondral bone marrow. Isolated areas of T2 hyperintensity can be identified in cartilage of patients with no reported history of trauma. In our experience, focal elevation of T2 at the articular surface is frequently associated with visible cartilage damage at arthroscopy. Less frequently, T2 elevation may be limited to the deeper layers of cartilage. In this setting the cartilage surface frequently appears normal at surgery. This is most often seen in thicker patellar cartilage where the cartilage is sufficiently thick to resolve the deep layer of cartilage. As illustrated in Figure 45-6, focal elevation in cartilage T2 can be associated with a focal blister or smooth contour abnormality of the overlying articular surface. Similar findings of focal swelling and alterations in the fibril density in the superficial zone of patellar cartilage have been reported in the electron microscopy literature, supporting the hypothesis that these lesions represent structural reorganization/degeneration of the collagen matrix. In contrast to focal elevation in T2 seen with grade I lesions, a diffuse increase in the T2 of cartilage occurs with aging.[19] This begins near the articular surface in the mid 40s, extending to the deeper layers of cartilage with increasing age.

In addition to T2 hyperintensity, which is frequently present in the acute setting, focal areas of decreased T2-weighted cartilage signal may be observed adjacent to sites of cartilage injury (Fig. 45-7). Decreased T2-weighted

TABLE 45-1   Classification Systems for Evaluation of Chondropathy

Description	Modified Outerbridge (MRI Evaluation)	Original Outerbridge (Surgical Evaluation)	Noyes Classification
Normal	Grade 0	Grade 0	Grade 0
Cartilage softening and swelling with an intact surface	Grade I: T2-weighted signal alteration with an intact articular surface	Grade I: Softening and swelling	Grade 1A: Moderate softening Grade 1B: Extensive softening with swelling of the articular surface
Superficial fragmentation and fissuring	Grade II: Extending less than 50% of depth	Fragmentation and fissuring equal to or less than 0.5 inch in diameter	Grade 2A: Surface irregularity less than one half of the cartilage thickness
Deep fragmentation and fissuring	Grade III: Surface irregularity extending to the deep 50% of the cartilage thickness	Fragmentation and fissuring greater than 0.5 inch in diameter	Grade 2B: Surface irregularity greater than one half of the cartilage thickness
Exposed bone	Grade IV	Grade IV	Grade 3A: Exposed bone Grade 3B: Cavitation or erosion of exposed bone

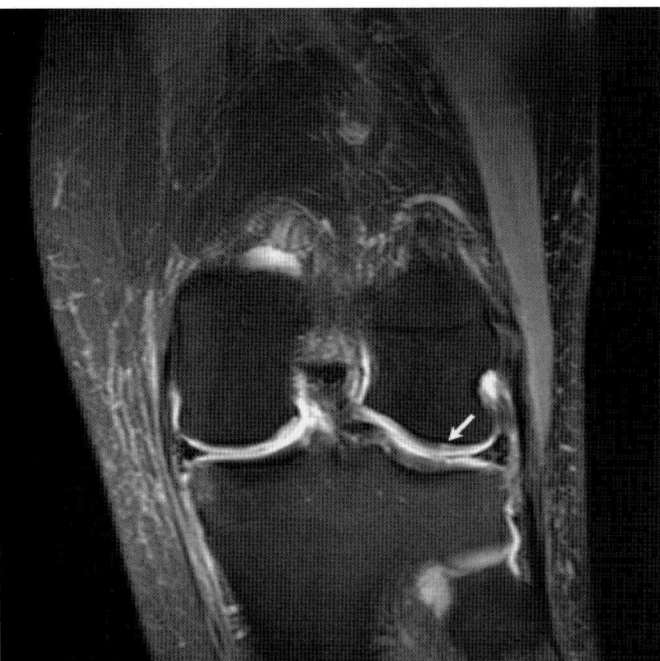

■ **FIGURE 45-6** Grade I lesion: 3T, coronal, fat-suppressed, PD-weighted MR image in a 54-year-old man with chronic knee pain demonstrates focal elevated signal intensity in the radial zone of the lateral femoral condyle (*arrow*) with an intact articular surface.

signal is generally not observed immediately after trauma but can develop several weeks after cartilage injury. The etiology of the decreased T2 signal intensity has not been determined but may reflect a hypertrophic healing

response or fragmentation of the collagen fibrils exposing additional water binding sites on collagen. Areas of low T2-weighted signal intensity are also observed with sites of chondrocalcinosis, particularly with gradient-echo techniques or with high magnetic field strengths.

A variation of the grade I cartilage lesion is cartilage delamination or debonding. This occurs when shear forces applied to the cartilage-bone interface injure the tidemark zone and disrupt collagen fibers that hold cartilage to the subchondral bone. In addition to shear force applied directly to the articular surface, high shear strain at the bone-cartilage interface develops with axial compression.[20] Cartilage delamination may not be readily apparent at arthroscopy because the articular surface is often intact.[21] In addition to biomechanical factors, recent evidence demonstrates that genetic factors influence the risk of cartilage delamination.[22]

MRI findings of cartilage delamination consist of linear T2 elevation at the bone-cartilage interface (Fig. 45-8). This is likely due to focal elevation in water content as well as to reduced collagen fibril anisotropy in the radial zone that occurs when cartilage is cleaved from bone.[23] These injuries are best seen on T2- or PD-weighted images with fat saturation. Direct MR arthrography has been used to assess acetabular cartilage delamination in the hip, which is a frequent finding in the presence of femoral acetabular impingement. With this technique, cartilage delamination is inferred by the presence of high signal on T1-weighted fat-suppressed images between bone and cartilage. In the knee, delamination injuries may be seen in the femoral condyle, frequently in cartilage adjacent to the posterior horn of the meniscus. In the

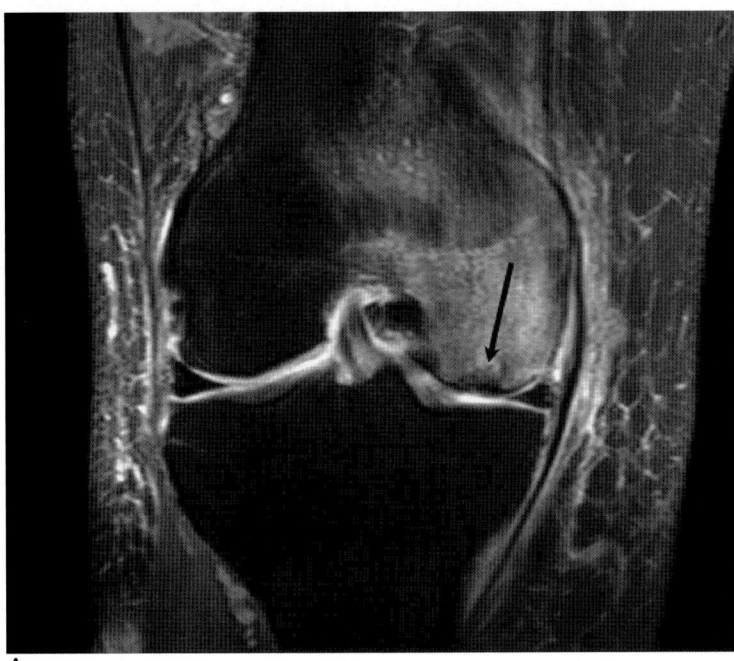

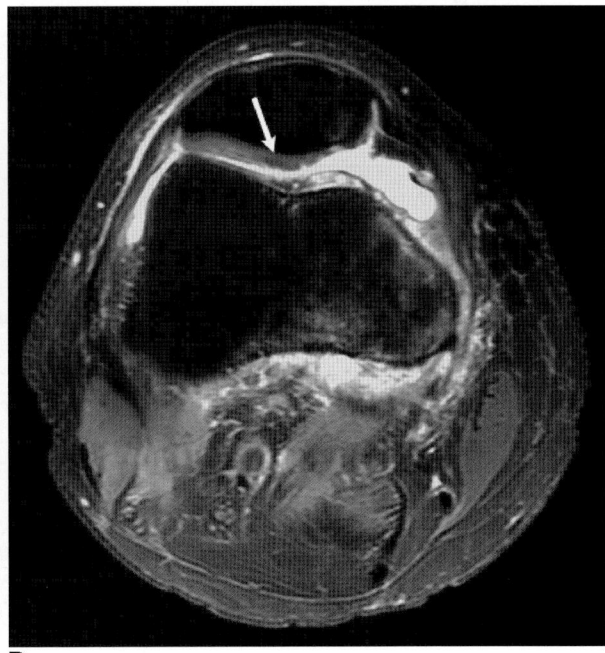

A

B

■ **FIGURE 45-7** **A,** A 3T, coronal, fat-suppressed, PD-weighted, TSE MR image of a 55-year-old man with medial and anterior knee pain demonstrates a subchondral insufficiency fracture (*arrow*) with collapse of the articular surface and an overlying full-thickness cartilage defect of the medial femoral condyle. Extensive marrow edema is present throughout the medial femoral condyle. **B,** Axial, fat-suppressed MR image demonstrates advanced cartilage loss of the medial patella facet. Focal areas of hypointense T2-weighted signal are present in the adjacent segments of cartilage on the median ridge (*arrow*).

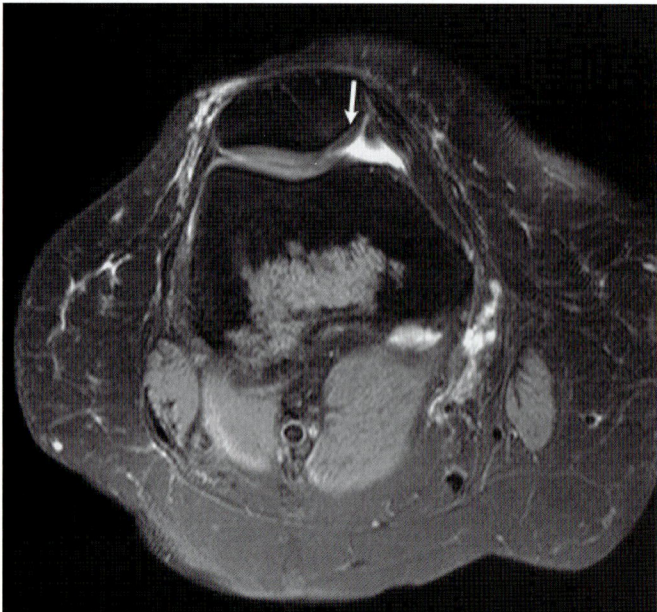

■ **FIGURE 45-8** A 3T, axial, fat-suppressed, PD-weighted, TSE MR image of 39-year-old woman with right knee pain. A full-thickness linear fissure extends to the bone interface near the median ridge. Linear T2-weighted hyperintensity is present at the bone-cartilage interface of the medial patella facet (*arrow*) with subtle marrow edema in the adjacent patella consistent with cartilage delamination.

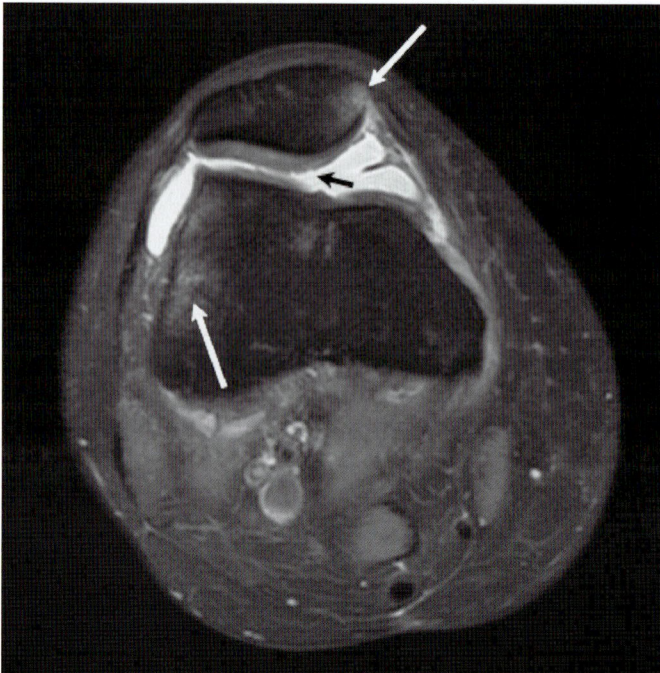

■ **FIGURE 45-9** Patella dislocation with chondral fissure (modified Outerbridge grade II) in a 33-year-old woman (*black arrow*). Note the characteristic pattern of marrow edema in the inferomedial patella and anterolateral femoral condyle seen after transient patellar dislocation (*white arrows*). Superficial fibrillation and fraying (Noyes 2A) were identified on the median ridge and medial patellar facet during surgery for patellar instability.

setting of patellar dislocation, shearing injury can lead to delamination injuries of the median patellar ridge and may be associated with full-thickness cartilage fissures or flap tears. Delamination injuries are also frequently observed in the femoral trochlea after blunt anterior knee trauma, frequently in association with patellar cartilage injury.

Grade II Lesions

Magnetic Resonance Imaging

Grade II lesions represent fissures, erosion, ulceration, or fibrillation involving the superficial 50% of cartilage thickness. There is no consensus in the MRI literature regarding terminology used to report cartilage lesions. Fissures represent linear clefts of the articular surface. They are most frequently observed after joint trauma, particularly in patellar cartilage. As seen in Figure 45-9, obliquely oriented fissures or flap tears can be seen after patellar dislocation, most frequently near the median ridge. The rate and magnitude of loading of the shear force influence the location of cartilage injury. When shear force is applied at high speed but with low energy, cracks are produced along the articular cartilage surface. At low speed and low energy, splits initially occur in the deeper layers. Ulceration of superficial cartilage blisters results in a small focal irregular crater (Fig. 45-10). Erosion refers to a smoothly marginated area of thinned cartilage and is frequently seen in older patients. Cartilage erosion is often identified in the posterior tibial plateau and femoral condyle, particularly in patients with chronic tears of the anterior cruciate ligament. Fibrillation or fraying of the articular surface appears

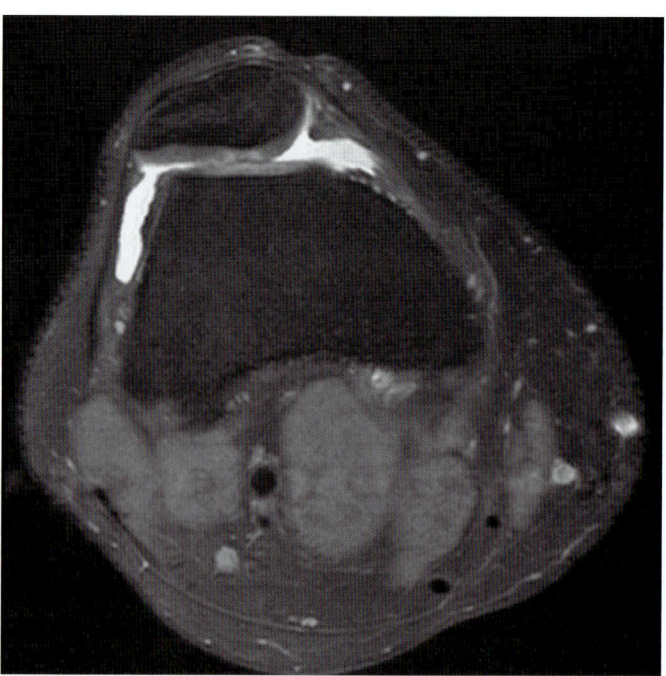

■ **FIGURE 45-10** Axial, PD-weighted, FSE MR image of a 31-year-old man with persistent anterior knee pain 4 months after a fall onto the patellofemoral joint. Partial-thickness ulceration is present in the median ridge of the patella extending to the deep 50% of cartilage (modified Outerbridge grade III).

visually as a fine velvety surface and is a common finding in subjects with OA. MRI has insufficient spatial resolution to resolve the individual fibrillations and they generally appear as an indistinct articular margin.

MRI has relatively poor sensitivity and accuracy in identifying grade II lesions when using arthroscopy as the gold standard. This is partly due to limited spatial resolution of MRI and partly due to the subjective nature in estimating lesion depth with arthroscopy. Because of greater contrast between the bright signal intensity of synovial fluid and intermediate signal intensity of cartilage, T2-weighted images have greater sensitivity in identifying superficial fibrillation. Magnetization transfer enhances the surface contrast resolution and can improve conspicuity of these lesions. Despite higher spatial resolution, on T1-weighted gradient-echo images the low signal intensity of fluid and resulting poor contrast decreases the conspicuity of superficial fibrillation.

Grade III Lesions

Magnetic Resonance Imaging

As illustrated in Figure 45-10, lesions that extend more than 50% of the depth of the articular cartilage but do not result in exposure of the underlying bone are classified as grade III lesions. In correlation with arthroscopy or surgical grading, both T1-weighted fat-suppressed SGE and PD-weighted TSE MRI have high diagnostic accuracy in identification of grade III lesions.

Grade IV Lesions

Magnetic Resonance Imaging

Full-thickness lesions with exposure of the underlying subchondral bone are classified as grade IV lesions. The margin of the lesion can suggest the mechanism of cartilage injury. Sharply marginated borders are characteristic of traumatic cartilage injuries, whereas shallow or irregular margins are features more characteristic of chronic degeneration. Abnormal signal intensity from the underlying bone marrow and central osteophytes are frequently associated with grade IV lesions. MRI has demonstrated high specificity and sensitivity for detection of grade IV defects.

Bone Marrow Lesions Associated with Cartilage Injury

Magnetic Resonance Imaging

Increased T2-weighted signal intensity from the subchondral bone marrow is a frequent finding in acute traumatic osteochondral injury (see Fig. 45-9), as well as the setting of chronic osteochondral injury (see Fig. 45-7) or OA (Fig. 45-11). Similar alterations in bone marrow signal intensity are observed after high-intensity exercise or with altered joint biomechanics. It is a nonspecific MRI finding but can be associated with pain and with internal derangement in the knee.

The characteristics of the MRI signal abnormality in the marrow are similar to those of water, which is dark on

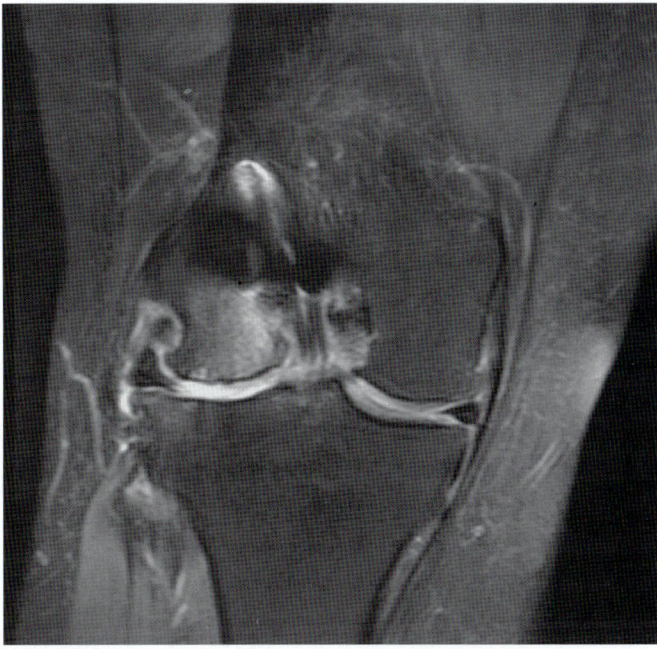

■ FIGURE 45-11 A 3T, coronal, fat-suppressed, PD-weighted FSE image of a 29-year-old woman with anterior cruciate ligament reconstruction and partial lateral meniscectomy 3 years before the examination. Extensive cartilage loss is present in the lateral compartment associated with a horizontal cleavage tear of the lateral meniscus, tibial osteophyte formation, femoral subluxation, and degenerative T2-weighted hyperintensity and cyst formation in the subchondral marrow.

short echo time sequences and bright on fluid-sensitive sequences such as fat-suppressed PD- or T2-weighted SE or FSE sequences or short tau inversion recovery (STIR) images. Because the abnormal signal closely follows water, this finding has been erroneously termed *bone marrow edema*. Correlation studies with histology indicate a mixture of tissue types contribute to the abnormal marrow signal. In the setting of acute trauma, areas of fluid-like signal are associated with regions of trabecular microfracture, hemorrhage, necrosis, and edema.[24] In this clinical setting the marrow findings represent a bone marrow contusion. Follow-up studies have shown that the abnormal marrow signal intensity can persist for several months after resolution of symptoms and is infrequently associated with long-term sequelae.[25] In contrast to lesions with an ill-defined reticular border, bone marrow contusions that have a well-demarcated margin that extends to the subchondral plate have a 50% likelihood of progressing to localized cartilage loss.[26] In the presence of OA or chronic focal osteochondral injury, the region of abnormal marrow signal has a heterogeneous histology consisting of necrosis, fibrosis, subchondral cysts, edema, hemorrhage, and granulation tissue.[27] In the setting of OA, the presence of subchondral marrow T2 hyperintensity is correlated with pain[28] and malalignment and has been shown to be prognostic of disease progression.[29] The presence of elevated T2-weighted signal in bone marrow may be a secondary indication of an overlying full-thickness articular cartilage defect. In correlation with arthroscopic grading of focal cartilage defects, the prevalence of subchondral marrow hyperintense T2-weighted signal is 1% for athroscopically normal cartilage, 10% for partial-thickness defects, and 53% for full-thickness articular cartilage defects.[30]

DIFFERENTIAL DIAGNOSIS

Laboratory tests are primarily used to exclude other causes of joint pain such as inflammatory or crystal-induced arthropathies as well as infection. Several serum and urinary biologic markers (biomarkers) are being explored as possible measures of disease severity and progression in clinical trials on OA. These may be used to either select or exclude subjects with preclinical stages of OA or may be used as an end point to monitor response to therapy. To be effective a biomarker must be valid (a true measure of the disease), reliable (provides a reproducible measure of disease severity), and responsive (capable of detecting significant differences in disease severity). In OA, biomarkers are being evaluated as indicators of cartilage matrix degradation or synthesis. Combinations of biomarkers are frequently employed to indicate loss of cartilage homeostasis in which there is an imbalance of matrix synthesis and breakdown products. Because of their high abundance in the cartilage matrix, type II collagen and aggrecan are major targets for biomarker development. Other matrix proteins such as cartilage oligomeric matrix protein (COMP) have been studied because of their proposed specificity for cartilage or serum markers of matrix metalloproteinases (MMPs) because of their critical role in matrix degradation. Markers from other joint tissues such as serum osteoclastin, a marker of new bone formation, and urinary type I collagen cross-links, a measure of bone turnover, may also have a role in OA. Currently, routine application of biomarkers has been limited by low sensitivity and specificity. This is partly due to the substantial dilutional effect that occurs when OA is confined to a single joint with relatively small cartilage volume. Greater specificity may be gathered by combining biologic markers with MR image markers of matrix degradation.[31]

SYNOPSIS OF TREATMENT OPTIONS

Medical Treatment

Current management of patients with OA and cartilage degeneration is focused on reducing disability by reducing pain and improving joint function. Although disease modification therapies for inflammatory arthropathies have been successful in reducing disease progression, disease-modifying OA drugs (DMOADs) are in preliminary stages of development and evaluation. Mild to moderate pain in patients is generally treated with over-the-counter analgesics such as acetaminophen, ibuprofen, or nonsteroidal anti-inflammatory drugs (NSAIDs); however, long-term use of these agents is limited by side effects. Opioid analgesics are reserved for more severe pain when NSAIDs are not tolerated or efficacious. Supplemental nutraceuticals such as glucosamine and chondroitin sulfate are commonly used in patients with OA. Although a recent multicenter trial suggested the combination of these supplements may have benefit in a subset of patients with moderate to severe knee pain, they were not found to be efficacious compared with placebo in controlling pain in OA in the general OA cohort.[32] Intra-articular injections of hyaluronic acid have had limited efficacy in large clinical trials. For short-term relief of pain, intra-articular injections of corticosteroids have been found to be moderately efficacious; however, the comparative efficacy decreases after 3 weeks.

Surgical Treatment

Surgical management of patients with OA or focal chondral defects consists of techniques to reduce symptoms, alter joint biomechanics, joint reconstruction, and a variety of new techniques targeted toward repair of focal cartilage lesions. Arthroscopic lavage has been shown to alleviate pain. This may occur through removal of inflammatory mediators in the synovial fluid; however, the mechanism for pain relief is unknown. For patients with unicompartmental arthritis and malalignment, osteotomies may be used to improve joint biomechanics. For patients with more severe forms of OA, joint reconstruction remains the mainstay of surgical therapy.

Given the growing evidence that focal cartilage defects represent a substantial risk factor for developing OA, more patients are undergoing surgical repair procedures to either restore cartilage function or decrease the rate of cartilage degradation. The techniques are limited to focal cartilage defects and are aimed at filling the articular void with tissue, preferably with biomechanical properties similar to native cartilage, which is integrated into adjacent native tissue. There are two general surgical approaches for cartilage repair: local stimulation techniques and transplantation techniques.

Local stimulation techniques such as Pridie drilling, microfracture, or abrasion arthroplasty are aimed at disrupting the subchondral cortical surface to induce bleeding. This process induces fibrocartilage production in the chondral defect and is considered palliative rather than reparative. The long-term clinical response of these techniques varies with the quality of the repair tissue, body habitus, age, and activity level. As demonstrated in Figure 45-12, the MRI initial postoperative examinations typically demonstrate subchondral hyperintensity on fluid-sensitive sequences. The initial tissue fill is usually less than that of the adjacent native tissue. Over time, the edema generally resolves and there is an increase in thickness of the reparative tissue. Failure is generally defined by a paucity of reparative tissue, chondral fissures, or gaps in the articular surface.

A variety of chondral transplantation techniques are available. Large defects may be treated with allografts, whereas autologous osteochondral grafts are reserved for smaller defects. With autologous osteochondral transplantation, small osteochondral cylinders or plugs are harvested from non–weight-bearing surfaces of the joint and then transferred into the prepared site of the cartilage defect. The intervening gaps between the osteochondral

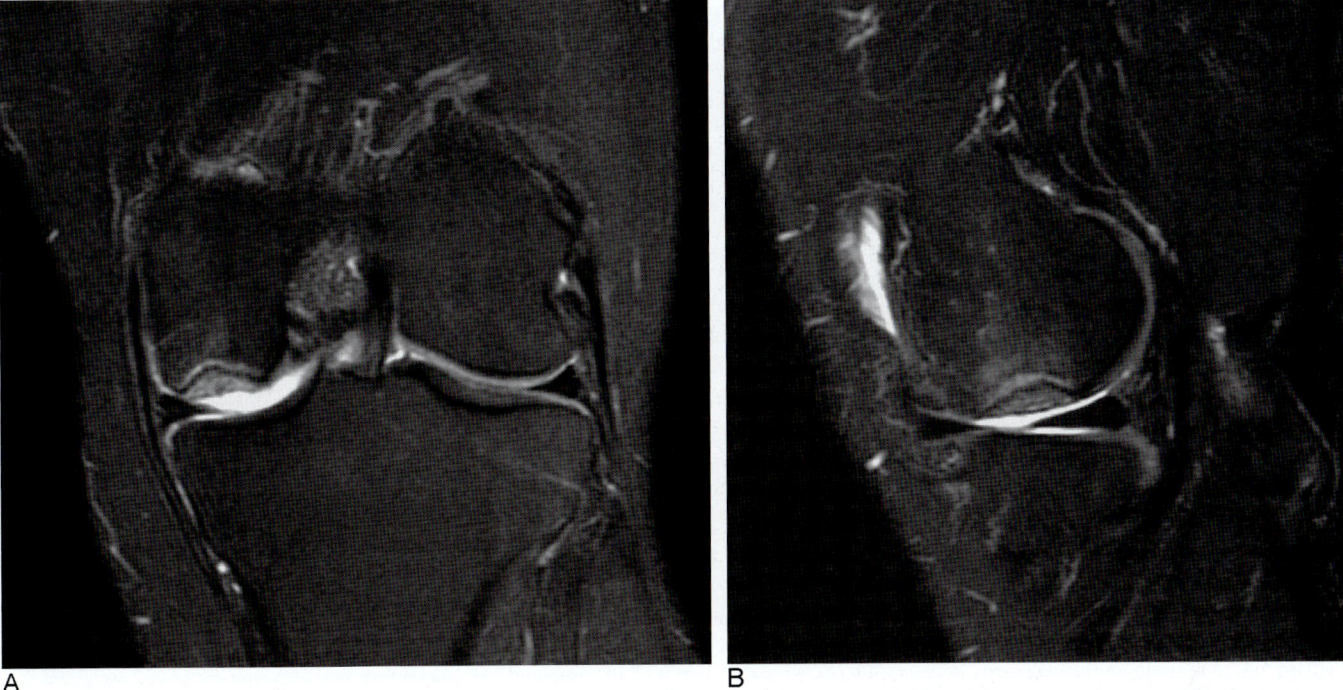

A　　　　　　　　　　　　　　　　　　　B

■ **FIGURE 45-12**　Microfracture repair. Coronal, fat-suppressed, PD-weighted FSE (**A**) and sagittal, fat-suppressed T2-weighted FSE (**B**) MR images from a 55-year-old man 5 months after microfracture repair for a focal osteochondral defect of the medial femoral condyle. The repair tissue is heterogeneously bright compared with native cartilage. A linear zone of marrow hyperintensity persists at the repair site.

grafts fill with fibrocartilage repair tissue. The goal is to produce a smooth surface that is congruent with the adjacent native cartilage. MRI can be used postoperatively to evaluate surface congruity and integration of the fibrocartilage repair tissue surrounding the osteochondral plugs. Cartilage in the osteochondral plugs retains the signal characteristics of the donor site. The fibrocartilage tissue has heterogeneously elevated signal intensity compared with the osteochondral plugs.

Autologous chondrocyte implantation (ACI) is an alternative transplantation technique. In contrast to autologous osteochondral transplantation this is a two-stage procedure. First, cartilage tissue is harvested from a non–weight-bearing articular surface. In the laboratory, chondrocytes are isolated and grown in culture to increase their numbers. In the second procedure the osteochondral defect is débrided and covered with a periosteal patch that is sealed with fibrin glue. The cultured chondrocytes are injected beneath the periosteal patch. A more recent variation is matrix-induced autologous chondrocyte implantations (MACI) in which chondrocytes are placed into a collagen scaffold, thereby providing stabilization to the repair tissue. In ACI, the repair tissue passes through three phases as it matures from implanted cells to tissue. During the initial 6 weeks the cells proliferate and expand to fill the defect. This is followed by the transitional phase, lasting approximately 6 months, in which cells produce an extracellular matrix and the repair tissue stiffens. In the final phase the tissue undergoes remodeling

and develops tissue properties resembling that of hyaline cartilage. The MRI appearance of the repair site changes during the maturation process. During the proliferative phase the tissue is of intermediate signal intensity on T1-weighted images and of high signal intensity on fluid-sensitive images. As the extracellular matrix develops and matures, the MRI appearance begins to resemble hyaline cartilage. Complications of ACI include failure to incorporate with the adjacent tissue, characterized by fluid-like signal intensity at the demarcation zones, and periosteal hypertrophy (Fig. 45-13) or delamination.

Cartilage repair techniques are an active area of research. There is ongoing research on cartilage tissue engineering using mesenchymal stem cells, tissue scaffolds, and growth factors to generate repair tissue that more closely resembles the biomechanical properties of native hyaline cartilage.

What the Referring Physician Needs to Know

- Location of cartilage injury
- Size and extent of cartilage lesion
- Presence or absence of subchondral marrow abnormalities
- Associated derangement of the joint (e.g., meniscal pathology, ligament tear)
- Presence or absence of joint effusion

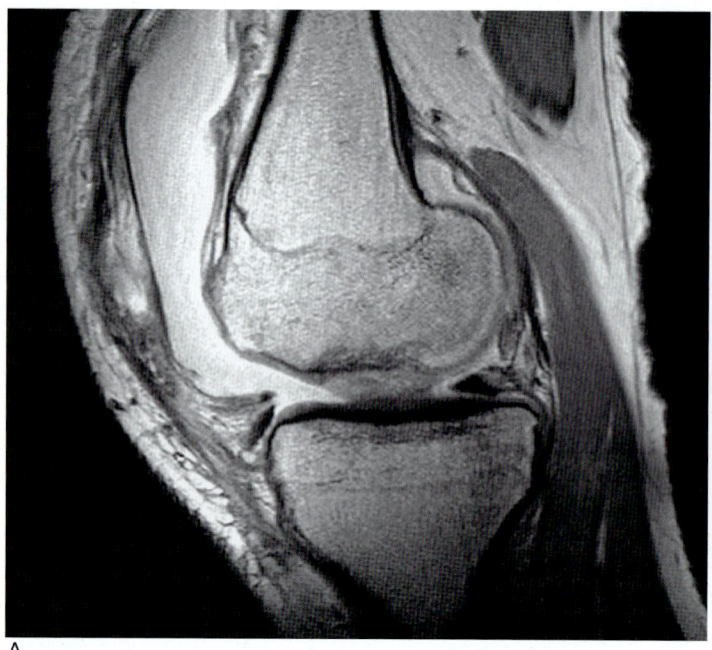
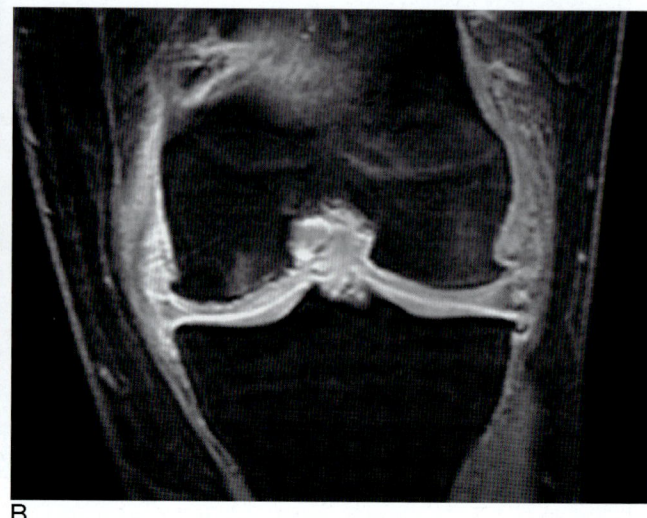

A   B

■ **FIGURE 45-13** Autologous chondrocyte implantation (ACI) repair. Sagittal 3T PD-weighted TSE (**A**) and coronal 3D water-excited T1-weighted gradient-echo (**B**) MR images of a 14-year-old girl 5 months after ACI repair. The sagittal image demonstrates heterogeneous signal of the reparative tissue, which is isointense to cartilage on the coronal image. There is thickening of the repair tissue compatible with hyperplasia of the periosteal flap.

SUGGESTED READINGS

Eckstein F, Glaser C. Measuring cartilage morphology with quantitative magnetic resonance imaging. Semin Musculoskelet Radiol 2004; 8:329–353.

Felson DT. An update on the pathogenesis and epidemiology of osteoarthritis. Radiol Clin North Am 2004; 42:1–9, v.

Felson DT, Lawrence RC, Dieppe PA, et al. Osteoarthritis: new insights: I. The disease and its risk factors. Ann Intern Med 2000; 133:635–646.

Gold GE, McCauley TR, Gray ML, Disler DG. What's new in cartilage? Radiographics 2003; 23:1227–1242.

Goodwin DW, Dunn JF. High-resolution magnetic resonance imaging of articular cartilage: correlation with histology and pathology. Top Magn Reson Imaging 1998; 9:337–347.

Mosher TJ, Dardzinski BJ. Cartilage MRI T2 relaxation time mapping: overview and applications. Semin Musculoskelet Radiol 2004; 8:355–368.

Recht MP, Goodwin DW, Winalski CS, White LM. MRI of articular cartilage: revisiting current status and future directions. AJR Am J Roentgenol 2005; 185:899–914.

Xia Y. Magic-angle effect in magnetic resonance imaging of articular cartilage: a review. Invest Radiol 2000; 35:602–621.

REFERENCES

1. Altman R, Asch E, Bloch D, et al. Development of criteria for the classification and reporting of osteoarthritis. Classification of osteoarthritis of the knee. Diagnostic and Therapeutic Criteria Committee of the American Rheumatism Association. Arthritis Rheum 1986; 29:1039–1049.

2. Felson DT. An update on the pathogenesis and epidemiology of osteoarthritis. Radiol Clin North Am 2004; 42:1–9.

3. Huberti HH, Hayes WC. Patellofemoral contact pressures: the influence of q-angle and tendofemoral contact. J Bone Joint Surg Am 1984; 66:715–724.

4. Jeffery AK, Blunn GW, Archer CW, Bentley G. Three-dimensional collagen architecture in bovine articular cartilage. J Bone Joint Surg Br 1991; 73:795–801.

5. Fullerton GD, Cameron IL, Ord VA. Orientation of tendons in the magnetic field and its effect on T2 relaxation times. Radiology 1985; 155:433–435.

6. Erickson SJ, Prost RW, Timins ME. The "magic angle" effect: background physics and clinical relevance. Radiology 1993; 188:23–25.

7. Morris GA, Freemont AJ. Direct observation of the magnetization exchange dynamics responsible for magnetization transfer contrast in human cartilage in vitro. Magn Reson Med 1992; 28:97–104.

8. Kim DK, Ceckler TL, Hascall VC, et al. Analysis of water-macromolecule proton magnetization transfer in articular cartilage. Magn Reson Med 1993; 29:211–215.

9. Henkelman RM, Stanisz GJ, Kim JK, Bronskill MJ. Anisotropy of NMR properties of tissues. Magn Reson Med 1994; 32:592–601.

10. Wolff SD, Chesnick S, Frank JA, et al. Magnetization transfer contrast: MR imaging of the knee. Radiology 1991; 179:623–628.

11. Yao L, Gentili A, Thomas A. Incidental magnetization transfer contrast in fast spin-echo imaging of cartilage. J Magn Reson Imaging 1996; 6:180–184.

12. Goodwin DW, Wadghiri YZ, Zhu H, et al. Macroscopic structure of articular cartilage of the tibial plateau: influence of a characteristic matrix architecture on MRI appearance. AJR Am J Roentgenol 2004; 182:311–318.

13. Lazovic-Stojkovic J, Mosher TJ, Smith HE, et al. Interphalangeal joint cartilage: high-spatial-resolution in vivo MR T2 mapping—a feasibility study. Radiology 2004; 233:292–296.

14. Roos EM, Dahlberg L. Positive effects of moderate exercise on glycosaminoglycan content in knee cartilage: a four-month, randomized, controlled trial in patients at risk of osteoarthritis. Arthritis Rheum 2005; 52:3507–3514.

15. Eckstein F, Glaser C. Measuring cartilage morphology with quantitative magnetic resonance imaging. Semin Musculoskelet Radiol 2004; 8:329-353.
16. Potter HG, Linklater JM, Allen AA, et al. Magnetic resonance imaging of articular cartilage in the knee: an evaluation with use of fast-spin-echo imaging. J Bone Joint Surg Am 1998; 80:1276-1284.
17. Outerbridge RE. The etiology of chondromalacia patellae. J Bone Joint Surg Br 1961; 43:752-757.
18. Noyes FR, Stabler CL. A system for grading articular cartilage lesions at arthroscopy. Am J Sports Med 1989; 17:505-513.
19. Mosher TJ, Liu Y, Yang QX, et al. Age dependency of cartilage magnetic resonance imaging T2 relaxation times in asymptomatic women. Arthritis Rheum 2004; 50:2820.
20. Wong M, Carter DR. Articular cartilage functional histomorphology and mechanobiology: a research perspective. Bone 2003; 33:1-13.
21. Levy AS, Lohnes J, Sculley S, et al. Chondral delamination of the knee in soccer players. Am J Sports Med 1996; 24:634-639.
22. Holderbaum D, Malvitz T, Ciesielski CJ, et al. A newly described hereditary cartilage debonding syndrome. Arthritis Rheum 2005; 52:3300-3304.
23. Keinan-Adamsky K, Shinar H, Navon G. The effect of detachment of the articular cartilage from its calcified zone on the cartilage microstructure, assessed by 2H-spectroscopic double quantum filtered MRI. J Orthop Res 2005; 23:109-117.
24. Rangger C, Kathrein A, Freund MC, et al. Bone bruise of the knee: histology and cryosections in 5 cases. Acta Orthop Scand 1998; 69:291-294.
25. Boks SS, Vroegindeweij D, Koes BW, et al. Follow-up of occult bone lesions detected at MR imaging: systematic review. Radiology 2006; 238:863-871.
26. Vellet AD, Marks PH, Fowler PJ, Munro TG. Occult posttraumatic osteochondral lesions of the knee: prevalence, classification, and short-term sequelae evaluated with MR imaging. Radiology 1991; 178:271-276.
27. Bergman AG, Willen HK, Lindstrand AL, Pettersson HT. Osteoarthritis of the knee: correlation of subchondral MR signal abnormalities with histopathologic and radiographic features. Skeletal Radiol 1994; 23:445-448.
28. Felson DT, Chaisson CE, Hill CL, et al. The association of bone marrow lesions with pain in knee osteoarthritis. Ann Intern Med 2001; 134:541-549.
29. Felson DT, McLaughlin S, Goggins J, et al. Bone marrow edema and its relation to progression of knee osteoarthritis. Ann Intern Med 2003; 139:330-336.
30. Kijowski R, Stanton P, Fine J, De Smet A. Subchondral bone marrow edema in patients with degeneration of the articular cartilage of the knee joint. Radiology 2006; 238:943-949.
31. King KB, Lindsey CT, Dunn TC, et al. A study of the relationship between molecular biomarkers of joint degeneration and the magnetic resonance-measured characteristics of cartilage in 16 symptomatic knees. Magn Reson Imaging 2004; 22:1117-1123.
32. Clegg DO, Reda DJ, Harris CL, et al. Glucosamine, chondroitin sulfate, and the two in combination for painful knee osteoarthritis. N Engl J Med 2006; 354:795-808.

46

Rheumatoid Arthritis

Marcy B. Bolster and Johnny U. V. Monu

Rheumatoid arthritis (RA) is a chronic and progressive inflammatory systemic disease that primarily affects the synovium and is characterized by destruction of bone and cartilage. The small joints of the hands and feet are typically affected, although the larger joints are also affected by the disease. Radiographic changes, characterized by joint space narrowing and marginal erosions, typically occur within the first 2 years of disease onset. The natural history of the disease involves progressive joint damage and disability. Newer therapies, however, appear to be having an impact on the radiographic disease progression.

ETIOLOGY

The etiology of RA is not well understood. Certain human leukocyte antigen (HLA) class II alleles or haplotypes have been associated with the development of RA. HLA-DR4 is the most frequently associated haplotype with the development of RA and is associated with its more severe form.

PREVALENCE AND EPIDEMIOLOGY

Rheumatoid arthritis occurs in approximately 1% of the U.S. population. Its incidence is 0.75 per 1000 adults per year.[1] RA occurs more frequently in women and has a 3:1 predilection for women as compared with men. The disease may present at any age, but the peak onset is in the fourth to sixth decades. Patients with RA are at an increased risk for the development of cardiovascular disease and have a high mortality rate related to its presence.[2] Additionally, patients with RA are at an increased risk for the development of certain malignancies, including lymphoma and leukemia.

CLINICAL PRESENTATION

Rheumatoid arthritis is an inflammatory, symmetric polyarthritis that typically involves the hands and feet, although all synovial joints are susceptible to disease. It may have a sudden, explosive onset, or it may have a more indolent course. Typical of the inflammatory arthritides,

the patient will experience joint swelling, erythema, warmth, and/or pain. The diagnosis of rheumatoid arthritis requires that the inflammatory polyarthritis be present for at least 6 weeks. As with other forms of inflammatory arthritis, the patient usually experiences prolonged stiffness on awakening, or morning stiffness, as well as stiffness after prolonged periods of immobility, termed *gelling*. The criteria for the diagnosis of RA include the following:

- Osteopenia
- Osteolysis
- Erosions
- Lax ligaments
- Subluxations

The laboratory abnormalities associated with rheumatoid arthritis include a serum rheumatoid factor (RF) that is positive in 85% of patients; however, at the time of presentation, the RF is positive in only 40% of patients. Frequently, the antinuclear antibody (ANA) is also positive. There is a newer autoantibody test termed the anti-citrullinated cyclic peptide (anti-CCP) that has a sensitivity of 65% but is highly specific for RA and, in combination with a positive RF, has a specificity of 95% for the diagnosis of RA.[3-5] The anti-CCP antibody may also be positive in patients many years before the development of RA. The

KEY POINTS

- Periarticular osteopenia may initially occur.
- There is a bilateral, symmetric disease pattern.
- Involvement of the small joints of the hands and feet is characteristic of RA.
- Anti-CCP antibody is associated with a worse prognosis and a higher likelihood of erosive disease.
- Marginal erosions progress centrally.
- RA is a disease of small joints; therefore, large joint effusions (i.e., of large joints or large volumes) are not characteristic.
- Ligamental laxity and rupture manifest as subluxations and dislocations.

inflammatory markers—erythrocyte sedimentation rate (ESR) and C-reactive protein (CRP)—are also typically elevated in patients with active disease. A normochromic, normocytic anemia may also be seen in patients with RA.

Subcutaneous nodules, also termed *rheumatoid nodules*, occur in approximately 25% of patients[6,7] but may not be present at the time of presentation. The nodules most commonly involve the extensor surfaces of the upper extremities, the joints of the hands, and the Achilles tendon. Pathologically, these nodules comprise a central area of fibrinoid necrosis surrounded by palisading histiocytes that do not have an inflammatory appearance.

IMAGING TECHNIQUES

Radiographs have remained the basis of imaging diagnosis.[8] Initial diagnostic studies should include radiographs of both joints or appendages, such as hands, wrists, feet, and ankles because the disease is typically bilaterally symmetric (Fig. 46-1).

Radionuclide scans using technetium-99 m–labeled methylene diphosphonate (^{99m}Tc-MDP) may show increased radioisotope uptake in the affected joints. The uptake reflects both increased synovial activity and increased bone turnover. The findings are nonspecific and do not necessarily reflect active inflammation. Gallium scanning may also be positive and reflects chronic inflammatory response. The scans also lack specificity.

Unusual or new symptoms, a change in the symptomatology, or failed response to treatment should trigger an additional evaluation with other modalities.

Ultrasonography and MRI should be used to evaluate and follow the course of established disease.[8-13] High field MRI is more sensitive than radiographs and CT scans in detecting erosions.[14,15] MRI also depicts other changes such as synovial proliferation, bursal enlargement, and bone inflammation or edema (Figs. 46-2 and 46-3). Bursal inflammation similarly may show enhancing synovium. The fluid distending the bursal space will not enhance immediately after intravenous contrast administration (see Fig. 46-3). Osteitis will be seen as abnormal high signal on T2-weighted images and will enhance after intravenous administration of a contrast agent.[16,17] There is a positive correlation between the number of enhancing bones and the severity of disease activity.[18] Some areas of bone marrow edema and enhancement will progress to cavitation and cyst formation.[18]

Joint swelling often due to the presence of effusion is more easily detectable in early disease using ultrasonography when compared with clinical examination.[19-23] Ultrasonography is more sensitive than radiographs and CT in detecting erosion. It is believed to be equally as sensitive as or more sensitive than MRI in detecting erosion.[14,16,17,24] On ultrasonography, erosion appears as a cortical defect usually greater than 2 mm in depth, with variable width and irregular floor. The subjacent marrow usually shows acoustic enhancement.[17,18] Some studies suggest that ultrasonography is more sensitive than MRI in detecting and evaluating synovitis.[12,25] Identification of various intra-articular structures and assessment of inflammatory activity in the disease process can be achieved with color Doppler imaging.[13,26,27]

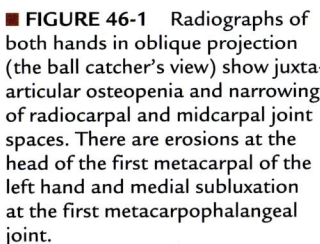

■ **FIGURE 46-1** Radiographs of both hands in oblique projection (the ball catcher's view) show juxta-articular osteopenia and narrowing of radiocarpal and midcarpal joint spaces. There are erosions at the head of the first metacarpal of the left hand and medial subluxation at the first metacarpophalangeal joint.

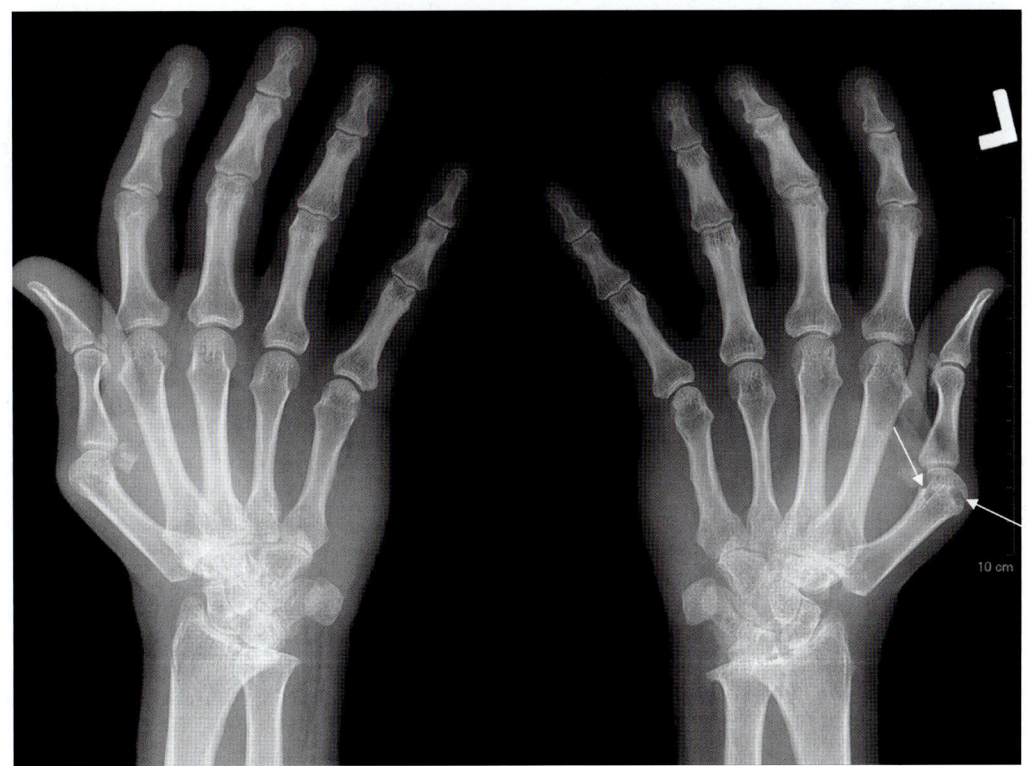

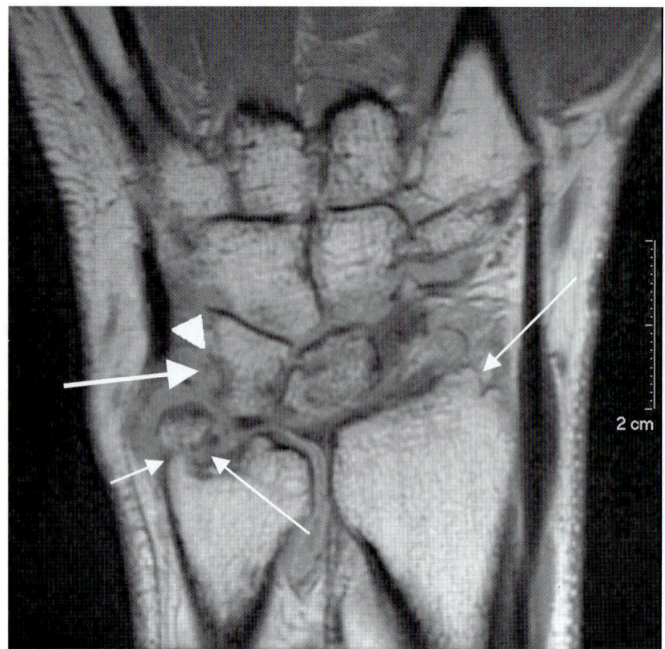

A

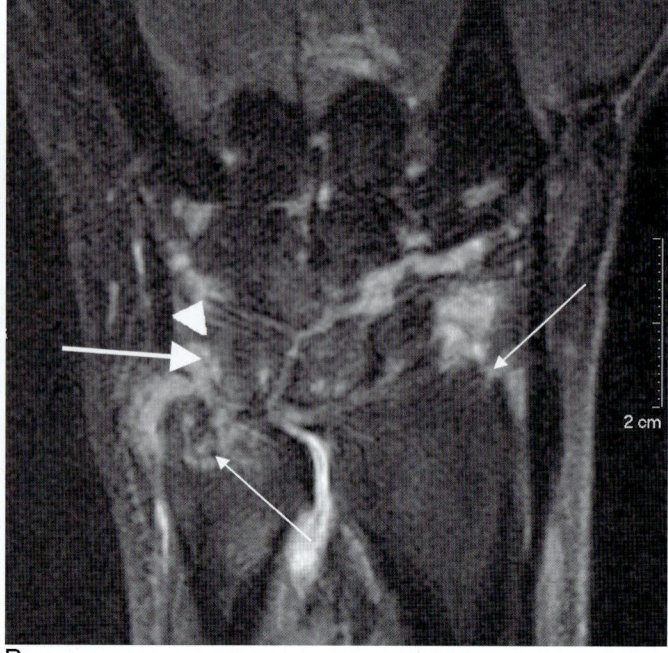

B

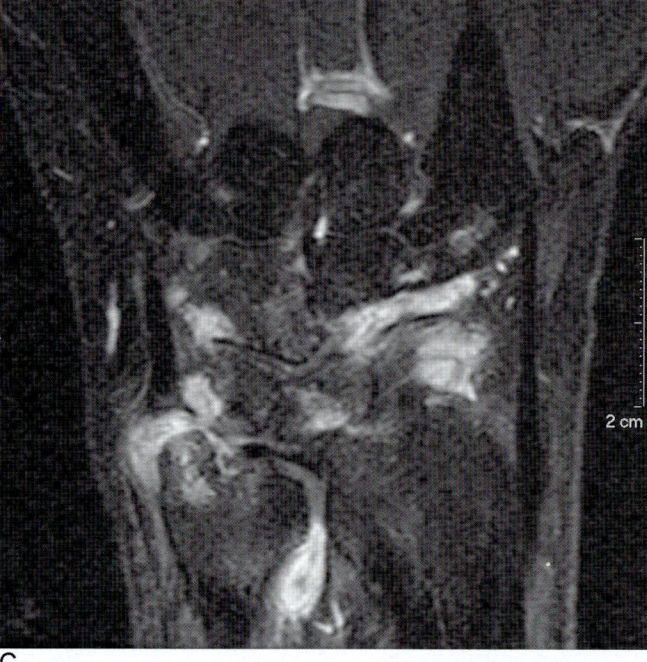

C

■ **FIGURE 46-2** Coronal proton density–weighted (**A**), fast spin-echo, fat-saturated, T2-weighted (**B**), and contrast-enhanced, fat-saturated, T1-weighted (**C**) MR images of the wrist show erosive change at the ulnar styloid (*large arrow*), radial styloid (*small arrows*), triquetrum (*arrowheads*), and hamate. On the T2-weighted and contrast-enhanced T1-weighted MR images, synovial expansion is seen as areas of abnormal mixed high and intermediate signal pattern in the radiocarpal, midcarpal, and distal radioulnar joints.

General Radiographic Observations

Joint Swelling

One of the earlier radiographic observations in RA is para-articular soft tissue swelling (Fig. 46-4). This is mostly from the presence of joint effusions and synovitis. Synovitis with attendant wrist swelling is commonly located around the flexor carpi ulnaris and extensor carpi radialis longus tendons. Soft tissue swelling is also frequently observed at the metacarpophalangeal, metatarsophalangeal, and proximal interphalangeal joints.

The soft tissue swelling may be subtle and inapparent on initial radiographs. Later in the course of the disease the soft tissue swelling may be due to the presence of rheumatoid nodules.[6]

The presence of large joint effusions and bursal fluid collections is a frequent observation in RA and another reason for joint swelling (see Fig. 46-4).[28-32] In fact, an unexplained large bursal fluid collection should prompt evaluation for RA or other inflammatory arthropathies. The source of the fluid collection is the synovitis related to RA.[30,32]

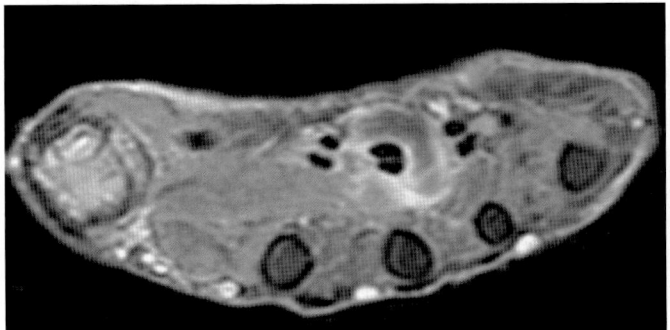

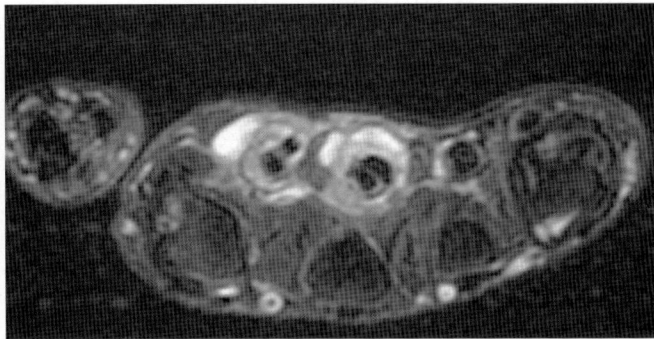

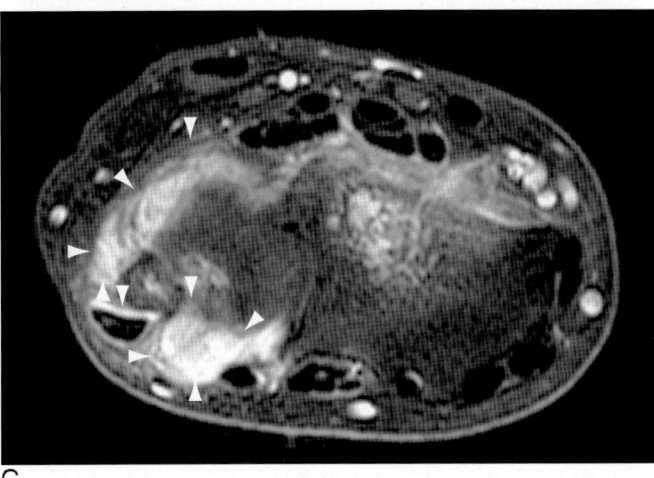

■ **FIGURE 46-3** Axial, fat-suppressed, contrast-enhanced, T1-weighted (**A**), fast spin-echo, T2-weighted (**B**), and fat-suppressed, contrast-enhanced, T1-weighted (**C**) MR images of the hand show abnormal signal surrounding the flexor tendons of the second and third digits in a patient with rheumatoid arthritis. This is consistent with tenosynovitis. The contrast medium–enhanced T1-weighted image shows extensive synovial enhancements seen as high signal around the ulna (*arrowheads*) at the distal radioulnar joint. The abnormal signal in the distal radius is due to inflammation (osteitis) and subarticular cyst formation.

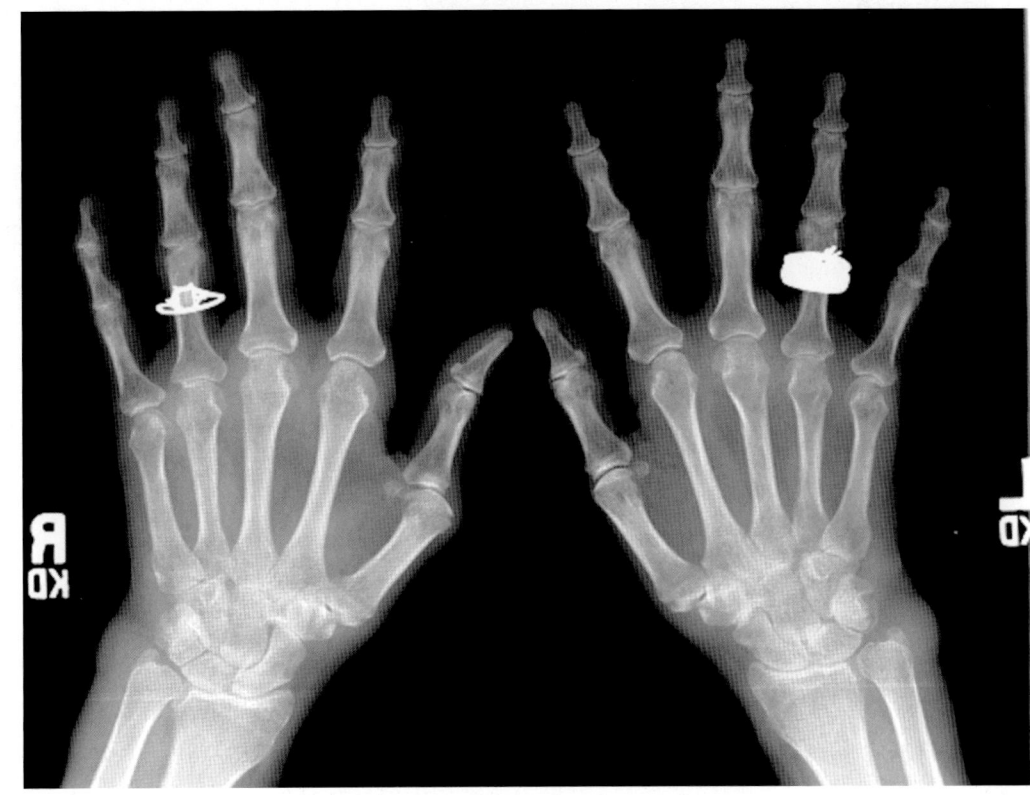

■ **FIGURE 46-4** Radiographs of both hands show focal soft tissue swelling over the ulnar styloid likely due to tenosynovitis in this region. There is subtle diffuse osteopenia and loss of joint space at the radiocarpal, midcarpal, and metacarpophalangeal joints. Erosions are present at the heads of the third and fifth left metacarpals. There is mild medial subluxation at the right first metacarpophalangeal joint.

Subluxations

Rheumatoid arthritis due to active synovitis and pannus formation weakens ligaments and tendons, making them susceptible to rupture. Ligament or tendon ruptures result in subluxations and dislocations (see Figs. 46-1 and 46-4). Spontaneous rupture of the extensor tendons and ligaments is frequent in RA.[33] Boutonnière deformities (Fig. 46-5), swan-neck deformities, and ulnar drift of the carpus, although not pathognomonic, are frequently seen in RA. These deformities result from selective involvement of the tendons and ligaments in the hands and feet. Nontraumatic massive rotator cuff tears with large shoulder joint effusions are often seen in RA. Subluxations and dislocations are late observations.

Osteopenia

A common observation is osteopenia.[34,35] The osteopenia is initially periarticular, is observed around the joints, and may be partly due to periarticular hyperemia. Ultimately, the osteopenia my become diffuse in long-standing RA (Fig. 46-6), particularly if the patient has taken long-term corticosteroid therapy.

Loss of Joint Space

Usually, concentric loss of joint space is seen as RA progressively affects a joint. The loss of joint space is due to progressive destruction of cartilage by the inflammatory exudates in the rheumatoid joint (see Figs. 46-1, 46-4 to 46-6).

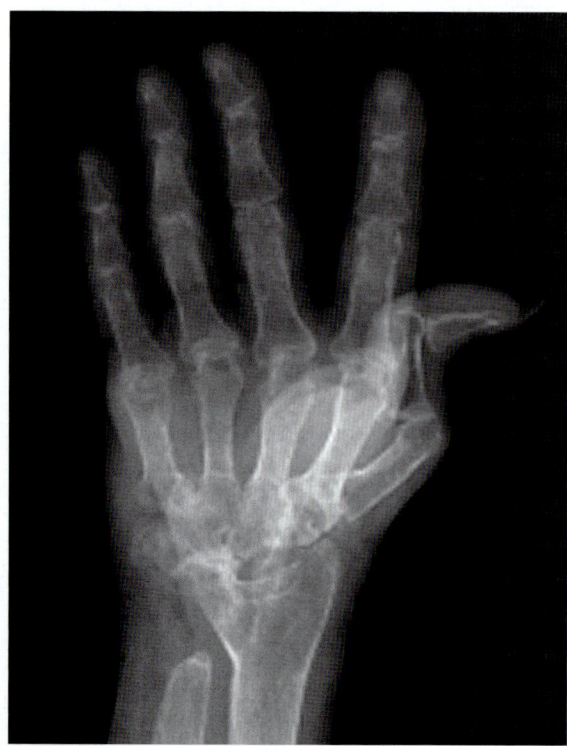

■ FIGURE 46-5 Severe chronic changes of rheumatoid arthritis in the hand. There is marked diffuse osteopenia. Note the complete collapse of the carpus. Osteolysis of the distal ulna is present. Flexion deformity at the metacarpophalangeal joint and dorsal subluxation at the interphalangeal joint of the thumb are present, and these create the appearance of the so-called hitchhiker's thumb.

Erosions

Erosions develop early and occur within the first 2 years of the disease. The erosion of RA may be marginal or central but typically starts from the margins and extends centrally (Figs. 46-7 and 46-8; see also Fig. 46-4). Erosions frequently involve the ulnar styloid such that in some cases the ulnar styloid is virtually absent due to osteolysis (see Figs. 46-5 and 46-8). Excessive central erosions may produce the "pencil-in-cup" deformity that is seen in more advanced cases at the metacarpophalangeal and metatarsophalangeal joints. Generally, erosions are seen proximally at these joints and at the proximal interphalangeal joints and less at the distal interphalangeal joints. Sites of tendon or ligament attachments (enthesis) may also show erosive activity (enthesopathy and enthesitis) (Figs. 46-9 and 46-10).

Osteolysis

Rheumatoid arthritis is essentially an atrophic process in which the body's ability to form bone is impaired. Thus, there is continued unimpaired bone resorption (osteopenia, osteolysis, and erosions) with little repair. In the wrist the loss of volume in the carpal bones results in various forms of carpal crowding and collapse (see Figs. 46-5, 46-7, and 46-8).

Osteitis

Osteitis or active bone inflammation will show as abnormal signal on T1- and T2-weighted images. The abnormal areas will enhance after intravenous administration of a contrast agent (see Fig. 46-3).

Subchondral Cysts

Subchondral cysts are common in RA. In the larger joints, such as the knee, the hip, the shoulder, the ankle, and the wrist, the subchondral cysts may be quite large and may be referred to as geodes (Figs. 46-7 and 46-11). It is believed that increased pressure in the joint due to synovitis forces synovial fluid through microfissures into the bones and by hydraulic pressure these small accumulations gradually enlarge into large subchondral cystic collections.

Osteonecrosis

Avascular necrosis and infarcts are not a usual manifestation of uncomplicated RA. Corticosteroids and cytotoxic drugs are often used in the management of RA, and these may predispose patients to bone infarction and avascular necrosis.

Selected Joints

Hands and Feet

Rheumatoid arthritis particularly affects the small joints of the hands and feet. In the hands there may be narrowing of the radiocarpal, midcarpal, and carpometacarpal joints. The metacarpophalangeal joints are narrowed, and the proximal interphalangeal joints are also narrowed. Disease changes in the distal interphalangeal joints,

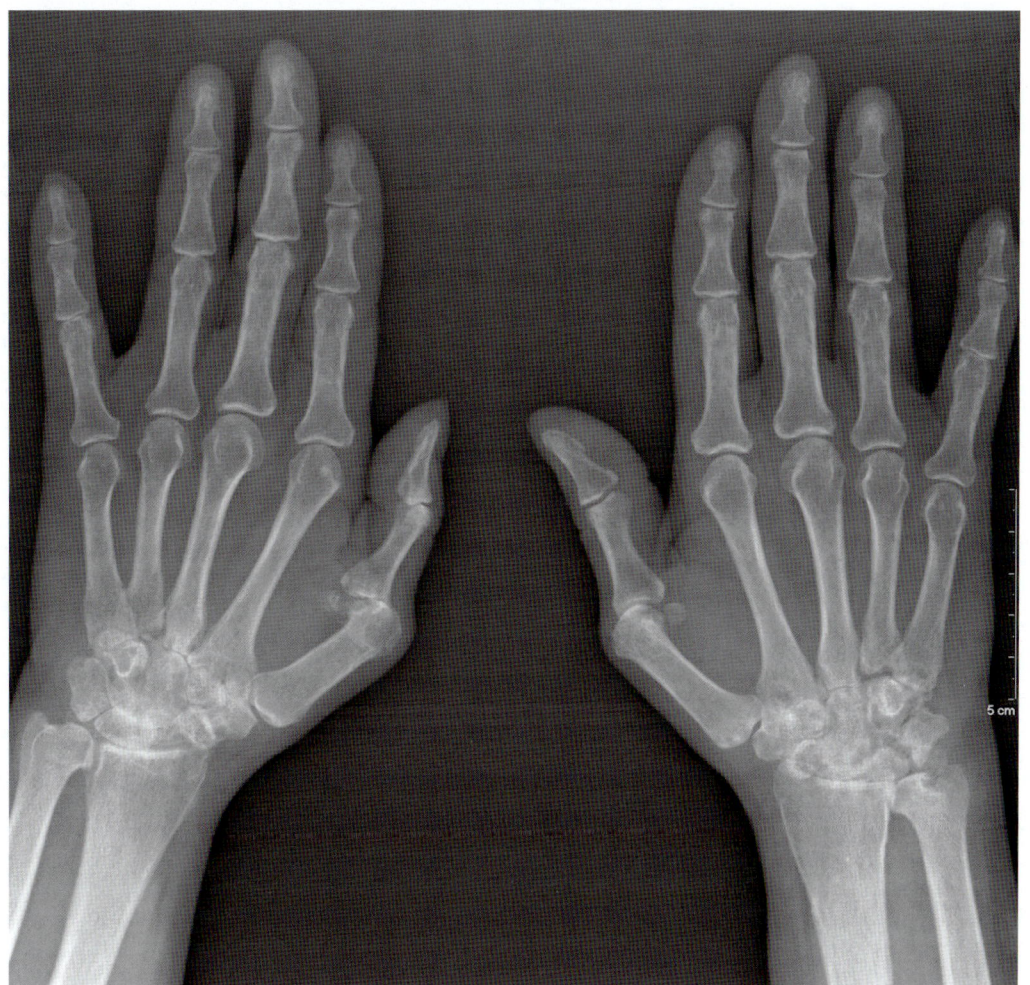

■ **FIGURE 46-6** Radiographs of both hands show changes of established rheumatoid arthritis. There is diffuse osteopenia. In the wrist there is carpal crowding, and collapse is worse on the left. Erosions are seen at the carpal bones, ulnar styloid, the bases of the metacarpals, and the first metacarpophalangeal joint. There is also medial subluxation at the first metacarpophalangeal joints of both hands.

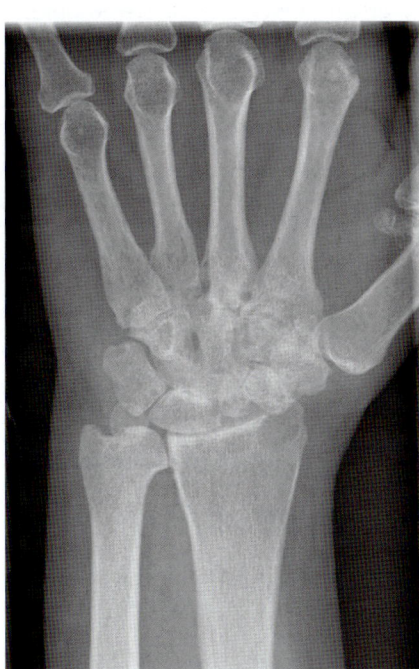

■ **FIGURE 46-7** Radiograph of the wrist in a patient with established rheumatoid arthritis. There is a large subchondral cyst (geode) in the distal radius and loss of joint space at the radiocarpal and midcarpal joints. Erosive change is seen at the head of the second metacarpal.

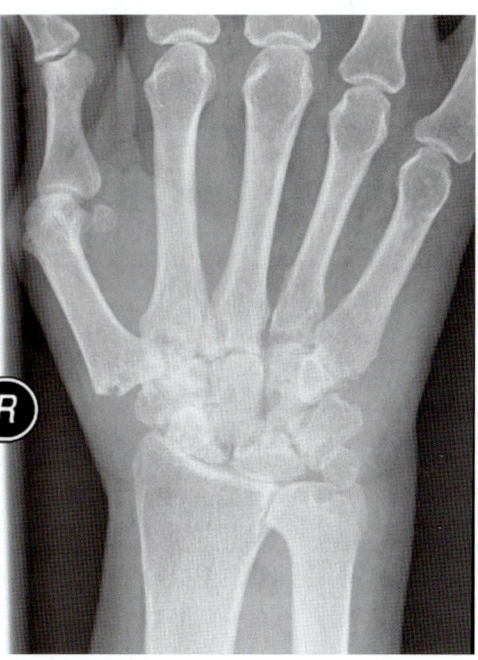

■ **FIGURE 46-8** Frontal radiograph of a wrist with severe changes of rheumatoid arthritis. There is resorption of, and a large subchondral cyst at, the ulnar styloid. There are erosions at the base of the ulnar styloid, lunate, triquetrum, hamate, and first metacarpal. Cysts are also seen at the bases of the second and third metacarpals.

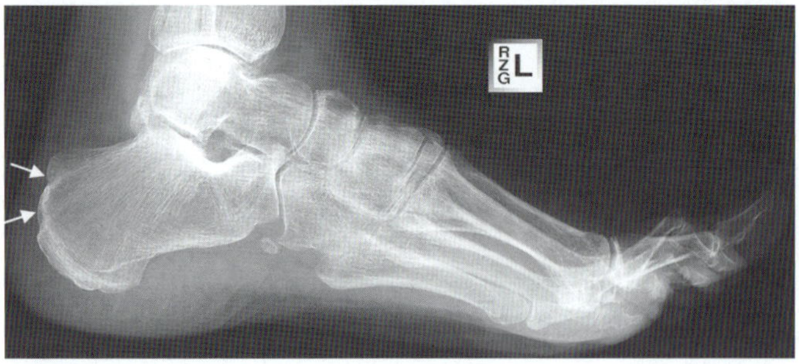

■ **FIGURE 46-9** Foot of a patient with rheumatoid arthritis shows early erosive changes in the posterior aspect of the calcaneus (*short arrows*). There is diffuse osteopenia.

although unusual, may occur later in the disease. Other changes that may be seen late in the disease include boutonnière deformity (flexion at the proximal interphalangeal joint and hyperextension at the distal interphalangeal joint), swan-neck deformity (hyperextension at the proximal interphalangeal joint and flexion at the distal interphalangeal joint), ulnar drift (occurs at the metacarpophalangeal joints), palmar subluxations at metacarpophalangeal joints, hitchhiker's thumb (flexion at the metacarpophalangeal joint and hyperextension at the interphalangeal joint) (see Fig. 46-5), and radial deviation at the wrist. A combination of radial subluxation at the wrist and ulnar drift at the metacarpophalangeal joints results in the zigzag hand seen in severe RA.

Erosion at the head of the fifth metatarsal is characteristic for RA. Other metatarsophalangeal joints are also commonly involved. Changes that may be found in the posterior aspect of the calcaneus include retrocalcaneal erosion (see Figs. 46-10 and 46-11) and bursitis.

Spine

Rheumatoid arthritis commonly affects only the cervical spine. In the spine as elsewhere there is remarkable paucity of osteophytes in untreated RA. The disc spaces are not usually directly affected by RA. The zygapophyseal joints are narrowed and may show erosive changes. The atlantoaxial joints may be widened or narrowed secondary to erosive and/or osteolytic changes in the odontoid (Figs. 46-12 to 46-14). Erosion of supporting structures leads to atlantoaxial instability as well as basilar invagination. Central canal narrowing is a prominent feature (see Figs. 46-13 and 46-14) and can lead to cervical cord injury. In the cervical spine, multilevel spondylolisthesis may create a stepladder appearance in the vertebral bodies (see Fig. 46-12). The presence of subaxial subluxations and absence of osteophytes is seen almost exclusively in RA. Often in such cases the disc spaces may be normal or minimally reduced in height.

MANIFESTATIONS OF THE DISEASE

Extra-articular Manifestations

Extra-articular disease manifestations occur in patients with RA. The extra-articular manifestations typically occur in conjunction with active joint disease and occur in patients with a positive RF titer. Other organ involvement that occurs in patients with RA include ocular, skin, peripheral nerve (mononeuritis multiplex), hematologic, pulmonary, and cardiac manifestations.

The ocular manifestations associated with RA include scleritis and episcleritis. The scleritis is characterized by an inflammatory infiltration of the sclera and may have associated nodular changes, which are pathologically identical

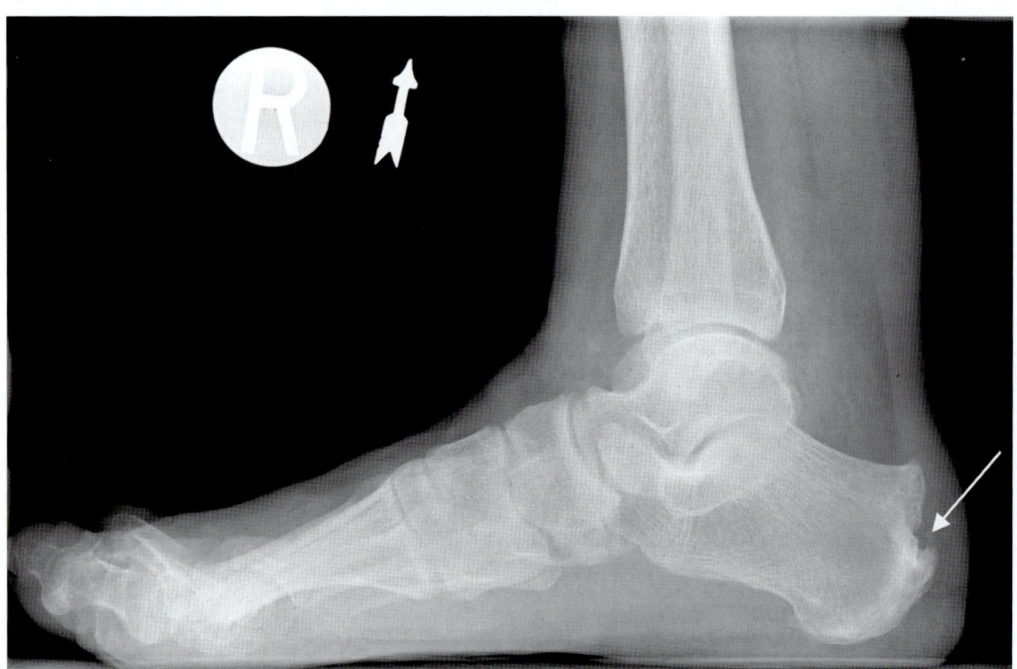

■ **FIGURE 46-10** Lateral radiograph of the foot in a patient with rheumatoid arthritis. There is diffuse osteopenia and erosion at the posterior aspect of the calcaneus (*arrow*).

What the Referring Physician Needs to Know

■ Rheumatoid arthritis is a symmetric inflammatory erosive polyarthritis typically involving the small joints of the hands and feet.

■ The larger joints such as the hips and knees may rarely be affected.

■ Early identification and treatment of the patient with rheumatoid arthritis helps slow disease progression.

■ There are many extra-articular manifestations of rheumatoid arthritis.

■ Newer therapies, including biologic agents, have had a large impact on slowing the progression of disease (clinically and radiographically) and have reduced resultant disability.

■ A significant cause of patient morbidity relates to infectious complications of therapy and an increased risk of cardiovascular disease in patients with rheumatoid arthritis.

SUGGESTED READINGS

Bohndorf K, Schalm J. Diagnostic radiography in rheumatoid arthritis: benefits and limitations. Baillieres Clin Rheumatol 1996; 10:399-407.

Tehranzadeh J, Ashikyan O, Dascalos J. Advanced imaging of early rheumatoid arthritis. Radiol Clin North Am 2004; 42:89-107.

Tehranzadeh J, Ashikyan O, Dascalos J. Magnetic resonance imaging in early detection of rheumatoid arthritis. Semin Musculoskelet Radiol 2003; 7:79-94.

REFERENCES

1. Doran MF, Pond GR, Crowson CS, et al. Trends in incidence and mortality in rheumatoid arthritis in Rochester, Minnesota, over a forty-year period. Arthritis Rheum 2002; 46:625-631.
2. Pincus T, Callahan LF. Taking mortality in rheumatoid arthritis seriously—predictive markers, socioeconomic status and comorbidity. J Rheumatol 1986; 13:841-845.
3. Tamai K, Yamato M, Yamaguchi T, Ohno W. Dynamic magnetic resonance imaging for the evaluation of synovitis in patients with rheumatoid arthritis. Arthritis Rheum 1994; 37:1151-1157.
4. Vallbracht I, Helmke K. Additional diagnostic and clinical value of anti-cyclic citrullinated peptide antibodies compared with rheumatoid factor isotypes in rheumatoid arthritis. Autoimmun Rev 2005; 4:389-394.
5. van Venrooij WJ, van de Putte LB. Early diagnosis of rheumatoid arthritis with a test based upon a specific antigen: cyclic citrullinated peptide. Ned Tijdschr Geneeskd 2003; 147:191-194.
6. Batalov AZ, Kuzmanova SI, Sapoundjiev LI. Intraarticular rheumatoid nodule detection in the knee joint using ultrasonography. Fol Med (Plovdiv) 2000; 42:27-29.
7. Kaye BR, Kaye RL, Bobrove A. Rheumatoid nodules: review of the spectrum of associated conditions and proposal of a new classification, with a report of four seronegative cases. Am J Med 1984; 76:279-292.
8. Bohndorf K, Schalm J. Diagnostic radiography in rheumatoid arthritis: benefits and limitations. Baillieres Clin Rheumatol 1996; 10:399-407.
9. Keen HI, Brown AK, Wakefield RJ, Conaghan PG. MRI and musculoskeletal ultrasonography as diagnostic tools in early arthritis. Rheum Dis Clin North Am 2005; 31:699-714.
10. Ostergaard M, Ejbjerg B, Szkudlarek M. Imaging in early rheumatoid arthritis: roles of magnetic resonance imaging, ultrasonography, conventional radiography and computed tomography. Best Pract Res Clin Rheumatol 2005; 19:91-116.
11. Ostergaard M, Gideon P, Sorensen K, et al. Scoring of synovial membrane hypertrophy and bone erosions by MR imaging in clinically active and inactive rheumatoid arthritis of the wrist. Scand J Rheumatol 1995; 24:212-218.
12. Stone M, Bergin D, Whelan B, et al. Doppler ultrasound assessment of rheumatoid hand synovitis. J Rheumatol 2001; 28:1979-1982.
13. Weidekamm C, Koller M, Weber M, Kainberger F. Diagnostic value of high-resolution B-mode and Doppler sonography for imaging of hand and finger joints in rheumatoid arthritis. Arthritis Rheum 2003; 48:325-333.
14. Alasaarela E, Suramo I, Tervonen O, et al. Evaluation of humeral head erosions in rheumatoid arthritis: a comparison of ultrasonography, magnetic resonance imaging, computed tomography and plain radiography. Br J Rheumatol 1998; 37:1152-1156.
15. Corvetta A, Giovagnoni A, Baldelli S, et al. Imaging of rheumatoid hand lesions: comparison with conventional radiology in 31 patients. Clin Exp Rheumatol 1992; 10:217-222, 1992.
16. Tehranzadeh J, Ashikyan O, Dascalos J: Advanced imaging of early rheumatoid arthritis. Radiol Clin North Am 2004; 42:89-107.
17. Tehranzadeh J, Ashikyan O, Dascalos J. Magnetic resonance imaging in early detection of rheumatoid arthritis. Semin Musculoskelet Radiol 2003; 7:79-94.
18. Conaghan PG, O'Connor P, McGonagle D, et al. Elucidation of the relationship between synovitis and bone damage: a randomized magnetic resonance imaging study of individual joints in patients with early rheumatoid arthritis. Arthritis Rheum 2003; 48:64-71.
19. Gibbon WW. Applications of ultrasound in arthritis. Semin Musculoskelet Radiol 2004; 8:313-328.
20. Grassi W, Filippucci E, Farina A, Cervini C. Sonographic imaging of the distal phalanx. Semin Arthritis Rheum 2000; 29:379-384.
21. Naredo E, Bonilla G, Gamero F, et al. Assessment of inflammatory activity in rheumatoid arthritis: a comparative study of clinical evaluation with grey scale and power Doppler ultrasonography. Ann Rheum Dis 2005; 64:375-381.
22. Szkudlarek M, Court-Payen M, Strandberg C, et al. Contrast-enhanced power Doppler ultrasonography of the metacarpophalangeal joints in rheumatoid arthritis. Eur Radiol 2003; 13:163-168.

23. Szkudlarek M, Court-Payen M, Jacobsen S, et al. Interobserver agreement in ultrasonography of the finger and toe joints in rheumatoid arthritis. Arthritis Rheum 2003; 48:955–962.

24. Hau M, Schultz H, Tony HP, et al. Evaluation of pannus and vascularization of the metacarpophalangeal and proximal interphalangeal joints in rheumatoid arthritis by high-resolution ultrasound (multidimensional linear array). Arthritis Rheum 1999; 42:2303–2308.

25. Guermazi A, Taouli B, Lynch JA, Peterfy CG. Imaging of bone erosion in rheumatoid arthritis. Semin Musculoskelet Radiol 2004; 8:269–285.

26. Taylor PC. Serum vascular markers and vascular imaging in assessment of rheumatoid arthritis disease activity and response to therapy. Rheumatology 2005; 44:721–728.

27. Teh J, Stevens K, Williamson L, et al. Power Doppler ultrasound of rheumatoid synovitis: quantification of therapeutic response. Br J Radiol 2003; 76:875–879.

28. Barbaric ZL, Young LW. Synovial cysts in juvenile rheumatoid arthritis. Am J Roentgenol Radium Ther Nucl Med 1972; 116:655–660.

29. Grassi W, De Angelis R, Lamanna G, Cervini C: The clinical features of rheumatoid arthritis. Eur J Radiol 1998; 27:S18–S24.

30. Watson JD, Ochsner SF. Compression of bladder due to "rheumatoid" cysts of hip joint. AJR Am J Roentgenol 1967; 99:695–696.

31. Weissman BN, Sledge CB. Orthopedic Radiology. Philadelphia, WB Saunders, 1986.

32. Grassi W, Tittarelli E, Blasetti P, et al. Finger tendon involvement in rheumatoid arthritis: evaluation with high-frequency sonography. Arthritis Rheum 1995; 38:786–794.

33. Birkett V, Ring EF, Elvins DM, et al. A comparison of bone loss in early and late rheumatoid arthritis using quantitative phalangeal ultrasound. Clin Rheumatol 2003; 22:203–207.

34. Madsen OR, Suetta C, Egsmose C, et al. Bone status in rheumatoid arthritis assessed at peripheral sites by three different quantitative ultrasound devices. Clin Rheumatol 2004; 23:324–329.

35. Jacobs CV, Fultz PJ, Totterman SMS, Condemi JJ. Extra-articular manifestations of rheumatoid arthritis. Postgrad Radiol 1995; 15:153–163.

36. Buskila D, Shnaider A, Neumann L, et al. Musculoskeletal manifestations and autoantibody profile in 90 hepatitis C virus–infected Israeli patients. Semin Arthritis Rheum 1998; 28:107–113.

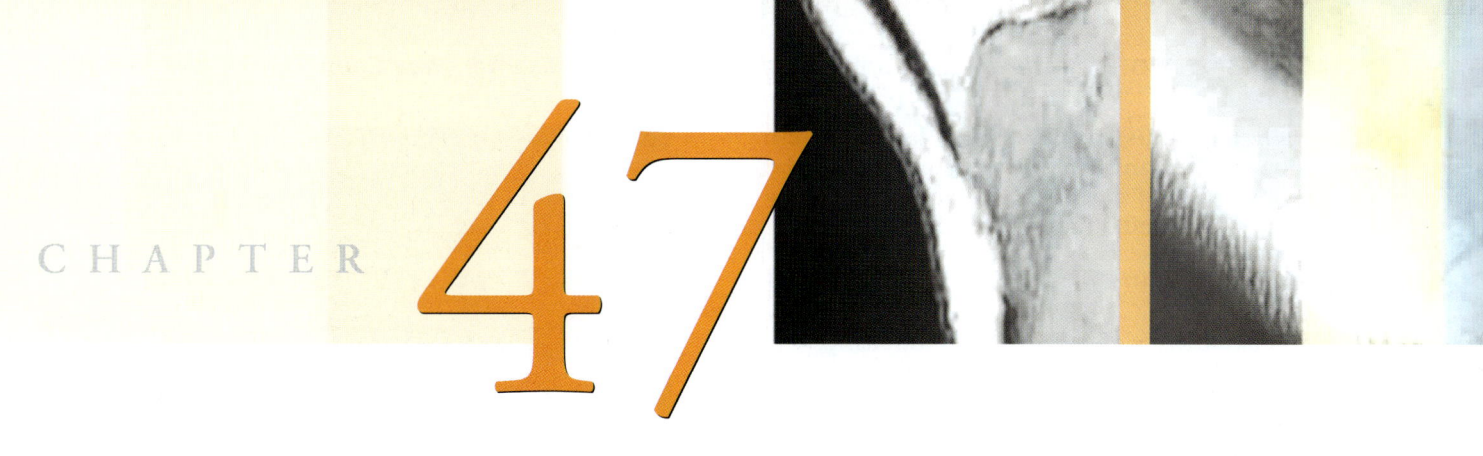

47

Psoriatic Arthritis and Psoriatic Spondylarthropathy

Karsten Jablonka and Jürgen Freyschmidt

Psoriatic arthritis (also known as psoriatic osteoarthropathy) is an autoimmune response disorder that belongs to the seronegative spondyloarthropathies. It is strongly associated with dermatologic psoriasis.

Psoriatic spondylarthropathy refers to the involvement of the axial skeleton in patients who suffer from psoriatic arthritis.

ETIOLOGY

The etiology of all clinical manifestations of psoriasis, psoriatic arthritis, and psoriatic spondylarthropathy seems to be a T cell–dependent tumor necrosis factor–mediated multifactorial autoimmune disorder.

PREVALENCE AND EPIDEMIOLOGY

Psoriasis has no known sex predilection. Its peak incidence is between 30 and 50 years of age. It has been estimated that between 1% and 6% of the population in Western countries have some clinical degree of psoriasis vulgaris. Up to 15% of these patients develop clinically and radiographically variable degrees of psoriatic arthritis. Other sites of involvement besides the skin and bones are the tendons at bony insertions, referred to as the entheses. Psoriatic spondylarthropathy accounts for almost 20% of the seronegative spondyloarthropathies. A genetic association via the HLA-B27 antigen has been identified. Among HIV-infected patients, psoriasis arthropathy is 40 times more common than in the general population.[1-5]

CLINICAL PRESENTATION

Dermatologic changes include erythematous macules with a silvery-white scale; nail changes (oil spots, pitting, crumbling), and sterile pustules. The changes can be very subtle, for instance, on the scalp.

Psoriatic arthritis and psoriatic spondylarthropathy are disorders resulting in inflammation of entheses (enthesitis) and erosion or destruction of joints; affected sites often exhibit bone proliferation. Patients may present with diffuse swelling of one or more digits (dactylitis).[6] In 20% to 30% of cases there are no psoriatic skin changes when arthritis sets in. After a sudden onset (pseudogout arthritis) the course of the disease usually waxes and wanes. Only rarely is the course of the disease primarily chronic.

IMAGING TECHNIQUES

Techniques and Relevant Aspects

Early changes in psoriatic arthritis are nonspecific. They are detectable using MRI and, to a certain extent, ultrasound. In early stages of the disease osseous changes

---

KEY POINTS

- Primary features are the combination of erosive and proliferative bone changes.
- If there is radiologic suspicion of psoriasis, a careful history (including family history) and a close dermatologic examination are necessary.
- Radiographic signs: erosive, mutilating, and ankylosing joint changes, mainly involving the hands and feet, with a typical axial, transverse, or mixed pattern of involvement; proliferative changes (periosteal ossification, protuberances); spondylarthritis with sacroiliitis, parasyndesmophytes, and enthesopathy.

(especially periostitis) are very subtle and require high-resolution radiographs. Findings in late stages of the disease are typical and diagnostic in most cases. They are sufficiently visualized on routine radiographs.[7-9]

Pros and Cons

In combination with observation of skin changes, radiographic examinations are sufficient in most cases. It can be argued that inflammatory changes naturally are better examined with MRI than on radiographs or CT. Once bony changes have occurred then radiographs are sufficient for detection of the typical changes of psoriatic arthritis. MRI is thought to help in the differentiation of psoriatic arthritis and rheumatoid arthritis; this statement is based on differing sites of edema (see later).

MANIFESTATIONS OF THE DISEASE

Peripheral Skeleton

Initial joint complaints are usually monarticular or oligoarticular. Typical sites of the skeletal disease are the entheses and articulations. There is a slight predilection for the great toe. Large joints are involved in fewer than 10% of cases.

In later stages, the distribution changes to being oligoarticular or polyarticular. Polyarticular disease is characterized by the distribution among the small joints of the fingers and toes. One manifestation of this condition is "sausage digit" (see later under Enthesitis).

Radiography

The basis of imaging psoriatic arthritis is conventional radiography. According to Freyschmidt, examinations should include views of both hands and feet, the lower thoracic spine, the lumbar spine, and other symptomatic regions or joints, in two projections.[3] Examinations of the hands and feet are preferably performed using high-resolution techniques. Very useful and convenient in this respect is the use of mammography systems.

Relatively early changes (Fig. 47-1) that can be visualized radiographically include the following:

- Spiculated or woolly sites of epiphyseal ossification on the distal phalanges, sometimes only visible by using a magnifying tool
- Acro-osteolysis
- Layered or periosteal ossifications on the shafts of tubular bones

Later signs in the appendicular skeleton (Fig. 47-2) include:

- Nondelineation of the subchondral plate
- Erosions
- Destructive changes
- Joint space narrowing
- Ankylosis
- Mutilations
- Protuberances (spicular ossifications at joint margins, especially at the bases of the distal phalanges)
- Insufficiency and stress fractures

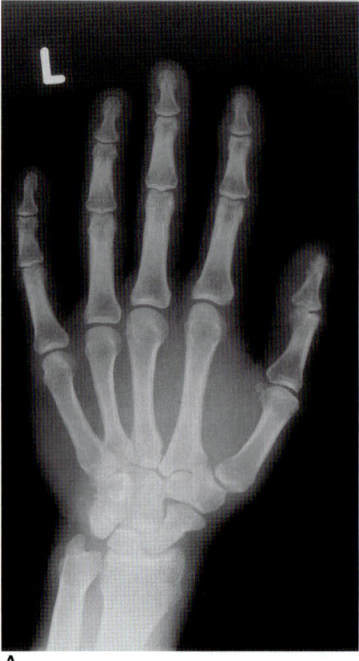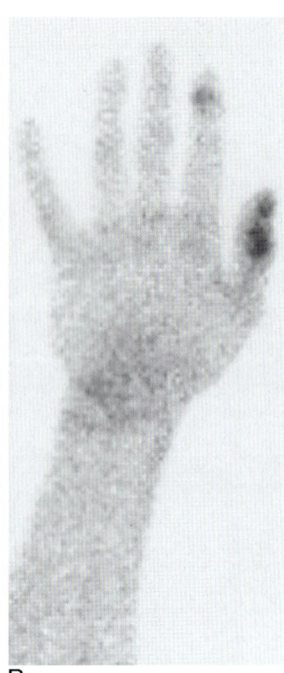

A   B

■ **FIGURE 47-1** Early manifestations of psoriatic arthritis of the peripheral skeleton. **A,** Anteroposterior radiograph of the hand. Note soft tissue swelling of the thumb and second digit, with fluffy bone proliferation of the terminal tuft of the thumb. **B,** Bone scintiscan of the same patient shows increased uptake in regions of involvement.

Most often the distal interphalangeal joints of the hands and feet are involved. The distribution of the visible changes is of key importance in the radiographic assessment and classification of the disease. The lesions tend to be asymmetric with an oligoarticular or polyarticular distribution. If all the joints of one finger or toe are involved, the pattern of involvement is called "axial" or "vertical." If all the distal interphalangeal joints of a hand or foot are affected, a "transverse" or "horizontal" pattern is present. There are also asymmetric mixed patterns.

Magnetic Resonance Imaging

Magnetic resonance imaging can detect erosions and early articular and entheseal inflammation significantly better than conventional radiography and CT.

Multidetector Computed Tomography

Computed tomography can be very useful as an adjunct to radiographs to verify the presence of osseous manifestations of psoriatic spondyloarthropathy, including erosions at the sacroiliac joints. When combined with intravenous contrast media administration, CT can characterize inflammatory tissue; however, this is inferior to MRI.

Ultrasonography

Ultrasonography is an effective tool to visualize joint effusions associated with psoriatic arthritis.

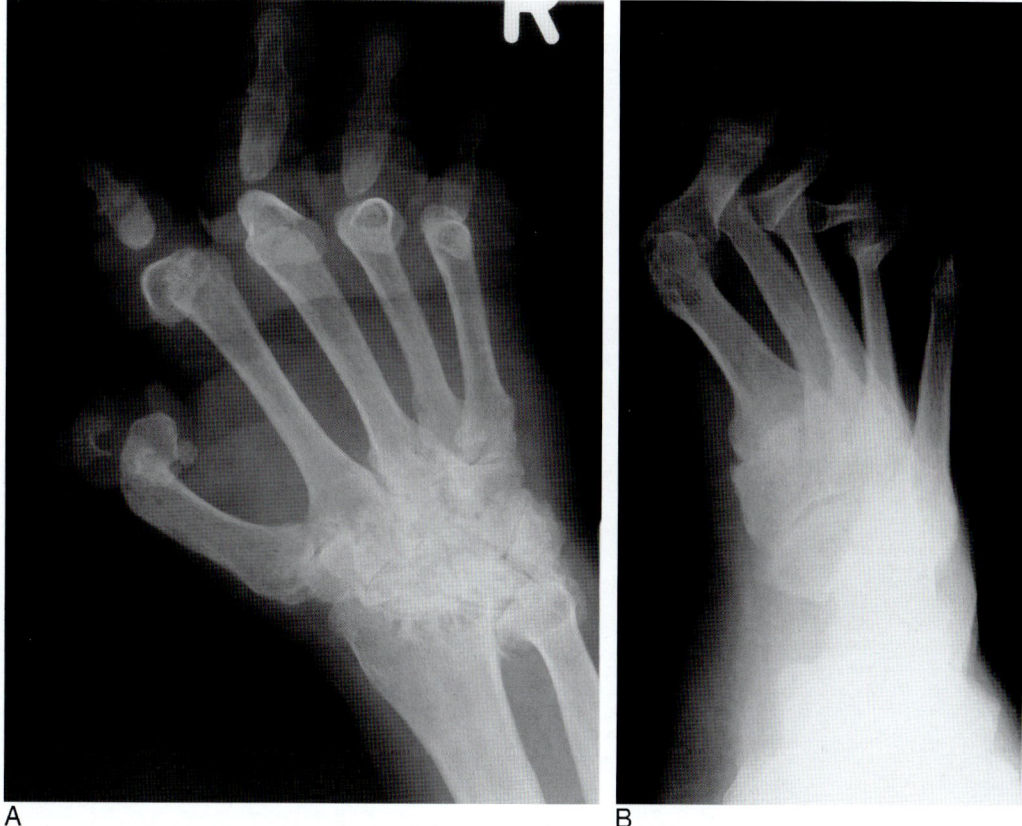

■ **FIGURE 47-2** Psoriatic arthritis with arthritis mutilans. **A,** Anteroposterior radiograph of the hand showing gross destruction of the proximal interphalangeal joints with rounded, whittled margins and, to a lesser degree, involvement of the metacarpophalangeal joints. Note also fusion of the carpus and distal interphalangeal joints. **B,** Radiograph of the foot showing similar changes.

Nuclear Medicine

Bone scintigraphy is a very convenient tool especially for claustrophobic patients for whom MRI is difficult. Because of its lack of specificity, findings should be compared with radiographs and clinical history. Nuclear bone scintiscans can be helpful in establishing the diagnosis, because they clearly define affected joints and make the pattern of involvement more obvious.

Classic Signs

On radiographs of the hands and feet:
- Erosive and coexistent osteoproliferative changes
- Joint space narrowing
- Arthritis mutilans with "pencil-in-cup" appearance
- Ankylosis

Axial Skeleton

Psoriatic spondylarthropathy is present if one or both sacroiliac joints and the spine are involved.

Radiography

Early signs of an evolving psoriatic spondylarthropathy are not detectable radiographically. Later, one half of the patients show signs of a (usually unilateral) sacroiliac joint involvement with erosions and sclerosis. Conventional radiographs of the spine show typical changes of the vertebra. The predilection site is the upper lumbar spine. Just as in rheumatoid arthritis, involvement of the cervical spine can lead to atlantoaxial instability.

Typical features seen in seronegative spondarthritis include:

- Marginal syndesmophytes
- Nonmarginal syndesmophytes
- Paravertebral ossification
- Destructive discovertebral lesion
- Romanus lesion ("shiny corners" or sclerosis of the anterosuperior end plate)
- Sacroiliitis

Magnetic Resonance Imaging

Magnetic resonance imaging is the best modality for visualizing ongoing inflammation (Fig. 47-3). With the possible exception of periosteal changes, all imaging features of psoriatic arthritis are visualized to a better advantage by

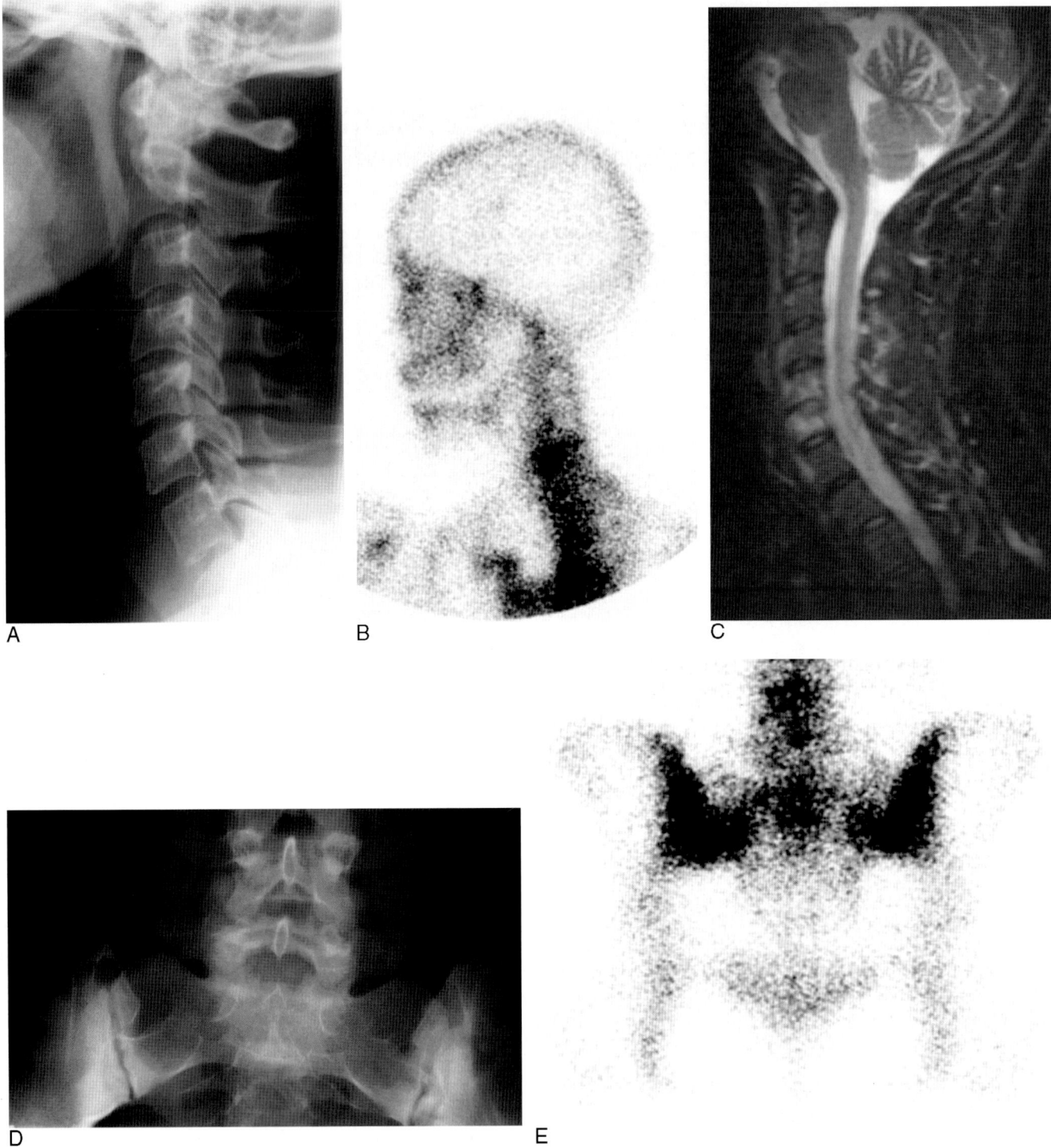

■ **FIGURE 47-3**   Psoriatic spondylarthritis. **A,** Lateral radiograph of the cervical spine. **B,** Bone scintiscan of cervical spine showing abnormal uptake in the lower cervical region. **C,** STIR MR image of the cervical spine showing edema of C5 and C6 vertebral bodies and multiple spinous processes. Findings can simulate infection. **D,** Radiograph of the same patient showing sacroiliitis. **E,** Corresponding bone scintiscan showing abnormal radiotracer uptake at the sacroiliac joints.

using MRI than by using any other modality. If instability of the craniocervical junction is suspected, MRI of the cervical spine is mandatory.

Multidetector Computed Tomography

If radiographs are insufficient to visualize psoriatic spondylarthropathy, CT can be very helpful.

Ultrasonography

Ultrasonography is a useful tool for observing inflammatory changes in patients with proven psoriatic arthritis.

Nuclear Medicine

Bone scintigraphy can be useful for documenting spinal or sacroiliac involvement (see Fig. 47-3) and for acquiring an overview of all sites involved around the body.

Classic Signs

Typical signs of seronegative spondylarthropathy include:
- Marginal syndesmophytes
- Nonmarginal syndesmophytes
- Paravertebral ossification
- Destructive discovertebral lesion
- Romanus lesion ("shiny corners" or sclerosis of the antero-superior end plate)
- Sacroiliitis

Entheses

Entheses are the regions of direct contact between bone and tendons, ligaments, or fascia.

Radiography

The findings in enthesitis vary. Enthesitis is typical of an extra-articular manifestation of a psoriatic arthropathy and spondylarthropathy (Fig. 47-4). An enthesopathy can cause polymorphic ossifications of insertions of tendons, ligaments, fascia, and articular capsules.

Massive swelling of the extra-articular soft tissues of a digit is termed *psoriatic dactylitis*.[6] The affected fingers or toes have a sausage-shaped appearance ("sausage digits").

Magnetic Resonance Imaging

Even in early stages of the disease, intense bone marrow edema closely related to entheses is typical. MRI is the best modality for examination of active inflammation of entheses, for instance, at the gluteal region.

Multidetector Computed Tomography

Computed tomography is not commonly indicated for psoriatic arthritis manifestations other than spinal and sacroiliac involvement. However, CT can show enthesial bone production with high detail, allowing for narrowing of the differential diagnosis especially when the disease is manifest in atypical locations (see Fig. 47-4).

Ultrasonography

Ultrasonography can give useful information on the extent of abnormality of the entheses. It is also capable of visualizing tenosynovitis that contributes to the diffuse, sausage-like swelling of involved fingers (dactylitis).

Nuclear Medicine

Bone scintigraphy can provide a useful overview regarding sites of entheseal, articular, and spinal involvement (see Fig. 47-4).

DIFFERENTIAL DIAGNOSIS

Psoriatic arthritis is probable if three or more of the following criteria are met, including at least one of criteria 5, 6, or 8. If rheumatoid factor is positive, two additional criteria must be fulfilled.

1. Involvement of the distal interphalangeal joints
2. Involvement of the metacarpophalangeal and interphalangeal joints of the same finger
3. Early involvement of the joints of the toes
4. Heel pain
5. Dermatologically confirmed psoriatic lesions of the skin or nails
6. Close relative with confirmed psoriasis
7. Negative rheumatoid factor
8. Radiographs of the hands and/or feet showing typical osteolytic changes along with bony proliferation and no periarticular osteoporosis
9. Clinical and/or radiographic involvement of the sacroiliac joints
10. Typical paravertebral ossifications on spinal radiographs

Evidence of Reiter's disease, ankylosing spondylitis, or polyarthritis of the fingers makes the diagnosis of psoriatic arthropathy unlikely.

Reiter's disease appears radiographically identical but is more common in the lower extremity. Quite often, the patient's history makes one diagnosis more likely than the other; Reiter's disease is seen in males, whereas psoriatic arthritis shows similar incidence in males and females; Reiter's disease also involves conjunctivitis and urethritis. Psoriatic arthritis also commonly involves the skin and nails with characteristic lesions.

Ankylosing spondylitis is characterized clinically by a stiff, painful back and radiographically by symmetric sacroiliitis and spinal syndesmophytes (bamboo spine). Paravertebral ossification can be a characteristic of late-stage psoriatic spondylarthropathy but is usually large, nonuniform, and asymmetric.

Laboratory tests usually are not diagnostic of psoriatic arthritis. The erythrocyte sedimentation rate is slightly elevated. The rheumatoid factor usually is negative; a positive test may signify a concomitant rheumatoid arthritis.

SYNOPSIS OF TREATMENT OPTIONS

Anti-inflammatory drugs are the basis of treatment. Immune modulators are being introduced. Surgical interventions can become necessary, including joint replacement and arthrodesis.

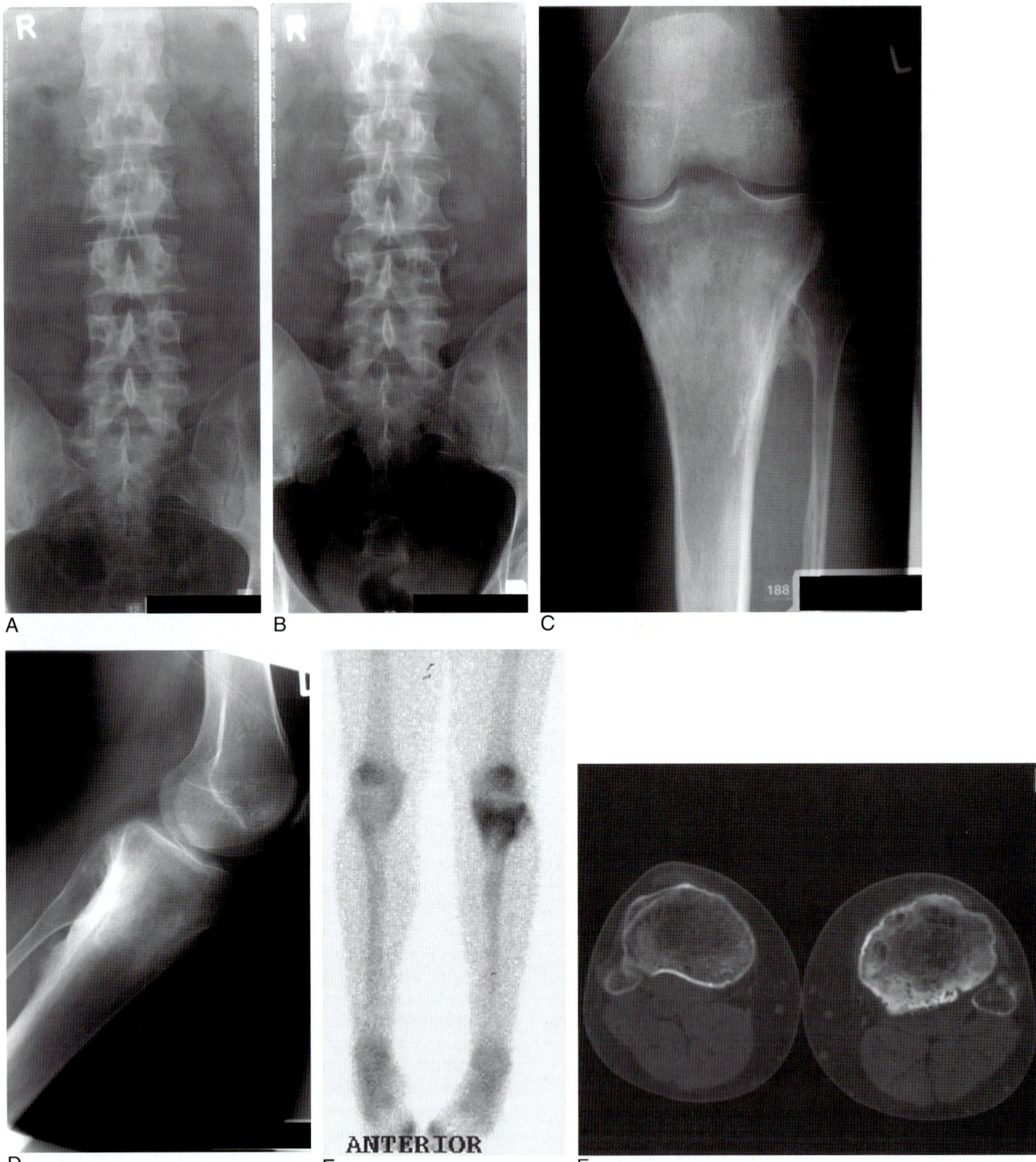

■ **FIGURE 47-4** Psoriatic spondylarthropathy: enthesopathy. **A,** Radiograph of the lumbar spine taken on initial presentation showing no parasyndesmophytes. **B,** Radiograph of the same patient taken 4 years later, now showing parasyndesmophytes. Note also sclerosis at the sacroiliac joints. **C,** Anteroposterior radiograph of the same patient showing enthesopathy of the tibia. **D,** Lateral radiograph with enthesopathy of the tibia particularly at the soleus origin; note reactive sclerosis of adjacent bone with proliferative bone formation. **E,** Bone scintiscan with uptake representing enthesopathy of the proximal tibia. **F,** CT image of the same patient showing reactive sclerosis.

What the Referring Physician Needs to Know

- Patients with psoriatic arthritis must be treated by specialists in this field.
- Radiographs are the baseline imaging modality.
- MRI, CT, ultrasonography, and bone scintigraphy are useful additional tools.

SUGGESTED READINGS

Evangelisto A, et al. Imaging in early arthritis. Best Pract Res Clin Rheumatol 2004; 18:927-943.

Kainberger F. Imaging of systemic rheumatoid diseases involving the musculoskeletal system. Radiologie 2004; 4:395-416.

Kassimos D, et al. The hand x-ray in rheumatology. Hosp Med 2004; 65(1).

Klecker RJ, et al. Imaging features of psoriatic arthritis and Reiter's syndrome: advanced imaging of arthritis. Semin Musculoskelet Radiol 2003; 7:115-126.

Myers W, et al. Common clinical features and disease mechanisms of psoriasis and psoriatic arthritis. Curr Rheumatol Rep 2004; 6:306-313.

Taylor WJ, et al. Operational definitions and observer reliability of the plain radiographic features of psoriatic arthritis. J Rheumatol 2003; 30:2645-2658.

Taylor WJ, et al. Development of diagnostic criteria for psoriatic arthritis: methods and process. Curr Rheumatol Rep 2004; 6:299-305.

Veale DJ, et al. Immunopathology of psoriasis and psoriatic arthritis. Ann Rheum Dis 2005; 64(Suppl II):ii26-ii29.

REFERENCES

1. Anandarajah AP, et al. Pathogenesis of psoriatic arthritis. Curr Opin Rheumatol 2004; 16:338-343.
2. Freyschmidt J. SKIBO-Diseases: Disorders affecting the skin and bones: A clinical, dermatologic, and radiologic synopsis. Heidelberg, Springer-Verlag Telos, 1998.
3. Freyschmidt J. Skeletterkrankungen. Heidelberg, Springer, 2003, pp 433-457.
4. Gladman DD, et al. Psoriatic arthritis: epidemiology, clinical features, course, and outcome. Ann Rheum Dis 2005; 64(Suppl II): ii14- ii17.
5. Moll JM, Haslock I, Macrae IF, Wright V. Associations between ankylosing spondylitis, psoriatic arthritis, Reiter's disease, the intestinal arthropathies, and Behçet's syndrome. Medicine 1974; 53:343-364.
6. Olivieri I, Barozzi L, Favaro L, et al. Dactylitis in patients with seronegative spondylarthropathy. Arthritis Rheum 1996; 39: 1524-1528.
7. Lingg G, et al. Insufficiency and stress fractures of the long bones occurring in patients with rheumatoid arthritis and other inflammatory diseases, with a contribution on the possibilities of computed tomography. Eur J Radiol 1997; 26:54-63.
8. Lingg G, et al. Bildgebende Verfahren bei der Arthritis psoriatica. Akt Rheumatol 2000; 25:123-131.
9. Totterman SMS. Magnetic resonance imaging of psoriatic arthritis: Insight from traditional and three-dimensional analysis. Curr Rheumatol Rep 2004; 6:317-321.

48

Reactive Arthritis

Daniel Nissman and Thomas L. Pope

Reactive arthritis is a postinfectious seronegative spondyloarthropathy (SNSA) syndrome characterized by a spectrum of specific musculoskeletal and extra-articular manifestations. The syndrome occurs after infection with specific organisms in two major settings: diarrheal illness and urogenital infection. The majority of patients have an underlying predisposing factor, either the presence of the human leukocyte antigen (HLA)-B27 or infection with the human immunodeficiency virus (HIV). Onset of symptoms is usually within 4 weeks of the triggering infection and usually after the triggering infection has resolved.

Like the other SNSA syndromes such as ankylosing spondylitis and psoriatic arthritis, reactive arthritis shares an association with HLA-B27 and a particular symptom-complex. Musculoskeletal complaints include joint pain from enthesitis and peripheral arthritis and back pain from sacroiliitis. Extra-articular complaints include conjunctivitis, urethritis, and a variety of mucocutaneous lesions.

The symptom triad of arthritis, conjunctivitis, and urethritis after a triggering infection is classically known as Reiter's syndrome even though Reiter was not the first to describe this triad. This triad was described previously in 1776 after a diarrheal illness and again in 1818 after a urogenital infection.[1] Reports of cases with similar features predate even these descriptions. Hans Reiter published a similar case in 1916, and the term *Reiter's syndrome* was coined in 1942 by Bauer and Engelman. The term *reactive arthritis* was suggested by Ahvonen in 1969 and is now the favored term.[2] Reasons for abandoning the reference to Reiter include the facts that he was not the first to describe the syndrome, he attributed the syndrome incorrectly to infection by a spirochete, and he was a very high ranking Nazi physician who personally authorized medical experiments on prisoners that led to many deaths in concentration camps, including 250 people from experimental typhus infection.[3,4]

ETIOLOGY

Reactive arthritis is unique among the SNSA syndromes in that it occurs after a clearly associated trigger—an enteric or urogenital infection. Enteric organisms that have a well-documented association with reactive arthritis include *Campylobacter, Salmonella, Shigella*, and *Yersinia* species. *Chlamydia trachomatis* is responsible for the vast majority of cases of reactive arthritis after a urogenital infection. Many other organisms, including parasites, and situations that trigger this syndrome have been reported. *Chlamydia pneumoniae, Ureaplasma urealyticum*, and *Giardia intestinalis* are examples. Reactive arthritis after intravesical instillation of bacille Calmette-Guérin (BCG) for bladder cancer has been reported.[5]

As a member of the SNSA syndromes there is a strong association with HLA-B27, although its presence is not necessary for the diagnosis. However, symptomatic disease is more likely in individuals with HLA-B27. An estimated 1% to 4% of individuals who are HLA-B27 negative will develop reactive arthritis, whereas 20% to 30% of individuals who are HLA-B27 positive will develop reactive arthritis.

An important subgroup of HLA-B27–negative individuals are those infected with HIV. Individuals who are positive for both HIV infection and HLA-B27 can experience particularly severe manifestations of reactive arthritis.

The exact pathogenesis of reactive arthritis is unknown. Factors that are important in its development include a triggering infection with specific types of bacteria and

---

KEY POINTS

- Reactive arthritis is an asymmetric, lower limb-predominant spondyloarthropathy that follows a triggering infection, usually within 4 weeks.
- Conjunctivitis, urethritis, and skin lesions may be associated.
- There is a strong association with HLA-B27 and HIV infection.
- Heel pain and back pain are the most common complaints.
- Radiographs of the spine, sacroiliac joints, and other affected joints are used to evaluate disease progression.
- MRI and CT can detect early sacroiliitis.
- Septic arthritis should be excluded first.

an altered immune response, manifested by either HLA-B27 positivity or HIV infection. Recent data suggest a central role for macrophages in the development of erosive disease. Subclinical intestinal inflammation has been associated with the entire spectrum of SNSA syndromes, including reactive arthritis. Mechanical factors may also be important but have not been sufficiently studied. Many other potential genetic factors beyond HLA-B27 positivity likely play a role.

All bacterial organisms definitively linked to reactive arthritis are gram-negative and are either obligate intracellular organisms or are capable of intracellular survival. Antigenic material from these organisms disseminates from the site of primary infection to other parts of the body where this material has been recovered from the joint fluid and synovium of affected joints. In the case of *Chlamydia*, entire living organisms have been recovered, but with an altered gene expression profile from those involved with active infection.[6] The antigenic material produced by these organisms persists in the tissues for long periods, especially material associated with chlamydial infection. These organisms all have a variety of means for evading the host immune response in addition to the capacity to live intracellularly, including the production of lipopolysaccharide (LPS), a proinflammatory molecule, and the ability to manipulate various cell membrane signaling molecules. The end result is a prolonged proinflammatory environment created by the presence and poor clearance of this antigenic material. These factors alone do not explain the manifestations of reactive arthritis because most people with primary infections with these organisms do not develop the disease.

The majority of individuals with symptomatic disease are either HLA-B27 positive or are infected with HIV, and the common thread between these is an altered T-cell response. HLA-B27 is part of the major histocompatibility complex machinery responsible for antigen presentation to CD8-positive T cells. The specific role that HLA-B27 plays in the pathogenesis of reactive arthritis is not known, although there are a number of hypotheses.[7,8] The HLA-B27 molecule folds more slowly than other HLA molecules and may become trapped in the endoplasmic reticulum. On the cell surface, the HLA-B27 molecule has the capacity to dimerize. Aberrant folding on the cell surface can cause part of the HLA-B27 molecule to occupy the antigen binding site. Through a variety of mechanisms, all these properties may lead to an elevated and prolonged inflammatory response. Antigenic mimicry may play a role as well. Peptides from HLA-B27 share sequence homology with antigens from *Chlamydia* and the reactive arthritis–associated enteric bacteria.

HIV infection significantly alters the T-cell response to infection in patients with reactive arthritis in an unknown manner. Early in HIV infection, the CD8-positive T cells are relatively spared. In end-stage disease, the symptoms of reactive arthritis disappear and are likely due to further alteration in the proportions of the various T-cell subtypes.

Tumor necrosis factor-α (TNF-α) is a proinflammatory cytokine that plays a key role in the inflammatory arthritis in the spondyloarthropathies. Anti-TNF-α therapeutics have shown benefit in arresting the progression of these diseases, although no specific studies have been performed in patients with reactive arthritis. Histologic analysis of samples obtained from sites of enthesitis has revealed a macrophage-predominant cellular infiltrate and not a T-cell–predominant infiltrate as previously expected.[9] Macrophages are the primary producers of TNF-α. The role of TNF-α and its potential modulation by HLA-B27 positivity and HIV infection is not understood.

Chronic intestinal inflammation has been observed in many patients with an SNSA syndrome, including individuals with reactive arthritis, particularly those with enteric-associated reactive arthritis. The degree of gut inflammation appears to follow the activity of the articular symptoms.[10] The exact nature of the association, however, is not clear. Does the gut inflammation predispose to reactive arthritis, or is it simply another extra-articular manifestation of the syndrome?

Finally, the musculoskeletal manifestations of reactive arthritis are most common in the lower extremity and particularly in the heel. These sites represent areas of increased stress when compared with the upper extremity. A single study demonstrated microfractures in the vicinity of the entheses that were not seen in the comparison population of patients with rheumatoid arthritis.[11] This trauma is also proinflammatory and may explain the lower limb predominance.

PREVALENCE AND EPIDEMIOLOGY

The incidence of reactive arthritis follows the prevalence of HLA-B27 in the geographic region of study. The Scandinavian countries have a particularly high prevalence of HLA-B27 in the general population (10% to 16%) and a correspondingly high incidence of reactive arthritis (10 to 28 per 100,000).[12,13] In Africa, where the SNSA syndromes are relatively unheard of, the prevalence of HLA-B27 is also very low. The prevalence of HLA-B27 in general Western populations is approximately 8%. A study examining the prevalence in Rochester, Minnesota, between 1950 and 1980 found a prevalence of 3.5 per 100,000 in men younger than age 50.[14] In individuals with reactive arthritis, the prevalence of HLA-B27 is nearly 50%.

Numbers regarding the incidence and prevalence of reactive arthritis should be regarded as very loose approximations of their real values. Many of the studies reporting these data use different criteria for making the diagnosis of reactive arthritis. Strict criteria requiring the presence of an extra-articular manifestation will be very specific but not very sensitive. Those using more lax criteria, such as monoarthritis after any infection, will have improved sensitivity but low specificity. A factor that could result in a substantial underestimation of the true incidence of reactive arthritis is that mild self-limited cases may never be recognized or may never come to the attention of health care personnel.

Overall, the disease is most common in those between 20 and 40 years old, with an overall slight male predominance that is attributed specifically to *Chlamydia*-associated reactive arthritis. Enteric infection–associated reactive arthritis, on the other hand, affects men and women with equal frequency.

Reactive arthritis is rare in children, but when it occurs it is almost always due to a gastrointestinal infection.[15,16]

Unlike adults in whom extra-articular manifestations often precede articular complaints, children usually express the articular complaints first. As in adults, the prevalence of HLA-B27 in children with reactive arthritis is likely near 50%, with reported prevalences ranging from near 0% to near 100%.

The incidence of reactive arthritis in elderly individuals hospitalized for arthritis is reported to be between 3% and 16%.[17] Reactive arthritis is thought to be rare in the elderly, but many of these patients have joint complaints related to osteoarthritis and other conditions, such as polymyalgia rheumatica, that may obscure the musculoskeletal findings in reactive arthritis.

Among HIV-infected individuals, the incidence of reactive arthritis is at least 10 times greater than for an individual of the general population. In sub-Saharan Africa, the incidence of reactive arthritis among HIV-infected individuals is extremely high but quite low among individuals not infected. The prevalence of SNSA in Zambia is 180 per 100,000 in HIV-infected individuals but only 15 per 100,000 in HIV-negative individuals.[18] At least one third of cases of SNSA are attributable to reactive arthritis. In one series, 94% of patients with reactive arthritis were HIV positive.[19]

A longitudinal cohort study examining rheumatic complications associated with HIV infection spanning the years 1989 to 2000 conducted at the Cleveland Clinic showed a dramatic drop in the incidence of reactive arthritis in HIV-infected individuals after the widespread use of highly active anti-retroviral therapy (HAART) (late 1995).[20] Studies following patients prior to 1995 failed to show significant changes in HIV-associated rheumatic complications even after the introduction of one- and two-drug therapies.[10]

Among individuals presenting with acute anterior uveitis, approximately 10% have reactive arthritis. Among individuals with a spondyloarthropathy in the same sample, acute anterior uveitis was twice as common in individuals with ankylosing spondylitis.[21]

CLINICAL PRESENTATION

Reactive arthritis represents a spectrum of disease after a gastrointestinal or urinary tract infection usually within 4 weeks. The predominant feature is an asymmetric lower limb–predominant oligoarthritis (four or fewer affected joints). The addition of extra-articular symptoms, including urethritis and conjunctivitis, represents more severe disease. The classic triad of symptoms of urethritis, conjunctivitis, and arthritis is only observed in up to 30% of patients. When extra-articular symptoms are present, they typically precede the arthritis.

A number of diagnostic criteria exist for reactive arthritis, ranging from very specific to more general in nature. Specific criteria include the American College of Rheumatology criteria that require the presence of at least one extra-articular manifestation. More general criteria, such as the Third International Working Group on Reactive Arthritis criteria, require only onset of an asymmetric oligoarthritis within 4 weeks of a documented infection. Practically, confidence in a diagnosis of reactive arthritis hinges on identification of an associated pathogen or a typical constellation of symptoms.

The vast majority of enteric infections that precede reactive arthritis are caused by certain subspecies of *Shigella, Salmonella, Yersinia*, and *Campylobacter. Chlamydia trachomatis* causes almost all cases of urogenital tract infections preceding reactive arthritis. However, a triggering infection is only identified in up to 60% of cases. Evaluation of joint fluid or the synovium of an affected joint reveals no living organisms, but polymerase chain reaction assays often identify genetic material from the triggering organism.

Because reactive arthritis is a member of the SNSA syndromes, serum rheumatoid factor and other antibodies found in association with the other rheumatic diseases are absent. Erythrocyte sedimentation rate, C-reactive protein, and levels of other acute-phase reactants are frequently elevated. Analysis of joint fluid reveals a predominant neutrophilia and no organisms on Gram stain.

Musculoskeletal Manifestations

The musculoskeletal manifestations of reactive arthritis include enthesitis, peripheral arthritis, and sacroiliitis in an asymmetric lower limb–predominant pattern of distribution. Enthesitis is the most common manifestation, with the Achilles tendon and plantar aponeurosis insertions on the calcaneus most frequently involved. Heel pain is very common in patients with reactive arthritis. Dactylitis results from inflammation of the entheses, and the synovial linings of the tendons and joints of an entire digit. When associated with significant swelling, the result is the "sausage digit," a characteristic but nonspecific feature of both reactive arthritis and psoriatic arthritis. Other sites associated with enthesitis in reactive arthritis include the iliac crests, ischial tuberosities, and the tibial tuberosities. Bursitis and enthesitis often occur simultaneously, particularly at the Achilles tendon insertion on the calcaneus.

The peripheral arthritis of reactive arthritis is asymmetric and nonmigratory and preferentially affects the large joints of the lower extremity. The most frequently involved joints are the knee, ankle, and metatarsophalangeal joints. Manifestations include erythema, swelling, and joint effusion. Often, only a single joint is affected, but it is not unusual for several to be affected simultaneously. Polyarthritis is rare. When the upper extremity is affected, the most common affected joints are the elbow, wrist, and the finger joints. Several studies have reported different distributions of arthritic symptoms for non-*Chlamydia* reactive arthritis and *Chlamydia*-associated reactive arthritis. The enteric form appears to affect the upper extremities more frequently than in the reactive arthritis triggered by *Chlamydia*.[22] *Chlamydia*-associated reactive arthritis is also more likely to be monoarticular than non-*Chlamydia* reactive arthritis.

Low back pain is a frequent symptom and due to spondylitis or sacroiliitis. Asymmetric sacroiliitis may present as low back and buttock pain. Owing to its asymmetric nature, this pain pattern may be confused for sciatica. Late in the disease process, the sacroiliitis may become symmetric.

Rarely, erosive disease of the temporomandibular and manubriosternal joints can occur.

Extra-articular Manifestations

Extra-articular symptoms are signs of a systemic disease process and most commonly involves the eyes, urogenital system, and skin. Rarely, cardiac involvement is present. Extra-articular symptoms are more common in *Chlamydia*-associated reactive arthritis. Systemic complaints of fatigue, fever, and weight loss are not uncommon.

Conjunctivitis is the most common ocular manifestation (30% to 60% of patients), followed by acute anterior uveitis (5%). When present, these ocular symptoms generally follow urethritis. The conjunctivitis is usually bilateral, whereas the uveitis is usually unilateral and if not treated may result in visual loss or blindness. The primary urogenital tract manifestation is urethritis. In men, prostatitis is common; and in women, localized inflammation of the reproductive tract, such as cervicitis, can be present. Cutaneous manifestations include keratoderma blennorrhagicum, circinate balanitis, and painless oral ulcers. Psoriatic skin and nail changes may be present in up to 15% of patients. Cardiac involvement is uncommon and can manifest as aortitis, valve abnormalities, myocarditis, or cardiac conduction abnormalities.

Natural History and Prognosis

The disease is generally self-limited and lasts from 3 to 5 months. Information regarding long-term sequelae of reactive arthritis is predominantly due to study of patients with enteric-associated reactive arthritis. Approximately 50% of individuals will have persistent mild musculoskeletal complaints for years after the acute syndrome and up to 15% progress to ankylosing spondylitis. Radiologic evidence of sacroiliitis is seen in up to 30%. Reactive arthritis after urogenital infection is prone to recurrence, perhaps due to repeated infections.

PATHOLOGY

Evaluation of the synovial fluid reveals macrophages containing entire phagocytized cells within their cytoplasm. The function of these cells appears to be to ingest apoptotic polymorphonuclear leukocytes to prevent them from spilling their proinflammatory contents into the synovial fluid. These cells are called Reiter cells but are not specific to reactive arthritis. Although more common in the SNSA syndromes, these cells have also been seen in the synovial fluid of patients with rheumatoid arthritis and crystal-induced arthritis.[23]

Histologic examination of synovial biopsy specimens in reactive arthritis reveals inflammatory changes that are nonspecific. Thickening of the synovial cell lining, inflammatory cell infiltration, and increased cellularity of the stroma are common findings. A macrophage-predominant infiltrate is present at the sites of enthesitis.[9]

IMAGING TECHNIQUES

The diagnosis of reactive arthritis is primarily clinical. Imaging is used to evaluate for progression of disease, evaluate difficult cases, and guide therapeutic interventions.

Radiography is the technique of choice in evaluating progression of disease. CT and MRI are used to evaluate patients early in the disease course when radiographs are normal. MRI and ultrasonography are used to evaluate the entheses. In the United States MRI is the preferred modality, whereas elsewhere in the world ultrasonography is the preferred modality, because it is less expensive. Image-guided intervention is predominantly performed using CT and ultrasonography, although MRI is gaining popularity as an image-guidance modality. Bone scintigraphy is sensitive but not as useful as MRI for evaluating extent of inflammatory changes. Standard techniques are used in the performance of all imaging studies with few exceptions.

The imaging appearances of all manifestations of reactive arthritis are indistinguishable from those of psoriatic arthritis. The only difference is that reactive arthritis preferentially affects the lower limbs and psoriatic arthritis preferentially affects the upper limbs. As a significant proportion of patients, up to 15%, with reactive arthritis progress to ankylosing spondylitis, features of ankylosing spondylitis may also be seen.

MANIFESTATIONS OF THE DISEASE

Spondylitis

In the spine, reactive arthritis causes asymmetric, coarse and thick paravertebral ossifications called parasyndesmophytes or nonmarginal syndesmophytes. In contrast to ankylosing spondylitis, these paravertebral ossifications are nonmarginal and originate away from the vertebral body end plate. The syndesmophytes of ankylosing spondylitis are thin, are symmetric, and involve the fibers of the annulus fibrosus. The lower thoracic and upper lumbar spine are preferred sites of involvement. According to one study, uroarthritis is more likely to have spine manifestations than enteroarthritis.[24]

The primary differential diagnosis is diffuse idiopathic skeletal hyperostosis, which can result in asymmetric, thick nonmarginal flowing osteophytes. The parasyndesmophytes of reactive arthritis are indistinguishable from those seen in psoriatic arthritis.

The finding of erosion at the peripheral attachment of the annulus fibrosus that subsequently heals resulting in bony sclerosis and, ultimately, remodeling that results in loss of the normal convexity of the anterior vertebral bodies is less likely to be seen in reactive arthritis than in ankylosing spondylitis.[25] Diffuse idiopathic skeletal hyperostosis is not associated with erosive disease.

Radiography

Radiographic evaluation of the spine in reactive arthritis consists of the standard anteroposterior and lateral views covering the region of interest. When radiographic changes are present, the asymmetric parasyndesmophytes are most common. Rarely, Romanus lesions (erosion at attachment site of the annulus fibrosus) and "shiny corners" (the resultant bony reaction to the erosion) may be seen. The Romanus lesion and the "shiny corner" are typical features of ankylosing spondylitis, however, and are rarely seen in reactive arthritis (Figs. 48-1 and 48-2).

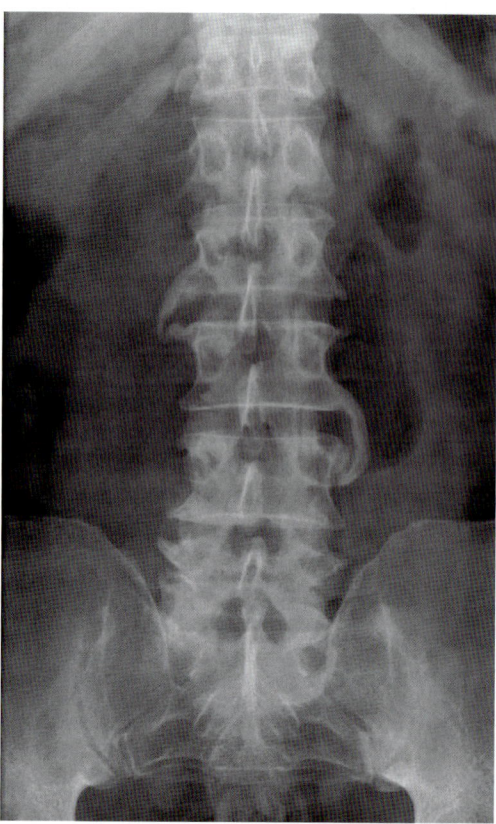

■ **FIGURE 48-1** Anteroposterior radiograph of the lumbar spine demonstrates isolated large nonmarginal syndesmophytes, one on either side of the spine.

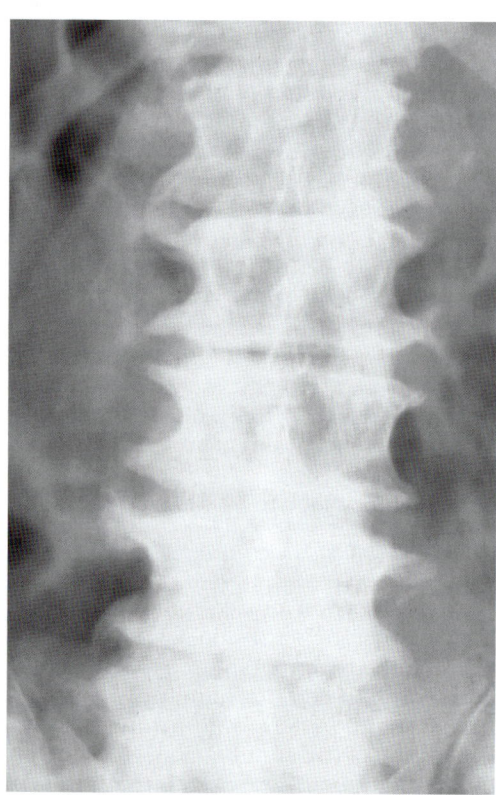

■ **FIGURE 48-2** A close-up anteroposterior view of the lumbar spine reveals bilateral asymmetric parasyndesmophytes with bridging on the right at L1-L2.

Magnetic Resonance Imaging

Magnetic resonance imaging findings are nonspecific and illustrate end-plate changes, edema, and signal dropout in the ossified syndesmophytes. Before the appearance of radiographic changes, however, MRI may help to identify early enthesitis and erosive disease.

Multidetector Computed Tomography

Computed tomography demonstrates similar findings as radiography but has greater sensitivity for early changes.

Nuclear Medicine

Bone scintigraphy shows increased radiotracer accumulation at sites of bone deposition, but the appearance is nonspecific.

Classic Signs

- Asymmetric parasyndesmophytes: nonmarginal thick syndesmophytes
- Romanus lesion and "shiny corner": more common in ankylosing spondylitis

---

Sacroiliitis

The sacroiliac joint is a curved joint composed of an upper ligamentous portion and a lower synovial portion. The inflammatory changes of interest occur in the lower aspect of the joint. Like psoriatic arthritis, the sacroiliitis of reac-

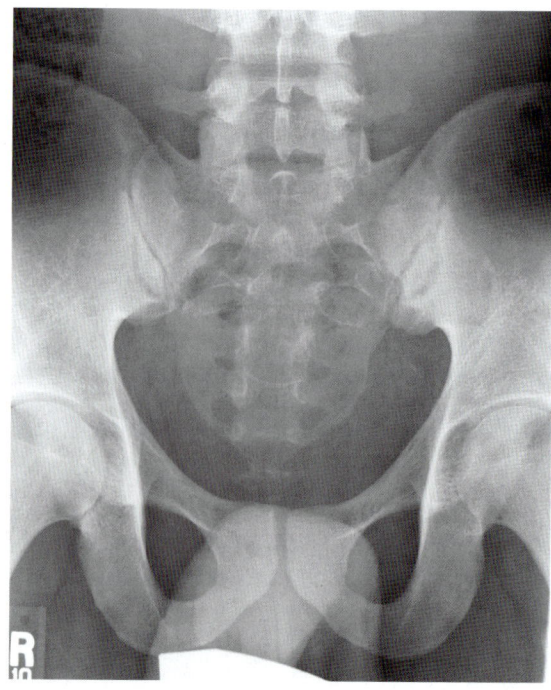

■ **FIGURE 48-3** Frontal view of the sacrum reveals sclerosis and joint space widening involving the left inferior sacroiliac joint compatible with sacroiliitis. *(Courtesy of Dr. Johnny Monu, University of Rochester, Rochester, NY.)*

tive arthritis is asymmetric but usually bilateral. Very early in the disease process, the sacroiliitis may be unilateral. Over time, however, involvement of both sacroiliac joints may become symmetric. Ankylosis is a late finding.

Radiography

The standard anteroposterior view of the sacrum is supplemented by a 15- to 25-degree cephalad view, the Ferguson view, which allows better visualization of the inferior sacroiliac joint. The progression of changes at the joint due to chronic inflammation begins with tiny erosions and periarticular sclerosis without joint space narrowing. Increased sclerosis on both sides of the joint follows and is associated with some widening of the joint. This process continues with increased production of bone that eventually crosses the joint, resulting in ankylosis (Figs. 48-3 to 48-5).

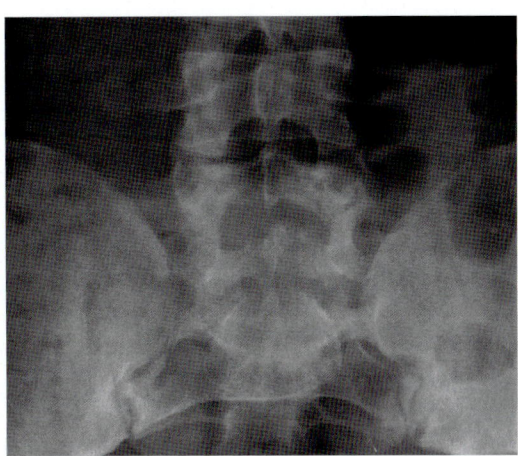

■ **FIGURE 48-4** Close-up view of the sacroiliac joints reveals marked asymmetric sacroiliitis on the right characterized by irregular joint space widening and subchondral sclerosis. See Figure 48-7 for CT of the sacroiliac joints in the same patient.

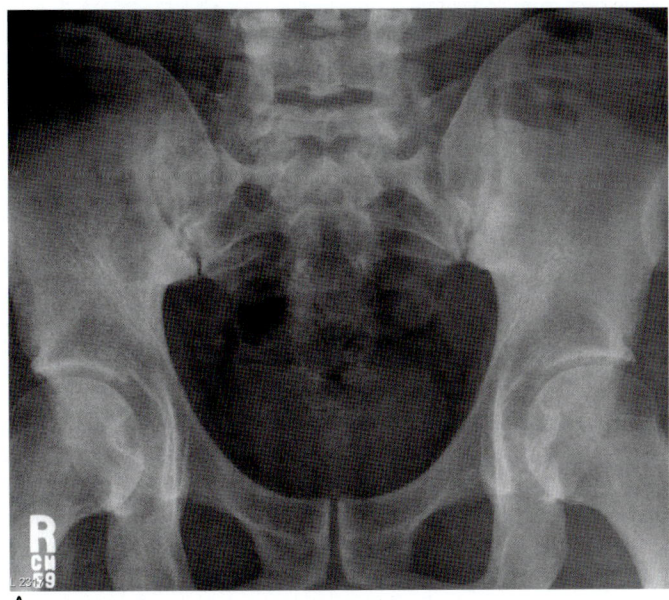

A

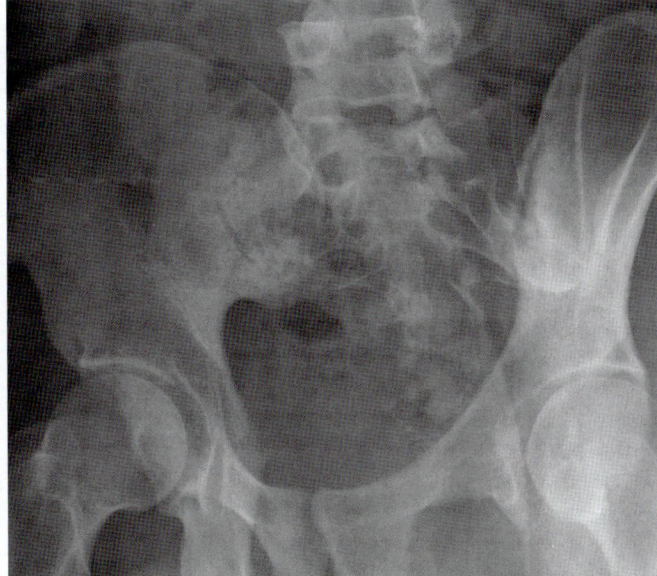

B

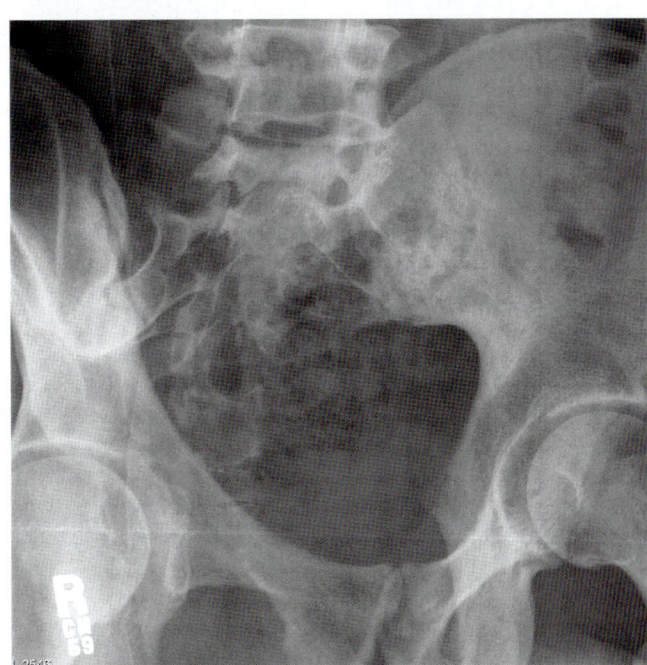

C

■ **FIGURE 48-5** Asymmetric sacroiliitis, left greater than right. **A,** Anteroposterior view. **B,** A 45-degree right postero-oblique image. **C,** A 45-degree left postero-oblique image.

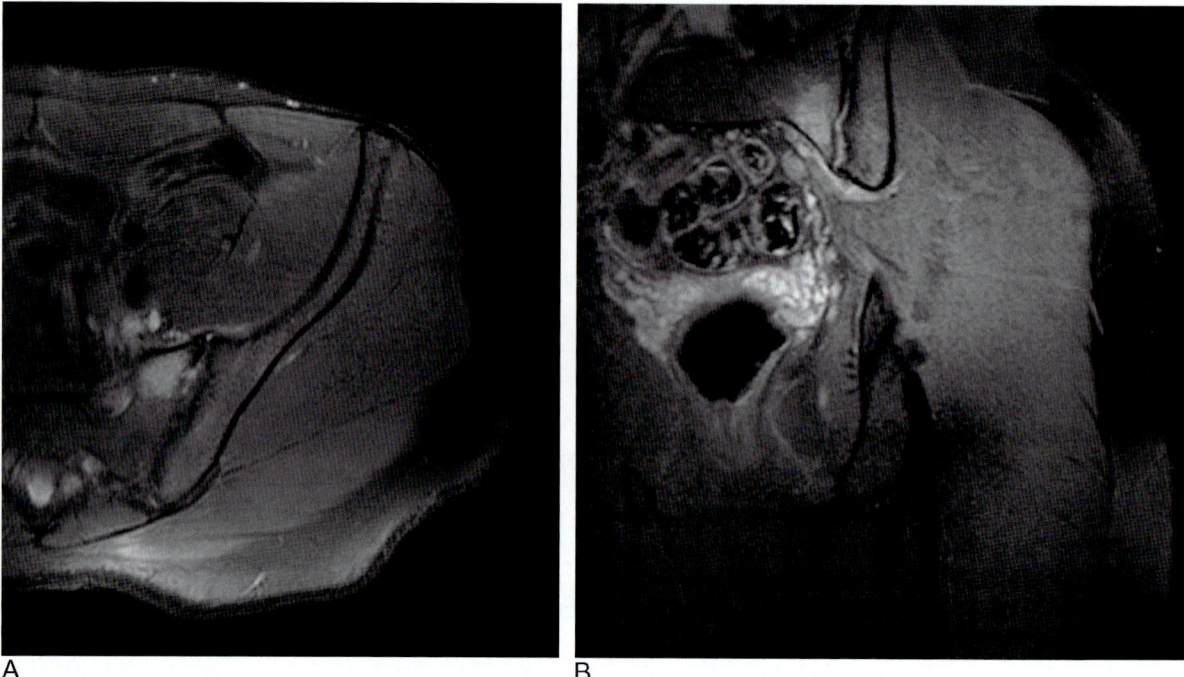

A   B

■ **FIGURE 48-6**   T2-weighted, fat-saturated axial (**A**) and coronal (**B**) MR images demonstrate increased signal intensity in the anterior aspect of the left sacroiliac joint, predominantly on the sacral side, compatible with sacroiliitis. *(Courtesy of Dr. Johnny Monu, University of Rochester, Rochester, NY.)*

Magnetic Resonance Imaging

Magnetic resonance imaging is the most sensitive method for the detection of sacroiliitis due to its ability to identify cartilage abnormalities and associated bone marrow edema.[26] The use of intravenous gadolinium contrast material can be helpful in identifying inflammation and after response to therapy (Fig. 48-6).

Multidetector Computed Tomography

The ability to image the sacroiliac joint in thin axial sections using CT is useful for eliminating the extensive overlap of the anterior and posterior sides of the joint that limits plain radiographic analysis. In very early cases or cases in which there is a question of osteitis condensans ilii versus sacroiliitis, CT may show small erosions and sclerosis when plain radiographs are normal or indeterminate (Fig. 48-7).

Nuclear Medicine

Bone scintigraphy is a sensitive technique for detecting sacroiliitis but is nonspecific and does not provide as much information as MRI.

Erosive Arthritis and Proliferative New Bone Formation

The arthritis of reactive arthritis is characterized by marginal erosions, proliferative new bone formation, joint space narrowing, and joint effusions. In the acute phase, periarticular osteopenia is usually present. Ankylosis is a finding in advanced disease. The joints of the foot are particularly affected, and the specific aspects of the disease

at those locations are mentioned separately. In the digits, significant soft tissue swelling can be present.

Radiography

Radiographic evaluation of the joints uses standard radiographic projections. Marginal erosions with fluffy periosteal reaction are classic, particularly in the digits. The erosions progress from the periphery of the joint toward the central subchondral bone. Proliferative periosteal reaction is particularly common in the small bones of the foot. Any joint of the lower extremity can be involved, usually in an asymmetric pattern.

The bones and joints of the forefoot are frequently involved in reactive arthritis (Fig. 48-8). Among the joints in the forefoot, the first metatarsophalangeal joint is most commonly affected. Ankylosis may occur between bones in the foot but less frequently than seen in the hand in patients with psoriatic arthritis.

The calcaneus is one of the most common sites of involvement with indistinct periosteal reaction on the inferior posterior surface leading to the formation of a plantar calcaneal spur with indistinct margins. A posterior superior calcaneal spur can also develop with similar characteristics.

The most common manifestation of reactive arthritis in the knee is a joint effusion.

When the upper extremities are affected, the pattern of involvement is identical to that seen in psoriatic arthritis (Fig. 48-9).

Magnetic Resonance Imaging

The MRI findings are nonspecific and are related to generic signs of inflammation. These include bone mar-

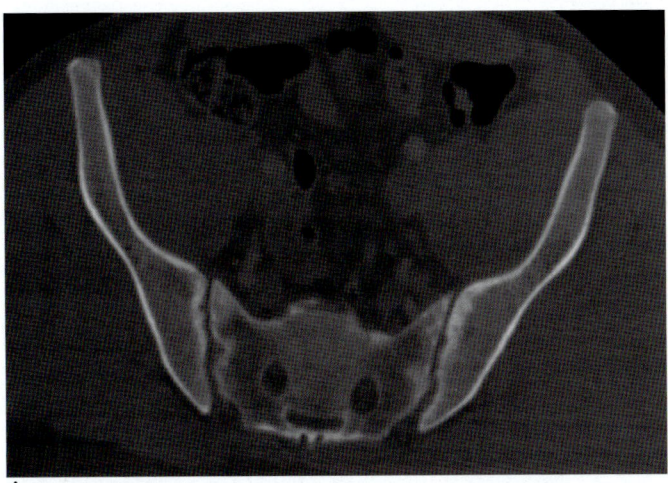

A

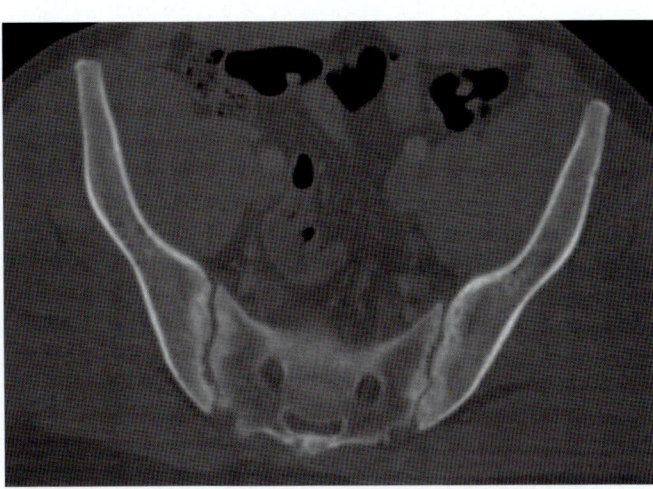

B

■ **FIGURE 48-7** A to C, Axial CT images at three levels of the lower sacroiliac joint demonstrate bilateral asymmetric (right greater than left) subchondral sclerosis, irregular joint space widening, and erosions.

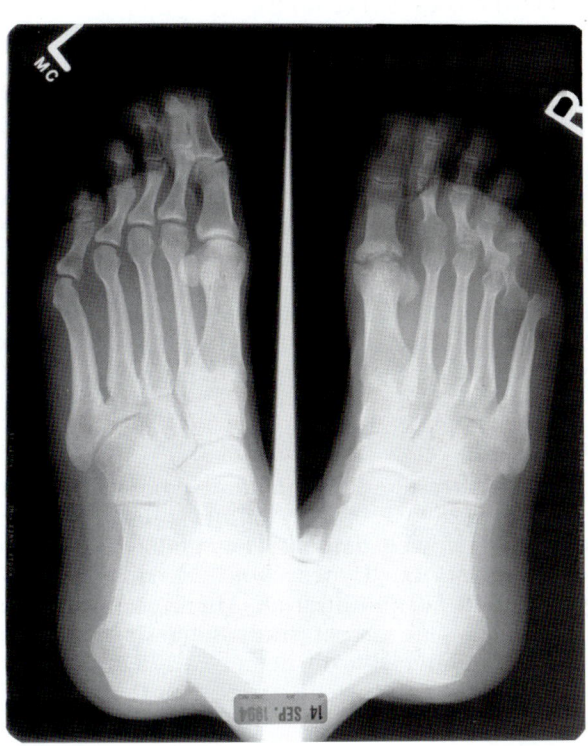

C

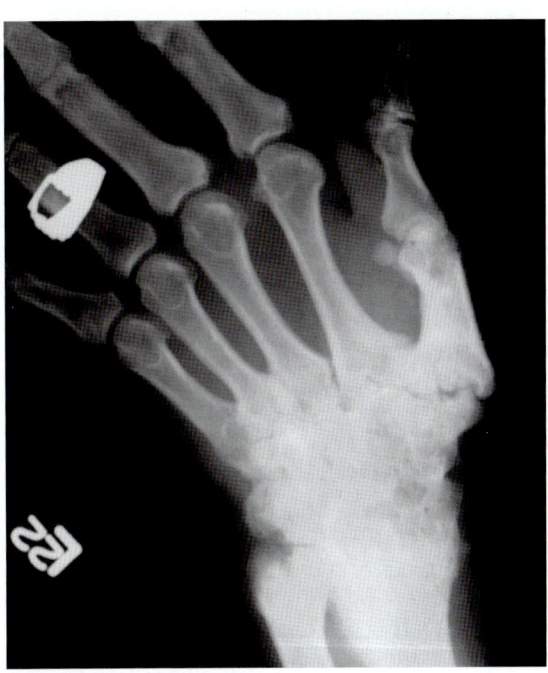

■ **FIGURE 48-8** Oblique radiographs of the feet reveal fluffy periosteal new bone with underlying erosions at the first metatarsophalangeal joint of the right foot. The left foot is unaffected. Incidental note is also made of medial dislocation of the left fifth metatarsophalangeal joint. *(Courtesy of Dr. Don Flemming, Penn State University, Hershey, PA.)*

■ **FIGURE 48-9** Posteroanterior radiograph of the left hand reveals fluffy periosteal new bone and erosive disease involving the entire carpus and the first carpometacarpal joint.

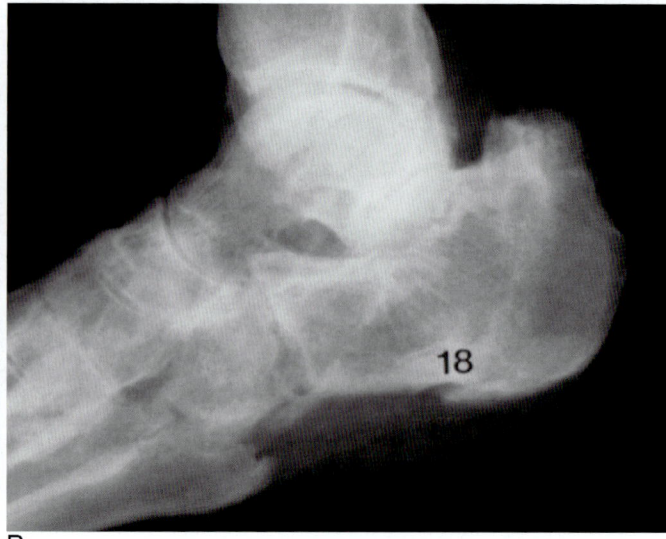

■ **FIGURE 48-10** A and B, Lateral radiographs of the calcaneus and midfoot in two patients reveal plantar and superior calcaneal spurs with an indistinct quality typical of the enthesopathic changes seen in reactive arthritis. Note the large enthesophyte involving the attachment site of the peroneus brevis tendon on the base of the fifth metacarpal.

row edema, joint fluid, and thickened soft tissue structures. Irregularities in marginal bone can be appreciated but are poorly resolved on MRI.

Multidetector Computed Tomography

Computed tomography is more sensitive than radiography for subtle erosions and periosteal reaction, primarily owing to its ability to eliminate overlapping structures. MRI, however, is more sensitive for inflammatory changes.

Ultrasonography

Ultrasonography does not have a role in the imaging of erosions and the proliferative new bone. However, it can detect the surrounding tissue edema and the presence of a joint effusion.

Nuclear Medicine

Bone scintigraphy with a bone-seeking agent can identify areas of bone turnover and therefore can be used to identify extent of disease, particularly in new cases.

Enthesitis

Enthesitis is one of the most frequent manifestations of reactive arthritis and is a feature of the SNSA syndromes as a whole. In reactive arthritis, any of the entheseal insertions on the foot may be involved. The most commonly affected sites are the Achilles tendon and plantar aponeurosis insertions on the posterior calcaneus. Retrocalcaneal bursitis is also frequently present.

MRI and ultrasonography are the imaging modalities of choice for evaluating the entheses. Enthesitis is associated with proliferative new bone formation. Therefore, radiography can detect long-term changes via calcium deposition and soft tissue swelling, but these are nonspecific.

Radiography

Radiographic findings in enthesitis are nonspecific. Tiny erosions and new bone formation may be seen. The inflammatory context, however, is not visualized. The presence of erosions can help to distinguish the enthesopathic changes of the SNSA syndromes from diffuse idiopathic skeletal hyperostosis (Fig. 48-10).

Magnetic Resonance Imaging

Evaluation of the enthesis is performed using T1-weighted, T2-weighted, and short tau inversion recovery (STIR) sequences. Findings include increased signal intensity on T2-weighted imaging, increased tendon thickness, and neighboring bone edema. In long-standing enthesitis, fatty infiltration is represented by intermediate-level signal on T1-weighted images.

For retrocalcaneal bursitis, MRI shows increased Achilles tendon thickness and fluid within the bursa. MRI is twice as sensitive for bursitis as ultrasonography.

Ultrasonography

Findings on ultrasound examination of enthesitis include thickening and loss of the uniform, linear echo pattern of the involved tendon. The tendon margins may become indistinct. Hyperechoic intratendinous foci may represent fatty infiltration. Microcalcifications can also be seen. One recent study suggests that ultrasonography is better able to detect early enthesitis than MRI.[27] Ultrasonography is also useful for the detection of subclinical enthesitis.[28]

For retrocalcaneal bursitis, ultrasonography shows increased Achilles tendon thickness and fluid within the bursa. However, ultrasonography is much less sensitive than MRI for bursitis at this location.

Dactylitis

Inflammation of an entire digit is termed *dactylitis* and can be due to any number of causes. When associated with significant soft tissue swelling, the result is a "sausage digit." Recent investigations into dactylitis secondary to the spondyloarthropathies reveal that this form of dactylitis is due to flexor tendon synovitis with marked adjacent soft tissue swelling.[29] Synovitis of the finger joints, however, is present in only up to 62% of cases. Depending on the digit involved, inflammation can extend to associated palmar bursae.

Imaging of dactylitis is primarily with MRI but it is seen on plain radiographs of the hands and feet when evidence of erosive arthritis is sought.

Radiography

Radiographic evaluation in dactylitis reveals only soft tissue swelling.

Magnetic Resonance Imaging

MRI demonstrates fluid in the flexor tendon sheaths of the affected digits. Surrounding soft tissue edema may also be seen. MRI is better than ultrasonography in detecting fluid in potentially involved joint capsules

Ultrasonography

Ultrasonography demonstrates fluid within the flexor tendon sheaths as well as thickening of the surrounding tissues. It can show fluid within the joints but not as well as MRI.

DIFFERENTIAL DIAGNOSIS

The primary differential diagnostic considerations include other postinfectious arthropathies and the other SNSA syndromes. Exclusion of a septic joint is the essential first step. Several particular postinfectious entities deserve special mention. These are poststreptococcal reactive arthritis, Poncet's disease, and the HIV-related arthropathies.

Poststreptococcal reactive arthritis is an acute sterile arthritis at a remote site associated with a positive throat culture or positive antistreptococcal antibody titers. The patient cannot satisfy the Jones criteria for acute rheumatic fever. Like reactive arthritis, the condition primarily affects the lower limbs and can be associated with an enthesitis. With the exception of uveitis, extra-articular symptoms typical for reactive arthritis have not yet been reported in association with this syndrome. Rash, vasculitis, and glomerulonephritis can occur in this and other poststreptococcal syndromes.

Poncet's disease is an aseptic arthritis that is associated with an active pulmonary tuberculosis. The knees, ankles, and elbows are preferred sites of involvement. Symptoms resolve after adequate treatment for tuberculosis.

HIV infection is associated with many conditions that lead to arthritic pain. HIV-associated arthropathy and painful articular syndrome are examples. Hypertrophic osteoarthropathy preferentially affects the lower limbs and can present as arthralgias. The prevalence of other rheumatic diseases is higher in those infected with HIV, which also need to be considered in the differential diagnosis.

Additional entities to be considered include Lyme disease, Whipple's disease, and syphilis.

The primary differential diagnosis for the imaging findings is the other SNSA syndromes, owing to the considerable overlap in manifestations.

SYNOPSIS OF TREATMENT OPTIONS

Medical Treatment

Treatment of reactive arthritis is supportive using nonsteroidal anti-inflammatory drugs and corticosteroids as needed for pain control. Intra-articular injections of corticosteroids can be used to control particularly severe localized pain. If the patient demonstrates progressive radiographic changes, treatment is similar to that of psoriatic arthritis, including the use of TNF-α inhibitors such as infliximab and etanercept.

Antibiotics play no role in the control or prevention of reactive arthritis with the possible exception of *Chlamydia*-associated reactive arthritis. In a single study, a course of lymecycline was shown to shorten the symptomatic period in patients with *Chlamydia*-associated reactive arthritis but not enteric-associated reactive arthritis.[30]

What the Referring Physician Needs to Know

- Aside from the asymmetric lower limb–predominant distribution, the imaging findings in reactive arthritis are common to the other spondyloarthropathies and particularly overlap with psoriatic arthritis.
- If it is important to document early sacroiliitis, MRI and CT may be useful.
- Radiographs of the spine, sacroiliac joints, and other affected joints are used to evaluate disease progression.
- Other inflammatory arthritides, including septic arthritis, should be excluded before considering a diagnosis of reactive arthritis.

SUGGESTED READINGS

Carter JD. Reactive arthritis: defined etiologies, emerging pathophysiology, and unresolved treatment. Infect Dis Clin North Am 2006; 20:827–847.

Petersel DL, Sigal LH. Reactive arthritis. Infect Dis Clin North Am 2005; 19:863–883.

REFERENCES

1. Leirisalo-Repo M. Reactive arthritis. Scand J Rheumatol 2005; 34:251–259.
2. Ahvonen P, Sievers K, Aho K. Arthritis associated with *Yersinia enterocolitica* infection. Scand J Infect Dis 1971; 3:37–40.
3. Panush RS, Wallace DJ, Dorff EN, Englemann EP. Retraction of the suggestion to use the term "Reiter's syndrome" sixty-five years later: the legacy of Reiter, a war criminal, should not be eponymic honor but rather condemnation. Arthritis Rheum 2007; 56:693–694.
4. Lu DW, Katz KA. Declining use of the eponym "Reiter's syndrome" in the medical literature, 1998–2003. J Am Acad Dermatol 2005; 53:720–723.
5. Tinazzi E, Ficarra V, Simeoni S, et al. Reactive arthritis following BCG immunotherapy for bladder carcinoma. Clin Rheumatol 2005; 24:425–427.
6. Zeidler H, Kuipers J, Kohler L. *Chlamydia*-induced arthritis. Curr Opin Rheumatol 2004; 16:380–392.
7. Kim T, Uhm W, Inman RD. Pathogenesis of ankylosing spondylitis and reactive arthritis. Curr Opin Rheumatol 2005; 17:400–405.
8. Vahamiko S, Penttinen MA, Granfors K. Aetiology and pathogenesis of reactive arthritis: role of non-antigen-presenting effects of HLA-B27. Arthritis Res Ther 2005; 7:136–141.
9. McGonagle D, Marzo-Ortega H, O'Connor P, et al. Histological assessment of the early enthesitis lesion in spondyloarthropathy. Ann Rheum Dis 2002; 61:534–537.
10. Mielants H, De Vos M, Cuvelier C, Veys EM. The role of gut inflammation in the pathogenesis of the spondyloarthropathies. Acta Clin Belg 1996; 51:340–349.
11. McGonagle D, Reade S, Marzo-Ortega H, et al. Human immunodeficiency virus associated spondyloarthropathy: pathogenic insights based on imaging findings and response to highly active antiretroviral treatment. Ann Rheum Dis 2001; 60:696–698.
12. Soderlin MK, Borjesson O, Kautiainen J, et al. Annual incidence of inflammatory joint diseases in a population based study in southern Sweden. Ann Rheum Dis 2002; 61:911–915.
13. Sieper J, Rudwaleit M, Khan MA, Braun J. Concepts and epidemiology of spondyloarthritis. Best Pract Res Clin Rheumatol 2006; 20:401–417.
14. Michet CJ, Machado EB, Ballard DJ, McKenna CH. Epidemiology of Reiter's syndrome in Rochester, Minnesota: 1950–1980. Arthritis Rheum 1988; 31:428–431.
15. Zivony D, Nocton J, Wortmann D, Esterly N. Juvenile Reiter's syndrome: a report of four cases. J Am Acad Dermatol 1998; 38:32–37.
16. Liao C, Huang J, Yeh K. Juvenile Reiter's syndrome: a case report. J Microbiol Immunol Infect 2004; 37:379–381.
17. Toussirot E, Wendling D. Late-onset ankylosing spondylitis and related spondyloarthropathies: clinical and radiological characteristics and pharmacological treatment options. Drugs Aging 2005; 22:451–469.
18. Njobvu P, McGill P, Kerr H, et al. Spondyloarthropathy and human immunodeficiency virus infection in Zambia. J Rheumatol 1998; 25:1553–1559.
19. Mijiyawa M, Oniankitan O, Khan MA. Spondyloarthropathies in sub-Saharan Africa. Curr Opin Rheumatol 2000; 12:281–286.
20. Calabrese LH, Kirchner E, Shrestha R. Rheumatic complications of human immunodeficiency virus infection in the era of highly active antiretroviral therapy: emergence of a new syndrome of immune reconstitution and changing patterns of disease. Semin Arthritis Rheum 2005; 35:166–174.
21. Linder R, Hoffman A, Brunner R. Prevalence of the spondyloarthropathies in patients with uveitis. J Rheumatol 2004; 31:2226–2229.
22. Ozgul A, Dede I, Taskaynatan MA, et al. Clinical presentations of chlamydial and non-chlamydial reactive arthritis. Rheumatol Int 2006; 26:879–885.
23. Selvi E, Manganelli S, De Stefano R, et al. CD36 and CD14 immunoreactivity of Reiter cells in inflammatory synovial fluids. Ann Rheum Dis 2000; 59:399–400.
24. Mannoja A, Pekkola J, Hamalainen M, et al. Lumbosacral radiographic signs in patients with previous enteroarthritis or uroarthritis. Ann Rheum Dis 2005; 64:936–939.
25. Helliwell PS, Hickling P, Wright V. Do the radiological changes of classic ankylosing spondylitis differ from the changes found in the spondylitis associated with inflammatory bowel disease, psoriasis, and reactive arthritis? Ann Rheum Dis 1998; 57:135–140.
26. Inanc N, Atagunduz P, Sen F, et al. The investigation of sacroiliitis with different imaging techniques in spondyloarthropathies. Rheumatol Int 2005; 25:591–594.
27. Kamel M, Eid H, Mansour R. Ultrasound detection of heel enthesitis: a comparison with magnetic resonance imaging. J Rheumatol 2003; 30:774–778.
28. Borman P, Koparal S, Babaoglu S, et al. Ultrasound detection of entheseal insertions in the foot of patients with spondyloarthropathy. Clin Rheumatol 2006; 25:373–377.
29. Olivieri I, Scarano E, Padula A, et al. Dactylitis, a term for different digit disease. Scand J Rheumatol 2006; 35:333–340.
30. Laasila K, Laasonen L, Leirisalo-Repo M. Antibiotic treatment and long term prognosis of reactive arthritis. Ann Rheum Dis 2003; 62:655–658.

49

Ankylosing Spondylitis

Corinna Schorn and Gerwin Lingg

ETIOLOGY

Ankylosing spondylitis (AS) is the prototype of the seronegative spondyloarthropathies, a moderately heterogeneous group of distinct entities composed of AS, psoriatic spondyloarthropathy, reactive spondyloarthropathy (Reiter's disease), enteropathic spondyloarthropathy in Crohn's disease and ulcerative colitis, and so-called undifferentiated spondyloarthropathy.[1] As such, it shares several characteristics with the latter diseases: the genetic background (HLA-B27), the promotion by genitourinary or gastrointestinal bacterial infection and its subsequent or persistent immunologic response, the typical sites of inflammatory involvement, and the peri-inflammatory and postinflammatory osseous proliferation.[2,3] However, there are some manifestations virtually unique to this disease.[4]

The exact etiology remains unclear, even though the role of some autoimmunologic effector mechanisms has been illuminated in recent years. Animal model studies as well as human studies address the humoral and cellular immunity to certain proteoglycans found in cartilage, fibrocartilaginous entheses, and intervertebral discs (aggrecan and versican). This immunity promotes the typical lesions found in AS.[5-7]

The pathophysiologic role of HLA B27 remains to be defined. This molecule is involved in the antigen-presenting process of T cell–mediated defense. It is currently hypothesized that cytotoxic T-cell autoreactivity is induced as a cross reactivity to bacteria-derived peptides or by mispresentation of arthritogenic self-peptides derived from cartilage. Several other less studied hypotheses exist.

PREVALENCE AND EPIDEMIOLOGY

The annual incidence of AS in the white population in the United States is approximately 6.6/100,000, with a prevalence of 0.1 (2%).[8] The male predominance is not as pronounced as classically suggested and is now accepted to be 2 to 5:1.[9] In some cases, the racial and ethnic variance is considerable. Specifically, AS rarely affects blacks and has a higher-than-average prevalence in Native Americans.

Unlike epidemiologic data about the prevalence of AS, data concerning HLA-B27 positivity are widely available for multiple ethnic groups. For example, 4% to 13% of Eurocaucasians are HLA-B27 positive, as are 20% to 40% of Native Americans and less than 1% of Japanese. For African blacks, HLA-B27 positivity is extremely rare.[10]

The prevalence of HLA-B27 in a population has a significant impact on the occurrence of AS. Nevertheless, HLA-B27–negative individuals may develop typical AS. The proportion of cases that are HLA-B27 negative is higher in populations with low HLA-B27 positivity. For Eurocaucasians, 90% to 95% of AS patients are HLA-B27 positive. Thus, HLA-B27 positivity can be considered as a risk factor for development of sacroiliitis and progression to AS.[11] However, HLA-B27 positivity is not the only genetic basis of disease predisposition, contributing 20% to 30% of the risk, and it is not a self-sufficient diagnostic criterion.[12] Certain subtypes of HLA-B27 may be only weakly disease associated, and additional HLA loci and non-HLA loci contribute, as do environmental factors.

The peak incidence of AS is in early adulthood or adolescence (mean 25 years). Disease onset after the age of 45 is rare. In 15% of AS patients, arthritis and enthesitis are present from childhood, with some delay of the vertebral symptoms.

KEY POINTS

- Diagnose sacroiliitis early and accurately with MRI or CT.
- Basic documentation should include radiographic images of the lumbar spine.
- Radiologic follow-up should be used sparingly.
- Consider osteoporosis and perform DEXA or QCT.
- Consider Andersson lesion type B in patients with considerable pain after minor trauma.

CLINICAL PRESENTATION

The key symptom of ankylosing spondylitis is inflammatory back pain. This pain is characterized mainly by late night or early morning attacks of low back pain; it is associated with morning stiffness, which improves with exercise, in a patient younger than the age of 40.[13] Onset of the relapsing attacks is insidious; periods of pain last for more than 3 months. Approximately 30% to 65% of patients with inflammatory back pain have sacroiliitis.[14,15] Buttock pain may alternate sides. All these categories of pain respond to NSAIDs.

Further in its course, the inflammatory process migrates up the vertebral column with some predilection for the thoracolumbar and cervical segments, leaving behind new bone formation and ankylosis and causing deteriorated posture. In late stages, thoracic and thoracolumbar deformity with severe kyphosis may severely handicap patients. The stiffness of the cervical spine hampers head turning, so that activities of daily living such as driving become difficult.

Apart from the vertebral complaints of pain and stiffness, symmetric or asymmetric synovitis/arthritis, mainly of the lower extremity or the proximal joints, may be present. Hips, shoulders, and knees are the most common locations affected by arthralgia and arthritis in AS.

Pain, swelling, and tenderness in the ankles and feet may occur at the plantar aspect, or more often at the distal Achilles tendon insertion, as a result of retrocalcaneal bursitis or enthesitis.

A characteristic extraskeletal symptom of AS is anterior uveitis.[16-18] In fact, the most frequent diagnosis in patients with anterior uveitis is AS.[19] In addition, patients often complain of fatigue.

Physical examination reveals tenderness at the sacroiliac joints (Mennell's sign).[20] Motion restriction of the vertebral column, as well as restricted chest expansion, occurs mainly as a result of the ankylosing condition but sometimes precedes actual bony ankylosis.[21-23] Flexion deformity of the hip joints occurs frequently, and in its early stage it is only appreciated with special tests, such as patient-supine, maximal flexion of the contralateral hip, in order to balance the compensatory hyperlordosis. In fixed-flexion deformity, the knee and hip of the affected side will involuntarily remain flexed as well.

LABORATORY FINDINGS

Elevated levels of erythrocyte sedimentation rate (ESR) and C-reactive protein (CRP) are seen but are nonspecific signs of inflammation. As stated, HLA-B27 is usually positive. However, a positive result does not indicate the presence of sacroiliitis and a negative result is not an exclusion criterion (see Prevalence earlier).

DIAGNOSIS

The modified New York Classification criteria for AS demand, in addition to radiographically proven sacroiliitis, at least one clinical manifestation of inflammatory back pain, vertebral motion restriction, and/or respiratory motion restriction. Average diagnostic delay is 5 to 9 years and is, in part, a result of the low sensitivity of radiographic imaging for early arthritis. There have been proposals for early clinical diagnosis, and the diagnosis of "undifferentiated spondyloarthropathy" has been introduced as a new subgroup in 1991, covering, in part, patients with subsequent development of AS.[1,24-26] New diagnostic approaches employ MRI, which provides high enough sensitivity to detect inflammatory changes.

PATHOPHYSIOLOGY

Anatomy

The junction of the sacrum with the iliac bone can be divided into two compartments. At the ventral portion there is a synovial joint with asymmetric cartilage lining. The diagnostic clues for sacroiliitis are located in this synovial portion. Posteriorly, there is a tight ligamentous junction containing the ligamenta sacroiliaca interossea dorsalia. This is referred to as the retroarticular space. The ligamentous attachments of the retroarticular space may be affected by degeneration or inflammatory disease.

The joint space of the synovial portion of the sacroiliac joint is oriented in varying angles. Consequently, on an anteroposterior view, the joint space is only partially visible, such that the laterally projected contours of the joint margins correspond to the ventral aspect and the medially visible parts correspond to the dorsal aspect of the joint space, respectively.

The joint facets are C shaped and in opposition to the C shape of the os sacrum. On cross-sectional images (CT as well as MRI), in paracoronal angulation, this may result in a display of joint space ventrally and dorsally and of retroarticular space in between for one or two dorsally located images.

A considerable amount of variation exists:

1. Segmental variants can occur with unilateral or bilateral accessory articulation of large transverse processes of the lowest lumbar vertebra with the sacral ala (hemilumbarization, hemisacralization, incomplete sacralization of L5, or incomplete lumbarization of S1). These accessory articulations are prone to premature degenerative disease and may be a reason for onset of low back pain in early and middle adulthood.
2. Some patients show a sulcus or even a canal at the dorsal surface of the posterior process of the iliac bone in close vicinity to the joint margin. On CT or MRI, this sulcus or canal will appear as a small groove and should not be confused with an erosion. To confirm diagnosis, this irregularity can be followed on multiple images.
3. The form of the joint facet itself is highly variable, with flat, curved, and wavy surfaces.

Pathology

Early features of sacroiliitis are *synovitis* and *subchondral bone marrow inflammation*. Synovitis in MRI is characterized by thickening and contrast enhancement in the synovial and capsular structures, reflecting these structures' hyperemia and vascular permeability. This feature is, however, not very conspicuous, because in the sacroiliac joint the capsule is tight and marginally attached, and therefore in tomographic techniques the capsule appears as merely a tiny dot-like structure at the joint margin.

Subchondral bone marrow inflammation—osteitis—in AS is highlighted in short tau inversion recovery (STIR) or spectral presaturation inversion recovery (SPIR) MR images and is described as "bone marrow edema"; rather, it is granulation tissue, or infiltration by inflammatory cells, and/or hyperemia. Contrast material uptake in the corresponding area is typical. On CT, neither synovitis nor early osteitis is visible. Later osteitis leads to sclerosis and is then visible on both CT and radiography. The sclerosis is cloudy and ill defined.

With further disease progression, the subchondral granulation tissue erodes through the joint cartilage into the joint space, penetrating the calcified zone of the cartilage and producing *central erosions*. On MRI, erosions appear as contrast-enhancing defects in the subchondral bone. Intra-articular granulation tissue is the reason for contrast enhancement in the joint space itself. The erosion process progresses to widespread destruction of the subchondral bone and cartilage. Bony erosions are easily visible in CT. On radiography, early erosions are inconspicuous due to superimposition. Blurring of the joint margins may be the only sign of early erosions. Later, discrete erosions become visible with loss of the subchondral white line and an appearance of a widened joint space.

Irregular endochondral ossification and subsequent replacement of subchondral bone and calcified cartilage by new bone leads to intra-articular ankylosis. CT is the best imaging tool for visualization of *osseous bridging and intra-articular ankylosis*. In late stages of complete or partial ankylosis, the inflammatory signs completely fade away, leaving behind normal lamellar bone that will eventually replace parts of the joint space. Therefore, in late stages, no contrast enhancement or bone marrow edema is found on MRI. On radiographs the sclerosis, which is a sign of periarticular osteitis, disappears.

In contrast to the intra-articular erosive and ankylosing arthritis of AS, osseous bridging of capsuloligamentous structures at the margin of the synovial sacroiliac joint (capsular ankylosis) is very common in elderly individuals. These ossifications are best visualized on CT, which clearly demonstrates the osseous encapsulation of an otherwise normal joint. On radiographs, superimposition effects lead to a faint sclerosis at the upper sacroiliac joint. This capsular ankylosis should not be mistaken for inflammatory disease.

In addition to affecting the synovial part of the sacroiliac junction, AS may cause enthesitis of the ligamenta sacroiliaca interossea in the retroarticular space. Pathology of ligamentous attachments may occur in degenerative disease as well; this is referred to as fibro-ostosis. In radiographic imaging, both degenerative and inflammatory enthesitis in the retroarticular space are occult, due to superimposition. In the synovial sacroiliac joints as well as in the hip joints, enthesitis does not appear to be prominent at any stage.[27]

The hallmark of AS, as well as its pathologic feature in many other locations is *enthesitis*.[28] It begins with an erosive phase, followed by a defective healing, with new bone formation resulting in a bony irregular prominence. The inflammatory hyperemia leads to hyperintensity on STIR images and contrast enhancement. The described bony irregular prominence forms a new enthesis, which corresponds to a radiographically visible spur.[29] As the inflammatory process relapses, the bony outgrowth can finally bridge, resulting in a capsular bony ankylosis, for example, at an apophyseal joint. At the intervertebral discs, the annulus fibrosus is affected by this type of bone-producing inflammation. The bony prominence corresponds to the well-known syndesmophyte. The final stage is a circularly ossified annulus fibrosus providing an osseous casing for the disc. When it is present at multiple levels it is referred to as a "bamboo spine." Additional or isolated central transdiscal ossification occurs as a result of either lack of motion or subsequent to the inflammatory process.

Typical enthesitis may take place in various locations: in joint capsules and intracapsular ligaments of large synovial joints, in the ligamentous structures of a synchondrosis (cartilaginous joints like symphysis, manubriosternal joint, intervertebral discs), and in overall ligamentous attachments.

BIOMECHANICS

The vertebral column provides both firm support for the body and considerable mobility for bending and torsion. These diametrically opposed tasks are achieved through the vertebral column's construction as a chain of small, joined elements. The junctions of the vertebrae regulate movement. The apophyseal joints are positioned symmetrically dorsal to the vertebral bodies. Because their facets are obliquely oriented, the apophyseal joints of both sides work together to provide hinge-like movements for ventral or lateral flexion/extension and sliding movement for axial torsion. The extent, limitation, and direction of movements are determined mostly by the angle between the joint spaces of the bilateral joints.

Ventrally, the annulus fibrosus attaches the adjacent vertebrae tightly, limiting the movement of the vertebrae, and encasing the nucleus pulposus. The latter functions like an elastic ball that distributes compressive forces (e.g., of weight bearing and bending) equally over the entire vertebral end plate.

The microarchitecture of a vertebral body, with its dense three-dimensional trabeculation of cancellous bone, adapts perfectly to weight bearing in different postures, such as inclining, reclining, axial torsion, and lateral flexion. In an immobile ankylosed spine, the weight bearing takes place in static segments. The nucleus pulposus no longer distributes the forces to the end plate nor from there to the cancellous bone. Instead, the cortical shell of the vertebrae, the syndesmophytic bridges, and the ossified columns of the apophyseal joints transmit the weight along the axial skeleton.

Bone is a living tissue, and its structure is remodeled due to mechanical requirements. Vertical load application in an immobile body segment is best adapted with cortical long bones. Thus, the structural remodeling of the primarily inflammatory ankylosed spine bears some resemblance to a long bone: the cancellous bone is eliminated and replaced by a fat-containing marrow canal. The cortical shell is reinforced and broadened. The end plates are partially reabsorbed, completing the bamboo-like appearance.

Because the typical vertebral microstructure is completely rearranged in the bamboo spine, the aspect of vertebral fractures, either due to trauma or in osteoporosis, differs from those in normal individuals. Specifically, the "bamboo spine" is infrequently affected by compression/wedge-shaped fractures but is relatively prone to slice and Chance fractures. A marked thoracolumbar kyphosis is a point of decreased mechanic stability and, together with osteoporosis, it is a risk factor for transvertebral or transdiscal fractures.

In an ankylosed spine, posture deterioration and stiffness attract the physician's attention and cause a great deal of discomfort to the patient. The thoracolumbar kyphosis in long-standing disease forces the patient to compensate by hyperextending the cervical spine (with consequent muscular pain) to provide forward vision. In addition, the shock-absorbing quality that is provided by the physiologic double S-form of the mobile vertebral column is lost; therefore, running, jumping, or skipping may produce discomfort.

IMAGING TECHNIQUES

Techniques and Relevant Aspects

The first-line method remains radiographic imaging despite its known low sensitivity for early arthritis.[30,31] There is no radiographic projection that provides a purely tangential view of the joint space, because of the curved shape of the joint facets. On anteroposterior views, only relatively short and individually different segments of the joint contours are outlined. In clinical practice, in back pain patients with suspected AS, anteroposterior and lateral views of the lumbar spine should be taken. The anteroposterior view must include the sacroiliac joints and their surroundings. Only in severe lumbosacral hyperlordosis may an additional Barsony (Ferguson) view be necessary.

Tomographic techniques such as MRI and CT show the complicated anatomy of the sacroiliac joint and are able to close the diagnostic gap between symptom onset and objective changes. CT images should be acquired primarily in paracoronal orientation, which is facilitated with the patient prone, and requires breath-hold technique. Three-millimeter slices using a helical scan with a pitch of approximately 1.5, 140 kVp, and 250 mAs are recommended. Obese patients may require a higher dose (mAs) to prevent a low signal-to-noise ratio. Multidetector CT provides a more comfortable examination in supine position, with slice thicknesses of 1 to 2.5 mm and multiplanar reformatted imaging in a paracoronal angulation.

Sacroiliac STIR or T2*- and T1-weighted MR images should be acquired in paracoronal (paratransversal) orientation tilted in plane with the sacrum and with long repetition time/echo time images in an oblique transverse plane perpendicular to the paracoronal images. For optimal visualization of the pathology, contrast-enhanced images are recommended, either with high-resolution technique and fat saturation or as a dynamic examination with a time resolution of 1 to 2 minutes to assess the activity of the inflammatory process.[32]

Pros and Cons

Radiography is known to be insensitive in early sacroiliitis. However, it is inexpensive, reliable, and quick; it provides the diagnosis in typical cases and gives additional information about lumbar inflammatory manifestations. Thus, radiographic imaging provides an advantageous overview of the disease spread and is useful to confirm or exclude other causes of back pain.

Bone scintigraphy is very sensitive to any osteoblastic process, but it lacks the specificity to fulfill the requirements for a powerful diagnostic tool in the diagnosis of sacroiliitis.

MRI uniquely combines a high degree of anatomic information and visualization of inflammatory activity. It is the best imaging tool for early diagnosis especially in young patients. CT shows equally high anatomic resolution and provides even better information about bony erosions and osseous bridges. It seems to be advantageous in middle-aged patients with marked sclerosis and for the differential diagnosis of diffuse idiopathic skeletal hyperostosis (DISH). Because arthritis is only detected when bony erosions or bridges are present, the sensitivity of CT for early diagnosis is inferior to that of MRI.

Controversies

Computed tomography of the sacroiliac joints is not an established procedure in all rheumatologic centers. Because of its superior sensitivity, MRI is most commonly preferred. Whether CT can serve as a powerful tool depends on the patient population; for example, it can be helpful in examining patients of middle or higher age with long-standing back pain. In these patients, the arthritis is usually advanced, producing unmistakable bony changes.

Studies of contrast uptake over time have been proposed to differentiate simple reactive bone marrow edema from osteitis. Reactive edema, due to causes such as degenerative disease or asymmetric weight bearing, is characterized by lower peak enhancement and slower uptake. Dynamic sequences are often optimized for speed rather than resolution; subsequent imaging of the joint with high resolution and fat saturation allows for better morphologic evaluation of the inflammatory features of the entire joint.

MANIFESTATIONS OF THE DISEASE

Sacroiliitis

The imperative diagnostic clue for AS is the radiographic proof of sacroiliitis (i.e., grade II bilaterally or grade III unilaterally). Radiologic grading is as follows[33,34]:

0: Without abnormality
1: With suspicious findings
2: With minor abnormalities
3: With definite abnormalities
4: With ankylosis

Radiography

Sacroiliitis is characterized by a triad of erosion, sclerosis, and the bony bridges that mark the beginning of ankylosis.[35] These three findings should be visible at the same time.

Erosions

The first aspect of sacroiliitis is a certain obscuration of the joint outlines, which is actually only in part due to erosion and in part due to bony bridging. Radiographically definite erosions mainly become visible as dentate ill-defined contours in the caudad portion of the joint. If the erosive component is prominent, a "string of pearls" appearance with pseudo-widening of the joint space may result (Fig. 49-1A and B).

Differential diagnosis of sacroiliac joint erosions comprises:

● Hyperparathyroidism in which sclerosis is not present
● Bacterial infection that is mostly unilateral and does not fulfill the triad
● (In cases of indistinct contours) the normal unfused physis in adolescence

Sclerosis

Rheumatic sacroiliitis is associated with various degrees of sclerosis. Typically it involves not only the caudad but also the middle portion of the joint. It is broad and woolly and more pronounced in the iliac bone (see Fig. 49-1A and B).

Differential diagnosis of sacroiliac sclerosis comprises:

● Osteitis condensans ilii, associated with childbirth, which is typically triangular in configuration, relatively well delineated, and often bilateral[36]
● Anterior capsular ossification in DISH, which produces a sclerosis in the cranial third of the joint

Bony Bridges and Ankylosis

Radiographs do not show individual bony bridges. Early bony bridging leads to blurring of the joint outlines and may be relatively difficult to detect, because only various parts of the joint space are visible even in normal individuals. Progressive partial ankylosis is detected easily in follow-up studies. Even if no previous examinations are available for comparison, partial ankylosis can be suspected when only minor parts of the joint contours

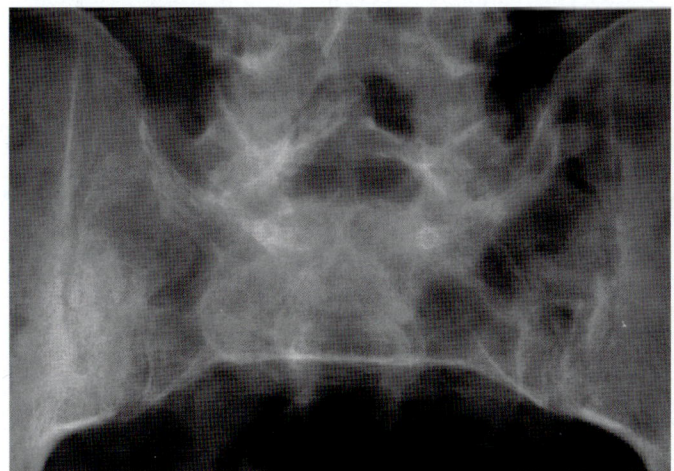

A

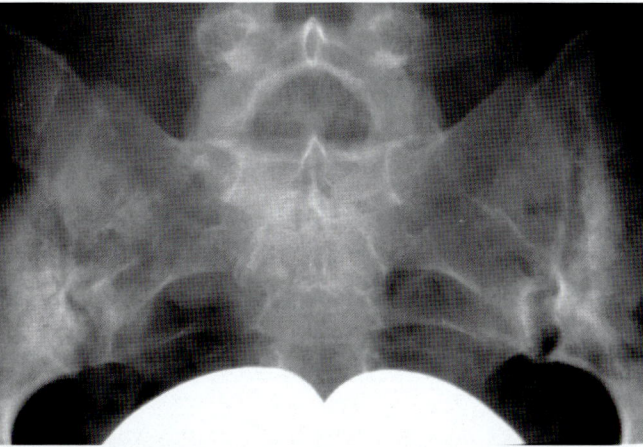

B

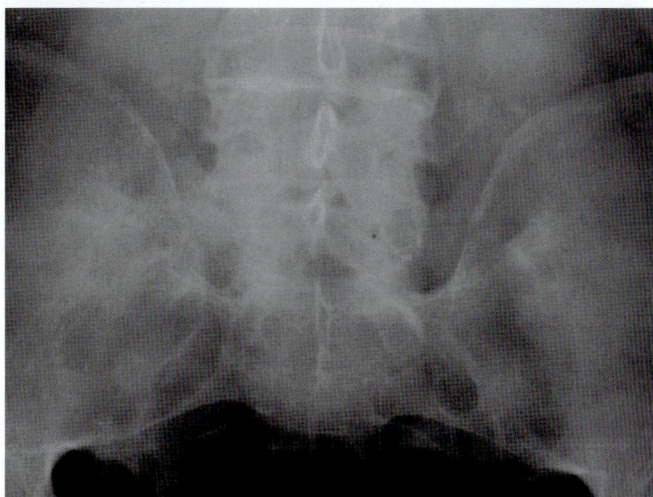

C

■ **FIGURE 49-1** Sacroiliitis is the hallmark of ankylosing spondylitis. The triad of sclerosis, erosion, and bony bridges is diagnostic. Early arthritis is often not very conspicuous on radiography. **A,** Asymmetric sclerosis and indistinct joint margins. **B,** Pseudodilatation and "string of pearls" erosions are typical. **C,** Late-stage sacroiliitis is characterized by complete ankylosis. The sclerosis fades away and normal bone replaces the entire joint. The ventral capsular insertion may be seen as a sclerotic triangle, which is known as the star sign.

are detected. Ankylosis is present when no joint space is visible (see Fig. 49-1C). In long-standing ankylosis, the sclerotic bone reaction fades away and normally structured bone replaces the joint.

Magnetic Resonance Imaging

The occurrence of STIR/T2-weighted hyperintense and T1-weighted hypointense zones in the marrow surrounding the sacroiliac joint, the so-called bone marrow edema, is a nonspecific sign in that it is associated with fracture, traumatic joint disruption, asymmetric weight bearing, degenerative disease, tumor, or inflammation. MRI is so sensitive to this process in AS, and the finding persists for so long after the inciting event, that it is not suitable for the estimation of disease activity. Nevertheless, it is one feature of sacroiliitis and adjacent osteitis and appears often as an indistinct rim around a center of para-articular sclerosis (Fig. 49-2).

On MRI, sclerosis appears as hypointensity on T2-weighted and T1-weighted images. It begins at the iliac side and may later affect the sacrum. The joint margins grow indistinct with increasing sclerosis. Bone marrow edema may be masked by extensive sclerosis. Sclerosis is a marker of chronicity and can be detected in degenerative disease as well.[32]

In chronic joint affliction, patchy areas of para-articular fat accumulation can be detected para-articularly in the sacrum and ilium (see Fig. 49-2). In sacroiliitis, para-articular fat accumulation is not as pronounced as after irradiation and it is more focal than in long-term corticosteroid medication. Para-articular fat accumulation may occur also in degenerative disease and with asymmetric weight bearing. The features of para-articular fat accumulation may be similar to the features of Modic type II disc degeneration.[37]

Bone marrow edema, sclerosis, and para-articular fat accumulation are typical but not specific for sacroiliitis. In sacroiliitis, all three signs often occur together and in middle and late stages are arranged in a certain pattern: the sclerosis is directly para-articularly located (with preference for the ilium) and is surrounded by an indistinct rim of bone marrow edema. Areas of fat accumulation are found in para-articular segments that are not affected by sclerosis or bone marrow edema, and there is some predilection for the sacrum.

Joint effusion (intra-articular fluid signal) may be present in sacroiliitis, in traumatic joint disruption, in fracture with joint affection, and in degenerative disease.

The diagnostic clue for sacroiliitis is the erosion that is a contrast material–enhancing defect of the subchondral bone. The diagnosis is certain when multiple erosions are

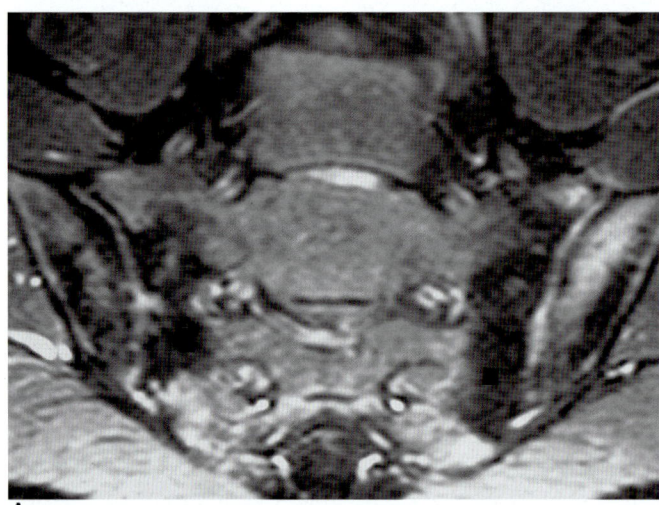

A

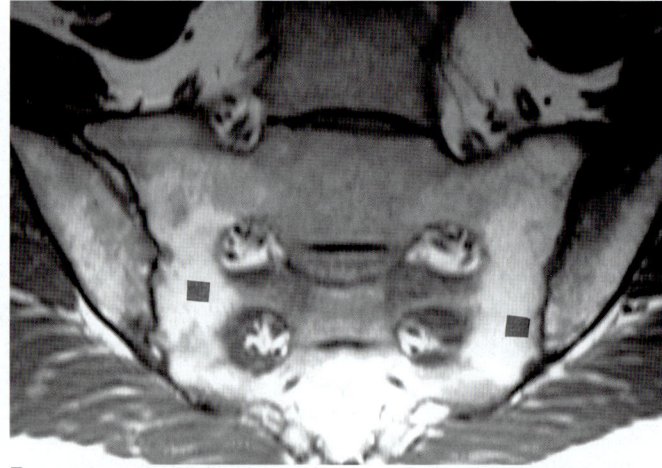

B

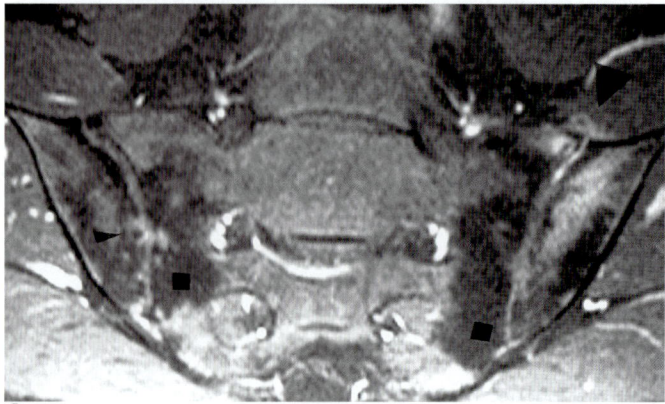

C

■ **FIGURE 49-2** MRI findings in sacroiliitis. Para-articular bone marrow edema in the left posterior iliac process (**A**, paracoronal STIR image), intra-articular fluid signal, erosions (**C**, *small arrowhead*, paracoronal contrast-enhanced T1-weighted, spin-echo, fat-saturated image), bony bridges, and capsular enhancement (**C**, *large arrowhead*) are typical for sacroiliitis. Fat accumulation (■) and sclerosis are signs of chronic disease and best visualized in short repetition time/echo time pulse sequences (**B**, T1-weighted turbo spin-echo image).

visible. Early arthritis is probable when two separate erosions are visible (see Fig. 49-2). A typical pitfall is to mistake vessels in the retroarticular space (especially in the dorsally located paracoronal images) for intra-articular lesions, but correct identification occurs on examining the next and prior images.

Typically, contrast enhancement is seen in the joint space itself, in the joint capsule, in erosions, and in the para-articular bone; the latter is considered to be juxta-articular osteitis. Retroarticular enhancement or pathologic T2 hyperintensity and contrast medium uptake in the posterior process of the iliac bone are not necessarily associated with sacroiliitis but are frequent in AS patients due to enthesitis. In patients with degenerative disease, these indicate ligamentous attachment disease.

Signs of bacterial infection that should *not* be mistaken for rheumatic sacroiliitis include enhancement of the periarticular soft tissue, especially ventrally; skip lesions of osseous enhancement; soft tissue fluid accumulations; and abscesses or sinus tracts.

Multidetector Computed Tomography

Computed tomography makes visible the complex anatomy of the sacroiliac joint. Careful consideration should be given to the discrimination of the retroarticular from the articular space. The articular space is identified by the two parallel lines of the subchondral bone with typical distance. In the more dorsally located images, the C shape of the joint leads to a projection phenomenon, with articular space (cranial and caudal) and retroarticular space in between (Fig. 49-3A). Contour irregularities of the os ilium and sacrum in the retroarticular space are normal but, if extensive, are called fibro-ostosis. Fibro-ostosis may be part of DISH.

As in radiographs, the triad erosions, bony bridges/ankylosis and sclerosis are the diagnostic clues for sacroiliitis. With tomography, the joint space is freely visible, and iliac erosions and bony bridges, as well as sclerosis,

are easily detected (see Fig. 49-3).[38,39] Sacral lesions tend to appear later in the disease course. Demineralization of the os sacrum is frequent in patients with long-standing AS.

Ultrasonography

Ultrasonography is not well established in the diagnostic pathway of sacroiliitis. In children, bulging ligamentous and capsular contours and hypoechoic articular structures may be found.

Nuclear Medicine

In the 1970s there were attempts to close the diagnostic gap between symptom onset and diagnosis of AS by means of scintigraphy.[40,41] To distinguish the normal registration of the sacroiliac joints from inflammatory disease, it had been necessary to develop a quantification technique. With this technique, the specificity for early arthritis of the sacroiliac joint in selected patients with HLA-B 27 and inflammatory back pain seemed to be acceptable. However, the subsequent development of CT offered complete display of the joint space without superposition effects, outstripping the scintigraphic efforts by far. The only advantage of scintigraphy over CT is the superior detection of the osteoblastic activity that may indicate sacroiliitis. At present, MRI equals scintigraphy in sensitivity and display of inflammatory features and exceeds it in revealing anatomic changes and specificity. The scintigraphic technique has developed over time as well, and single positron emission CT (SPECT) has been found to be useful in revealing inflammatory foci of the complete spine in AS patients.[42,43] Even special techniques like immunoglobulin G scintigraphy have been tried for diagnosis of AS, but in clinical practice nuclear medicine is of limited use for the primary diagnosis of sacroiliitis, especially because MRI is widely available. Nevertheless, bone scintigraphy can show inflammatory foci of the complete skeleton and therefore can direct the following workup to these foci.

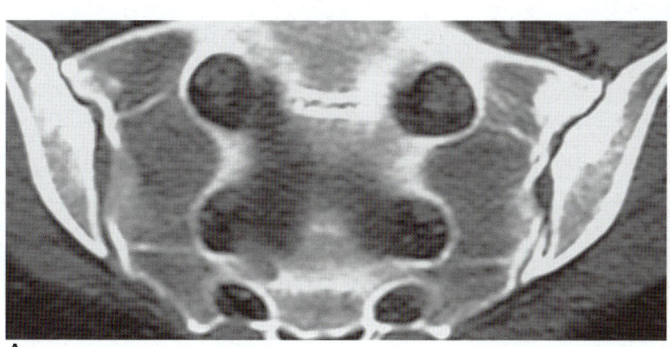
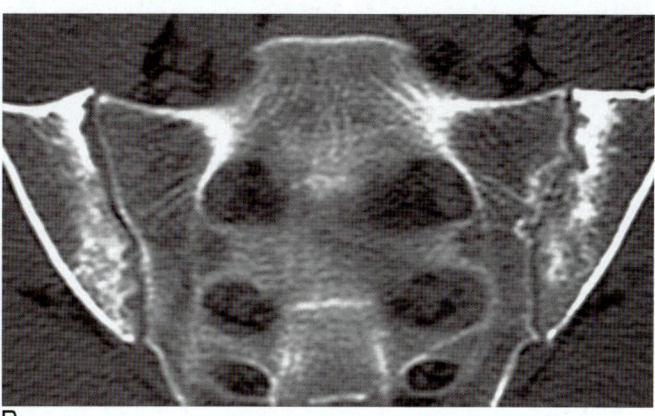

A   B

■ **FIGURE 49-3** CT findings in sacroiliitis. Differential diagnosis of para-articular sclerosis is the so-called hyperostosis triangularis ossis ilii (HTI), which is typically sharply delineated and triangular (**A**). Diagnostic pitfall is a section phenomenon of the retroarticular space that is due to the C shape of the articular surface. Thus, in paracoronal angulation there are often images with articular space ventrally and dorsally and retroarticular space in between that may simulate intra-articular erosion (**A**). Some patients show a sulcus in the proximity of the joint space, which should not be mistaken for an erosion (**A**). In arthritis, erosions are intra-articularly located and produce a dentate joint contour. Bony bridges develop intra-articularly, too. Para-articular woolly sclerosis may be of variable amount (**B**, same patient as Figure 49-1B).

Positron Emission Tomography/Computed Tomography

The combination of PET/CT is not universally available and is exceptionally expensive. Therefore, it is not in the routine diagnostic pathway for sacroiliitis.

Arthroscopy

Arthroscopy is not performed for the diagnosis of sacroiliitis.

Classic Signs

■ Radiography: Triad of sclerosis, erosions, and bony bridging/ankylosis
■ MRI: Joint effusion, adjacent bone marrow edema, para-articular sclerosis, periarticular fat accumulation, contrast material uptake in the joint space, erosions, para-articular bone (osteitis), capsular structures

---

VERTEBRAL MANIFESTATIONS

Vertebral manifestations in AS include:

● Syndesmophytes
● Apophyseal joint ankylosis

● Discovertebral inflammation (spondylitis marginalis, Romanus lesion, Andersson lesion A = discitis, rheumatic spondylodiscitis)
● Square vertebra, barrel-shaped vertebra
● Enthesitis and ligament ossification.

Radiography

The characteristic feature of spine involvement in AS is the syndesmophyte, which grows from the vertebral body corner in the exact position of the anulus fibrosus (Figs. 49-4A and 49-5). This is in contrast to its degenerative counterpart, the spondylophyte, which originates from the lateral or ventral aspect of the vertebral body near the corner. The syndesmophyte progressively bridges the intervertebral space circularly. Multisegmental involvement of complete circular annulus fibrosus ossification is called "bamboo spine" and is typical of the late stages of AS. The affected discs often show dystrophic calcification. Ankylosis of the spine mostly develops in a kyphotic posture of the thoracolumbar region. If the inflammatory process takes place in primarily degenerated discs, the form of the syndesmophyte may be modified, with a more bulging contour corresponding to a mixture of spondylophyte and syndesmophyte. Sometimes, syndesmophytic growth begins consecutively in a Romanus lesion. Syndesmophytes are best visualized by radiography.

Discovertebral inflammation (discitis, rheumatic spondylodiscitis) is another typical manifestation in AS. According to Cawley, three types are possible:

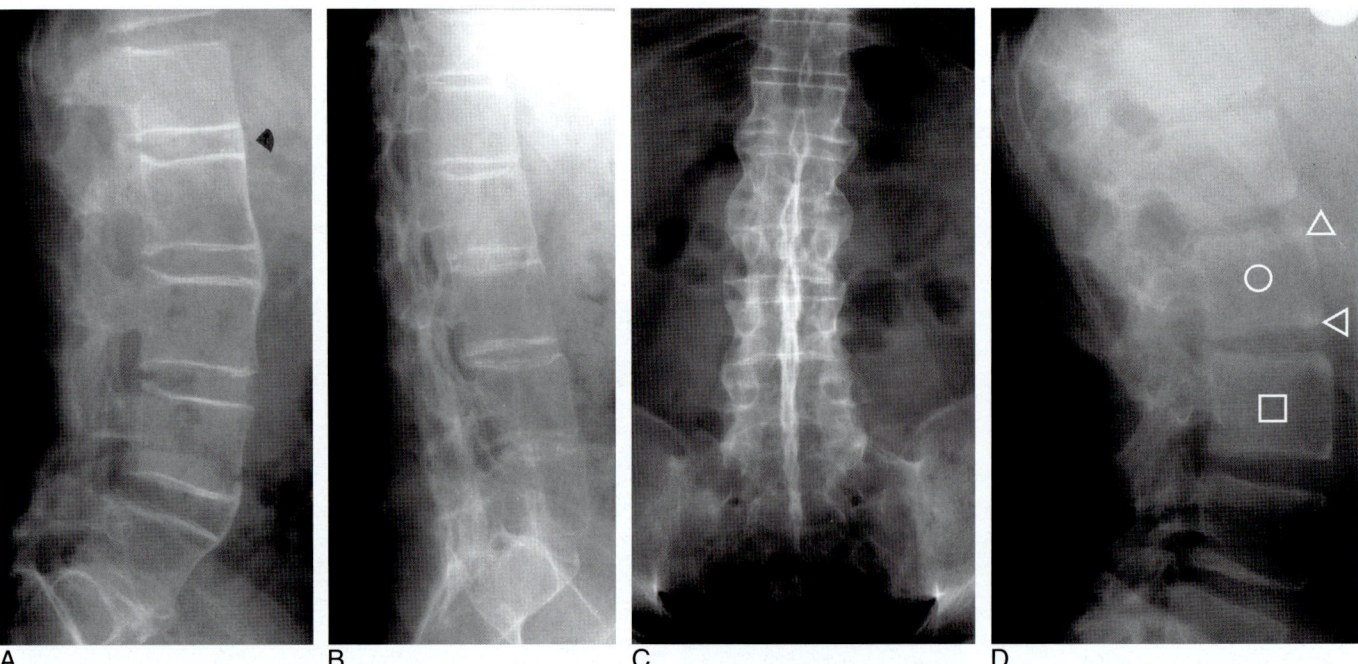

A   B   C   D

■ **FIGURE 49-4** Radiographic findings in ankylosing spondylitis. The syndesmophyte is the characteristic intervertebral osteophyte in ankylosing spondylitis. **A,** In contrast to the spondylophyte in degenerative disease, it grows vertically, as shown in this lateral view of the lumbar spine in a 32-year-old man with a 10-year history of ankylosing spondylitis (*arrowhead*). **B,** Especially in adolescent-onset ankylosing spondylitis the apophyseal joint ankylosis is pronounced with broad bands of ossification in this lateral view in a 45-year-old man with approximately 30 years of symptoms who was diagnosed at the age of 28. **C,** This ossification produces the so-called trolley track sign in the anteroposterior view. **C,** Dagger sign refers to multisegmental ossification of the interspinous ligaments. **D,** Square vertebra (□) and barrel-shaped anterior vertebral aspect (○) are additional characteristic features of ankylosing spondylitis. Multisegmental vertebral corner sclerosis is often detected in the thoracolumbar junction segments. Without erosion it is called "shiny corner" (△). A Romanus lesion consists of a vertebral corner sclerosis with an erosion of the vertebral end plate also corresponding to a Cawley lesion type II.

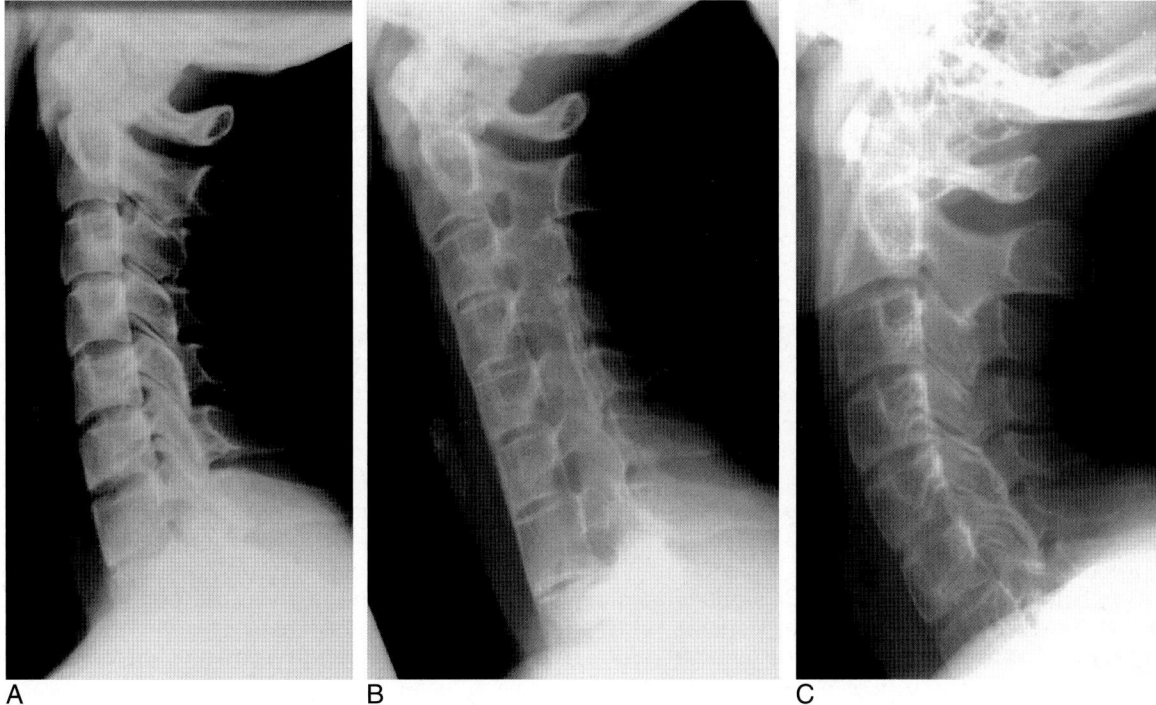

A   B   C

■ **FIGURE 49-5** Radiography of the spine in ankylosing spondylitis. Cervical involvement is very frequent and leads to significant movement restriction. Syndesmophytes as well as apophyseal joint ankylosis may develop over years. **A,** The lateral view of the cervical spine in a 25-year-old woman with onset of ankylosing spondylitis shows square vertebrae and apophyseal joint space narrowing as a sign of minor cervical inflammatory affection. **B,** Example of complete multisegmental ankylosis by means of syndesmophytes and apophyseal joint arthritis. **C,** Barrel-shaped vertebrae are characteristic and may develop not exclusively in the lumbar spine.

Type I: localized central lesions (cartilaginous nodules)
Type II: localized peripheral lesions (Romanus lesions)
Type III: extensive central and peripheral lesions (fracture with pseudarthrosis, Andersson lesion B)

The Romanus lesion is confined to the anterior upper or inferior corner of the vertebra and occurs mainly in the lumbar region. It is characterized by a triangular sclerosis and an erosion of the anterior vertebral end plate and corresponds to Cawley type II (see Fig. 49-4D). Similar lesions at the posterior vertebral corners are referred to as spondylitis marginalis. A faint sclerosis at the anterior vertebral corner (a minimal variant of the Romanus lesion) has been termed "shining corner." Romanus lesions tend to resolve over years and "heal" with syndesmophyte formation. They are found mainly in younger patients.

Erosions or destructions of the subdiscal bone resemble spondylodiscitis and are called Andersson lesion type A or inflammatory type. Unlike the destruction caused by bacterial spondylitis, the destruction in rheumatic disease remains mild, focal, and unchanged for months or even years. In clinical practice, the diagnosis is based on plain films. The predilection site of rheumatic spondylodiscitis in AS is the thoracolumbar region. Typically it is found in the first decade of the disease. Approximately in 10% of AS patients radiographs show end-plate erosions, depending on the age of the patient. However, MRI is much more sensitive for rheumatic discitis; in fact, mild manifestations are often radiographically occult.[44,45] The lesions are in most cases asymptomatic; therefore, MRI is not necessarily indicated.

In the past, the Andersson lesion type B was described in connection with the rheumatic spondylodiscitis (Andersson lesion type A) due to a certain radiographic similarity.[46] Today it is considered to correspond to a malunion or nonunion of a transdiscal insufficiency fracture in a multisegmental vertebral column ankylosis. Consequently it is found in late-stage disease. It is a rare but grave diagnosis. Risk factors for the development of an Andersson lesion type B are osteoporosis, marked thoracolumbar kyphosis, and (minimal or repeating) trauma. The predilection site is the thoracolumbar region. The lesions are painful, and patients report a newly arisen mobility after a minor trauma. The prognosis for local control is moderate. Primarily the lesion can be very difficult to detect, especially if no previous films are available (e.g., in case of a formerly complete, now incomplete syndesmophytic bridging). The dorsal vertebral elements are usually involved. A transverse lamina fracture is most conspicuous in an anteroposterior projection. The lateral projection may show unisegmental dehiscence of the spinous processes. In Andersson lesion type B, vertebral end-plate destruction is a result of fragment resorption and appears as subchondral bone defects or erosions in radiographic images. In long-standing nonunion, the destruction of the subdiscal bone is much more pronounced than in Andersson lesion type A. The surrounding sclerosis is a reactive feature and its extent depends on the mobility in the fracture/pseudarthrosis.

Square vertebra and barrel-shaped vertebra are the result of inflammatory and osteoproliferative affection of the ventral vertebral aspect (see Fig. 49-5C).

Apophyseal joint ankylosis is the result of either a capsular ossification due to enthesitis or of an erosive arthritis. On radiographs this feature is not very conspicuous, especially in early involvement. Then it is responsible forthose cases with considerable vertebral column movement restriction and relatively unremarkable radiographic results. In late stages, broad ossification bands over the dorsolateral aspect of the vertebral column are seen. In the anteroposterior view they correspond to two parallel bands of sclerosis, a phenomenon called the tramlines sign (see Figs. 49-4B and C and 49-5).

Subaxial cervical spine involvement is very frequent and may precede thoracic involvement. In contrast to rheumatoid arthritis, involvement of the craniocervical junction in AS is relatively uncommon. In patients with complete syndesmophytic and apophyseal joint ankylosis of the cervical spine, the rest of cervical mobility is provided in C0-C2. Nevertheless, there are patients with atlantoaxial ligament destruction typically followed by ventral subluxation of the atlas. *Subluxation* is defined as a distance between the anterior arch of the atlas and the anterior contour of the odontoid process exceeding 3 mm. In AS patients with this deformity, the risk for subsequent myelopathy seems to be higher than in rheumatoid arthritis and the risk increases with the degree of subluxation.

Ligament ossifications such as of the ligamentum interspinale and ligamentum iliolumbale occur in late stages of ankylosing spondylitis. Predilection sites is the ligamenta interspinalia, in which polysegmental ossification is called the "dagger sign."

Magnetic Resonance Imaging

Magnetic resonance imaging is the most sensitive and accurate diagnostic tool for discovertebral inflammation, but because it lacks therapeutic relevance, it is not routinely indicated. Individually MRI may be employed for differential diagnosis of localized pain when radiographic imaging results are equivocal or for detection of inflammation before TNFα-blockage.

Romanus lesions are characterized by triangular bone marrow edema of the anterior upper vertebral corner and by an erosion. The erosion consists of a small defect of the ventral vertebral end plate. After administration of a contrast agent the defect and the adjacent subdiscal bone show considerable enhancement. In chronic lesions, T2 hyperintensity and contrast agent uptake completely fade away. T1-weighted images display fat accumulation of the bone marrow in a typically triangular configuration at the anterior upper or lower vertebral corner. In long-standing disease, multilevel triangular fat accumulation at the vertebral corners is common (Fig. 49-6).

Andersson lesions type A resemble Schmorl's nodes of Scheuermann's disease with central end-plate defects and a rim of adjacent bone marrow edema. There is usually moderate contrast material enhancement in the subdiscal bone, in the erosion, and in the disc itself (see Fig. 49-6).

Andersson lesions type B typically cause massive edema of the bone marrow and perivertebral soft tissue. The fracture line is hyperintense in STIR images. Bone fragments of the end plates appear as dotted hypointense structures in all pulse sequences. The posterior elements are involved, and fractures of the apophyseal joint processes, or of the lamina and spinous process, are highlighted. Intensive contrast material enhancement is displayed in the surroundings of the fracture.

Costotransversal and costovertebral joint arthritis give rise to persistent thoracolumbar pain and cause respiratory movement restriction. In radiographic images, this feature is mostly occult; therefore, MRI is the best method for assessing these joints. One drawback, however, is that standard MR images of the thoracic spine may result in false-negative readings. In sagittal angulation, the far lateral images show the adjacent bone marrow edema and effusion of the costovertebral joints as a faint, rounded, ill-defined hyperintensity at the upper third of the vertebral body. Transversal images show bone marrow edema/osteitis in the vertebral body and the caput costae, joint effusion, synovial hypertrophy, and contrast medium enhancement (see Fig. 49-6).

Syndesmophytes are not conspicuous in MRI. The new bone formation appears just as hypointense as the normal annulus fibrosus. Rarely, active inflammatory foci are seen as tiny dots of contrast material enhancement.

Enthesitis of the ligamenta interspinalia are highlighted in STIR images and in contrast enhanced studies as hyperintensities in the ligamentous attachments and in the adjacent bone (see Fig. 49-6).

Multidetector Computed Tomography

Computed tomography shows spinal manifestations as well as other modalities do, but because it lacks therapeutic impact, it is rarely necessary when radiography is available. In some cases of Andersson lesions type B, helical scans with sagittal multiplanar reformatted images may be employed. The fracture line, bony defects, reactive sclerosis, and dorsal element involvement can be easily assessed.

Ultrasonography

For vertebral manifestations, ultrasonography is not beneficial.

Nuclear Medicine

In bone scintigraphy and SPECT, abnormalities of the thoracic and lumbar vertebral spine are frequently identified in patients with AS. Most often, facetal joint uptake is found at multiple sites. The other common site of uptake is in the vertebral bodies. These hot spots usually correspond to inflammatory foci such as capsular ossifying enthesitis or arthritis of the apophyseal joints and Romanus/Andersson lesions type A, respectively.[43] Scintigraphy may be helpful in the early detection of pseudarthrosis (Andersson lesion B) when MRI is not available or is contraindicated.[47]

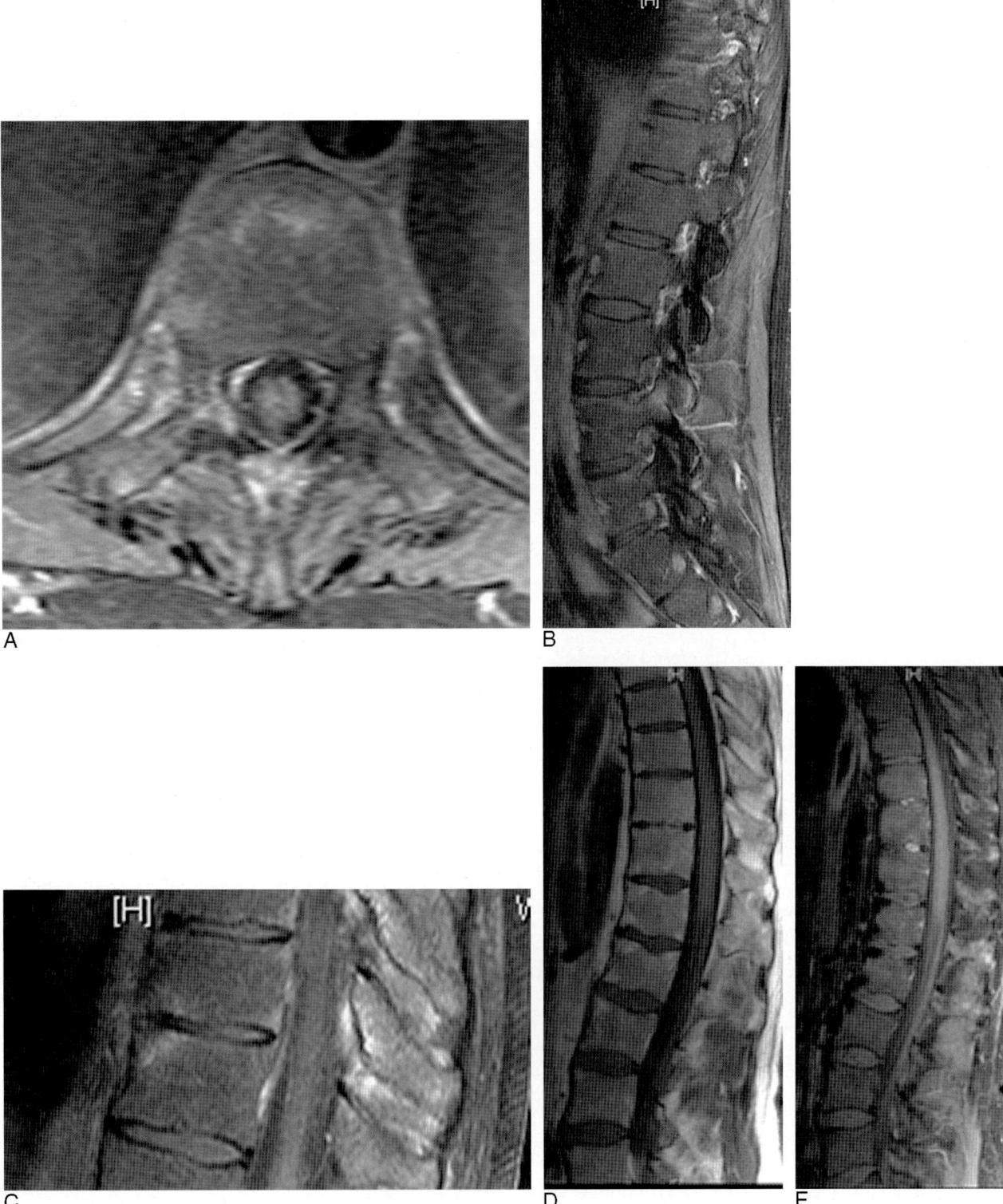

■ **FIGURE 49-6**   MRI of vertebral involvement in ankylosing spondylitis. **A,** Transverse T1-weighted fat-saturated, contrast-enhanced MR image of the costovertebral joints shows intraosseous contrast enhancement (osteitis), erosions and synovitis in costovertebral arthritis. **B,** Multisegmental apophyseal joint arthritis in the chronic stage is characterized by hypointensity due to sclerosis and absence of uptake of contrast material. In active arthritis (L3/4), enhancement is present (sagittal T1-weighted, fat-saturated, contrast-enhanced). **C,** Romanus' lesions (discovertebral inflammatory affection type Cawley II) show triangular enhancement of the upper or lower vertebral body corner (T1-weighted, fat-saturated, contrast enhanced). Note enhancement in and between the spinous processes represents enthesitis. In the chronic stage of Romanus lesions the enhancement fades away and is replaced by fat signal, a phenomenon that is frequently multisegmental (precontrast [D] and postcontrast [E] T1-weighted images).

Classic Signs

SYNDESMOPHYTES

■ Radiography: marginal intervertebral osteophyte
■ MRI: inconspicuous

ROMANUS LESIONS

■ Radiography: triangular sclerosis of the anterior upper vertebral corner (Cawley II) and end-plate erosion
■ MRI:
❑ Active: STIR hyperintense/contrast-enhancing erosion at the anterior upper vertebral corner
❑ Chronic: triangular fat accumulation in the vertebral corner

ANDERSSON LESION A

■ Radiography: central vertebral end-plate defect, minor involvement occult
■ (Cawley I) MRI:
❑ Enhancing central end-plate defects (often multilevel)
❑ Discal enhancement
❑ Subdiscal bone marrow edema and enhancement

ANDERSSON LESION B

■ Radiography: transdiscal insufficiency fracture/malunion (Cawley III), transverse lamina fracture
❑ In early stages, inconspicuous
❑ In late stages, considerable destruction and sclerosis
■ MRI: hyperintense fracture line (STIR/T2) adjacent edema, and contrast enhancement

APOPHYSEAL JOINT ANKYLOSIS

■ Radiography: at early stages, inconspicuous; at late stages, broad ossification, trolley track sign

COSTOTRANSVERSAL AND COSTOVERTEBRAL ARTHRITIS

■ Radiography: occult
■ MRI: edema in bone marrow and in capsular structures; contrast enhancement in capsule, osteitis, erosions

ENTHESITIS OF LIGAMENTA INTERSPINALIA

■ Radiography: polysegmental ossification: "dagger sign"
■ MRI: hyperintensity/enhancement at the ligamentous attachments

Extravertebral Skeletal Manifestations

The inflammatory involvement of proximal joints is very frequent in AS. The most frequent site of involvement is the hip joint, followed by the shoulder and knee. Nevertheless, peripheral synovitis/erosive arthritis is well known. The overall characteristic of AS is the presence of enthesitis, which may be found near virtually any joint. Bursitis with involvement of the adjacent bone is also typical (e.g., at the Achilles tendon insertion). Synchondritis (inflammatory involvement of cartilaginous joints) is a frequent symptom at the manubriosternal junction or clinically silent at the symphysis pubis.

Radiography

In AS, the predilection sites of arthritis are the hips, knees, and shoulders. Periarticular demineralization, joint effusion, and diffuse joint space narrowing are the radiologic signs of arthritis. In contrast to rheumatoid arthritis, erosions are seldom seen. In a considerable number of patients, the radiographic signs of arthritis are not very conspicuous and premature degenerative disease (osteophyte formation) is the most prominent finding. In fact, concentric joint space diminution combined with osteophytosis is characteristic of hip disease in AS (Fig. 49-7).[48] Sometimes the inflammatory process is aggressive, and marked destruction develops in a few years. Postarthritic ankylosis at end stage is well known but not very frequent.

The small joints of the hands and feet as well as of the wrists are affected less frequently than large joints. The distribution tends to be asymmetric. In comparison, rheumatoid arthritis predominantly affects the lower extremity and the distal interphalangeal joints. Periarticular osteoporosis, soft tissue swelling, joint space narrowing, erosion, and destruction occur (see Fig. 49-7C). Sometimes postarthritic ankylosis can appear very soon after arthritic onset.

Enthesitis (fibro-ostitis, inflammatory affection of the ligamentous, tendinous, and capsular insertions) is the most characteristic sign of seronegative rheumatic disease. The predilection sites are the tubera ischiadica, trochanter, plantar calcaneal surface, triceps insertion, and patella, but enthesitis may affect virtually any attachment. Radiographically, the cortical lining disappears and an ill-defined erosion develops, forming a small groove. Subsequently, osteoproliferation with new bone formation in the groove and the surroundings takes place. The process relapses, and erosive and proliferative features are seen at the same time.

Symphysitis with erosion and prominent sclerosis is common. Further evaluation by other techniques is not necessary. Inflammatory involvement of the manubriosternal synchondrosis is characterized by soft tissue swelling, bony sclerosis, fuzzy contours, and erosions.

Bursitis compromising the underlying bone is most often seen at the Achilles tendon insertion (bursa subachillea), bursa trochanterica, and iliopsoas bursa. Soft tissue swelling is found in the typical places (see Fig. 49-7D). Pressure erosions of the bone and inflammatory destructions, as well as new bone formation, are possible. In fact, they are very common at the os calcis.

Magnetic Resonance Imaging

Magnetic resonance imaging is very sensitive and accurate for the detection of enthesitis, arthritis, and bursitis. Nevertheless, in clinical practice it is not really necessary for the diagnosis.

The characteristic feature of enthesitis is the edema (T2/STIR hyperintensity) and contrast medium enhancement in the surroundings of a capsular, ligamentous, or tendinous attachment. The ligament or tendon is often thickened and attenuated. The adjacent bone often shows signs of osteitis. Typical sites of affection seen in musculoskeletal MRI are the plantar calcaneal surface, the Achilles tendon insertion (often with associated bursitis), the tibial apophysis, the tubera ischiadica, the scapular triceps insertion, and similar structures.

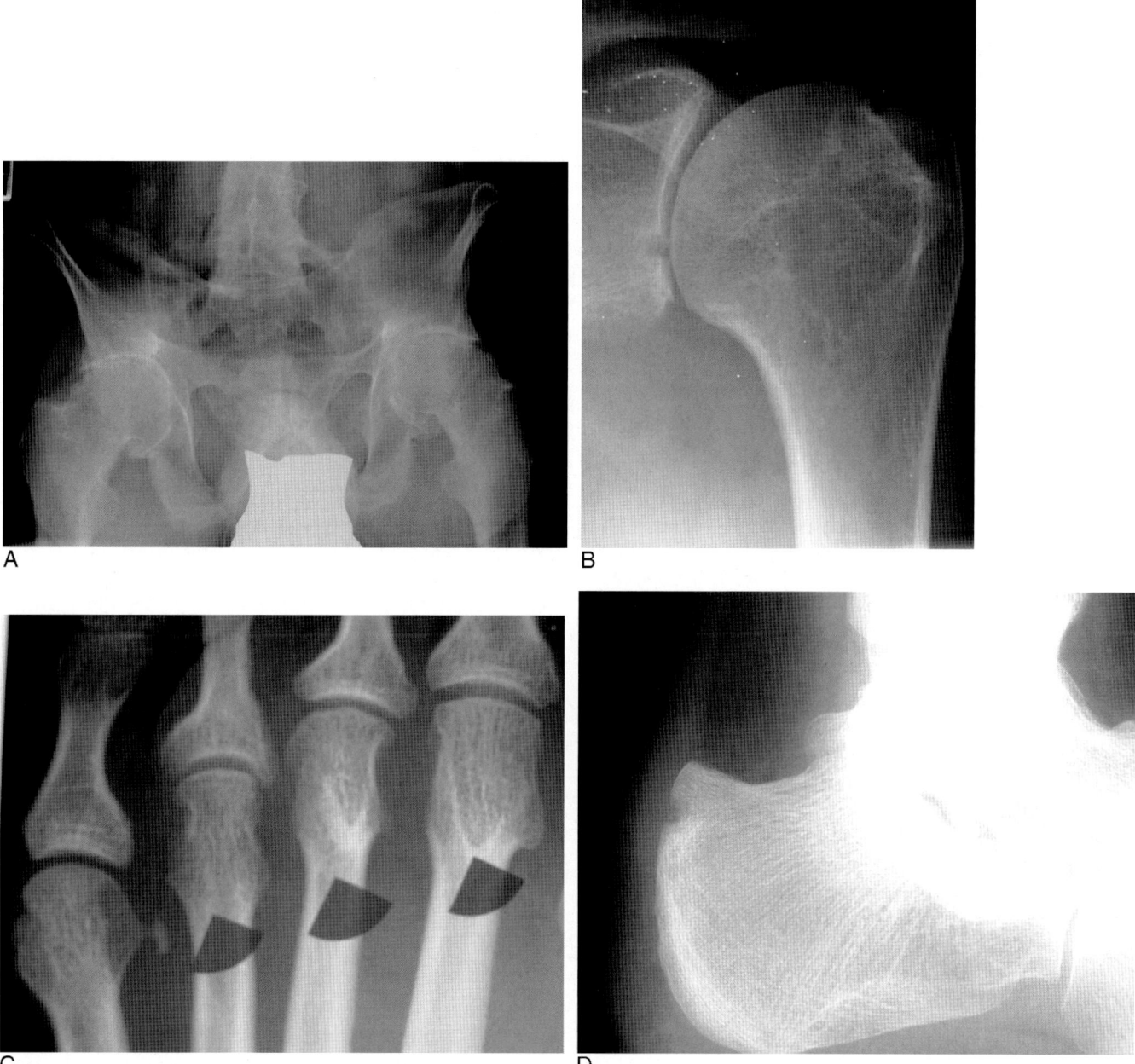

■ **FIGURE 49-7** Arthritis and enthesitis in ankylosing spondylitis. Proximal joint arthritis with involvement of hips and shoulders is typical. **A,** Arthritis often results only in mild premature degenerative disease with concentric joint space narrowing as a sign of cartilage destruction. Note the typical posture of the pelvis in a patient with ankylosing spondylitis and considerable fibro-ostosis of the ischial tuberosities. **B,** The shoulder is the second most frequent location of proximal joint involvement. Joint space narrowing and premature degenerative osteoarthritis are common. Erosions are found primarily marginal at the humeral head and at the glenoid, later in the central part of the joint. Peripheral arthritis is less frequent. In contrast to rheumatoid arthritis, it is more often asymmetric in distribution and also affects the distal small joints. **C,** In a number of patients, however, imaging features of peripheral arthritis do not differ from those of rheumatoid arthritis as shown in this 38-year-old man with metatarsophalangeal arthritis and long-standing ankylosing spondylitis. **D,** In retrocalcaneal bursitis, soft tissue swelling at the Achilles tendon insertion and a typical pressure erosion of the dorsal aspect of the calcaneus are present as shown in this 49-year-old man with an approximate 30-year history of ankylosing spondylitis.

In active arthritis, thickening and contrast medium enhancement in the synovial membrane and capsule as well as joint effusion are typical. The synovial membrane may show focal or diffuse thickening, nodules, or massive proliferations with intermediate signal in T1-weighted images. In rheumatoid arthritis, pannus is found with moderate frequency and extent. Various degrees of pannus activity are recognized according to their signal intensity: STIR/T2 hyperintensity and contrast medium uptake characterize active pannus; T2 hypointensity and lack of enhancement correspond to fibrous pannus. Erosions are contrast-enhancing focal defects of the subchondral bone. They can be recognized earlier than in radiographic imaging in the same predilection sites (bare areas, joint margins). In long-standing disease, secondary degenerative disease with smoothing of the eroded contours and spur formation occurs.

Bursitis, at the Achilles tendon insertion or the iliopsoas, for example, is characterized by an effusion that appears as a localized fluid collection surrounded by contrast-enhancing synovial lining in typical location.

Synchondritis manubriosternalis may be imaged by means of MRI. Respiratory motion and flow artifacts from the large vessels and heart may obscure the images if not carefully omitted. Coronal and sagittal angulations are recommended. STIR/T2 hyperintensity and contrast medium enhancement of the bone marrow of the manubrium and of the corpus sterni corresponding to osteitis, and of the intrathoracic and extrathoracic soft tissue, are typical, as are erosions of the cartilaginous joint itself.

Computed Tomography

Synchondritis manubriosternalis and arthritis of the sternoclavicular joints are easily imaged by means of CT with additional sagittal and coronal, curved multiplanar reformatted imaging. Bony erosions, sclerosis, and adjacent soft tissue swelling are typical. If the sclerosis and new bone formation are tremendous, the differential diagnosis of SAPHO syndrome arises. For SAPHO syndrome, the findings of ossification of the costoclavicular ligaments, cartilaginous ribs, and surrounding soft tissue and sclerosis and broadening of the affected bones are typical.

Ultrasonography

Especially in enthesitis and bursitis, ultrasonography is advantageous. Bursitis is characterized by fluid accumulation in typical locations. The echogenicity is mostly equivalent to fluid. However, fibrinous contents floating, or constant isoechogenic structures, are frequent. Isoechogenicity (with consequent difficulties for detection and evaluation) is possible. Enthesitis is characterized by thickening of the tendon or ligament and by hypoechogenicity and structure inhomogenity at the attachment and its surroundings.

Nuclear Medicine

Bone scintigraphy shows inflammatory foci as hot spots. It demonstrates the extent, activity, and sites of involvement. It may direct the diagnostic workup of certain foci. The therapeutic impact, however, remains limited.

Positron Emissions Tomography/Computed Tomography

The combination of PET/CT is not established in the routine diagnostic workup of AS.

Arthroscopy

Arthroscopy is not performed for diagnostic workup but as a therapeutic tool to perform a synovectomy (see later).

Classic Signs

ENTHESIS
- Radiography: fuzzy contoured grooves and osseous proliferations at muscular, ligamentous, capsular or tendon attachment sites
- MRI: Thickening and structure inhomogeneity of ligament or tendon; STIR/T2 hyperintensity, T1 intermediate signal/contrast enhancement in the preinsertional ligament or tendon, the surroundings, and the adjacent bone
- Ultrasonography: thickening and structure inhomogeneity/hypoechogenicity of the preinsertional ligament or tendon and in the surroundings

ARTHRITIS
- Radiography: joint effusion, periarticular demineralization, joint space narrowing, erosions, destruction. Secondary premature degenerative osteoarthritis
- MRI: joint effusion, thickening, T1-weighted intermediate signal and contrast enhancement of the synovial membrane, nodules, intra-articular pannus, erosions of the joint surface
- Ultrasonography: joint effusion, synovial thickening, pannus, erosions

BURSITIS
- Ultrasonography: fluid accumulation, echogenic structures

SYNCHONDRITIS MANUBRIOSTERNALIS
- Radiography: sclerosis, erosions
- CT: sclerosis, erosions, soft tissue swelling
- MRI: erosions, osteitis, soft tissue swelling

Osteoporosis

Despite the relatively young age of the patients and the male predominance, the incidence of osteoporosis in AS patients is high (18%-62%).[49,50] It increases in prevalence with patient age, disease duration, severity of vertebral involvement, and peripheral arthritis.[51] Unlike osteoporosis in rheumatoid arthritis patients, osteoporosis in AS patients is confined mostly to the axial skeleton. Osteoporosis significantly increases the risk of vertebral compression fractures as well as transdiscal and transvertebral insufficiency fractures (Andersson lesion B).[52] Therefore, AS patients should be considered as a high-risk group who will eventually need regular spinal bone mineral density (BMD) scans and therapy. However, measuring bone density is challenging. Dual-energy x-ray absorptiometry (DEXA) of the lumbar spine is affected by superposition due to syndesmophyte formation, sclerotic Romanus lesions, and apophyseal joint ankylosis with excessive bone formation especially in patients at risk (Fig. 49-8).[53,54] There have been different approaches to overcome this disadvantage, such as DEXA measurement of the hip, lateral projection DEXA of the third lumbar vertebra, quantitative CT (QCT), peripheral quantitative CT (pQCT), and calcaneal quantitative ultrasonography (QUS).[55-57] For DEXA measurement of the hip, the possibility of periarticular osteoporosis due to coxitis should be kept in mind. Lateral projection DEXA of only one vertebra has its limits for estimation of fracture risk of the whole axial

skeleton and is of minor reliability. Peripheral QCT allows no estimation of axial skeleton fracture risk in patients with AS.[50] QCT is unique in its ability to detect selectively cancellous bone loss without superimposition. It is much more sensitive, and therefore can be of use in detecting demineralization earlier than with other methods. In patients with AS, the loss of cancellous bone is often tremendous when lumbar affection is present (see Fig. 49-8). The fracture risk, however, is not increased to the same extent. Estimations of fracture risk by means of BMD measurements are based on normal microarchitecture and macroarchitecture of the spine. In longstanding AS, ankylosis of the dorsal elements (often with extensive bone formation and syndesmophytic growth, with bridging of the disc space as well as broadening

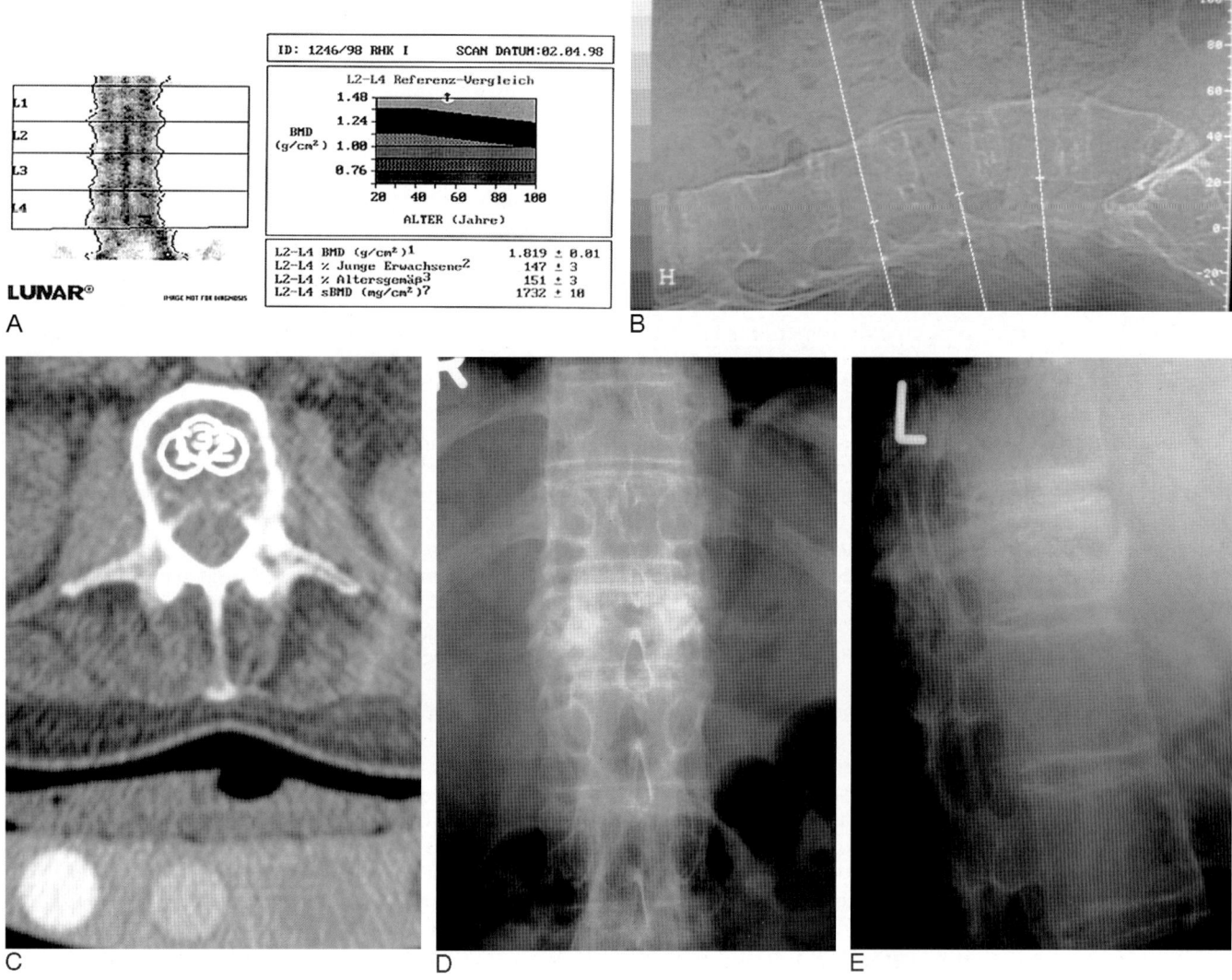

■ **FIGURE 49-8** Bone mineral density in AS. BMD measurement in a patient with long-standing disease and complete syndesmophytic ankylosis of the lumbar spine. **A,** The DEXA measurement of the lumbar spine displays high values. This result is probably not valid because of overlying syndesmophytes. **B** and **C,** Quantitative CT reveals a marked osteoporosis of the cancellous bone with 14 mg/mL hydroxyapatite equivalent. Such a very low BMD in the quantitative CT measurement is not uncommon in patients with ankylosing spondylitis. Sometimes the values are even negative owing to nearly complete transformation into fat. The cortical shell is in contrast broad and dense, reflecting new bone formation. Thus, the low BMD value does not represent the same fracture risk as in postmenopausal osteoporosis. For the fracture risk estimation in patients with ankylosing spondylitis apart from the BMD measurement factors that must be taken into consideration include the thoracolumbar kyphosis, the extent or absence of coarse new bone formation, the presence of spinal inflammatory activity, the peripheral joint affection, and a corticosteroid medication. **D** and **E,** Transvertebral fractures after minor trauma in a 46-year-old patient with a 30-year history of ankylosing spondylitis.

of the cortical shell of the vertebra) is present. The micro-architecture and macroarchitecture are completely altered, so that the formation of the vertebral bodies mimics that of the long bones. Hence, the weight and power transmission in the ankylosed vertebral column is different from that of normal individuals. Abnormal ossification contributes to load-bearing capacity.[58] This leads to different fracture mechanisms in trauma and to the unusual transdiscal or transvertebral form of AS-typical insufficiency fractures (Fig. 49-8D and E).

In spite of these limitations for clinical practice, BMD assessment by means of lumbar DEXA in patients with only minor radiographic abnormalities, by means of hip DEXA in patients without coxitis, and by means of QCT in patients with severe vertebral and hip affection will give sufficient information for estimation of fracture risk and decisions about therapy.

DIFFERENTIAL DIAGNOSIS

Low back pain in early adulthood may arise from degenerative disease (e.g., spondylolysis with spondylolisthesis), disc degeneration with protrusion, or asymmetric segmental variants.

In some patients nighttime attacks of low back pain and sacroiliac tenderness result from degenerative disease with enthesopathy of the dorsal sacral and iliac surface. Because radiographic imaging has a low negative predictive value for early diagnosis, tomographic techniques should be employed. Retroarticular fibro-ostosis is a relatively common finding in these patients. Stiffness of the lumbar and thoracic spine in elderly patients is commonly seen in DISH.

On radiography, the differential diagnosis of sacroiliitis comprises degenerative disease in DISH or triangular sclerosis, asymmetric weight bearing, the normal joints, and, in cases of pseudodilatation, hyperparathyroidism. Infectious arthritis of the sacroiliac joint is mainly unilateral and causes considerable destruction with minor sclerosis. Syndesmophytes can be distinguished from degenerative intervertebral osteophytes by their marginal growth. Andersson lesions should not be mistaken for bacterial spondylitis.

With sacroiliac CT, retroarticular fibro-ostosis and marginal sacroiliac irregularities may be a pitfall and should be carefully localized to distinguish them from erosions.

On sacroiliac MRI, bone marrow edema, joint effusion, para-articular fat accumulations, and sclerosis are unspecific features and may occur in degenerative osteoarthritis, asymmetric weight bearing, or post-traumatically. For the diagnosis of arthritis, central erosions of the joint surface should be visible. Bacterial sacroiliitis is characterized by soft tissue abnormalities, abscesses, sinus tracts, and skip lesions. Abnormalities in sacral insufficiency fractures are found medial to the joint space. The fracture line is usually visible in T1-weighted images.

On lumbar MRI, Andersson lesions B may resemble spondylitis. One should note the fracture line in the dorsal elements and the absence of epidural collections or paravertebral abscesses. Schmorl's nodes and Andersson lesions A have a striking resemblance to each other; some authors suggest that their pathogenesis is identical. Scheuermann's disease may be included in the differential diagnosis.

For the diagnosis of AS, the sacroiliitis is absolutely necessary. Patients with AS may show additional features of Scheuermann's disease. There is no therapeutic impact from additional diagnosis of Scheuermann's disease in a patient with AS.

On a scintiscan, tracer uptake in the sacroiliac region is not easy to interpret. In addition to normal conditions, it may indicate premature degeneration in the obese and in multipara or indicate asymmetric weight bearing due to scoliosis and sacroiliitis. Hot spots in the facetal joints or vertebrae are equivocal. Facetal hypertrophy, degenerative spurs, and other bone remodeling conditions may be the cause.

SYNOPSIS OF TREATMENT OPTIONS

Physiotherapy

Physiotherapy is the most important element in the therapeutic management of AS.[59] Symptom relief is achievable with exercise.[60] Because lifelong regular exercise is mandatory, major educational effort and constant reinforcement is crucial. Thus, from the moment of accurate diagnosis, the patient should undergo both an intensive educational program and a physiotherapeutic program. A thorough understanding of the disease and its management is the basis for building and maintaining the impetus for maximal self-care and appropriate lifestyle.

In the beginning, the patient should be referred for physiotherapy. The objective of the initial phase is to restore as much movement as possible. Hydrotherapy is particularly valuable.[61] A dedicated exercise regimen must be taught to the patient. It must include not only exercises for mobilization of the vertebral column and joints but also breathing exercises for better chest expansion. Passive stretching may help even in patients with long-standing disease. Because regaining lost movement causes discomfort in this early phase, pain relief should be attempted to allow full mobilization. Pulsed short wave, local heat or cold, interferential therapy, local ultrasonography, or transcutaneous nerve stimulation may be employed and adapted to the individual. Drug therapy will support these efforts. Psychologic training can lead to the development of pain-control strategies.[62]

The initial phase of therapy yields especially striking improvements in mobility and pain relief. This initial phase should be used to persuade the patients to establish long-term management habits. Lifelong maintenance of appropriate lifestyle and daily exercise is crucial for disease management. In the chronic phase, maximal self-care should be attempted and drugs should be cautiously prescribed. The objectives are to reduce pain and stiffness by self-management; to maintain symptom relief, posture, and movement; and to enable full work capacity. Educational efforts have an extraordinary impact on the success of disease management in the chronic phase. Understanding, help, and support of the family members is important. For that reason, the family should also receive educational advice. Joining self-help groups may support these efforts. Repeated supervision of the exercises by a physiotherapist has been proven to improve the persistence of a home exercise program.[62]

Medical Treatment

Pain relief is the primary goal of most patients. Pain is difficult to estimate, and many patients add analgesics without prescription, without knowledge of the treating physician. Analgesic medication is needed especially in the initial phase to allow maximal mobilization. Nonsteroidal anti-inflammatory drugs (NSAIDs) such as indomethacin, diclofenac, or naproxen are the first choice. Local problems of enthesitis may be addressed with local corticosteroid injections if needed.

In the chronic phase, drug therapy should be minimal and exercise should be used as the first choice to reduce pain. If no relief is achieved despite appropriate exercise, NSAIDs can support the regimen.

Systemic therapy with corticosteroids for short-term control of severe symptoms is effective. Long-term corticosteroid medication is not recommended for AS patients. Local corticosteroid injections for peripheral joints and enthesitis can be helpful. The risk for tendon rupture as a complication is increased by local corticosteroid application.

Despite their use in cases of RA, disease-modifying anti-rheumatic drugs (DMARDs) are not entirely proven to be valuable for AS. With sulfasalazine there is evidence of short-term efficacy in peripheral synovitis. The use of sulfasalazine should be considered in patients with poor response to physical treatment and NSAIDs and persistent inflammatory activity as evident by laboratory results. Low dose therapy with methotrexate appears to have an effect on peripheral joints and spinal disease but should be used only in cases of severely active and unremittingly progressive disease. Tumor necrosis factor-α blockade studies are promising in a hope for genuine disease retardation. Its efficacy seems to be very encouraging. Currently, it is indicated only in severe active cases and progressive cases and otherwise uninfluenced early cases. Its exact role in the medical management of AS remains to be defined.

Surgical Treatment

Synovectomy is performed for local control of lingering inflammatory activity unresponsive to drug therapy, such as inflammation in the knee or the ankle joint. The objective is to avoid destruction of the cartilage, bone, capsule, ligaments, and tendons. The procedure is usually performed arthroscopically in early stages or as open synovectomy in advanced cases.

Endoprosthetic reconstruction is the predominant procedure in advanced joint destruction and severe postinflammatory degenerative osteoarthritis. It is performed very frequently at the hip or knee. For the hip, cementless replacement offers good long-term results in the young patient population in which necessity of frequent revision surgery must be anticipated. For the knee, bicondylar resurfacing prostheses in cases of stable ligaments or constrained prostheses for instable ligaments or varus/valgus malalignment are available.

Spinal surgery for posture improvement may be indicated in select patients with severe kyphosis and consequent alteration of their forward vision. The procedure is associated with considerable risk of neurologic damage and should therefore only be performed in highly specialized centers.

The upper cervical segments remain mostly unaffected in AS and provide a rest of movement. In some cases, however, atlantoaxial subluxation occurs. The risk for subsequent myelopathy is higher in AS than in rheumatoid arthritis, in which this deformity is much more common. Severe headache and occipital numbness are two of the symptoms of impending neurologic damage. In these patients, cervical fusion is required.

What the Referring Physician Needs to Know

- Early accurate, confident diagnosis of sacroiliitis
- Vertebral manifestation and extent of ankylosis
- Presence of Andersson lesion type B (transdiscal insufficiency fracture)
- Enthesitis/arthritis of proximal or peripheral joints

SUGGESTED READINGS

Resnick D, Niwayama G. Ankylosing spondylitis. In Resnick D, Niwayama G eds). Diagnosis of Joint and Bone Disorders, 2nd ed. Philadelphia, WB Saunders, 1988, pp 1103–1170.

Russell AS, van der Linden S, van der Heijde D, et al. Ankylosing spondylitis. In Hochberg MC, Silman AJ, Smolen JS, et al (eds). Rheumatology. Amsterdam, Elsevier, 2003, pp 1145–1224.

REFERENCES

1. Dougados M, van der Linden S, Juhlin R, et al. The European spondyloarthropathy study group preliminary criteria for the classification of spondyloarthropathy. Arthritis Rheum 1991; 34:1218–1227.
2. Moll JM, Wright V. New York clinical criteria for ankylosing spondylitis. Ann Rheum Dis 1973; 32:354–363.
3. Moll JM, Haslock I, McRae IF, Wright V. Associations between ankylosing spondylitis, psoriatic arthritis, Reiter's disease, the intestinal arthropathies, and Behçet's syndrome. Medizine 1974; 53:343–364.
4. Helliwell PS, Hickling P, Wright V. Do the radiological changes of classic ankylosing spondylitis differ from the changes found in the spondylitis associated with inflammatory bowel disease, psoriasis and reactive arthritis? Ann Rheum Dis 1998; 57:135–140.
5. Zhang Y, Guerassimov A, Leroux JY, et al. Arthritis induced by proteoglycan aggrecan G1 domain in *BALB/c* mice: evidence for T-cell involvement and the immunosuppressive influence of keratan sulfate on recognition of G and B cell epitopes. J Clin Invest 1998; 101:1678–1686.
6. Mikecz K, Glant TT, Baron M, Poole AR. Isolation of proteoglycan-specific T Lymphocytes from patients with ankylosing spondylitis. Cell Immunol 1988; 112:55–63.

7. Glant T, Mikecz K, Arzoumanian A, Poole AR. Proteoglycan-induced arthritis in *Balb/c* mice. Arthritis Rheum 1987; 30:201-212.
8. Carter ET, McKenna CH, Brian DD, Kurland LT. Epidemiology of ankylosing spondylitis in Rochester, Minnesota 1935-1973. Arthritis Rheum 1979; 22:365-370.
9. van der Linden SJ, van der Heijde S. Ankylosing spondylitis: clinical features. In Yu D (ed). Spondyloarthropathies. Rheum Dis Clin North Am 1998; 24:663-676.
10. Khan MA. HLA and ankylosing spondylitis. In Calabro JJ, Carson Dick W (eds). Ankylosing Spondylitis: New Clinical Applications. Lancaster, MTP, 1987, pp 23-44.
11. Mielants H, Veys EM, Goemaere S, et al. A prospective study of patients with spondyloarthropathy with special reference to HLA-B27 and to gut histology. J Rheumatol 1993; 20:1353-1358.
12. van der Linden SM, Valkenburg HA, De Jong BM, Cats A. The risk of developing ankylosing spondylitis in HLA-B27 positive individuals: a comparison of relatives of spondylitis patients with the general population. Arthritis Rheum 1984; 27:241-249.
13. Calin A, Kaye B, Sternberg M, et al. The prevalence and nature of back pain in an industrial complex: a questionnaire and radiographic and HLA analysis. Spine 1980; 5:201-205.
14. Underwood MR, Dawes P. Inflammatory back pain in primary care. Br J Rheumatol 1995; 34:1074-1077.
15. Brandt J, Bollow M, Haberle J, et al. Studying patients with inflammatory back pain and arthritis of the lower limbs clinically and by magnetic resonance imaging: most but not all patients with sacroiliitis have spondyloarthropathy. Rheumatology 1999; 38:831-836.
16. Linssen A, Feltkamp TE. B27 positive diseases versus B27 negative diseases. Ann Rheum Dis 1988; 47:431-439.
17. Derhaag DJ, De Waal LP, Linssen A, Feltkamp TE. Acute anterior uveitis and HLA-B27 subtypes. Invest Ophthalmol Vis Sci 1988; 29:1137-1140.
18. van der Linden SM, Rentsch HU, Gerber N, et al. The association between ankylosing spondylitis, acute anterior uveitis and HLA-B27: the results of a Swiss family study. Br J Rheumatol 1988; 27(Suppl 2):39-41.
19. Paivonsalo-Hietanen T, Vaahtoranta-Lehtonen H, Tuominen J, Saari KM. Uveitis survey at the University Eye Clinic in Turku. Acta Ophthalmol Copenh 1994; 72:505-512.
20. Mennell JB. Physical Treatment by Movement, Manipulation and Massage. London, Churchill Livingstone, 1977, p 328.
21. Schober P. Lendenwirbelsäule und Kreuzschmerzen. Münch Med Wochenschr 1937; 84:336-428.
22. Moll JMH, Wright V. An objective study of chest expansion. Ann Rheum Dis 1972; 31:1-8.
23. Archer IA, Moll JM, Wright V. Chest and spinal movement in ankylosing spondylitis. Rheumatol Rehabil 1974; 13:30-31.
24. Cats A, van der Linden SJ, Goei The HS, Khan MA. Proposals for diagnostic criteria of ankylosing spondylitis and allied disorders. Clin Exp Rheumatol 1987; 5:167-171.
25. Mau W, Zeidler H, Mau R, et al. Outcome of possible ankylosing spondylitis. Clin Rheumatol 1987; 6(Suppl 2):60-66.
26. Mau W, Zeidler H, Mau R, et al. Clinical features and prognosis of patients with possible ankylosing spondylitis: results of a 10-year follow up. J Rheumatol 1988; 15:1109-1114.
27. Francois FJ, Gardner DL, Degrave EJ, Bywaters EGL. Histopathologic evidence that sacroiliitis in ankylosing spondylitis is not merely enthesitis. Arthritis Rheum 2000; 4:2011-2024.
28. Ball J. Enthesopathy of rheumatoid and ankylosing spondylitis. Ann Rheum Dis 1971; 30:213-223.
29. Benjamin M, Rufai A, Ralphs JR. The mechanism of formation of bony spurs (enthesophytes) in the Achilles tendon. Arthritis Rheum 2000; 43:576-583.
30. Forrester DM. Imaging of the sacroiliac joints. Radiol Clin North Am 1990; 28:1055-1072.
31. Dale K, Vinje O. Radiography of the spine and sacroiliac joints in ankylosing spondylitis and psoriasis. Acta Radiol Diagn 1985; 26:145-159.
32. Bollow M, Braun J, Hamm B, et al. Early sacroiliitis in patients with spondyloarthropathy: evaluation with dynamic gadolinium-enhanced MR imaging. Radiology 1995; 194:529-536.
33. Bennett PH, Burch TA. New York symposium on population studies in the rheumatic diseases: new diagnostic criteria. Bull Rheum Dis 1968; 17:453-458.
34. van der Linden SJ, Valkenburg HA, Cats A. Evaluation of diagnostic criteria for ankylosing spondylitis: a proposal for modification of the New York criteria. Arthritis Rheum 1984; 27:361-368.
35. Dihlmann W. Radiologic Atlas of Rheumatic Diseases. Stuttgart, Thieme, 1986.
36. Resnick D, Niwayama G, Goergen TG. Comparison of radiographic abnormalities of the sacroiliac joint in degenerative disease and ankylosing spondylitis. AJR Am J Roentgenol 1977; 128:189-196.
37. Modic MT, Masaryk TJ, Ross JS, Carter JR. Imaging of the degenerative disk disease. Radiology 1988; 168:177-186.
38. Carrera WF, Foley WD, Kozin F, et al. CT of sacroiliitis. AJR Am J Roentgenol 1981; 136:41-46.
39. Fam AG, Rubenstein JD, Chin-Sang H, Leung FY. Computed tomography in the diagnosis of early ankylosing spondylitis. Arthritis Rheum 1985; 28:930-937.
40. Lentle BC, Russell AS, Percy JS, Jackson FI. Scintigraphic findings in ankylosing spondylitis. J Nucl Med 1977; 18:524-528.
41. Lentle BC, Russell AS, Percy JS, Jackson FI. The scintigraphic investigation of sacroiliac disease. J Nucl Med 1977; 18:529-533.
42. Jacobsson H, Larsson SA, Vesternkold L, Lindvall N. The application of single photon emission computed tomography to the diagnosis of ankylosing spondylitis of the spine. Br J Radiol 1984; 57:133-140.
43. Ryan PJ, Gibson T, Fogelman I. Spinal bone SPECT in chronic symptomatic ankylosing spondylitis. Clin Nucl Med 1997; 22:821-824.
44. Kenny JB, Hughes PL, Whitehouse GH. Discovertebral destruction in ankylosing spondylitis: the role of computed tomography and magnetic resonance imaging. Br J Radiol 1990; 63:448-455.
45. Wienands K, Lukas P, Albrecht HJ. Clinical value of MR tomography of spondylodiscitis. Z Rheumatol 1990; 49:356-360.
46. Dihlmann W, Delling C. Disco-vertebral destructive lesions (so-called Andersson lesions) associated with ankylosing spondylitis. Skeletal Radiol 1978; 3:10-15.
47. Peh WC, Hoh WY, Luk KD. Application of bone scintigraphy in ankylosing spondylitis. Clin Imaging 1997; 21:54-62.
48. Resnick D, Niwayama G: Ankylosing spondylitis. In Resnick D, Niwayama G (eds). Diagnosis of Joint and Bone Disorders, 2nd ed. Philadelphia, WB Saunders, 1988, pp 1103-1170.
49. Mitra D, Elvins DM, Speden DJ, Collin AJ. The prevalence of vertebral fractures in mild ankylosing spondylitis and their relationship to bone mineral density. Rheumatology 2000; 39:85-89.
50. Bessant R, Keat A. How should clinicians manage osteoporosis in ankylosing spondylitis? J Rheumatol 2002; 29:1511-1519.
51. Ralston SH, Urquhart GD, Brzeski M, Sturrock RD. Prevalence of vertebral compression fractures due to osteoporosis in ankylosing spondylitis. BMJ 1990; 3:563-565.
52. Devogelaer JP, Maldague B, Malghem J, et al. Appendicular and vertebral bone mass in ankylosing spondylitis: a comparison of plain radiographs with single- and dual-photon absorptiometry and with quantitative computed tomography. Arthritis Rheum 1992; 35:1062-1067.
53. Donnelly S, Doyle DV, Denton A, et al. Bone mineral density and vertebral compression fracture rates in ankylosing spondylitis. Ann Rheum Dis 1994; 53:117-121.
54. Sivri A, Kilinc S, Gokce-Kutsal Y, Ariyre KM. Bone mineral density in ankylosing spondylitis. Clin Rheumatol 1996; 15:51-54.
55. Karberg Z, Zochling J, Sieper J, et al. Bone loss is detected more frequently in patients with ankylosing spondylitis with syndesmophytes. J Rheumatol 2005; 32:1290-1298.
56. Gilgil E, Kacar C, Tuncer T, Butun B. The association of syndesmophytes with vertebral bone mineral density in patients with ankylosing spondylitis. J Rheumatol 2005; 32:292-294.
57. Jansen TL, Aarts MH, Zanen S, Bruyn GA. Risk assessment for osteoporosis by quantitative ultrasound of the heel in ankylosing spondylitis. Clin Exp Rheumatol 2003; 21:599-604.
58. Andresen R, Werner HJ, Schober HC. Contribution of the cortical shell of the vertebrae to mechanical behaviour of the lumbar vertebrae with implications for predicting fracture risk. Br J Radiol 1998; 71:759-765.
59. Kraag G, Stokes B, Groh J, et al. The effects of comprehensive home physiotherapy and supervision on patients with ankylosing spondylitis—a randomised controlled trial. J Rheumatol 1990; 17:228-233.
60. Wynn Parry CB. Physical measures of rehabilitation. In Moll JMH (ed). Ankylosing Spondylitis. Edinburgh, Churchill Livingstone, 1980, pp 214-226.
61. Tishler M, Brostovski Y, Yaron M. Effect of spa therapy on patients in Tiberias with ankylosing spondylitis. Clin Rheumatol 1995; 1:21-25.
62. Haslock I. Ankylosing spondylitis: management. In Hochberg MC, Silman AJ, Smolen JS, et al (eds). Rheumatology. Amsterdam, Elsevier, 2003, pp 1211-1224.

50

Progressive Scleroderma

Karsten Jablonka and Jürgen Freyschmidt

ETIOLOGY

Progressive scleroderma (progressive systemic sclerosis) is one of the collagen vascular diseases, which makes it one of the systemic autoimmune disorders. Collagen vascular diseases include:

- Progressive systemic sclerosis (progressive scleroderma)
- Systemic lupus erythematosus
- Polymyositis and dermatomyositis
- Sjögren's syndrome
- Jo-1 syndrome
- Mixed connective tissue disease (Sharp's syndrome)
- Undifferentiated inflammatory systemic connective tissue disease
- Relapsing polychondritis

These diseases have in common a fibrinoid degeneration of the connective tissues. Typical features are clinical overlap phenomena and non–organ-specific autoantibodies.

PREVALENCE AND EPIDEMIOLOGY

Scleroderma is a rare disease with an estimated prevalence of about 1 new case per 100,000 persons per year. The peak incidence is between 30 and 50 years of age. About 90% of patients are female.

CLINICAL PRESENTATION

Clinical features include an insidious onset with Raynaud's phenomenon, shrinking of skin, especially of the fingertips (Madonna fingers) and the face (microstomia), and swallowing difficulties as a result of an immobilization of the esophagus or the small bowel. A claw-like deformity of the hands and "rat-bite" mutilations of the fingertips may occur. Soft tissue calcifications are common. These deposits can ulcerate through the skin. The sclerosis leads to a restricted mobility of the affected skin, including the tongue (Fig. 50-1). Other clinical features are poikiloderma, telangiectases, and alopecia; pulmonary arterial hypertension; pleurisy; and a pulmonary fibrosis.

The myocardial abnormalities that are associated with systemic sclerosis usually are subclinical. Pericarditis may develop. Vasculitis in the kidneys can lead to infarctions, hypertension, and loss of function. A distinct group of mostly female patients suffers from typical features of organ involvement of systemic sclerosis but show only limited or no skin involvement. Diffuse involvement of the skin is more typical for male patients.[1,2]

PATHOPHYSIOLOGY

Pathology

Activation of T cells, monocytes, and macrophages leads to a production of cytokines, stimulating fibroblast proliferation and leading to increased collagen synthesis. Additionally endothelial cell damage leads to intimal proliferation, which accounts for an occlusive vasculopathy. Ultimately, infarcts and necrosis occur in the skin, bone (typically osteolytic lesions), kidneys, and other organs.[3,4]

Variants of classic progressive systemic sclerosis are:

- Localized scleroderma (morphea): localized cutaneous sclerosis without involvement of internal organs
- CRESTA syndrome stands for calcinosis, Raynaud's phenomenon, esophageal dysfunction, sclerodactyly, telangiectasia, and arthritis (this supposedly has a better prognosis)
- Secondary progressive systemic sclerosis as a result of exposure to chemicals or certain drugs such as solvents, polyvinyl chloride, bleomycin, and many others.

KEY POINTS

- Hardening and retraction of skin
- Soft tissue calcifications
- Organ infarctions
- Soft tissue and bone necrosis

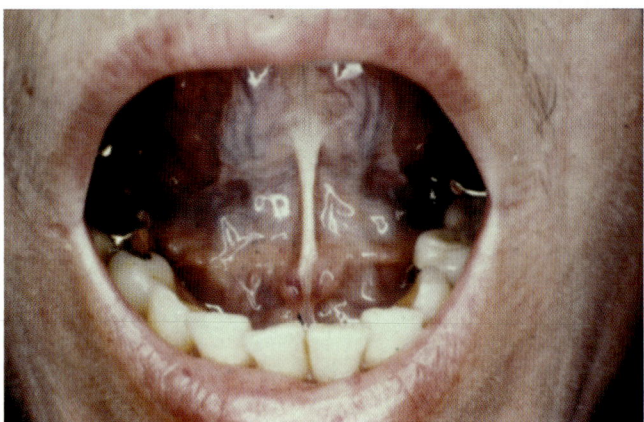

■ **FIGURE 50-1** Sclerosis of the frenulum of the tongue.

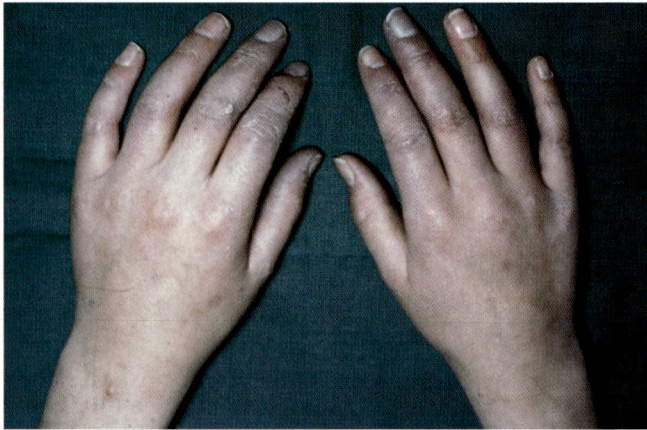

■ **FIGURE 50-2** Raynaud phenomenon of the first through third distal phalanges of the left hand and the second and third distal phalanges on the right, with fingertip necrosis and ulcerating calcification of the third distal phalanx on the left.

IMAGING TECHNIQUES

In typical cases of scleroderma the clinical diagnosis is straightforward. Radiography is the modality of choice to depict soft tissue calcifications and locate possible future ulcerations. Shrinking of soft tissues, especially the fingertips, is also detectable on radiographs.

MRI has been utilized for its ability to show sites of active inflammation that eventually will form necrosis and calcification. Organ involvement is visualized using an upper gastrointestinal series or abdominal CT or MRI.

MANIFESTATIONS OF THE DISEASE

Radiography

Flexion contracture is present in more than 90% of patients. The most prominent feature is a typical interstitial calcinosis (Thibierge-Weissenbach syndrome). Another feature is a diffuse osteoporosis of the hands with resorption of the distal phalanges and terminal tufts. Additionally, the bones of the wrist sometimes show fine osteolytic or cystic lesions.

Definition of atrophy of the soft tissues of the fingertips[5] has been described as when the distance from the edge of soft tissue of the fingertip to the end of the distal phalanx is less than 20% of the width of the base of the distal phalanx. In healthy individuals this ratio is at least 25% (Figs. 50-2 to 50-4).

Osteolytic foci and erosions may be seen in other skeletal regions (Figs. 50-5 and 50-6).

Computed Tomography

Computed tomography is advantageous to localize soft tissue calcifications and to characterize possible erosions and osteolytic foci.

Magnetic Resonance Imaging

Contrast-enhanced MRI is capable of showing sites of "active disease" with signs of edema that in the later stages of the disease will evolve into the chronic phase ("sclerosing disease").[6]

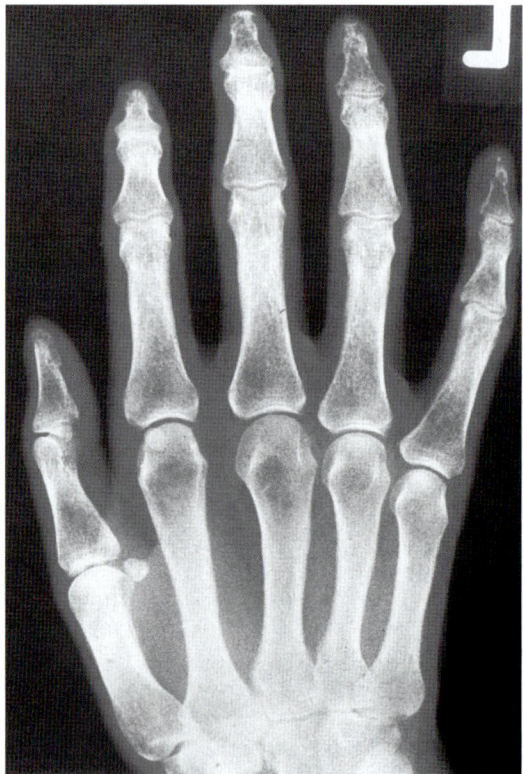

■ **FIGURE 50-3** Fingertip necrosis, with retraction of the fingertips.

Classic Signs

- Interstitial calcinosis (Thibierge-Weissenbach syndrome)
- Resorption of distal phalanges and terminal tufts
- May occur in other sites (e.g., ribs and spine)

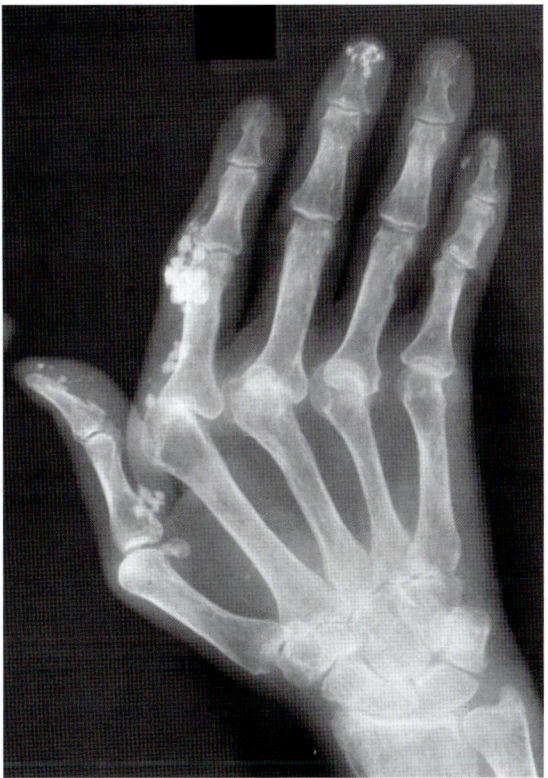

■ **FIGURE 50-4**   Soft tissue calcifications of the fingers (with ulnar deviation).

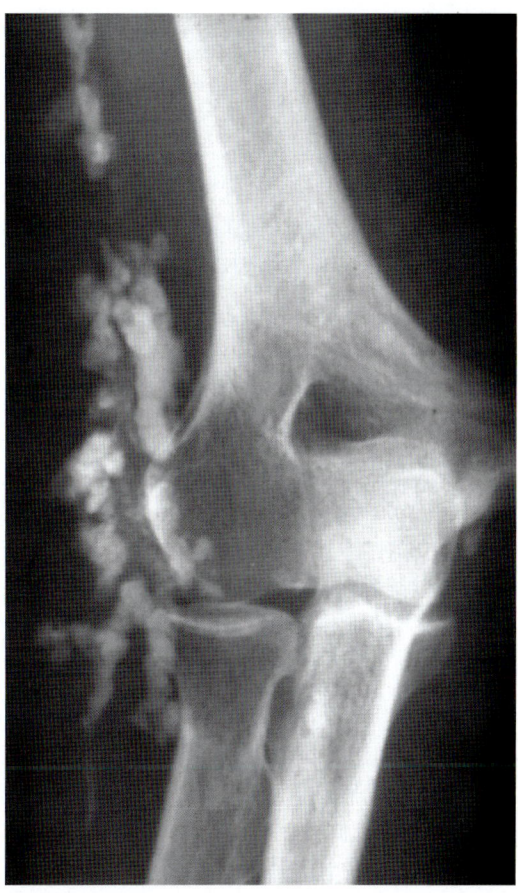

■ **FIGURE 50-6**   Soft tissue calcifications at the elbow.

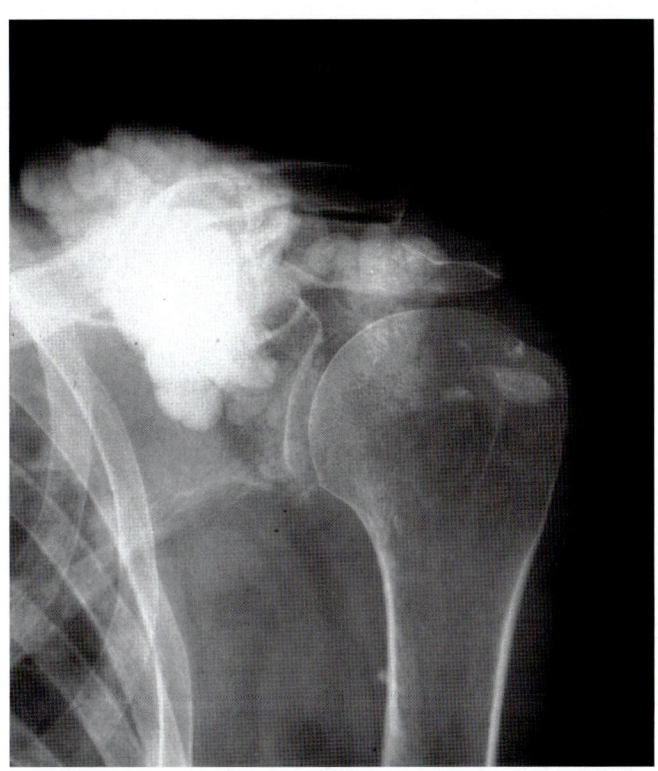

■ **FIGURE 50-5**   Soft tissue calcifications at the shoulder.

DIFFERENTIAL DIAGNOSIS

Scleroderma is generally a clinical diagnosis. The Raynaud phenomenon, which is painful blanching of the skin of the face (especially the nose and ears), hands (especially the fingers), and feet (especially the toes), alternating with blueness and redness that is often induced by temperature variations, especially in combination with swallowing difficulties and organ infarction, makes the diagnosis straightforward. It is much more difficult to establish the diagnosis in patients with limited cutaneous (musculoskeletal) involvement.[7] In less well-defined cases the primary differential diagnosis is composed of the other collagen vascular diseases.

Laboratory tests are not very sensitive for detection of progressive scleroderma. On the other hand, anti-centromeric antibodies and antibodies against the chromosomal antigen Scl-70 are highly specific. Of all the known antibodies that are related to scleroderma, anti-topoisomerase I antibodies seem to have the greatest association with digital joint deformity and distal osteolysis.[8,9]

SYNOPSIS OF TREATMENT OPTIONS

Medical Treatment

The search for an effective therapy for patients with progressive systemic sclerosis has been frustrating. Until now the most widely used drug has been nifedipine. Iloprost seems to have potential. Methotrexate, cyclophosphamide, and other anti-inflammatory drugs are also being evaluated.[3]

Surgical Treatment

The goals of surgery for advanced progressive systemic sclerosis affecting the hand are pain relief through sympathectomy and increased perfusion, improving mobility through resection arthroplasty, and repositioning the digit to provide a functional position for fusion.

What the Referring Physician Needs to Know

- Like other collagen vascular diseases, progressive systemic sclerosis involves specialists of different medical fields, especially dermatology, vascular surgery, immunology, rheumatology, gastroenterology, and orthopedic surgery.
- The disease is characterized by inflammatory and fibrotic changes of the skin, synovial membranes, and internal organs (gastrointestinal tract, lungs, kidneys, heart) that result from excessive production of collagens and from obliterative changes in small blood vessels.
- Late in the course of the disease radiologically visible changes occur.[10]

SUGGESTED READINGS

Bassett LW, Blocka KL, Furst De, et al. Skeletal findings in progressive systemic sclerosis (scleroderma). AJR Am J Roentgenol 1981; 136:1121–1126.

Bogoch ER, Gross DK. Surgery of the hand in patients with systemic sclerosis: outcome and considerations. J Rheumatol 2005; 32:642–648.

Hanlon R, King S. Overview of the radiology of connective tissue disorders in children. Eur J Radiol 2000; 33:74–84.

Leighton C. Drug treatment of scleroderma. Drugs 2001; 61:419–427.

LeRoy EC, Black C, Fleischmajer R, et al. Scleroderma (systemic sclerosis): classification, subsets and pathogenesis. J Rheumatol 1989; 15:202–205.

REFERENCES

1. Coghlan JG, Mukerjee D. The heart and pulmonary vasculature in scleroderma: clinical features and pathobiology. Curr Opin Rheumatol 2001; 13:495–499.
2. Pinstein ML, Sebes JI, Leventhal M, Robertson JT. Case report 579: Progressive systemic sclerosis (PSS) with cervical cord compression syndrome: osteolysis and bilateral facet arthropathy. Skeletal Radiol 1989; 18:603–605.
3. Faggioli P, Giani L, Mazzone A. Possible role of iloprost (stable analog of PG12) in promoting neoangiogenesis in systemic sclerosis. Clin Exp Rheumatol 2006; 24:220–221.
4. Vlachoyiannopoulos PG, Drosos AA, Wiik A, Moutsopoulos HM. Patients with anticentromere antibodies, clinical features, diagnoses and evolution. Br J Rheumatol 1993; 32:297–301.
5. Yune HY, Vix VA, Klatte EC. Early fingertip changes in scleroderma. JAMA 1971; 215:1113–1116.
6. Bonél H, Messer G, Seemann M, et al. [MRI of the fingers in patients with systemic scleroderma: early results of contrast-enhanced examinations on a dedicated MRI system.] Radiologe 1997; 37:794–801. German.
7. Poormoghim H, Lucas M, Fertig N, Medsger TA Jr. Systemic sclerosis sine scleroderma: demographic, clinical, and serologic features and survival in forty-eight patients. Arthritis Rheum 200; 43:444–451.
8. Ferri C, Bernini L, Cecchetti R, et al. Cutaneous and serologic subsets of systemic sclerosis. J Rheumatol 1991; 18:1826–1832.
9. Jacobsen S, Halberg P, Ullman S, et al. Clinical features and serum antinuclear antibodies in 230 Danish patients with systemic sclerosis. Br J Rheumatol 1998; 37:39–45.
10. Pope JE, Ouimet JM, Krizova A. Scleroderma treatment differs between experts and general rheumatologists. Arthritis Rheum 2006; 55:138–145.

CHAPTER

51

Systemic Lupus Erythematosus

Corinna Schorn and Gerwin Lingg

ETIOLOGY

Despite the explosion of the molecular genetic research in the past decades the etiology of this prototype auto-immune disease is still elusive. A confusing complexity of serologic, immunopathologic, and genetic phenomena have been described, most of which are likely to be secondary effects. The current main hypotheses for the initiation of autoimmune response propose a defect in the clearance of apoptotic cells (cells undergoing programmed cell death).[1] Apoptotic cells release nucleosomes and histones, the typical autoantigens in systemic lupus erythematosus (SLE), from the nucleus into the cytoplasm. Ultraviolet irradiation leads to cell surface expression of lupus autoantigens of dying keratocytes.[2]

Because apoptosis is a normal physiologic event, this means it is controlled by immunotolerance: SLE is only manifested when apoptosis is combined with certain autoimmune characteristics. The precise susceptible condition is unknown and probably varies from one affected individual to another. Consequently, a considerable genetic heterogeneity with variable relationships and occasional multiple associations in differing populations and clinical phenotypes exist. A number of genes are important for characterization of the disease risk: class II HLA genes, complement component genes/tumor necrosis factor, and immunoglobulin receptor genes.[3-9] However, there is a high frequency of associated alleles in the normal population suggesting complex factor composition, incomplete penetrance, and environmental influences.

HLA genes have an important role in the immune response. The products of class II genes (DR, DQ, DP) present peptides from the extracellular milieu to CD4+ helper cells. Excessive or poorly controlled T-helper cells are involved in the activation and differentiation of auto-antibody-forming B cells.[10] The cellular dysfunction is influenced by genetic and hormonal factors and probably triggered by viruses, particularly retroviral products, ultraviolet radiation, and certain drugs. The result is an excessive autoantibody formation with characteristics of a secondary immune response (polyclonal IgG) resembling properties of antibodies to foreign antigens. Complement deficiency decreases the ability to eliminate immune complexes both from circulation and from tissues. The immune complex deposition causes tissue damage, vasculitis, and glomerulonephritis.

PREVALENCE AND EPIDEMIOLOGY

The characterization of serologic phenomena in the past century with better recognition of mild cases transformed SLE from a rare fulminant disease to a relatively common entity with a wide range of manifestations and a chronic course. The racial/ethnic and gender differences in incidence and prevalence are considerable. For the U.S. white population incidence rates are reported to be approximately 0.5 and 3.5 per 100,000 for men and women, respectively, which is similar to the European rates.[11,12] The incidence is increased in African Americans, reaching 1.5 and 10 per 100,000 for men and women, respectively.

KEY POINTS

- Musculoskeletal complaints are common in SLE, but imaging often remains unremarkable.
- Typical lupus-associated findings include
  - Symmetric nonerosive polyarthritis of the small joints
  - Jaccoud-like arthropathy (joint deformities in absence of joint destruction)
  - Myositis, which is (in contrast to myalgia) not frequent but which indicates a dismal outcome
- Disease complications and treatment associated findings include:
  - Osteonecrosis, mostly of the hip but also in unusual or multiple sites
  - Bone infarctions
  - Tendon rupture
  - Septic arthritis
- Rarely, in more or less typical SLE, destructive arthritis or tuftal resorption and soft tissue calcifications may occur.

1153

Prevalence is 15 and 50 per 100,000. Interestingly in Africa the disease is rare. Asian populations seem to exhibit increased prevalence rates compared with Caucasians.

The peak onset of the disease is in early and middle adulthood, in the child-bearing years of women, although it may begin at any age.[13] Mortality rates for SLE patients are increased by a factor of 3 to 5 compared with the general population. Risk factors for SLE-related mortality include older age at disease onset; male sex; African American ethnicity, which is eventually linked with low socioeconomic status; disease severity at the time of diagnosis; and especially renal and central nervous system involvement.[14] Early diagnosis and modern treatment options have contributed to improvement in the survival rate over the past 50 years, which is now approaching 70% over 20 years.[15,16]

CLINICAL PRESENTATION

Various symptoms and symptom combinations are seen depending on organ systems involved.[17] Nonspecific complaints include weakness, fever, malaise, fatigue, loss of appetite, and weight loss. Major abnormalities affect the skin, musculoskeletal system, central and peripheral neural systems, kidneys, lungs, and cardiovascular system.

Skin manifestations with photosensitivity are very common. Patients present typically with a malar rash with butterfly appearance or a discoid rash with keratotic scaling. Musculoskeletal involvement constitutes the most common presenting manifestation. The spectrum ranges from weakness, myalgia, and arthralgia to myositis and joint deformities. Morning stiffness, pain, tenderness, soft tissue swelling, and moderate joint effusion are associated with symmetric polyarthritis. Arthritis affects commonly the small joints of the hand, the wrists, and the knees with a migratory, relapsing or chronic deforming course. Tenosynovitis and spontaneous tendon ruptures occur. In late stages, especially with prolonged corticosteroid medication, localized arthralgia may be the result of osteonecrosis. This most commonly affects the hips but may involve any joint. Multiple or unusual sites of involvement are characteristic for SLE. Myalgia and weakness are equivocal complaints that may be from joint disease, fibromyalgia, medications, or sometimes true myositis.

Neuropsychiatric disorders with cerebral thrombotic vasculopathy as well as peripheral neuropathy may occur. Cognitive dysfunction, personality changes, seizures, ataxia, hemiplegia, and chorea are possible symptoms.[18] Frequently, patients complain about headache. However, it is difficult to determine in which cases headaches are part of the disease spectrum.[19]

Renal involvement can lead to proteinuria and hematuria, hypertension, nephrotic or nephritic syndrome, progressive glomerulonephritis, and chronic renal failure.[20] Pulmonary symptoms include pleurisy with effusion, pneumonia, vasculitis, fibrosis, and atelectasis. Cardiovascular disease comprises cardiomyopathy, pericarditis, endocarditis, and vasculitis. Peripheral thrombophlebitis or vasculitis may occur. Gastrointestinal manifestations include peritonitis, pancreatitis, perihepatitis, and intestinal involvement. Splenomegaly and lymphadenopathy are less frequent.

Patients are prone to infections, probably due to secondary effects of the immune related disease and immunosuppressive medication.

Serologic findings include anemia, leukopenia, abnormalities of the plasma proteins (hyperglobulinemia, hypalbuminemia), positive rheumatoid factor, cryoglobulinemia, and low serum complement activity. More specific signs are LE cells and antinuclear factors. Recent development of advanced immunologic tests have significantly improved the diagnostic evaluation.[21] Genetic studies reveal an association to major histocompatibility complex HLA-DR2, HLA-DR3, and HLA-B8.

Patients with SLE have multiple risk factors for osteoporosis. Lupus disease–associated damage, renal involvement, corticosteroid medication, low body mass index, and especially older age are associated with reduced bone mineral density. In addition, vitamin D deficiency is common. Osteoporosis with vertebral fractures develops in 4% to 20% of SLE patients, and osteopenia occurs in 40% to 50%.[22,23] This is a significant comorbidity and mandates routine bone mineral density evaluation in SLE patients with multiple risk factors.

PATHOLOGY

Systemic lupus erythematosus manifests in multiple organs. Prominent pathologic features are the generalized immunocomplex deposition that forms, for example, the lupus band (a feature of immunofluorescence), vasculitis, and a thrombotic microangiopathy. Hematoxylin (LE) bodies are a characteristic but not very frequent finding in various tissues. They correspond to basophilic lumpy structures consisting of chromatin and immunoglobulin. The LE cell is a phagocyte with ingested LE-body material, an in-vitro phenomenon.

The histo/immunopathology reflects the basic mechanisms of tissue injury. For example, in the skin the immunoglobulins are deposited at the dermal-epidermal junction and may be found in normal or affected skin. Ultraviolet irradiation leads to increased apoptosis of keratinocytes with subsequent nuclear debris and immune complex precipitation. In acute lesions in the upper regions of the dermis a vascular, perivascular, and periappendageal inflammation and mononuclear cell infiltration is prominent. Liquefactive degeneration of the basal cell layer of the dermis and fibrinoid necrosis is present.

The universal immune complex deposition in the walls of small arteries and arterioles with or without inflammatory response and facultatively necrotizing vasculitis is very characteristic for SLE. Similar aspects may be found in multiple organs. Renal involvement with mesangial deposits and hypercellularity or proliferative, sclerosing, or membranous features has major impact on the disease course, and the World Health Organization classification of glomerulonephritis allows prognostic conclusions. Interestingly, most cerebral involvement constitutes thrombotic lesions associated with anticardiolipin or antiphospholipid antibodies, and only a minority correspond to vascular inflammation.

Compared with these major findings in multiple organs the musculoskeletal disease appears relatively unremarkable. Histologic examination of the synovium in acute lupus arthritis reveals perivascular inflammatory cell infiltrates, mild synovial cell proliferation, and mild fibrinous deposition. In the chronic stage the synovial cell proliferation may increase, but usually it remains moderate compared with rheumatoid arthritis. Features of tenosynovitis are similar to those in arthritis. Tendon ruptures, however, do not exhibit inflammatory changes but indicate degenerative disease. In myositis, histopathology reveals atrophy, microtubular inclusions, and mononuclear cell infiltrates.

BIOMECHANICS

The typical deforming arthropathy in lupus is characterized by ulnar drift of the digits, swan-neck (hyperextension of the proximal interphalangeal joint and flexion of the distal interphalangeal joint) and boutonnière deformities (flexion of the proximal interphalangeal joint and hyperextension of the distal interphalangeal joint), and hyperextension of the interphalangeal joint of the thumb and is known as Jaccoud's hand. Destruction and laxity of the metacarpophalangeal joint connective tissues with ulnar slippage of the extensor tendon is the main reason for the ulnar drift.[24] The initiation of the swan-neck deformity takes place in the metacarpophalangeal joint. Primarily, the deformities are nonfixed and reversible at the patient's own efforts with normal active flexion. In later stages, adhesions between the extensor tendons on the dorsum of the proximal interphalangeal joint fix the later band to the middle slip insertion, leading to fixed swan-neck deformity.[25] The boutonnière deformity, in contrast to the swan-neck deformity, begins at the proximal interphalangeal joint itself with swelling followed by elongation of the central slip, subluxation of the later bands, and contracture of the retinacular ligament.[26]

Patients with Jaccoud hands suffer from instability of the metacarpophalangeal joints, pain, weakness, and loss of dexterity. The grip function is severely hampered when the thumb/index finger opposition for the pinch grip is lost. Daily activities such as buttoning and writing become obstacles for affected patients.

IMAGING TECHNIQUES

Radiography is the method of choice for evaluation of symptomatic joints. Anteroposterior views of the hands and feet should be taken using high-resolution technique. These images must guarantee display of soft tissues and bony structures at the same time to assess for fusiform articulosynovitis.

In cases of osteonecrosis, radiographic images do not provide early diagnosis. Additional methods such as MRI or nuclear bone scan may be necessary. For tendon disease, ultrasonography is advantageous.

MRI for myositis is performed with short tau inversion recovery (STIR), spectral presaturation inversion recovery (SPIR), or T2-weighted turbo spin-echo, fat saturated and T1-weighted spin-echo pulse sequences in coronal and axial planes mostly of the thigh or calf. Usually, contrast medium–enhanced sequences do not provide additional information.

MANIFESTATIONS OF THE DISEASE

Musculoskeletal Manifestations

Musculoskeletal involvement is only one part of the disease spectrum. Features directly associated with lupus include the following:

● Symmetric polyarthritis
● Jaccoud-like arthropathy (deformity of the hand in the absence of destructive arthritis).

Disease complications and treatment sequelae comprise:

● Osteonecrosis
● Spontaneous tendon weakening and rupture
● Septic arthritis due to immunologic impairment and/or immunosuppressive therapy

Soft tissue calcifications and tuftal resorption or destructive arthritis are features sometimes associated with SLE and, if pronounced, may be signs of an overlap syndrome with scleroderma or rheumatoid arthritis, respectively.

Radiography

Symmetric polyarthritis is very common (90% of patients). The predilection sites are the small joints of the hand and feet, the wrists, knees, and shoulders. Synovial soft tissue swelling especially at the proximal interphalangeal and metacarpophalangeal joints is frequent. Periarticular demineralization may progress to diffuse osteoporosis. In contrast to findings in rheumatoid arthritis, no joint space narrowing, marginal erosion, or destruction occurs. Sometimes small subchondral cysts are visible and are thought to correspond to micronecrotic foci.

In long-standing disease 4% to 50% of patients develop a *Jaccoud-like arthropathy* also known as deforming nonerosive arthropathy that is characterized by reducible joint deformities (Fig. 51-1). Because deformities are reduced by the radiographer the radiographic image is to some degree insensitive. Swan-neck deformities, boutonnière deformities, and hyperextension of the interphalangeal joint as well as ulnar deviation of the metacarpophalangeal joint is typical. Unless associated with rheumatoid arthritis usually no joint destruction occurs. If present, joint space narrowing is not a result of cartilage destruction but a sign of atrophy and erosions are not caused by pannus invasion but by pressure in subluxation.

SLE patients are prone to epiphyseal *osteonecrosis* and metaphyseal/diaphyseal bone infarction with a frequency of 5% to 40%.[27,28] Avascular necrosis is not strongly associated with corticosteroid therapy or disease-related vasculitis, but it is more frequent in such cases.[29] Often atypical (metacarpal and metatarsal heads, carpals), multiple, or symmetric sites are affected—a feature relatively suggestive for SLE.[30] Nevertheless, the femoral head is the most frequent site of manifestation. The radiologic appearance of avascular necrosis does not differ in patients with and without SLE. Subchondral fracture, depression, fragmentation of the osseous surface, sclerosis, and cyst formation are signs of avascular necrosis. Secondarily, degenerative osteoarthritis leads to osteophyte formation, cartilage loss, sclerosis, and cyst formation of the opposing joint surface.

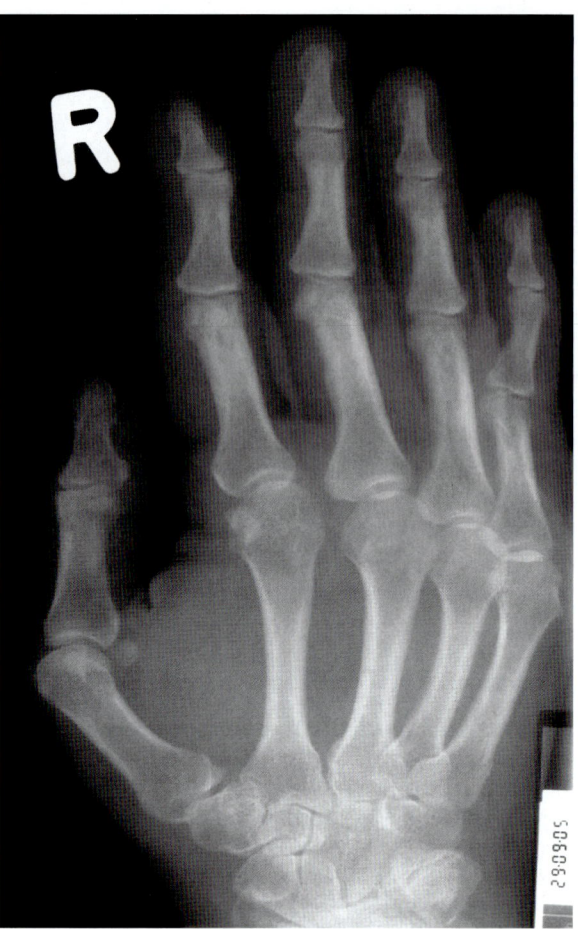

■ **FIGURE** 51-1 Radiographic imaging of the hand in systemic lupus erythematosus. Because deformities of the finger joints are corrected by the radiographer, they may become apparent only when they are fixed. Therefore, the swan-neck deformities and increased flexion of the metacarpophalangeal joints displayed in this patient are not an early sign of Jaccoud's hand. There are no erosions despite the advanced deformity, a feature very suggestive of SLE, but the clinical diagnosis usually precedes this finding. In general the radiographic appearance of the hands remains unremarkable in SLE despite considerable clinical symptoms.

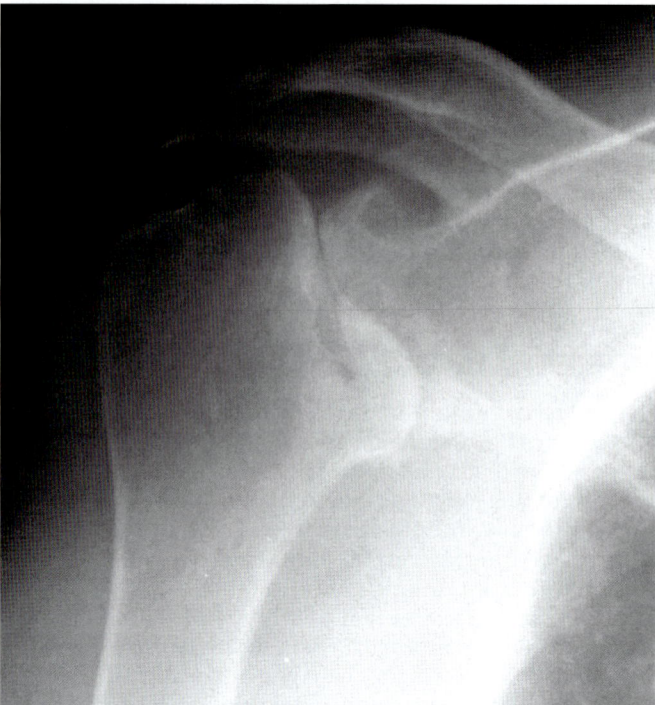

■ **FIGURE** 51-2 Osteonecrosis of the humeral head. There is a large defect of the humeral head resulting from necrosis and resorption of the necrotic fragments. In this late stage, the contours are smooth and well defined and secondary degenerative disease takes place.

Magnetic Resonance Imaging

Spontaneous tendon weakening and rupture is much more frequent in SLE patients than in degenerative disease. Its features do not differ from those in normal individuals, and likewise it is mostly associated with local or systemic corticosteroid therapy. The best imaging techniques are ultrasound and MRI. An acute and subacute rupture is characterized by surrounding fluid, edema, and tendon sheath effusion. The tendon is attenuated, and in complete rupture the retracted end is curled and wavy (Fig. 51-3). Incomplete rupture is characterized by intermediate signal intensity on T1-weighted images, intratendinous dots or stripes of fluid signal, decreased or increased diameter, or deformity.

MRI is much more sensitive for a *vascular necrosis* than radiographic imaging. In SLE, epiphyseal osteonecrosis often occurs in unusual sites. The features, however, do not differ from osteonecrosis in otherwise normal individuals. Geographically shaped or triangular bone marrow edema is seen in ARCO (Association Recherche Circulation Osseous) stage I, followed by demarcation by the so-called double-line sign in ARCO stage II (serpiginous line of hypointensity on T1-weighted images and hyper/hypointense double line on T2-weighted images at the margin of the necrotic area). An insufficiency fracture of the affected epiphyseal area is called a crescent sign, representing ARCO stage III. In stage IV, deformity and secondary degenerative osteoarthritis have taken place. The necrotic area itself may exhibit various signal characteristics from fat to sclerosis or fluid components.

Myalgia is reported in up to 40% of patients, but only 4% develop *myositis* with pain, diffuse tenderness, weakness, atrophy, and elevated muscle enzymes. Myositis is a risk factor for dismal outcome.[32] In some patients it may

Radiographic imaging is not positive in early cases; in fact, a normal radiograph in patients with hip pain and corticosteroid therapy should raise the suspicion for osteonecrosis (Fig. 51-2) and additional imaging (MRI or bone scan) should be performed.

Bone infarctions present as serpiginous lines of calcification centrally in the metaphysis and/or diaphysis of long bones surrounding and surrounded by apparently normal bone. If the calcified rim of the osteonecrosis is not entirely visible, especially in smaller bones, wavy lines of sclerotic shadows are seen.

Soft tissue calcification and tuftal resorption have been described in SLE patients, but these features may be a sign of an overlap syndrome with scleroderma. Diffuse linear, streaky, plaque-like, or nodular calcifications are found subcutaneously or periarticularly, sometimes associated with skin lesions.[31]

Septic arthritis and osteomyelitis as complications of SLE show similar features as in standard cases.

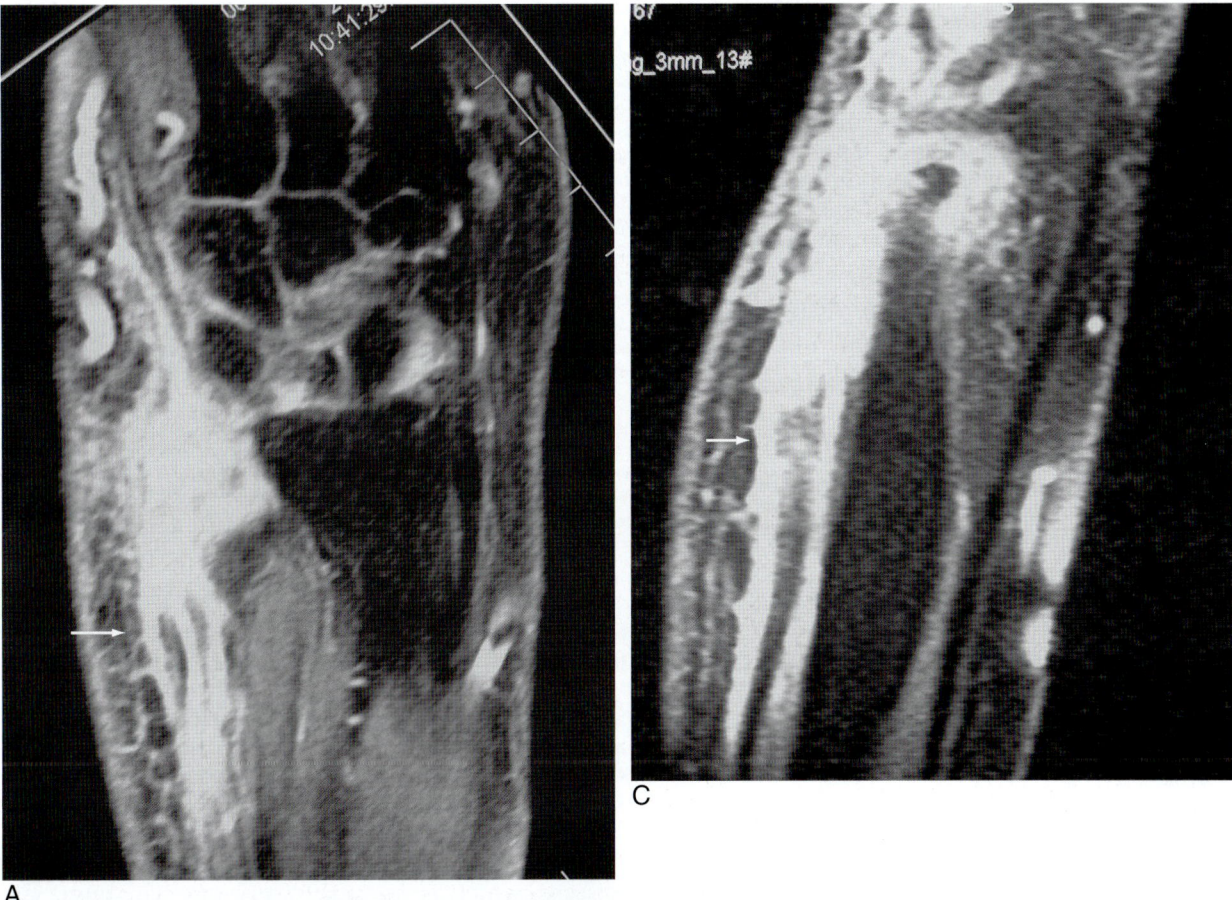

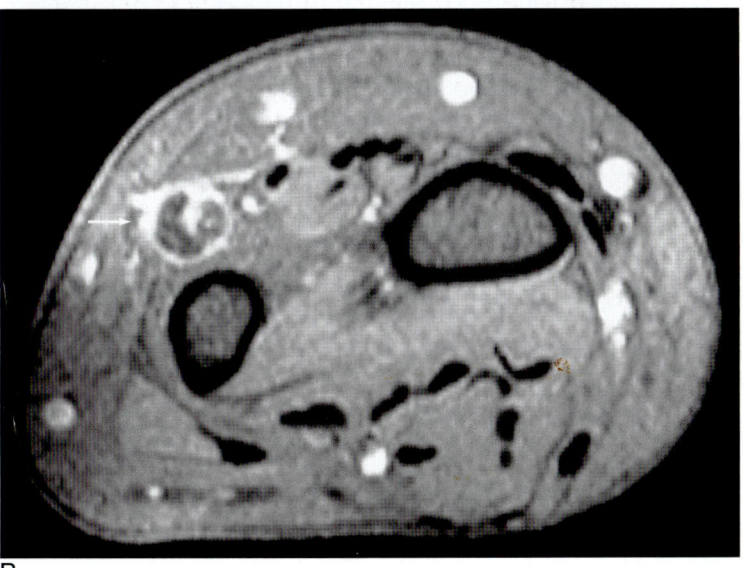

■ **FIGURE 51-3** Spontaneous tendon rupture. Pain and swelling at the ulnar styloid process primarily raised suspicion of tenosynovitis. Coronal (**A**), transverse (**B**), and sagittal (**C**) planes show the retracted extensor carpi ulnaris tendon end curling inside the synovial sheath (*arrow*).

be part of an overlap syndrome. MRI is sensitive to muscle edema and fatty atrophy. Contrast medium enhancement may be seen in affected muscles.

Multidetector Computed Tomography

Computed tomography is not in the routine diagnostic algorithm for SLE musculoskeletal manifestations.

Ultrasonography

For *spontaneous tendon rupture* in most cases ultrasonography is an excellent diagnostic method. An acute and subacute rupture is characterized by surrounding fluid, edema, and tendon sheath effusion. The tendon pattern is inhomogeneous, and in complete rupture the retracted end is curled and wavy.

Nuclear Medicine

Hip pain despite normal radiography in SLE patients with or without corticosteroid therapy is typical for osteonecrosis of the femoral head. MRI and nuclear medicine are powerful tools for definitive diagnosis. ^{99m}Tc-methylene diphosphonate triphasic bone scintigraphy reveals arterial hypoperfusion and a cold area in the femoral head. SPECT is considered to be positive when a cold defect is detected with or without presence of adjacent increased uptake (cold spot within a hot spot).[33] Later stages may show a hot spot within a hot spot.

Classic Signs

- Nonerosive polyarthritis: synovial soft tissue swelling, demineralization
- Deforming arthropathy (Jaccoud's hand): ulnar drift of the digits, swan-neck and boutonnière deformities
- Avascular necrosis: commonly affecting the hips, characteristically multiple or unusual sites
  - Radiographic: early—occult; late—subchondral fracture, fragmentation
  - MRI: well-defined epiphyseal region of signal alteration sharply demarcated by the double-line sign (ARCO classification)
  - Bone scan: triangular area of hypoperfusion
- Bone infarctions: radiographs/MRI—metaphyseal and/or diaphyseal serpiginous lines
- Spontaneous tendon ruptures: ultrasound/MRI—edema, retracted tendon end in complete ruptures, thickened attenuated tendon in incomplete ruptures
- Septic arthritis: radiographic—patchy demineralization, rapid destruction

DIFFERENTIAL DIAGNOSIS

Some of the most common symptoms of SLE are completely nonspecific. The changeable nature and the intermittently relapsing multiplicity of features make the diagnosis challenging. Primarily established for research purposes, the classification criteria serve as helpful for the diagnosis, although by no means describing the complete disease spectrum (Table 51-1).[34] Positivity for at least 4 of the 11 criteria allows classification of a patient as having SLE.

Serologic features are widely used to confirm a clinical diagnosis, but antibodies cannot be used alone to diagnose autoimmune disease. The LE cell phenomenon was primarily considered to be lupus specific. Now it is clear that it can be present in some other autoimmune conditions, for example, in 16% of patients with rheumatoid arthritis. Nevertheless, it is positive in 50% to 70% of lupus patients. Antinuclear antibodies (ANA) are highly important in the diagnosis of SLE. A negative ANA test makes the diagnosis of SLE unlikely. Some of the antibodies seen in SLE are specific for certain subgroups: anti-dsDNA antibodies and anti-Sm are highly specific for SLE, anti-histone is common in drug-induced lupus, and anti-Ro and anti-La occur in SLE and Sjögren's disease. Almost all sera containing

TABLE 51-1   1997 Revised Criteria for Diagnosis of Systemic Lupus Erythematosus
Malar rash
Discoid rash
Photosensitivity
Oral ulcers
Arthritis (two or more peripheral joints)
Serositis
Renal disorders (proteinuria, cellular casts)
Neurologic disorders (seizures, psychosis)
Hematologic disorders (hemolytic anemia, leukopenia, lymphopenia, thrombopenia)
Immunologic disorders (antibodies to native DNA, anti-Sm, antiphospholipid)
Antinuclear antibodies

Data from Hochberg MC. Updating the American College of Rheumatology revised criteria for the classification of systemic lupus erythematosus. Arthritis Rheum 1997; 40:1725.

anti-Sm also contain anti-RNP. The converse, however, anti-RNP without anti-Sm, is typical for mixed connective tissue disease. Anti-ssDNA antibodies are produced in infections and other autoimmune disorders. Antibody levels are not appropriate for monitoring disease activity.

Most *imaging features* of SLE, especially the musculoskeletal afflictions (e.g., nonerosive polyarthritis or osteonecrosis), are highly nonspecific. Nonerosive deforming arthropathy was primarily described in poststreptococcal disease, which is nowadays very rare. Therefore, the Jaccoud hand is considered to be a sign of SLE; but it is no early manifestation, and radiographic imaging is insensitive to reducible deformities. Usually the diagnosis is known or suspected from clinical and serologic criteria and imaging is performed to exclude destructive arthritis or complications.

Musculoskeletal complaints such as arthralgia and myalgia are frequent constitutional symptoms, along with fever, malaise, and fatigue, and can occur alone or may accompany organ flares. In this setting it is important to bear in mind the differential diagnosis of an infectious disease.

SYNOPSIS OF TREATMENT OPTIONS

Medical Treatment

Nonsteroidal Anti-inflammatory Drugs

For lupus-associated constitutional symptoms such as musculoskeletal complaints in the acute phase, NSAIDs are often effective and if not may be combined with low-dose corticosteroid therapy. Adverse effects of NSAIDs may mimic features of SLE, such as nephritis, liver enzyme abnormalities, or neuropsychiatric symptoms. If there is doubt, NSAIDs should be discontinued before assuming a flare.

Corticosteroids

Corticosteroids are promptly efficacious for resolving the inflammatory activity of a lupus flare. For control of arthralgia and myalgia, low-dose therapy in addition to NSAIDs is frequently necessary. High-dose therapy is reserved for life- or organ-threatening active disease. After disease control, dose tapering and finally total discontinuation should be attempted. However, many patients require maintenance therapy to prevent flares. In this case antimalarial agents or, in more severe cases, immunosuppression should be considered.

Antimalarial Agents

Antimalarial agents are commonly used for chronic therapy for repeatedly recurrent or persistent constitutional symptoms especially when corticosteroids cannot be discontinued. These agents have complex immunomodulatory effects, and the response is to be expected with a delay of several weeks. The combination of different antimalarial agents (hydroxychloroquine, chloroquine, quinacrine) is synergistic. Smoking significantly decreases the efficacy of these drugs.

A special adverse effect, the hemolytic anemia in glucose-6-phosphate dehydrogenase deficiency, mandates screening before administration, especially in people of African descent. The toxic effect on the retina is of major concern and is dose and duration dependent. Because early lesions are reversible, careful follow-up with ophthalmologic examinations is mandatory.

Immunosuppressive Agents

Azathioprine

If corticosteroid discontinuation is not possible, azathioprine may be used as a corticosteroid-sparing drug. Additionally, it is used for patients with repeated flares. Women of child-bearing age need effective contraception because of its teratogenic effects. Nevertheless, for the fetus the risk of a lupus flare is considerable, and for this reason azathioprine is not necessarily discontinued during pregnancy.

Methotrexate

Methotrexate is useful in lupus arthritis and also in corticosteroid-sparing and antimalarial- resistant constitutional disease. However, lupus patients seem to be more prone to adverse effects, such as hepatopathy compared with patients with rheumatoid arthritis. Teratogenic effects must be considered.

Surgical Treatment

Numerous procedures are available for the operative correction of the Jaccoud hand, such as realignment of the ulnarly drifted digits by soft tissue rebalancing and extensor centralization or, in later stages with fixed deformity and articular surface damage, arthroplasty. The choice of the surgical procedure is dependent on the ability for passive correction, state of the articular cartilage, and/or presence of additional deformities. Boutonnière deformities do not limit the hand function to the same degree as swan-neck deformities and ulnar drift of the digits.[35]

The goal of surgical deformity correction is the induction of pain relief and re-creation of balance of forces with improvement of the grip function.[36] However, late recurrence remains a problem.[37,38]

What the Referring Physician Needs to Know

- Typical deformities of the hands may be inconspicuous on radiographic images because they are routinely reduced by radiographers.
- Destructive arthritis, tuftal resorption, and calcifications may be signs of an overlap syndrome.
- Patchy demineralization and rapid joint destruction are suggestive of infectious arthritis.
- Discrepancy between considerable joint pain, especially at the hip joints, and unremarkable radiography may be a sign of osteonecrosis and calls for MRI or bone scan.

SUGGESTED READINGS

Gladman DD, Urowitz MB. Connective tissue disorders: Systemic lupus erythematosus. In Hochberg MC, Silman AJ, Smolen JS, et al (eds). Rheumatology, 3rd ed. St. Louis, Mosby, 2003, pp 1285–1430.

Resnick D. Systemic lupus erythematosus. In Resnick D, Niwayama G (eds). Diagnosis of Joint and Bone Disorders, 2nd ed. Philadelphia, WB Saunders, vol 2, 1988.

REFERENCES

1. Gaipl US, Voll RE, Sheriff A, et al. Impaired clearance of dying cells in systemic lupus erythematosus. Autoimmun Rev 2005; 4:189–194.
2. LeFeber WP, Norris DA, Ryan SR, et al. Ultraviolet light induces binding of antibodies to selected nuclear antigens on cultured human keratinocytes. J Clin Invest 1984; 74:1545–1551.
3. Merrill JT, Buyon JP. The role of biomarkers in the assessment of lupus. Best Pract Res Clin Rheumatol 2005; 19:709–726.
4. Takeuchi T, Tsuzaka K, Abe T, et al. T cell abnormalities in systemic lupus erythematosus. Autoimmunity 2005; 38:339–346.
5. Arnett FC, Reveille JD, Moutsopoulos HM, et al. Ribosomal P autoantibodies in systemic lupus erythematosus: Frequencies in different ethnic groups and clinical immunogenetic associations. Arthritis Rheum 1996, 39:1833–1839.
6. Steinsson K, Jonsdottir S, Arason GJ, et al. Ann Rheum Dis 1998; 57:503–505.
7. Hong GH, Kim HY, Takeuchi F, et al. Association of complement C4 and HLA-DR alleles with systemic lupus erythematosus in Koreans. J Rheumatol 1994; 21:442–447.
8. Howard PF, Hochberg MC, Bias WB, et al. Relationship between C4 null genes, HLA-D region antigens and genetic susceptibility to systemic lupus erythematosus in Caucasian and black Americans. Am J Med 1986; 81:187–193.
9. Reveille JD, Moulds JM, Ahn C, et al. Systemic lupus erythematosus in three ethnic groups: I. The effects of HLA class II, C4, and CR1 alleles, socioeconomic factors, and ethnicity at disease onset. LUMINA Study Group. Lupus in minority populations, nature versus nurture. Arthritis Rheum 1998; 41:1161–1172.

10. Crow MK. Cellular immunology. In Hochberg MC, Silman AJ, Smolen JS, et al. Rheumatology, 3rd ed. St. Louis, Mosby, 2003, pp 1347-1358.

11. Hochberg MC. The incidence of systemic lupus erythematosus in Baltimore, Maryland, 1970-77. Arthritis Rheum 1985; 28:80-86.

12. McCarty DJ, Manzi S, Medsger TA, et al. Incidence of systemic lupus erythematosus: race and gender differences. Arthritis Rheum 1995; 38:1260-1270.

13. Petri M. Epidemiology of systemic lupus erythematosus. Best Pract Res Clin Rheumatol 2002, 16:847-858.

14. Waard MM, Pyun E, Studenski S. Long-term survival in systemic lupus erythematosus: patient characteristics associated with poorer outcomes. Arthritis Rheum 1995; 38:274-283.

15. Abu-Shakra M, Urowitz MB, Gladman DD, Gough J. Mortality studies in systemic lupus erythematosus: results from a single centre: II. Predictor variables for mortality. J Rheumatol 1995; 22:1265-1270.

16. Petri M, Genovese M. Incidence of and risk factors for hospitalisations in systemic lupus erythematosus: a prospective study of the Hopkins Lupus Cohort. J Rheumatol 1992; 19:1559-1565.

17. Haq I, Isenberg DA. How does one assess and monitor patients with systemic lupus erythematosus in daily clinical practice? Best Pract Res Clin Rheumatol 2002; 16:181-194.

18. Hermosillo-Romo D, Brey RL. Neuropsychiatric involvement in systemic lupus erythematosus. Curr Rheumatol Rep 2002; 4:337-344.

19. Cuadrado MJ, Sanna G. Headache and systemic lupus erythematosus. Lupus 2003; 12:943-946.

20. Balow JE. Clinical presentation and monitoring of lupus nephritis. Lupus 2005; 14:25-30.

21. Esdaile JM, Joseph L, Abrahamowicz M, et al. Routine immunologic tests in systemic lupus erythematosus: is there a need for more studies. Comment in: J Rheumatol 1996; 23:1891-1896.

22. Leventhal GH, Dorfman HD. Aseptic necrosis of bone in systemic lupus erythematosus. Semin Arthritis Rheum 1974; 4:73-93.

23. Siemsen JK, Brook J, Meister L. Lupus erythematosus and vascular bone necrosis: a clinical study of three cases and review of the literature. Arthritis Rheum 1962; 5:492-501.

24. Bielefeld T, Neumann DA. The unstable metacarpophalangeal joint in rheumatoid arthritis: anatomy, pathomechanics and physical rehabilitation considerations. J Orthop Sports Phys Ther 2005; 35:502-520.

25. Heywood AW. The pathogenesis of the rheumatoid swan neck deformity. Hand 1979; 11:176-183.

26. Ferlic DC. Boutonnière deformities in rheumatoid arthritis. Hand Clin 1989; 5:215-222.

27. Abeles M, Urman JD, Rothfield NF. Aseptic necrosis of bone in systemic lupus erythematosus: relationship to corticosteroid therapy. Arch Intern Med 1978; 138:750-754.

28. Urman JD, Abeles M, Houghton AN, Rothfield NF. Aseptic necrosis presenting as wrist pain in SLE. Arthritis Rheum 1977; 20:825-828.

29. Budin JA, Feldmann F. Soft tissue calcifications in systemic lupus erythematosus. Am J Roentgenol 1975; 124:358.

30. Dayal NA, Isenberg DA. SLE/myositis overlap: are the manifestations of SLE different in overlap disease. Lupus 2002; 11:293-298.

31. Bultink IE, Lems WF, Kostense PJ, et al. Prevalence of and risk factors for low bone mineral density and vertebral fractures in patients with systemic lupus erythematosus. Arthritis Rheum 2005; 52:2044-2050.

32. Pineau CA, Urowitz MB, Fortin PJ, et al. Osteoporosis in systemic lupus erythematosus: Factors associated with referral for bone mineral density studies, prevalence of osteoporosis and factors associated with reduced bone density. Lupus 2004; 13:436-441.

33. Ryu JS, Kim JS, Moon DH, et al. Bone SPECT is more sensitive than MRI in the detection of early osteonecrosis of the femoral head after renal transplantation. J Nucl Med 2002; 43:1006-1011.

34. Hochberg MC. Updating the American College of Rheumatology revised criteria for the classification of systemic lupus erythematosus. Arthritis Rheum 1997; 40:1725.

35. Boyer MI, Gelberman RH. Operative correction of swan-neck and boutonniere deformities in the rheumatoid hand. J Am Acad Orthop Surg 1999; 7:92-100.

36. Wood VE, Ichtertz DR, Yahiku H. Soft tissue metacarpophalangeal reconstruction for treatment of rheumatoid hand deformity. J Hand Surg 1989: 14:163-174.

37. Burezq H, Polyhronopoulos GN, Beaulieu S, et al. The value of radial collateral ligament reconstruction and abductor digiti minimi release in metacarpophalangeal joint arthroplasty. Ann Plast Surg 2005; 54:397-401.

38. Dell PC, Renfree KJ, Below Dell R. Surgical correction of extensor tendon subluxation and ulnar drift in the rheumatoid hand: long-term results. J Hand Surg 2001; 26:560-564.

CHAPTER 52

Mixed Connective Tissue Disease

Corinna Schorn and Gerwin Lingg

ETIOLOGY, EPIDEMIOLOGY, AND PREVALENCE

The distinctiveness of the connective tissue diseases is less pronounced than the classification system implies. In practice there is a continuous spectrum of symptom combinations, merging features of various entities. Mixed connective tissue disease (MCTD) is the prototype of an overlap syndrome, combining features of systemic lupus erythematosus (SLE), systemic scleroderma (SSc), polymyositis (PM), and rheumatoid arthritis (RA). As described by Sharp and colleagues, MCTD constitutes a likewise separate entity and is now, despite previous debate, a commonly used label for the anti-U1-RNP–associated disease spectrum.[1-6]

The etiology underlying this special symptom combination is unknown. There are several hypotheses, such as the induction of autoantibodies due to molecular mimicry after retrovirus infection (or Epstein-Barr virus infection) or defects in the clearance of apoptotic cells similar to SLE concepts. The exact prevalence and incidence rates are unknown but estimated to be approximately one of every four SLE patients. The female predominance is nearly 10-fold. Genetic studies show mostly HLA-DR4 and HLA-Dw4 association, a genetic background that is different from that of SLE patients.[7]

CLINICAL PRESENTATION

Due to the overlapping nature, MCTD does not present a constant clinical picture. Especially in the early disease course the diagnosis often remains limited to undifferentiated connective tissue disease (UCTD). This term, however, has received its own definition and can self-sufficiently serve as a basis for patient care.[8,9] In patients with Raynaud's phenomenon, factors have been defined that have prognostic significance for the future development of a specific connective tissue disease.[10] Most patients with UCTD and anti-U1 RNP develop MCTD.[11]

Nonspecific signs such as fatigue, weight loss, and fever are often associated with more specific manifestations, the latter including:

- Puffy hands
- Raynaud's phenomenon
- Keratoconjunctivitis sicca
- Arthralgia, unexplained polyarthritis
- Myalgia, myositis
- Skin symptoms: rash, sclerodactyly
- Serositis
- Central nervous system symptoms, peripheral neuropathy
- Fibrosing alveolitis and pulmonary hypertension
- Esophageal dysfunction
- Adenopathy, hematologic disorders

Presentation with symptoms of two or more well-defined connective tissue diseases (SLE, SSc, RA, PM) is typical. Even the characteristic of swollen hands may incorporate features of more specific diseases: erythema of the dorsum of the proximal interphalangeal joint and metacarpophalangeal joint like in PM or sclerodactyly and fixed finger flexion like in SSc. The disease course may be stable over many years or progress to one of the

---

KEY POINTS

- In early disease the most prominent finding on radiographs of the hands may be the soft tissue swelling. If present, more specific radiographic signs may appear slightly atypical, owing in part to the combination of features of two different connective tissue diseases and in part to an unusual involvement or an irregular distribution of the polyarthritis compared with RA.
- Prognosis is not always favorable. One should especially search for pulmonary hypertension with or without fibrosing alveolitis at regular follow-up evaluations and treat myositis efficiently.

well-defined connective tissue diseases in later stages (i.e., evolving into more or less typical SLE, SSc, PM, or RA).

Serologic findings include raised erythrocyte sedimentation rate (ESR) and elevated C-reactive protein (CRP), which are nonspecific signs of inflammation. The presence of antibodies against U1 ribonucleoprotein (anti-U1-RNP) is fundamental for the diagnosis and has been initially stressed to be specific.[4,12-15] Nowadays it is known that high titers can also be found in 40% of patients with SLE, as well as some cases of SSc, RA, PM and other overlapping syndromes.[16-19] IgG and complement levels are usually high. In addition to clinical overlap, serologic overlap has also been recognized. Antinuclear antibodies (ANA) and rheumatoid factor (Waaler-Rose as well as enzyme-linked immunosorbent assay) may be found in patients with MCTD, and anti-ds-DNA and anti-Sm suggest SLE.

Sharp and colleagues initially described a favorable prognosis. However, this notion has been disproven; myositis as well as fibrosing alveolitis and pulmonary hypertension are potentially fatal, and therefore the overall prognosis is worse than that for SLE.[7,20-22]

MANIFESTATIONS OF THE DISEASE

Multiple classification criteria sets have been proposed owing to the variability of the disease presentation and course. Alarcón-Segovia's criteria have been accepted for the definition of MCTD and include only five clinical criteria.[23] Prerequisite is a high titer of anti-U1 RNP; however, the exact levels for assays commonly used have not been described. Clinical criteria are swollen hands, Raynaud's phenomenon, acrosclerosis, synovitis, and myositis. According to Alarcón-Segovia, MCTD can be diagnosed with reasonable specificity and sensitivity when in addition to the serologic marker, three clinical criteria are present. If the criteria of swollen hands, Raynaud's phenomenon, and acrosclerosis are positive, one of the other two criteria is additionally necessary. Fulfillment of the criteria of another connective tissue disease (RA, SLE, SSc, PM) in a patient with positive diagnosis of MCTD should not be considered an association but refers to the nature of MCTD being an overlap syndrome itself.

RADIOGRAPHY

Radiographically the overlapping nature of the disease is once more confirmed.[24,25] Bone and soft tissue abnormality often resemble SSc. Joint involvement is more variable and shows features of RA or SLE, sometimes with a slightly atypical pattern ranging from mild effusion to mutilating arthritis.

Diffuse soft tissue swelling of the hand and periarticular or diffuse osteoporosis are nonspecific signs. RA features such as synovitis, joint space narrowing, marginal erosions that progress to destruction, and deformities with predilection for the metacarpophalangeal and proximal interphalangeal joints, wrist, and metatarsophalangeal and interphalangeal joints can be seen. Slightly atypical RA manifestations have been stressed to be typical for MCTD, that is, asymmetric involvement, distal interphalangeal joint involvement, and postarthritic capitate-trapezoid ankylosis.[26,27] Deformity without joint destruction is some

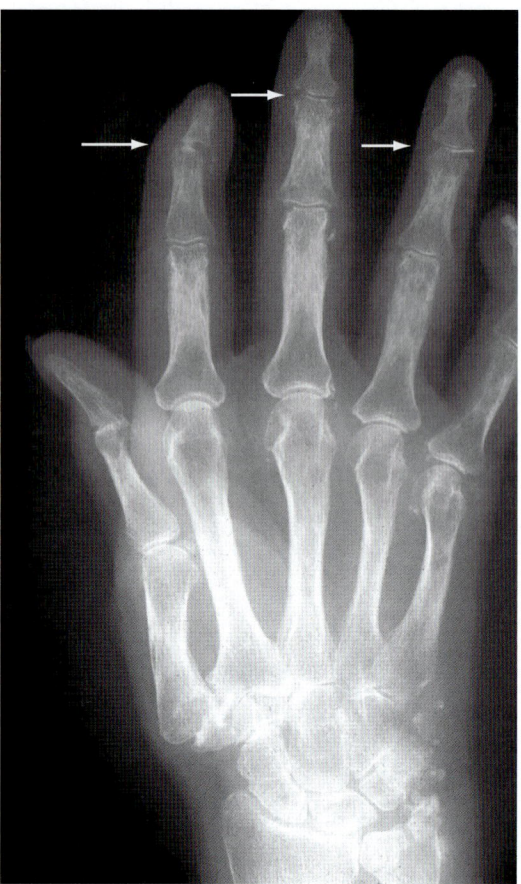

■ **FIGURE 52-1** Mixed connective tissue disease. Anteroposterior view of the hand shows periarticular demineralization (*arrows*). Soft tissue loss of the tip of the index finger, soft tissue calcification, and bandlike destruction of the distal interphalangeal joints resemble the features of scleroderma. Carpal involvement and soft tissue swelling due to tenosynovitis of the extensor carpi ulnaris are similar to the findings in rheumatoid arthritis. (*Courtesy of Dr. Kapp, Schlangenbad, Germany.*)

hint of the SLE component. Osteonecrosis of the femoral head, condyles, diaphysis, carpal bones, and metacarpal heads may occur with or without corticosteroid therapy. SSc-like involvement includes soft tissue atrophy and calcification, tuft resorption, and band-like distal interphalangeal joint destruction (Fig. 52-1). Punctate, linear, or extensive soft tissue calcification with predilection for the fingertips and periarticular as well as subcutaneous location is not uncommon (Fig. 52-2).

SYNOPSIS OF TREATMENT OPTIONS

Treatment depends entirely on the pattern of clinical involvement. For arthralgia and arthritis as well as constitutional symptoms nonsteroidal anti-inflammatory agents are used and, if needed, combination with low-dose corticosteroid therapy has been shown to be effective. It is very important to monitor and treat the serious manifestations of myositis as well as fibrosing alveolitis and pulmonary hypertension. For more severe disease, immunosuppressive drugs such as cyclophosphamide are used, followed by maintenance therapy with drugs such as azathioprine.

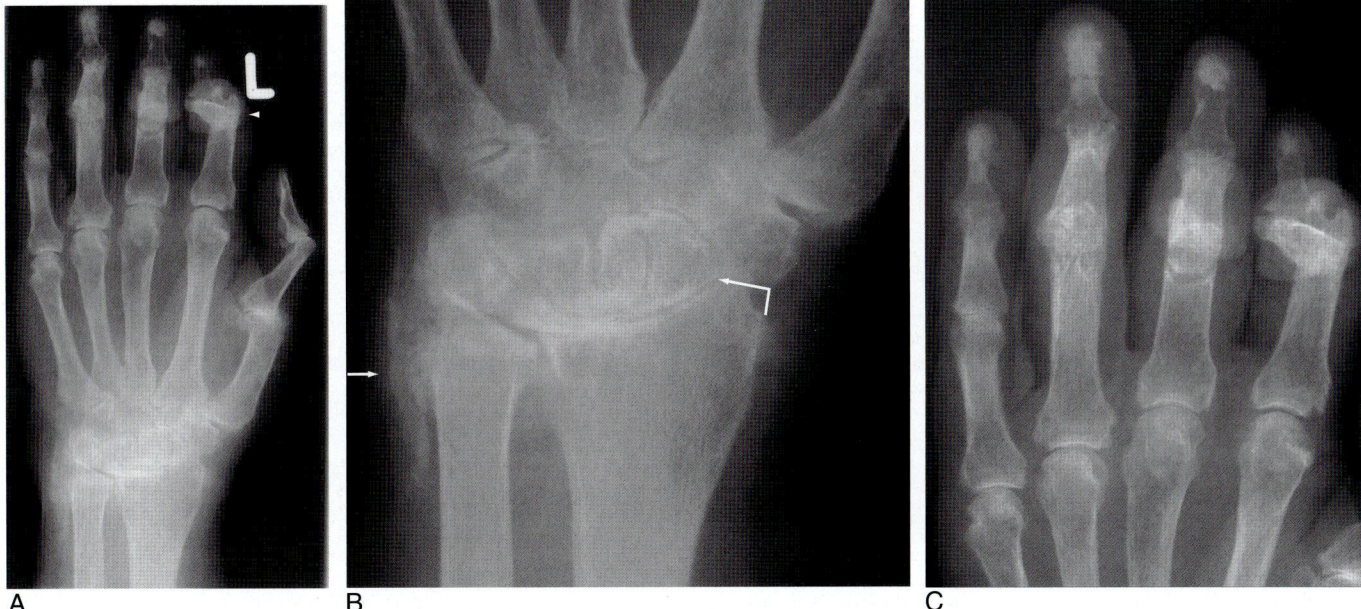

■ FIGURE 52-2   Mixed connective tissue disease. **A** to **C**, Late stage with subcutaneous calcifications (**B**, *arrow*) and atypical erosive arthritis. The arthritis affects the carpals with joint space narrowing and postarthritic instability (*bent arrow* indicates the tilted scaphoid) and secondary degenerative osteoarthritis with subchondral sclerosis. The metacarpophalangeal joints show small erosions similar to rheumatoid arthritis; the proximal and distal interphalangeal joints are already severely deformed (**A**, *arrowhead*). Atypical distal interphalangeal joint arthritis is present with erosions in the third and fourth fingers and ankylosis in the fifth finger. Note the sclerosis of the unguicular processes, which is unspecific but relatively frequent in systemic lupus erythematosus.

Classic Signs

- Nonspecific signs are the most common finding.
- Polyarthritis ranges from nonerosive to a mutilating course, but only sometimes with unusual involvement or distribution compared with RA.

- Mixture of radiologic symptoms belonging to two or more "classic" connective tissue diseases is very typical but not regularly seen.

SUGGESTED READINGS

Mixed connective tissue disease and collagen vascular overlap syndromes. In Resnick D: Diagnosis of Joint and Bone Disorders, 4th ed. Philadelphia, WB Saunders, 2002, vol 2, pp 1249–1259.

Venables PJW. Overlap syndromes. In Hochberg MC, Silman AJ, Smolen JS, et al (eds): Rheumatology, 3rd ed. St. Louis, Mosby, 2003, pp 1573–1580.

REFERENCES

1. Sharp GC, Irwin WS, Tan EM, et al. Mixed connective tissue disease: an apparently distinct rheumatic disease syndrome associated with a specific extractable nuclear antigen. Am J Med 1972; 52:148–159.
2. Maddison PJ. Mixed connective tissue disease: overlap syndromes. Baillieres Best Pract Res Clin Rheumatol 2000; 14:111–124.
3. Hoffman RW, Greidinger EL. Mixed connective tissue disease. Curr Opin Rheumatol 2000; 12:386–390.
4. Nimelstein SH, Brady S, McShane D, Holman HR. MCTD: a subsequent evaluation of the original 25 patients. Medicine 1980; 59:239–248.
5. Reichlin M: Problems in differentiating SLE and MCTD. N Engl J Med 1976; 295:1194–1195.
6. Gendi NST, Welsh KI, Van Venrooij WJ, et al. HLA type as a predictor of mixed connective tissue disease differentiation. Arthritis Rheum 1995; 38:259–266.
7. Ruuska P, Hämeenkorpi R, Forsberg S, et al. Differences in HLA antigens between patients with mixed connective tissue disease and systemic lupus erythematosus. Ann Rheum Dis 1992; 51:52–55.
8. Alarcón GS, Williams GV, Singer JZ, et al. Early undifferentiated connective tissue disease: I. Early clinical manifestation in a large cohort of patients with undifferentiated connective tissue disease compared with cohorts of well established connective tissue disease. J Rheumatol 1991; 18:1332–1339.

9. Clegg DO, Williams HJ, Singer JZ, et al. Early undifferentiated connective tissue disease: II. The frequency of circulating antinuclear antibodies in patients with early rheumatic diseases. J Rheumatol 1991; 18:1340-1343.

10. Kallenberg CGM: Connective tissue disease in patients presenting with Raynaud's phenomenon alone. Ann Rheum Dis 1991; 50:666-667.

11. Lundberg I, Hedfors E. Clinical course of patients with anti-RNP antibodies: a prospective study of 32 patients. J Rheumatol 1991; 18:1511-1519.

12. Alarcón-Segovia D, Villareal M. Classification and diagnostic criteria for mixed connective tissue disease. In Kasukawa R, Sharp GC (eds). Mixed Connective Tissue Disease and Antinuclear Antibodies. Amsterdam, Elsevier, 1987, pp 33-40.

13. Kasukawa R, Tojo T, Miyawaki S: Preliminary diagnostic criteria for classification of mixed connective tissue disease. In Kasukawa R, Sharp GC (eds). Mixed Connective Tissue Disease and Antinuclear Antibodies. Amsterdam, Elsevier, 1987, pp 41-47.

14. Sharp GC. Diagnostic criteria for classification of MCTD. In Kasukawa R, Sharp GC (eds). Mixed Connective Tissue Disease and Antinuclear Antibodies. Amsterdam, Elsevier, 1987, pp 23-32.

15. Alarcón-Segovia D, Cardiel MA. Comparison between 3 diagnostic criteria for connective tissue disease: Study of 593 patients. J Rheumatol 1989; 16:328-334.

16. Sharp GC, Irwin WS, May CM. Association of antibodies to ribonucleoprotein and Sm with mixed connective tissue disease, systemic lupus erythematosus and other rheumatic diseases. N Engl J Med 1976; 29:1149-1154.

17. Leibfarth JH, Perselin RH. Characteristics of patients with serum antibodies to serum extractable nuclear antigens. Arthritis Rheum 1976; 9:851-856.

18. Farber SJ, Bole GG. Antibodies to components of extractable nuclear antigens. Arch Intern Med 1976; 136:425-431.

19. Lemmer JP, Curry NH, Mallory JH. Clinical characteristics and course in patients with high titer anti-RNP antibodies. J Rheumatol 1982; 9:536-542.

20. Cooke CL, Lurie HI: Case report: Fatal gastrointestinal hemorrhage in mixed connective tissue disease. Arthritis Rheum 1977; 20:1421-1426.

21. Weiss TD, Nelson JS, Woosley RM, et al. Transverse myelitis in mixed connective tissue disease. Arthritis Rheum 1978; 21:982-986.

22. Jones MB, Osterholm RK, Wilson RB, et al. Fatal pulmonary hypertension and resolving immune-complex glomerulonephritis in mixed connective tissue disease. Am J Med 1978; 65:855-862.

23. Amigues JM, Cantagrel A, Abbal M, Mazieres B. Comparative study of 4 diagnosis criteria sets for mixed connective tissue disease in patients with anti-RNP antibodies. J Rheumatol 1996; 23:2055-2062.

24. Resnick D. Mixed connective tissue disease and collagen vascular overlap syndromes. In: Resnick D, Niwayama G (eds): Diagnosis of Joint and Bone Disorders, 2nd ed. Philadelphia, WB Saunders. 2002, vol 2, pp 1342-1352.

25. Udoff EJ, Genant HK, Kozin F, Ginsberg M. Mixed connective tissue disease: The spectrum of radiographic manifestations. Radiology 1977; 124:613-618.

26. Bennett RM, O'Connel DJ: The arthritis of mixed connective tissue disease. Ann Rheum Dis 1978; 37:397-403.

27. Halla JT, Hardin JG. Clinical features of the arthritis of mixed connective tissue disease. Arthritis Rheum 1978; 21:497-503.

CHAPTER 53

Juvenile Idiopathic Arthritis

Karl Johnson

ETIOLOGY

Juvenile idiopathic arthritis (JIA) represents a heterogeneous group of autoimmune disorders that begin in childhood and involve persistent inflammation of one or more joints. It is a disorder of unknown etiology, but in a minority of cases there is an association with rheumatoid factor and human leukocyte antigen (HLA)-B27.

The JIA classification of childhood arthropathies unifies and replaces the criteria of juvenile rheumatoid arthritis (JRA), used by the American College of Rheumatology, and juvenile chronic arthritis (JCA), used by the European League Against Rheumatism. The purpose of this new classification is to be able to identify disease entities of true etiologic and pathologic homogeneity. The different subclassifications of JIA and the corresponding JRA and JCA equivalents are shown in Table 53-1.[1-5]

PREVALENCE AND EPIDEMIOLOGY

The incidence of JIA is 6 to 12 per 100,000, with a prevalence of approximately 1 in 1,000. Overall, females are more affected than males.[1]

CLINICAL PRESENTATION

The diagnosis of JIA is a clinical one, in which there is persisting arthritis for at least 6 weeks in a child younger than the age of 16 years in whom there is no known underlying cause. Other symptoms include general fatigue, weight loss, fevers, and generalized systemic ill health. There may be associated lymphadenopathy, pericarditis, hepatosplenomegaly, dermatologic features, pleuritis, interstitial lung disease, and uveitis.[1,5]

PATHOPHYSIOLOGY

Anatomy

The disease can affect any joint. Extra-articular sites include the eye (uvea), chest, heart, and skin. Systemic symptoms may be widespread and generalized.[5-8]

Pathology

Within the joint the primary pathologic process is autoimmune-related synovial proliferation. There is associated soft tissue swelling and effusion. This is a hypervascular process that can result in periarticular osteopenia, localized bone overgrowth, and remodeling. If left untreated, the synovial proliferation will cause cartilage thinning and bone erosions. Involvement of adjacent soft tissues and ligaments can cause joint deformity and loss of function. Initially, the hypervascularity can cause accelerated localized growth, but in the patient with more chronic disease there is reduction in growth.[7-10]

IMAGING TECHNIQUES

Techniques and Relevant Aspects

Radiographs of an involved joint are useful as a primary imaging investigation to exclude other causes of joint disease such as dysplasias, tumors, and other localized pathologic processes such as Legg-Calvé-Perthes disease.

The radiographic features are osteopenia, periarticular swelling, epiphyseal overgrowth, loss of joint space, and erosions. There may be subluxation of the joint and periosteal new bone formation in bone adjacent to the joint.[5,6,9,10]

Ultrasonography will demonstrate hypoechoic joint effusions with thickened mixed echogenic synovial lining of the joint. Synovial cysts and inflammatory changes

---

KEY POINTS

- Sepsis needs to be excluded in all children with an inflamed joint.
- MRI with gadolinium enhancement is most sensitive in detecting synovial hypertrophy.

TABLE 53-1 Classification of Different Subtypes of Juvenile Idiopathic Arthritis and Comparison with Previous Classification Systems

Characteristic	JIA (ILAR)	JCA (EULAR)	JRA (ACR)	Adult Equivalent
Age at onset	<16 yr	<16 yr	<16 yr	
Minimum duration of symptoms	6 wk	3 mo	6 wk	
Subtypes	Systemic arthritis	Systemic-onset JCA	Systemic-onset JRA	Adult Still's disease
	Oligoarthritis	Oligoarticular	Pauciarticular JCA	
	Persistent			
	Extended		Pauciarticular to polyarticular JCA	
	Polyarthritis	Polyarticular JRA	Polyarticular JCA	
	RhF negative	(RhF does not alter classification)	Juvenile rheumatoid arthritis (JRA)	
	RhF positive			Rheumatoid arthritis
	Enthesitis-related Arthritis	Excluded	Juvenile spondyloarthropathies (including Juvenile ankylosing spondylitis, juvenile psoriatic arthritis, Reiter's syndrome, arthropathies of inflammatory bowel disease)	
	Psoriatic arthritis	Excluded		Psoriatic arthritis
	Other			

ILAR, International League of Associations for Rheumatology; EULAR, European League Against Rheumatism; ACR, American College of Rheumatology; RhF, rheumatoid factor.
Modified from Johnson K, Gardiner-Medwin J. Childhood arthritis: classification and radiology. Clin Radiol 2002; 57:47–58.

in adjacent tendons may be observed. Ultrasonography may also detect cartilage thinning and bone erosions.[11-15]

MRI is useful to detect synovial hypertrophy, marrow edema, erosions, and cartilage damage.[7,8]

T1-weighted MR images will show erosions as hypointense defects in the cortex at the joint margin, which may be surrounded by low-signal-intensity subchondral sclerosis and marrow edema. With post-gadolinium, T1-weighted MR sequences the inflamed synovium will show intense enhancement. Post-gadolinium, fat-saturated, T1-weighted MR sequences are the most sensitive in detecting synovial hypertrophy because the signal from the adjacent fatty marrow will be suppressed. Volume measurements of the enhanced synovium may be useful in monitoring disease progress.[16-19]

T2-weighted MR sequences will show hyperintense marrow edema, tenosynovitis, and joint effusions. Synovium is often similar in signal intensity to the adjacent effusion, which can make its detection difficult.[8] However, with proper windowing, fluid can be differentiated from synovial proliferation.

Proton density–weighted, fast spin-echo, fat-saturated MR sequences will show high-signal-intensity cartilage. The synovial hypertrophy is slightly less hyperintense when compared with joint effusion.[20]

T2 mapping sequences of the cartilage may provide early information about cartilage damage and erosive changes.[21,22]

Pros and Cons

Radiographs are a simple and inexpensive method to detect damage around the joints and are useful at the time of diagnosis to exclude other causes of joint damage. They are indicated if there has been a significant change in the patient's symptoms or joint function. Unfortunately, they are relatively insensitive in detecting intra-articular

changes and pre-erosive damage, and the routine use of radiographs for the diagnosis and follow-up of JIA is not indicated.[5,9,23,24]

Both ultrasonography and MRI are more sensitive in detecting effusions, synovial hypertrophy, synovial cysts, and joint abnormalities than clinical examination.[6] Ultrasonography may be difficult in the smaller child with a painful joint because it may not be possible to obtain a satisfactory acoustic window.

MRI is more sensitive than ultrasonography in detecting intra-articular damage and synovial hypertrophy deep within a joint.[6] It is useful for assessing the sacroiliac joints. Post-gadolinium, T1-weighted, fat-saturated MR sequences are the most sensitive detector of synovial hypertrophy.[5,18]

MANIFESTATIONS OF THE DISEASE

Appendicular Skeleton Involvement

The carpal and interphalangeal joints are common sites of involvement (Fig. 53-1). The disease involvement is often bilateral, but it may not be completely symmetric. Soft tissue swelling and pain are early features whereas erosions, subluxation, and joint damage can cause significant long-term morbidity problems. Radial deviation at the wrist joint is a characteristic feature of JIA compared with ulnar deviation, which is seen in adults.[8,9,25]

The knee joint is one of the most common joints involved in JIA. It is particularly amenable to evaluation with MRI. Initially, the joint may be swollen with restriction of movement and pain. If the disease is not treated, significant functional disability and valgus or varus deformity can result.

The initial hypervascularity around the joint can cause generalized metaphyseal widening and epiphyseal overgrowth. In the long bones there may be accelerated

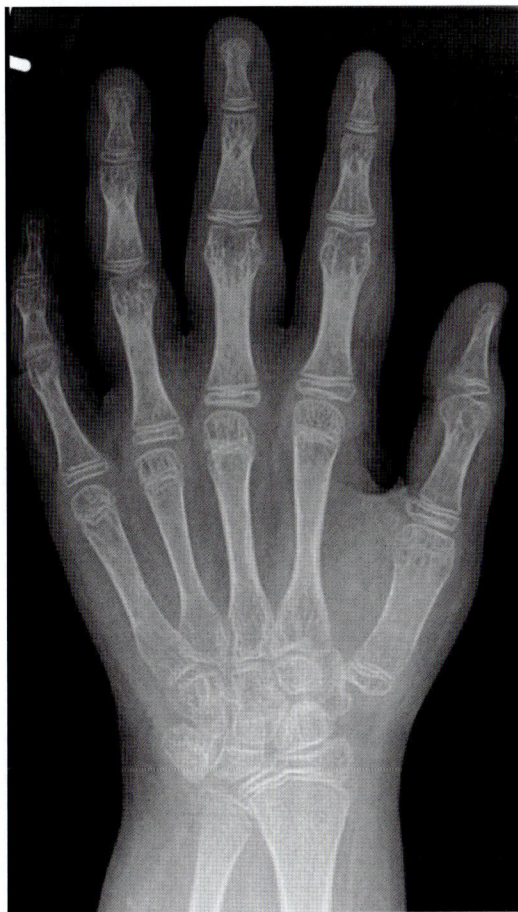

■ **FIGURE 53-1** Anteroposterior radiograph of the left hand. There is extensive periarticular osteopenia with some metaphyseal widening and generalized loss of joint space around the carpal bones. Bone density is significantly reduced. Note erosions within the carpal bones.

Radiography

In the hand and wrist initially there is soft tissue swelling around the interphalangeal joints that may be associated with metaphyseal widening and periarticular osteopenia. Periosteal new bone formation may occur along the phalanges, and this is particularly associated with psoriatic arthropathy. Localized growth disturbance and alteration in the normal chronologic appearance of the ossification centers of the carpal bones is not uncommon. With more advanced disease there is a generalized loss of joint space that will lead to the crowding of the carpal bones. The carpal bones may become square and angulated and eventually ankylosed.[5,9,24,25,28]

In the knee joint hypervascularity can result in squaring of the patella, metaphyseal widening, and bony overgrowth. This can lead to the characteristic appearance of a widened intercondylar notch. The knee is a common site for erosive damage, and there can be displaced bony fragments within the joint that may result in locking.[9]

Comparison radiographs of the limbs may show limb-length discrepancies and asymmetric ossification of the carpal and tarsal bones. Radiographs of the left hand are useful for determining bone age as it corresponds to chronologic age.

Magnetic Resonance Imaging

Initially with early disease there is lymphadenopathy and joint effusion associated with the synovial hypertrophy, and MRI is optimal for evaluation; contrast-enhanced images are particularly useful for documenting the presence of synovitis (Figs. 53-2 and 53-3). There is often prominent synovial proliferation within the joint and adjacent tendon sheaths. Disease progression can cause cartilage loss and erosions with thinning and atrophy of the fibrocartilage structures and ligaments.[29-32] MRI is useful in detecting synovial involvement of the adjacent tendons.

Multidetector Computed Tomography

Radiographs are generally adequate for evaluation of osseous findings; CT utilizes a high radiation dose and should be minimized in pediatric patients.

longitudinal growth that initially will cause increased limb length but, unfortunately, will eventually result in premature fusion of the growth plates and, ultimately, a relative reduction in limb length. In both the hands and feet there can be an acceleration in the normal ossification pattern of the carpal and tarsal bones. With chronic disease there is generalized reduction in growth and height. Pain and restriction of movement will cause some muscle atrophy.[26,27]

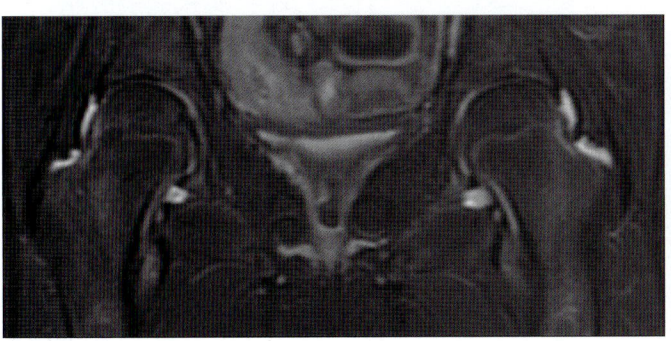
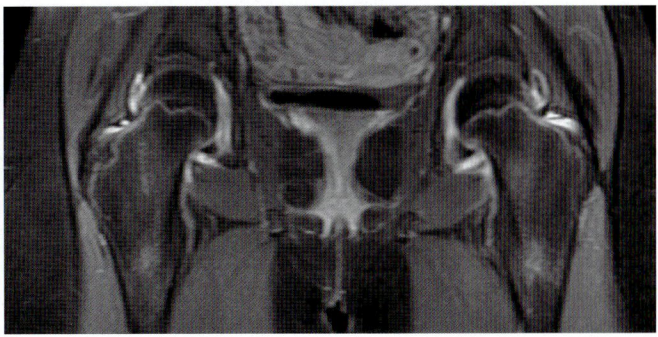

A   B

■ **FIGURE 53-2** Coronal STIR **(A)** and post-gadolinium, fat-saturated, T1-weighted **(B)** MR images of the hips. On the STIR image there is high signal intensity around both hip joints. This may represent either synovium or fluid. The post-gadolinium image demonstrates the presence of fluid and synovium.

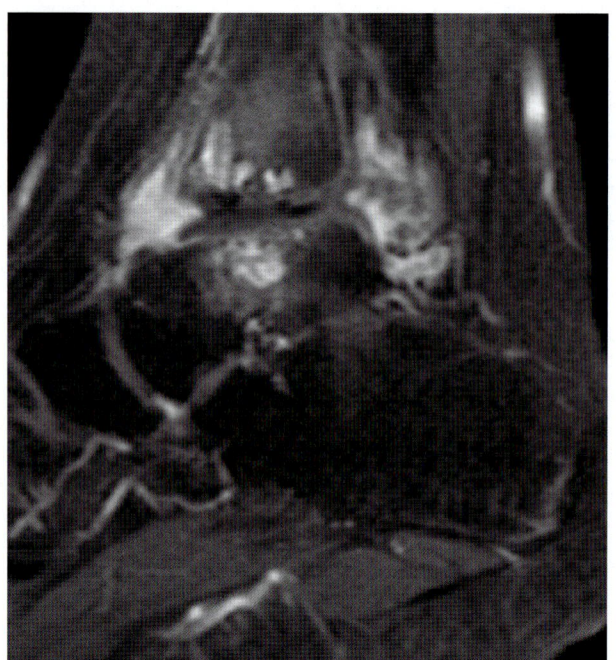

■ **FIGURE 53-3** Sagittal, T1-weighted, post-gadolinium, fat-saturated MR image of the ankle. There is extensive synovial hypertrophy around the ankle joint. There are enhancing subchondral synovial deposits within the distal tibia and enhancing marrow around the ankle joint. Note the significant loss of joint space.

Ultrasonography

Ultrasonography is useful as a noninvasive, widely available, rapid tool to document joint effusion and synovitis.

Classic Signs

- Joint narrowing and fusions
- Synovitis/effusions
- Overgrowth of bone
- Enlarged ("ballooned") epiphyses
- Limb-length discrepancy

MANIFESTATIONS OF THE DISEASE

Axial Skeleton Involvement

Involvement of the cervical spine is more common in children with a positive rheumatoid factor, whereas lumbar involvement is more common in HLA-B27–positive cases. There is an increased incidence of scoliosis in JIA. Prolonged corticosteroid treatment and uncontrolled disease can lead to osteopenia and vertebral collapse.[5,8,9] Involvement of the mandible and temporomandibular joint can lead to severe facial asymmetry and micrognathia. Involvement of the temporomandibular joint can cause restriction of movement and functional disability.[33-35]

Radiography

In the cervical spine there is squaring of the vertebral bodies and loss of intervertebral disc height with scle-

rosis around the facet joints. Ankylosis of the facet and apophyseal joints can occur that will cause significant restriction of joint movement (Fig. 53-4). Conversely, erosions of the odontoid with involvement of the adjacent ligaments will result in atlantoaxial subluxation and instability of the cervical spine. There is widening of the distance between the odontoid and anterior body of C1 to greater than 5 mm on a lateral radiograph, with alteration in this distance on flexion and extension views.[36,37]

In the lumbar spine there is squaring of the vertebral bodies. There may be prominent osteophyte formation, which can lead to ankylosis and movement restriction.

The sacroiliac joints are not uncommonly involved. Radiographs will demonstrate sclerosis and irregularity of the joint margins. Ankylosis is a late feature.

There is a characteristic finding of antegonial notching of the mandible (concave on the undersurface of the mandible). Generalized micrognathia and joint erosions are not uncommon.[33]

Magnetic Resonance Imaging

Synovial enhancement is typically seen around the odontoid and facet joints. Around the sacroiliac joints there is often marked marrow edema, which is most obviously seen on short tau inversion recovery (STIR) sequences. Enhancement of the sacroiliac joints can occur.[38,39] Erosions, cartilage thinning, and flattening of the temporomandibular joint surface with loss of the intra-articular disc occur. Synovial hypertrophy within the joint can be seen on post-gadolinium MR sequences.[40]

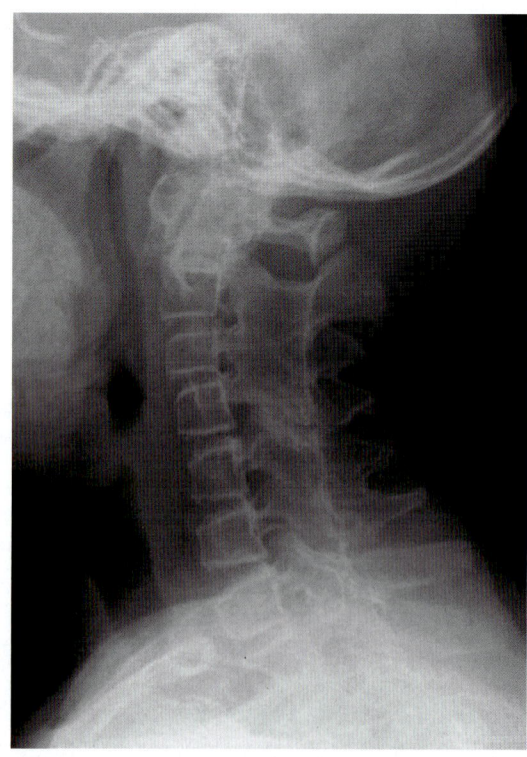

■ **FIGURE 53-4** Lateral radiograph of the cervical spine. There is squaring of the vertebral bodies. Note the extensive ankylosis of the facet joints posteriorly and widening of the space anterior to the odontoid.

Classic Signs

- Facet fusions and spinal deformity
- Atlantoaxial instability

DIFFERENTIAL DIAGNOSIS

The important differential diagnosis that needs to be excluded is sepsis. This can only be totally excluded after joint aspiration and culture, which should be undertaken in all cases in which sepsis is clinically suspected. Reactive arthritis is in the differential diagnosis but does not typically last 6 weeks. Malignancy (particularly neuroblastoma and leukemia in the younger child) needs to be considered in all cases but is a rare cause for joint inflammation.

JIA may be associated with raised antinuclear antibody, rheumatoid factor, and IgM levels.

Both pigmented villonodular synovitis and hemophilic arthropathy are associated with hemorrhage within the joint, which is seen as low signal hemosiderin deposition on all MR sequences that will be accentuated on gradient-echo sequences.

Malignant infiltration of the bone typically extends beyond the growth plate, which would be unusual in JIA. This would be seen as altered marrow signal on T1- and T2-weighted sequences.

SYNOPSIS OF TREATMENT OPTIONS

Medical management is aimed at symptom control, preventing disease progression, maintaining joint function, and promoting the child's independence. Nonsteroidal anti-inflammatory drugs along with localized corticosteroid joint injections are often the first-line treatments. Methotrexate is the primary drug used for disease modification, with the new anti-tumor necrosis factor receptors as second-line therapy.

What the Referring Physician Needs to Know

- Sepsis needs to be excluded in all cases.
- Radiographs are poor at monitoring disease progression.
- MRI is the most sensitive in the detection of synovial hypertrophy.

SUGGESTED READINGS

Azouz EM. Arthritis in children: conventional and advanced imaging. Semin Musculoskelet Radiol 2003; 7:95–102.

Cohen PA, Job-Deslandre CH, Lalande G, Adamsbaum C. Overview of the radiology of juvenile idiopathic arthritis (JIA). Eur J Radiol 2000; 33:94–101.

Johnson K. Imaging of juvenile idiopathic arthritis. Pediatr Radiol 2006; 36:743–758.

Miller ML. Use of imaging in the differential diagnosis of rheumatic diseases in children. Rheum Dis Clin North Am 2002; 28:483–492.

REFERENCES

1. Andersson Gare B. Juvenile arthritis—who get it, where and when? A review of current data on incidence and prevalence. Clin Exp Rheumatol 1999; 17:367–374.
2. Gare B, Fasth A. The natural history of juvenile chronic arthritis: a population based cohort study: II. Outcome. J Rheumatol 1995; 22:308–319.
3. Petty RE, Southwood TR. Classification of childhood arthritis: divide and conquer. J Rheumatol 1998; 25:1869–1870.
4. Foeldvari I, Bidde M. Validation of the proposed ILAR classification criteria for juvenile idiopathic arthritis. J Rheumatol 2000; 27:1069–1072.
5. Johnson K, Gardner-Medwin J. Childhood arthritis: classification and radiology. Clin Radiol 2002; 57:47–58.
6. Cohen PA, Job-Deslandre CH, Lalande G, et al. Overview of the radiology of juvenile idiopathic arthritis (JIA). Eur J Radiol 2000; 33:94–101.
7. Gylys-Morin VM. MR imaging of pediatric musculoskeletal inflammatory and infectious disorders. Magn Reson Imaging Clin North Am. 1998; 6:537–559.
8. Buchmann RF, Jaramillo D. Imaging of articular disorders in children. Radiol Clin North Am 2004; 42:151–168.
9. Ansell BM, Kent PA. Radiological changes in juvenile chronic polyarthritis. Skeletal Radiol 1977; 1:129–144.
10. Oen K, Reed M, Malleson PN, et al. Radiologic outcome and its relationship to functional disability in juvenile rheumatoid arthritis. J Rheumatol 2003; 30:832–840.
11. Lamer S, Sebag GH. MRI and ultrasound in children with juvenile chronic arthritis. Eur J Radiol 2000; 33:85–93.
12. Sureda D, Quiroga S, Arnal C, et al. Juvenile rheumatoid arthritis of the knee: evaluation with US. Radiology 1994; 190:403–406.
13. El-Miedany YM, Housny IH, Mansour HM. Ultrasound versus MRI in the evaluation of juvenile idiopathic arthritis of the knee. Joint Bone Spine 2001; 68:222–230.
14. Fedrizzi MS, Ronchezel MV, Hiliaro MOE, et al. Ultrasonography in the early diagnosis of hip joint involvement in juvenile rheumatoid arthritis. J Rheumatol 1997; 24:1820–1825.
15. Cellerini M, Salti S, Trapani S, et al. Correlation between clinical and ultrasound assessment of the knee in children with mono-articular or pauciarticular juvenile rheumatoid arthritis Pediatr Radiol 1999; 29:117–123.
16. Barnewolt CE, Chung T. Techniques, coils, pulse sequences, and contrast enhancement in pediatric musculoskeletal MR imaging. Magn Reson Imaging Clin North Am 1998; 6:441–453.
17. Senac MO Jr, Deutsch D, Bernstein BH, et al. MR imaging in juvenile rheumatoid arthritis. AJR Am J Roentgenol 1998; 150:873–878.

18. Herve-Somma CMP, Sebag GH, Prieur A-M, et al. Juvenile rheumatoid arthritis of the knee: MR evaluation with Gd-DPTA. Radiology 1992; 182:93-98.

19. Graham TB, Laor T, Dardzinski BJ. Quantitative magnetic resonance imaging of the hands and wrists of children with juvenile rheumatoid arthritis. J Rheumatol 2005; 32:1811-1820.

20. Jaramillo D, Shapiro F. Growth cartilage: normal appearance, variants and abnormalities. Magn Reson Imaging Clin North Am 1998; 6:455-471.

21. Kight AC, Dardzinski BJ, Laor T, et al. Magnetic resonance imaging evaluation of the effects of juvenile rheumatoid arthritis on distal femoral weight-bearing cartilage. Arthritis Rheum 2004; 50:901-905.

22. Mosher TJ, Dardzinski BJ. Cartilage MRI T2 relaxation time mapping: overview and applications. Semin Musculoskelet Radiol 2004; 8:355-368.

23. Martel W, Holt JF, Cassidy JT. Roentgenologic manifestations of juvenile rheumatoid arthritis. Am J Roentgenol Radium Ther Nucl Med 1962; 88:400-423.

24. Reed MH, Wilmot DM. The radiology of juvenile rheumatoid arthritis: a review of the English language literature. J Rheumatol Suppl 1991; 31:2-22.

25. Chaplin D, Pulkki T, Saarimaa A, et al. Wrist and finger deformities in juvenile rheumatoid arthritis. Acta Rheumatol Scand 1969; 15:206-223.

26. Ansell BM, Bywaters EG. Growth in Still's disease. Ann Rheum Dis 1956; 15:295-319.

27. Simon S, Whiffen J, Shapiro F. Leg-length discrepancies in monoarticular and pauciarticular juvenile rheumatoid arthritis. J Bone Joint Surg Am 1981; 63:209-215.

28. Maldonado-Cocco JA, Garcia-Morteo O, Spindler AJ, et al. Carpal ankylosis in juvenile rheumatoid arthritis. Arthritis Rheum 1980; 23:1251-1255.

29. Eich GF, Halle F, Hodler J, et al. Juvenile chronic arthritis: imaging of the knees and hips before and after intraarticular steroid injection. Pediatr Radiol 1994; 24:558-563.

30. Doria AS, Kiss MH, Lotito AP, et al. Juvenile rheumatoid arthritis of the knee: evaluation with contrast enhanced color Doppler ultrasound. Pediatr Radiol 2001; 31:524-531.

31. Gylys-Morin VM, Graham TB, Blebea JS, et al. Knee in early juvenile rheumatoid arthritis: MR imaging findings. Radiology 2001; 220:696-706.

32. Johnson K, Wittkop B, Haigh F, et al. The early magnetic resonance imaging features of the knee in juvenile idiopathic arthritis. Clin Radiol 2002; 57:466-471.

33. Larheim TA, Dale K, Tveito L. Radiographic abnormalities of the temporomandibular joint in children with juvenile rheumatoid arthritis. Acta Radiol 1981; 22:277-284.

34. Larheim TA, Hoyeraal HM, Stabrun AE, Hannaes HR. The temporomandibular joint in juvenile rheumatoid arthritis. Scand J Rheumatol 1982; 11:5-12.

35. Ronchezel MV, Odete M, Hilario OE, et al. Temporomandibular joint and mandibular growth alterations in patients with juvenile rheumatoid arthritis. J Rheumatol 1995; 22:1956-1961.

36. Thompson GH, Khan MA, Bilenker RM. Spontaneous atlanto-axial subluxation as a presenting manifestation of juvenile ankylosing spondylitis. Spine 1982; 7:78-79.

37. Foster HE, Carins RA, Burnell RH, et al. Atlantoaxial subluxation in children with seronegative enthesopathy and arthropathy syndrome: 2 case reports and a review of the literature. J Rheumatol 1995; 22:548-551.

38. Bollow M, Braun J, Biedermann T, et al. Use of contrast-enhanced MR imaging to detect sacroiliitis in children. Skeletal Radiol 1998; 27:606-616.

39. Bollow M, Biedermann T, Kannenberg J, et al. Use of dynamic magnetic resonance imaging to detect sacroiliitis in HLA-B27 positive and negative children with juvenile arthritides. J Rheumatol 1998; 25:556-564.

40. Kuseler A, Pederson TK, Herlin T, et al. Contrast enhanced magnetic resonance imaging as a method to diagnose early inflammation changes in the temporomandibular joint in children with juvenile chronic arthritis. J Rheumatol 1998; 25:1406-1412.

54

Idiopathic Inflammatory Myopathy

Lawrence Yao and Lisa G. Rider

ETIOLOGY

The idiopathic inflammatory myopathies (IIM) include polymyositis (PM), dermatomyositis (DM), and sporadic inclusion-body myositis (sIBM). The IIM are thought to be cell-mediated, systemic autoimmune disorders, although a specific autoantigen has not been identified. Autoantibodies are often present in DM and PM and are of value in the classification and prognosis of subgroups of IIM, but they do not have a well-established pathogenic role.[1] Genetic and environmental factors may contribute to the development of these diseases.[1]

PREVALENCE AND EPIDEMIOLOGY

The IIM are rare. These illnesses are three to five times more frequent in adults than children, with an annual incidence of 10 to 20 new cases per million population. PM constitutes 10% to 40% of adult IIM and 10% of juvenile IIM, whereas DM constitutes 30% to 60% of adult IIM and 85% of juvenile IIM, depending on the referral population.[2] sIBM constitutes 15% to 30% of adult IIM.[2] PM and DM are more common in females, whereas sIBM predominates in older adult males.

CLINICAL PRESENTATION

Disease onset is usually more acute in DM than in PM, whereas sIBM is characterized by an indolent disease onset.[2] Symmetric proximal muscle weakness is the primary presenting symptom in PM and DM. In sIBM, weakness is greater in the distal than proximal muscles and more asymmetric than in PM.

In DM, the characteristic cutaneous findings of heliotrope rash or Gottron's papules may precede muscle involvement by up to 6 months. Myalgia and tenderness can occur and are more common in DM. Extramuscular involvement, particularly dysphagia, may be present in all three forms of IIM. Arthritis, dysphonia, interstitial lung disease, a number of other photosensitive and non-photosensitive rashes, myocarditis, and intestinal manifestations are often part of the illness.[3]

PM and DM may occur in association with other connective tissue diseases, most commonly scleroderma and systemic lupus erythematosus and less commonly with rheumatoid arthritis.[2] Adult-onset DM and PM have a potential association with malignancy, particularly within 2 years of diagnosis[4]; the frequency and spectrum of tumor types parallel those found in the general population.[5] All adults with DM and PM should undergo screening and surveillance for occult malignancy.[6]

The Bohan and Peter diagnostic criteria for PM and DM[7] are still widely used and include proximal and symmetric muscle weakness; elevated serum levels of muscle enzymes; myopathic pattern on electromyography; and characteristic findings on muscle biopsy. Three criteria

KEY POINTS

- Fluid-sensitive MR images depict the important features of edema-like signal in muscle, fascia, and subcutis in the IIM.
- T1-weighted MR images demonstrate muscle atrophy and fatty infiltration, consistent with myofiber damage in chronic IIM.
- MRI findings, although nonspecific, can be helpful in establishing a diagnosis of idiopathic inflammatory myopathy and selecting a site for muscle biopsy.
- MR spectroscopy and contrast-enhanced ultrasonography may yield metabolic or functional information in patients with active myositis.
- Calcinosis is best detected by plain radiographs, although MRI may demonstrate subcutaneous inflammation in patients with DM that is a precursor to calcinosis.

are necessary for a diagnosis of probable PM, and four criteria are required for a definite diagnosis of PM. The diagnosis of DM requires a fifth criterion of characteristic rashes. sIBM is reliably distinguished from PM only by muscle biopsy but should be suspected when symptoms are refractory to standard immunosuppressive therapy.

PATHOPHYSIOLOGY

Anatomy

Any skeletal muscle can be involved in IIM. Disease distribution is usually bilateral and fairly symmetric in proximal appendicular or axial muscle groups in DM and PM, whereas in sIBM the distal muscle groups and quadriceps are most often involved. Occasionally, cardiac or smooth muscle may also be affected.

Pathology

The characteristic findings of IIM on muscle biopsy are inflammatory infiltrates, muscle fiber necrosis, and muscle fiber regeneration. In DM the inflammation tends to be perivascular, whereas in PM it tends to be endomysial. Muscle hyperintensity on T2 or short tau inversion recovery (STIR) MR images may reflect endomysial, perimysial, perifascicular, or perivascular inflammation, as well as muscle necrosis and phagocytosis. Less inflammation of involved muscle is present in cases of sIBM than in PM or DM. The characteristic finding of IBM on biopsy is that of muscle vacuoles rimmed by granular material, and on electron microscopy it is the presence of cytoplasmic, tubulofilamentous inclusion bodies.

IMAGING TECHNIQUES

Magnetic Resonance Imaging

Techniques and Relevant Aspects

T2-weighted MRI sequences depict increased signal intensity in affected muscles of patients with inflammatory myopathy.[8,9] These changes in signal intensity can be described as "edema-like" and are typically widespread but patchy in distribution (Fig. 54-1). Edema-like muscle signal intensity is also readily detected on STIR sequences, even at relatively short echo times, by virtue of fat signal suppression and concomitant T1 prolongation in areas of inflammation.

Fat suppression enhances the detection of muscle abnormalities in IIM on T2-weighted imaging.[10] Because spectral fat saturation may fail when static magnetic field homogeneity is poor, STIR imaging is preferred for survey studies done with a large field of view.

Non–fat-suppressed, T1-weighted imaging is valuable for identification of fatty involution of muscle, a conspicuous marker of disease damage (Fig. 54-2). Contrast-enhanced MRI does not appear to improve depiction of muscle disease in IIM.[8]

Step table capabilities on MR scanners now facilitate MR surveys of the whole body. Because detection of inflammatory myopathy does not require high spatial resolution, a total-body survey, typically using a STIR sequence, is a viable diagnostic strategy in cases of suspected myopathy. This approach may reveal truncal disease that precedes disease in appendicular sites that are more typically surveyed by MRI.[11]

Pitfalls (Pros and Cons)

Exercise creates signal changes in work-loaded muscles on STIR or T2-weighted imaging that may simulate inflammatory disease.[12] Muscle strain injuries or delayed-onset muscle soreness (DOMS) also manifests edema-like signal intensity changes on MRI but should be distinguishable on clinical grounds.

Signal variations in muscle groups on STIR or T2-weighted imaging may also reflect normal differences in muscle fiber type predominance. Slow-twitch muscles are characterized by longer T1 relaxation,[13] and muscle groups with greater type I muscle fiber predominance may exhibit T2 prolongation with aging.[14]

The findings of myopathy on MRI tend to be difficult to quantify. Technical differences in scan acquisition can also alter the apparent intensity or conspicuousness of diseased muscle on MRI. For this reason, MR acquisition parameters should be rigorously standardized in longitudinal evaluations of myopathy. Postprocessing techniques, as applied to STIR imaging, may aid the quantification of disease in PM.[15] T2 mapping also has potential value as an objective marker of active disease in IIM.[16]

Controversies

Although MRI arguably has greater diagnostic value in cases of suspected IIM than electromyography or serum enzyme measurements, MRI findings have not been formalized as a diagnostic criterion for IIM. The cost of MRI, and lack of standardized methods for acquiring and interpreting MRI, have limited the application of MRI in the study of IIM.[17] MRI evaluation before muscle biopsy, however, has become routine at many tertiary care centers.

MANIFESTATIONS OF THE DISEASE

Myositis

Magnetic resonance imaging may contribute to the diagnosis of PM and DM, particularly in cases in which standard criteria are equivocal. Characteristic MRI findings of extensive muscle inflammation can help confirm a diagnosis, particularly if they are symmetric. Other diagnostic imaging modalities, although potentially helpful, are not widely used in the routine evaluation of suspected IIM.

Disease distribution in IIM is usually bilateral and fairly symmetric in the thigh and hip girdle muscles. The pattern of muscle involvement shown by MRI has some value in distinguishing between the IIM. In PM, anterior and posterior compartment involvement are equally likely in the thigh, whereas in DM the adductor muscles and quadriceps, particularly the vastus lateralis, are predilected.[18] Edema-like muscle signal changes may be more common, and muscle atrophy less common, in DM as compared with PM.[8]

The pattern of MRI findings may also aid distinction of sIBM from PM. Muscle atrophy is more prominent on presentation in cases of sIBM. In the thigh, anterior

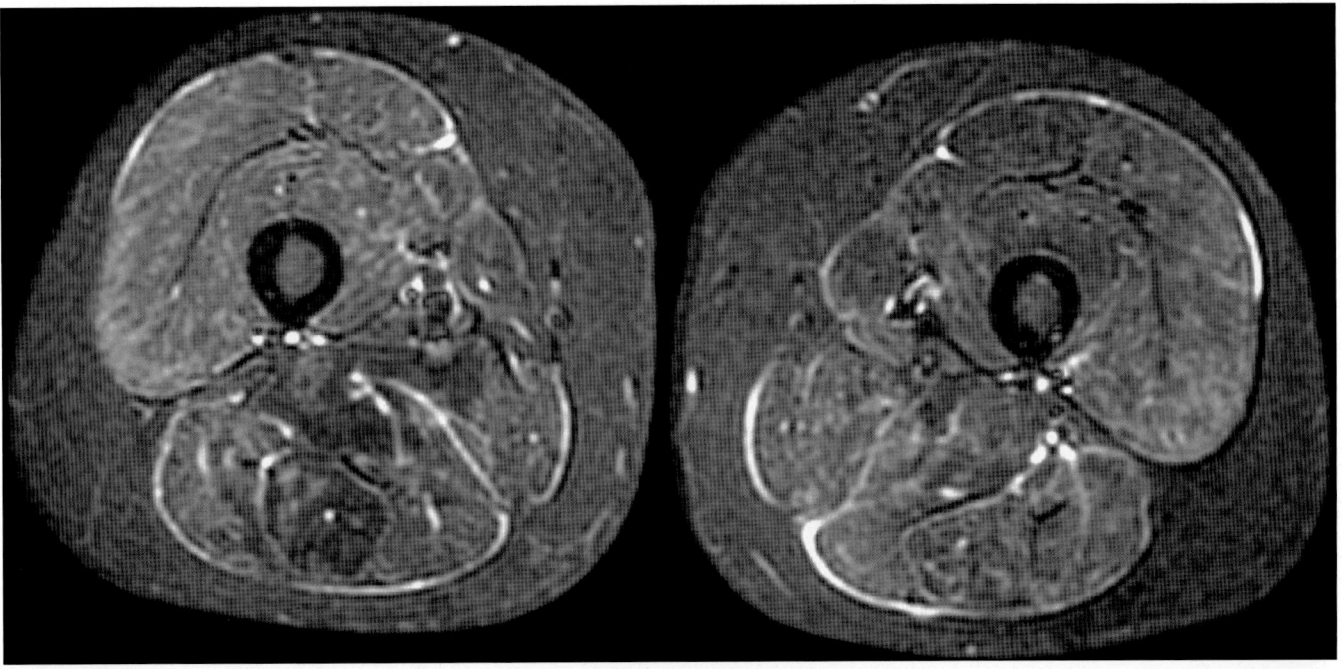

A

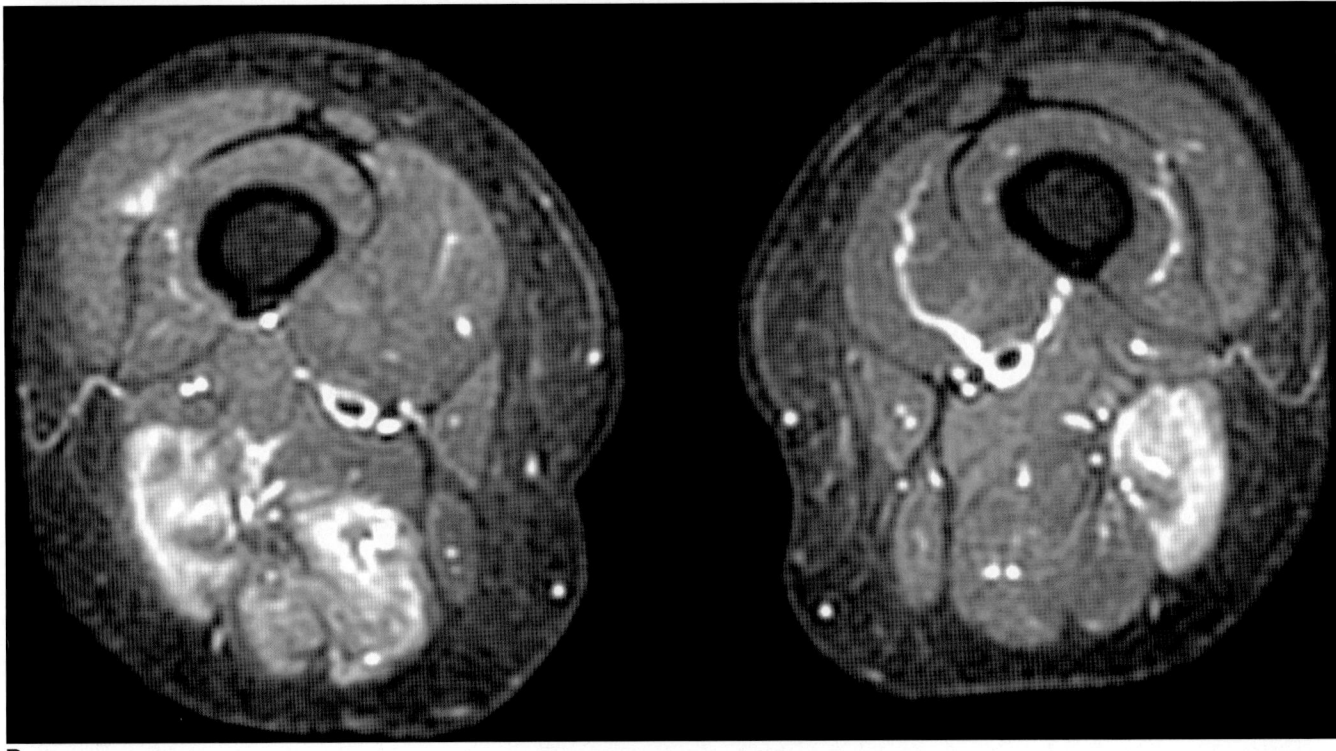

B

■ **FIGURE 54-1** **A,** Axial short tau inversion recovery (STIR) image of polymyositis depicts characteristic, diffuse, edema-like signal in the affected thigh muscles bilaterally. There are some areas of muscle sparing in the right hamstring and adductor muscles. There are also features of fasciitis. **B,** Axial STIR image of polymyositis showing a more localized pattern of muscle inflammation, preferentially involving the hamstring musculature in this case.

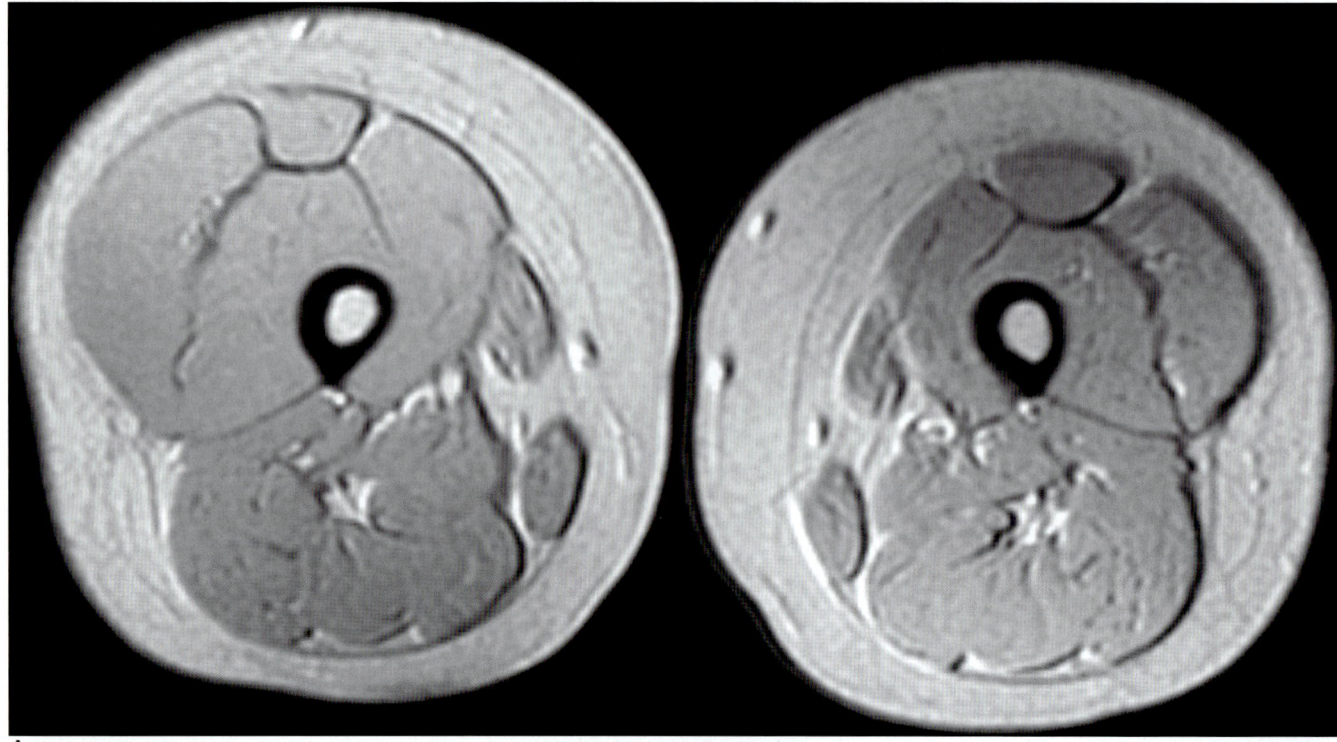

A

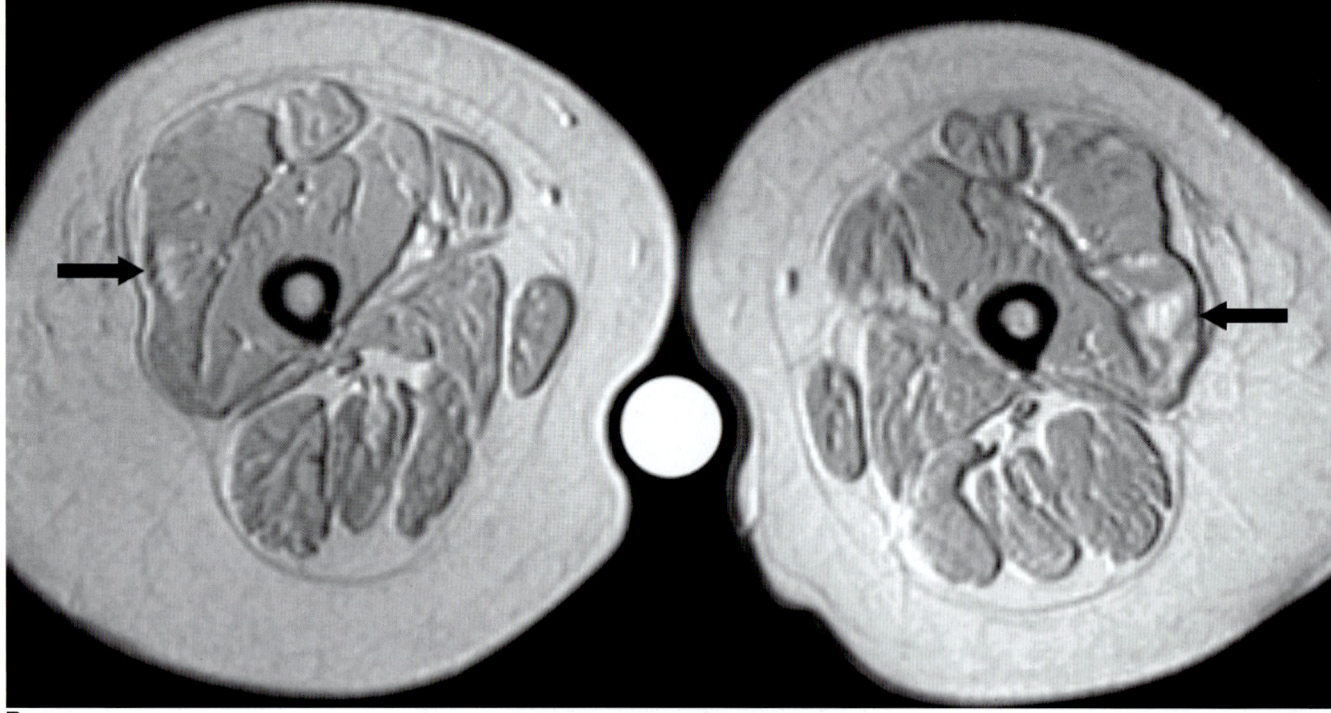

B

■ **FIGURE 54-2** **A,** Axial T1-weighted gradient-echo image depicts global muscle loss in the quadriceps musculature of the left thigh in a patient with juvenile dermatomyositis. **B,** Axial T1-weighted gradient-echo image in chronic polymyositis showing global muscle loss as well as fatty involution of multiple muscles bilaterally, most notably in the vastus lateralis muscles (*arrows*).

compartment atrophy predominates in sIBM and can be pronounced, occasionally with rectus femoris sparing. Predominant posterior compartment disease in the thigh or a myofascial pattern of inflammation is more indicative of PM.[19,20] In sIBM, triceps sura and particularly medial head gastrocnemius involvement predominates in the leg; deep flexor involvement predominates in the forearm, with sparing of the superficial flexors.

MRI may also be useful for selecting a location for muscle biopsy. Because of the heterogeneous pattern of muscle involvement in inflammatory myopathy, a blind muscle biopsy may be negative or inconclusive in IIM. The false-negative rate for a blind muscle biopsy is as high as 20% in DM.[21] Muscle regions exhibiting increased signal on STIR or T2-weighted imaging are more appropriate for histologic and biochemical sampling in cases of suspected inflammatory myopathy, whereas areas of fatty involution of muscle should be avoided during biopsy. MRI may be a cost-effective procedure in guiding biopsy.[22]

Magnetic Resonance Imaging

Edema-like muscle signal on MRI may be a useful indicator of active disease in PM and DM.[8,9,23] These signal changes likely reflect an increase in extracellular water. MRI findings of muscle edema correlate with diminished muscle strength[18] but do not correlate with serum muscle enzyme levels, another measure of disease activity.[8,19] The extent and degree of muscle edema shown by fluid-sensitive MRI sequences may serve as a gauge of disease activity, which may be useful to determine the efficacy of treatment.[18,24,25] This information may help guide decisions at critical therapeutic junctures. Similarly, MRI may serve as an outcome measure in clinical trials that study disease interventions in inflammatory myopathy.[26]

Muscle damage in inflammatory myopathy may result in either diminished muscle volume or fatty involution of muscle, features that are well demonstrated by T1-weighted MRI. These changes are markers of more advanced or chronic disease.

Computed Tomography

Contrast-enhanced CT is a viable alternative to MRI in the evaluation of inflammatory myopathy when the suspected etiology is infectious and to exclude pyomyositis or abscess formation.

Ultrasonography

Muscle echogenicity is altered in cases of inflammatory myopathy, but these changes are difficult to quantify with respect to extent and severity.[27] Fatty involution and muscle edema both alter the echogenicity of muscle, limiting the ability of ultrasonography to differentiate disease activity from disease damage. Increased muscle vascularity, however, may be detected in DM and PM with power Doppler ultrasonography.[28] An increase in muscle perfusion can also be potentially quantified in these patients with the use of ultrasound contrast agents.[29]

Magnetic Resonance Spectroscopy

Phosphorus-31 MR spectroscopy may reveal abnormalities in high-energy phosphate metabolites, both at rest and, more notably, in response to exercise, in cases of DM and PM. In cases of DM, ^{31}P MR spectroscopy may show abnormalities in oxidative metabolism in response to exercise in muscle that appears normal on standard MRI.[30] The utility of proton MRS has not been well established in IIM.[31]

Nuclear Medicine

Gallium-67 and technetium-99m pyrophosphate scintigraphy can detect sites of disease involvement in DM and PM.[32] These techniques have the advantage of whole-body coverage and can identify cardiac as well as skeletal muscle disease but are not very sensitive.

Fasciitis

MRI can establish the involvement of the deep fascia and contiguous epimysium as a primary or associated finding in cases of suspected inflammatory myopathy. In cases of DM, MRI may reveal disease isolated to the deep fascial region. The finding of isolated fascial disease, particularly if localized, may suggest alternative diagnoses such as eosinophilic fasciitis.[33] On occasion, in PM and DM, disease may preferentially involve muscle fibers deep to epimysium, a so-called myofascial pattern.[8,23] In such cases, or in cases with severe myositis, a specific diagnosis of fasciitis is difficult to establish.

Magnetic Resonance Imaging

Fascial disease is manifested on MRI by fascial or perifascial hyperintensity on fluid-sensitive sequences (Fig. 54-3). Edema-like signal in the deep subcutis may accompany fasciitis and can indicate associated panniculitis (Fig. 54-4). Chemical shift may create artifactual hyperintensity along fascial boundaries, however, particularly if receiver bandwidth is low. The clue to this artifact is that it occurs in a consistent direction and is seen along muscle boundaries that are perpendicular to the axis of frequency encoding. This artifact can pose a diagnostic pitfall in limited or localized fasciitis. This diagnosis is facilitated by targeted MRI studies performed at high resolution (see Fig. 54-3) and by the use of intravenous contrast media.

Calcinosis

Calcinosis may accompany DM, particularly in juvenile-onset disease. Calcinosis may serve as a useful end point in evaluation of DM, whereas the prevention of calcinosis may improve function. In chronic cases of DM, mass-like collections containing milk of calcium may occur along the fascia or within muscle,[34] resembling the findings in tumoral calcinosis or calcific myonecrosis.

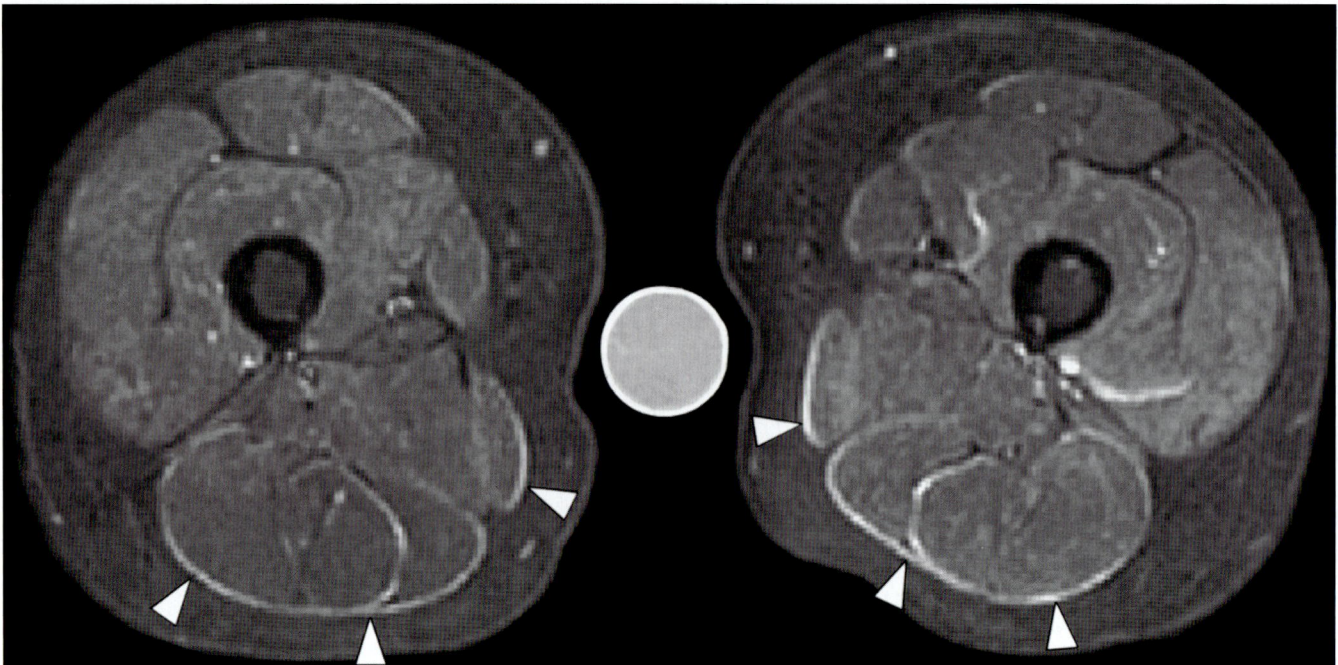

A

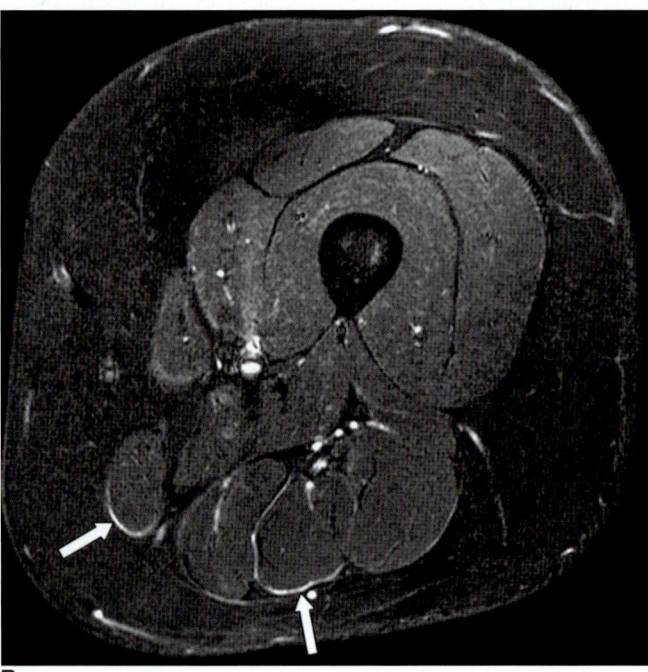

B

■ **FIGURE 54-3** **A,** Axial STIR image in juvenile dermatomyositis shows no substantial muscle disease but linear hyperintensity along the fascia of the posterior compartment musculature bilaterally (*arrows*), indicative of fasciitis. **B,** Higher-resolution axial STIR image in another patient with juvenile dermatomyositis demonstrates localized, linear hyperintensity along the fascia of the gracilis and semimembranosus (*arrows*), indicative of fasciitis. Frequency-encoding axis is right to left in this case, excluding chemical shift artifact as an explanation for these localized findings at the muscle boundary.

Radiography

Radiography remains the most efficient means of confirming the presence of soft tissue calcinosis (Fig. 54-5).

Magnetic Resonance Imaging

In DM or PM, MRI may reveal patchy or diffuse areas of edema-like signal in the subcutis (see Fig. 54-4). Particularly in DM, these findings may indicate "panniculitis" and may constitute another marker of active disease.

In DM, these areas of panniculitis may be a precursor to subcutaneous calcinosis.[35]

Computed Tomography

Compared with radiography, CT more sensitively depicts the extent, location, and severity of calcinosis in cases of DM, distinguishing subcutaneous from fascial and muscle calcification. The added radiation exposure of CT, however, precludes its routine application in evaluation of these patients.

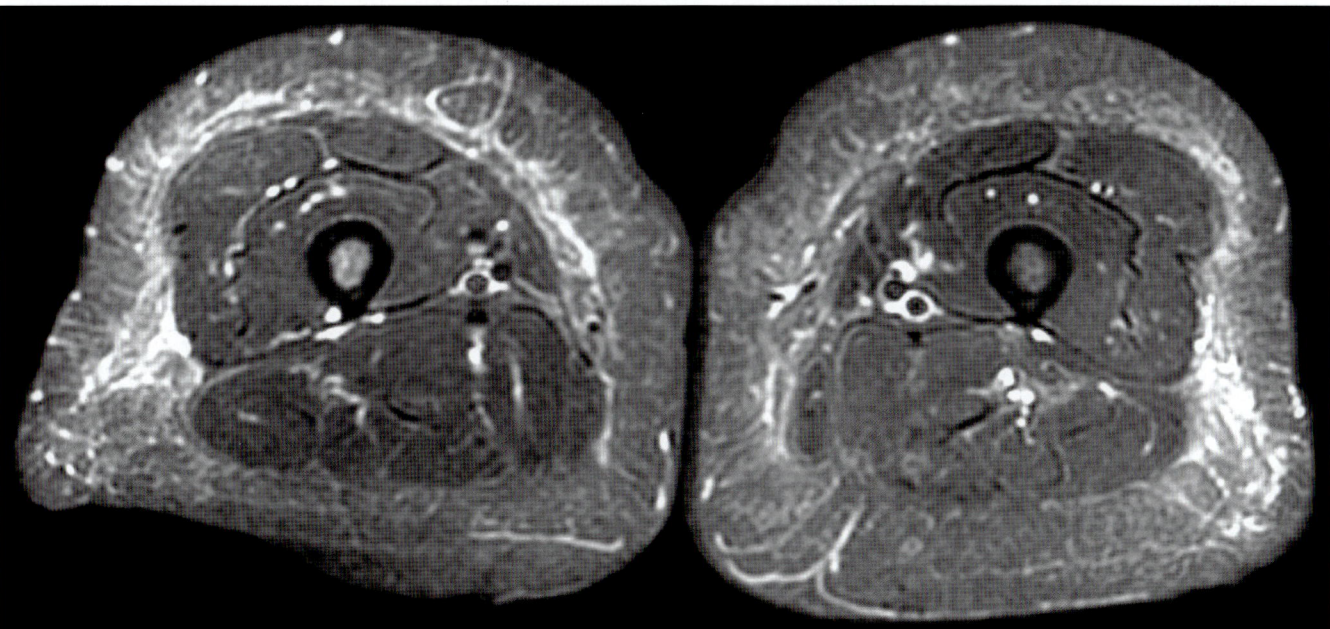

■ **FIGURE 54-4** Subcutaneous inflammation in idiopathic inflammatory myopathy. Axial STIR image in polymyositis shows extensive, edema-like signal intensity in the deep subcutis of the thighs and only minimal increased signal intensity along some fascial boundaries, such as the left gracilis.

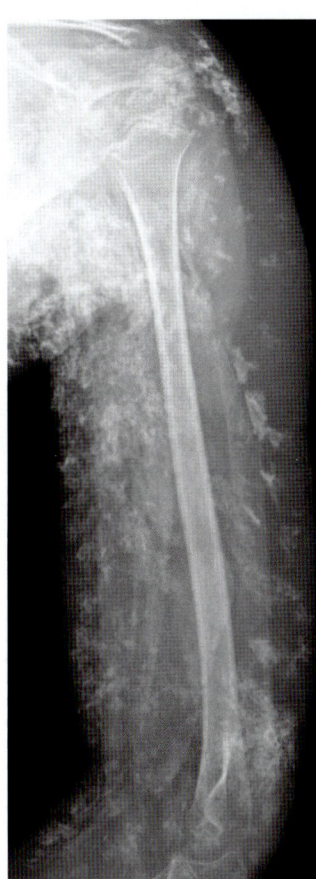

■ **FIGURE 54-5** Advanced calcinosis. Radiograph of the arm of a girl with juvenile dermatomyositis shows extensive amorphous and wispy calcification corresponding to subcutaneous calcinosis. Sheet-like calcification outlining muscles corresponds to deep fascial calcification.

DIFFERENTIAL DIAGNOSIS

The differential diagnosis for the IIM is quite broad, including many entities that are also rare. It may include muscular dystrophies, infectious myopathies, metabolic myopathies, endocrine myopathies, and drug-associated myopathies.

The muscle findings in IIM that are revealed by MRI are nonspecific. The extent and severity of muscle findings shown by MRI, however, have some differential diagnostic value. Drug-associated and endocrine myopathies, for example, are typically associated with milder or minimal muscle signal alterations on MRI. Chronic, noninflammatory myopathies often exhibit fatty involution of muscle, but, in distinction to the atrophy seen with IIM, relative muscle volume tends to be preserved.[36]

The diagnosis of metabolic and congenital myopathies is largely dependent on careful analysis of family history, clinical presentation, and laboratory findings, including specialized biochemical and molecular tests. The MR findings in metabolic myopathies can be similar to those in PM, with fatty involution of muscle and edema-like signal in remaining muscle. These conditions also occur in a patchy, often asymmetric distribution, with a proximal limb predominance. A clue to metabolic myopathy and muscular dystrophy on MRI, however, is that edema-like muscle signal is typically not encountered on MRI without concomitant muscle atrophy.[36]

The pattern of specific muscle involvement in the various myopathies is quite varied and is therefore of limited differential diagnostic value. One exception may be the mitochondrial myopathies that can selectively involve the sartorius and gracilis, in contradistinction to the relative sparing of these muscles in IIM, muscular dystrophy, and congenital myopathy.[37]

MRI may localize a muscle abnormality to one muscle or one muscle group, which may suggest an alternate diagnosis in cases of myopathy. Localized muscle inflammation, with muscle enlargement, can be seen in focal myositis, a self-limited but occasionally relapsing condition that is difficult to distinguish from PM on biopsy.[38] In focal myositis, MRI is useful in differentiating the condition from a mesenchymal neoplasm. Localized muscle signal changes simulating inflammation may also occur secondary to peripheral neuropathy. When a central stellate region of diminished signal intensity is noted within an area of edema-like muscle signal on fluid-sensitive MRI sequences, sarcoid myopathy should enter the differential diagnosis.[39]

SYNOPSIS OF TREATMENT OPTIONS

Medical Treatment

Corticosteroids are the mainstay of initial therapy for the IIM and improve muscle strength, normalize muscle enzymes, and reverse findings of muscle edema on MRI.[1] Immunosuppressive agents are used as second-line therapy, both for patients with a partial response to corticosteroids, and as corticosteroid-sparing agents in patients with intolerable corticosteroid side effects. These adjunctive agents include methotrexate, azathioprine, intravenous immunoglobulin, cyclosporine, and cyclophosphamide. Recent reports support a role for mycophenolate mofetil, particularly for refractory skin disease; tacrolimus, particularly for patients with interstitial lung disease; and anti–tumor necrosis factor-α therapies and the anti-B cell monoclonal antibody rituximab, both as experimental agents for patients with refractory severe disease. Current therapies in sIBM at best slow the rate of muscle deterioration rather than improve muscle strength.[40]

Surgical Treatment

Surgery does not have a role in the routine management of IIM. Operative intervention is occasionally required in DM patients for painful or disfiguring calcinosis lesions, subcutaneous infection, or complications from bowel ischemia.

What the Referring Physician Needs to Know

- MRI of the thigh and hip girdle musculature can aid diagnosis and guide biopsy in cases of suspected IIM.
- Longitudinal MRI evaluation of the thigh muscles can gauge treatment effect and disease damage in IIM.

SUGGESTED READINGS

Adams E, Chow CK, Premkumar A, Plotz PH. The idiopathic inflammatory myopathies: spectrum of MR imaging findings. RadioGraphics 1995; 15:563–574.

Christopher-Stine LM, Plotz PH. Adult inflammatory myopathies. Best Pract Res Clin Rheumatol 2004; 18:331–344.

Fleckenstein JL. Muscle weakness and myalgia: MR imaging investigation. MRI Clin North Am 1995; 3:773–803.

Fleckenstein JL, Reimers CD. Inflammatory myopathies: radiologic evaluation. Radiol Clin North Am 1996; 34:427–439.

Mastaglia FL, Garlepp MJ, Phillips BA, Zilko PJ. Inflammatory myopathies: clinical, diagnostic and therapeutic aspects. Muscle Nerve 2003; 27:407–425.

Mastaglia FL, Phillips BA. Idiopathic inflammatory myopathies: epidemiology, classification, and diagnostic criteria. Rheum Dis Clin North Am 2002;28:723–741.

Park JH, Olson NJ. Utility of magnetic resonance imaging in the evaluation of patients with inflammatory myopathies. Curr Rheumatol Rep 2001; 3:334–345.

Reimers CD, Finkenstaedt M. Muscle imaging in inflammatory myopathies. Curr Opin Rheumatol 1997; 4:475–485.

Rider LG. Outcome assessment in the adult and juvenile idiopathic inflammatory myopathies. Rheum Dis Clin North Am 2002; 28:935–977.

REFERENCES

1. Christopher-Stine LM, Plotz PH. Adult inflammatory myopathies. Best Pract Res Clin Rheumatol 2004; 18:331–344.

2. Rider LG, Targoff IN. Single organ systems and autoimmunity: muscle diseases. In Lahita RG, Chiorazzi N, Reeves WH (eds). Textbook of Autoimmune Diseases. Philadelphia, Lippincott-Raven, 2000, pp 429–474.

3. Spiera R, Kagen L. Extramuscular manifestations in idiopathic inflammatory myopathies. Curr Opin Rheumatol 1998; 10:556–561.

4. Buchbinder R, Forbes A, Hall S, et al. Incidence of malignant disease in biopsy-proven inflammatory myopathy: a population-based cohort study. Ann Intern Med 2001 134:1087–1095.

5. Hill CL, Zhang Y, Sigurgeirsson B, et al. Frequency of specific cancer types in dermatomyositis and polymyositis: a population-based study. Lancet 2001; 357:96–100.

6. Chen YJ, Wu CY, Shen JL. Predicting factors of malignancy in dermatomyositis and polymyositis: a case-control study. Br J Dermatol. 2001; 144:825–831.

7. Bohan A, Peter JB. Polymyositis and dermatomyositis. N Engl J Med 1975; 292:344–347.

8. Reimers CD, Schedel H, Fleckenstein JL, et al. Magnetic resonance imaging of skeletal muscles in idiopathic inflammatory myopathies of adults. J Neurol 1994; 241:306–314.

9. Schedel H, Reimers CD, Vogl T, Witt TN. Muscle edema in MR imaging of neuromuscular diseases. Acta Radiol 1995; 36:228–232.

10. Hernandez RJ, Keim DR, Chenevert TL, et al. Fat-suppressed MR imaging of myositis. Radiology 1992; 182:217–219.

11. O'Connell MJ, Powell T, Brennan D, et al. Whole-body MR imaging in the diagnosis of polymyositis. AJR Am J Roentgenol 2002; 179:967–971.

12. Summers RM, Brune AM, Choyke PL, et al. Juvenile idiopathic inflammatory myopathy: Exercise-induced changes in muscle at short inversion time inversion-recovery MR imaging. Radiology 1998; 209:191–196.

13. Houmard JA, Smith R, Jendrasiak GL. Relationship between MRI relaxation time and muscle fiber composition. J Appl Physiol 1995; 78:807-809.
14. Hatakenaka M, Ueda M, Ishigami K, et al. Effects of aging on muscle T2 relaxation time: difference between fast- and slow-twitch muscles. Invest Radiol. 2001; 36:692-698.
15. Bartlett ML, Ginn L, Beitz L, et al. Quantitative assessment of myositis in thigh muscles using magnetic resonance imaging. Magn Reson Imaging 1999; 17:183-191.
16. Maillard SM, Jones R, Owens C, et al. Quantitative assessment of MRI T2 relaxation time of thigh muscles in juvenile dermatomyositis. Rheumatology (Oxford) 2004; 43:603-608.
17. Miller FW, Rider LG, Chung YL, et al., International Myositis Outcome Assessment Collaborative Study Group. Proposed preliminary core set measures for disease outcome assessment in adult and juvenile idiopathic inflammatory myopathies. Rheumatology (Oxford). 2001; 40:1262-1273.
18. Hernandez RJ, Sullivan DB, Chenevert TL, Keim DR. MR imaging in children with dermatomyositis: Musculoskeletal findings and correlation with clinical and laboratory findings. AJR Am J Roentgenol 1993; 161:359-366.
19. Dion E, Cherin P, Payan C, et al. Magnetic resonance imaging criteria for distinguishing between inclusion body myositis and polymyositis. J Rheumatol 2002; 29:1897-1906.
20. Phillips BA, Cala LA, Thickbroom GW, et al. Patterns of muscle involvement in inclusion body myositis: clinical and magnetic resonance imaging study. Muscle Nerve 2001; 24:1526-1534.
21. Pachman LM, Hayford JR, Chung A, et al. Juvenile dermatomyositis at diagnosis: clinical characteristics of 79 children. J Rheumatol 1998; 25:1198-1204.
22. Schweitzer ME, Fort J. Cost-effectiveness of MR imaging in evaluating polymyositis. AJR Am J Roentgenol 1995; 165:1469-1471.
23. Adams E, Chow CK, Premkumar A, Plotz PH. The idiopathic inflammatory myopathies: spectrum of MR imaging findings. RadioGraphics 1995; 15:563-574.
24. Fraser DD, Frank JA, Dalakas M, et al. Magnetic resonance imaging in the idiopathic inflammatory myopathies. J Rheumatol 1991; 18:1693-1700.
25. Park JH, Vital TL, Ryder NM, et al. Magnetic resonance imaging and P-31 magnetic resonance spectroscopy provide unique quantitative data useful in the longitudinal management of patients with dermatomyositis. Arthritis Rheum 1994; 37:736-746.
26. Adams EM, Pucino F, Yarboro C, et al. A pilot study: use of fludarabine for refractory dermatomyositis and polymyositis, and examination of endpoint measures. J Rheumatol 1999; 26:352-360.
27. Meng C, Adler R, Peterson M, Kagen L. Combined use of power Doppler and gray-scale sonography: a new technique for the assessment of inflammatory myopathy. J Rheumatol 2001; 28:1271-1282.
28. Meng C, Adler R, Peterson M, Kagen L. Combined use of power Doppler and gray-scale sonography: a new technique for the assessment of inflammatory myopathy. J Rheumatol 2001; 28:1271-1282.
29. Weber MA, Krix M, Jappe U, et al. Pathologic skeletal muscle perfusion in patients with myositis: detection with quantitative contrast-enhanced US—initial results. Radiology 2006; 238:640-649.
30. Park JH, Olsen NJ, King L, et al. Use of magnetic resonance imaging and P-31 magnetic resonance spectroscopy to detect and quantify muscle dysfunction in the amyopathic and myopathic variants of dermatomyositis. Arthritis Rheum 1995; 38:68-77.
31. Chung YL, Smith EC, Williams SC, et al. In vivo proton magnetic resonance spectroscopy in polymyositis and dermatomyositis: a preliminary study. Eur J Med Res 1997; 2:483-487.
32. Buchpiguel CA, Roizemblatt S, Pastor EH, et al. Cardiac and skeletal muscle scintigraphy in dermato- and polymyositis: clinical implications. Eur J Nucl Med 1996; 23:199-203.
33. Baumann F, Bruhlmann P, Andreisek G, et al. MRI for diagnosis and monitoring of patients with eosinophilic fasciitis. AJR Am J Roentgenol 2005; 184:169-174.
34. Samson C, Soulen RL, Gursel E. Milk of calcium fluid collections in juvenile dermatomyositis: MR characteristics. Pediatr Radiol 2000; 30:28-29.
35. Kimball AB, Summers RM, Turner M, et al. Magnetic resonance imaging detection of occult skin and subcutaneous abnormalities in juvenile dermatomyositis: implications for diagnosis and therapy. Arthritis Rheum 2000; 43:1866-1873.
36. Fleckenstein JL. Muscle weakness and myalgia: MR imaging investigation. MRI Clin North Am 1995; 3:773-803.
37. Fleckenstein JL, Haller RG, Girson MS, Peshock RM. Focal muscle lesions in mitochondrial myopathy: MR imaging evaluation. J Magn Reson Imaging 1992; 2(Suppl):121.
38. Smith AG, Urbanits S, Blaivas M, et al. Clinical and pathologic features of focal myositis. Muscle Nerve 2000; 23:1569-1575.
39. Otake S, Banno T, Ohba S, et al. Muscular sarcoidosis: findings at MR imaging. Radiology 1990; 176:145-148.
40. Griggs RC. The current status of treatment for inclusion-body myositis. Neurology 2006; 66(2 Suppl 1):S30-32.

55

Hemochromatosis

Mini N. Pathria

ETIOLOGY

Hemochromatosis is a common underdiagnosed disorder of excess iron storage in tissue.[1] The disorder is categorized into primary and secondary forms. Primary hemochromatosis is inherited as an autosomal recessive disorder; approximately 10% of the population is heterozygous for the disorder and asymptomatic.[2] Causes of secondary hemochromatosis include iron overload from refractory anemias associated with ineffective hematopoiesis, multiple transfusions, and dietary iron overload.

PREVALENCE AND EPIDEMIOLOGY

Primary hemochromatosis is one of the most common inherited diseases, with a homozygote frequency of at least 1 in 300 people of northern European descent.[3,4] The specific gene defect responsible for 80% to 100% of cases of primary hemochromatosis are homozygotes for a *C282Y* mutation of the *HFE* gene residing on chromosome 6.[4] The *HFE* gene mutation modifies proteins that reside in the duodenum, resulting in increased absorption of iron.[1] Less common gene mutations associated with primary hemochromatosis include defects in the *HFE2* gene on chromosome 1, responsible for juvenile-onset hemochromatosis, other mutations related to the *HFE* gene, and defects unrelated to the *HFE* gene.[1,3]

Hemochromatosis is diagnosed by measuring fasting serum transferrin saturation and ferritin, coupled with genetic testing.[1] CT and MRI of the liver are used for noninvasive evaluation of disease severity and may obviate the need for liver biopsy.[1] In hemochromatosis, iron deposition in the viscera results in increased parenchymal density of the liver and spleen on CT.[5] MRI is more sensitive, showing decreased signal within the liver on both T1- and T2-weighted sequences due to the T2 shortening effect of intracellular iron production.[6,7]

CLINICAL PRESENTATION

Clinical symptoms are more profound in primary hemochromatosis than in the secondary form. Symptoms develop only after protracted excessive iron accumulation, typically between the ages of 40 and 60. It is estimated that the body's normal iron stores of 3 to 4 g have to be increased to 20 to 40 g before symptoms develop.[4] Homozygotes may remain asymptomatic or show variable symptomatology related to gene penetrance, diet, use of iron supplements, and blood loss from conditions such as donation, menstruation, and bowel disease.[1,2] Symptomatic disease is 8 to 10 times more common in men than in women, presumably owing to the protective iron-wasting effect of menstruation. The characteristic clinical triad consists of bronze cutaneous pigmentation, diabetes mellitus, and hepatomegaly. Other common manifestations include arthropathy, cardiac disease, and hypogonadism. There is an increased risk for cirrhosis and hepatocellular carcinoma, particularly in older patients who drink heavily.[1] Treatment with intermittent phlebotomy can arrest symptoms and allow for a normal life expectancy.[1]

MANIFESTATIONS OF THE DISEASE

Musculoskeletal symptoms are common in patients with hemochromatosis. Characteristic musculoskeletal disorders associated with the disease are osteoporosis, arthralgia and stiffness, chondrocalcinosis, and a peculiar structural arthropathy that shares features with both osteoarthritis and the arthropathy related to calcium

KEY POINTS

- Primary hemachromatosis is one of the most common inherited disorders.
- The characteristic clinical triad consists of bronze cutaneous pigmentation, diabetes mellitus, and hepatomegaly.
- The typical arthropathy present in 25% to 50% of patients is "hook-like" excrescences on the radial side of the metacarpal heads.
- Chondrocalcinosis may be identified in up to 60% of patients with hemachromatosis.
- Involvement of the large joints is less common and may be difficult to distinguish from osteoarthritis.

pyrophosphate dehydrate (CPPD) crystal deposition.[8] Osteoporosis is present in up to 58% of patients with primary hemochromatosis and is generally asymptomatic, although vertebral body deformity and fractures may develop in severe cases. Fatigue, joint pain, stiffness, and acute attacks of arthritis without any structural arthropathy affect the majority of patients with overt hemochromatosis and are often an early but nonspecific manifestation of the disease.[2,9]

Radiography

There is a high frequency of CPPD crystal deposition in patients with hemochromatosis. Chondrocalcinosis is visible radiographically in up to 60% of patients. While it has been suggested by some authors that all patients with significant amounts of chondrocalcinosis undergo screening for hemochromatosis, the indications for screening remain controversial.[3] Chondrocalcinosis tends to develop late in the disease course and probably has limited value in screening for the disorder.[9] The distribution of CPPD is identical to that seen in the idiopathic form of pyrophosphate deposition, with deposition primarily in the knee, pubic symphysis, and triangular fibrocartilage (Fig. 55-1). Para-articular calcification is less frequent than in other forms of CPPD deposition.[8] It has been suggested that there is a stronger correlation between the severity of arthropathy and the degree of chondrocalcinosis in patients with hemochromatosis as compared with patients with idiopathic CPPD deposition.[8]

In 1964, Schumacher reported that hemochromatosis was associated with a specific structural arthropathy that is estimated to develop in 25% to 50% of patients.[10] Arthropathy characteristically develops after long-standing disease, although it may rarely precede other manifestations.[9] It is more common in the primary form of hemochromatosis than in secondary forms and does not appear to reverse significantly with phlebotomy therapy.[1] The structural arthropathy shows a predilection for involvement of the metacarpophalangeal (MCP) joints, particularly the second and third. Arthropathy starts in the MCP joints in two thirds of patients with structural arthritis.[4] Articular space narrowing and subchondral sclerosis are associated with peculiar hook-like excrescences on the radial side of the metacarpal heads (Fig. 55-2). The noninflammatory arthropathy is not associated with erosions.

Involvement of large joints is less common and typically develops subsequent to the development of symptomatic MCP arthropathy. The hip, knees, and shoulders are most

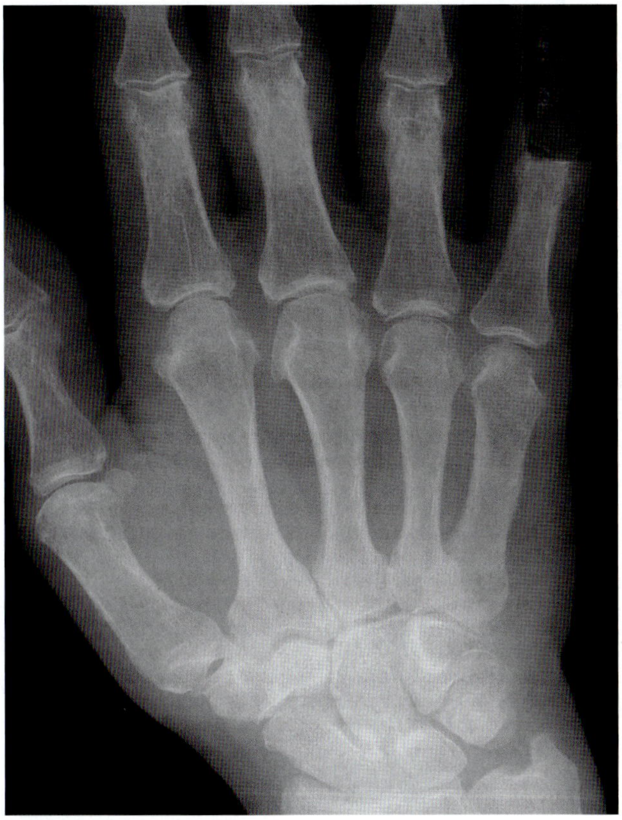

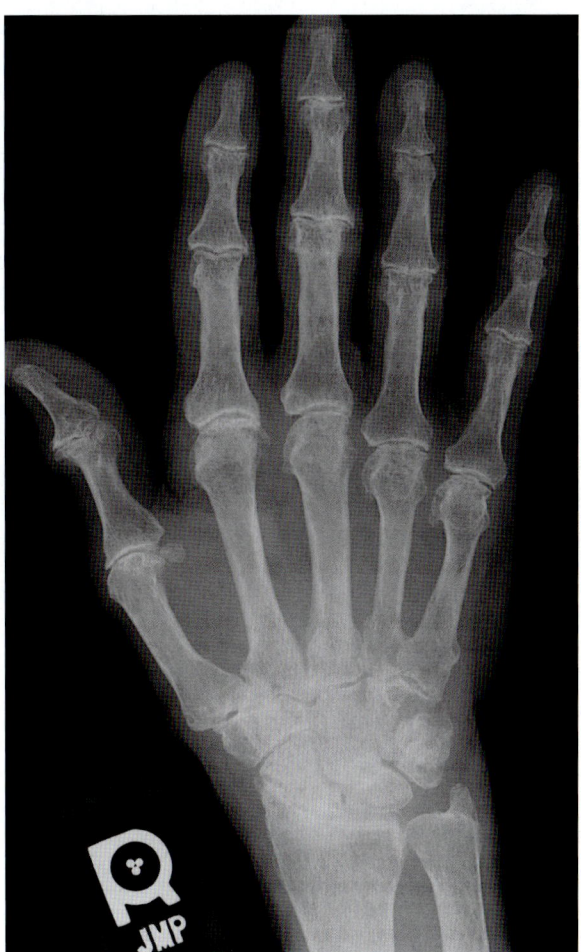

■ **FIGURE 55-2** Anteroposterior view of the hand demonstrates extensive arthropathy throughout the carpus and fingers. There is articular space narrowing and osteophyte formation, particularly at the second through fifth MCP joints. Note the prominent radial-sided hook-like osteophytes at the MCP joints.

■ **FIGURE 55-1** Anteroposterior view of the hand shows chondrocalcinosis within the triangular fibrocartilage and arthropathy at the second and third MCP joints.

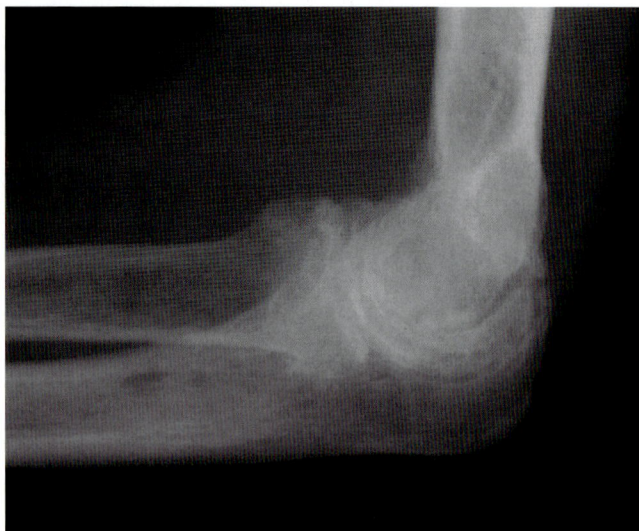

■ **FIGURE 55-3** Lateral view of the elbow shows an effusion and arthropathy with severe articular space narrowing and relatively little osteophyte formation.

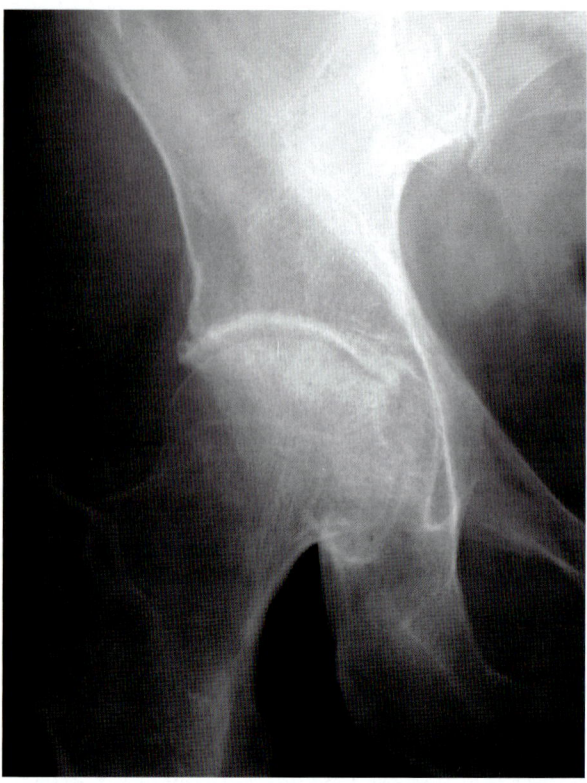

■ **FIGURE 55-4** Anteroposterior view of the right hip shows superomedial articular space narrowing with subchondral cyst formation within the femoral head. There is subtle irregularity and flattening of the head above the fovea.

frequently affected. In the large joints it is difficult to distinguish the arthropathy of hemochromatosis from osteoarthritis, although the articular space loss tends to be more uniform and osteophyte formation less prominent in hemochromatosis (Fig. 55-3).[8]

Magnetic Resonance Imaging

On MRI, a characteristic but nonspecific finding of the arthropathy of hemochromatosis is the presence of prominent subchondral cysts. The etiology of the subchondral cysts is related to stripping of cartilage from bone in its deepest layer with cartilage ingrowth and fibrous tissue proliferation in the subchondral region.[11] Flattening and subchondral sclerosis of the femoral head may develop, simulating osteonecrosis (Fig. 55-4).[11] Iron deposition within the affected joints may occasionally be identified on MRI, although most cases of arthropathy due to hemochromatosis do not demonstrate visible siderosis of the synovium.[11]

What the Referring Physician Needs to Know

■ Distribution of articular involvement
■ Severity of joint disease

REFERENCES

1. McCarthy GM, Crowe J, McCarthy CJ, et al. Hereditary hemochromatosis: a common, often unrecognized, genetic disease. Cleve Clin J Med 2002; 69:224–237.
2. Jordan JM. Arthritis in hemochromatosis or iron storage disease. Curr Opin Rheumatol 2004; 16:62–66.
3. Timms AE, Sathananthan R, Bradbury L, et al. Genetic testing for haemochromatosis in patients with chondrocalcinosis. Ann Rheum Dis 2002; 61:745–747.
4. Limdi JK, Crampton JR. Hereditary haemochromatosis. Q J Med 2004; 97:315–324.
5. Georgiades CS, Neyman EG, Francis IR, et al. Typical and atypical presentations of extramedullary hemopoiesis. AJR Am J Roentgenol 2002; 179:1239–1243.
6. Tani I, Kurihara Y, Kawaguchi A, et al. MR imaging of diffuse liver disease. AJR Am J Roentgenol 2000; 174:965–971.
7. Ben Salem D, Cercueil JP, Ricolfi F, Krause D. Case 75: Erythropoietic hemochromatosis. Radiology 2004; 233:116–119.
8. Resnick D. Hemochromatosis and Wilson's disease. In Resnick D (ed). Diagnosis of Bone and Joint Diseases, 4th ed. Philadelphia, WB Saunders, 2001, pp 1658–1670.
9. Mathews JL, Williams HJ. Arthritis in hereditary hemochromatosis. Arthritis Rheum 1987; 30:1137–1141.
10. Schumacher HR Jr. Hemochromatosis and arthritis. Arthritis Rheum 1964; 7:41–50.
11. Papakonstantinou O, Mohana-Borges AV, Campell L, et al. Hip arthropathy in a patient with primary hemochromatosis: MR imaging findings with pathologic correlation. Skeletal Radiol 2005; 34:180–184.

CHAPTER 56

Ochronosis

Claire Coggins and Curtis Hayes

ETIOLOGY

Ochronosis is the bluish-black discoloration that can be seen in connective tissues of patients with alkaptonuria, a rare disorder caused by the absence of homogentisic acid oxidase. The absence of this enzyme causes a buildup of homogentisic acid (HGA) in connective tissues, including the sclera, cornea, articular cartilage, intervertebral discs, tendons, and ligaments. The accumulated HGA is polymerized and oxidized, causing the characteristic pigmentation of the connective tissue.[1] HGA or its oxidized form, benzoquinone, is also thought to physically bind to the connective tissue, thereby altering its structure.[2-4]

PREVALENCE AND EPIDEMIOLOGY

Ochronosis is a rare disorder, with a reported incidence between 1 in 250,000 and 1 in 1 million. The disease is hereditary, with an autosomal recessive pattern of inheritance. It affects both men and women, with a slight male predilection, and is typically asymptomatic until adulthood.[4-6]

CLINICAL PRESENTATION

Ochronosis may be discovered accidentally in infancy, with darkening of urine in diapers with exposure to air. Otherwise, patients present with pigmentation of sclerae and auricles around age 20 to 30. The musculoskeletal manifestation of this process is termed *ochronotic arthropathy,* which is the most common clinical feature of alkaptonuria.[7,8] Ochronotic arthropathy typically presents as pain and limitation of motion in the hip, knee, shoulder, or spine and usually occurs after age 40 in patients with this disease and often progresses to complete disability in older patients.[4]

PATHOPHYSIOLOGY

There is blue-black pigmentation of connective tissue, including sclera, cornea, tracheal cartilage, bronchial cartilage, heart valves, articular cartilage, tendons, and ligaments.[9-13]

Microscopically, there is intercellular and intracellular deposition of a pigment that chemically resembles melanin.[12] Because of the pigment deposition and the altered structure, the connective tissues become progressively weak and brittle, leading to inflammation, degeneration, and fragmentation.[14-16] Over time, the weakened intervertebral discs and hyaline cartilage are destroyed, resulting in narrowing of the disc and joint spaces.

BIOMECHANICS

Because of the pigment deposition, collagen-rich tissues throughout the body lose elasticity, and therefore lose resistance to mechanical stress.[17,18]

IMAGING TECHNIQUES

In most cases, routine radiography of the spine or peripheral joints will demonstrate the manifestations of ochronotic arthropathy. MRI may show damage to the fibrocartilaginous structures not seen with routine radiography.

KEY POINTS

- Ochronotic arthropathy is the musculoskeletal manifestation of ochronosis.
- Ochronotic arthropathy typically presents as pain and limited range of motion in the spine and large joints after age 40 in patients with ochronosis.
- Characteristic radiographic findings in the spine include widespread disc calcification, loss of lordosis, vacuum discs, and progressive disc narrowing.
- Characteristic radiographic findings in the peripheral skeleton include early degenerative change in the large joints with relative lack of osteophyte formation and prominent intra-articular bodies.

MANIFESTATIONS OF THE DISEASE

Radiography

In the spine there are several characteristic radiographic findings in patients with ochronosis. The thoracic and lumbar spine are involved but the cervical spine is typically spared. The classic radiographic finding in ochronosis is widespread disc calcification. The calcification occurs primarily in the anulus fibrosus and is thought to be due to dystrophic calcification of the abnormal connective tissue.[7,19] Radiographs of the spine also typically demonstrate disc space narrowing, progressive disc ossification, loss of the normal lumbar lordosis, vertebral osteoporosis, and vacuum discs.[7,18,20] In patients with long-standing disease there is progressive kyphosis, obliteration of the disc spaces, and marginal intervertebral bridges, resembling syndesmophytes of ankylosing spondylitis (Figs. 56-1 and 56-2).[21,22]

In the extraspinal sites, the changes of ochronotic arthropathy are very similar to those of osteoarthritis. Joint narrowing, subchondral sclerosis, and intra-articular bodies are often seen in the knee, hip, and shoulder. However, there is typically a relative lack of osteophyte formation (Fig. 56-3). The knee is the most common extraspinal site of involvement.[7] In the knee, the joint narrowing is often more pronounced in the lateral compartment or similar in the medial and lateral compartments.[7] Joint narrowing, mild osteophyte formation, and subchondral sclerosis are also seen at other sites, including the pubic symphysis and sacroiliac joints (see Figs. 56-2A and 56-3).

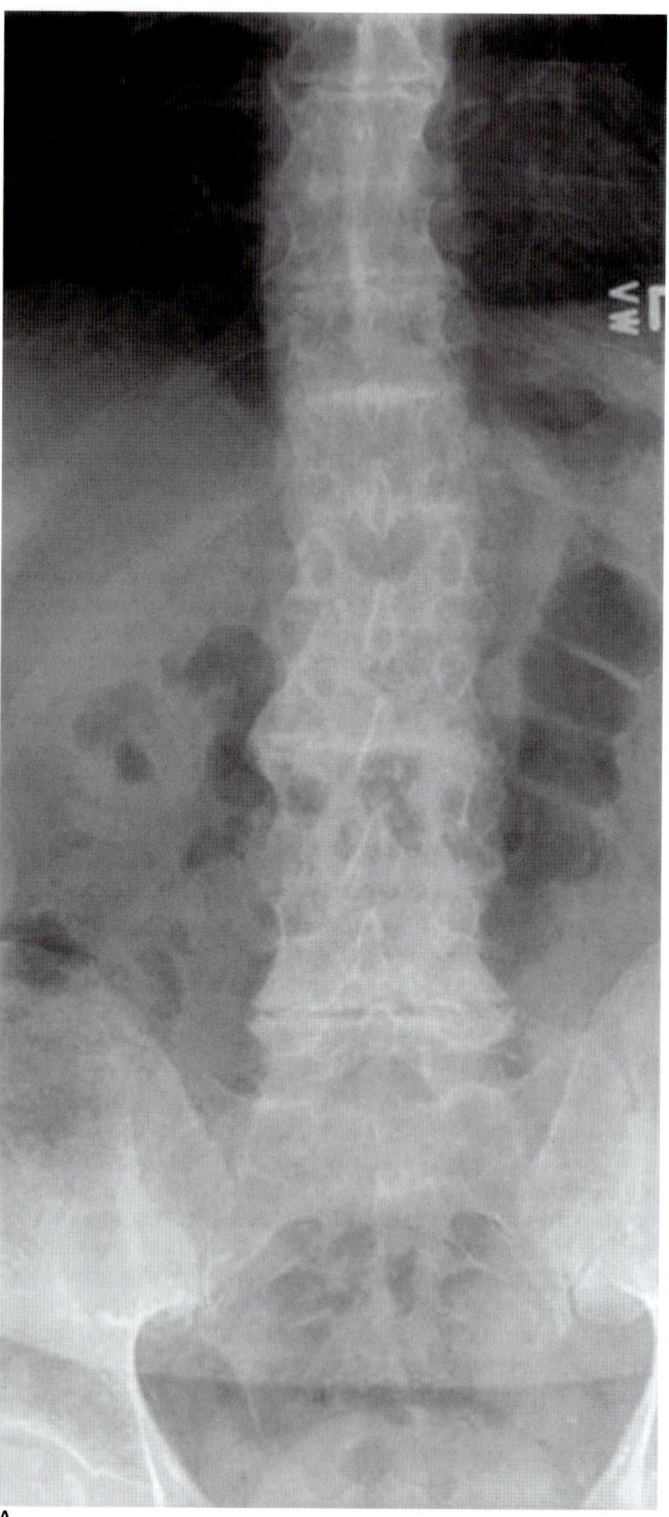

A

■ FIGURE 56-1　Lateral chest radiograph of a 69-year-old man demonstrates straightening of the thoracic spine, multilevel disc calcification, and thin osseous bridging, resembling syndesmophyte formation. *(Courtesy of Eric A. Bogner, MD, New York, NY.)*

■ FIGURE 56-2　Ochronosis. Anteroposterior radiograph (**A**).

(Continued)

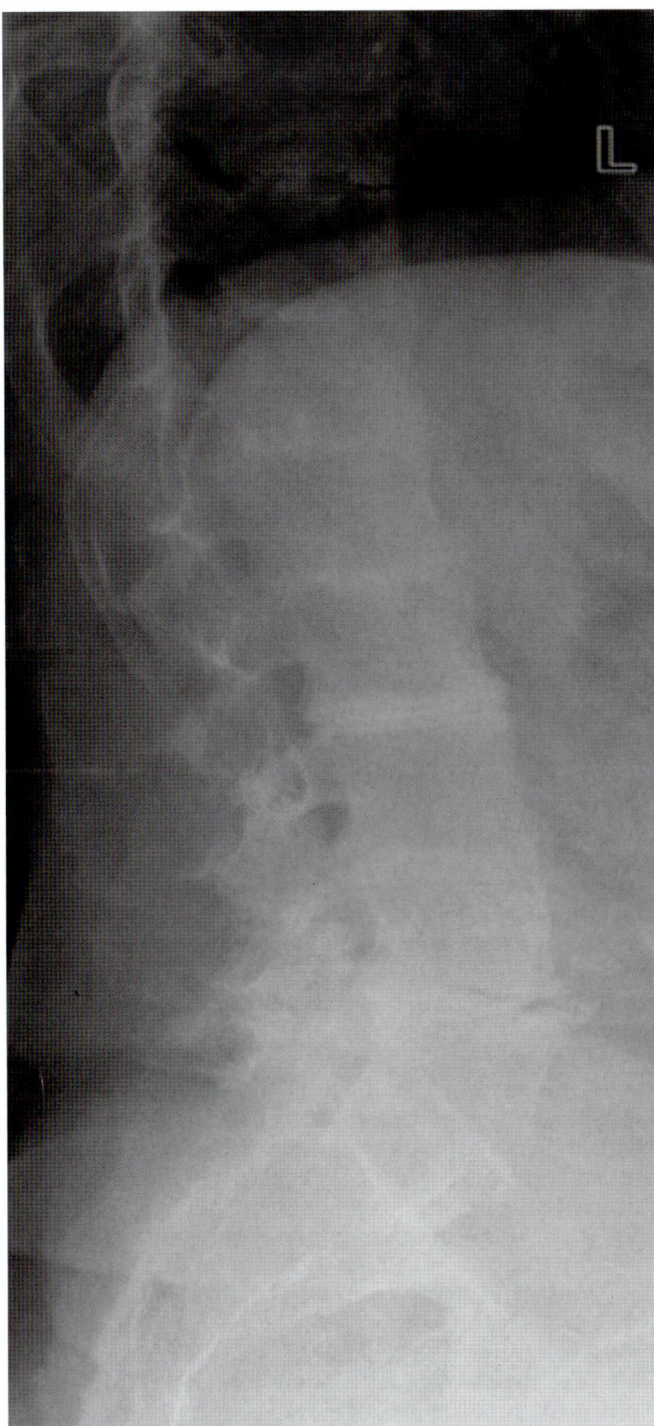

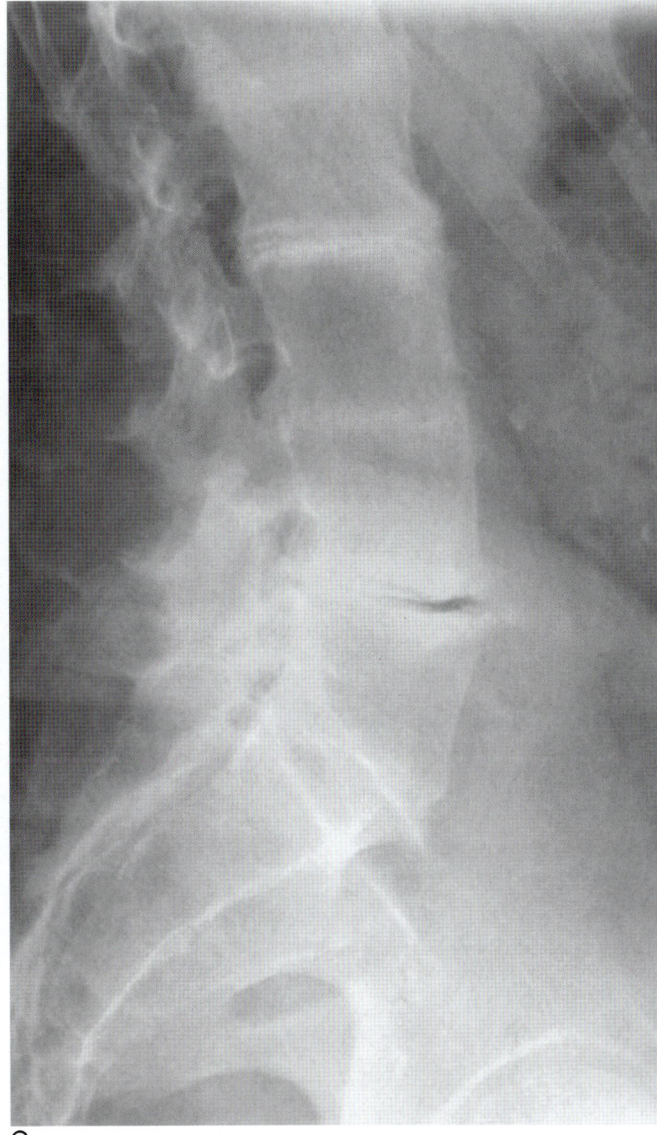

■ **FIGURE 56-2—Cont'd** Lateral (**B**) and coned-down lateral (**C**) radiographs of the lumbar spine in a 54-year-old man demonstrate multilevel disc calcification and disc space narrowing, as well as loss of lumbar lordosis and fine osseous bridging. There is a vacuum disc at L4-L5. The sacroiliac joints are narrowed with associated subchondral sclerosis, but no joint fusion is seen.

Magnetic Resonance Imaging

Magnetic resonance imaging of the spine demonstrates similar findings to those on radiographs, including loss of lordosis, disc narrowing, and degenerative end-plate changes. MRI may also demonstrate loss of signal intensity in the intervertebral disc on T2-weighted images, owing to disc desiccation and/or calcification.[22] In addition, spine MRI often shows thickening of the longitudinal ligaments.[4]

In the large joints, MRI may demonstrate damage to the fibrocartilaginous structures, such as menisci and labra, not seen on radiography. MRI is also more sensitive for detection of intra-articular bodies.[18] With increasing use of MRI, changes in tendons and ligaments in patients with ochronosis are identified more frequently. Thickening of the tendons and rupture of tendons and ligaments with minimal or no trauma are characteristic findings.[6,23,24]

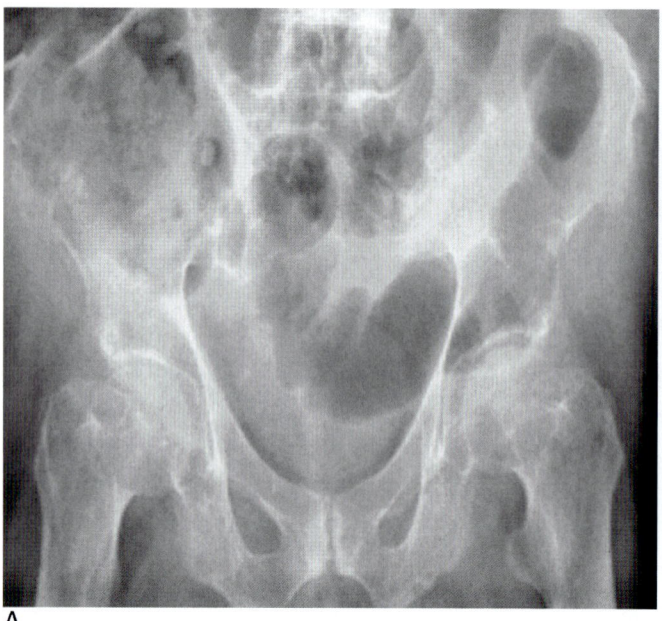
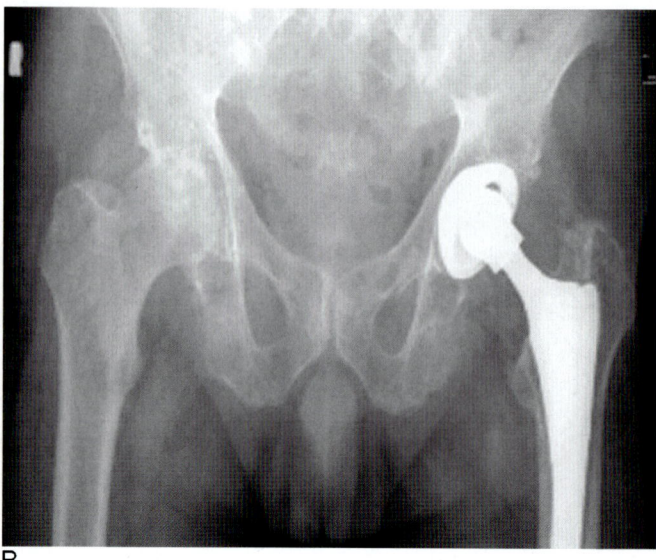

■ **FIGURE 56-3** **A,** Frontal view of the hips from an obstruction series performed for abdominal pain in a 66-year-old man (same patient as in Fig. 56-1) demonstrates fragmentation and sclerosis of the pubic symphysis and osteopenia, but there is preservation of the hip joint spaces. **B,** Three years later there is obliteration of the superolateral right hip joint space with associated subchondral sclerosis and relative lack of osteophyte formation. The patient has undergone left hip arthroplasty for ochronotic arthropathy. The sacroiliac joints and pubic symphysis also demonstrate narrowing and sclerosis. *(Courtesy of Eric A. Bogner, MD, New York, NY.)*

Arthroscopy

Findings at arthroscopy include darkly pigmented articular cartilage, loose bodies, and synovial hyperplasia.

Classic Signs

SPINE/AXIAL SKELETON

- Widespread disc degeneration and calcification
- Loss of lumbar lordosis
- Prominent vacuum discs
- Vertebral osteopenia
- Narrowing and calcification of symphysis pubis and sacroiliac joints

PERIPHERAL SKELETON

- Early degenerative change in knees, shoulders, and hips
- Relative lack of osteophyte formation
- Prominent intra-articular bodies

DIFFERENTIAL DIAGNOSIS

Clinical presentation of ochronotic arthropathy in the spine and large joints is similar to that of ankylosing spondylitis. In the spine, patients experience stiffness, pain, and loss of lumbar lordosis. In the large joints, patients often experience pain and decreased range of motion.[4]

Radiographically, ochronotic arthropathy in the spine may be difficult to distinguish from ankylosing spondylitis.

In both ankylosing spondylitis and ochronosis there may be loss of lordosis, disc calcification, and end-plate changes. However, although there may be mild narrowing and subchondral sclerosis of the sacroiliac joints in ochronosis, there is rarely severe involvement or fusion of the sacroiliac joints, helping to distinguish the two entities. Additionally, there is typically severe facet joint involvement in ankylosing spondylitis, a finding not commonly seen in ochronosis. Disc calcification has also been noted with hyperparathyroidism, hemochromatosis, amyloidosis, and diffuse idiopathic skeletal hyperostosis. However, associated radiographic changes and clinical findings can help to distinguish these entities from ochronosis.

In the peripheral joints, ochronotic arthropathy may be indistinguishable from osteoarthritis. Findings that can suggest ochronotic arthropathy over osteoarthritis include advanced degenerative changes for the patient's age, a relative lack of osteophyte formation in relation to joint loss, prominence of intra-articular bodies, lack of hand involvement, and severe glenohumeral joint involvement, an uncommon finding in osteoarthritis without a history of prior trauma (Fig. 56-4).[7] The diagnosis of ochronotic arthropathy is ensured by the excretion of HGA in the urine.

SYNOPSIS OF TREATMENT OPTIONS
Medical Treatment

There is currently no effective preventive treatment for ochronotic arthropathy.[25] Patients are treated symptomatically, with analgesics, physical therapy, and dietary restriction of tyrosine and phenylalanine.[25,26]

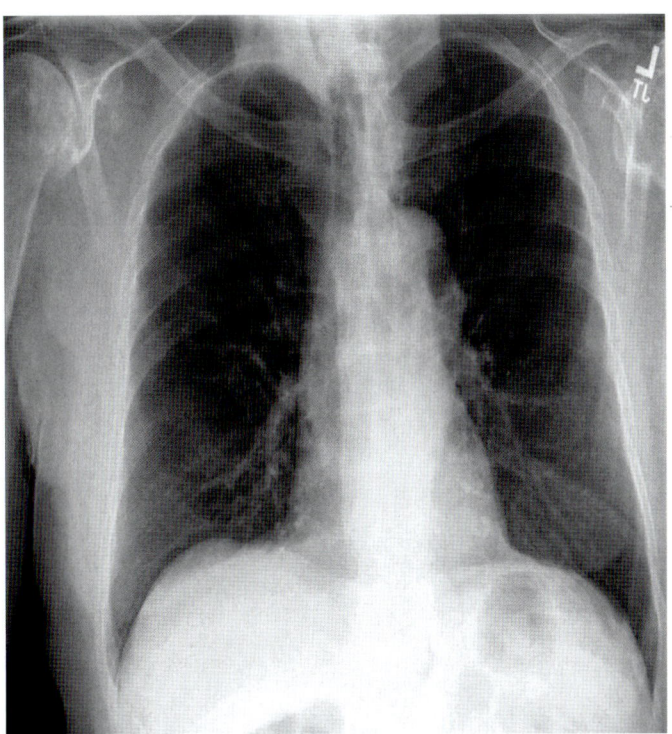

■ FIGURE 56-4 Frontal chest radiograph of the same patient in Figure 56-1 demonstrates marked narrowing and subchondral sclerosis of the right glenohumeral joint, with relative lack of osteophyte formation. *(Courtesy of Eric A. Bogner, MD, New York, NY.)*

Surgical Treatment

Surgical joint replacement or tendon repair is performed when indicated.[6,25,27]

What the Referring Physician Needs to Know

■ The diagnosis of ochronotic arthropathy should be considered in patients with widespread disc degeneration and calcification in the thoracolumbar spine and/or premature degenerative change in the knee, hip, or shoulders with relative lack of osteophyte formation.

■ Ochronotic arthropathy can be difficult to distinguish, both clinically and radiographically, from ankylosing spondylitis in the spine and from osteoarthritis in the peripheral joints. If ochronosis is suspected, the presence of HGA in the urine ensures the diagnosis.

■ Although there is currently no specific therapy for ochronosis, early detection and symptomatic treatment may increase the quality of life in patients with this rapidly progressive disease.

SUGGESTED READINGS

Borman P, Bodur H, Ciliz D. Ochronotic arthropathy. Rheumatol Int 2002; 21:205-209.

Hamdi N, Cooke T, Hassan B. Ochronotic arthropathy: case report and review of the literature. Int Orthop 1999; 23:122-125.

Keller J, Macaulay W, Nercessian O, Jaffe I. New developments in ochronosis: review of the literature. Rheumatol Int 2005; 25:81-85.

REFERENCES

1. Cortina R, Moris C, Astudillo A, et al. Familial ochronosis. Eur Heart J 1995; 16:285-286.
2. Ellaway CJ, Holme E, Standing S, et al. Outcome of tyrosinaemia type III. J Inherit Metab Dis 2001; 24:824-832.
3. La Du B. Alkaptonuria. In Royce RM, Steinman B (eds). Connective Tissue and its Heritable Disorders, Molecular, Genetic, and Medical Aspects, 2nd ed. New York, Wiley-Liss, 2002, pp 809-825.
4. Perrone A, Impara L, Bruni A, et al. Radiographic and MRI findings in ochronosis. Radiol Med (Torino) 2005; 110:349-358.
5. Sahin G, Milcan A, Bagis S, et al. A case of ochronosis: upper extremity involvement. Rheumatol Int 2001; 21:78-80.
6. Manoj Kumar RV, Rajasekaran S. Spontaneous tendon ruptures in alkaptonuria. J Bone Joint Surg Br 2003; 85:883-886.
7. Resnick D. Alkaptonuria. In Resnick D. Diagnosis of Bone and Joint Disorders, 4th ed. Philadelphia, WB Saunders, 2002, pp 1678-1691.
8. Kocyigit H, Gurgan A, Terzioglu R, Gurgan U. Clinical, radiographic and echocardiographic findings in a patient with ochronosis. Clin Rheumatol 1998; 17:403-406.
9. Poulsen V. Uber Ochronose bei Menschen und Tieren. Beitr Pathol Anat. 1910; 48:437.

10. Puhr L. Uber Ochronose. Virchows Arch 1926; 260:130.
11. Lichtenstein L, Kaplan L. Hereditary ochronosis; pathologic changes observed in two necropsied cases. Am J Pathol 1954; 30:99-125.
12. Cooper J, Moran T. Studies on ochronosis: I. Report of case with death from ochronotic nephrosis. AMA Arch Pathol 1957; 64:46-53.
13. Seradge H. Ochronotic stenosing flexor tenosynovitis—case report. J Hand Surg 1981; 6:359-360.
14. Selvi E, Manganelli S, Mannoni A, et al: Chronic ochronotic arthritis: clinical, arthroscopic, and pathologic findings. J Rheumatol 2000; 27:2272-2274.
15. La Du B Jr. Alkaptonuria and ochronotic arthritis. Mol Biol Med 1991; 8:31-38.
16. Mestan M, Bustin G, Wagner L. Chiropractic care and ochronotic arthropathy. J Manipulative Physiol Ther 1999; 22:473-477.
17. Albers S, Brozena S, Glass L, Fenske N. Alkaptonuria and ochronosis: case report and review. J Am Acad Dermatol 1992; 27:609-614.

18. Borman P, Bodur H, Ciliz D. Ochronotic arthropathy. Rheumatol Int 2002; 21:205-209.
19. Lagier R, Sitaj S. Vertebral changes in ochronosis. Ann Rheum Dis 1974; 33:86-92.
20. Kostka D, Sitaj S, Niepel G. [The prevalence of the vacuum phenomenon and its pathognomonic importance in ochronotic diskopathy.] Fortschr Geb Rontgenstr Nuklearmed 1965; 102:62-68.
21. Kabasakal Y, Kiyici I, Ozmen D, et al. Spinal abnormalities similar to ankylosing spondylitis in a 58-year-old woman with ochronosis. Clin Rheumatol 1995; 14:355-357.
22. Hamdi N, Cooke T, Hassan B. Ochronotic arthropathy: case report and review of the literature. Int Orthop 1999; 23:122-125.
23. Phorphutkul C, Introne W, Perry M, et al. Natural history of alkaptonuria. N Engl J Med 2002; 347:2111-2121.
24. Nas K, Gur A, Akdeniz S, et al. Ochronosis: a case of severe ochronotic arthropathy. Clin Rheumatol 2002; 21:170-172.
25. Keller J, Macaulay W, Nercessian O, Jaffe I. New developments in ochronosis: review of the literature. Rheumatol Int 2005; 25:81-85.
26. Suzuki Y, Oda K, Yoshikawa, et al. A novel therapeutic trial of homogentisic aciduria in a murine model of alkaptonuria. J Hum Genet 1999; 44:79-84.
27. Carrier D, Harris C. Bilateral hip and bilateral knee arthroplasties in a patient with ochronotic arthropathy. Orthop Rev 1990; 19:1005-1009.

57

Diffuse Idiopathic Skeletal Hyperostosis and Ossification of the Posterior Longitudinal Ligament

Curtis Hayes and Claire Coggins

Diffuse idiopathic skeletal hyperostosis (DISH), a term proposed by Resnick[1,2] is the widely accepted name describing a common disorder affecting mostly elderly persons characterized by increased bone formation at multiple sites in the spine and peripheral skeleton. Although the radiographic changes of DISH may be florid, clinical symptoms are often mild or absent, hence the importance of the imaging appearance in establishing this diagnosis.

Ossification of the posterior longitudinal ligament (OPLL), both symptomatic and asymptomatic, occurs in association with DISH and independently.[3]

ETIOLOGY

The cause of DISH is uncertain. DISH has been tenuously associated with several risk factors, most notably diabetes mellitus and hyperinsulinemia, hyperuricemia, obesity, and other endocrine abnormalities.[4,5,7] Other issues of possible importance include mechanical, trauma, dietary, environmental, and genetic factors.

The precise cause of OPLL is also unknown. Trauma, fluoride or vitamin A toxicity, diabetes mellitus, inherited factors, and prior infection have been proposed as causative, but no single factor has been definitively confirmed.[8]

PREVALENCE AND EPIDEMIOLOGY

DISH is common in the elderly. In one large population study, 25% of men and 15% of women older than age 50 years showed radiographic changes of DISH based on chest radiographs.[9] In men older than age 80 years, the prevalence was 35%.[9] The prevalence is lower in African Americans, Native Americans, and Asians.[9,10] Because prevalence data are usually based on radiographic criteria relating to the spine, it is likely that the overall prevalence of DISH is higher than reported.

OPLL was initially believed to have a striking predilection in Japanese persons, thought to occur with a frequency of 1.0% to 1.7% among those with cervical spine disorders.[11,12] More recently, reports indicate a more widespread ethnic and geographic distribution of this disease.[13,14] The diagnosis of OPLL is usually established between 50 and 60 years of age. OPLL is more common in men than women. It is a relatively common occurrence in patients with conditions associated with hyperostosis of the spine, especially DISH.[3]

CLINICAL PRESENTATION

For multiple reasons, establishing strong causal associations between radiographic changes and clinical symptoms in DISH is difficult. In the elderly, minor or nonspecific symptoms are sometimes disregarded as age related or attributed to other musculoskeletal diseases that frequently coexist with DISH. Spine-related symptoms such as pain and stiffness are usually mild with DISH and may be no greater than in the general population.[15] Symptoms relating to DISH involving the peripheral skeleton are also ambiguous. Local pain, tendinosis, and swelling are considered common peripheral symptoms by Resnick.[16] Bone changes of DISH in the pelvis may be asymptomatic.[17] Although

spaces, producing flowing ossification of variable thickness. Advanced spinal changes consist of massive flowing ossification, frequently with large, irregular bony masses at the level of the disc. Peripheral pathologic changes of DISH include hyperostosis at entheses, para-articular osteophytosis, and conspicuous ligament ossification. Adjacent tendons show degenerative changes of tendinosis.

The bony growth in OPLL consists of mature cortical bone, most predominantly along the midline of the posterior vertebral bodies. It is uncertain whether the mechanism of bone formation involves endochondral ossification versus some other initiator of bone formation. Ultimately, the ligament ossification encroaches on the adjacent spinal cord, producing cord compression, infarction, and demyelination.[8]

IMAGING TECHNIQUES

In most cases, the diagnosis of DISH is established on the basis of routine radiography of the spine or peripheral skeleton. On occasion, CT may aid in differentiating DISH from other diseases affecting the spine and pelvis, such as ankylosing spondylitis or other spondyloarthropathies.

Although advanced cases of OPLL are easily recognized on routine radiography, the linear ossification in early cases is more easily demonstrated with cross-sectional imaging. CT clearly delineates the calcified ligament, whereas MRI is useful in assessing both the extent of the ossification and the status of the adjacent spinal cord.[31]

uncommon, cervical dysphagia, stridor, and aspiration are potentially serious symptoms attributed to DISH affecting the cervical spine.[18,19] Extensive DISH in the cervical spine may lead to difficult intubation.[20] The most severe potential complication of DISH are fractures through the fused levels, which have been reported after minor trauma.[3,21-24] Most common in the cervical spine, such fractures may displace markedly, with disastrous consequences. Painful pseudarthrosis has been reported, particularly in the thoracic and lumbar regions.[25,26]

Patients with OPLL may be asymptomatic or experience neck pain and/or neurologic symptoms, including lower or upper extremity motor and sensory abnormalities. Neurologic symptoms are more common in cases in which the ligament thickening decreases the spinal canal by greater than 60%[27] or the sagittal diameter less than 8mm.[28] Neurologic symptoms may progress slowly or arise precipitously after trauma.[29,30]

PATHOPHYSIOLOGY

Resnick characterizes the pathology of thoracic spine bone formation in DISH into three types.[16] Type I are ligamentous calcifications within fibers of the anterior longitudinal ligament, independent of disc abnormalities. Type II changes occur in association with disc abnormalities, especially involving the anulus fibrosis. These changes are identical to those found in spondylosis deformans. Type III changes are early ossification at the enthesis of the anterior longitudinal ligament along the midanterior aspect of the vertebral body. Ossification eventually bridges the disc

MANIFESTATIONS OF THE DISEASE
Radiography

In the spine, radiographic findings of DISH are most common in the thoracic region (Fig. 57-1). Multilevel ossification along the anterior and lateral aspect of the vertebral bodies bridging several disc spaces is typical. The thickness and irregularity of the ossification varies from thin and delicate, mimicking ankylosing spondylitis,[2] to over 2 cm in thickness.[2] In the cervical spine, involvement is more common in the lower levels, especially C4 through C7 (Fig. 57-2). Massive ossifications may cause dysphagia. Ossification of the stylohyoid ligament and other entheses may be seen. Lumbar changes are most common in the upper levels, with variable thickness flowing ossification, frequently with pointed excrescences at the disc spaces. There may also be hypertrophy and close apposition of the spinous processes. Osteopenia is not a feature of DISH.[32,33] In fact, bone mineral density has been reported to be spuriously elevated due to the ossifications in DISH.[34]

Resnick describes three radiographic diagnostic criteria for DISH:[16] (1) flowing calcification and ossification along at least four contiguous vertebral levels, (2) relative preservation of disc space height, and (3) absence of apophyseal joint ankylosis, erosions, or intra-articular fusion. These criteria are important in enabling differentiation of DISH from common degenerative disc diseases and from ankylosing spondylitis and other spondyloarthropathies. Strict adherence to these criteria likely results in lower sensitivity for mild disease.

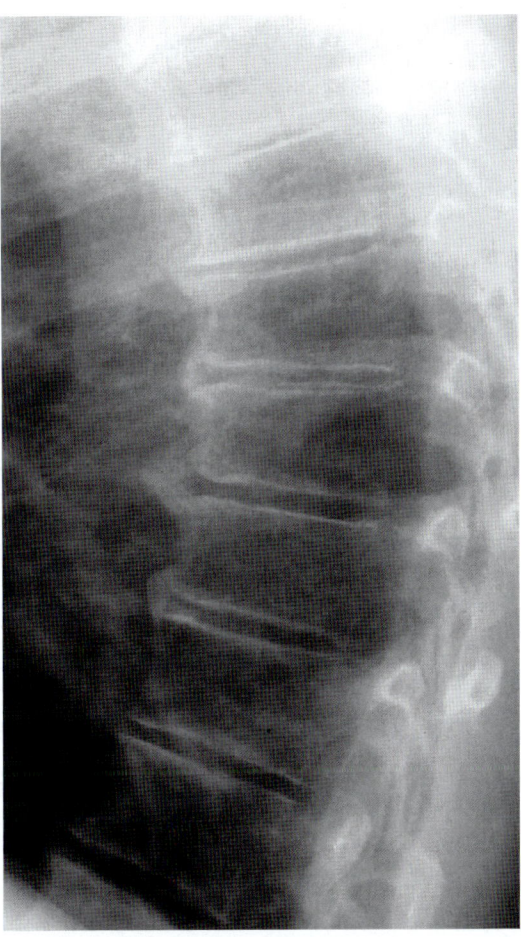

■ **FIGURE 57-1** Lateral radiograph of thoracic spine showing typical changes of DISH, with flowing ossification extending four or more consecutive levels.

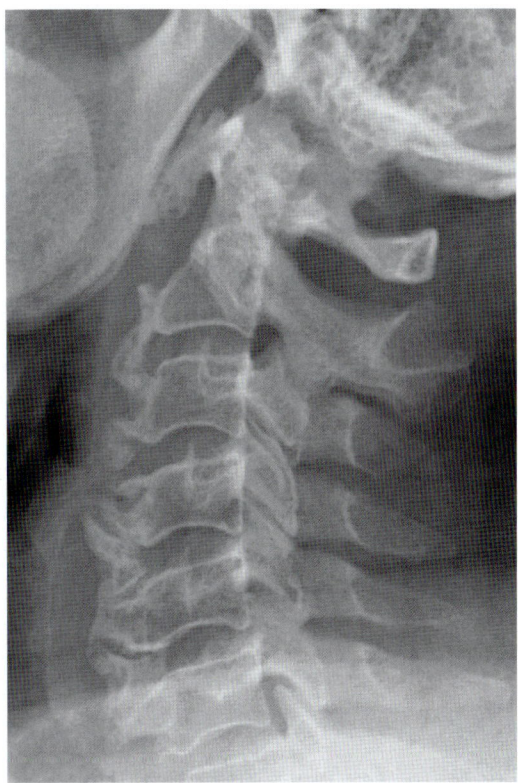

■ **FIGURE 57-2** Lateral radiograph showing typical DISH, with massive ossification along the anterior cervical spine and preservation of the disc spaces.

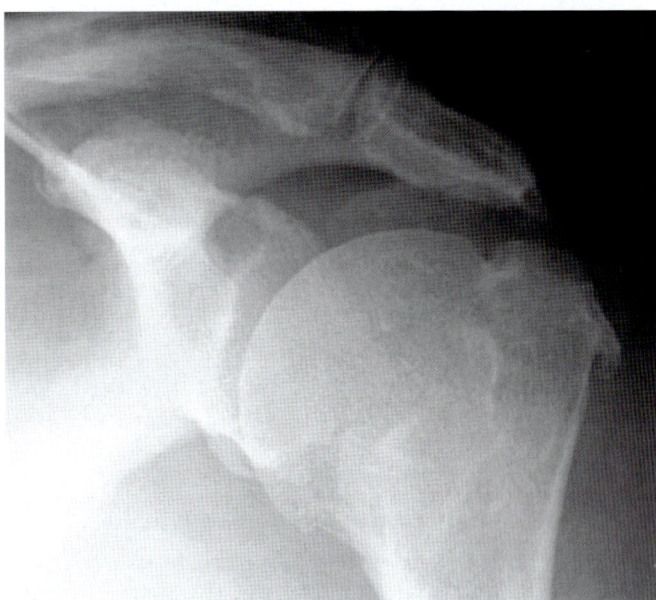

■ **FIGURE 57-3** Pronounced ossification at multiple entheses around the shoulder, typical of peripheral findings with DISH.

In the peripheral skeleton, numerous sites of tendon and ligament attachment (entheses) may be affected by typical excessive bone formation with DISH. Around the shoulder, findings include excrescences arising from the acromion and coracoid process, coracoacromial and coracoclavicular ligament ossifications, and hypertrophic bone formation at the deltoid tuberosity (Fig. 57-3).

At the elbow, the olecranon process and epicondyles frequently show enthesophytes. Around the pelvis, bone excrescences are often seen arising along the iliac crests, iliac spines, ischial tuberosities, and trochanters and along the posterior proximal femur (Fig. 57-4). These excrescences are well formed and sharply marginated, which aids in distinguishing them from the fuzzy excrescences more typical of spondyloarthropathies. Bridging ossification at the superior aspect of the sacroiliac joints is also common. Anterior bridging ossification in the midportion of the sacroiliac joint may appear as a sclerotic focus when viewed en face, mimicking a blastic metastasis.

In cases of OPLL, radiographic findings include both continuous and segmental patterns of calcification, usually involving the midcervical region (Fig. 57-5). Severe canal stenosis is more likely with the continuous variety.[35] The thickness of the ossified ligament is variable. The width of the disc spaces is usually preserved, and changes of DISH are frequently present. Involvement of the cervical spine is most common, although thoracic and lumbar involvement is possible.

Magnetic Resonance Imaging

Magnetic resonance imaging may have limited utility in assessing rare spinal complications of DISH, such as fractures or pseudarthrosis of the spine.[36]

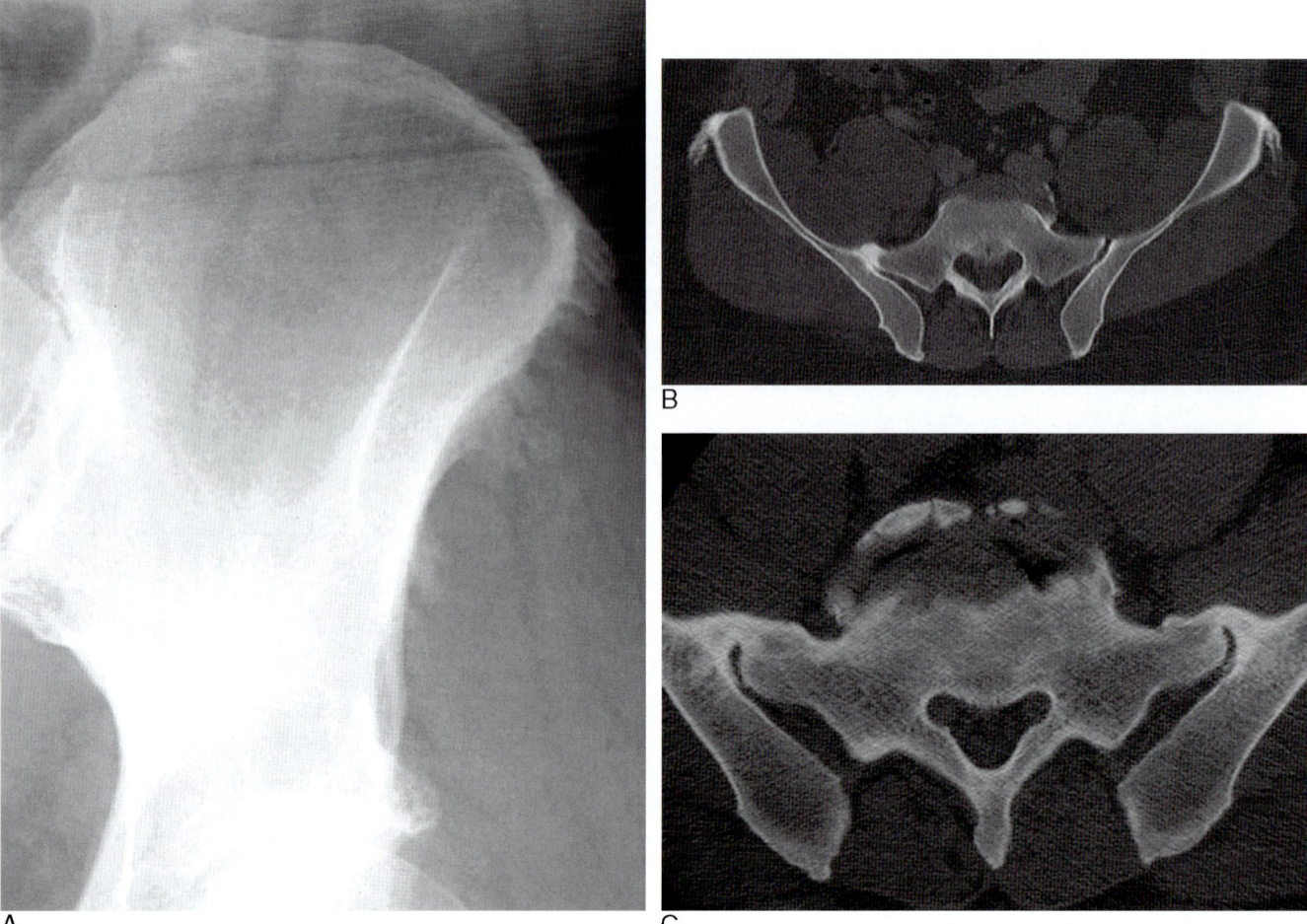

■ **FIGURE 57-4** Findings of DISH at the pelvis. **A,** Radiograph showing sharply marginated but irregular ossification at multiple entheses. **B,** CT image through upper pelvis shows bone formation at entheses. **C,** CT image through upper sacroiliac joints shows bridging ossification at anterior aspect of joints. Note that the remainder of the sacroiliac joints are unaffected, distinguishing DISH from ankylosing spondylitis.

With OPLL, MRI identifies thickening of the posterior longitudinal ligament with great sensitivity, although it may be difficult to distinguish a thickened ligament from true ossification (Fig. 57-6). MRI is also useful in assessing the adjacent spinal cord compromise or edema.

Multidetector Computed Tomography

Multidetector CT has a limited role in assessing DISH. MDCT may be particularly useful in assessing fractures and pseudarthoses (Fig. 57-7). In cases in which ankylosing spondylitis or other spondyloarthopathy is considered in the differential diagnosis, MDCT may be useful in assessing the status of the apophyseal joint of the spine and sacroiliac joints for intra-articular fusion and erosions.

MDCT precisely delineates the extent of involvement and canal compromise in OPLL (Fig. 57-8). It is more sensitive than conventional radiography in detecting minor degrees of ossification, especially the segmental variety.

Classic Signs

DISH
- Flowing ossification along at least four contiguous vertebral levels
- Relative preservation of disc height
- Absence of apophyseal joint ankylosis or erosion
- Prominent, sharply marginated bony excrescences arising at ligament and tendon attachments (entheses)

OPLL
- Continuous or segmental ossification along the posterior vertebral body of one or several levels, most often involving the cervical spine

DIFFERENTIAL DIAGNOSIS

Several diseases may result in radiographic changes similar to those of DISH. Because it is common in the elderly, DISH often coexists with other degenerative spine

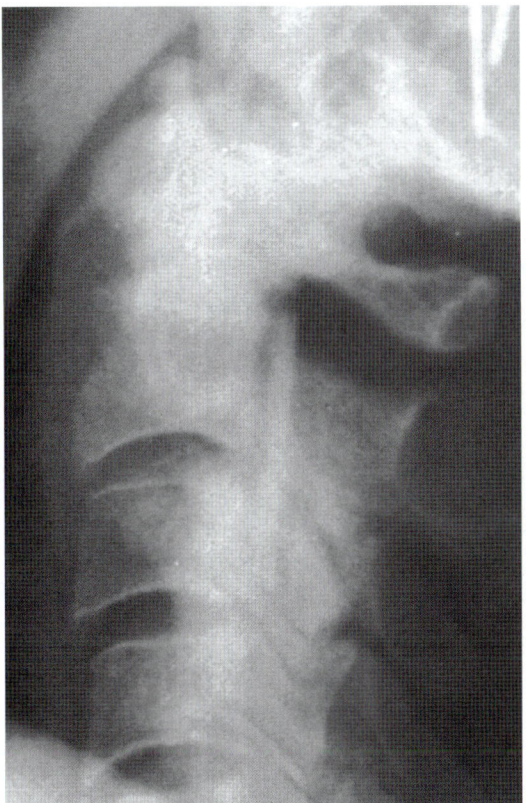

■ **FIGURE 57-5** Lateral radiograph showing continuous pattern of OPLL involving two levels of the upper cervical spine.

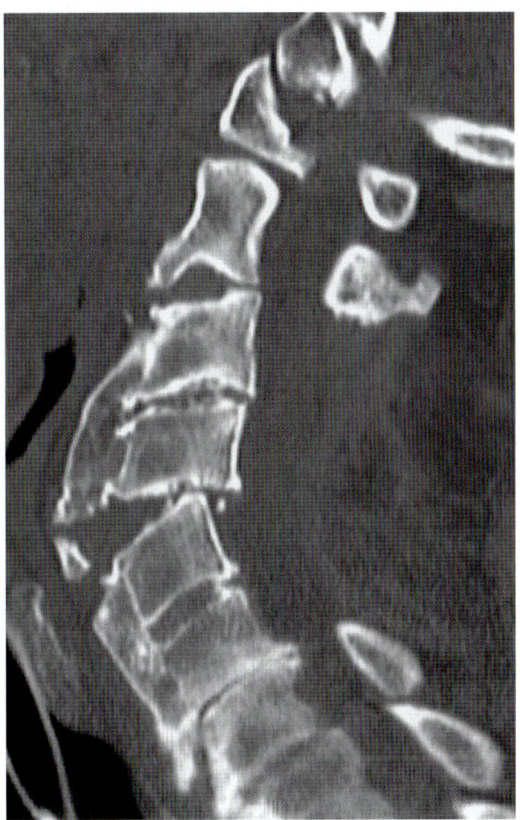

■ **FIGURE 57-7** Sagittal reformatted MDCT image showing hyperextension fracture with subluxation through C4–C5 level in patient with massive DISH. Such injuries may occur after relatively trivial trauma in such patients.

■ **FIGURE 57-6** MRI of OPLL. **A,** T1-weighted image showing extensive thickening of the posterior longitudinal ligament. **B,** T2-weighted image showing marked irregular thickening of the posterior longitudinal ligament over multiple cervical segments, with pronounced narrowing of the canal.

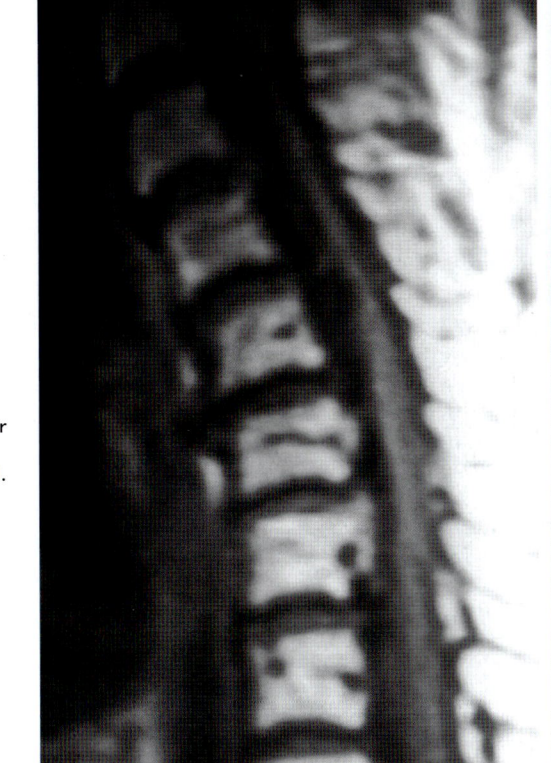

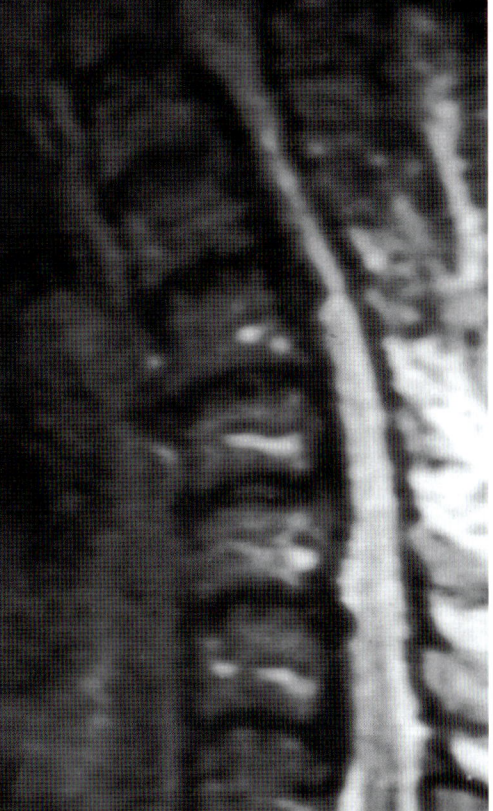

A

B

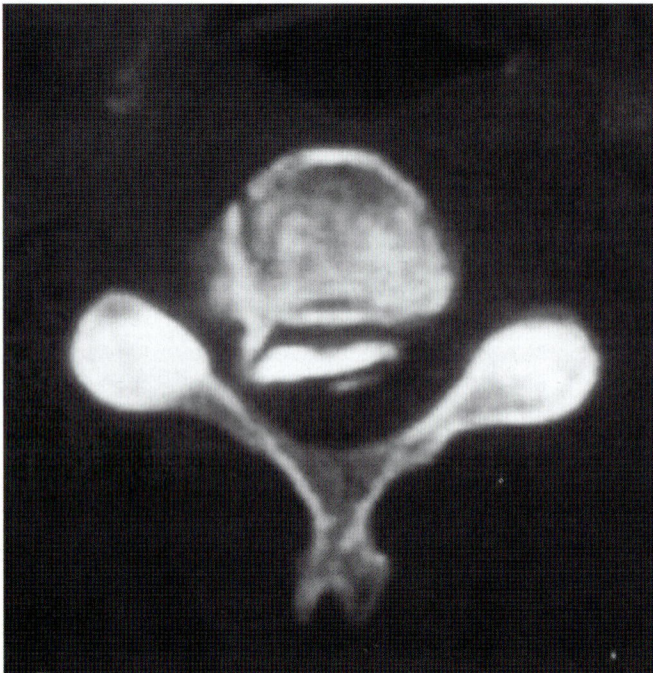

A

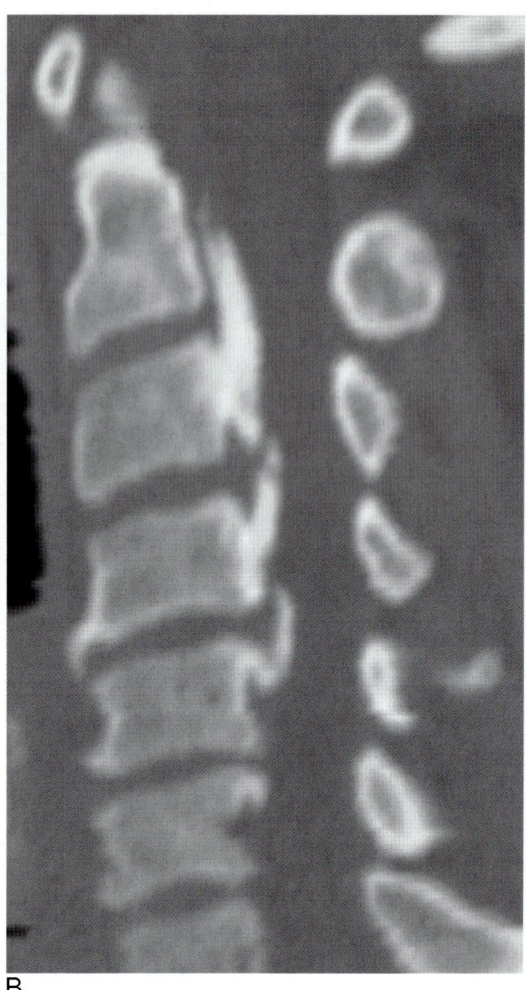

B

■ **FIGURE 57-8** CT of OPLL of the cervical spine. **A,** Axial CT image showing typical ossification of the posterior longitudinal ligament. **B,** Sagittal reformatted MDCT image shows extent of ossification, both continuous and segmental patterns.

diseases. Other conditions associated with bony excrescences in the spine include degenerative disc diseases (spondylosis deformans, intervertebral osteochondrosis), ankylosing spondylitis and other spondyloarthopathies, trauma, neuropathic arthropathy, acromegaly, hypoparathyroidism, fluorosis, and ochronosis. Differentiating features of degenerative disc disease include disc space narrowing, vertebral end-plate sclerosis, and disc vacuum phenomenon. With ankylosing spondylitis, the bridging ossifications are typically gracile and are accompanied by apophyseal and sacroiliac joint changes, erosions, or intra-articular fusion. With Reiter and psoriatic arthritis, the calcifications are typically asymmetric and more prominent laterally than anteriorly.

In the peripheral skeleton, bony excrescences related to repetitive trauma and chronic overuse may locally mimic the typical enthesophytes of DISH.

The imaging appearance of OPLL is usually characteristic.

SYNOPSIS OF TREATMENT OPTIONS

Medical Treatment

Treatment of DISH is generally symptomatic. Physical therapy and massage are aimed at relieving stiffness whereas nonsteroidal anti-inflammatory drugs or local corticosteroid injections are used to treat pain.

Patients with OPLL do not necessarily develop progressive myelopathy. In a 10-year follow-up study, 55 (17%) of 323 patients without myelopathy at presentation developed myelopathy.[27] Risk factors for evolution of myelopathy in OPLL include greater than 60% compromise of the canal by ossification, sagittal canal diameter less than 8 mm, and increased cervical range of motion.[27]

Surgical Treatment

Surgical treatment in DISH is reserved for complications such as fracture or pseudarthrosis. Preoperative knowledge of DISH may prevent surgical complications such as difficult intubation[20] and aspiration.[18] Whether DISH predisposes patients undergoing total joint replacement to develop postoperative heterotopic ossification is debated.[37,38]

Surgical approaches to OPLL include anterior, posterior, and combined approaches and may require extensive procedures involving multiple levels.[39] Surgical sites may involve the cervical,[39] thoracic,[40] or lumbar spine.[41]

What the Referring Physician Needs to Know

- DISH is most often a radiologic diagnosis, because symptoms are mild and nonspecific.
- Complications of DISH are rare but include fracture through fused levels and dysphagia or aspiration due to cervical spine involvement.
- Radiographic changes of DISH must be differentiated from ankylosing spondylitis and spondyloarthropathy by lack of apophyseal and sacroiliac joint erosions or fusion.

- OPLL is best evaluated with CT (for ossification) and MRI (for evaluation of cord).
- OPLL is more likely to progress to myelopathy if there is canal compromise of 60%, a sagittal canal diameter of 8 mm, or increased cervical range of motion.

SUGGESTED READINGS

Resnick D. Degenerative diseases of the vertebral column. Radiology 1985; 156:3–14.

Resnick D, Niwayama G. Radiographic and pathologic features of spinal involvement in diffuse idiopathic skeletal hyperostosis (DISH). Radiology 1976; 119:559–568.

REFERENCES

1. Resnick D, Shaul SR, Robins JM. Diffuse idiopathic skeletal hyperostosis (DISH): Forestier's disease with extraspinal manifestations. Radiology 1975; 115:513–524.
2. Resnick D, Niwayama G. Radiographic and pathologic features of spinal involvement in diffuse idiopathic skeletal hyperostosis (DISH). Radiology 1976; 119:559–568.
3. Resnick D, Guerra J, Robinson CA, Vint VC. Association of diffuse idiopathic skeletal hyperostosis (DISH) and calcification and ossification of the posterior longitudinal ligament. AJR Am J Roentgenol 1978; 131:1049–1053.
4. Julkunen H, Knekt P, Aromaa A. Spondylosis deformans and diffuse idiopathic skeletal hyperostosis (DISH) in Finland. Scand J Rheumatol 1981; 10:193–203.
5. Kiss C, Szilagyi M, Paksy A, Poor G. Risk factors for diffuse idiopathic skeletal hyperostosis: a case-control study. Rheumatology 2002; 41:27–30.
6. Sarzi-Puttini P, Atzeni F. New developments in our understanding of DISH (diffuse idiopathic skeletal hyperostosis). Curr Opin Rheumatol 2004; 16:287–292.
7. Sencan D, Elden H, Nacitarhan V, et al. The prevalence of diffuse idiopathic skeletal hyperostosis in patients with diabetes mellitus. Rheumatol Int 2005; 25:518–521.
8. Resnick D. Calcification and ossification of the posterior spinal ligaments and tissues. In Resnick D. Diagnosis of Bone and Joint Disorders, 4th ed. Philadelphia, WB Saunders, 2002, vol 2, pp 1504–1516.
9. Weinfeld RM, Olson PN, Maki DD, Griffiths HJ. The prevalence of diffuse idiopathic skeletal hyperostosis (DISH) in two large American Midwest metropolitan hospital populations. Skeletal Radiol 1997; 26:222–225.
10. Kim SK, Choi BR, Kim CG, et al. The prevalence of diffuse idiopathic skeletal hyperostosis in Korea. J Rheumatol 2004; 31:2032–2035.
11. Onji Y, Akiyama H, Shimomura Y, et al. Posterior paravertebral ossification causing cervical myelopathy: report of eighteen cases. J Bone Joint Surg Am 1967; 49:143.
12. Yokoi K. Ectopic calcifications in the epidural space. Orthop Surg 1963; 14:1262.
13. Trojan DA, Pouchot J, Pokrupa R, et al. Diagnosis and treatment of ossification of the posterior longitudinal ligament of the spine: report of eight cases and literature review. Am J Med 1992; 92:296–306.
14. Heller JG, Johnston RB, Goodrich A. Ossification of the posterior longitudinal ligament: a report of nine cases in non-Oriental patients. Skeletal Radiol 1994; 23:601–606.
15. Schlapbach P, Beyeler C, Gerber NJ, et al. Diffuse idiopathic skeletal hyperostosis (DISH) of the spine: a cause of back pain? A controlled study. Br J Rheumatol 1989; 28:299–303.
16. Resnick D. Diffuse idiopathic skeletal hyperostosis. In Resnick D. Diagnosis of Bone and Joint Disorders, 4th ed. Philadelphia, WB Saunders, 2002, vol 2, pp 1476–1503.
17. Fahrer H, Barandum R, Gerber NJ, et al. Pelvic manifestations of diffuse idiopathic skeletal hyperostosis (DISH): are they clinically relevant? Rheumatol Int 1989; 8:257–261.
18. Giddings CE, Caulfield HM, Dorward NL. Diffuse idiopathic skeletal hyperostosis resulting in dysphagia and aspiration pneumonia. Br J Neurosurg 2003; 17:467–468.
19. Castellano DM, Sinacori JT, Karakla DW. Stridor and dysphagia in diffuse idiopathic skeletal hyperostosis (DISH). Laryngoscope 2006; 116:341–344.
20. Crosby ET, Grahovac S. Diffuse idiopathic skeletal hyperostosis: an unusual cause of difficult intubation. Can J Anaesth 1993; 40:54–58.
21. Paley D, Schwartz M, Cooper P, et al. Fractures of the spine in diffuse idiopathic skeletal hyperostosis. Clin Orthop Relat Res 1991; 267:22–32.
22. Hendrix RW, Melany M, Miller F, Rogers LF. Fracture of the spine in patients with ankylosis due to diffuse idiopathic skeletal hyperostosis: clinical and imaging findings. AJR Am J Roentgenol 1994; 162:899–904.
23. Burkus KJ, Denis F. Hyperextension injuries of the thoracic spine in diffuse idiopathic skeletal hyperostosis. J Bone Joint Surg Am 1994; 76:237–243.
24. Sreedharan S, Li YH. Diffuse idiopathic skeletal hyperostosis with cervical spinal cord injury—a report of 3 cases and a literature review. Ann Acad Med Singapore 2005; 34:257–261.
25. Quagliano PV, Hayes CW, Palmer WE. Vertebral pseudoarthrosis associated with diffuse idiopathic skeletal hyperostosis. Skeletal Radiol 1994; 23:353–355.
26. Miyamoto K, Shimizu K, Arimoto R, et al. Spontaneous symptomatic pseudoarthrosis at the T11–T12 intervertebral space with diffuse idiopathic skeletal hyperostosis: a case report. Spine 2003; 28:E320–E322.
27. Matsunaga S, Sakou T, Taketomi E, Komiya S. Clinical course of patients with ossification of the posterior longitudinal ligament: a minimum 10-year cohort study. J Neurosurg 2004; 100(3 Suppl Spine):245–248.
28. Koyanagi I, Imamura H, Fujimoto S, et al. Spinal canal size in ossification of the posterior longitudinal ligament of the cervical spine. Surg Neurol 2004; 62:286–291.

29. Pouchet J, Watts CS, Esdaile JM, Hill RO. Sudden quadriplegia complicating ossification of the posterior longitudinal ligament and diffuse idiopathic skeletal hyperostosis. Arthritis Rheum 1987; 30:1069-1072.
30. Wimberley DW, Vaccaro AR, Goyal N, et al. Acute quadriplegia following closed traction reduction of a cervical facet dislocation in the setting of ossification of the posterior longitudinal ligament: case report. Spine 2005; 30:E433-E438.
31. Hirai T, Korogi Y, Yamashita Y, et al. Ossification of the posterior longitudinal ligaments: evaluation with MRI. J Magn Reson Imaging 1998; 8:398-405.
32. Sahin G, Polat G, Bagis S, et al. Study of axial bone mineral density in postmenopausal women with diffuse idiopathic skeletal hyperostosis related to type 2 diabetes mellitus. J Womens Health 2002; 11:801-804.
33. Di Franco M, Mauceri MT, Sili-Scavalli A, et al. Study of peripheral bone mineral density in patients with diffuse idiopathic skeletal hyperostosis. Clin Rheumatol 2000; 19:188-192.
34. Schwartz JB, Rackson M. Diffuse idiopathic skeletal hyperostosis causes artificially elevated lumbar bone mineral density measured by dual x-ray absorptiometry. J Clin Densitometry 2001; 4:385-388.
35. Yamashita Y, Takahashi M, Matsuno Y, et al. Spinal cord compression due to ossification of the ligaments: MR imaging. Radiology 1990; 175:843-848.
36. Le Hir PX, Sautet A, Le Gars L, et al. Hyperextension vertebral body fractures in diffuse idiopathic skeletal hyperostosis: a cause of intravertebral fluidlike collections on MR imaging. AJR Am J Roentgenol 1999; 173:1679-1683.
37. Bundrick TJ, Cook DE, Resnik CS. Heterotopic bone formation in patients with DISH following total hip replacement. Radiology 1985; 155:595-597.
38. Iorio R, Healy WL. Heterotopic ossification after hip and knee arthroplasty: risk factors, prevention, and treatment. J Am Acad Orthop Surg 2002; 10:409-416.
39. Epstein N. Diagnosis and surgical management of cervical ossification of the posterior longitudinal ligament. Spine J 2002; 2:436-449.
40. Matsuyama Y, Yoshihara H, Tsuji T, et al. Surgical outcome of ossification of the posterior longitudinal ligament (OPLL) of the thoracic spine: implication of the type of ossification and surgical options. J Spinal Disord Tech 2005; 18:492-497.
41. Tamura M, Machida M, Aikawa D, et al. Surgical treatment of lumbar ossification of the posterior longitudinal ligament: report of two cases and description of surgical technique. J Neurosurg Spine 2005; 3:230-233.

CHAPTER

58

Gout

Lee F. Rogers and Sachin Dheer

ETIOLOGY

Gout is a disease with manifestations relating directly from the deposition of monosodium urate monohydrate crystals or uric acid from hyperuricemic body fluids. In humans, urate is a nonmetabolized byproduct of purine metabolism and is excreted via the kidneys (two thirds) and gastrointestinal tract (one third). The development of gout is related to both polygenic inheritance (specifically, the inability of one's kidneys to increase urate secretion in response to an acute load) and environmental factors, particularly the ingestion of red meat, seafood, and alcohol (especially beer, which contains a high level of purines).[1]

PREVALENCE AND EPIDEMIOLOGY

Gout has been recognized since antiquity by its distinctive acute attacks. The disease is even mentioned in the Bible. Asa, of the line of David, enjoyed a highly lauded 41-year reign as King of Judah but toward the end suffered from painful feet, since attributed as likely due to gout. This was recorded in II Chronicles 16:12 as follows: "Asa...was diseased in his feet, until his disease was exceeding great: yet in his disease he sought not to the Lord, but to the physicians." Surprisingly, this is recorded as fact without editorial comment.

The Greeks referred to the acute attacks as "podagra" from the Greek words *pous* for "foot" and *agra* for "attack." Hippocrates had described the disease in the 5th century BC. In a treatise published in 1683, Thomas Sydenham[2] provided the now classic clinical description of gout. By the latter half of the 18th century gout was so well recognized that the genteel, "gouted" gentry were frequently lampooned by London caricaturists to the delight of their viewing public (Fig. 58-1).

Gouty arthritis accounts for approximately 5% of all symptomatic arthropathies and is the most common inflammatory arthropathy in men older than the age of 40 years. Gout has a prevalence of approximately 20 per 1000 patients, and an annual incidence of 1 to 2 per 1000 patients. Ten times as many individuals have asymptomatic

hyperuricemia (defined as > 6 mg/dL in women and > 7 mg/dL in men). Both the incidence and prevalence of gout have doubled in the United States and Europe in the past 40 years. This is believed to be due to both aging of the population and changes in lifestyle. In fact, 75% of patients with gout have metabolic syndrome X (central obesity, hypertension, hyperglycemia, hypertriglyceridemia, and low high-density lipoproteins). Gout is particularly prevalent in Maori and Polynesian populations.[1]

CLINICAL PRESENTATION

Manifestations of gout include arthropathy, tenosynovitis, bursitis, noninfectious cellulitis, soft tissue deposits (tophi), renal disease, and urinary tract calculi.

KEY POINTS

- Gout is a relatively common cause of arthritis, particularly in middle-aged to older males, and has an increasing incidence in Western populations.
- The radiographic findings of gouty arthropathy typically manifest after 6 or more years of the disease being present.
- Characteristic radiologic findings include sharply defined erosions with "hooked" margins and calcified, asymmetric, periarticular tophi. The disease is usually monarticular or oligoarticular, with a strong propensity to involve the appendicular skeleton, especially the first metatarsophalangeal joint.
- Soft tissue involvement includes bursitis, especially of the olecranon bursa.
- Advanced imaging, such as CT and MRI, is infrequently used in the evaluation of gout. Notable exceptions include spinal involvement in symptomatic patients and, rarely, in the evaluation of intra-articular masses.
- Ultrasonography is not typically used to evaluate gout but is becoming more common, and some observations regarding the ultrasound appearance of tophi have been made.

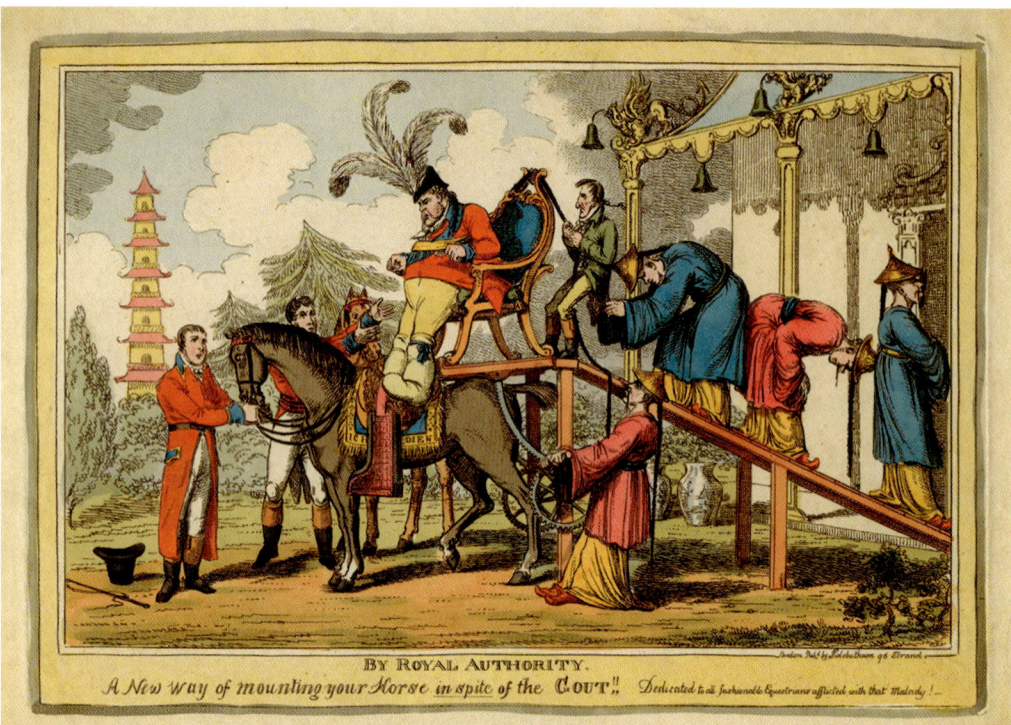

■ **FIGURE 58-1** Anonymous drawing, "By Royal Authority," depicting a nobleman afflicted with gout being hoisted onto his horse. *(© Yale University, Harvey Cushing/John Hay Whitney Medical Library.)*

Gout progresses through four stages: asymptomatic hyperuricemia, acute gouty arthritis, intercritical gout (periods without symptoms, ranging from months to years), and chronic, tophaceous gout.

Acute gouty arthropathy is intensely painful and most commonly involves the first metatarsophalangeal joint. In the drawing in Figure 58-2, an 18th century cartoonist, James Gillray, is said to have captured a patient's perception of distress from an acute attack of podagra. Acute attacks may also occur in the other peripheral joints and rarely present as tenosynovitis, bursitis, or cellulitis. Acute attacks often subside spontaneously, sometimes with resultant pruritus or desquamation. Repeated attacks may then progress to involve multiple joints. In some

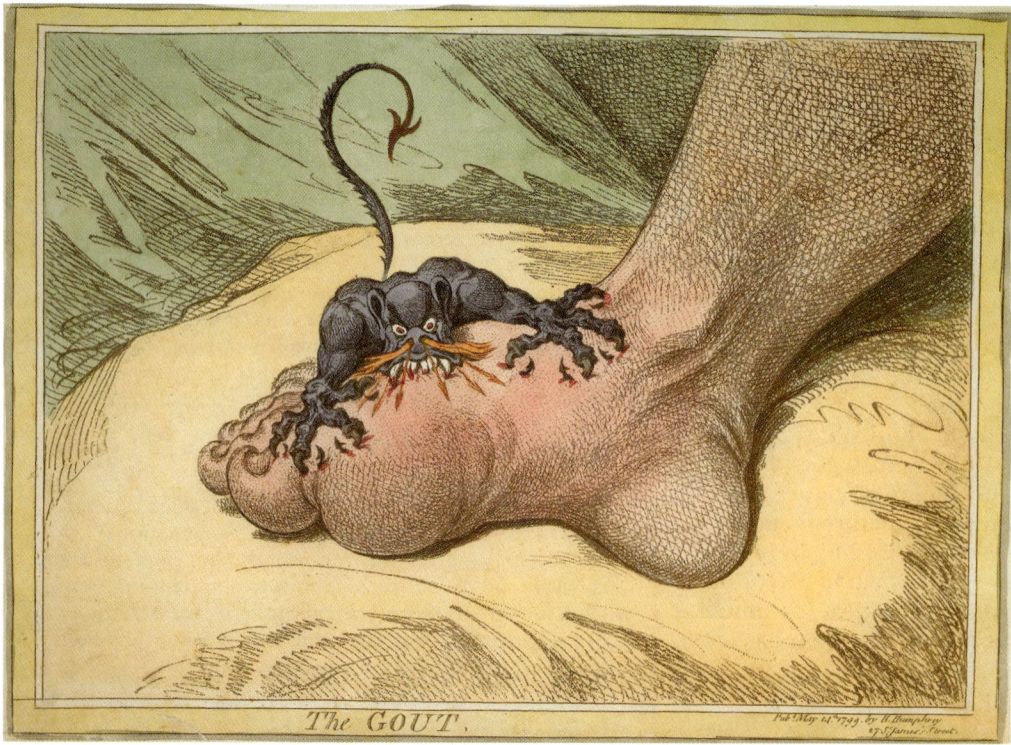

■ **FIGURE 58-2** James Gillray's (1757-1825) "The Gout," an insightful caricature depicting the agonies of those who suffer an acute attack of podagra. *(Courtesy of Princeton University, Princeton, NJ.)*

individuals, the disease becomes chronic without full relief from symptoms. Before the advent of effective therapy, 60% of patients ultimately developed tophi. Tophi are much rarer today and present as subcutaneous soft tissue deposits, which are primarily periarticular, peritendinous, and periligamentous in location. Tophi can occur anywhere, and in rare cases tophi have been reported within the eyes,[1] larynx (Fig. 58-3),[3] parotid gland,[4] bowel wall (Fig. 58-4),[5] and heart.[1]

PATHOPHYSIOLOGY

Anatomy

The disease is characteristically monarticular or oligoarticular and typically asymmetric, both within any given joint and in comparison with the opposite side of the body. Although gout may affect any joint, the disease most frequently involves the appendicular skeleton. In order of decreasing frequency, the feet, hands and wrist, elbows, and knees are involved. The spine is involved uncommonly, but disease in this location carries significant implications due to the presence of the spinal cord.[6]

Pathology

Tophi are collections of urate crystals and amorphous urate surrounded by a chronic inflammatory reaction consisting of giant cells, histiocytes, and fibrosis (Fig. 58-5).[7]

The tophaceous deposits occur within the intra-articular synovium and cartilage, the tendinous and capsular insertions in proximity to joints, and the bones adjacent to joints. Occasionally, tophaceous deposits accumulate with the substance of tendons[8] and may lead to tears in, or ruptures of, the affected tendon.[9]

Tophi often present as small, whitish plaques or nodules in the helix of the ear where they serve as a ready source of the distinctive needle-shaped monosodium urate crystals. Simply scraping the nodules and viewing the scrapings under a polarized light microscope aids in establishing the diagnosis of gout.

Tophi also arise in bursae, particularly the olecranon bursa, where they may be associated with underlying erosion of the olecranon (Fig. 58-6). Superficial subcutaneous tophi may ulcerate and exude urate crystals as a gritty, chalky substance.

Analysis of the synovial fluid in patients with gouty arthritis typically demonstrates needle-shaped, negatively birefringent monosodium urate crystals within neutrophils under polarizing light microscopy. Serum uric acid levels may also be elevated, although only in 60% of patients during an acute attack.[1,7]

MANIFESTATIONS OF THE DISEASE

Findings of gout do not occur until the disease has been present for as long as 6 to 8 years.[10] Therefore, a "negative radiograph" does not rule out the possibility of gout.

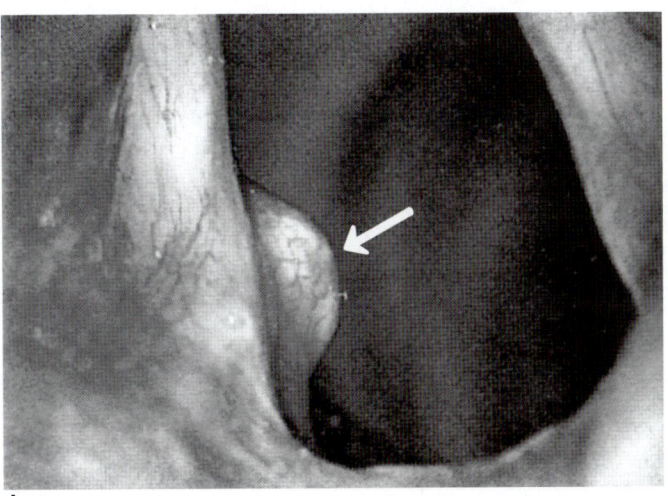

A

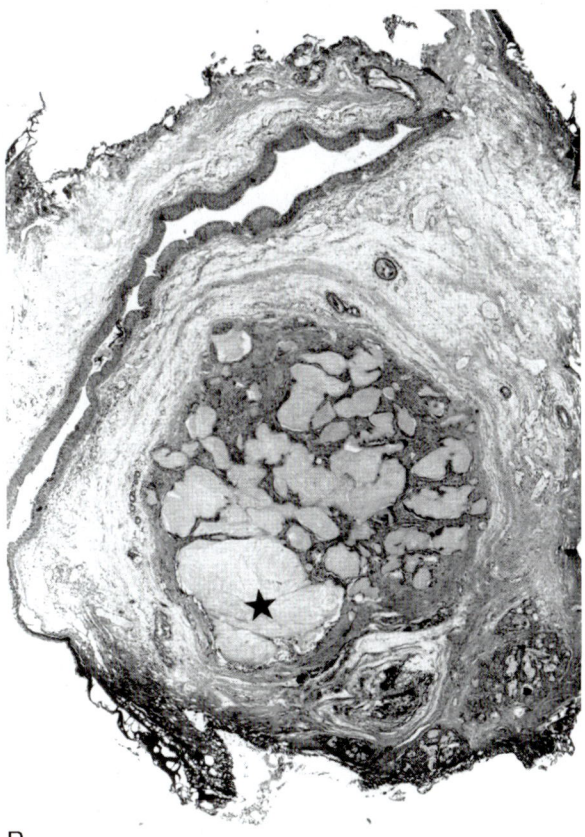

B

■ **FIGURE 58-3**   Gouty tophus involving the subglottic larynx.
A, Laryngoscopic view of a submucosal subglottic lesion (*arrow*).
B, Hematoxylin and eosin–stained pathologic specimen viewed under 20× magnification demonstrates a confluence of urate crystals (*star*) and surrounding inflammatory reaction. (*From Habermann W, Kiesler K, Eherer A, et al. Laryngeal manifestation of gout: a case report of subglottic gout tophus. Auris Nasus Larynx 2001; 28:265–267.*)

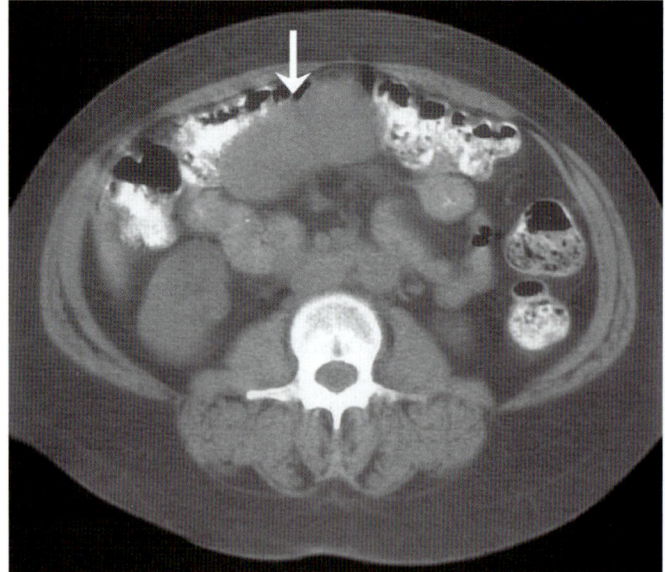

A

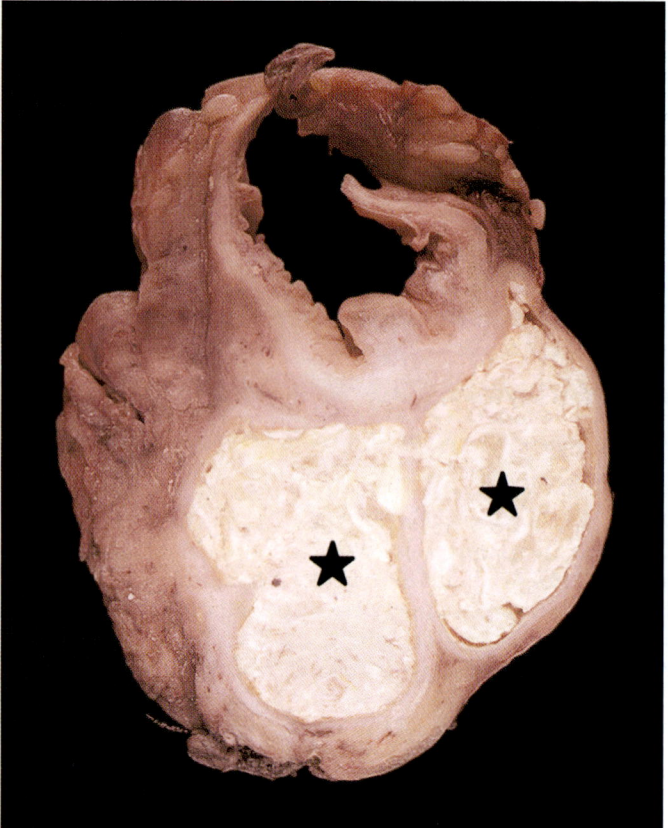

B

■ FIGURE 58-4 Gouty tophus involving the colonic wall. Interestingly, this patient had no other signs or symptoms of gout. **A,** CT scan with contrast enhancement shows a homogeneous, soft tissue density mass involving the wall of the transverse colon (*arrow*). **B,** Gross pathologic specimen cut in transverse demonstrates a subserosal tophi filled with characteristic white, chalky material (*stars*). *(From Wu H, Klein M, Stahl R, Sanchez M. Intestinal pseudotumorous gouty nodulosis: a colonic tophus without manifestation of gouty arthritis. Hum Pathol 2004; 35:897–899.)*

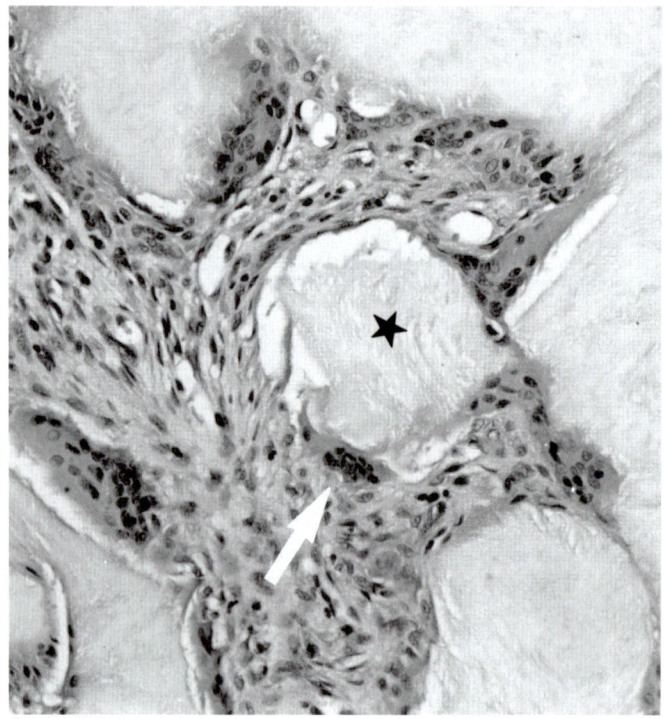

A

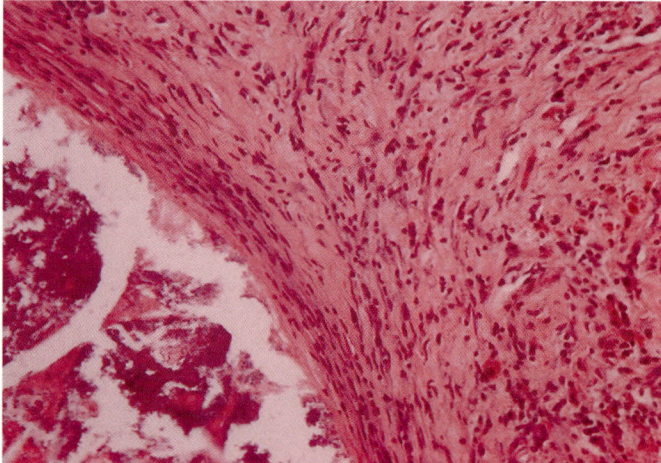

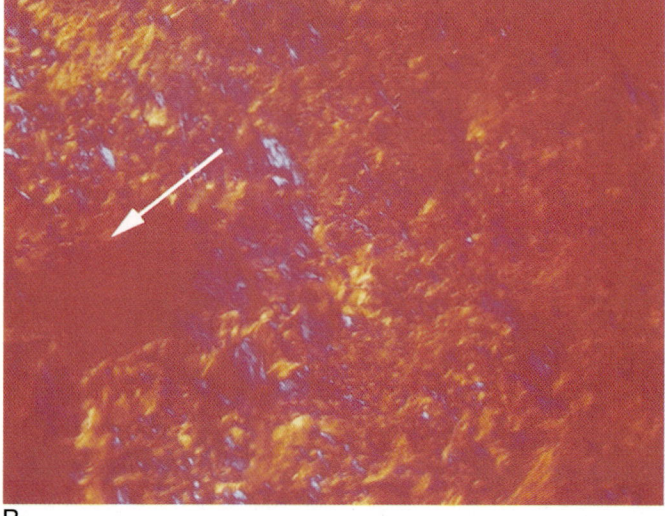

B

■ FIGURE 58-5 Histologic appearance of gouty tophi. **A,** Hematoxylin and eosin–stained 40× magnification of a gouty tophus demonstrates urate crystals (*star*) and surrounding inflammation, including a multinucleated giant cell (*arrow*). **B,** Polarized light microscopy (*bottom*) of a tophus reveals needle-shaped, strongly negative birefringent crystals that appear as bright areas. The *arrow* refers to the axis of compensator slow ray. The nonpolarized hematoxylin and eosin–stained specimen (*top*) is shown for comparison. *(**A** from Habermann W, Kiesler K, Eherer A, et al. Laryngeal manifestation of gout: a case report of subglottic gout tophus. Auris Nasus Larynx 2001; 28:265–267; **B** from Wu H, Klein M, Stahl R, Sanchez M. Intestinal pseudotumorous gouty nodulosis: a colonic tophus without manifestation of gouty arthritis. Hum Pathol 2004; 35:897–899.)*

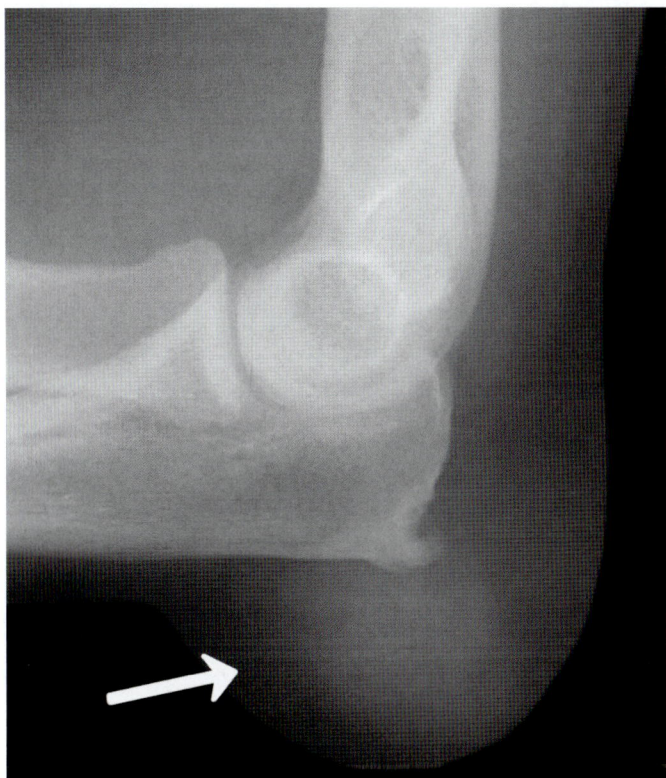

■ FIGURE 58-6 Gouty olecranon bursitis in a 55-year-old man. A rounded soft tissue mass (*arrow*) containing "cloud-like" calcifications surrounds the olecranon. The elbow joint is normal. Olecranon bursitis is a common finding in gout.

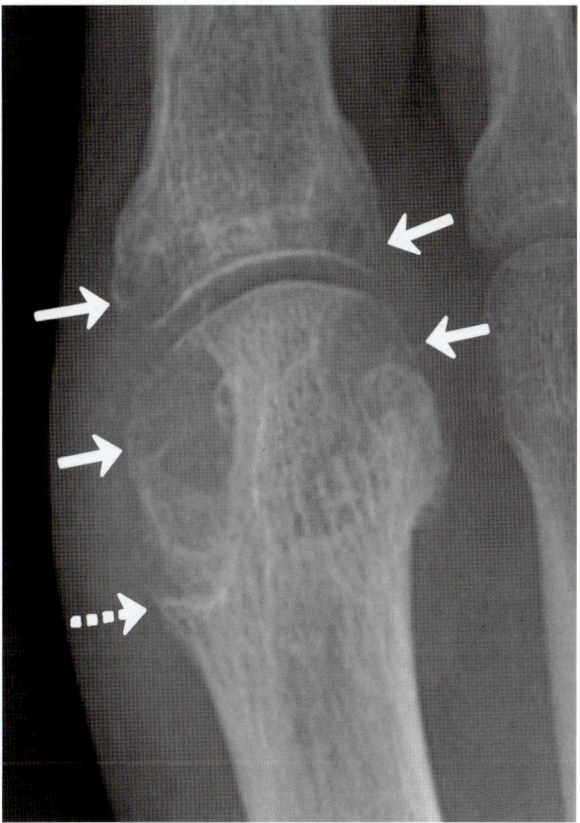

■ FIGURE 58-7 Classic radiographic findings of gout in a 69-year-old man. Note the asymmetric, well-marginated erosions in the head of the first metatarsal and lesser erosions in the opposing phalanx (*solid arrows*). The medial erosions are characteristically larger than the lateral erosions. There is a "hook" sign on the inferior margin of the large medial erosion of the head of the metatarsal (*dashed arrow*). The joint space is preserved, and there is no osteopenia.

The principal features of the disease are periarticular marginal erosions, asymmetric periarticular soft tissue masses representing tophi with or without calcification, preservation of the joint space, and an absence of osteoporosis (Fig. 58-7).

Characteristically, the bones maintain a normal density without evidence of osteoporosis. Disuse osteoporosis does not develop, because the joints are relatively free of symptoms between acute exacerbations.

The joint space is often well maintained despite the presence of sizable erosions (Fig. 58-8). Eventually, deposition of urate crystals within the articular cartilage results in degeneration of the articular cartilage, which narrows the joint space (Fig. 58-9). However, narrowing of the joint space does not occur early nor is it generally severe.

Periarticular Erosions and Tophi

Radiography

The margins of erosions caused by tophaceous deposits are typically rather sharply defined and sclerotic, variable in size, and asymmetric. The slow accumulation of urate crystals in tophi allows time for reactive bone to form on the surface of the tophaceous deposits. Tophaceous deposits at the margin of the joint give rise to periosteal reaction, which forms an overhanging edge—the "hook" sign, a characteristic hook- or spur-like projection of cortical bone at the peripheral margin of the erosion

(Fig. 58-10).[11] When viewed en face, erosions may have a distinctive, round or oval, broadened, sclerotic bony margin that might be called a "ring" sign (Fig. 58-11).

Tophi produce soft tissue masses that are characteristically asymmetric and often contain milky, cloud-like, or irregular, chalky calcification. Intraosseous tophi may extend well beyond the articular surface and, when calcified, superficially mimic either a bone infarct or enchondroma (Fig. 58-12).

If the tophaceous deposit is entirely within bone, it may have the appearance of a cyst. Tophi may become so large that they destroy the entire end of a phalanx or metatarsal or metacarpal, often sparing a thin segment of the joint surface (Fig. 58-13). An entire phalanx, sesamoid, or carpal bone may be destroyed by an even larger tophaceous deposit (Fig. 58-14).

The first metatarsophalangeal joint is the most common joint affected by gout, in 75% to 90% of cases, and is usually the first (in approximately 60% of cases) and most severely involved. Involvement of the first metatarsophalangeal joint is so characteristic of gout that whenever arthritis is encountered in this location, gout should be the primary diagnostic consideration until a thorough analysis of the findings proves otherwise. Hallux valgus may be present but is an intercurrent abnormality and not a manifestation of gout.[10]

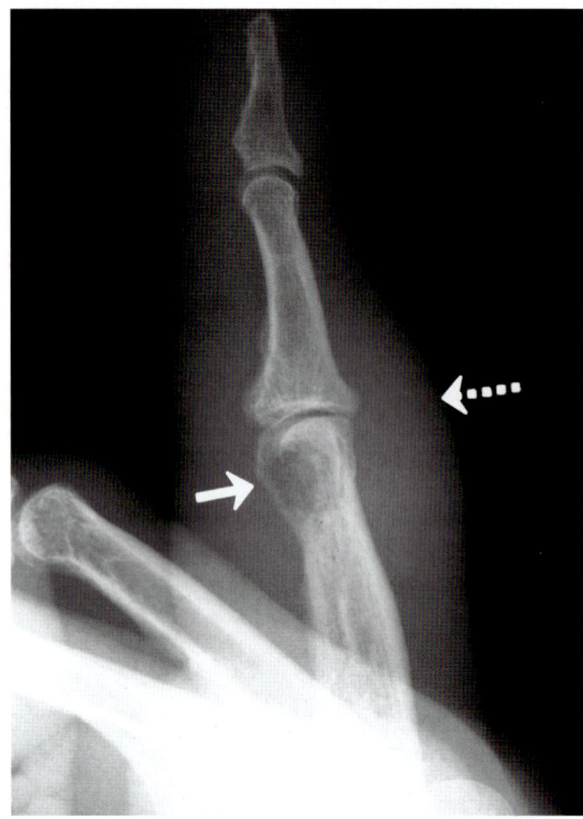

■ **FIGURE 58-8**   A large periarticular erosion is noted at the volar aspect of the proximal phalanx (*solid arrow*). The adjacent joint space is preserved, there is no osteopenia, and a tophus is evident on the extensor surface (*dashed arrow*).

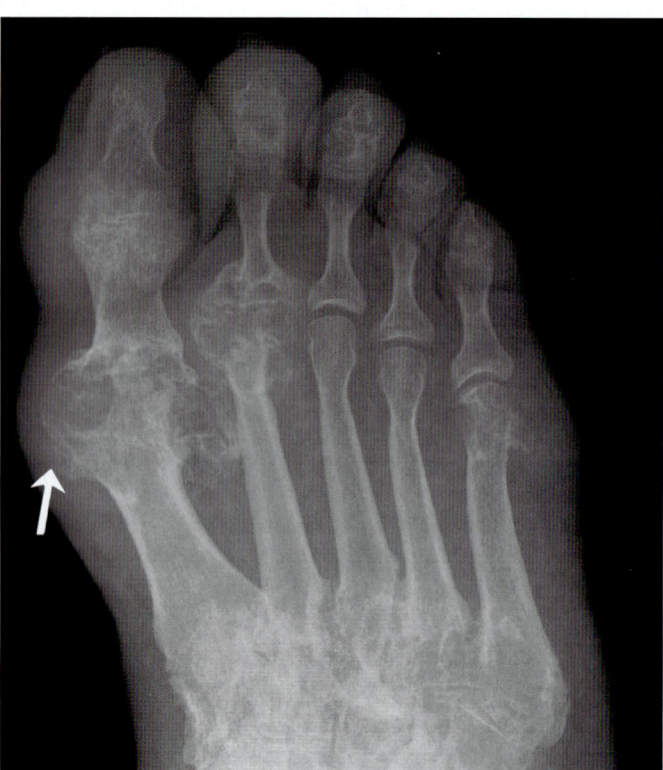

■ **FIGURE 58-10**   Oblique radiograph of the foot in a patient with advanced gouty arthropathy. A large, "hooked" erosion is present at the medial aspect of the first metatarsophalangeal joint (*arrow*). Erosive changes with joint space narrowing, a late finding, are noted at the first interphalangeal joint, second and fifth metatarsophalangeal joints, and Lisfranc's joint.

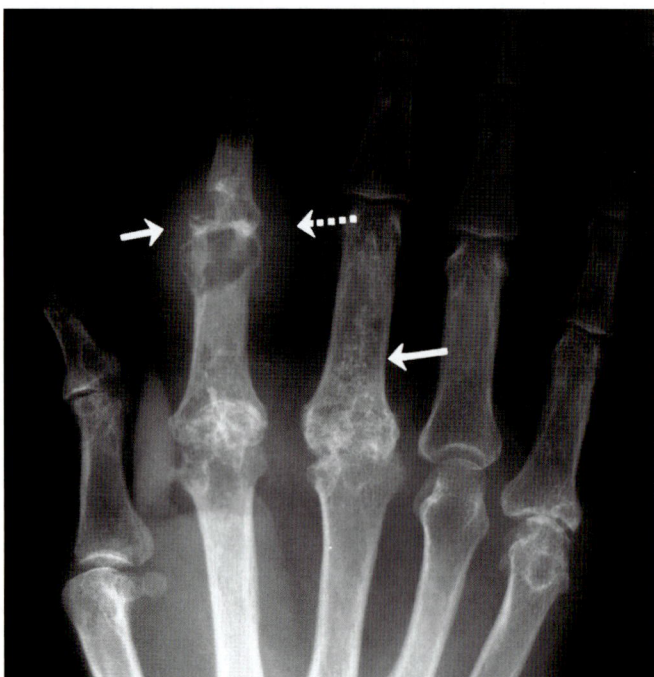

■ **FIGURE 58-9**   More advanced gout in the hand demonstrates soft tissue tophi (*dashed arrow*), particularly in the second digit, sharply marginated erosions, and joint space narrowing (*short solid arrow*), which is the result of cartilage destruction from long-standing and repeated episodes of inflammation secondary to the intra-articular deposition of urate crystals. Joint space narrowing is also noted in the first interphalangeal and second, third, and fifth metacarpophalangeal joints. Sclerotic density within the second through fourth proximal phalanges and second middle phalanx represents intraosseous extension of tophi (*long solid arrow*).

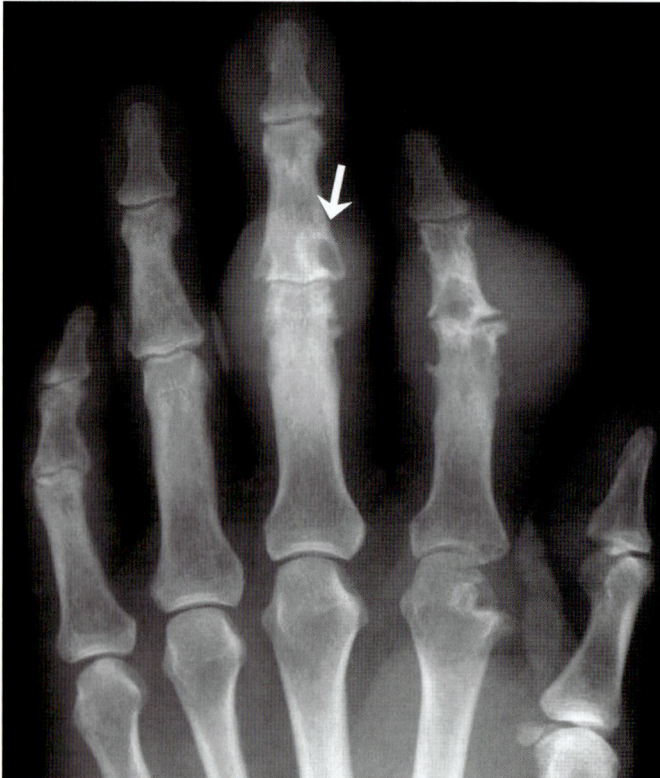

■ **FIGURE 58-11**   Far-advanced gout in the hand of a 55-year-old man. Note the asymmetry of the joint involvement. The asymmetric nature of the soft tissue masses (tophi) is more easily appreciated in the hand than in the foot. Note also the normal bone density. A "ring" sign is seen in the base of the middle phalanx of the middle finger (*arrow*). This is an erosion seen en face.

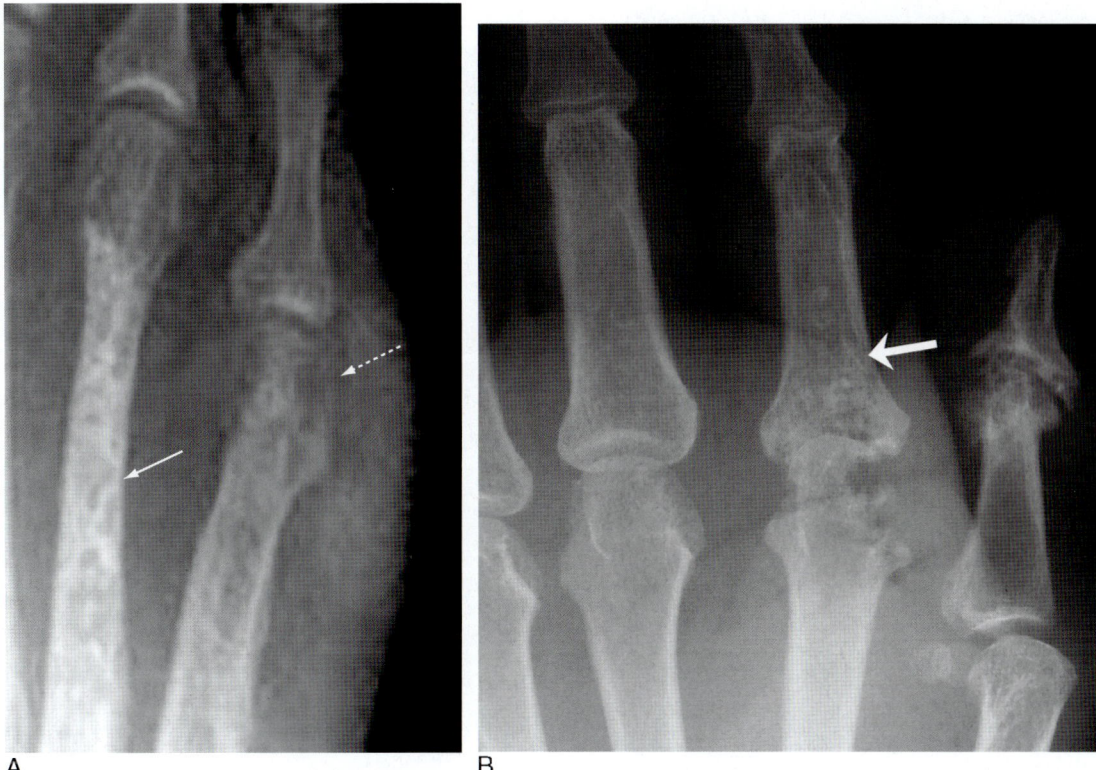

■ **FIGURE 58-12** **A,** Intraosseous tophus in the fourth metatarsal in a 58-year-old woman. Note the peculiar pattern of calcification within the medullary canal (*solid arrow*). A tophus with cloud-like calcification overlies the lateral margin of the fifth metatarsophalangeal joint (*dashed arrow*). **B,** A less dramatic example of intraosseous tophus in the second proximal phalanx of a patient with gout (*solid arrow*). There is increased bone density, mimicking an enchondroma. However, it is important to recognize this manifestation of gout. A well-marginated erosion with overhanging edges ("hook sign") is also noted at the radial aspect of the second metatarsophalangeal joint.

Erosions are more frequent on the medial and posterior aspects of the head of the first metatarsal than elsewhere. Smaller erosions are usually noted on the opposing margins of the proximal phalanx (see Fig. 58-7). Tophi commonly are found in the surrounding soft tissues medial to the joint and often contain characteristic hazy or cloud-like calcifications. They may also be found within the underlying sesamoids, particularly the medial sesamoid (Fig. 58-15).[12]

The fifth metatarsophalangeal joint is the next most commonly involved, as evidenced by typical erosions and surrounding tophi seen as asymmetric soft tissue masses lateral to the joint (Fig. 58-16). The second, third, and fourth metatarsophalangeal joints are less commonly involved.

The interphalangeal joints of the great toe are the most commonly affected interphalangeal joint, but multiple joints of other toes can be affected in an asymmetric fashion. The ends of phalanges can be largely replaced by tophaceous deposits, leaving only a short, thin segment of the joint surface. Rarely, an entire phalanx is destroyed by a tophus.

Involvement of the tarsometatarsal joints are particularly common and may be associated with erosions of the intermetatarsal joints at the base of the metatarsals (see Fig. 58-16). Tophi may extend into and thicken the soft tissues of the foot (Fig. 58-17).

Gouty involvement of the ankle is less common; however, typical marginal erosions are occasionally noted about the ankle joint. Tophi may, at times, be found in the Achilles or other tendons about the ankle.

Gout in the knee is usually manifest by tophi and marginal erosions of the femur and tibia (Fig. 58-18) at or about the joint line and at the superior border of the patella and may even involve bipartite patella.[13] When large erosions occur they may result in a pathologic fracture of the patella.

Tophi accumulate anterior to the patella and within and about the prepatellar bursa.[13] Tophi may also arise with the joint or a popliteal or Baker's cyst in the absence of other evidence of disease about the knee.[14] These popliteal cysts may spontaneously rupture. Intra-articular tophi may occur.[15]

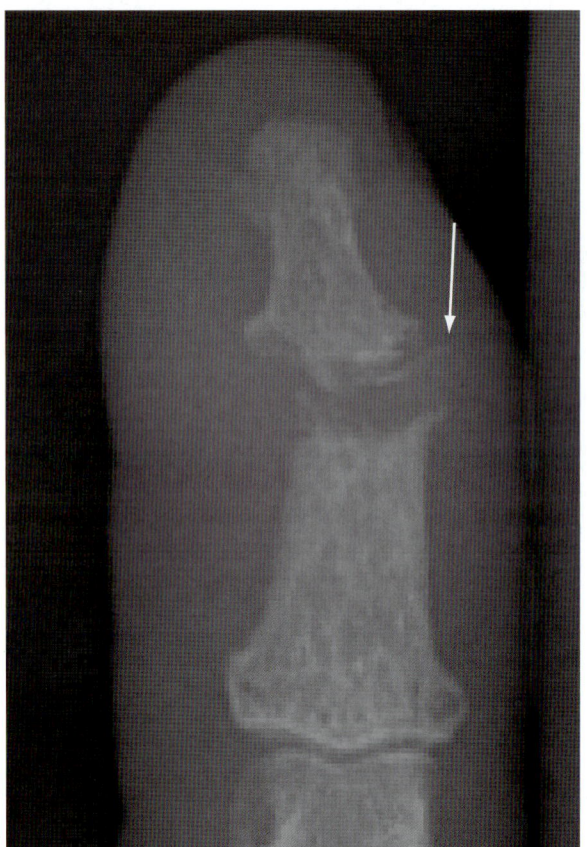

■ **FIGURE 58-13** Destruction of the head of the middle phalanx of the index finger in a 70-year-old man from a large erosion in a relatively small joint. Note the residual fragment of the joint surface and partial preservation of the joint space (*arrow*). The bone density is preserved without osteopenia.

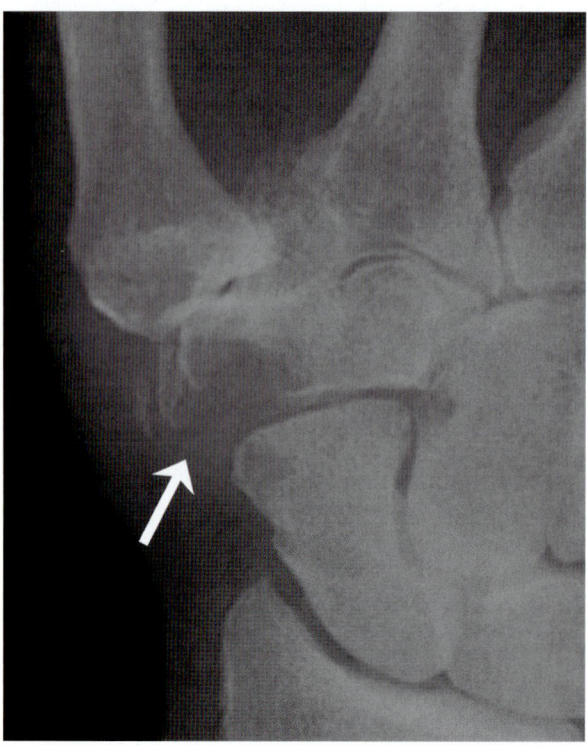

■ **FIGURE 58-14** Large erosion almost completely destroys the trapezium (*arrow*) in this 89-year-old man. The scaphotrapezial joint space is preserved.

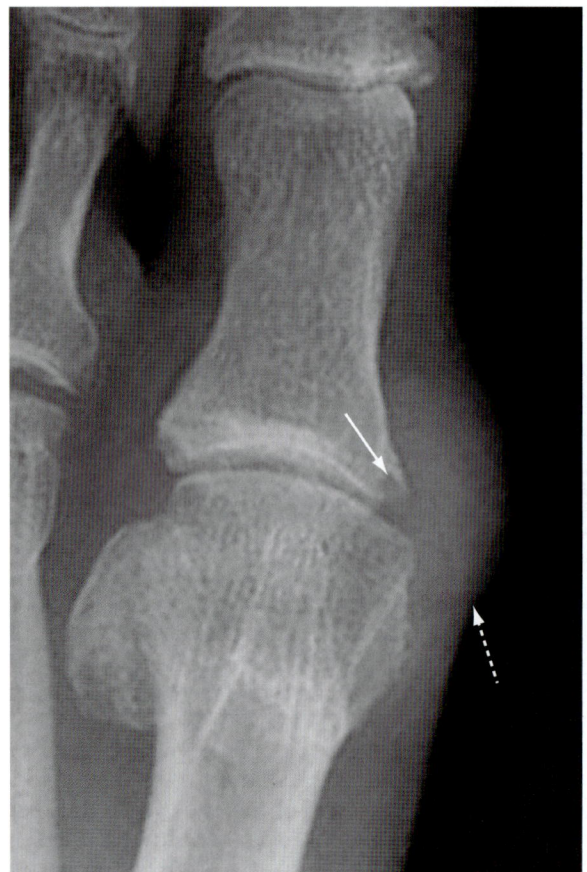

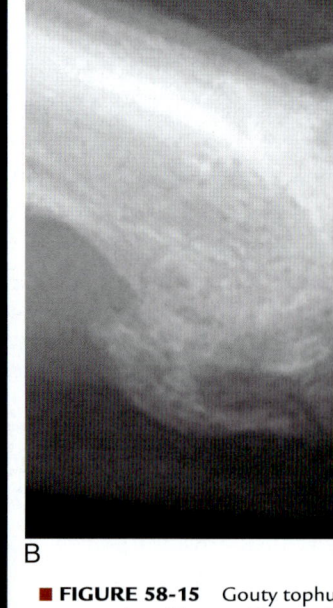

■ **FIGURE 58-15** Gouty tophus involving the tibial sesamoid of the great toe in a 48-year-old man. **A,** There is a tophus medial to the first metatarsophalangeal joint containing faint, cloud-like calcification (*dashed arrow*). Note the small erosion of the medial margin of the proximal phalanx at the joint line (*solid arrow*) and lack of erosion of the head of the first metatarsal. Closer inspection reveals an absence of the underlying medial sesamoid bone. **B,** Lateral view reveals that the medial sesamoid is significantly eroded and largely replaced by the tophaceous deposit (*arrow*).

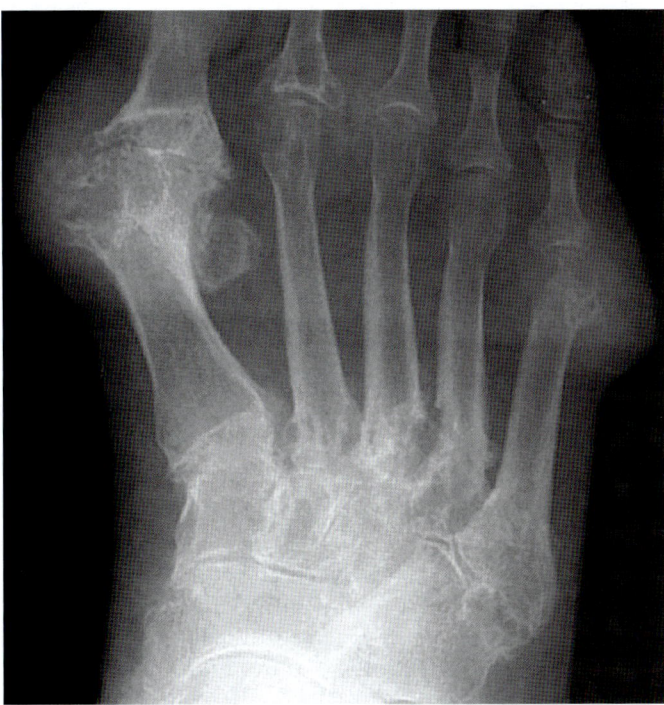

■ **FIGURE 58-16** A typical case of long-standing gout in an older man. The first metatarsophalangeal joint is destroyed by a large tophus arising medially in the head of the first metatarsal. Destruction of the articular surface is a late finding. Note the more classic appearing findings in the adjacent second metatarsophalangeal joint where the joint space is preserved. A tophus also overlies the lateral margin of the fifth metatarsophalangeal joint with erosions of the head of the metatarsal. Note the pattern of cloud-like calcifications in the tophi. Note also typical findings of gout in the metatarsal tarsal joints.

Chondrocalcinosis may also be noted in less than 10% of patients with gout. Whether this is a true manifestation of gout or related to simultaneous calcium pyrophosphate dihydrate (CPPD) disease is unclear. The incidence of chondrocalcinosis in gout approaches the incidence of chondrocalcinosis encountered in the general age-related population, thus clouding the relationship between chondrocalcinosis and gout. Simultaneous CPPD disease and gout seems a more likely explanation for the occurrence of chondrocalcinosis in those with gout.

Gouty tophi have been reported in the quadriceps tendon, as have ruptures of the quadriceps tendon.[8]

Imaging abnormalities in the hip are rarely noted in gout.

Asymmetric soft tissue masses, periarticular erosions of the proximal interphalangeal joints, distal interphalangeal joints, and metacarpophalangeal joints with preservation of joint space and normal bone density are the hallmarks of gout in the hands.[10] The asymmetric nature of soft tissue masses and joint involvement are often more easily recognized in radiographs of the hands than in the feet (see Fig. 58-11).

Erosions may involve any bone of the carpus and be seen as marginal erosions or well-defined, cyst-like lesions within the carpal bones (Fig. 58-19). Tophaceous deposits may become so large that they destroy the greater portion if not all of the carpal bones (see Fig. 58-14). Tophi may

accumulate in any part of the joint, including the carpal tunnel.[16] Intraosseous tophi may have large extraosseous components that present as soft tissue masses on the dorsal or volar surface of the wrist.

Erosions may involve the distal ulna and its styloid process as well as the joint margins of the radius. Erosions or subchondral cysts may be noted at the margins of the joint but are less common than olecranon bursitis. Olecranon bursitis is common in gout and presents as a soft tissue mass with or without calcification overlying the dorsal surface of the olecranon with or without erosion of the posterior cortex of the ulna (see Fig. 58-6).[10] In fact, a patient who presents with bilateral olecranon bursitis is said to have gout until proven otherwise.

Gout tends to spare the shoulder joints. Tophaceous deposits may occur within the rotator cuff.[17] Soft tissue masses with bony erosion are occasionally encountered in either the glenohumeral or acromioclavicular joints. Tophaceous deposits in the outer margin of the clavicle give rise to a peculiar, although characteristic, splaying or expansion of the outer end of the clavicle that should suggest the diagnosis of gout (Fig. 58-20).

Spinal involvement is less common than appendicular skeletal involvement; and there is currently debate as to whether gout is evenly distributed within the cervical, thoracic, and lumbar portions of the spine or has a predilection for the lower thoracic and lumbar spine. Tophaceous deposits may accumulate in the epidural space, intervertebral discs, and facet joints, resulting in subchondral cysts and erosion.[6] Such changes in the intervertebral disc may mimic infectious spondylitis. Tophaceous deposits may also lead to spinal cord or nerve root compression.[18] Patients with an established history of gout who present with signs or symptoms of spinal cord or nerve root compression should be evaluated for tophaceous spinal involvement. At the same time, it is extremely unlikely that a patient would present with spinal involvement as the initial or only manifestation of gout. CT and MRI[19] are required to identify such changes with any degree of certainty (Figs. 58-21 and 58-22).

Larger cystic and subchondral erosions may occur on either or both sides of the sacroiliac joints in gout (Fig. 58-23). Smaller such erosions are problematic because they are more likely due to osteoarthritis in the older patients in which gout is encountered.

Magnetic Resonance Imaging

Magnetic resonance imaging is not routinely used in the evaluation of gout. Disease in the axial skeleton with neurologic findings is a clear indication for MRI. Gouty tophi are uniformly of intermediate to low signal intensity on T1-weighted images (Fig. 58-24A and B) and somewhat variable in appearance on T2 weighted sequences, usually demonstrating heterogeneously low to intermediate and sometimes even high signal intensity (see Fig. 58-24C). Cases in which tophi demonstrate high T2 signal are thought to represent a relatively high water content. Small foci of persistently low signal that do not enhance have been noted as well, corresponding to calcification, fibrosis, or hemosiderin within the tophi. Contrast enhancement of tophi is either uniform or heterogeneous and peripheral (see Fig. 58-24D). Multiple patterns of

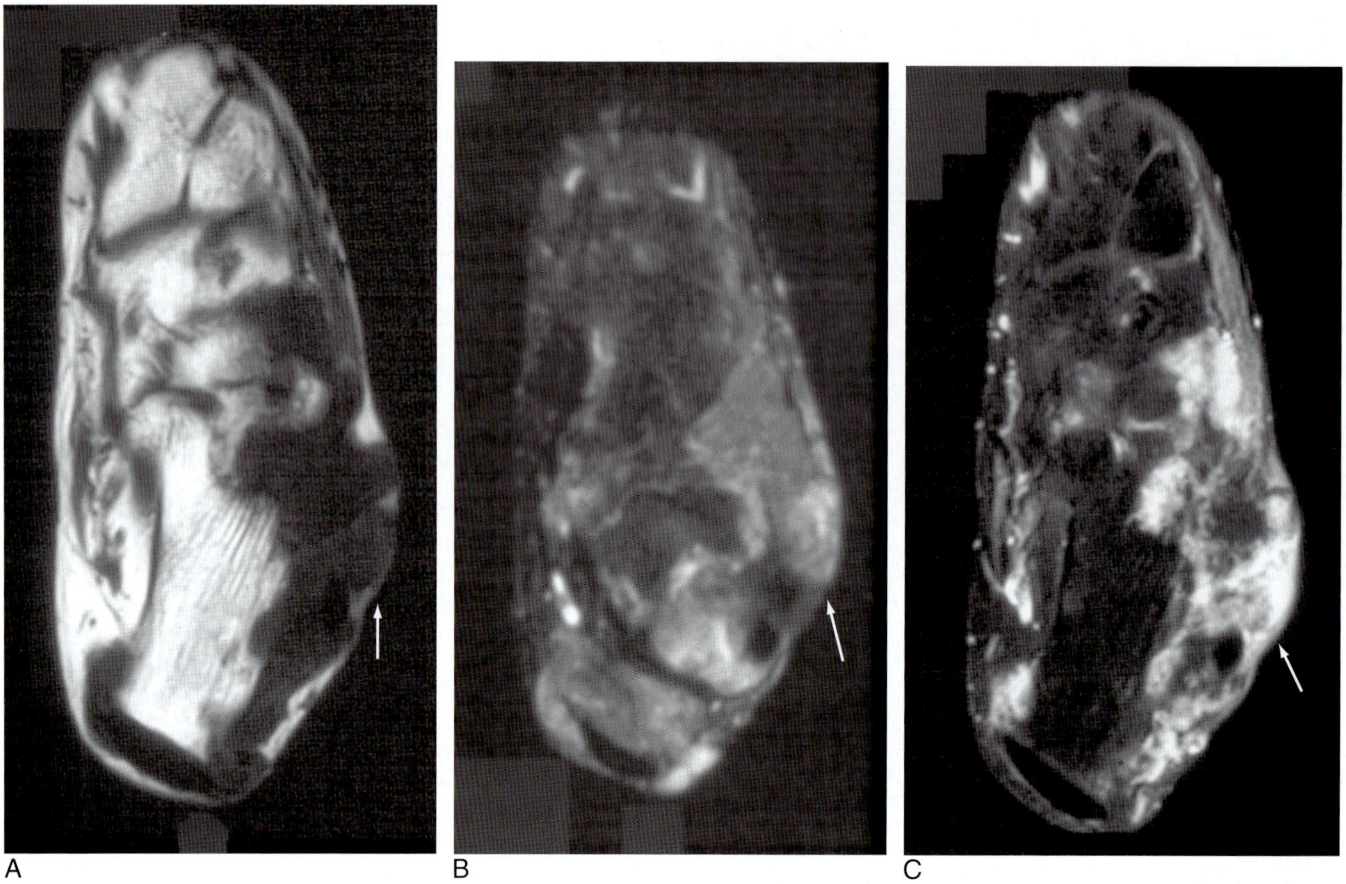

A   B   C

■ **FIGURE 58-17** MRI of gout in the foot of a 64-year-old man. A large, firm subcutaneous mass is palpable along the lateral aspect of the calcaneus and cuboid bones. **A,** T1-weighted MR image. Note the uniformly low density, lobulated mass representing a large gouty tophus that erodes the lateral margin of the calcaneus and replaces the majority of the cuboid bone (*arrow*). **B,** T2-weighted MR image. The tophus is low to intermediate in signal (*arrow*). **C,** T1-weighted MR image with gadolinium enhancement. Note the rather uniform high signal within the tophus (*arrow*) as is characteristic of gout. *(Case courtesy of Jamshid Tehranzadeh, MD, Irvine, CA.)*

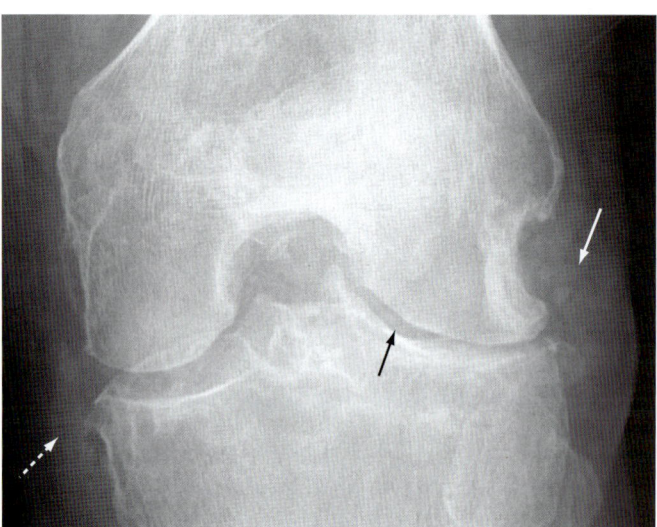

■ **FIGURE 58-18** Gout of the knee in a 58-year-old man. There is a faintly calcified tophus extending along the lateral margin (*solid arrow*) of the lateral femoral condyle, across the joint. Less obvious tophus is noted medially (*dashed arrow*). Chondrocalcinosis is present in the lateral meniscus (*black arrow*). Chondrocalcinosis is frequently seen in conjunction with gout, although the exact relationship between the two is not known. The medial and lateral compartments are narrowed, with marginal spur formation, due to osteoarthritis.

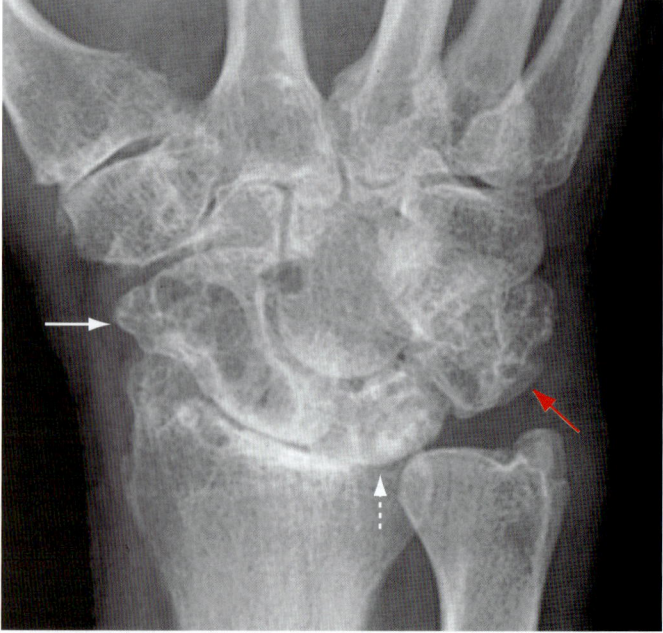

■ **FIGURE 58-19** Gout in the carpal bones of a 60-year-old man. Cyst-like lesions of varying size are noted within multiple carpal bones, particularly the scaphoid (*solid arrow*), lunate (*dashed arrow*), and triquetrum (*red arrow*). These represent intraosseous tophi. The bone mineral density and joint spaces are maintained.

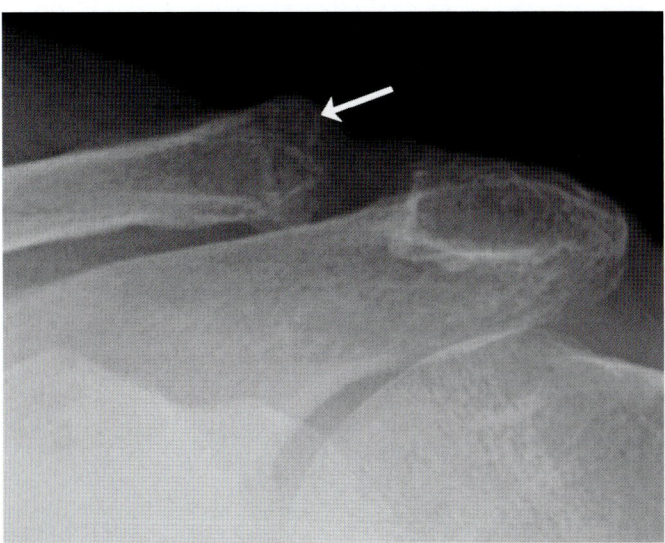

■ FIGURE 58-20 Gout in the lateral clavicle and acromioclavicular joint in a 62-year-old man. Note the marked widening of the acromioclavicular joint and expansion of the outer end of the clavicle bordered by faint line of sclerosis (*arrow*).

enhancement may be seen within the same patient, and even the same tophus, and are believed to be due to vascularized reactive tissue within the tophus and granulation tissue surrounding the tophus. Occasionally, tophi may be nonenhancing, in which case they demonstrate low signal on both T1- and T2-weighted sequences.[20]

Multidetector Computed Tomography

Computed tomography has a limited role in the diagnosis and evaluation of gout. However, it is useful for imaging in the rare gouty involvement of the spine (see Fig. 58-21) because the findings on radiographs are either subtle or nonexistent in such cases. CT is, of course, more sensitive than radiography to the presence of calcification in tophaceous deposits and, as a result, may aid in characterizing an intra-articular soft tissue mass.[21] One study has reported a mean CT density of 160 Hounsfield units within tophi.[22]

Ultrasonography

Ultrasonography is also not typically used in evaluating gout. However, with the increasing use of musculoskeletal ultrasonography, especially in evaluating hand pain, it is

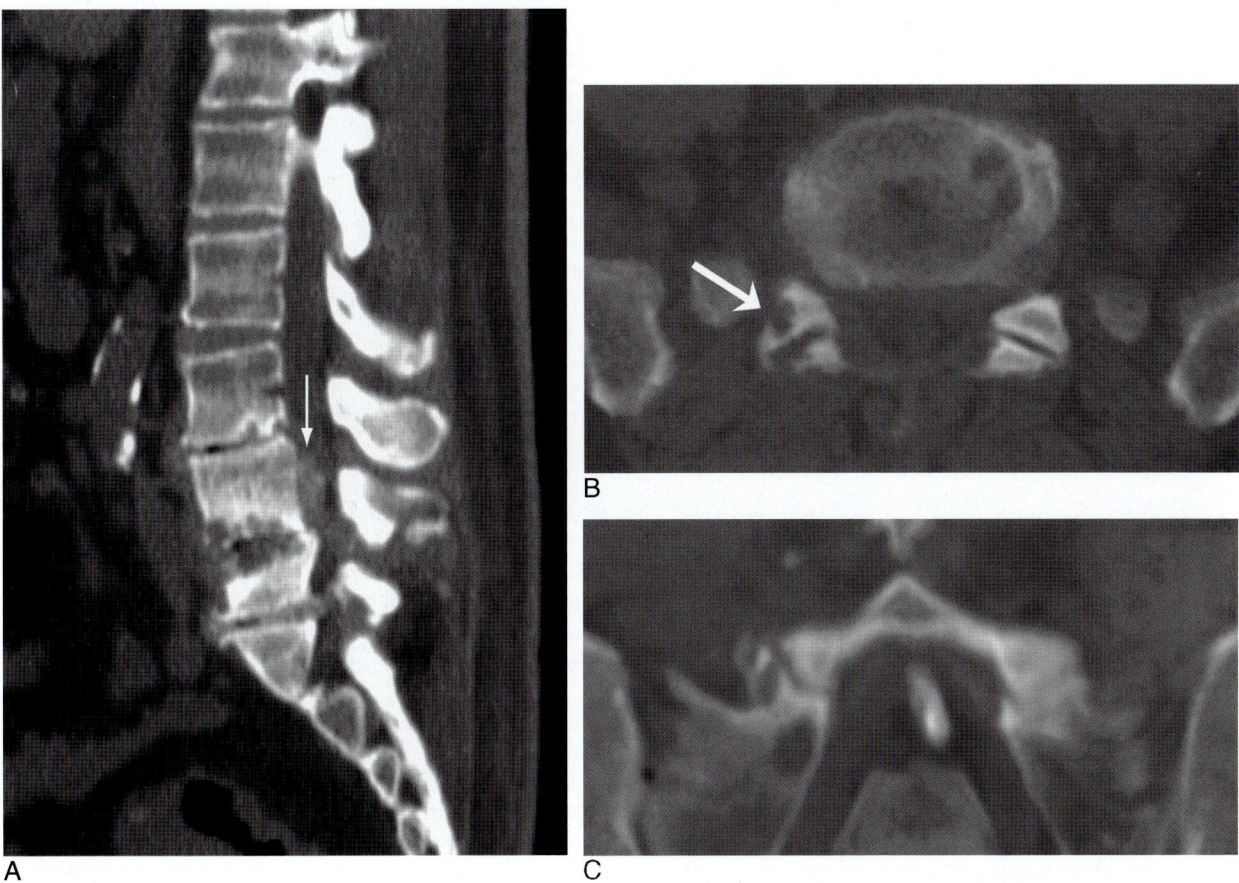

■ FIGURE 58-21 Two cases of gout in the lumbar spine, demonstrated on CT. **A,** Sagittal reformatted CT images show end-plate erosion from L3–4 through L5-S1. Note the epidural dense soft tissue posterior to L4 (*arrow*), compatible with tophus. This patient had a known history of gout and back pain. **B,** The axial CT scan in a different patient shows a well-defined lucent lesion in the right superior facet (*arrow*). **C,** Coronal reconstruction of the CT in **B** shows ovoid lucent lesions in the right side of the body of the first sacral segment and right S1 superior facet. Both lesions were attributed to gout without pathologic proof. The patient responded to conservative treatment with colchicine and uricosuric agents. *(Case courtesy of Joachim Seeger, MD, Tucson.)*

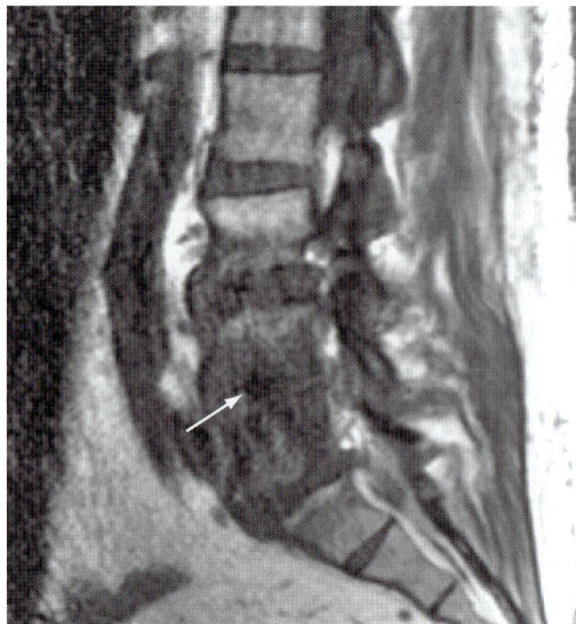

A

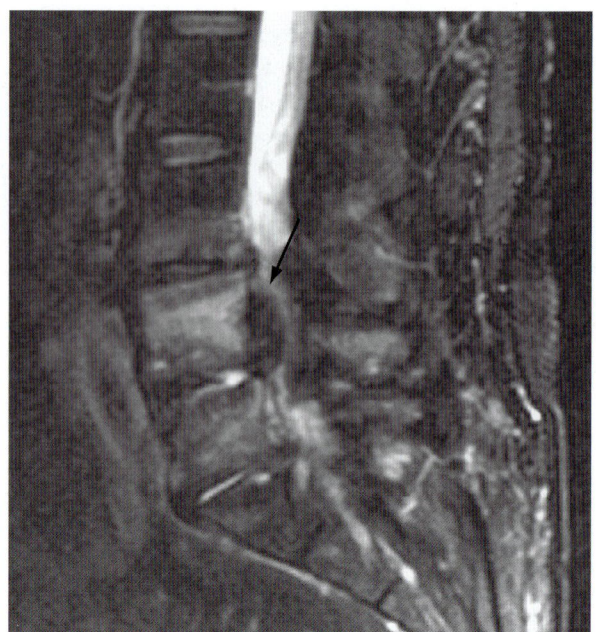

B

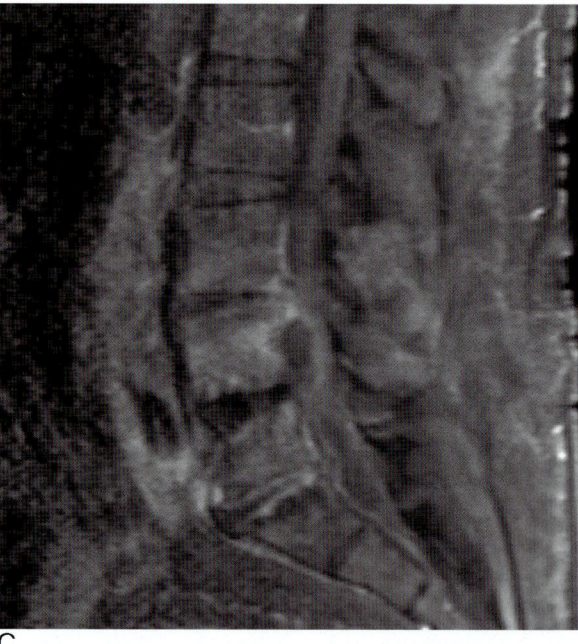

C

■ **FIGURE 58-22** MRI of the lumbar spine of the same patient in Figure 58-21A. **A,** Sagittal T1-weighted MR image shows low signal intensity in the L4–5 disc space and adjacent vertebral bodies (*arrow*). **B,** Corresponding T2-weighted MR image shows edema with the L4 and L5 vertebral bodies. Epidural soft tissue noted on the CT at the L4 level is of low density, compatible with tophus (*arrow*). **C,** Corresponding gadolinium-enhanced, fat-saturated, T1-weighted MR image shows mild vertebral body enhancement, no significant disc enhancement, and peripheral epidural tophus enhancement at L4 (*arrow*).

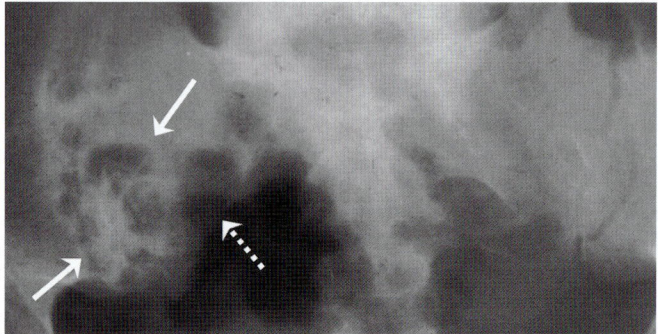

■ **FIGURE 58-23** Gouty arthritis of the right sacroiliac joint in a 65-year-old man. The right sacroiliac joint is widened with well-marginated erosions (*solid arrows*). Larger cystic areas with sclerotic margins are present in the adjacent right sacral ala (*dashed arrow*). The left sacroiliac joint is normal.

important to know the sonographic appearance of gouty arthritis. Erosions are well defined and may demonstrate significant shadowing from overhanging edges. Tophi are homogeneous and hypoechoic, sometimes demonstrating punctate calcifications, which are hyperechoic and result in posterior acoustic shadowing (Fig. 58-25).[23] Some authors have also observed hyperechoic, hypervascular rims surrounding tophi on color or power Doppler imaging. Vascularity is sometimes also seen within the tophus, although not to the same extent as the periphery.[22]

Nuclear Medicine

Very little attention has been given to the appearance of gouty arthritis on radionuclide imaging. Affected areas show increased activity on technetium-99m–labeled

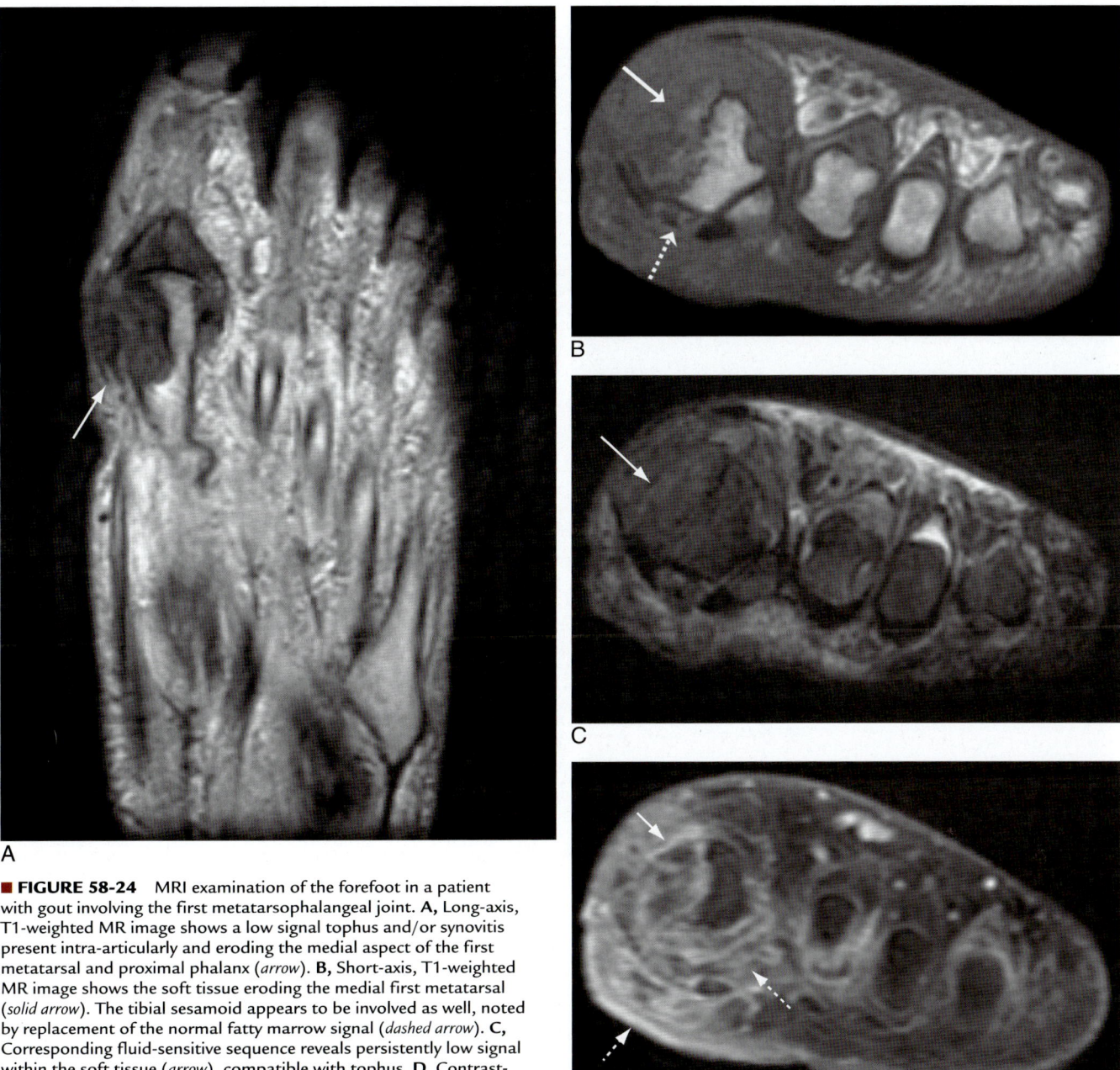

A

B

C

D

■ **FIGURE 58-24** MRI examination of the forefoot in a patient with gout involving the first metatarsophalangeal joint. **A,** Long-axis, T1-weighted MR image shows a low signal tophus and/or synovitis present intra-articularly and eroding the medial aspect of the first metatarsal and proximal phalanx (*arrow*). **B,** Short-axis, T1-weighted MR image shows the soft tissue eroding the medial first metatarsal (*solid arrow*). The tibial sesamoid appears to be involved as well, noted by replacement of the normal fatty marrow signal (*dashed arrow*). **C,** Corresponding fluid-sensitive sequence reveals persistently low signal within the soft tissue (*arrow*), compatible with tophus. **D,** Contrast-enhanced MR image demonstrates peripheral enhancement of the tophus (*solid arrow*) and surrounding, ill-defined subcutaneous and peritendinous soft tissue enhancement (*dashed arrows*), indicating an accompanying inflammatory response.

methylene diphosphonate bone scintiscans, secondary to the localized periosteal and inflammatory reaction. This is nonspecific and may also be seen with infection, fracture, or neoplasm. Gout is sometimes included in the differential diagnosis when activity is noted in the region of the first metatarsophalangeal joint.[24]

Positron Emission Tomography/Computed Tomography

Combined PET/CT is not usually performed for evaluation of gouty arthritis. However, one would expect to note hypermetabolic activity due to the intense inflammatory reaction associated with urate deposition. Like other radionuclide imaging, this is nonspecific.[24]

Arthroscopy

Arthroscopists have noted a "pearly" or "chalky" white appearance to gouty tophi with surrounding hyperemia, or enlarged vessels, at arthroscopy, that corresponds to findings noted on gross pathologic and histologic evaluation (Fig. 58-26). Arthroscopy is not routinely performed

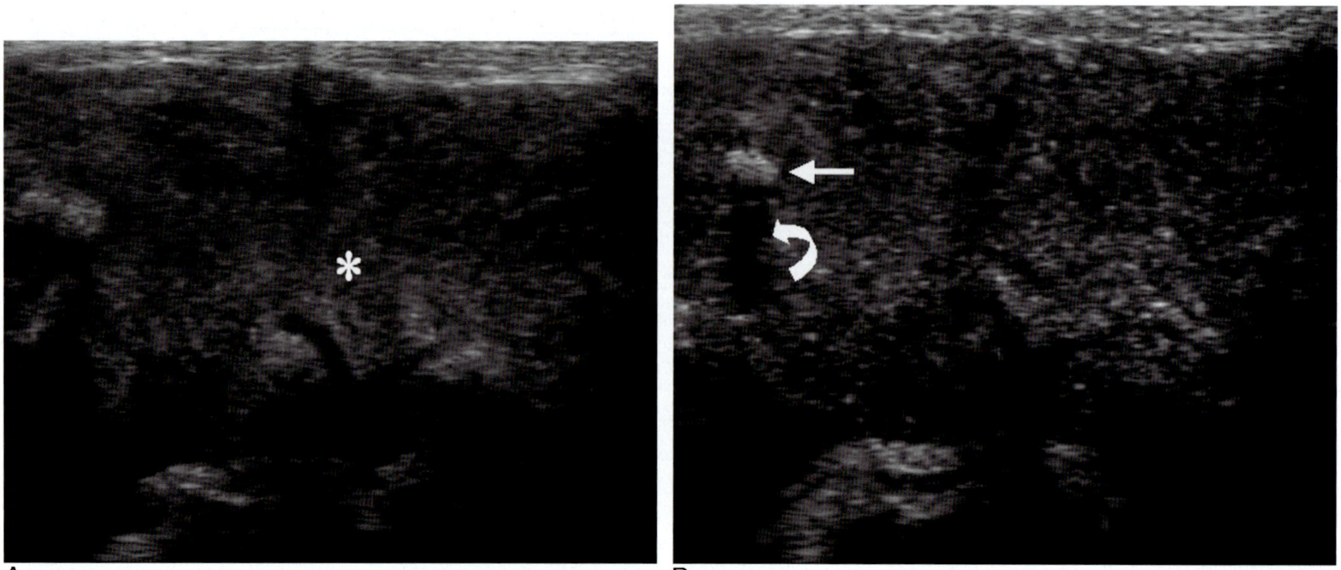

■ **FIGURE 58-25** Ultrasound images of the first metatarsophalangeal joint in a patient with gout. **A,** Homogeneous appearance of the tophus (*asterisk*). **B,** Punctate, hyperechoic calcification (*straight arrow*) with posterior shadowing (*curved arrow*). If small enough, some calcifications will not shadow. *(From Grassi W, Meenagh G, Pascual E, Filippucci E. "Crystal clear"—sonographic assessment of gout and calcium pyrophosphate deposition disease. Semin Arthritis Rheum 2006; 36:197–202.)*

in the diagnosis or treatment of gout, and the few reported cases of its arthroscopic appearance are due to a mistaken diagnosis or otherwise confounding clinical situation (Fig. 58-27).[25,26]

Classic Signs

- Sharply marginated periarticular erosions, most commonly of the first metatarsophalangeal joint, but also occurring elsewhere in the appendicular skeleton, such as the Lisfranc joints, elbow, and ankle.
- Overhanging edges (i.e., the "hook sign") at the margin of the erosions, representing a benign-appearing, chronic periosteal reaction. Erosions viewed en face appear cyst-like (i.e., the "ring sign").
- Soft tissue tophi, which may be periarticular, intra-osseous, peritendinous, or periligamentous. Tophi give rise to the characteristic erosions over the course of years.
- Tophi may contain calcium and are, therefore, sometimes dense on radiographs and CT. The MRI appearance of tophi is less uniform: low to intermediate on T1-weighted images and heterogeneously low, intermediate, or high on T2-weighted images. Surrounding inflammatory changes are common.
- Tophi may show homogeneous, heterogeneous peripheral or, rarely, no enhancement. Nonenhancing tophi tend to be of low signal intensity on both T1- and T2-weighted sequences.
- The ultrasound appearance of tophi is homogeneously hypoechoic, sometimes with a hyperechoic rim. If calcifications are present, punctate hyperechoic foci with acoustic shadowing are present. Doppler interrogation reveals peripheral and, to a lesser extent, internal flow.

DIFFERENTIAL DIAGNOSIS

Clinically, the differential diagnosis of an acute, monarticular arthropathy should always include infectious arthritis. Another important consideration is the clinical syndrome of pseudogout, due to CPPD deposition, which is primarily excluded on the basis of laboratory testing. Other differential considerations could be bursitis, cellulitis, tenosynovitis, hemarthrosis, rheumatoid arthritis (the uncommon nodular and even rarer palindromic variant), sarcoid arthropathy, and xanthomatosis.

When gouty arthropathy is far advanced, it may be confused radiographically with rheumatoid arthritis because of marginal erosions and soft tissue swelling. In general, rheumatoid arthritis is symmetric and accompanied by osteoporosis, whereas gout is typically asymmetric and the bone mineral density is normal.

The difference in distribution of the marginal erosions and the appearance of the soft tissue swelling provide the key to the differential diagnosis. Characteristically, in rheumatoid arthritis there is periarticular osteoporosis and symmetric involvement of the proximal interphalangeal joints, metacarpophalangeal joints, and radiocarpal joints, and the soft tissue swelling about the joints is symmetrical. In contrast, gouty arthritis initially involves the feet, specifically the metatarsophalangeal or interphalangeal joints of the great toe; joint involvement is asymmetric, tophaceous deposits appear as asymmetric soft tissue masses; and there is no evidence of osteoporosis.

Rheumatoid arthritis also affects a similar age group, but has a female, rather than male, predilection. Pannus in rheumatoid arthritis progresses from a hypervascular to fibrotic composition and, as a result, may have intermediate signal on T1-weighted images and heterogeneously low or high signal on T2-weighted images and enhancement similar to gout owing to the associated inflammatory

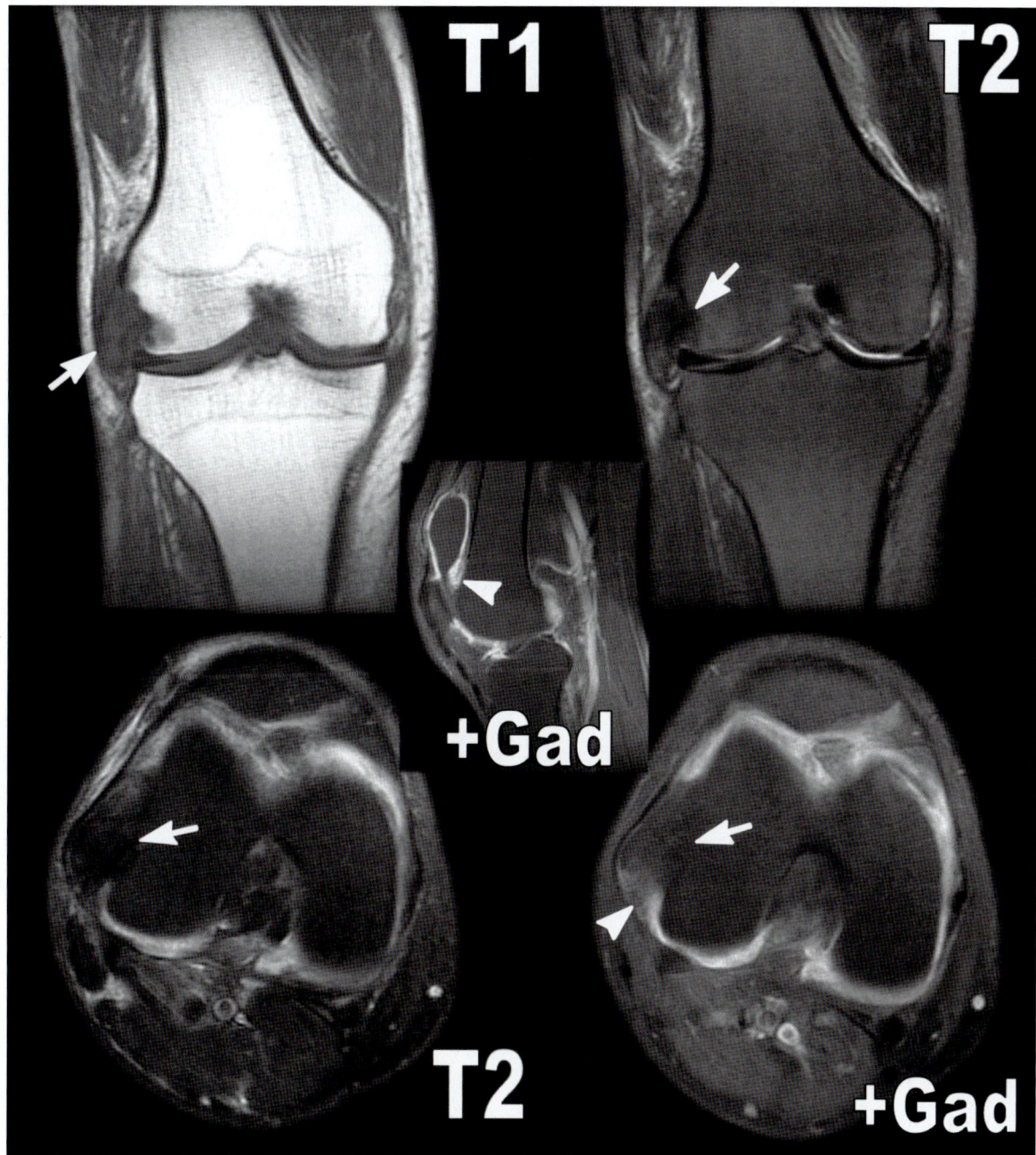

A

■ **FIGURE 58-26** MRI and arthroscopic correlation in a 53-year-old man with knee pain and limited range of motion. **A,** Contrast-enhanced MRI reveals an intra-articular soft tissue mass with intermediate T1- and low T2-weighted signal (*arrows*) with peripheral enhancement (*arrowhead*). This was interpreted as suggestive of a synovial tumor, and arthroscopy was performed.

(Continued)

response. In these cases, clinical history, laboratory values and radiographic correlation should be helpful.

The presence of gout does not spare one from other bone or articular diseases. Gout occurs in older individuals, and those with gout are subject to the same diseases of aging as those without gout. Therefore, gout may appear in those with osteoarthritis, chondrocalcinosis or pseudogout, rheumatoid arthritis, and even seronegative rheumatoid disease. Two, or more, of these diseases may be encountered in the same patient.

Chondrocalcinosis and pseudogout from CPPD deposition sometimes occurs concurrently with gout (Fig. 58-28). In these cases, synovial crystal analysis is quite useful. CPPD crystals are characteristically needle shaped or rhomboidal, as opposed to monosodium urate crystals, which are only needle shaped and do not show negative birefringence like monosodium urate crystals (Fig. 58-29).[7]

Gouty arthritis in the spine may have a similar radiographic appearance to discovertebral infection. However,

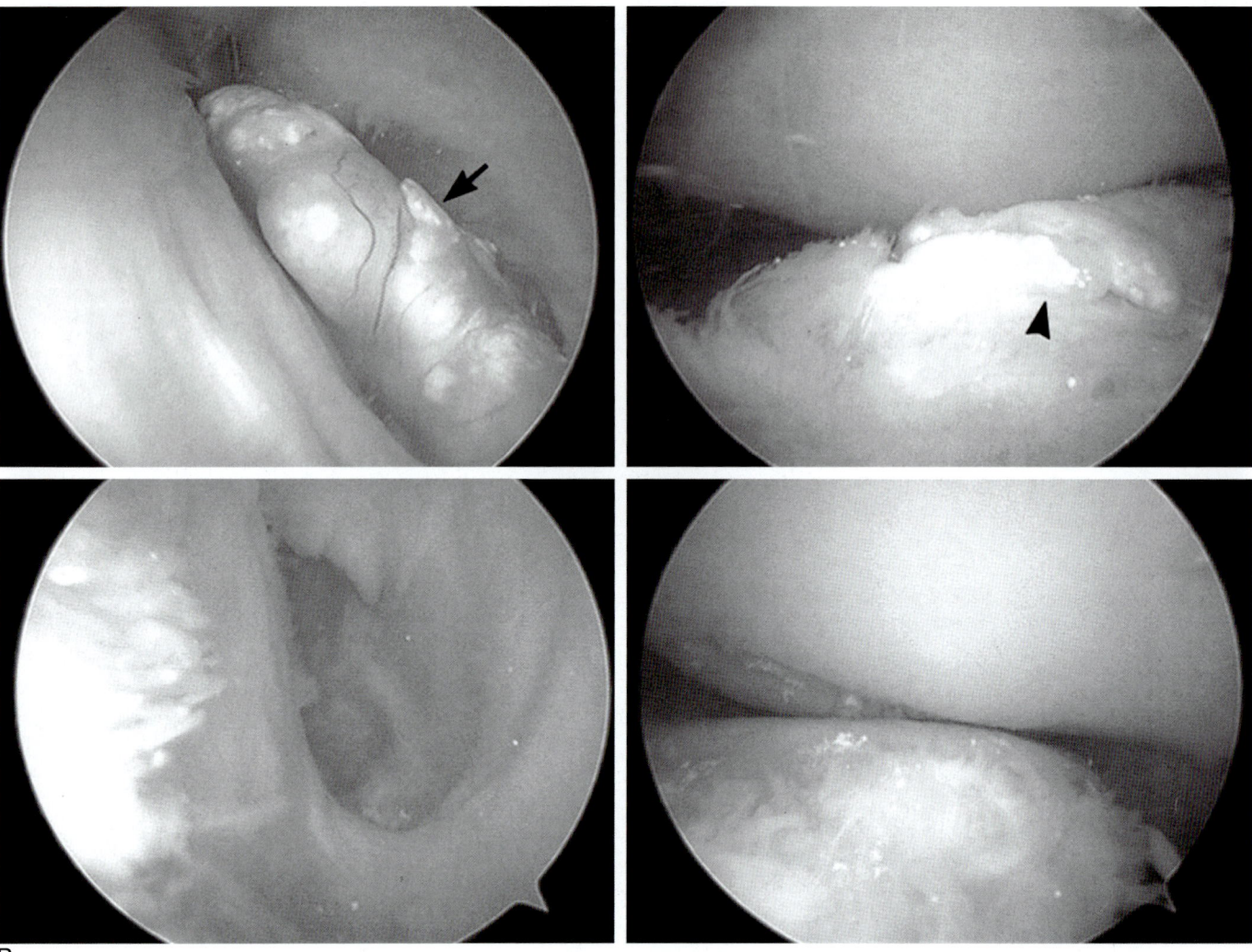

B

■ **FIGURE 58-26—Cont'd** **B,** Four intraoperative views from the subsequent arthroscopy reveal chalky white deposits (*arrow* and *arrowhead*) in the medial femoral condyle, compatible with tophi. These were excised and confirmed pathologically. Hyperemia and engorged vessels were also noted during arthroscopy. *(From Li TJ, Lue KH, Lin ZI, Lu KH. Arthroscopic treatment for gouty tophi mimicking an intra-articular synovial tumor of the knee. Arthroscopy 2006; 22:910e1–910e3.)*

the clinical symptoms, and CT and MRI appearances are usually distinct. The hallmark of discovertebral infection on T2-weighted MT images is high signal intensity within the disc and usually the vertebral body, features that are not typical for gout. On CT, gouty erosions are typically sharply marginated and involve the synovial joints, which is unusual for discovertebral infection. Finally, tophi on CT demonstrate increased density, which would be unusual for infection, which usually has a low-density fluid component.

Other entities that exhibit erosive changes and/or relatively low T1 and T2 signal on MRI include dialysis-related amyloid spondyloarthropathy, CPPD deposition, pigmented villonodular synovitis, giant cell tumor of the tendon sheath, and benign soft tissue neoplasms such as xanthomas and fibromas.[20]

Amyloid arthropathy in dialysis patients has a similar radiographic, CT, and MRI appearance to gout; but, in contradistinction to gout, it is most common in the spine.

There is also a long-standing history of dialysis in these patients. Pigmented villonodular synovitis is typically monarticular, occurs in the knees and hips (locations less common for gout), usually occurs in a younger age group (most commonly age 20 to 45 years), and has no sex predilection. Giant cell tumor of the tendon sheath, the extra-articular form of pigmented villonodular synovitis, is also usually isolated, occurs in a younger age group than gout, and may or may not be associated with pain. Benign soft tissue neoplasms do not demonstrate surrounding inflammatory changes or the typical arthropathy associated with gout. Clinical history, laboratory testing, and radiographs should again be utilized.

SYNOPSIS OF TREATMENT OPTIONS

Medical Treatment

Acute attacks are usually first treated with nonsteroidal anti-inflammatory drugs; however, aspirin is avoided because

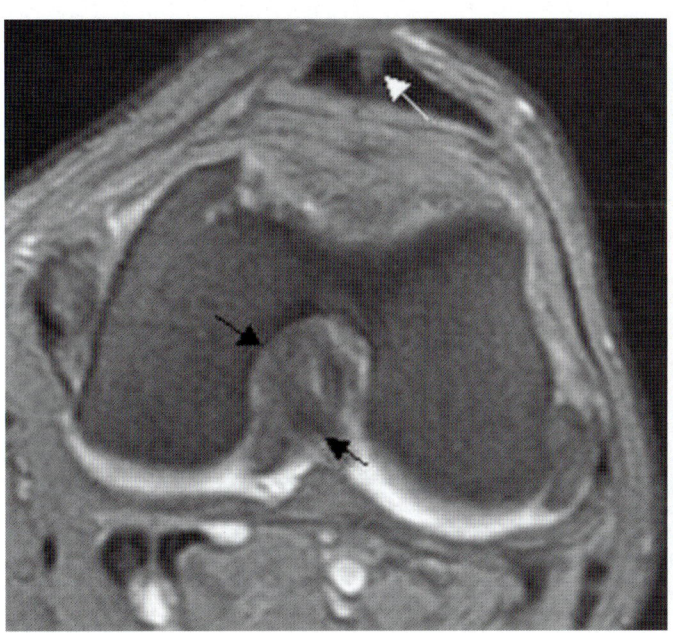
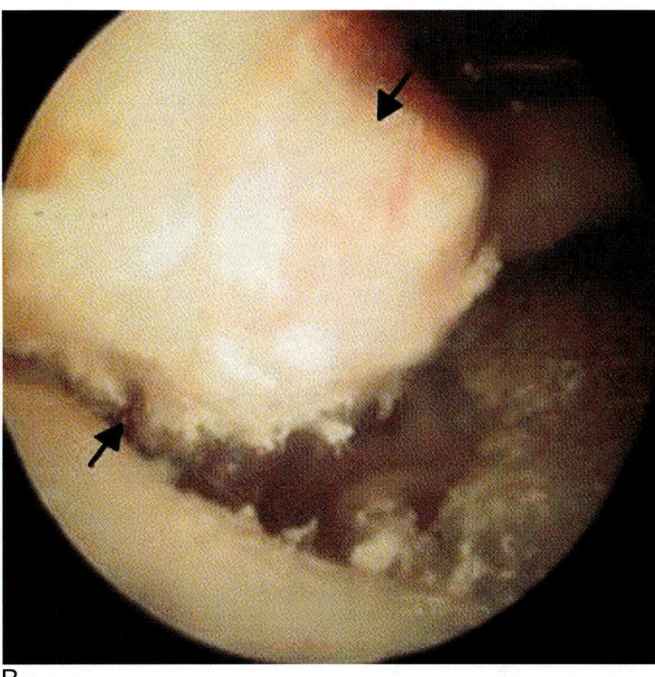

A   B

■ **FIGURE 58-27** MRI and arthroscopic correlation in a 49-year-old man with knee pain. **A,** Axial T2-weighted MRI shows a low signal mass-like lesion in the region of the anterior cruciate ligament (*black arrows*), believed to be a tumor. A small patellar erosion is also present (*white arrow*). **B,** Intraoperative pictures obtained during arthroscopy show grossly hypertrophic tissue at the base of the anterior cruciate ligament (*black arrows*). This was resected. Pathologic examination was consistent with gouty tophus. *(From Melloni P, Valls R, Yuguero M, Saez A. An unusual case of tophaceous gout involving the anterior cruciate ligament. Arthroscopy 2004; 20:e117–e121.)*

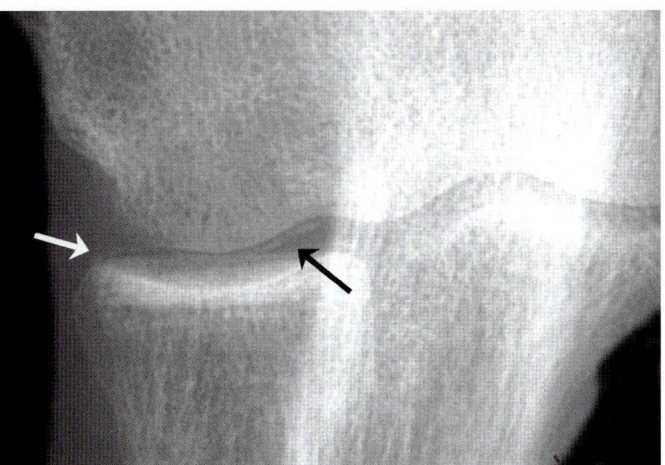

■ **FIGURE 58-28** Anteroposterior view of the elbow, coned down to the radiocapitellar joint, shows chondrocalcinosis (*white and black arrows*). This patient was also being treated for symptomatic olecranon bursitis due to gout. The association between calcium pyrophosphate dihydrate deposition and gout is unclear.

it results in uric acid retention in high doses. Alternatives include selective cyclooxygenase-2 inhibitors. Oral colchicine is also used; however, it has a low therapeutic index and side effects (nausea, diarrhea, and abdominal pain) usually develop before the resolution of an acute attack. Allopurinol and other uricosuric agents should only be started after the resolution of an acute attack because they may prolong or precipitate an acute episode. Diuretics, which raise serum urate levels, and salicylates should be avoided. Dietary modification is needed.[1]

Surgical Treatment

Surgical treatment is extremely uncommon and is reserved for severe complications related to gout arthropathy, such as skin breakdown with osteomyelitis and tissue necrosis in patients with peripheral vascular disease. Obviously, such complications were more common in the years before effective medical therapy and an understanding of the pathophysiology involved.[27]

What the Referring Physician Needs to Know

- Imaging, particularly with radiography, serves as a supportive tool in the diagnosis of gout. Radiographs may exclude other inflammatory arthropathies or causes of swelling and pain or alert the clinician to consider gout as a diagnosis.
- In cases in which gout is already diagnosed, imaging is crucial in determining the presence of complications such as spinal cord/nerve impingement, tendon tear, and articular erosions.

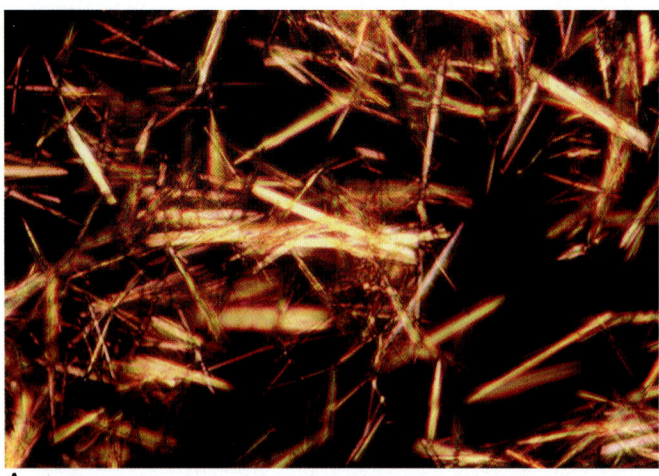

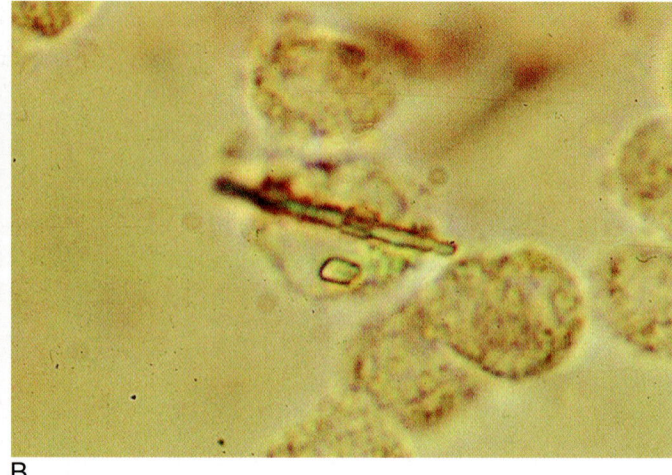

A   B

■ **FIGURE 58-29** Light microscopic analysis of crystals obtained from synovial fluid in two patients with painful synovitis. **A,** Polarized light microscopy at 1000× shows abundant needle-shaped, strongly negative birefringent crystals, compatible with monosodium urate. **B,** Polarized light microscopy at 1000× shows rhomboidal and needle-shaped crystals without negative birefringence, compatible with calcium pyrophosphate deposition. *(From Pascual E, Jovani V. Synovial fluid analysis. Best Pract Res Clin Rheumatol 2005; 19:371–386.)*

SUGGESTED READINGS

Forrester DM, Brown JC. The Radiology of Joint Disease, 3rd ed. Philadelphia, WB Saunders, 1987.

Gentili A. Advanced imaging of gout. Semin Musculoskelet Radiol 2003; 7:165–174.

Monu JU, Pope TL Jr. Gout: a clinical and radiologic review. Radiol Clin North Am 2004; 42:169–184.

Nuki G. Gout. Medicine 2006; 34:417–423.

Resnick D. Gouty arthritis. In Resnick D (ed). Diagnosis of Bone and Joint Disorders, 4th ed. Philadelphia: WB Saunders, 2002, pp 1519–1559.

Schlesinger N, Schumacher HR Jr. Update on gout. Arthritis Rheum 2002; 47:563–565.

Wise CM. Crystal-associated arthritis in the elderly. Clin Geriatr Med 2005; 21:491–511.

REFERENCES

1. Nuki G. Gout. Medicine 2006; 34:417–423.
2. Sydenham T. A Treatise on Gout and Dropsy. The Works of Thomas Sydenham, M.D. Volume II. RG Latham (trans). London, Sydenham Society, 1850, p 119.
3. Habermann W, Kiesler K, Eherer A, et al. Laryngeal manifestation of gout: a case report of subglottic gout tophus. Auris Nasus Larynx 2001; 28:265–267.
4. Al Saab F. Rare gout manifestation of head and neck. Otol Head Neck Surg 2004; Vol 131:298–299.
5. Wu H, Klein M, Stahl R, Sanchez M. Intestinal pseudotumorous gouty nodulosis: a colonic tophus without manifestation of gouty arthritis. Hum Pathol 2004; 35:897–899.
6. Pfister AK, Schlarb CA, O'Neal JF. Vertebral erosion, paraplegia, and spinal gout. AJR Am J Roentgenol 1998; 171:1430.
7. Pascual E, Jovani V. Synovial fluid analysis. Best Pract Res Clin Rheumatol 2005; 19:371–386.
8. Bond JR, Sim FH, Sundaram M. Radiologic case study: gouty tophus involving the distal quadriceps tendon. Orthopedics 2004; 27:90–92.
9. Lagoutaris ED, Adams HB, DiDomenico LA, Rothenberg RJ. Longitudinal tears of both peroneal tendons associated with tophaceous gouty infiltration: a case report. J Foot Ankle Surg 2005; 44:222–224.
10. Watt I, Middlemiss H. The radiology of gout. Clin Radiol 1975; 26:27–36.
11. Martel W. The overhanging margin of bone: a roentgenologic manifestation of gout. Radiology 1968; 91:755–756.
12. Mair SD, Coogan AC, Speer KP, Hall RL. Gout as a source of sesamoid pain. Foot Ankle Int 1995; 16:613–616.
13. Kobayashi K, Deie M, Okuhara A, et al. Tophaceous gout in the bipartite patella with intra-osseous and intra-articular lesions: a case report. J Orthop Surg 2005; 13:199–202.
14. Levitin PM, Keats TE. Dissecting synovial cyst of the popliteal space in gout. AJR Am J Roentgenol 1975; 124:32–33.
15. Chen CKH, Yeh LR, Pan H-B, et al. Intra-articular gouty tophi of the knee: CT and MRI imaging in 12 patients. Skeletal Radiol 1999; 28:75–80.
16. Chen CKH, Chung CB, Yeh LR, et al. Carpal tunnel syndrome caused by tophaceous gout: CT and MR imaging features in 20 patients. AJR Am J Roentgenol 2000; 175:655–659.
17. O'Leary ST, Goldberg JA, Walsh WR. Tophaceous gout of the rotator cuff: a case report. J Shoulder Elbow Surg 2003; 12:200–201.
18. Diaz A, Porhiel V, Sabatier P, et al. Tophaceous gout of the cervical spine, causing cord compression: case report and review of the literature. Neurochirurgie 2003; 49:600–604.
19. Miller LJ, Pruett SW, Losada R, et al. Tophaceous gout of the lumbar spine: MR findings. J Comput Assist Tomogr 1996; 20:1004–1005.
20. Yu JS, Chung C, Recht M, et al. MR imaging of tophaceous gout. AJR Am J Roentgenol 1997; 168:523–527.
21. Sheldon PJ, Forrester DM, Learch TJ. Imaging of intraarticular masses. RadioGraphics 2005; 25:105–119.
22. Gerster JC, Landry M, Dufresne L, Meuwly JY. Imaging of tophaceous gout: computed tomography provides specific images compared with magnetic resonance imaging and ultrasonography. Ann Rheum Dis 2002; 61:52–54.
23. Grassi W, Meenagh G, Pascual E, Filippucci E. "Crystal clear"—sonographic assessment of gout and calcium pyrophosphate deposition disease. Semin Arthritis Rheum 2006; 36:197–202.
24. Mettler FA, Guiberteau MJ. Essentials of Nuclear Medicine Imaging, 3rd ed. Philadelphia, Elsevier Saunders, 2006.
25. Li TJ, Lue KH, Lin ZI, Lu KH. Arthroscopic treatment for gouty tophi mimicking an intra-articular synovial tumor of the knee. Arthroscopy 2006; 22:910e1–910e3.
26. Melloni P, Valls R, Yuguero M, Saez A. An unusual case of tophaceous gout involving the anterior cruciate ligament. Arthroscopy 2004; 20:e117–e121.
27. Savory W. A Lecture on gout in some of its relations to surgery. Lancet 1894; 1:74–79.

CHAPTER

59

Crystal-Related Arthritis

Iain Watt

A number of crystals are associated with joint disease (Fig. 59-1). The major culprits are calcium pyrophosphate dihydrate and hydroxyapatite (basic calcium phosphate). The focus in this chapter is on the disorders associated with crystal deposition in and around joints, except for true gout, which is discussed in Chapter 58.

CALCIUM PYROPHOSPHATE DIHYDRATE DEPOSITION

Etiology

The discovery of crystals in synovial fluid that were not urate by McCarty and colleagues in the 1960s prompted a review of diseases apparently associated with crystals in joints.[1,2] The same finding had been described previously in the Czech Republic as chondrocalcinosis polyarticularis (familiaris).[3] Subsequently, two slightly different crystals were identified: calcium pyrophosphate dihydrate (CPPD), in about 3.3% of cadavers, seen radiographically as linear or punctate deposits, and dicalcium phosphate dihydrate (DCPD), which produced diffuse punctate deposits in a further 2.3%. Subsequently, a number of clinical and radiologic disorders became associated with these crystals, resulting in some confusion of terminology. These crystals will be grouped together as CPPD in this chapter.

Prevalence and Epidemiology

CPPD crystals may be found in or around joints in a number of circumstances:

1. *Chondrocalcinosis.* Deposits of crystals that are radiopaque may be seen pathologically, arthroscopically, or radiologically as cartilage calcification. Such calcification is not always due to CPPD (including DCPD), although it is the major cause. Chondrocalcinosis is an age-related phenomenon; about 25% of otherwise normal people 85 and older will exhibit it.[4] Furthermore, they may have no more joint symptoms than others

without chondrocalcinosis. CPPD crystals are present as a normal constituent of hyaline cartilage[5] and may have an important role in high stress zones in the subarticular region. They occur at all ages, the crystal area being age related. For unknown reasons, chondrocalcinosis is particularly prevalent in those joints with both hyaline cartilage and fibrocartilage within them (e.g., the knee and wrist).

2. *Pseudogout.* Episodes of crystal shedding occur in some patients with chondrocalcinosis. Because of an apparent, although inaccurate, likeness with gout this phenomenon became known as pseudogout. However, the clinical features of pseudogout are distinct from true gout. First, the common joints of involvement are the knee or wrist (compared with the great toe metatarsophalangeal joint). Second, the patients are often older women (compared with middle-aged men).

3. *Pyrophosphate arthropathy.* A form of osteoarthritis-like disease was described in some patients with "the pseudogout syndrome" by Martel and associates.[6] Subsequently called pyrophosphate arthropathy it became a disease in its own right.[7] The concept of this as a distinct clinical entity has been challenged in recent

> ### KEY POINTS
>
> - Chondrocalcinosis is equivalent to calcium pyrophosphate dihydrate (CPPD) deposition in hyaline and fibrocartilage.
> - CPPD deposition is often asymptomatic.
> - CPPD deposition may be associated with a number of metabolic conditions as well as old age.
> - CPPD deposition can be associated with osteoarthritis development and prominent subchondral cysts, referred to as "pyrophosphate arthropathy" or "CPPD arthropathy."
> - Some patients experience recurrent synovitis related to CPPD deposition, referred to as "pseudogout."

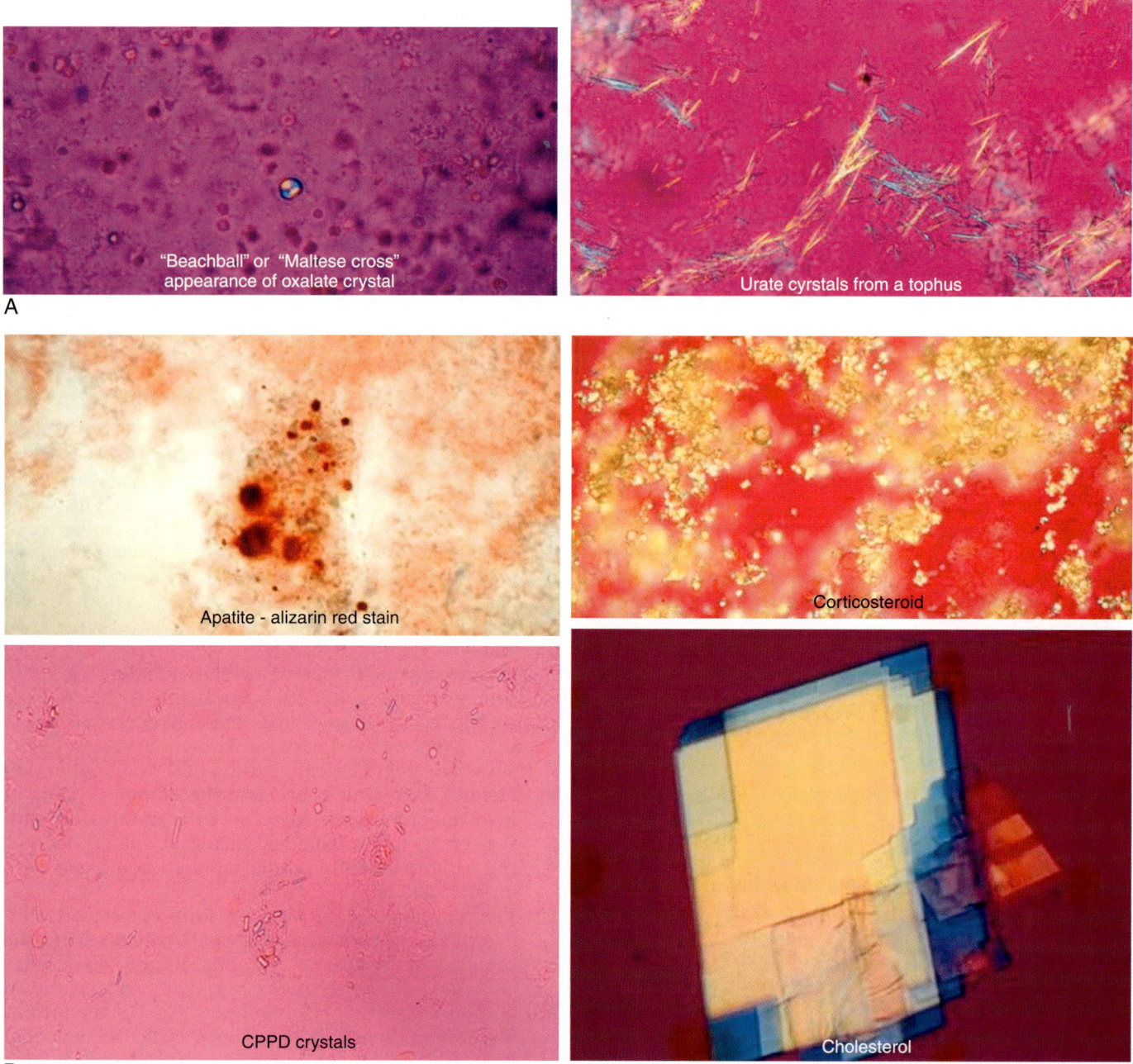

"Beachball" or "Maltese cross" appearance of oxalate crystal

Urate cyrstals from a tophus

A

Apatite - alizarin red stain

Corticosteroid

CPPD crystals

Cholesterol

B

■ **FIGURE 59-1** Example of crystals as seen in the crystal laboratory. **A,** Typical oxalate (*left*) and urate (*right*) crystals. **B,** Examples of hydroxyapatite, cholesterol, intra-articular corticosteroid injection material, and calcium pyrophosphate. (*Courtesy of Professor Michael Doherty, University of Nottingham.*)

years, but in this chapter the term *pyrophosphate arthropathy* will be used to describe a variant of hypertrophic osteoarthritis found in conjunction with CPPD crystals in synovial joints. The relationship between CPPD and the arthropathy is not fully clarified. Debate persists as to whether pyrophosphate arthropathy is truly an entity, distinct from osteoarthritis, or merely a hypertrophic variant of osteoarthritis in which the crystals of CPPD occur that are not necessarily the primary pathogenic cause.

Clinical Presentation

The various manifestations of CPPD occur in both sexes, mainly in middle-aged and elderly patients. Chondrocalcinosis as such is totally asymptomatic and often an incidental finding at radiography or surgery. Classically, crystal shedding causes attacks of pseudogout. These acute or subacute self-limited attacks of arthritis involve one or more joints and last from 1 day to several weeks. They may be provoked by trauma, surgery, intra-articular injections, or systemic illness. The exact mechanism is unknown, but shedding of the superficial zones of hyaline cartilage, in which the crystals are deposited, seems to be likely. Because the distribution of involvement reflects those joints with fibrocartilage in them, the knee is the most common site.

The onset of episodes of arthropathy can be variable, and a number of clinical patterns have been suggested, including pseudorheumatoid disease (35% to 60%) in which chronic large joint arthritis occurs with acute inflammatory episodes; pseudo-osteoarthritis (10% to 35%) as chronic arthritis without acute exacerbations; asymptomatic joints (10% to 20%) and pseudo-Charcot disease (0% to 2%) in which joints resemble neuropathic osteoarthropathy without the neuropathy.[2] From this, it is clear that CPPD does not have a distinct clinical pattern.

Whereas chondrocalcinosis polyarticularis (familiaris) is, by definition, a hereditary disorder unassociated with other disease processes, the majority of cases of CPPD appear to be sporadic. However, CPPD deposition is increased in some metabolic disorders, particularly primary hyperparathyroidism and hemochromatosis, when the onset of symptoms and signs occurs at a younger age. Many other diseases have been described in association with CPPD but no definite linkage with them has been proven. These include diseases that are themselves more common in middle-aged or older people, such as osteoarthritis, diffuse idiopathic skeletal hyperostosis, hypertension, atherosclerosis, and diabetes mellitus.

The relationship with idiopathic osteoarthritis is difficult to assess and lies at the heart of deciding whether pyrophosphate arthropathy actually exists or if it is a subset of osteoarthritis with hypertrophic and perhaps modified features (see later).

Other metabolic disorders such as gout have a higher frequency of CPPD crystals occurring in the same joint, and a proportion of gout patients have chondrocalcinosis. Hyperparathyroidism, especially the primary disease, has a well-documented incidence of chondrocalcinosis, which is usually asymptomatic; interestingly, such patients do not develop structural changes of osteoarthritis. Many do not suffer acute pseudogout attacks. Other coexistent or precipitating conditions include hemochromatosis in which about 40% develop a joint disease resembling pyrophosphate arthropathy. Lastly, hypomagnesemia is associated with CPPD deposition because pyrophosphatase activity depends on the presence of magnesium ions.

The only documented condition in which a negative relationship exists with CPPD is rheumatoid arthritis.[8] The incidence of chondrocalcinosis radiographically and CPPD in joint fluid is reduced in rheumatoid arthritis, but those few patients who do get both have erosions that are far less aggressive than usual, characterized by a patchy, asymmetric distribution, retained bone density, prominent osteophytes, and few, well-corticated erosions. This observation led to the suggestion that CPPD is a marker of a hypertrophic bone response to joint injury. Another study showed that CPPD deposition occurred more frequently in a knee that had undergone meniscectomy compared with the other, unoperated knee. Furthermore, the degree of osteoarthritis in the operated knee on the Kellgren and Lawrence scale was greater when CPPD was present. This supported the view that trauma can provoke chondrocalcinosis but also that osteophyte formation may be enhanced.[9] A follow-up study looked at osteoarthritis of the hand in these patients after meniscectomy. It was found that the degree of osteoarthritis of the knee was worse if the patient had osteoarthritis of the hand. In other words, an underlying systemic predisposition to osteoarthritis was provoked locally by surgery to the knee and enhanced if CPPD was present.[10]

Pathology

CPPD crystals are deposited mainly in hyaline and fibrocartilage. In more advanced cases they are found in all the tissues of a joint as well as periarticular structures, including tendons. No abnormality is found in serum or urine, but inorganic pyrophosphate levels in synovial fluid are increased markedly during an episode of pseudogout, especially as it subsides. It is thought that the excess of inorganic pyrophosphate in cartilage results from overproduction by aging chondrocytes. The cause and/or mechanism is not known presently. The role of extracellular pyrophosphatase may be important because this enzyme may be inhibited by divalent ions, such as iron, calcium, and copper, perhaps explaining the accumulation of CPPD crystals in articular cartilage in hemochromatosis, hyperparathyroidism, and Wilson's disease.

Similarly, the mechanism of crystal shedding is unknown. CPPD crystals injected subcutaneously or into joints produce an acute inflammatory response. Thus, the pathogenesis of acute synovitis may be due simply to crystal shedding. Because the crystals lie in the subarticular region of hyaline cartilage and the radiologically visible chondrocalcinosis may disappear during an attack of pseudogout, it seems probable that the crystals are shed as the result of superficial hyaline cartilage damage. It has been shown that the crystals shed during pseudogout attacks are structurally different with a greater proportion of monoclinic, larger crystals than those found in the more chronic disease. The latter tend to be smaller, triclinic crystals.[11]

The structural joint changes associated with CPPD crystal deposition are those of osteoarthritis, including hyaline cartilage fibrillation and erosion, subchondral sclerosis with thickened trabeculae, multiple growth arrest line, and multiple "cysts." The cysts are larger and more numerous than conventional osteoarthritis. Collapse of cysts may underlie the reported increase in bony fragmentation and the multiple intra-articular osteochondral bodies found either loose within the joint cavity or embedded in synovium. Overall, the findings are of a hypertrophic variant of osteoarthritis with a predilection for subchondral cystic lesions.

As described earlier, it is not unusual to find pyrophosphate arthropathy in conjunction with Forestier's disease or diffuse idiopathic skeletal hyperostosis. A meticulous paleopathologic study confirmed the apparent association between osteophytosis and enthesophytosis and coined the expression "bone formers."[12] This suggestion, that

CPPD marks a bone-forming predisposition, has drawn much attraction, especially because centrally measured bone density is normal or high in patients with it.[13]

Manifestations of the Disease

Because CPPD deposition results in radiographically visible calcification of certain structures, radiographs are the primary modality for their characterization. In fact, on modalities such as MRI, chondrocalcinosis can be inapparent or even misleading, occasionally simulating meniscal tear.

Radiography

Articular and Periarticular Calcification—Chondrocalcinosis

As indicated previously, articular and periarticular calcification is most commonly seen in those joints with both fibrocartilage and hyaline cartilage within them (Fig. 59-2). Hence, the knees and wrists are most commonly involved. Anteroposterior radiographs of the knees alone will detect calcification in approximately 90% of these patients.[14] Calcification is linear or punctate in hyaline cartilage but may be granular in fibrocartilage (Fig. 59-3). Fibrocartilaginous calcification is most common in the menisci of the knee and triangular cartilage of the wrist, although no joint is exempt, including the shoulder, elbow, and hip (Fig. 59-4). In more severe cases, calcification may involve synovium, especially the suprapatellar pouch, capsule, or entheses around the joint (Fig. 59-5). Tendon calcification typically involves the Achilles, triceps, or quadriceps. Such calcification appears thin and linear. Chondrocalcinosis on a radiograph is usually due to CPPD, but both CPPD and calcium hydroxyapatite can occur together.

On occasion, it is possible to demonstrate crystal shedding concurrent with a clinical episode of pseudogout (Fig. 59-6A). Joint aspiration reveals turbid, yellow fluid that may be misinterpreted as pus due to sepsis (see Fig. 59-6B). Pseudogout almost always involves the knee or wrist (Fig. 59-7), unlike true gout, which in 80% of cases involves the feet.

Occasionally, CPPD may present as a solitary space-occupying lesion known variously as tophaceous pseudogout or tumoral CPPD. These are most common in the digits and may present as an acute attack similar to tophaceous gout.[15] Spinal lesions have been recorded associated with cord compression on rare occasions.[16]

Structural Changes in Joints—"Pyrophosphate Arthropathy"

Not surprisingly, this most commonly involves those joints with a predilection for CPPD deposition. Hence the knee and the wrist are typically affected. In the original description of this form of arthritis occurring in pseudogout syndrome five differences from conventional osteoarthritis were noted.[6] This was subsequently reviewed and confirmed by Martel and colleagues,[17] who again emphasized the following points:

1. *Unusual articular distribution*. Whereas knee and hip disease is typical in osteoarthritis, involvement of other sites is less commonly affected by osteoarthritis, such as the wrist and elbow. However, the wrist is frequently involved in injury in older patients and elbow osteoarthritis is well recognized by archeologists, if not by clinicians, because it appears to be largely asymptomatic.[18]

2. *Unusual intra-articular distribution*. Compared with osteoarthritis the intra-articular distribution of

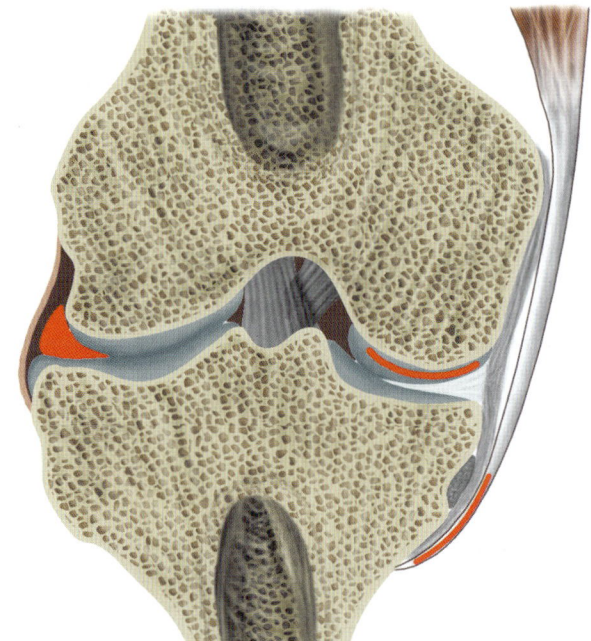

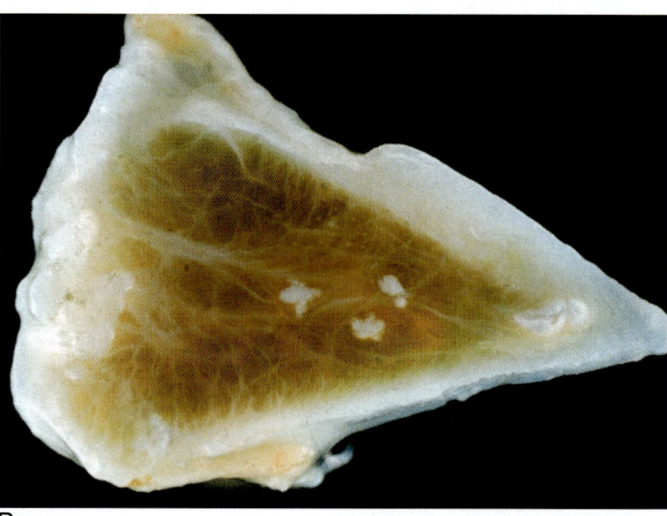

■ **FIGURE 59-2** **A,** Typical distribution of intra-articular deposition of calcium pyrophosphate. Note the meniscal, hyaline cartilage, and entheseal sites of deposition. **B,** A section through a meniscus confirms the linear superficial deposition as well as the deeper granular foci.

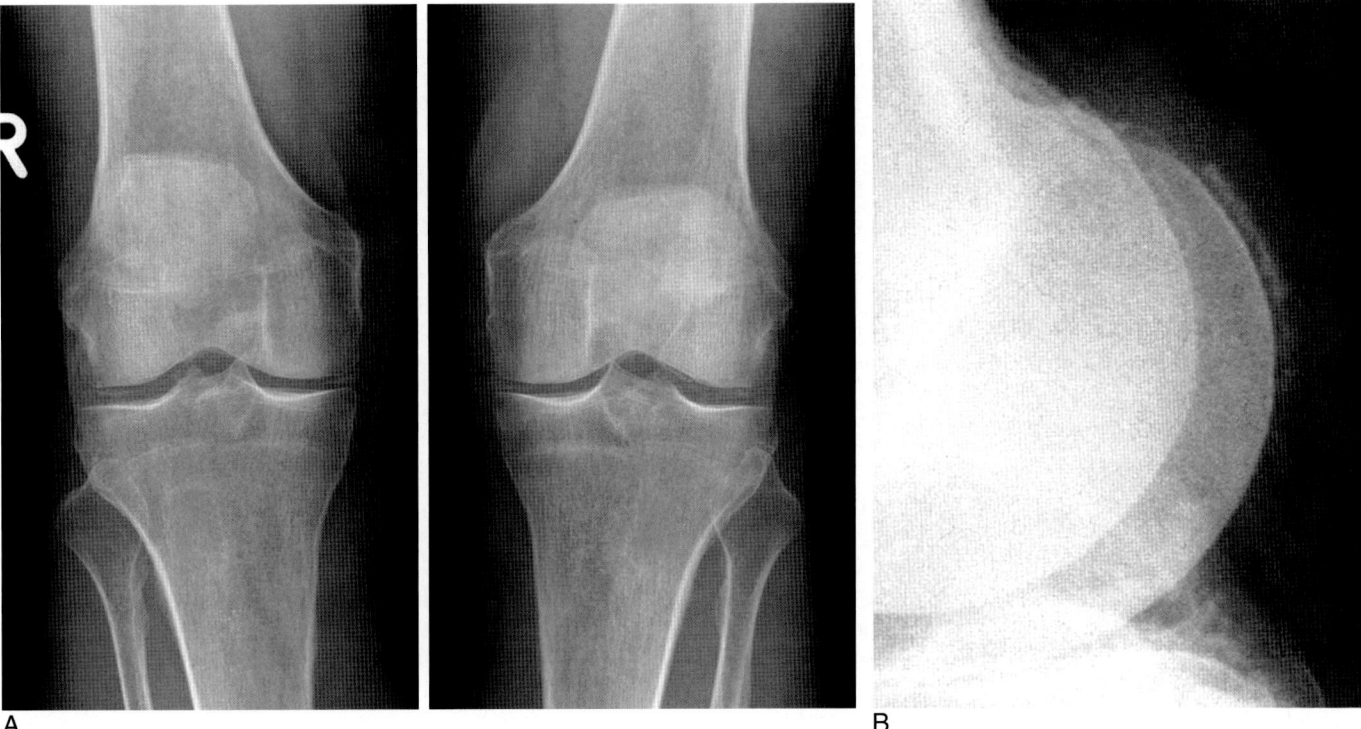

A   B

■ **FIGURE 59-3** **A,** Typical pyrophosphate deposition on knee radiographs. The frontal view conforms to the line drawing in Figure 59-2A. **B,** Note the linear nature on the lateral view.

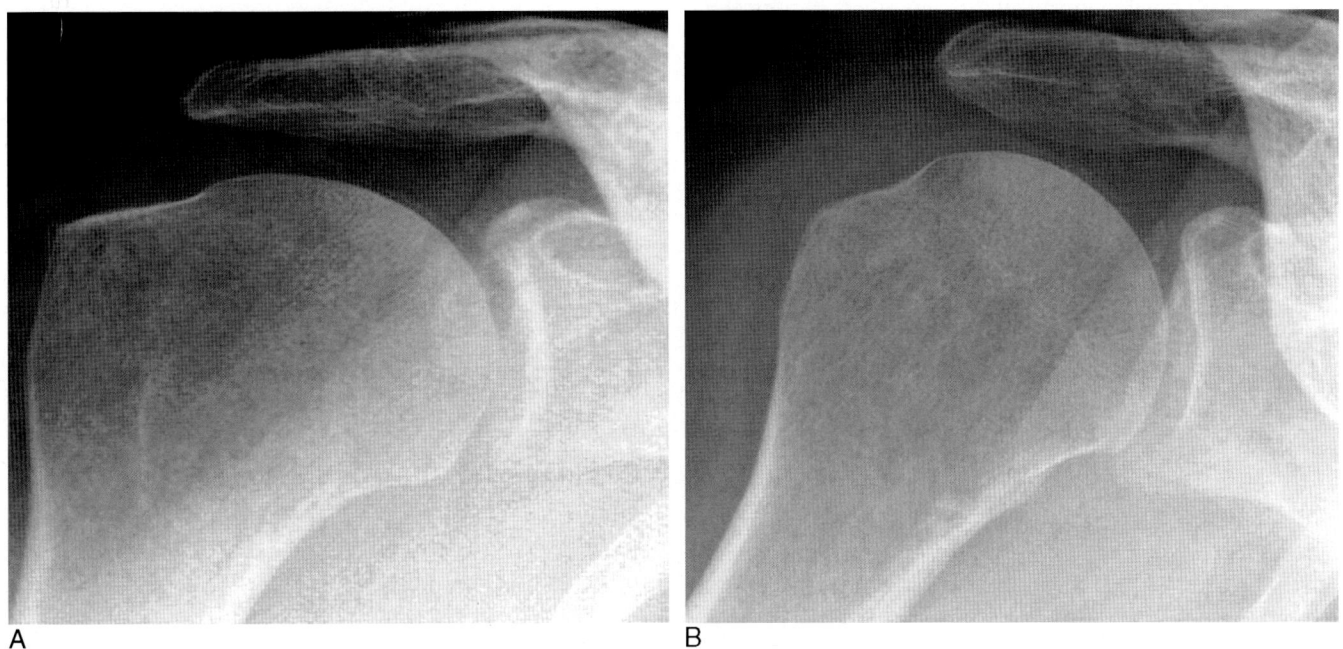

A   B

■ **FIGURE 59-4** **A and B,** Hyaline cartilage chondrocalcinosis in the shoulder joint.

pyrophosphate arthropathy may be considered unusual. Thus, particular involvement of the scaphotrapezial joint of the wrist or the patellofemoral compartment of the knee is cited (Fig. 59-8). One study confirms a higher prevalence of scaphotrapezial joint degeneration in a group of patients with chondrocalcinosis of the wrist,

confirmed either radiographically or on joint aspiration, compared with conventional osteoarthritis.[19] However, again looking at archeological materials, 500 years ago osteoarthritis of the patellofemoral joint was the norm whereas tibiofemoral osteoarthritis seems to be a more recent disease.[20]

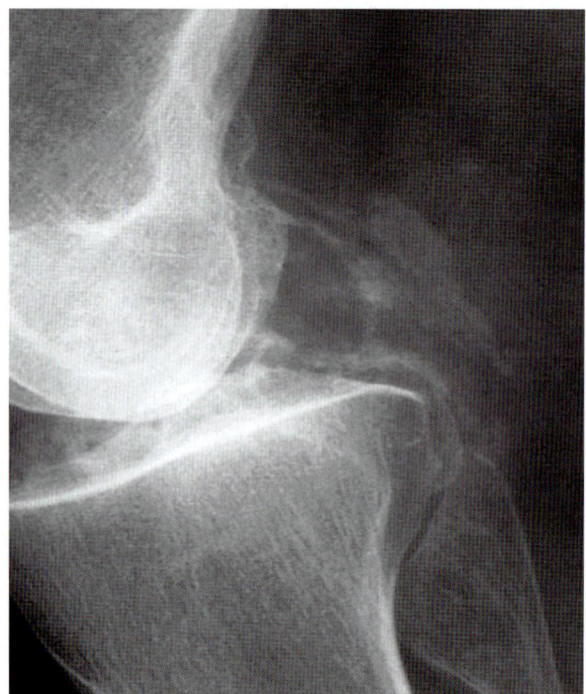

■ FIGURE 59-5 In cases in which deposition is heaviest, entheseal and capsular calcification may be seen outside the confines of the joint.

3. *Prominent subchondral cyst formation.* Lesions are often numerous, large, and well demarcated with a sclerotic border but often somewhat ill defined. However, this is not unique to CPPD and also may be seen in hemochromatosis, Wilson's disease, or even chronic bleeding states such as hemophilia (Fig. 59-9).
4. *Pyrophosphate arthropathy.* This may be associated with subchondral bone collapse and fragmentation, perhaps due to collapse of the cysts and the release of multiple intra-articular osseous bodies.

5. *Variable osteophyte formation.* In some patients, large osteophytes are typical (Fig. 59-10). In others, a polished, eburnated bony surface may be seen. However, both occur in conventional osteoarthritis and, again, are used by archeologists as the features that permit them a diagnosis of osteoarthritis. They may represent different aspects of joint failure and repair.
6. *Synovial calcification.* This is said to be common but may be due to calcium hydroxyapatite as well as CPPD deposition, particularly if advanced degenerative changes were present (see section on calcium hydroxyapatite).

Subsequently, Resnick and coworkers[14] reviewed 85 patients with probable or definite CPPD deposition and they came to a number of conclusions:

1. No definite relationship was found between the presence and distribution of pyrophosphate arthropathy and the diagnostic level of confidence.
2. No definite relationship existed between the clinical pattern of arthritis and the presence of articular calcification or arthropathy.
3. Articular calcification was slightly more frequent in symptomatic compared with asymptomatic joints. No definite relationship was found between joint symptoms and the type of cartilage calcification (fibrocartilage vs. hyaline cartilage).
4. The frequency and extent of local calcification and arthropathy did not correlate with the successful crystal recovery during joint aspiration.
5. Arthropathy was consistently more common, although not more severe, in joints with calcification. No relationship was found between the site of chondrocalcinosis (fibrocartilage versus hyaline cartilage) and the presence and severity of arthropathy.

Both from the spectrum of clinical presentation and the uncertainties expressed earlier, pyrophosphate arthropathy

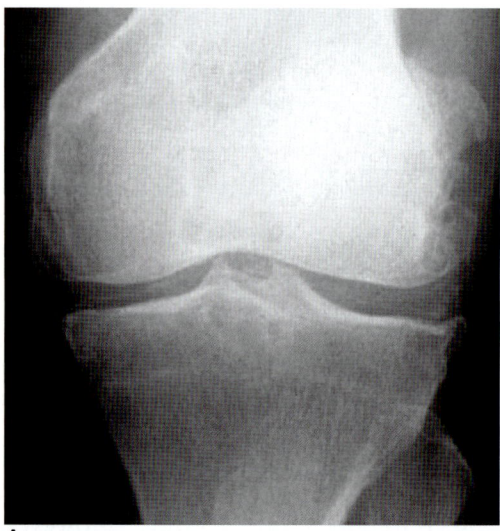
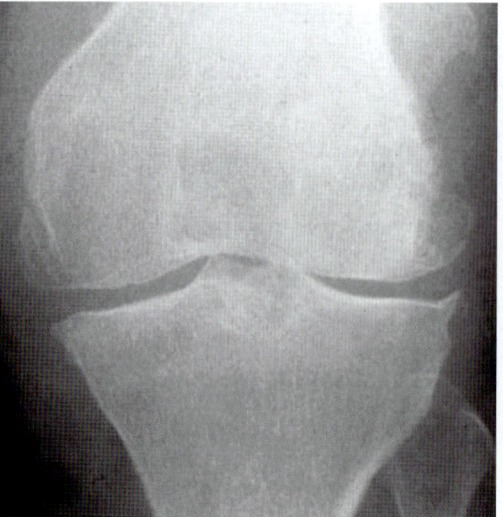
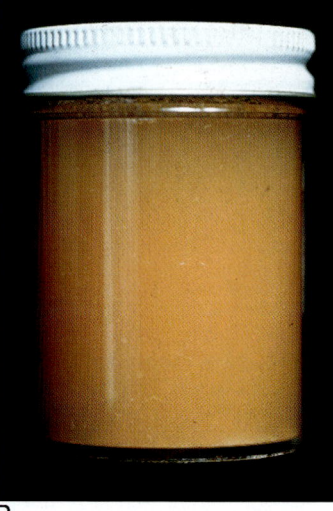

A   B

■ FIGURE 59-6 Crystal shedding associated with clinical pseudogout. **A,** Two views of the left knee of a middle-aged man who sustained two episodes of pseudogout in the 6 months between these radiographic examinations. Note that on the second examination (*right*) not only is the calcification less marked but also the joint space width is reduced. Often pseudogout occurs as the superficial layers of hyaline cartilage are shed, the crystals being released from them. **B,** Joint aspiration from this patient's second episode of pseudogout shows the pus-like nature of the fluid.

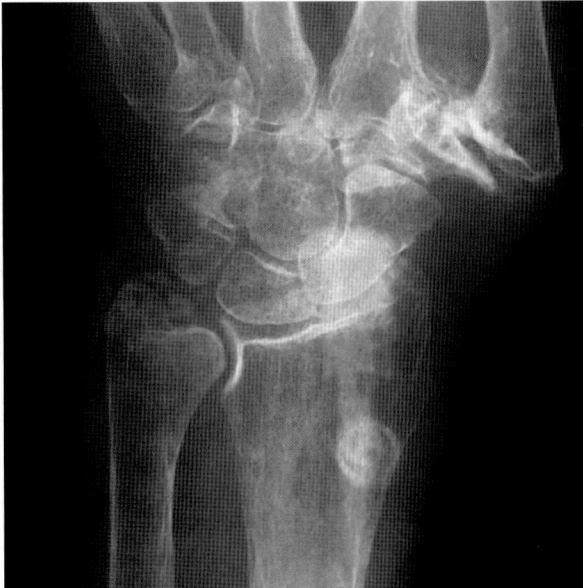

■ **FIGURE 59-7** A typical case of pseudogout. An elderly woman, in the hospital for another reason, has a venous cannula in her forearm. Note the chondrocalcinosis in the triangular fibrocartilage. Clinically she was suspected of having sepsis in the wrist, but the correct diagnosis was pseudogout.

seems to be a diagnosis without finite definitions. The view that it represents a hypertrophic variant of osteoarthritis is gaining ground in which the crystals are epiphenomena rather than the cause of disease. Furthermore, CPPD may be protective of joint damage because most patients with CPPD deposition who have been followed for several years

have done well clinically, with the degree of calcification and arthropathy generally remaining unchanged.[21] In that study, after a mean of 4.6 years, symptoms had improved in 41% of joints and were unchanged in another 33%. Radiographic worsening of osteoarthritis was found in only 16%, whereas chondrocalcinosis had increased in 52%. More recently, two studies have shed doubt on the role of CPPD in the genesis of osteoarthritis changes at all. In one study[22] it was suggested that the relative risk of CPPD over conventional osteoarthritis was as little as 4%, and another found a strong relative risk for osteophyte formation with CPPD but not joint space narrowing,[23] hence the growing concept that CPPD is a marker of bone formation in joints, the entheses, and systemically.

Other Radiologic Findings

Joint effusion and soft tissue swelling occur during episodes of pseudogout. Aspiration of joint fluid produces a turbid, yellow specimen that has a high white blood cell count and may be mistaken for septic arthritis. Chronic joint effusions are, as usual, associated with popliteal cysts.

Stress fractures in neighboring bones, especially the upper tibia, occur and are associated with angular deformities[24] but are not unique to CPPD and are noted in conventional osteoarthritis and rheumatoid disease.

Carpal collapse may occur secondary to radiocarpal osteoarthritis, particularly the so-called scapholunate advanced collapse (SLAC) wrist. This type of osteoarthritis occurs spontaneously or after trauma and is one of the most common patterns of degenerative joint disease in the wrist with or without CPPD deposition.[25]

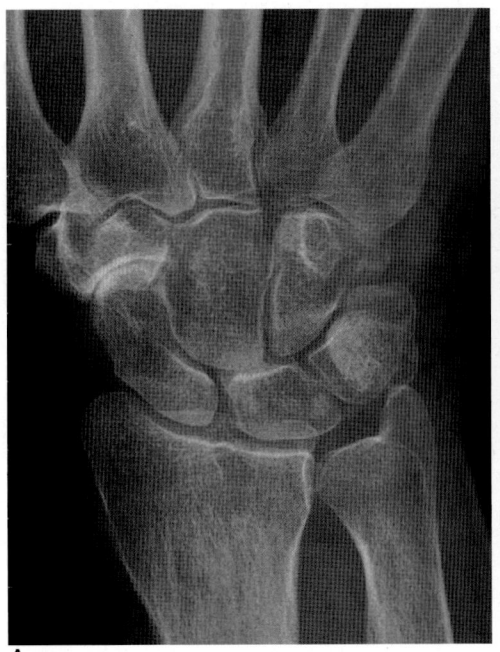
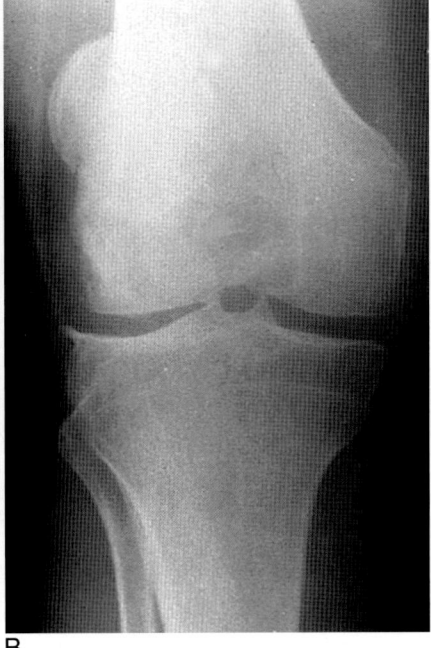
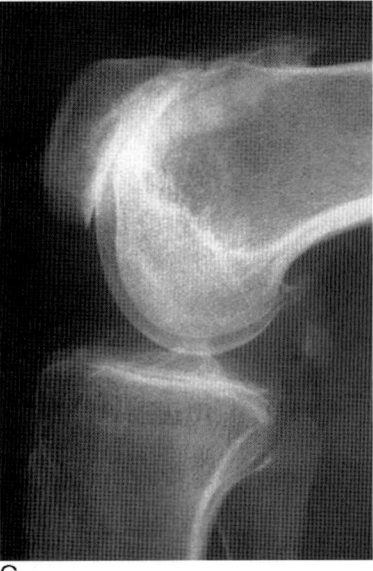

A   B   C

■ **FIGURE 59-8** Example of patients with osteoarthritis in which somewhat atypical joint involvement has occurred and consideration needed to be given to pyrophosphate arthropathy as a diagnosis. **A,** Patient does indeed have unusual scaphotrapezial osteoarthritis with chondrocalcinosis of the triangular fibrocartilage. **B** and **C,** However, this is a case of severe patellofemoral osteoarthritis with virtually normal tibiofemoral compartments. No pyrophosphate could be found on joint aspiration. Is the apparent association between atypical joint involvement and pyrophosphate real or simply part of the spectrum of osteoarthritis?

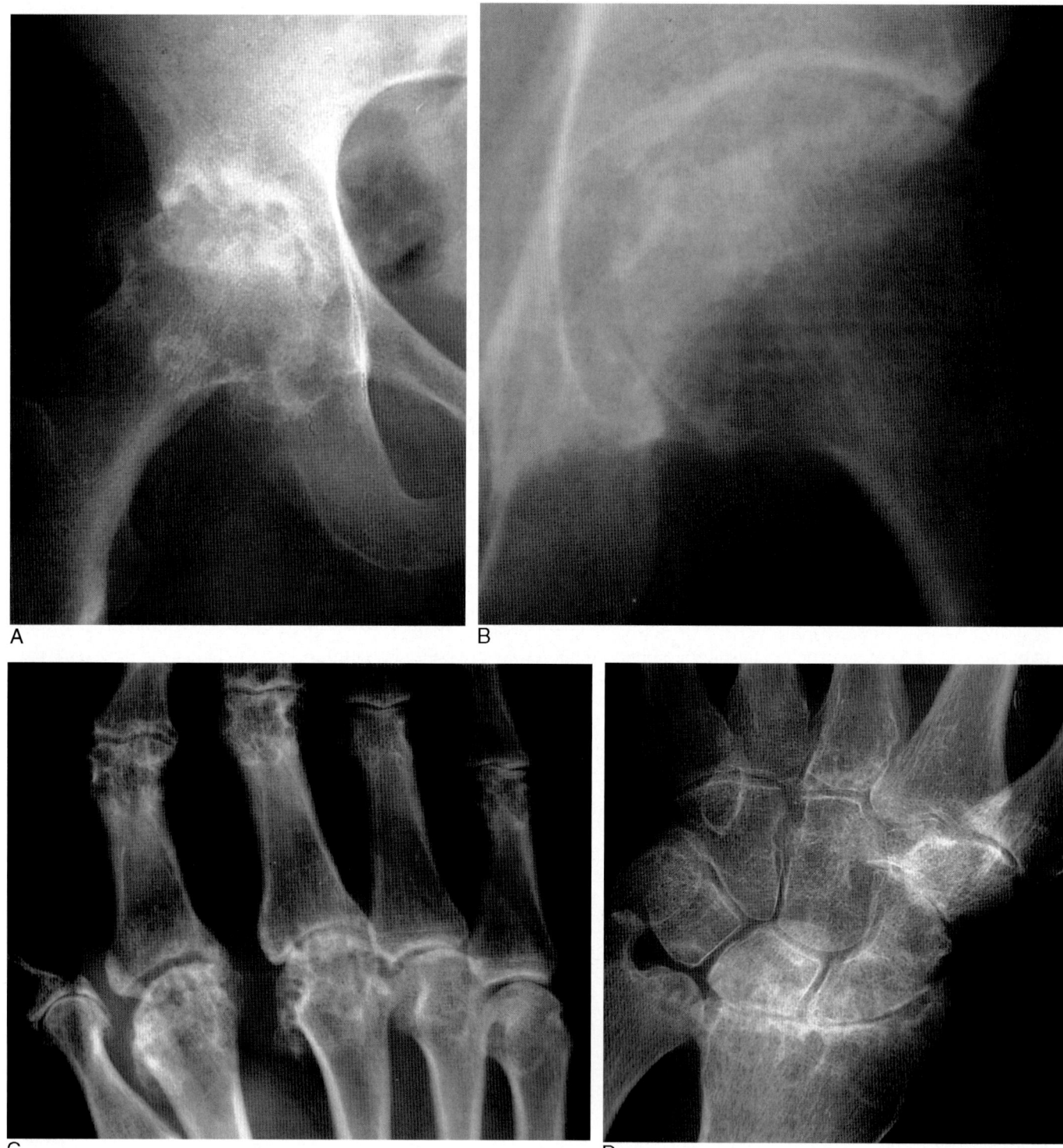

■ FIGURE 59-9 Multiple subchondral radiolucencies ("cysts") occur in a number of conditions involving iron and calcium metabolism. These lesions occur in conjunction with pyrophosphate deposition (**A**) and hemochromatosis (**B**). Further examples of the latter are shown involving the metacarpophalangeal joints (**C**) and the wrist (**D**).

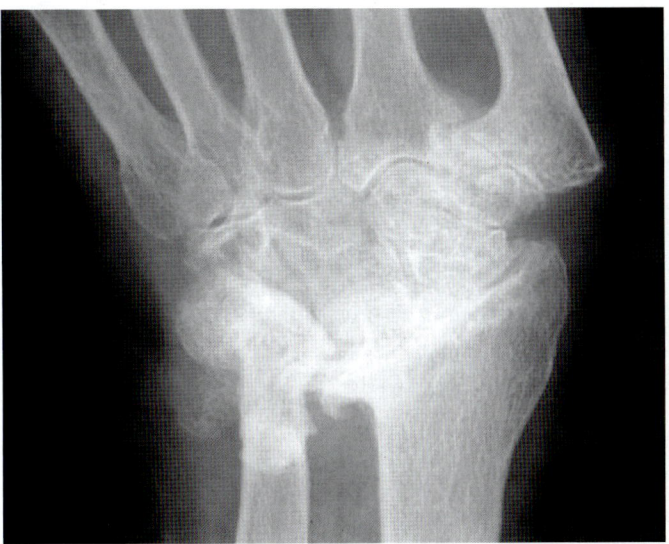

A

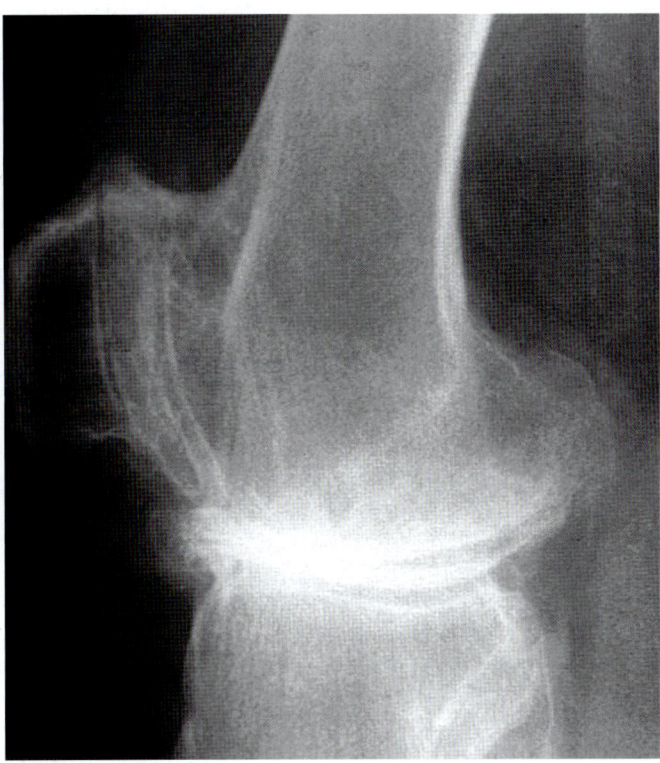

B

■ **FIGURE 59-10** Marked osteophyte formation in the knee (**A**) and the wrist (**B**). These huge osteophytes are a marker of hypertrophic osteoarthritis and are part of the spectrum of CPPD.

Metacarpophalangeal (MCP) joint involvement has been emphasized as a feature of pyrophosphate arthropathy, especially affecting the index and middle fingers. Conventional osteoarthritis, particularly the erosive type, has a greater predilection for the interphalangeal joints and indeed the MCP joints are often omitted from scoring atlases of osteoarthritis. Hemochromatosis also involves the MCP joints, often with well-marked subchondral cysts and also extending across the MCP joint row to the ring and little fingers.[26]

Intervertebral discal calcification is thought to be an incidental finding without clinical significance, with deposits typically being in the outer fibers of the annulus fibrosus.[27] The nucleus pulposus generally is not involved. CPPD may be seen, especially on CT, in other spinal tissues, including the ligamentum flavum, especially in the cervical region. Calcification has been recorded also in association with type 2 odontoid fractures. In all nine cases reported erosion of the odontoid process was present as well as deposits of CPPD in the transverse ligament. It is unclear whether the CPPD contributed to the fracture, but the suggestion that the deposits might threaten the cervical cord is important.[28]

Magnetic Resonance Imaging

Magnetic resonance imaging has no specific role in the diagnosis or assessment of CPPD. Indeed, a meticulous histologic study in cadavers confirmed that MRI was insensitive to the presence of CPPD deposits in the knee, even when they were widespread. The best site for visualization of the low-signal, rather granular deposits was the femoral condyles compared with other intra-articular structures.[29] Granted that the femoral condyles have the thickest hyaline cartilage in the body, this does not seem a particularly clinically relevant finding beyond noting that CPPD may produce these changes if a radiograph is not at hand when it is being interpreted. Additionally, the presence of CPPD in the meniscus has been suggested to simulate surfacing signal of a meniscal tear on MRI.

Multidetector Computed Tomography

Computed tomography is highly sensitive to the presence of calcification due to chondrocalcinosis, but it can be seldom justified to diagnose it. Usually, calcification is an incidental finding or concurrent with another pathologic process as described in cervical trauma.[28]

Ultrasonography

Ultrasonography in the evaluation of CPPD has been reported rarely, for example in the evaluation of the Achilles tendon and plantar fascia.[30] It may reveal asymptomatic deposits and show a high correlation with radiography. Typically linear in distribution, CPPD is shown as intratendinous, hyperechoic lesions parallel to the tendon fibrillar structure, with acoustic shadowing most obvious on the transverse scans. A high incidence of Achilles tendinopathy (14.9% of heels) and retrocalcaneal bursitis (7.0%) was found in comparison with none in osteoarthritis control subjects.[30] Other studies have used ultrasound to assess chondrocalcinosis in the knee and wrist with successful results, but the clinical relevance is difficult to gauge.

Synopsis of Treatment Options

The role of CPPD in health and disease remains controversial. It may be that two distinct "diseases" exist. In one, crystals are shed from hyaline cartilage, for whatever reason, and are more monoclinic and attacks of pseudogout occur. In the other, predominantly triclinic crystals are present and may act as a marker of a systemic predisposition to a hypertrophic response to joint injury. That injury may be meniscectomy or primary osteoarthritis. Certainly, the association between CPPD and other forms of exuberant bone formation, such as ossification of the posterior longitudinal ligament and diffuse idiopathic skeletal hyperostosis suggest a genetic predisposition. Indeed, a family predisposition has been identified with abnormalities on chromosomes 5 and 8 that supports the concept that "bone formers" are real.[31]

HYDROXYAPATITE AND BASIC CALCIUM PHOSPHATE

Etiology

Apart from monosodium monourate and CPPD, other crystals have been identified in and around joints that are associated with inflammatory episodes. Identified as calcium hydroxyapatite (HA) and calcium orthophosphate dihydrate, they, in common with monosodium urate and CPPD, produce an acute inflammatory response when injected into a joint or even subcutaneously. Calcium hydroxyapatite is the most common form of calcium in

bone and is associated with most of the pathologic deposits of calcium in the body. Typically, the crystals are found in foci of periarticular calcification, which results in bursitis and other periarticular inflammatory conditions. Their roles in intra-articular pathology have been recognized more recently. Identification of HA crystals, or other basic calcium phosphates (BCP), is not simple and requires electron microscopic techniques or x-ray diffraction analysis owing to their size and complexity of form (75 to 250 nm in length). In joint fluid, larger clumps may be identified using a stain (alizarin red S) and ordinary light microscopy. Because a spectrum of BCP crystals often coexists it is convenient to lump them together as HA but to recognize that individual subtypes may be identified as specific to particular clinical presentation in the future. Furthermore, HA may coexist with CPPD and/or monosodium urate monohydrate crystals.

The etiology is unknown. Ischemia has been suggested with secondary necrosis. For example, the classic site of calcification in the rotator cuff of the shoulder is the zone where vascular supply is scantiest, approximately 1.5 cm from its insertion. HA is deposited also in abnormal collagen, as in the collagen vascular diseases. Furthermore, as the inducers and inhibitors of calcification are becoming identified, as in vascular and muscle diseases, speculation increases that the deposition of HA is purely passive, secondary to the production of proteins and other products that nucleate calcification.[32]

Prevalence and Epidemiology

Recurrent painful episodes that are associated with periarticular calcific deposits in tendons and soft tissues have a variety of names, including peritendinitis calcarea, calcific tendinitis, peritendinitis, and bursitis. Usually monoarticular, the most frequent site is the shoulder. Patients are typically middle aged, are of either sex, and present with acute pain and tenderness on pressure. Occasionally younger patients, including children, may be affected. The disease may be chronic and sometimes incapacitating. However, calcification may be found radiographically in entirely asymptomatic patients or even in the asymptomatic contralateral limb of a patient in pain. Patients may attribute onset of the disorder to an episode, or episodes, of trauma. Manual workers are at greater risk than sedentary workers.[33] Interestingly, the frequency of involvement of a given joint is paralleled by its physiologic range of movement. Hence, the shoulder is the most common site.[34] Laboratory investigation is usually noncontributory.

Clinical Presentation

A number of distinct clinical syndromes are identified in which HA is a feature:

● Calcification in tendons or ligaments: "calcific periarthritis"
● Episodes of acute transient synovitis
● Calcification in soft tissues associated with the collagen vascular group of disorders and other diseases
● Association with a rapidly progressive form of osteoarthritis

Pathology

Histologic evaluation reveals granular, milky or cheesy deposits of calcified material in fibrous tissue associated with necrosis and surrounding inflammatory changes. All fibrous structures including tendons, capsule, ligaments, and bursae may be involved.

Manifestations of the Disease

Radiography

Calcification in Ligaments and Tendons

Radiographic findings depend on the age of the lesion. Initially, the deposits appear low density, cloud-like, poorly defined, and without trabeculation (Fig. 59-11). Most lesions are ovoid, although they may be triangular or linear.[35] Older lesions are denser, more opaque, and better defined, usually without an associated bone lesion. However, when the lesions are large or situated very close to bone, cystic lesions and reactive sclerosis may occur. At follow up in most patients the sequence of evolution just described is obvious. In others, the focus or foci of calcification may remain static for long periods of time, often correlating poorly with patient symptoms. Some patients suffer an acute attack of pain,[36] and a radiograph will reveal that some of the calcific material has been extruded into an adjacent bursa or joint, causing an acute synovitis (see later).

Typical sites of radiologic involvement include the shoulder and hip regions. Other foci are uncommon (Figs. 59-12 and 59-13). In most instances, radiographs are sufficient to make a diagnosis and monitor progress if considered necessary. Occasional findings include the presence of erosion of bone deep to the insertion of the affected tendon. Usually, this is the pectoralis major or gluteus maximus.[35,37]

1. *The shoulder.* All of the major tendons around the shoulder may be involved, but the rotator cuff remains the most usual. Lesions are more common on the dominant right side but are often bilateral, even if not symptomatic. The supraspinatus tendon is the most frequent site of calcification, usually close to the tendinous insertion on the greater tuberosity. Because the lesion may be projected over bone if the area is not suitably profiled, views on internal and external rotation may be necessary. Axial views are also helpful. Supraspinatus calcification is best seen on external rotation whereas infraspinatus calcification is in profile on internal rotation. Calcification may be seen also in the long head of the biceps tendon in the bicipital groove. Calcification occurs at the pectoralis major

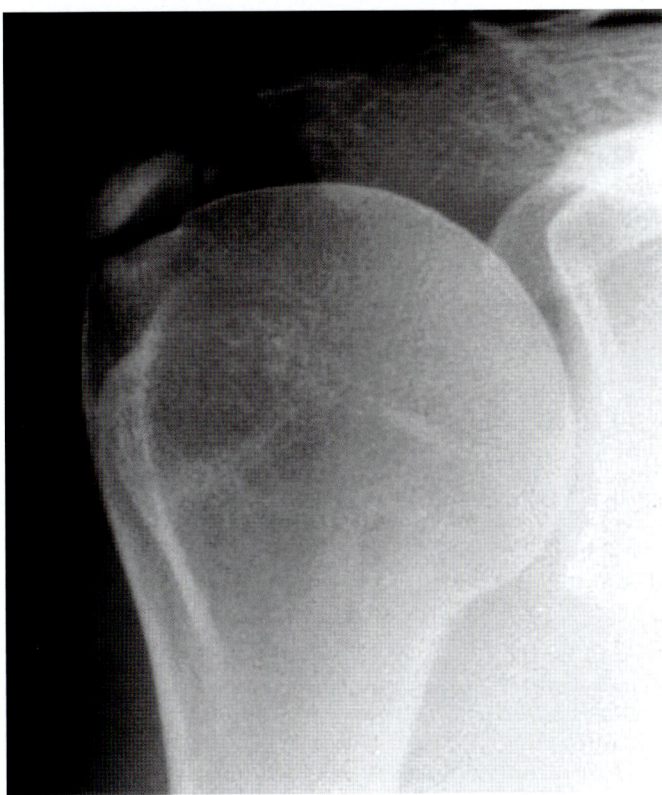

■ **FIGURE 59-11** Acute calcific periarthritis of the shoulder. An extensive area of low density calcification is present in the region of the lateral aspect of the supraspinatus tendon. The patient presented with acute shoulder pain, especially at night and on abduction of the shoulder.

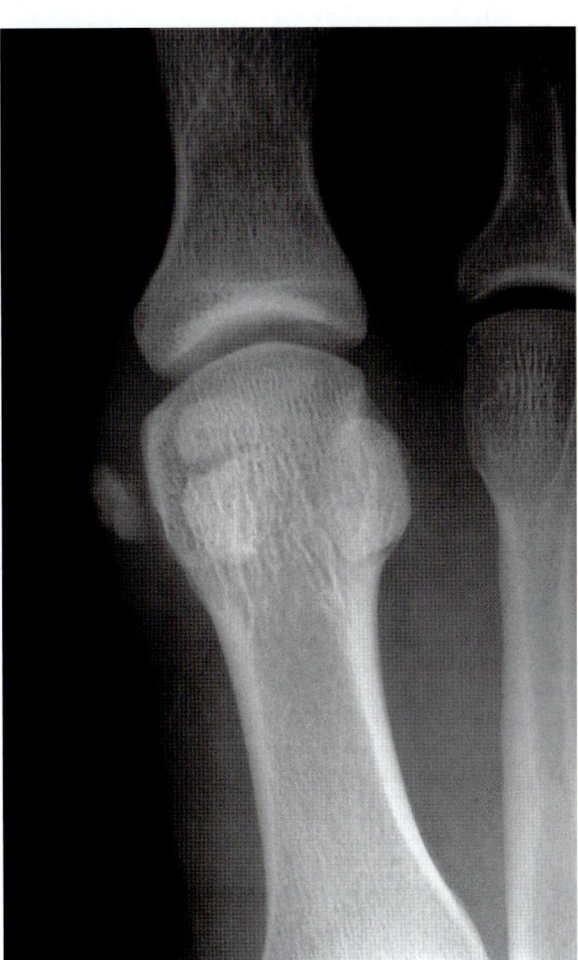

■ **FIGURE 59-12** Calcific periarthritis of the great toe. This lesion had been present longer and is better defined and denser. The site is unusual for calcific periarthritis, and the possibility of true gout might have been considered clinically. BCP crystals were aspirated, however.

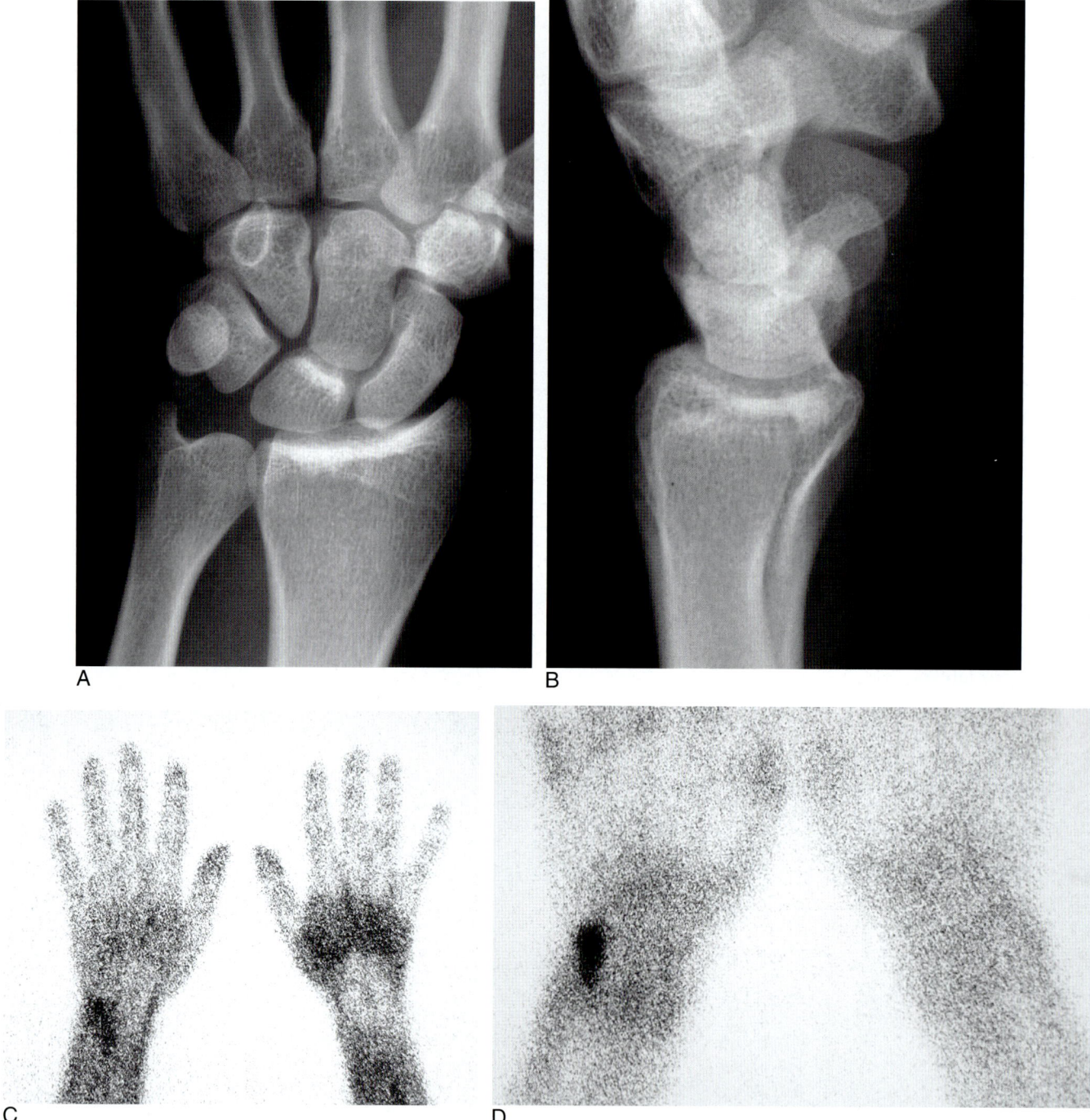

■ **FIGURE 59-13** Calcific periarthritis involving the flexor carpi ulnaris tendon. **A** and **B,** Radiographs reveal ill-defined, low-density calcification. Consideration clinically was given to palm space infection and a bone scan was requested. **C,** The perfusion phase confirmed a focal inflammatory lesion that is avid for the radiopharmaceutical on the delayed scan (**D**). Confirmation of the diagnosis was achieved by aspiration and identification of BCP crystals.

insertion, occasionally with cortical erosion. Rupture of crystals from the rotator cuff may result in an acute, transient synovitis, either in the subdeltoid bursa or the shoulder joint itself. Granular calcification, being heavier than joint fluid, tends to precipitate to the most dependent area, appearing as a lenticular, calcified zone. However, the presence of calcification in the rotator cuff carries prognostic significance about cuff tears. In an

arthrographic study, an inverse relationship was found between the size of the calcific deposit on radiographs and the finding of a cuff tear.[38]

2. *The pelvis.* Calcific deposits are common at the gluteal insertions on the greater trochanter and adjacent bursae. Radiopacities occur also next to the acetabular margin when differentiation from so-called normal variants such as an os acetabulum may be difficult. Such foci

may be associated with symptomatic pain that resolves as the lesion disappears.

3. *The hand and wrist.* Calcification of tendons and periarticular structures of the hand are well recognized. As anticipated, symptoms include pain and swelling; the flexor carpi ulnaris (near the pisiform) and flexor carpi radialis (on the volar aspect of the wrist joint) are particularly involved (see Fig. 59-13). Sometimes the appearances can be subtle and require careful scrutiny (Fig. 59-14).

4. *Other joints.* These are less frequently involved and include the elbow (collateral ligaments) and triceps insertion and the foot, particularly around the great toe when confusion may arise with the misdiagnosis of gout. However, HA deposition typically affects young women as opposed to middle-aged men.

5. *The spine.* Foci of calcification in the neck typically occur in the longus colli muscle and tendon in middle-aged patients, commonly affecting the superolateral tendons (Fig. 59-15). The calcification is seen usually anterior to the anterior tubercle of the atlas and the second, third, and fourth cervical vertebrae. Prevertebral soft tissue swelling may be present. The patient usually presents with acute neck and occipital pain, and dysphagia may be a major complaint.[39] As elsewhere, calcification may

be asymptomatic. The calcification is usually transient and self-limiting with resorption in 1 or 2 weeks. Calcification of the ligamentum flavum, especially in the cervical spine, may occur in middle-aged or elderly patients, who may have pain and neurologic complaints due to cord compression. At the other end of the age spectrum discal calcification in the cervical spine occurs in children who present with acute neck pain and low-grade fever. The etiology is unknown and the process is self-limiting unless the disc contents rupture dorsally into the neural canal when, very rarely, cord compression can occur.

Episodes of Acute Transient Synovitis

Hydroxyapatite crystals are associated with an acute inflammatory response when liberated into a synovial cavity. The crystals are shed usually from rupture of an adjacent collection in a tendon. For example, crystals in the rotator cuff may be shed either into the subdeltoid bursa, initiating an acute bursitis, or into the shoulder joint (Fig. 59-16). Such episodes are short lived and self limiting. Clinically, differentiation from any other cause of acute synovitis may be difficult. Because the patients are usually of the same age group as those with gout or pseudogout the etiology may be overlooked. The joint of involvement should lead to a correct diagnosis, being not usually the great toe (gout) or knee or wrist (pseudogout). However, it must be emphasized that HA deposition may occur in association with both or either of these other crystals and the diagnosis may be complicated. Ultimately, the exact diagnosis requires aspiration of joint or bursal fluid and examination in a crystal reference laboratory.

Radiographic findings may include the presence of residual calcification left behind in the tendon of origin (e.g., the rotator cuff). Crystals within the affected bursa or joint are heavier than synovial fluid and may be demonstrated by erect images of the appropriate area. Such fluid-fluid levels may be overlooked on supine images.

Calcification due to HA in Soft Tissues Other Than Joints

Many other disorders are associated with soft tissue deposition of BCP. Many relate to abnormalities of calcium and/or phosphorus metabolism, particularly renal osteodystrophy and renal dialysis. Others include hypoparathyroidism, sarcoidosis, hypervitaminosis D, and the milk-alkali syndrome. In all of these the calcification is essentially metastatic. A second group of disorders exist in which the underlying etiology relates to primarily abnormal collagen or soft tissue components. Such dystrophic calcification is a feature of locally damaged tissue, as in frostbite or the Ehlers-Danlos syndrome. It is more generalized in the collagen vascular diseases, including scleroderma, dermatomyositis, and tumoral calcinosis (Fig. 59-17).

Rapidly Progressive Osteoarthritis

The presence of HA crystals within joints has been documented since the 1970s when Dieppe and coworkers described six patients with HA crystals in their joints,

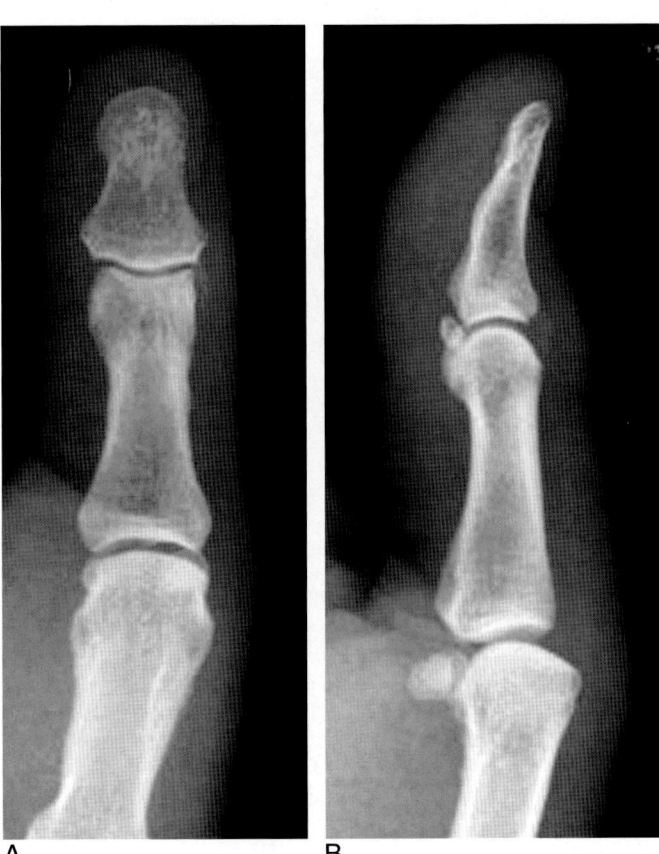

■ FIGURE 59-14 **A** and **B,** This patient presented with acute pain in the thumb, adjacent to the interphalangeal joint. Note the subtle, low-density calcification confirming the diagnosis of calcific periarthritis in this atypical anatomic site. The symptoms resolved with anti-inflammatory therapy.

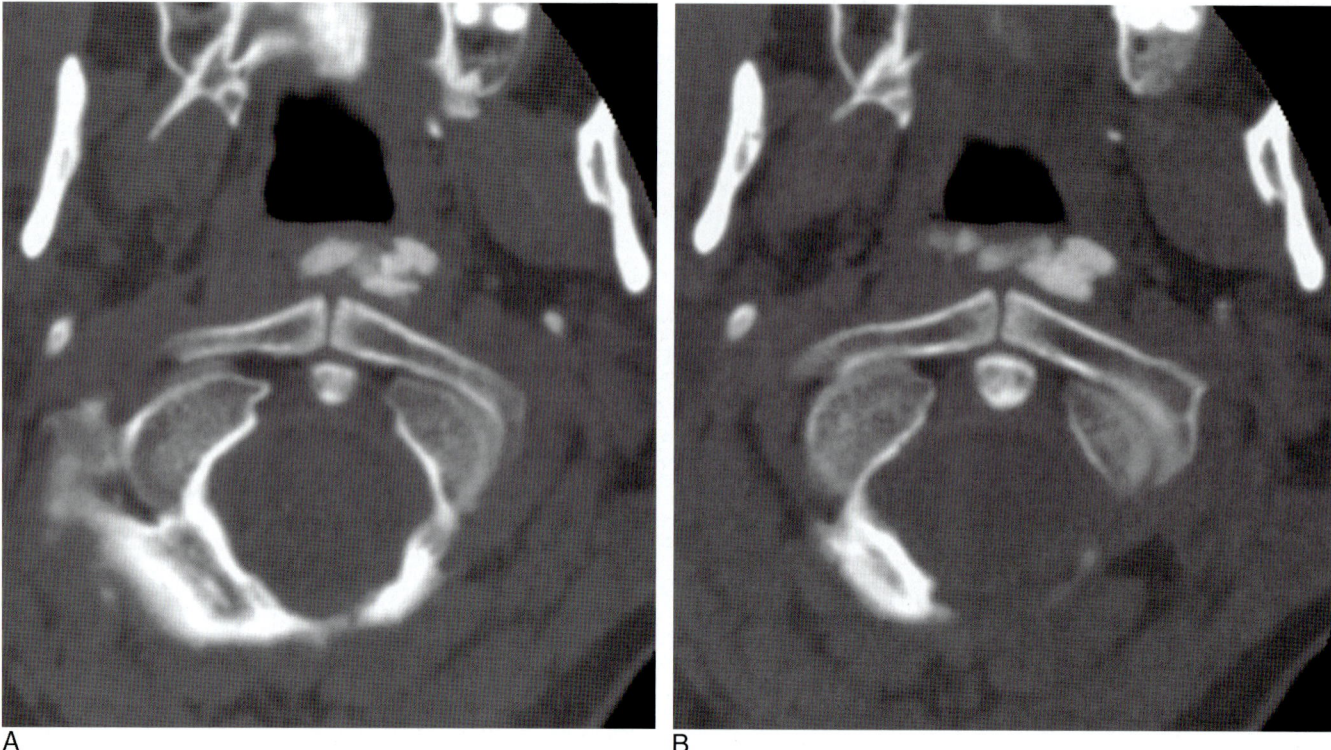

■ **FIGURE 59-15**   **A** and **B**, Acute calcification in the longus coli tendons shown on two consecutive CT scans at the level of C1. Note the coincidental bipartite anterior arch of C1. The patient had classic retropharyngeal pain and dysphagia at presentation.

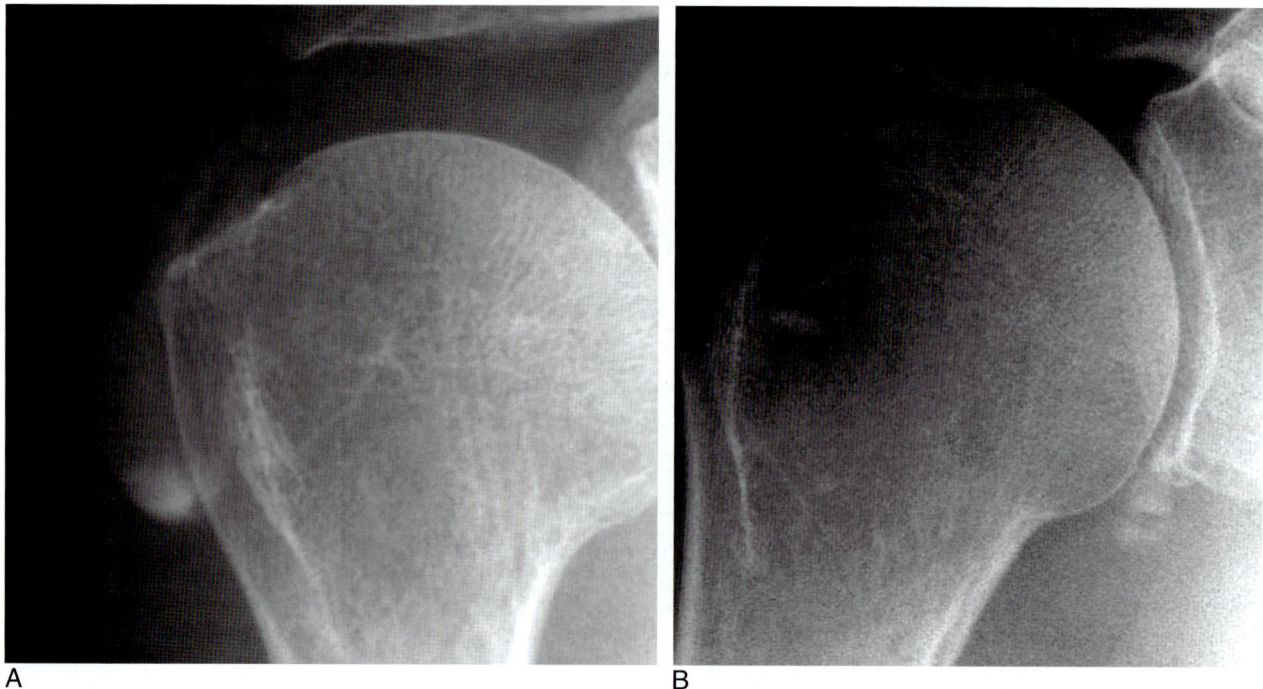

■ **FIGURE 59-16**   **A,** Acute synovitis resulted from the rupture of crystals of BCP from the rotator cuff into the subdeltoid bursa. Note the fluid level as the heavier BCP crystalline material sank to the bottom of the bursal effusion on an erect view. **B,** A similar event had occurred in this patient when the BCP ruptured into the shoulder joint itself. Again, a fluid level has formed.

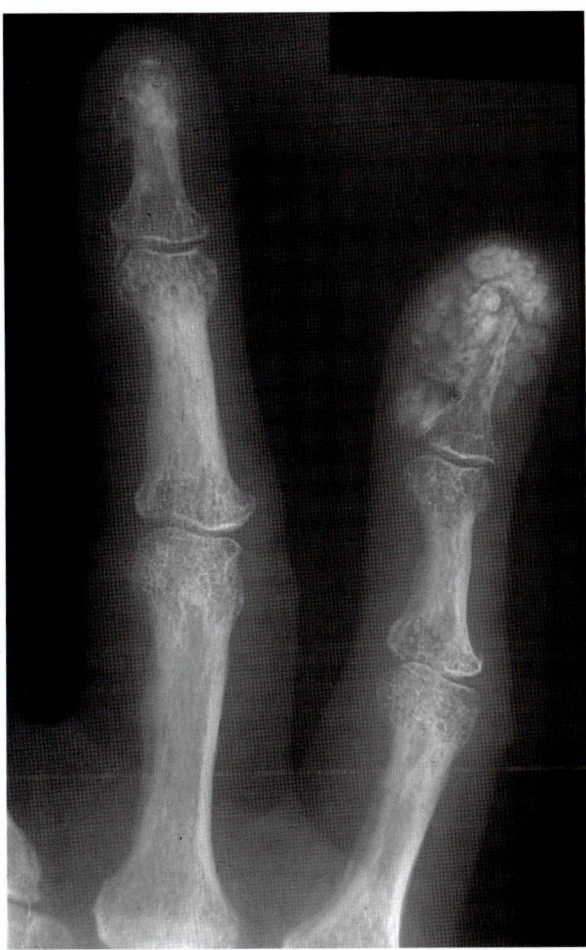

■ **FIGURE 59-17** Calcinosis cutis of uncertain etiology. This patient probably suffered from a collagen vascular disorder. Note the extensive and ill-defined masses of cloud-like calcification in the soft tissues of this little finger.

three of whom had acute inflammatory episodes with joint effusions.[40] Radiographs revealed findings of "generalized osteoarthritis with radiopaque material in or around the joints." Injection of HA crystals into the pleural cavity or subcutaneously in animals and humans was associated with an acute inflammatory reaction, leading these investigators to suggest the existence of a new arthropathy—calcium HA crystal deposition disease. Subsequently, McCarty and colleagues described the presence of microspheroids containing HA crystals by means of scanning electron microscopy of samples of synovial fluid from elderly women who had painful shoulders with decreased mobility and stability.[41] Such patients also had disruption of the rotator cuff. Synovial fluid in their report contained activated collagenase and neutral protease. This syndrome became known as "Milwaukee shoulder." Subsequently, a further paper by this group reported that these enzymes were detectable in some, but not all, of their 30 cases.[42] However, HA is a normal component of joint fluid and may be shown by staining the fluid with alizarin red whereas it is present in marked excess in patients with a Milwaukee shoulder. Furthermore, the presence of the collagenase and protease could not be confirmed by others.[43] Synovial fluid in this form of

rapidly destructive arthritis contains abundant collagen fragments, suggesting that the crystalline spheroid and the fragments are derived from "bone dust" as the joint fails.[44] The concept can be and has been applied to other sites, including the knee and hip, and the names apatite-associated destructive arthritis[44] and rapidly progressive (or atrophic) osteoarthritis have become popular.

Patients are usually elderly women, who are often osteopenic and present with considerable joint swelling and variable degrees of pain affecting their dominant arm.

Radiographic findings are related to the findings of joint opacification and destruction. Although chondrocalcinosis may be due to HA, in severe cases calcified material representing HA containing spheroids and debris usually causes amorphous or cloud-like radiodense areas within the joint (Fig. 59-18). However, large amounts of HA may be present in a joint that is not opacified. It is the structural joint damage that is most striking in these patients. When first described in the shoulder the major findings were of severe loss of joint space, bone destruction, intra-articular osseous debris, joint disorganization, and deformity. Furthermore, osteophytosis, subchondral sclerosis, and cyst formation are notable by their relative infrequency. Coexistent rotator cuff disease adds to joint instability and permits migration of the humeral head superiorly, with narrowing of the subacromial space and marked bone attrition of the undersurface of the acromion, the lateral aspect of the clavicle, and glenoid fossa (Fig. 59-19). Such severe changes have been termed *cuff arthropathy* in the belief that the primary failure lies in the rotator cuff, followed by secondary joint failure.[45]

Apart from the shoulder, other joints are involved, especially the knee (approximately 50% of cases). Here, the lateral tibiofemoral compartment is typically involved, unlike "conventional" osteoarthritis (Fig. 59-20). As in the shoulder, joint space narrowing, collapse of the articular surfaces of the tibia and femur, valgus angulation, and a large noninflammatory joint effusion are evident. The patellofemoral compartment also may be affected. Overall, the rapidly destructive nature of the arthropathy may raise the possibility of septic arthritis or a neuropathic joint. In all cases it is important to recall that both chondrocalcinosis and the confirmed presence of CPPD crystals may be found. The relationship between these crystals and the etiology of the associated joint disease remains controversial. That they may coexist only serves to complicate the issue. Current conventional wisdom is that the crystals are markers of joint pathology and not the prime cause (Fig. 59-21).

Magnetic Resonance Imaging

Hydroxyapatite and basic calcium phosphates are often observed on MR images as low signal on all sequences at the site of deposition; however, in the setting of superimposed inflammation, edema and enhancement of surrounding soft tissues as well as adjacent bursitis, tenosynovitis, and joint synovitis may be observed[36]; unless radiographic correlation is made, this can lead to misinterpretation as infection, injury, or even tumor.

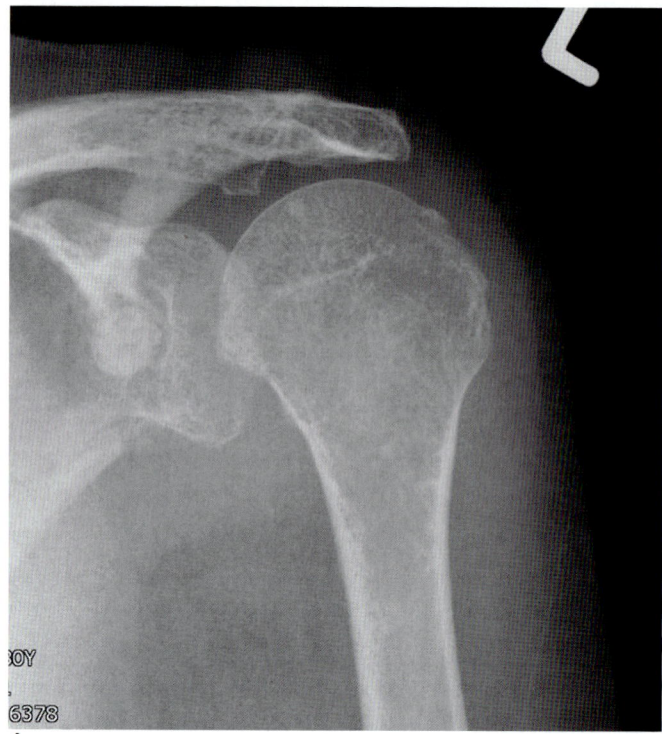

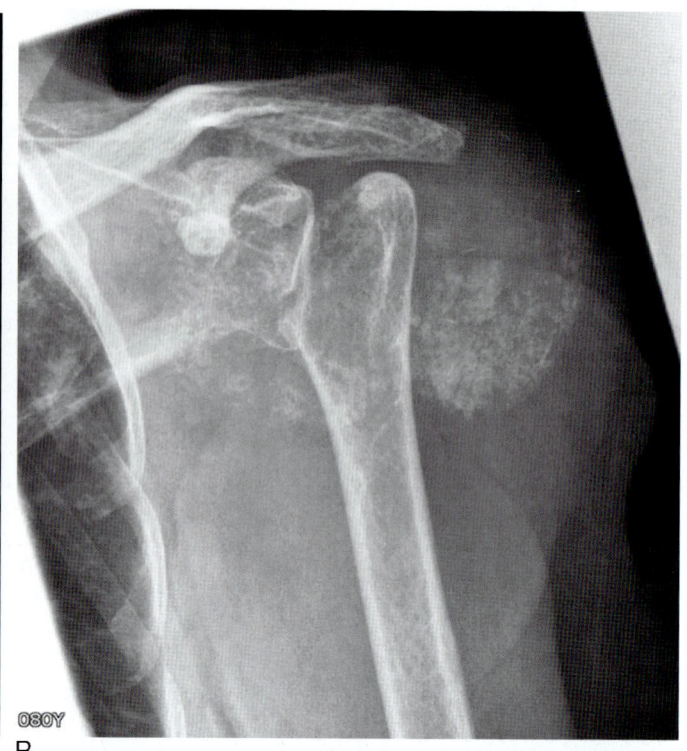

■ **FIGURE 59-18** Rapidly destructive osteoarthritis in an elderly female. **A,** The presentation image suggests a joint effusion but little else to predict the massive fragmentation and loss of bone that was shown 5 months later (**B**). **C,** The loss of bone, fragmentation, and extensive debris are well shown on the CT image. No suggestion of any other pathologic process was found.

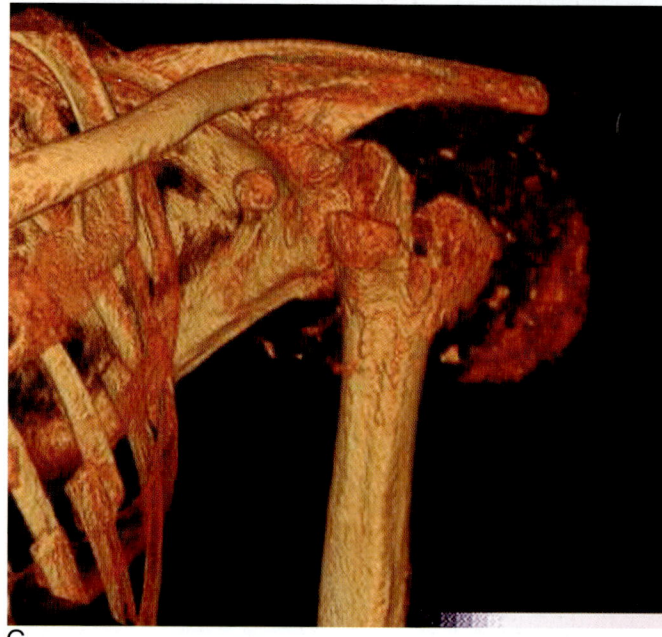

Multidetector Computed Tomography

Computed tomography is seldom indicated for diagnosis of pathology related to crystal deposition. However, CT is more sensitive for detection of calcification and can better localize deposition compared with radiographs. Additionally, rarely, the deposition results in erosion of adjacent bone, which can simulate tumor; CT is helpful to document the presence of intraosseous calcium.

Ultrasonography

With transient synovitis related to HA/BCP deposition, ultrasound examination may reveal acute synovitis with rather turbid, reflective joint fluid.

Nuclear Medicine

The deposition of HA/BCP and acute inflammation can cause uptake on bone scintigraphy in the affected area

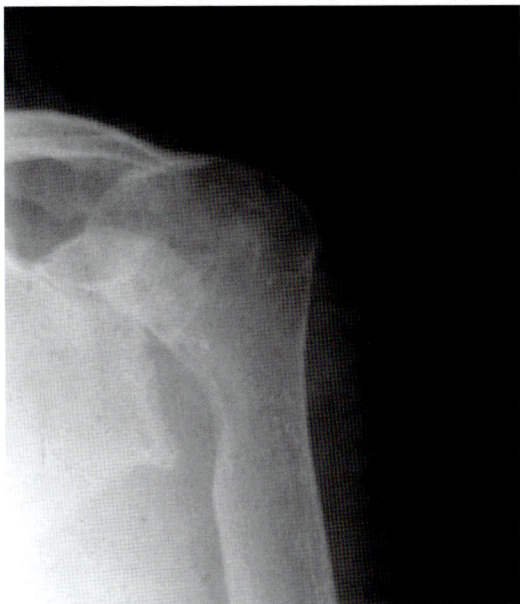
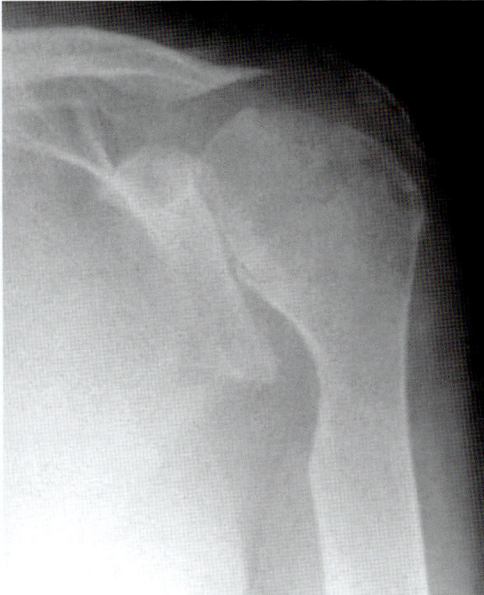

■ **FIGURE 59-19** Rapidly destructive osteoarthritis in another elderly female. Note the instability of the shoulder joint on two consecutive images, the atrophy of bone, and the lack of secondary repair phenomena (no new bone, osteophyte, or sclerosis).

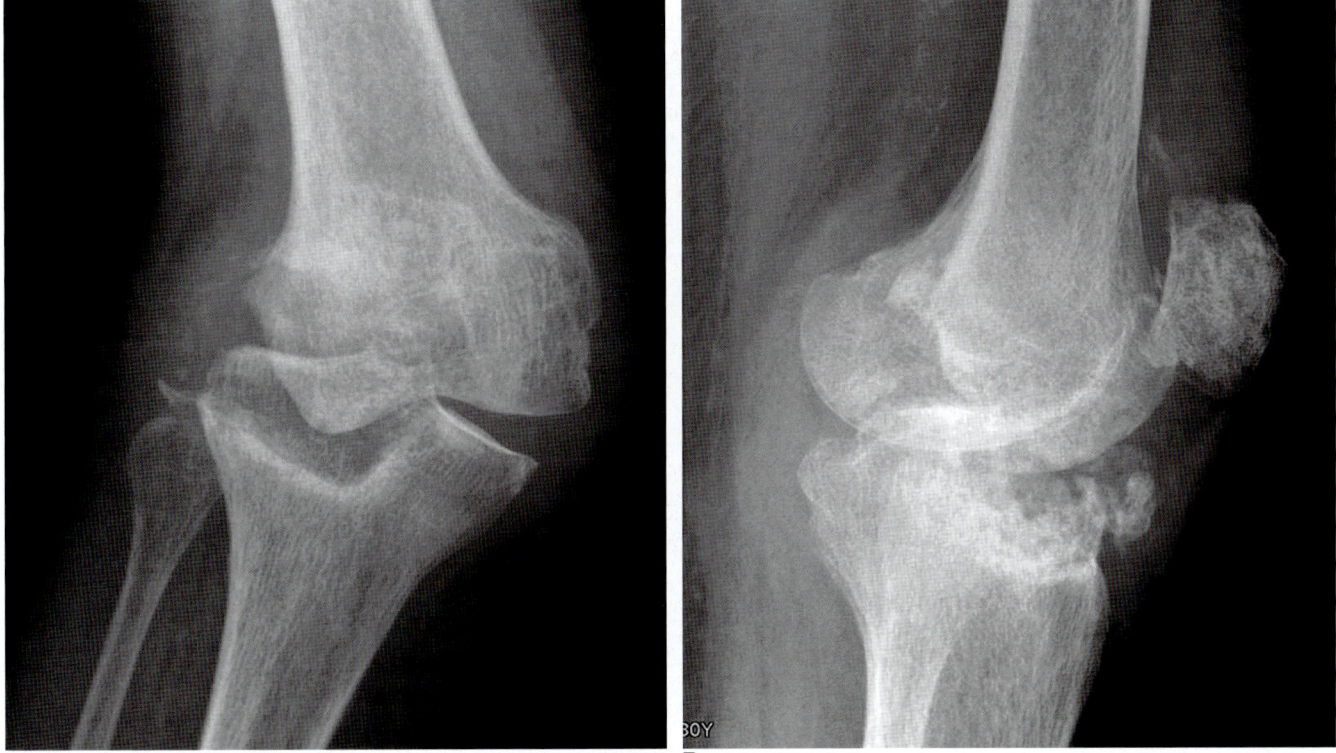

A   B

■ **FIGURE 59-20** **A,** Rapidly destructive osteoarthritis affecting the lateral tibiofemoral joint compartment. This is the same patient as in Figure 59-8. **B,** Note particularly the destruction of the tibial plateau, the valgus deformity, the large joint effusion, and the lack of secondary bone repair.

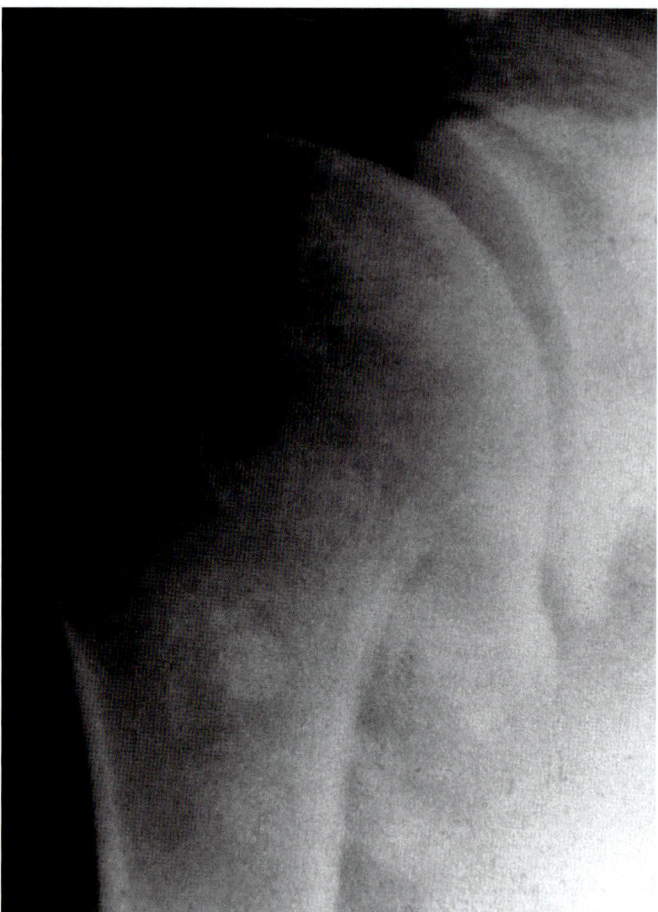

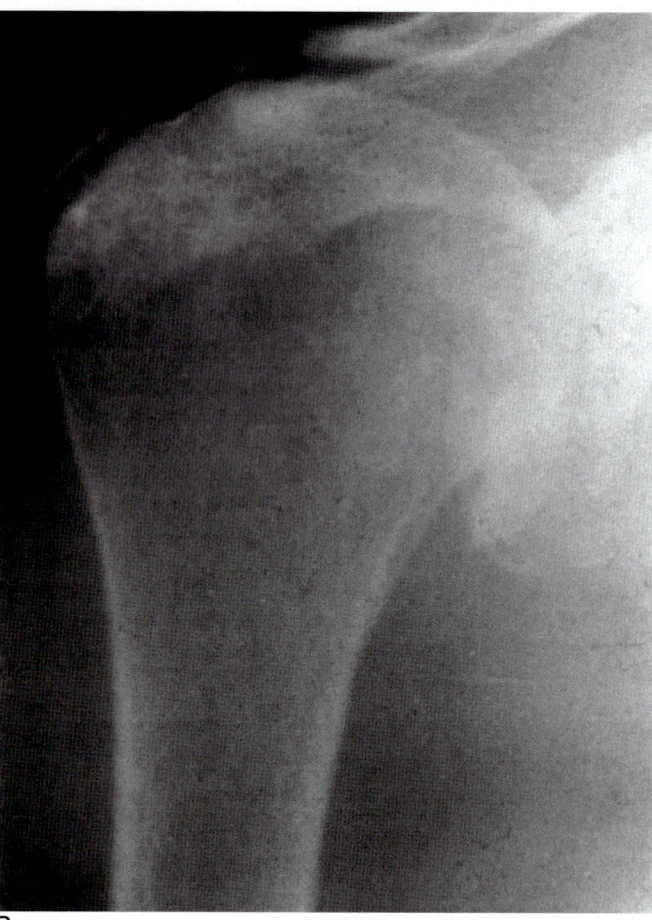

A   B

■ **FIGURE 59-21**   What is the role of crystals in arthritis? **A,** This elderly woman had a stiff shoulder with marked osteophytosis and some sclerosis. Joint aspiration contained abundant CPPD crystals but no excess of BCP. One year later, she had increasing pain. **B,** The radiograph now shows atrophic changes, the osteophytes and sclerosis are no longer present, and a large joint effusion is shown in the subdeltoid bursa. Aspiration at this time showed scanty CPPD crystals but now abundant BCP collections. What caused the switch from hypertrophic to atrophic osteoarthritis is unclear, but the crystals seem to be a marker of disease process rather than the prime etiology.

in a nonspecific fashion and therefore can be a source of confusion unless findings are correlated with those of radiographic examinations. On occasion, skeletal scintigraphy may have been undertaken to exclude bone disease or infection. The scintigraphic changes of calcific periarthritis can be striking (see Fig. 59-13).

Classic Signs

- Globular calcification within tendons and bursae
- Adjacent soft tissue swelling/hyperemia with edema and enhancement seen with acute inflammation; clinically presents as severe pain, occasionally accompanied by a low-grade fever.
- Calcium often resorbs after the acute attack.

Differential Diagnosis

Other crystals apart from monosodium urate (see Chapter 58), CPPD, and calcium HA may be associated with soft tissue, bone, and joint abnormalities. These include cholesterol crystals that are found in joint fluid in patients with rheumatoid arthritis and osteoarthritis and may be associated with low-grade synovitis; corticosteroid preparations, which when injected into joints are accompanied by a mild synovial inflammatory response; and calcium oxalate crystals, which arise in both primary and secondary oxalosis, the latter most typically occurring as a complication of chronic renal disease.

Cholesterol

Crystals of cholesterol are common findings in synovial fluid microscopically seen as stacked rectangular or rhomboid plates with a defective corner. They measure 5 to 10 μm and while they may be found in almost any joint aspirate are most frequently found in rheumatoid arthritis and, less commonly, osteoarthritis. Cholesterol crystals are not a feature of synovial fluid in patients with hyperlipoproteinemia. The etiology is unknown; transient synovitis occurs secondary to phagocytosis when cholesterol crystals are injected intra-articularly. The resulting cholesterol granulomas, synovial lining cell hyperplasia, and synovial fibrosis suggest that cholesterol crystals may result in a genuine, albeit low-grade, synovitis in vivo.

Corticosteroids

A number of intra-articular corticosteroid products are available for injection that may persist for some time. Subsequent joint aspiration may reveal crystals that may be mistaken for urate or CPPD using polarizing light microscopy. Some crystals are large, round edged, and clumped together. Others are tiny, with positive birefringence (similar to CPPD crystals), or larger, needle shaped, and negatively birefringent (similar to urate crystals).

Experimental intra-articular injection of these products may be associated with a white blood cell exudative response. The resulting inflammation is less than that occurring after injection of sodium urate or CPPD crystals but may account for transient flares of synovitis seen about 24 hours after intra-articular injection in clinical practice.

Calcium Oxalate (Oxalosis)

Calcium oxalate crystals may be deposited either as the result of a rare hereditary process or, more commonly, secondary to chronic renal disease.

Primary oxalosis is an autosomal recessive trait in which glycolic aciduria is secondary to the absence of one of two enzymes. The resulting excessive production of oxalate crystals causes accumulation in the kidneys particularly either as nephrolithiasis or nephrocalcinosis, resulting in progressive renal failure. Deposition also occurs in the small arteries, eyes, soft tissues, and bone. Both sexes are affected; clinical onset is usually before the age of 5 years due to renal disease. Routine radiographs may reveal small, contracted kidneys with parenchymal calcification due to crystal deposition in the renal tubules (Fig. 59-22). Renal glomeruli are normal.

Bony changes comprise poorly defined, dense metaphyseal bands in the long bones with abnormal tubulation (Fig. 59-23). Alternating radiolucent and radiodense bands may occur in flat bones, and the spine may resemble the "rugger-jersey" appearance of renal osteodystrophy (Fig. 59-24). In the later stages of the disease features of secondary hyperparathyroidism and osteomalacia due to renal osteodystrophy may complicate the presentation (Fig. 59-25).

Secondary oxalosis complicates other diseases, especially renal disorders. Ingestion of excessive oxalate or substances that are metabolized to oxalate (rhubarb, ethylene glycol), thiamine, and pyridoxine deficiencies that inhibit glyoxylate metabolism and increase production of oxalate and intestinal malabsorption or steatorrhea

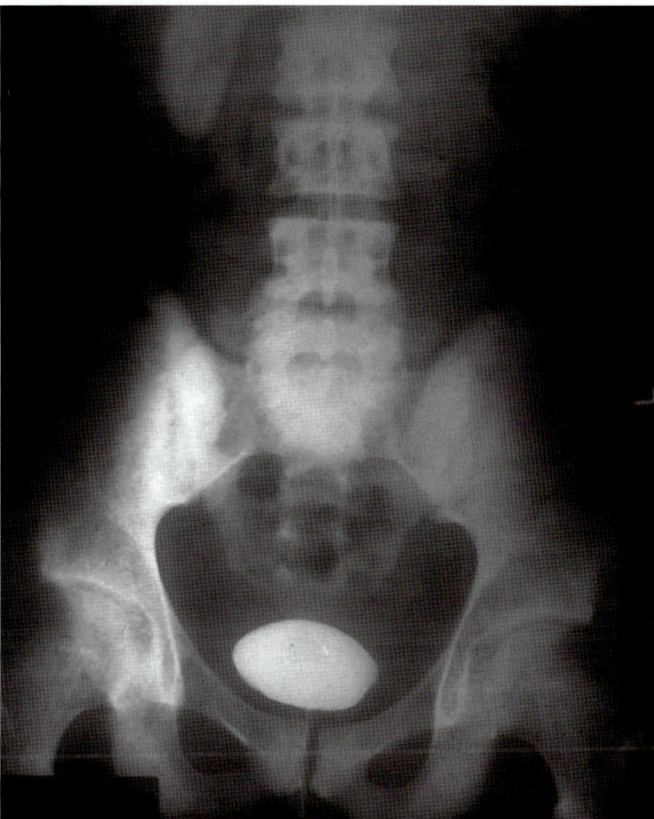

■ **FIGURE 59-22** Primary oxalosis. An abdominal radiograph reveals a shrunken, calcified kidney, sclerotic bone, and wide irregular sacroiliac joints due to secondary hyperparathyroidism. Contrast medium is present in the bladder.

also are recognized causes. Resultant crystal deposition in bone and soft tissues may cause joint effusions, pain, and stiffness, typically involving the knees, wrists, and MCP and interphalangeal joints. The term *oxalate gout* has been used. Bony manifestations are of a more subtle diffuse sclerosis than that of the primary disorder (Fig. 59-26).

Chondrocalcinosis, as well as calcification in the joint capsule and tendons, can arise due to oxalate deposition as well as that due to CPPD and occasionally hydroxyapatite. Furthermore, the picture may be complicated by secondary hyperparathyroidism and amyloid deposition. Secondary oxalosis is a disorder to be borne in mind when dealing with a patient in renal failure or in a known risk group.

Synopsis of Treatment Options

Medical Treatment

Treatment of acute calcific tendinosis, bursitis, and periarthritis consists of supportive care and nonsteroidal anti-inflammatory drugs (NSAIDs). Rapid response to NSAIDs within 1 or 2 days is typical. Occasionally, needle aspiration is performed; a large-gauge (e.g., 18-gauge) needle should be used because the consistency has been likened

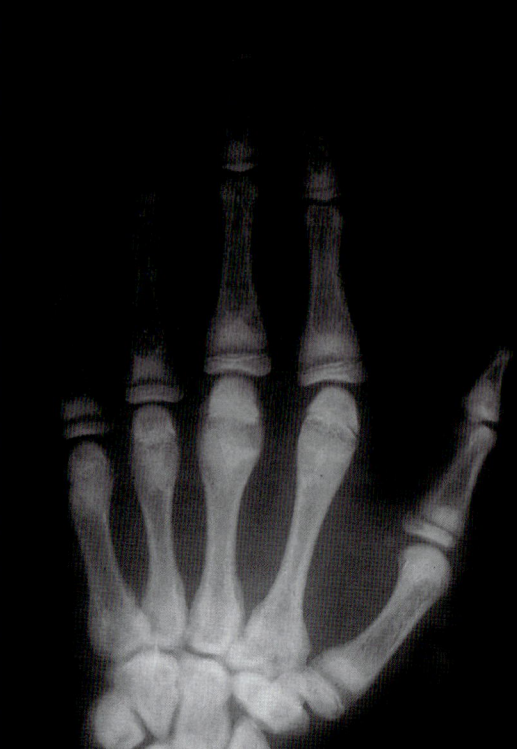
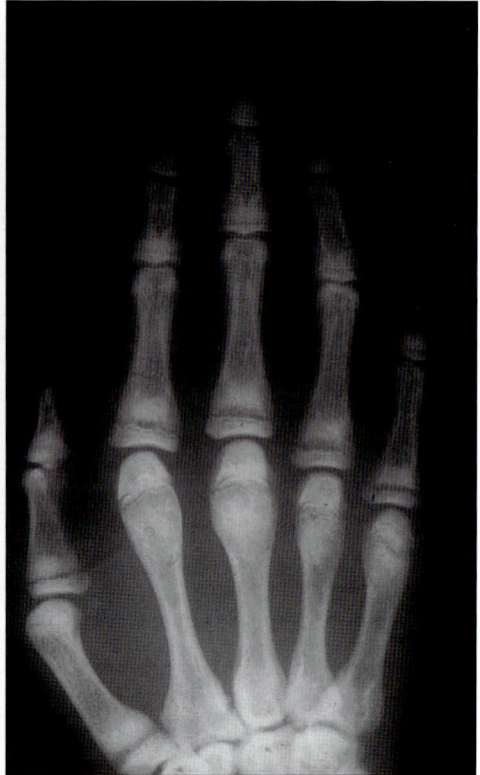

■ **FIGURE 59-23** Primary oxalosis. The skeleton is sclerotic with ill-defined bands of radiolucency at the former metaphyses. Note the slightly abnormal tubulation of bone.

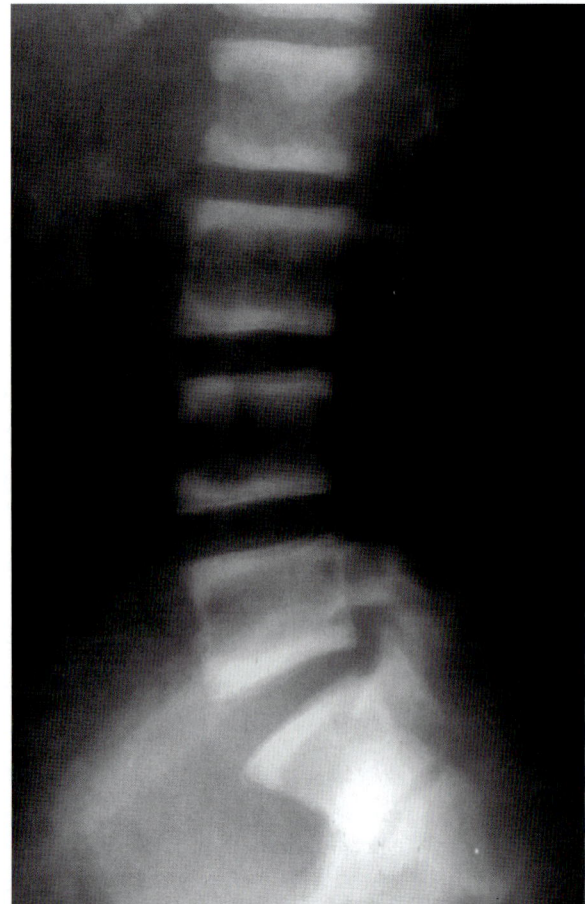

■ **FIGURE 59-24** Primary oxalosis. The dense sclerotic bands in the lumbar vertebrae resemble those of hyperparathyroidism but are more marked and associated with abnormal bone tubulation.

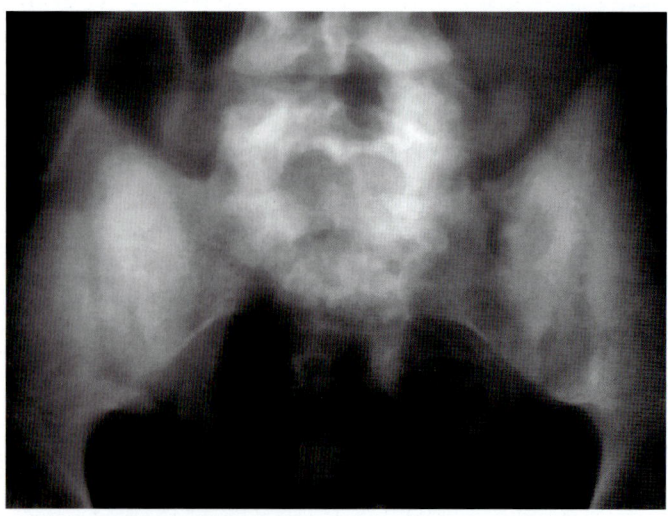

■ **FIGURE 59-25** Primary oxalosis. A localized view of the sacroiliac joints demonstrates the wide, irregular nature of the joint margins due to secondary hyperparathyroidism in another patient.

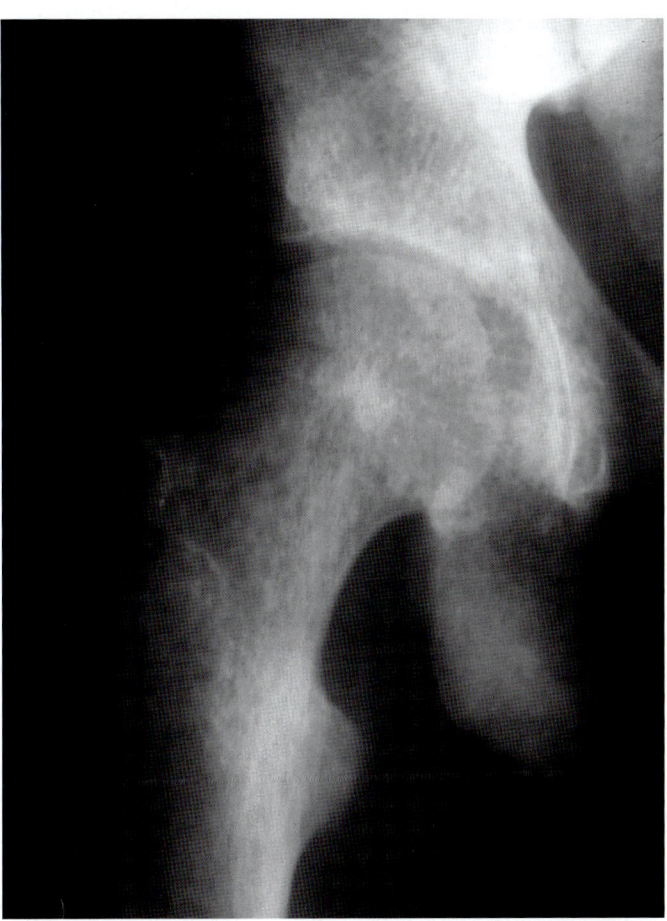

■ **FIGURE 59-26** Secondary oxalosis. Note the diffuse, ill-defined sclerosis of bone in this patient with renal failure. It would be difficult, from this image alone, to be totally sure of the primary etiology.

to that of toothpaste. Ultrasonography is helpful in needle guidance. In addition, irrigation of the site has been suggested using two needles within the deposit, with injection of saline through one and aspiration through the other.

Surgical Treatment

Surgical management is generally not indicated for acute crystal deposition disease.

What the Referring Physician Needs to Know

■ Identification of HA/BCP as cause of acute inflammatory clinical presentation, as opposed to infection

---

SUGGESTED READINGS

Choi MH, MacKenzie JD, Dalinka MK. Imaging features of crystal-induced arthropathy. Rheum Dis Clin North Am 2006; 32:427–446, viii.

Bencardino JT, Hassankhani A. Calcium pyrophosphate dihydrate crystal deposition disease. Semin Musculoskelet Radiol 2003; 7:175–185.

Steinbach LS, Resnick D. Calcium pyrophosphate dihydrate crystal deposition disease: imaging perspectives. Curr Probl Diagn Radiol 2000; 29:209–229.

Hayes CW, Conway WF. Calcium hydroxyapatite deposition disease. RadioGraphics 1990; 10:1031–1048.

Garcia GM, McCord GC, Kumar R. Hydroxyapatite crystal deposition disease. Semin Musculoskelet Radiol 2003; 7:187–193.

REFERENCES

1. McCarty DJ, Hollander JL. Identification of urate crystals in gouty synovial fluid. Ann Intern Med 1961; 54:452–460.
2. McCarty DJ, Kohn NN, Faires JS. The significance of calcium pyrophosphate crystals in synovial fluid of arthritis patients: the "pseudogout" syndrome. Ann Intern Med 1962; 56:711–737.
3. Zitnan D, Sitaj S. Chondrocalcinosis polyarticularis (familiaris): roentgenological and clinical analysis. Cesk Rentgenol 1960; 14:27–34.
4. Timms AE, Zhang Y, Russell RG, Brown MA. Genetic studies of disorders of calcium crystal deposition. Rheumatology 2002; 41:725–727.
5. Scotchford CA, Greenwald S, Ali SY. Calcium phosphate crystal distribution in the superficial zone of human femoral head articular cartilage. J Anat 1992; 181:293–300.
6. Martel W, Champion CK, Thompson GR, et al. A roentgenologically distinctive arthropathy in some patients with the pseudogout syndrome. AJR Am J Roentgenol 1970; 109:587–605.
7. Steinbach LS, Resnick D. Calcium pyrophosphate dihydrate crystal deposition disease revisited. Radiology 1996; 200:1–9.
8. Doherty M, Dieppe P, Watt I. Low incidence of calcium pyrophosphate dihydrate crystal deposition in rheumatoid arthritis, with modification of radiographic features in coexistent disease. Arthritis Rheum 1984; 27:1002–1009.
9. Doherty M, Watt I, Dieppe P. Localised chondrocalcinosis in post-meniscectomy knees. Lancet 1982; 1:1207–1210.
10. Doherty M, Watt I, Dieppe P. Influence of primary generalised osteoarthritis on development of secondary osteoarthritis. Lancet 1983; 2:8–11.

11. Swan A, Heywood B, Chapman B, et al. Evidence for a causal relationship between the structure, size and load of calcium pyrophosphate dihydrate crystals, and attacks of pseudogout. Ann Rheum Dis 1995; 54:825-830.

12. Rogers J, Shepstone L, Dieppe P. Bone formers: osteophyte and enthesophyte formation are positively correlated. Ann Rheumatic Dis 1997; 56:85-90.

13. Dequeker J. The inverse relationship between osteoporosis and osteoarthritis. Adv Exp Med Biol 1999; 455:419-422.

14. Resnick D, Niwayama G, Georgen TG, et al. Clinical, radiographic and pathologic abnormalities in calcium pyrophosphate dihydrate deposition disease (CPPD): pseudogout. Radiology 1977; 122:1-15.

15. Yamakawa K, Iwasaki H, Ohjimi Y, et al. Tumoral calcium pyrophosphate dihydrate crystal deposition disease. Pathol Res Pract 2001; 197:499-506.

16. Rivera-Sanfeliz G, Resnick D, Haghighi P, et al. Tophaceous pseudogout. Skeletal Radiol 1996; 25:699-701.

17. Martel W, McCarter DK, Solsky MA, et al. Further observations on the arthropathy of calcium pyrophosphate crystal deposition disease. Radiology 1981; 141:1-15.

18. Doherty M, Preston B. Primary osteoarthritis of the elbow. Ann Rheum Dis 1989; 48:743-747.

19. Stucki G, Hardegger D, Böhni U, Michel BA. Degeneration of the scaphoid-trapezium joint: a useful finding to differentiate calcium pyrophosphate deposition disease from osteoarthritis. Clin Rheumatol 1999; 18:232-237.

20. Rogers J, Dieppe P. Is tibiofemoral osteoarthritis in the knee a new disease? Ann Rheum Dis 1994; 53:612-613.

21. Doherty M, Dieppe P, Watt I. Pyrophosphate arthropathy: a prospective study. Br J Rheumatol 1993; 32:189-196.

22. Felson DT. The epidemiology of knee osteoarthritis: results from the Framingham osteoarthritis study. Semin Arthritis Rheum 1990; 20(Suppl):42-50.

23. Neame RL, Carr AJ, Muir K, Doherty MD. Community prevalence of chondrocalcinosis and evidence that correlation with osteoarthritis is through a shared association with osteophyte. Rheumatology 2002; 41(Suppl 1):19-20.

24. Ross DA, Dieppe PA, Watt I, Newman JH. Tibial stress fracture in pyrophosphate arthropathy. J Bone Joint Surg Br 1983; 65:474-477.

25. Chen C, Chandnini VP, Chang HS, et al. Scapholunate advanced collapse: a common wrist abnormality in calcium pyrophosphate crystal deposition disease. Radiology 1990; 177:459-461.

26. Adamson TC III, Resnik CS, Guerra J Jr, et al. Hand and wrist arthropathies of hemochromatosis and calcium pyrophosphate deposition disease: distinct radiographic features. Radiology 1983; 147:377-381.

27. Berlemann U, Gries NC, Moore RJ, et al. Calcium pyrophosphate dihydrate deposition in degenerate lumbar discs. Eur Spine J 1998; 7:45-49.

28. Kakitsubata Y, Boutin RD, Theodorou DJ, et al. Calcium pyrophosphate dihydrate crystal deposition in and around the atlantoaxial joint: association with type 2 odontoid fractures in nine patients. Radiology 2000; 216:213-219.

29. Abreu M, Johnson K, Chung CB, et al. Calcification in calcium pyrophosphate dihydrate (CPPD) crystalline deposits in the knee: anatomic, radiographic, MR imaging, and histologic study in cadavers. Skeletal Radiol 2004; 33:392-398.

30. Falsetti P, Frediani B, Acciai C, et al. Ultrasonographic study of Achilles tendon and plantar fascia in chondrocalcinosis. J Rheumatol 2004; 31:2242-2250.

31. Timms AE, Zhang Y, Russell RG, Brown MA. Genetic studies of disorders of calcium crystal deposition. Rheumatology 2002; 41:725-729.

32. Giachelli CM. Inducers and inhibitors of biomineralization: lessons from pathological calcification. Orthod Craniofacial Res 2005; 8:229-231.

33. Wright V, Haq AM. Periarthritis of the shoulder: I. Aetiological considerations with particular reference to personality factors. Ann Rheum Dis 1976; 35:213-219.

34. Gondos B. Observations on periarthritis calcarea. AJR Am J Roentgenol 1957; 77:93-108.

35. Hayes CW, Conway WF. Calcium hydroxyapatite deposition disease. RadioGraphics 1990; 10:1031-1048.

36. Bui-Mansfield LT, Moak M. Magnetic resonance appearance of bone marrow edema associated with hydroxyapatite deposition disease without cortical erosion. J Comput Assist Tomogr 2005; 29:103-107.

37. Kraemer EJ, El-Khoury GY. Atypical calcific tendinitis with cortical erosions. Skeletal Radiol 2000; 29:690-696.

38. Jim YF, Hsu HC, Chang CY, et al. Coexistence of calcific tendinitis and rotator cuff tear; an arthrographic study. Skeletal Radiol 1993: 22:183-185.

39. De Maeseneer M, Vreugde S, Laureys S, et al. Calcific tendinitis of the longus colli muscle. Head Neck 1997; 19:545-548.

40. Dieppe PA, Crocker P, Huskisson EC, Willoughby DA. Apatite deposition disease: a new arthropathy. Lancet 1976; 1:266-268.

41. McCarty DJ, Cheung HS, Halverson PB, Garancis JC. "Milwaukee shoulder" syndrome: microspherules containing hydroxyapatite, acetic collagenase and neutral protease in patients with rotator cuff defects and glenohumeral osteoarthritis. Semin Arthritis Rheum 1981; 11(Suppl 1): 119-121.

42. Halverson PB, Carrera GF, McCarty DJ. Milwaukee shoulder syndrome: fifteen additional cases and a description of contributing factors. Arch Intern Med 1990; 150:677-682.

43. Dieppe PA, Cawston T, Mercer E, et al. Synovial fluid collagenase in patients with destructive arthritis of the shoulder joint. Arthritis Rheum 1988; 31:882-890.

44. Dieppe P, Doherty M, MacFarlane D, et al. Apatite associated destructive arthritis. Br J Rheumatol 1984; 23:84-91.

45. Neer CS 2nd, Craig EV, Fukuda H. Cuff-tear arthropathy. J Bone Joint Surg Am 1983; 65:1232-1244.

CHAPTER 60

Neuropathic Osteoarthropathy

Sandra Moore

Neuropathy results from functional abnormalities or structural insults to the axons (sensory, motor, or combined), the myelin, or both. The insensate neuropathic joint is liable to arthrosis, fractures, alignment deformities, abnormal function, ulcer, and infection. Predilection for skeletal location is influenced by whether the insult is central or peripheral and the degree to which sensory, motor, and/or autonomic function is insulted. Because diabetic pedal neuroarthropathy (Charcot foot) is commonly encountered by radiologists, the presentation and pathogenesis of this entity is emphasized.

ETIOLOGY

Neuropathy may be inherited, congenital, or acquired. Inherited neuropathies include hereditary sensory and autonomic neuropathy, sporadic sensory neuropathy, and Charcot-Marie-Tooth disease. Congenital insensitivity to pain (familial dysautonomia with and without anhidrosis) is a well-known but uncommon neuropathy of unknown etiology. Acquired peripheral neuropathy results from neural insult secondary to trauma, cancer, many common drugs including corticosteroids, human immunodeficiency virus infection, nutritional deficiencies, alcoholism, syphilis, vascular and metabolic diseases including diabetes mellitus types 1 and 2, and/or infection affecting the peripheral nerves. Central causes for neuropathy include stroke, syringomyelia, tumor, spinal cord injury, and meningomyelocele.

PREVALENCE AND EPIDEMIOLOGY

Over 100 types of peripheral neuropathy have been described. Charcot-Marie-Tooth disease has a prevalence of 1 in 2500.[1] Syphilis was the disease most commonly associated with neuroarthropathy until antibiotic control in the mid 1930s. In some underdeveloped countries, Hansen's disease (leprosy) persists as a major cause of neuroarthropathy (see Chapter 68). The longer lifespan of diabetics due to insulin treatment permits the development of chronic complications, with diabetes presently the most common cause of neuroarthropathy in developed countries. There are an estimated 20 million diabetics in the United States,[2] with pedal neuropathy detectable in about 7.5% at disease onset and 30% overall. Only 0.1% to 2.5% progress to Charcot changes, which are more common in patients of advanced age, with longer disease duration, with poor glycemic control, and with ocular and renal damage.

CLINICAL PRESENTATION

Different neuropathic conditions have predilection for specific joints. In the upper extremity, syringomyelia is the most common cause for Charcot joint, usually of the shoulder, but occasionally the elbow or hand. The finding of shoulder girdle neuroarthropathy should elicit a search for cord abnormality (Fig. 60-1).[3,4] Congenital insensitivity

---

KEY POINTS

- Different neuropathic conditions have predilection for specific joints. In the upper extremity, syringomyelia is the most common cause of Charcot joint. Vertebral Charcot spine is usually seen in the setting of insult to the spinal cord. Lower extremity neuroarthropathy is manifest most commonly in diabetics and alcoholics.
- Charcot joint changes require intact vascularity. Regarding diabetic pedal complications, patients with vasculopathy and neuroarthropathy are different cohorts. Ulcers over bony exostoses are the conduit of infection in Charcot foot; cognizance of the patterns of collapse assists localization and specificity. If there is no ulcer, osteomyelitis is unlikely.

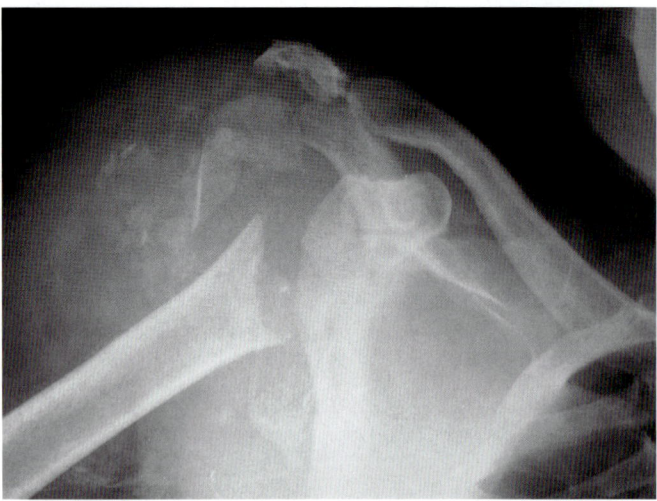

■ **FIGURE 60-1** A middle-aged man presented with shoulder pain. Anteroposterior radiograph shows effusion, fracture, fragmentation, and dislocation of the humeral head. The sharp margination of the shaft fragment is characteristic of Charcot shoulder. A cervical MRI revealed a syrinx.

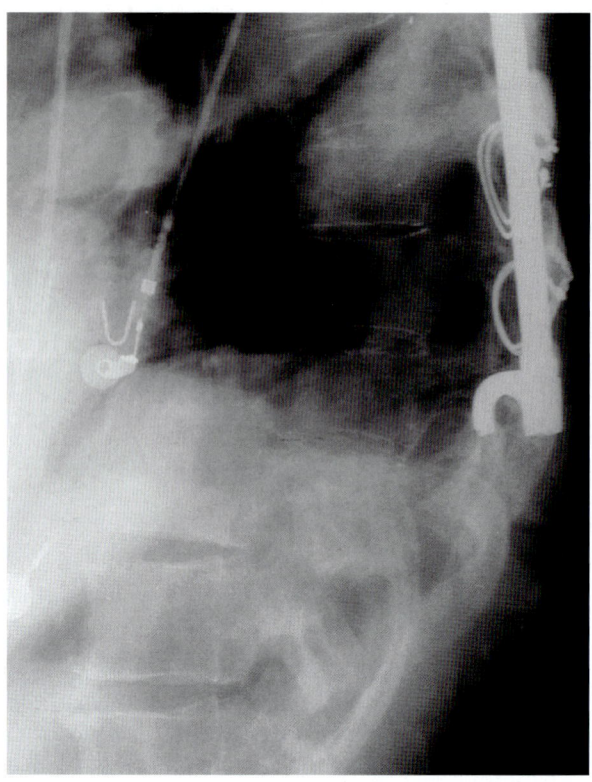

■ **FIGURE 60-2** Vertebral Charcot joint with fracture and frank vertebral dislocation, just caudal to the level of stabilization hardware.

to pain can involve multiple joints (lower extremity > upper extremity) and the spine. Syphilitic and alcoholic neuropathies affect the weight-bearing joints of the lower extremity, most commonly the knee. Alcoholic pedal neuroarthropathy manifests in the forefoot.[5] The inherited nerve disorder of Charcot-Marie-Tooth disease (type 1 demyelization, type 2 axonal) is manifested by progressive motor and sensory neuropathy due to damage to the peroneal nerve. Fatty replacement and atrophy of calf and pedal flexor and extensor muscles results in high arch and claw-toe deformities.[6] Diabetic neuroarthropathy usually affects the ankle and tarsus and, less commonly, the metatarsophalangeal joints. Large-joint Charcot involvement does occur in diabetes, although uncommonly.[7] The neuroarthropathy of Hansen's disease commonly involves the feet or hands, resembling other conditions with sensory deficit, such as frostbite and scleroderma. Vertebral involvement is seen with cord pathologic processes such as meningomyelocele, congenital insensitivity to pain,[8] syphilis, and, rarely, diabetes. If the spine is fused, Charcot changes usually are seen just caudal to the lowest fused level (Fig. 60-2).[3]

With congenital insensitivity to pain, trivial trauma may result in fracture or epiphyseal detachment. Beginning at birth, manifestations include fractures, dislocations, Charcot joints, osteonecrosis, and osteomyelitis, most commonly of femur, tibia, metatarsals, and spine (Fig. 60-3).[9,10] In the chronic setting, the extremities may be shortened due to premature epiphyseal fusion.

Diabetic Pedal Neuropathy

Pedal neuropathy is often asymmetric in diabetics, with the acutely affected foot edematous, with or without pain. Chronic motor neuropathy produces muscle atrophy resulting in alignment deformities.[11,12] If neuropathy is unchecked, Charcot changes may ensue. The acute Charcot foot will be hot and edematous with

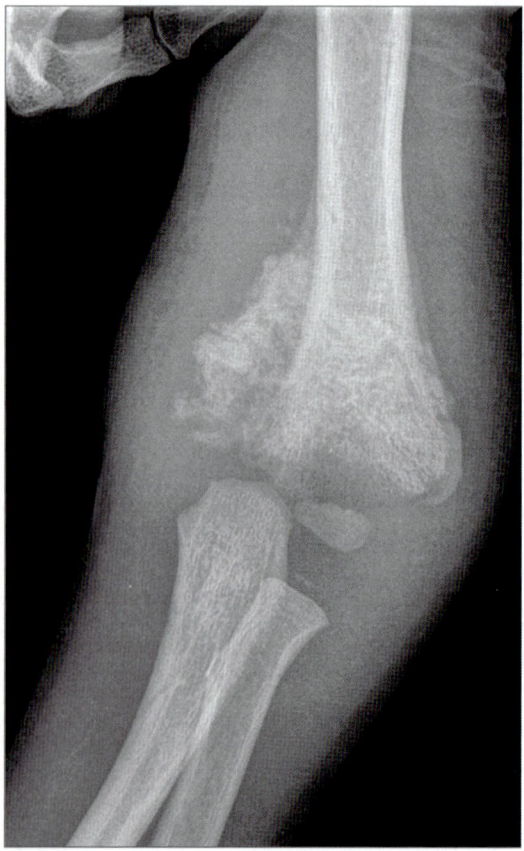

■ **FIGURE 60-3** Congenital insensitivity to pain. Anteroposterior radiograph shows comminuted fracture of the distal humerus with fragmentation and exuberant callus formation. The known context of congenital insensitivity to pain militates against a diagnosis of tumor. *(Courtesy of Gary Gold, MD, Stanford University, Palo Alto, CA.)*

palpable pulses and is clinically worrisome for cellulitis or even osteomyelitis. The mean skin temperature increases from 2° to 5° C in the Charcot joint as compared with the contralateral foot.[13] Rearfoot valgus, forefoot adductus, and hypermobile joints are common. Diabetic ischemic ulcers usually occur at the toes or the plantar aspect of the first and fifth metatarsal heads[14] and are shallow, erythematous, and painful and do not bleed. In contradistinction, diabetic neuropathic ulcers are fungating and callused, may bleed, can be painless, and typically occur over midfoot and hindfoot bony protuberances.

PATHOPHYSIOLOGY

Jean Martin Charcot posited that neuropathic arthropathy (usually luetic in the 1860s) resulted from damage to the central nervous system and "trophic" peripheral centers controlling the nutrition of bones and joints. His concepts are no longer in currency, but Charcot's name continues as the descriptor for neuropathic osteoarthopathy. Two theories—the neurovascular and the neurotraumatic—elucidate the pathophysiology of neuroarthropathy. According to the neurovascular theory, in the absence of neural stimulus to the extremities, sympathetic tone is compromised. This results in vasodilatation and hyperemia in the soft tissues *and* marrow, predisposing to osteopenic subchondral bone liable to pathologic fractures.[15] The fractures can heal with exuberant and bizarre callus formation. Diabetic Charcot changes require intact vascularity. Therefore, diabetic persons with vasculopathy and neuroarthropathy are nearly mutually exclusive cohorts, although there are case examples of persons with vasculopathy developing neuropathy after a revascularization procedure.[16]

The neurotraumatic theory explains neuroarthropathy as the result of diminished proprioception and loss of normal sensory feedback, with progressive joint destruction from repeated trauma. The patient may be unaware of the problem and add insult to injury by continuing to use the joint.

Most likely, both neurotraumatic and neurovascular causes are collusive in the diabetic neuropathic foot. Furthermore, hyperglycemia causes adverse effects on nerve metabolism, perineural vasoconstriction, and hypoxia. It is not understood why Charcot foot is often unilateral and occurs only in a small subset of diabetics.

Anatomy

Regarding pedal neuroarthropathy, the foot can be divided longitudinally into medial and lateral columns, with the medial column involved earlier and more frequently by neuroarthropathy. In diabetics, the forefoot is more often involved with ischemia and the midfoot and hindfoot are more often involved with neuroarthropathy. The *weight-bearing line* is drawn from the calcaneal tuberosity to the sesamoids on lateral radiographs taken with the patient bearing weight. If the pedal arch collapses and a bony structure extends below this line (i.e., rocker-bottom deformity), the overlying soft tissues may ulcerate (Fig. 60-4).

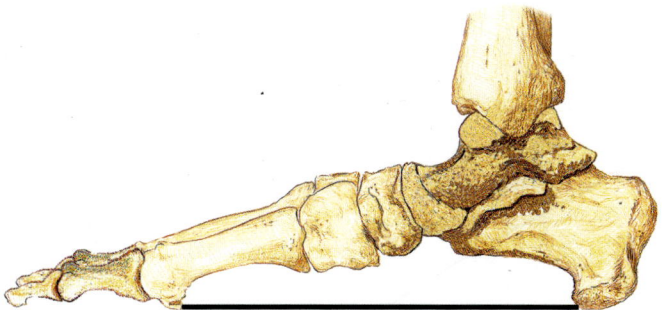

■ **FIGURE 60-4** The weight-bearing line is drawn on a standing lateral view of the foot between the plantar aspect of the calcaneus and the sesamoid bones. Any bone extending below this line in the setting of arch collapse comprises a "rocker" exostosis.

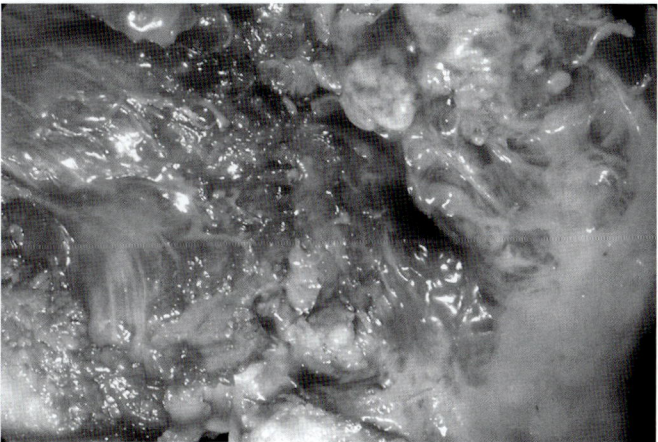

■ **FIGURE 60-5** Gross specimen of a Charcot joint (knee) shows bone and cartilage fragments embedded in the synovium. (*Courtesy of German Steiner, MD, Hospital for Joint Diseases, New York, NY.*)

Pathology

The gross Charcot foot specimen has bone fragments embedded in synovium (Fig. 60-5). On histologic study the specimen may demonstrate calcium, cartilage, and shards of bone lining the deep layers of the synovium. This is termed *detritic synovitis* and may also be seen with osteonecrosis, calcium pyrophosphate deposition disease, psoriatic arthritis, and osteoarthritis. Biopsy may be performed to confirm infected Charcot foot or differentiate Charcot foot from tumor (e.g., chondrosarcoma is occasionally initially considered in Charcot shoulder), but biopsy and histologic analysis are infrequently performed now to diagnose an uninfected Charcot joint.

BIOMECHANICS

Regarding pedal neuroarthropathy, in advanced Charcot joint disease, the plantar arch (medial > lateral) may collapse, resulting in a rocker-bottom deformity. There are several orthopedic classification systems for evaluation of patterns of pedal collapse. The classification system developed by Schön and colleagues[17] delineates four midfoot and hindfoot patterns that are readily discernable on radiographs and cross-sectional studies:

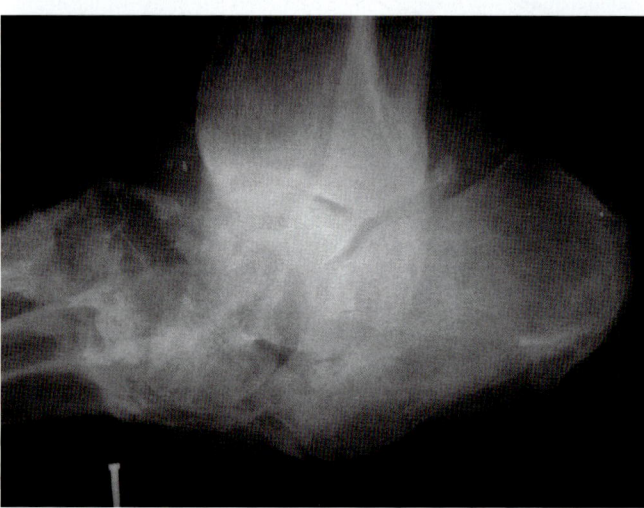

A

B

■ **FIGURE 60-6** **A,** Lateral radiograph of the foot demonstrates the Lisfranc pattern of arch collapse (Schön pattern I) with fracture-dislocation at the tarsometatarsal joints. The cuboid bone protrudes below the weight-bearing line. **B,** Lateral view of the foot demonstrates the transtarsal pattern of arch collapse (Schön pattern IV) with down-turned talar head, dislocated from the navicular. There is reversal of the normal calcaneal pitch, with anterior calcaneus and cuboid fragment "rocker" exostoses.

Class I: Lisfranc pattern at the tarsometatarsal joints (Fig. 60-6A)
Class II: Naviculocuneiform pattern
Class III: Chopart/perinavicular pattern
Class IV: Transverse tarsal pattern (see Fig. 60-6B) with plantargrade talar head, subluxed or dislocated from the navicular bone.

As the pedal arches collapse, weight bearing transfers to bone protruding below the weight-bearing line, the plantar-prominent "rocker." The pathogenesis of ulcer formation is not fully understood but may be related to ischemia and subcutaneous tissue breakdown over these plantar exostoses, allowing the ingress of pathogens. Awareness of the collapse patterns helps the radiologist localize the site of infection.

IMAGING TECHNIQUES

Techniques and Relevant Aspects

Imaging of a suspected neuropathic joint should always begin with routine standard radiographs and comparison with results of examinations if available. Because radiographs

may be misleading, if there is clinical concern for infection either an MR scan or a nuclear medicine study may be requested.

Controversies

Marrow edema in the setting of neuropathy or Charcot joint may enhance after the intravenous administration of gadolinium. If osteomyelitis is considered, the demonstration of marrow enhancement on routine MRI does not increase specificity. Gadolinium enhancement does improve sensitivity for secondary signs of osteomyelitis, including ulcer, adjacent sinus tracts and abscesses; and enhancement may help differentiate necrosis and abscess from vascularized tissue.[18]

MANIFESTATIONS OF THE DISEASE

Radiography

In the setting of a warm erythematous neuropathic joint, the radiologist may be asked to exclude superimposed infection. Radiographs may be negative or show soft tissue swelling and osteopenia. If Charcot derangement ensues, radiographs reveal classic findings of joint disorganization, dislocation, debris, and destruction. Charcot changes may occur gradually or catastrophically with derangement within days of minor trauma, such as a twisted ankle. Charcot osteoarthropathy evolves from the acute osteopenic phase (which mimics infection) to the bone-forming phase, characterized by exuberant repair, osteosclerosis, and bony fragmentation. A chronic neuroarthropathic joint shows derangement, bony hypertrophy, eburnation, and subchondral cysts. With offloading and casting, the hyperemia abates and the joint may be stabilized, but ulcers can develop over bony protuberances (see Chapter 65, Diabetic Pedal Infection).

Radiographs can be misleading in all phases of Charcot joint deformity, because the "bag of bones" may be so fragmented and indistinctly marginated that infection can be overcalled.

Magnetic Resonance Imaging

Magnetic resonance imaging is the anatomic gold standard for evaluating the neuropathic joint. It reveals edema due to neuropathic vasodilatation in the subcutaneous soft tissues, the muscles, and the bone marrow. Before the development of frank Charcot joint disease, marrow edema seen on MRI is presumed to be due to medullary hyperemia. This is called the "ghost sign" and in the absence of ulcer or other signs of soft tissue infection does *not* imply osteomyelitis (Fig. 60-7). If the neuropathic joint collapses, interpretation of MRI is challenging. There are significant overlapping MRI findings between acute Charcot foot and infection, including effusions, adventitial bursae, and extensive soft tissue and bone marrow edema. The marrow edema in noninfected neuroarthropathy has an *articular* epicenter (Fig. 60-8), whereas osteomyelitis has a *marrow* epicenter, involving fewer bones (Fig. 60-9).[18] It should be stressed that, in adults, pedal infection is introduced transcutaneously in more than 90% of cases. If there is no ulcer, osteomyelitis is unlikely, despite the

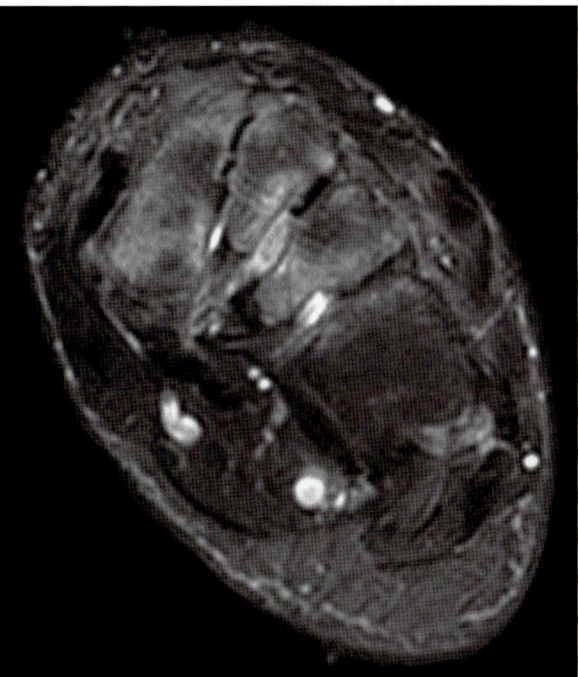

■ FIGURE 60-7   Short-axis, T2-weighted, fat-saturated MR image of the midfoot shows marrow edema of the cuneiforms. In the absence of secondary soft tissue findings of infection, this comprises the MRI "ghost sign" and reflects medullary hyperemia, not osteomyelitis.

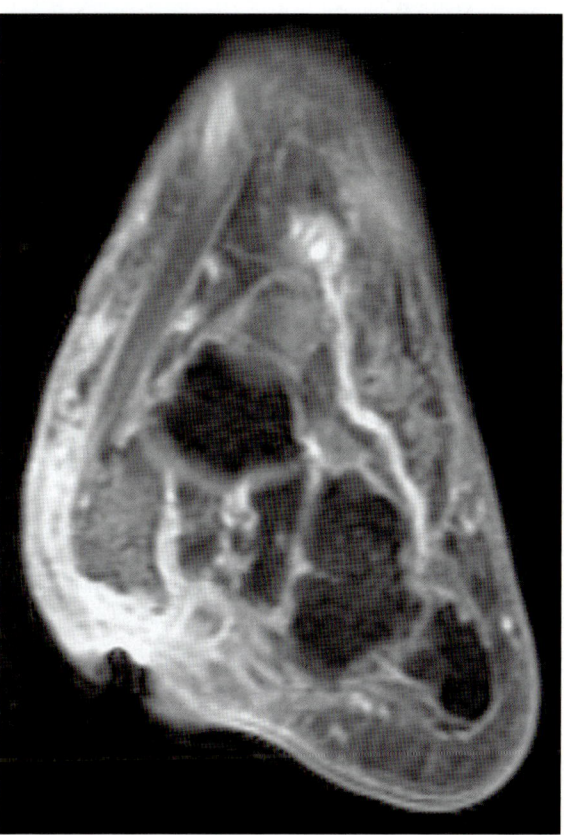

■ FIGURE 60-9   T1-weighted, fat-saturated, postcontrast, short-axis image of the midfoot shows an ulcer and tract directly underlying an edematous and enhancing first cuneiform. This bone protrudes below the weight-bearing line. Regardless of the presence of marrow edema in the adjacent bones due to Charcot foot collapse, the association of the tract and ulcer to the first cuneiform raises suspicion of osteomyelitis in this bone. *(Courtesy of Mark Schweitzer, NYU Medical Center, New York City.)*

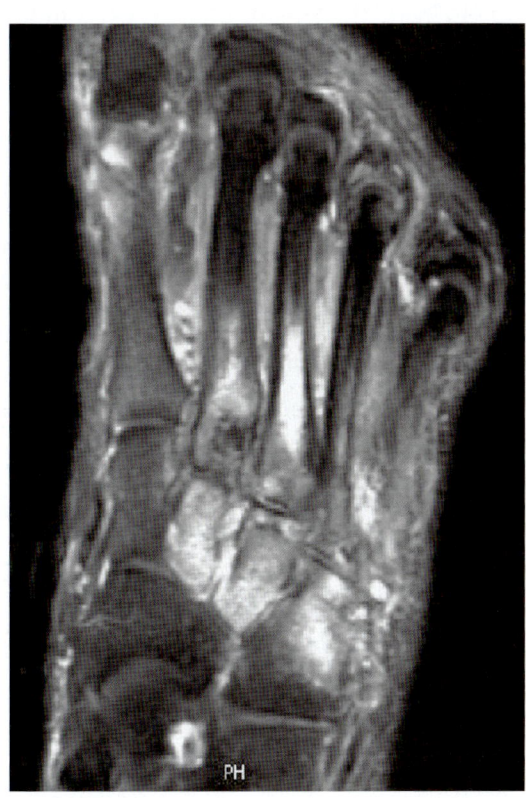

■ FIGURE 60-8   Acute Charcot foot. Inversion recovery MR image parallel to the plantar surface shows small subchondral fracture lines and marrow edema pattern with an articular epicenter.

frankly disconcerting marrow edema that is seen in acute Charcot foot. A close assessment of the marrow edema and arch collapse patterns, in concert with a search for "rocker" exostoses and associated secondary soft tissue findings, allows for a more confident and accurate differentiation. This directs a more conservative débridement.

Multidetector Computed Tomography

Computed tomography can be useful for evaluating subtle flake fractures, such as an early Lisfranc fracture-dislocation. It is of limited utility in differentiating the uninfected from the infected Charcot joint, but contrast enhancement helps with abscess localization. CT is useful to diagnose the extensive perivertebral bone fragments characteristic of spinal Charcot deformity but not expected in infection or neoplasm.

Nuclear Medicine

The nuclear medicine test of choice to differentiate between Charcot joint and superinfected Charcot deformity is combined indium-111-labeled leukocyte/technetium-99m sulfur colloid scan.

Classic Signs

- Neuropathy (before the development of a Charcot joint)—soft tissue edema
- Acute Charcot joint: Hyperemic, osteopenic bone is predisposed to fracture, leading to deformity, joint derangement, and bony fragmentation, with an articular epicenter.
- Chronic Charcot joint: Soft tissue swelling and marrow edema may subside. A stabilized osteoarthritic Charcot joint eventually shows bony ankylosis, subchondral cysts, alignment deformities, and exostoses that predispose to ulcer formation (Fig. 60-10).
- Infected Charcot joint (acute or chronic): Cutaneous ulcer over a bony exostosis or "rocker" prominence may track to bone or joint, leading to septic arthritis and/or osteomyelitis. This results in characteristic MRI findings of synovial and osseous infection. In the acute setting, this is difficult to tease from the "backdrop" of neuropathic edema and joint disorganization, but knowledge of collapse patterns and likely "rocker" location can direct the search for the likeliest site(s) of infection.

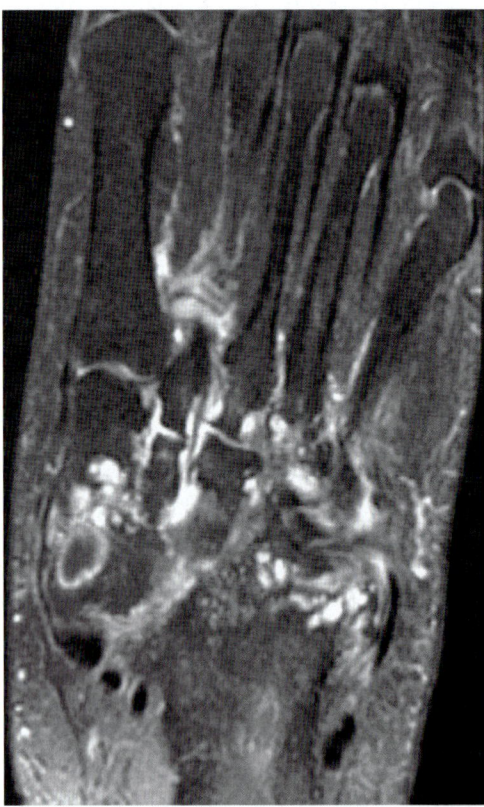

■ **FIGURE 60-10** Chronic Charcot foot. T1-weighted, fat-saturated MR image parallel to the plantar surface after intravenous administration of gadolinium. Hyperemia has subsided, but hindfoot derangement, subchondral cysts, and synovial enhancement are present. Rocker-bottom deformity may predispose to ulcers and infection.

A Charcot joint will show either no focal white cell accumulation or white cell activity correlating to the distribution of marrow as imaged by ^{99m}Tc sulfur colloid. Osteomyelitis will show focal white cell accumulation *without* corresponding marrow activity.[19]

DIFFERENTIAL DIAGNOSIS

Neuroarthropathy may mimic, and be misdiagnosed as, cellulitis, osteomyelitis, gout, severe osteoarthritis, and, rarely, matrix-producing tumor. Spinal Charcot deformity may resemble discitis or even neoplasm. Delay in diagnosis is common.

Peripheral nerve function is tested with Semmes-Weinstein monofilaments, which test perception of sensation with different thickness filaments and distances between filaments applied to the skin. Electrodiagnostic testing (velocity and electromyography) may be required to establish the etiology and level of a neural insult. Dermal thermography of Charcot foot is assessed with a handheld, infrared thermometer.

SYNOPSIS OF TREATMENT OPTIONS

Medical Treatment

Since the mid 1990s the trend for treating the acute Charcot joint has been immobilization and non–weight bearing with casting or bracing to halt the cascading joint destruction. If an ulcer is present, infection should be excluded. Débridement is kept as minimal as feasible. A surgical shoe, brace, or total contact cast is used to offload an ulcer. Nonoperative treatment is preferred, but up to 50% of patients with Charcot deformities eventually undergo surgery for ulcer recurrence or painful arthropathy.

Surgical Treatment

Salvage arthrodesis is becoming the procedure of choice over amputation.[20,21] Arthrodesis provides for corrective reshaping of deformities and elimination of instability. Internal fixation is performed if there is no ulcer, and external fixation (with pins at a distance from the infection site) is done if there is ulceration. The goal is stability and remodeling of the deformity not joint function, that is, an ambulating flat foot.

What the Referring Physician Needs to Know

- The critical question posed to the radiologist in the setting of neuroarthropathy and ulcer is: Are the deep soft tissues and/or bones infected?

SUGGESTED READINGS

Brower AC, Allman RM. The neuropathic joint: a neurovascular bone disorder. Radiol Clin North Am 1981; 19:571-580.

Gupta RA. A short history of neuropathic arthropathy. Clin Orthop Relat Res 1993; 296, 43-49.

Hartemann Huertier A, The Charcot foot. Lancet 2002; 360:1776-1779.

Jones EA, Manaster BK, May DA, Disler MD. Neuropathic osteoarthropathy: diagnostic dilemmas and differential diagnosis. RadioGraphics 2000; 20:S279-S293.

Ledermann HP, Morrison WB, Schweitzer M. MR image analysis of pedal osteomyelitis. Radiology 2002; 223:747-755.

Ledermann HP, Morrison WB. Differential diagnosis of pedal osteomyelitis and diabetic neuroarthropathy: MR imaging. Semin Musculoskel Radiol 2005; 9:272-328.

REFERENCES

1. National Institute of Neurological Disorders and Stroke. Charcot-Marie-Tooth Fact Sheet. NIH 07-4897, 2007.
2. www.cdc.gov/diabetes/statistics
3. Jones EA, Manaster BK, May DA, Disler MD. Neuropathic osteoarthropathy: diagnostic dilemmas and differential diagnosis. RadioGraphics 2000; 20:S279-S293.
4. Tristano AG, Willson ML, Montes De Oca I. Axillary vein thrombosis as a manifestation of rapidly progressive neuropathic arthropathy of the shoulder associated with syringomyelia. Mayo Clin Proc 2005; 80:416-418.
5. Thornhill IIL, Richter RW, Shelton ML, Johnson CA. Neuropathic arthropathy (Charcot forefeet) in alcoholics. Orthop Clin North Am 1973; 1:7-20.
6. Stilwell G, Kilcoyne RF, Sherman JL. Patterns of muscle atrophy in the lower limbs in patients with Charcot-Marie-Tooth disease as measured by magnetic resonance imaging. J Foot Ankle Surg 1995; 34:593-596.
7. Lambert AP, Close CF. Charcot neuroarthopathy of the knee in type 1 diabetes: treatment with TKA. Diabet Med 2002; 19:338-341.
8. Ingram CM, Harris MB, Dehne R. Charcot spinal arthropathy in congenital insensitivity to pain. Orthopedics 1996; 19:251-255.
9. Gherlinzoni F, Gherlinzoni G. Neurogenic joint disease secondary to congenital insensitivity to pain. Ital J Orthop Traumatol 1982; 8:487-492.
10. Greider TD. Orthopedic aspects of congenital insensitivity to pain. Clin Orthop Relat Res 1983; (172):177-185.
11. Bus SA, Yang QX, Wang JH, et al. Intrinsic muscle atrophy and toe deformity in the diabetic neuropathic foot: a magnetic resonance imaging study. Diabetes Care 2002; 25:1444-1450.
12. Greenman RL, Khaodhiar L, Lima C, et al. Foot small muscle atrophy is present before the detection of clinical neuropathy. Diabetes Care 2005; 28:1425-1430.
13. Archer AG, Roberts VC, Watkins PJ. Blood flow patterns in diabetic neuropathy. Diabetologia 1984; 27:563-567.
14. Ledermann HP, Morrison WB, Schweitzer M. MR image analysis of pedal osteomyelitis. Radiology 2002; 223:747-755.
15. Brower AC, Allman RM. The neuropathic joint: a neurovascular bone disorder. Radiol Clin North Am 1981; 19:571-580.
16. Edelman SV, Kosofsky EM, Paul RA, Kozak GP. Neuroarthropathy (Charcot's joint) in diabetes mellitus following revascularization surgery. Arch Intern Med 1987; 147:1504-1508.
17. Schön LC, Easley ME, Weinfeld SB. Charcot neuroarthropathy of the foot and ankle. Clin Orthop 1998; (349):116-131.
18. Ledermann HP, Morrison WB. Differential diagnosis of pedal osteomyelitis and diabetic neuroarthropathy: MR imaging. Semin Musculoskelet Radiol 2005; 9:272-283.
19. Palestro CJ, Megta HH, Patel M, et al. Marrow vs. infection in the Charcot joint: indium-111 leukocyte and technetium-99m sulfur colloid scintigraphy.
20. Cooper PS. Application of external fixators for management of Charcot deformities of the foot and ankle. Foot Ankle Clin 2002; 7:207-254.
21. Herbst SA. External fixation of Charcot arthropathy. Foot Ankle Clin 2004; 9:596-609.

Infection

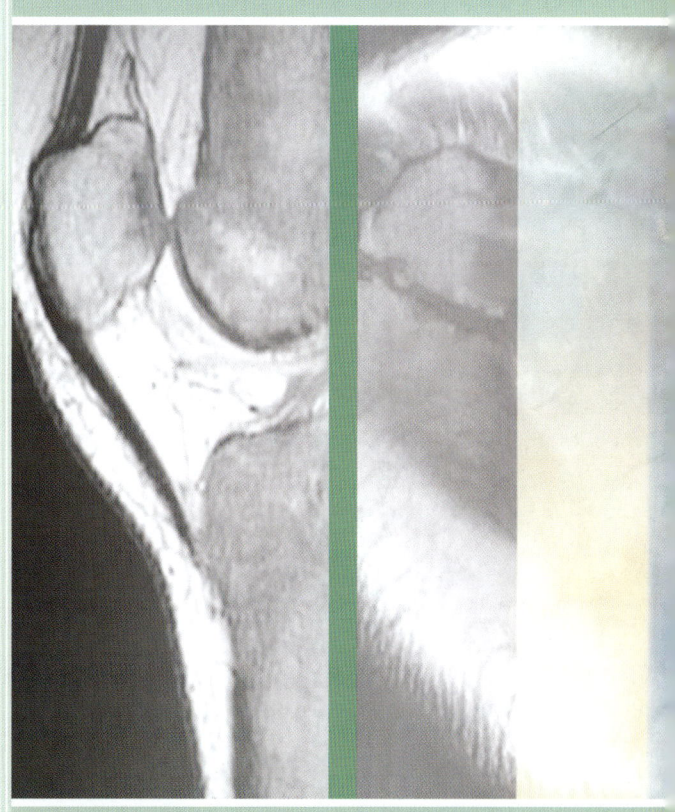

61

Soft Tissue Disease: Cellulitis, Pyomyositis, Abscess, Septic Arthritis

David Wilson and Bridget Atkins

Infections of the soft tissues range clinically from indolent low-grade conditions to fulminant disease that may be life threatening within a matter of hours. A wide range of organisms can produce an infection, although there are common culprits. Clinical confusion may occur because the presentation may mimic tumor or degenerative disease and vice versa. Infection should always be in the mind of those involved in diagnosis of musculoskeletal disorders. Antibiotics provide an important part of the treatment, but in many cases drugs alone are inadequate to deal with the disease. It may be necessary to perform surgery to remove dead and necrotic tissue and allow drainage of deep cavities. Resistance to antibiotic regimens is an increasing problem, and the recognition of failure of response to antibiotic therapy is an important part of the diagnostic process.

ETIOLOGY

Organisms may be introduced into the body by a variety of means, depending on environmental, organism, and host factors. These routes include inhalation, direct inoculation (often by trauma or surgery), and ingestion. These can be followed by further local invasion, hematogenous or lymphatic spread, and thereby invasion of organisms into regions of the body where their presence is damaging. Once the organism has reached the location where infection might develop, the chance of establishing infection depends on organism factors and the host's local and systemic immunity. Poor vascular supply, dead or damaged tissue, collections of blood or lymph, and foreign implanted material including endoprostheses all increase the risk of infection. Tumors are also destructive and produce necrotic areas within them that may be the center of secondary sepsis.

Systemic disorders and immune suppression not only change the individual's susceptibility but also affect the way in which infection manifests and which organisms are the likely cause. Imaging plays a fundamental role in the diagnosis, assessment, treatment, management, and follow-up of patients with soft tissue and bone infection.

PREVALENCE AND EPIDEMIOLOGY

Staphylococcus aureus infection is the most common cause of soft tissue infection throughout the world. However, there are regional variations in the incidence and causative organism. For example, abscesses due to melioidosis are typically seen in rice field workers and *Mycobacterium marinum* is a hazard to those who keep tropical fish.

KEY POINTS

- There are a variety of manifestations of soft tissue infection that overlap and merge in some cases.
- Imaging is useful to define the extent of disease, and this is most accurately achieved by MRI.
- Ultrasonography is particularly effective at distinguishing abscess cavities from edematous tissue.
- MRI has supplanted sinography in the definition of sinus tracts and cavities.
- Image-guided biopsy is useful to confirm the diagnosis and determine the causative organisms.
- Repeat MRI examination is a useful way to follow progress of therapy.

CLINICAL PRESENTATION

Given the wide variety of organisms and means of infections, there are many ways in which soft tissue infection may present. The clinical entities described here are not really separate diseases but more an emphasis of one part of the spectrum. One may lead to the next, and two or more may be present in the same case.

PATHOLOGY

In the early stages of infection when the organism is establishing itself there will be an acute associated inflammatory response leading to soft tissue edema and opening of normal vascular channels with increased blood flow to the affected area. The patient will complain of swelling, pain, and heat if the site is superficial. There is likely to be a systemic response with a febrile illness. Subsequent progress depends on the location and nature of the organisms involved. Some infections lead to rapid tissue destruction and necrosis. This, in turn, leads to systemic toxicity and severe ill health. Septicemic shock, hypotension, and tachycardia may result. In other infections in which the growth rate is slower there may be local destruction of tissue with abscess formation. At first microcavities containing pus will occur, but these may coalesce into larger collections. These abscesses, in turn, may spread and penetrate adjacent structures. They may perforate the skin and discharge through a sinus track. They may enter joint spaces or abdominal viscera. When soft tissue infections are located adjacent to bone they may excite a periosteal reaction and cause underlying bone edema. Those that are particularly destructive may cause erosion of the bone cortex. Infections that begin within or enter joints can cause early damage to the articular cartilage, which intrinsically has a poor blood supply. This destruction is likely to be irreversible. Joint effusion will occur early, either due to pus within the joint or, more commonly, a reactive effusion. Joint space narrowing occurs late because the early manifestation of cartilage involvement will be edema. Secondary osteomyelitis may be due to direct spread of the organism into the adjacent bone. This implies penetration of the articular cartilage and joint capsule if the infection arose primarily within the joint. Osteomyelitis is infection arising principally in bone. However, sometimes it will present as a soft tissue infection due to cortical penetration and spread into the adjacent structures.

Chronic infection is when the disease process reaches a stable state or one that is changing very slowly. Here the combination of reactive changes to the infection will be seen with the acute structure or residual necrosis. Chronic abscess cavities may be associated with fibrous reaction in the adjacent soft tissue. Cloacae and sinus tracks may become lined by epithelium. In the very long term, areas of chronic infection may be complicated by amyloid formation and rarely by malignant change.

IMAGING TECHNIQUES

Imaging is pivotal in the diagnosis and management of soft tissue and bone infections. The appropriate investigation depends on the clinical presentation.

Soft Tissue Swelling with Erythema

In acute cellulitis and in abscess formation radiographs may show no abnormality. Later in the disease there may be subtle periosteal reaction and large abscesses may cause bone damage. The only circumstance in which early radiography is contributory is when gas-forming organisms are present (e.g., in clostridial myonecrosis) because the gas may be identified. However, these patients are critically ill and clinical features will be more important in the initial assessment. Tissue crepitus is occasionally palpable. The radiologist is unlikely to add to the clinician's view of the severity of the case by finding gas in the immune-competent patient. Ultrasound examination is useful to discriminate cavitating abscess formation from diffuse cellulitis. Areas of fluid collection may be aspirated both to obtain a microbiologic diagnosis and to alleviate pressure from an abscess cavity. The ultrasound appearances will be of a hypoechoic area that may appear as clear fluid or alternatively could contain particulate matter. The adjacent soft tissues will have increased blood flow on Doppler imaging.

MRI is useful for assessing the extent of edema and the size of any abscess cavity. It is the definitive way of determining whether an abscess communicates with a joint. MRI is particularly useful in determining the extent of sinus tracks and the involvement of adjacent bones and has virtually replaced sinography. Although ultrasonography can be used as described earlier, the majority of patients suspected of having an infection should have MRI as the initial examination after radiography.

Unexplained Pain with or without Fever

In the assessment of acute osteomyelitis, radiographs may be normal or may show some patchy and localized osteopenia in the region of the infection. The finding of periosteal reaction is a specific one but is not often present in the early stages. Ultrasonography is of less value unless periosteal edema is detected with increased blood flow on power Doppler imaging. This constellation of ultrasound findings is useful in this setting. Unfortunately, patients with acute osteomyelitis may not exhibit this finding. Therefore, the combination of ultrasonography and MRI is the best way to discriminate soft tissue infection from bone infection (Fig. 61-1).

The combination of rapid and slow growth in the same patient are features that suggest a lesion is infectious rather than tumorous in origin.

Nuclear medicine studies have a minor role to play in the assessment of infection and would probably only be of value when MRI is not available. This technique is less specific than MRI and no more likely to show up areas of edema. The patients normally present with pain in a specific location, and so a limited examination of that area by MRI is appropriate. Furthermore, the epiphyseal regions of the younger child with active growth will show increased radionuclide accumulation on the nuclear medicine study, and this finding may be misleading or confusing. Bone scintigraphy may show areas of uptake in soft tissue infection due to the increased vascular supply and areas of necrosis. A central area of activity void suggests an

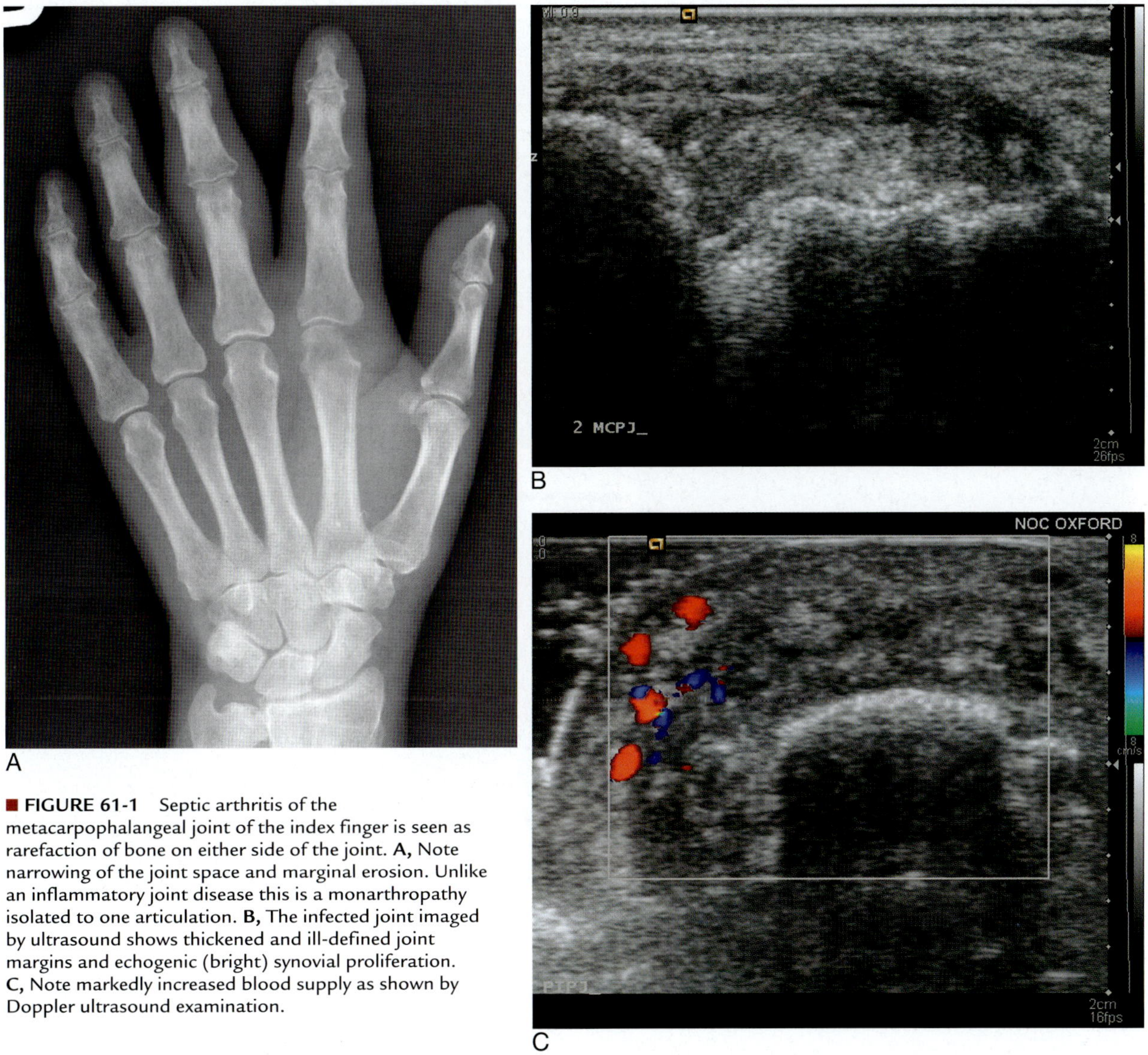

■ FIGURE 61-1 Septic arthritis of the metacarpophalangeal joint of the index finger is seen as rarefaction of bone on either side of the joint. **A,** Note narrowing of the joint space and marginal erosion. Unlike an inflammatory joint disease this is a monarthropathy isolated to one articulation. **B,** The infected joint imaged by ultrasound shows thickened and ill-defined joint margins and echogenic (bright) synovial proliferation. **C,** Note markedly increased blood supply as shown by Doppler ultrasound examination.

abscess. More specific techniques to show infected areas including gallium citrate– and indium chloride–labeled white blood cell scintigraphy. These studies are more specific and have an occasional role in complex cases.

MANIFESTATIONS OF THE DISEASE

Cellulitis

This is an acute inflammatory response due to a soft tissue infection and is most commonly caused by *S. aureus or Streptococcus pyogenes* (group A streptococcus). Other organisms are possible offenders depending on the environmental exposure. The infection is usually acquired by inoculation (e.g., via athlete's foot), although in about half of cases the actual route is unclear. Edema, redness, and swelling may spread throughout the affected limb, producing pain and dysfunction. The patient is likely to have a fever and will feel systemically unwell. Cellulitis may spread in a progressive "wild fire" fashion and sometimes

by a lymphatic spread producing red lines or marks in the distribution of the inflamed lymph tracks. Reactive nodes will be seen in drainage areas. The infection may also spread along tendon sheaths and be relatively confined to these cavities (Fig. 61-2). Today cellulitis is most commonly treated actively and acutely with antibiotics and the more advanced stages of the disease are rare. Prior to antibiotic therapy, soft tissue infection of this type was often lethal. Indeed, the introduction of penicillin to treat patients with acute streptococcal cellulitis produced miraculous results for the times.

Abscess

Abscesses may occur as the result of a variety of soft tissue infections. They are probably more commonly associated with infection due to inoculation (Fig. 61-3). *S. aureus* is the most common cause of an abscess, particularly if it is acquired by a hematogenous route. This includes methicillin-resistant *S. aureus* (MRSA), particularly if the patient

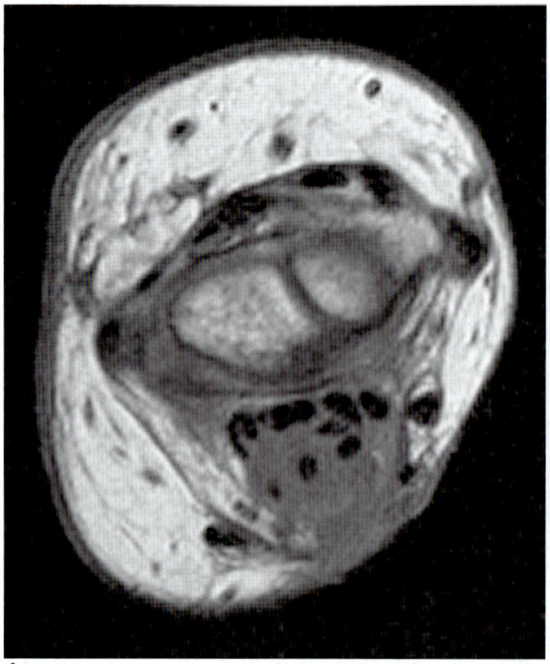

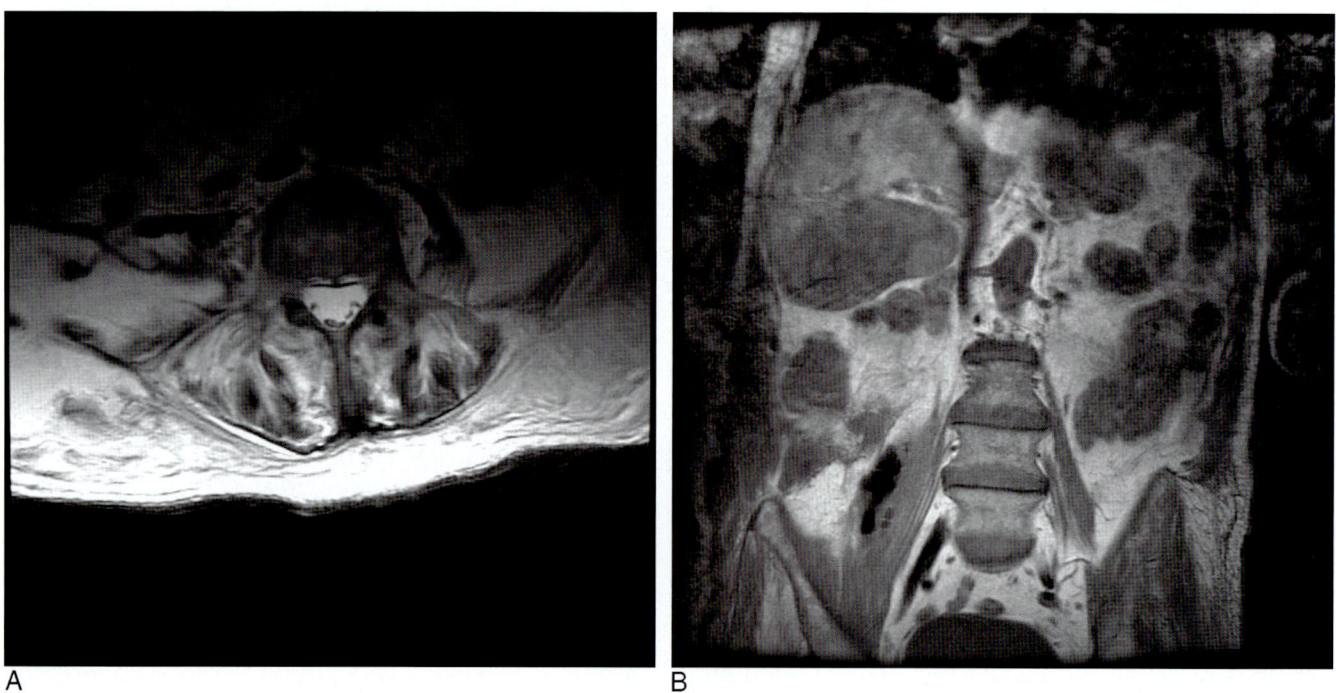

■ **FIGURE 61-2**   Soft tissue infection may involve the tendon sheaths. In this case of *Staphylococcus aureus* tenosynovitis the patient was unable to tolerate the high field magnet. **A,** This open MR image shows swelling around the carpal tunnel. **B,** Ultrasound examination shows extensive tenosynovitis and distortion of the tendon sheath, which is filled with thickened echogenic synovial tissue. **C,** Axial ultrasound image shows marked Doppler signal from the intense vascular reaction.

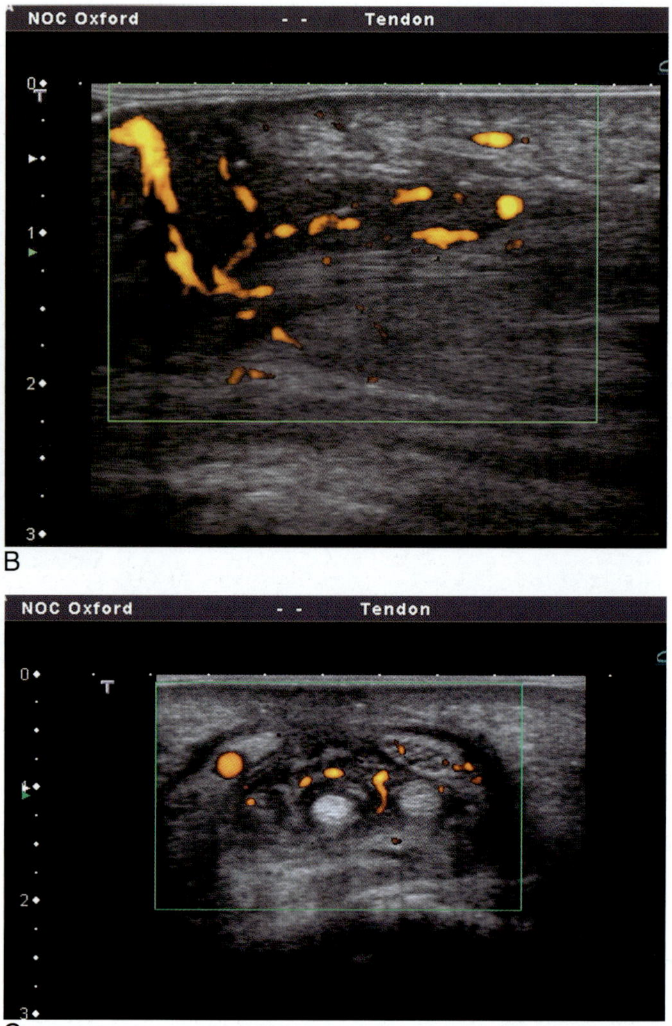

■ **FIGURE 61-3**   **A,** Axial T2-weighted MR image shows a mass in the right psoas muscle that extends through the posterolateral abdominal wall. **B,** T1-weighted MR image shows that the abscess contains gas. This could be the result of gas-forming organisms, perforation of a viscus, a sinus tract to the skin, or severe central necrosis. In this case, necrosis resulted from a methicillin-resistant *Staphylococcus aureus* infection.

has frequent contact with the health care environment. Organisms including bowel flora may also be the source of infection. When abscesses are established, particularly within the sinus tracks, multiple secondary infections may occur, producing a mixed growth on culture.

Impetigo

Impetigo is the cutaneous and subcutaneous reaction to *S. aureus* or *Streptococcus pyogenes* infection and is more common in children than in adults. It can be bullous or nonbullous and results in crusting lesions often around the mouth and nose.

Acute Septic Arthritis

Joint infections may occur at any age. Irritable hip is a clinical condition in children in the 4- to 12-year age range and is most often due to a benign transient synovitis with no apparent cause and no serious sequelae. Unfortunately, imaging (ultrasonography and MRI), although sensitive to the detection of joint effusion, cannot determine its nature because pus looks like transudate on MRI and ultrasonography (Figs. 61-4 and 61-5). Therefore, the small but important minority of cases with septic arthritis may be overlooked. Some patients with sepsis have normal body temperature, normal hematologic investigations, and small joint effusions. The only safe course is to aspirate all effusions found in acutely painful joints and to send the aspirate for urgent microscopy and culture. Fortunately, in many instances, this will also alleviate the symptoms.

In the adult patient, debility from other conditions such as systemic arthropathy may mask the signs and symptoms of septic arthritis and a similarly cautious approach must be taken. *S. aureus*, *Streptococcus pneumoniae*, and β-hemolytic streptococci are common

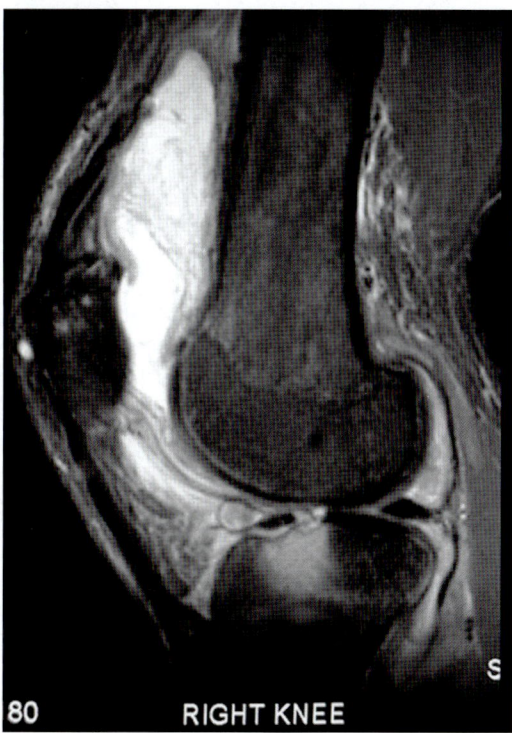

■ FIGURE 61 5 Septic arthritis of the knee caused by infection with *Pseudomonas*. Note the large effusion and the bone marrow edema in the proximal tibia. If these cases are not treated aggressively and rapidly, severe joint destruction is inevitable.

causes of acute septic arthritis in the adult, but *Neisseria gonorrhoeae* is also a possible factor if there is a relevant sexual history. Effusions should be aspirated and samples sent for microscopy and culture. When gout or pyrophosphate arthropathy is suspected, microscopy for crystals should be requested. Microorganisms in a joint are highly destructive, and permanent damage to the articular surfaces occurs quickly so early therapy is mandatory. Simple aspiration is rarely sufficient, and formal surgical drainage should be combined with antibiotic therapy. In acute prosthetic joint septic arthritis, diagnostic aspiration is also the initial investigation of choice.

Chronic Septic Arthritis

It is imperative to obtain the microbiologic organism before starting therapy in the case of chronic septic arthritis. In this situation, obtaining a prior environmental and travel history may help. A synovial biopsy for histology (including fungal and acid-fast bacillus stains) should be considered along with microscopy and culture requesting the inclusion of mycobacteria and fungi. It may also be important to consult a microbiologist in unusual cases.

In chronic prosthetic joint infection, the infection is often caused by native skin organisms such as coagulase-negative staphylococci. These microbacteria can also be a contaminant in the aspiration, so aseptic technique when sampling is imperative. Infection eventually results in loosening of the prosthesis, which can be detected on radiographs as a lucency developing at the bone/prosthesis or bone/cement interface.

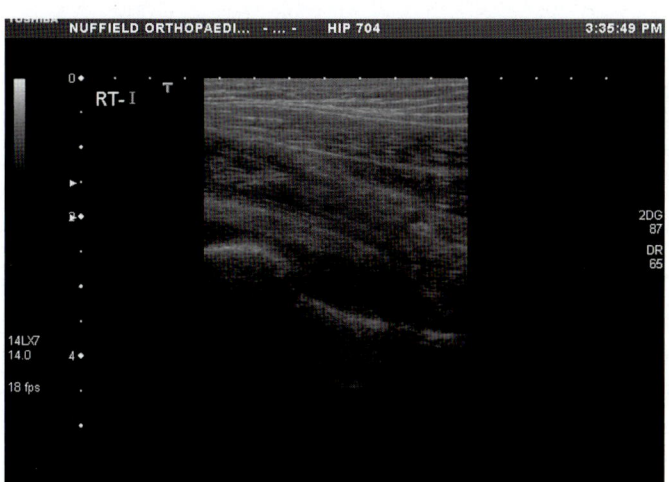

■ FIGURE 61-4 Ultrasound examination of the hip in a child shows an echo-free joint effusion. The appearance of a benign transient synovitis can be identical to that of an aggressive septic arthritis. There are no secure clinical or laboratory indicators of infection to help differentiate the two. Therefore, ultrasound-guided aspiration is the best way to exclude infection and at the same time immediately relieve the patient's pain.

Radiologically, it is difficult to distinguish aseptic from septic loosening. Around 15% of loosening is due to infection, and the presence of rapidly progressive lysis or periosteal reaction is highly suggestive of this diagnosis. In cases of suspected infection, synovial biopsy under ultrasound or periprosthetic biopsy of lucent areas may be helpful adjunct procedures in addition to synovial fluid aspiration. Ideally, several samples using separate instruments should be sent. However, this is usually only possible when open biopsies are performed in the operating room; and, in such cases, samples should be sent for both histology and microbiology. It is crucial to mention the presence of a prosthetic device to the microbiology laboratory so that the correct tests can be requested and to avoid skin contaminants as being interpreted as the infecting organism (Fig. 61-6).

Pyomyositis

Although once thought to be a disease of tropical countries, pyomyositis is being increasingly observed throughout the world. Patients usually present with a short history of fever and have localized pain and tenderness on passive movement of the muscle. Inflammatory markers are usually raised. In the typical example, there is diffuse infection of a muscle or muscle group, leading to edema and enlargement of the muscle. Soft tissue fluid collections may follow. *S. aureus* is the most common infecting organism. Clostridial myonecrosis (gas gangrene) is a very acute, life-threatening infection accompanied by systemic signs of severe toxicity. It can follow surgery or trauma, and early surgical débridement is often the only chance for survival (Figs. 61-7 and 61-8).

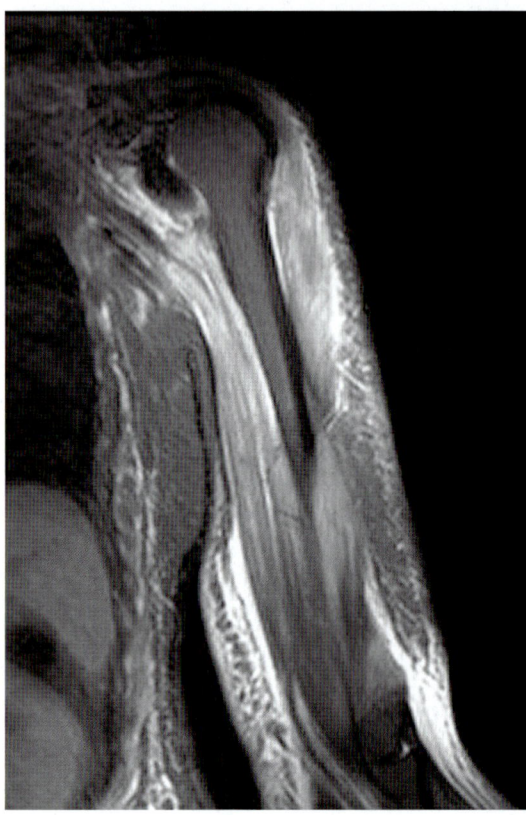

■ **FIGURE 61-7** Muscle infection is rare but dramatic on MRI. Pyomyositis is seen as edema and swelling within a muscle group. Later necrosis and abscess formation may change the imaging appearances.

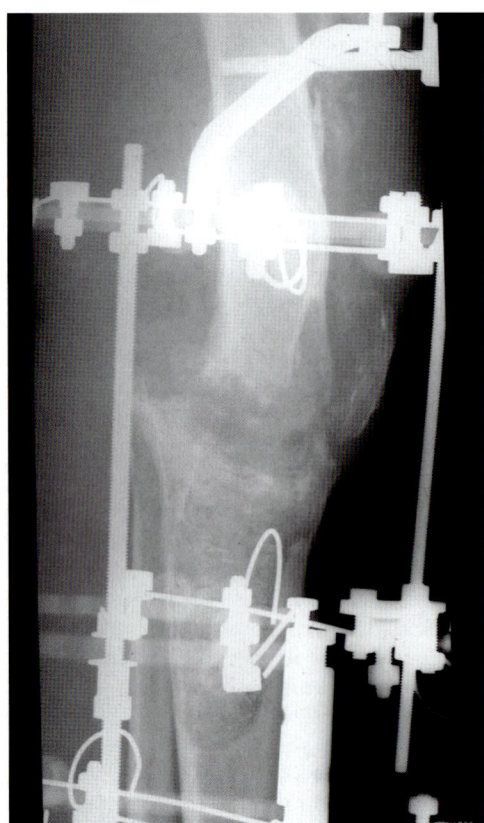

■ **FIGURE 61-6** When an implant becomes infected it is necessary to remove the metal, débride dead tissue, and begin antibiotic treatment. After removal of the implant and treatment for infection it may be possible to revise the implant or, as in this case, attempt a fusion.

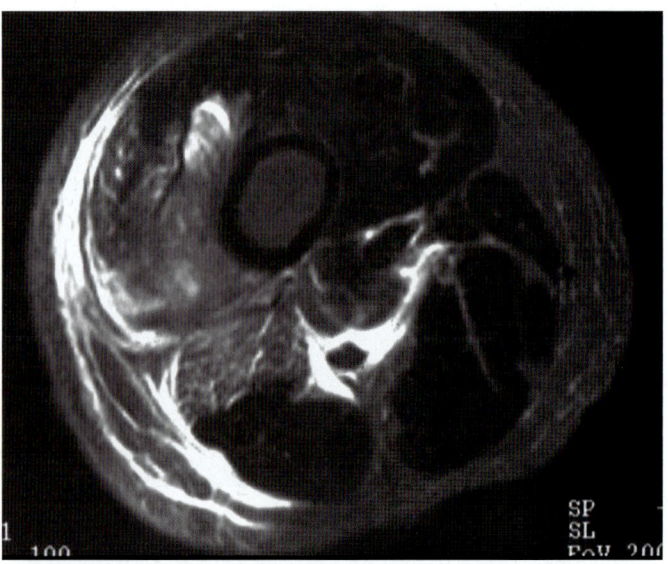

■ **FIGURE 61-8** Pyomyositis of the thigh with perhaps less dramatic muscle involvement than was seen in the case of necrotizing fasciitis. The distinction between these conditions is dependent on clinical presentation and speed of progression.

Necrotizing Fasciitis

This is a rapidly destructive disease that is associated with group A streptococcal infections but may often be the consequence of polymicrobial infection with a variety of gram-positive, gram-negative, aerobic and anaerobic bacteria. It results in rapid tissue destruction and has been called "flesh-eating disease" in the lay press. A form of necrotizing fasciitis involving the scrotal fascia in males is termed *Fournier's gangrene*. Necrotizing fasciitis usually requires radical surgery and is often life threatening (Fig. 61-9).

Tuberculosis

Although most infections are due to *S. aureus* or *Streptococcus pyogenes, Mycobacterium tuberculosis* is probably the third most common infecting organism worldwide. Tuberculosis typically produces a low-grade infection that leads to abscess formation without a pyrexial illness, the so-called cold abscess. It may be slowly destructive and produce lytic lesions as part of the tissue reaction of caseation. These lesions may mimic a malignant processes in bone. Typically, tuberculosis may cross joint spaces and, in the spine, spread across disc spaces. However, it may present in a myriad of fashions and is known for its ability to mimic other disorders. Several mycobacteria other then tuberculosis ("atypical mycobacteria") can cause soft tissue infections and/or ulceration. For example, *Mycobacterium marinum* has been reported to cause a nodular lymphadenitis as a consequence of inoculation of the skin in individuals cleaning tropical fish tanks.

Fungal Infections

Fungi most often affect those who are immune compromised. In these circumstances they may produce a variety of signs and symptoms. A travel and exposure history in a competent host may raise the possibility of a dimorphic fungal infection, usually acquired by inhalation followed by dissemination to other sites. Fungal infection should be considered whenever the bacteriologic findings do not fit the clinical picture. Most cases should be discussed with a local microbiologist because a tissue diagnosis is usually crucial.

MANIFESTATIONS OF THE DISEASE

The imaging of soft tissue infections is similar for each of the previously mentioned clinical manifestations.

Ultrasonography

Ultrasonography is useful for assessing the progress of cavitating abscesses because reasonably accurate measurements can be taken, particularly with extended field of views. Ultrasonography is also useful for discriminating fluid from edematous soft tissues, which may be a more difficult distinction on MRI.

Magnetic Resonance Imaging

For staging the extent and following the progress of infection of both soft tissue and bone, MRI is the definitive technique. Axial, coronal, and sagittal planes should be obtained with a combination of T1-weighted and fluid

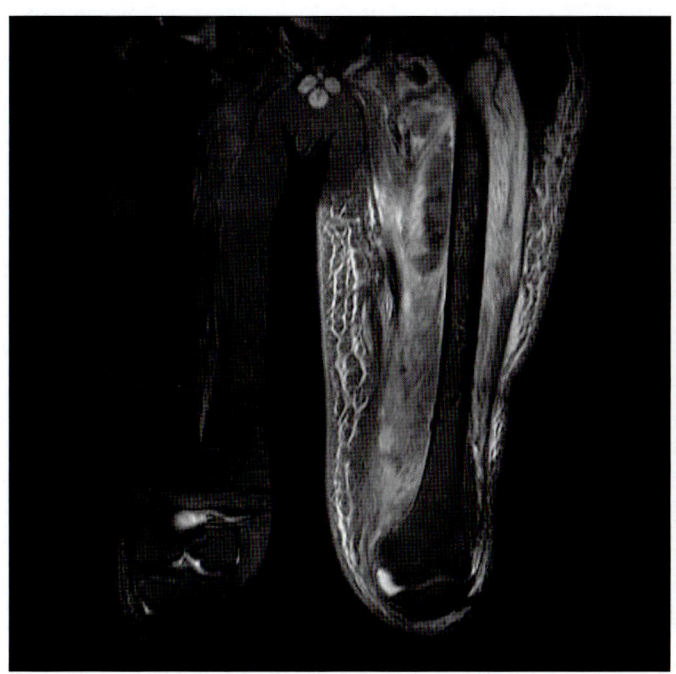
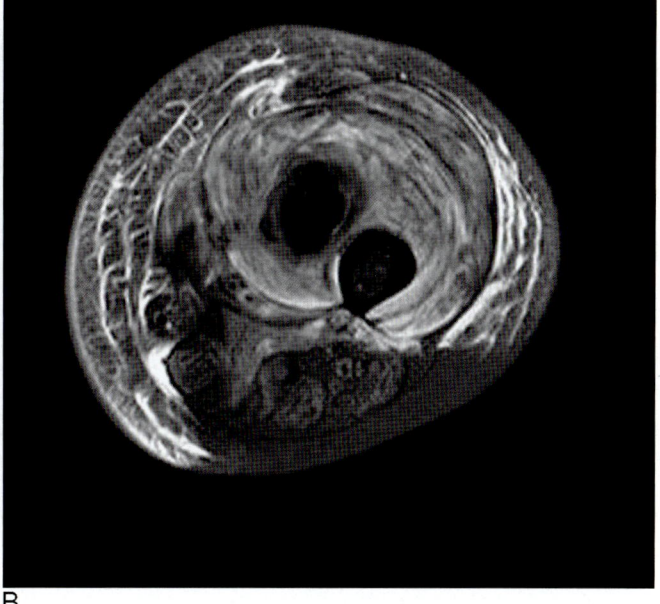

A   B

■ **FIGURE 61-9** Extensive muscle and soft tissue necrosis in a case of severe necrotizing fasciitis. **A,** Coronal FSTIR MR image shows the extent of tissue damage. **B,** Axial MR image.

sensitive sequences such as T2-weighted images with fat suppression or, alternatively, a short tau inversion recovery (STIR) sequence (see Fig. 61-3B). Intravenous gadolinium is rarely of diagnostic discriminatory use, because all infective processes lead to increased blood flow.

Image-Guided Biopsy

Aspiration or fine-needle biopsy is a simply performed technique, but the results are often unrewarding. The most accurate culture specimens are obtained from the margins of a lesion where tissue is not necrotic using a cutting needle or open biopsy. Imaging is important in selecting the location for biopsy in all cases and in guiding the needle when a percutaneous route is attempted. The best imaging for the purpose will be one that shows the abnormal area clearly and allows real-time guidance of the needle. Ultrasonography is likely the easiest and best method of guidance, although CT and even MRI guidance can be utilized by individuals without experience or access to the appropriate ultrasound techniques to perform the procedure.

SYNOPSIS OF TREATMENT OPTIONS

Medical Treatment

Antibiotic therapy is best targeted to the specific organism. However, treatment should optimally be delayed until the exact organism and its antibiotic sensitivities have been identified by the methods described earlier, except in the most life-threatening situations.

Surgical Treatment

Excision, drainage, and removal of dead and necrotic tissue is essential. The timing and extent of surgical intervention will depend on a team approach with advice from clinical microbiologists, imagers, and surgeons.

SUGGESTED READINGS

Atkins BL, Bowler IC. The diagnosis of large joint sepsis. J Hosp Infect 1998; 40:263-274.

Atkins BL, Gottlieb T, Shaw D. Soft tissue, bone and joint infections. Med J Aust 2002; 176:609-615.

Atkins BL, Berendt AR. Prosthetic joint infection. In Bulstrode C, Buckwalter J, Carr A, et al (eds). Oxford Textbook of Orthopaedics and Trauma. Oxford, Oxford University Press, 2002, pp 1443-1454.

Mandell GL, Bennett JE, Dolin R (eds). Mandell's Principles and Practice of Infectious Diseases. Edinburgh, Elsevier Churchill Livingstone, 2005.

62

Infection in the Appendicular Skeleton (Including Chronic Osteomyelitis)

Shah H. M. Khan and Hans L. Bloem

Infection of bone or bone marrow can be characterized using various definitions that reflect the interaction between the causative organism and the host's response (Box 62-1). The clinical diagnosis is relatively straightforward in the late stages of osteomyelitis. However, despite the tremendous advancement in the imaging of bone infection, the challenge remains to detect and diagnose osteomyelitis at an early stage. The implication of early diagnosis is that early treatment can be instituted that significantly increases the cure rate and reduces the complications and associated morbidity. A clear understanding of the clinical, radiologic, and biochemical background is paramount in early diagnosis, thus enabling rapid and effective treatment as well as diagnosing activity of chronic osteomyelitis. The focus of this chapter is on effective use of imaging in dealing with these aspects of osteomyelitis based on an understanding of information displayed using conventional and advanced imaging techniques.

ETIOLOGY

Bacteria are the most common cause of osteomyelitis, but viruses, fungi, and protozoa are reported to be causative agents, particularly in the immunocompromised patient. The bacterial pathogens vary with age and also with certain groups of patients (Table 62-1). However, the predominant cause of osteomyelitis is *Staphylococcus aureus*.

Haemophilus influenzae and group B streptococcus are common causes of osteomyelitis in children, whereas gram-negative bacteria such as *Escherichia coli* and anaerobes are found in adult and diabetic cases. *Staphylococcus epidermidis* osteomyelitis is common in intravenous drug abusers and those with joint implants. *Salmonella* osteomyelitis is frequently seen in patients with sickle cell disease, although *S. aureus* is still the most common cause in this group.[1]

S. aureus adheres to bone by expressing receptors (adhesins) for components of bone matrix (fibronectin, laminin, collagen, and bone sialoglycoprotein) and cartilage. It also elaborates fibronectin-binding adhesins, which enables it to attach to surgically implanted devices in bone.[2]

PREVALENCE AND EPIDEMIOLOGY

Acute hematogenous osteomyelitis is predominantly a disease of children (85% of cases occur in children), whereas the post-traumatic or contiguous-focus type of osteomyelitis is more common in adults and adolescents. Contiguous-focus osteomyelitis forms about half of all cases of osteomyelitis.

According to the literature, the incidence of acute osteomyelitis in the developed world is 1 case per 5000 children. Data on the incidence or prevalence of acute and chronic osteomyelitis in adults are not available. The incidence is thought to be much lower with widespread use of antibiotics.

The risk of chronic osteomyelitis after an episode of acute osteomyelitis is 5% to 25%.

Appendicular osteomyelitis is predominantly a disease of the lower limbs, accounting for about 90% of cases, and the remaining 10% occur in the upper limbs. The most common bones affected are the tibia (50%) and the femur (30%).

CLINICAL PRESENTATION

The main factors that determine clinical presentation are virulence of the infective pathogen, the dose of the inoculum, and the immune status of the host. Traditionally,

BOX 62-1   Definitions

Acute osteomyelitis: abrupt-onset infection
Subacute osteomyelitis: subacute presentation
Brodie's abscess: abscess cavity (type of subacute osteomyelitis)
Chronic osteomyelitis: late-stage infection with marked host reaction
Sequestrum: dead or necrotic bone
Involucrum: new bone formation following onset of healing process
Cloaca: opening in involucrum
Garré's osteomyelitis: sclerosing osteomyelitis

TABLE 62-1   Common Organisms Seen in Different Age Groups and Some Special Conditions

Age/Subtype	Organisms
Infants	*Staphylococcus aureus,* group B streptococcus, *Escherichia coli, Enterobacter*
Children	*S. aureus,* group A streptococcus, *Haemophilus influenzae*
Adults	*S. aureus,* coagulase-negative *Staphylococcus, Pseudomonas, E. coli, Serratia*
Diabetic foot	Polymicrobials: *S. aureus, Streptococcus,* enterococcus, *Proteus,* anaerobes
Brodie's abscess	Coagulase-positive *S. aureus, Streptococcus, Pseudomonas, Kingella*
Sickle cell disease	*S. aureus, Salmonella*

osteomyelitis has been subdivided into acute, subacute, and chronic on the basis of speed of onset and course of the infection.

Acute osteomyelitis commonly occurs in children. It is rapid in onset and may present as systemic toxicity. This is especially seen in children in the bacteremic phase of the infection. Nonetheless, almost 50% of cases may not manifest any of the acute systemic features. The bones most commonly affected are the tibia, the femur, and the humerus. The patient presents with pain and unwillingness to use the affected limb and as an unwell and irritable child. Redness, swelling, and warmth due to acute inflammatory response may be seen in the affected part. However, this is also seen in bone tumors. The laboratory results may indicate an elevated white blood cell count and increased levels of inflammatory markers such as erythrocyte sedimentation rate (ESR) and C-reactive protein, but the absence of such changes does not exclude the diagnosis. The blood cultures are positive in only 50% of cases.

The presentation of subacute osteomyelitis or Brodie's abscess is more insidious. This may be secondary to inadequate treatment or low virulence of the organism. The disease may have been present for several months. Indolent pain is the predominant presentation, which may be worse after activity. Swelling may be present, but redness is normally not seen. Effusion in the adjacent joint and some atrophy of the muscles may be noted. Systemic toxicity is conspicuously absent. Subacute osteomyelitis is more common in adolescent boys, with the knee and ankle being the sites of predilection.

Subacute osteomyelitis may progress to chronic osteomyelitis, which generally presents as recurrent attacks of acute inflammation over a period of more than 6 weeks to many years. Pain is the predominant presenting symptom. Occasionally, a discharging sinus may be the presenting complaint in an otherwise asymptomatic patient. On examination, the bone may feel thickened and a number of skin scars from old healed sinuses may be seen. Anemia and generalized malnourishment may be noticed in long-standing cases. A previous history of acute osteomyelitis, trauma, or orthopedic implants that was complicated by infection is often present.

PATHOPHYSIOLOGY

The infection of bone can occur by one of four main routes: hematogenous, spread from contiguous source, direct implantation, and postoperative infections.

The infection has a predilection for growing ends of appendicular bones. The infective pathogen tends to lodge at the metaphyseal vessels in acute hematogenous infection. These metaphyseal vessels have slow but turbulent flow of blood, reduced leukocytes, as well as impaired phagocytic ability, which are conducive to proliferation of infective organisms.

Anatomy

The anatomy of the vasculature of the appendicular long bones varies with age. The metaphyseal and epiphyseal vessels are distinct and separated by the growth plate in children, but communication is present in infants and adults after the fusion of the growth plate. Therefore, infection can easily extend into the epiphyseal region in the infants and adults. Infection in the epiphyseal region can potentially spread to the joint, causing septic arthritis. In some joints, such as the hip or shoulder, where the metaphysis lies within the capsule, septic arthritis can occur from a breach of the metaphyseal cortex.

Pathology

Acute hematogenous osteomyelitis commonly affects children and is relatively uncommon in healthy adults, but it can occur in immunocompromised individuals or intravenous drug abusers. The metaphyses, especially around the knee, are sites of predilection. These are sites of rapid growth and are also more prone to trauma in children. The onset of infection triggers the inflammatory response with influx of leukocytes and exudate formation. The intraosseous pressure is raised due to edema within the rigid medullary cavity, producing thrombosis of vessels. This further exacerbates and spreads the infective process. Ultimately, the exudates track through the haversian canals of the cortex, which is particularly thin at the metaphysis. The spread of inflammatory exudates to the subperiosteal region elevates the periosteum. This causes periosteal vessel thrombosis, leading to cortical necrosis. The enzymes released by the bacteria, polymorphonuclear cells, and dying tissues further contribute to the local bone marrow and cortical necrosis.

The elevation of the periosteum also triggers the osteoblasts to produce new bone, which manifests as periosteal reaction. This response is earlier and more florid in children but is delayed and somewhat patchy in adults. In children, the periosteum is loosely attached and thus can be easily peeled off, manifesting as an early periosteal reaction, whereas in adults it is more firmly attached. This periosteal new bone formation is also well seen radiographically when using MRI and ultrasonography.

Necrotic bone fragment bereft of vascularization is dense relative to vascularized bone. The vascularized bone undergoes demineralization due to the inflammatory response. Areas of infected bone also undergo destruction due to osteoclastic action. These are seen as patchy osteopenic areas on plain radiographs, whereas the devascularized bone fragment, which is referred to as a sequestrum, stands out as a dense bony fragment within patchy osteopenia on radiographs and CT. The sequestrum is of low signal intensity on all pulse sequences on MRI (Fig. 62-1). The dead sequestrum can harbor infective organisms. These may be difficult to eradicate unless the sequestrum is removed and the infective area is thoroughly cleaned and débrided. Therefore, the presence of sequestrum has the potential to make the infection chronic with risk of future acute exacerbations.

The periosteal new bone formation that takes place is referred to as involucrum and attempts to contain the infection. This tends to surround the infected area and

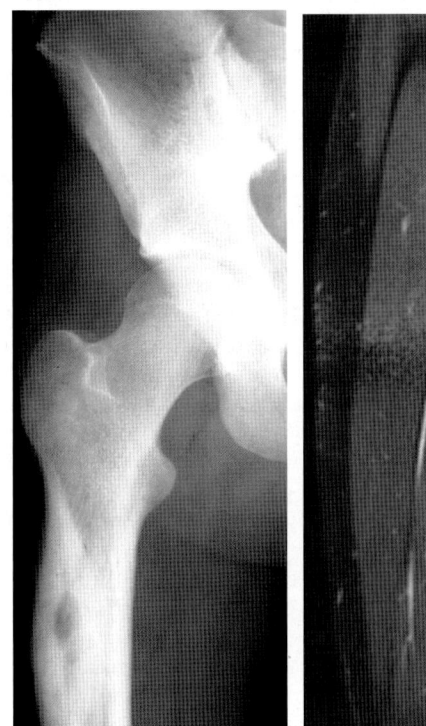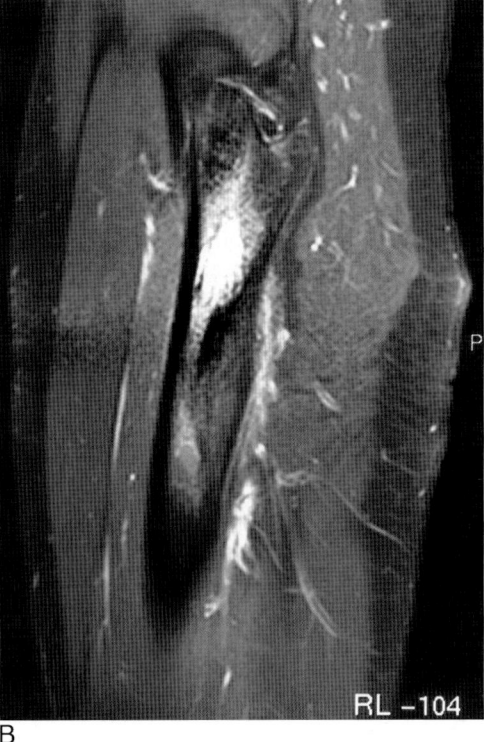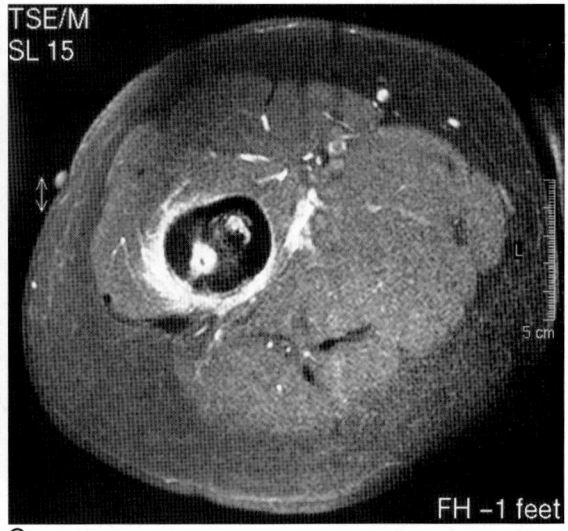

A   B   C

■ **FIGURE 62-1** Osteomyelitis mimicking osteoid osteoma. This patient had nonspecific symptoms of pain in the thigh. **A,** The initial radiograph showed a lucent lesion in the proximal femur with marked surrounding sclerosis. Subtle density is seen within the lucent lesion. This was suspected to be an osteoid osteoma, but osteomyelitis was considered in the differential diagnosis. Sagittal (**B**) and axial (**C**) T1-weighted, fat-suppressed, gadolinium-enhanced MR images demonstrate high signal intensity in the marrow with a small nonenhancing lesion of low signal intensity noted within. The nonenhancing lesion is a sequestrum within infected marrow, a classic feature of osteomyelitis. Note the breach of the cortex in the axial image (**C**) with periosteal reaction.

has pathologically a soft spongy texture. If the infection is controlled, then the involucrum undergoes remodeling and bridges the gap in the cortex.

If the infection is not adequately controlled, then the infective exudates may breach through the involucrum, producing an opening called a cloaca. The pus may then accumulate in the soft tissues to form abscesses before tracking through the soft tissues to break through the skin as a sinus. The cloaca may be seen on plain radiographs but is difficult to detect unless a sinogram is performed before the examination. The sinogram can delineate the soft tissue track of the sinus and abscesses as well as indicate the sites of the cloacae (Fig. 62-2). Sinography is now less frequently undertaken because the cloaca and soft tissue abscesses and fistulous track may be exquisitely seen on MRI (Fig. 62-3). CT can delineate the cloacae and abscesses in the soft tissues as rim-enhancing collections.

When the infection is adequately controlled and healing has taken place, the infected marrow undergoes cystic changes with fatty infiltration and the bony cortex undergoes remodeling.

BIOMECHANICS

The biomechanical significance of osteomyelitis is that the infected bone is not strong and is prone to pathologic fractures. This is a particular problem of long-standing chronic osteomyelitis.

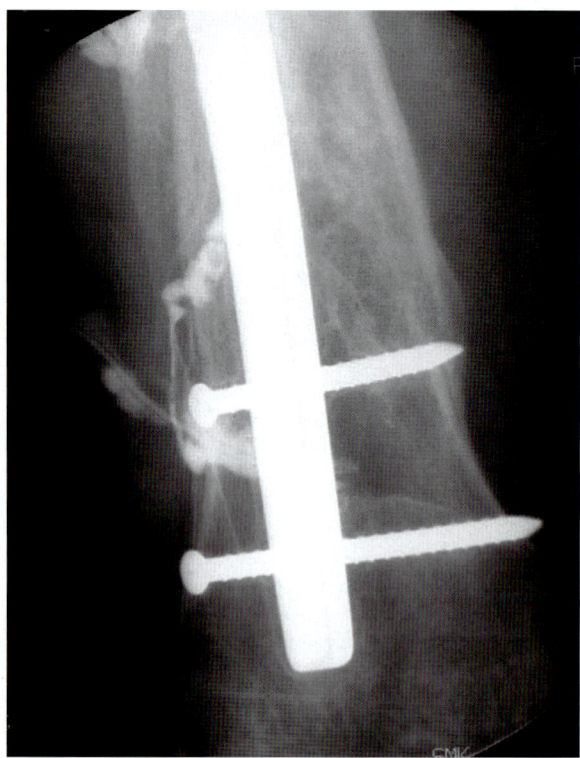

■ **FIGURE 62-2** Sinogram. A 73-year-old woman presented with discharging sinus about 3 years after internal fixation of a femoral shaft fracture. Sinogram demonstrates the catheter extending into the femur with contrast medium seen at multiple sites along the bone. This demonstrates communication between the bone and a soft tissue abscess as well as multiple cloacae.

IMAGING TECHNIQUES

Osteomyelitis is a potentially treatable disease, but early diagnosis is critical to avoid extensive damage and morbidity. Although clinical findings combined with laboratory results and imaging findings are unambiguous in most cases, there are a significant number of cases in which the diagnosis may not be clear, especially in children. In addition, the differentiation from other conditions such as tumors and fractures that have completely different management pathways means that the imaging has to be tailored with close cooperation between various disciplines.

Techniques and Relevant Aspects

In suspected cases of osteomyelitis, a baseline radiograph is essential. Although the radiographic changes of acute osteomyelitis may lag behind by 10 to 14 days, the radiograph can exclude other causes and, more pertinently, serve as a means of assessing progress after treatment. Both bone scintigraphy and MRI are equally sensitive in detection of infection in the bone. However, MRI is able to detect infection earlier and also affords precise anatomic localization and soft tissue contrast in three dimensions, which makes it more specific than nuclear imaging. MRI using a short tau inversion recovery (STIR) sequence is a very cost-effective method of screening for osteomyelitis.

CT is useful in the assessment of osteomyelitis, particularly in detecting early bone destruction or the presence of small sequestrum, which may not be evident on other imaging methods. It is very helpful in the assessment of atypical bones, such as clavicle, sternum, and pelvis, and may provide useful information especially when coupled with 3D reconstruction. CT is commonly used in the assessment of the spinal disease when overlapping bones may elude detection of small infective foci. CT also enables precise localization for biopsy and aspirations of infected bone or abscesses.

Ultrasonography has a complementary role in the investigation of osteomyelitis. It is extremely useful in detecting soft tissue abscesses but in children can also detect the elevation of periosteum and subperiosteal collections. It is the first line of investigation in joint effusions, particularly in the hips of children. It also affords guided aspiration but avoids the risk of radiation, as is the case with CT. Note that if a periosteal reaction is not detected using ultrasonography then the diagnosis of osteomyelitis is not excluded.

Newer imaging techniques of positron emission tomography (PET) are proving to be useful, with current literature suggesting improved detection, particularly in cases of chronic osteomyelitis. However, they remain less specific than MRI. Other techniques occasionally used are sinography, which can delineate the track in the soft tissue extending to the infected bone (see Fig. 62-2).

Pro and Cons (Table 62-2)

After a baseline radiograph, MRI is preferred for imaging of osteomyelitis owing to its superior soft tissue contrast

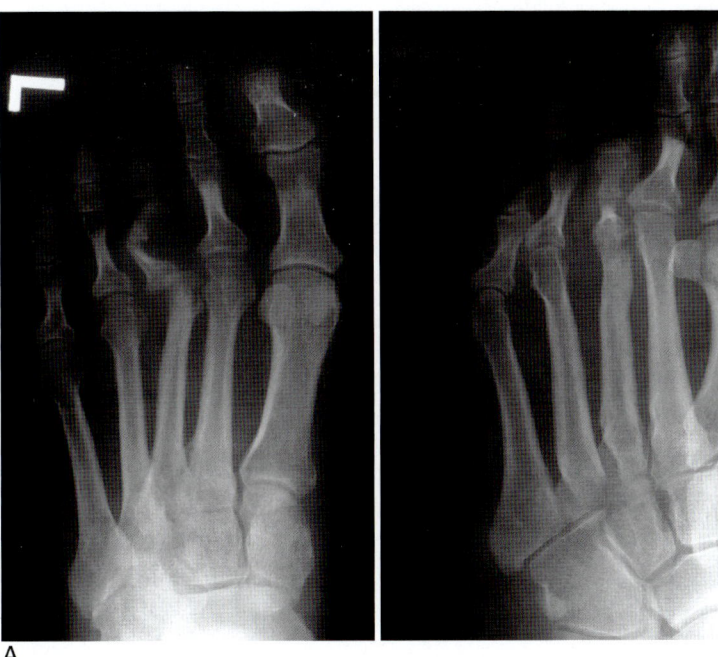

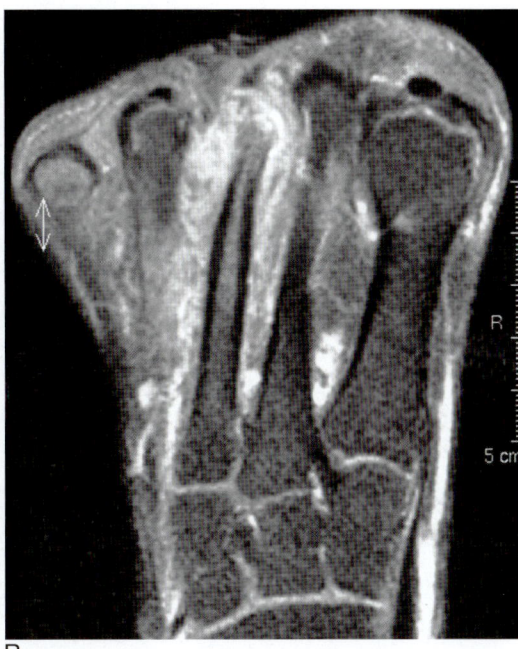

A B

■ **FIGURE 62-3** Chronic osteomyelitis. **A,** Plain radiograph shows erosion in the metatarsal head of the third toe. Bony remodeling with thickening of the cortex of the metatarsal shaft is noted. **B,** Axial T1-weighted fat-suppressed MR sequence with gadolinium chelate demonstrates erosion of the metatarsal head of the third toe with marrow edema and soft tissue enhancement that is likely to represent extension of infection into the soft tissue. **C,** T2-weighted MR sequence with fat suppression clearly demonstrates the soft tissue abscess adjacent to the infected third metatarsal.

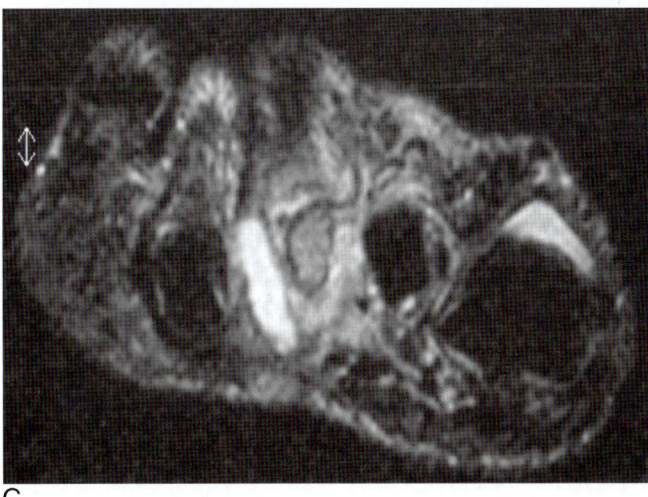

C

and ability to demonstrate 3D anatomy. It also enables preoperative planning. Although both the sensitivity and specificity is over 90%, it can be nonspecific and the clinical context along with laboratory results are important in reaching an exact diagnosis. Nuclear medicine is sensitive in detecting infection but has a relatively low specificity and the anatomic localization can be difficult. However, negative bone scintigraphy virtually excludes an infection. Because scintigraphy easily images the whole body it is extremely useful in assessing multiple sites of infection, as can occur in chronic recurrent multifocal osteomyelitis.

Early studies using PET have demonstrated higher sensitivity and specificity than nuclear medicine and MRI, being particularly useful in chronic osteomyelitis. In chronic osteomyelitis, white blood cell–labeled scans are useful in detecting recurrence and have reasonable specificity.

CT is useful in delineating small sequestrum especially in chronic osteomyelitis, and it can also detect early bone destruction.

Controversies

In cases of chronic osteomyelitis the diagnosis can be difficult. MRI is very sensitive and can show abnormal areas due to tissue edema and increased perfusion, but this may persist for up to 12 months after treatment of infection or after surgery, making it less specific. In the absence of abscess or sequestrum and other morphologic signs of osteomyelitis the detection of recurrent infection can be difficult. This may be further compounded by the presence of metal implants and the associated degradation of image quality on MRI.

Recent meta-analysis reviewing the accuracy of diagnosis in chronic osteomyelitis showed fluorodeoxy-

TABLE 62-2 Pros and Cons of the Various Imaging Modalities

Imaging Modality	Pros	Cons
Radiography	Useful baseline	Low sensitivity Lags behind the pathology by 7–14 days
Ultrasonography	Can detect soft tissue abscess and subperiosteal collection, particularly in pediatric cases Image guided aspiration	Cannot assess sequestrum and intraosseous pathology
Computed tomography	Assessment of atypical bones such as sternum, pelvis and spine Accurately detects subtle changes of bony destruction, sequestrum, and periosteal reaction Enables guided aspirations and biopsies	Soft tissue contrast is not as good as MRI Degree of marrow involvement cannot be adequately assessed
Magnetic resonance imaging	Excellent soft tissue contrast and exquisite anatomic detail High sensitivity and specificity of over 90% in detection of osteomyelitis	Can still be nonspecific, particularly in the setting of chronic complex osteomyelitis and neuroarthropathy
Nuclear medicine	Can assess the whole body, which is useful in multiple site involvement High negative predictive value	Low specificity in children and elderly Low resolution
Positron emission tomography	High accuracy in chronic osteomyelitis	Limited availability Expensive

glucose-labeled PET (FDG-PET) to be the most accurate, with a sensitivity of 96% and specificity of 91%. On the other hand, the sensitivity was 84% and specificity 60% for MRI. The accuracy of leukocyte scintigraphy was reasonably high for the peripheral skeleton, with sensitivity of 84% and specificity of 80%. However, these figures reduced significantly when accuracy for both axial and peripheral skeleton was combined.[3]

It is likely that both MRI and PET have complementary roles. MRI provides morphologic and anatomic assessment and PET assesses the functional aspect, thus enabling the distinction of infected areas in chronic osteomyelitis.

MANIFESTATIONS OF THE DISEASE

Understanding of the previously described pathophysiology makes it easy to understand and predict the imaging findings irrespective of the technique used.

Radiography

Radiographic signs of osteomyelitis are delayed by 7 to 14 days behind the disease process. Radiographs are often negative at the initial stage because the destruction of more than 60% of trabecular bone is necessary before osteomyelitis can be detected reliably.

However, the earliest sign observed may be effacement of fat planes with diffuse soft tissue swelling. Epiphyseal, metaphyseal, or diaphyseal ill-defined radiolucencies corresponding to the osseous destruction are seen on radiographs of the mature skeleton. Endosteal scalloping, intracortical lucencies or tunneling, and poorly defined subperiosteal bony defects are also seen. Mild periostitis is usually associated, but periosteal reaction is more prominently observed in the immature skeleton on radiographs (see Fig. 62-4A). In virulent infection the periosteal reaction may be irregular and similar to periosteal reaction seen in bone sarcoma. Periosteal reaction implies increased intramedullary pressure. When intramedullary pressure does not increase because cortical bone is not intact as a result of fracture or surgery, then periosteal reaction may be absent.

In subacute osteomyelitis a lucent lesion is seen that is normally located in the epiphysis or the metaphysis, and it may be associated with a linear track. Periosteal reactions may be subtle or even absent (Fig. 62-5A).

In the chronic stages of osteomyelitis there is extensive bony remodeling with considerable radiodensity and contour irregularity. Cystic changes may occur within the sclerotic area and sequestra are common (see Fig. 62-1A).

Patchy osteopenic areas may herald acute exacerbations and may be associated with periosteal reaction. Dense sequestrum may be seen standing among the altered bone, but this is generally difficult to detect. Cloacae, which are defects in the involucrum, are also difficult to detect on plain radiographs. A sequestrum was visible in only 9% of cases in one series. The sensitivity increases with serial review of radiographs to 14% and specificity of 70%.[4] Differentiating active from inactive chronic osteomyelitis can be extremely difficult. The extensive bony remodeling and osteosclerosis of the chronic osteomyelitis may obscure changes of reactivation. Radiographically, signs of reactivation are new areas of destruction, thin linear periostitis, and sequestration (Figs. 62-6A and 62-7B; see also Fig. 62-3A). In cases with prostheses, lucency at the cement-prosthesis or cement-bone interface in cemented prostheses or at the prosthesis-bone interface in uncemented prostheses is suggestive, but not specific, for infection. This may be associated with evidence of movement of the prosthesis and extensive destruction or even fracture of the bone.

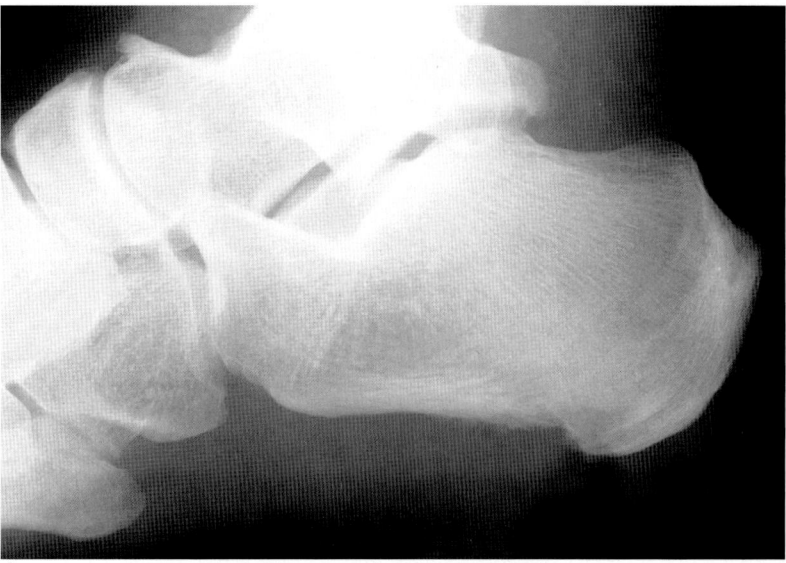

A

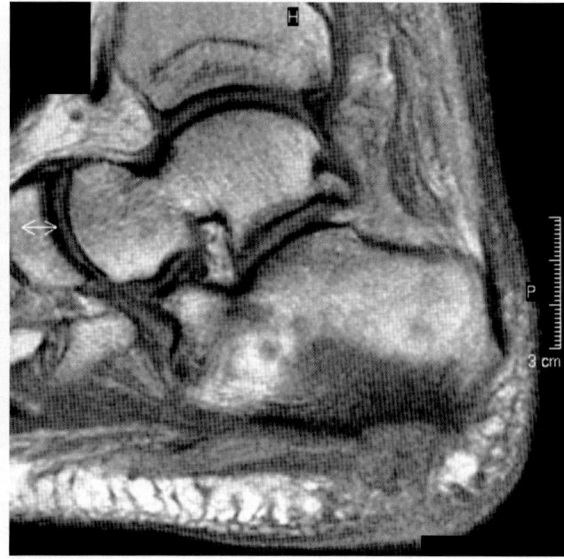

B

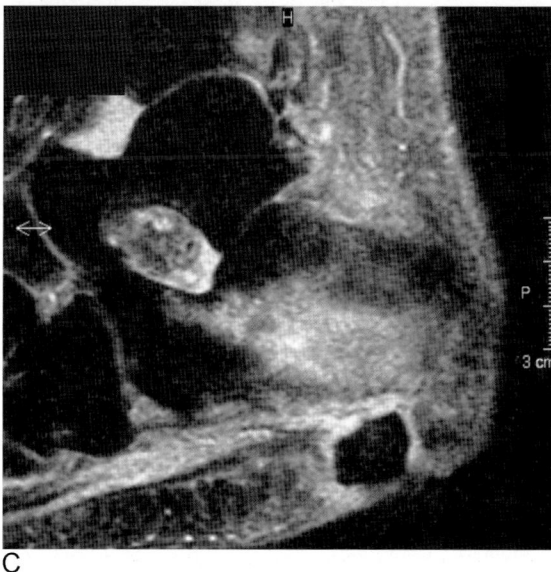

C

■ **FIGURE 62-6** Osteomyelitis in a diabetic. **A,** Lateral plain radiograph of the ankle shows cortical erosion on inferior aspect of calcaneus. A deep heel ulcer is delineated by the air extending up to the calcaneus. T1-weighted (**B**) and T1-weighted, fat suppressed, gadolinium-enhanced (**C**) MR images of the calcaneus demonstrate low signal intensity in the calcaneal marrow with marked enhancement after gadolinium administration. Erosion of the inferior cortex of calcaneus is seen in the base of the deep ulcer of the heel. Note the enhancement of the lining of the ulcer.

the sequestrum never demonstrates enhancement (see Fig. 62-6). Marrow abscesses may show rim enhancement. Enhancement is also seen along the sinus tract as well as granulation lining of soft tissue abscesses. The marrow may remain abnormal in treated osteomyelitis, trauma, tumor, and neuroarthropathy. Distinguishing osteomyelitis from neuroarthropathy becomes particularly important in the setting of diabetic foot, which is discussed in detail elsewhere in this text. However, there are secondary MRI findings that augment confidence in diagnosing infection. These are presence of a deep ulcer adjacent to abnormal bone, associated cortical discontinuity, and soft tissue abscess or sinus tract demonstrating enhancement.[7]

MRI is effective in monitoring treatment, especially in subacute and chronic osteomyelitis. When the patient responds well to treatment, clinical improvement precedes changes on MR images. These changes consist of decreased high signal intensity areas on T2-weighted images, decrease of enhancement, disappearance of abscess cavities, and return of yellow bone marrow seen on T1-weighted images. Return of yellow bone marrow is a late, but very specific sign of healing.

Computed Tomography

Computed tomography is quite useful in demonstrating early cortical destruction that may not be evident on other imaging methods. It is possible to unravel a sequestrum that may be enveloped by grossly remodeled bone in chronic osteomyelitis. Soft tissue or marrow abscesses may demonstrate rim enhancement after contrast agent administration. Subtle periosteal new bone formation may be evident. Gas within the infected bone is considered to be the earliest sign seen on CT.

With the advent of multislice CT with multiplanar reconstruction, CT plays a very useful role in the imaging of infections involving the irregular bones and joints such

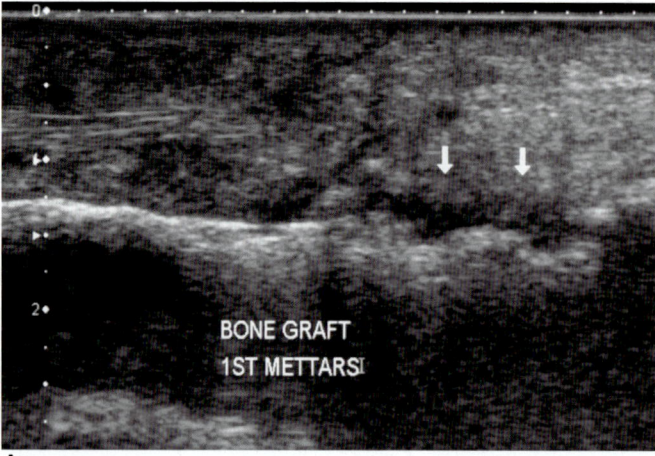

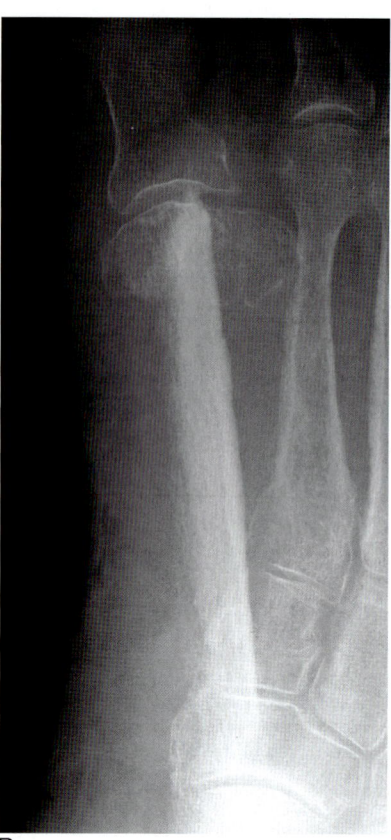

■ **FIGURE 62-7** **A,** Sonogram of the foot of patient with a discharging sinus who had bone grafting after resection of the first metatarsal for tumor. Erosion of the cortical outline of the bone graft is noted. A small amount of pericortical collection is seen in keeping with a small abscess. **B,** Subsequent radiograph confirmed osteomyelitis. Extensive erosive changes are seen in the bone graft, also in keeping with osteomyelitis.

as the sternoclavicular joint, pelvis, and spine (see Figs. 62-4B and 62-5B). It is particularly useful as image guidance enabling aspiration or biopsy.[8]

However, CT is limited by inability to accurately distinguish between suppuration, reactive granulation tissue, edema, and fibrosis.[9]

Ultrasonography

Ultrasonography is useful in the assessment of the soft tissue component of the infection. Being noninvasive and easily accessible, it enables rapid assessment of joints for effusion, which may be seen in septic arthritis. Soft tissue abscess can be confidently diagnosed on ultrasonography (see Fig. 62-7A). In children, it is possible to visualize elevation of the periosteum and the underlying collection before mineralization of the periosteum. This is useful in the early stages of acute osteomyelitis when plain radiographs may be normal, although the absence of this sign does not exclude the disease. Ultrasonography plays a particularly valuable role in assessment of the possible soft tissue causes of pain or swelling, which are factors in the differential diagnosis of osteomyelitis, which includes cellulitis, thrombophlebitis, bursitis, hematoma, tenosynovitis, or subcutaneous abscess. Ultrasonography is very useful in enabling guided aspiration and biopsy of collections or joint effusion.[10]

Nuclear Medicine

Nuclear medicine is a functional imaging modality that assesses bone turnover, which increases in the presence of infection. Conventional bone scintigraphy uses technetium-99m–labeled methylene diphosphonate (^{99m}Tc-MDP) and ^{99m}Tc-labeled hydromethylene diphosphonate (^{99m}Tc-HMDP), which are sensitive in detecting osteomyelitis. The uptake of the ^{99m}Tc-phosphonate complex depends on the perfusion and vascular permeability of the infected bone. The images are acquired at 4 hours because optimal target to background ratio is achieved at about 3 hours after injection of the radionuclide. Triple-phase bone scintigraphy is commonly used in investigation of osteomyelitis. The vascular and blood pool phases are useful in assessing the hyperemia and inflammation. There is generally increased uptake in all three phases of the bone scintigraphy in osteomyelitis. However, this is not very specific and may be abnormal in fracture, tumor, treated osteomyelitis, and neuroarthropathy (see Fig. 62-8B). Occasionally, photopenia may be seen in osteomyelitis. This may be due to aggressive infection, subperiosteal pus, or joint effusion.[11] Bone scintigraphy has been found to have a mean sensitivity of 85% to 93% and specificity of 43% to 54%.[12]

The sensitivity is lower in children and the elderly. In children, the epiphyses are active on bone scintigraphy

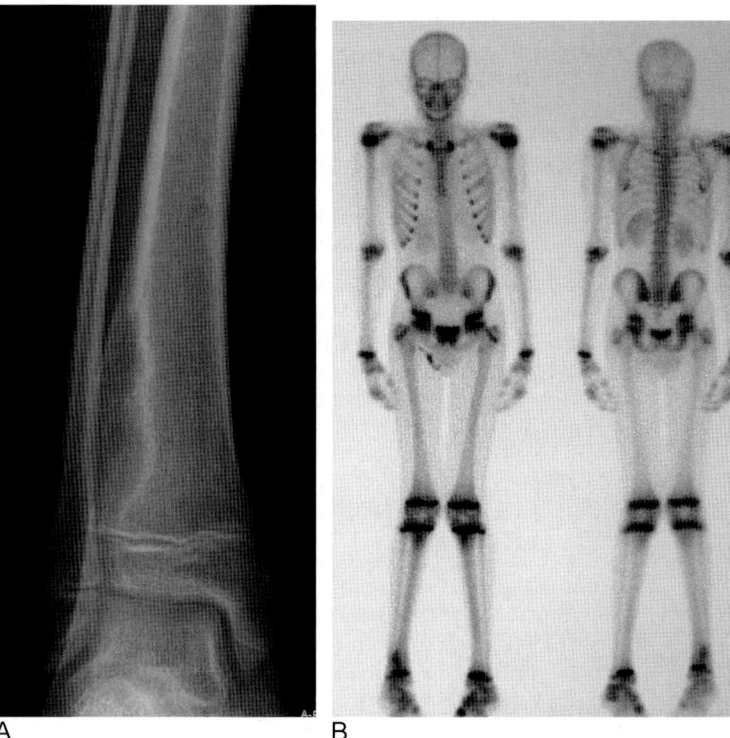

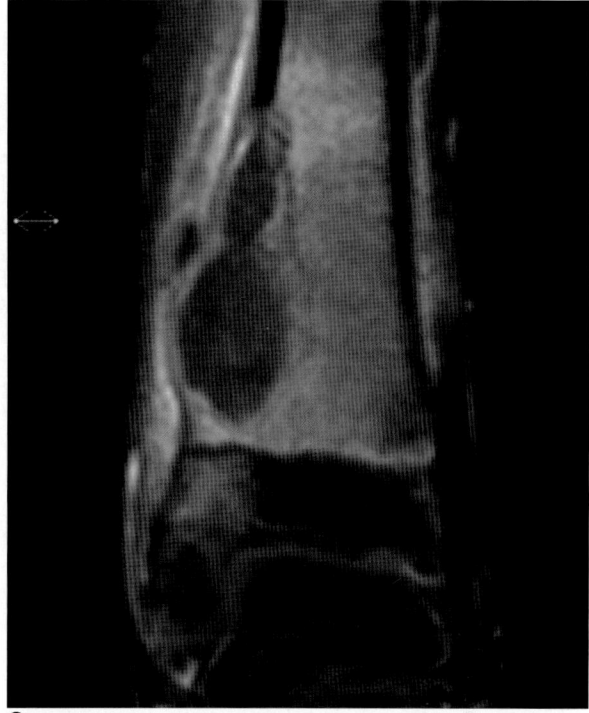

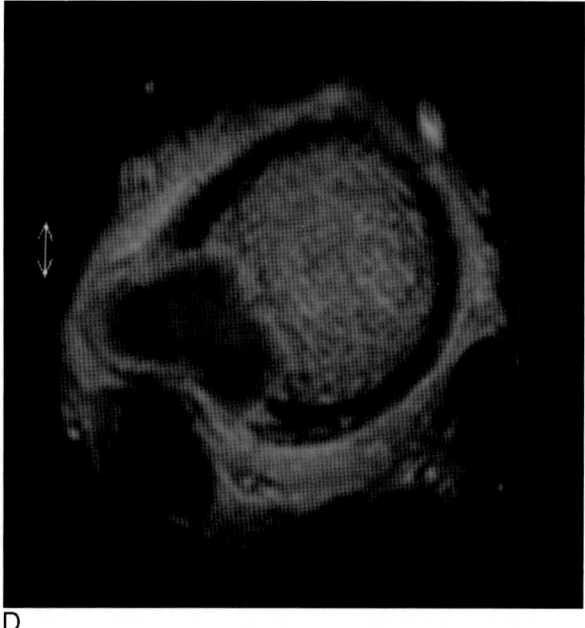

■ **FIGURE 62-8** Brodie's abscess mimicking a tumor. This patient was suspected to have an osteosarcoma but results of the MRI cast doubt on the diagnosis. The diagnosis was confirmed to be Brodie's abscess after a second biopsy because the first was not conclusive. **A,** Lucent expanded lesion seen in the distal tibia with sclerotic margin. **B,** Anterior and posterior bone scans demonstrate intense uptake in the distal tibia. This is nonspecific because increased uptake is seen in both tumor and osteomyelitis. Note the intense uptake seen normally at the epiphyses. Coronal (**C**) and axial (**D**) T1-weighted, fat-suppressed, gadolinium-enhanced MR images show typical penumbra sign with intense enhancement of the inner granulation ring. Marked surrounding bone marrow edema also demonstrates enhancement.

and may obscure sites of infection in the metaphysis, which limits its usefulness. However, scintigraphy enables examination of the whole skeleton, which is particularly useful for multiple sites involvement as can occur in chronic recurrent multifocal osteomyelitis.

Radionuclide imaging is also limited by poor resolution, which restricts the ability to accurately pinpoint the lesion. This may be overcome to a certain extent by employing single photon emission computed tomography (SPECT). Nevertheless, bone scintigraphy may be important in the workup of patients suspected of having osteo-

myelitis. A negative scan can exclude osteomyelitis with a sensitivity that is greater than 90%.

In chronic osteomyelitis, bone scintigraphy may be abnormal despite adequate treatment making distinction of active infection from inactive disease difficult. However, white blood cell scans are considered superior to bone scintigraphy and gallium-67 scans in the assessment of chronic osteomyelitis. Accuracy figures for white blood cell scans in literature indicate a higher specificity of 78% to 91%, particularly in difficult cases of chronic osteomyelitis. White blood cell scintigraphy entails labeling separated autologous granulocytes with indium-111 or ^{99m}Tc-labeled hexamethylpropylene amine oxime (^{99m}Tc-HMPAO). Granulocytes are preferentially tagged and infiltrate areas of chronic infections as part of the inflammatory response. Therefore, it is possible to detect a focus of infection by increased uptake of the radionuclides. The images are acquired 24 hours after injection. Significant radiation dose remains a concern with indium-111, particularly in children. White blood cell scans have a higher specificity in infections of appendicular bones than in the axial skeleton, owing to false-positive uptake in the normal red marrow of spine.

In-vivo agents are also available that consist of technetium-99m labeled with monoclonal murine antigranulocyte antibodies against the surface antigen NCA-95. This has the same accuracy as in-vitro white blood cell agents but is easier to use.[8]

Gallium scans are useful in chronic infections that are very difficult to diagnose. However, this examination is associated with significant radiation dose to the patient and is falling out of favor.

Positron Emission Tomography

Positron emission tomography uses ^{18}F-fluorodeoxyglucose as an agent that mimics glucose. This can be used to study the metabolic function depending on the degree of glycolysis. Infection is associated with increased glycolysis, and hence there is increased uptake. It is particularly useful in the assessment of infection in the spine and in complex cases of osteomyelitis.

Extensive research is being carried out to assess the usefulness of PET in osteomyelitis. Preliminary studies indicate that in metal implant infection, FDG-PET is not hampered by metal artifact as is the case with CT and

MRI, but its usefulness in the diagnosis of a failed joint prosthesis is debatable.

The accuracy of PET in diagnosis of musculoskeletal infections was 94% compared with 81% for combined bone and leukocyte scan. It demonstrated the ability to distinguish areas of hematopoiesis in the axial skeleton from foci of infection, which are difficult to tell apart using imaging.[13]

Recent meta-analysis assessing the diagnostic accuracy of all available imaging found PET to be the most accurate, with a sensitivity of 96% and a specificity of 91%. However, the anatomic localization can be a problem with PET. This can be easily remedied with combined PET/CT. Nevertheless, there is currently limited availability of PET scanners.

DIFFERENTIAL DIAGNOSIS (Table 62-3)

The main differential diagnoses are trauma and tumors. It is essential that these be distinguished, because the management is very different. Acute osteomyelitis can occasionally pose a problem in distinguishing it from osteosarcoma or Ewing's tumor and fracture. Chronic osteomyelitis may be difficult to distinguish from osteoid osteoma (in particular intracortical abscess), fracture, and osteosarcoma (see Figs. 62-1 and 62-8).

The clinical symptoms and signs of warm, red, and painful swelling seen in acute osteomyelitis are also seen in tumors such as osteosarcoma and Ewing's sarcoma. This is further complicated by the preponderance of all three conditions in children. Tumors may manifest as systemic toxicity, such as pyrexia.

Toddlers may present with unwillingness to use the affected limb. A history of trauma may not always be available in children.

In children, acute osteomyelitis is common and generally has an acute onset with systemic features. Tumors tend to be more indolent in presentation. A recent history of sinus or other infections needs to be elicited because this may be the cause of osteomyelitis.

Radiographic findings may be normal in osteomyelitis, early greenstick fracture, and tumors. Although both osteomyelitis and osteosarcoma may demonstrate destruction at the metaphysis with periosteal reactions there are important differences. The tumor is associated with soft tissue mass that may show variable degree of ossification and/or calcification. The periosteal reaction

---

Classic Signs

- Osteolysis is most prominent in acute osteomyelitis.
- Reactive sclerosis is most prominent in chronic osteomyelitis.
- Irregular periosteal reaction is most prominent in acute osteomyelitis.
- Regular periostitis and thickened cortex are most prominent in chronic osteomyelitis.
- Periosteal reaction may be absent when the medullary canal is not intact (after surgery).
- Brodie's abscess
- Sequestrum
- Involucrum
- Cloaca
- Four-ring appearance on MRI, with high signal intensity on T1-weighted images of the ring surrounding the central area
- Unminerilized periosteal reaction is seen on MRI and ultrasonography.
- Inflammatory changes outside periosteum are seen on MRI or ultrasonography.
- Presence of low signal sequestrum within an abscess or abnormal marrow is highly suggestive of acute osteomyelitis or acute exacerbation of chronic osteomyelitis.

TABLE 62-3 Differential Diagnosis of Osteomyelitis
Cellulitis
Septic arthritis
Fracture
Benign bone tumors
Eosinophilic granuloma
Osteoid osteoma
Malignant bone tumors
Osteosarcoma
Ewing's sarcoma
Crystal arthropathy

in tumors tends, as in acute osteomyelitis, to be spiculated and associated with Codman's triangle, whereas in chronic osteomyelitis it is typically linear, multilamellar, or solid. The presence of a soft tissue mass is readily seen on MRI, enabling distinction from osteomyelitis.

Occasionally, greenstick or spiral fractures may not be detectable on initial radiographs but may become evident in subsequent films. However, these fractures can be detected on MRI as a break in the cortex with a low signal fracture line surrounded by edema on T2-weighted images even when radiographs are normal. Similarly, insufficiency fractures can mimic osteomyelitis.

Distinguishing chronic osteomyelitis from osteoid osteoma is usually possible on radiographs, CT, and MRI. The nidus of the osteoid osteoma, depending on the degree of mineralization, is intermediate to high signal intensity on MRI, whereas the sequestrum is always of low signal intensity on all pulse sequences. The nidus demonstrates marked enhancement, unlike the sequestrum (see Fig. 62-1). CT may play a complementary role in delineating the nidus, which will be surrounded by an extensive sclerotic reaction.

SYNOPSIS OF TREATMENT OPTIONS

The aim of treatment is eliminating the organism, stopping the spread of infection, and avoiding destruction, deformity, and associated morbidity. Complications such as growth disturbance and fractures should be kept to a minimum. Reconstructive surgery in case of deformities will require complete eradication of the infective organism.

Good preoperative preparation, operating theaters with laminar flow, and use of prophylactic antibiotics have greatly reduced infection rates.

In any bone surgery, prophylactic antibiotics should be administered intravenously 30 minutes before skin incision and for no longer than 24 hours after the operation.

Patients with open bone injuries should receive a first- or second-generation cephalosporin intravenously, which should be given for 24 to 48 hours. If postoperative infection develops, then appropriate antibiotics guided by culture growth should be administered. In complex open fractures, therapy with broad-spectrum antibiotics for longer periods of 4 to 6 weeks is recommended.[14]

Medical Treatment

Antibiotics may be adequate treatment in early hematogenous osteomyelitis. Antibiotic treatment should be started promptly whenever there is a suspicion of osteomyelitis, but prior blood culture and/or bone biopsy must be obtained. Antibiotics effective against the common pathogens may be administered initially. *S. aureus* is the most common etiologic agent, and the antibiotics that are effective against this organism include flucloxacillin, nafcillin, cefuroxime, and cefazolin. Ciprofloxacin, gentamicin, and vancomycin are used in methicillin-resistant infections. Courses of antibiotics are generally given intravenously in the acute phase, lasting up to a week, and then replaced by oral antibiotics for the next 6 weeks. This can

be changed to more appropriate antibiotics depending on the result of the culture.[15]

Hyberbaric oxygen therapy has been shown to augment healing of infected bone by improving leukocyte activity, particularly in osteomyelitis associated with reduced vascularity.[16]

Surgical Treatment

Surgical treatment is indicated for cases not responding to medical therapy or when there is clear evidence of bone necrosis and abscess formation.

The main principles of surgical management of osteomyelitis include the following[17]:

- Débridement is done to resect necrotic bone and soft tissues, ensuring adequate drainage.
- External fixation is performed for stabilization. This is useful in difficult cases of chronic osteomyelitis complicated by nonunion or malunion.
- Reconstruction is done by filling of bony and soft tissue defects with bone grafts and free muscle or fasciocutaneous flaps transfer to provide vascularity.
- Amputation is reserved for cases with poor vascularity, as occurs in diabetic foot. The level of amputation is determined by the vascularity of the viable tissues proximal to the site of infection.

Recent advances using microvascular techniques involving fibular grafts and a composite osteocutaneous iliac flap reduce the duration of bone union and period of immobilization.[18]

In infection involving joint prosthesis, it is best to remove the prosthesis. There are two common approaches. In the two-stage exchange arthroplasty, surgical débridement of infected bone and soft tissues is carried out after removal of the infected prosthesis. This is followed by a period of 4 to 6 weeks of antibiotics therapy, and antibiotic-impregnated beads may be left in situ. Revision surgery is subsequently carried out. In the one-stage procedure a new prosthesis is placed after removal of the infected prosthesis at one sitting. However, antibiotics containing cement are used to reduce recurrence of infection. Nonetheless, the two-stage procedure has less risk of recurrent infection than the one-stage procedure.

What the Referring Physician Needs to Know

- Can osteomyelitis be excluded based on normal radiograph or is the radiograph taken too early to exclude osteomyelitis?
- Is sarcoma excluded as an alternative diagnosis?
- What is the best advanced imaging method in case of a nonspecific finding?
- Is there an abscess?
- Is there a sequestrum?
- What is the best advanced imaging method to produce answers to planning treatment in chronic osteomyelitis?

ACKNOWLEDGMENT

We are grateful to Mr. J. L. Barrie, Consultant Orthopaedic Surgeon, Royal Blackburn Hospital, United Kingdom, for valuable help with this manuscript.

SUGGESTED READINGS

Bureau NJ, Chhem RK, Cardinal E. Musculoskeletal infections: US manifestations. RadioGraphics 1999; 19:1585–1592.

Crim JR, Seeger LL. Imaging evaluation of osteomyelitis. Crit Rev Diagn Imaging 1994; 35:201–256.

Lew DP, Waldvogel FA. Osteomyelitis. N Engl J Med 1997; 336:999–1007.

Marti-Bonmati L, Aparisi F, Poyatos C, Vilar J. Brodie abscess: MR imaging appearance in 10 patients. J Magn Reson Imaging 1993; 3:543–546.

Morrison WB, Schweitzer ME, Batte WG, et al. Osteomyelitis of the foot: relative importance of primary and secondary MR imaging signs. Radiology 1998; 207:625–632.

Sammak B, Abd EB, Al Shahed M, et al. Osteomyelitis: a review of currently used imaging techniques. Eur Radiol 1999; 9:894–900.

Schauwecker DS. The scintigraphic diagnosis of osteomyelitis. AJR Am J Roentgenol 1992; 158:9–18.

Tehranzadeh J, Wong E, Wang F, Sadighpour M. Imaging of osteomyelitis in the mature skeleton. Radiol Clin North Am 2001; 39:223–250.

Termaat MF, Raijmakers PG, Scholten HJ, et al. The accuracy of diagnostic imaging for the assessment of chronic osteomyelitis: a systematic review and meta-analysis. J Bone Joint Surg Am 2005; 87:2464–2471.

Unger E, Moldofsky P, Gatenby R, et al. Diagnosis of osteomyelitis by MR imaging. AJR Am J Roentgenol 1988; 150:605–610.

REFERENCES

1. Resnick D, Niwayama G. Osteomyelitis, septic arthritis, and soft tissue infection: mechanisms and situations. In Resnick D (ed). Diagnosis of Bone and Joint Disorders. Philadelphia, WB Saunders, 2004, pp 2354–2418.

2. Lew DP, Waldvogel FA. Osteomyelitis. Lancet 2004; 364:369–379.

3. Termaat MF, Raijmakers PG, Scholten HJ, et al. The accuracy of diagnostic imaging for the assessment of chronic osteomyelitis: a systematic review and meta-analysis. J Bone Joint Surg Am 2005; 87:2464–2471.

4. Tumeh SS, Aliabadi P, Weissman BN, McNeil BJ. Disease activity in osteomyelitis: role of radiography. Radiology 1987; 165:781–784.

5. Morrison WB, Schweitzer ME, Bock GW, et al. Diagnosis of osteomyelitis: utility of fat-suppressed contrast-enhanced MR imaging. Radiology 1993; 189:251–257.

6. Grey AC, Davies AM, Mangham DC, et al. The "penumbra sign" on T1-weighted MR imaging in subacute osteomyelitis: frequency, cause and significance. Clin Radiol 1998; 53:587–592.

7. Morrison WB, Schweitzer ME, Batte WG, et al. Osteomyelitis of the foot: relative importance of primary and secondary MR imaging signs. Radiology 1998; 207:625–632.

8. Sammak B, Abd EB, Al Shahed M, et al. Osteomyelitis: a review of currently used imaging techniques. Eur Radiol 1999; 9:894–900.

9. Gold RH, Tong DJF, Crim JR, Seeger LL. Imaging the diabetic foot. Skeletal Radiol 1995; 24:563–571.

10. Bureau NJ, Chhem RK, Cardinal E. Musculoskeletal infections: US manifestations. RadioGraphics 1999; 19:1585–1592.

11. Schauwecker DS. The scintigraphic diagnosis of osteomyelitis. AJR Am J Roentgenol 1992; 158:9–18.

12. Larcos G, Brown ML, Sutton RT. Diagnosis of osteomyelitis of the foot in diabetic patients: value of ^{111}In-leukocyte scintigraphy. AJR Am J Roentgenol 1991; 157:527–531.

13. de Winter F, Vogelaers D, Gemmel F, Dierckx RA. Promising role of 18-F-fluoro-D-deoxyglucose positron emission tomography in clinical infectious diseases. Eur J Clin Microbiol Infect Dis 2002; 21:247–257.

14. Bamberger DM. Diagnosis and treatment of osteomyelitis. Compr Ther 2000; 26:89–95.

15. Healy B, Freedman A. Infections. BMJ 2006; 332:838–841.

16. Kindwall EP. Uses of hyperbaric oxygen therapy in the 1990s. Cleve Clin J Med 1992; 59:517–528.

17. Tetsworth K, Cierny G III. Osteomyelitis débridement techniques. Clin Orthop Relat Res 1999; (360):87–96.

18. Zweifel-Schlatter M, Haug M, Schaefer DJ, et al. Free fasciocutaneous flaps in the treatment of chronic osteomyelitis of the tibia: a retrospective study. J Reconstr Microsurg 2006; 22:41–47.

63

Spinal Infection

Bernhard Tins and Victor Cassar-Pullicino

ETIOLOGY

Spinal infection is still a potentially lethal disease with several causes. The three most commonly encountered routes of infection are hematogenous spread, direct spread, and direct inoculation, which is usually iatrogenic.

Arterial hematogenous spread can be due to an infectious focus anywhere in the body. This can be responsible for pyogenic as well as nonpyogenic infections and is the most common source of infection. Venous spread is unusual.

The second main cause of spinal infection is direct spread from an infectious focus adjacent to the spine. Spread from infection in the pelvic, perirenal, pleural, and pharyngeal areas is particularly common.

The third main group of spinal infections results from direct inoculation. These are usually due to iatrogenic infections, that is, infection of the spine after a medical intervention. This can be after spinal surgery but is also seen after discography, myelography, facet joint injection, and epidural anesthesia and also after minor interventions such as paraspinal injections of trigger points or acupuncture. It may be seen as a consequence of vertebroplasty.

The most common infectious agent is *Staphylococcus aureus,* which is encountered in about 60% of cases. Apart from *S. aureus,* virtually any infectious agent may cause spinal infection. Bacterial infections are much more common than fungal or parasitic infections. After *Staphylococcus* and *Mycobacterium tuberculosis,* commonly found infectious agents are *Escherichia coli* and, in immunocompromised patients, gram-negative bacteria; intravenous drug users often suffer *Pseudomonas* infections.[1-5]

PREVALENCE AND EPIDEMIOLOGY

Spontaneous spinal infection most commonly occurs in the elderly and the immunocompromised individual. Recognized risk factors are advanced age, male gender, immunosuppression, intravenous drug abuse, human immunodeficiency virus infection/AIDS, diabetes mellitus, sickle cell disease, use of corticosteroids, chemotherapy, rheumatologic or immunologic disease, hepatic or renal failure, malnutrition, myelodysplastic disease, and other severe systemic diseases. The increased frequency of tuberculosis in developed as well as underdeveloped countries and the increased number of chronically debilitated patients all contribute to a greater incidence of spinal infection.[6-9]

The peak age for spinal infection is in the sixth and seventh decades of life, and more than 50% of patients with spinal infection are older than 50 years of age. Spinal infection represents 2% to 8% of all cases of osteomyelitis.

Spinal involvement in tuberculosis occurs in about 50% of all tuberculosis cases when there is musculoskeletal involvement, although musculoskeletal involvement in tuberculosis overall is not common and occurs in only 1.5% to 3% of patients infected with *M. tuberculosis*. However, about a third of the world's population harbors tuberculosis and this results in a significant prevalence of infections.

Spinal infections due to nonpyogenic and nontuberculous agents such as brucellosis or fungal infections are comparatively rare in the Western world.

Iatrogenic spinal infections occur in up to 4% of all spinal surgery patients and represent up to 30% of all cases of spinal infection. The use of preoperative antibiotic prophylaxis dramatically decreases the risk of postoperative infection by about a factor 10.

KEY POINTS

- MRI is the imaging method of choice.
- Bone marrow edema is evident.
- Bone destruction occurs.
- The infection is often centered around the intervertebral disc, but any part of the spine can be affected.
- Phlegmon and abscess formation are best imaged with contrast agent enhancement.
- Epidural involvement is a surgical emergency; the whole spine needs to be imaged.

The incidence and pathway of spinal infection differs according to age as the blood supply changes (see later). Infants have a direct vascular supply to the intervertebral disc up to the age of about 6 months.

The area most commonly affected by infection is the lumbar spine, followed by the thoracic spine, and then the cervical spine.

Polymicrobial spondylodiscitis (concurrent infection with more than one infectious agent) is typically seen after surgery. Its incidence is as high as 50% of all cases. Otherwise, polymicrobial spondylodiscitis is unusual and seen overall in less than 2.5% of cases.

CLINICAL PRESENTATION

The clinical presentation of spinal infection is highly varied and ranges from asymptomatic to critically ill patients. The severity and type of signs and symptoms depend on the part of the spine infected, the type of organism, and the host's immune response. The clinical symptoms are usually nonspecific. Back pain, which is often localized, coupled with local tenderness, increased body temperature with raised C-reactive protein, and erythrocyte sedimentation rate is common. Leukocytosis can be present but is an unreliable sign.

The back pain caused by spinal infection often worsens with standing and activity and is improved by not bearing weight. Pain can occur at night with varying severity. The varied and often vague symptoms make it difficult to differentiate spinal infection from simple mechanical back pain.[10-12]

Involvement of the epidural space results in clinical deterioration and the onset of neurologic symptoms and signs.

The clinical diagnosis of spinal infection poses a particular challenge in patients with underlying preexisting disease.

In patients with prior chronic back pain a change in the type or quality of pain can be a sign of spinal infection. However, this finding is nonspecific and more often is due to deterioration of mechanical back pain. In patients who have had back surgery, recurrence of pain may be the only indicator of clinical infection.

Biopsies and blood cultures aid the diagnosis and help to identify the infective pathogen but do not exclude spinal infection if they are negative! The yield of positive cultures varies greatly and is reported in the literature to be between 50% and 90% for biopsies and 25% and 60% for blood cultures. However, the combination of both tests can result in diagnostic yields of up to 96%! If a spinal biopsy sample is taken, the infected end plate (not the disc) usually results in the highest yield. More samples result in a higher diagnostic yield. Antibiotic therapy before biopsy or blood culture results in poorer diagnostic yields.

The diagnosis of spinal infection is often delayed by 2 to 3 months. This potential delay is important because good clinical outcome depends on early diagnosis!

PATHOPHYSIOLOGY

Anatomy

The understanding of the disease process in spinal infection requires a good knowledge of spinal anatomy.

In infants younger than 6 months old there is a direct vascular supply to the intervertebral disc so that direct hematogenous infection can occur.

As infants age the direct vascular supply disappears but there are still focal areas of vascular channels in the cartilaginous end plate of the vertebral bodies that are seen to an age of 5 to 7 years. These enable hematogenous deposition of pathogens into the immediate vicinity of the intervertebral disc.

Finally, in the normal adult the vertebral body end plate poses a considerable barrier to bloodborne infection. However, in severe degenerative disc disease, blood vessels can secondarily invade the intervertebral disc and direct hematogenous infection can occur.

In the adult, the spinal column is surrounded by a dense anastomotic network of arteries formed by segmental vessels and their branches. These segmental arteries enter the spinal canal through the intervertebral foramina. Nutrient arteries enter the vertebral body from inside as well as outside the vertebral canal. The terminal branches of the nutrient arteries are end arterioles. This predisposes to embolic infarctions in the richly vascularized paradiscal area of the vertebrae.

The metaphyseal anterolateral part of the vertebral body, adjacent to the cartilaginous end plates, has a particularly dense vascular supply. This area is often the starting point of infection by oxygen-loving *M. tuberculosis,* but it is also the site of most change in inflammatory spondyloarthropathies and the origin of degenerative osteophytes.

The paravertebral venous plexus is valveless, but whether the venous plexus contributes significantly to the spread of infection remains unclear.

Pathology

In the most commonly encountered cases of hematogenous spinal infection the primary infected area is often the anterolateral paradiscal area of the vertebral body as a consequence of the increased vascular supply to this area. Initially, an inflammatory, edematous bone marrow reaction occurs. Bone destruction, paravertebral spread, and involvement of the adjacent intervertebral disc follow.

The pattern of spread of a spinal infection is partly dictated by the location of the initial infection and the aggressiveness and type of the infectious agent (Fig. 63-1). Pathogens producing proteolytic enzymes (e.g., *S. aureus*) quickly spread into adjacent structures. The vertebral body end plate and the intervertebral disc are not effective barriers. Disc involvement in infection with pyogenic pathogens is most often seen after 1 to 3 weeks and usually leads to involvement of an intervertebral disc and the two adjacent vertebrae. Disc destruction leads to loss of disc height. The concurrent end-plate destruction becomes clearer with time. At 8 to 12 weeks after the onset of spinal infection reactive bony sclerosis is observed.

When spread to adjacent tissues takes place there will be edema, phlegmon (diffuse inflammatory mass), and abscess formation.

Pathogens that do not produce proteolytic enzymes (such as *M. tuberculosis*) typically spread slowly and

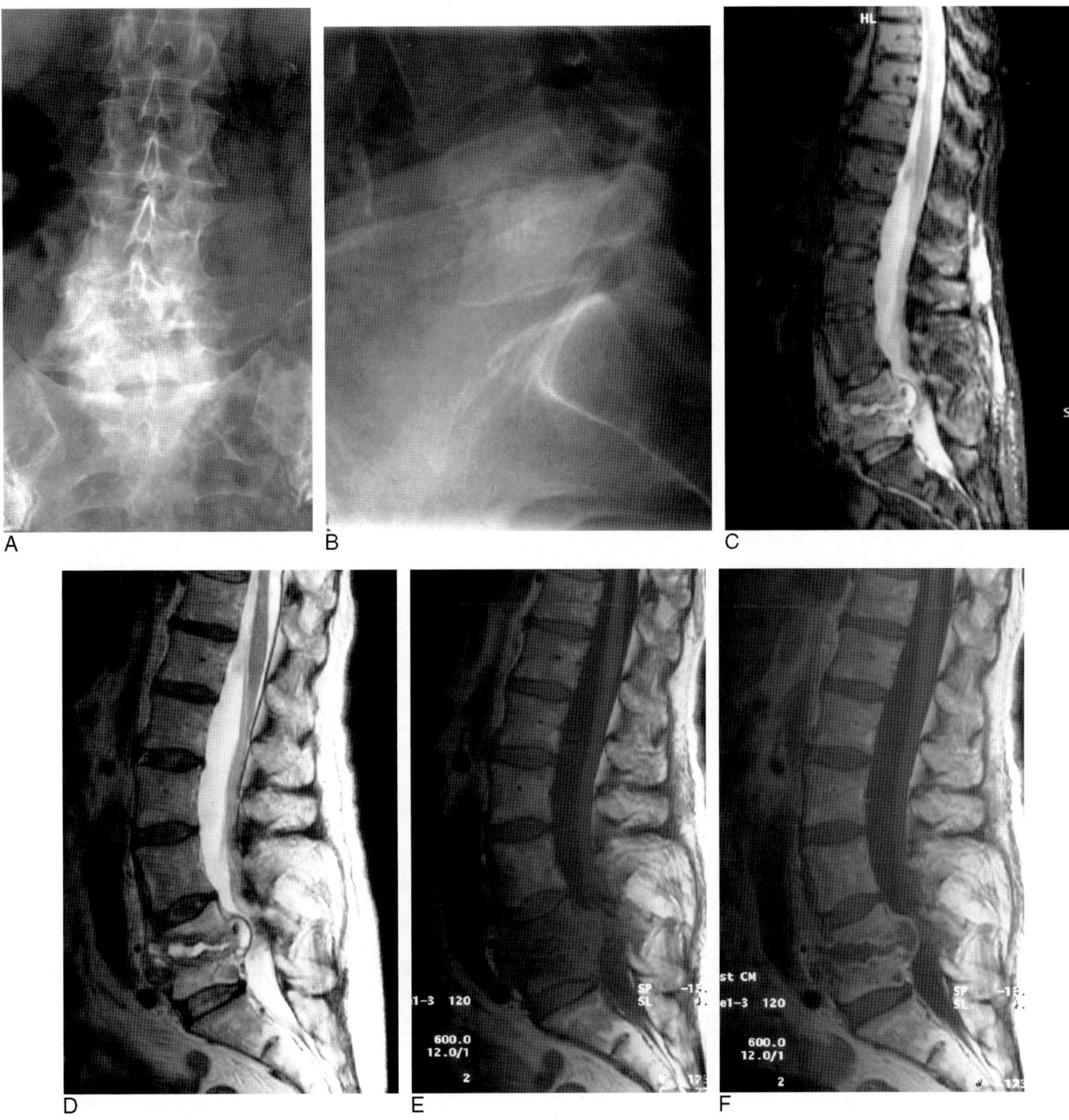

■ **FIGURE 63-1** A 75-year-old woman presented with worsening severe back pain. Radiographs (**A** and **B**) demonstrate L4-L5 disc and vertebral end-plate destruction with focal kyphosis. STIR (**C**), T2-weighted (**D**), and T1-weighted precontrast (**E**) and postcontrast (**F**) MR images show vertebral high signal intensity in STIR, less marked signal increase with T2 weighting, and signal decrease with T1 weighting. Note the increased signal intensity after contrast medium administration in the remnants of L4 and L5 vertebral bodies and a rim-enhancing abscess centered onto the L4–5 disc space bulging posteriorly into the spinal canal. Note also the improved depiction of edema on STIR as compared with T2-weighted images. These are typical findings of spondylodiscitis.

insidiously (Fig. 63-2). Complications of the infection such as fistulating abscesses (either along fascial spaces or even into peritoneum or pleura) or gibbus formation can be the presenting features. The intervertebral disc can be spared completely or may be involved very late in the disease process. Apparent loss of disc height can be due to disc herniation into vertebral bodies through weakened end plates rather than disc involvement by the infection. Involvement of paravertebral tissue can be in the form of a phlegmon or abscess formation. Abscess can spread underneath the paraspinous ligaments, elevating them and even leading to compromise of the vertebral vascular supply, ultimately causing avascular necrosis of the vertebrae.

In spinal infection by direct inoculation there is usually a relevant clinical history either of penetrating trauma or an iatrogenic intervention. The localization of the infection is obviously dependent on the history.

The most serious complications of spinal infection are epidural or meningeal and spinal cord involvement. Epidural phlegmon or abscess formation can lead to rapid deterioration with permanent disability or death if not treated early (Fig. 63-3; see also Fig. 63-1). Epidural abscesses frequently demonstrate discontinuous spread within the spinal canal; and if epidural infection is noted, the whole of the spine should be imaged. Epidural involvement constitutes a surgical emergency!

Involvement of the subdural space with meningitis or direct involvement of the spinal cord is relatively rare.

IMAGING TECHNIQUES

Techniques and Relevant Aspects

Radiography

Radiography is often the first examination performed in a patient with back pain. The first radiographic signs of spondylodiscitis are loss of disc height, vertebral end-plate destruction, and possibly paraspinal soft tissue masses (see Figs. 63-1 and 63-3). New bone formation or paraspinal calcification may also be observed. With advanced destruction, spinal deformity may occur.[13-15]

A diagnostic approach solely based on radiographs is inaccurate because of the poor sensitivity particularly for early infection and spinal infection other than spondylodiscitis and because of its poor specificity. Destruction of the vertebral end plate is the most specific sign of spinal infection but is seen at the earliest several weeks (4 to 6 weeks) into a pyogenic infection. Loss of disc height is nonspecific, and its most common cause is degenerative disc disease. Paraspinal masses are not often identified on radiographs and, if observed, are not specific for infection.

If children are affected, the radiographic changes develop significantly faster. Loss of disc height may be seen after a few days to 2 weeks, end-plate erosion/destruction may be noted after a few weeks, and reactive bone sclerosis may be observed after 1 month.

Magnetic Resonance Imaging

Magnetic resonance imaging is the examination of choice in cases of suspected or established spinal infection. Its sensitivity, specificity, and accuracy have been reported as 96%, 92%, and 94%, and these are the best values for any imaging.[16-29] In addition, MRI is the ideal method for evaluation of epidural and paraspinal spread, facilitating medical and surgical management. Other imaging methods are superior only in postoperative imaging (nuclear medicine) or in the assessment of an early bony response (CT).

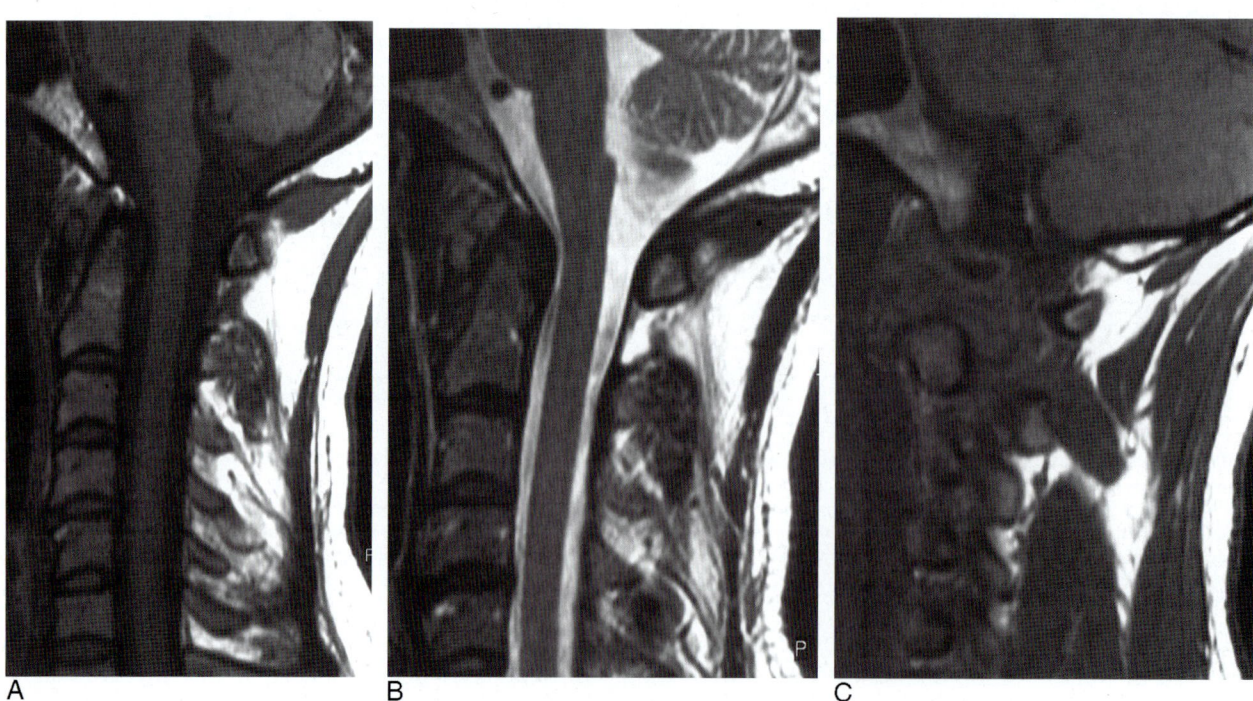

A   B   C

■ FIGURE 63-2 A 31-year-old man presented with complaints of persistent neck pain. An initial MRI of the cervical spine was reported as normal. The T1-weighted (**A**) and T2-weighted (**B**) midline slices demonstrate subtle abnormal signal in relation to the anterior aspect of the atlantodental articulation. Parasagittal slices (**C**) demonstrated a soft tissue mass between the lateral masses of C1 and C2. This was not appreciated at the time. Axial images were acquired from the C2-3 interforaminal level caudally and did not include the area of abnormality.

(Continued)

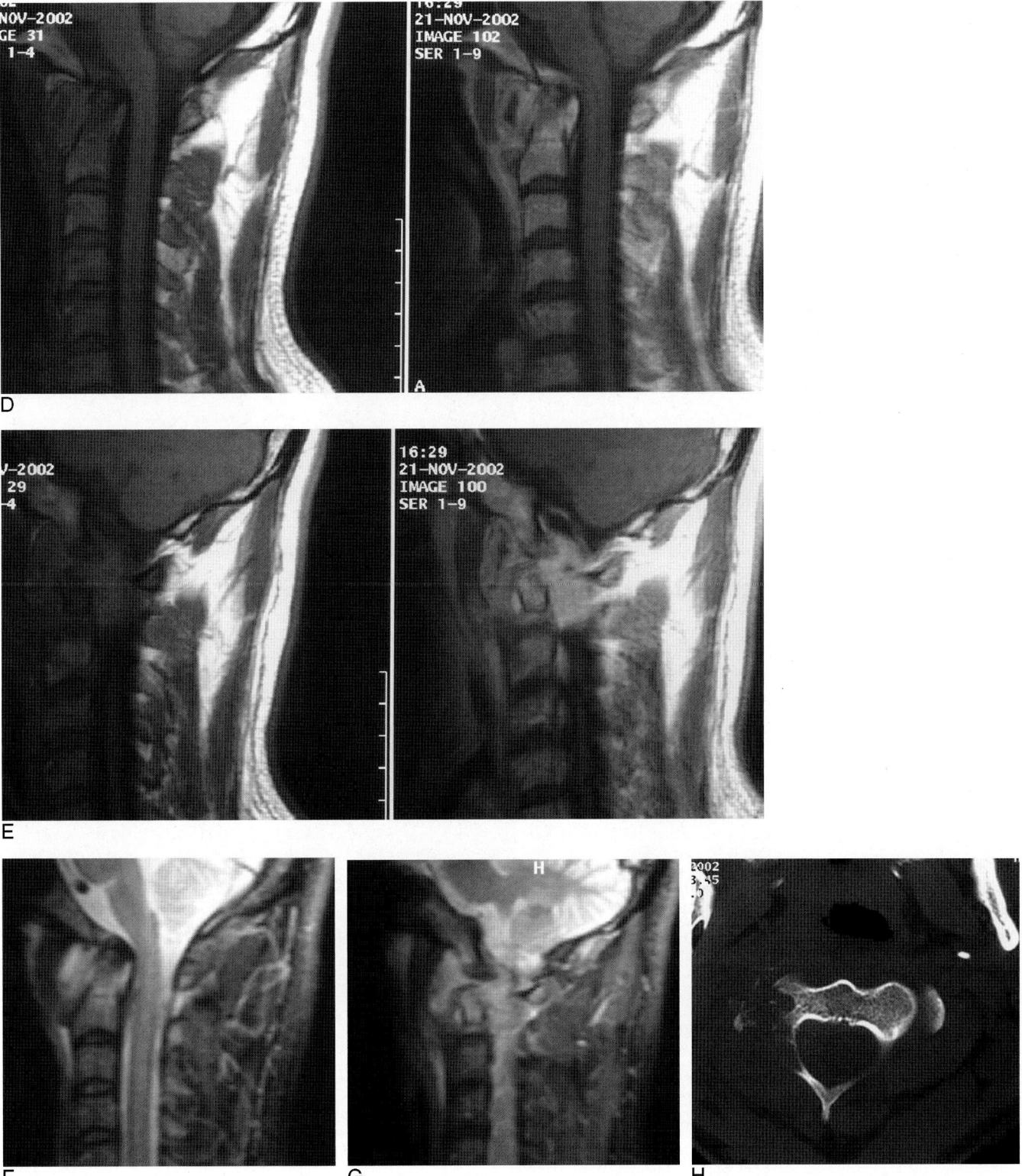

■ **FIGURE 63-2—Cont'd**   A repeat examination due to persistent severe pain 5 months later with T1-weighted precontrast (**D**) and postcontrast (**E**) and STIR (**F** and **G**) MR images demonstrate abscess formation in relation to the anterior aspect of the atlantodental articulation; the laterally extending inflammatory soft tissue mass is much better demonstrated after contrast medium enhancement and in STIR weighting. CT (**H**) shows a soft tissue mass with calcific debris and bone destruction. *Mycobacterium tuberculosis* was isolated in culture. Spinal infection can be missed even on MRI, especially when not presenting in a typical fashion. *M. tuberculosis* infection is more likely not to present as typical spondylodiscitis.

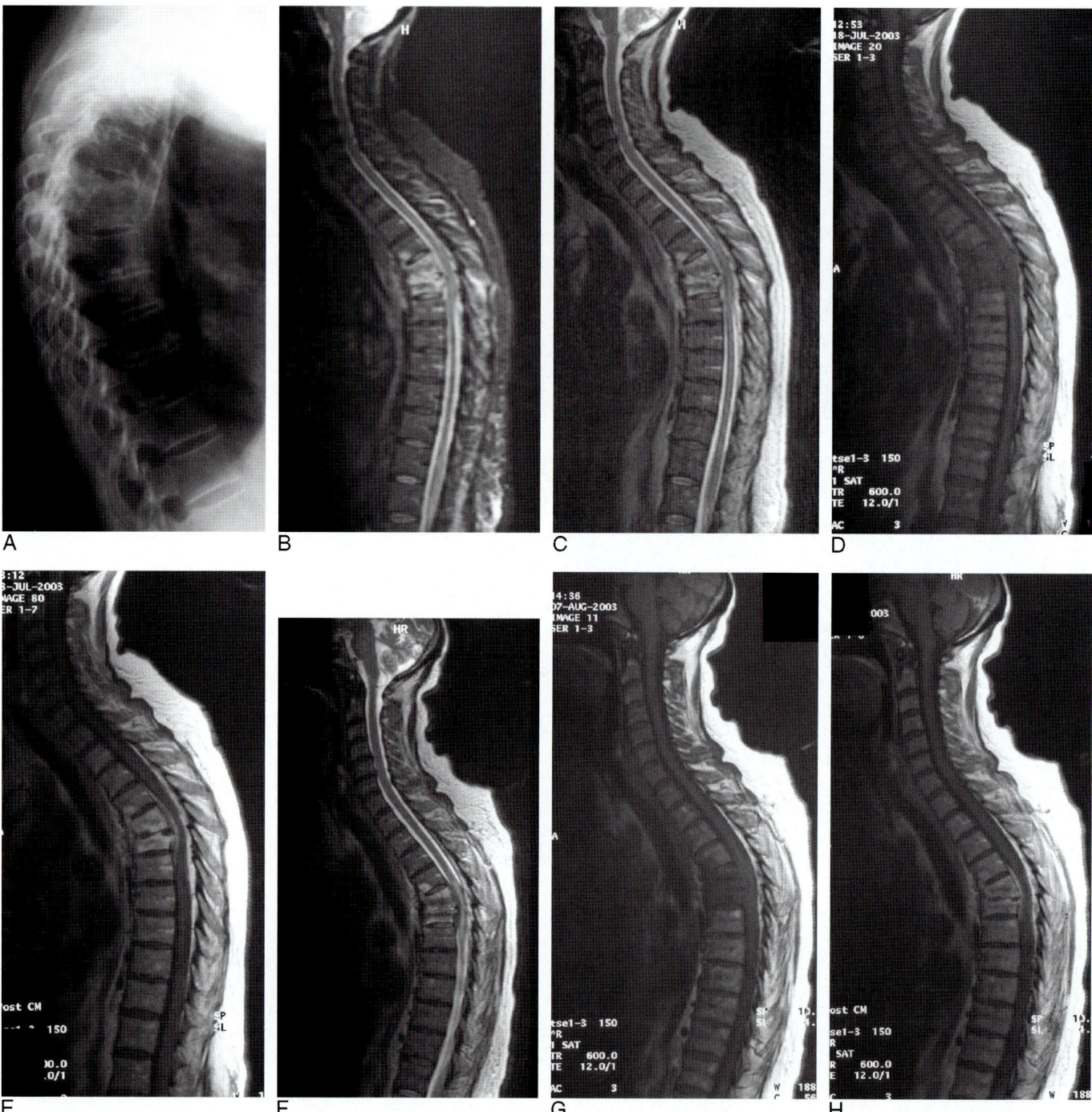

■ **FIGURE 63-3** A 69-year-old woman presented with pyogenic infection at T5–6 with epidural abscess formation. **A,** Lateral radiograph demonstrates disc and end-plate destruction. MRI shows bone marrow edema and epidural abscess formation causing cord compression on STIR (**B**), T2-weighted (**C**), T1-weighted (**D**), and contrast-enhanced T1-weighted (**E**) images. The epidural abscess is best appreciated on the T2-weighted image in **C**. Note also the involvement of the anterior inferior edge of T4 vertebral body. Antibiotic drug therapy was begun. One month later, T2-weighted (**F**), T1-weighted (**G**), and T1-weighted contrast-enhanced (**H**) images show that the epidural abscess has decreased in size but the spinal cord shows abnormally high signal intensity on T2 weighting. The patient now was paraplegic.

(Continued)

Bone marrow edema (shown by high short tau inversion recovery [STIR], high T2-weighted, fat saturated, low T1-weighted signal) is the hallmark of spinal infection (see Figs. 63-1 and 63-3). Via the disc the adjacent vertebral body is often also involved early in spondylodiscitis. The infected intervertebral disc loses the low T2-weighted signal intranuclear cleft and displays a very high T2-weighted signal intensity in its entire body. The disc height is usually reduced early but can sometimes appear widened due to erosion of the adjacent vertebral end plate. Contrast agent enhancement helps differentiate nonenhancing disc fragments from inflammatory tissue because normal disc does not enhance.

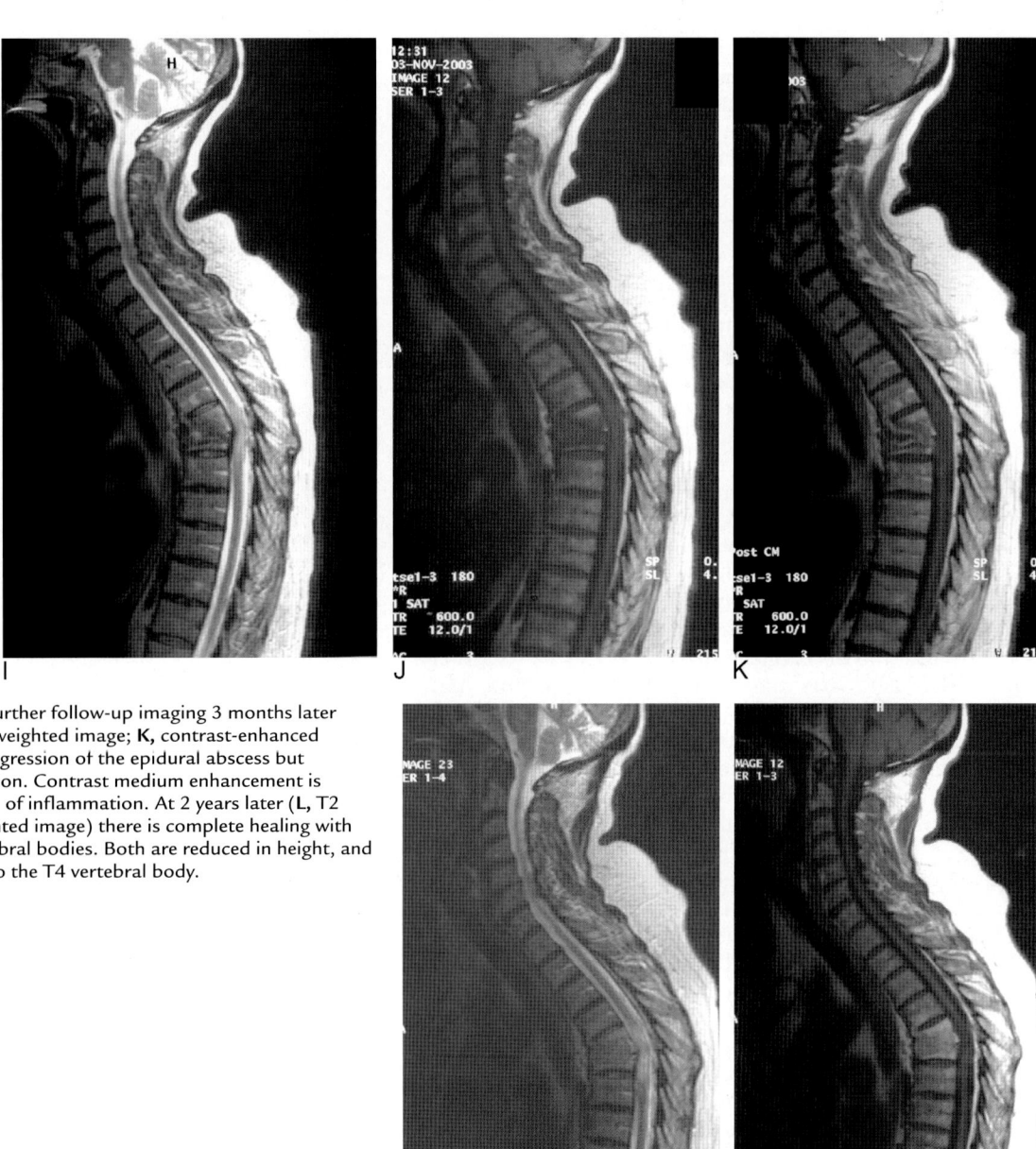

■ **FIGURE 63-3—Cont'd** Further follow-up imaging 3 months later (**I**, T2 weighted image; **J**, T1-weighted image; **K**, contrast-enhanced T1-weighted image) shows regression of the epidural abscess but progression of bone destruction. Contrast medium enhancement is reduced, indicating reduction of inflammation. At 2 years later (**L**, T2 weighted image; **M**, T1-weighted image) there is complete healing with fusion of the T5 and T6 vertebral bodies. Both are reduced in height, and there is also anterior fusion to the T4 vertebral body.

Infection of the spinal canal and the posterior elements is imaged most accurately by MRI. Epidural involvement in spinal infection is indicated by a decrease in T1-weighted signal intensity of epidural fat; increase in T2-weighted signal can be difficult to appreciate without fat suppression. STIR or fluid-attenuated inversion recovery (FLAIR) imaging is more sensitive. Abnormal fluid collections usually demonstrate higher T1-weighted and lower T2-weighted signal intensity than cerebrospinal fluid, but phlegmon as well as abscess collections can show mixed signal on T1- and T2-weighted images. The use of contrast agents permits reliable differentiation of phlegmon and abscesses. Collections show rim enhancement only whereas phlegmon shows uniform contrast enhancement. Diffusion-weighted imaging also has been shown to help in the diagnosis of collections because they exhibit markedly hyperintense signal against adjacent tissue and appear dark on apparent diffusion coefficient (ADC) maps. Meningitis can be diagnosed by observing abnormal contrast enhancement. If enhancement is nodular or "shaggy," it suggests granulomatous disease (including tuberculosis). Involvement of the spinal cord is indicated by an increase in T2-weighted signal intensity, abnormal contrast enhancement, and, if severe, vacuolization.

In cases of proven epidural involvement the whole spine has to be imaged because there is often very extensive involvement of the spinal canal with areas of relative sparing.

Paravertebral involvement can occur as phlegmon, diffuse infection of tissue, or abscess. Care must be taken to image paravertebral infection in its entirety because otherwise fistulas and tracking abscesses can be overlooked.

Once a spinal infection has been diagnosed and treatment begun there is no clear body of opinion as to the role of imaging in clinically uncomplicated cases.

MRI findings of healing are the decrease in contrast enhancement, reduction of edema and abscess size, and beginning normalization of the signal pattern, which is seen a few weeks to months after the start of treatment.

The absence of contrast medium enhancement and return of the spine to a normal signal pattern are both sure signs of complete healing of a spinal infection. However, the reverse is not true. Persistence of contrast medium enhancement in the intervertebral disc as opposed to the vertebral body is more common. The signal pattern of the bone marrow can revert to normal, but sclerosis and fibrosis can lead to low T1- and T2-weighted signal patterns. If fatty marrow replacement occurs, high T1-weighted signal will be seen (see Fig. 63-3).

Surgical implants can cause artifact and make image interpretation more difficult or impossible.

The imaging protocols for MRI of spinal infection are straightforward. Sagittal imaging should include edema-sensitive sequences such as STIR or T2-weighted, fat-saturated images. If a reliable fat-saturation technique is not available T2-weighted spin-echo imaging (TR > 2000 ms; TE 100–200 ms) is advised. Fast spin-echo imaging should not be used in these cases because edema may not be reliably diagnosed. Contrast medium enhancement is more clearly seen on T1-weighted, fat-saturated images. Abnormal areas should be assessed in sagittal and axial planes and particularly for axial imaging an enlarged field of view may be necessary to demonstrate paraspinal involvement. If epidural infection is seen, whole-spine imaging with contrast medium enhancement is mandatory.

Diffusion-Weighted Imaging

Diffusion-weighted imaging of spinal abnormalities can be used as an adjunct in select cases. Sometimes the imaging features of spinal infection and malignancy are very similar and confident diagnosis is not possible. Paraspinal abscesses are hyperintense compared with adjacent tissue in diffusion-weighted imaging and low signal on the ADC map. Usually the ADC of neoplastic lesions is significantly lower than that of infection.

Computed Tomography

Computed tomography of the spine is not normally the examination of choice for diagnosis of spinal infection. CT has relatively poor soft tissue contrast and cannot demonstrate the earliest sign of spondylitis, which is bone marrow edema. It usually can demonstrate paraspinal masses and abscesses but not as well as MRI.[30] CT can show loss of disc height, although the differentiation of degeneration and infection can be difficult. Epidural phlegmon and even epidural abscess formation are not well imaged or differentiated using CT.

CT is well suited to demonstrate bone destruction and bony reaction in the form of sclerosis. It also is the best imaging method to show calcification and gas in soft tissue. CT best allows the assessment of an early healing response (new bone formation) after successful treatment of spondylodiscitis. It can demonstrate sclerosis of the remaining bone cortex and marrow at about 6 weeks after the onset of infection whereas these changes are only clearly appreciated on MRI at around 12 weeks after the onset. CT is valuable for the imaging of postoperative infections.

Ultrasonography

Ultrasonography plays little role in the diagnosis of spinal infection, although its use in children has been suggested. It is sometimes used intraoperatively especially for localizing epidural abscess collections, and it is sometimes of value in differentiating paravertebral abscesses from diffusely solid phlegmon. It has been used to guide percutaneous drainage of abscesses.

Nuclear Medicine

Nuclear medicine techniques include technetium-99m–labeled bone scintigraphy and infection-specific techniques, such as labeled white cells, labeled antibody fragments, ciprofloxacin, gallium, and also positron emission tomography.[31-33] All these methods offer good sensitivity but poor specificity and anatomic resolution even when combined with single photon emission computed tomography. For the initial diagnosis these techniques have been superseded by MRI, but they are still sometimes useful in the imaging of postoperative infection.

Pros and Cons

MRI is the imaging method of choice for spinal infection. Cost considerations may play a role, and MRI may not be possible in all patients with back pain.

The only feature in favor of radiography is its almost universal availability. The problem with radiographs is poor or absent sensitivity for any spinal infection other than destructive spondylodiscitis. Radiographs can play a role in monitoring complications.

CT is well suited to assess bone response to spinal infection and can be performed under virtually any circumstances. Disadvantages are the poor depiction of soft tissues when compared with MRI and that it uses ionizing radiation.

Nuclear medicine techniques (including positron emission tomography) offer reasonable sensitivity but poor specificity and poor anatomic detail.

Ultrasonography does not play any significant role in the initial diagnosis of spinal infection.

Controversies

There are no real controversies in the imaging of spinal infection. The main caveat in imaging of spinal infection is to image the whole spine when spinal infection has been diagnosed so as to not miss epidural or other multi-level involvement.

MANIFESTATIONS OF THE DISEASE

Infection with *Mycobacterium tuberculosis*

Infection with *M. tuberculosis* is the most common granulomatous disease of the spine, and spinal tuberculosis accounts for half of all cases of musculoskeletal tuberculosis. In developed countries, musculoskeletal tuberculosis affects mainly the elderly and is thought to be due to reactivation of an old focus of tuberculosis; however, it may be seen in immigrants of any age who are in otherwise good health when they come from countries with a high prevalence of tuberculosis. In underdeveloped countries, children and young adults are primarily affected and the disease tends to be more aggressive.

Tuberculous spinal infection usually presents as relatively mild symptoms and progresses slowly, often leading to a long delay before diagnosis (see Fig. 63-2). Spinal tuberculosis is usually due to hematogenous spread from a focus in the lung or the genitourinary tract.

The thoracolumbar junction or lumbar spine is most commonly affected. The more cranial parts of the spine are more often infected with tuberculous infection than pyogenic infection.

Spinal tuberculosis typically starts in the well-vascularized anterolateral edge of a vertebral body. It can spread underneath the longitudinal ligaments to adjacent vertebral bodies and can cause vascular compromise with avascular necrosis and subsequent vertebral body collapse. Central abscess formation within the vertebral body is relatively common whereas bone sclerosis is less common and florid than for pyogenic infection, although in chronic cases reactive new bone formation can be considerable.

Arachnoiditis, meningitis, and infection of the spinal cord occur more frequently in tuberculosis of the spine than other spinal infections. Often there is no associated spondylitis.

Erosion of the vertebral body end plate can cause disc herniation into the vertebral body and loss of disc height without actual infection of the disc.

Large paravertebral abscesses are commonly seen in tuberculosis of the spine. They are often symmetric and tend to be larger than in pyogenic infections. Abscesses can track long distances, and sinuses are frequently seen in the groin, buttock, and chest. If an abscess is calcified, this is very suggestive of tuberculosis; if an air-fluid level is seen, then tuberculosis is virtually excluded (provided that there is no sinus connecting to the skin surface or gas-containing structures).

Vertebral body destruction is common in spinal tuberculosis (up to 73%), and this makes spinal deformity with gibbus or vertebra plana and neurologic compromise more common than in other infections. Kyphotic deformities tend to be more severe in the thoracic spine.

Neurologic compromise rarely occurs due to bony collapse alone. It is either due to associated subluxation/dislocation or occurs in the acute disease as the result of epidural involvement.

Involvement of the posterior elements is common in spinal tuberculosis and seen in more than 40% of cases. This leads to an increased incidence of neurologic complications and a more difficult differential diagnosis, especially against neoplasia. Isolated infection of the posterior elements is rare (<2%).

After treatment, progression of destructive change is regularly seen and can last up to 14 months. This is significantly longer than for pyogenic infection.

Radiography

The radiographic findings are largely nonspecific. There is usually less reactive sclerosis of bone, and abscess calcification is more frequent than in pyogenic infections.

Magnetic Resonance Imaging

The signal pattern of vertebral osteomyelitis due to tuberculosis is the same as in other infections or inflammation with edema-like signal, that is, signal decrease in T1-weighted imaging and increase in T2-weighted imaging, although in the vertebral body a mixed pattern can be seen in both types of images.

In cases of suspected tuberculous meningitis the entire spine should be imaged and, if positive, the brain should be examined as well.

Multidetector Computed Tomography

Computed tomographic findings are nonspecific. Bone destruction but also reactive bone sclerosis is quite well imaged by CT. CT is also well suited to demonstrate soft tissue calcification (see Fig. 63-2).

Ultrasonography

Ultrasonography does not play a significant role in the diagnosis of spinal tuberculosis.

Nuclear Medicine

Nuclear medicine techniques can be used for screening of the skeleton in generalized infectious processes, but the specificity is limited.

Positron Emission Tomography/Computed Tomography

There is a limited role for the assessment of tuberculous abscesses, but the activity of a tuberculous abscess can be assessed by fluorodeoxyglucose (FDG)-labeled PET. High activity of the entire abscess indicates a hot abscess; uptake only of the abscess rim indicates a cold abscess.

Classic Signs: Tuberculosis of the Spine

- Insidious onset, protracted clinical course
- Locally less aggressive than pyogenic infection but of long duration
- Bone destruction and disc involvement relatively slow but can be very extensive
- Bone sclerosis relatively little early in disease compared with pyogenic infection
- Bone collapse with gibbus formation and spinal instability
- Extensive soft tissue spread and abscess formation with fistulation more common
- Multilevel involvement possibly with disc sparing
- Soft tissue calcification

Pyogenic Infection

There is no single sign that would allow a reliable differentiation of pyogenic from tuberculous infection. The clinical presentation of pyogenic spinal infections is usually much more acute than that of spinal tuberculosis. The distribution of pyogenic spinal infections is similar to that in tuberculosis; the lumbar spine is most commonly affected, followed by the thoracic, the cervical, and the sacral spine. Most pyogenic infections are caused by *S. aureus,* but almost any bacterium can be found. The infection usually starts in the well-perfused anterolateral vertebral edge. Proteolytic enzymes help to quickly spread the infection to the intervertebral disc. The early spread to discs with loss of disc height and disc herniation is more suggestive of pyogenic infection than of tuberculosis. Loss of disc height is seen 1 to 3 weeks after the onset of infection, and reactive bone sclerosis is seen after 8 to 12 weeks (at about 6 weeks with CT). Pyogenic infection spreads usually to contiguous vertebral bodies (see Fig. 63-3), as opposed to tuberculosis or fungal infection in which skip lesions are more common. Intravertebral and paravertebral abscesses are generally smaller than in tuberculosis and more often asymmetric. Involvement of the posterior elements is rare.

Significant bony destruction with kyphosis, scoliosis, or neurogenic compromise is rare.

S. aureus is by far the most commonly pathogen found in spinal infections, reported in more than 55% of published cases. *Pseudomonas aeruginosa* is common in intravenous drug abusers. *Salmonella* infections occur fairly frequently in patients with sickle cell disease and elderly men with infections of the genitourinary tract, although *S. aureus* remains the most common cause of spine infection in these groups. In patients with sickle cell disease, avascular necrosis is in the differential diagnosis of early infection. Sickle cell disease does not affect the intervertebral discs, and spinal involvement is more commonly seen in the less well perfused middle area of the end plates than in the anterolateral area preferred by infection. Bacteria of the *Proteus* group are frequently seen in urinary tract infections and can lead to spinal infections. There is no particular distinguishing feature to any of the pathogens discussed so far.

Brucellosis is caused by the gram-negative coccobacillus *Brucella*. In Western countries it is seen in people employed in animal husbandry. It is also transmitted by unprocessed goat and camel milk and hyperendemic in parts of Latin America and the Middle East. Brucellosis mimics tuberculosis in its clinical behavior and the imaging features. It is diagnosed by culture or serology. Spinal brucellosis is often indolent and has a predilection for the lumbar spine and can cause step-like deformities; a so-called parrot's beak appearance is strongly suggestive of spinal brucellosis. If only sclerosis is seen, the appearances can strongly resemble degenerative change on radiography. Spinal brucellosis can be focal or diffuse; in the diffuse form disc involvement and paraspinal abscesses are seen.

Syphilis can affect the musculoskeletal system, usually in the tertiary phase of acquired syphilis, and is due to tabes dorsalis with a Charcot arthropathy of the lower limbs and spine. The denervation leads to vertebral subluxation-dislocation with sclerosis and destruction and can mimic tuberculosis of the spine.

Radiography

Generally, radiography is nonspecific in spinal infection. Loss of disc height and destruction of the adjacent vertebral body end plates is the presentation of classic spondylodiscitis. Bone destruction occurs more rapidly than in tuberculosis.

Magnetic Resonance Imaging

The MRI findings are not specific for a particular pathogen. Edema-like signal indicates the osteomyelitis.

Multidetector Computed Tomography

Computed tomography is best suited to show the bony destruction associated with pyogenic infections. Sclerosis can be the first sign of a healing response.

Ultrasonography

Ultrasonography has little part in the diagnosis or the monitoring of spinal infection.

Nuclear Medicine

Nuclear medicine findings are nonspecific. Bone scan and more inflammation-specific techniques all show increased activity, but the specificity is poor.

Positron Emission Tomography/Computed Tomography

As with other nuclear medicine techniques, PET suffers from limited specificity. The specificity is increased by the combination of PET and CT, but it remains unreliable.

Classic Signs: Pyogenic Spine Infection

- Often acute onset and rapid clinical course
- Locally aggressive
- Bone destruction and disc involvement relatively early
- More bone sclerosis than in tuberculosis
- Skip lesion less common
- Abscess formation more local, fistulation not typical
- Soft tissue calcification not typical
- Classic spondylodiscitis: centered around intervertebral disc with loss of disc height and destruction of the adjacent bony end plates

---

DIFFERENTIAL DIAGNOSIS

The main symptom of spinal infection is back pain. If accompanied by fever, as is the case in two thirds of patients with spinal infection, then infection or neoplasia must be suspected.

The back pain is usually relieved by lying down and is aggravated by activity. These features make it difficult to differentiate back pain caused by spinal infection from that caused by mechanical back problems.[34-35]

If spinal infection presents with neurologic problems, any cause of cord or nerve root compromise has to be considered.

Useful laboratory parameters are raised erythrocyte sedimentation rate and C-reactive protein levels, but in chronic tuberculosis the C-reactive protein value can be normal.

The list of differential diagnoses is reasonably long, but in practice the diagnosis of spinal infection is not usually difficult.

In atypical presentations of preexisting or coexisting other disease the diagnosis can be difficult and might not always be possible with a high degree of confidence. The approach for the differential diagnosis is to start with the pertinent imaging features to discuss which further diseases need to be considered.

Collapsed Vertebral Body

The most common cause for a collapsed vertebral body in the elderly is osteoporosis. It also occurs in infection, tumor, and trauma; and the collapse can obscure the more typical findings in these disease entities. Infection can lead to vertebral body collapse, although this is rare. Paravertebral soft tissue involvement is not common in osteopenic collapse and is more suggestive of a neoplastic disease or infection.

Single Vertebral Body Edema

Vertebral body edema in a single vertebra can be a sign of (early) infection, benign or malignant infiltration, trauma, or various rarer abnormalities, such as chronic multifocal recurrent osteomyelitis. The differentiation is often difficult. Assessment of the rest of the skeleton can be of help. Biopsy is often necessary.

Disc and End-Plate Changes

Fluid- or edema-like signal in the intervertebral disc and destruction and edema-like signal in the adjacent end plate are signs of spondylodiscitis. However, these features can also be seen in degenerative change of the spine with end-plate edema, neuroarthropathy (Charcot disease of the spine), erosive osteochondrosis, inflammatory spondyloarthropathies, long-term hemodialysis, and, rarely, sarcoidosis and other granulomatous diseases of the spine.

Features allowing differentiation are the presence of gas in the disc in degenerative disease (extremely rare in infection) and the absence of paravertebral abscesses or significant soft tissue masses (suggests noninfective cause), although minor paravertebral soft tissue involvement is sometimes seen with noninfectious granulomatous disease.[36-39]

Destructive Soft Tissue Mass

A destructive soft tissue mass in the spine can be due to tumor or spinal infection. The presence of a phlegmon or abscess formation is a strong marker of spinal infection. If there is only a focal mass present, a malignant tumor is more likely than infection. Whereas most often the intervertebral discs are spared by tumors, rarely they can be involved; for example by multiple myeloma, lymphoma, chordoma, eosinophilic granuloma, aneurysmal bone cyst, and giant cell tumors. Involvement of the posterior elements is typical but not pathognomonic for spinal neoplasia. Paravertebral involvement with tumor or hemorrhage is also seen, although the paravertebral fat is often displaced whereas in infection it is edematously infiltrated. Subligamentous spread is not seen with tumors.

SYNOPSIS OF TREATMENT OPTIONS

Medical Treatment

Medical treatment is the treatment of choice in the absence of neurologic symptoms (or presence of only minimal symptoms) and in the absence of significant spinal deformity or instability. This is the case in about 75% of patients with spinal infection. The mainstay of medical treatment is antibiotic therapy. If the offending pathogen has been identified by blood culture or biopsy, specific treatment can be instituted. Otherwise, broadband antibiotic treatment covering the most likely pathogens including *S. aureus* is indicated. Depending on the personal circumstances of the patient, the treatment has to be adjusted to cover rarer infections that occur more frequently in a particular patient group, such as drug users (*Pseudomonas*) or those with sickle cell disease (*Salmonella*). Underlying medical problems that might have predisposed the patient for a spinal infection or are the likely source of hematogenous seeding should be addressed (e.g., urinary or respiratory tract problems leading to repeated bouts of infection).

The recommendations for the duration of antibiotic therapy vary, as do the recommendations for the length of intravenous treatment. There is no conclusive evidence as to when it is appropriate to switch from intravenous to oral antibiotics. Generally, intravenous antibiotics are recommended as long as the patient is clinically ill (i.e., pyrexial), and some authors recommend that antibiotics are only given intravenously. The recommendations regarding the length of treatment vary from 1 to 4 weeks to 3 months. For infection with *M. tuberculosis* the treatment recommendations vary between 3 to 18 months. Obviously this is oral treatment.

Surgical Treatment

Surgical treatment of spinal infection is indicated in the presence of neurologic symptoms, spinal instability or significant deformity. It is sometimes performed for spinal infections unresponsive to medical treatment. Epidural abscess formation is a surgical emergency![40,41]

The aim of surgery is thorough débridement ensuring good vascularity and spinal stability.

Generally, an anterior approach is preferred because it is easier to achieve or maintain spinal stability; however, depending on the location of the infection a posterior or a combined approach can be necessary.

The use of surgical implants is controversial. Surgical instrumentation seems less of a problem with regard to infection when the anterior approach is used. Similarly, it is controversial whether surgical implants need to be removed in cases of infected postoperative spines. Removal of implants potentially removes the harborer of infection but causes instability, which, in turn, favors the persistence of infection. Persistence of infection is more common with stainless steel implants than with titanium implants, owing to the formation of a pseudocapsule around the steel implant. Pyogenic infections are more likely to lead to bony fusion than tuberculosis, which is more likely to lead to permanent instability.

The treatment of epidural abscesses relies critically on preoperative imaging to decompress all abscesses. Endoscopic surgery may then be possible.

What the Referring Physician Needs to Know

- Type of pathogen and sensitivity to antibiotics
- Location and extent of infection
- Neurologic symptoms or instability warrant surgical referral.
- Epidural abscess formation is a surgical emergency.

SUGGESTED READINGS

Calderone RR, Larsen JM. Overview and classification of spinal infections. Orthop Clin North Am 1996; 27:1-8.

Dagirmanjian A, Schils J, McHenry MC. MR imaging of spinal infections. Magn Reson Imaging Clin North Am 1999; 7:525-538.

Early SD, Kay RM, Tolo VT. Childhood diskitis. J Am Acad Orthop Surg 2003; 11:413-420.

Gillams AR, Chaddha B, Carter AP. MR appearances of the temporal evolution and resolution of infectious spondylitis. AJR Am J Roentgenol 1996; 166:903-907.

Hsieh PC, et al. Surgical strategies for vertebral osteomyelitis and epidural abscess. Neurosurg Focus 2004; 17:E4.

Khan IA, Vaccaro AR, Zlotolow DA. Management of vertebral diskitis and osteomyelitis. Orthopedics 1999; 22:758-765.

Love C, et al. FDG PET of infection and inflammation. RadioGraphics 2005; 25:1357-1368.

Quinones-Hinojosa A, et al. General principles in the medical and surgical management of spinal infections: a multidisciplinary approach. Neurosurg Focus, 2004; 17:E1.

Rankine JJ, et al. Therapeutic impact of percutaneous spinal biopsy in spinal infection. Postgrad Med J 2004; 80:607-609.

Rothman SL. The diagnosis of infections of the spine by modern imaging techniques. Orthop Clin North Am 1996; 27:15-31.

Tins BJ, Cassar-Pullicino VN. MR imaging of spinal infection. Semin Musculoskelet Radiol 2004; 8:215-229.

REFERENCES

1. Hopkinson N, Stevenson J, Benjamin S. A case ascertainment study of septic discitis: clinical, microbiological and radiological features. Q J Med 2001; 94:465-470.
2. Butler JS, Shelly MJ, Timlin M, et al. Nontuberculous pyogenic spinal infection in adults: a 12-year experience from a tertiary referral center. Spine 2006; 31:2695-2700.
3. Priest DH, Peacock JE Jr. Hematogenous vertebral osteomyelitis due to *Staphylococcus aureus* in the adult: clinical features and therapeutic outcomes. South Med J 2005; 98:854-862.
4. Nolla JM, Ariza J, Gomez-Vaquero C, et al. Spontaneous pyogenic vertebral osteomyelitis in nondrug users. Semin Arthritis Rheum 2002; 31:271-278.
5. Honan M, White GW, Eisenberg GM. Spontaneous infectious discitis in adults. Am J Med 1996; 100:85-89.
6. Carragee EJ. Pyogenic vertebral osteomyelitis. J Bone Joint Surg Am 1997; 79:874-880.
7. Colmenero JD, Jimenez-Mejias ME, Sanchez-Lora FJ, et al. Pyogenic, tuberculous, and brucellar vertebral osteomyelitis: a descriptive and comparative study of 219 cases. Ann Rheum Dis 1997; 56:709-715.
8. Williams RL, Fukui MB, Meltzer CC, et al. Fungal spinal osteomyelitis in the immunocompromised patient: MR findings in three cases. AJNR Am J Neuroradiol 1999; 20:381-385.
9. Cahill DW, Love LC, Rechtine GR. Pyogenic osteomyelitis of the spine in the elderly. J Neurosurg 1991; 74:878-886.
10. Perronne C, Saba J, Behloul Z, et al. Pyogenic and tuberculous spondylodiskitis (vertebral osteomyelitis) in 80 adult patients. Clin Infect Dis 1994; 19:746-750.
11. Alothman A, Memish ZA, Awada A, et al. Tuberculous spondylitis: analysis of 69 cases from Saudi Arabia. Spine 2001; 26:E565-E570.
12. Gasbarrini AL, Bertoldi E, Mazzetti M, et al. Clinical features, diagnostic and therapeutic approaches to haematogenous vertebral osteomyelitis. Eur Rev Med Pharmacol Sci 2005; 9:53-66.
13. Smith AS, Blaser SI. Infectious and inflammatory processes of the spine. Radiol Clin North Am 1991; 29:809-827.
14. Stabler A, Reiser MF. Imaging of spinal infection. Radiol Clin North Am 2001; 39:115-135.
15. Sharif HS, Aideyan OA, Clark DC, et al. Brucellar and tuberculous spondylitis: comparative imaging features. Radiology 1989; 171:419-425.
16. Modic MT, Feiglin DH, Piraino DW, et al. Vertebral osteomyelitis: assessment using MR. Radiology 1985; 157:157-166.
17. Thrush A, Enzmann D. MR imaging of infectious spondylitis. AJNR Am J Neuroradiol 1990; 11:1171-1180.
18. Maiuri F, Iaconetta G, Gallicchio B, et al. Spondylodiscitis: clinical and magnetic resonance diagnosis. Spine 1997; 22:1741-1746.
19. Dagirmanjian A, Schils J, McHenry MC. MR imaging of spinal infections. Magn Reson Imaging Clin North Am 1999; 7:525-538.
20. Ruiz A, Post MJ, Sklar EM, Holz A. MR imaging of infections of the cervical spine. Magn Reson Imaging Clin North Am 2000; 8:561-580.
21. Dagirmanjian A, Schils J, McHenry M, Modic MT. MR imaging of vertebral osteomyelitis revisited. AJR Am J Roentgenol 1996; 167:1539-1543.
22. Post MJ, Sze G, Quencer RM, et al. Gadolinium-enhanced MR in spinal infection. J Comput Assist Tomogr 1990; 14:721-729.
23. Post MJ, Quencer RM, Montalvo BM, et al. Spinal infection: evaluation with MR imaging and intraoperative US. Radiology 1988; 169:765-771.
24. Sharif HS. Role of MR imaging in the management of spinal infections. AJR Am J Roentgenol 1992; 158:1333-1345.
25. Smith AS, Weinstein MA, Mizushima A, et al. MR imaging characteristics of tuberculous spondylitis vs vertebral osteomyelitis. AJR Am J Roentgenol 1989; 153:399-405.
26. Michael AS, Mikhael MA. Spinal osteomyelitis: unusual findings on magnetic resonance imaging. Comput Med Imaging Graph 1988; 12:329-331.

27. Gillams AR, Chaddha B, Carter AP. MR appearances of the temporal evolution and resolution of infectious spondylitis. AJR Am J Roentgenol 1996; 166:903-907.

28. Sharif HS, Clark DC, Aabed MY, et al. Granulomatous spinal infections: MR imaging. Radiology 1990; 177:101-107.

29. Ahmadi J, Bajaj A, Destian S, et al. Spinal tuberculosis: atypical observations at MR imaging. Radiology 1993; 189:489-493.

30. De Backer AI, Mortele KJ, Vanschoubroeck IJ, et al. Tuberculosis of the spine: CT and MR imaging features. JBR-BTR 2005; 88:92-97.

31. Palestro CJ, Kim CK, Swyer AJ, et al. Radionuclide diagnosis of vertebral osteomyelitis: indium-111-leukocyte and technetium-99m-methylene diphosphonate bone scintigraphy. J Nucl Med 1991; 32:1861-1865.

32. Adatepe MH, Powell OM, Isaacs GH, et al. Hematogenous pyogenic vertebral osteomyelitis: diagnostic value of radionuclide bone imaging. J Nucl Med 1986; 27:1680-1685.

33. El-Maghraby TA, Moustafa HM, Pauwels EK. Nuclear medicine methods for evaluation of skeletal infection among other diagnostic modalities. Q J Nucl Med Mol Imaging 2006; 50:167-192.

34. Kapeller P, Fazekas F, Krametter D, et al. Pyogenic infectious spondylitis: clinical, laboratory and MRI features. Eur Neurol 1997; 38:94-98.

35. Le Page L, Feydy A, Rillardon L, et al. Spinal tuberculosis: a longitudinal study with clinical, laboratory, and imaging outcomes. Semin Arthritis Rheum 2006; 36:124-129. Epub 2006 Jul 13.

36. Wolansky LJ, Heary RF, Patterson T, et al. Pseudosparing of the endplate: a potential pitfall in using MR imaging to diagnose infectious spondylitis. AJR Am J Roentgenol 1999; 172:777-780.

37. De Roos A, Kressel H, Spritzer C, Dalinka M. MR imaging of marrow changes adjacent to end plates in degenerative lumbar disk disease. AJR Am J Roentgenol 1987; 149:531-534.

38. Lucio E, Adesokan A, Hadjipavlou AG, et al. Pyogenic spondylodiskitis: a radiologic/pathologic and culture correlation study. Arch Pathol Lab Med 2000; 124:712-716.

39. Fouquet B, Goupille P, Gobert F, et al. Infectious discitis diagnostic contribution of laboratory tests and percutaneous discovertebral biopsy. Rev Rhum Engl Ed 1996; 63:24-29.

40. Hadjipavlou AG, Mader JT, Necessary JT, Muffoletto AJ. Hematogenous pyogenic spinal infections and their surgical management. Spine 2000; 25:1668-1679.

41. Mann S, Schutze M, Sola S, Piek J. Nonspecific pyogenic spondylodiscitis: clinical manifestations, surgical treatment, and outcome in 24 patients. Neurosurg Focus 2004; 17:E3.

64

Complications of Infection

Francesca Beaman and Laura Bancroft

ETIOLOGY

Musculoskeletal infection may occur in a myriad of clinical settings, including systemic infection or illness, blunt or penetrating trauma, or iatrogenic causes. Infection is both a primary complication and a medium through which deleterious effects may impact bone, muscle, neurovascular, and soft tissue environments as well as implanted materials. Infectious complications may occur if there is delayed diagnosis of an infection, inadequate antimicrobial treatment of a confirmed infection, or compromise of the patient's soft tissues or bones by an offending organism despite appropriate treatment. Complications of infection may be subdivided into those that (1) require percutaneous or surgical drainage; (2) result in tendon failure; (3) result in joint destruction, ankylosis, or deformity; (4) result in hardware failure that requires revision surgery; (5) require myocutaneous flap coverage of a defect caused by infection; and (6) require amputation.

PREVALENCE AND EPIDEMIOLOGY

The pathophysiology of musculoskeletal infection has been extensively discussed in the preceding chapters on infection. Complications related to infection have multiple causes but are more prevalent in patients undergoing arthroplasty and in diabetic patients.

At least 250,000 joint replacements are performed annually, with infection rates estimated to be 1% to 2% for primary joint replacement and 3% to 4% for revision surgery.[1] In a composite review of complications of total shoulder arthroplasties in the literature over an 18-year period, there was an average 0.5% rate of infection in unconstrained arthroplasties and a 2.9% rate in constrained arthroplasties.[2] Mankin and colleagues reviewed a series of 945 patients who received massive cadaveric allografts and showed that 12.8% of these patients experienced infectious complications.[3] The highest frequency of infection was seen in patients with soft tissue tumors, irradiated sites, stage IIB tumors, or surgeries consisting of an allograft arthrodesis.[3] Allograft infections may be

secondary to contamination with exogenous microorganisms or to microbes present within the tissue at the time of harvest.[4]

The diabetic population is particularly susceptible to musculoskeletal infection, especially that involving the feet (see Chapter 65). Nontraumatic lower limb amputations most commonly afflict patients with diabetes, with more than 82,000 amputations performed in the United States annually in diabetic patients for infection.[5]

CLINICAL PRESENTATION

Complications of musculoskeletal infection are varied, but most patients with musculoskeletal infections will present with pain. In the setting of arthroplasty, persistent rest or night pain or progressive stiffness should raise the concern for deep infection.[6] Systemic pathology such as deep vein thrombosis must be considered when patients develop sudden swelling of an infected extremity, and if septic pulmonary emboli develop they can be life threatening.[7] Deep vein thrombosis can be detected quickly and noninvasively with ultrasonography, and pulmonary emboli can be evaluated with enhanced CT, ventilation/perfusion scanning, or pulmonary angiography. When restricted to the musculoskeletal system, complications of infection include spread of infection, failure of soft tissues, infection requiring additional intervention (drainage, surgical débridement, revision, or amputation), permanent joint destruction/ankylosis, prosthesis failure, graft removal, and tumor.

IMAGING TECHNIQUES

The evaluation for possible complications of musculoskeletal infection begins with radiography, which can identify osseous (erosions, lysis) and soft tissue (gas, foreign bodies) abnormalities. CT is more sensitive in detecting subtle osseous changes and focal abscesses. MRI is quite helpful in evaluating subtle soft tissue and osseous complications, but it may be degraded by artifacts related to metallic hardware. Ultrasonography may detect complications of fluid collections and is a rapid and widely available modality for use in

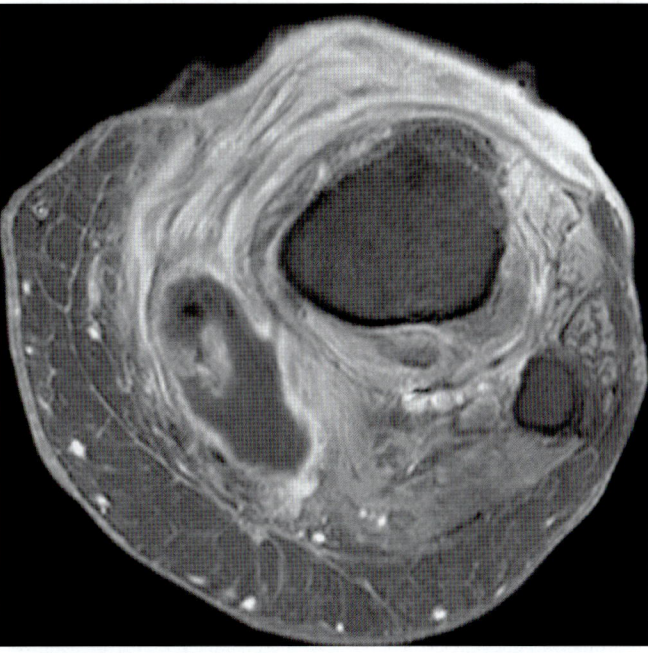

■ **FIGURE 64-1** Gastrocnemius myocutaneous flap abscess requiring surgical drainage and débridement. Axial T1-weighted enhanced fat-suppressed MR image through an infected rotational flap demonstrates an irregular, nonenhancing focus in the posteromedial calf. Flap was originally placed for coverage of defect after sarcoma resection.

guided therapy for such complications, such as soft tissue biopsy and fluid collection drainage. It has also been shown to be useful in the diagnosis and treatment (corticosteroid, phenol injection) of stump neuromas.[8,9] Nuclear scintigraphy is invaluable for the diagnosis of primary musculoskeletal infection but is not particularly useful in the evaluation of secondary complications. Preliminary research on fluorodeoxyglucose-labeled positron emission tomography (FDG PET) indicates that FDG accurately detects musculoskeletal infection.[10,11] PET scans also can detect hypermetabolic processes, such as tumors occurring secondary to chronic osteomyelitis or draining sinus tracts.

MANIFESTATIONS OF THE DISEASE

Infection Requiring Percutaneous/Surgical Drainage

Abscess formation and tissue necrosis resulting in a fluid-like necrotic cavity are not uncommon infectious complications and often require urgent intervention (Fig. 64-1). Percutaneous musculoskeletal interventions are widely performed, minimally invasive procedures well established as both diagnostic and therapeutic tools, particularly in those patients who cannot undergo surgical intervention.[12] Percutaneous interventions may be performed with fluoroscopic, CT, or US guidance (Fig. 64-2). (Infectious spondylitis is discussed in detail in Chapter 63.)

Infection Resulting in Tendon Failure

Musculoskeletal infections may affect native or graft tendons directly or via contiguous spread from local soft

tissues or bone resulting in graft laxity, partial tearing, or complete rupture (Fig. 64-3). Infections associated with tissue allograft implants occur due to transmitted diseases within the graft, intraoperative contamination, or postoperative hematogenous seeding.[13,14] Infections transmitted through allografts include those caused by human immunodeficiency virus, hepatitis B and C virus, and other viruses, bacteria, and fungi.[3] Complications related to these infections include allograft failure, sepsis, liver disease requiring transplantation, and death.[5] Reports of anterior cruciate ligament graft infections have led to graft débridement, graft removal (Fig. 64-4), sepsis, and death.[15] In a series of 331 patients who underwent anterior cruciate ligament reconstruction, the infection rate for patients who received aseptically processed allografts was 4.4%, compared with no patients who received autografts or sterile allografts.[15] All infections occurred at the tibial fixation site of the graft, and use of a supplementary staple increased the risk of infection 10-fold.[15] Patients may have pain and delayed recovery after infected anterior cruciate ligament reconstruction.[16]

Infection Resulting in Joint Destruction/Ankylosis/Deformity

Permanent destructive joint changes may be secondary to musculoskeletal infections that are either not treated, are treated suboptimally, or are unresponsive to therapy. Pyogenic infections tend to damage joints more rapidly because of the ability to produce proteases, whereas atypical organisms (e.g., tuberculosis and fungi) are more indolent. Once an infection destroys the articular

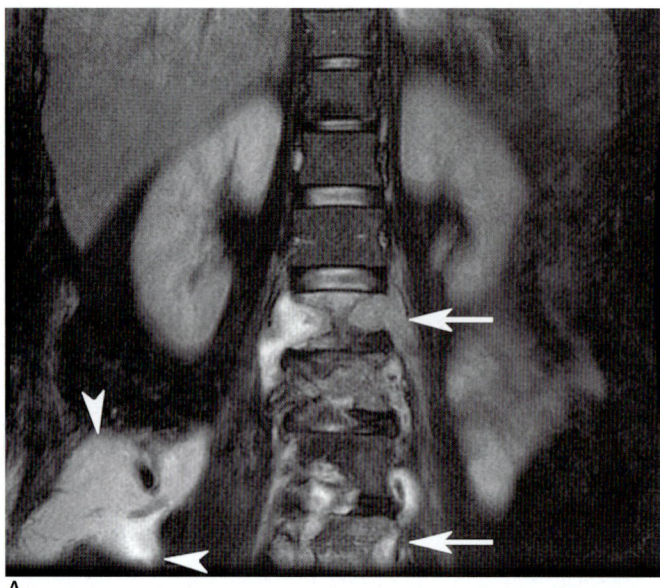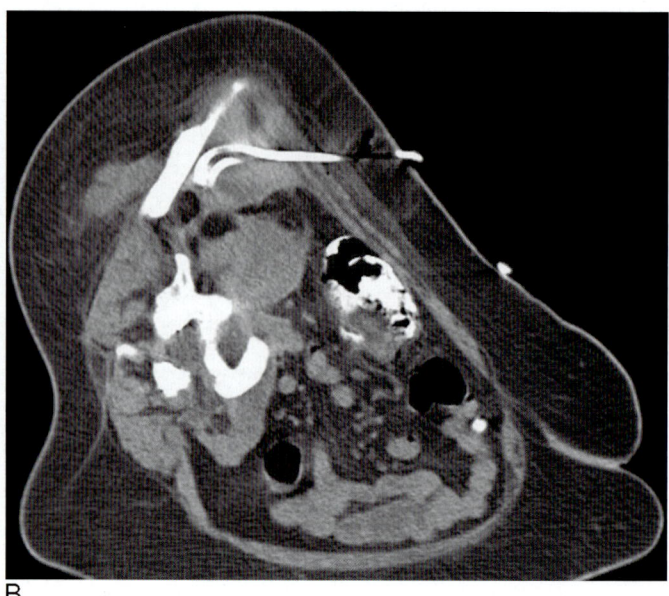

A   B

■ **FIGURE 64-2** Blastomycosis of the spine with iliacus abscess requiring percutaneous drainage. **A,** Fast spin-echo T2-weighted fat-suppressed coronal MR image from the thoracolumbar spine demonstrates abnormally increased signal within multiple vertebral bodies and disc spaces (*arrows*). Note the irregular hyperintense fluid collection along the right iliacus muscle (*arrowheads*). **B,** CT image with patient in the left lateral position obtained during placement of percutaneous drainage catheter into abscess.

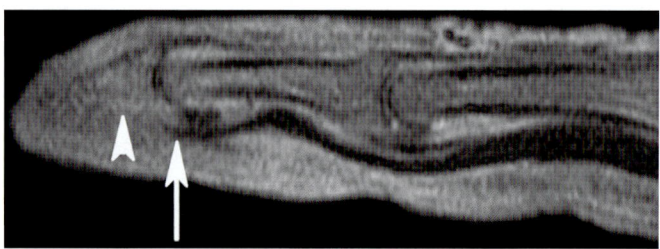

■ **FIGURE 64-3** Rupture of the flexor digitorum profundus tendon secondary to osteomyelitis. Sagittal T1-weighted enhanced fat-suppressed MR image through the index finger demonstrates an avulsed flexor digitorum profundus tendon (*arrow*) and associated abnormal enhancement throughout the distal phalanx. Note loss of the volar cortex of the distal phalanx (*arrowhead*).

cartilage, it can lead to permanent impairment of the joint. Arthritis, fibrous or osseous ankylosis (Fig. 64-5), and angular deformities (Fig. 64-6) of the joints can occur. Tuberculous spondylitis is classic for resulting in a severe kyphotic deformity of the thoracolumbar spine (Fig. 64-7). In addition, infection may cause complete osteolysis of the dens with resulting atlantoaxial subluxation.[17]

Surgical fusion may be warranted in extreme cases of advanced joint destruction caused by infection. Fusion may be performed in cases of previously infected native joints or those that have undergone prior arthroplasty placement and removal. Patients experience discomfort/pain, restricted mobility, and, possibly, social limitations.[18] Joint replacement in cases of partially or

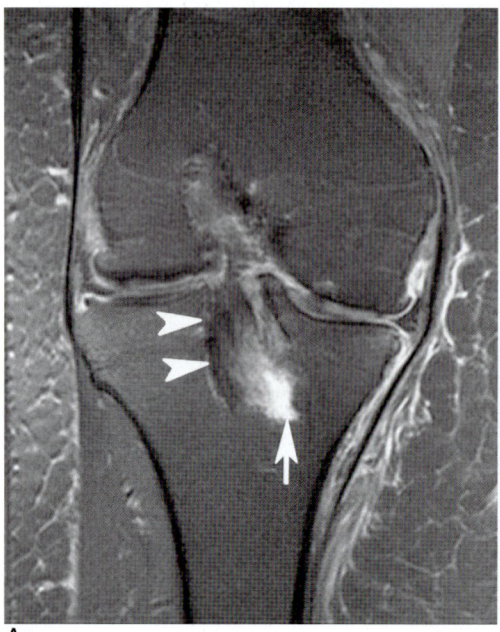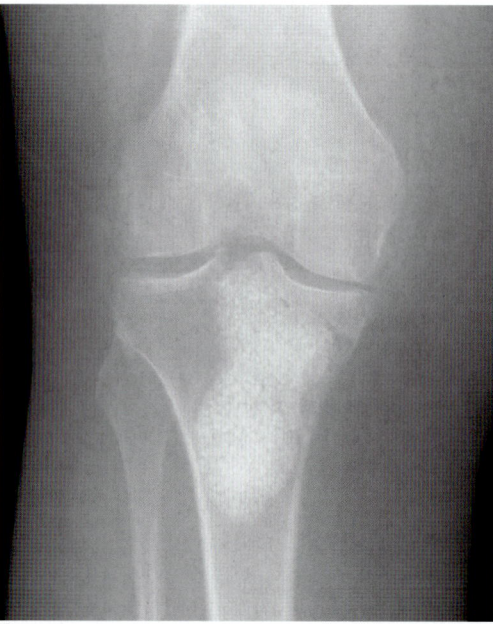

A   B

■ **FIGURE 64-4** Infected anterior cruciate ligament (ACL) graft requiring removal. **A,** Coronal T1-weighted enhanced fat-suppressed MR image through the knee demonstrates abnormal enhancement (*arrow*) surrounding the intact ACL graft (*arrowheads*). **B,** Anteroposterior radiograph of the knee demonstrates antibiotic-laden cement in the ACL tunnel, after infected graft removal.

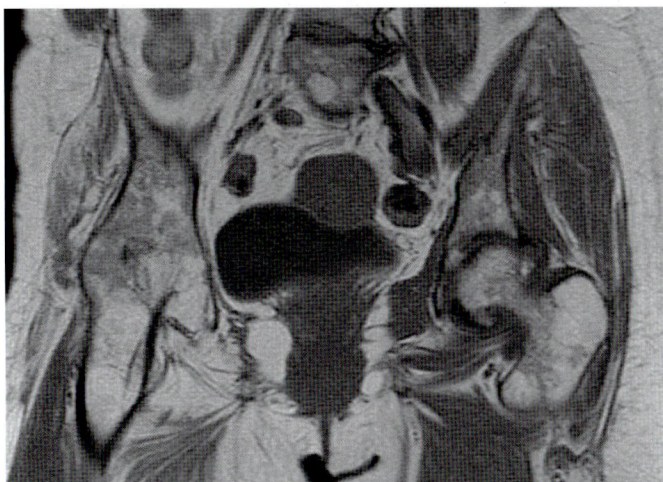

■ **FIGURE 64-5** Autofusion of right hip after tuberculous infection. Coronal T1-weighted MR image through the pelvis demonstrates ankylosis of the right hip joint, with obliteration of the joint space and continuous red and yellow marrow.

completely ankylosed knees secondary to infection has a poor prognosis, with complication rates ranging from 12.5% to 57%.[18,19] Reported complications include superficial and deep infection, supracondylar femoral fracture, transient palsy of the common peroneal nerve, stiffness requiring manipulation, delayed wound healing, recurrent hemarthrosis, myositis ossificans, persistent pain requiring arthrodesis, aseptic loosening, avulsion of the patellar tendon or tibial tubercle, and rupture of the quadriceps tendon.[18] Severe soft tissue contractures occurring in patients with ankylosed joints may necessitate more extensive surgery, such as lengthening of the quadriceps tendon or tibial tuberosity transfer.[18] In a series of 58 patients undergoing primary total hip arthroplasty after late infectious sequelae of the hip there were few overall complications, which included only one case of recurrent infection, two femoral fractures occurring during surgery, and one periprosthetic fracture; 1 patient had a tran-

sient nerve palsy, and another experienced postoperative deep vein thrombosis.[20] Lim and Park believed the clinical results supported their theory that the clinical results were not influenced by the type of infection but rather by the age of the patient at the onset of the infection and the extent of the preoperative anatomic deformity.[20]

Infectious Hardware Failure Requiring Revision Arthroplasty

Infection is a painful, potentially fatal condition that can complicate joint instrumentation and arthoplasty. Diagnosis can be difficult.[21] Periprosthetic infections may necessitate removal of hardware if there are signs of septic loosening, component dissociation, or osteomyelitis (Fig. 64-8). Molecular diagnostic strategies have been implemented to enhance the treatment of musculoskeletal infections. Molecular-based assays are used as tests for the genomic detection of certain pathogens.[22]

Infected joint arthroplasty often requires surgical removal, with current options including a two-stage procedure arthroplasty, débridement, and retention of the prosthesis or a Girdlestone arthroplasty.

In two-stage procedures, the use of beads and antibiotic-impregnated cement spacers has lowered infection rates.[23] In turn, complications of antibiotic-impregnated cement for joint arthroplasty include weakening of the cement and development of antibiotic-resistant bacteria.[23] Débridement and retention of the prosthesis may be performed in the treatment of prosthetic infection.[24] In a series of 99 cases of prosthetic joint infection there was a 2-year survival rate free of treatment failure of 60%; treatment failure was most commonly associated with the presence of a sinus tract and duration of symptoms for more than 8 days.[24] Open débridement may be best suited in the treatment of an acute infection in the early postoperative period or of an acute hematogenous infection at the site of a secure and functional prosthesis.[6]

Removal of a joint prosthesis for infection, such as a Girdlestone procedure, may leave a patient with a functional disability and wheelchair bound. Patients can

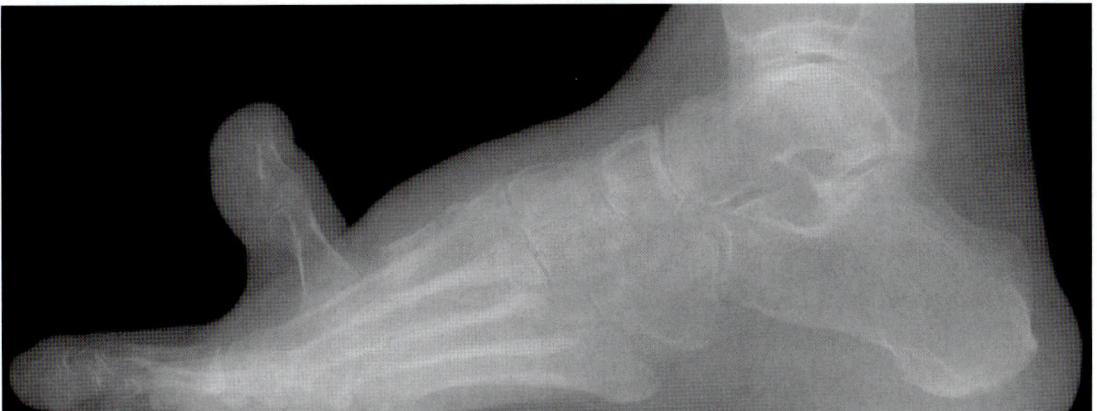

■ **FIGURE 64-6** Infected hallux valgus repair resulting in multiple surgeries, hyperextended hallux, and ultimate amputation. Lateral radiograph of the foot demonstrates a hyperextended great toe after history of removal of MTP Silastic implant, débridement, placement of antibiotic-impregnated spacer, and failed plate and screw fixation. Patient subsequently had first ray amputation.

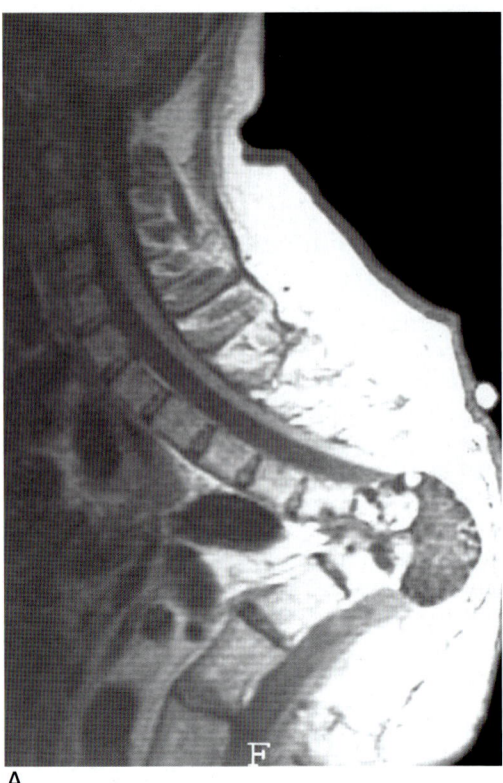
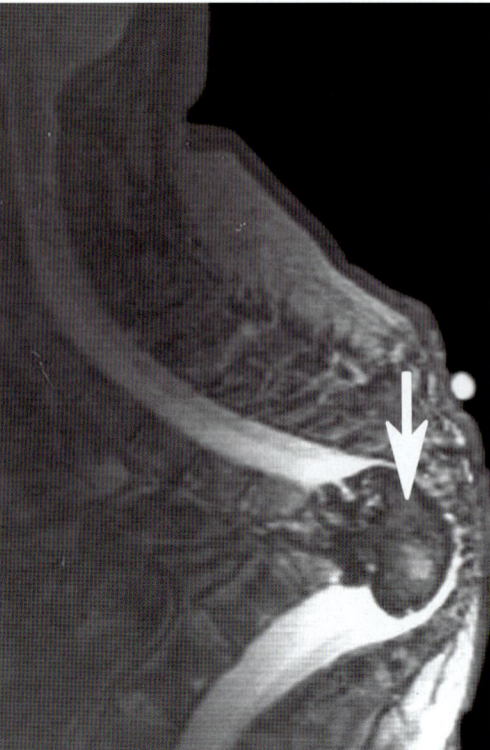

A   B

■ FIGURE 64-7   Gibbus deformity secondary to tuberculous spondylitis. Coronal T1-weighted (*left*) and fast spin-echo T2-weighted fat-suppressed (*right*) MR images through the thoracolumbar junction demonstrate marked kyphotic deformity and low signal intensity paraspinal calcification (*arrow*), resulting in cord compromise.

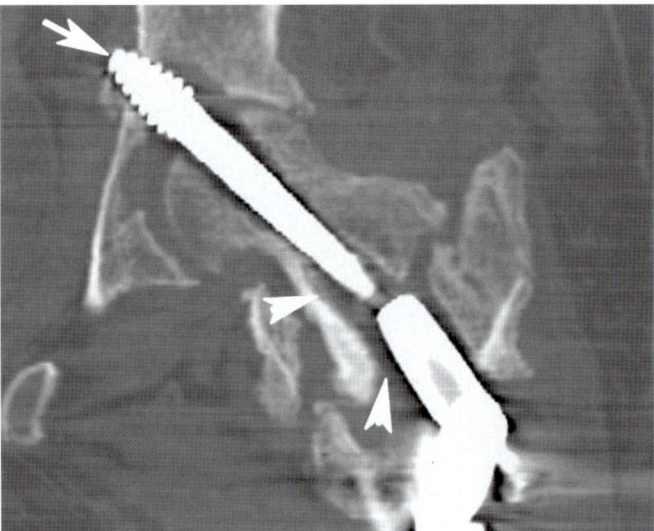

■ FIGURE 64-8   Dissociated, migrated dynamic hip screw and nonunion of femoral neck fracture. Coronal reconstructed CT image through the left hip demonstrates migration of the hip screw through the acetabulum and into the lateral pelvis (*arrow*). Note the osteolysis about the screw (*arrowheads*) and nonunion of femoral fracture fragments.

have pain, large discrepancy in leg length, instability, and poor function.[25] Studies have shown a considerable rate of complications related to reimplantation after Girdlestone arthoplasty.[26,27] In a series of 44 patients undergoing reimplantation after Girdlestone arthroplasty, 98% of patients were free of infection, but 11% had subsequent dislocations and 39% had a persistent limp.[27] In a series of 39 hip arthroplasties placed after Girdlestone procedures, the functional outcome of patients was difficult to predict; microbial culture, patient age, duration of Girdlestone arthroplasty, and number of preceding surgeries did not correlate with functional outcome after conversion.[26] Complications include residual/recurrent infection, delayed soft tissue closure necessitating surgical revision, hip dislocation, trochanteric nonunion, perioperative wound drainage, sciatic or femoral nerve palsy, deep vein thrombosis, periprosthetic fracture, hematoma, heterotopic ossification, persistent limp, and heparin-induced thrombocytopenia.[26,27]

In a multi-institutional study involving patients undergoing revision knee arthroplasty, patients who had revisions for periprosthetic infection had lower function scores and were unable to return to normal activities of daily living.[28] When comparing patient satisfaction and outcome after septic versus aseptic revision total knee arthroplasty, patients in the septic cohort had inferior functional results but reported an equal degree of satisfaction with the results of their treatment.[28] Infection has been reported in the literature to occur in up to 3.9% of patients after shoulder arthroplasty.[2] In patients requiring revision shoulder arthroplasty for infection, additional reported complications include further revision for periprosthetic humeral fracture, acromial pseudarthrosis after transacromial surgery, and recurrent dislocations.[29]

Several methods are available for the treatment of musculoskeletal infection. Periprosthetic infection can be treated with local antibiotic delivery vehicles such as antibiotic-loaded bone cement (ALBC). ALBC is the gold standard for local antibiotic delivery, because it can deliver high concentrations of antibiotics (e.g., gentamicin and tobramycin) to avascular areas that are inaccessible by systemic antibiotics (Fig. 64-9).[30,31] However, complications of antibiotic-impregnated cement include renal failure in patients with poor renal function, impeded osteoblast function and bone regeneration, weakened cement, and generation of antibiotic-resistant bacteria in infected implant sites.[23,30] Polymethyl methacrylate beads have been used successfully for the treatment of osteomyelitis for management of dead space but are rarely advocated in the treatment of infected knee or hip arthroplasty.[30,32] This is because the beads can become surrounded by dense scar tissue and be extremely difficult to remove. However, block ALBC spacers are effective and maintain the length and shape of the effective joint space.[30] In addition, infected hip arthroplasties may be removed and a prosthesis composed of antibiotic-laden cement (PROSTALAC) may be placed at the same time, thus minimizing the number of surgeries. Intraoperatively, the PROSTALAC is prepared by putting the metal core of the arthroplasty within a mold and pouring antibiotic-impregnated cement into it; metal and polyethylene cover only the articulating surfaces.[1,33]

Infectious Complications Requiring a Myocutaneous Flap

Myocutaneous flaps are commonly used in orthopedic reconstructive surgery employed in the reconstruction after surgical treatment for sarcoma of an extremity and for wound coverage to prevent or help eradicate wound infection.[34,35] They are most frequently used for soft tissue coverage, such as after tumor resection, but they may also be employed after extensive surgical débridement for osteomyelitis (Fig. 64-10).[34] Vascularized flaps serve many functions, including closing dead space, reestablishing a cutaneous envelope, and providing a blood supply, factors that are all necessary in decreasing the risk of postoperative infection.[34-36] Flaps may also be selected to provide a degree of function as well as tissue coverage.[34]

Infectious Complications Requiring Amputation

Nontraumatic lower limb amputations most commonly afflict diabetic patients with infection.[5] Amputations may also be necessary in cases of chronically infected total joint prosthesis, which may cause recalcitrant pain and draining sinus tracts (Figs. 64-11 and 64-12). Complications of lower limb amputations include pain from a multitude of causes, including aggressive bone edge, heterotopic ossification, recurrent osteomyelitis, fluid collections, cancers, neuromas, and traumatic bone lesions. Deep vein thrombosis, lymphedema, and scar/keloids and soft tissue inflammation associated with prostheses are also known

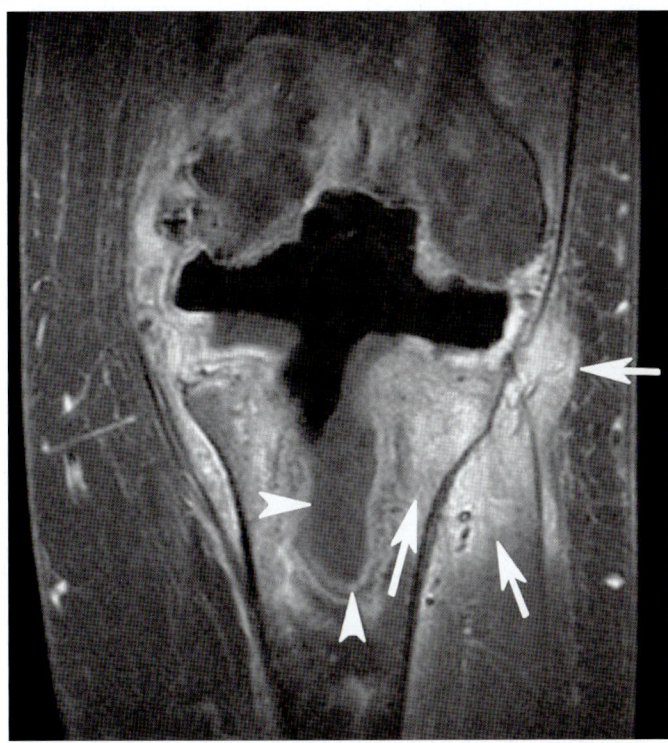

■ **FIGURE 64-9** Antibiotic-impregnated cement spacer placed after removal of infected total knee arthroplasty. Coronal T1-weighted enhanced MR image of the knee demonstrates cement (signal void) within the defect (*arrowheads*) previously occupied by the knee arthroplasty. Note the extensive enhancement of the actively infected marrow and extraosseous soft tissues (*arrows*).

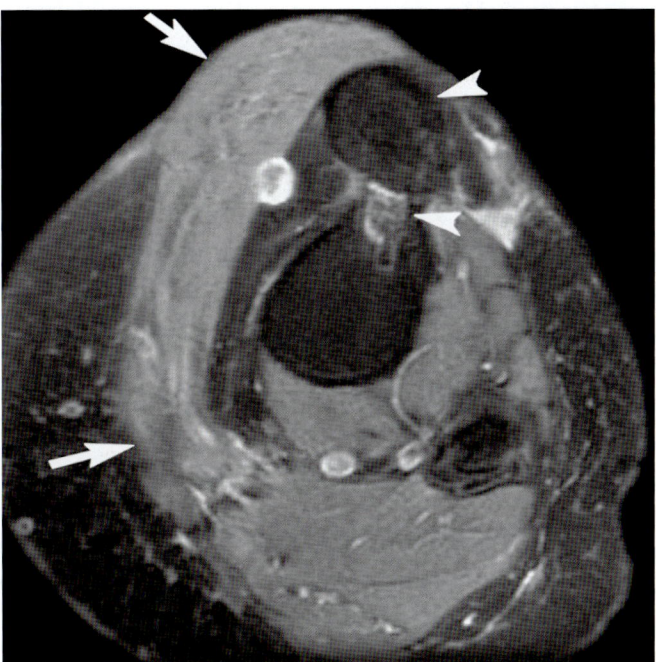

■ **FIGURE 64-10** Gastrocnemius flap placed for coverage of osteomyelitis defect. Axial fast spin-echo T2-weighted fat-suppressed MR image through the proximal calf demonstrates a rotated myocutaneous flap (*arrows*) covering deformed proximal tibia (*arrowheads*) resulting from prior osteomyelitis.

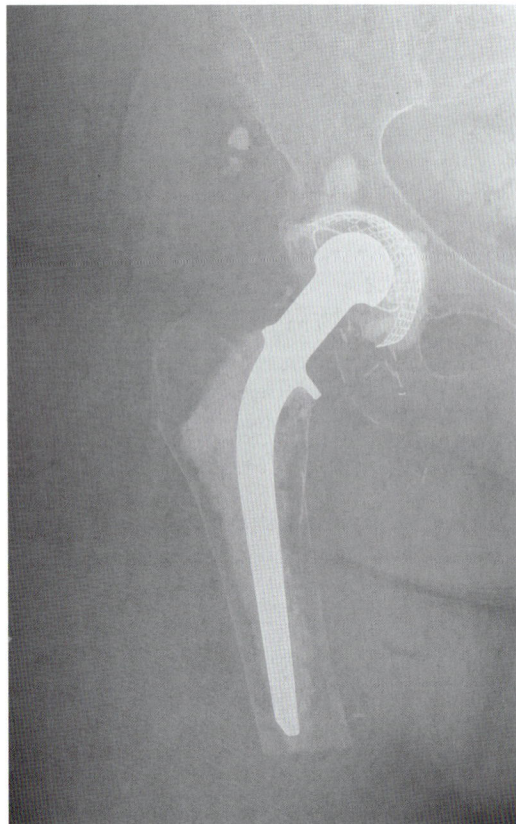

■ **FIGURE 64-11** Amputation for chronically infected total knee arthroplasty, recalcitrant pain, and draining sinus tract. After multidepartmental consultation, patient elected for amputation of her leg below her total hip arthroplasty and above the chronically infected total knee arthroplasty. She cited her inability to live with excruciating pain and the social drawbacks of a continuously draining anterior knee wound.

complications of amputations, which were performed for infection.[37]

Two additional well-recognized scenarios in which amputation is warranted are development of carcinoma from chronic osteomyelitis or ulcer and in cases of stump (traumatic) neuromas. Recurrent infection despite aggressive medical therapy does occur, particularly in the diabetic foot (see Chapter 65).

Chronic osteomyelitis associated with a draining sinus tract is a well-documented risk scenario resulting in the development of carcinoma in a small percentage of patients. Men are markedly more affected than women.[38] The lower extremity is involved in 85% of cases, with the tibia affected most commonly, followed by the femur and the foot.[38,39] Squamous cell carcinoma is the most common type of malignancy that occurs secondary to chronic ulceration, also called Marjolin's ulcer.[39] Other types of malignancies include fibrosarcoma, myeloma, lymphoma, plasmacytoma, angiosarcoma, rhabdomyosarcoma, and malignant fibrous histiocytoma (undifferentiated pleomorphic sarcoma).[38,39] In this scenario, the squamous cell carcinoma is generally low grade. Despite low-grade malignancy, these lesions are typically treated with amputation so that the carcinoma and infection may both be eradicated. Signs that raise the suspicion for malignancy include pain, foul or bloody discharge, enlarging mass, and progressive bone destruction.[38] Malignant change typically occurs after a long latency period of 20 to 50 years, but there have been cases reported ranging from 1 to 71 years.[38] Local recurrence and metastases are not uncommon complications that must be monitored on subsequent imaging.

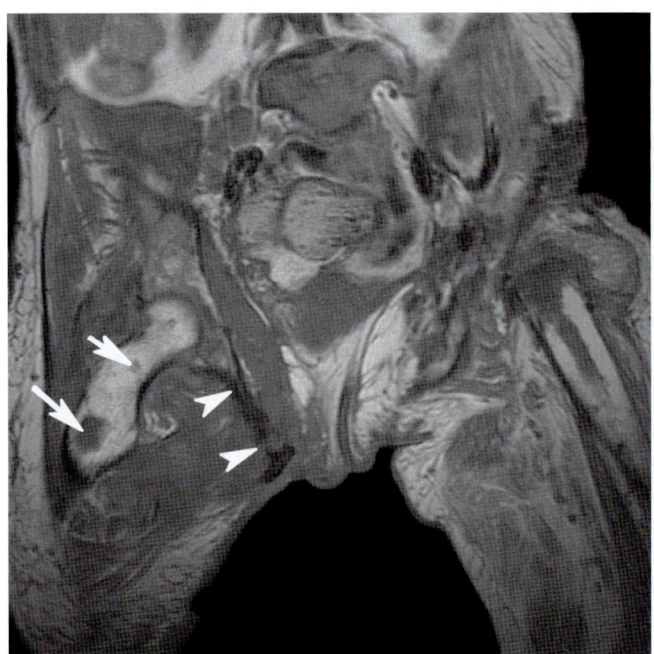
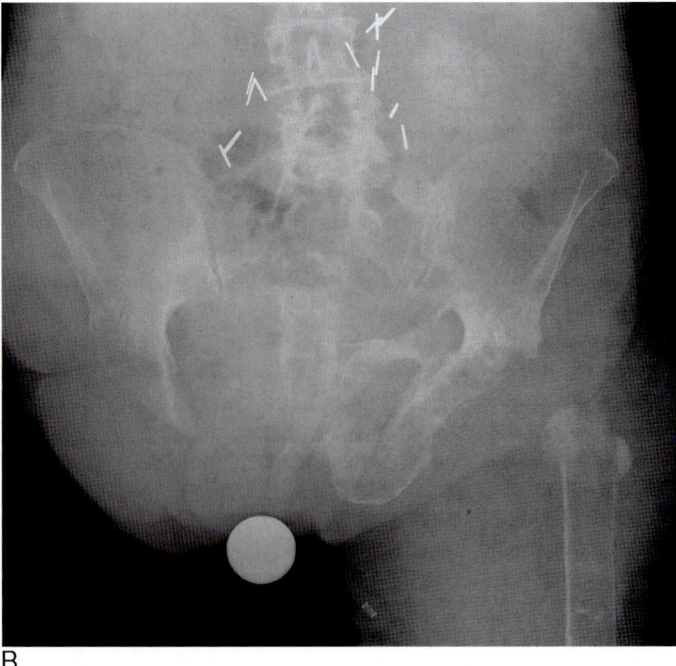

A   B

■ **FIGURE 64-12** Hemipelvectomy and Girdlestone arthroplasty performed for infection. **A,** Coronal T1-weighted MR image through the pelvis delineates a sinus tract (*arrowheads*) extending from the right perineum into the distended, infected right hip joint. Multifocal marrow-replacing lesions in the proximal right femur correlate to surgically confirmed osteomyelitis (*arrows*). Note the left-sided Girdlestone arthroplasty and residual left femoral marrow abnormality. **B,** Anteroposterior pelvic radiograph demonstrates extensive postsurgical change after right hemipelvectomy, left-sided Girdlestone arthroplasty, and débridement of the osseous pelvis.

Stump neuromas are disorganized proliferations of nerve fascicles that occur after amputations for infection or other causes. They are relatively common and can be a cause of stump pain.[8] Stump neuromas can occur either at the end of a transected nerve (terminal neuroma) or along the course of the nerve (spindle neuroma). Neuromas occur when an injured nerve attempts to repair itself. In the case of a terminal neuroma, the proximal axons overgrow and form an extremely sensitive bulbous overgrowth. Spindle neuromas occur from a stretching injury or are due to compression by local scar tissue. Neuromas generally present within 1 to 12 months after surgery and can enlarge for 2 to 3 years.[8] Stump neuromas are typically a fusiform mass or focal enlargement visualized along the stretched portion of a nonterminal nerve or a terminal, transected nerve terminating in a bulbous shape.[37,40] Neuromas typically have intermediate (similar to skeletal muscle) signal on T1-weighted images and intermediate to high signal on T2-weighted images.[34,38] They often have heterogeneous signal intensity, which is best appreciated on T2-weighted images.[40] Ultrasonography has been useful in both identifying lesions and guiding therapy. Stump neuromas are oval, hypoechoic nodules that are in direct continuity with the nerve. They can be either well-defined or irregular. Ultrasonographically guided neuroma injection with corticosteroids can confirm accurate localization within the neuroma by direct visualization and with patient report of "exquisite tenderness."[8] Injections can also be guided into the nerve just proximal to the neuroma.[9] Other injected agents include phenol, *Clostridium botulinum* toxin, glycerol, and alcohol.[9]

SYNOPSIS OF TREATMENT OPTIONS
Medical

- Anticoagulants are utilized for infectious complications of deep vein thrombosis and pulmonary emboli.
- Otherwise, the complications presented in this chapter require more than mere medical therapy.

Surgical

- Complications of spread of infection are treated with débridement or amputation.
- Abscesses may be drained percutaneously using CT or US guidance; alternatively, complex or inaccessible cases may be addressed surgically.
- Ruptured tendons are repaired after eradication of the infection either by primary repair or tendon transfer.
- Tendinous grafts that fail due to complications of infection are evaluated for rupture of the graft, associated septic arthritis, and osteomyelitis. The graft is either débrided if intact or revised after eradication of infection. Any diseased soft tissues or bone is débrided.
- Joints that are destroyed, ankylosed, or angulated by complications of infection are treated with either surgical fusion or joint replacement after eradication of infection.
- Infected hardware often requires surgical removal. Current options for infected prosthesis include a two-stage arthroplasty, débridement and retention of the prosthesis, or Girdlestone arthroplasty.

SUGGESTED READINGS

Boutin RD, Pathria MN, Resnick D. Disorders in the stumps of amputee patients: MR imaging. AJR Am J Roentgenol 1998; 171:497-501.

DeBacker AI, Mortele KJ, Vanhoenacker FM, Parizel PM. Imaging of extraspinal musculoskeletal tuberculosis. Eur J Radiol 2006; 57:119-130.

Fitzgerald RH. Infected total hip arthoplasty: diagnosis and treatment. J Am Acad Orthop Surg 1995; 3:249-262.

Henrot P, Stines J, Walter F, et al. Imaging of the painful lower limb stump. Radiographics 2000; 20:219-235.

Kothari NA, Pelchovitz DJ, Meyer JS. Imaging of musculoskeletal infections. Radiol Clin North Am 2001; 29:653-671.

Love C, Palestro CJ. Radionuclide imaging of infection. J Nucl Med Technol 2004; 2:47-57.

McCarthy JJ, Dormans JP, Kozin SH, Pizzutillo PD. Musculoskeletal infections in children: basic treatment principles and recent advancements. Instr Course Lect 2004; 54:515-28.

Moore SL, Rafii M. Advanced imaging of tuberculosis arthritis. Semin Musculoskel Radiol 2003; 7:143-153.

Nelson CL, McKaren AC, MacLaren SG, et al. Is aseptic loosening truly aseptic? Clin Orthop Relat Res 2005; 437:25-30.

Restrepo S, Vargas D, Riascos R, Cuellar H. Musculoskeletal infection imaging: past, present, and future. Curr Infect Dis Rep 2005; 7:365-372.

REFERENCES

1. Gee R, Munk PL, Keogh C, et al. Radiography of the PROSTALAC (prosthesis with antibiotic-loaded acrylic cement) orthopedic implant. AJR Am J Roentgenol 2003; 180:1701-6170.
2. Cofield RH, Edgerton BC. Total shoulder arthroplasty: complications and revision surgery. Instr Course Lect 1990; 39:449-462.
3. Mankin HJ, Hornicek FJ, Raskin KA. Infection in massive bone allografts. Clin Orthop Relat Res 2005; 432:210-216.
4. Patel R, Trampuz A. Infections transmitted through musculoskeletal-tissue allografts. N Engl J Med 2004; 350:2544-2546.
5. Centers for Disease Control and Prevention. National Diabetes Fact Sheet: General Information and National Estimates on Diabetes in the United States, 2002. Atlanta, U.S. Department of Health and Human Services, Centers for Disease Control and Prevention, 2003.
6. Leone JM, Hanssen AD. Management of infection at the site of a total knee arthroplasty. J Bone Joint Surg Am 2005; 87:2336-2348.
7. Walsh S, Phillips F. Deep vein thrombosis associated with pediatric musculoskeletal sepsis. J Pediatr Orthop 2002; 22:329-332.
8. Ernberg LA, Adler RS, Lane J. Ultrasound in the detection and treatment of a painful stump neuroma. Skeletal Radiol 2003; 32:306-309.

9. Gruber H, Kovacs P, Peer S, et al. Sonographically guided phenol injection in painful stump neuroma. AJR Am J Roentgenol 2004; 182:952-954.

10. Crymes WB, Demos H, Gordon L. Detection of musculoskeletal infection with ¹⁸F-FDG PET: review of the current literature. J Nucl Med Technol 2004; 32:12-15.

11. Love C, Tomas MB, Tronco GG, Palestro CJ. FDG PET of infection and inflammation. RadioGraphics 2005; 25:1357-1368.

12. Thanos L, Mylona S, Kalioras V, et al. Percutaneous CT-guided interventional procedures in musculoskeletal system (our experience). Eur J Radiol 2004; 50:273-277.

13. Septic arthritis following anterior cruciate ligament reconstruction using tendon allografts—Florida and Louisiana, 2000. MMWR Morb Mortal Wkly Rep 2001; 50:1081-1083.

14. Update: allograft-associated bacterial infections—United States, 2002. MMWR Morb Mortal Wkly Rep 2002; 51:207-210.

15. Crawford C, Kainer M, Jernigan D, et al. Investigation of postoperative allograft-associated infections in patients who underwent musculoskeletal allograft implantation. Clin Infect Dis 2005; 41:195-200.

16. Viola R, Marzano N, Vianello R. An unusual epidemic of *Staphylococcus*-negative infections involving anterior cruciate ligament reconstruction with salvage of the graft and function. Arthroscopy 2000; 16:173-177.

17. Busche M, Bastian L, Riedemann NC, et al. Complete osteolysis of the dens with atlantoaxial luxation caused by infection with *Staphylococcus aureus*. Spine 2005; 30:369-374.

18. Bae DK, Yoon KH, Kim HS, Song SJ. Total knee arthroplasty in stiff knees after previous infection. J Bone Joint Surg Br 2005; 87:333-336.

19. Naranja RJ, Lotke OA, Oagnano MW, Hanssen AD. Total knee arthroplasty in a previously ankylosed or arthrodesed knee. Clin Orthop Relat Res 1996; 331:234-237.

20. Lim SJ, Park YS. Modular cementless total hip arthroplasty for hip infection sequelae. Orthopaedics 2005; 28:1063-1068.

21. Panousis K, Grigoris P, Butcher I, et al. Poor predictive value of broad-range PCR for the detection of arthroplasty infection in 92 cases. Acta Orthop 2005; 76:341-346.

22. Tarkin IS, Dunman PM, Garvin KL. Improving the treatment of musculoskeletal infections with molecular diagnostics. Clin Orthop Relat Res 2005; 437:83-88.

23. Joseph TN, Chen AL, DeCesare PE. Use of antibiotic-impregnated cement in total joint arthroplasty. J Am Acad Orthop Surg 2003; 11:38-47.

24. Marculescu CE, Berbari EF, Hanssen AD, et al. Outcome of prosthetic joint infections treated with débridement and retention of components. Clin Infect Dis 2006; 42:471-478.

25. Ilyas I, Morgan DA. Massive structural allograft in revision of septic hip arthroplasty. Int Orthop 2001; 24:319-322.

26. Rittmeister ME, Manthei L, Hailer NP. Prosthetic replacement in secondary Girdlestone arthroplasty has an unpredictable outcome. Int Orthop 2005; 29:145-148.

27. Charlton WP, Hozack WJ, Teloken MA, et al. Complications associated with reimplantation after Girdlestone arthroplasty. Clin Orthop Relat Res 2003; 407:119-126.

28. Barrack RL, Rorabeck C, Sawhney J, Woolfrey M. Patient satisfaction and outcome after septic versus aseptic revision total knee arthroplasty. J Arthroplasty 2000; 15:990-993.

29. Ince A, Seemann K, Frommelt, et al. One-stage exchange shoulder arthroplasty for peri-prosthetic infection. J Bone Joint Surg Br 2005; 87:814-818.

30. Hanssen AD. Local antibiotic vehicles in the treatment of musculoskeletal infection. Clin Orthop Relat Res 2005; 437:91-96.

31. Wang J, Calhoun JH, Mader JT. The application of bioimplants in the management of chronic osteomyelitis. Orthopedics 2002; 25:1247-1252.

32. Mohanty SP, Kumar MN, Murthy NS: Use of antibiotic-loaded polymethyl methacrylate beads in the management of musculoskeletal sepsis—a retrospective study. J Orthop Surg (Hong Kong) 2003; 11:73-39.

33. Meek R, Dunlop D, Garbuz D, et al. Patient satisfaction and functional status after aseptic versus septic revision total knee arthroplasty using the PROSTALAC articulating spacer. J Arthroplasty 2004; 19:874-879.

34. Fox MG, Bancroft LW, Peterson JJ, et al. MR imaging appearance of myocutaneous flaps commonly used in orthopedic reconstructive surgery. AJR Am J Roentgenol 2006; 187:800-806.

35. Mitra A, Mitra A, Harlin S. Treatment of massive thoracolumbar wounds and vertebral osteomyelitis following scoliosis surgery. Plast Reconstr Surg 2004; 113:206-213.

36. Heitmann C, Higgins LD, Levin LS. Treatment of deep infections of the shoulder with pedicled myocutaneous flaps. J Shoulder Elbow Surg 2004; 13:13-17.

37. Henrot P, Stines J, Walter F, et al. Imaging of the painful lower limb stump. RadioGraphics 2000; 20:S219-S235.

38. McGrory JE, Pritchard DJ, Unni KK, et al. Malignant lesions arising in chronic osteomyelitis. Clin Orthop Relat Res 1999; 362:181-189.

39. Smith J, Mello LF, Noguiera Neto NC, et al. Malignancy in chronic ulcers and scars of the leg (Marjolin's ulcer): a study of 21 patients. Skeletal Radiol 2001; 30:331-337.

40. Murphey MD, Smith WS, Smith SE, et al. Imaging of musculoskeletal neurogenic tumors: radiologic-pathologic correlation. RadioGraphics 1999; 19:125-1280.

CHAPTER

65

Diabetic Pedal Infection

William Morrison and H. P. Ledermann

ETIOLOGY

Although hematogenous spread is the most common cause of osteomyelitis in most other areas of the body, contiguous spread and direct implantation are more common in the foot and ankle.[1] Direct implantation can occur from puncture wounds or deep lacerations, open fractures, and surgery or injection procedures. However, the vast majority of osteomyelitis involving the foot and ankle in diabetic patients occurs through contiguous spread from adjacent ulceration and subsequent soft tissue infection.[2]

PREVALENCE AND EPIDEMIOLOGY

Diabetes affects approximately 15 million people in the United States.[3] Of these, 15% to 20% will suffer a foot-related complication requiring hospitalization (predominantly for ischemia or infection) at some point in their lives. These complications may necessitate amputation; diabetes is the main reason for nontraumatic lower extremity amputation, which is 15 to 40 times more common in diabetics than in nondiabetics. Annually in the United States more than 80,000 lower extremity amputations are performed on diabetic patients, each with a hospital stay averaging 14.7 days, resulting in over 1 billion dollars of immediate health care expense; rehabilitation, prosthetics or other mobility assistance devices, home nursing, and lost work productivity further stress the health care system. In addition to decreased quality of life, it has been shown that after pedal amputation there is a 50% incidence of serious complication involving the contralateral foot within 2 years, resulting in a 50% to 66% incidence of amputation within 5 years. This reflects the systemic nature of the disease but appears to also be related to shifting of weight-bearing onto the intact extremity after the initial surgery. As a result, over the past decade there has been increasing emphasis on managing these patients earlier in their disease course[4]; these interventions include ulcer prevention and care and revascularization procedures. Once infection is suspected, aggressive medical and surgical management is instituted. Surgical

care includes débridement of devascularized tissue and partial, foot-sparing amputation intended to preserve functionality.

CLINICAL PRESENTATION

In the diabetic foot, infection typically begins due to a skin break, which may be due to minor trauma, such as a puncture wound or toenail cutting, or may be due to breakdown of skin callus. Callus forms over areas of friction, locations of which are somewhat predictable. Callus is seen commonly adjacent to the first and fifth metatarsal heads (Fig. 65-1A), particularly in the setting of hallux valgus. Callus is also common adjacent to the calcaneus and the medial and lateral malleoli and over the dorsum of the toes, particularly when clawtoe deformity is present.[5] Other deformities cause callus in atypical locations; for example, in the setting of neuropathic disease or posterior tibial tendon dysfunction, the foot can obtain a rocker-bottom deformity, in which case callus may be

---

KEY POINTS

- Most commonly, osteomyelitis occurs due to contiguous spread from ulcerated callus
- Radiographic findings are often delayed by as much as 2 weeks, presenting as soft tissue swelling and bone lucency/destruction.
- Three-phase bone scintigraphy is highly sensitive for diagnosis of osteomyelitis, but uptake may be nonspecific; labeled white blood cell scanning improves specificity.
- MRI has high sensitivity and specificity and provides good anatomic definition; it serves as a useful preoperative "road map."
- Gadolinium contrast in MRI is useful to characterize soft tissue pathology, including cellulitis, abscess, septic tenosynovitis, and devitalization.
- Neuropathic osteoarthropathy can simulate osteomyelitis clinically and on imaging, especially in the acute form or in the setting of neuropathic fracture.

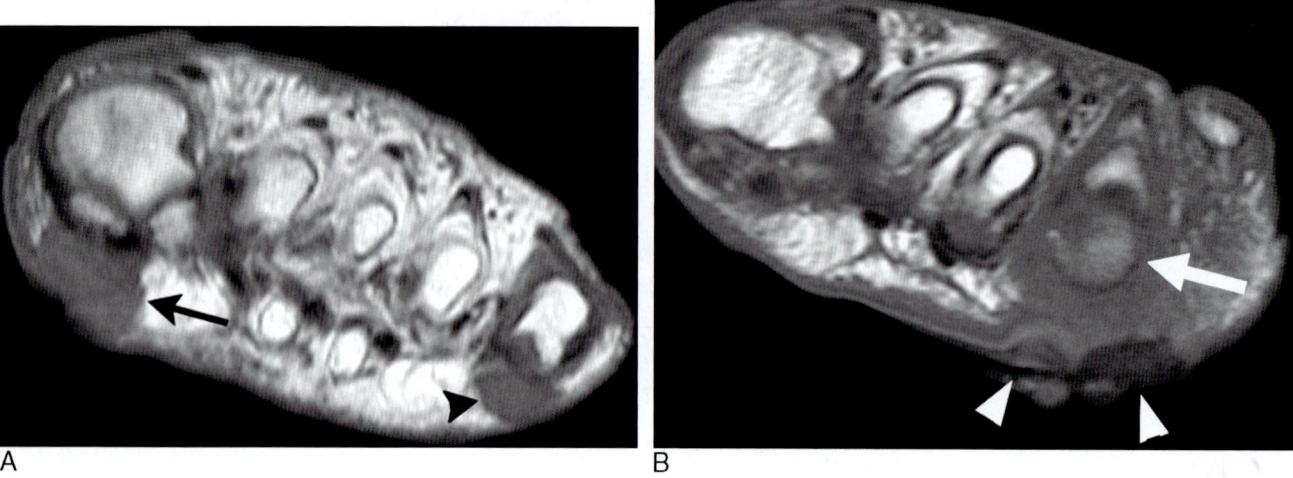

■ **FIGURE 65-1** Callus and ulceration. **A,** T1-weighted MR image shows typical location of callus formation, under the first (*arrow*) and fifth (*arrowhead*) metatarsal heads. **B,** T1-weighted MR image shows ulcerated callus (*arrowheads*) with typical heaped-up edges. Note replacement of marrow fat in the underlying metatarsal head (*arrow*) representing osteomyelitis occurring due to contiguous spread.

seen at the plantar aspect of the midfoot.[2] These areas of callus and subsequent callus breakdown correspond to the most common areas of infection in the diabetic foot and ankle, and these locations should be evaluated with particular attention, especially on cross-sectional imaging studies such as MRI (see Fig. 65-1B).

Vascular disease is very common in diabetic patients (Fig. 65-2). Resultant baseline ischemia creates a setting in which cuts or other minor injuries heal slowly or not at all. Calluses in ischemic areas break down. This situation promotes formation and progression of foot ulceration. Immunopathy, also a feature of diabe-

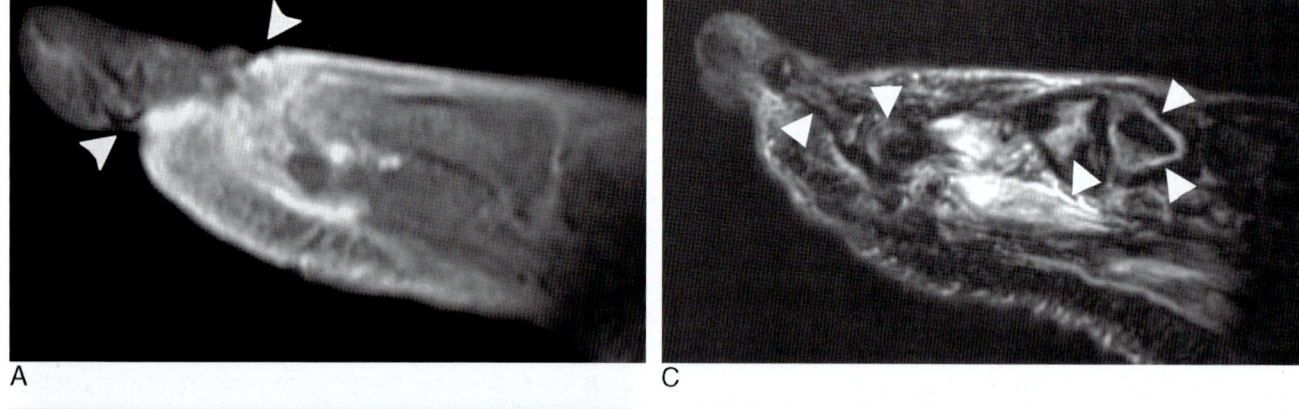

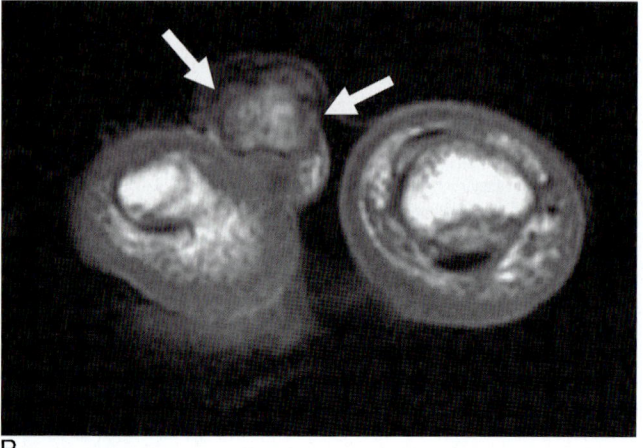

■ **FIGURE 65-2** Effects of ischemic disease in the diabetic foot. **A,** Subacute devitalization of the great toe: contrast-enhanced MRI. T1-weighted fat-suppressed sagittal image shows sharp demarcation (*arrowheads*) of contrast enhancement. Note discrete rim enhancement at the border of necrotic tissue. **B,** Chronic devitalization (gangrene). Short-axis T1-weighted image through the toes demonstrates loss of soft tissue (*arrows*) at the second toe representing a chronically gangrenous digit. **C,** Bone infarction. Sagittal T2-weighted fat-suppressed image shows well-defined areas of high signal (*arrowheads*) consistent with chronic bone infarction in this patient with severe chronic pedal ischemia but no infection.

tes, coupled with vascular disease and diminished sensation, leads to wound infection that is typically caused by more than one organism; progression of infected ulcers results in soft tissue abscesses, sinus tracts, septic tenosynovitis, and, eventually, septic arthritis and osteomyelitis. More advanced ischemia may cause gangrene, particularly at the digits and forefoot, referred to as "dry" gangrene if noninfected and "wet" gangrene if superinfected. With severe chronic ischemia, infarcts may also be seen in the bone marrow.

Neuropathy is also a feature of diabetic disease (Fig. 65-3). Sensory neuropathy leads to diminished perception of minor foot trauma, including cuts, ulcers, blisters, and friction-related skin breakdown, tendon and

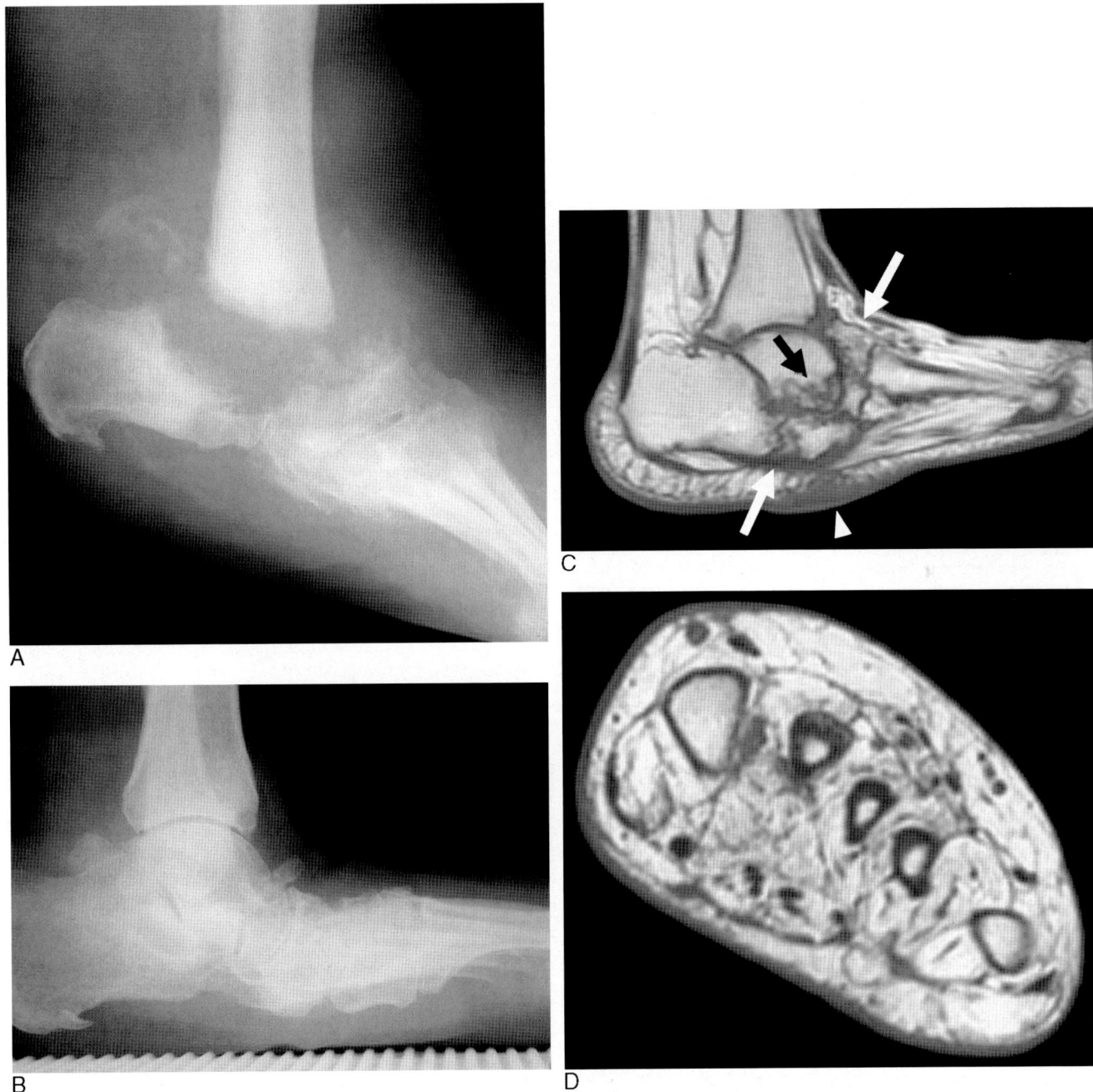

■ **FIGURE 65-3** Effects of neuropathic disease in the diabetic foot. **A,** Total destruction of the ankle and hindfoot in a patient with mixed atrophic and hypertrophic form of neuropathic osteoarthropathy. In the acute phase this often simulates infection clinically and on imaging examinations. **B,** Lateral radiograph of the ankle shows chronic hypertrophic neuropathic osteoarthropathy of the midfoot and hindfoot with collapse of the arch and rocker-bottom deformity. **C,** Sagittal T1-weighted MR image demonstrates deformity of the midfoot and hindfoot, with collapse, subluxation, and disorganization of the tarsal bones (*arrows*) and bone proliferation, characteristic of chronic neuropathic disease. Note rocker-bottom deformity; skin thickening and subcutaneous low signal (*arrowhead*) beneath the cuboid represent callus formation. **D,** Muscle atrophy. T1-weighted short-axis MR image through the metatarsal bones shows fatty atrophy of the intrinsic foot muscles in a patient with long-standing diabetes mellitus.

ligament injury, joint injury, and fractures.[6] Along with ischemic disease, neuropathy contributes to formation and progression of skin wounds and infection. Articular injury with diminished sensation and ischemia can result in an aggressive-appearing, deforming arthropathy referred to as neuropathic osteoarthropathy, or Charcot arthropathy.[7] Tendon injury and ischemia can also lead to tendinopathy and tear. Foot deformity occurs due to tendon dysfunction and articular deformity; in particular, arch collapse can cause a rocker-bottom deformity of the foot. Diabetic neuropathy also affects the peripheral motor nerves, causing diffuse muscle atrophy and muscle imbalance that contributes to deformity.[4] Foot deformity alters weight bearing and distribution of plantar pressures[4]; also, deformity causes footwear to fit poorly. These factors lead to abnormal friction with subsequent callus formation and ulceration. Autonomic

dysfunction also occurs; this, combined with vascular fragility, ischemia, and reduced muscular activity, results in deposition of fluid in the soft tissues. On physical examination diffuse swelling of the foot can be seen. Edema within confined compartments of the foot increases intracompartmental pressures and can accentuate the ischemic cascade.

ANATOMY

The foot has been found to be composed of distinct myofascial compartments (Fig. 65-4A). The plantar aspect of the foot is divided by the muscle groups into medial, central, and lateral compartments, which extend from the metatarsophalangeal joints to the heel. The deep aspect of the central compartment has access to the lower calf via the long flexors that pass the ankle. If infection

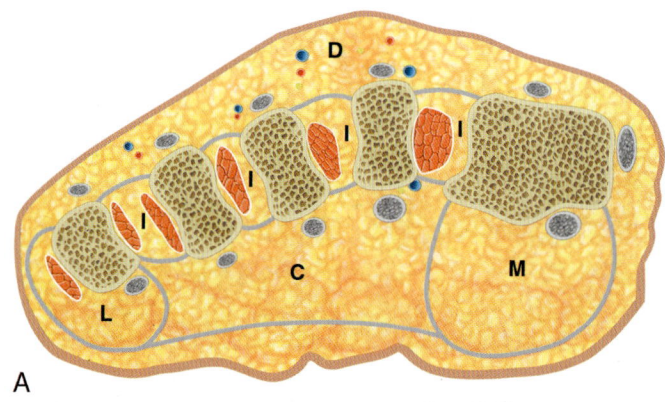

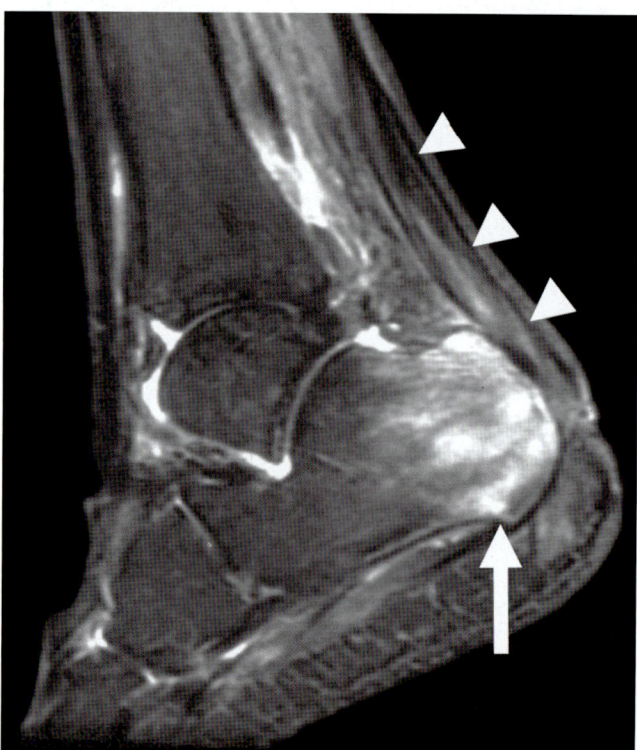

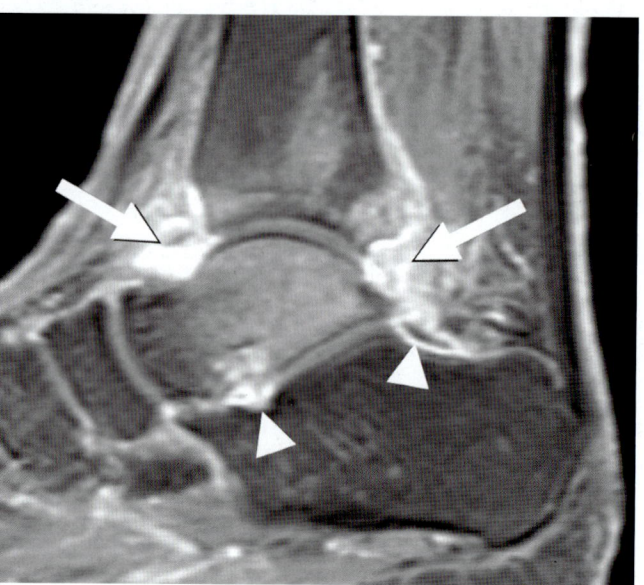

■ **FIGURE 65-4** Spread of infection; anatomic considerations. **A,** Fascial compartments of the foot. At the plantar aspect of the foot are the medial (M), central (C), and lateral (L) compartments; the deep aspect of the central compartment has access to the lower leg above the ankle and is a potential source of spread of infection. The interosseous (I) compartments are located between the metatarsal shafts, bounded superiorly by the dorsal (D) subcutaneous compartment. **B,** Tendinous spread of infection on MRI. STIR image shows osteomyelitis of the calcaneus (*arrow*) with infection extending proximally along the Achilles tendon (*arrowheads*) to the myotendinous junction. **C,** Articular spread of infection. Postcontrast, fat-suppressed, T1-weighted MR image shows communication of the ankle (*arrows*) and subtalar (*arrowheads*) joints with propagation of infection depicted by enhancing synovium. Enhancement of the tibia and talus is indicative of underlying osteomyelitis.

involves this deep fascial compartment, care must be taken to ensure that the process has not spread proximally. Interosseous compartments exist between the metatarsal bones as well. This compartmental anatomy, studied in cadavers, has been used to suggest patterns of spread of pedal infection. In actuality, in the diabetic foot the myofascial compartmental anatomy is not a good predictor of extent of spread.[8] This may be due to variability of compartmental interconnections or due to ischemia and injury in diabetics causing pathologic communications. Spread of infection in diabetics tends to follow a centripetal pattern from the source rather than spreading proximally preferentially along myofascial planes.[8] However, proximal spread is always a consideration that should be taken into account when interpreting imaging studies. Tendons and their sheaths are another route for proximal spread of infection, and spread via this route should be evaluated on cross-sectional imaging studies, particularly MRI (see Fig. 65-4B). Another anatomic consideration is that in many cases there is communication of the tibiotalar joint and posterior facet of the subtalar joint; involvement of one with septic arthritis often leads to rapid involvement of the other, with potential for development of extensive osteomyelitis (see Fig. 65-4C).

IMAGING TECHNIQUES

Techniques and Relevant Aspects

There are a number of factors that make it difficult to propose a uniform algorithm for diagnosis of infection in the diabetic foot. First, access to advanced imaging modalities varies geographically, as does reader expertise. Radiologist and referring clinician preference vary, often related to training. Treatment of patients with aggressive surgical management (limb-sparing surgery) versus conservative surgery (definitive amputation) versus medical therapy varies depending on severity of disease as well as the surgeon's training and the patient's underlying condition. Aggressive surgical management may necessitate acquisition of a "road map" of the patient's pathologic process to achieve success, versus other treatment options that require only a positive or negative diagnosis. Venous access and extremity perfusion obviously influence the success of diagnostic examinations that require injection.

Pros and Cons

Radiography is generally the first examination ordered when infection in the diabetic foot is suspected; radiographs provide excellent overview of anatomy, and the modality is widely available, which facilitates follow-up examinations as well as evaluation of postoperative changes. However, radiographs are insensitive to osteomyelitis in early stages and cannot determine the extent of involvement of osseous or soft tissue disease. Therefore, whether negative or positive, generally additional imaging is necessary.

Ultrasonography is useful for identifying soft tissue fluid collections, joint effusions, and tendon sheath fluid

and can even detect periosteal elevation and cortical interruption associated with infection. Power Doppler imaging may be useful for detecting areas of cellulitis, synovitis, and relative hyperemia. The most obvious limitation of ultrasonography is evaluation of the osseous structures beyond the cortical margin. Also, ultrasonography is a targeted examination without the anatomic overview provided by other modalities. Therefore, beyond answering specific questions about fluid collections, or targeting areas for aspiration, ultrasonography has played a limited role in evaluation of infection in the diabetic foot.

CT provides more anatomic definition than radiographs and can detect abscess formation (when contrast medium is used) as well as periostitis and cortical erosion, but it remains limited in determining the extent of involvement within the bone as well as in the soft tissues; given these limitations as well as associated expense, its use as a clinical tool for this purpose has also been limited. Biopsies that require imaging can generally be performed utilizing fluoroscopy. The advanced capabilities of multidetector CT may increase the use of CT for evaluation of pedal infection in the future.

Nuclear medicine examinations include technetium-99m three-phase bone scintigraphy, gallium-67 scan, and labeled white blood cell scan. Three-phase bone scintigraphy remains widely popular as a sensitive tool for detection of osteomyelitis in the diabetic foot. However, uptake can occur owing to other processes, resulting in bone turnover, including injury and neuropathic osteoarthropathy.[9] Also, in cases of severe ischemia, uptake may be artifactually low. Gallium scan, although commonly used for detection of inflammatory processes around the body, has shown limitations in the diabetic foot. Instead, when there is a question of infection versus other process, labeled white blood cells (using indium-111 or technetium-99m) have been used.[10] Tracer is taken up preferentially by inflammatory tissue. One limitation of scintigraphic methods in general is that the anatomic resolution is low, making these techniques less useful as preoperative anatomic "road maps."

MRI has become popular for evaluation of infection in the diabetic foot in regions where access to high-quality MRI units is available. Soft tissue and bone marrow pathology can be detected with high sensitivity, similar in most settings to scintigraphic methods. High contrast between different tissue types as well as inflammatory versus non-inflammatory tissue combined with anatomic definition has made this modality useful to surgeons interested in acquiring a "road map" of pathologic tissue before surgery.[11-13] Additionally, with intravenous contrast administration it is possible to evaluate areas of devitalization that may require débridement.[14] A multitude of articles in the radiologic and clinical literature have documented the use of MRI for evaluation of osteomyelitis of the foot and ankle. Sensitivity ranges from 77% to 100%, and specificity ranges from 79% to 100% in the larger studies; those that include at least 25 patients are summarized in Table 65-1. Superimposed factors such as prior surgery, neuropathic osteoarthropathy, or other inflammatory disease, such as rheumatoid arthritis, may lower the specificity of MRI.[15]

TABLE 65-1	Magnetic Resonance Imaging for Evaluation of Osteomyelitis of the Foot and Ankle				
Author/Year	No. Patients/No. with Histology or Culture Proven	Sensitivity	Specificity	Accuracy	Comments
Croll, 1996	27/21	88%	100%	95%	1.5 T, No gadolinium
Levine, 1994	27/18	77%	100%	90%	1.5 T, No gadolinium
Morrison, 1995	59/41	82% diabetic 89% nondiabetic	80% diabetic 94% nondiabetic	89% overall	1.5 T, gadolinium and fat, saturated (N = 53)
Weinstein, 1993	47/32	100%	81%	95%	0.5 T (N = 20) 1.5 T (N = 27) No gadolinium
Nigro, 1992	44/34	100%	95%	98%	1.5 T, No gadolinium
Wang, 1990	50/32	99%	81%	94%	0.5 T (N = 23) 1.5 T (N = 27) No gadolinium
Ledermann, 2002	158/158	90%	79%	103 TP, 37 TN, 11 FN, 10 FP	1.5 T, All gadolinium

Note: Only studies that include at least 25 patients are listed. TP, true positive; TN, true negative; FN, false negative; FP, false positive.

Controversies

There has been controversy in the literature regarding the relative utility of scintigraphic methods and MRI for evaluation of infection in the diabetic foot. Comparison studies are sparse and generally include a small number

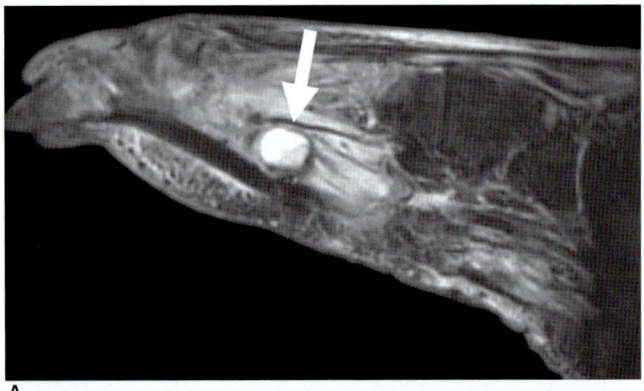

A

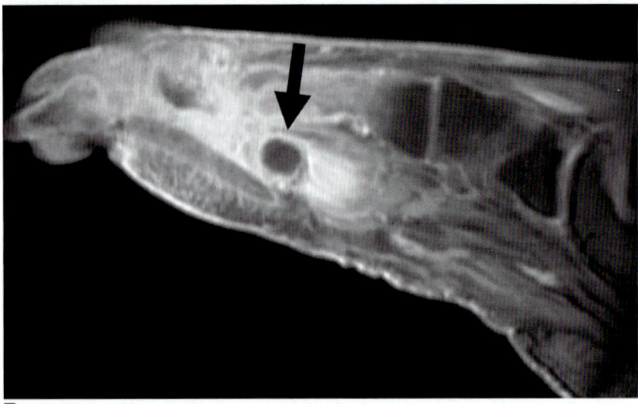

B

■ **FIGURE 65-5**   Abscess. **A,** Sagittal, T2-weighted, fat-suppressed MR image shows focal fluid signal (*arrow*) representing an abscess in the deep plantar soft tissues. **B,** Sagittal, contrast-enhanced, fat-suppressed, T1-weighted MR image demonstrates thick rim enhancement of the abscess (*arrow*) with surrounding soft tissue enhancement consistent with cellulitis.

of patients; additionally, articles are often written from a preferential perspective. Both modalities are excellent overall for diagnosis of osteomyelitis, and both have limitations. Three-phase bone scintigraphy is highly sensitive for osseous involvement[16] but exhibits relatively low specificity in complicated settings such as neuropathic disease, trauma, and postoperative situations.[17] Labeled white blood cell scanning increases specificity but generally is performed in conjunction with three-phase bone scintigraphy. MRI provides excellent anatomic depiction of disease and is highly sensitive for osteomyelitis as well. Specificity, as with scintigraphic methods, decreases in the setting of underlying complications such as neuropathic disease. MRI is especially useful to serve as a surgical planning tool[11-13,18] to determine the extent of soft tissue and bone pathology, and to characterize soft tissue structures involved by infection and necrosis.

Regarding use of gadolinium in MRI, some studies recommend intravenous contrast[15] whereas others believe it to be unnecessary.[19] It remains controversial whether addition of a contrast-enhanced sequence improves the accuracy of MRI for the diagnosis of osteomyelitis. However, it is not disputed that contrast enhancement improves detection of soft tissue infection.[13] It differentiates cellulitis from diabetic soft tissue edema and improves evaluation of the extent of soft tissue disease (Fig. 65-5). It helps detect sinus tracts and abscesses,[20] and it is the only way to delineate areas of devitalization or necrosis.[14] Therefore, administration of a contrast agent can provide useful information, especially if the patient is being considered for surgical management.

MANIFESTATIONS OF THE DISEASE

Radiography

For patients with clinical suspicion of pedal infection, radiographs are typically the initial radiologic examination obtained (Fig. 65-6). For the foot, in addition to anteroposterior and lateral views, oblique views are use-

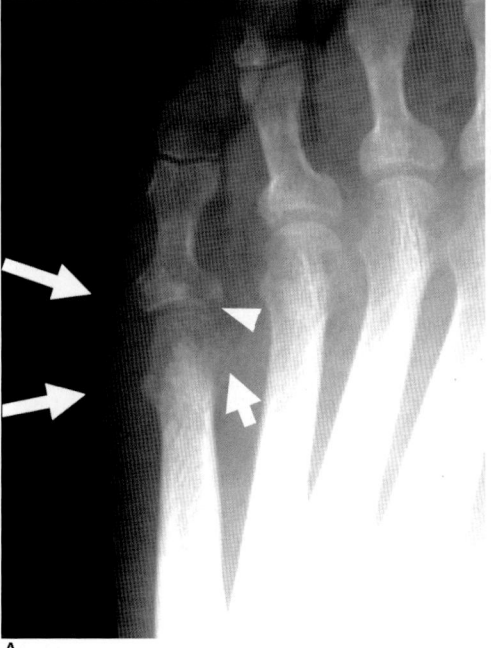
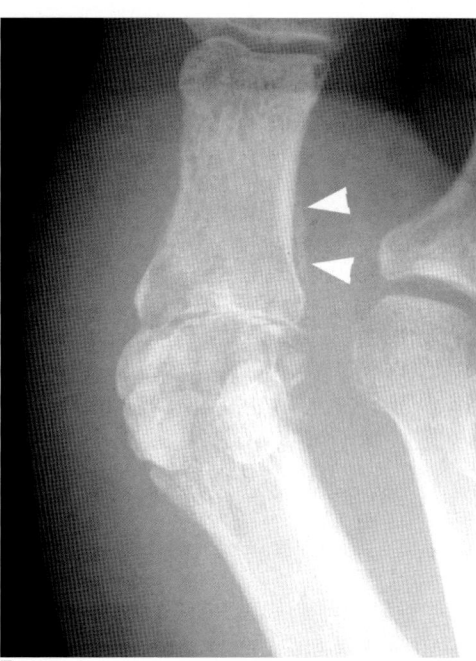

A
B

■ **FIGURE 65-6** Diabetic pedal infection: radiographic appearance. **A,** Early osteomyelitis. Anteroposterior radiograph of the lateral forefoot shows soft tissue swelling (*long arrows*) with rarefaction (lucency) of the fifth metatarsal head (*short arrow*). Note erosion at the proximal phalanx (*arrowhead*) associated with slight narrowing of the MTP joint, likely representing underlying septic arthritis. **B,** Osteomyelitis and septic arthritis— late. Anteroposterior radiograph of the medial forefoot shows marked narrowing of the first MTP joint with adjacent bone destruction and soft tissue swelling. Note periostitis (*arrowheads*) along the proximal phalanx.

ful for evaluation of the digits and metatarsals. Oblique views are also helpful at the ankle to visualize subtle areas of periostitis and bone rarefaction.

Early infection is seen as soft tissue swelling, representing cellulitis. In diabetic feet, skin ulceration is commonly seen, with interruption of the skin margin that may be apparent if imaged tangentially. Seen en face, ulceration results in a focal, rounded area of relative lucency surrounded by soft tissue swelling. Soft tissue

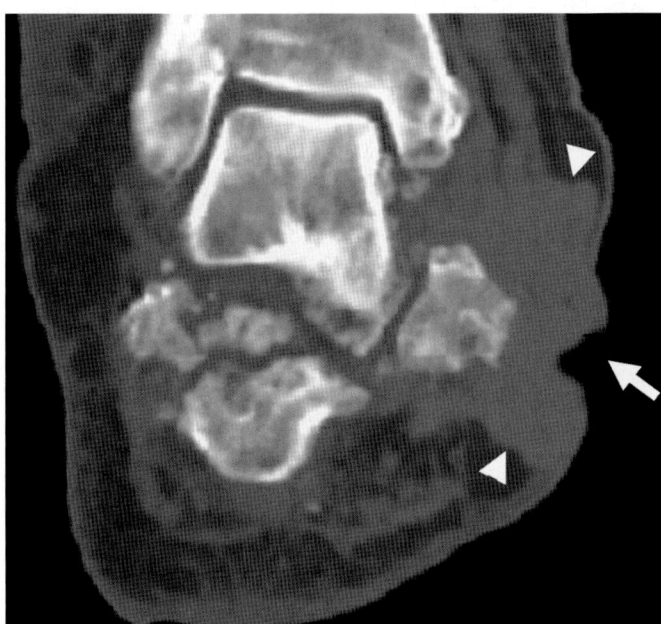

■ FIGURE 65-7 Osteomyelitis. Coronal reformatted multidetector CT image shows neuropathic changes in the hindfoot with disorganization. Note medial cutaneous ulcer (*arrow*) and soft tissue swelling (*arrowheads*) representing cellulitis leading to bone.

swelling is nonspecific, and abscess cannot be differentiated from mere cellulitis. Occasionally, soft tissue gas is observed, characterized by tiny foci of soft tissue lucency, typically adjacent to a skin ulcer. This does not necessarily imply presence of a gas-forming organism but more commonly results from communication of an abscess or area of devitalized tissue with an ulcer. Septic arthritis is characterized in the early stages by joint effusion, which may be visible at the ankle in the form of anterior capsular distention and in the toes as fusiform (symmetric) soft tissue swelling around joints of the toes. Effusion in joints of the midfoot is difficult to detect on radiographs. In later stages, septic arthritis appears similar to other inflammatory arthropathies, with marginal erosions and diffuse joint narrowing (Fig. 65-7). As the disease progresses to osteomyelitis, frank bone destruction is seen. Radiographic changes of osteomyelitis can be delayed as much as 2 weeks after onset of infection; therefore, sensitivity is poor. When visible radiographically, osteomyelitis results in focal rarefaction, or decreased density of bone, followed by periostitis and frank bone erosion or destruction. Periostitis may not be seen in the tarsal bones or the phalanges, however. Despite low utility for diagnosing osteomyelitis, radiographs nevertheless help define postoperative anatomy; identify soft tissue calcification, gas, and foreign bodies; and characterize the pattern and distribution of arthritis, including neuropathic osteoarthropathy. Radiographs obtained while bearing weight are useful to evaluate foot deformities. Therefore, radiographs can be helpful in conjunction with other modalities.

Magnetic Resonance Imaging (Table 65-2)

If the primary site of infection is known, coil selection and imaging planes should be tailored; for example, an

TABLE 65-2 Magnetic Resonance Signal Characteristics of Conditions Affecting the Diabetic Foot

	T1	T2	T1 Post Contrast	Comments
Marrow Signal				
Osteomyelitis	Low	High	High	Adjacent soft tissue infection
Infarction	Low sharp margins	High rim well defined	Marginal	Enhancement
Neuropathic				
Acute	Low	High	High	To differentiate from osteomyelitis, see Table 66-3
Chronic	Normal to low	Normal to high	Subchondral enhancement	
Soft Tissue Signal				
Devitalization	Normal to low	High diffusely	Regional absence of enhancement	Osteomyelitis, abscesses; cellulitis may not enhance
Diabetic edema	Normal to slightly low	High diffusely	Little enhancement	Associated with muscle atrophy
Cellulitis	Low regionally	High diffusely	Enhancement	Regionally
Callus	Focally low subcutaneously	Low to intermediate	Focal enhancement	Blends with skin signal
Ulcer	Low	High	Marginal enhancement of crater	Focal discontinuity of skin signal
Sinus tract	Low	Linear high	"Tram-track" linear enhancement	Connects to skin or abscess
Abscess	Low		focal fluid	Rim enhancement

extremity coil designed for the knee is generally excellent for imaging the ankle but often results in suboptimal examination of the toes. For toe imaging, 3-inch or 5-inch surface coils are preferred. However, if the main concern is extent of proximal spread, the small surface coils may not provide adequate coverage. A minimum of two planes should be acquired to best depict the area of concern; plane selection should also be tailored to the situation. For the forefoot and metatarsals, short-axis images should be included because the narrow bones easily volume average in long-axis planes. However, for flexed or deformed toes, sagittal images are very useful. Long-axis images provide an excellent visualization of the bones of the midfoot as well as depiction of anatomic extent of infection. Sagittal images are optimal for evaluation of deformities of the midfoot arch. Spin-echo, T1-weighted images should be acquired to evaluate anatomy as well as subcutaneous fat and marrow fat. Edema and fluid signal is best evaluated using fat-suppressed, fast spin-echo, T2-weighted images. Use of fat suppression is important; otherwise, edema in the bone marrow and soft tissues will blend with signal from fat. If fat suppression is not available or is heterogeneous, short tau inversion recovery (STIR) images should be acquired. Fat suppression is also important when acquiring post-contrast T1-weighted images.[15] Obtaining both precontrast and postcontrast fat-suppressed images can be useful to evaluate relative tissue vascularity and differentiate true enhancement from heterogeneous fat suppression. This can be facilitated by use of a T1-weighted, fast gradient-echo sequence instead of a conventional spin-echo sequence to shorten scan time.

Callus is seen as focal cutaneous and subcutaneous soft tissue prominence; the skin and subcutaneous signal often blends imperceptibly, although a rounded subcutaeous focus may be observed. Calluses have low signal intensity on T1-weighted images but show variable signal intensity on T2-weighted images based on the degree of granulation tissue and vascularity.[2] More vascular calluses demonstrate higher T2 signal and enhance diffusely

after gadolinium administration. The chronic friction that leads to callus formation can also result in adventitial bursitis, seen as a focus of fluid, usually thin and elongated or ovoid, in the subcutaneous tissues adjacent to a callus; if the focus is well defined without adjacent soft tissue inflammation, it can be confidently attributed to friction-related bursitis rather than abscess. Contrast-enhanced sequences can be useful to exclude surrounding inflammation.

In ulcerated callus (Fig. 65-8), typically a large skin defect is seen with rounded or "heaped up" margins, surrounded by vascular callus. The ulcer usually enhances at the margin, unless the surrounding tissue is devitalized. Minor skin disruption or superficial skin erosion without underlying callus is more difficult to detect and may only be visualized as a focal discontinuity of skin signal. Wound breakdown can also occur in postoperative patients. Any

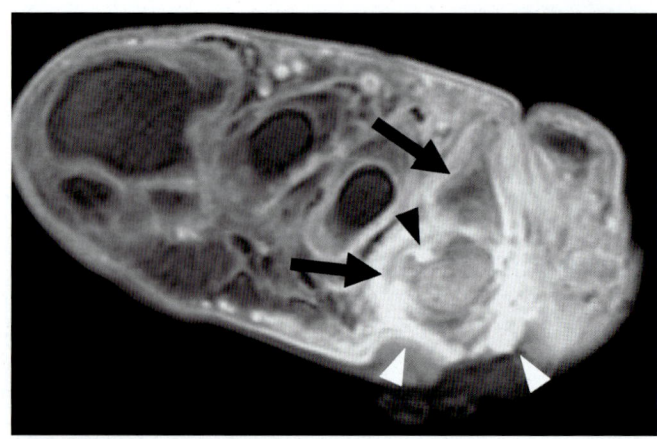

■ **FIGURE 65-8** Ulceration. Short-axis, contrast-enhanced, fat-suppressed, T1-weighted MR image shows enhancement at the base of the ulcer (*white arrowheads*). There is enhancement of the underlying soft tissues representing cellulitis. Note also enhancement of the metatarsal head and phalanx (*arrows*) indicating osteomyelitis. Erosion at the metatarsophalangeal joint (*black arrowhead*) represents septic arthritis.

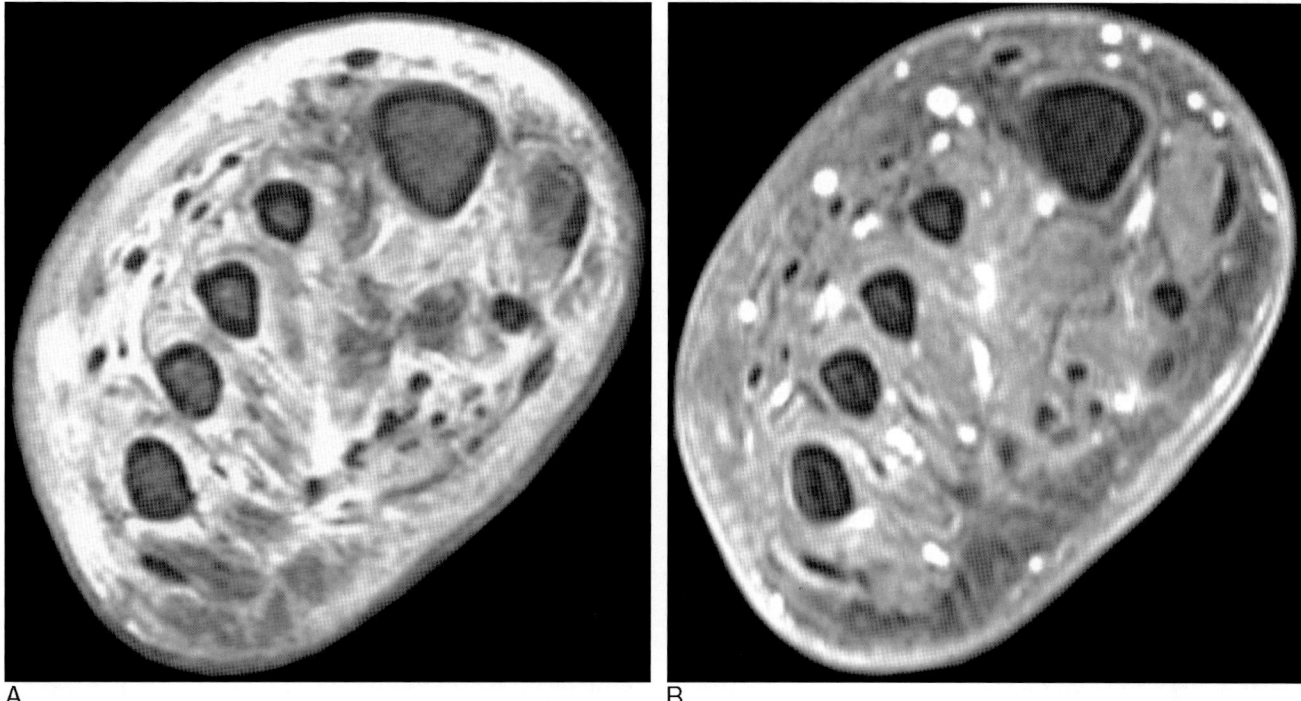

A   B

■ FIGURE 65-9 Pedal edema in the diabetic foot. **A,** T2-weighted, fat-suppressed MR image of the forefoot in a diabetic patient reveals diffuse subcutaneous and muscular edema. **B,** After administration of a contrast agent there is no enhancement of the edematous areas; this is consistent with typical diabetic pedal edema related to ischemia and neuropathic disease not cellulitis.

form of skin interruption may serve as a route for soft tissue infection. Deep ulceration is especially important to identify because there is a high association with underlying osteomyelitis.[21]

Soft tissue edema, observed within muscles, subcutaneous fat, or both, is very common on MR images of diabetic feet and should not be mistaken for cellulitis (Fig. 65-9). Subcutaneous fat signal is usually not replaced, as it is with cellulitis. On gadolinium-enhanced images, diabetic edema shows minimal enhancement, unlike cellulitis, which enhances brightly. In advanced diabetes, the muscles of the foot are typically atrophied, with decreased size and fatty infiltration. The atrophied muscles often appear edematous on T2-weighted images.

Cellulitis is seen as replacement of the normal fat signal in subcutaneous tissues on T1-weighted images, with high signal (though less than fluid) on T2-weighted or STIR images and diffuse enhancement after contrast agent administration. The margins are generally poorly defined. Gas can also be seen within areas of cellulitis in diabetic feet and is particularly common adjacent to ulcers or in devitalized areas. Abscesses appear as a focal collection of signal approximating fluid on T2-weighted or STIR images, with thick rim enhancement on postcontrast T1-weighted images.[22] Sinus tracts (Fig. 65-10A) are characterized by a thin, discrete line of fluid signal extending through the soft tissues. On postcontrast images, sinus tracts, like abscesses (see Fig. 65-10B), stand out due to enhancement of the

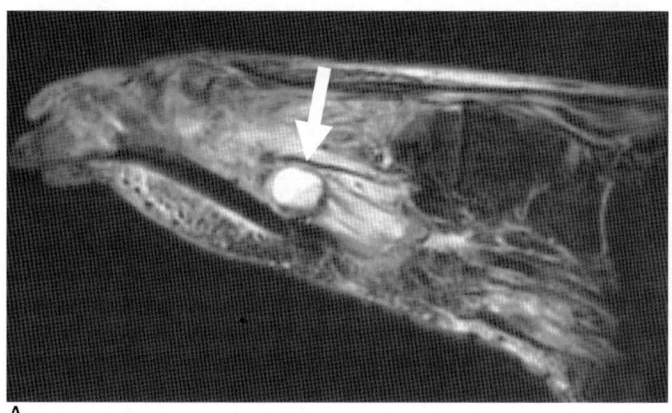
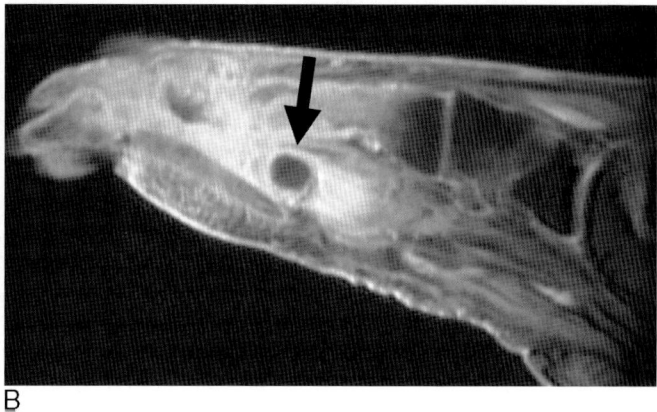

A   B

■ FIGURE 65-10 Sinus tract. **A,** Short-axis, T2-weighted, fat-suppressed MR image shows diffuse soft tissue edema with focal signal near fluid intensity in the fifth digit (*arrow*) extending to the skin margin. **B,** Short-axis, contrast-enhanced, fat-suppressed T1-weighted MR image demonstrates enhancing cellulitis of the fifth digit; thick rim enhancement of the central fluid collection (*arrow*) represents an abscess surrounding the phalanx. Thin, linear rim enhancement consistent with sinus tracts extends from this collection to the skin.

hyperemic margins.[23] Sinus tracts are visualized as parallel lines of enhancement in a "tram-track" configuration.[21]

In a septic joint (Fig. 65-11), an effusion is usually seen. However, the fluid may drain through a sinus tract or decompress into a tendon sheath before imaging, leaving only a small amount in the joint. Synovial thickening and enhancement is seen on postcontrast images. Marginal erosions and reactive subchondral edema are common[24]; if the marginal erosions are small, and if edema is confined to a thin rim beneath the cortex, it is not indicative of secondary osteomyelitis. However, if the edema or enhancement related to septic arthritis extends deeper into the medullary bone, osteomyelitis should be considered.[24] In septic tenosynovitis, MRI reveals fluid within the tendon sheath that is disproportionate to that in other sheaths; on T2-weighted images the fluid may appear complex. Although mechanical tenosynovitis is common in the foot and ankle, septic tenosynovitis should be suspected if these changes are associated with surrounding soft tissue infection. Contrast enhancement may also help identify involved tendons.[25] Postcontrast images show a thick rim of enhancement around the tendon representing the proliferative, inflamed synovium.

Osteomyelitis (see Fig. 65-11) is characterized by altered bone marrow signal, with low signal (loss of the normal fat signal) on T1-weighted images, edema on T2-weighted or STIR images, and enhancement on postgadolinium T1-weighted images.[15] Other MRI findings in cases of osteomyelitis may include cortical disruption and periostitis. Periostitis is seen as a thin, linear pattern of edema and enhancement surrounding the outer cortical margin that will appear thickened if the periostitis is chronic.

Recognition of abnormal bone marrow signal in the appropriate clinical setting results in high sensitivity for diagnosis of osteomyelitis; however, other entities can mimic this alteration of the bone marrow signal, including fracture, tumor, active inflammatory arthritis or neuropathic disease, infarction, or recent postoperative change.[15,26] These other processes usually have different morphology than osteomyelitis; recognition of these patterns often enables differentiation. For example, identification of a fracture line, a discrete lesion, adjacent arthritis or neuropathic disease, or postoperative metal artifact improves specificity; correlation with radiographs and clinical history is also important. Another consideration is that over 90% of the time osteomyelitis of the foot and ankle is a result of contiguous spread through the skin[1]; therefore, the majority of cases of osteomyelitis also have some manifestation of adjacent soft tissue disease, such as skin ulceration, cellulitis, soft tissue abscess, or a sinus tract. These findings can be thought of as "secondary signs" of osteomyelitis, recognition of which can also improve specificity.[21]

Devitalization

Changes related to ischemia (see Fig. 65-2) should be taken into account when interpreting MRI of the diabetic foot. Documentation of the presence and extent of ischemic and devitalized areas can facilitate surgical planning for débridement and limited, foot-sparing amputations. If precontrast and postcontrast MR images are acquired, ischemia and devitalization of the foot can be detected as focal or regional lack of soft tissue contrast enhancement.[14] Devitalization, which may be called foot "infarction," is seen as a focal area of nonenhancement with a sharp cutoff; the surrounding soft tissues typically show increased enhancement representing reactive, hypervascular tissue. Only contrast-enhanced images allow reli-

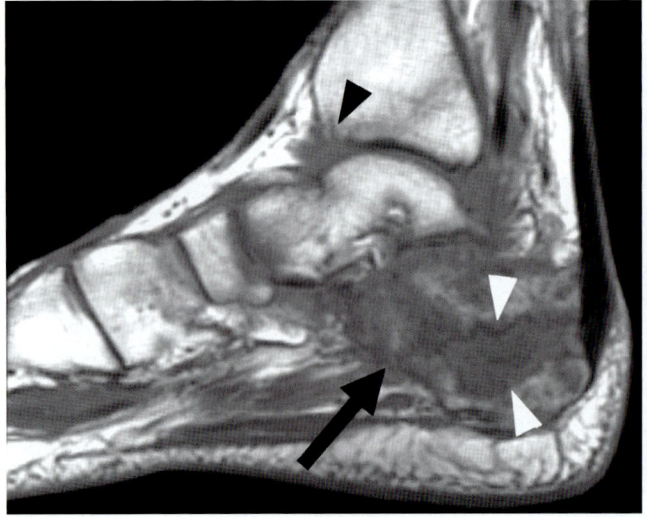
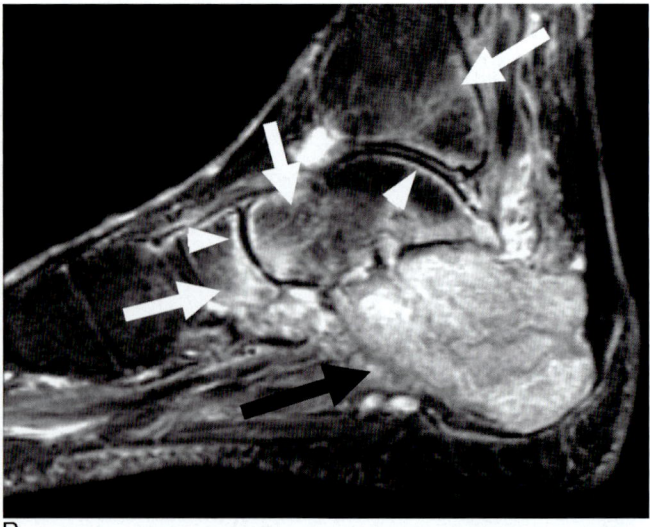

A   B

■ **FIGURE 65-11** Septic arthritis and osteomyelitis. **A,** Sagittal, T1-weighted MR image reveals low signal in the calcaneus (*arrow*) representing osteomyelitis with a central focus of lower signal (*white arrowheads*) proven to be an intraosseous abscess. There is septic arthritis of the subtalar joint and ankle joint as well as the talonavicular joint, with an erosion evident at the anterior ankle joint margin (*black arrowhead*). **B,** Sagittal, T2-weighted, fat-suppressed MR image shows diffuse edema in the infected calcaneus (*black arrow*) with effusions and thin subchondral edema (*arrowheads*) in the ankle, subtalar, and talonavicular joints representing hyperemia related to septic arthritis. Edema extending deeper into the medullary bone (*white arrows*) is consistent with osteomyelitis.

able recognition of gangrenous tissue because T2- and T1-weighted images reveal uncharacteristic signal alterations.[14] Noninfected gangrene is characterized by regional soft tissue loss, particularly affecting the distal digits; T1 and T2 signal may be normal within these areas, although subtle edema signal may be seen. Soft tissue air, seen as small foci of signal void, may be seen within areas of devitalization and is often a sign of superimposed infection; however, this does not generally imply presence of a gas-forming organism ("gas gangrene") but is usually related to communication of devitalized soft tissue with overlying skin ulceration, allowing air to enter.

Additional considerations regarding diabetic vascular disease should be noted when interpreting MRI examinations for suspected infection; underlying infection, including osteomyelitis, cellulitis, and abscess would not be expected to enhance within necrotic areas.[14] In this setting, signal characteristics on T1- and T2-weighted images should be primarily relied on for diagnosis of soft tissue and osseous infection. If intravenous contrast is provided, the radiologist should be familiar with the appearance of devitalized tissue to reduce false-negative readings for infection.

Bone infarction may also be seen within regions of chronic pedal ischemia. The MRI pattern is similar to that of bone infarction in other areas of the body; longitudinally oriented regions of signal abnormality are observed in the central medullary cavity, generally with a serpentine pattern and a sharp, well-defined margin. Internal signal intensity is variable, with fat signal, fibrous signal (low T1 and T2), or edema-type signal. Although high signal intensity on T2-weighted images is seen at the margins, the classic rim of high and low T2 signal "double line sign" may not be evident in the small bones of the foot. The sharp margins, characteristic morphology, and normal surrounding marrow help distinguish infarction from infection.

Evaluation of Extent of Involvement

Extent of infection in soft tissue and bone is usually fairly well delineated on postcontrast MR images. However, infection does not tend to remain confined by fascial planes; it spreads centripetally from the inoculation site and readily spreads into and across joints, through tendons, and across fascial compartments.[8] Although tendon involvement appears to be common in areas of soft tissue infection, this does not appear to be a common mode of proximal spread.[25] Nevertheless, soft tissue involvement is often more extensive than the osseous disease, so the radiologist should carefully examine the soft tissues extending proximally from the source of infection; if this tissue is not débrided, the patient may fail the foot-sparing procedure and require more extensive amputation.

Multidetector Computed Tomography

The protocol for MDCT of pedal infection is the same as that for injury and other diseases; high-resolution and high-quality multiplanar reformatted images are optimized by acquiring thin sections with high kVp and overlap (e.g., low pitch), which results in high photon flux. Contrast may be given intravenously using standard doses to detect abscess formation.

Regarding evaluation of pathology, similar findings as on radiographs will be observed. This includes soft tissue swelling in the early stages of infection with little to no osseous changes. If intravenous contrast medium is administered, soft tissue enhancement reflecting cellulitis will be seen, with fluid collections demonstrating rim enhancement indicating abscess formation. In later stages of infection, as osteomyelitis sets in, periostitis and rarefaction of bone will be seen. Eventually, frank bone destruction ensues. Septic arthritis is seen as joint effusion, articular narrowing, and marginal erosions. Evaluation of soft tissue and osseous extent is limited. Because of this and delay in demonstration of bone involvement, CT does not add much information over radiographs. However, if anatomic information is needed and MRI cannot be obtained, or if there are metal implants present, MDCT may be useful.

Ultrasonography

Use of a high-frequency transducer offers excellent depiction of soft tissue anatomic detail, and ultrasonography can be useful for answering specific questions, such as whether there is a fluid collection in the subcutaneous tissues that may represent a drainable abscess. Fluid collections (Fig. 65-12) are seen as focal regions of hypoechogenicity. Detection of joint effusions and tendon sheath fluid can also be seen, but these findings are common also in absence of infection. Infected fluid collections and effusions often have complex internal characteristics. Also, use of power Doppler can demonstrate hyperemia of the synovium and surrounding tissues, suggesting inflammation. Although ultrasonography cannot visualize the marrow compartment, a focused examination can demonstrate cortical breakthrough and periosteal elevation. However, owing to availability of other modalities that offer a more comprehensive evaluation, use of ultrasonography for this purpose has been limited.

Nuclear Medicine

Nuclear medicine examinations are performed commonly for evaluation of pedal infection. Three-phase bone scintigraphy is highly sensitive for detection of osteomyelitis, which is seen as regional radiotracer uptake on the early phases and concentration in the underlying bone marrow on the delayed phase.[27] When there is no increased uptake the test is excellent for excluding presence of osteomyelitis, except in the setting of severe vascular disease. However, other processes resulting in hyperemia and bone turnover can also result in a positive test, and, consequently, specificity is low.[15,28] Labeled white blood cell examination has higher specificity and is generally interpreted in conjunction with the three-phase bone scintiscan.

Three-Phase Bone Scintigraphy

The uptake in three-phase bone scintigraphy is related to blood flow and osteoblastic activity. A three-phase bone scintiscan consists of an initial blood flow or angiographic phase obtained immediately after injection of 25 mCi of ^{99m}Tc-labeled methylene diphosphonate, a blood pool phase obtained within 5 minutes after injection, and a delayed phase, 4 to 6 hours after injection

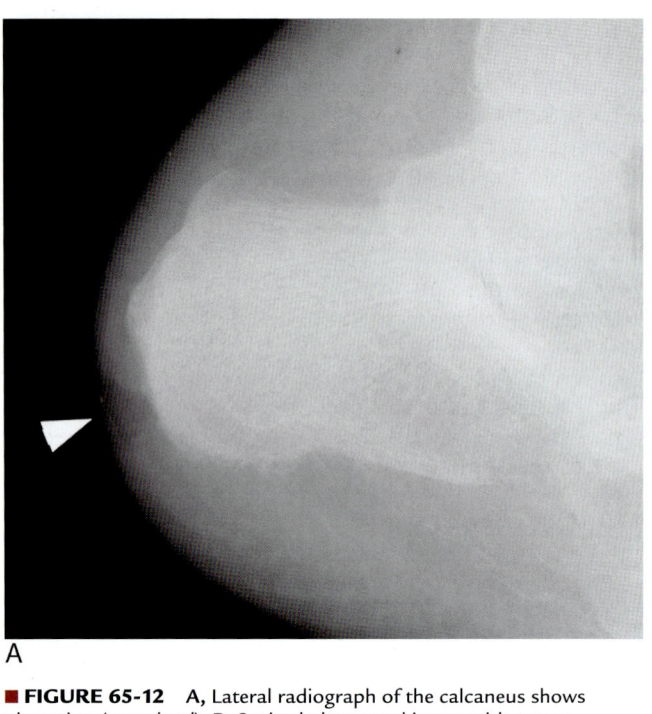

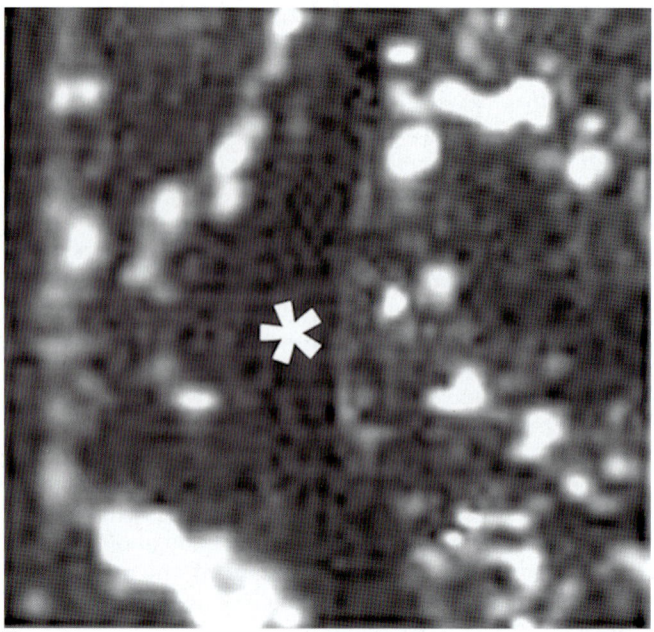

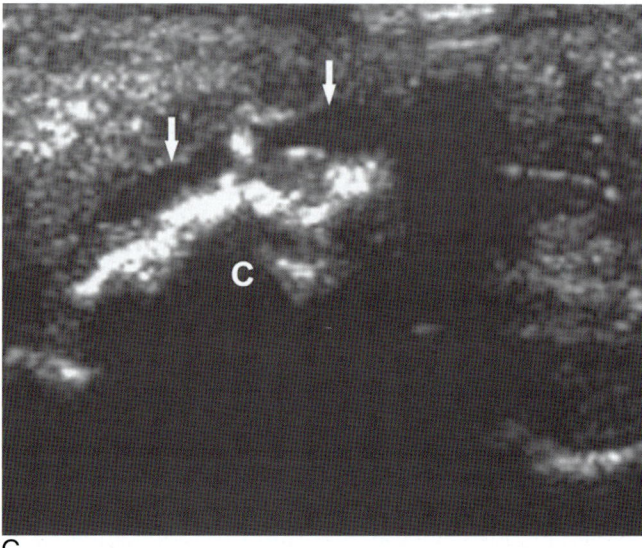

■ **FIGURE 65-12** **A,** Lateral radiograph of the calcaneus shows ulceration (*arrowhead*). **B,** Sagittal ultrasound image with power Doppler adjacent to the ulcer shows a thin, anechoic fluid collection (*asterisk*) with surrounding hyperemia. **C,** Transverse image shows fluid collection (*arrows*) extending laterally around the calcaneus (C).

(Fig. 65-13). An additional static image may be acquired after 24 hours ("fourth phase"). The first phase depicts vascular perfusion and is generally increased in the setting of inflammation, although ischemic disease in diabetic feet may cause delay in vascular uptake. In areas of inflammation, capillaries dilate, causing increased blood flow and blood pooling, which is captured on the second phase. The third phase depicts relative bone turnover, which is increased in infection but also in many other disorders.[15,29] Therefore, uptake localized to bone on the delayed phase is nonspecific, but if associated with increased uptake on the vascular and blood pool phases it is presumed to reflect inflammatory bone turnover; and in the setting of suspected infection the test is highly sensitive for diagnosis of osteomyelitis. Cellulitis, abscess, and other soft tissue infections typically show increased uptake on the first two phases that fails to concentrate in bone on the third phase. Occasionally, there is persistent blood pool distribution of tracer, especially in ischemic feet, which can be suspected if there is poorly defined tracer distribution. The fourth phase image, acquired after 24 hours, showing residual tracer concentrated in bone, can help distinguish osteomyelitis from overlying cellulitis in this setting. Severe ischemia results in lack of tracer uptake and may lead to appearance of photopenic regions or relative lack of uptake that can cause a false-negative examination. Chronic osteomyelitis or partially treated infection may not show characteristic uptake on the first two phases. Another consideration is that osteomyelitis may demonstrate tracer uptake for a long period of time after treatment. Bone turnover and hyperemia caused by neuropathic osteoarthropathy, trauma, recent surgery, or inflammatory arthropathy can also appear

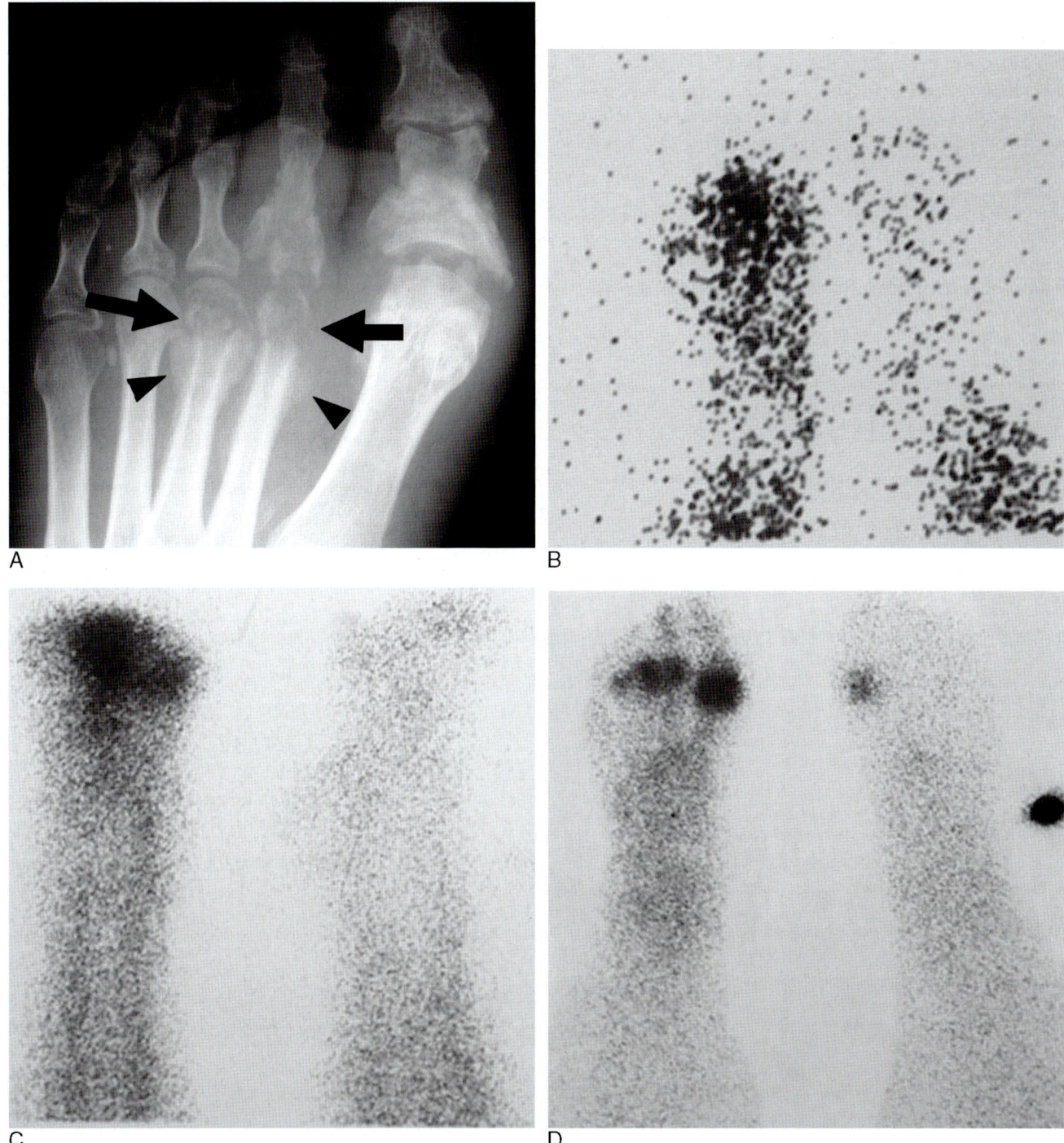

■ **FIGURE 65-13** Acute osteomyelitis. **A,** Anteroposterior radiograph of the forefoot shows bone rarefaction and destruction, predominantly at the second and third metatarsal heads (*arrows*). Thick periostitis (*arrowheads*) is seen more proximally. Vascular phase (**B**), blood pool phase (**C**), and delayed phase (**D**) scintiscans of the same patient as in A show hyperemia with late concentration of radiotracer at the metatarsophalangeal joints consistent with osteomyelitis.

similar to infection, leading to false-positive examination. Reported sensitivities range from 75% to 100% in the literature. Specificity is lower as a result of vascular insufficiency and complicating neuroarthropathy (Fig. 65-14). In the setting of underlying complicating conditions such as this, where there is nonspecific uptake on the delayed phase, corresponding uptake on a labeled white blood cell scan increases specificity.

Labeled White Blood Cell Scan

White blood cell scanning is based on accumulation of labeled leukocytes in infected tissue (Fig. 65-15). This involves withdrawing approximately 50 mL of autologous blood with a leukocyte count of approximately 5,000/ mL; leukocytes are collected by centrifuge, exposed to indium-111 oxine, and reinjected intravenously. Images

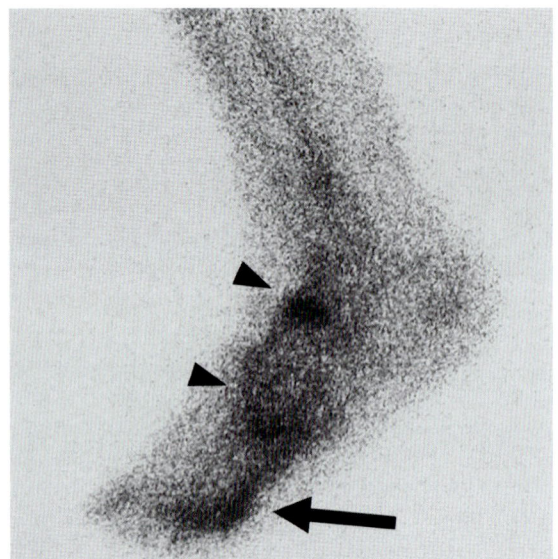

■ FIGURE 65-14 Osteomyelitis and neuropathic disease. Delayed phase of a three-phase ⁹⁹ᵐTc-MDP bone scintiscan in the lateral projection shows uptake concentrating in the bones of the lateral forefoot (*arrow*), representing osteomyelitis. Uptake in the midfoot and hindfoot (*arrowheads*) is present due to underlying neuropathic disease.

are obtained at 2 to 4 hours as well as at 24 hours. Images obtained at 24 hours normally show significant activity only in the liver, spleen, and red marrow. Focal uptake in the foot, which does not contain appreciable amounts of red marrow, is generally indicative of infection.[30] Drawbacks include the low count rate, cost of the radiopharmaceutical preparation, complexity of the labeling, and lack of bony landmarks. It may be difficult to separate soft tissue from bone infection, both of which will accumulate leukocytes. However, if there is a positive three-phase bone scintiscan with delayed uptake in the same region a diagnosis of osteomyelitis can be made. Previous treatment with antibiotics may reduce leukocyte accumulation, and, as with three-phase bone scintigraphy, ischemia can also prevent uptake. Noninfectious inflammatory conditions such as rheumatoid arthritis and hyperemic conditions such as acute neuropathic disease can occasionally show uptake as well. Leukocytes may also be labeled with ⁹⁹ᵐTc-hexa-methylpropyleneamine oxime (HMPAO). Its advantage is that the radionuclide is more readily available and the energy window is more advantageous, improving image quality. Reported sensitivities of labeled white blood cell scanning range from 75% to 100%, and specificities range

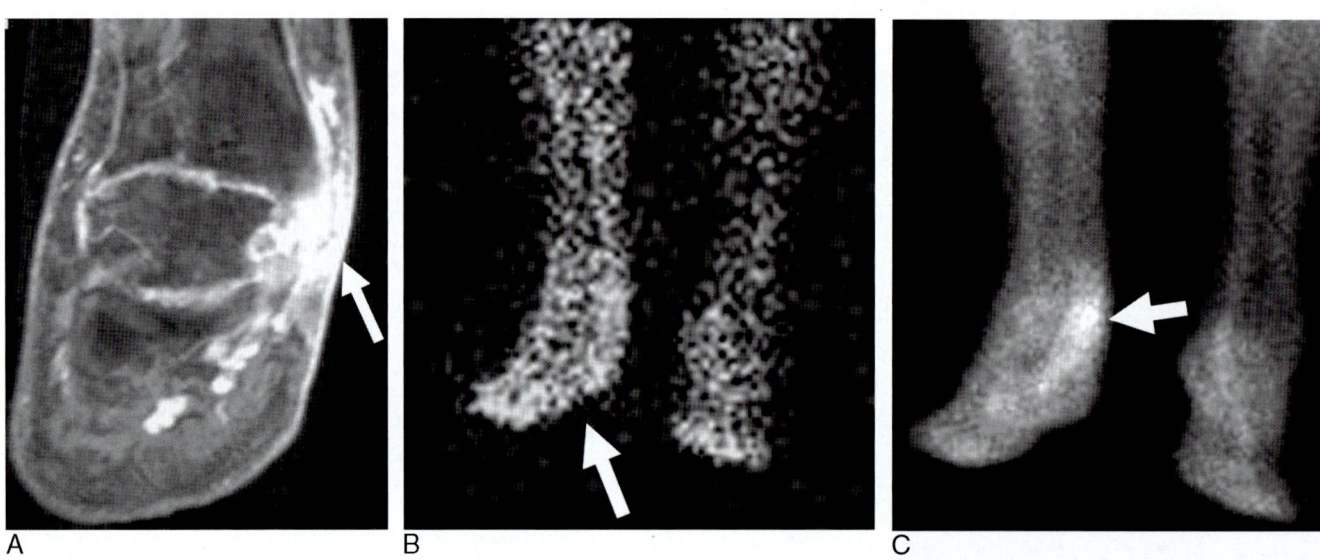

A   B   C

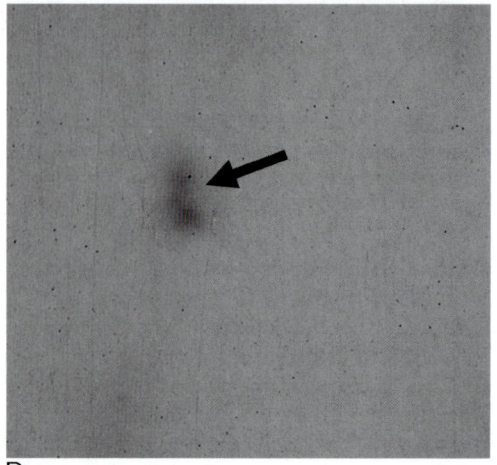

D

■ FIGURE 65-15 Osteomyelitis. **A,** Coronal, postcontrast, T1-weighted, fat-suppressed MR image of the ankle shows enhancement (*arrow*) in the medial soft tissues and medial malleolus. **B,** Vascular phase of a three-phase bone scintiscan shows increased uptake (*arrow*) in the right foot and ankle. **C,** Delayed phase of three-phase bone scintiscan demonstrates focal uptake concentrating in the region of the medial malleolus (*arrow*). **D,** Labeled white blood cell scan confirms infection with uptake concentrating in the medial ankle (*arrow*).

from 69% to 100%. Combined with three-phase bone scintigraphy, specificity increases to 90% to 100%.

Gallium Scanning

Gallium scanning is based on the localization of gallium-67 citrate in areas of osteomyelitis resulting from direct leukocyte and bacterial uptake, lactoferrin and transferrin binding (proteins mediating inflammation), increased vascularity, and increased bone turnover. Five millicuries of gallium-67 citrate is administered intravenously. Delayed images of the feet are obtained at 48 hours, at which time concentration of tracer in bone is observed with osteomyelitis. Gallium is also taken up by bone at sites of remodeling, such as fracture and arthritis, decreasing specificity. Like labeled white blood cell scanning, gallium scans are usually interpreted in conjunction with three-phase bone scanning. However, with similar limitations in specificity as bone scanning, labeled white blood cell scanning is generally preferred as a secondary method.

Positron Emission Tomography/ Computed Tomography

Positron emission tomography has shown promise for imaging infection, related to increased metabolism of glucose in areas of inflammation. However, to date, no large studies have been performed to test its efficacy in the diabetic foot.

DIFFERENTIAL DIAGNOSIS

Clinically, the main differential diagnosis for diabetic foot infection is early neuropathic osteoarthropathy and various inflammatory arthropathies such as gout. These entities present as foot swelling and erythema, and often blood leukocyte count and erythrocyte sedimentation rate are noncontributory unless there is associated sepsis. Similarly, low-grade or even high-grade temperature is nonspecific. This explains to a certain degree the reliance on imaging tests for accurate and prompt diagnosis.

Neuropathic Osteoarthropathy

This aggressive, deforming arthritis results from a combination of repetitive microtrauma and macrotrauma to the articular surfaces and supporting ligaments, peripheral neuropathy with impaired perception of injury, and ischemia with poor healing.[6] Neuropathic disease of the foot tends to present as a mixed pattern of proliferation and erosion, as opposed to atrophic (primarily erosive) and hypertrophic (mostly proliferative) manifestations seen elsewhere in the body. Neuropathic osteoarthropathy in the foot and ankle is most common at the Lisfranc (tarsometatarsal) joint but has been reported in many different joints. Multiple joints in a region are often involved, reflecting the regional instability that is characteristic of the disease.

The acute form (Fig. 65-16) presents clinically as a warm, swollen, erythematous foot that clinically mimics infection.[7] On radiographs there may be little or no deformity, with only diffuse soft tissue swelling present. Owing to marked hyperemia, scintigraphic examinations may be falsely positive. On MR images there is diffuse soft tissue edema.[31] On postcontrast images, the joint capsule and juxta-articular soft tissues enhance but the subcutaneous tissues typically show little enhancement.[32] Joint effusion is common. Bone marrow edema and enhancement is typically centered in the subchondral bone, reflecting the articular pattern of disease. However, in more severe cases, prominent edema and enhancement can extend well into the periarticular medullary bone.[32] This is especially the case in the setting of neuropathic fracture. This marrow signal pattern and associated periarticular soft tissue abnormality can simulate infection.

The chronic form (Fig. 65-17) shows more typical imaging characteristics recognized as neuropathic arthropathy; joint deformity is common, with subluxation or even dislocation, which often involves multiple joints. Subchondral cysts and bone proliferation are prominent, with "debris" or intra-articular bodies. Bone density is usually preserved. In later stages of disease, adjacent bones can become necrotic

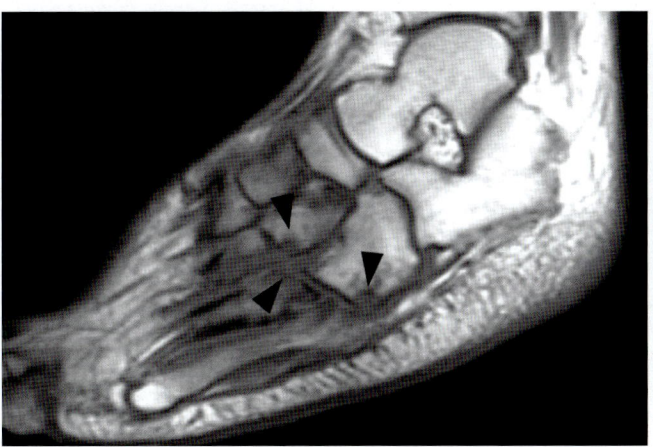
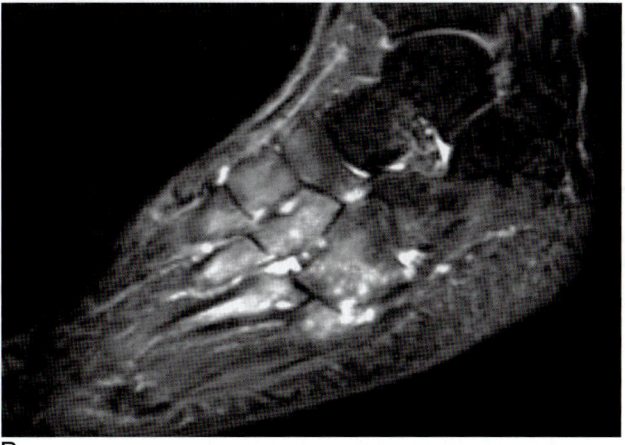

A   B

■ **FIGURE 65-16** Acute neuropathic osteoarthropathy. **A,** Sagittal, T1-weighted MR image shows marginal erosions (*arrowheads*) at the Lisfranc joint and intertarsal joints. Note that the surrounding subcutaneous fat is preserved, a finding that would be unlikely in the setting of infection. **B,** Sagittal, T2-weighted, fat-suppressed MR image of the same patient shows bone marrow edema with extensive regional distribution around the Lisfranc and intertarsal joints that contain small effusions.

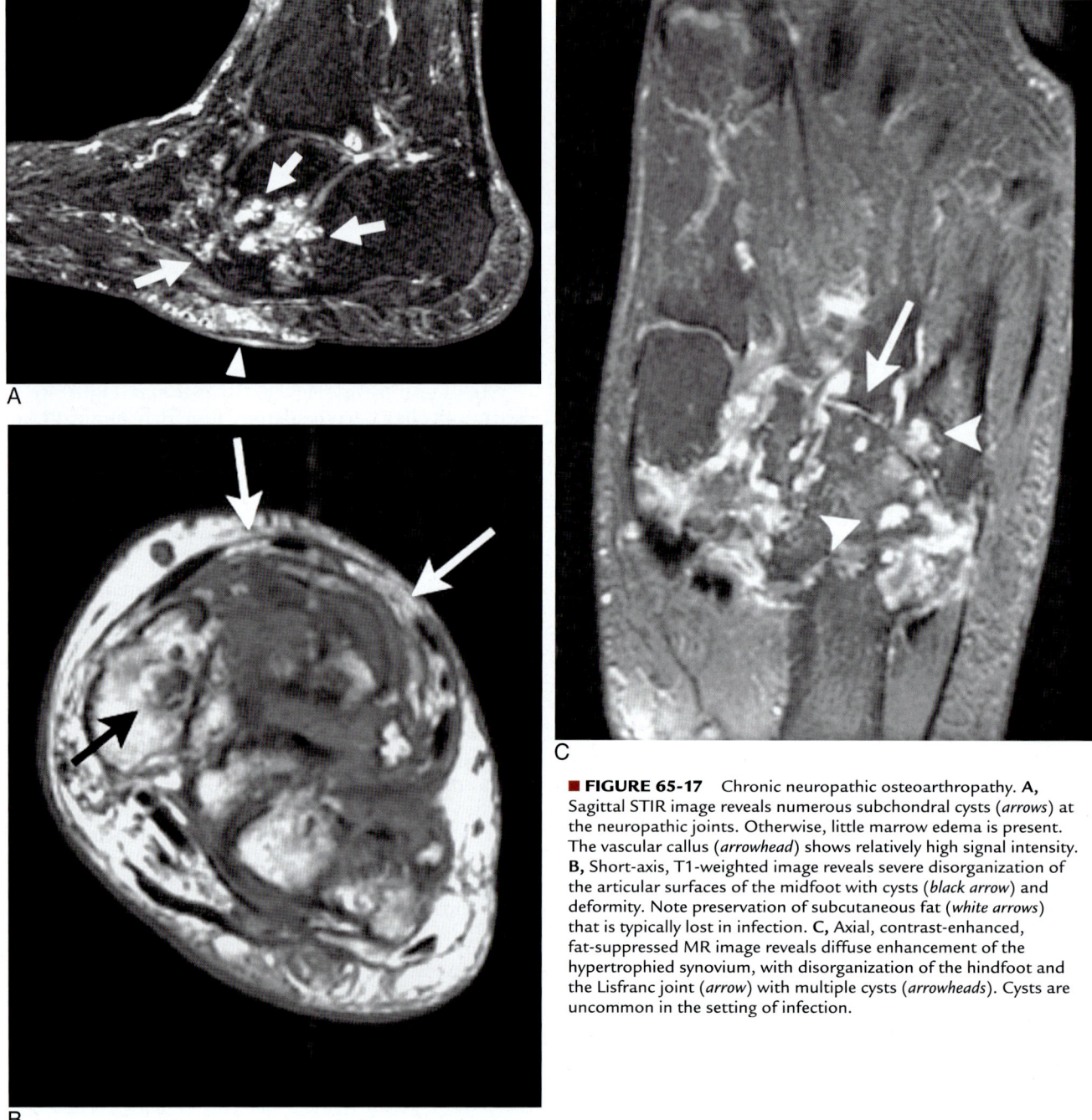

■ **FIGURE 65-17** Chronic neuropathic osteoarthropathy. **A,** Sagittal STIR image reveals numerous subchondral cysts (*arrows*) at the neuropathic joints. Otherwise, little marrow edema is present. The vascular callus (*arrowhead*) shows relatively high signal intensity. **B,** Short-axis, T1-weighted image reveals severe disorganization of the articular surfaces of the midfoot with cysts (*black arrow*) and deformity. Note preservation of subcutaneous fat (*white arrows*) that is typically lost in infection. **C,** Axial, contrast-enhanced, fat-suppressed MR image reveals diffuse enhancement of the hypertrophied synovium, with disorganization of the hindfoot and the Lisfranc joint (*arrow*) with multiple cysts (*arrowheads*). Cysts are uncommon in the setting of infection.

and collapse or resorb.[33] The overall pattern is one of disorganization and deformity of the bones. Neuropathic disease of the Lisfranc joint typically results in superolateral subluxation of the metatarsals, leading to a rocker-bottom deformity in which the cuboid becomes a weight-bearing structure. Imaging characteristics are more characteristic of a chronic, degenerative arthritis, although recurrent episodes of acute disease may result in bone marrow and periarticular edema and enhancement on MRI and uptake on scintigraphic methods.

Differentiation of osteomyelitis and neuropathic osteoarthropathy can be difficult, because both can demonstrate marrow abnormality, joint effusion, and surrounding soft tissue edema.[32] However, there are some rules one may use to help differentiate these entities on MR images (Table 65-3). The first consideration is that the vast majority of cases of osteomyelitis of the foot and ankle are due to contiguous spread. Therefore, a bone marrow abnormality without adjacent skin ulceration, sinus tract, or soft tissue inflammation is less likely to represent infection.[21] This is especially useful when there are extensive bone marrow signal abnormalities; in this setting infection is unlikely if the subcutaneous tissues are uninvolved.

Another consideration is that neuropathic osteoarthropathy is a predominantly articular process; because it is a manifestation of instability, often multiple joints in a

TABLE 65-3 Differentiation of Osteomyelitis from Neuropathic Osteoarthropathy

	Osteomyelitis	Neuropathic	Comments
Typical Location	Toes (tips, dorsum)	Lisfranc joint	In the setting of foot deformity
	Metatarsal heads (especially first, fifth)	Chopart joint—calcaneus	
	Malleoli	Osteomyelitis can occur at atypical locations	
Distribution	Focal, local centripetal spread	Multiple joints in a region	
	Pattern of edema/enhancement	Predominant involvement of one bone	Epicenter in joint and subchondral bone
Deformity	Uncommon (unless there is underlying neuropathic disease)	Common	
Soft Tissues	Adjacent ulcer, cellulitis, sinus tract	Enhancement limited to juxta-articular soft tissues; skin, subcutaneous tissues intact	Diffuse subcutaneous edema typical in diabetic feet

region are similarly affected (e.g., the entire Lisfranc joint, Chopart joint, or multiple adjacent metatarsophalangeal joints). This finding and other articular manifestations of neuropathic disease (subluxation, cysts, necrotic debris) are not as common in infection.[23] Also, marrow changes associated with neuropathic osteoarthropathy can be extensive (especially at the midfoot) but tend to be centered at a joint and subarticular bone and are present on both sides of the joint fairly equally. Osteomyelitis shows more diffuse marrow involvement, and unless there is primary septic arthritis the marrow changes are generally greater on one side of the joint.[32]

Location of disease is also important. Osteomyelitis occurs predominantly at the metatarsal heads, the toes, the calcaneus, and the malleoli, a distribution that mirrors that of friction, callus, and ulceration. Neuropathic osteoarthropathy by far is most common at the Lisfranc and Chopart joint. However, if there is foot deformity, contiguous spread of infection can occur at atypical sites (e.g., the cuboid in cases of rocker-bottom deformity).

Classic Signs

RADIOGRAPHY/COMPUTED TOMOGRAPHY

- Early: soft tissue swelling
- Middle: periostitis, bone rarefaction
- Late: bone destruction

MAGNETIC RESONANCE IMAGING

- T1: replacement of marrow fat
- T2/STIR: marrow edema
- Gadolinium: marrow enhancement
- Look for associated soft tissue pathology (e.g., ulcer) reflecting contiguous spread.

NUCLEAR MEDICINE

- Three-phase bone scintiscan: tracer uptake on all phases, concentrating in bone on delayed phase
- Gallium-67 and labeled white blood cells: tracer accumulation corresponding to bone uptake on delayed phase of three-phase bone scintiscan

Gout and Other Inflammatory Arthropathies

Gout may simulate osteomyelitis on clinical examination as well as on imaging studies.[34] On physical examination, patients have swelling, erythema, and occasionally associated skin break and drainage. Radiographically, erosions are often seen, which may be periarticular or marginal, and there is often associated joint narrowing. Uptake is common on three-phase bone scintigraphy owing to the hyperemia and bone turnover. Migration of white blood cells may result in a false-positive indium scan as well. On MRI, findings can be identical to infection, with joint effusion and soft tissue fluid collections with thick rim enhancement, as well as marrow edema and enhancement. Gouty tophi are generally of low signal on T1- and T2-weighted images, which can be a discriminating factor.[34,35] Clinical suspicion of the diagnosis may be required with subsequent aspiration and fluid analysis. For similar reasons, rheumatoid arthritis and other inflammatory arthropathies can mimic infection. History and disease distribution is an important factor when considering a differential diagnosis for suspected pedal infection.

SYNOPSIS OF TREATMENT OPTIONS

Medical Treatment

Medical therapy for diabetic foot infection is based on aggressive therapy for skin callus and ulceration to promote healing combined with débridement of necrotic tissue and intravenous antibiotic treatment targeted toward multiorganism infection; generally, 6 weeks or longer is provided for osteomyelitis, with a shorter period for cellulitis. Assessment is made of vascularity; ischemia will lead to poor healing and propagation of infection. If vascular disease is mainly proximal rather than microvascular, the patient may benefit from angioplasty or an arterial bypass procedure. After treatment the patient is reassessed for improvement, after which a decision is made whether to perform amputation. Long-term follow-up includes treatment of foot deformity, fitting of specialized footwear, and early treatment of calluses and skin breaks. Underlying acute neuropathic disease may be treated with casting.

Surgical Treatment

Surgical treatment may be as simple as débridement of devitalized or phlegmonous tissue and decompression/drainage of abscesses as well as infected fascial, tendon, and joint compartments. For more diffuse infection or in the presence of severe ischemia, definitive transmetatarsal, hindfoot, or below-knee amputation may be performed. In appropriate patients with localized infection and adequate blood supply, a partial, foot-sparing amputation may be considered, with the goal being to preserve as much viable tissue as possible.

What the Referring Physician Needs to Know

- Radiographs are insensitive for osteomyelitis in the diabetic foot.
- MRI and three-phase bone scintigraphy are both highly sensitive for osteomyelitis.
- Neuropathic osteoarthropathy can simulate osteomyelitis on all modalities.
- Radiotracer-labeled white blood cell scanning adds specificity compared with three-phase bone scintigraphy and may be needed to distinguish neuropathic disease from infection.
- MRI is useful for determining precise extent of involvement for preoperative planning.
- Contrast-enhanced MRI can be used to diagnose soft tissue complications such as abscess, septic tenosynovitis, sinus tract, and devitalization.
- Percutaneous bone biopsy for diagnosis of suspected osteomyelitis should not transgress infected soft tissue; similarly, joints should not be aspirated for diagnosis through infected tissue.

SUGGESTED READINGS

Ahmadi ME, Morrison WB, Carrino JA, et al. Neuropathic arthropathy of the foot with and without superimposed osteomyelitis: MR imaging characteristics. Radiology 2006; 238:622–631.
Berendt AR, Lipsky B. Is this bone infected or not? Differentiating neuro-osteoarthropathy from osteomyelitis in the diabetic foot. Curr Diab Rep 2004; 4:424–429.
Craig JG, Amin MB, Wu K, et al. Osteomyelitis of the diabetic foot: MR imaging—pathologic correlation. Radiology 1997; 203:849–855.
El-Maghraby TA, Moustafa HM, Pauwels EK. Nuclear medicine methods for evaluation of skeletal infection among other diagnostic modalities. Q J Nucl Med Mol Imaging 2006; 50:167–192.
Morrison WB, Ledermann HP. Work-up of the diabetic foot. Radiol Clin North Am 2002; 40:1171–1192.

Nigro ND, Bartynski WS, Grossman SJ, et al. Clinical impact of magnetic resonance imaging in foot osteomyelitis. J Am Podiatr Med Assoc 1992; 82:603–615.
Snyder RJ, Cohen MM, Sun C, Livingston J. Osteomyelitis in the diabetic patient: diagnosis and treatment: I. Overview, diagnosis, and microbiology. Ostomy Wound Manage 2001; 47:18–22, 25–30.
Snyder RJ, Cohen MM, Sun C, Livingston J. Osteomyelitis in the diabetic patient: diagnosis and treatment: II. Medical, surgical, and alternative treatments. Ostomy Wound Manage 2001; 47:24–30, 32–41.
Wang A, Weinstein D, Greenfield L, et al. MRI and diabetic foot infections. Magn Reson Imaging 1990; 8:805–809.
Yu JS. Diabetic foot and neuroarthropathy: magnetic resonance imaging evaluation. Top Magn Reson Imaging 1998; 9:295–310.

REFERENCES

1. Ledermann HP, Morrison WB, Schweitzer ME. MR image analysis of pedal osteomyelitis: distribution, patterns of spread, and frequency of associated ulceration and septic arthritis. Radiology 2002; 223:747–755.
2. Morrison WB, Ledermann HP, Schweitzer ME. MR imaging of the diabetic foot. Magn Reson Imaging Clin North Am 2001; 9:603–614.
3. Boulton AJ, Vileikyte L. The diabetic foot: the scope of the problem. J Fam Pract 2000; 49(11 Suppl):S3–S8.
4. Lavery L Gazewood JD. Assessing the feet of patients with diabetes. J Fam Pract 2000; 49(Suppl):S9–S16.
5. Sumpio BE. Foot ulcers. N Engl J Med 2000; 343:787–793.
6. Jeffcoate W, Lima J, Nobrega L. The Charcot foot. Diabet Med 2000; 17:253–258.
7. Rajbhandari SM, Jenkins RC, Davies C, Tesfaye S. Charcot neuroarthropathy in diabetes mellitus. Diabetologia 2002; 45:1085–1096.
8. Ledermann HP, Morrison WB, Schweitzer ME. Is soft-tissue inflammation in pedal infection contained by fascial planes? MR analysis of compartmental involvement in 115 feet. AJR Am J Roentgenol 2002; 178:605–612.

9. Schauwecker DS. Differentiation of infected from noninfected rapidly progressive neuropathic osteoarthropathy [published erratum appears in J Nucl Med 1995 Oct;36(10):1757] [see comments]. J Nucl Med 1995; 36:1427–1428.
10. Seabold JE, Flickinger FW, Kao SC, et al. Indium-111-leukocyte/technetium-99m-MDP bone and magnetic resonance imaging: difficulty of diagnosing osteomyelitis in patients with neuropathic osteoarthropathy. J Nucl Med 1990; 31:549–556.
11. Nigro ND, Bartynski WS, Grossman SJ, Kruljac S. Clinical impact of magnetic resonance imaging in foot osteomyelitis. J Am Podiatr Med Assoc 1992; 82:603–615.
12. Horowitz JD, Durham JR, Nease DB, et al. Prospective evaluation of magnetic resonance imaging in the management of acute diabetic foot infections. Ann Vasc Surg 1993; 7:44–50.
13. Morrison WB, Schweitzer ME, Wapner KL, et al. Osteomyelitis in feet of diabetics: clinical accuracy, surgical utility, and cost-effectiveness of MR imaging. Radiology 1995; 196:557–564.
14. Ledermann HP, Schweitzer ME, Morrison WB. Nonenhancing tissue on MR imaging of pedal infection: characterization of necrotic tissue and associated limitations for diagnosis

of osteomyelitis and abscess. AJR Am J Roentgenol 2002; 178:215–222.

15. Morrison WB, Schweitzer ME, Bock GW, et al. Diagnosis of osteomyelitis: utility of fat-suppressed contrast-enhanced MR imaging [see comments]. Radiology 1993; 189:251–257.

16. Crim JR, Seeger LL. Imaging evaluation of osteomyelitis. Crit Rev Diagn Imaging 1994; 35:201–256.

17. Boutin RD, Brossmann J, Sartoris DJ, et al. Update on imaging of orthopedic infections. Orthop Clin North Am 1998; 29:41–66.

18. Durham JR, Lukens ML, Campanini DS, et al. Impact of magnetic resonance imaging on the management of diabetic foot infections. Am J Surg 1991; 162:150–153.

19. Craig JG, Amin MB, Wu K, et al. Osteomyelitis of the diabetic foot: MR imaging—pathologic correlation. Radiology 1997; 203:849–855.

20. Ledermann HP, Morrison WB, Schweitzer ME. Pedal abscesses in patients suspected of having pedal osteomyelitis: analysis with MR imaging. Radiology 2002; 224:649–655.

21. Morrison WB, Schweitzer ME, Batte WG, et al. Osteomyelitis of the foot: relative importance of primary and secondary MR imaging signs. Radiology 1998; 207:625–632.

22. Dangman BC, Hoffer FA, Rand FF, O'Rourke EJ. Osteomyelitis in children: gadolinium-enhanced MR imaging. Radiology 1992; 182:743–747.

23. Morrison WB, Ledermann HP. Work-up of the diabetic foot. Radiol Clin North Am 2002; 40:1171–1192.

24. Graif M, Schweitzer ME, Deely D, Matteucci T. The septic versus nonseptic inflamed joint: MRI characteristics. Skeletal Radiol 1999; 28:616–620.

25. Ledermann HP, Morrison WB, Schweitzer ME, Raikin SM. Tendon involvement in pedal infection: MR analysis of frequency, distribution, and spread of infection. AJR Am J Roentgenol 2002; 179:939–947.

26. Gold RH, Tong DJ, Crim JR, Seeger LL. Imaging the diabetic foot. Skeletal Radiol 1995; 24:563–571.

27. Weinstein D, Wang A, Chambers R, et al. Evaluation of magnetic resonance imaging in the diagnosis of osteomyelitis in diabetic foot infections. Foot Ankle 1993; 14:18–22.

28. Seabold JE, Nepola JV, Conrad GR, et al. Detection of osteomyelitis at fracture nonunion sites: comparison of two scintigraphic methods. AJR Am J Roentgenol 1989; 152:1021–1027.

29. Larcos G, Brown ML, Sutton RT. Diagnosis of osteomyelitis of the foot in diabetic patients: value of 111In-leukocyte scintigraphy. AJR Am J Roentgenol 1991; 157:527–531.

30. Maurer AH, Millmond SH, Knight LC, et al. Infection in diabetic osteoarthropathy: use of indium-labeled leukocytes for diagnosis. Radiology 1986; 161:221–225.

31. Marcus CD, Ladam-Marcus VJ, Leone J, et al. MR imaging of osteomyelitis and neuropathic osteoarthropathy in the feet of diabetics. RadioGraphics 1996; 16:1337–1348.

32. Ahmadi ME, Morrison WB, Schweitzer ME, et al. Neuropathic arthropathy of the foot with and without superimposed osteomyelitis: MR imaging characteristics. Radiology 2006; 238:622–631.

33. Clouse ME, Gramm HF, Legg M, Flood T. Diabetic osteoarthropathy: clinical and roentgenographic observations in 90 cases. Am J Roentgenol Radium Ther Nucl Med 1974; 121:22–34.

34. Weishaupt D, Schweitzer ME, Alam F, et al. MR imaging of inflammatory joint diseases of the foot and ankle. Skeletal Radiol 1999; 28:663–669.

35. Morrison WB, Ledermann HP, Schweitzer ME. MR imaging of inflammatory conditions of the ankle and foot. Magn Reson Imaging Clin North Am 2001; 9:615–638.

66

Pediatric Infections

Helen Williams

Musculoskeletal infection in children is a relatively common occurrence. However, unless there are superficial signs of infection such as swelling and redness of the overlying skin it can be difficult to diagnose because the symptoms and signs are often nonspecific in children. The diagnostic challenge is further compounded by difficulties assessing the child who due to distress, age, or level of development may be unable to assist in localizing the region causing the symptoms.

Prompt recognition of bone and joint infection is essential to prevent complications such as joint destruction, alteration of growth, or onset of chronic infection, which can lead to persisting skeletal deformity with significant and ongoing associated morbidity. Imaging has an important role in the management of a child with suspected musculoskeletal infection. It is used for confirmation of the diagnosis, to localize and define the extent of infection, and to help determine appropriate medical or surgical treatment. However, when a clinical diagnosis of joint or superficial soft tissue infection is clear, unnecessary imaging delays definitive management. Children should not be unnecessarily exposed to ionizing radiation, particularly when there are acceptable alternative methods such as ultrasonography and MRI. Bone scintigraphy and CT now have a limited role, although the choice of imaging method depends to some extent on local expertise and accessibility. Although MRI is a highly sensitive and relatively specific technique for the diagnosis of musculoskeletal infection, availability is often limited and young children who are unable to cooperate for MRI will require sedation or general anesthesia to obtain a high-quality scan. The need for accurate diagnostic information needs to be balanced with the inherent risks of sedation and anesthesia in such cases.

SOFT TISSUE INFECTION

Cellulitis

Cellulitis is diffuse infection of the skin and subcutaneous soft tissues. Causative organisms include *Staphylococcus aureus* and *Streptococcus* species. Clinical signs of cellulitis are common to all ages, and the diagnosis is usually obvious. However, the extent of infection and involvement of deeper soft tissues or bone is difficult to determine clinically, and imaging has a particular role. Uncomplicated cellulitis is treated with antibiotics, but an abscess requires surgical drainage. Radiographs are generally not helpful, although soft tissue swelling may be apparent. On ultrasound examination, infected skin and subcutaneous tissues appear thickened with increased echogenicity. Subcutaneous edema may be present with thin anechoic or hypoechoic strands of fluid between fatty lobules in the interlobular septa. This causes a "cobblestone" appearance.[1] There may also be increased vascularity of the soft tissues using color Doppler imaging. Focal tissue inflammation without abscess formation (phlegmon) appears as a focal area of increased echogenicity. Abscess formation may be overlooked when using ultrasonography if the contents of the abscess cavity are isoechoic or hyperechoic to surrounding tissues. Swirling of the contents by exerting pressure on the transducer and lack of vascularity are indicators of necrosis and liquefaction[1] (Figs. 66-1 and 66-2).

In children with cellulitis, CT and MR are not routinely employed unless there is suspicion of deep soft tissue infection with abscess. When practical, MRI is the method of choice for these patients. Because CT confers a high radiation dose its use should be restricted to children in whom MRI is contraindicated or unavailable. CT examination of children with cellulitis will show thickening of the skin and subcutaneous tissue with increased attenuation of fat, which may appear septated. Abscesses are rim-enhancing collections that often contain septa and have varying wall thickness. MRI demonstrates infected tissues as decreased signal intensity on T1-weighted sequences and increased signal intensity on T2-weighted and short tau inversion recovery (STIR) sequences. Abscesses are focal fluid intensity collections with surrounding or rim enhancement after intravenous administration of gadolinium-diethylene-triamine-pentaacetic acid (Gd-DTPA). MRI is also indicated to differentiate soft tissue infection from osteomyelitis because it will show abnormalities in bone as well as muscles and supportive tissues (Fig. 66-3).

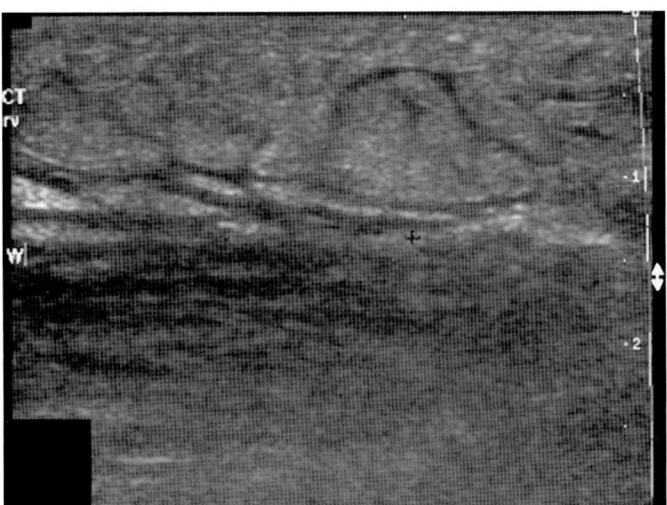

■ **FIGURE 66-1** Sonogram showing "cobblestone" appearance of the edematous subcutaneous soft tissues in a patient with cellulitis.

Pyomyositis

Pyomyositis is a primary bacterial infection of skeletal muscle that is not secondary to contiguous infection of skin, bone, or other soft tissue. It usually affects adults between 20 and 40 years of age and is rarely seen in children. Pyomyositis in children occurs almost exclusively in tropical or subtropical climates, although it has infrequently been reported in children in temperate climates.[2] Muscles around the hip and pelvis are commonly affected at all ages so that diseases of the joint or bones may be

suspected. *Staphylococcus aureus* is the usual pathogen. Muscle enlargement with focal intramuscular inflammatory changes are observed using MRI. The inflamed muscle is of low signal intensity on T1-weighted sequences and high signal intensity on T2-weighted and STIR sequences. Enhancement of the area after intravenous Gd-DTPA is characteristic. Abscess formation may occur.

Necrotizing Fasciitis

Necrotizing fasciitis is a rapidly progressive, deep-seated bacterial infection of the subcutaneous soft tissues that may involve any area of the body. An increased frequency is seen in patients with peripheral vascular disease, intravenous drug users, alcoholics, diabetics, and immunosuppressed patients, but it also occurs in young, previously healthy patients, including children. The disease often has a fulminant course accompanied by multiple organ failure and shock. It is associated with a high mortality rate, estimated to lie within 25% to 75%.[3] Mortality rates in children and previously healthy patients tend to be lower.

After the inoculation of the bacterial infection the process spreads along fascial planes leading to necrosis of the superficial muscle fascia, deeper layers of the dermis, and surrounding tissues. In children, the most frequent cause is secondary to infection with group A β-hemolytic streptococcus, either after surgery or as a result of trauma, burns, minor cuts, or insect bites. Patients with eczema are also predisposed to introduction of infection if the skin is broken. In newborns, necrotizing fasciitis may complicate omphalitis (infection of the umbilical stump) or circumcision. Necrotizing fasciitis is also described

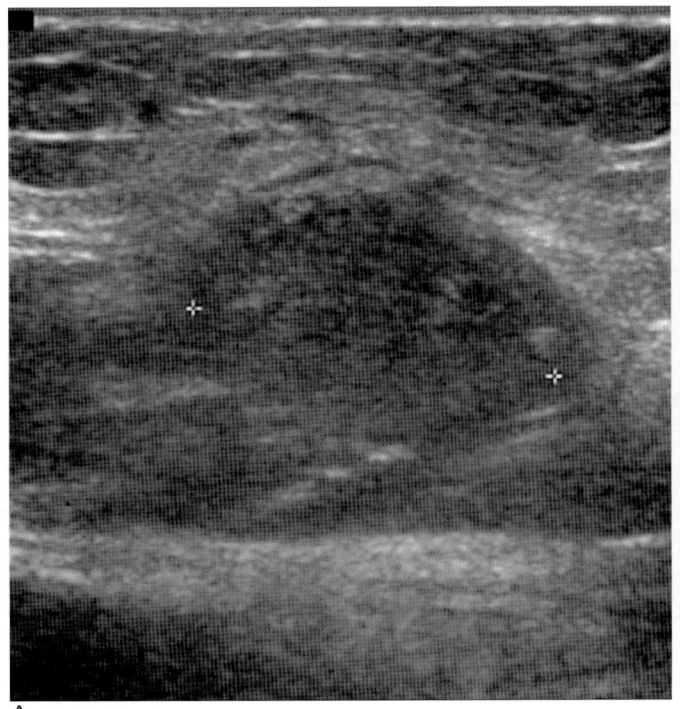

A

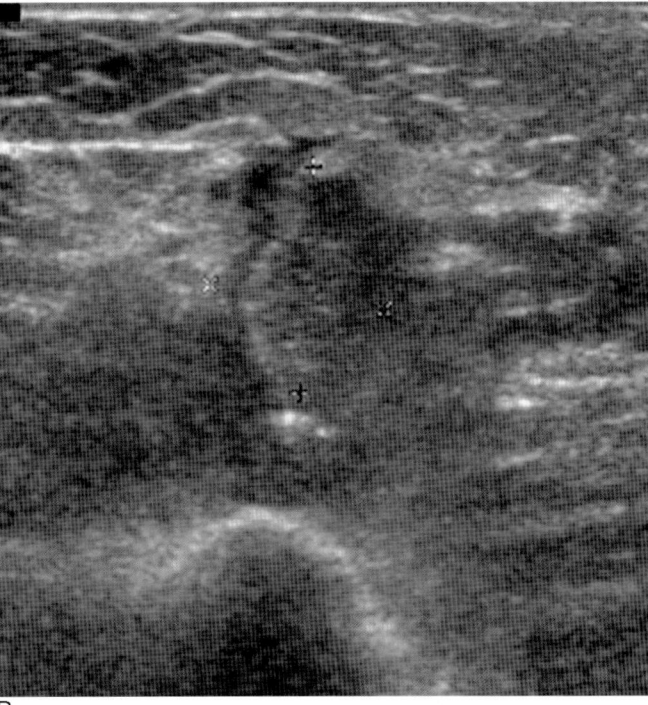

B

■ **FIGURE 66-2** **A** and **B,** Sonograms showing small abscess in the arm of a child with chronic osteomyelitis of the humerus after a fracture. The contents of the abscess are hypoechoic to the surrounding tissues with internal echoes.

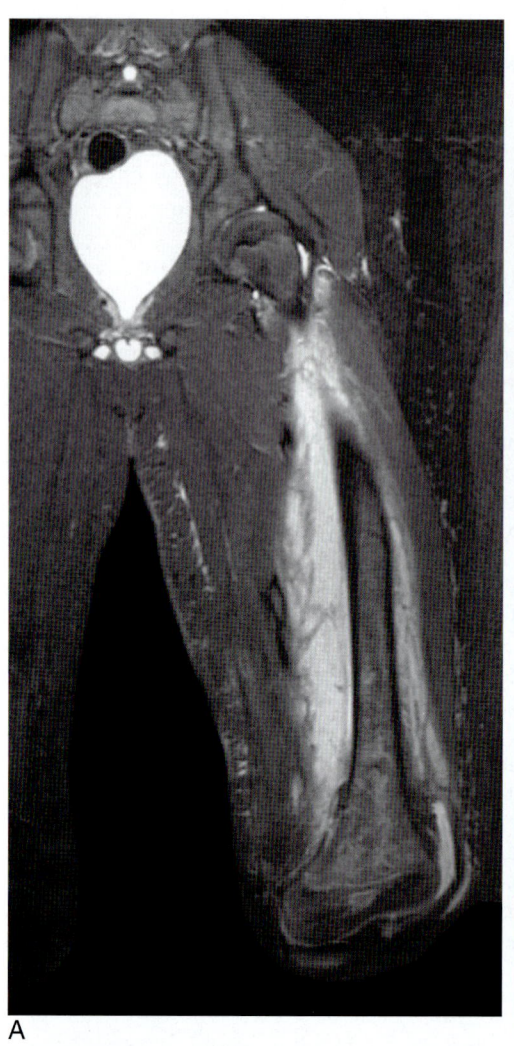

A

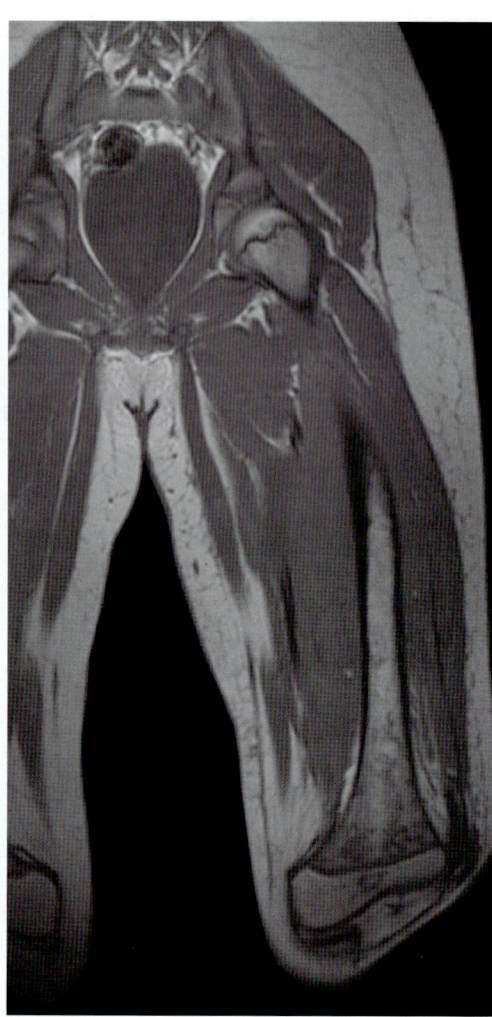

B

■ **FIGURE 66-3** STIR coronal MR image (**A**), T1-weighted coronal MR image (**B**), post-contrast T1-weighted fat-saturated axial MR image (**C**), and post-contrast T1-weighted fat-saturated axial MR image (**D**), in a 10-year-old boy with extensive abscess associated with osteomyelitis of the left femur.

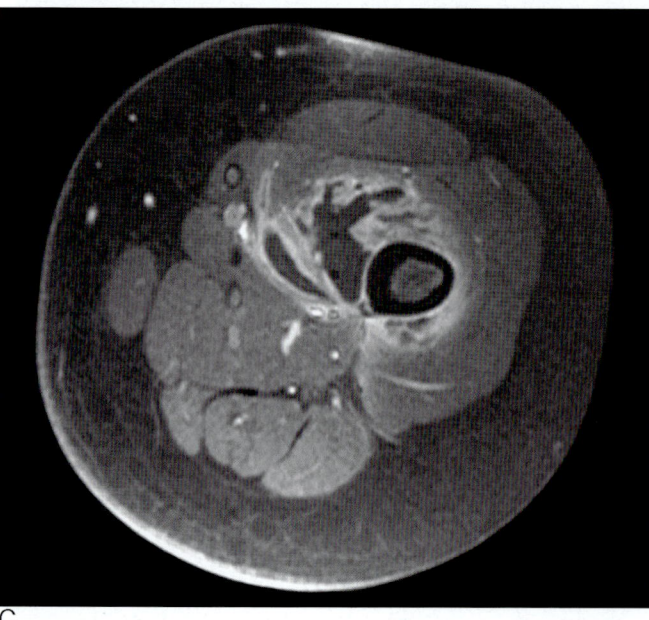

C

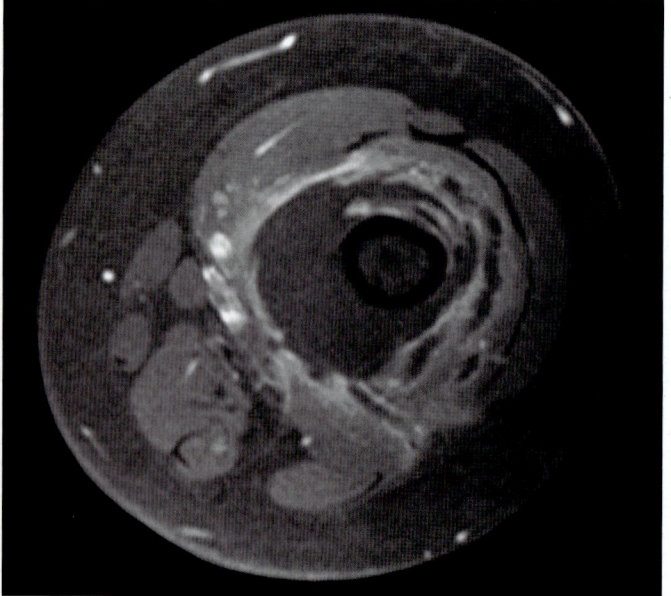

D

as a complication of varicella infection.[4] A polymicrobial form of the disease has occurred with increased frequency after surgery and in patients with diabetes or peripheral vascular disease. Gas gangrene is a myonecrotic disease caused by clostridial infection that quickly leads to systemic toxicity and shock. It is associated with trauma or crush injury.[3]

In children, necrotizing fasciitis often presents 1 to 4 days after trauma with soft tissue swelling and pain near the affected area. Patients may be initially well. When associated with varicella infection the symptoms typically begin 3 to 4 days after the onset of the rash. Infants and toddlers may be irritable, and walking children may limp or be reluctant to bear weight. There may be severe pain on movement of the affected extremity. As the disease progresses, induration and edema of the soft tissues is rapidly followed by blistering. Spreading infection leads to necrosis and results in a dusky appearance of the skin with production of thick foul-smelling fluid. The differential diagnosis of necrotizing fasciitis includes cellulitis and pyomyositis.

The diagnosis of necrotizing fasciitis is primarily clinical. Imaging studies may be supportive but should not delay surgical intervention to remove necrotic tissue. Radiographs may show gas or soft tissue edema but are otherwise nonspecific. MRI is the preferred cross-sectional method because it can show extension of inflammation along fascial planes and demonstrates areas of inflammation and necrosis.

Osteomyelitis

Approximately half of cases of osteomyelitis in children occur in those younger than the age of 5 years, with a higher incidence in boys.[3] In infants and children, most cases result from hematogenous spread of organisms after an acute episode of bacteremia. The manifestations of osteomyelitis in this group vary, determined by the normal developmental changes affecting the vascular anatomy of bones and cartilage. Osteomyelitis due to direct inoculation with organisms from infection of adjacent soft tissues or after trauma or surgery occurs with much less frequency in children when compared with adults. Osteomyelitis secondary to vascular insufficiency is rare in children.

In infants up to approximately 12 months of age, diaphyseal vessels extend through the metaphysis and penetrate the cartilaginous growth plate to reach the epiphysis. This results in higher incidence of epiphyseal and joint infection in newborns and young infants.[5] From 8 to 18 months of age, with increasing ossification of the epiphysis the transphyseal vessels disappear. By 18 months of age, the diaphyseal vessels no longer penetrate the growth plate. They terminate in the metaphysis where they form slow-flowing venous sinusoids and lakes. This is an ideal environment for bloodborne organisms to proliferate, which accounts for the typical metaphyseal location of long bone osteomyelitis in childhood. Metaphyseal equivalents such as the femoral trochanter are similarly affected. After growth plate closure, vascular continuity between the epiphysis and metaphysis is restored so that epiphyseal and/or joint infections are again potential sites of focal infection via a bloodborne route (Fig. 66-4).

Staphylococcus aureus is the most common cause of acute osteomyelitis in infants and children, accounting for 80% to 90% of cases,[6,7] followed by β-hemolytic streptococcus, *Streptococcus pneumoniae*, *Escherichia coli*, and *Pseudomonas aeruginosa*. Before the widespread introduction of vaccination against *Hemophilus influenzae* this agent was also a common causative organism.

In neonates, the most common causative organism is *Staphylococcus aureus,* followed by β-hemolytic *Streptococcus* and gram-negative coliforms. Fungal infection and that from *Pseudomonas* species usually arise from penetrating injuries, although *Aspergillus* osteomyelitis can occur as a result of contiguous extension from adjacent tissue (e.g., in chronic lung infection where the organism may extend to involve the ribs and spine). Boys with chronic granulomatous disease have an increased tendency to develop this complication.[8] Infection with *Salmonella* species is more frequent in patients with sickle cell anemia because microinfarctions of the bowel wall allow organisms to enter the bloodstream via the gastrointestinal tract; however, these patients are more commonly affected by the same organisms that affect children without the hemoglobinopathy.[9] Diaphyseal location of infection is more common in patients with sickle cell anemia, and a diagnosis of osteomyelitis should be suspected when symptoms of an acute vaso-occlusive

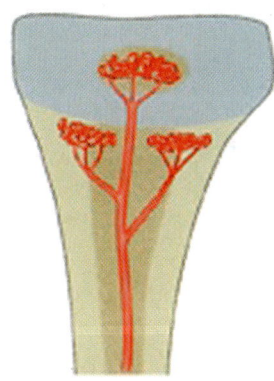 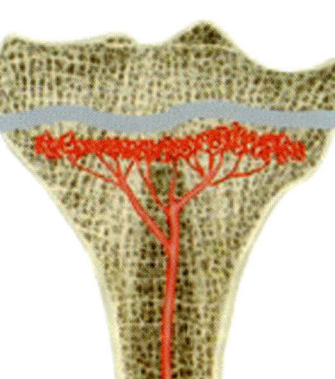 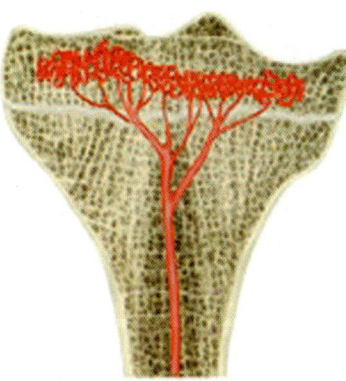

A   B   C

■ **FIGURE 66-4** Diagram showing the blood supply to distal long bones at different ages. **A,** Neonate. **B,** From 8 to 18 months until epiphyseal closure. **C,** After epiphyseal closure and in adulthood.

crisis persist despite treatment. Mycobacteria (especially *M. tuberculosis*) disseminate to the skeleton via a hematogenous route, with vertebral infection being the most frequent manifestation, although localization of infection in a phalanx (spina ventosa) is not unusual (Fig. 66-5).[10]

Osteomyelitis usually involves a single bone, and any bone can be affected. In children, the most frequent sites of infection are the metaphyses of the distal femur and proximal tibia, followed by the distal humerus, distal radius, proximal femur, and proximal humerus.[11] Flat bones, vertebrae, the calcaneus, and the ileum are affected in up to 25% of cases. Infants and children with evolving osteomyelitis often present with nonspecific signs of illness, with fever, irritability, and anorexia. As the disease becomes established, pseudoparalysis of the affected limb occurs and pain is observed with passive movement. Walking children with involvement of the lower limb may limp or refuse to bear weight. Decreased use of an affected upper limb is a frequent presentation. A reduced range of motion with accompanying local tenderness, redness, and swelling may be observed on clinical examination; however, localization can be difficult in younger children. The erythrocyte sedimentation rate, C-reactive protein, and white blood cell count are usually elevated but may be normal. Blood cultures are positive in up to 55% of affected children.[3] Neonates with bone or joint infection may not appear toxic, and serologic markers for infection may not be elevated because of inability to mount a significant inflammatory reaction.

These factors contribute to delayed presentation and increased complication rates.

Acute bony infection results in cellular infiltration, vascular engorgement and marrow edema. As infection spreads throughout the intramedullary cavity there may be extension to the cortex via the haversian and Volkmann's canals, where infection can extend to the subperiosteal space and surrounding soft tissues. Abscesses can develop in the intramedullary space, between cortex and periosteum (subperiosteal space) and in the soft tissues. If the metaphysis is intra-articular (i.e., in the hip, knee, elbow, or shoulder), rupture of a metaphyseal abscess results in septic arthritis.

Pelvic osteomyelitis typically affects older children. Any pelvic bone can be involved, but the ilium is most commonly affected, possibly due to its rich blood supply. Symptoms are often nonspecific and include hip, buttock, back, or abdominal pain; inability or reluctance to bear weight; and pelvic tenderness or restricted hip movement. Fever may be absent. Symptoms are often attributed to other diseases, such as septic arthritis of the hip or appendicitis, and the diagnosis is often delayed.[12]

Acute Osteomyelitis

The radiographic signs of osteomyelitis do not develop until 7 to 10 days after the onset of infection; therefore, a normal radiograph does not exclude acute osteomyelitis. Although not sensitive for diagnosis in the early stages of

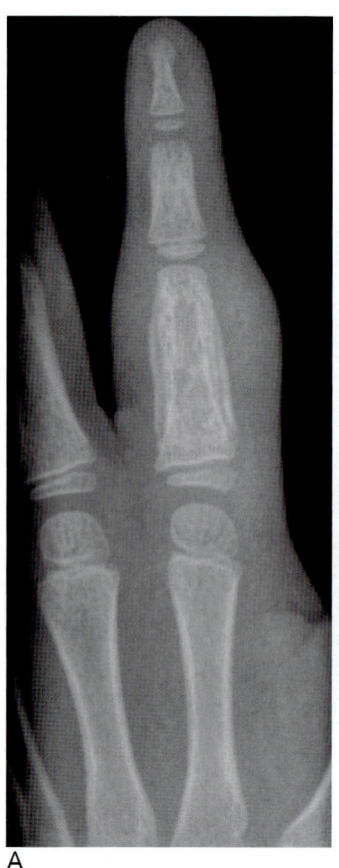
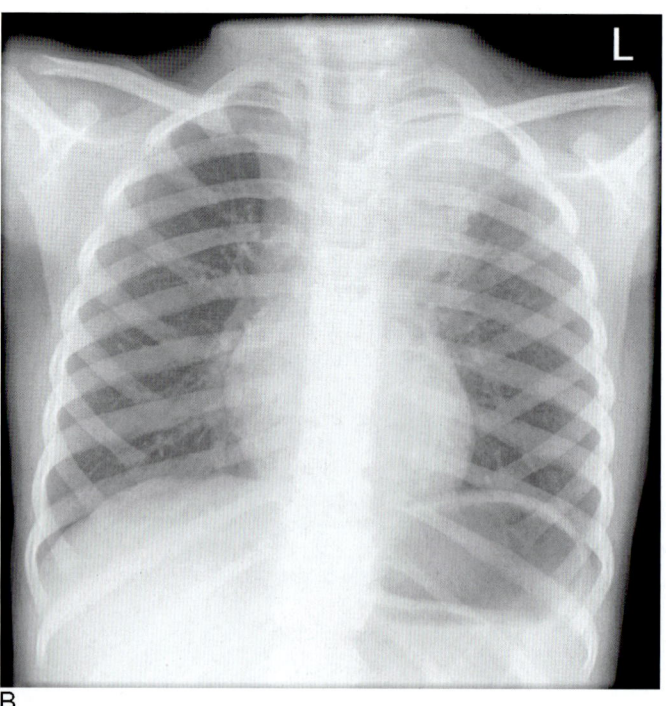

■ **FIGURE 66-5** **A,** Chronic TB osteomyelitis "spina ventosa" affecting the proximal phalanx of the left index finger. The patient was a 5-year-old Somalian immigrant with active pulmonary tuberculosis who presented with a swollen painful finger. **B,** Chest radiograph of the same patient shows left upper lobe consolidation subsequently proven to be tuberculosis. The patient had no respiratory symptoms.

infection, radiography is usually the initial imaging study, and its main role is to exclude other conditions such as fracture or tumor that may mimic infection (Fig. 67-6).

The earliest signs of osteomyelitis visible on radiographs are associated soft tissue swelling and distortion and obliteration of fat planes, which may be apparent within 48 hours of onset. After several days, hyperemia and infiltration of the bone marrow result in increased bony resorption and osteolysis. Loss of 30% to 50% of bone mineral density is required for this to be detected on radiographs, and changes can be easily overlooked, particularly in the absence of appropriate clinical information. Later, extension of infection through the cortex may be detected because of cortical destruction or periosteal elevation with new bone formation, which is seen 7 to 10 days after the onset of infection (Fig. 66-7).

MRI is the most useful imaging method for the diagnosis of suspected osteomyelitis in children, owing to its high sensitivity and specificity.[11] Lack of ionizing radiation, high resolution, and the ability of MRI to demonstrate changes in soft tissue and cartilage also make it ideal for the detection of infection in the immature skeleton. MRI availability is often limited, particularly in hospitals without facilities for sedation and anesthesia of children. In these circumstances, young children with suspected acute osteomyelitis or joint infection are often best managed in a center with specialist pediatric orthopedic and radiology services.

A combination of unenhanced T1- and T2-weighted sequences including T2 weighting with fat saturation or STIR sequences should be employed. STIR sequences are particularly sensitive for detecting marrow edema, which is often the earliest sign of osteomyelitis. Affected marrow demonstrates decreased signal intensity on T1-weighted sequences and increased signal intensity on T2-weighted and STIR sequences. The presence of normal hematopoietic marrow in children can be confused with marrow edema, so it is important to be aware of its distribution at different ages.[13] Bone marrow edema generally has higher signal intensity than hematopoietic marrow on T2-weighted and STIR sequences. Gd-DTPA–enhanced images should always be obtained in children with suspected osteomyelitis or septic arthritis. Fat suppression after enhancement increases conspicuity of abnormal enhancing tissue in the marrow, cortex, and soft tissues, indicating areas of active inflammation. The typical appearance of an abscess independent of location or patient age is of peripheral enhancement with a nonenhancing central fluid collection. Well-defined areas that do not enhance with intravenous Gd-DTPA are suggestive of necrosis or abscess formation. Periosteal elevation and subperiosteal collections are detected by MRI before they are evident on radiographs.

Ultrasonography may detect periosteal elevation, subperiosteal collections, and swelling of the overlying soft tissues in association with osteomyelitis, but absence of these signs does not exclude osteomyelitis. The use of ultrasonography in diagnosing osteomyelitis is limited by its inability to penetrate bone. CT is particularly good at demonstrating cortical changes and is the best method for detecting intraosseous gas, foreign bodies, sequestrum, and involucrum formation in chronic osteomyelitis. It can also be used to direct biopsy in chronic osteomyelitis. However, it does not allow accurate assessment of involvement of unossified/cartilaginous structures or changes within the bone marrow, both of which are well demonstrated using MRI. CT should not be used as a routine diagnostic investigation in children with suspected acute osteomyelitis (Figs. 66-8 and 66-9).

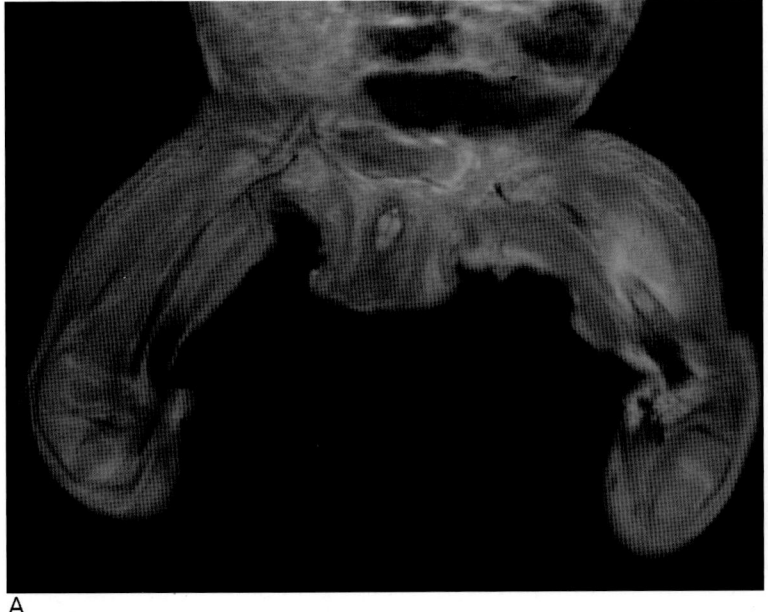
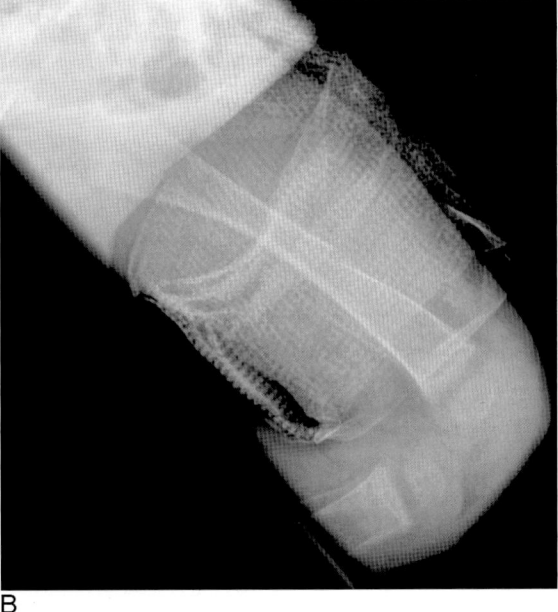

A

B

■ **FIGURE 66-6** **A,** Post-contrast T1-weighted coronal MR image of the thighs. The enhancement of the soft tissues and the bone marrow edema centered around the midfemoral shaft were misinterpreted as infective changes in this 6-month-old child who was not moving his left leg.
B, Radiograph of the femur in the same patient shows pathologic fracture of the femoral shaft. This patient had multiple congenital abnormalities and rickets associated with liver disease.

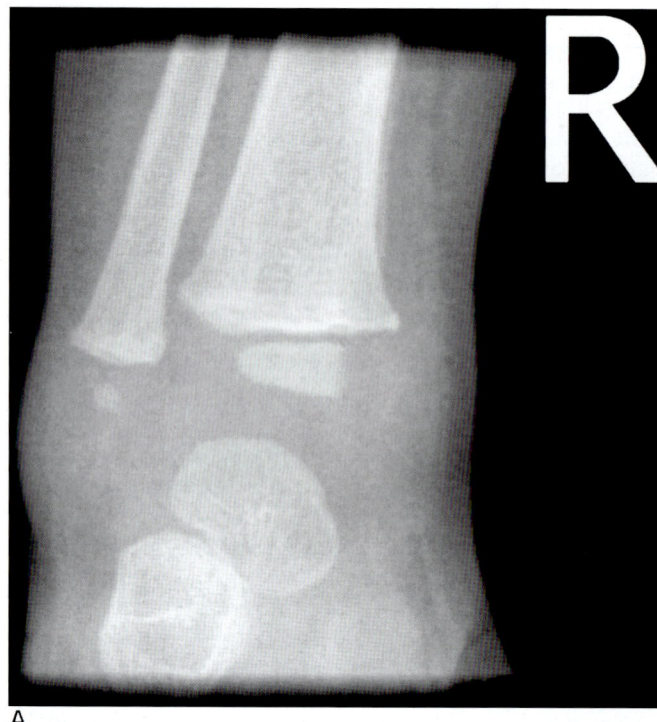

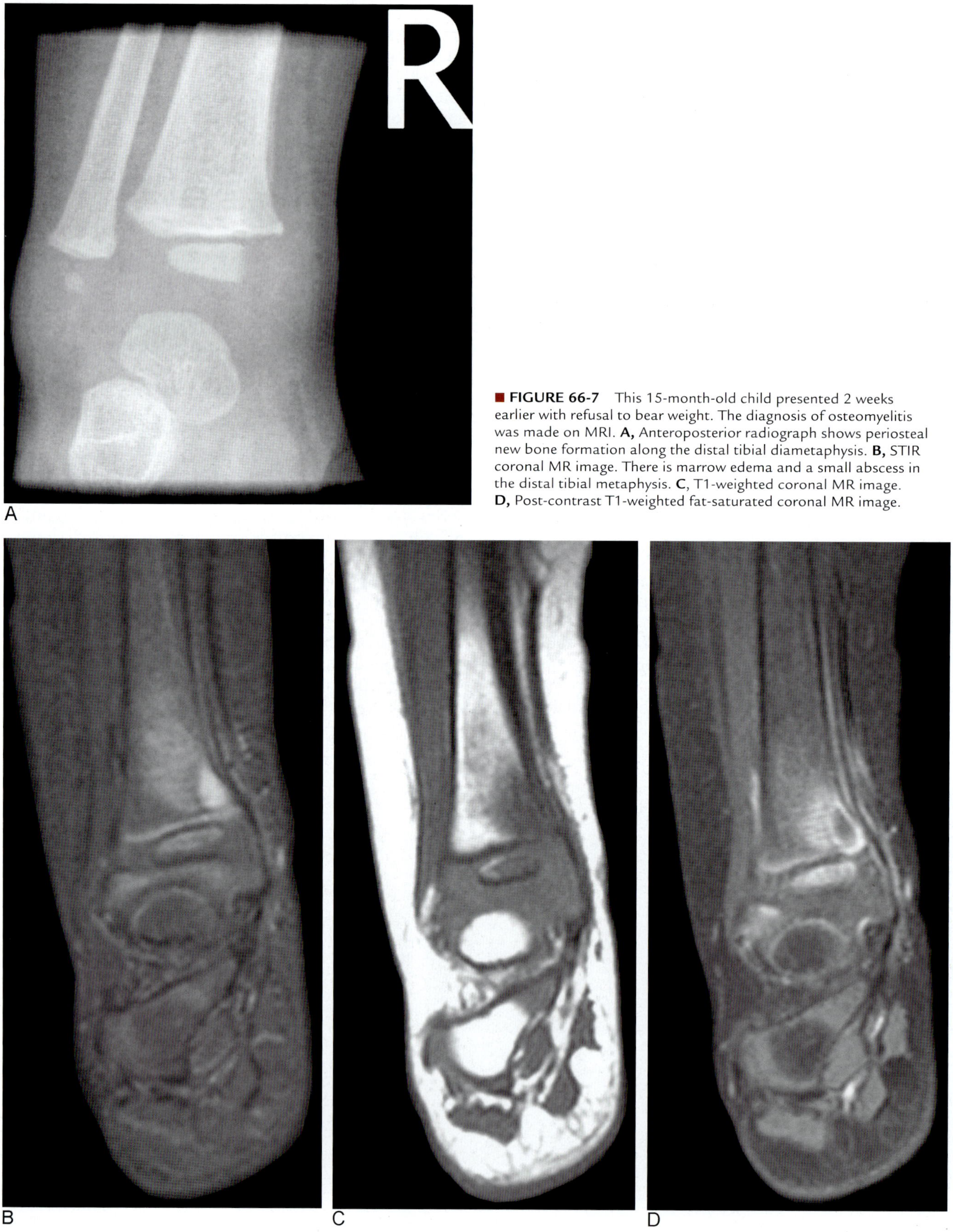

A

B

C

D

■ **FIGURE 66-7** This 15-month-old child presented 2 weeks earlier with refusal to bear weight. The diagnosis of osteomyelitis was made on MRI. **A,** Anteroposterior radiograph shows periosteal new bone formation along the distal tibial diametaphysis. **B,** STIR coronal MR image. There is marrow edema and a small abscess in the distal tibial metaphysis. **C,** T1-weighted coronal MR image. **D,** Post-contrast T1-weighted fat-saturated coronal MR image.

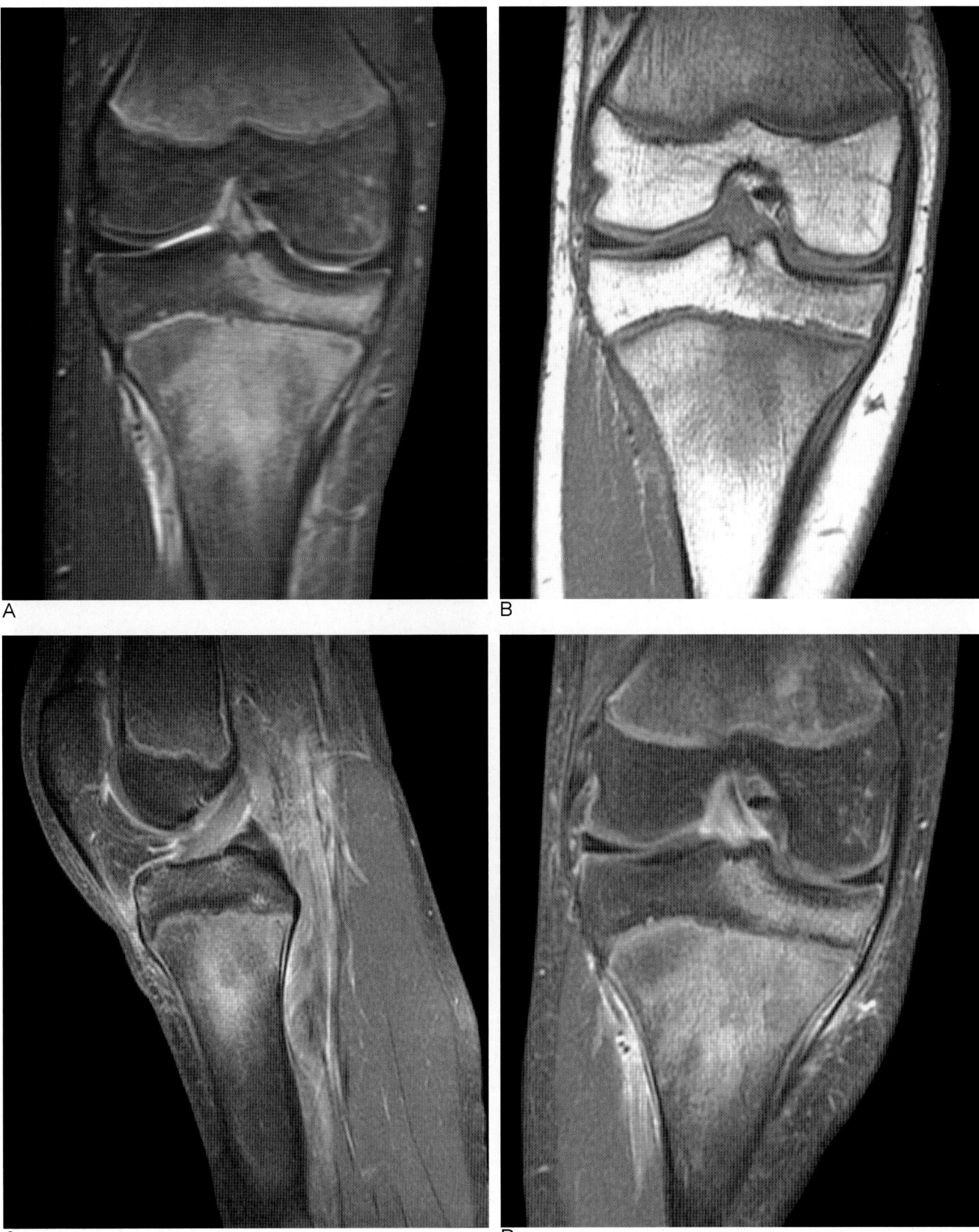

■ **FIGURE 66-8** A 13-year-old boy presented with osteomyelitis of the proximal tibia. Radiographs were normal. **A,** STIR coronal MR image of right knee. This sequence demonstrates high signal (marrow edema) intensity in the epiphysis and metaphysis and metaphyseal periosteal elevation. **B,** Bone marrow edema is also evident on T1-weighted coronal sequence. There is enhancement of these areas and the surrounding soft tissues on post-contrast T1-weighted fat-saturated sagittal (**C**) and coronal (**D**) MR images.

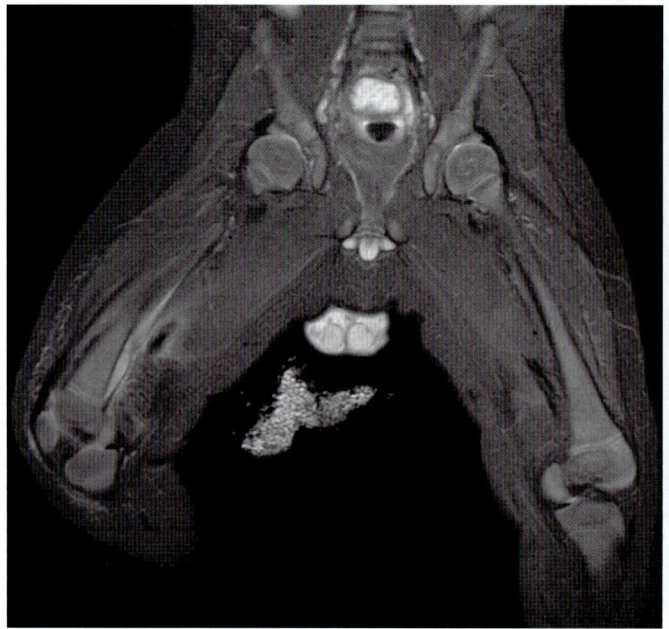

A

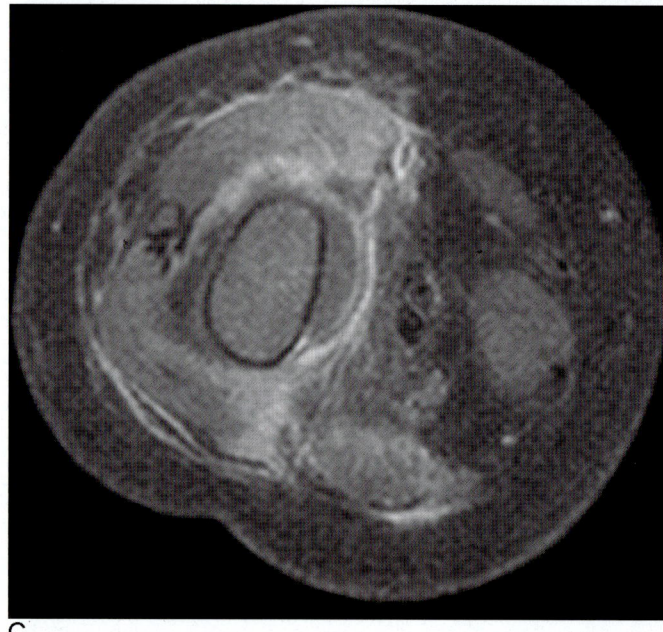

B

C

■ **FIGURE 66-9** This 6-month-old child was not moving the right leg but the site of pathology was difficult to localize clinically. Radiographs were normal. **A,** STIR, coronal, oblique MR images of both femurs. There is a subperiosteal collection associated with osteomyelitis of the distal right femur and marked inflammatory changes in the surrounding soft tissues that are edematous and enhance after intravenous instillation of contrast agent. **B,** Post-contrast T1-weighted fat-saturated coronal oblique MR image shows a subperiosteal collection related posteriorly to the distal right femoral metaphysis and narrow tract containing pus in the underlying bone. **C,** Post-contrast T1-weighted fat-saturated axial MR image of distal right femur shows the subperiosteal collection and associated myositis.

Bone scintigraphy using technetium-99m methylene diphosphonate (^{99m}Tc-MDP) is highly sensitive for the detection of bone infection and may be positive in 24 to 48 hours after onset of disease.[14] Abnormal bone scintigraphy alone is nonspecific and must always be interpreted in context of clinical and laboratory findings in addition to other imaging. It can occasionally be difficult to differentiate a focus of increased epiphyseal or metaphyseal uptake from normal increased uptake by the physeal cartilage in children. However, the main disadvantage of ^{99m}Tc-MDP bone scintigraphy is its high radiation dose, which is of particular relevance in pediatric practice. Detection of radiographically occult osteomyelitis using scintigraphy should be reserved for selected patients in whom MRI is

contraindicated or not available. In selected cases, bone scintigraphy may also be used for the detection of clinically occult infection. The single most important use of ^{99m}Tc-MDP scintigraphy in the era of MRI remains the detection of multiple sites of bone infection. However, whole-body STIR imaging may prove to be an effective and acceptable nonionizing alternative to replace scintigraphy in the future for the detection of multifocal osteomyelitis in children (Fig. 66-10).[15]

Subacute and Chronic Osteomyelitis

Subacute osteomyelitis was first described by Garre in 1893 as a sclerosing, nonsuppurative form of osteomyelitis. It is

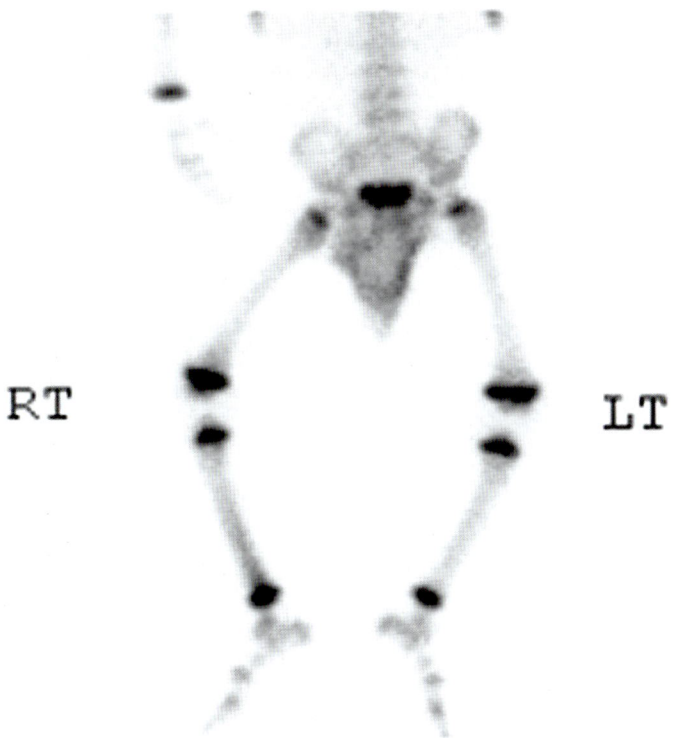

■ **FIGURE 66-10** Single phase radioisotope bone scan. There is increased uptake in the distal right tibial diaphysis, metaphysis, and physis in this 6-month-old child with osteomyelitis (same patient as Fig. 66-6).

still debated whether this represents a distinct entity or is a variant of chronic recurrent multifocal osteomyelitis.[16] Furthermore, the original paper described the sequel of osteomyelitis in the preantibiotic era. Predisposing factors for the development of subacute osteomyelitis in children include increased host resistance, decreased bacterial virulence, and previous antibiotic treatment. Typically, there is an insidious onset of symptoms with absence of systemic signs and varying degrees of bone pain. Blood cultures are rarely positive, and the yield from culture of biopsy specimens is lower than with acute osteomyelitis. The radiologic findings can mimic various benign or malignant bone tumors and nonpyogenic infections; therefore, histologic confirmation may be necessary in such cases to avoid a delay in diagnosis.[17]

Brodie's abscess is a specific type of subacute osteomyelitis characterized by a central area of suppurative bone necrosis walled off by fibrous tissue. In these patients the white blood cell count and erythrocyte sedimentation rate are frequently normal, and radiographs may remain normal until a late stage, making diagnosis more difficult.[18] Brodie's abscesses are more frequent in the metaphyses of long bones, particularly the tibia, but involvement of the carpal or tarsal bones and diaphyses of long bones may occur. Typical radiographic features are common in all age groups and consist of an elongated lucent lesion with surrounding rim of sclerosis and ill-defined transition zone between normal and abnormal marrow. There is variable accompanying periosteal new bone formation. However, subacute bone infection may be so small that it is radiographically occult. MRI has a role in such patients, and those with radiographic evidence of subacute and chronic bone infection because it can accurately define the extent of the abscess and subperiosteal and epiphyseal involvement not visualized on radiographs.[19]

Chronic osteomyelitis is present when symptoms have persisted for more than 1 month before treatment or when there is bone infection at least 1 month after surgery or existing osteomyelitis is inadequately treated. Clinically, there is low-grade fever and drainage of pus from the affected site. Both CT and MRI may demonstrate sequestrum and involucrum in these patients with chronic sinus tracts. Using MRI, sequestra are nonenhancing with low signal intensity on all pulse sequences. Sinus tracts are typically linear or curvilinear areas of hyperintensity on T2-weighted images owing to fluid in the sinus tract. The sinus may enhance after intravenous Gd-DTPA but not in all cases.

Chronic Recurrent Multifocal Osteomyelitis

Chronic recurrent multifocal osteomyelitis (CRMO) is an unusual form of chronic nonsuppurative inflammatory bone disease involving multiple sites, characterized by multiple exacerbations and spontaneous remissions. The cause is uncertain but it may be immunologically mediated, and there is evidence of genetic susceptibility in family studies. An unidentified infective agent has also been suggested as the cause. The condition occurs mainly in children and adolescents, and lesions are common in tubular bones, the clavicle, and, less frequently, the spine and pelvic bones; the occurrence in other locations is rare. The disease may be associated with cutaneous lesions similar to the SAPHO syndrome.[20] Radiographic appearance of CRMO suggests subacute or chronic osteomyelitis but can mimic tumors such as Ewing's sarcoma. Histopathology and laboratory findings are nonspecific, and bacterial culture is usually negative. CRMO is diagnosed in patients with a characteristic clinical course after exclusion of bacterial infection and tumor. Scintigraphy and MRI have an important role in diagnosis.[21] Some children affected by chronic nonbacterial osteomyelitis do not have multiple lesions or a recurrent course, and these children have a better prognosis (Fig. 66-11).[22]

ORTHOPEDIC COMPLICATIONS OF MENINGOCOCCAL SEPTICEMIA

Meningococcal septicemia is a devastating, life-threatening illness that primarily affects children. The causative organism, *Neisseria meningitides,* contains an endotoxin that sets up a cascade of events resulting in complement activation, release of inflammatory mediators, a diffuse vasculitis, and disseminated intravascular coagulation. Vascular occlusion, hemorrhage, and necrosis can occur in any organ, including the skeleton, during the illness. Those who develop purpura fulminans characterized by shock, multiple organ failure, and large areas of ecchymoses have a higher incidence of complications and decreased rate of survival.[23] Although mortality has decreased due to improvements in medical management, survivors have a high incidence of long-term sequelae secondary to the disease processes that occur as part of

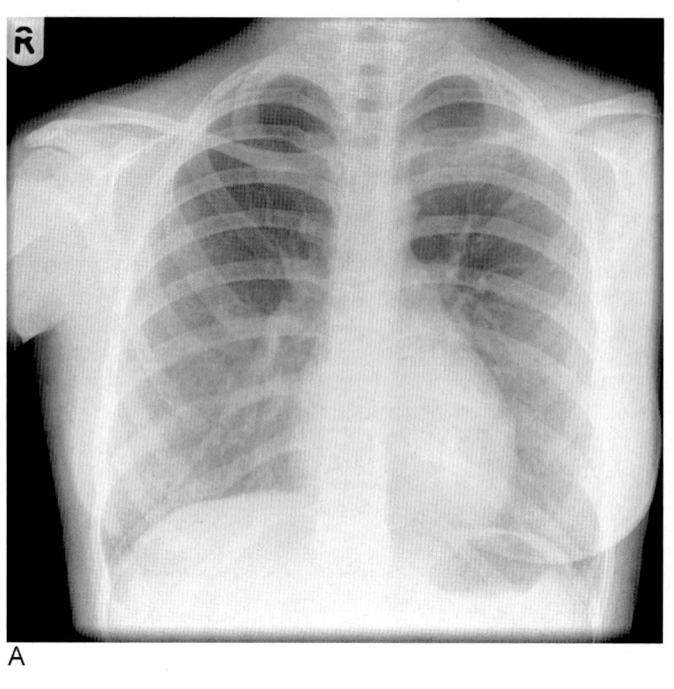

A

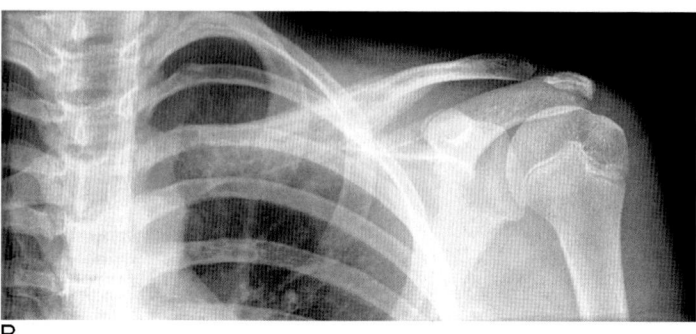

B

ANT PELVIS

ANT KNEES

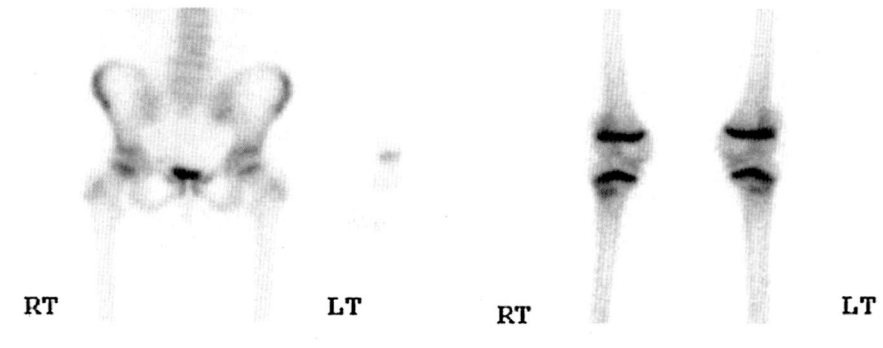

RT   LT   RT   LT

ANT FEET

ANT THORAX

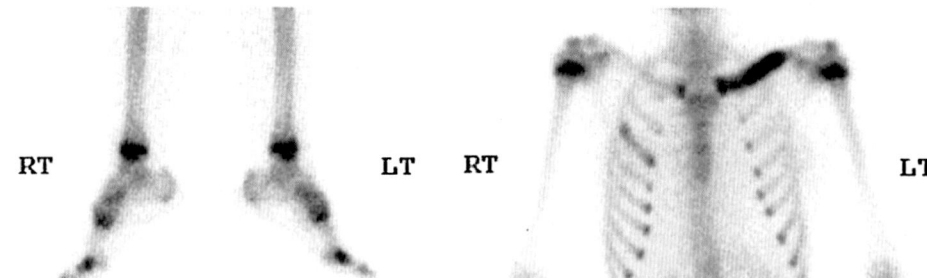

RT   LT   RT   LT

127

C

■ FIGURE 66-11 A, Postero-anterior chest radiograph shows expanded right third anterior rib and left clavicle with periosteal new bone formation in an 11-year-old patient with chronic recurrent multifocal osteomyelitis. B, Left clavicle. C, Single-phase radio-isotope bone scan shows increased uptake in the left clavicle and right third rib. There were no other lesions.

the acute illness. Orthopedic complications may be seen both acutely and chronically, related to soft tissue ischemic injury and the effects of the disease on the vasculature of growing bone and cartilage. During the acute illness, necrosis of skin, muscle, and other soft tissues may necessitate fasciotomy, surgical débridement, skin grafting, or amputation and are managed accordingly. In the acute phase, a vascular occlusive process renders all areas of the developing skeleton, both bone and cartilage variably ischemic. Subsequently, a discrete inflammatory response is also seen in the trabecular bone of the marrow space and in the subperiosteal space, with formation of abscesses in the metaphyseal loop area.[24] These two processes contribute to growth plate injury, which may not manifest until long after the acute disease has been treated. Growth abnormalities are related to microvascular damage to the physis with formation of osseous physeal bridges, resulting in partial or complete growth arrest. Multiple sites may be affected; and as with soft tissue injury, the lower limbs are affected more than the upper limbs.[23] Growth plate arrest leads to cessation of growth and limb shortening if complete and to angular deformity often with limb shortening in cases of partial arrest, which is more common.[23] Affected patients often require corrective surgery, including osteotomy and epiphysiodesis. Ischemic contractures may require soft tissue releases (Figs. 66-12 and 66-13).

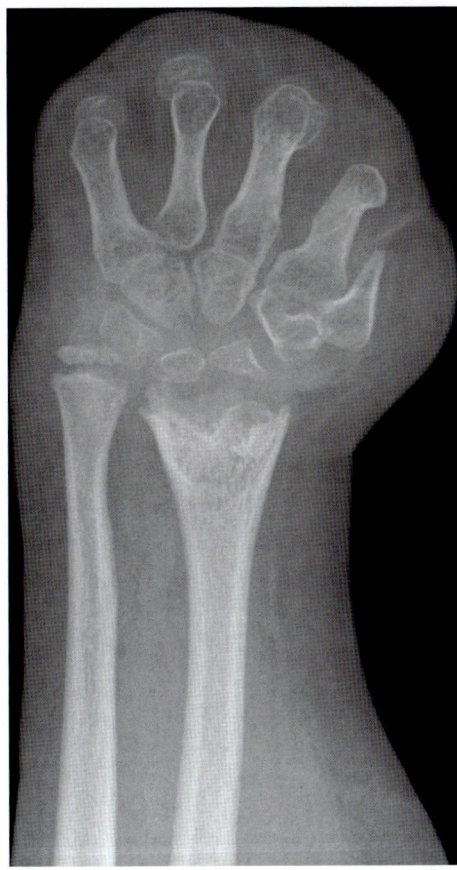

■ FIGURE 66-12 Amputations and carpal and chronic growth plate injury in an 8-year-old patient after meningococcal septicemia.

SEPTIC ARTHRITIS

Septic arthritis can occur at any age, but the peak incidence is in children younger than 3 years of age. Usually a single joint is involved, and the most common sites are the hip, knee, shoulder, elbow, and ankle. Hematogenous seeding of bacteria to the joint is the most common cause because the synovial membrane is highly vascular. Synovial fluid serves as an ideal culture medium for bacteria arriving via the hematogenous route, but infection can also spread to the joint from adjacent osteomyelitis or after trauma or surgery. *S. aureus* is the most common pathogen, followed by group A streptococcus and *S. pneumoniae*. Group B streptococcus and gram-negative coliforms are important causes in neonates. *Neisseria gonorrhoeae* should be considered in sexually active adolescents presenting with acute arthritis.[3] In common with acute osteomyelitis, *H. influenzae* joint infection has almost been eradicated following introduction of widespread vaccination. Bacterial septic arthritis is a recognized complication following varicella (chickenpox) infection in children.[25]

The presentation is similar to that of acute osteomyelitis, with an increased incidence of nonspecific signs in young children. Affected neonates may present later owing to failure to mount an effective immune reaction, and dislocation of the hip is a well-recognized presentation of septic arthritis in this age group. Older children have more localized pain with fever and decreased range of movement of the affected joint. Patients tend to keep the joint in a position that maximizes intracapsular volume and comfort. Knees are held moderately flexed, and hips are kept flexed, abducted, and externally rotated. Joint swelling helps to differentiate the condition clinically from acute osteomyelitis. Progression of the disease is rapid, with the diagnosis usually being made within 72 hours of the onset of symptoms. The cornerstone of diagnosis is the evaluation of aspirated joint fluid, although blood cultures may help to identify the pathogen when synovial fluid culture is negative.

Acute joint infection is a pediatric orthopedic emergency. Delay in diagnosis and treatment may lead to rapid cartilage destruction due to proteolytic degradation by inflammatory exudate. Increased pressure within the infected joint increases the likelihood of joint subluxation, ischemia, and avascular necrosis. Other complications of osteomyelitis include fracture, slipped epiphysis, and premature physeal fusion and chronic infection. All of these complications increase morbidity, particularly if there is skeletal deformity or joint dysfunction. When there is good clinical and serologic evidence of joint sepsis, imaging should not delay surgical treatment.

Radiographic examination of a suspected septic joint should always be performed to obtain an overview of joint morphology. There may be radiographic signs of joint effusion, although this is a nonspecific finding and failure to detect an effusion radiographically does not reliably exclude effusion or joint sepsis. Distortion of soft tissue planes may be apparent on radiographs, but this is nonspecific and more likely to be due to varied positioning of the limbs. Widening of the joint space may be due to cartilage edema or dislocation and is rarely the result

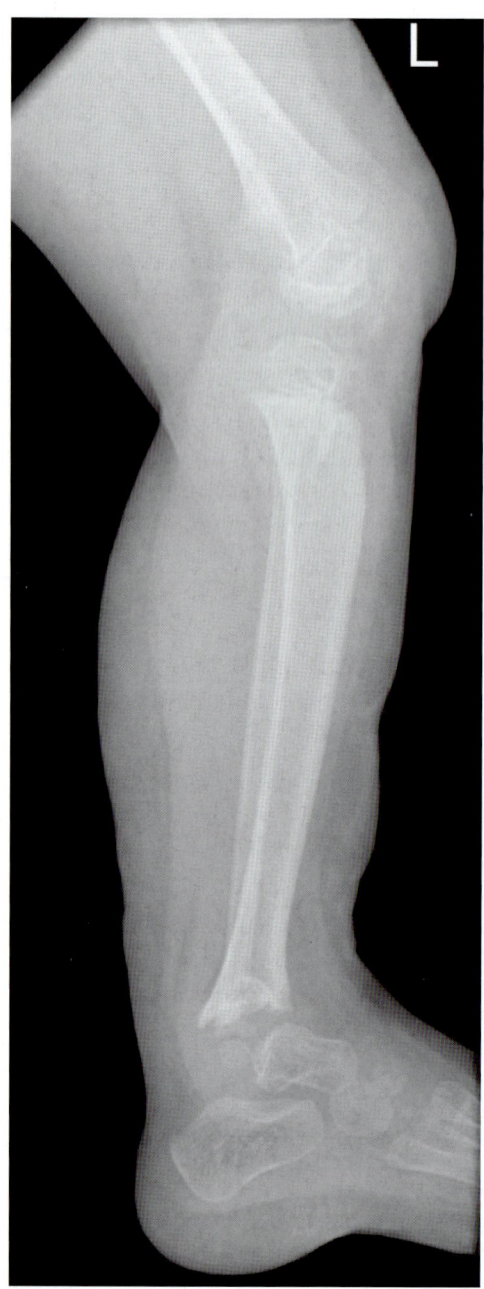

A

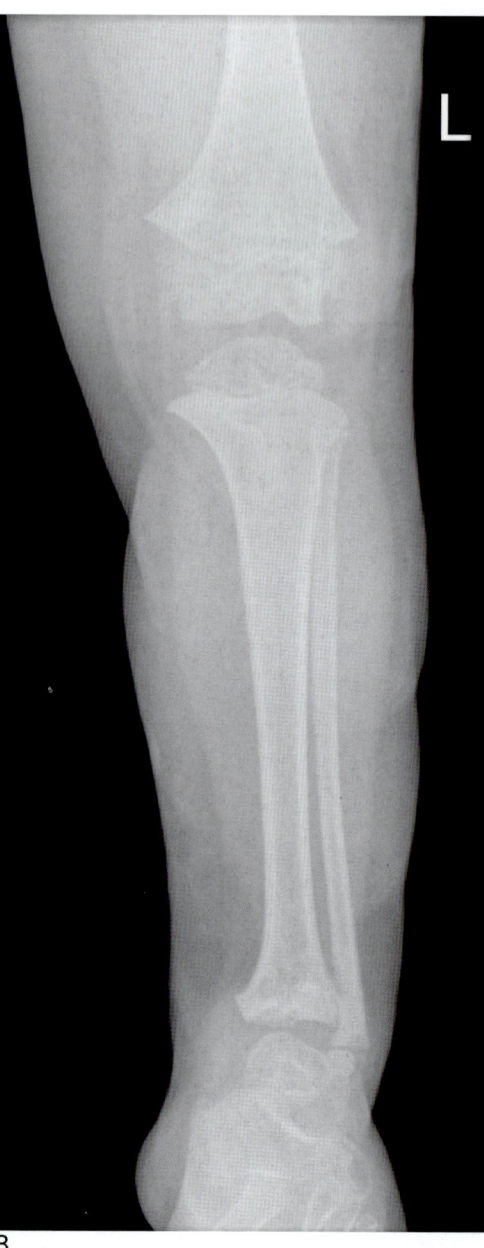

B

■ **FIGURE 66-13**   Lateral (**A**) and anteroposterior (**B**) radiographs of the left leg in a 3-year old who had meningococcal septicemia at 20 months of age. The physes of all the long bones have been affected.

of an effusion. Fluid prefers to collect in the lax compartments of a joint and only leads to misalignment when under considerable pressure. Radiographs are frequently normal in a patient with acute septic arthritis.

Ultrasonography is highly sensitive for the detection of joint effusion and can be used to guide aspiration to obtain fluid for microscopic examination. However, absence of a joint effusion on ultrasonography does not exclude joint infection.[26] Furthermore, when an effusion is present the amount and echogenicity of the fluid cannot be used as a reliable predictor for infection because it could indicate other causes of inflammation, such as transient synovitis or inflammatory arthropathy. In a child with clinical and biochemical signs of joint infection, negative ultrasonographic findings should be treated with extreme caution (Figs. 66-14 and 66-15).

Further preoperative imaging should be performed only if the diagnosis is in doubt or to detect coexisting osteomyelitis with abscess formation, which may require drainage. MRI is extremely sensitive for the detection of joint effusions and inflammatory changes in the synovium and other soft tissues; however, such changes must be interpreted in the context of clinical and biochemical evidence of joint sepsis because other inflammatory conditions such as transient synovitis and juvenile idiopathic arthritis can have similar appearances. More advanced features of septic arthritis such as cartilage destruction may be detected in addition to coexisting osteomyelitis. There in no role for CT in children with suspected septic arthritis except in selected cases such as postoperatively or after trauma and to detect intraarticular radiopaque foreign bodies. Bone scintigraphy has no role in the diagnosis of septic arthritis in children.

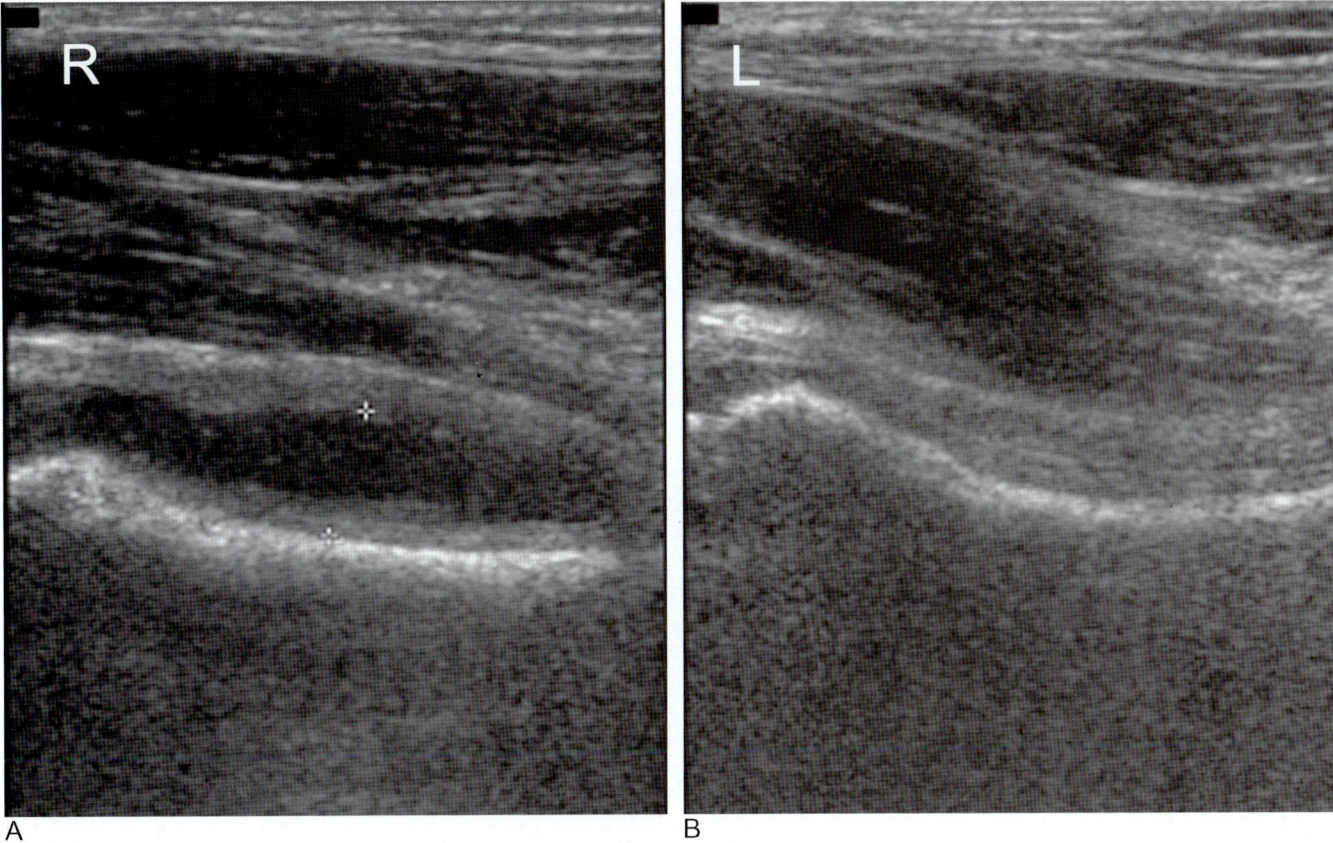

■ FIGURE 66-14   A, Sonogram in an 8-year old with septic arthritis shows right hip joint effusion. **B,** Normal sonogram of left hip for comparison.

VERTEBRAL OSTEOMYELITIS AND DISCITIS

Vertebral osteomyelitis and discitis are uncommon diagnoses in children but are quite different both in terms of severity and prognosis compared with adult-onset forms of the disease. Childhood spondylodiscitis is often a benign, self-limiting condition that responds to conservative management. In discitis, inflammation is restricted to the disc, whereas in spondylodiscitis both the disc and adjacent bony structures are involved. Blood supply to the disc and cartilaginous vertebral end plate in children is different from in adults, and this could predispose to infectious agents settling in and around the disc and may also explain the characteristic good prognosis for recovery and lack of long-term complications. The vertebral blood supply undergoes involution from numerous anastomotic channels in the vertebral end plate that communicate with the disc in the fetus, infant, and young child up to around the seventh year of life, to end arteries seen in the adolescent and adult. The nucleus pulposus of the disc contains no blood or lymphatic vessels at any age, but blood vessels are present in the anulus fibrosus up to 20 years of age.[27] Isolated inflammation of the disc can occur in childhood owing to persistence of this vascular supply to the disc that disappears later in life. Although discitis can occur at any age in childhood there is a higher incidence in toddlers and a second subtler peak in late childhood to

early adolescence. Vertebral osteomyelitis, in contrast, has a peak in adolescence and in the age group older than age 50 years.[28]

Childhood spondylodiscitis frequently presents in a nonspecific way; symptoms are often mild, making it difficult to diagnose. A common presenting symptom is refusal to walk or sit. Limping, gait disturbance, hip or leg pain, and a need to hold onto objects for support are also typical. Back pain is a common symptom in all age groups. Patients with discitis can also present with fever or abdominal pain. Restricted spinal mobility and loss of lumbar lordosis may be found on clinical examination. Biochemical markers of inflammation are usually only slightly raised, and blood cultures are usually negative.

Discitis can affect any spinal level but occurs with more frequency in the thoracic and lumbar spine. Usually only one disc space is affected. Involvement of more than one level can be seen in infection with *Mycobacterium tuberculosis*. Radiographic signs of discitis may not be seen until 3 to 8 weeks after the onset of symptoms when loss of disc height and end-plate irregularity are seen. Bone scintigraphy can be positive within 1 week of the onset of symptoms, but this test cannot differentiate between other causes of back pain. The diagnostic imaging method of choice is MRI. Characteristic findings of loss of disc height and abnormal disc signal intensity with accompanying vertebral end plate irregularity are best

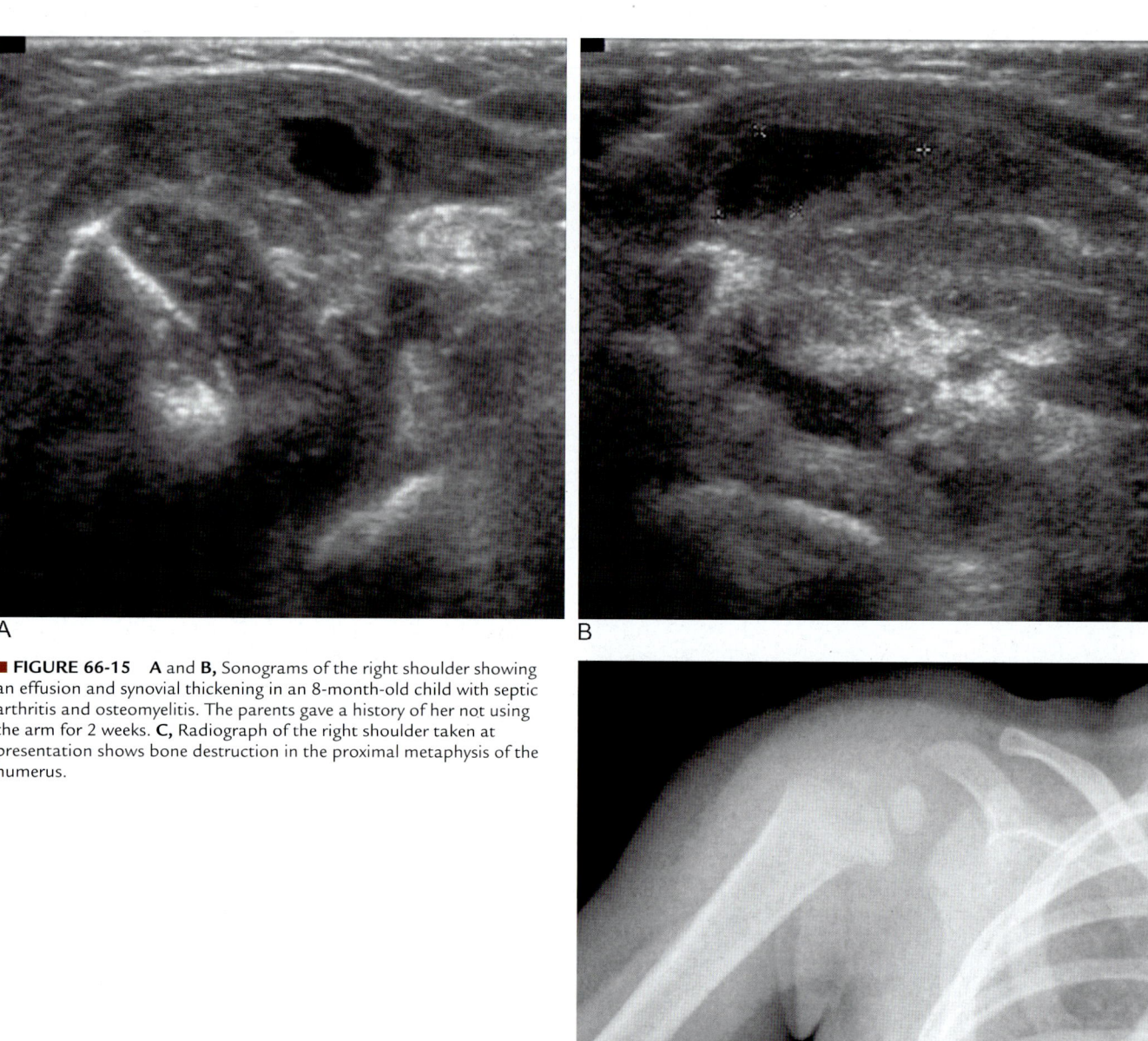

■ FIGURE 66-15 **A** and **B,** Sonograms of the right shoulder showing an effusion and synovial thickening in an 8-month-old child with septic arthritis and osteomyelitis. The parents gave a history of her not using the arm for 2 weeks. **C,** Radiograph of the right shoulder taken at presentation shows bone destruction in the proximal metaphysis of the humerus.

seen on T2-weighted sequences. Abnormal enhancement of the disc and adjacent vertebral bodies is frequently demonstrated with Gd-TPA enhancement. Enhanced scans may also demonstrate paravertebral inflammatory masses and abscesses in addition to other complications that may require surgery such as nerve root compromise secondary to disc protrusion (Figs. 66-16 and 66-17).

Most authors propose an infective cause for discitis; however, most cultures, including vertebral and disc biopsy specimens are sterile and some patients recover without antimicrobial treatment. Trauma and an inflammatory pro-

cess of unknown cause have also been implicated in the cause of discitis. This uncertainty makes decisions about treatment more difficult, although the usual choice is antistaphylococcal antibiotics and spinal splinting or traction and bed rest. Biopsy is usually reserved for patients not responding to antibiotic treatment and in whom tuberculous, fungal, or other infections are suspected or in immunocompromised patients. Some centers do not routinely prescribe antibiotics unless there are signs of systemic toxicity. In contrast, vertebral osteomyelitis is thought to occur due to organisms lodging in the low flow vertebral end

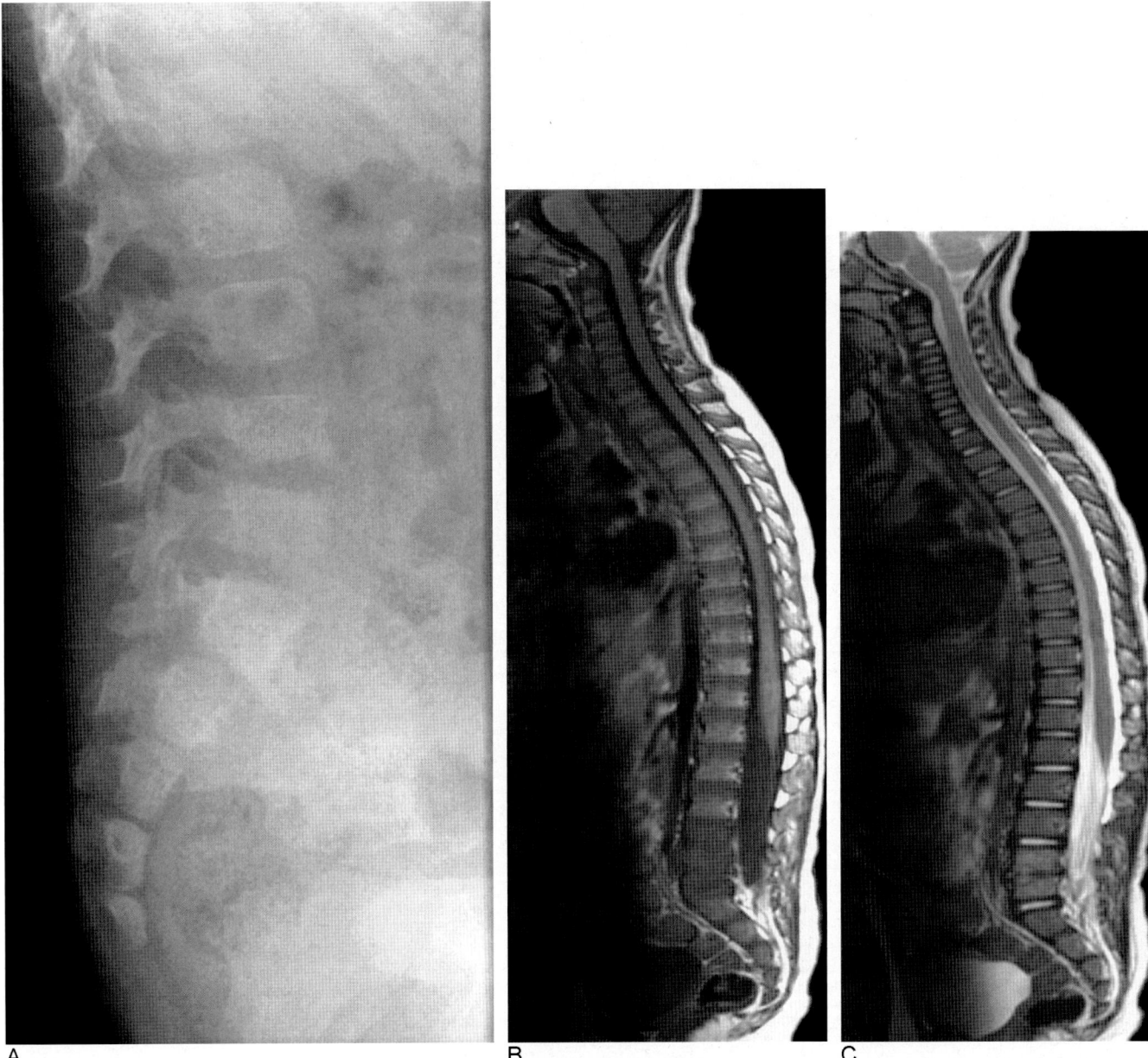

■ **FIGURE 66-16** A 2-year-old child presented with juvenile discitis. **A,** Lateral lumbosacral radiograph shows end-plate irregularity at the L4–5 disc space. All blood cultures were negative. T1-weighted (**B**) and T2-weighted (**C**) sagittal MR images of the spine showing L4-5 disc space narrowing and marrow edema in the adjacent vertebral bodies. There is a small soft tissue mass anterior to the spine level centered on the disc space.

vessels close to the cartilaginous end plate. In both conditions, association with a prior septic condition is uncommon.

Childhood spondylodiscitis has a good prognosis, and long-term functional deficit is rare.[27] Restricted spinal movement, kyphosis, and back pain occur in a minority of patients after previous documented spondylodiscitis. Persistent radiographic abnormalities are typical and vary from mild disc space narrowing to high-grade disc space narrowing and partial or complete bony ankylosis. Kyphosis may also be detected radiographically.

The main differential for childhood spondylodiscitis is tuberculous spondylitis. In contrast to childhood spondylodiscitis, patients with tubercular spondylitis frequently present with abnormal neurology and bladder or bowel symptoms, although the onset of the illness is usually insidious, which helps to differentiate it from pyogenic vertebral osteomyelitis. Vertebral body and disc involvement are found on MRI, usually accompanied by a paraspinal soft tissue mass or abscess. The mass characteristically has smooth margins and rim enhancement with intravenous contrast agents.[10] Tuberculous infection of the spine is via the hematogenous route and is thought to begin in the anterior part of the vertebral body adjacent to the superior or inferior end plates. The disc is only secondarily affected at a later stage, and infection spreads to involve adjoining disc spaces by the subligamentous route or by penetration of the subchondral end plate. The posterior elements of the vertebrae are less commonly affected.

Scheuermann's disease usually affects multiple levels of the spine, but if it presents with involvement of a single level there can be diagnostic uncertainty because it is

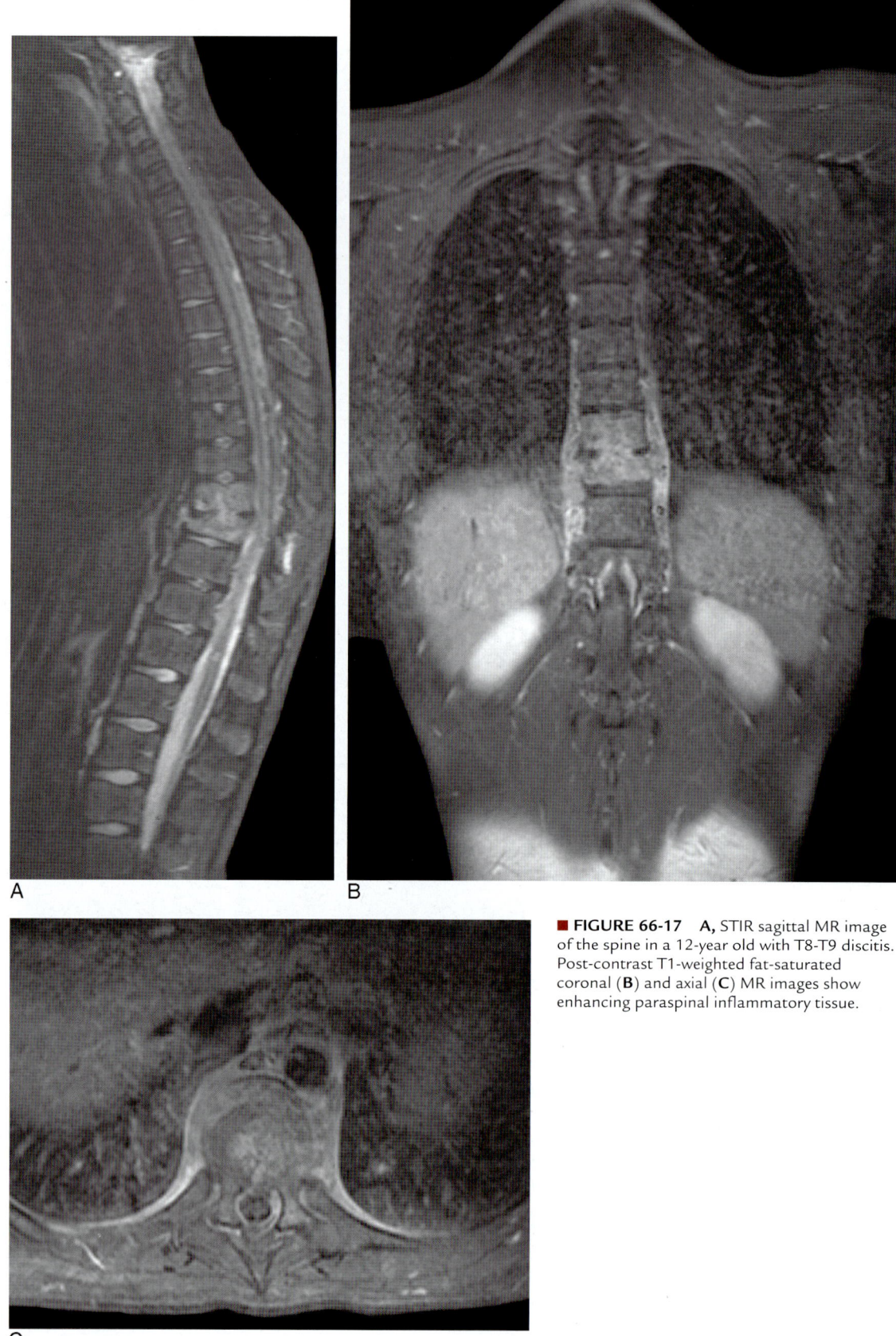

■ **FIGURE 66-17** **A,** STIR sagittal MR image of the spine in a 12-year old with T8-T9 discitis. Post-contrast T1-weighted fat-saturated coronal (**B**) and axial (**C**) MR images show enhancing paraspinal inflammatory tissue.

sometimes accompanied by disc space narrowing and end-plate destruction resembling that of childhood spondylodiscitis. The radiographic features of Langerhans cell histiocytosis can resemble spondylodiscitis, but MRI demonstrates that the process is restricted to the vertebral body, sparing the intervertebral disc.[29] Progressive ventral fusion of the vertebral end plates is thought to be caused by abnormality of the anterior fibers of the anulus fibrosus, which results in incomplete fusion of the spine at multiple levels and can lead to progressive kyphosis. These changes can resemble the sequelae of childhood spondylodiscitis.

CONGENITAL INFECTION

Congenital infections occur when the organism is transmitted from mother to fetus through the placenta. Nonspecific changes may be seen in the long bones with congenital viral infections such as rubella and cytomegalovirus. Transverse bands of lucency in the metaphyses or a "celery stalk" appearance is noted in which longitudinally oriented bands of increased and decreased density are seen extending from the metaphysis into the diaphysis. Growth plate irregularity may also be seen with cytomegaloviral infection. The changes may be due to alterations in bone formation and tend to be transient, with resolution over the first few weeks of life (Fig. 66-18).

Congenital syphilitic infection with the organism *Treponema pallidum* leads to multiple osseous abnormalities if the fetus survives. The organism localizes in the perichondrium, periosteum, cartilage, bone marrow, and sites of endochondral ossification. Osseous manifestations can be divided into early and late lesions.[30] Early lesions develop up to 2 years of age and include osteochondritis or metaphysitis, diaphyseal osteomyelitis, or osteitis and periostitis. Osteochondritis is characterized by symmetric metaphyseal irregularity and destruction. Metaphysitis, owing to direct spirochetal invasion of the metaphysis, may result in epiphyseal separation from proliferation of granulation tissue. Osteitis or diaphyseal osteomyelitis occurs with extension of the metaphyseal infection into the diaphysis. Irregular lytic cortical and medullary lesions are often associated with solid or lamellar periosteal new bone formation. Periostitis may occur alone, usually in the long bones, but can also affect flat bones. The early manifestations of the disease regress even without treatment, but it can recur (Fig. 66-19).

Late lesions occur in children older than 2 years of age. Lytic bone lesions, endosteal bony proliferation, and periosteal new bone formation are typical. A characteristic lesion is the "sabre" shin with anterior bending of the bone.

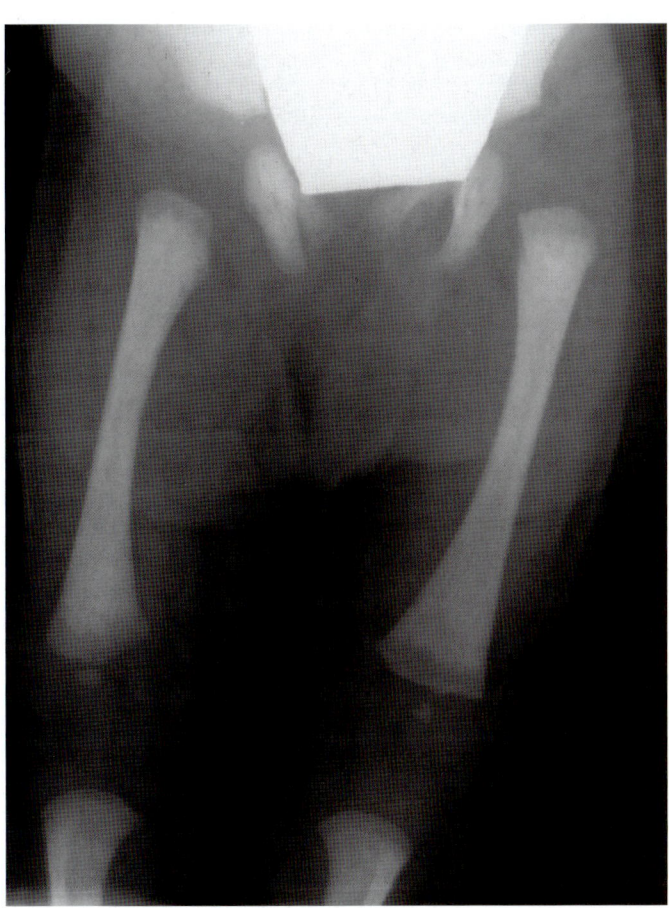

■ **FIGURE 66-18** Transverse lucent metaphyseal bands in the long bones of an 8-day-old infant with congenital rubella infection. Maternal infection occurred at 6 weeks' gestation.

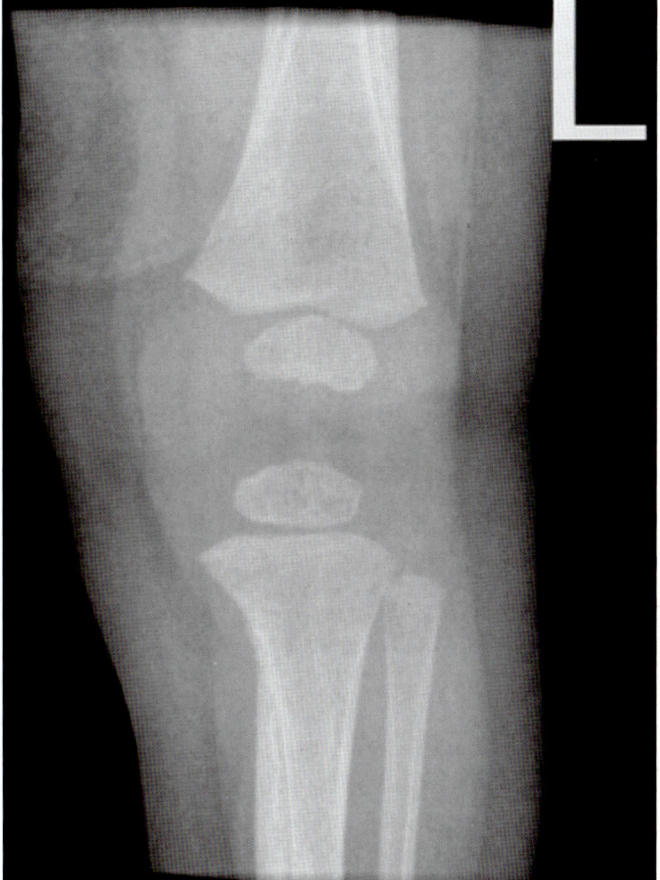

■ **FIGURE 66-19** Anteroposterior radiograph of left knee of a 5-month-old child with congenital syphilis. There is thick, organized periosteal new bone formation along the long-bone diaphyses. Presentation was in the neonatal period with hepatosplenomegaly.

REFERENCES

1. Loyer EM, DuBrow RA, David CL, et al. Imaging of superficial soft-tissue infections: sonographic findings in cases of cellulitis and abscess. AJR Am J Roentgenol 1996; 166:49–52.

2. Peckett WRC, Butler-Manuel A, Apthorp LA. Pyomyositis of the iliacus muscle in a child. J Bone Joint Surg Br 2001; 3:103–105.

3. Frank G, Mahoney HM, Eppes SC. Musculoskeletal infections in children. Pediatr Clin North Am 2005; 52:1083–1106.

4. Clark P, Davidson D, Letts M, et al. Necrotizing fasciitis secondary to chickenpox infection in children. Can J Surg 2002; 46:9–14.

5. Asmar BI. Osteomyelitis in the neonate. Infect Dis Clin North Am 1992; 6:117–132.

6. Nelson JD. Acute osteomyelitis in children. Infect Dis Clin North Am 1990; 4:513–522.

7. Karwowska A, Davies H, Jadavji T. Epidemiology and outcome of osteomyelitis in the era of sequential intravenous-oral therapy. Pediatr Infect Dis J 1998; 17:1021–1026.

8. Schmit P, Glorion C. Osteomyelitis in infants and children. Eur Radiol 2004(Suppl 4); 14:L44–L54.

9. Thanni LO, Ogunfowora OB, Olanrewaju DM. Hemoglobinopathy and pattern of musculoskeletal infection in children. J Natl Med Assoc 2004; 96:224–228.

10. Teo HE, Peh WC. Skeletal tuberculosis in children. Pediatr Radiol 2004; 34:853–860.

11. Kothari NA, Pelchovitz DJ, Meyer JS. Imaging of musculoskeletal infections. Radiol Clin North Am 2001; 39:653–671.

12. Davidson D, Letts M, Khoshhal K. Pelvic osteomyelitis in children: a comparison of decades from 1980–1989 with 1990–2001. J Pediatr Orthop 2003; 23:514–521.

13. Foster K, Chapman S, Johnson K. MRI of the marrow in the paediatric skeleton. Clin Radiol 2004; 59:651–673.

14. Treves ST, Connolly LP, Kirkpatrick JA, et al. Bone. In Treves ST (ed). Pediatric Nuclear Medicine, 2nd ed. New York, Springer-Verlag, 1995, pp 233–301.

15. Mentzel HJ, Kentouche K, Sauner D, et al. Comparison of whole-body STIR-MRI and ^{99m}Tc-methylene-diphosphonate scintigraphy in children with suspected multifocal bone lesions. Eur Radiol 2004; 14:2297–2302.

16. Segev E, Hayek S, Lokiec F, et al. Primary chronic sclerosing (Garre's) osteomyelitis in children. J Pediatr Orthop B 2001; 10:360–364.

17. Rasool MN. Primary subacute haematogenous osteomyelitis in children. J Bone Joint Surg Br 2001; 83:93–98.

18. Kozlowski K. Brodie's abscess in the first decade of life: report of eleven cases. Pediatr Radiol 1980; 10:33–37.

19. Pöyhiä Y, Azouz EM. MR imaging evaluation of subacute and chronic bone abscesses in children. Pediatr Radiol 2000; 30:763–768.

20. Earwaker JW, Cotten A. SAPHO: syndrome or concept? Imaging findings. Skeletal Radiol 2003; 32:311–327.

21. Jurik AG. Chronic recurrent multifocal osteomyelitis. Semin Musculoskeletal Radiol 2004; 8:243–53.

22. Girschick HJ, Raab P, Surbaum S, et al. Chronic non-bacterial osteomyelitis in children. Ann Rheum Dis 2005; 64:279–285.

23. Belthur MV, Bradish CF, Gibbons PJ. Late orthopaedic sequelae following meningococcal septicaemia: a multicentre study. J Bone Joint Surg Br 2005; 87:236–240.

24. Grogan DP, Love SM, Ogden JA, et al. Chondro-osseous growth abnormalities after meningococcemia: a clinical and histopathological study. J Bone Joint Surg Am 1989; 71:920–928.

25. Konyves A, Deo SD, Murray JRD, et al. Septic arthritis of the elbow after chickenpox. J Pediatr Orthop B 2004; 13:114–117.

26. Gordon JE, Huang M, Dobbs M, et al. Causes of false-negative ultrasound scans in the diagnosis of septic arthritis of the hip in children. J Pediatr Orthop 2002; 22:312–316.

27. Kayser R, Mahlfeld K, Greulich M, Grasshoff H. Spondylodiscitis in childhood: results of a long-term study. Spine 2005; 30:318–323.

28. Fernadez M, Carrol CL, Baker CJ. Discitis and vertebral osteomyelitis in children: An 18-year review. Pediatrics 2005; 105:1299–1304.

29. Kayser R, Mahlfeld K, Grasshoff H. The Langerhans granulomatosis of the spine in childhood—a differential diagnosis of the spinal osteomyelitis. Klin Pediatr 1998; 210:1–6.

30. Sachdev M, Bery K, Chawla S. Osseous manifestations in congenital syphilis: a study of 55 cases. Clin Radiol 1982; 33:319–323.

67

Human Immunodeficiency Virus Infection and Acquired Immunodeficiency Syndrome

Sandra Moore and Theodoros Katsivas

Human immunodeficiency virus (HIV) infection is prevalent worldwide and is almost universally fatal if left untreated, leading to, and being the etiologic agent of, the acquired immunodeficiency syndrome (AIDS). Initial reports of cases of men who have sex with men in major U.S. cities in 1981, presenting with malignancies and/or infections associated with severe immunosuppression, were quickly followed by the definition of what we know today as AIDS. The Centers for Disease Control and Prevention (CDC) has published the current case definition criteria, which include three different categories of clinical conditions and three categories of quantification of CD4-positive T lymphocytes, the primary cellular immunologic marker of the infection (Table 67-1).[1]

Many of the central nervous system, thoracic, and abdominal presentations in HIV/AIDS are familiar to radiologists, but musculoskeletal manifestations are less common and not as well known. Radiologists should be aware of, and vigilant in, diagnosing the musculoskeletal disorders associated with HIV/AIDS, because these may be the initial presentation or may significantly affect the quality of life. They may complicate advanced disease and/or be highly aggressive. Musculoskeletal manifestations include infections with opportunistic and common pathogens, HIV or treatment effects on the musculoskeletal system, arthritis, myositis, and HIV/AIDS-related neoplasms. People living with HIV/AIDS undergoing highly active antiretroviral therapy (HAART) regimens may present with musculoskeletal manifestations differing from those in individuals who are either unable to obtain, adhere to, or tolerate those regimens. The musculoskeletal side effects and complications of treatment are controversial but may include significant marrow abnormalities, myopathy, fat redistribution, and osteoporosis or osteopenia.

As our understanding of HIV/AIDS matures and as new treatments become available, the medical community is progressing from regarding HIV/AIDS as a stigmatizing, sexual behavior–related illness to what HIV actually represents—a devastating viral pandemic that urgently needs to be addressed at all levels of social life worldwide. It is important that radiologists in developed countries do not respond to the major strides made in treating HIV/AIDS with complacency and amnesia.

PREVALENCE AND EPIDEMIOLOGY

HIV is estimated to have caused 65 million human infections and 25 millions deaths worldwide so far, according to World Health Organization and the Joint AIDS United Nations program (UNAIDS) data, as of the end of 2006. Currently, there are about 39.5 million people living with HIV/AIDS, of which 17.7 million are women, with an estimated worldwide prevalence of infection of 1%. In the United States, there are an estimated 1.2 million people living with HIV/AIDS,[2] the majority of whom are homosexuals; unprotected sex between men remains the dominant mode of transmission, followed by unprotected heterosexual sex and use of nonsterile injecting equipment. An estimated 25% of people living with HIV/AIDS in the United States are not aware of their serology status. One of the striking facets of the epidemic in the United States is the concentration of HIV infections among ethnic minorities. Despite constituting 12% of the country's population, African Americans accounted for 50% of new AIDS diagnoses in 2001 to 2004 and Hispanics (14% of the U.S. population) accounted for 20% of AIDS cases for the same period.

As well as racial and ethnic disparity in developed countries, global geographical disparity is apparent in that 63% of all cases of people living with HIV/AIDS are located in

KEY POINTS

- Musculoskeletal infection in people living with HIV/AIDS is most commonly from the same pathogens seen in noninfected patients.
- The most common musculoskeletal infection in people living with HIV/AIDS is septic arthritis.
- The most serious musculoskeletal infections in people living with HIV/AIDS are acute osteomyelitis and necrotizing fasciitis.
- The most important risk factor for musculoskeletal infections in people living with HIV/AIDS is intravenous drug use.
- Risk of tuberculous reactivation in people living with HIV/AIDS is 7% to 10% per year.
- Average delay from presentation to diagnosis in osteoarticular musculoskeletal tuberculosis is 16 to 19 months.
- The most common aseptic musculoskeletal manifestation in people living with HIV/AIDS is arthralgias (up to 45%).
- The most common noninfectious arthritis in people living with HIV/AIDS is reactive arthritis.
- Differentiation between HIV-related psoriatic and reactive arthritis cannot be made on the basis of radiographic appearance.

TABLE 67-1 CDC Definition of CD4 Lymphocyte Count and Clinical Categories of HIV Infection*

Categories of CD4 Cell Counts
Category 1: greater than or equal to 500 cells/mm³
Category 2: 200–499 cells/mm³
Category 3: less than 200 cells/mm³
Clinical Categories
Category A
Asymptomatic HIV infection
Persistent generalized lymphadenopathy
Acute (primary) HIV infection
Category B
Bacillary angiomatosis
Candidiasis, oropharyngeal (thrush)
Candidiasis, vulvovaginal; persistent, frequent, or poorly responsive to therapy
Cervical dysplasia (moderate or severe)/cervical carcinoma in situ
Constitutional symptoms, such as fever (38.5°C) or diarrhea lasting greater than 1 month
Hairy leukoplakia, oral
Herpes zoster (shingles), involving at least two distinct episodes or more than one dermatome
Idiopathic thrombocytopenic purpura
Listeriosis
Pelvic inflammatory disease, particularly if complicated by tubo-ovarian abscess
Peripheral neuropathy
Category C
Candidiasis of bronchi, trachea, or lungs
Candidiasis, esophageal
Cervical cancer, invasive
Coccidioidomycosis, disseminated or extrapulmonary
Cryptococcosis, extrapulmonary
Cryptosporidiosis, chronic intestinal (>1 month's duration)
Cytomegalovirus disease (other than liver, spleen, or nodes)
Cytomegalovirus retinitis (with loss of vision)
Encephalopathy, HIV-related
Herpes simplex: chronic ulcer(s) (>1 month's duration); or bronchitis, pneumonitis, or esophagitis
Histoplasmosis, disseminated or extrapulmonary
Isosporiasis, chronic intestinal (>1 month's duration)
Kaposi sarcoma
Lymphoma, Burkitt's (or equivalent term)
Lymphoma, immunoblastic (or equivalent term)
Lymphoma, primary, of brain
***Mycobacterium avium* complex or *M. kansasii*, disseminated or extrapulmonary**
***Mycobacterium tuberculosis*, any site (pulmonary or extrapulmonary)**
***Mycobacterium*, other species or unidentified species, disseminated or extrapulmonary**
Pneumocystis jiroveci (*carinii*) pneumonia
Pneumonia, recurrent
Progressive multifocal leukoencephalopathy
Salmonella septicemia, recurrent
Toxoplasmosis of brain
Wasting syndrome due to HIV

*Categories A3, B3, C1, C2, and C3 meet the case definition for AIDS.
Musculoskeletal entities associated with HIV/AIDS **are in boldface type**.

sub-Saharan Africa, an area where there were 72% of all AIDS-related deaths in 2006.[2] The epidemic continues to intensify in Africa, and there are alarming signs that prevalence rates are escalating in East Asia, Eastern Europe, and Central Asia. High risk behaviors such as unprotected sex between men, unprotected paid sex, and needle sharing are important in these new areas.

CLINICAL PRESENTATION

The clinical presentations of the musculoskeletal disorders encountered in people living with HIV/AIDS are comparable to those seen in those who are not infected with HIV. However, people living with HIV/AIDS may demonstrate atypical sites of involvement, incomplete presentations of arthritis, advanced findings at presentation, and/or infection with uncommonly encountered organisms.

PATHOPHYSIOLOGY

HIV is one of the human retroviruses of the Lentivirus family. There are solid data that HIV has been acquired by humans from primate cross-species transmission.[3-5] HIV type 1 has spread globally whereas type 2 remains mostly confined to western Africa.

After exposure to HIV, a symptomatic mononucleosis-like illness termed primary HIV infection occurs in 1 to 4 weeks in more than half the patients; however, clinical immunodeficiency or AIDS develops after a long period of clinical latency that follows primary HIV infection. Clinical latency is a dynamic period in which active viral replication occurs and immunologic abnormalities begin to emerge, notably quantitative and qualitative defects in the CD4-positive T-lymphocyte pool. The average length of the latency period in adults is approximately 10 years

without treatment. Opportunistic infections as listed in the case definition (Table 67-1) are the hallmarks of progression to AIDS and usually happen with a CD4-positive count <200 cells/mm³.

HIV impairs T-lymphocyte response, rendering the patient vulnerable to myriad diseases and disorders that may involve the musculoskeletal system. Many of the pathophysiologic mechanisms of the musculoskeletal disorders seen with AIDS are not well understood but probably reflect complex interactions between immuno-suppression, the HIV virus, and immunologic, genetic, environmental, and treatment factors.

Anatomy

HIV-associated lipodystrophy syndrome consists of a combination of metabolic abnormalities (hyperlipidemia and insulin resistance) and morphologic changes, including subcutaneous fat atrophy (lipoatrophy), abdominal fat accumulation (lipohypertrophy), or mixed lipoatrophy/lipohypertrophy patterns. Focal fat deposition has also been described. Advanced age may be a factor, although lipodystrophy has been described in pediatric patients with HIV/AIDS.[6] These findings are more advanced in individuals with a low CD4 count and long duration of antiretroviral therapy, although the cause of the change in fat distribution is not well understood and the affects of highly affective antiretroviral therapy (HAART) with specific agents are debated.[7,8] Clinical assessment of lipodystrophy is usually based on history and physical examination. Individuals on antiretroviral treatment regimens are monitored for early detection of fat redistribution, with alteration in the drug regimen as needed. No uniform standard criteria exist for establishing or grading lipodystrophy. Dual-energy x-ray absorptiometry (DEXA), CT, and/or MRI have been used to characterize the fat redistribution and may provide an objective means for follow-up but at present are mostly employed in research settings. Studies of insulin-sensitizing agents are underway. Surgical interventions include liposuction, lipotransfer, and filling agents.

HIV wasting syndrome is defined as involuntary weight loss of more than 10% of baseline body weight plus either chronic diarrhea or chronic weakness, and documented fever, in the absence of a concurrent illness or condition other than HIV infection.

Despite the fact that the incidence of new wasting has declined, loss of weight is common in HIV-infected patients, even in populations with widespread access to HAART, and severely affects people living with HIV/AIDS in the nonprivileged parts of the world ("slimming disease"). Classic wasting must be differentiated from lipodystrophy/lipoatrophy and from the rapid weight loss often observed in lactic acidosis. Cachexia may be demonstrated on cross-sectional imaging, but imaging is not helpful.

Inflammation of Hoffa's fat pad in patients has been described in people living with HIV/AIDS. The MRI appearance is nonspecific, and the etiology is unclear.[9]

Pathology

Individuals with HIV/AIDS may demonstrate altered marrow signal on MRI. In addition to possible marrow neoplasm or infection, patients with advanced HIV/AIDS often have multifactorial hematopoietic dysfunction.[10] Late in the course of HIV this can manifest with low serum iron and "reticuloendothelial iron blockade," with increased ferritin, and with storage iron in the marrow macrophages, despite low to normal serum levels of iron and total iron-binding capacity. On T1-weighted MR images, red marrow may appear isointense or lower in signal intensity than

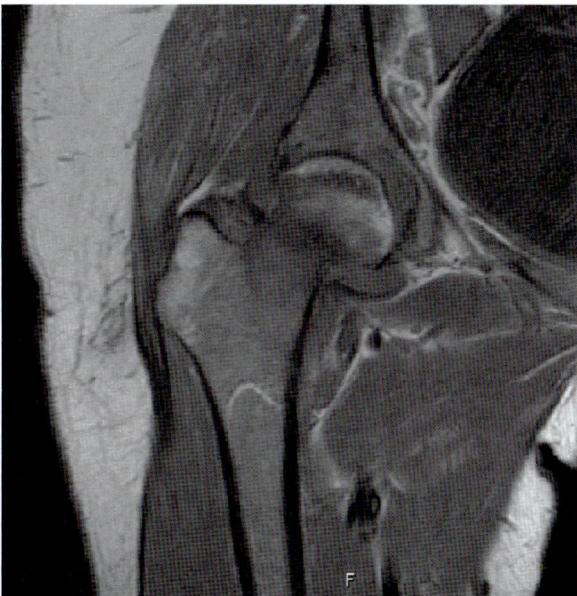

■ **FIGURE 67-1** T1-weighted coronal MR image of the right hip in a young woman with AIDS. In addition to avascular necrosis with femoral head collapse and a femoral neck fracture, abnormal low signal intensity throughout the right hemipelvis and proximal femur indicates anemia of chronic disease with reticuloendothelial iron blockade. The fat signal within the trochlear apophysis and the femoral epiphysis is relatively spared.

disc and muscle (Fig. 67-1). This reflects the normocytic/normochromic anemia of chronic disease in people living with HIV/AIDS. Additionally, there might be secondary hemosiderosis due to repeated blood transfusions.

Patients with advanced cachexia (due to HIV/AIDS, anorexia, malabsorption) may develop serous atrophy, which is gelatinous transformation of marrow. At imaging, multiple gelatinous foci, eventually coalescing, replace marrow fat. On MRI, serous atrophy changes show intramedullary bright signal on fluid-sensitive sequences and, in contradistinction to metastatic disease, begin in the appendicular skeleton, progressing axially.[11]

IMAGING TECHNIQUES

Techniques and Relevant Aspects

The imaging workup of musculoskeletal complaints in people living with HIV/AIDS is identical to the routine imaging evaluation of any other individuals with infection, joint disease, or tumor; however, the differential considerations are expanded. Especially in the setting of infection, which may be aggressive and/or life threatening in people living with HIV/AIDS, the radiologist's diagnostic reflexes must be acute.

Radiography

Imaging for musculoskeletal complaints in people living with HIV/AIDS usually begins with plain radiographs. In the setting of suspected infection radiographs may reveal soft tissue swelling, gas, and cortical indistinction and/or destruction. In acute osteomyelitis radiographs may lag behind clinical findings by up to 2 weeks; therefore, cross-sectional or nuclear medicine imaging may be warranted. Radiographic examination of fasciitis and muscle infection is limited in its sensitivity but may reveal swelling and blurring of soft tissue planes and, in some cases, soft tissue gas. The usual radiographic findings of septic arthritis include soft tissue swelling and joint effusion, with or without erosions and cartilage loss. Arthrocentesis is usually required to establish the diagnosis. An indolent history of a swollen boggy joint, with calcifications and associated fluid collections (abscess, bursitis, tenosynovitis) favors the diagnosis of infection with *Mycobacterium tuberculosis*.[12] In the setting of fungal or tubercular involvement of joints, plain film findings of effusion and periarticular osteopenia are subtle and not pathognomonic. This radiographic appearance may be mistaken for rheumatoid arthritis. Because tubercular exudate is not proteolytic, cartilage loss and erosions develop late.

Findings on radiographs of HIV/AIDS-related spondyloarthropathies (psoriatic and reactive arthritis) are comparable to those seen in cohorts without HIV/AIDS. With both entities the feet are involved more often than the hands.

Radiographs of musculoskeletal tumors such as non-Hodgkin's lymphoma may demonstrate suggestive but nonspecific findings such as periosteal reaction, frank or subtle osteolysis, sclerosis, and paraosseous soft tissue mass. Kaposi sarcoma in the extremities may present as soft tissue swelling and mass. Kaposi sarcoma uncommonly invades bone, which is potentially a differentiating point from bacillary angiomatosis. Bacillary angiomatosis is an infection that can present as foci of osteomyelitis in 25% of cases, with radiographic appearance of multifocal well- or indistinctly-marginated lytic lesions with cortical and medullary involvement.

Cross-Sectional Imaging

Radiographic findings are delayed in the setting of acute osteomyelitis and are limited for the examination of soft tissue infection and masses. Therefore, if there is clinical suspicion, cross-sectional imaging is often employed. Cross-sectional imaging can demonstrate the compartments involved, allowing the radiologist to distinguish between superficial infection such as cellulitis, which is usually treated medically, from deeper infection at the fascial, subfascial, and osseous level, which may require surgical intervention.[13] CT has the advantage of being expedient, available, and rapidly performed in emergency settings. It is useful for revealing calcifications (e.g., in musculoskeletal tuberculosis), multiple osteolytic lesions (e.g., in bacillary angiomatosis), and soft tissue gas and abscesses and discretely depicts the sequestra in active, chronic osteomyelitis.

MRI provides better tissue contrast than CT in the study of muscles, joint structures, tumors, and marrow. MRI, however, may not be as available as CT in the urgent setting. CT and MRI are often complementary (for example, for the examination of musculoskeletal tuberculosis and bone tumors). With musculoskeletal infection the axial images best delineate the compartment(s) involved, from the surface to the deep structures, from skin to bone. If either tumor or infection is suspected, contrast enhancement with CT or MRI increases conspicuity of lesions, including delineation of tracts, collections, and extent of soft tissue involvement. Enhanced MR images can be used to differentiate vascularized from devitalized and/or necrotic tissue. It is always necessary to ascertain that the patient has adequate renal function and/or glomerular filtration rate before contrast medium administration. Abscesses in any compartment, bursitis, and tenosynovitis are well depicted on axial images, with the conspicuity of the capsule or pseudocapsule increased by the administration of a contrast agent. Cross-sectional imaging is useful to plan and guide aspiration and drainage. Either CT or MRI is employed to study pyomyositis, which manifests as muscle edema and small abscesses.

The excellent tissue contrast of MRI makes this a sensitive method for the examination of marrow abnormalities, including infections. The MRI finding of marrow edema is nonspecific and is also seen with trauma, tumor, and metabolic disorders. The primary findings of geographic low T1-weighted signal intensity of the marrow, periosteal reaction, and cortical disruption and the secondary findings of ulcers, tracts, phlegmons, and abscesses in the vicinity of bone involvement support the diagnosis of osteomyelitis. Bacillary angiomatosis is a specific form of osteomyelitis seen in people living with HIV/AIDS. On MRI this is manifested as vascularized soft tissue masses, occasionally with osteolytic lesions, showing low signal intensity on T1-weighted images and high signal on T2-weighted images.

Nuclear Scintigraphy

Three-phase technetium-99m methylene diphosphonate (MDP) scintigraphy is a sensitive technique for the detection of osteoblastic metastases and skeletal infection but has limited specificity and suboptimal resolution. Scintigraphy with gallium-67 and/or indium-111–labeled white blood cells may complement bone scintigraphy and often increases specificity for osteomyelitis. Gallium scintigraphy is more sensitive than indium scintigraphy for imaging infection of the spine. Indium-111 white blood cell scans can be combined with sulfur colloid imaging for improved specificity in cases in which normal bone marrow distribution has been altered (e.g., postsurgical imaging or superinfection in a neuroarthropathic foot).

Positron Emission Tomography

Positron emission tomography with fluorodeoxyglucose (FDG-PET) is an important imaging tool in the evaluation of malignancy. In the assessment of the patient with non-Hodgkin's lymphoma, FDG-PET is both sensitive and specific for evaluation of nodal disease. However, specificity is limited in lesions of the bone marrow in patients receiving colony-stimulating factors. Infectious and inflammatory conditions may also demonstrate significant uptake of FDG. This method is of limited specificity in the assessment of infected prostheses, but initial studies have shown potential use in the assessment of vertebral osteomyelitis. FDG-PET or PET/CT may potentially assume increasing importance in examining musculoskeletal infection in the future as scanners will become more available and the imaging findings in infection are further being refined.[14]

Ultrasonography

Ultrasonography can play an important role in the imaging workup of musculoskeletal disorders in people living with HIV/AIDS. This technique has the advantage of being portable and practical at the bedside and allows for real-time and dynamic imaging (e.g., tendon disorders). Ultrasonography can be used to define the extent and depth of involvement with infection and to demonstrate abscesses, bursae, and tenosynovitis. Its use is limited for the examination of marrow infection or infiltration, but it can depict cortical breakthrough and periostitis. If a baseline MRI had been performed to evaluate osteomyelitis or soft tissue infection, ultrasonography is useful for follow-up response to treatment. Ultrasonography can be employed to guide aspiration and biopsy of infectious and neoplastic lesions. Power Doppler imaging can elucidate the vascularity of lesions.

Pros and Cons

In the urgent or emergent setting in people living with HIV/AIDS, the fastest and most available cross-sectional modality (CT) usually is chosen over the optimal soft tissue contrast of MRI. MRI and CT are complementary in many circumstances; for example, in assessment of vertebral tuberculosis MRI can be performed when the patient is adequately stabilized to undergo scanning.

Controversies

Although MRI and ^{99m}Tc-MDP plus indium-111 white blood cell scanning have comparable sensitivity and specificity for osteomyelitis, the overall cost of MRI may be less when the possibility of an extended hospital stay for additional scintigraphic imaging is considered.

MANIFESTATIONS OF THE DISEASE

Musculoskeletal Infection

Infection is the most common musculoskeletal presentation in people living with HIV/AIDS and in most cases encompasses the same manifestations seen with individuals without immune compromise but may be atypical in presentation and more aggressive. As in the non–HIV-infected population, the most common pathogen is *Staphylococcus aureus,* but other opportunistic organisms may be encountered (Fig. 67-2).[15] (See also Chapter 62 for further discussion of specific opportunistic agents that may involve the musculoskeletal system.)

Cellulitis, carbuncles, and furuncles represent invasion of pathogens into the deeper layers of the skin, usually from local trauma or inflammation and rarely from hematogenous or contiguous spread of infection.[16] About 3% of all HIV admissions are related to cellulitis. The most common implicated organism (>50% of cases) is *S. aureus,* including methicillin-resistant *S. aureus* (MRSA) strains, which have increased in incidence over the past 4 years in people living with HIV/AIDS.[17] MRSA strains cause a rapidly progressive and exquisitely painful suppurative infection; patients often complain of a "spider bite." Other pathogens include *Pseudomonas* species, *Escherichia*

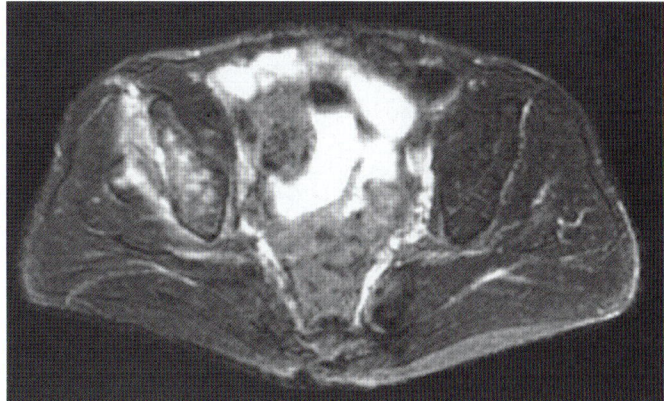

■ FIGURE 67-2 Axial T2-weighted MR image in a 49-year-old man with previously unsuspected AIDS, with right iliac osteomyelitis, indicated by marrow edema with a paraosseous tract, extending to an abscess cavity. The differential diagnosis included pyogenic, musculoskeletal tuberculosis, and fungal infection. *Nocardia* infection was established by bone biopsy, which yielded branching filamentous bacillary organisms. The majority of cases of osteomyelitis with *Nocardia* are presumed to be from direct extension of local soft tissue infection. Bone involvement from hematogenous dissemination is considered rare.

coli and other gram-negative organisms, *Streptococcus pyogenes,* and *Mycobacterium* species. *Helicobacter cinaedi* can cause a multifocal cellulitis and bacteremia,[18] while in about 40% of cases polymicrobial infection is present. In the setting of cellulitis with clinical concern for deeper involvement, cross-sectional imaging is helpful to characterize or exclude deep/subfascial infection. Treatment consists of surgery for incision and drainage of large abscess cavities or débridement of necrotic tissue, along with oral or parenteral antibiotics, preferably with activity against *Staphylococcus,* including MRSA.

Abscesses, Bursitis, Tenosynovitis

Most abscesses are the result of suppuration of a community-acquired cellulitis or of hematogenous spread of bacterial infection. The organisms involved are as those cited earlier for cellulitis, and treatment requires prompt incision and drainage by the surgical team or drainage by a large-bore catheter inserted under CT guidance, which is a priority because most appropriate antibiotics even administered intravenously are not as effective within abscess cavities (Fig. 67-3). In the setting of profound immunocompromise, tenosynovitis may permit infection to track extensively within an extremity (Fig. 67-4). When suppurative tenosynovitis is encountered, imaging should encompass an adequate field of view to ensure that all foci of infection are detected. Septic bursitis is usually due to *S. aureus* (especially in intravenous drug users) or *Streptococcus* species, presenting most commonly in the prepatellar, trochanteric, or olecranon bursae. Incision and drainage along with antibiotics is effective therapy.

Necrotizing Fasciitis

Necrotizing fasciitis is commonly preceded by trauma or intravenous drug use in people living with HIV/AIDS. It is a rapidly progressive infection accompanied by severe

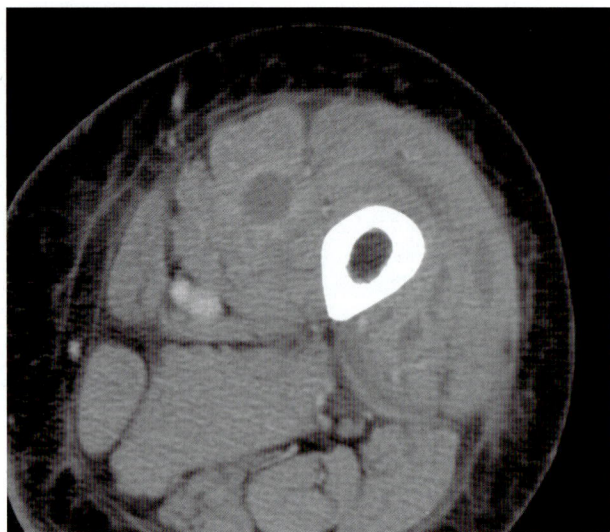

■ **FIGURE 67-3** Pyomyositis. Axial CT image (with contrast) of the left thigh demonstrates intramuscular abscesses with enhancing margins in the vastus lateralis and medialis muscles and intermuscular fluid collections between the vastus intermedius and rectus muscles.

systemic toxicity, caused by mixed aerobic and anaerobic infection, including *Clostridium* species with gas formation along fascial planes, and can be fatal if not promptly diagnosed and treated. Clinically, the patient's pain is out of proportion to the objective findings of fever and brawny edema. When employed, imaging should be expedient but should not delay surgical exploration if the diagnosis is suspected (Fig. 67-5). Cross-sectional imaging demonstrates fascial thickening with or without enhancement, fluid along fascial septa, muscle edema, occasional soft tissue gas, and associated collections. Necrotic muscle is low in attenuation on CT. Lack of enhancement is seen on MRI in nonviable foci. Antibiotics are not effective unless the necrotic tissue is extensively débrided; hyperbaric oxygen therapy may provide some benefit.

Pyomyositis

Although bacterial myositis was formerly considered rare outside the tropics the incidence has been rising recently in the West because this is a fairly common entity in people living with HIV/AIDS. Pyogenic myositis is most com-

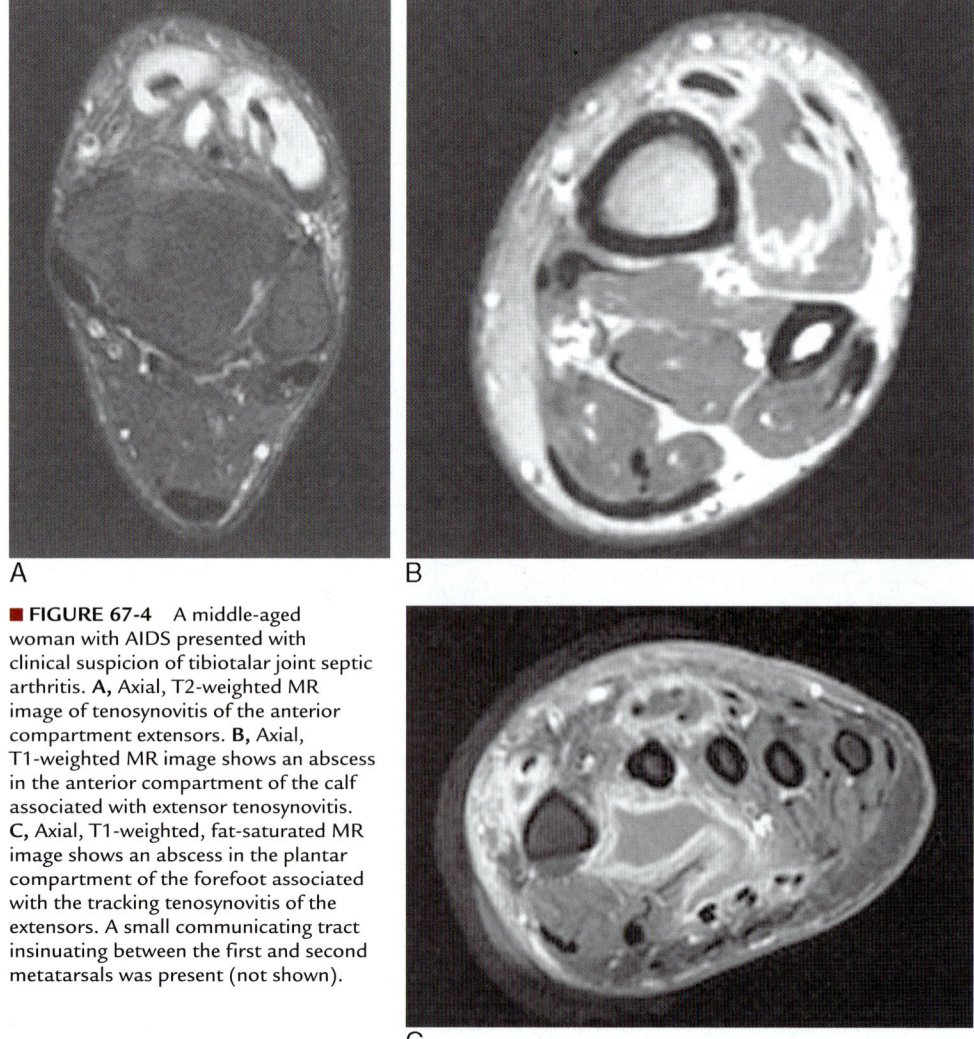

A

B

C

■ **FIGURE 67-4** A middle-aged woman with AIDS presented with clinical suspicion of tibiotalar joint septic arthritis. **A,** Axial, T2-weighted MR image of tenosynovitis of the anterior compartment extensors. **B,** Axial, T1-weighted MR image shows an abscess in the anterior compartment of the calf associated with extensor tenosynovitis. **C,** Axial, T1-weighted, fat-saturated MR image shows an abscess in the plantar compartment of the forefoot associated with the tracking tenosynovitis of the extensors. A small communicating tract insinuating between the first and second metatarsals was present (not shown).

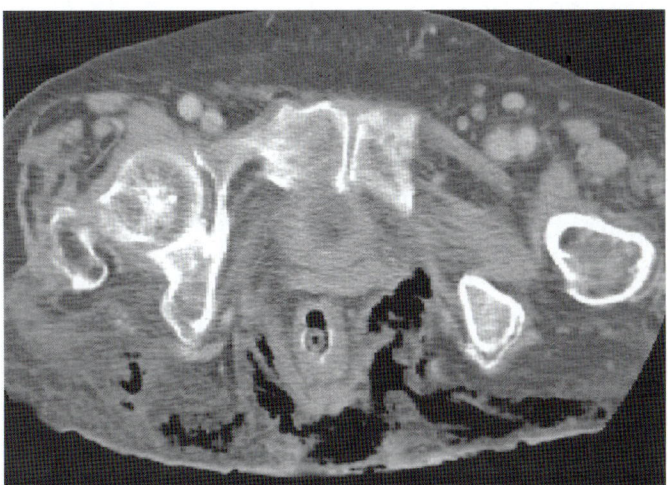

■ FIGURE 67-5 A middle-aged woman with profound sepsis presented with clinical suspicion of appendicitis. Axial CT image of the pelvis with enhancement shows necrotizing fasciitis, with gas tracking within the soft tissues of the buttocks, ischiorectal fossae, and paraspinal muscles and fascia.

monly seen in the thigh or buttocks, most commonly in the quadriceps muscles. In people living with HIV/AIDS, pyomyositis is mostly seen in males (95% of cases) with CD4 count less than 100 cells/mm³; pyomyositis is also seen in the context of diabetes or other systemic illnesses. Pyomyositis is characterized as a multifocal suppurative abscess-forming infection of the muscles presenting as local tenderness and stiffness ("woody induration"), associated with fever, leukocytosis, and systemic symptoms. The skin and subcutis are relatively unaffected. Initially, there is a stage of inflammatory myositis followed by myonecrosis and abscess formation. A history of preceding intravenous drug abuse, local trauma, or exercise is

common. Intravenous antibiotics are effective if instituted early. Blood cultures are positive in 20% to 50% of patients; by far the most common pathogen isolated is *S. aureus,* followed by *Streptococcus* and *Salmonella* species. *M. tuberculosis* and numerous opportunistic organisms have been described.[19-21] CT of pyogenic myositis shows muscle enlargement and decreased attenuation of edematous muscle; contrast enhancement may reveal intramuscular collections/abscesses. MRI better depicts the muscle edema, and contrast reveals the microabscesses (Fig. 67-6). MRI or CT is helpful in defining the extent of infection and guiding the drainage of the infected areas, and ultrasonography is useful for follow-up. Treatment is surgical drainage and long-term therapy with appropriate antibiotics.

Septic Arthritis

The most common predisposing factor in the Western world is intravenous drug use, followed by hemophilia. It presents as monarthritis in more than two thirds of the cases, involving a peripheral joint (knee, wrist, hip, shoulder, sternoclavicular joint, ankle and metacarpophalangeal joints), but the spine is also affected in a third of cases. The most commonly implicated organisms are *S. aureus* in 30%, atypical mycobacteria (*M. haemophilum, M. kansasii, M. avium complex, M. terrae*), *Salmonella* species, *Streptococcus* species (including *S. pneumoniae*), fungi, and *M. tuberculosis* (Fig. 67-7). In cases of prosthetic joint infections, an indolent organism such as coagulase-negative *Staphylococcus* is most commonly implicated. Fever, leukocytosis-localizing signs of inflammation, and extreme pain are common, especially with native joint infections. Septic arthritis is usually hematogenous in people living with HIV/AIDS owing to intravenous drug abuse; blood cultures are posi-

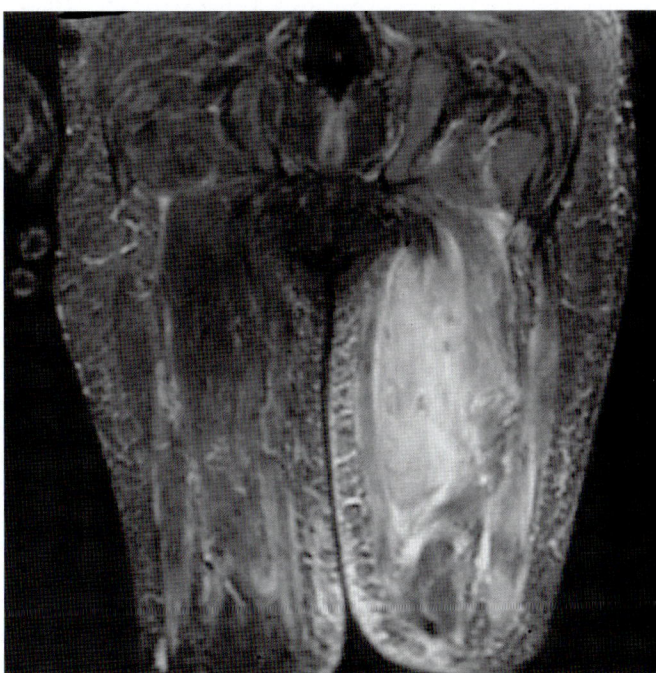

A

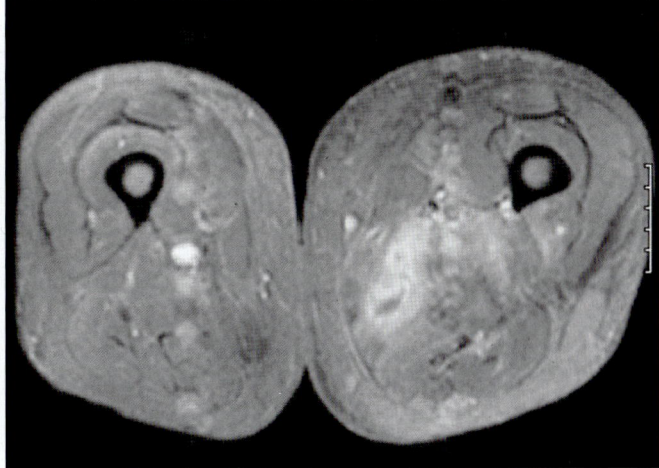

B

■ FIGURE 67-6 A young patient with AIDS presented with fever and swelling of the left thigh. **A,** Coronal inversion recovery MR image shows extensive edema in the adductor compartment. **B,** Axial, T1-weighted MR image with fat saturation, after intravenous administration of gadopentetate dimeglumine, shows enhancement of the adductor brevis muscle and a small abscess collection with enhancing margins.

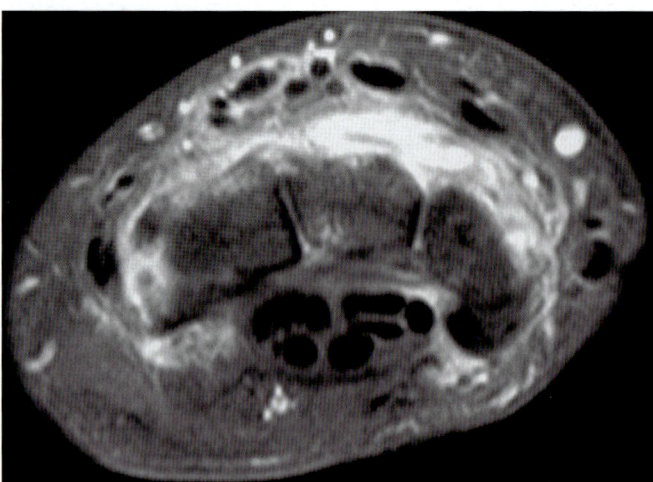

■ **FIGURE 67-7** Musculoskeletal tubercular septic joint. Axial, T2-weighted MR image of the wrist demonstrates wrist effusion, synovitis, small bone erosions, and tenosynovitis.

tive in about 40% of cases. It is not clear whether people living with HIV/AIDS have a higher incidence of septic arthritis or if the septic arthritis is related to concomitant risk factors (e.g., intravenous drug abuse); however, the spectrum of pathogens is more diverse in HIV infection and the prognosis can be worse.

Imaging is important to assess the extent of infection and the number of associated abscess cavities that need to be drained and to assist in aspiration of difficult-to-access spaces; occasionally, joints can be irrigated via a catheter placed by interventional radiology.

Ultrasonography is useful for the assessment of associated bursitis and tenosynovitis.

The diagnosis of septic arthritis is confirmed by analysis of the synovial fluid, which is critical for Gram stain and cultures (60% are positive) to guide intravenous antibiotic therapy. Since in most cases rapid destruction of the joint space can ensue, prompt arthrotomy and irrigation of the affected joint is essential. In prosthetic joint infections, removal of the prosthesis and interval placement of antibiotic-laced spacers is usually warranted to manage the infection.[22,23]

Osteomyelitis (Nontuberculous)

Acute osteomyelitis often involves the axial skeleton in people living with HIV/AIDS, usually presenting in patients with lower CD4 counts than those with septic arthritis. Infecting organisms can reach the bone by hematogenous dissemination, contiguous spread, and trauma/wound/direct inoculation. Atypical mycobacteria are commonly isolated, followed by *S. aureus* (most often associated with intravenous drug use), *Streptococcus* species, *Candida*, other fungi including endemic ones (*Coccidioides immitis*) and gram-negative organisms. Because blood cultures are positive only in 20%, bone biopsy, open débridement, and cultures may be needed to guide therapy.

Acute bacterial osteomyelitis of the spine usually presents as discitis extending subsequently to adjacent vertebral bodies, in contradistinction to tuberculous spondylitis, which involves the disc late. MRI is helpful in identifying the extent of infection of marrow and in the surrounding tissues and to follow response to treatment. Bone scintigraphy can be sensitive but is not specific for infection, and gallium scanning may be employed. Depending on the infecting organisms and extent of involvement, osteomyelitis can be difficult to treat and carries a mortality rate of about 20%.[24]

Cases of bacillary angiomatosis have been described in patients with AIDS since the early 1980s. The causative organisms are *Bartonella henselae* and *B. quintana,* which also cause cat scratch disease and trench fever. Cats are the main host, and fleas are the vector. The patient presents with fever, anemia, hepatosplenomegaly, characteristic reddish skin papules, and hemangioendothelial lesions of varying size and number. The lymph nodes, central nervous system, eyes, gastrointestinal tract, and gingiva may be involved. About 25% of cases also demonstrate underlying painful nonsclerotic osteolysis, usually without sclerosis. The skin and subcutaneous lesions resemble Kaposi sarcoma. Diagnosis is made by serology for *Bartonella* and verified by biopsy; Warthin-Starry silver stain is required for histologic confirmation. Treatment is with antibiotics.[25]

Tuberculous Osteomyelitis, Spondylitis, Spondylodiscitis

Mycobacterium tuberculosis and *M. bovis* (the two most common causes of tuberculosis) infect approximately one third of the global human population, with 2 million deaths annually as a result of tuberculosis complications.[26] The HIV epidemic and its impact on tuberculosis epidemiology, the emergence of multidrug-resistant strains, malnutrition, poverty, and increasing urban population concentration are all factors that make the control of tuberculosis difficult to achieve. The World Health Organization declared tuberculosis a global public health emergency in 1993, focusing on implementation of directly observed therapy. Humans are the only reservoir for *M. tuberculosis;* transmission of musculoskeletal tuberculosis occurs by inhalation of infectious respiratory droplet nuclei, causing primary infection, which can later reactivate. In non–HIV-infected individuals, the risk of reactivation is 5% to 15% overall, versus 7% to 10% per year for people living with HIV/AIDS. Musculoskeletal tuberculosis is the most common opportunistic infection in HIV-seropositive individuals in many countries. People living with HIV/AIDS co-infected with musculoskeletal tuberculosis have a higher rate of conversion to active disease than non–HIV-infected individuals, a shorter period of incubation, and more atypical and extrapulmonary manifestations of musculoskeletal tuberculosis, including musculoskeletal involvement, which is found in 3% to 5% of patients with tuberculosis. The majority (30%–50%) of musculoskeletal tuberculosis cases involve the spine (tuberculous spondylitis/Pott's disease), with the lower thoracic area involved more than the lumbar region and the least involvement of the cervical and sacral areas. Transmission is usually hematogenous but can also be due to contiguous disease or lymphatic spread from tuberculous pleuritis. In contradistinction to pyogenic

Classic Signs

- About one fourth of cases of bacillary angiomatosis demonstrate underlying osteolytic bone involvement, usually without sclerosis.
- Osteoarticular musculoskeletal tuberculosis infection has a nonspecific radiographic appearance, but periarticular osteopenia, calcifications, abscesses and tenosynovitis *with clinical history of indolence* support this diagnostic consideration.

spinal infection, which initially presents as discitis with adjacent vertebral body involvement, tuberculous spondylitis characteristically insinuates along the anterior longitudinal ligament and then infiltrates the vertebral body. With time, spread to the adjacent disc and vertebrae occurs. Paraspinal "cold" abscesses develop in 50%, which can track along tissue planes and present as masses in remote areas (supraclavicular, inguinal, popliteal, posterior iliac). Aspiration of abscesses yield a paucity of bacilli, but biopsy can reveal bone marrow granulomas in about 75% of cases. In uncomplicated cases of Pott's disease, response rates to systemic chemotherapy and bed rest until pain resolves exceeds 90%. Surgical intervention including laminectomy is helpful for neurologic complications and for advancing defects and/or significant spinal instability.

Extravertebral tuberculous infection can occur in any bone or joint (most commonly in the large weight-bearing joints) and should be considered in people living with HIV/AIDS, particularly with low CD4 count, indolent history of bone or joint involvement, and atypical soft tissue or skeletal lesions. The findings of periarticular osteopenia, soft tissues abscess, and calcifications support this diagnosis. Diagnostic delay with osteoarticular tuberculosis is the unfortunate norm. Radiologists need to bear in mind that tuberculosis is 200 times more likely to occur in people living with HIV/AIDS and to have atypical, extrapulmonary and disseminated manifestations of tuberculosis than in noninfected individuals.

Related Inflammatory Conditions: Arthritides, Polymyopathies

A number of arthritides and arthralgias including entities that may be unfamiliar to radiologists are seen in people living with HIV/AIDS.[27-32] These include HIV-associated arthritis, painful articular syndrome (severe pain, short duration, self-limited, usually of the knees), and acute symmetric polyarthropathy. These show minimal changes at radiography and may not be imaged. Classification of arthritis in people living with HIV/AIDS can be difficult because these patients often present with incomplete or atypical manifestations of rheumatologic disease.

Psoriatic Arthritis

The incidence of psoriatic arthritis (with or without psoriatic skin changes) is 10 to 40 times more common in people living with HIV/AIDS than in the noninfected population, with a reported prevalence of 1% to 32%,[33] but severity is often greater and progresses with the disease. The cause of psoriatic arthritis in this population is not well understood. Radiographic evidence of spinal or sacroiliac joint involvement is rare. Nail changes and radiographic findings of digital "pencil in cup" deformities, single-ray involvement, erosions, and proliferative periosteal reaction may be seen. HIV-related psoriatic arthritis presents most commonly in the foot and ankle with enthesopathy and dactylitis but minimal synovitis and effusions.

Reactive Arthritis

Reactive arthritis, formerly known as Reiter's disease, was the first rheumatologic manifestation associated with AIDS and is the most common aseptic arthritis seen in people living with HIV/AIDS, with an estimated prevalence of 5% to 10%. It is commonly associated with enteric pathogen infections. In people living with HIV/AIDS the classic triad of arthritis, urethritis, and conjunctivitis is the exception. There is no consensus of the role of HIV in the development of reactive arthritis. An asymmetric oligoarthritis of the lower extremity more so than upper extremity joints is seen, with involvement of ankle and foot most common. Plantar fasciitis, dactylitis, and enthesopathies (e.g., calcaneus, epicondyles) are demonstrated on radiographs. As for psoriatic arthritis, synovitis is uncommon. Differentiation between HIV-related psoriatic and reactive arthritis cannot be performed on the basis of radiographic appearance.[34] Treatment is with nonsteroidal anti-inflammatory agents.

Acute Symmetric Polyarthritis

Acute symmetric polyarthritis is characterized by acute onset, negative rheumatoid factor, and proliferative periosteal new bone formation. Radiographic manifestations are similar to those of rheumatoid arthritis and include alignment abnormalities of the digits, erosions, joint space narrowing, and periarticular osteopenia. Periosteal proliferation is highly suggestive of this HIV-associated arthritis and is the differentiating feature from rheumatoid arthritis.

Nonspecific Arthralgias

Nonspecific arthralgias are the most common noninfectious musculoskeletal complaint in people living with HIV/AIDS, occurring in up to 45% of patients; they often accompany primary HIV but are also seen in latency. They usually respond to mild analgesics and anecdotally improve after virologic suppression with HAART. A more severe painful syndrome of oligoarticular intermittent pain requiring narcotics for relief has also been described, occasionally associated with syphilitic infection in people living with HIV/AIDS.

Inflammatory Conditions of Muscle

Idiopathic inflammatory polymyositis, which is often seen early in the course of HIV infection (prevalence < 1%), is of unknown pathogenesis but is hypothesized to be due to viral invasion of muscle versus an autoimmune response. Patients present with heliotrope rash, bilateral proximal muscle weakness and soreness, and elevated levels of creatine phosphokinase (CPK). The diagnosis is suggested by electromyography and muscle edema without discrete/rim-enhancing collections on MRI and is verified by muscle fiber biopsy.[35]

Rhabdomyolysis is manifested as abnormal release of creatine kinase and myoglobin from insulted muscle cells into the circulation. In people living with HIV/AIDS, rhabdomyolysis may be due to the HIV itself or may be secondary to bacteremia and sepsis or to alcohol and substance abuse. Common findings include the detection of pigments in urine in association with diffuse myalgia, muscle swelling, weakness, pain, and elevated CPK levels, along with some degree of hematuria. MRI may be used to exclude infectious causes of muscle pain such as abscess and pyomyositis. Treatment is supportive and aimed at protection of the kidneys.

Inclusion-body myositis and nemaline myopathy are rare conditions, presenting as muscle weakness and wasting in people living with HIV/AIDS; the biopsy shows characteristic findings.

Diffuse infiltrative lymphocytosis syndrome, a rare condition in people living with HIV/AIDS, usually presents as painless parotid enlargement (with sicca syndrome in 60% of cases), associated with polymyositis, lymphocytic infiltration of muscles, and inflammatory myopathy. Treatment is based on HAART and corticosteroids.

Related Musculoskeletal Neoplasms

Kaposi sarcoma is the most common AIDS-associated neoplasm, previously seen in up to 20% of people living with HIV/AIDS, with recent decreasing incidence considered a direct result of HAART.[36-39] Kaposi sarcoma is usually seen in people living with HIV/AIDS with CD4 counts less than 200 cells/mm³ and in endemic form in HIV-negative individuals in the Mediterranean area. Kaposi sarcoma is a vascular-endothelial tumor related to infection with human herpesvirus type 8 (HHV8), which usually presents as multifocal hyperpigmented skin lesions. These can progress to involve the lymph nodes, mucosa of the gastrointestinal and respiratory tract, lungs, liver, and spleen and may involve contiguous muscle and bone. Bone involvement is not as common as with bacillary angiomatosis or non-Hodgkin's lymphoma. Kaposi sarcoma involving bone must be differentiated from bacillary angiomatosis and tuberculous osteitis, which they resemble radiographically with nonspecific findings of erosion and osteolysis. On MRI, lobulated subcutaneous lesions are seen that rarely extend to involve muscle and bone; Kaposi sarcoma lesions do not enhance as intensely as those of bacillary angiomatosis (Fig. 67-8). Kaposi sarcoma will uptake thallium but not gallium, which suggests the diagnosis.[40] Biopsy is necessary for definitive diagnosis.

Non-Hodgkin's lymphoma is considered one of the criteria for the diagnosis of AIDS and is the second most common neoplasm in people living with HIV/AIDS, occurring late in the disease course and associated with a low CD4 count. In this patient population, non-Hodgkin's lymphoma is more advanced and aggressive at presentation and associated with greater extranodal involvement than in non–HIV-infected individuals. Bone is affected in 20% to 30% of cases, usually lytic lesions of the long bones of the lower extremities and axial skeleton.[41] On radiographs and CT, extensive osteolysis, sclerosis, periosteal reaction, and pathologic fractures may be seen. MRI reveals any medullary infiltration and associated soft tissue masses. Biopsy is necessary for definitive diagnosis. Treatment is with chemotherapy and radiotherapy; the disease usually follows an aggressive course, with median survival at 12 months. Occasionally, adjacent or isolated muscle infiltration occurs; systemic symptoms (fever, weight loss, night sweats) are common. Other tumors that are seen in people living with HIV/AIDS that may infiltrate and/or metastasize to bone include multiple myeloma, lung, anal and cervical carcinomas, and Burkitt's lymphoma.

Kaposi sarcoma rarely invades bone, potentially a differentiating point from bacillary angiomatosis.

Musculoskeletal Complications of Antiretroviral Therapy

Zidovudine myopathy and *toxic mitochondrial myopathies* related to other nucleoside-analogue reverse-transcriptase inhibitors (NRTIs) present as proximal muscle weakness after several months of NRTI treatment; the myopathy is most likely related to mitochondrial toxicity of this class of agents. Biopsy shows multifocal necrotizing myopathy without inflammatory infiltrate, and the mitochondria reveal structural abnormalities at electron microscopy. Imaging is nonspecific. Treatment is withdrawal of the offending agent.

Immune reconstitution inflammatory syndrome presents as an adverse effect of HAART usually within 8 to 12 weeks of treatment initiation. It is believed to be due to immune restoration due to HAART and intensification of the inflammatory reaction to a preexisting opportunistic infection. Associated opportunistic infections can be musculoskeletal tuberculosis, *Mycobacterium avium* disease, cytomegalovirus end-organ disease, hepatitis B or C flares, and so on. Patients may present with fever, diffuse lymphadenopathy, and worsening of opportunistic infection symptoms. Although radiographic imaging can assist with diagnosis of lymphadenopathy (because intense contrast enhancement suggests increased nodal vascularity such as in acute infection, Kaposi sarcoma, and lymphomas), a muscle biopsy is required for diagnosis. Treatment is with corticosteroids, and, if needed, cessation of HAART.

Rarely described as a side effect of long-term protease inhibitor treatment in the shoulder joints, adhesive capsulitis presents as soreness and progressive restriction in range of motion of the shoulders; it subsides gradually with discontinuation of the offending agent.

Miscellaneous Musculoskeletal Manifestations

Avascular Necrosis

The cause of *avascular necrosis* (AVN) among people living with HIV/AIDS is not well understood; the incidence

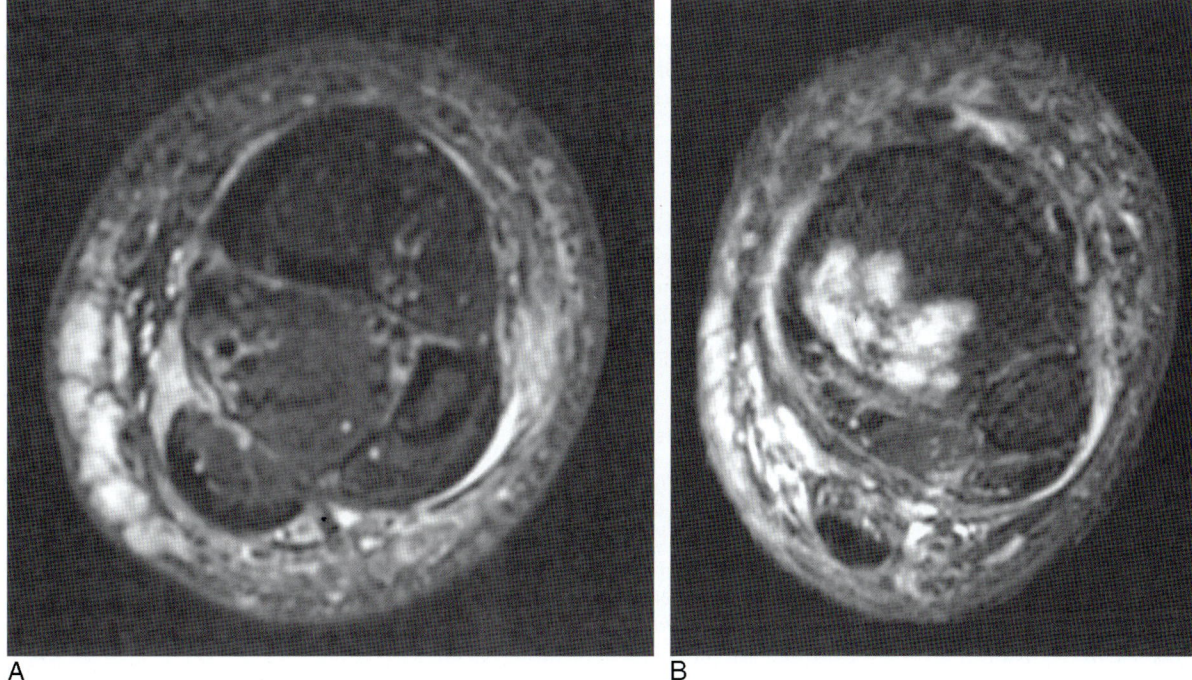

■ FIGURE 67-8 A young man presented with AIDS and skin lesions of Kaposi sarcoma. **A,** Axial, T2 weighted MR image with fat saturation shows a lobulated mass with fluid signal intensity in the posterior medial subcutaneous soft tissues of the distal calf. **B,** Axial, T2-weighted MR image with fat saturation demonstrates subcutaneous Kaposi sarcoma lesions with infiltration into the distal tibia. Osseous involvement is uncommon with Kaposi sarcoma.

has increased in the past few years in people living with HIV/AIDS but not in the general population.[42] Children with HIV/AIDS also demonstrate increased incidence of Legg-Calvé-Perthes disease.[43] Large, weight-bearing joints are involved, the lower extremity more than the upper extremity. AVN is often multiarticular and usually presents as pain with ambulation and eventually at rest. Causes advanced include corticosteroid use, hyperlipidemia, alcoholism, "hypercoagulable" state, hypergammaglobulinemia, protein S deficiency, and antiphospholipid antibodies.[44] There is poor correlation with CD4 count and suggestive but conflicting evidence of implication of HAART in the pathogenesis of AVN.[45] Advanced AVN can be detected on radiographs. MRI is the most sensitive method for detecting early changes. The management of AVN depends on stage and the clinical treatment philosophy, ranging from observation and avoidance of weight bearing in early cases to decompression and, in advanced cases, femoral capping or joint replacement (Fig. 67-9).

Osteopenia and Osteoporosis

A high prevalence (45%–70%) of decreased bone mineral density has been reported in HIV-infected individuals.[46] The cause has not been established; hypothesized causes implicate the HIV virus, protease inhibitors, nucleoside-related mitochondrial toxicity or lactic acidosis, development of lipodystrophy, immune reconstitution, nutritional and hormonal factors, prior AIDS-related wasting, and immobility. Dual-energy x-ray absorptiometry (DEXA) scans have been utilized for diagnosis and follow-up but

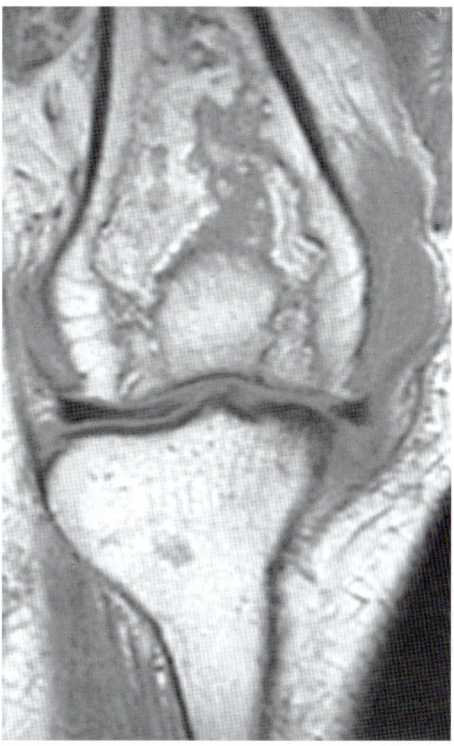

■ FIGURE 67-9 Coronal, T1-weighted MR image of the knee in a patient infected with HIV and experiencing knee pain shows extensive osteonecrosis/avascular necrosis of the distal femur, evidenced by a large lesion with geographic borders extending from the diaphysis to the articular surface. There is a minimal lateral condyle articular contour irregularity. A small infarct is present in the proximal tibial metaphysis.

are not well standardized in people living with HIV/AIDS. The management and follow-up of people living with HIV/AIDS with low bone density remains controversial, but calcium and vitamin D supplementation along with bisphosphonates is used.

Hypertrophic Osteoarthropathy

People living with HIV/AIDS with pulmonary infections such as *Pneumocystis jiroveci* or other pneumonitides may develop hypertrophic osteoarthropathy. Wavy periosteal reaction along the lower extremity tubular bones first involves the diaphysis but eventually can become more irregular and extend to the metaphysis and epiphysis.

Myositis Ossificans Circumscripta

Myositis ossificans circumscripta is focal, nonmalignant heterotopic bone and/or cartilage formation in soft tissues and muscles, which may be seen in people living with HIV/AIDS, usually with antecedent trauma/insult.

The appearance on radiographs, cross-sectional images, and scintiscans of hypertrophic osteoarthropathy and myositis ossificans is identical with findings in patients without HIV/AIDS.

SYNOPSIS OF TREATMENT OPTIONS

Further curbing of the rates of the HIV epidemic will be difficult because prevention strategies are usually underused or partially effective, a vaccine is not available, and treatment cannot so far eradicate the virus. Therefore, managing the mortality and suffering associated with the pandemic needs to be addressed primarily through provision of effective treatment. Since 1996, potent antiretroviral agents became available in the privileged parts of the world, allowing for effective and durable virologic suppression and immunologic benefits in HIV infection. As of the end of 2006, 22 agents have been approved by the U.S. Food and Drug Administration (FDA) for treatment of HIV infection, in four major therapeutic classes: (1) nucleoside and nucleotide reverse transcriptase inhibitors, (2) non-nucleotide reverse transcriptase inhibitors, (3) protease inhibitors, and (4) fusion inhibitors. Presently, there are novel agents undergoing advanced-phase clinical trials that are expected to enter the therapeutic armamentarium soon in all the above and in newer classes. Access to treatment and care has greatly increased in recent years, and the number of people living with HIV/AIDS who have access to care and treatment in nonprivileged countries in 2006 is finally surpassing those in privileged ones. The benefits of HAART are dramatically significant and well documented in both settings.[47] However, access to HAART in the areas that need it most is still significantly limited because of cost, lack of infrastructure and knowledge base for its use, local conflicts, and stigma, hence the underachievement of most of the global efforts for antiretroviral rollout so far.

What the Referring Physician Needs to Know

- In the setting of infection, the clinician needs to assess the presence and extent of deep soft tissue and/or bone involvement.
- Imaging is sought to detect the presence of a gas-forming infection, abscess, myositis, necrosis, or underlying osteomyelitis.

ACKNOWLEDGMENT

The authors would like to thank Kent Friedman, MD, Doohi Lee, MD, and Jamshid Tehranzadeh, MD, for their assistance in assembling this chapter.

SUGGESTED READINGS

Belzunegui J, Gonzalez C, Lopez L, et al. Osteoarticular and muscle infectious lesions in patients with the human immunodeficiency virus. Clin Rheumatol 1997; 16:450–453.

Bureau NJ, Cardinal E. Imaging of musculoskeletal and spinal infections in AIDS. Radiol Clin North Am 2001; 39:343–355.

Lane N. Rheumatologic and Musculoskeletal Manifestations of HIV. HIV InSite Knowledge Base (web publication), October 1998, pp 1–14.

Major NM, Tehranzadeh J. Musculoskeletal manifestations of AIDS. Radiol Clin North Am 1997; 35:1167–1189.

Marquez J, Candia L, Restrepo CS, Espinoza LR. HIV-associated musculoskeletal involvement: the AIDS reader. 2004; 14:175–179, 183–184.

Restrepo CS, Martinez S, Lemos JA, Carillo JA. Imaging manifestations of Kaposi sarcoma. RadioGraphics 2006; 26:1169–1185.

Restrepo CS, Lemos DF, Gordillo H, et al. Imaging findings in musculoskeletal complications of AIDS. RadioGraphics 2004; 24:1029–1049.

Tehranzadeh J, Raymon RT, Steinbach L. Musculoskeletal disorders associated with HIV infection and AIDS: I. Infectious musculoskeletal conditions. Skeletal Radiol 2004; 33:249–259.

Tehranzadeh J, Raymon RT, Steinbach, L. Musculoskeletal disorders associated with HIV infection and AIDS: II. Non-infectious musculoskeletal conditions. Skeletal Radiol 2004; 33:331–320.

Tehranzadeh J, O'Malley P, Rafii M. The spectrum of osteoarticular and soft tissue changes in patients with human immunodeficiency virus (HIV) infection: Crit Rev Diagn Imaging 1996; 37:305–347.

Tehranzadeh J, O'Malley P, Rafii M. The spectrum of osteoarticular and soft tissue changes in patients with human immunodeficiency virus (HIV) Infection. Crit Rev Diagn Imaging 1996; 37:305–347.

Vassilopoulos D, Chalasani P, Jurado RL, et al. Musculoskeletal infections in patients with human immunodeficiency virus infection. Medicine 1997; 76:284–294.

REFERENCES

1. Centers for Disease Control. 1993 revised classification system for HIV infection and expanded surveillance case definition for AIDS among adolescents and adults. MMWR Morbid Mortal Wkly Rep 1992; 41(RR-17):1–19.
2. WHO/UNAIDS website: http://www.who. int/hiv/mediacentre/2006_EpiUpdate_en.pdf
3. Gao F, Bailes E, Robertson DL, et al. Origin of HIV1 in the chimpanzee Pan troglodytes troglodytes. Nature 1999; 397:436–441.
4. Gurtler L. [SIV as a source of HIV: On the origin of human immunodeficiency viruses from non-human primates.] Bundesgesundheitsblatt Gesundheitsforschung Gesundheitsschutz 2004; 47:680–684. German.
5. Keele BF, Van Heuverswyn F, Li Y, et al. Chimpanzee reservoirs of pandemic and nonpandemic HIV-1. Science 2006; 313:523–526.
6. Leonard EG, McComsey GA. Metabolic complications of antiretroviral therapy in children. Pediatr Infect Dis J 2003; 22:77–84.
7. Monier PL, Wilcox R. Metabolic complications associated with the use of highly active antiretroviral therapy in HIV-1 infected adults. Am J Med Sci 2004; 328:48–56.
8. Mallon PW, Carr A, Cooper DA. HIV-associated lipodystrophy: description, pathogenesis, and molecular pathways. Curr Diab Rep 2002; 2:116–124.
9. Torshizy H, Pathria M, Chung C. Inflammation in Hoffa's fat pad in the setting of HIV: magnetic resonance findings in 6 patients. Skeletal Radiol 2007; 36:35–40.
10. Tripathi AK, Misra R, Kalra P, et al. Bone marrow abnormalities in HIV disease. J Assoc Physicians India 2005; 53:705–710.
11. Mehta K, Gascon P, Robboy S. The gelatinous bone marrow (serous atrophy) in patients with acquired immunodeficiency syndrome: evidence of excess sulfated glycosaminoglycan. Arch Pathol Lab Med 1992; 116:504–508.
12. Leigh Moore S, Rafii M. Advanced imaging of tuberculosis arthritis. Semin Musculokelet Radiol 2003;7:143–153.
13. Wu CM, Davis F, Fishman EK. Musculoskeletal complications of the patient with acquired immunodeficiency syndrome (AIDS): CT evaluation. Semin Ultrasound CT MRI 1998; 19:200–208.
14. Love C, Tomas MB, Palestro CJ. FDG PET of infection and inflammation. RadioGraphics 2005; 25:1357–1368.
15. Moore S, Jones S, Lee J. *Nocardia* osteomyelitis in the setting of previously unknown HIV infection. Skeletal Radiol 2005; 34:58–60.
16. Manfredi R, Calza L, Chiodo F. Epidemiology and microbiology of cellulitis and bacterial soft tissue infection during HIV disease: a 10-year survey. J Cutan Pathol 2002; 29:168–172.
17. Mathews WC, Caperna JC, Barber RE, et al. Incidence of and risk factors for clinically significant methicillin-resistant *Staphylococcus aureus* infection in a cohort of HIV-infected adults. J Acquir Immune Defic Syndr 2005; 40:155–160.
18. Kiehlbauch JA, Tauxe RV, Baker CN, Wachsmuth IK. *Helicobacter cinaedi*-associated bacteremia and cellulitis in immunocompromised patients. Ann Intern Med 1994; 121:90–93.
19. Crum NF. Bacterial pyomyositis in the United States. Am J Med 2004; 117:420–428.
20. Pretorius ES, Hruban RH, Fishman EK. Tropical pyomyositis: imaging findings and a review of the literature. Skeletal Radiol 1996; 25:576–579.
21. Small LN, Ross JJ. Tropical and temperate pyomyositis. Infect Dis Clin North Am 2005; 19:981–989, x–xi.
22. Small LN, Ross JJ. Suppurative tenosynovitis and septic bursitis. Infect Dis Clin North Am 2005; 19:991–1005, xi.
23. Zalavras CG, Dellamaggiora R, Patzakis MJ, et al. Septic arthritis in patients with human immunodeficiency virus. Clin Orthop Relat Res 2006; 451:46–49.
24. Weinstein MA, Eismont FJ. Infections of the spine in patients with immunodeficiency virus. J Bone Joint Surg Am 2005; 87:604–609.
25. Pape M, Kollaras P, Mandraveli K, et al. Occurrence of *Bartonella henselae* and *Bartonella quintana* among human immunodeficiency virus infected patients. Ann NY Acad Sci 2005; 1063:299–301.
26. World Health Organization: Global Tuberculosis Control: Surveillance, Planning, Financing. WHO Report 2005 (WHO/HTM/TB/2005.349). Geneva, WHO, 2005.
27. Havlir DV, Barnes PF. Tuberculosis in patients with human immunodeficiency virus infection. N Engl J Med 1999; 340:367.
28. Berman A, Cahn P, Perez H, et al. HIV infection associated arthritis: clinical characteristics. J Rheumatol 1999; 26:1158–1162.
29. Marquez J, Restrepo CS, Candia L, et al. Human immunodeficiency virus-associated rheumatic disorders in the HAART era. J Rheumatol 2004; 31:741–746.
30. Mody GM, Parke FA, Reveille JD. Articular manifestations of human immunodeficiency virus infection: best practice & research. Clin Rheumatol 2003; 17:265–287.
31. Solinger AM. Rheumatic manifestations of human immunodeficiency virus. Curr Rheumatol 2003; 5:205–209.
32. Cuellar ML. HIV infection-associated inflammatory musculoskeletal disorders. Rheum Dis Clin North Am 1998; 24:403–421.
33. Plate AM, Boyle BA. Musculoskeletal manifestations of HIV infection. AIDS Read 2003; 13:62–72.
34. Teranzadeh J, Tran M. Musculoskeletal imaging in AIDS. In: Medical Radiology—Diagnostic Imaging and Radiation Oncology: Radiology of AIDS. A Practical Approach. Berlin, Springer, 2001, pp 169–197.
35. Authier FJ, Gherardi RK. [Muscular complications of human immunodeficiency virus (HIV) infection in the era of antiretroviral therapy.] Rev Neurol (Paris) 2006; 162:71–81. French.
36. Cattelan AM, Calabro ML, De Rossi A, et al. Long-term clinical outcome of AIDS-related Kaposi's sarcoma during highly active antiretroviral therapy. Int J Oncol 2005; 27:779–785.
37. Cattelan AM, Calabro ML, De Rossi A, et al. Acquired immunodeficiency syndrome related Kaposi's sarcoma regression after highly active antiretroviral therapy: biologic correlates of clinical outcome. J Natl Cancer Inst Monogr 2001; (28):44–49.
38. Restrepo CS, Martinez S, Lemos JA, Carillo JA. Imaging manifestations of Kaposi's sarcoma. RadioGraphics 2006; 26:1169–1185.
39. Schwartz RA. Kaposi's sarcoma: an update. J Surg Oncol 2004; 87:146–151.
40. Turoglu HT, Akisik MF, Naddaf SY, et al. Tumor and infection localization in AIDS patients: Ga- 67 and Tl-201 findings. Clin Nucl Med 1998; 23:446–459.
41. Little RF, Gutierrez M, Jaffe ES, et al. HIV-associated non-Hodgkin lymphoma: incidence, presentation, and prognosis. JAMA 2001; 285:1880–1885.
42. Tehranzadeh J, Raymon RT, Steinbach L. Musculoskeletal disorders associated with HIV infection and AIDS: II. Non-infectious musculoskeletal conditions. Skeletal Radiol 2004; 33:331–320.
43. Gaughan DM, Mofenson LM, Hughes MD, et al. Pediatric AIDS Clinical Trials Group Protocol 219 Team. Osteonecrosis of the hip (Legg-Calvé-Perthes disease) in human immunodeficiency virus-infected children. Pediatrics 2002; 109:E74-E4.
44. Allison GT, Bostrom MP, Glesby MJ. Osteonecrosis in HIV disease: epidemiology, etiologies, and clinical management. AIDS 2003; 17:1–9.
45. Mary-Krause M, Billaud E, Poizot-Martin I, et al. Risk factors for osteonecrosis in HIV-infected patients: impact of treatment with combination antiretroviral therapy. AIDS 2006; 20:1627–1635.
46. Delaunay C, Loiseau-Peres S, Benhamou CL. Osteopenia and human immunodeficiency virus. Joint Bone Spine 2002; 69:105–108.
47. Sow PS, Otieno LF, Bissagnene E, et al. Implementation of an antiretroviral access program for HIV-1-infected individuals in resource-limited settings: clinical results from 4 African countries. J Acquir Immune Defic Syndr 2006; 69:105–108.

CHAPTER

68

Atypical Mycobacterial Infection

Mihra S. Taljanovic

Mycobacterial Infection

In the 1950s the atypical mycobacteria were recognized as human pathogens. They are morphologically similar to *Mycobacterium tuberculosis* but have different colonial characteristics. Because there is no evidence of human-to-human transmission, the atypical mycobacteria do not pose public health hazards.[1,2]

ETIOLOGY

The mycobacterial organisms known to cause musculoskeletal system infections in humans are: *M. avium-intracellulare* (found in soil, water, swine, cattle, birds, and fowl), *M. xenopi* (found in water), *M. malmoense* (reservoir unknown), *M. haemophilium* (reservoir unknown), *M. ulcerans* (reservoir unknown), *M. terrae* (found in soil and water), *M. triviale* (found in soil and water), *M. gastri* (found in soil and water), *M. kansasii* (found in water, cattle, and swine), *M. marinum* (found in fish and water), *M. simiae* (found in primates and possibly water), *M. asiaticum* (found in primates), *M. scrofulaceum* (found in soil, water, and moist or liquid foodstuffs), *M. szulgai* (reservoir unknown), *M. fortuitum* (found in soil, water, animals, and marine life), *M. chelonae* (found in soil, water, animals, and marine life), *M. abscessus* (found in soil, water, animals, and marine life), *M. smegmatis* (found in soil, water, animals, and marine life), *M. phlei* (found in grass and hay), and *M. nonchromogenicum* (found in grass and hay). Most osseous infections, however, are caused by *M. kansasii* and *M. scrofulaceum,* followed in frequency by *M. avium-intracellulare* and *M. fortuitum.*[1]

PREVALENCE AND EPIDEMIOLOGY

Atypical mycobacteria account for 0.5% to 30% of all mycobacterial infections. The rate of clinical infection by atypical mycobacteria is low, because they colonize rather than invade the host. The infection of skin and lungs is most common. The involvement of the musculoskeletal system occurs in 5% to 10% of patients with atypical mycobacterial infections. Although the atypical mycobacterial infections are more commonly seen in elderly and immunocompromised patients, they can occur in a normal host.[1-18] In patients with AIDS, the atypical mycobacteria usually produce musculoskeletal infections in advanced stages of disease.[10,11]

CLINICAL PRESENTATION

Musculoskeletal infections caused by atypical mycobacteria resemble those caused by *M. tuberculosis,* although they tend to have a milder course. However, in children, atypical mycobacterial infections can be more aggressive and can result in gross disturbance. Presenting symptoms are nonspecific and include local pain and swelling, joint stiffness, low-grade fever, sweats, chills, anorexia, malaise, and weight loss. The diagnosis is frequently delayed, with average diagnosis from the onset of symptoms up to 10 months. With the disseminated infection, osseous manifestations are common.[1,2]

KEY POINTS

■ The infection is indolent.
■ Imaging characteristics are similar to those for infection with *M. tuberculosis.*
■ Antimycobacterial chemotherapy and surgical removal of the lesion are recommended.

In patients with mycobacterial spondylitis, local tenderness, pain, and limitation of spinal mobility are the presenting symptoms, whereas constitutional symptoms such as fever, malaise, and weight loss may also occur. On neurologic examination, evidence of compressive neuropathy with or without paralysis may be revealed.[1]

Dermal inoculation of atypical mycobacteria can result in soft tissue infection including skin ulcers, cellulitis, cutaneous granulomas, deep necrotizing infection, and abscesses. Septic myositis, polymyositis, septic bursitis, septic tenosynovitis, and carpal tunnel syndrome can also occur. The presenting symptoms are nonspecific and include pain, swelling, erythema, warmth, stiffness, and functional compromise.[1,7,12,18]

PATHOPHYSIOLOGY

Mechanisms of musculoskeletal infection include hematogenous spread and contamination after injury or surgery. In particular, atypical mycobacterial strains usually acquired by trauma are *M. fortuitum*, *M. chelonae*, and *M. marinum*. The gastrointestinal tract is also suggested as a portal of entry because some of the atypical mycobacteria are found in the mouth of normal persons.[1,2]

Granulomatous lesions with or without caseation are typical, but a spectrum of abnormalities can occur. The diagnosis is made by aspiration, tissue sampling, and culturing. In case the cultures are negative, DNA amplification and subsequent determination of the nucleic acid sequence have reportedly been helpful in identifying the pathogen (Figs. 68-1 and 68-2).[1,2,6]

IMAGING TECHNIQUES

Radiologic imaging techniques used in the diagnosis of atypical mycobacterial infections are radiography, CT, MRI, nuclear medicine scans, and ultrasonography.

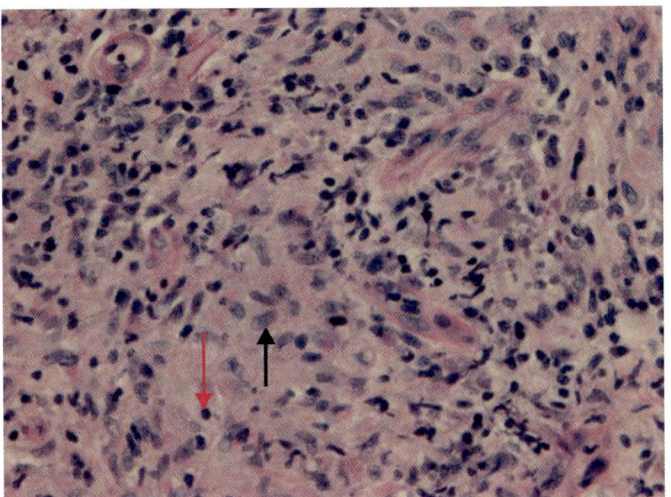

■ **FIGURE 68-1** *Mycobacterium avium-intracellulare.* Note the epithelioid cells (*black arrow*), the lack of good circumscription of the granuloma at its margin, and the small number of lymphocytes (*pink arrow*), which have failed to form a well-defined peripheral cuff. These are the hallmarks of a poorly formed granuloma characteristic of the immunocompromised patient. (Hematoxylin and eosin stain.) *(Courtesy of Anna Graham, MD, Tucson, AZ.)*

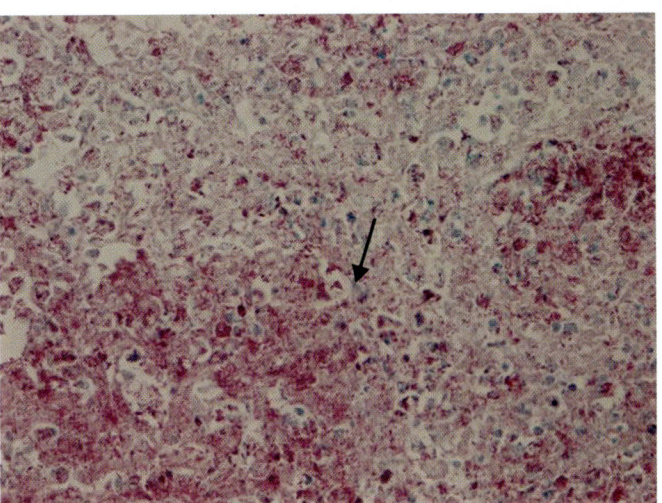

■ **FIGURE 68-2** *Mycobacterium avium-intracellulare.* Note the huge number of bright rose-pink bacilli that have been engulfed by macrophages (*black arrow*). This finding of enormous numbers of bacilli being phagocytosed by macrophages is a common finding in immunodeficient patients. (Acid-fast bacillus stain.) *(Courtesy of Anna Graham, MD, Tucson, AZ.)*

MANIFESTATIONS OF THE DISEASE

Osteomyelitis and septic arthritis caused by atypical mycobacteria resemble acute pyogenic infections but have a more indolent course. Muscles, bursae, and tendon sheaths can also be affected. Atypical mycobacteria can also cause carpal tunnel syndrome.[1-18] Penetrating trauma results in cutaneous and/or deep soft tissue infection and can also result in septic arthritis.[12,18]

Most cases of atypical mycobacterial infections in the musculoskeletal system are recognized in a subacute stage of osteomyelitis.[1-2]

Radiography

Radiography should be the initial imaging modality in evaluation of any musculoskeletal infection. The differentiation of tuberculous and atypical mycobacterial musculoskeletal infection is not possible in the majority of cases.[1-2,10]

Early radiographic findings include soft tissue swelling related to inflammatory changes, followed by bone involvement. Radiographic characteristics of atypical mycobacterial musculoskeletal infections have not been well delineated for each group. Multiple lesions predominate over solitary lesions, the metaphyses and diaphyses of long bones are commonly involved, and discrete lytic lesions may have sclerotic margins. Osteoporosis may not be as prominent as in tuberculous infection, there may be a tendency for development of abscesses and sinus tracts, and articular disease can simulate tuberculosis or rheumatoid arthritis.[1,2]

Atypical mycobacterial osteomyelitis shares similar morphologic abnormalities with tuberculous spondylitis (Pott's disease).[1,2]

The findings in mycobacterial osteomyelitis of the spine may include involvement of one or several contiguous vertebral bodies that may result in kyphosis, destruction of the intervening discs, absence of reactive sclerosis, and formation of soft tissue abscesses, usually containing calcifications. Soft tissue abscesses may extend into the epidural space or may spread into adjacent soft tissue structures. The infection may include a single end plate or noncontiguous levels.[1,2,9]

The triad of Phemister, consisting of osteoporosis, peripheral marginal erosions, and slowly progressing destruction of articular cartilage, characterizes mycobacterial arthritis. If untreated, mycobacterial arthritis can result in severe osseous destruction and fibrous ankylosis. Less frequently, a linear periostitis and bone proliferative changes may be seen.[1-2]

Magnetic Resonance Imaging

Magnetic resonance imaging is regarded as the most sensitive imaging method for the early detection of osteomyelitis and may show the absolute extent of the inflammatory process, thus contributing to preoperative planning. Infected areas demonstrate decreased signal intensity on T1-weighted sequences and increased signal intensity on T2-weighted and short tau inversion recovery (STIR) sequences. T1-weighted imaging with fat saturation after the intravenous administration of a gadolinium-based contrast medium may allow detection and delineation of the extent of epidural involvement in spinal infection, may indicate whether the infection is limited to soft tissues or to bones and joints, and may show the absolute extent of the inflammatory process and delineate abscesses, thus contributing to preoperative planning (Figs. 68-3 to 68-6).[1-2,20]

Multidetector Computed Tomography

Computed tomography is superior to radiography in depicting early cortical erosions, bone fragmentation, small fluid collections, cloacae, bone sequestra, and increased intraosseous density that corresponds to the accumulation of pus replacing bone marrow fat. Contrast-enhanced CT may also facilitate visualization of abscesses and necrotic tissue, may provide supplemental diagnostic information regarding paraspinal and intraspinal extension of infection, and may characterize the extent of bone and disc involvement, which may be not be visible on radiography. In addition, CT can be used to facilitate percutaneous biopsy of infected areas (Figs. 68-5 and 68-6).[1-2,19]

Ultrasonography

Ultrasonography may be used in diagnosis of atypical mycobacterial soft tissue infection and septic joint. It can be used to guide percutaneous aspiration, biopsy, or drainage of the infected soft tissue structures or joints. Ultrasonography has a limited value in diagnosis of osteomyelitis.[1]

Nuclear Medicine

Technetium-99m methylene diphosphonate (^{99m}Tc-MDP) scintigraphy may be useful in differentiating cellulitis from subjacent osteomyelitis. It is also useful in evaluation of multifocal infection. In patients with cellulitis, accumulation of the radionuclide in the infected area is increased during the angiographic and blood pool images of a three-phase scintiscan, whereas in patients with osteomyelitis a focal increase in the accumulation of the radionuclide is evident in all three phases of the scintiscan. ^{111}In-labeled leukocytes may be helpful in differentiating cellulitis from osteomyelitis.[1,20,21]

Positron Emission Tomography/ Computed Tomography

The value of positron emission tomography (PET) in evaluation for atypical skeletal mycobacterial infection has not been determined.

DIFFERENTIAL DIAGNOSIS

Musculoskeletal infections by atypical mycobacteria are clinically indistinguishable from those of tuberculosis, and diagnosis is usually delayed. Information regarding specific occupational history, recreational activities, and geographic region is important.[1-18]

Early radiographic findings of atypical mycobacterial osteomyelitis may be inconspicuous. Differential diagnosis includes acute pyogenic or fungal osteomyelitides, malignant bone tumors, neuropathic osteoarthropathy, reflex sympathetic dystrophy, transient regional osteoporosis, stress fractures, and healing fractures.[1]

Imaging findings of atypical mycobacterial arthritis are nonspecific. The differential diagnosis generally includes different types of synovial arthropathy, including tuberculous, pyogenic and fungal arthritides, inflammatory and metabolic arthritides, as well as pigmented villonodular synovitis, idiopathic synovial osteochondromatosis, and idiopathic chondrolysis.[1]

The differential diagnosis for mycobacterial spondylitis includes pyogenic or fungal infections, primary and metastatic tumors of the spine, and sarcoidosis.[1]

Imaging findings of atypical mycobacterial soft tissue infections are nonspecific with a broad differential diagnosis that includes tuberculous, pyogenic, and fungal infections and rheumatologic diseases. In atypical mycobacterial tenosynovitis the differential diagnosis also includes giant cell tumor of the tendon sheath.[1]

SYNOPSIS OF TREATMENT OPTIONS
Medical Treatment

Patients with tuberculosis caused by atypical mycobacteria are treated by regimens containing amikacin, a fluoroquinolone, rifabutin, clarithromycin, or clofazimine, to which they are more susceptible, along with other standard chemotherapeutic drugs. The outcome of treatment in patients with mycobacterial infections is more favorable in previously healthy individuals than in patients with underlying disease.[22]

Surgical Treatment

Antimycobacterial chemotherapy alone usually is not sufficient. Whenever possible, surgical débridement of infected tissue followed by chemotherapy is recommended.[22,23]

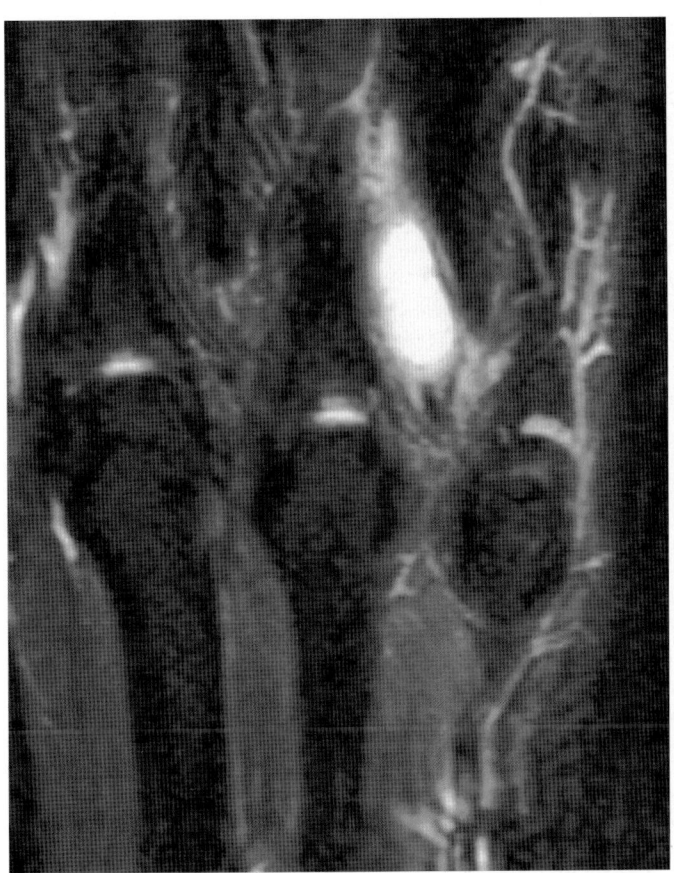

A

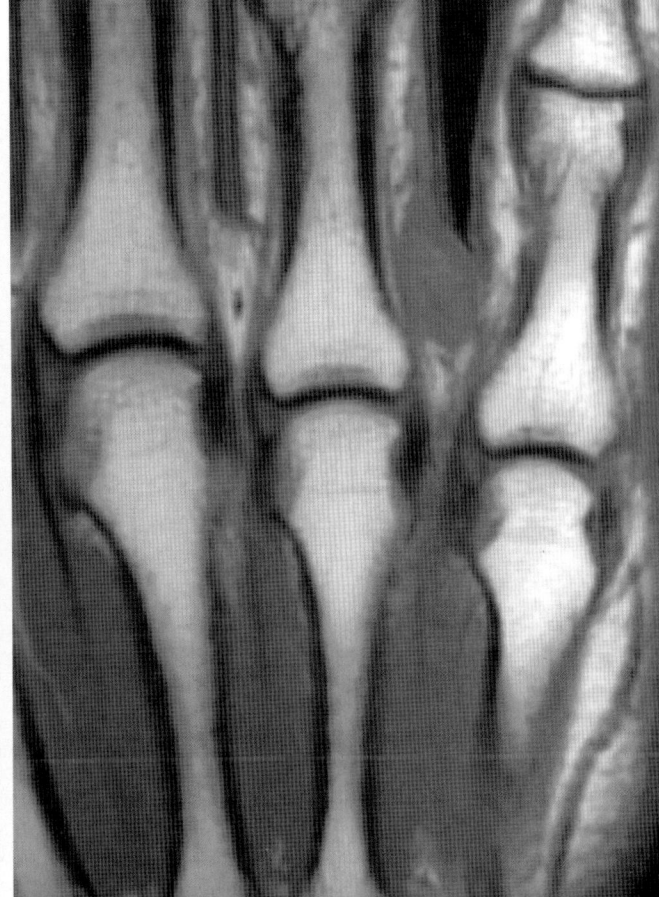

B

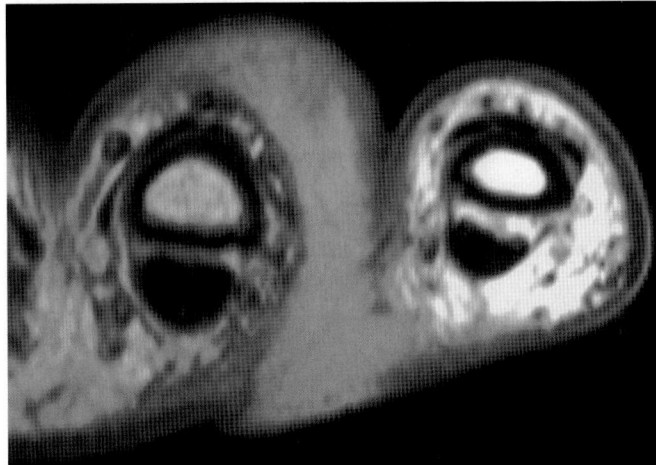

C

■ **FIGURE 68-3** *Mycobacterium marinum* infection in a fish-tank worker. **A,** Coronal T2-weighted image with fat saturation shows a well-circumscribed soft tissue lesion of high signal intensity adjacent to the ulnar aspect of the proximal fourth phalanx compatible with and proven to be a soft tissue abscess. The lesion demonstrates intermediate signal intensity on coronal (**B**) and axial (**C**) T1-weighted images. Note extension of the lesion to the skin at both dorsal and palmar aspects on the axial image. *(Courtesy of T. Berquist, MD, Jacksonville, FL.)*

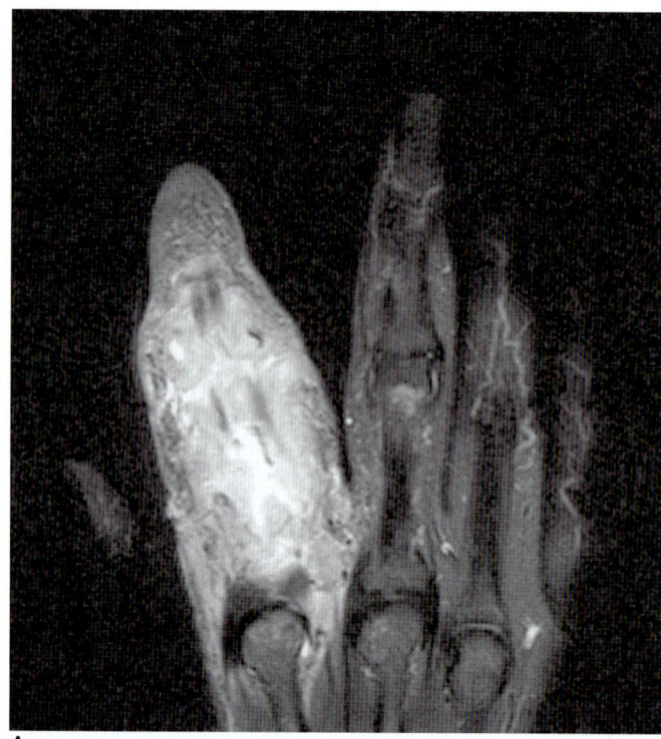

A

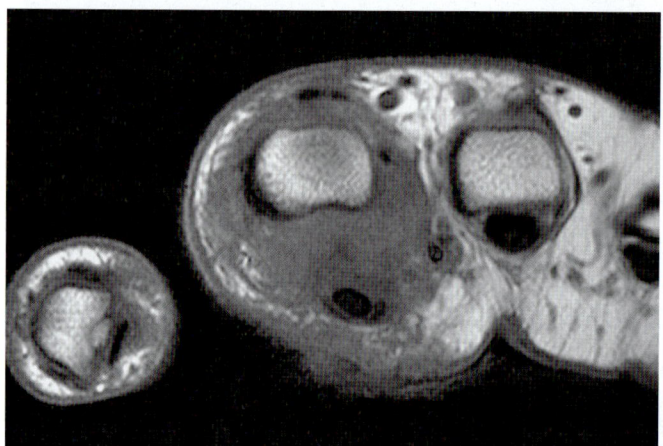

B

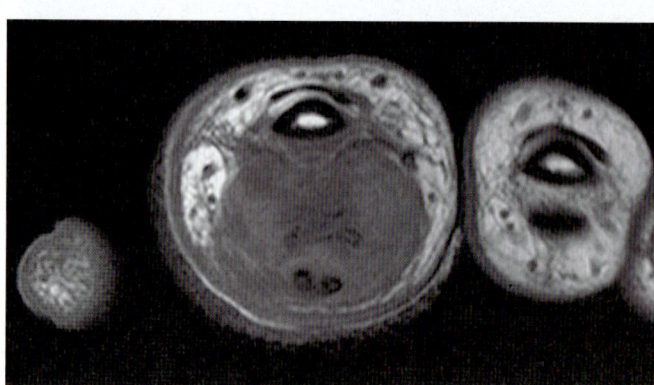

C

■ FIGURE 68-4 *Mycobacterium kansasii* infection after animal bite. **A,** Coronal T2-weighted image with fat saturation shows soft tissue swelling and increased signal intensity involving the flexor tendon sheath of the index finger consistent with tenosynovitis. **B** and **C,** Axial T1-weighted images show intermediate signal intensity within and about the distended flexor tendon sheath. **D,** Sagittal T1-weighted image with fat saturation after the intravenous administration of gadolinium-based contrast agent shows significant enhancement of the affected soft tissues with areas of nonenhancement compatible with fluid/pus. *(Courtesy of Ruth Ceulemans, MD, Chicago, IL.)*

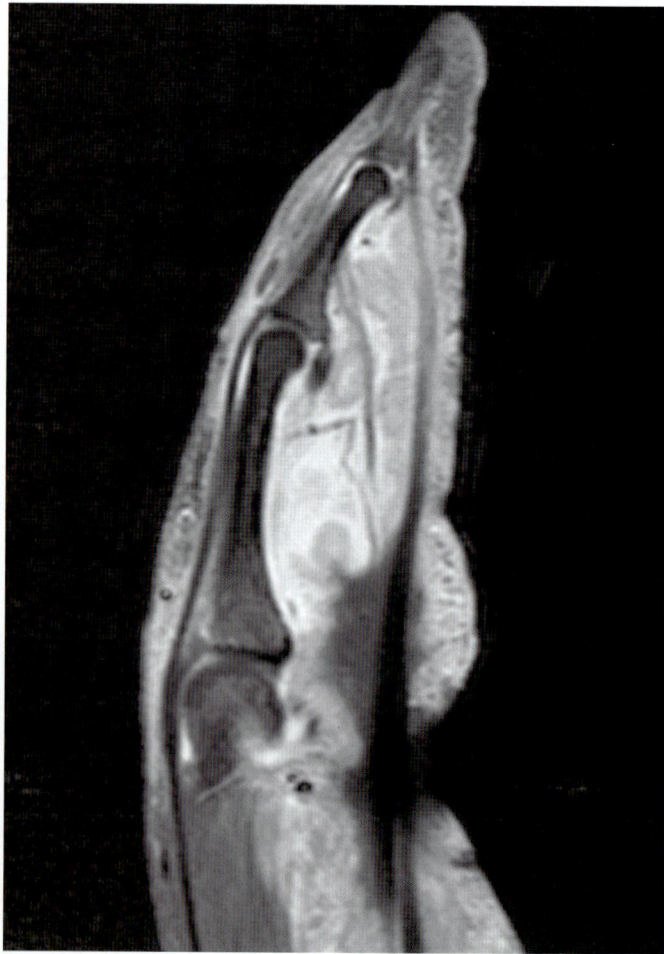

D

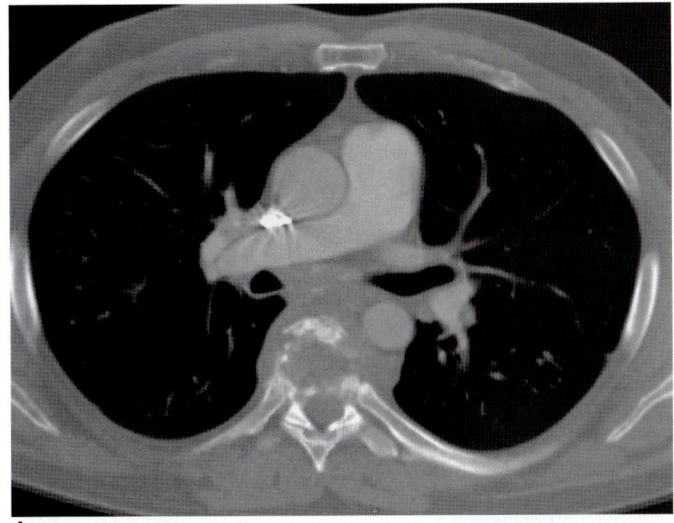

■ **FIGURE 68-5** *Mycobacterium avium-intracellulare* infection.
A, Axial CT image of the chest shows destructive changes involving the T7 vertebral body compatible with osteomyelitis. Note perispinal soft tissue thickening consistent with an abscess. T1-weighted (**B**), T2-weighted (**C**), and proton density–weighted (**D**) sagittal images of the thoracic spine in the same patient show signal abnormality involving the T7 and T8 vertebral bodies and T7–T8 disc space consistent with discitis and osteomyelitis. Note epidural extension of infection. *(Courtesy of J. Alcala, MD, Tucson, AZ.)*

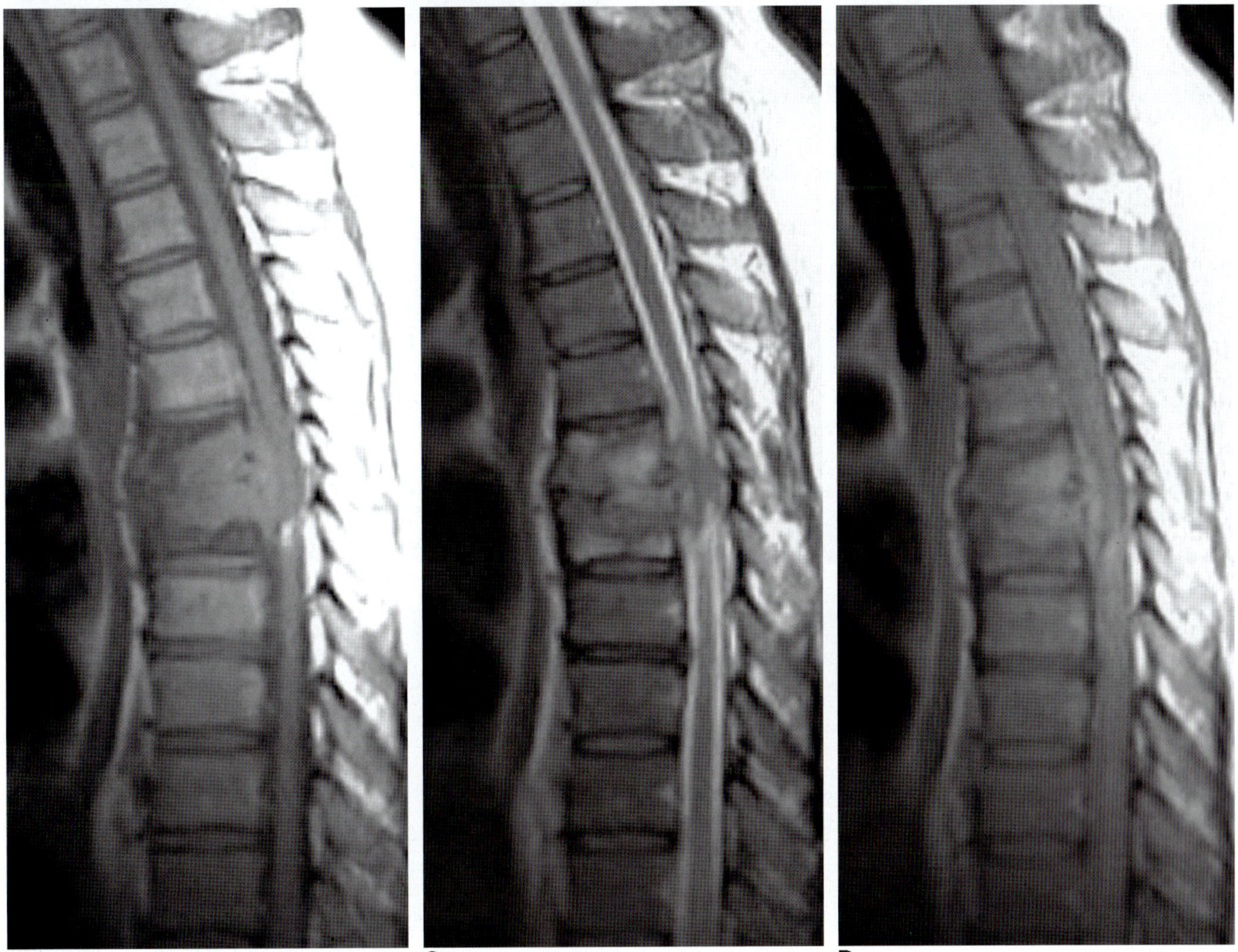

A

B

C

D

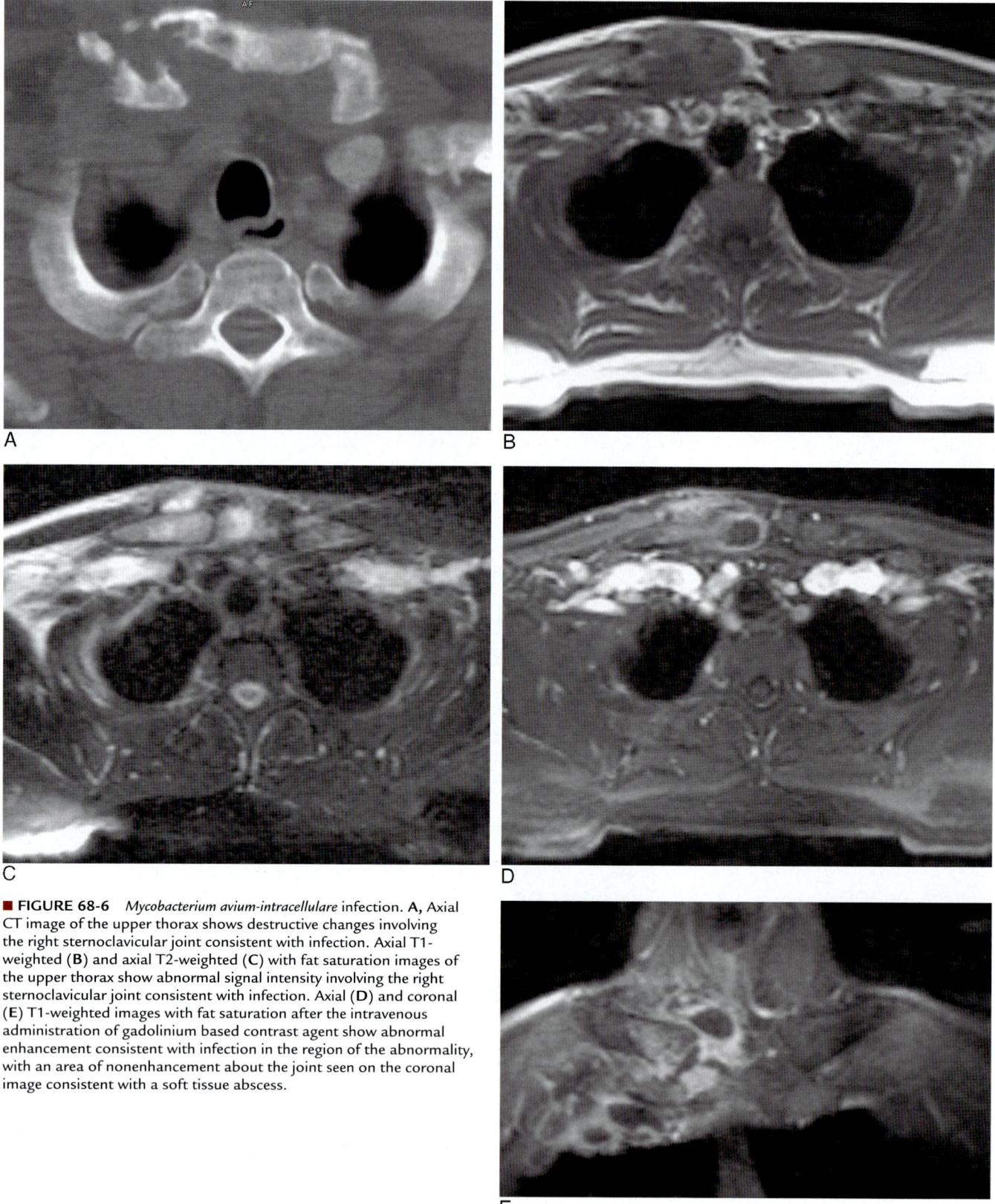

■ **FIGURE 68-6** *Mycobacterium avium-intracellulare* infection. **A,** Axial CT image of the upper thorax shows destructive changes involving the right sternoclavicular joint consistent with infection. Axial T1-weighted (**B**) and axial T2-weighted (**C**) with fat saturation images of the upper thorax show abnormal signal intensity involving the right sternoclavicular joint consistent with infection. Axial (**D**) and coronal (**E**) T1-weighted images with fat saturation after the intravenous administration of gadolinium based contrast agent show abnormal enhancement consistent with infection in the region of the abnormality, with an area of nonenhancement about the joint seen on the coronal image consistent with a soft tissue abscess.

What the Referring Physician Needs to Know

- There is no evidence of human-to-human transmission.
- The course of infection is usually indolent.
- Imaging characteristics are similar to those seen with *M. tuberculosis*.
- Tissue diagnosis is necessary.
- Antimycobacterial chemotherapy alone usually is not sufficient, and surgical removal of the lesion is recommended.

SUGGESTED READING

Theodorou DJ, Theodorou SJ, Kakitsubata Y, et al. Imaging characteristics and epidemiologic features of atypical mycobacterial infections involving the musculoskeletal system. AJR Am J Roentgenol 2001; 176:341–349.

REFERENCES

1. Theodorou DJ, Theodorou SJ, Kakitsubata Y, et al. Imaging characteristics and epidemiologic features of atypical mycobacterial infections involving the musculoskeletal system. AJR Am J Roentgenol 2001; 176:341–349.
2. Resnick D. Osteomyelitis, septic arthritis, and soft tissue infection: organisms. In Resnick D (ed). Diagnosis of Bone and Joint Disorders, 4th ed. Philadelphia, WB Saunders, 2002, pp 2510–2624.
3. Wolinsky E. Mycobacterial diseases other than tuberculosis. Clin Infect Dis 1992; 15:1–12.
4. Wolinsky E. Nontuberculous mycobacteria and associated diseases. Am Rev Respir Dis 1979; 119:107–159.
5. Hofer M, Hirschel B, Kirshner P, et al. Brief report: disseminated osteomyelitis from *Mycobacterium ulcerans* after a snakebite. N Engl J Med 1993; 328:1007–1009.
6. Marchevsky A, Damsker B, Green S, Tepper S. The clinico-pathological spectrum of nontuberculous mycobacterial osteoarticular infections. J Bone Joint Surg Am 1985; 67:925–29.
7. Kelly P, Weed L, Lipscomb P. Infections of tendon sheaths, bursae, joints and soft tissues by acid-fast bacilli other than tubercle bacilli. J Bone Joint Surg Am 1963; 45:327–336.
8. Rougraff B, Reeck C, Slama T. *Mycobacterium terrae* osteomyelitis and septic arthritis in a normal host. Clin Orthop 1989; 238:308–310.
9. Miller W, Perkins M, Richardson W, Sexton D. Pott's disease caused by *Mycobacterium xenopi*: case report and review. Clin Infect Dis 1994; 19:1024–1028.
10. Tehranzadeh J, Ter-Oganesyan RR, Steinbach LS. Musculoskeletal disorders associated with HIV infection and AIDS: I. Infectious musculoskeletal conditions. Skeletal Radiol 2004; 33:249–259. Epub 2004 Mar 18.
11. Nalaboff KM, Rozenshtein A, Kaplan MH. Imaging of *Mycobacterium avium-intracellulare* infection in AIDS patients on highly active antiretroviral therapy: reversal syndrome. AJR Am J Roentgenol 2000; 175:387–390.
12. Mateo L, Rufi G, Nolla JM, Alcaide F. *Mycobacterium chelonae* tenosynovitis of the hand. Semin Arthritis Rheum 2004; 34:617–622.
13. Corrales-Medina V, Symes S, Valdivia-Arenas M, Boulanger C. Localized *Mycobacterium avium* complex infection of vertebral and paravertebral structures in an HIV patient on highly active antiretroviral therapy. South Med J 2006; 99:174–177.
14. Girard DE, Bagby GC Jr, Walsh JR. Destructive polyarthritis secondary to *Mycobacterium kansasii*. Arthritis Rheum 1973; 16:665–669.
15. Loddenkemper K, Enzweiler C, Loddenkemper C, et al. Granulomatous synovialitis with erosions in the shoulder joint: a rare case of polyarthritis caused by *Mycobacterium kansasii*. Ann Rheum Dis 2005; 64:1088–1090.
16. van der Werf TS, Stienstra Y, Johnson RC, et al. *Mycobacterium ulcerans* disease. Bull World Health Org 2005; 83:785–791. Epub 2005 Nov 10.
17. Butorac R, Littlejohn GO, Hooper J. Mycobacterial disease in the musculoskeletal system. Med J Aust 1987; 147:388–391.
18. Barton A, Bernstein RM, Struthers JK, O'Neill TW. *Mycobacterium marinum* infection causing septic arthritis and osteomyelitis. Br J Rheumatol 1997; 36:1207–1209.
19. Sharif H, Morgan J, Shahed M, Al Thagafi M. Role of CT and MR imaging in the management of tuberculous spondylitis. Radiol Clin North Am 1995; 33:787–804.
20. Gilday D, Paul D, Paterson J. Diagnosis of osteomyelitis in children by combined blood pool and bone imaging. Radiology 1975; 117:331–335.
21. Schauwecker D. Osteomyelitis: diagnosis with In-111-labeled leukocytes. Radiology 1989; 171:141–146.
22. Shembekar A, Babhulkar S. Chemotherapy for osteoarticular tuberculosis. Clin Orthop Relat Res 2002; (398):20–26.
23. Noonburg GE. Management of extremity trauma and related infections occurring in the aquatic environment. J Am Acad Orthop Surg 2005; 13:243–253.

Brucellosis

Human brucellosis (also known as undulant fever, Mediterranean fever, Malta fever, Cyprus fever, Gibraltar fever, or typhomalarial fever) is a systemic zoonotic infection caused by gram-negative coccobacilli of the *Brucella* genus. This infection is typically transmitted by ingestion of unpasteurized milk or milk products. Brucellosis can also be transmitted through skin contact with infected tissues or secretions. Human-to-human transmission is unusual but has been reported. Brucellosis can affect any organ system.[1-3]

ETIOLOGY

The causative organisms include more virulent *B. melitensis* and *B. suis*, less virulent *B. abortus* and *B. canis*,[1] and sometimes *B. ovis*.[3] Various polymerase chain reaction/restriction fragment length polymorphisms are used for identification of *Brucella* species and biotypes.[4]

PREVALENCE AND EPIDEMIOLOGY

Brucellosis is a worldwide disease with 500,000 new cases annually. It is more prevalent in the Mediterranean basin, Arabian peninsula, Indian subcontinent, and parts of Mexico and Central and South America. This reportable disease most often affects young or middle-aged predominantly male adults and has a low incidence rate in children and the elderly. Brucellosis is an occupational risk among farmers, laboratory personnel, and veterinarians and can occur in several family members, especially with the common source of infected food.[1,5]

CLINICAL PRESENTATION

The causative organisms localize in tissues of the reticuloendothelial system, such as the liver, spleen, lymph nodes, and bone marrow. The first symptoms of brucellosis usually appear 1 to 4 weeks after inoculation. Any organ system can be affected. The presenting symptoms of brucellosis are nonspecific and include fatigue, fever, loss of appetite, nausea, and diarrhea and are more common in the acute stage of disease. Weight loss, palpitations, and osteoarticular symptoms are more common in the chronic stage of brucellosis, whereas sweating, headache, abdominal pain, psychiatric disorders, cutaneous lesions, and pulmonary symptoms are equally common in acute, subacute, and chronic stages.[1,2]

An elevated erythrocyte sedimentation rate, anemia, elevated level of serum C-reactive protein, and elevated transaminase levels are observed. The diagnosis is made by serologic testing with rising serum agglutination titer or by clinical symptoms combined with a positive blood culture. Culture of the organisms from the tissues, joint, or bursal aspirate confirms the diagnosis.[1,2]

Osteoarticular involvement is the most common complication of chronic brucellosis, and its incidence varies significantly in the literature, ranging from 5% to greater than 85%.[3] Bones, joints, and bursae can be involved. The most common form of musculoskeletal brucellosis is brucellar spondylodiscitis, with the most frequent involvement that of the lumbar spine. Other regions of the spine and multiple sites of spinal involvement may be encountered. Subligamentous spread of disease is not a characteristic of spinal brucellosis. With spinal disease an acute clinical onset and rapid progression of radiologic findings are observed.[1-3]

Brucellar arthritis is usually monoarticular or pauciarticular, with the hip and knee joints the most frequently involved peripheral joints. Unilateral or bilateral involvement of sacroiliac joints is common. Sternoclavicular joints can also be involved. Osteomyelitis can affect the long, short, and flat bones. It is frequently chronic, and the bony structures may be secondarily infected by staphylococci.[2] Avascular necrosis secondary to brucellosis is extremely rare and has been reported in the femoral head.[1] The most commonly affected bursa is the prepatellar bursa.[2]

PATHOPHYSIOLOGY

Histologic examination of the synovial membrane reveals granulomatous tissue, cellular infiltration with large or small mononuclear cells, and granulomatous formation. Bone biopsy specimens may show granulomatous osteomyelitis.[2] Noncaseating granulomatous tissue and chronic inflammation are characteristic histologic features of spinal brucellosis.[3]

IMAGING TECHNIQUES
Radiography

Radiographic findings of brucellar spondylodiscitis resemble those of pyogenic or tuberculous infection and include destructive changes of the affected vertebrae

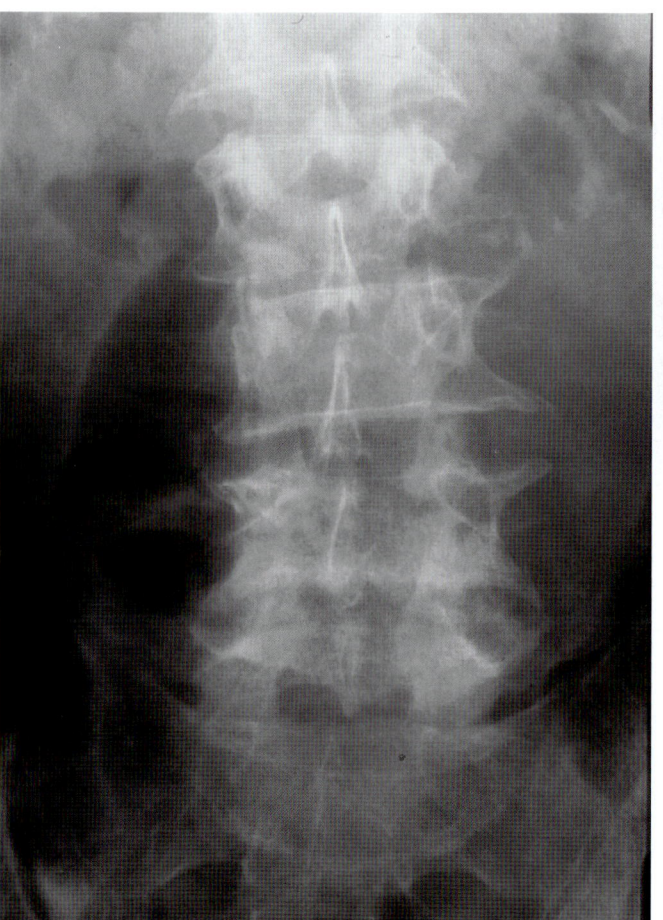

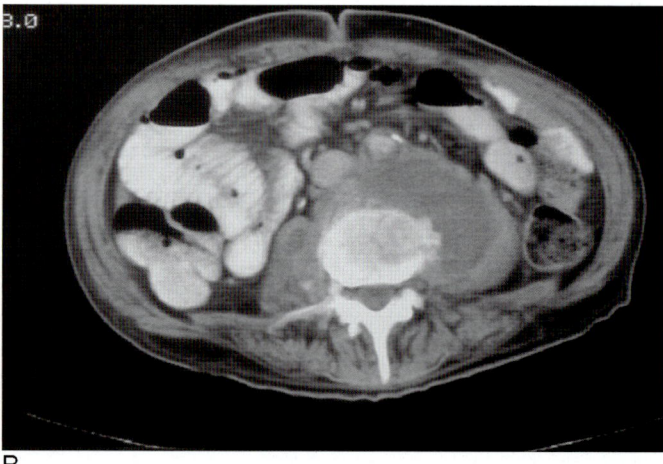

B

■ **FIGURE 68-7** Brucellar spondylodiscitis. **A,** Frontal radiograph of the lumbar spine shows destructive changes at the inferior end plates of L1 and L2 on the left, destructive changes at the superior end plate of L5, and less extensive destruction at the adjacent inferior end plate of L4 on the left. Note mild intervertebral disc space narrowing at the L1–L2 and L4–L5 levels and parrot beak–like end plate osteophytes at multiple levels on the left. Note also a large left paraspinal mass consistent with soft tissue abscess. **B,** Axial CT image through the upper lumbar spine in the same patient shows destructive changes of a vertebral body, more pronounced on the left, with an associated large paraspinal abscess larger on the left. *(Courtesy of Raymond Carmody, MD, Tucson, AZ.)*

A

and intervertebral discs, sclerosis, paravertebral abscess formation, and healing with bony fusion and osteophytosis. Large parrot beak–like osteophytes can be seen with spinal brucellosis (Fig. 68-7A). In early disease initial radiographs may be normal and the diagnosis can be delayed. The earliest radiographic finding is epiphysitis of the anterosuperior angle of the vertebra. Osteoporosis, large soft tissue abscesses, and paraspinal calcifications are more common in tuberculosis than in brucellosis. Brucellar spondylodiscitis shows less disc space loss and more common bony ankylosis of the affected vertebrae than is seen in tuberculous infection. A peripherally located gas within the intervertebral disc can be seen in brucellar infection.[1-3]

Radiologic findings of sacroiliitis include poor definition of the cortex, narrowing or widening of the joint space, erosive changes, sclerosis, and ankylosis.[6] With involvement of peripheral joints, joint effusion, periarticular soft tissue swelling, and joint space narrowing can be observed that may be associated with osteomyelitis. Initial radiographs are frequently unremarkable. In patients with periarticular brucellosis soft tissue swelling is seen on radiographs.[6]

Magnetic Resonance Imaging

Magnetic resonance imaging is the study of choice in the diagnosis and evaluation of the extent of disease in brucellar spondylodiscitis and osteomyelitis. Vertebral destruction, epidural abscesses, spinal cord, and nerve root compression are nicely demonstrated by MRI. Involvement of the apophyseal joints is common. Abnormal signal in vertebral bodies without morphologic changes and enhancement of the facet joints after intravenous gadolinium-based contrast agent injection have been identified as specific MRI features of brucellar spondylitis. The lesions display low signal intensity on the T1-weighted images, high signal intensity on the fluid-sensitive sequences, and enhancement on the postcontrast images. Postcontrast images are useful in delineation of paraspinal and intraosseous abscesses.[1-3,6] MRI is the study of choice in the evaluation of brucellar arthritis, osteomyelitis, and periarticular soft tissue infection.[6]

Multidetector Computed Tomography

Computed tomography is useful in evaluation of brucellar spondylodiscitis (see Fig. 68-7B). However, it has been reported that some cases were initially misdiagnosed as lumbar disc herniation or tuberculosis.[3] CT is also useful in evaluation of brucellar arthritis and osteomyelitis.[6]

Ultrasonography

Ultrasonography may be utilized in evaluation of joint effusions, synovitis, and bursitis caused by brucellar infection and may provide guidance for fluid aspiration.[2]

Nuclear Medicine

Radionuclide bone scintigraphy with ^{99m}Tc-MDP is useful in the evaluation of osteoarticular brucellosis and shows increased radiotracer uptake in the affected regions. Bone scintigraphy is particularly useful in searching for multifocal disease.[1,6,7] However, scintigraphy is not very useful in determining the outcome of brucellar musculoskeletal infection, because the abnormal radiotracer uptake persists for a long time.[6]

Positron Emission Tomography/Computed Tomography

Utility of PET/CT in evaluation of brucellar musculoskeletal infection is to be determined. There is a case report suggesting the usefulness of PET scanning in detection of skeletal brucellar infection in a patient with human immunodeficiency virus infection.[8]

SYNOPSIS OF TREATMENT OPTIONS
Medical Treatment

Osteoarticular brucellosis is treated with a combination of two or three antibiotics, including ciprofloxacin, doxycycline, tetracycline, rifampicin, and streptomycin, with median duration of therapy of 6 to 8 weeks. If the patient does not respond to the usual treatment regimen or the disease relapses, longer treatment of 3 to 6 months or different regimens are sometimes needed.[1,3,6]

Surgical Treatment

In the patients with spinal involvement and spinal instability or radiculopathy, surgery is performed.[1,3,9]

SUGGESTED READING

Pourbagher A, Pourbagher MA, Savas L, et al. Epidemiologic, clinical, and imaging findings in brucellosis patients with osteoarticular involvement. AJR Am J Roentgenol 2006; 187:873–880.

REFERENCES

1. Pourbagher A, Pourbagher MA, Savas L, et al. Epidemiologic, clinical, and imaging findings in brucellosis patients with osteoarticular involvement. AJR Am J Roentgenol 2006; 187:873–880.
2. Resnick D. Osteomyelitis, septic arthritis, and soft tissue infection: organisms. In Resnick D (ed). Diagnosis of Bone and Joint Disorders, 4th ed. Philadelphia, WB Saunders, 2002, pp 2510–2624.
3. Turgut M, Turgut AT, Kosar U. Spinal brucellosis: Turkish experience based on 452 cases published during the last century. Acta Neurochir (Wien) 2006; 148:1033–1044. Epub 2006 Sep 8.
4. Al Dahouk S, Tomaso H, Prenger-Berninghoff E, et al. Identification of *Brucella* species and biotypes using polymerase chain reaction–restriction fragment length polymorphism (PCR-RFLP). Crit Rev Microbiol 2005; 31:191–196.
5. Pappas G, Papadimitriou P, Akritidis N, et al. The new global map of human brucellosis. Lancet Infect Dis 2006; 6:91–99.
6. Geyik MF, Gur A, Nas K, et al. Musculoskeletal involvement of brucellosis in different age groups: a study of 195 cases. Swiss Med Wkly 2002; 132:98–105.
7. Aydin M, Fuat Yapar A, Savas L, et al. Scintigraphic findings in osteoarticular brucellosis. Nucl Med Commun 2005; 26:639–647.
8. Zaknun JJ, Zangerle R, Gabriel M, Virgolini I. ^{18}FDG-PET for monitoring disease activity in an HIV-1 positive patient with disseminated chronic osteomyelitic brucellosis due to *Brucella melitensis*. Eur J Nucl Med Mol Imaging 2005; 32:630.
9. Tezer M, Ozturk C, Aydogan M, et al. Noncontiguous dual segment thoracic brucellosis with neurological deficit. Spine J 2006; 6:321–324.

Cat-Scratch Disease

Cat-scratch disease was first described by Debré and colleagues in 1931 in Paris, and it was first recognized by physicians in the United States in 1932. The first published American case of cat-scratch disease was reported by Greer and Keefer in 1951, and the first large series of 160 patients was reported by Daniels and MacMurray in 1954.[1]

Cat-scratch disease most often presents as a self-limited benign, localized lymphadenopathy near the site of organism inoculation. A skin papule at the sight of inoculation often occurs before the development of adenopathy. Typically, the incubation period is 3 to 10 days. Cat-scratch disease generally occurs in young immunocompetent individuals and infrequently causes serious illness. However, 5% to 10% of patients, especially immunocompromised individuals, develop disseminated disease. In addition to the lymphatics, infection can affect the central nervous system, eyes, liver, spleen, bone, and lungs. Erythema nodosum and thrombocytopenia purpura also have been reported. Current data suggest that cat-scratch disease can result from a cat scratch or bite as well as possibly from a flea bite. Rare cases have been reported after exposure to a dog.[1-4]

ETIOLOGY

Bartonella henselae, a soil-borne protobacterium (also known as *Rochalimaea henselae*) that is a gram-negative coccobacillus, is currently believed to be the most common cause of cat-scratch disease. The disease is rarely linked to another soil-borne protobacterium, *Afipia felis.* *B. henselae* can cause bacillary angiomatosis in the immunocompromised patients, especially in those with human immunodeficiency virus infection.[1]

PREVALENCE AND EPIDEMIOLOGY

The overall incidence of cat-scratch disease in the United States is unknown. This is not a reportable disease, and few cases require hospitalization. However, in an analysis of three national databases, it was concluded that there are more than 2,000 patients hospitalized annually with the diagnosis of cat-scratch disease or 0.77 to 0.86/100,000 hospital discharges. Also based on these data it was estimated that in the United States there are 22,000 ambulatory patients with cat-scratch disease annually or 9.3/100,000 population. It occurs slightly more often in males than in females.[1,5]

KEY POINTS

■ Although cat-scratch disease is usually self-limited, localized regional lymphadenopathy can occur near the inoculation site.
■ Dissemination and skeletal lesions can occur.

Although cat-scratch disease may be associated with significant morbidity, no deaths have been reported to have been caused by this disease in immunocompetent patients. This infection appears to confer lifelong immunity because reports of recurrences of clinical cat-scratch disease are rare.[1]

Clinically, well flea-infested, *B. henselae*–bacteremic cats, primarily kittens, are a major reservoir for this organism and humans become naturally infected through direct and indirect contact with infected cats. Direct human-to-human transmission of *B. henselae* infection has not been reported.[1]

CLINICAL PRESENTATION

A history of contact with a cat, usually a kitten, in the previous 1 to 2 weeks is common in individuals with cat-scratch disease. The classic history of an individual with cat-scratch disease is a local rash followed by lymphadenopathy. The rash, which is present in more than 90% of infected patients, consists of one or more red papules that are 0.5 cm or less in diameter and appear at the site of inoculation, which often is a cat scratch or bite. Single lymph node involvement occurs in more than one half of patients. Frequently painful lymphadenitis usually persists for 4 to 6 weeks but can last 1 year or more. The lymphadenopathy in the decreasing order of frequency is observed in the axillary and epitrochlear, the cervical and submandibular, the inguinal and femoral, and the preauricular, postauricular, and supraclavicular chains. Adenopathy that involves more than one anatomic site may be accompanied by constitutional symptoms. Occasionally, the affected lymph nodes can suppurate. Fever of unknown origin and fatigue are observed in one third of patients. Parinaud oculoglandular syndrome occurs in 2% to 3% of patients. Central nervous system findings occur in 5% of patients. Disseminated illness is more common in immunocompromised patients. It is manifested by persistent spiking fever, hepatosplenomegaly, and abdominal pain associated with diffuse granulomatous disease of liver and spleen.[1]

PATHOPHYSIOLOGY

The pathologic response to infection with *B. henselae* varies significantly with the status of the host immune system. In immunocompetent patients the response is granulomatous and suppurative. In immunocompromised hosts the response is vasculoproliferative.[1]

Organisms are not seen in routinely stained tissue preparations. Diagnostic tests include a *B. henselae* antibody test, a silver impregnation Warthin-Starry stain, polymerase chain reaction, and DNA sequence analysis. In silver-stained lymph nodes, argyrophilic, non–acid-fast, pleomorphic bacilli may be seen.

The primary inoculation site and involved lymph nodes show a central area of avascular necrosis surrounded by lymphocytes. Histiocytes and giant cells often are present. Histologic findings in individuals with cat-scratch disease progress over time. Lymphoid hyperplasia, reticular cell hyperplasia, and arteriolar proliferation are followed by granulomas with central necrosis. Later, microabscesses appear.[1]

IMAGING TECHNIQUES

Magnetic resonance imaging is the most sensitive imaging modality in evaluation of musculoskeletal cat-scratch disease. The other imaging modalities include radiography, CT, PET/CT, ultrasonography, and nuclear medicine imaging.[2-4,6-13]

MANIFESTATIONS OF THE DISEASE

Bartonella henselae infection usually occurs early in children and young adults, is generally asymptomatic, and in most cases revolves spontaneously in 2 to 4 months. It may, however, produce a wide spectrum of clinical symptoms, the most frequent feature being cat-scratch disease. Disseminated atypical *B. henselae* infection may follow cat-scratch disease after a symptom-free period or may present de novo, mimicking a wide range of clinical disorders.[1-16]

Radiography

Radiography in patients with lymph node enlargement shows soft tissue swelling, mass, or both. Bone lesions may develop remote from the inoculation site, involving the axial and appendicular skeleton. The radiographic appearance of bone lesions is nonspecific and resembles other lytic lesions, such as eosinophilic granuloma or malignancies. The lesions are generally lytic, although associated sclerosis and periosteal reaction have been described.[1,2,6,7]

Magnetic Resonance Imaging

Magnetic resonance imaging is a useful modality for evaluation of both lymphadenopathy and rare skeletal lesions. An enlarged lymph node, which is typically seen in the axillary and epitrochlear regions, demonstrates heterogeneous low signal intensity on the T1-weighted images and high signal intensity on the fluid-sensitive sequences. On the T1-weighted images after intravenous administration of gadolinium-based contrast medium, peripheral enhancement of the lesion may be seen with nonenhancement of a central necrotic region. Diffuse heterogeneous enhancement of the infected lymph nodes can also be observed. Surrounding soft tissue edema is common (Fig. 68-8).[6-8] Bone lesions demonstrate intermediate-to-low signal intensity on the T1-weighted images and high signal intensity on the fluid-sensitive sequences (Fig. 68-9).[9-10]

Multidetector Computed Tomography

On the CT images enlarged lymph nodes appear often ill defined and may display a central low attenuation consistent with necrosis. Extensive soft tissue edema in an efferent lymphatic distribution is observed. Skeletal lesions demonstrate the same characteristics as on radiographs.[2,6,7]

Ultrasonography

Ultrasonography can be used in evaluation of lymphadenopathy and soft tissue edema as well as liver and splenic lesions.[2,6,8]

Nuclear Medicine

On bone scintigrams, the lesions demonstrate increased radionuclide uptake.[2-4,13]

Positron Emission Tomography/Computed Tomography

A PET/CT scan shows increased radiotracer uptake in the affected lymph nodes.[11]

Classic Signs

- Rash at the inoculation site
- Regional lymphadenopathy
- Nonspecific lytic lesions on radiography and CT that can be accompanied by sclerosis and periosteal reaction
- Nonspecific low signal intensity on the T1-weighted, increased signal intensity on the fluid-sensitive, and variable enhancement on the T1-weighted post-contrast MR images
- Increased radiotracer uptake on bone scintiscans and PET scan.

DIFFERENTIAL DIAGNOSIS

Cat-scratch disease may produce a wide spectrum of clinical symptoms that can mimic multiple other diseases.[1]

Adenopathy observed with cat-scratch disease may mimic a variety of bacterial or fungal infections as well as malignancies. Lytic lesions observed on radiography and CT have a broad differential diagnosis, including eosinophilic granuloma, malignancies, and bacterial and fungal infections.[1-4,6-16]

SYNOPSIS OF TREATMENT OPTIONS

Medical Treatment

In most patients who are immunocompetent, cat-scratch disease is self-limited and symptoms resolve in 2 to 4 months. Effective antibiotics used in treating cat-scratch disease include rifampin, ciprofloxacin, trimethoprim-sulfamethoxazole, and gentamicin. Clarithromycin, azithromycin, and tetracycline are likely to be effective. Although data are lacking, patients with cat-scratch disease who are treated should receive treatment for 10 to 14 days. Immunocompromised patients may require much longer courses of therapy.[1]

Surgical Treatment

In a patient with lymphadenopathy and skeletal lesions caused by cat-scratch disease, surgical treatment is typically not indicated. If needed, biopsy is performed. In a few cases in which the diagnosis was not initially recognized and simulated soft tissue sarcoma and osteomyelitis, surgical drainage and evacuation of the suppurated lymph node was performed. In one case, irrigation and débridement of spinal infection was performed. The patients recovered without sequelae.[15,16]

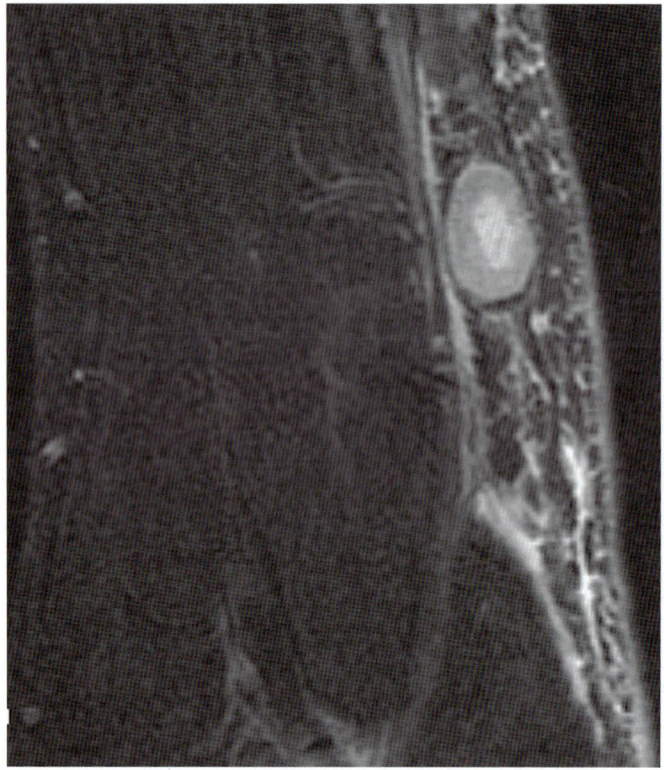

A

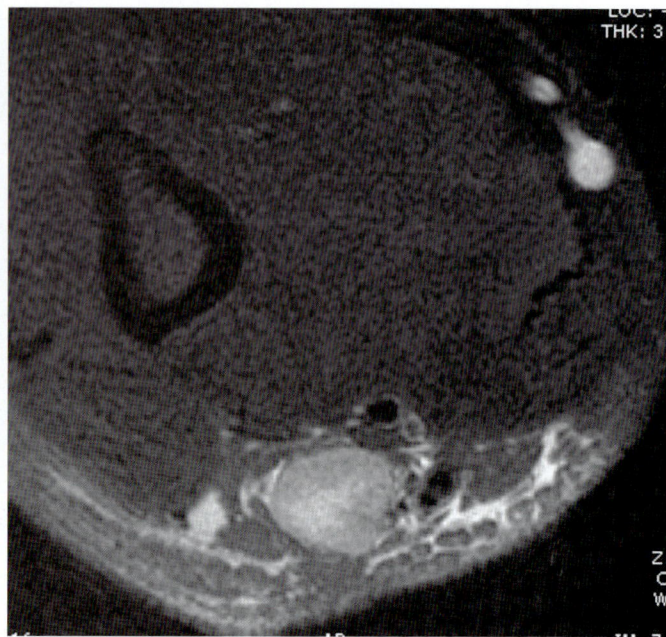

B

■ **FIGURE 68-8** A 39-year-old otherwise healthy man presented with cat-scratch disease. Coronal STIR (**A**) and T2-weighted axial (**B**) with fat saturation MR images of the elbow show enlarged epitrochlear lymph node of heterogeneous increased and centrally higher signal intensity within the medial subcutaneous soft tissues of the elbow. Note streaky areas of increased signal intensity in the adjacent subcutaneous soft tissues consistent with edema. Axial T1-weighted (**C**) image shows intermediate-to-low signal intensity in the regions of abnormalities.

(Continued)

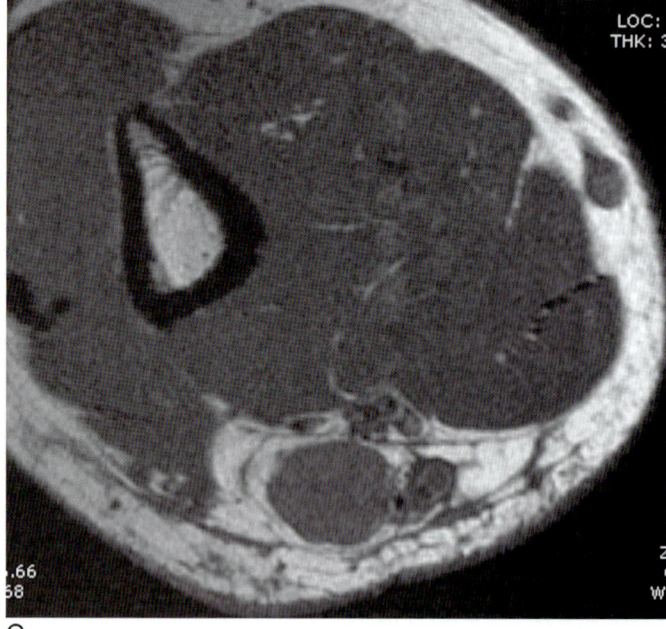

C

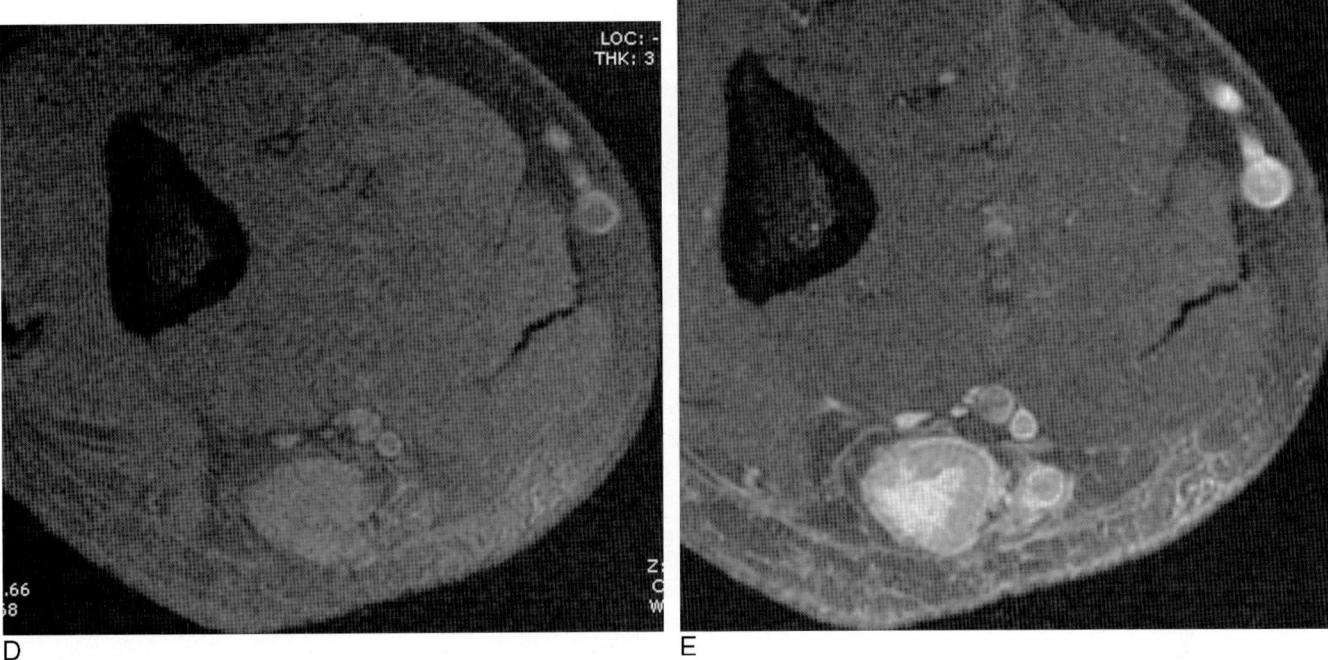

D   E

■ **FIGURE 68-8—Cont'd** (**D**) T1-weighted axial image with fat saturation and axial T1-weighted (**E**) image with fat saturation after intravenous administration of gadolinium-based contrast agent show heterogeneous enhancement in the regions of abnormalities, with prominent enhancement of the central part of the lymph node on the postcontrast image.

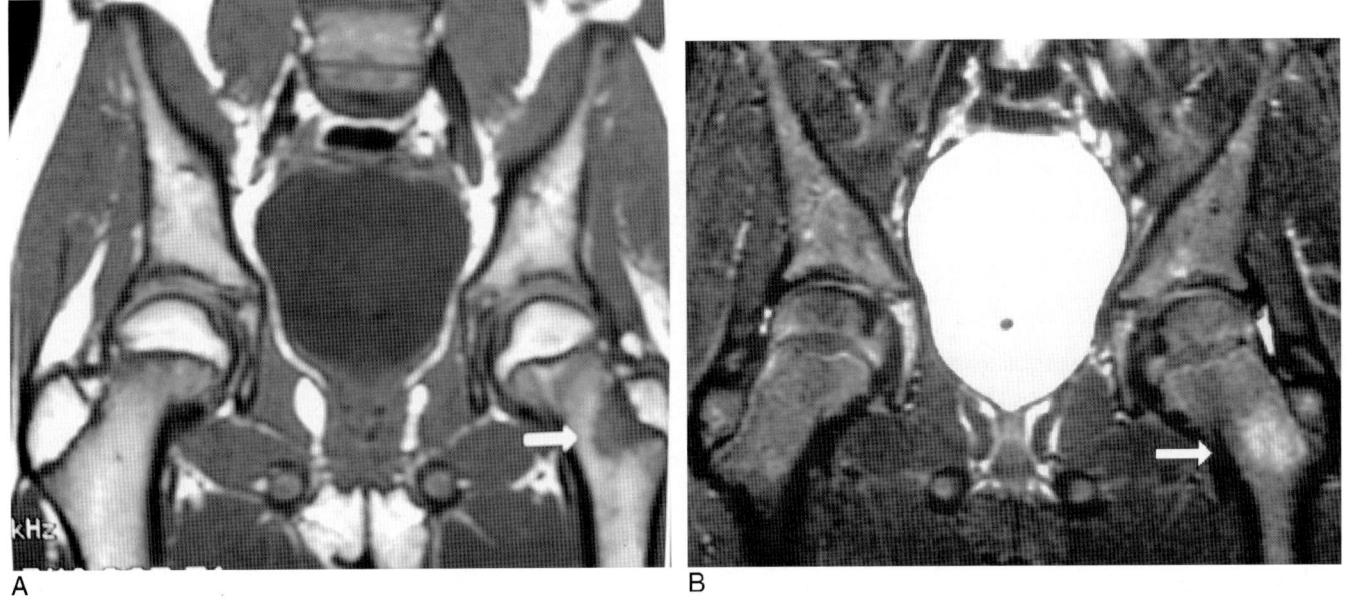

A   B

■ **FIGURE 68-9** Cat-scratch disease with multiple osseous lesions in a child. **A,** Coronal T1-weighted image of the pelvis shows a lesion of intermediate-to-low signal intensity in the region of the left femoral neck. **B,** The lesion demonstrates high signal intensity on the coronal STIR image.

(Continued)

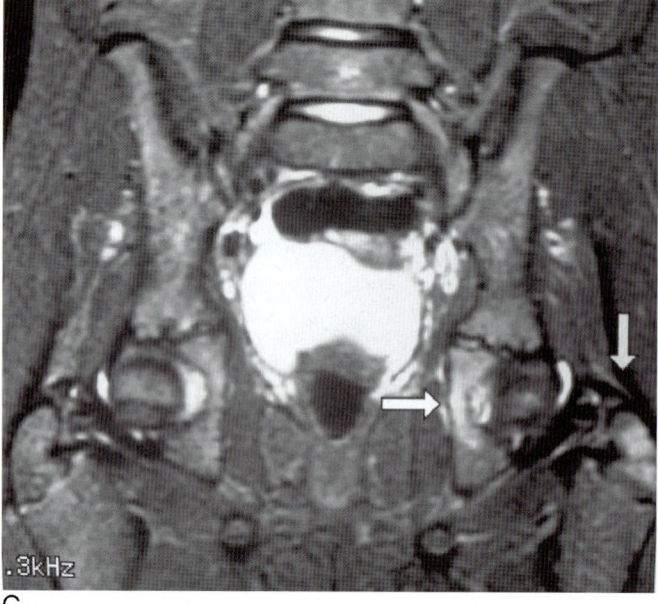

C

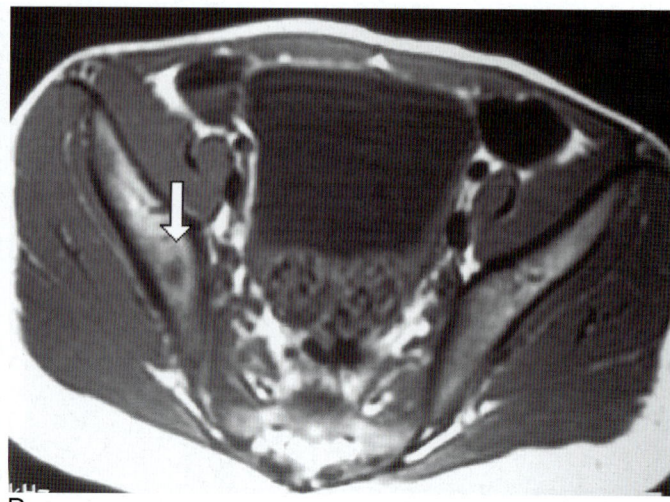

D

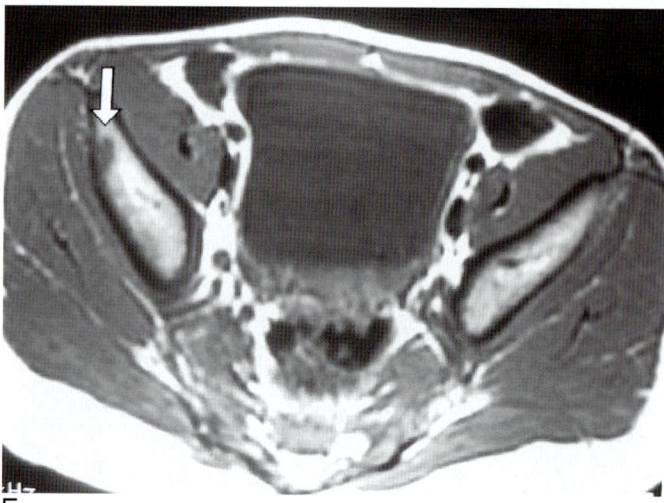

E

■ **FIGURE 68-9—Cont'd   C,** Note multiple additional lesions of similar signal intensity in the left acetabulum on the coronal STIR image and on the axial T1-weighted images (**D** and **E**) in the right iliac bone. *(Courtesy of Hilary Umans, MD, Bronx, NY.)*

What the Referring Physician Needs to Know

- Commonly there is a history of recent contact with a cat.
- Most often a self-limited rash appears at the site of organism inoculation and benign and localized lymphadenopathy is evident near the inoculation site.
- Lytic skeletal lesions and dissemination are uncommon.

SUGGESTED READINGS

Bass JW, Vincent JM, Person DA. The expanding spectrum of *Bartonella* infections: II. Cat-scratch disease. Pediatr Infect Dis J 1997; 16:163–79.

Dong PR, Seeger LL, Yao L, et al. Uncomplicated cat-scratch disease: findings at CT, MR imaging, and radiography. Radiology 1995; 195:837–839.

REFERENCES

1. Bass JW, Vincent JM, Person DA. The expanding spectrum of *Bartonella* infections: II. Cat-scratch disease. Pediatr Infect Dis J 1997; 16:163–179.
2. Hopkins KL, Simoneaux SF, Patrick LE, et al. Imaging manifestations of cat-scratch disease. AJR Am J Roentgenol 1996; 166:435–438.
3. Fretzayas A, Papadopoulos NG, Moustaki M, et al. Unsuspected extralymphocutaneous dissemination in febrile cat scratch disease. Scand J Infect Dis 2001; 33:599–603.
4. Keret D, Giladi M, Kletter Y, Wientroub S. Cat-scratch disease osteomyelitis from a dog scratch. J Bone Joint Surg Br 1998; 80:766–767.
5. Jackson LA, Perkins BA, Wenger JD. Cat scratch disease in the United States: an analysis of three national databases. Am J Public Health 1993; 83:1707–1711.
6. Resnick D. Osteomyelitis, septic arthritis, and soft tissue infection: organisms. In Resnick D (ed). Diagnosis of Bone and Joint Disorders, 4th ed. Philadelphia, WB Saunders, 2002, pp 2510–2624.
7. Dong PR, Seeger LL, Yao L, et al. Uncomplicated cat-scratch disease: findings at CT, MR imaging, and radiography. Radiology 1995; 195:837–839.

8. Gielen J, Wang XL, Vanhoenacker F, et al. Lymphadenopathy at the medial epitrochlear region in cat-scratch disease. Eur Radiol 2003; 13:1363–1369.

9. LaRow JM, Wehbe P, Pascual AG. Cat-scratch disease in a child with unique magnetic resonance imaging findings. Arch Pediatr Adolesc Med 1998; 152:394–396.

10. Hipp SJ, O'Shields A, Fordham LA, et al. Multifocal bone marrow involvement in cat-scratch disease. Pediatr Infect Dis J 2005; 24:472–474.

11. Jeong W, Seiter K, Strauchen J, et al. PET scan-positive cat scratch disease in a patient with T cell lymphoblastic lymphoma. Leuk Res 2005; 29:591–594.

12. Rolain JM, Chanet V, Laurichesse H, et al. Cat scratch disease with lymphadenitis, vertebral osteomyelitis, and spleen abscesses. Ann N Y Acad Sci 2003; 990:397–403.

13. Bruckert F, de Kerviler E, Zagdanski AM, et al. Sternal abscess due to *Bartonella (Rochalimaea) henselae* in a renal transplant patient. Skeletal Radiol 1997; 26:431–433.

14. Massei F, Gori L, Macchia P, Maggiore G. The expanded spectrum of bartonellosis in children. Infect Dis Clin North Am 2005; 19:691–711.

15. Bernini PM, Gorczyca JT, Modlin JF. Cat-scratch disease presenting as a paravertebral abscess: a case report. J Bone Joint Surg Am 1994; 76:1858–1863.

16. Nimityongskul P, Anderson LD, Sri P. Cat-scratch disease: orthopaedic presentation. Orthop Rev 1992; 21:55–59.

Fungal and Higher Bacterial Infections

There are approximately 100,000 species of fungi and as many species not yet discovered as estimated by mycologists. Many have a worldwide distribution, but some are seen in predominantly endemic areas. All are dimorphic with a free mycelial form that produces infectious spores that when inhaled are converted to yeast-like pathogens. Signs of infection are usually mild with chronic evolution and delay in diagnosis common; however, all fungi are more virulent in an immunocompromised host.

Interpretation of these cases requires knowledge of predisposing factors, imaging findings, and appropriate index of clinical suspicion. The final diagnosis often requires tissue sampling. Here the emphasis is on the musculoskeletal findings caused by fungal infections including coccidioidomycosis, North American blastomycosis, South American blastomycosis, cryptococcosis, sporotrichosis, histoplasmosis, aspergillosis, candidiasis, mucormycosis, maduromycosis and higher bacterial infections including actinomycosis and nocardiosis.[1,2]

ETIOLOGY, PATHOPHYSIOLOGY, PREVALENCE AND EPIDEMIOLOGY, CLINICAL PRESENTATION, PATHOLOGY, AND DIFFERENTIAL DIAGNOSIS

Coccidioidomycosis

Coccidioidomycosis (valley fever) is a systemic infection caused by the soil fungus *Coccidioides immitis* and *Posadasii*, and is endemic in northern Mexico and the southwest part of the United States, including Texas, New Mexico, Arizona, California, and parts of South America.[1,2] It is saprophytic but highly infective. It exists in the mycelial form within the soil and becomes infective when the airborne arthrospores are inhaled. In the infected host, the arthrospore develops into spherule, which may contain a few to several hundred endospores. Each endospore may then enlarge to spherule form (Fig. 68-10). The endospore-spherule cycle in the host continues indefinitely unless altered by an immune reaction or the endospore is extruded from the tissue. The extruded endospore may germinate in the soil within a week to produce hyphae and the mycelial-arthrospore cycle. There is no known human-to-human or animal-to-human transmission. The lungs are the primary focus of infection, but less than 40% of patients have a symptomatic disease. Of these, less than 1% of patients develop disseminated disease, which is often fatal and may involve any organ, including skin, lymphatics, lungs, osseous structures, liver, kidneys, and central nervous system.[3]

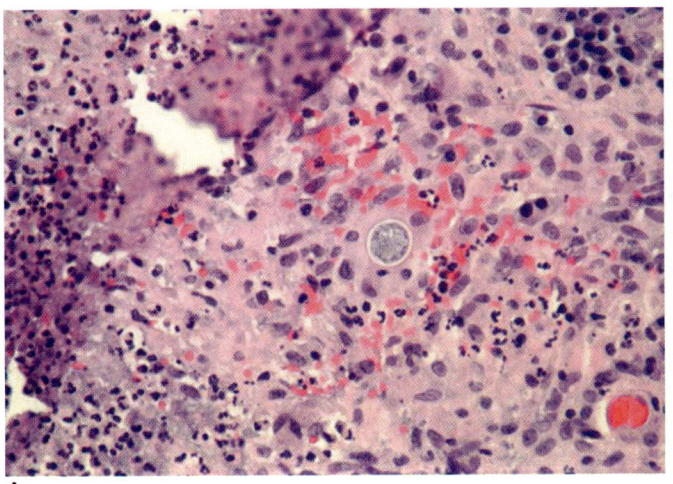
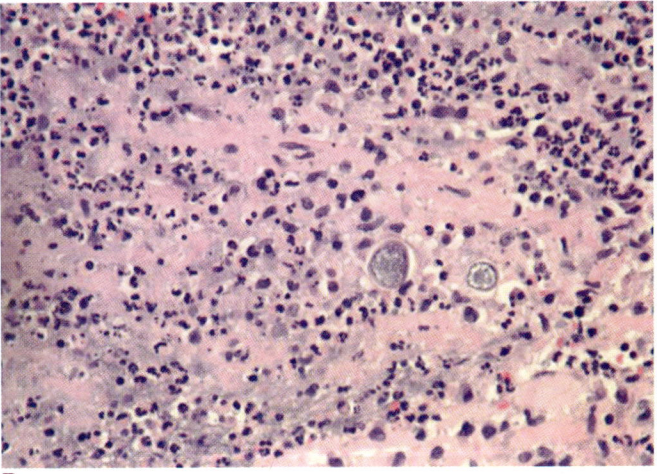

A   B

■ **FIGURE 68-10** **A** and **B**, *Coccidioides immitis* spherules with light microscopy (40×). Inflammatory reaction is present, which includes segmented neutrophils, epithelioid cells, and rare eosinophils. *(Courtesy of Anna Graham, MD, Tucson, AZ.)*

Skeletal coccidioidomycosis is seen in 10% to 50% of patients with disseminated disease.[1] It is frequently multicentric and may involve almost any bone, although the axial skeleton is more frequently involved.[4] At least three risk factors have been described that may lead to disseminated coccidioidomycosis: ethnicity (Filipino, African-American, Native American, Hispanic), gender (male > female), and immunosuppression.[1] All age groups can be affected, but patients younger than age 5 years or older than age 50 years are more likely to develop disseminated disease. Symptoms and signs can be prominent and include pain, swelling, and draining abscess.[2] Skeletal involvement can be seen as osteomyelitis or septic arthritis. A self-limited migratory sterile polyarthritis ("desert rheumatism") occurs as a hypersensitivity syndrome in 33% of cases. Septic arthritis usually occurs due to direct extension from an adjacent bone and rarely due to hematogenous spread. The most commonly involved joints are ankles and knees.[1] Coccidioidal bursitis, tenosynovitis, and soft tissue abscesses can occur.[2]

A positive serology test is diagnostic.[5] Biopsy reveals granulomatous lesions similar to tuberculosis with monocytes, giant cell epithelial cells, necrosis, and caseation. Differentiation requires isolation of the causative organism.[2]

The differential diagnosis includes lytic metastatic disease, multiple myeloma, Kaposi's sarcoma, and other fungal or mycobacterial infections.[2,4]

During 2003–2004, the number of reported cases of coccidioidomycosis increased 32%. In 2004, 6,449 cases of coccidioidomycosis were reported, yielding a national average of 4.1 cases for every 100,000 persons. The majority of these cases occurred in California and Arizona. Increases are probably attributable to recent changes in land use, demographics, and climate in endemic areas, although there may be increased physician awareness and testing.[6]

North American Blastomycosis

Blastomycosis is caused by the fungus *Blastomyces dermatitidis* and is most common in the southeastern United States, the Ohio-Mississippi Valley area, and the Mid-Atlantic states. It is also endemic to part of Africa. The primary infection is often pulmonary,[1] but the skin may be a portal entry for infection in some cases after cutaneous injuries.[2] Hematogenous dissemination may occur to lungs and other organs. The most common sites for dissemination include skin, skeletal structures, and the genitourinary tract.[1] An abscess can develop in the subcutaneous soft tissue and spread to the other viscera, lymph nodes, and skeletal structures. The peak age is between 20 and 50 years, but both males and females may be affected at any age.[2]

Osteomyelitis is seen in 14% to 60% of patients with disseminated blastomycosis, which can be the result of hematogenous seeding or direct extension from the adjacent soft tissues. The most common sites of skeletal involvement are the vertebrae, skull, ribs, and distal half of the extremities, but any bone can be affected. In the long bones the infection typically begins in the epiphysis or subarticular region.[1] Metaphyses of the long bones and small bones are also frequently involved. Blastomycotic septic arthritis is common after dissemination, with most frequent involvement of the elbows, knees, and ankles.[1] The presentation of blastomycosis clinically and radiographically is nonspecific and often mistaken for a neoplasm. Delay in diagnosis is common. Patients with osseous blastomycosis may present as pain, swelling, abscesses, septic joints, and draining sinuses.[7] The osseous lesions may also be asymptomatic.[8]

The definite diagnosis is made through identification of *B. dermatitidis* in body fluids, tissue, or cultured material. Serologic testing is available but not reliable.[7]

Histologic examination reveals round and broad-based budding yeast with an associated pyogranulomatous reaction. Another important finding is thermal dysmorphism on cultures.[7]

South American Blastomycosis

South American blastomycosis is caused by the fungus *Blastomyces (Paracoccidioides) brasiliensis*. The disease is endemic to South America and parts of Mexico and Central America. The causative fungi invade the pharynx and then spread locally or hematogenously to the other body sites. The musculoskeletal involvement is similar to that of North American blastomycosis.[2]

Cryptococcosis

Cryptococcosis (torulosis, European blastomycosis, Busse-Buschke disease) is a worldwide fungal infection caused by the encapsulated fungus *Cryptococcus neoformans,* a fungus that has an unusual predilection for the central nervous system.[2] The causative fungus can be found in the respiratory tract, intestinal tract, or skin in healthy individuals or can be recovered from the soil, pigeon droppings, or fruit. The disease starts after inhalation of *C. neoformans* aerosolized spores to the lungs with possible hematogenous spread to the brain, meninges, visceral organs, bones, and joints. Cryptococcosis is the fourth most life-threatening infection in patients with AIDS. It can also be seen in the other immunocompromised patients and patients with chronic diseases, including leukemia, lymphoma, Hodgkin's disease, sarcoidosis, tuberculosis, diabetes mellitus, and transplant patients. Less often this disease occurs in otherwise healthy individuals.[1,2] Neurologic manifestations include dizziness, ataxia, diplopia, headache, and convulsions; and the disease is frequently lethal.[2]

In the patients with disseminated disease, skeletal involvement occurs in 5% to 10% of cases. The most common site of skeletal involvement is the spine. The other common locations are pelvis, ribs, skull, tibia, and bones about the knees.[1,2] Bony prominences can be involved. A single site of infection can be present, but the disease can also be multifocal. Occasionally, the infection can be implanted into bone during soft tissue injury.[2]

Cryptococcal septic arthritis is rare and usually is a result of extension from the adjacent bone. This can later result in destructive changes of the involved joint. Bursal infections or tenosynovitis are rare.[2]

The adults are affected more frequently than children. The patients present with swelling and pain.[2]

For definitive diagnosis a tissue sample is needed.[9-11] The diagnosis can also be made by positive serology.[11]

The granulomatous infection caused by *C. neoformans* is similar to that of sarcoidosis, and differentiation between the two disorders may be difficult. There is striking paucity of cellular reaction. The absence of suppuration and necrosis is typical.[2]

Sporotrichosis

Sporotrichosis is a chronic fungal infection caused by *Sporothrix schenckii*. This fungus resides as a saprophyte on vegetation and in soil. It can invade the human body through a skin wound or a thorn puncture. Sporotrichosis is a recognized occupational hazard of florists and farmers in whom the dominant upper limb is commonly affected. Human disease can also result from animal bites from rats, mice, gophers, and parrots.[2,12] Most of the time this infection is limited to the skin and subcutaneous soft tissues, but hematogenous dissemination that includes bones and joints can occur. The disease starts with an erythematous, ulcerated or varicose nodule on the skin with common subsequent nodular lymphangitic spread. Extracutaneous sporotrichosis results from the hematogenous spread from the primary inoculation site or from inhalation of conidia. Disseminated disease is more common and can be fatal in immunocompromised patients.[2,13] Sporotrichosis is seen worldwide but mainly in warm and tropical areas.[1]

The skeletal involvement includes osteomyelitis or septic arthritis. The osteomyelitis progresses slowly and can affect a single location or be multifocal. The most commonly involved bones are tibia, fibula, femur, humerus, and short tubular bones of hands and feet. Both large and small extremity joints can be involved. Involvement of the synovial bursae can be present. Indolent tenosynovitis usually about the wrist and ankle can be observed.[1]

Skeletal findings of sporotrichosis are similar to those seen in tuberculosis and other fungal disorders, but involvement of small joints of hands and feet is more common.[1]

The definite diagnosis is made by fungal culture. The organisms are rarely seen in the biopsy specimens owing to their small number.[13,14]

Histoplasmosis

Histoplasmosis is an infection caused by a dimorphic fungus *Histoplasma capsulatum*, which is present in the United States predominantly in the Ohio and Mississippi river valleys as well as in certain areas of Central or South America, or *H. capsulatum var. dubosii*, present in Africa. Both species cause the same disease. *H. capsulatum* is a soil fungus.[1,15]

The disease usually starts in lungs after inhalation of fungal spores, but the gastrointestinal tract can be portal entry in some patients. The fungi proliferate in the reticuloendothelial system.[2] The vast majority of human infections are self limited and asymptomatic.[15] The disease can spread hematogenously to other organs, including bones.

Skeletal involvement is more common with *H. capsulatum var. dubosii* infection with predilection to flat and small tubular bones.[1] The radiologic findings are similar to those in tuberculosis and sarcoidosis.[1,2]

With *H. capsulatum* infection children are infected more commonly than adults. Joints as well as bones can also be affected. Sometimes, joint involvement is a result of hypersensitivity reaction to *H. capsulatum*. Tenosynovitis caused by this fungus can occur.[2,15] Fasciitis and myositis caused by this organism have also been reported.[16]

With histoplasmosis caused by *H. capsulatum var. dubosii*, granulomatous ulcerating and papular skin lesions can be associated with bone and joint involvement in as many as 80% of patients. The disease is frequently multifocal, predominantly involving the flat bones, but the spine and tubular bones can be involved.[2]

The diagnosis can be made with antigen testing from urine or blood. Fungal cultures from the affected tissues are also useful.[17] With the involvement of bone marrow, noncaseating granulomas are seen in histologic specimens. Histologic findings of histoplasmosis are similar to those in sarcoidosis and tuberculosis.[2]

Aspergillosis

Aspergillosis is a fungal disease defined as any other illness other than mycotoxicosis caused by various *Aspergillus* species. These fungi are ubiquitous and include the human upper respiratory tract, but disease is uncommon. The severe and invasive form of aspergillosis is typically seen in immunocompromised patients, in whom it represents an opportunistic infection with a high mortality rate.[1,18] The most common causative organism is *A. fumigatus*.[1]

Skeletal involvement is rare and usually occurs due to hematogenous dissemination, which is more common in adults or due to direct invasion of pulmonary disease into the chest wall, which is more common in children.[2] Vertebral, rib, or sternal involvement follows after respiratory infection, but the other skeletal sites can be involved.[1,2,19] Aspergillous spondylitis can occur in both immunocompetent and immunocompromised patients of any age. This is generally related to a contiguous spread of pulmonary disease, with the thoracic spine most commonly involved. Spinal involvement resembles tuberculous spondylitis. Contiguous spread of this infection is also observed in the orbital bones. Involvement of the appendicular skeleton is rare. Aspergillous arthritis is rare and usually associated with osteomyelitis.[2]

The diagnosis can be made with serology, but the result can be false negative.[18] The definite diagnosis is made by fungal culture.[19]

Candidiasis

Candidiasis (moniliasis) is a fungal infection caused by several species of *Candida*. The major causative organism is *C. albicans*. Other pathogenic *Candida* species include *C. tropicalis, C. guilliermondii, C. krusei, C. lusitanie, C. rugosa, C. pseudotropicalis, C. parapsilosis, C. glabrata,* and *C. lambica*.[2] This fungus is common in the normal human flora and presumably resides on the mucous membranes. Candidiasis represents an opportunistic infection that is mainly seen in patients with indwelling catheters, in intravenous drug abusers, and in immuno-compromised patients.[1-2]

In disseminated disease, involvement of bones and joints is uncommon and occurs in 1% to 2% of patients. Candidal osteomyelitis can affect any age group. The most commonly involved bones are the pelvis, sternum, and scapula. The ribs, spine, and tubular bones of the extremities can also be involved. Spine infection can occur from the direct extension of a contiguous infection or secondary to hematogenous seeding, with involvement of the lumbar spine most common. Candidal osteomyelitis cannot be differentiated from other bacterial or fungal infections by imaging.[1,2]

Septic arthritis caused by *C. albicans* can occur by hematogenous spread, owing to direct invasion from infected adjacent osseous or soft tissue structures, or from joint replacement surgery. The most commonly affected joint is the knee.[1] Monarticular involvement is more common than polyarticular involvement.

Candidal pyomyositis is rare.[20,21] Septic bursitis can also occur. Osteoarticular candidiasis is seen in approximately one third of heroin addicts with most typical osteochondral involvement.[2]

Systemic candidiasis is an iatrogenic disease of modern neonatal intensive care that deserves urgent attention for its prevention as well as effective treatment to minimize neonatal morbidity and mortality. The sources of candidiasis in neonatal intensive care units are often endogenous following colonization of the newborns with fungi. About 10% of these newborns are colonized in the first week of life, and up to 64% are colonized by 4 weeks of hospital stay. Disseminated candidiasis presents very much like bacterial sepsis and can involve multiple organs such as the kidneys, brain, eyes, liver, spleen, bones, joints, meninges, and heart.[22]

Confirming the diagnosis by laboratory tests is difficult, and a high index of suspicion is required. The definitive diagnosis of fungemia can be made only by recovering the organism from blood or other sterile body fluids.[22] With the bone or joint involvement the diagnosis is made by isolation of the organism from joint aspirate or sampled material.[2]

Mucormycosis

Mucormycosis is the most acute, fulminant, and fatal of all fungal infections in humans. It is also known as zygomycosis and phycomycosis. This infection is caused by fungi of the class Zygomycetes and order Mucorales, usually including the genera *Rhizopus*, *Absidia*, *Mortierella*, and *Mucor*. The organisms exist in soil and air.[23]

The frequency of mucormycosis has been increasing over the past 10 years; infections have been identified in up to 6.8% of patients at autopsy. The most common route of transmission for Zygomycetes fungi is inhalation of spores from the environment. Patients at highest risk for infections caused by Mucorales fungi include those with profound immunosuppression or diabetes, intravenous drug abusers, premature infants, those receiving deferoxamine, and recipients of bone marrow transplants. Mucormycosis commonly presents as rhinocerebral or pulmonary disease; gastrointestinal presentations also occur.[24] The preexisting disease influences the port of entry, but usually the lesions start from the paranasal sinuses.[1] Hematogenous dissemination of the disease can also occur.[2] Clinical manifestations of invasive mucormycosis are tissue necrosis and subsequent thrombosis. Common features of pulmonary disease include fever, dyspnea, hemoptysis, and cavitation upon radiologic examination.[24]

From the paranasal sinuses, the infection extends to the adjacent structures: to the lateral wall of the middle turbinate, the hard palate, the ethmoidal sinus, maxillary sinuses, orbit, retrobulbar region, and sphenoidal sinus. Intracranial extension and maxillary sinus thrombosis can occur.[1] Imaging shows destructive osteolytic lesions in the involved osseous structures, but in chronic cases osteosclerosis is also evident.[2]

The differential diagnosis of mucormycosis includes other types of osteomyelitis and neoplasm.[2]

Involvement of other osseous structures is rare and reported in spine,[23] femur, and cuboid bones.[2]

The Zygomycetes are easily identified in a tissue sample by the presence of predominantly aseptate (pauciseptate) wide, ribbon-like hyphae and of tissue necrosis and angioinvasion. The diagnosis can be made by fungal culture, but the result is frequently false negative.[25]

Overall, disease with the Mucorales tends to be fulminant and is uniformly fatal if not aggressively treated. Even with appropriate surgical and medical management, the vast majority of patients are expected to die of this disease process.[25]

Maduromycosis

Maduromycosis (mycetoma) is a chronic, granulomatous, subcutaneous, inflammatory disease caused by the true fungi of the Eumycetes class or the filamentous bacteria of the Actinomycetes. These infections are most prevalent in India, sub-Saharan Africa, the southern part of the Arabian Peninsula, and central and South America.[1,26] The disease was named after the Madura District of India, where it was described for the first time by Gill in 1842.[27]

The causative organisms are present in the soil and may enter the subcutaneous tissue by traumatic inoculation. Mycetoma commonly affects the feet in adults aged 20 to 40 years who are usually male. Both forms of mycetoma present as a progressive, subcutaneous swelling, but actinomycetoma has a more rapid course. After soft tissue contamination, the causative organism may penetrate the underlying muscles, tendons, bones, and joints. Multiple nodules develop that may suppurate and drain through sinuses, discharging grains during the active phase of the disease with subsequent contiguous involvement of the bones. Sinus tracts arising from the affected bones are common.[1,2,26] Infections of the hands, arms, legs, or scalp are less common. In the United States the most frequent cause of Madura foot is *Petriellidium boydii* (*Monosporium apiosermum*), although *Aspergillus*, *Penicillium*, *Madurella*, *Cephalosporium*, *Streptomyces*, and *Phialophora* can be causative organisms. Outside the United States, *Nocardia* species (*N. brasiliensis*, *N. madurae*) may cause this disease.[2]

The diagnosis may involve radiology, cytology, culture, histology, immunodiagnosis, and serology. Mycetoma lesions can be diagnosed by fine-needle aspiration biopsy and cytology. They are characterized by the presence of polymorphous inflammatory cells consisting of neutrophils, lymphocytes, plasma cells, histiocytes, macrophages, and foreign-body giant cells and grains. There is no known human-to-human or animal-to-human transmission.[26]

Actinomycosis

Actinomycosis is an uncommon noncontagious suppurative infection caused by gram-positive filamentous obligate or facultative anaerobic bacteria of the *Actinomyces* species, which belong to the normal flora of the intestinal tract and oral cavity. The most common causative organism is *A. israelii*.[2,28] These organisms represent higher bacteria and are frequently misclassified as fungi. Some of the other human *Actinomyces* pathogens are *A. bovis, A. naeslundii, A. viscous,* and *A. odontolyticus.*[2]

In tissues, *Actinomyces* aggregate into microcolonies and grow in a radial configuration, with the peripheral layer of organisms having club-shaped ends. These microcolonies form the characteristic sulfur granules. Actinomycosis is frequently associated with other organisms.[28]

Actinomycosis is usually seen in debilitated patients or in devitalized tissue. Trauma is important in the inoculation of the organism into the soft tissue.[2] Foreign body aspiration or ingestion, such as teeth or fish bone, is another predisposing factor.[2,29] The usual localizations of this disease are cevicofacial, pulmonary, or gastrointestinal.[2] The cevicofacial location is the most common and is seen 40% to 55% of patients.[30] Contiguous spread of this disease is more common than hematogenous.[28] There is a tendency for fistulization, and soft tissue abscesses also can occur.[31,32]

Musculoskeletal actinomycosis is more commonly the result of the direct spread of disease rather than hematogenous seeding.[2,28] Bone infection ranges between 1% and 15% in all patients with actinomycosis.[31] The most commonly involved bones are the mandible, the axial skeleton, as well as the major joints of the appendicular skeleton, but other bones can be involved.[2,33,34] The lesions can occur after extraction of a tooth or after a human bite.[2]

Diagnosis of skeletal actinomycosis is difficult and is often delayed until an advanced stage of the disease. The diagnosis is made by the isolation of the causative organism from the sampled biopsy material as well as the isolation of the sulfur granules, which are characteristic histologic findings. Successful isolation requires culturing multiple samples in enriched media under anaerobic conditions in the presence of carbon dioxide.[28]

Nocardiosis

Nocardia are gram-positive organisms that belong to the aerobic Actinomycetes. Human *Nocardia* pathogens include *N. asteroides, N. brasiliensis, N. farcinica,* and *N. caviae.*[2]

Humans are infected via the respiratory tract or gastrointestinal tract or through skin trauma. Immunocompromised patients and patients with chronic diseases are more susceptible to this disease. Pulmonary infection may extend into the chest wall. Skin infection may extend into the adjacent soft tissue and lead to cellulitis and soft tissue abscesses. Primary infection of the bursae is rare.[2] The most common sites of nocardiosis are the lungs, followed by the central nervous system and soft tissues. The other extrapulmonary sites are rare.[35,36]

Bones and joints are more commonly affected by contiguous extension from the adjacent tissues or rarely by hematogenous seeding.[2,35] The tubular and flat bones and the spine can be affected.[2]

The clinical and radiologic manifestations of musculoskeletal nocardiosis are nonspecific and resemble those of *Mycobacterium tuberculosis* and fungal infections.[35]

The diagnosis is made by identification of branching filaments in tissue specimens, Gram staining, and culture.[37]

MANIFESTATIONS OF THE DISEASE

Radiography

Coccidioidomycosis

Radiographs frequently show multiple lytic osseous lesions with permeative borders or well-defined punched-out lytic lesions with or without sclerotic borders. There is predilection to the metaphyses of long tubular bones and bone protuberances. In the tubular bones of hands and feet diaphyseal lesions are common. Soft tissue swelling and periosteal reaction and periostitis can be present, but sequestration is uncommon. Sclerosis is an attempt to heal or contain the lesion. The intervertebral discs are relatively spared, and vertebral body collapse is an uncommon and late manifestation.[2] In patients with septic arthritis osteoporosis, joint space narrowing and bone destructive changes are similar to those seen in other granulomatous infections (Figs. 68-11 to 68-15).[1]

North American Blastomycosis

Early in the disease process there may be no visible osseous radiographic abnormalities or there could be faint osteopenia in the involved location. Later an area of lucency is seen with either ill-defined or well-defined borders.[8] The radiographic appearance can be variable, but an eccentric lytic lesion without sequestrum or periosteal reaction is common. However, a periosteal reaction also can be present. The lesions are often mistaken for benign or malignant bone tumors.[7] Skeletal lesions can appear moth-eaten and can be associated with osteoporosis. Sclerotic margins can also be seen as well as an area of cortical erosion beneath the soft tissue abscesses.[2] The metaphyseal lesions tend to be eccentric, well circumscribed, and lytic.[8] In the spine the blastomycotic infection resembles tuberculosis (Figs. 68-16 and 68-17).[2]

Cryptococcosis

The skeletal lesions may be lytic with well-defined margins and mild surrounding sclerosis. Aggressive periosteal

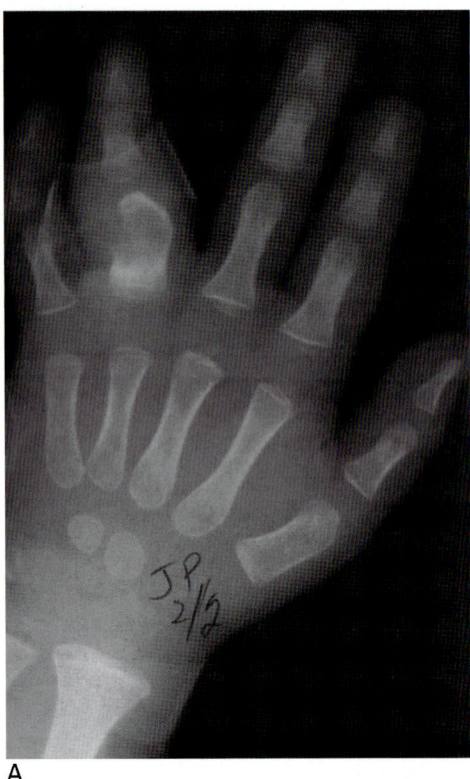

A

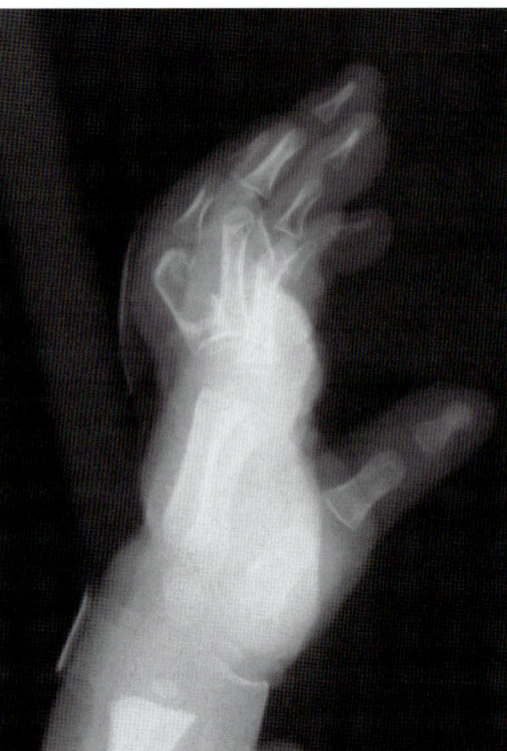

B

■ **FIGURE 68-11** Frontal (**A**) and lateral (**B**) radiographs of the hand in a child with disseminated coccidioidomycosis show an expansile lytic lesion involving the proximal phalanx of the fourth digit with associated cortical breakthrough at the ulnar aspect. *(Courtesy of George Barnes, MD, Tucson, AZ.)*

reaction is infrequent. Spinal cryptococcosis resembles pyogenic infection with more frequent paravertebral abscesses and extradural cryptococcal granulomas.[1] Extradural granulomas can cause myelopathy and cauda equina syndrome.[2] There can be extension of the vertebral body infection into the pedicle or adjacent rib.[1] Lytic lesions without a sclerotic margin and with associated soft tissue swelling can also be seen (Fig. 68-18).[11]

Sporotrichosis

Skeletal lesions are lytic or patchy or have a motheaten appearance, usually without periosteal reaction.[1,2] The findings with joint involvement include joint effusion, periarticular soft tissue swelling, joint space loss, and destructive changes (Fig. 68-19).[1-2,14]

Histoplasmosis

The radiographic findings of skeletal histoplasmosis are similar to those of sarcoidosis and tuberculosis.[1] With skeletal involvement destructive lesions are seen.[38]

With *H. capsulatum var. dubosii* infection cystic lytic areas in the affected osseous structures are most typical.[2] In the spine, *H. capsulatum var. dubosii* shows radiographic changes consistent with spondylodiscitis, with or without paravertebral abscesses.[39]

Aspergillosis

The radiographic features of skeletal aspergillosis resemble those of tuberculosis. Spinal involvement includes osseous and intervertebral disc destruction and paraspinal masses. If there is involvement of other skeletal sites or joints, destructive changes of typical osteomyelitis with or without associated periostitis can be seen. With septic joints, periarticular osteopenia, joint space loss, and erosive changes are observed (Fig. 68-20).[2]

Candidiasis

In vertebral osteomyelitis caused by *Candida* there are erosive and destructive changes and possible intervertebral disc involvement. Extension into the paravertebral soft tissues or spinal canal can occur.[1,40]

With candidal arthritis, radiography shows massive soft tissue swelling, joint effusion, joint space narrowing, erosions, bone collapse, and fragmentation (Fig. 68-21).[1]

Mucormycosis

Radiography may show destructive osteolytic and later osteosclerotic changes.[2] In the early phase of mucormycosis the radiographic changes of spondylodiscitis can be subtle and show only mild focal osteopenia[2] if compared with other unaffected vertebrae.[23]

Maduromycosis

The many findings in maduromycosis of the foot include soft tissue swelling, bone scalloping and cortical erosions, aggressive periostitis, coarse trabeculation, sclerosis and mottling, cavitary lesions, and, in advanced disease, intra-articular osseous fusion leading to an appearance of

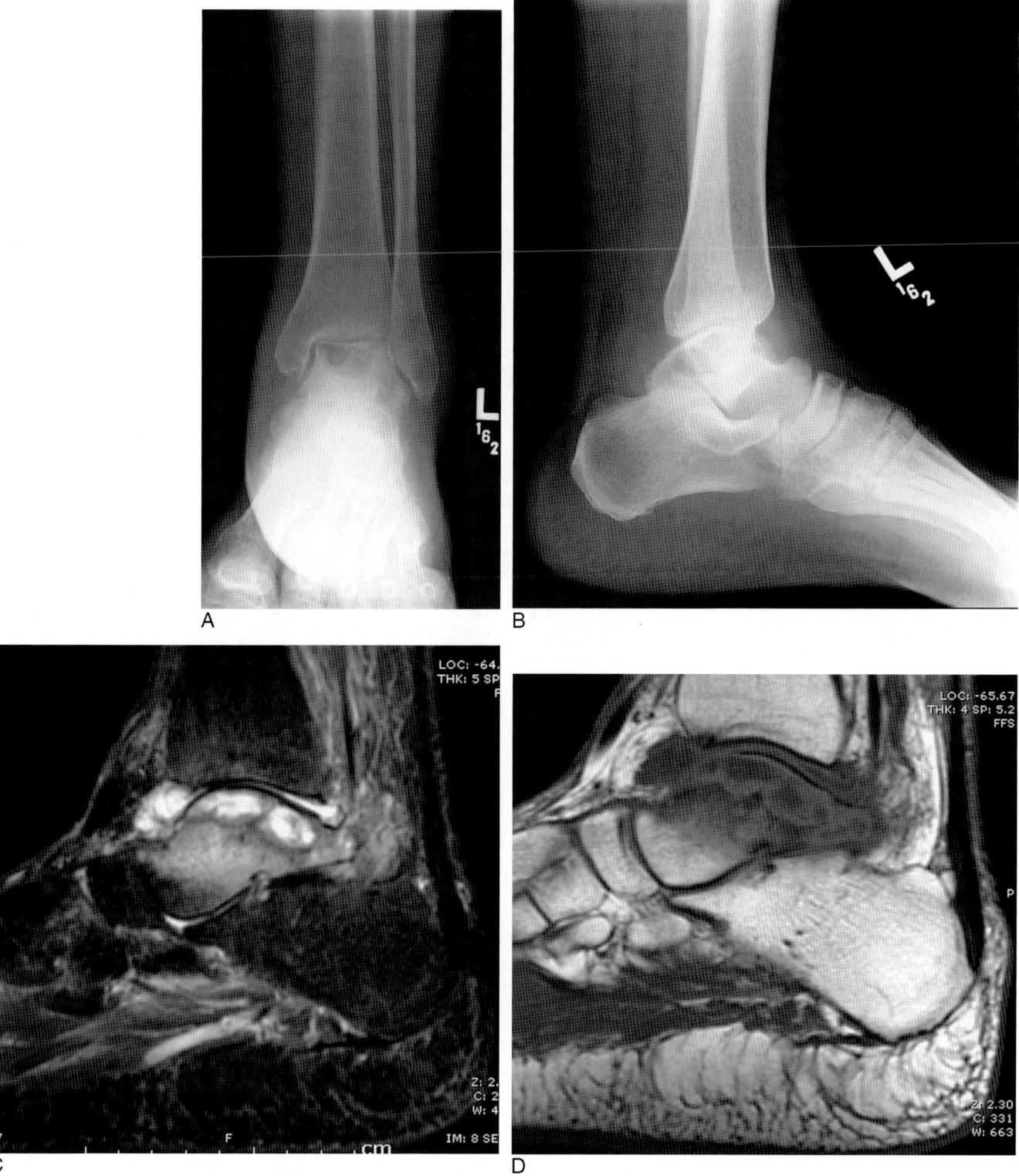

■ **FIGURE 68-12** Frontal (**A**) and lateral (**B**) radiographs of the left ankle in a 54-year-old male patient with disseminated coccidioidomycosis infection show lytic lesions in the talar trochlea and medial and lateral malleoli. Note a large synovial-fluid complex in the ankle joint seen in the lateral projection. Sagittal STIR MR image (**C**) shows a lobulated lesion of abnormal, predominantly increased signal intensity involving the talar trochlea with associated bone marrow edema extending into the talar body and a large synovial fluid complex in the ankle joint. The region of abnormality shows intermediate-to-low signal intensity on the sagittal T1-weighted MR image (**D**).

(Continued)

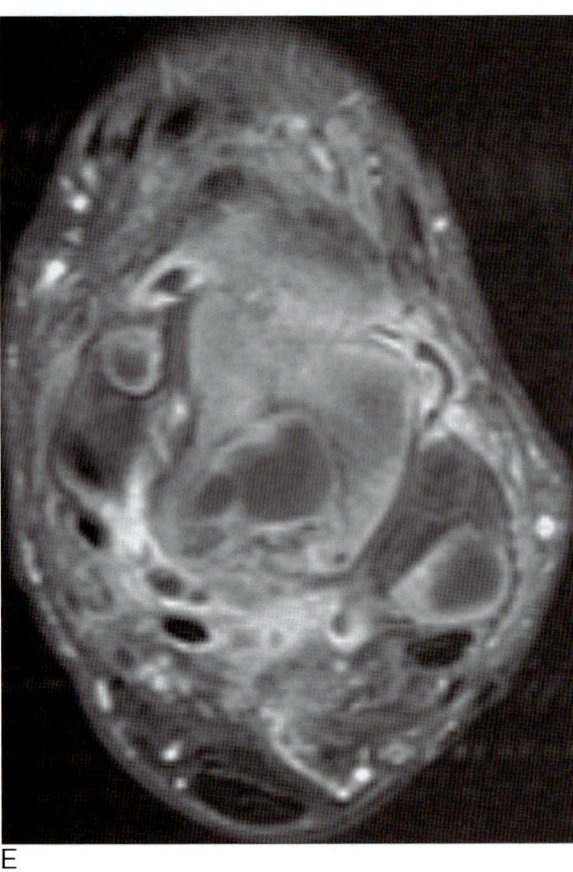

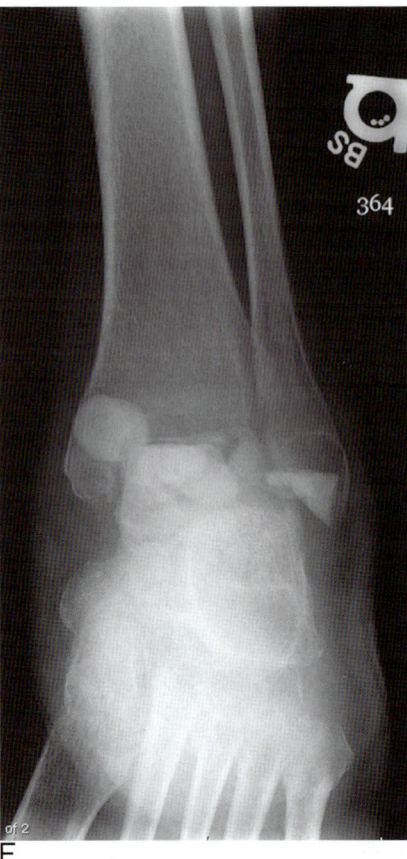

E

F

■ **FIGURE 68-12—Cont'd E,** Axial T1-weighted MR image with fat saturation shows abnormal enhancement in the region of abnormalities with rim-enhancing abscesses in the talar trochlea and medial and lateral malleoli. Note thick synovial enhancement in the ankle joint. **F,** Postoperative frontal radiograph of the ankle after surgical débridement in the same patient shows amphotericin B–impregnated cement in the talar trochlea and medial and lateral malleoli.

melting snow.[1,2,26,41] Bone cavities are larger, fewer, and better defined in eumycetoma when compared with actinomycetoma. These cavities are filled with solid masses of grains and fibrous tissues, providing a bone support. Because of this phenomenon pathologic fractures in mycetoma are rare. Radiographic findings in the skull are purely sclerotic, with dense bone formation and loss of trabeculation. In advanced maduromycosis, osteoporosis is seen that occurs secondary to disuse and compression of the bone and its blood supply by a mycetoma (see Fig. 68-22 and 68-23A).[26]

Actinomycosis

Skeletal actinomycosis is characterized by a combination of osteolysis and osteosclerosis.[2,28] With rib involvement, bony proliferation may be extensive, with the combination of severe osteosclerosis, cutaneous sinus tracts, and pleuritis suggestive of actinomycosis.[2] Infection of the spine may be a result of invasion from the adjacent mediastinal or retroperitoneal foci. Multiple vertebrae are usually involved that demonstrate lytic lesions with surrounding sclerosis. The intervertebral discs are usually spared. Posterior elements are frequently affected, and with involvement of the thoracic spine there is frequent involvement of the adjacent ribs. Paravertebral abscesses may be present but are usually smaller and without calcifications when compared with tuberculous abscesses. Vertebral body collapse and gib-

bus deformities are less common than in tuberculosis. Neurologic complications associated with spinal cord involvement can occur.[2]

Nocardiosis

Radiographic finding of nocardiosis are nonspecific and resemble those that are seen in tuberculosis and fungal infections.[35]

Magnetic Resonance Imaging

Coccidioidomycosis

Magnetic resonance imaging reveals lesions of intermediate-to-low signal intensity on the T1-weighted images and increased signal intensity on the T2-weighted and STIR sequences.[4] The MR signal characteristics are nonspecific. Intraosseous and soft tissue abscesses show rim enhancement. MRI is particularly useful in finding the local osseous and soft tissue extent of disease and spinal involvement.[2] In septic arthritis, enhancement of the synovial proliferation usually indicates active disease (see Figs. 68-12C to E, 68-13C to E, and 68-15A to C).[42]

North American Blastomycosis

Magnetic resonance imaging is helpful in evaluation of local osseous and soft tissue extension of the lesion. MRI

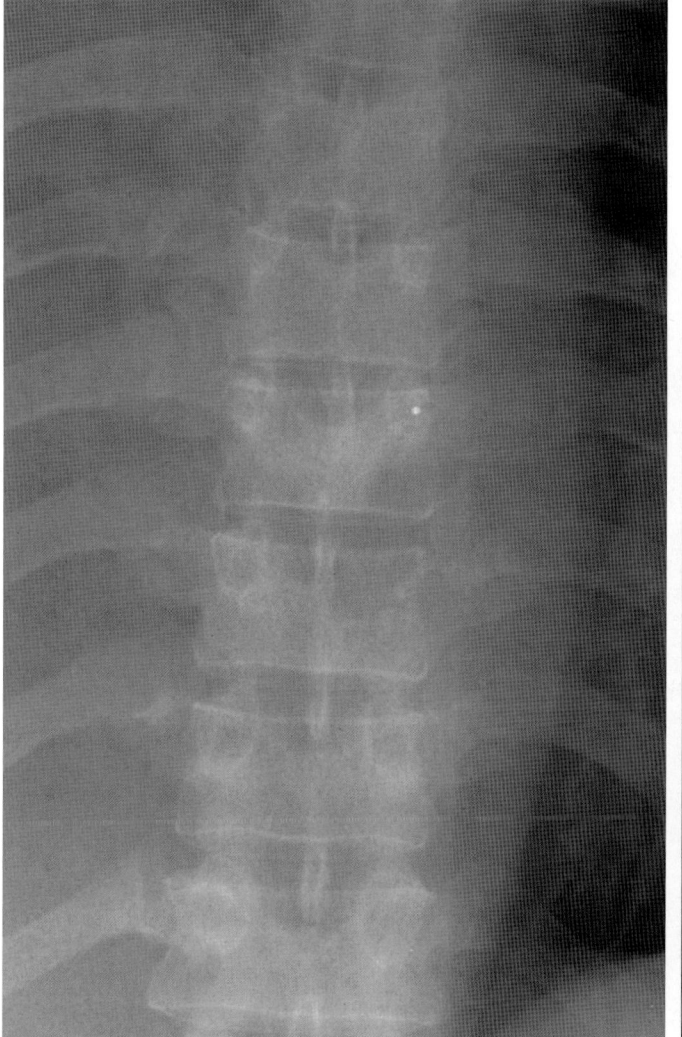

A

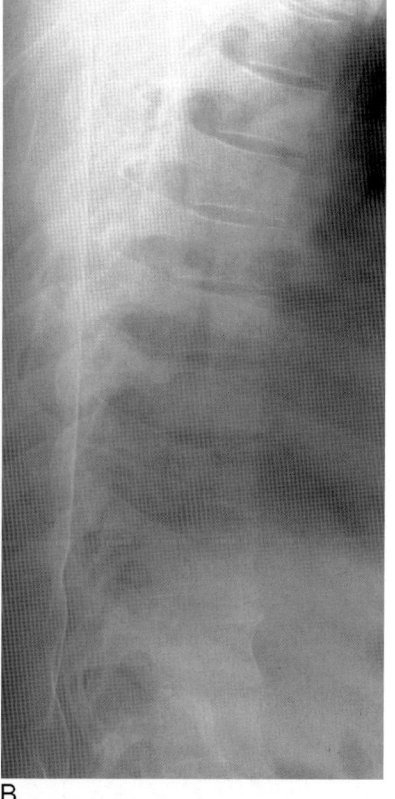

B

■ **FIGURE 68-13** Frontal (**A**) and lateral (**B**) radiographs of the thoracic spine in a 50-year-old male patient with disseminated coccidioidomycosis infection and paraplegia show destructive lytic lesions involving the left side of the two lower thoracic vertebrae including the vertebral bodies and posterior elements. Note preservation of the disc space. **C,** Sagittal STIR MR image in the same patient shows destructive lesions of intermediate-increased signal intensity involving the posterior aspect of the two lower thoracic vertebral bodies and their posterior elements with extension into the spinal canal and the posterior soft tissues. Note associated bone marrow edema in the lower vertebral body. Only the posterior aspect of the disc space is affected.

(Continued)

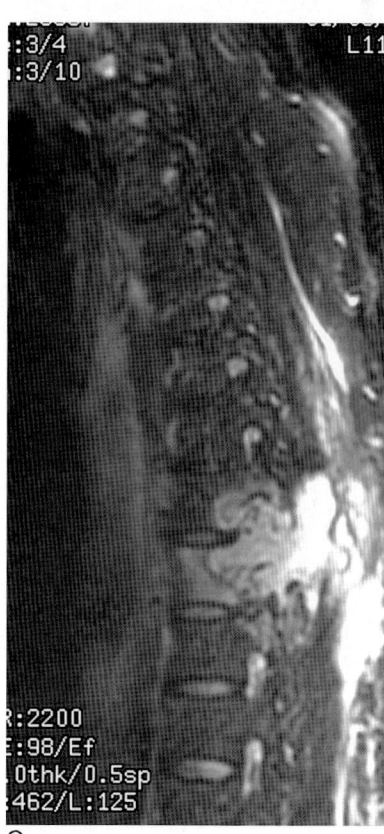

C

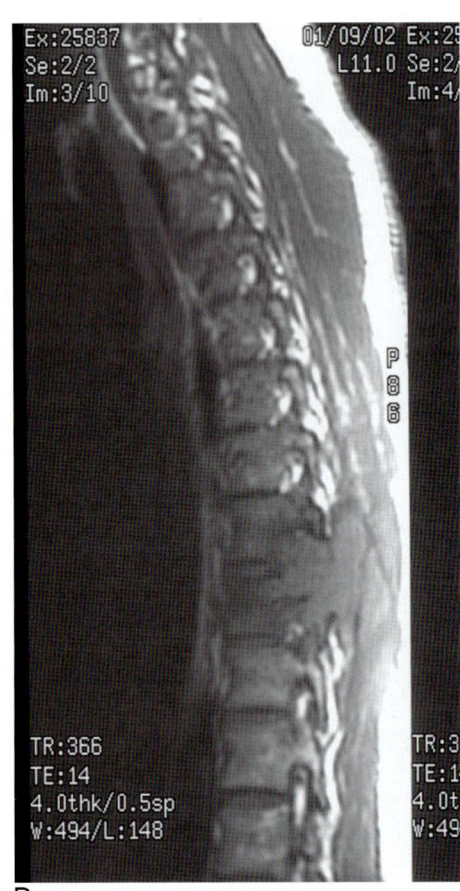

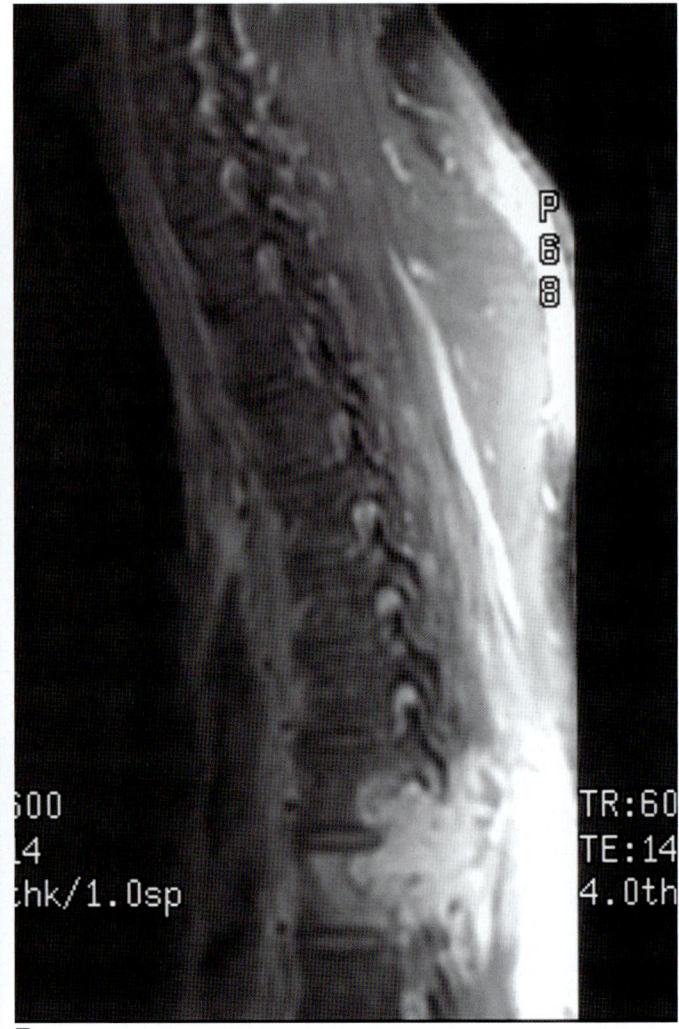

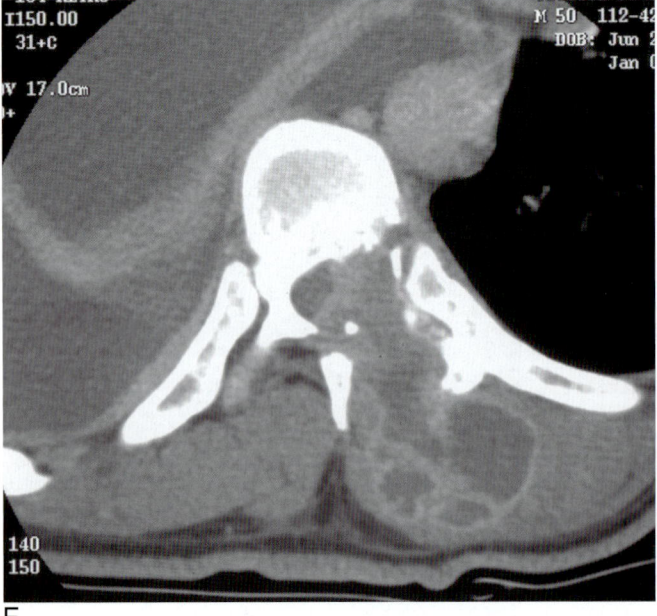

■ **FIGURE 68-13—Cont'd** **D,** Sagittal T1-weighted image demonstrates intermediate-to-low signal intensity in the regions of abnormality. **E,** Sagittal T1-weighted fat-saturated image after the intravenous administration of gadolinium-based contrast agent shows prominent enhancement in the region of abnormality with small intrinsic areas of nonenhancement consistent with osteomyelitis associated with intraosseous and soft tissue abscesses. **F,** Axial CT image of the lower thoracic spine after intravenous contrast agent administration in the same patient shows a destructive lytic lesion involving the posterior left aspect of the lower thoracic vertebral body and the posterior elements with associated rim-enhancing epidural abscess that extends into the posterior paravertebral soft tissues. *(Courtesy of Ray Carmody, MD, Tucson, AZ.)*

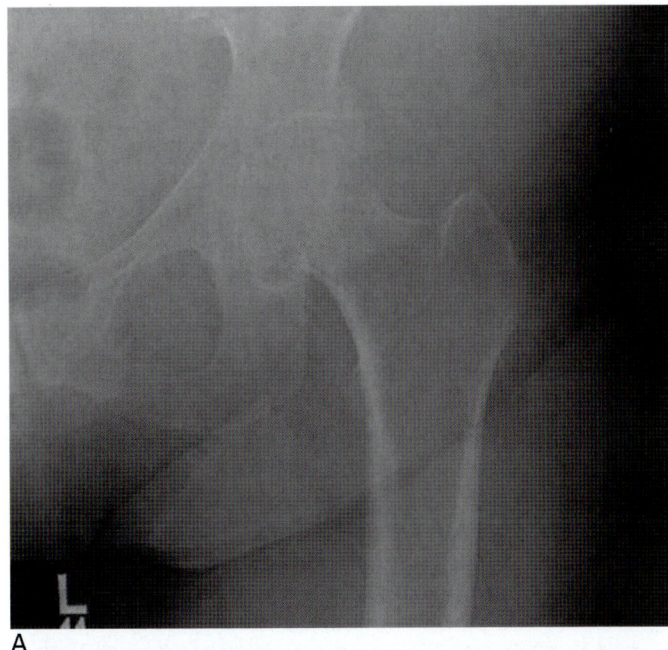

A

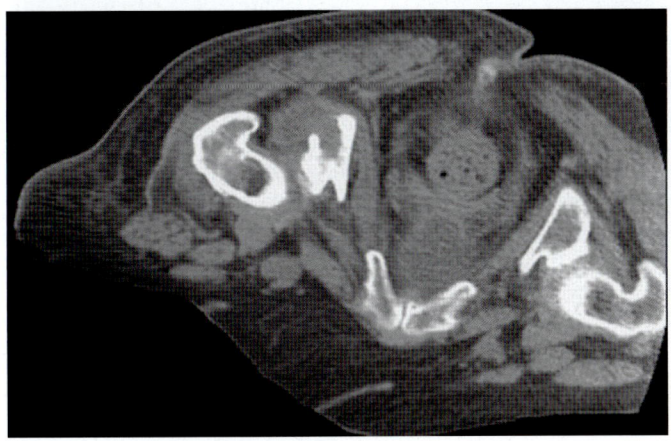

B

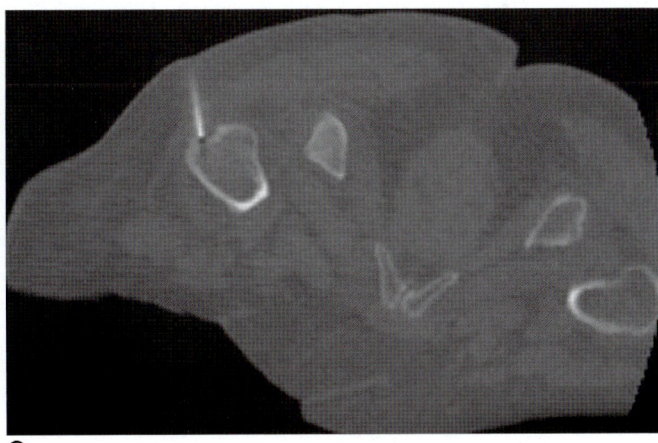

C

■ **FIGURE 68-14** A 65-year-old white woman presented with coccidioidomycosis in the left greater trochanter and left ischial tuberosity. **A,** Frontal radiograph of the left hip shows ill-defined lytic lesions involving the left greater trochanter and ischial tuberosity. **B,** CT image of the lower pelvis with the patient in prone position shows a destructive lesion with associated soft tissue mass in the left ischial tuberosity. **C,** Axial CT image of the lower pelvis with the patient in prone position shows a destructive lesion at the periphery of the left greater trochanter. Note biopsy needle within the lesion. Anteroposterior (**D**) and posteroanterior (**E**) technetium-99m methylene diphosphonate bone scintiscans of the pelvis show increased radiotracer uptake in the left ischial tuberosity and greater trochanter.

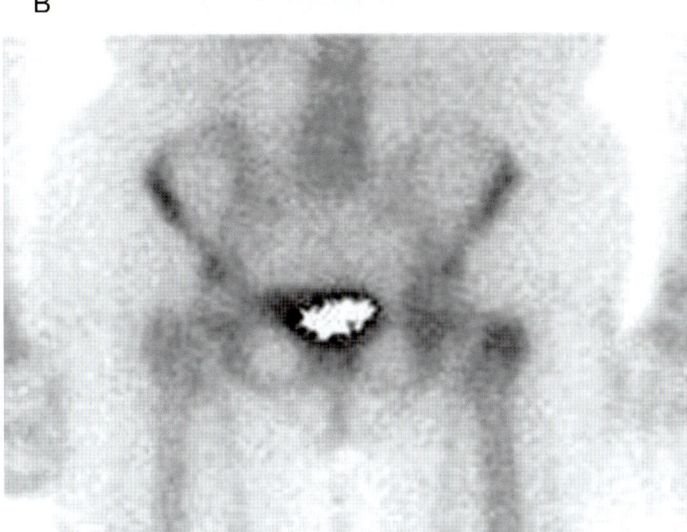

D

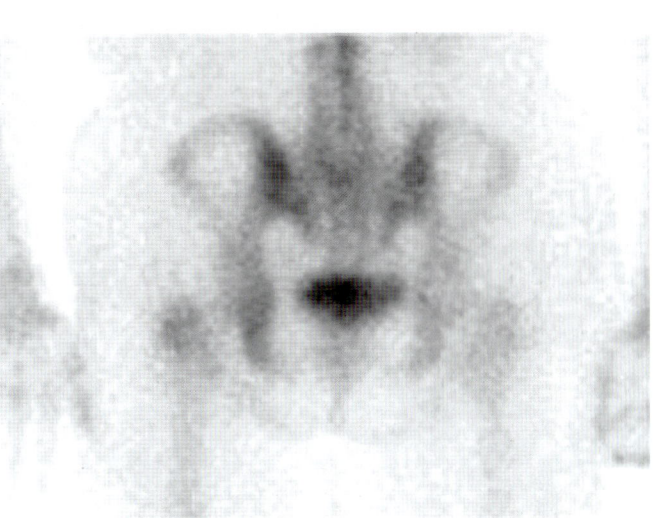

E

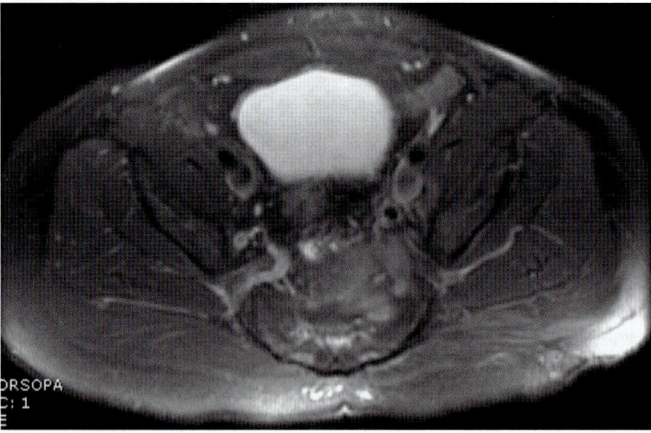

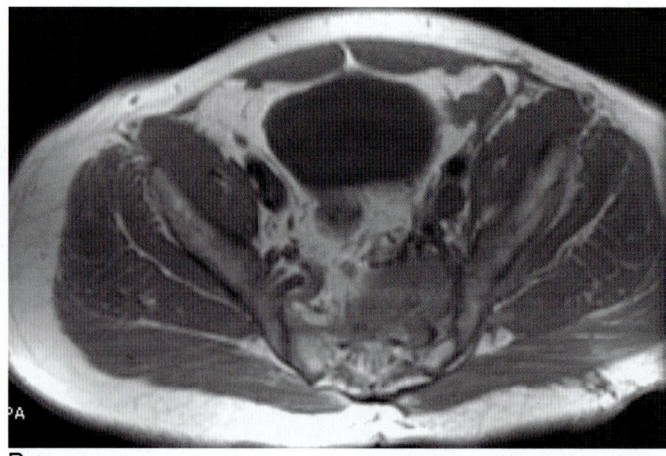

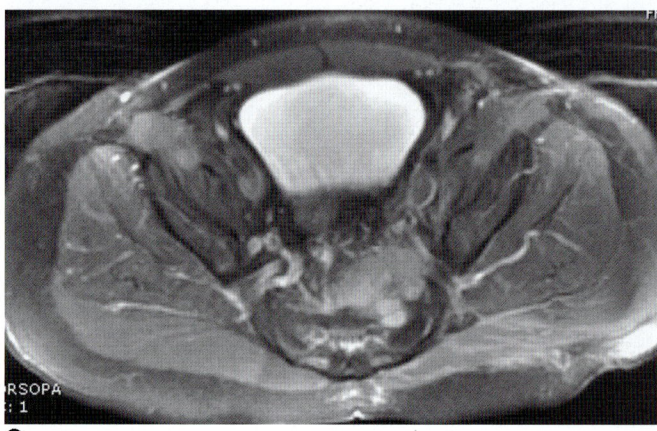

■ **FIGURE 68-15** **A,** Axial T2-weighted MR image with fat saturation of the pelvis in a 45-year-old male patient with disseminated coccidioidomycosis shows a destructive lesion of intermediate-increased signal intensity involving the anterior and central and left aspect of the sacrum with associated soft tissue mass. **B,** The lesion is of intermediate signal intensity on the T1-weighted axial MR image. **C,** Moderate enhancement is seen on the T1-weighted axial MR image with fat saturation after intravenous administration of gadolinium-based contrast agent.

findings are nonspecific and include increased signal intensity on the T2-weighted images and decreased signal intensity on the T1-weighted images.[7]

Cryptococcosis

Magnetic resonance imaging is useful in detection and evaluation of local extent of cryptococcal osteomyelitis and soft tissue abscesses.[10] The lesions can demonstrate enhancement on the postcontrast images (Fig. 68-24).[9]

Sporotrichosis

Magnetic resonance imaging can be utilized in evaluation of soft tissue or skeletal lesions. The findings are nonspecific.[12,43]

Histoplasmosis

Magnetic resonance imaging may be utilized in evaluation of musculoskeletal histoplasmosis, for both osseous and soft tissue infection. However, there is no relevant literature on MRI of osseous lesions. The findings of soft tissue infections are nonspecific.[15,16]

Aspergillosis

Magnetic resonance imaging is the study of choice for evaluation of the local extent of skeletal aspergillosis, especially with cranial and facial involvement.[44] The findings seen with involvement of peripheral skeletal structures and joints are nonspecific[2] (see Fig. 68-20B-D). The MRI appearance of aspergillous spondylitis is also nonspecific and resembles that of tuberculous infection.[45]

Candidiasis

Magnetic resonance imaging is very useful in delineation of the extent of candidal osteomyelitis. The signal characteristics are nonspecific with enhancement on the postcontrast images, as in other fungal or bacterial infections.[1,40,46]

Mucormycosis

Magnetic resonance imaging is the modality of choice in evaluation of the local extent of this devastating disease, especially with common rhinocerebral involvement[1,47] or rare spinal involvement.[23] With the involvement of

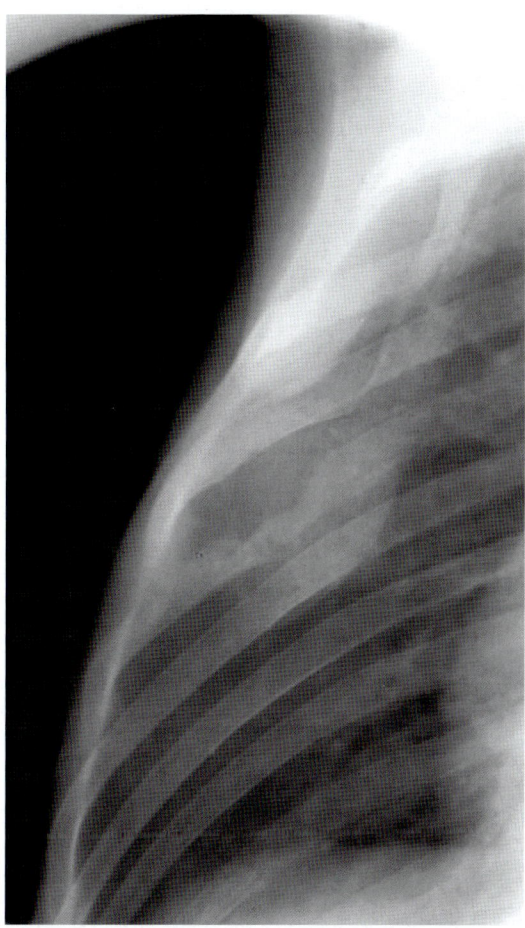

■ FIGURE 68-16 Frontal radiograph of the right hemithorax in a patient with blastomycosis shows a destructive lesion involving the lateral chest wall with associated soft tissue mass. *(Courtesy of Richard Daffner, MD, Pittsburgh, PA.)*

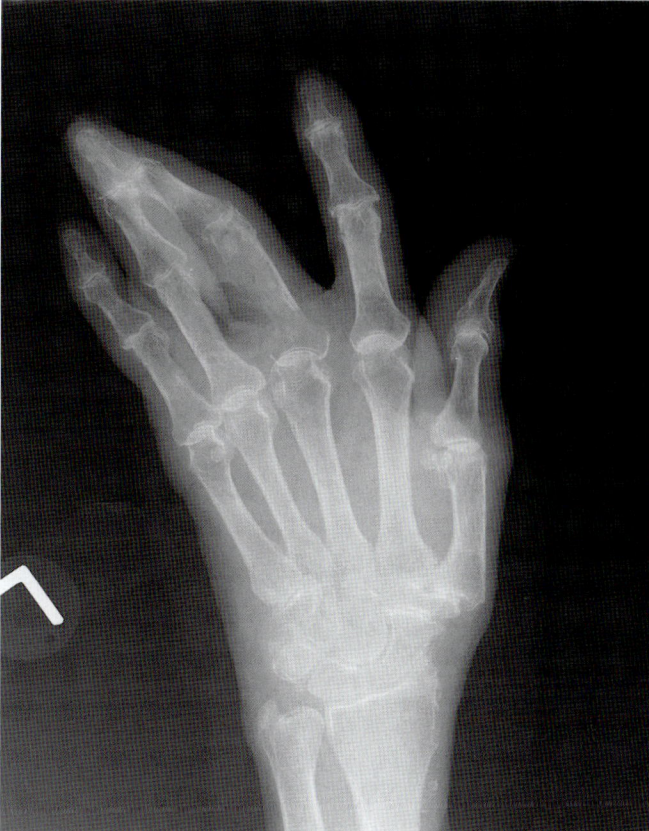

■ FIGURE 68-18 An 85-year-old patient presented with cryptococcal osteomyelitis and septic arthritis of the proximal third interphalangeal joint. Frontal radiograph of the hand shows destructive lytic lesions involving the proximal and, to a lesser extent, middle phalanges of the third digit with associated septic arthritis and soft tissue swelling. Note a large soft tissue ulcer at the ulnar aspect of the proximal phalanx. *(Courtesy of Ruth Ceulemans, MD, Chicago, IL.)*

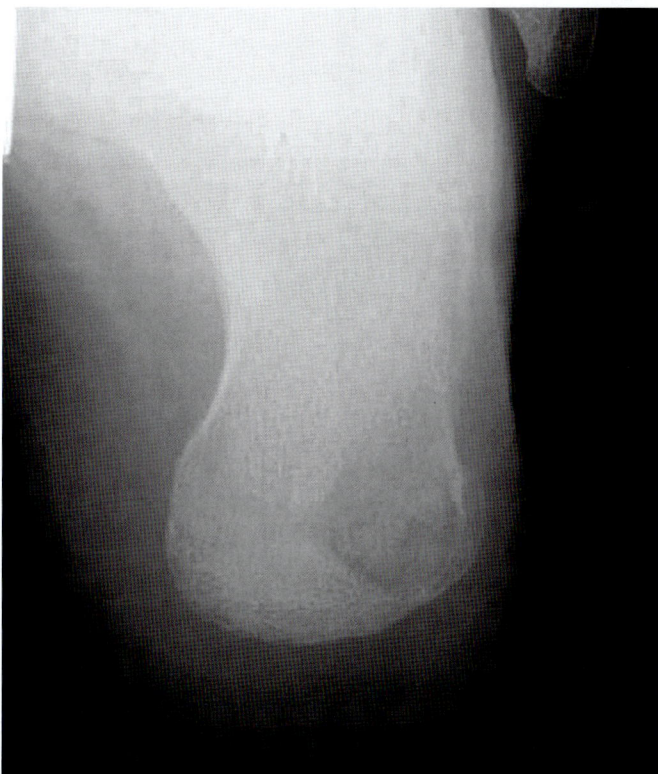

B

■ FIGURE 68-17 Blastomycosis osteomyelitis. Axial (**A**) and lateral (**B**) radiographs of the calcaneus show a destructive lesion in the calcaneal tuber. *(Courtesy of Richard Daffner, MD, Pittsburgh, PA.)*

A

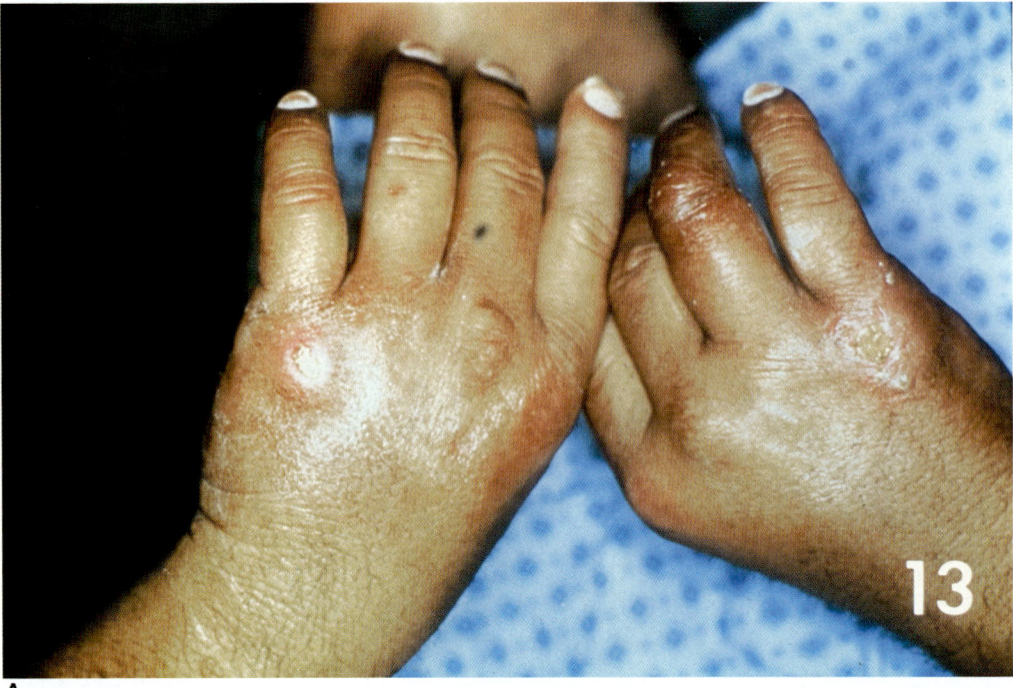

A

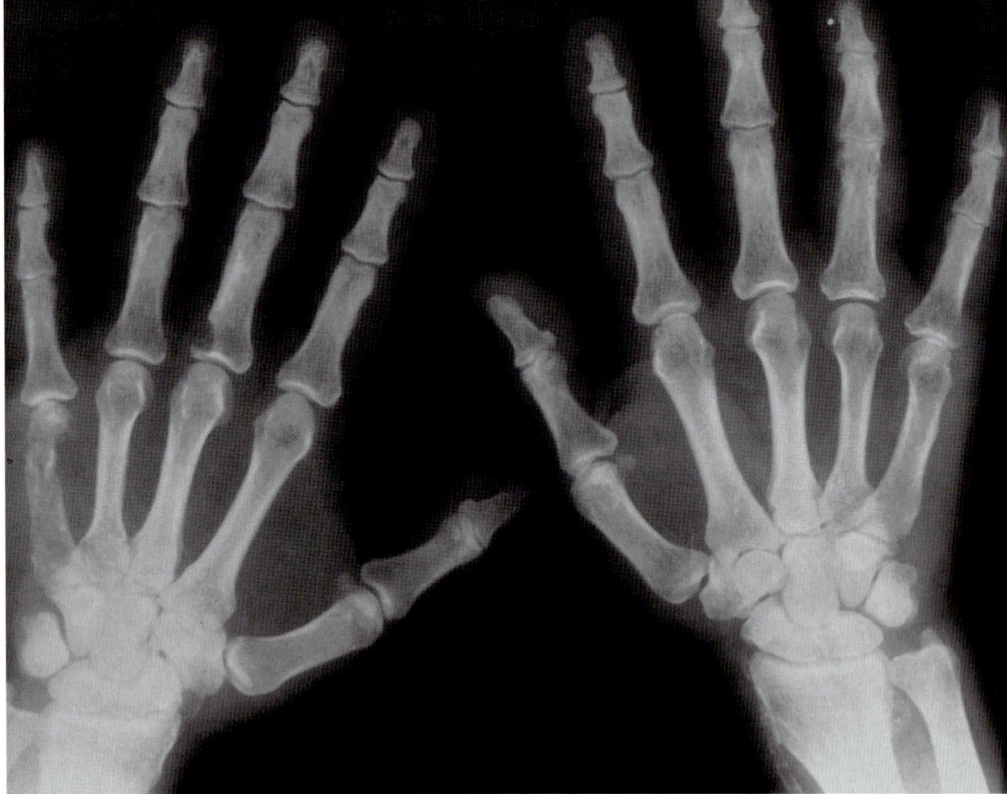

B

■ **FIGURE 68-19** Sporotrichosis osteomyelitis in a florist. **A,** Gross photograph of the hands shows bilateral soft tissue nodules and ulcers. **B,** Frontal radiograph of the hands shows a destructive lesion involving the entire left fifth metacarpal bone with associated pathologic fracture through the metacarpal neck. An additional destructive lesion is seen involving the ulnar aspect of the base of the left third proximal phalanx. *(Courtesy of George Barnes, MD, Tucson, AZ.)*

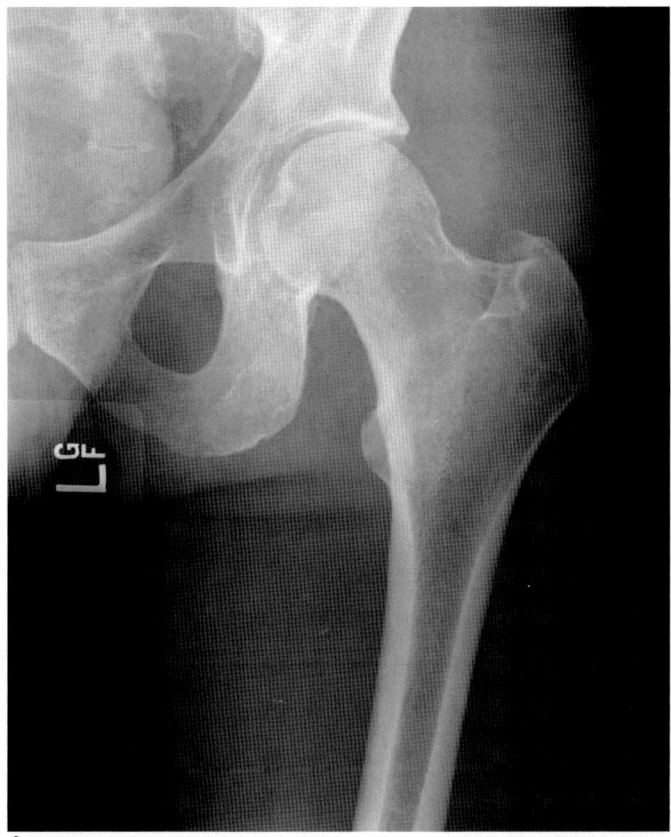

A

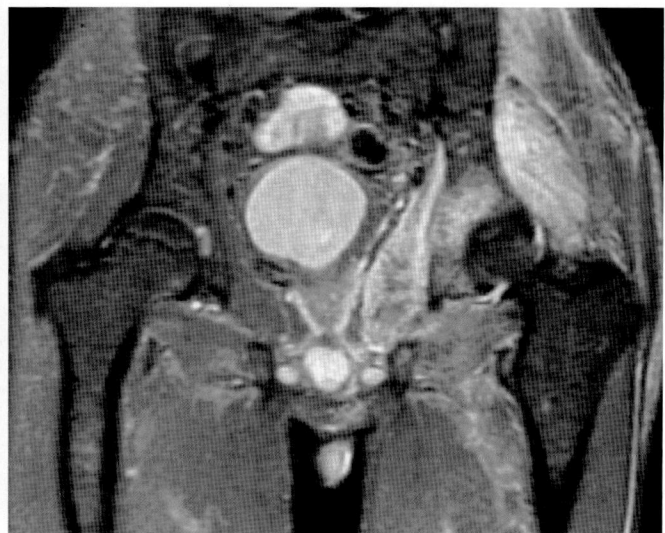

B

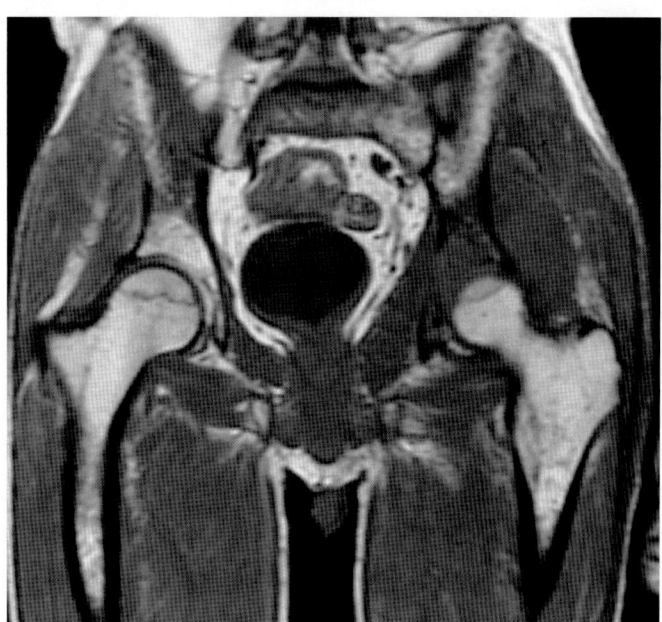

C

■ **FIGURE 68-20** Osteomyelitis resulting from aspergillosis with extension into the soft tissues. **A,** Frontal radiograph of the left hip shows an ill-defined lytic lesion involving the left acetabulum and superior pubic ramus. Note the associated soft tissue mass. **B,** Coronal STIR MR image of the pelvis shows an extensive lesion of predominantly increased signal intensity involving the left acetabulum and the superior pubic ramus with associated large soft tissue component about the medial pelvic wall and the periphery of the left acetabulum. Note the edema in the adjacent gluteal, pelvic floor, and adductor musculature. Some mass effect to the urinary bladder is present. **C,** Coronal T1-weighted MR image of the pelvis shows intermediate signal intensity in the regions of abnormality.

(Continued)

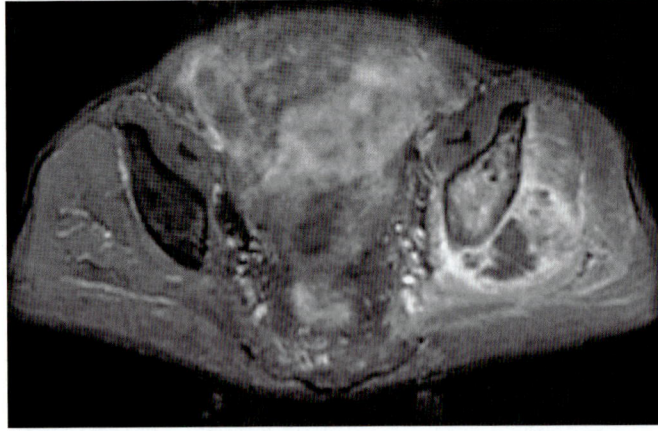

D

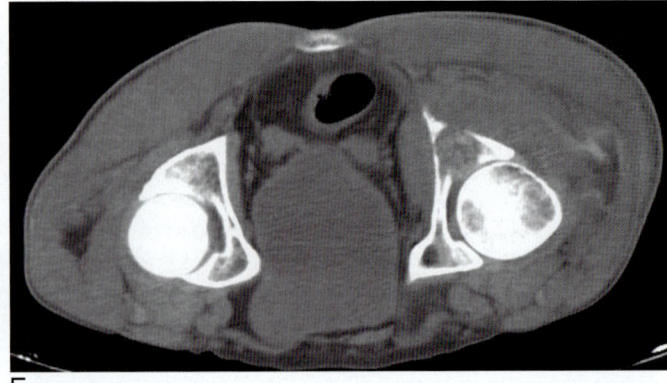

E

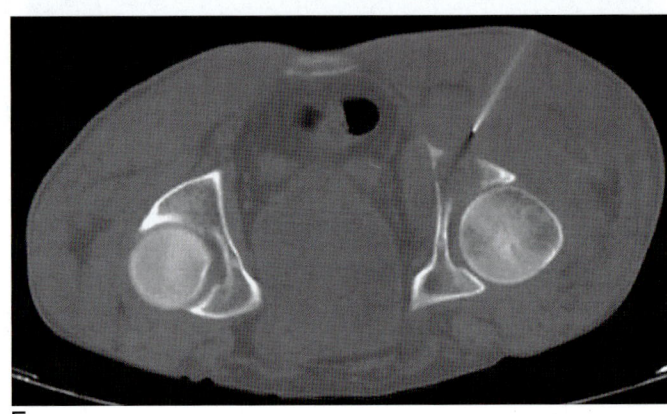

F

■ **FIGURE 68-20—Cont'd** **D,** Axial T1-weighted MR image with fat saturation after intravenous administration of gadolinium-based contrast agent shows enhancement in the affected areas and a rim-enhancing abscess posterior to the left hip in the left gluteal musculature. **E** and **F,** Axial CT images of the hips with the patient in prone position show a destructive lytic lesion involving the posterior aspect of the left acetabulum with areas of cortical breakthrough and associated soft tissue component. In **F,** note a biopsy needle within the soft tissue mass at the posterior aspect of the left hip. *(Courtesy of Hilary Umans, MD, Bronx, NY.)*

paranasal sinuses the MRI findings are similar to those of bacterial sinusitis. Necrosis of the turbinates, palate, or face and invasion of ophthalmic and carotid arteries are known complications of advanced mucormycosis.[1] In mucormycotic spondylodiscitis MRI shows local osseous and soft tissue extent of disease. The signal characteristics are nonspecific.[23]

Maduromycosis

Magnetic resonance imaging investigation is superior to the other imaging techniques in the evaluation of mycetoma and the assessment of therapy.[41] MRI allows good visualization of soft tissue involvement and bone destruction. T1-weighted images demonstrate decreased signal intensity of the affected bones and the adjacent soft tissues, findings suggestive of chronic osteomyelitis. Some enhancement is observed on the postcontrast images. T2-weighted and STIR sequences reveal increased signals in the affected regions[27,41] (see Fig. 68-23B-D).

In 80% of patients small low signal intensity lesions can be seen on both T1-weighted and T2-weighted images consistent with grains, which seem to differentiate mycetoma from other infections and tumorous lesions. MRI is useful in evaluation of healing.[41]

Actinomycosis

The MRI findings and signal characteristics are non-specific and resemble those of pyogenic, tuberculous, and other atypical infections. Decreased signal intensity on T1-weighted images and increased signal intensity on fluid-sensitive sequences are observed. Postcontrast images show enhancement in the affected regions.[28-30,48]

Nocardiosis

Magnetic resonance imaging findings of nocardiosis are nonspecific and resemble those that are seen in tuberculosis and fungal infections.[35]

Multidetector Computed Tomography

Coccidioidomycosis

Computed tomographic findings parallel those found on radiography. This imaging modality is effective in further assessment of the local extent of coccidioidomycosis in those with skeletal and soft tissue involvement (see Figs. 68-13F and 68-14B and C).[4]

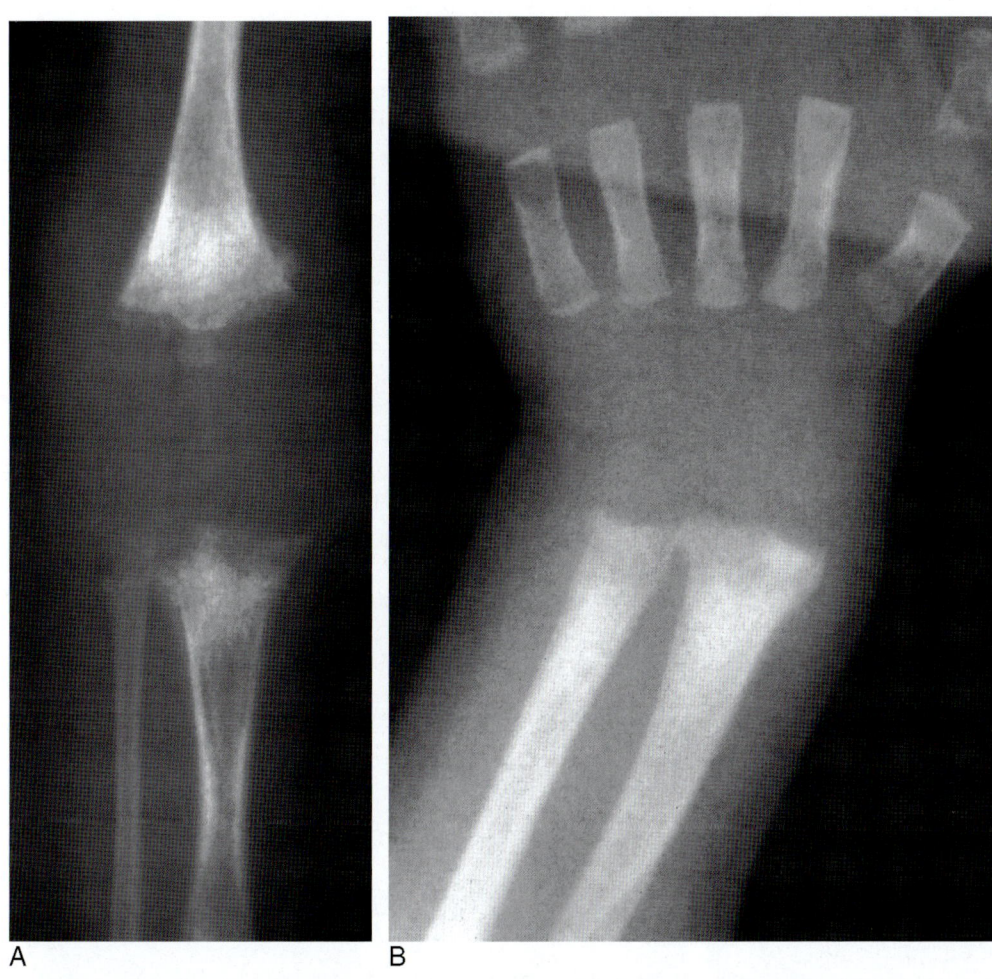

■ **FIGURE 68-21** Disseminated candidiasis with multifocal osteomyelitis and septic knee. **A,** Frontal radiograph of the knee in a 4-week-old male newborn shows bone destruction and sclerosis with associated periostitis involving the distal femur, proximal-to-mid tibia, and proximal fibula. **B,** Frontal radiograph of the wrist shows ill-defined lytic lesions involving the distal radial and ulnar metaphyses. *(Courtesy of George Barnes, MD, Tucson, AZ.)*

A   B

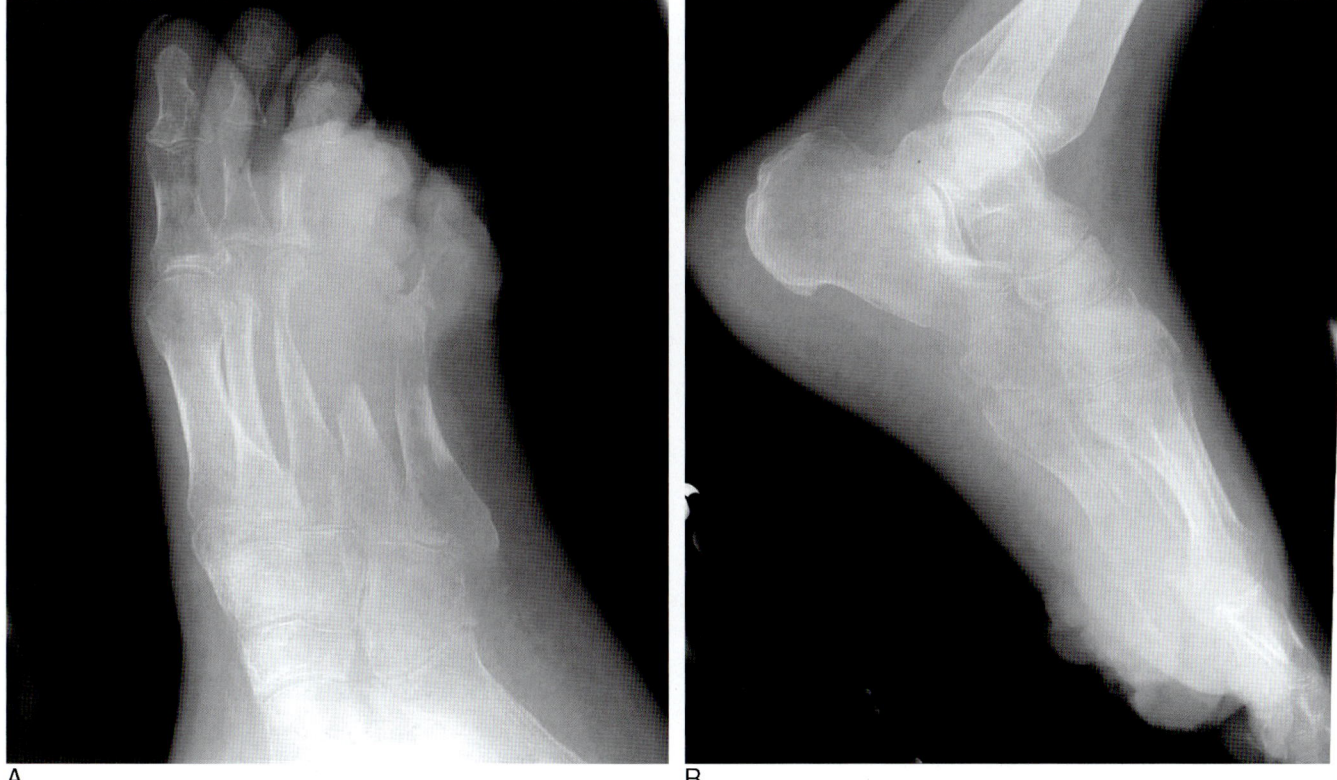

A   B

■ **FIGURE 68-22** Madura foot in a veteran patient. Oblique (**A**) and lateral (**B**) radiographs of the right foot show extensive destructive changes involving multiple bones at the lateral aspect of the foot with soft tissue ulcers and swelling. *(Courtesy of Richard Daffner, MD, Pittsburgh, PA.)*

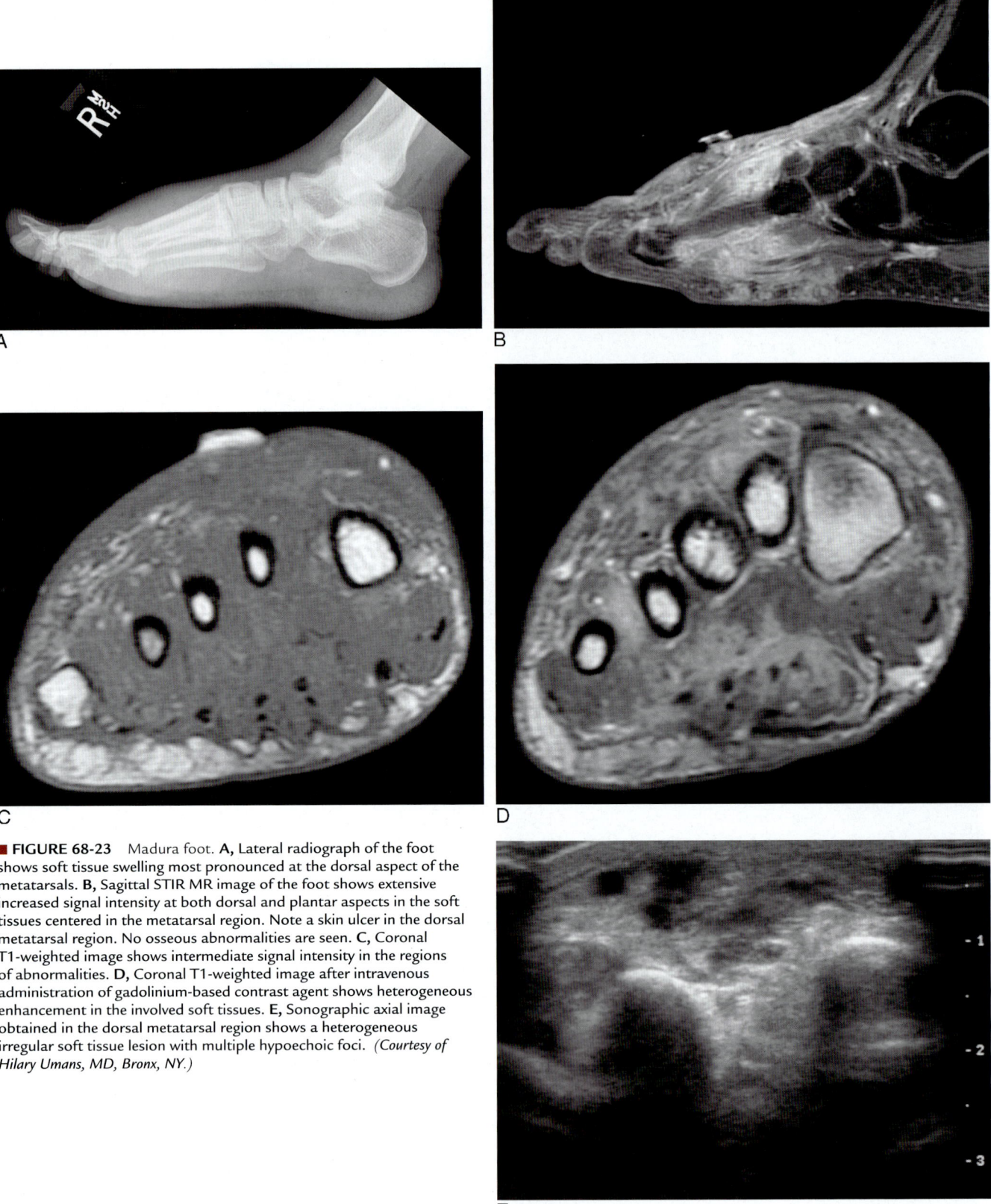

■ **FIGURE 68-23** Madura foot. **A,** Lateral radiograph of the foot shows soft tissue swelling most pronounced at the dorsal aspect of the metatarsals. **B,** Sagittal STIR MR image of the foot shows extensive increased signal intensity at both dorsal and plantar aspects in the soft tissues centered in the metatarsal region. Note a skin ulcer in the dorsal metatarsal region. No osseous abnormalities are seen. **C,** Coronal T1-weighted image shows intermediate signal intensity in the regions of abnormalities. **D,** Coronal T1-weighted image after intravenous administration of gadolinium-based contrast agent shows heterogeneous enhancement in the involved soft tissues. **E,** Sonographic axial image obtained in the dorsal metatarsal region shows a heterogeneous irregular soft tissue lesion with multiple hypoechoic foci. *(Courtesy of Hilary Umans, MD, Bronx, NY.)*

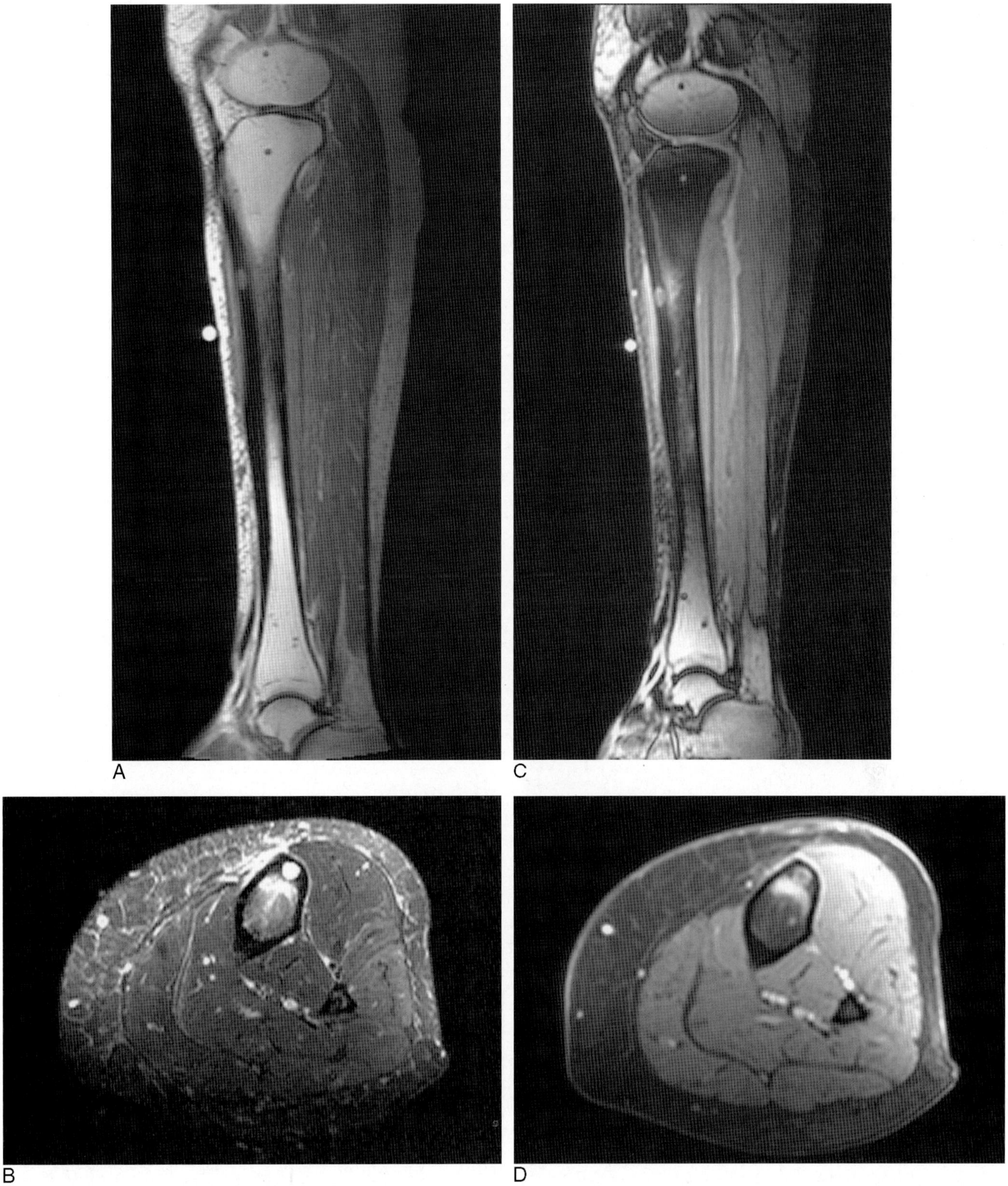

A

C

B

D

■ **FIGURE 68-24** Cryptococcal osteomyelitis with cortical abscess. **A,** Sagittal T1-weighted MR image of the leg shows a small lesion of intermediate signal intensity in the anterior tibial cortex with a larger area of associated periostitis and medullary edema also of intermediate signal intensity. **B,** Axial T2-weighted image with fat saturation shows increased signal intensity in the region of abnormality. Sagittal (**C**) and axial (**D**) T1-weighted images with fat saturation after intravenous administration of gadolinium-based contrast agent show enhancement of the region of abnormality with rim enhancement of the intracortical abscess. *(Courtesy of Ruth Ceulemans, MD, Chicago, IL.)*

North American Blastomycosis

Computed tomography is helpful in further characterization of radiographic findings and assessment of local skeletal and soft tissue extension of the lesion.[7]

Cryptococcosis

Computed tomography is useful in further characterization of radiographic findings and assessment of bone and soft tissue extension of the cryptococcal musculoskeletal lesions (Fig. 68-25).[9,11]

Sporotrichosis

Computed tomography can be utilized to characterize destructive skeletal and soft tissue lesions as well as other organ involvement.[13,49]

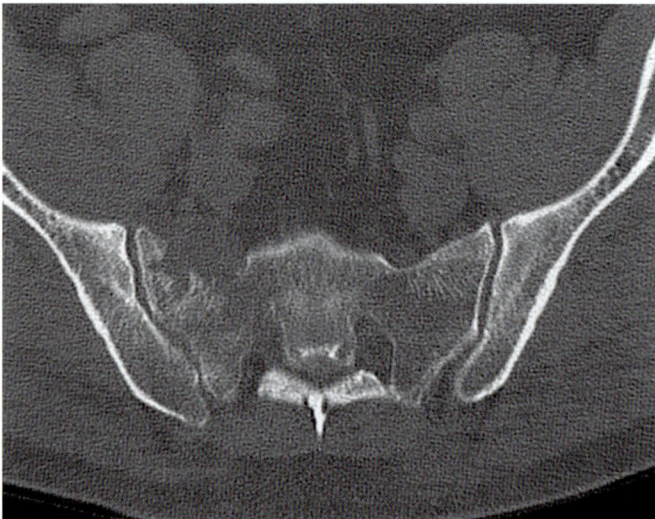

■ **FIGURE 68-25** A 25-year-old man presented with cryptococcal osteomyelitis involving the sacrum. Axial CT image of the pelvis shows a destructive lytic lesion involving the anterior aspect of the right sacrum with associated osteomyelitis. *(Courtesy of Richard Daffner, MD, Pittsburgh, PA.)*

Histoplasmosis

Radiographic findings of skeletal histoplasmosis are similar to those of sarcoidosis and tuberculosis.[1] CT parallels and further characterizes the radiographic findings.[39]

Aspergillosis

Computed tomography of skeletal aspergillosis parallels those seen on radiographs[19] with better characterization of local extension (Fig. 68-26).[44-45]

Candidiasis

Computed tomographic findings of candidal osteomyelitis parallel those seen on radiographs and better delineate osseous destruction and extension into the soft tissues and spinal canal.[1,40,46]

Mucormycosis

Computed tomography is a useful imaging modality in evaluation of local osseous and soft tissue extent of mucormycosis.[23,47]

Maduromycosis

Computed tomography is helpful in visualization of bone destruction, periosteal reaction, and soft tissue involvement in maduromycosis.[41]

Actinomycosis

Computed tomography is a helpful imaging modality in evaluation of local extent of skeletal and soft tissue actinomycosis (Fig. 68-27).[2,31,48]

Nocardiosis

The CT findings of nocardiosis are nonspecific and resemble those that are seen in tuberculosis and fungal infections.[35]

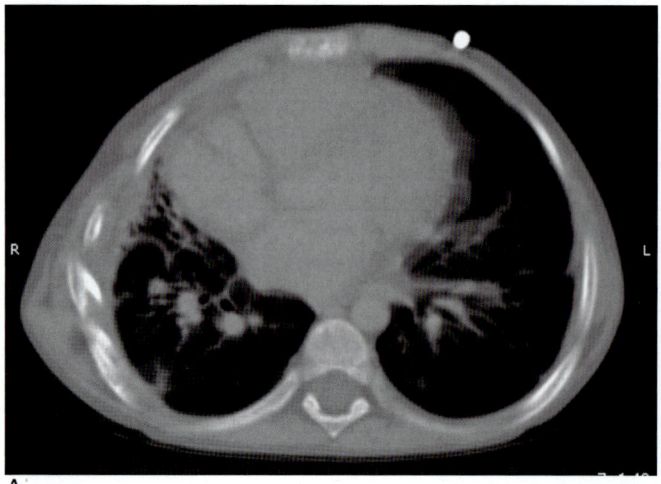
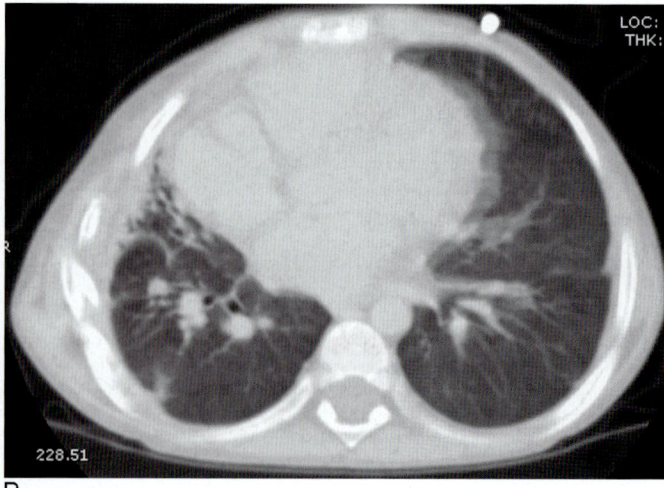

■ **FIGURE 68-26** A and B, Axial CT images of the chest in a child with invasive aspergillosis show pulmonary lesions in the right lung base with extension into the pleura and chest wall. Note destructive lesions involving multiple ribs.

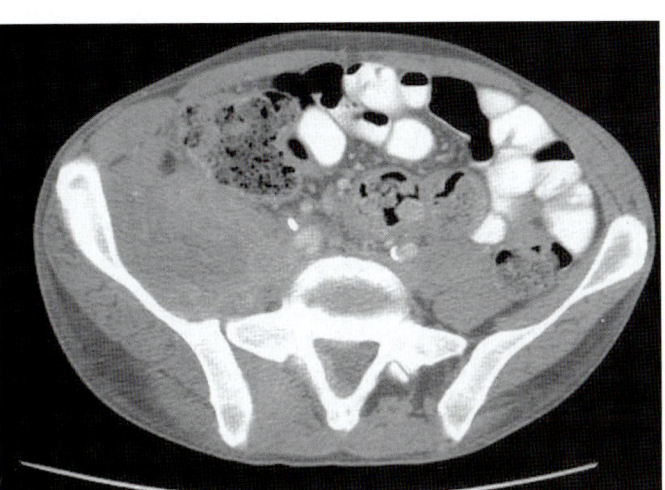

■ **FIGURE 68-27** Actinomycosis involving the iliopsoas muscle. Axial CT image of the pelvis shows a large abscess involving the right iliopsoas muscle. *(Courtesy of Jennifer Weaver, MD, Ann Arbor, MI.)*

Ultrasonography

The literature on sonographic evaluation of musculoskeletal fungal infections is limited. In a case report of soft tissue blastomycosis of the forearm in a child, ultrasound could not distinguish an inflammatory mass from a soft tissue tumor, including malignancy, and the diagnosis was made by biopsy.[50]

Ultrasonography is a useful imaging modality in diagnosis of mycetoma. Eumycetoma is characterized by the numerous sharp bright hyperechoic echoes produced by the black grains. Multiple thick-walled cavities are seen without acoustic enhancement. In actinomycetoma, the findings are similar but the grains are less distinct (see Fig. 68-23E).[26]

Nuclear Medicine

Coccidioidomycosis

Radionuclide bone scanning either with ^{99m}Tc-MDP or gallium-67 radiopharmaceutical agents is a sensitive method for detection of disseminated musculoskeletal coccidioidomycosis. Gallium scan delineates well the soft tissue involvement (see Fig. 68-14D and E).[2,4]

North American Blastomycosis

Scanning with ^{99m}Tc-MDP is useful in evaluation of skeletal blastomycosis and shows increased radiotracer uptake in the affected osseous structures.[7]

Cryptococcosis

Bone scintigraphy shows increased radiotracer uptake in the cryptococcal skeletal lesions and is helpful in evaluation of multifocal involvement.[9,11]

Sporotrichosis

Three-phase ^{99m}Tc-MDP and gallium-67 bone scintigraphy is useful in evaluation of the extent of sporotrichosis. Increased radiotracer uptake in the affected regions can be seen.[14,51,52]

Histoplasmosis

There is no relevant English literature on the use of bone scintigraphy in musculoskeletal histoplasmosis.

Aspergillosis

Technetium bone scintigraphy shows increased radiotracer uptake in the skeletal lesions of invasive aspergillosis.[19]

Candidiasis

Technetium bone scintigraphy shows increased radiotracer uptake in candidal osteomyelitis.[46] A gallium scan was reported as useful in the detection of early candidal septic arthritis and soft tissue abscess.[21,53]

Mucormycosis

There is no recent English literature on the use of bone scintigraphy in the evaluation of mucormycosis. Scinticans typically show increased radiotracer uptake in any inflammatory involvement of the skeleton.[54,55]

Maduromycosis

Three-phase technetium scintigraphy reveals increased radiotracer uptake in the mycetoma lesions. It is very helpful in assessment of the healing process characterized by normalization of radiotracer uptake on follow-up studies.[41]

Actinomycosis

The technetium bone scan is a sensitive examination that may show abnormal radionuclide uptake in an affected area in an early stage of the skeletal actinomycosis, before obvious radiographic findings.[28]

Nocardiosis

Nuclear medicine scans may show nonspecific increased uptake in the regions of nocardial osteomyelitis.[37]

Positron Emission Tomography/ Computed Tomography

The utility of PET and PET/CT imaging in musculoskeletal fungal and higher bacterial infections has yet to be determined.

SYNOPSIS OF TREATMENT OPTIONS
Medical Treatment

Coccidioidomycosis

Osteomyelitis secondary to coccidioidomycosis remains a rare but difficult disease to treat, with a lifelong risk of recurrence. A combined medical and surgical approach has been shown to be effective, and medical therapy alone with intravenous amphotericin B followed by suppressive azole therapy may be effective in selected patients (see Fig. 68-12F).[56]

Blastomycosis

Treatment with amphotericin B and ketoconazole, in conjunction with operative treatment, is very effective.[8] Current medications also include itraconazole and fluconazole. Osteomyelitis caused by *B. dermatitidis* requires at least 1 year of medical therapy.[7]

Cryptococcosis

The therapeutic protocol for treatment of cryptococcal osteomyelitis has not yet been defined. Most authors advocate a combined medical and surgical treatment. Medical treatment includes amphotericin B, fluconazole, and itraconazole.[9-11]

Sporotrichosis

Amphotericin B is recommended for the treatment of systemic infection caused by *S. schenckii*. However, because of toxicity, frequent relapses, and the resistance of some strains, newer drugs may be more effective. Itraconazole is effective in cutaneous and lymphocutaneous sporotrichosis, but data on their efficacy in systemic infections are scarce.[13,57]

Histoplasmosis

Itraconazole is now considered the therapy of choice for chronic histoplasmosis.[15,58] Combined medical and surgical treatments are utilized if needed.[39]

Aspergillosis

Optimum treatment of aspergillous osteomyelitis involves débridement and antifungal treatment with amphotericin B, although this drug has relatively poor bone penetration and a high incidence of side effects. Oral itraconazole has been used as a single agent in patients with invasive and osseous aspergillosis. It has been limited to improvement and not cure in many cases. It is usually very well tolerated and is therefore a good alternative to intravenous treatment.[19]

Candidiasis

Amphotericin B continues to be the mainstay of therapy for systemic fungal infections including candidiasis, but its use is limited because of the risks of nephrotoxicity and hypokalemia. Newer formulations of amphotericin B, namely, the liposomal and the lipid complex forms, have become available and have been reported to have less toxicity. Fluconazole, a triazole that has far less toxicity, has been used with some success. It has the additional advantage of being available as an oral formulation.[22,59] With candidal osteomyelitis surgical débridement and or resection combined with medical therapy may be needed.[60]

Mucormycosis

The standard treatment is a combination of amphotericin B therapy, surgical débridement, and reversal of the underlying disease or immunosuppression. Posaconazole, a new triazole antifungal, has been used successfully in a number of cases that did not respond to amphotericin B.[24]

Maduromycosis

Actinomycetoma is amenable to treatment by antibiotics, preferably by combined drug therapy for long periods. Eumycetoma is usually treated by aggressive surgical excision combined with medical treatment.[26]

Therapy for actinomycetoma is given over a long period and in higher doses because the microorganisms are locked in fibrous tissue. The mean duration of treatment is 1 year. The cure rate varies from 60% to 90%. The commonly used drugs include a combination of streptomycin sulfate and dapsone. If there is no response in a few months or if there are persistent side effects, then dapsone is replaced by co-trimoxazole. An excellent therapeutic response to amikacin sulfate alone or in combination with co-trimoxazole has been reported.

In resistant cases other drugs such as rifampicin, sulfadoxine-pyrimethamine (Fansidar), and sulfonamides have been tried. Because the actinomycetoma has an ill-defined border a margin of healthy tissue should be excised with the lesion.[26]

In many centers, surgery is still the most acceptable line of treatment for eumycetoma. Aggressive surgical excision, debulking, or amputation in advanced cases has been carried out. Medical treatment of the patients with eumycetoma may continue for periods ranging from a few months to many years. Ketoconazole or itraconazole is utilized. When the lesion becomes well localized and encapsulated, it can be easily removed surgically. There is no justification for mutilating surgery or amputation before trying medical treatment.[26]

Actinomycosis

Penicillin is considered the best therapeutic agent in the treatment of the musculoskeletal actinomycosis and is generally given for 6 to 12 months. Others drugs, including cephalosporins, erythromycin, and cyclines, are also effective.[28] With the treatment of complicated cases with spinal infection, the use of an external fixator may be of benefit in conjunction with medical therapy.[48]

Nocardiosis

Sulfamethoxazole-trimethoprim is an effective antibiotic agent for the treatment of nocardiosis.[35] Different subspecies show variable susceptibility to amikacin, the third generation of cephalosporins, imipenem/meropenem, and sulfur-based antimicrobial agents.[37]

SUGGESTED READING

Arkun R. Parasitic and fungal disease of bones and joints. Semin Musculoskelet Radiol 2004; 8:231–242.

REFERENCES

1. Arkun R. Parasitic and fungal disease of bones and joints. Semin Musculoskelet Radiol 2004; 8:231–242.
2. Resnick D. Osteomyelitis, septic arthritis, and soft tissue infection: organisms. In Resnick D (ed). Diagnosis of Bone and Joint Disorders, 4th ed. Philadelphia, WB Saunders, 2002, pp 2510–2624.

3. McGahan JP, Graves DS, Palmer PE, et al. Classic and contemporary imaging of coccidioidomycosis. AJR Am J Roentgenol 1981; 136:393-404.
4. Zeppa MA, Laorr A, Greenspan A, et al. Skeletal coccidioidomycosis: imaging findings in 19 patients. Skeletal Radiol 1996; 25:337-343.
5. Bronnimann DA, Galgiani JN. Coccidioidomycosis. Eur J Clin Microbiol Infect Dis 1989; 8:466-473.
6. Centers for Disease Control and Prevention (CDC) and Jajosky RA, Hall PA, Adams DA, et al. Summary of notifiable diseases—United States, 2004. MMWR Morb Mortal Wkly Rep 2006; 53:1-79.
7. Saiz P, Gitelis S, Virkus W, et al. Blastomycosis of long bones. Clin Orthop Relat Res 2004; (421):255-259.
8. MacDonald PB, Black GB, MacKenzie R. Orthopaedic manifestations of blastomycosis. J Bone Joint Surg Am 1990; 72:860-864.
9. Armonda RA, Fleckenstein JM, Brandvold B, Ondra SL. Cryptococcal skull infection: a case report with review of the literature. Neurosurgery 1993; 32:1034-1036; discussion 1036.
10. Zanelli G, Sansoni A, Ricciardi B, et al. Muscular-skeletal cryptococcosis in a patient with idiopathic CD4+ lymphopenia. Mycopathologia 2001; 149:137-139.
11. Raftopoulos I, Meller JL, Harris V, Reyes HM. Cryptococcal rib osteomyelitis in a pediatric patient. J Pediatr Surg 1998; 33:771-773.
12. Patramanis GM, Rosengarten JL. MR imaging appearance of cutaneous sporotrichosis. AJR Am J Roentgenol 1999; 172:1697.
13. Yang DJ, Krishnan RS, Guillen DR, et al. Disseminated sporotrichosis mimicking sarcoidosis. Int J Dermatol 2006; 45:450-453.
14. Kumar R, van der Smissen E, Jorizzo J. Systemic sporotrichosis with osteomyelitis. J Can Assoc Radiol 1984; 35:83-84.
15. Cucurull E, Sarwar H, Williams CS 4th, Espinoza LR. Localized tenosynovitis caused by *Histoplasma capsulatum*: case report and review of the literature. Arthritis Rheum 2005; 53:129-132.
16. Voloshin DK, Lacomis D, McMahon D. Disseminated histoplasmosis presenting as myositis and fasciitis in a patient with dermatomyositis. Muscle Nerve 1995; 18:531-535.
17. Stevens DA. Diagnosis of fungal infections: current status. J Antimicrob Chemother 2002; 49(Suppl 1):11-9.
18. Trullas JC, Cervera C, Benito N, et al. Invasive pulmonary aspergillosis in solid organ and bone marrow transplant recipients. Transplant Proc 2005; 37:4091-4093.
19. Allen D, Ng S, Beaton K, Taussig D. Sternal osteomyelitis caused by *Aspergillus fumigatus* in a patient with previously treated Hodgkin's disease. J Clin Pathol 2002; 55:616-618.
20. Tsai SH, Peng YJ, Wang NC. Pyomyositis with hepatic and perinephric abscesses caused by *Candida albicans* in a diabetic nephropathy patient. Am J Med Sci 2006; 331:292-294.
21. Oster MW, Gelrud LG, Lotz MJ, et al. Psoas abscess localization by gallium scan in aplastic anemia. JAMA 1975; 232:377-379.
22. Rao S, Ali U. Systemic fungal infections in neonates. J Postgrad Med 2005; 51(Suppl 1):S27-S29.
23. Chen F, Lu G, Kang Y, et al. Mucormycosis spondylodiscitis after lumbar disc puncture. Eur Spine J 2006; 15:370-376. Epub 2005 Nov 18.
24. Brown J. Zygomycosis: an emerging fungal infection. Am J Health Syst Pharm 2005; 62:2593-2596.
25. Greenberg RN, Scott LJ, Vaughn HH, Ribes JA. Zygomycosis (mucormycosis): emerging clinical importance and new treatments. Curr Opin Infect Dis 2004; 17:517-525.
26. Fahal AH. Mycetoma: a thorn in the flesh. Trans R Soc Trop Med Hyg 2004; 98:3-11.
27. Ispoglou SS, Zormpala A, Androulaki A, Sipsas NV. Madura foot due to *Actinomadura madurae*: imaging appearance. Clin Imaging 2003; 27:233-235.
28. Voisin L, Vittecoq O, Mejjad O, et al. Spinal abscess and spondylitis due to actinomycosis. Spine 1998; 23:487-490.
29. Yamada H, Kondo S, Kamiya J, et al. Computed tomographic demonstration of a fish bone in abdominal actinomycosis: report of a case. Surg Today 2006; 36:187-189.
30. Stewart AE, Palma JR, Amsberry JK. Cervicofacial actinomycosis. Otolaryngol Head Neck Surg 2005; 132:957-959.
31. Aldamiz-Echebarria San Sebastian M, Vesga Carasa JC, Aspiazu Alonso-Urquijo A, et al. [An ischiorectal abscess due to *Actinomyces*]. Rev Clin Esp 1992; 190:258-260. Spanish.
32. Langloh JT, Lauerman WC. Primary actinomycosis of the quadriceps. J Pediatr Orthop 1987; 7:222-223.
33. Pinilla I, Martin-Hervas C, Gil-Garay E. Primary sternal osteomyelitis caused by *Actinomyces israelii*. South Med J 2006; 99:96-97.
34. Mah E, Stanley P, McCombe DB. Actinomycosis infection of the finger. Hand Surg 2005; 10:285-288.
35. Moore SL, Jones S, Lee JL. *Nocardia* osteomyelitis in the setting of previously unknown HIV infection. Skeletal Radiol 2005; 34:58-60. Epub 2004 Nov 13.
36. Malani AK, Gupta C, Weigand RT, et al. Thigh abscess due to *Nocardia farcinica*. J Natl Med Assoc 2006; 98:977-979.
37. Larobina M, McLean C, Davis BB. Clinical-pathologic conference in general thoracic surgery: disseminated nocardiosis presenting as Pancoast syndrome. J Thorac Cardiovasc Surg 2004; 127:568-571.
38. Berdeaux DH, Grogan TM, Pond GD. Disseminated histoplasmosis diagnosed by computed tomography directed needle biopsy of an adrenal mass. Comput Radiol 1985; 9:101-104.
39. N'dri Oka D, Varlet G, Kakou M, et al. [Spondylodiscitis due to *Histoplasma dubosii*. Report of two cases and review of the literature]. Neurochirurgie 2001; 47:431-434. French.
40. Miller DJ, Mejicano GC. Vertebral osteomyelitis due to *Candida* species: case report and literature review. Clin Infect Dis 2001; 33:523-530. Epub 2001 Jul 20.
41. Czechowski J, Nork M, Haas D, et al. MR and other imaging methods in the investigation of mycetomas. Acta Radiol 2001; 42:24-26.
42. Lund PJ, Nisbet JK, Valencia FG, Ruth JT. Magnetic resonance imaging in coccidioidal arthritis. Skeletal Radiol 1996; 25:661-665. Skeletal Radiol 1996; 25:661-665.
43. Zacharias J, Crosby LA. Sporotrichal arthritis of the knee. Am J Knee Surg 1997; 10:171-174.
44. Gotze G, Bloching M, Hainz M, Knipping S. [Invasive aspergillosis of the skull base with orbit infiltration]. HNO 2006; (Epub ahead of print) German.
45. Alkhunaizi AM, Amir AA, Al-Tawfiq JA. Invasive fungal infections in living unrelated renal transplantation. Transplant Proc 2005; 37:3034-3037.
46. Gursel T, Kaya Z, Kocak U, et al. *Candida* vertebra osteomyelitis in a girl with factor X deficiency. Haemophilia 2005; 11:629-632.
47. Mnif N, Hmaied E, Oueslati S, et al. [Imaging of rhinocerebral mucormycosis]. J Radiol 2005; 86(9 pt 1):1017-1020. French.
48. Fenichel I, Caspi I. The use of external fixation for the treatment of spine infection with *Actinomyces bacillus*. J Spinal Disord Tech 2006; 19:61-64.
49. Kumar R, Kaushal V, Chopra H, et al. Pansinusitis due to *Sporothrix schenckii*. Mycoses 2005; 48:85-88.
50. Albert MC, Zachary SV, Alter S. Blastomycosis of the forearm synovium in a child. Clin Orthop Relat Res 1995; (317):223-226.
51. Anees A, Ali A, Fordham EW. Abnormal bone and gallium scans in a case of multifocal systemic sporotrichosis. Clin Nucl Med 1986; 11:663-664.
52. Patange V, Cesani F, Phillpott J, Villanueva-Meyer J. Three-phase bone and Ga-67 scintigraphy in disseminated sporotrichosis. Clin Nucl Med 1995; 20:909-912.
53. Bittini A, Dominguez PL, Martinez Pueyo ML, et al. Comparison of bone and gallium-67 imaging in heroin users' arthritis. J Nucl Med 1985; 26:1377-1381.
54. Zwas ST, Czerniak P. Head and brain scan findings in rhinocerebral mucormycosis: case report. J Nucl Med 1975; 16:925-927.
55. Meyer RD. Scan findings in rhinocerebral mucormycosis. J Nucl Med 1977; 18:96.
56. Holley K, Muldoon M, Tasker S. *Coccidioides immitis* osteomyelitis: a case series review. Orthopedics 2002; 25:827-831; discussion 831-832.
57. Winn RE, Anderson J, Piper J, et al. Systemic sporotrichosis treated with itraconazole. Clin Infect Dis 1993; 17:210-217.
58. Meier JL. Mycobacterial and fungal infections of bone and joints. Curr Opin Rheumatol 1994; 6:408-414.
59. Masood A, Sallah S. Chronic disseminated candidiasis in patients with acute leukemia: emphasis on diagnostic definition and treatment. Leuk Res 2005; 29:493-501. Epub 2004 Dec 30.
60. Armstrong N, Schurr M, Helgerson R, Harms B. Fungal sacral osteomyelitis as the initial presentation of Crohn's disease of the small bowel: report of a case. Dis Colon Rectum 1998; 41:1581-1584.

Hydatid Disease (Echinococcosis)

ETIOLOGY

Hydatid disease (echinococcosis, hydatidosis) is a parasitic infection caused by the larval stage of two species of the tapeworm *Echinococcus*: *E. granulosus* (cystic hydatid disease) and *E. multilocularis* (alveolar hydatid disease). *E. granulosus* is endemic in sheep-raising areas worldwide, whereas *E. multilocularis* is limited to certain areas of Central Europe, Canada, and Alaska. Few cases of infections due to *E. oligarthrus* (polycystic hydatid disease) have also been reported in South America. Rare cases of *E. vogelii* are also reported.[1,2]

The intermediate hosts of the larval stage of *E. granulosus* are usually sheep, but they can also be found in cattle, hogs, and other domestic livestock and, occasionally, humans. The definitive hosts are dogs, foxes, and other carnivores that harbor the adult tapeworm in the small intestine. The carnivore becomes infected by ingesting the larval form of the intermediate host. The intermediate host becomes infected by ingesting eggs passed in the carnivore feces. The larval stages are referred to as hydatid cysts.[2]

Current data, based on genome patterns, generally support previous characterizations based on morphologic and biologic criteria, although at least 10 genetically distinct populations exist within the complex until recently denoted *E. granulosus*. It is important to recognize that important biologic differences exist between populations presently identified in many texts as *E. granulosus*, the causative agent of cystic echinococcosis, and that these may account for local differences in patterns of transmission and clinical and public health significance of the disease.[3]

PREVALENCE AND EPIDEMIOLOGY

In many endemic regions, incidence rates of cystic echinococcosis range from 5 to 20 per 100,000 population. Most urban populations are at low risk, but in rural endemic areas diagnostic incidence is significantly higher. The rates based on clinically diagnosed cases underestimate the burden of infection, but surveys of populations in endemic areas using ultrasonographic diagnostic techniques often measure cystic echinococcosis prevalences of 2% to 6%, which are manyfold higher than evident from clinically diagnosed cases. Consistently highest prevalence is found among populations involved with sheep raising, thus emphasizing the predominant public health importance of *E. granulosus*.[3]

E. multilocularis is largely confined to life cycles involving foxes and arvicolid rodents in ecosystems generally separate from humans; therefore, exposure of humans to *E. multilocularis* is relatively less common than exposure of humans to *E. granulosus*, the cause of cystic echinococcosis. However, domestic dogs or cats may become infected when they eat infected wild rodents, and infected pets are an important source of infection for humans.

The incidence of diagnosed disease in humans remains low, between 0.02 and 1.4 per 100,000 worldwide or larger in endemic regions. The known distribution and prevalence of infection in foxes and coyotes has increased in the United States and now extends from Montana to western Ohio. Exposure of humans appears rare.[3]

A network of collaborating groups working on echinococcosis was created through the auspices of the World Health Organization (Informal Working Group on Echinococcosis) and has facilitated the production of guidelines on disease treatment and control.[3]

CLINICAL PRESENTATION

The most commonly affected organ by *E. granulosus* is the liver. The skeletal structures are rarely involved.

The presenting symptoms of skeletal echinococcosis are nonspecific and variable and include pain, swelling, functional impairment, muscle wasting, nerve root pain, and fracture. General health is usually unaffected. The men and women seem equally affected. This disease is rare in children.[1,4]

KEY POINTS

- Hydatid disease (echinococcosis, hydatidosis) is a parasitic infection caused by the larval stage of two species of the tapeworm: *Echinococcus granulosus* (cystic hydatid disease) and *Echinococcus multilocularis* (alveolar hydatid disease).
- *E. granulosus* is endemic in several areas (mostly sheep-raising) worldwide, whereas *E. multilocularis* is limited to certain areas of Central Europe, Canada, and Alaska.
- The intermediate hosts of the larval stage of *E. granulosus* are usually sheep, but they can also be cattle, hogs, and other domestic livestock and, occasionally, humans.
- The definitive hosts of *E. granulosus* are dogs, foxes, and other carnivores that harbor the adult tapeworm in the small intestine. The carnivore becomes infected by ingesting the larval form of the intermediate host.
- The intermediate host becomes infected by ingesting eggs passed in the carnivore feces. The larval stages are referred to as hydatid cysts.
- Human infection by *E. granulosus* occurs when eggs passed in dog feces are accidentally swallowed through consumption of contaminated food or water. Embryos liberated from the eggs penetrate the intestinal mucosa and enter the portal venous system and the liver where they are trapped and become hydatid cysts, with less common involvement of other organs including the musculoskeletal system.
- Imaging should start with radiographs. CT and MRI are very valuable imaging modalities in evaluation of local extent of disease.
- Serologic tests are useful for confirming the presumptive imaging diagnosis of *E. granulosus*.
- The treatment of skeletal echinococcosis is surgical and similar to oncologic therapy.
- For the skeletal lesions, the World Health Organization suggests adjuvant chemotherapy with mebendazole or albendazole for at least 2 years after surgery. The efficiency of the medical treatment remains debated.

Skeletal lesions caused by *E. granulosus* occur by hematogenous seeding. The parasite spreads along cancellous trabeculae and through the medullary canal. Because no adventitia is formed in bone, the cysts enlarge and give rise to daughter cysts that may spread to adjacent bones. Skeletal hydatid lesions are usually polycystic. The disease can remain asymptomatic for a protracted period of time. Because of the rigid structure of cortical bone, hydatid cysts tend to grow slowly and rarely exceed 2 cm in diameter but can be significantly larger. The growing cysts lead to bone destruction and deformity, and in some cases, to cortical erosion, pathologic fracture, or compressive myelopathy with vertebral lesions. Secondary infection may also occur.[2] The most frequently involved skeletal structure is the spine in 35% of cases, followed by the pelvis in 21% of cases, the femur in 16% of cases, and the tibia in 10% of cases. The ribs, skull, scapula, humerus, fibula, and tarsal bones are less frequently involved.[5] Spinal lesions typically appear multiloculated, usually with epidural and paraspinal extension.[6] Muscles are rarely involved.[7] Hydatid synovitis can occur usually due to secondary extension from the adjacent bone or infrequently after hematogenous spread.[8] Concomitant hepatic involvement can be seen with the skeletal echinococcosis.[9]

Complications associated with skeletal echinococcosis include pathologic fracture, secondary infection especially with staphylococci, and rupture into the spinal canal with neurologic impairment including paraplegia.[1,10]

Eosinophilia is seen in 25% to 45% of patients.[1] Serologic tests are useful for confirming presumptive imaging diagnosis of *E. granulosus*. However, the limitations of serodiagnosis in cystic echinococcosis must be understood to correctly interpret the findings. Specific confirmation of reactivity can be obtained by demonstrating echinococcal antigens by immunodiffusion (arc 5) procedures or immunoblot assays (8-, 16-, 21-kDa bands). These latter serodiagnostic markers are the most *E. granulosus*-specific criteria described, but even they may be detected in serum of patients with other forms of echinococcosis and 5% to 10% of patients with *T. solium* cysticercosis.[3]

Alveolar echinococcosis closely mimics hepatic carcinoma and is a challenge to diagnose. Serologic tests are usually positive at high titers and highly specific antigens and have been identified and synthesized that, when used in serologic assays, are highly sensitive and specific for diagnosis of alveolar echinococcosis and can distinguish this infection from other forms of echinococcosis. Antibodies of the IgG1 and IgG4 isotypes are the most sensitive IgG responses in alveolar echinococcosis, and monitoring of these isotypes tended to correlate with active versus inactive disease and successful treatment. In seronegative patients polymerase chain reactions for detection of echinococcal-specific RNA or DNA, in closed- or open-biopsy specimens, have been developed and may confirm the diagnosis.[3] Fewer cases of alveolar echinococcosis of the bone were reported. Most common involvement was of the spine, soft tissues, and sternum from contiguous spread of disease from the liver. Distant metastases to the bone and soft tissue structures can also occur. Endovesicular daughter cysts are never observed.[11]

PATHOPHYSIOLOGY

Human infection by *E. granulosus* occurs when eggs passed in dog feces are accidentally swallowed through consumption of contaminated food or water. Embryos liberated from the eggs penetrate the intestinal mucosa and enter the portal venous system and the liver where they are trapped and become hydatid cysts (70%–75% of all cases). Some larvae reach the lungs (15%–25%) and develop into pulmonary hydatid cyst disease. Infrequently (10%), cysts form in the brain, skeletal muscles, bones, kidneys, spleen, or other tissues. In 20% of patients the disease is multifocal. Bone involvement varies between 0.5% and 4%.[2]

The histologic and gross pathologic features of skeletal echinococcosis differ from those seen in the other organs. The wall of the cyst has three layers: the inner germinal layer that gives rise within the cyst to scoleces (the infectious embryonic tapeworms), brood cysts, and daughter cysts; the intermediate layer that consists of an acellular laminated membrane; and the outer granulomatous adventitial layer that is produced by the host, in contrast to the other two layers that come from the parasite. Cysts developed in bones lack the adventitial layer that is typically seen with the visceral organ involvement. As the lesion grows, secondary/daughter cysts are seen. This gives a multifocal appearance, which is related to apposing walls of the daughter cysts. In pathologic specimens the cystic spaces tend to be larger with *E. granulosus* than with *E. multilocularis*.[1,2]

IMAGING TECHNIQUES

Imaging should start with radiographs. CT and MRI are very valuable imaging modalities in evaluation of local extent of disease. Ultrasonography and bone scintigraphy may also be used.

MANIFESTATIONS OF THE DISEASE
Radiography

The most common radiologic manifestation of skeletal hydatid disease is a lucent expansile lesion with cortical thinning. Single or multiple expansile lytic lesions containing trabeculae can be seen. With associated cortical interruption an adjacent soft tissue mass with calcifications can be noted. Calcifications represent dystrophic changes in dead parasites. In early stages there is no sclerosis or periosteal reaction. Osteosclerosis may be seen in the later stages of disease. A periosteal reaction is not seen unless there is a pathologic fracture (Fig. 68-28).[1,10,12]

Magnetic Resonance Imaging

Magnetic resonance imaging is helpful in verifying the extent of the disease, texture of the cyst, degree of medullary involvement, and viability of the cyst. On T1-weighted images there is a mixed morphologic appearance. High signal intensity content of the cyst may correlate with high cell or protein content, which is suggestive of extensive parasite-host reaction. Daughter cysts are more hypointense than the parent cyst on T1-weighted images. The

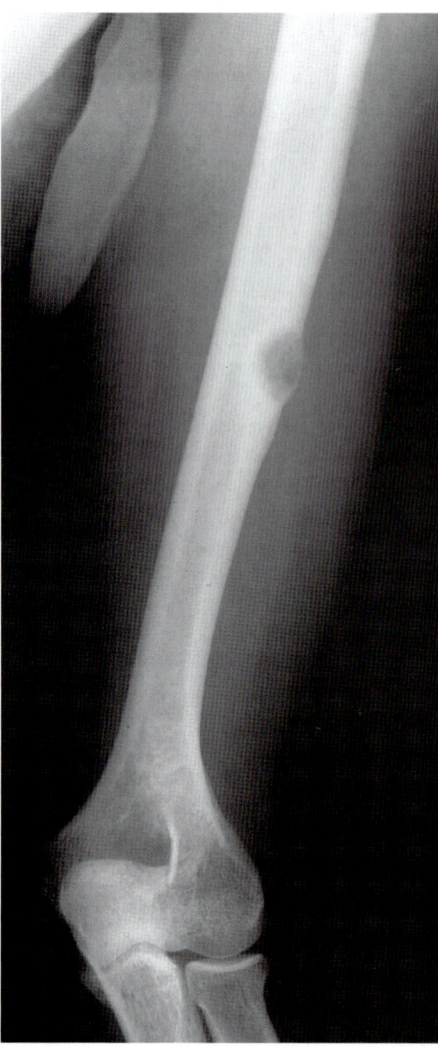

■ **FIGURE 68-28** Frontal radiograph of the humerus shows an eccentrically located mildly expansile bubbly lytic lesion with internal trabeculae involving the mid diaphysis in a Bosnian patient with hydatid disease. Note cortical thinning and sclerotic rim at the inner margin of the lesion. *(Courtesy of Department of Radiology, UMC Sarajevo, Bosnia & Herzegovina.)*

cyst wall or capsule is seen as a low intensity rim, which shows enhancement after intravenous administration of gadolinium. On T2-weighted imaging the daughter cysts are of slightly higher signal intensity than the parent cyst. Signal intensities may change with coexisting infection, calcification, or hemorrhage. With spinal involvement extradural spread of the hydatid cysts through a widened neural foramen into the muscle planes may result in the appearance of a "bunch of grapes." The T2- weighted sequence indicates whether a cyst is viable. A decrease in hyperintensity and an increase is hypointensity from a collapsed cyst wall is suggestive of a succumbed cyst. MRI may show endovesicular daughter cysts, which are frequently observed in hepatic disease but are rare in musculoskeletal manifestations of this disease.[1,9,10,12]

Patients with musculoskeletal lesions of cystic echinococcosis typically have cystic structures in adjacent soft tissues. These cysts morphologically resemble abscesses, with peripheral enhancement on the post-contrast T1-weighted fat-saturated images and variable signal intensities on T1-weighted MR images. The absence of calcifications or endovesicular daughter cysts does not exclude the diagnosis of cystic echinococcosis (Fig. 68-29A-G).[9]

Multidetector Computed Tomography

Computed tomography is a useful imaging modality in evaluation of skeletal hydatid disease. Single or multiple cystic lesions can be of variable size and typically are well defined, with no contrast enhancement, no daughter cysts, and no germinal membrane detachment. They may display a honeycomb appearance, cortical thinning or cortical destruction, pathologic fracture, and soft tissue mass.[5] CT may show endovesicular daughter cysts, which are frequently observed in hepatic disease but are rare in musculoskeletal manifestations of this disease (Figs. 68-29H-I and 68-30).[9]

Ultrasonography

Ultrasonography has a limited value in evaluation of musculoskeletal hydatid disease and may be utilized to show the extraosseous extension of the lesions into the adjacent soft tissues or to evaluate rare soft tissue lesions.[4,7]

Nuclear Medicine

The literature related to utility of nuclear medicine bone scans in evaluation of musculoskeletal echinococcosis is limited. Scanning with ^{99m}Tc-MDP scan may demonstrate increased uptake particularly at the peripheral borders.[13]

Positron Emission Tomography/ Computed Tomography

Positron emission tomography using (^{18}F) fluorodeoxy-glucose (FDG) has been developed for the follow-up of the patient with inoperable *E. multilocularis* liver disease who has undergone long-term therapy with a benzimidazole. This approach seems very promising to assess inflammatory activity and thereby to indirectly depict parasitic activity. PET/CT can evaluate the morphologic and functional aspects of the disease and assess the efficacy of treatment.[14] The utility of PET and PET/CT imaging in musculoskeletal hydatid disease is to be determined.

DIFFERENTIAL DIAGNOSIS

The differential diagnosis of skeletal echinococcosis is broad and includes plasmacytoma, brown tumor of hyperparathyroidism, cartilaginous neoplasms, fibrous dysplasia, metastatic disease, hemophiliac pseudotumor, giant cell tumor, aneurysmal bone cyst, and lymphoma. The differential diagnosis for spinal lesion includes chronic pyogenic and tuberculous osteomyelitis.[1,12]

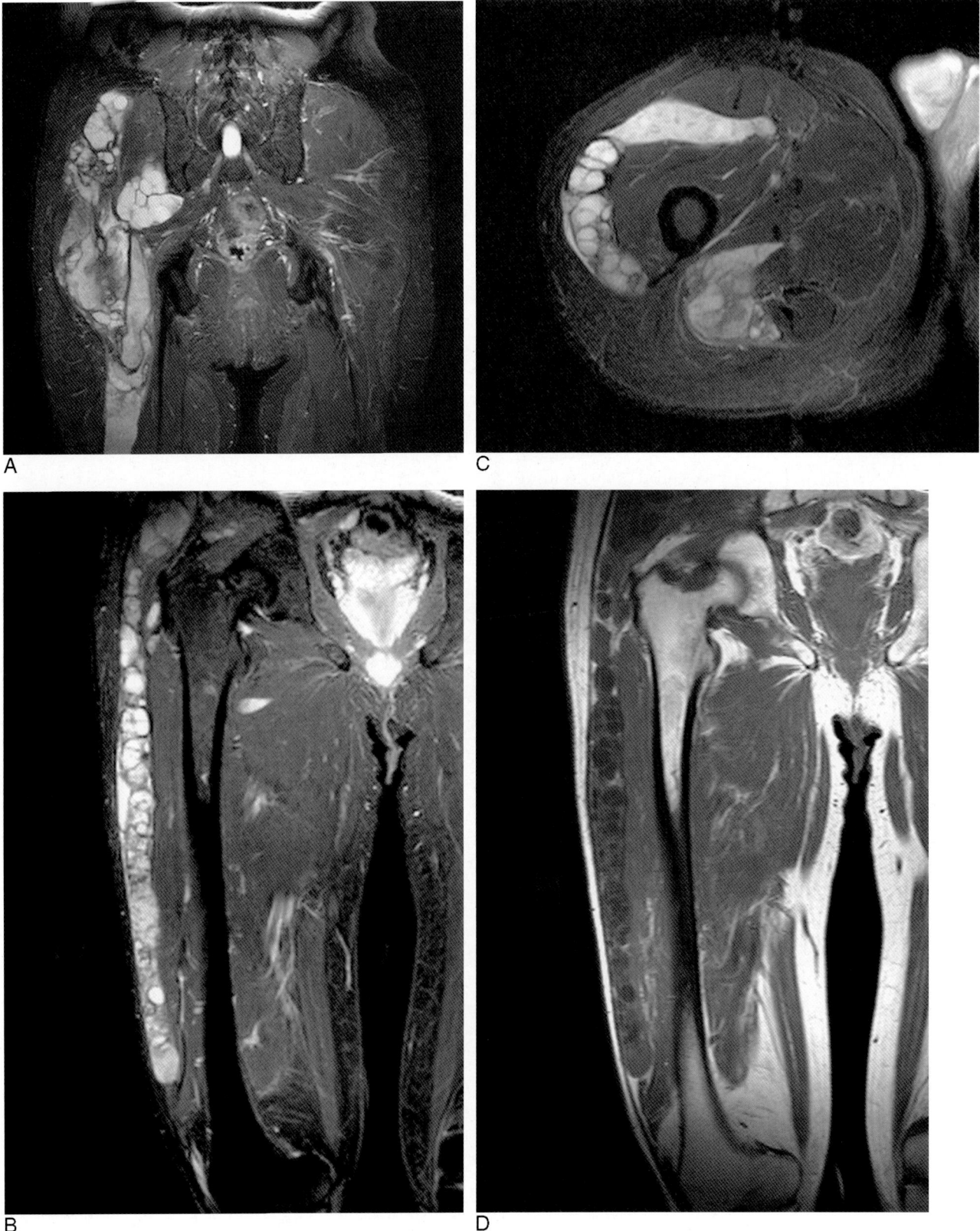

■ **FIGURE 68-29** Coronal (**A** and **B**) and axial (**C**) fluid-sensitive images with fat saturation, coronal (**D**) and axial

(Continued)

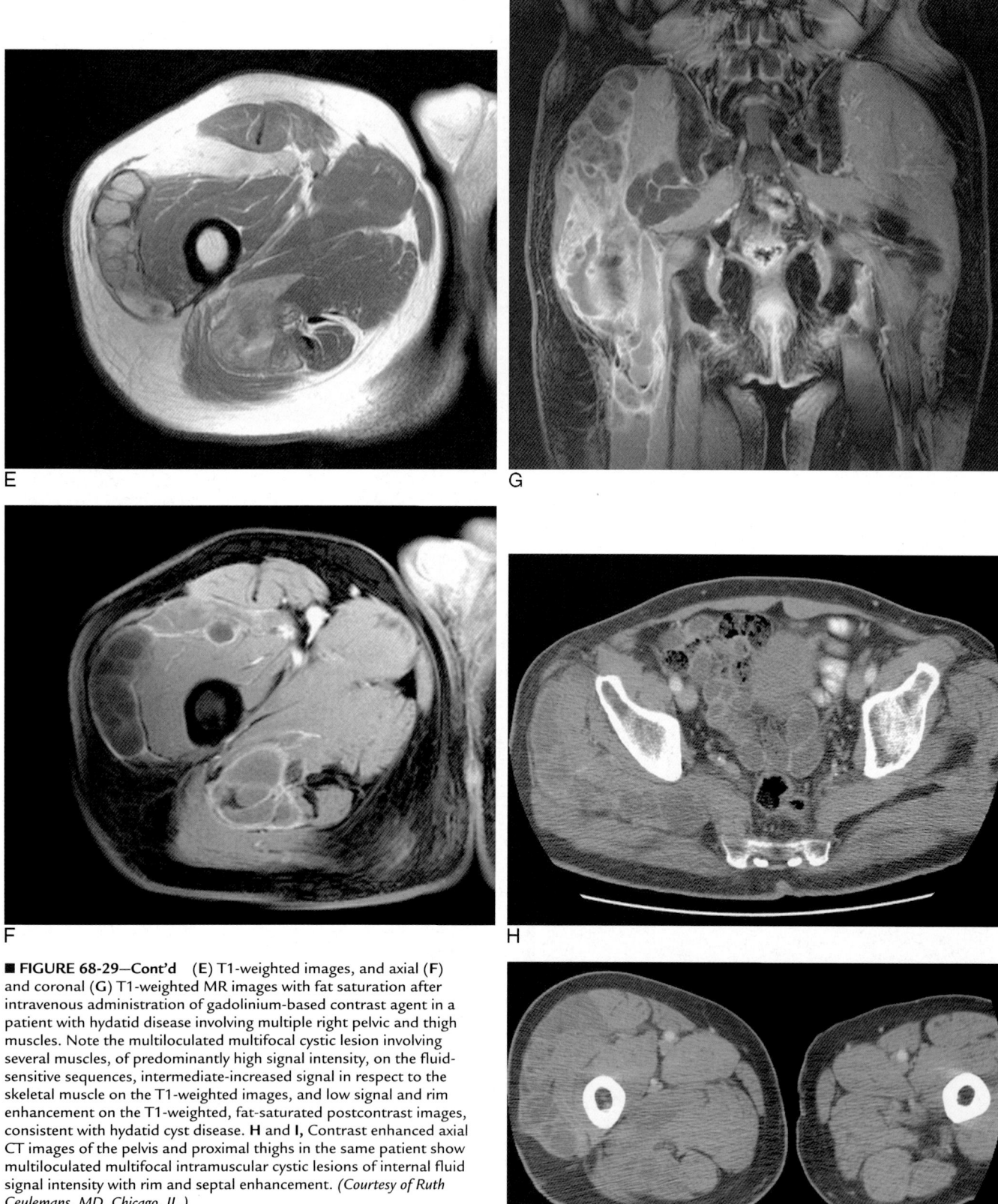

■ **FIGURE 68-29—Cont'd** (**E**) T1-weighted images, and axial (**F**) and coronal (**G**) T1-weighted MR images with fat saturation after intravenous administration of gadolinium-based contrast agent in a patient with hydatid disease involving multiple right pelvic and thigh muscles. Note the multiloculated multifocal cystic lesion involving several muscles, of predominantly high signal intensity, on the fluid-sensitive sequences, intermediate-increased signal in respect to the skeletal muscle on the T1-weighted images, and low signal and rim enhancement on the T1-weighted, fat-saturated postcontrast images, consistent with hydatid cyst disease. **H** and **I,** Contrast enhanced axial CT images of the pelvis and proximal thighs in the same patient show multiloculated multifocal intramuscular cystic lesions of internal fluid signal intensity with rim and septal enhancement. (*Courtesy of Ruth Ceulemans, MD, Chicago, IL.*)

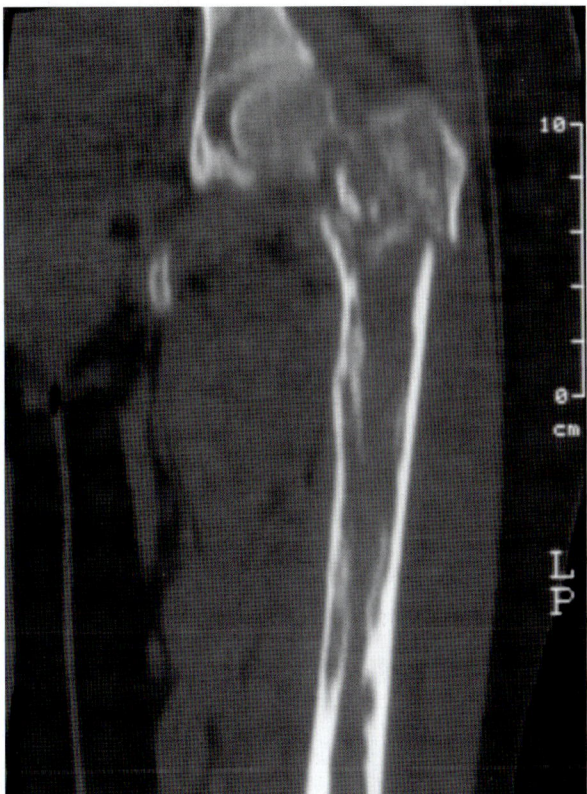

■ **FIGURE 68-30** Coronal reformatted CT image of the femur shows an intraosseous cystic/lytic lesion involving the midproximal femoral diametaphysis with associated cortical thinning and pathologic fracture through the femoral neck, intertrochanteric, and subtrochanteric region in a Bosnian patient. (*Courtesy of Department of Radiology, UMC Sarajevo, Bosnia & Herzegovina.*)

SYNOPSIS OF TREATMENT OPTIONS

Medical Treatment

Since the 1970s, with introduction of the derivates of the benzimidazoles, medical treatment has been attempted. For the skeletal lesions, the World Health Organization suggests adjuvant chemotherapy with mebendazole or albendazole for at least 2 years after surgery. In cases in which only a palliative treatment is possible, the anthelminthic drug administration can be continuous. However, its efficiency remains debated.[2,15,16]

Progress in developing effective vaccination against infection with oncospheres and immunotherapy of the metacestode has been reviewed by Lightowlers and others. Vaccination may provide an additional tool for control and prevention of this infection.[17]

Surgical Treatment

Skeletal echinococcosis is treated surgically. The treatment is similar to oncologic therapy The surgical approach requires preoperative cross-sectional imaging for the evaluation of local extent of the lesion and its relationship to adjacent structures. Curettage carries the risk

of anaphylaxis and implantation during surgery. A local recurrence rate of 70% to 80% has been reported. Radical resection of the involved segment and bone grafting is now recommended.[2,15]

SUGGESTED READINGS

Schantz PM. Progress in diagnosis, treatment and elimination of echinococcosis and cysticercosis. Parasitol Int 2006; 55(Suppl):S7-S13. Epub 2006 Jan 4.
Merkle EM, Schulte M, Vogel J, et al. Musculoskeletal involvement in cystic echinococcosis: report of eight cases and review of the literature. AJR Am J Roentgenol 1997; 168:1531-1534.

REFERENCES

1. Resnick D. Osteomyelitis, septic arthritis, and soft tissue infection: organisms. In Resnick D (ed). Diagnosis of Bone and Joint Disorders, 4th ed. Philadelphia, WB Saunders, 2002, pp 2510-2624.
2. Papanikolaou A, Antoniou N, Pavlakis D, Garas G. Hydatid disease of the tarsal bones: a case report. J Foot Ankle Surg 2005; 44:396-400.
3. Schantz PM. Progress in diagnosis, treatment and elimination of echinococcosis and cysticercosis. Parasitol Int 2006; 55(Suppl): S7-S13. Epub 2006 Jan 4.
4. Loudiye H, Aktaou S, Hassikou H, et al. Hydatid disease of bone: review of 11 cases. Joint Bone Spine 2003; 70:352-355.
5. Tuzun M, Hekimoglu B. CT findings in skeletal cystic echinococcosis: CT findings in skeletal cystic echinococcosis. Acta Radiol 2002; 43:533-538.
6. Mellado JM, Perez del Palomar L, Camins A, et al. MR imaging of spinal infection: atypical features, interpretive pitfalls and potential mimickers. Eur Radiol 2004; 14:1980-1989.
7. Mseddi M, Mtaoumi M, Dahmene J, et al. [Hydatid cysts in muscles: eleven cases]. Rev Chir Orthop Reparatrice Appar Mot 2005; 91:267-271. French.
8. Vallianatos PG, Tilentzoglou AC, Seitaridis SV, Mahera HJ. Echinococcal synovitis of the knee joint. Arthroscopy 2002; 18: E48.
9. Merkle EM, Schulte M, Vogel J, et al. Musculoskeletal involvement in cystic echinococcosis: report of eight cases and review of the literature. AJR Am J Roentgenol 1997; 168:1531-1534.
10. Raut AA, Nagar AM, Narlawar RS, et al. Echinococcosis of the rib with epidural extension: a rare cause of paraplegia. Br J Radiol 2004; 77:338-341.
11. Merkle EM, Kramme E, Vogel J, et al. Bone and soft tissue manifestations of alveolar echinococcosis. Skeletal Radiol 1997; 26:289-292.
12. Morris BS, Madiwale CV, Garg A, Chavhan GB. Hydatid disease of bone: a mimic of other skeletal pathologies. Australas Radiol 2002; 46:431-434.
13. Yildirim M, Varoglu E, Gursan N, et al. Unusual localization of hydatid cyst: bone scintigraphy, brain SPECT, and magnetic resonance imaging findings. Clin Nucl Med 2002; 27:449-450.
14. Bresson-Hadni S, Delabrousse E, Blagosklonov O, et al. Imaging aspects and non-surgical interventional treatment in human alveolar echinococcosis. Parasitol Int 2006; 55(Suppl):S267-272. Epub 2006 Jan 5.
15. Zlitni M, Ezzaouia K, Lebib H, et al. Hydatid cyst of bone: diagnosis and treatment. World J Surg 2001; 25:75-82.
16. Diedrich O, Perlick L, Kraft CN, Sommer T. [Orthopedic aspects of osseous echinococcosis—radiologic diagnosis, current surgery and drug therapy aspects]. Z Orthop Ihre Grenzgeb 2001; 139:261-266. German.
17. Lightowlers MW, Lawrence SB, Gauci CG, et al. Vaccination against hydatidosis using a defined recombinant antigen. Parasit Immunol 1996; 18:457-462.

Leprosy

Leprosy (Hansen's disease) is an infectious disease characterized by a long incubation period. It takes a chronic course with involvement of the skin, mucous membranes, and peripheral nervous system. Leprosy has been eliminated at the national level in 113 of the 122 countries in which it was a public health problem in 1985. It is still encountered in India, Brazil, Myanmar, Madagascar, Mozambique, Nepal, and Tanzania, where the prevalence rates still exceeded 1 per 10,000 at the beginning of 2004.[1,2]

ETIOLOGY

The causative agent, *Mycobacterium leprae*, is a nonmotile, non–spore-forming, microaerophilic bacterium that usually forms slightly curved or straight rods. It has a predilection for Schwann cells, where the organism multiplies unimpeded by organism-specific host immunity, resulting in destruction of myelin, secondary inflammatory changes, and destruction of the nerve architecture.[3,4]

PREVALENCE AND EPIDEMIOLOGY

The number of reported cases of leprosy in the United States peaked at 361 in 1985 and has declined since 1988. In 2004, 105 cases of leprosy were reported in the United States. Eighty-five percent of detected cases are in immigrants, in whom this disease may mimic many common dermatologic and neurologic entities, leading to delay of diagnosis.[4-6]

Despite being infrequent in the United States, leprosy is not uncommon in areas of Africa, South America, and Asia. In 1991, the World Health Organization adopted a resolution establishing a goal of eliminating leprosy as a public health problem by the year 2000, which meant reducing the prevalence to 1 case or fewer per 10,000 population. In some countries where the leprosy is endemic, such as India and Brazil, this goal could not be reached by the year 2000 and a new goal for elimination of this disease was pushed to the year 2005 but was not reached.[5]

CLINICAL PRESENTATION

Leprosy is best understood as two conjoined diseases. The first is a chronic mycobacterial infection that elicits an extraordinary range of cellular immune responses in humans. The second is a peripheral neuropathy that is initiated by the infection and the accompanying immunologic events. *M. leprae* remains nonculturable, and for over a century leprosy has presented major challenges in the fields of microbiology, pathology, immunology, and genetics; it continues to do so today.[3]

This disease is more common in men than women and can affect any age group, although more commonly individuals younger than 20 years of age are affected. Prodromal symptoms include malaise, fever, drowsiness, rhinitis, and profuse sweating.

According to the microscopic appearance leprosy is divided into four principal types: *lepromatous*, *tuberculoid*, *dimorphous*, and *intermediate*, with variable clinical manifestations. Typically the tuberculoid type of disease is less progressive than the lepromatous type.[1]

Currently, the WHO recommends counting external lepromatous lesions to distinguish paucibacillary from multibacillary disease, with fewer than five lesions being classified as paucibacillary and five or more lesions as multibacillary.[3]

The clinical manifestations vary among these types of leprosy. The tuberculoid type is typically less progressive than the lepromatous type. In tuberculoid leprosy, the skin and nerves are principally affected, whereas in lepromatous leprosy a more acute and generalized process may be evident. In lepromatous (multibacillary) leprosy, skin nodules, papules, macules, and diffuse infiltrations are bilaterally symmetric and usually numerous and extensive. Involvement of the nasal mucosa may lead to crusting and obstructed breathing and epistaxis; ocular involvement leads to iritis and keratitis.

In tuberculoid (paucibacillary) leprosy, skin lesions are single or few, sharply demarcated, anesthesic or hypoesthesic, and bilaterally asymmetric; involvement of peripheral nerves tends to be severe. Borderline leprosy has features of both polar forms and is more labile. Indeterminate leprosy is characterized by hypopigmented maculae with ill-defined borders; if untreated, it may progress to tuberculoid, borderline, or lepromatous disease. Lymphadenopathy is seen in all types of leprosy, although it is more prominent in the lepromatous type. In patients with prominent neurologic findings (neuritic variety), lepromatous granulation tissue forms about the nerves, leading to their thickening, tenderness, and paresthesias. Muscular atrophy and contractures may occur, as well as subsequent mutilations and secondary infections.[1,7]

Mycobacterium leprae has a predilection for the cooler appendages of the body with characteristic involvement of the small bones of the hands and feet. Bone lesions in patients with leprosy are usually due to trauma and secondary bacterial infection superimposed on denervated tissues.[8] The cardinal diagnostic features of leprosy

---

KEY POINTS

- This infectious disease is caused by *Mycobacterium leprae* and characterized by a long incubation period.
- It has been eliminated at the national level in 113 of the 122 countries but is still encountered in India, Brazil, Myanmar, Madagascar, Mozambique, Nepal, and Tanzania.
- The infection probably enters the body through the skin and mucous membranes, especially nasal mucosa. The causative organisms are disseminated via the bloodstream and the lymphatics and localize in the skin, the nerves, and, in advanced cases, in the viscera.
- It has a predilection for the cooler appendages of the body with characteristic involvement of the small bones of the hands and feet.
- It is curable but requires long-term multidrug therapy.

are anesthetic skin lesions, neuropathy, and positive skin smears for the bacilli. However, patients may rarely present without skin lesions in pure neuritic leprosy.[4]

Articular inflammatory manifestations involving small joints, large joints, or both and sacroiliitis may exist in patients with different forms of leprosy and can follow a chronic course.[9] Erythema nodosum is seen in leprosy and is associated with arthritis. Soft tissue swelling of the hands (swollen hand syndrome) with intra- and extra-articular inflammation in response to organisms and granulomatous reaction and subcutaneous nodules has been described.[1]

The frequency, nature, and importance of vascular lesions in leprosy are debated. Occasionally, soft tissue calcifications involving the nerves can be seen. As in chronic osteomyelitis with soft tissue sinuses, leprosy with cutaneous ulcerations may be associated with development of secondary malignancy, specifically squamous cell carcinoma of the skin.[1]

Leprosy is diagnosed by finding lepromatous bacilli in typical histologic lesions.[1]

The lepromin skin test is not approved by the U.S. Food and Drug Administration and is not recommended or provided for diagnostic use in the United States. This test provides a measure of the individual's ability to mount a granulomatous response against a mixture of lepromatous antigens. Responses to lepromin are not specific, and many individuals who have never been exposed to *M. leprae* will develop a positive lepromin reaction. Rapid molecular type assays (polymerase chain reaction analysis) of tissues for *M. leprae* now provide a valuable means for identifying this organism.[3]

PATHOPHYSIOLOGY

Patients affected with leprosy typically have a history of prolonged contact with the bacilli, but the exact mode of the transmission is not clear. The infection probably enters the body through the skin and mucous membranes, especially nasal mucosa. The *M. leprae* organisms are disseminated via the bloodstream and the lymphatics and localize in the skin, the nerves, and in advanced cases in the viscera. The incubation period is estimated to vary from 3 to 6 years.[1]

In the lepromatous type of disease the bacilli are numerous with paucity of cellular reaction. Skin lesions have a widespread symmetric distribution. Macrophages, containing fat droplets, leprae cells, and numerous bacilli, are distinctive. In the tuberculoid type of disease the bacilli are less numerous but they initiate a severe granulomatous reaction similar to tuberculosis and sarcoidosis. Asymmetrically distributed skin macules are seen. The dimorphous type is uncommon with microscopic features of both lepromatous and tuberculoid types. In the intermediate type a few bacilli stimulate a slight cellular reaction in the perivascular and perineural areas, with the pathologic features not prominent enough to allow classification into tuberculoid or lepromatous types.[1]

The histologic characteristics of involved joints in leprosy are similar to those in other neuropathic osteoarthropathies including serous joint effusion, villous proliferation of the synovial membrane, erosive and proliferative changes of cartilage, sclerosis and eburnation of bone, fragmentation, and osseous excrescences.[1]

IMAGING TECHNIQUES

Imaging should start with radiography. MRI, nuclear medicine bone scintiscans, ultrasonography, and CT may be useful in detection of occult musculoskeletal abnormalities associated with leprosy or in further characterization of known lesions.

MANIFESTATIONS OF THE DISEASE
Radiography

The skeleton is directly involved by leprosy in 3% to 5% of cases, typically involving the small bones of hands and feet. The radiographic findings comprise periostitis, osteitis, and osteomyelitis. Metaphyses of the phalanges are commonly involved, and metacarpal and metatarsal involvement is less frequent. Radiographs show soft tissue swelling, osteoporosis, endosteal thinning, enlargement of nutrient foramina, and destructive osseous lesions with a cystic or honeycombing appearance. With healing, the definition of the involved bones increases with remaining residual deformity. Destruction of the alveolar process and anterior nasal spine of the maxilla results in direct lepromatous involvement of the bone, and secondary infection is sometimes referred to as the rhinomaxillary or Bergen syndrome. In the long tubular bones symmetric periostitis of the tibia, fibula, and distal portion of the ulna may be noted. The constellation of erythematous skin lesions, pain, and periostitis in the lower extremity has been called "red leg."[1]

With less common hematogenous dissemination to bone, intramedullary foci of infection are seen including the tubular bones of the extremities and the ribs. The lesions are usually epiphyseal or metaphyseal in the long tubular bones, but medullary involvement can occur. The disease progresses slowly, but the cortex and periosteum can be violated. Periostitis and sclerosis are not prominent.[1]

Lepromatous arthritis is not common and may result from direct intra-articular extension or, less commonly, from hematogenous dissemination. Radiographs demonstrate joint effusion with associated soft tissue swelling. Small joints, large joints, or both can be affected, including the sacroiliac joints. The ankles, knees, wrists, finger joints, and the elbows are affected in decreasing frequency.[1,9]

The skeletal abnormalities occurring on a neurologic basis are much more frequent and severe than those produced by direct leprous infiltration of the bone. Motor denervation due to leprous infection of peripheral nerves results in neuropathic osteoarthropathy in 20% to 70% of hospitalized patients and contributes to deformities such as clawhand and clawtoes. This is sometimes associated with the development of concentric bone atrophy. Absorption of bone in leprosy manifests as a decrease in bone length and width and results in a tapered appearance at the end of the bone, which has been likened to a licked candystick. When complicated by repeated microtrauma, secondary bacterial infection, or both, digits may be resorbed (Figs. 68-31 and 68-32).[1,8]

Magnetic Resonance Imaging

Magnetic resonance imaging is able to detect abnormalities of the nerves in leprosy. Active reversal reaction of peripheral nerves is indicated by an increased T2 signal and gadolinium enhancement. These signs are suggestive of rapid progression of nerve damage and poor prognosis unless antireactional treatment is started.[10]

One study revealed significant MRI changes in clinically asymptomatic neuropathic feet in patients with leprosy. The most striking were the changes located in the region of the first metatarsophalangeal (MTP) joint. These changes ranged from degradation and interruption of the subcutaneous fat to effusion/synovitis in the first MTP joint, indicating that MRI may play an important role in detecting feet at risk and may influence clinical decision-making. Another study showed that MRI could play an important role in detecting osteomyelitis in leprosy patients with long-standing neuropathic feet.[11,12]

MRI findings of symmetric flexor and extensor tendons synovitis with pitting edema of the hands and feet

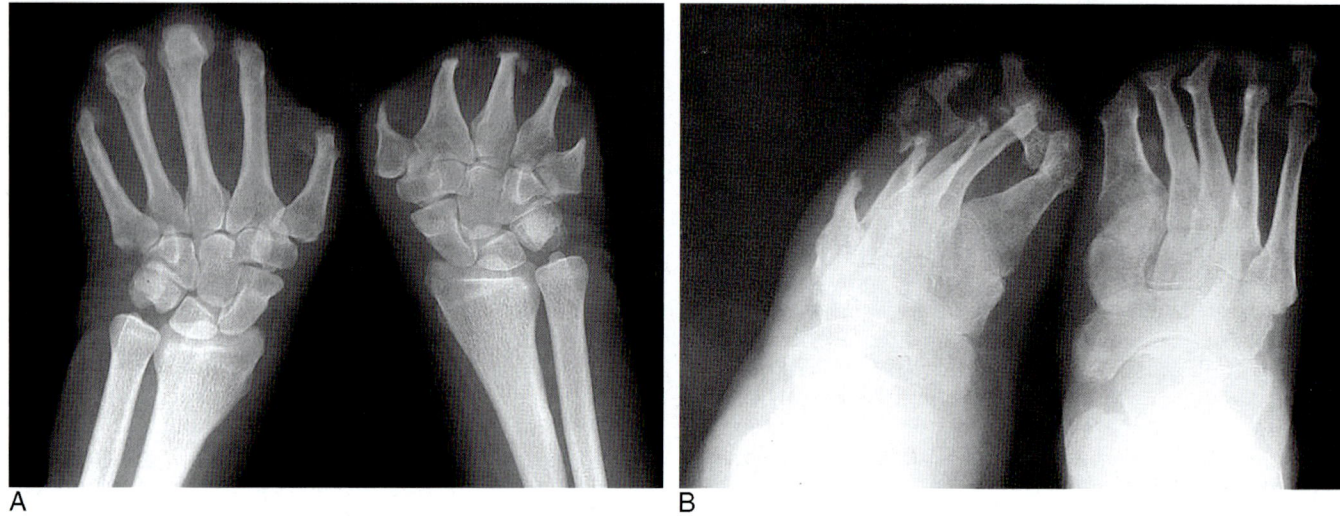

A   B

■ **FIGURE 68-31** Frontal radiograph of the hands (**A**) and frontal radiograph of the feet (**B**) show neuropathic lesions in a patient with leprosy. Note concentric bone atrophy in the hands and feet with tapered osseous structures and osteolysis involving multiple digits. *(Courtesy of Michael Pitt, MD, Birmingham, AL.)*

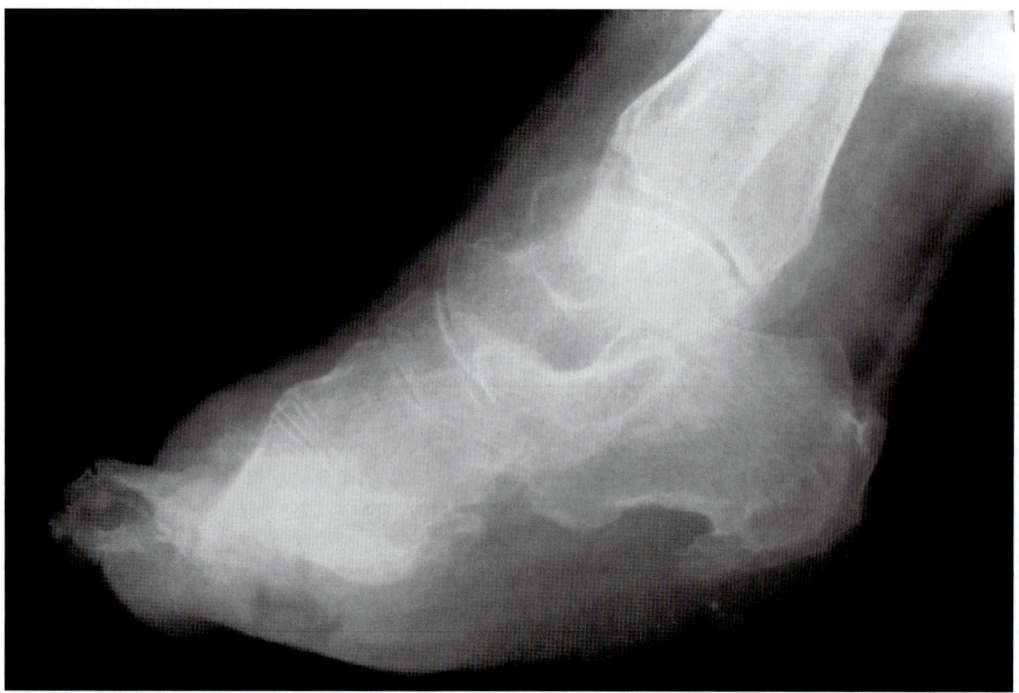

■ **FIGURE 69-32** Lateral radiograph of the foot and ankle in a patient with leprosy shows tapered appearance of the digits with associated soft tissue swelling, lack of the soft tissues about the digits, and an ulcer at the plantar aspect of the forefoot. *(Courtesy of Department of Radiology, UMC Sarajevo, Bosnia & Herzegovina.)*

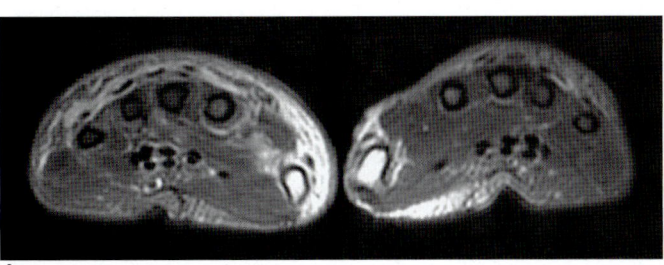 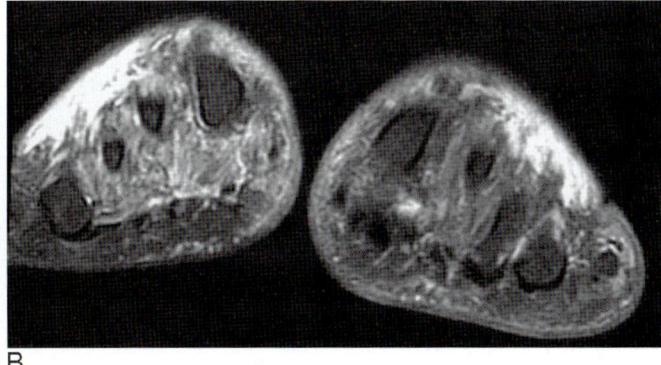

■ **FIGURE 68-33** Axial T2-weighted MR images with fat saturation of the hands (**A**) and of the feet (**B**) in a patient with leprosy show soft tissue edema predominantly involving the dorsal subcutaneous tissues. *(Courtesy of Claudia Helling, MD, Buenos Aires, Argentina.)*

were described in a patient with skin lesions and border-line tuberculoid leprosy (Fig. 68-33).[13]

Multidetector Computed Tomography

In the past, CT was reported as a useful imaging modality for evaluation of peripheral nerve lesions in patients with leprosy.[14] CT findings of the paranasal sinuses in patients with leprosy comprise nonspecific mucosal thickening that may mimic chronic sinusitis. The diagnosis of leprosy requires biopsy.[15]

Ultrasonography

Ultrasonography can be utilized to demonstrate normal peripheral nerves as well as their pathology, including leprosy. The lesions of tuberculoid leprosy appear hypoechoic on ultrasound examination.[16] Active reversal reactions of peripheral nerves are indicated by endoneural color flow signals, suggesting rapid progression of nerve damage and a poor prognosis unless antireactional treatment is started.[10]

Nuclear Medicine

Bone scintigraphy may be useful to determine disease activity in cases of mutilation caused by leprosy. It seems to be superior to conventional radiography and may enable bone biopsies to be avoided.[17]

Radionuclide bone scans in patients with leprosy show scan patterns simulating hypertrophic osteoarthropathy and diffuse arthritis consistent with a primary disease process.[18]

Gallium-67 imaging shows diffuse moderate radiotracer uptake over the entire skin surface except in the face, where it shows homogeneous, diffuse, and marked uptake in a series of 12 untreated patients with multibacillary disease. Internal organ involvement was variable. The pattern of body skin ("skin outlining") and facial skin ("beard distribution") may be distinct for untreated patients with multibacillary leprosy.[17] In one patient with borderline leprosy, gallium-67 showed increased radiotracer uptake in the subcutaneous tissues of the face and thighs.[19] In patients with lepromatous leprosy with an erythema nodosum leprosum, gallium-67 may reveal multiple patchy areas of radiotracer uptake in the skin of the face, trunk, arms, and thighs.[20]

In the reactive phase of leprosy, on the bone scan, erythema nodosum can cause a symmetric double stripe sign bilaterally involving the distal tibiae similar to those seen in hypertrophic osteoarthropathy.[21]

SYNOPSIS OF TREATMENT OPTIONS

Medical Treatment

Several effective antimicrobial agents are now available to treat leprosy, and this infection is curable. Long-term multidrug therapy with dapsone, clofazimine, and rifampin has been very practical and successful for treatment of leprosy. However, even with this powerful drug combination the overall number of newly registered cases has not fallen consistently, and drug resistance still occurs.[3]

Bacillus Calmette-Guérin vaccine provides a low but measurable degree of protection against *M. leprae*, but a highly effective, specific vaccine has not yet been developed.[3]

Surgical Treatment

Deformities in leprosy are the consequence of impairments of nerve function. The aim of reconstructive surgery on the hand in patients with leprosy is to augment its capabilities for the activities of daily living and for safe vocations and to restore form and structure adequately to accelerate the patient's integration into society.[2]

SUGGESTED READING

Scollard DM, Adams LB, Gillis TP, et al. The continuing challenges of leprosy. Clin Microbiol Rev 2006; 19:338–381.

REFERENCES

1. Resnick D. Osteomyelitis, septic arthritis, and soft tissue infection: organisms. In Resnick D (ed). Diagnosis of Bone and Joint Disorders, 4th ed. Philadelphia, WB Saunders, 2002, pp 2510–2624.
2. Anderson GA. The surgical management of deformities of the hand in leprosy. J Bone Joint Surg Br 2006; 88:290–294.
3. Scollard DM, Adams LB, Gillis TP, et al. The continuing challenges of leprosy. Clin Microbiol Rev 2006; 19:338–381.

4. Ooi WW, Srinivasan J. Leprosy and the peripheral nervous system: basic and clinical aspects. Muscle Nerve 2004; 30:393–409.
5. Centers for Disease Control and Prevention (CDC) and Jajosky RA, Hall PA, Adams DA, et al. Summary of notifiable diseases—United States, 2004. MMWR Morb Mortal Wkly Rep 2006; 53:1–79.
6. Ooi WW, Moschella SL. Update on leprosy in immigrants in the United States: status in the year 2000. Clin Infect Dis 2001; 32:930–937.
7. Case Definition Leprosy. Epidemiol Bull 2002; 23(No. 2).
8. Jones EA, Manaster BJ, May DA, Disler DG. Neuropathic osteoarthropathy: diagnostic dilemmas and differential diagnosis. RadioGraphics 2000; 20(Spec No):S279–S293.
9. Cossermelli-Messina W, Festa Neto C, Cossermelli W. Articular inflammatory manifestations in patients with different forms of leprosy. J Rheumatol 1998; 25:111–119.
10. Martinoli C, Derchi LE, Bertolotto M, et al. US and MR imaging of peripheral nerves in leprosy. Skeletal Radiol 2000; 29:142–150.
11. Maas M, Slim EJ, Akkerman EM, Faber WR. MRI in clinically asymptomatic neuropathic leprosy feet: a baseline study. Int J Lepr Other Mycobact Dis 2001; 69:219–224.
12. Maas M, Slim EJ, Heoksma AF, et al. MR imaging of neuropathic feet in leprosy patients with suspected osteomyelitis. Int J Lepr Other Mycobact Dis 2002; 70:97–103.
13. Helling CA, Locursio A, Manzur ME, et al. Remitting seronegative symmetrical synovitis with pitting edema in leprosy. Clin Rheumatol 2006; 25:95–97.
14. Barbancon O, Rath S, Alqubati Y. Hansen's disease: computed tomography findings in peripheral nerve lesions. Ann Radiol (Paris) 1989; 32:579–581.
15. Srinivasan S, Nehru VI, Bapuraj JR, et al. CT findings in involvement of the paranasal sinuses by lepromatous leprosy. Br J Radiol 1999; 72:271–273.
16. Fornage BD. Peripheral nerves of the extremities: imaging with US. Radiology 1988; 167:179–182.
17. Braga FJ, Araujo EB, Camargo EE, et al. Gallium scintigraphy in Hansen's disease. Eur J Nucl Med 1991; 18:866–869.
18. Goergen TG, Resnick D, Lomonaco A, O'Dell CW Jr. Radionuclide bone-scan abnormalities in leprosy: case reports. J Nucl Med 1976; 17:788–790.
19. Mouratidis B, Lomas FE. Gallium-67 scintigraphy in borderline lepromatous leprosy. Australas Radiol 1993; 37:270–271.
20. Peng NJ, Wang JH, Hsieh SP, et al. Ga-67 and Tc-99m HMPAO labeled WBC imaging in erythema nodosum leprosum reaction of leprosy. Clin Nucl Med 1998; 23:248–250.
21. Datz FL. Erythema nodosum leprosum reaction of leprosy causing the double stripe sign on bone scan: case report. Clin Nucl Med 1987; 12:212–214.

Lyme Disease

Lyme disease caused by the spirochete *Borrelia burgdorferi* is the most common vector-born illness in the United States and is *transmitted* to humans by the bite of infected blacklegged ticks.[1]

ETIOLOGY

The causative organism *Borrelia burgdorferi* normally lives in small animals. Certain species of ticks, *Ixodes dammini (scapularis)* or related ticks, transmit disease among the animals and to humans. In the northeastern and north-central United States the deer tick *Ixodes scapularis* transmits Lyme disease. In the Pacific coastal United States the disease is spread by the tick *Ixodes pacificus.*

Deer are an important host in transmitting ticks, but they do not become infected with Lyme disease. There is no known human-to-human transmission.[1,3-5]

PREVALENCE AND EPIDEMIOLOGY

Lyme disease was first identified as a distinct entity in the United States in 1975. It was named after the town in Connecticut in which it was first encountered. In 2004, 19,804 cases of Lyme disease were reported, yielding a national average of 6.8 cases for every 100,000 persons. In the 12 states where Lyme disease is most common, the average was 27.4 cases for every 100,000 persons. Nearly 80% of cases are reported between May and August. Lyme disease has a global distribution and has been detected on all continents except Antarctica. This disease occurs in both adults and children, with a slight male predominance.[1-4]

CLINICAL PRESENTATION

Clinical manifestations usually appear 1 week after a tick bite, although they may be delayed for several weeks. The disease begins with a distinctive skin lesion: *erythema chronicum migrans*. This lesion appears as a macule or papule in the area of a previous tick bite, most often on the trunk or proximal portion of the extremities, and expands to an annular lesion with an intensely red border, which may be pruritic or burning. The skin lesion resolves in a period of weeks. The cutaneous manifestations are not constant and are not always remembered by the patient. Other signs and symptoms commonly associated with the early stage of this disease include fever, chills, myalgias, arthralgias, headache, stiff neck, and exhaustion.[3,4]

Articular involvement may develop from 2 weeks to 2 years after infection or onset of systemic symptoms, making attribution to Lyme disease difficult. After several months, approximately 60% of patients with untreated infection will begin to have intermittent bouts of arthritis, with severe joint pain and swelling. Large joints are most often affected, particularly the knees in 80% of patients. Other areas involved include shoulders, elbows, ankles, hips, wrists, small joints of the extremities, and the temporomandibular joints. Recurrent, brief attacks (weeks or months) of objective joint swelling in one or more joints are sometimes followed by chronic arthritis in one or

---

KEY POINTS

- Lyme disease is the most common vector-borne illness in the United States and is transmitted to humans by the bite of infected blacklegged ticks.
- The causative organism is *Borrelia burgdorferi*.
- Erythema chronicum migrans is a characteristic skin lesion and usually the first manifestation of disease.
- Articular involvement may develop from 2 weeks to 2 years after infection or onset of systemic symptoms, making diagnosis of Lyme disease difficult.
- Most patients can be cured with a few weeks of oral antibiotics.

more joints. Approximately 10% of patients develop Lyme carditis typically 4 weeks after onset of disease. In addition, up to 5% of untreated patients may develop chronic neurologic complaints months to years after infection. These include shooting pains, numbness or tingling in the hands or feet, and problems with concentration and short-term memory.[1,3,4]

Nonspecific laboratory findings include mild leukocytosis, increased sedimentation rate, and minimally increased serum levels of transaminases. Increased total serum IgM occurs in 33% of patients, which if persistent in untreated patients is a predictor for later manifestations of Lyme disease.[3]

A two-test approach for active disease and for previous infection using a sensitive enzyme immunoassay (EIA) or immunofluorescent assay (IFA) followed by a Western immunoblot is the algorithm of choice. All specimens positive or equivocal by a sensitive EIA or IFA should be tested by a standardized Western immunoblot. Specimens negative by a sensitive EIA or IFA need not be tested further. When Western immunoblot is used during the first 4 weeks of disease onset (early Lyme disease), both immunoglobulin M (IgM) and immunoglobulin G (IgG) procedures should be performed. A positive IgM test result alone is not recommended for use in determining active disease in patients with illness greater than 1 month's duration because the likelihood of a false-positive test result for a current infection is high for these patients. If a patient with suspected early Lyme disease has a negative serology, serologic evidence of infection is best obtained by testing of paired acute- and convalescent-phase serum samples. Serum samples from patients with disseminated or late-stage Lyme disease almost always have a strong IgG response to *B. burgdorferi* antigens.[5]

PATHOPHYSIOLOGY

Blacklegged ticks live for 2 years and have three feeding stages: larvae, nymph, and adult. When a young tick feeds on an infected animal, the tick takes the bacterium into its body along with the blood meal. The bacterium then lives in the gut of the tick. The infected tick transmits disease to its new host. Sometimes the new host is a human.[3,4]

Although adult ticks often feed on deer, these animals do not become infected. Deer are nevertheless important in transporting ticks and maintaining tick populations.[3]

Lyme disease acquired during pregnancy may lead to infection of the placenta and possible stillbirth, but no negative effects on the fetus have been found when the mother receives appropriate antibiotic treatment. There are no reports of Lyme disease transmission from breast milk.[4,6]

The Lyme disease bacteria can live in blood that is stored for donation. As a precaution, the American Red Cross and the U.S. Food and Drug Administration ask that individuals with chronic illness due to Lyme disease do not donate blood. Lyme disease patients who have been treated with antibiotics and have recovered can donate blood beginning 12 months after the last dose of antibiotics was taken.

There is no credible evidence that Lyme disease can be transmitted through air, food, water, or from the bites of mosquitoes, flies, fleas, or lice.

Aspiration of the affected joints reveals inflammatory synovial fluid with or without eosinophilia. The causative organism is occasionally isolated from the blood, skin, cerebrospinal fluid, and synovial membrane of affected patients, which suggests hematogenous spread of disease. Biopsy of the synovial membrane reveals hypertrophy, vascular proliferation, and cellular infiltration with mononuclear cells and scattered lymphoid follicles. In chronic arthritis the histology of the synovial membrane reveals pannus formation similar to rheumatoid arthritis. It is possible that Lyme arthritis that is initially infectious later evolves to an antigen-induced arthritis. HLA-DR2 and DR4 antigens are found more often with chronic Lyme arthritis.[4]

IMAGING TECHNIQUES

Radiography should be the initial imaging modality in evaluation of any type of arthritis including Lyme arthritis. The local extent of disease including the joint effusion and articular and periarticular inflammation is best further characterized by MRI. Bone scintiscans are most helpful for detection of polyarticular involvement. CT and ultrasonography may also have a role in the diagnosis of Lyme arthritis. The role of positron emission tomography in the diagnosis and evaluation of Lyme arthritis is to be determined.

MANIFESTATIONS OF THE DISEASE

Radiography

Radiographic findings of Lyme arthritis are nonspecific. The most common finding is joint effusion, typically involving the large joints, most commonly the knee (Fig. 68-34A-B). A large joint effusion may lead to a rupture of the joint capsule with dissection of the joint fluid into the periarticular soft tissue planes, which about the knee can resemble thrombophlebitis. Periarticular soft tissue swelling is frequently present. This finding is frequently associated with edema of the infrapatellar fat pad. Erosive changes are not common but can occur in advanced disease. Subchondral cystic changes with typical thin sclerotic margins may be detected. Juxta-articular osteoporosis may occur and vary from mild to severe. Proliferative enthesopathic changes with associated calcifications or ossifications at the sites of capsular or ligamentous attachments may be seen. Symmetric joint space loss with associated loss of articular cartilage can be seen in the advanced disease. Chondrocalcinosis may occasionally occur.[3,4,7]

Magnetic Resonance Imaging

Magnetic resonance imaging is a useful imaging modality for detection of Lyme arthritis. The findings are nonspecific. Joint effusion, synovitis, myositis, adenopathy, and occasionally subcutaneous edema, popliteal cysts and hemarthrosis are observed. T1-weighted fat-suppressed images after intravenous administration of a contrast agent are most helpful in determining the severity of synovitis (see Fig. 68-34C to E). In advanced disease erosive

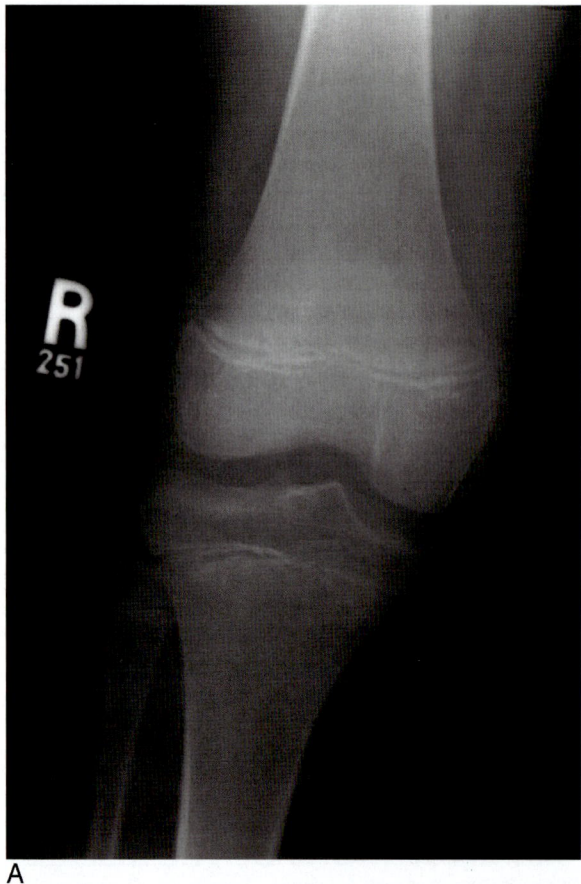

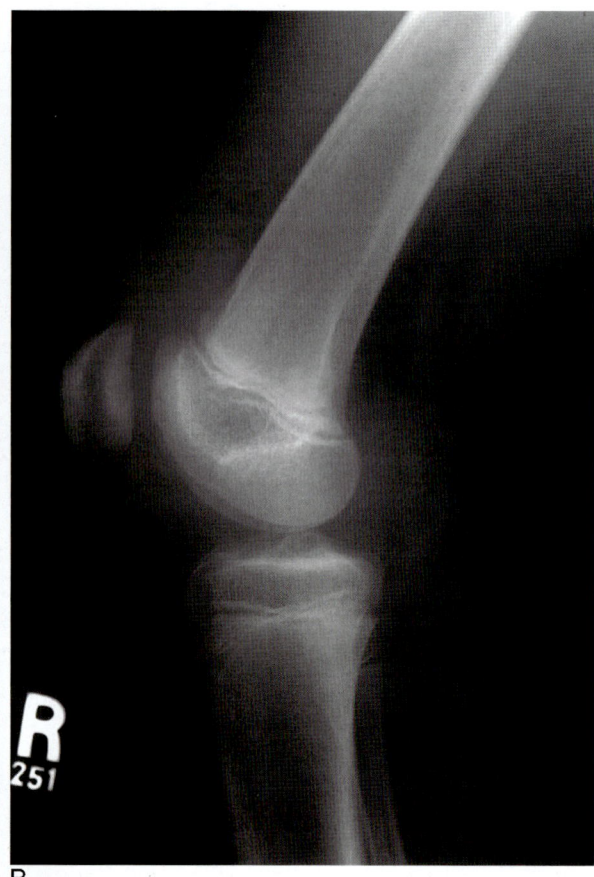

A

B

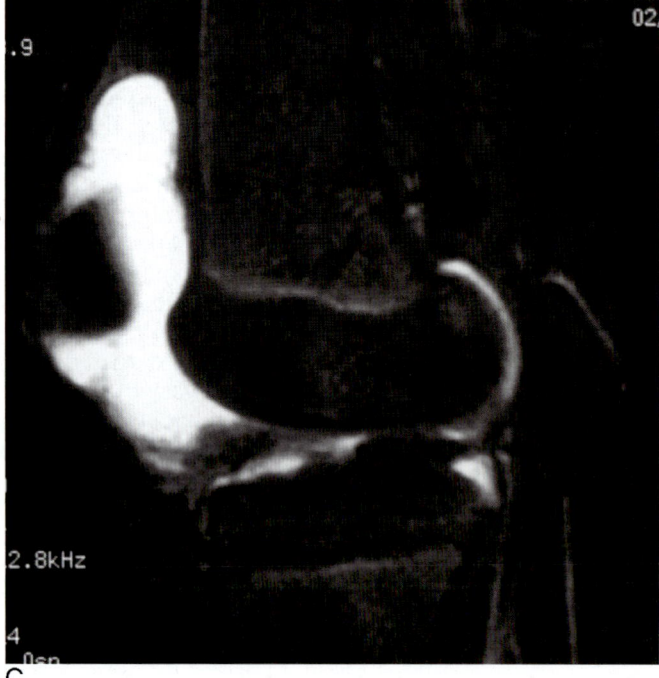

C

■ **FIGURE 68-34** Frontal (**A**) and lateral (**B**) radiographs of a knee in a 10-year-old girl with Lyme arthritis show a large joint effusion seen on the lateral projection and no evidence of erosions. Sagittal STIR (TR 4616, TE 75, TI 110) (**C**),

(Continued)

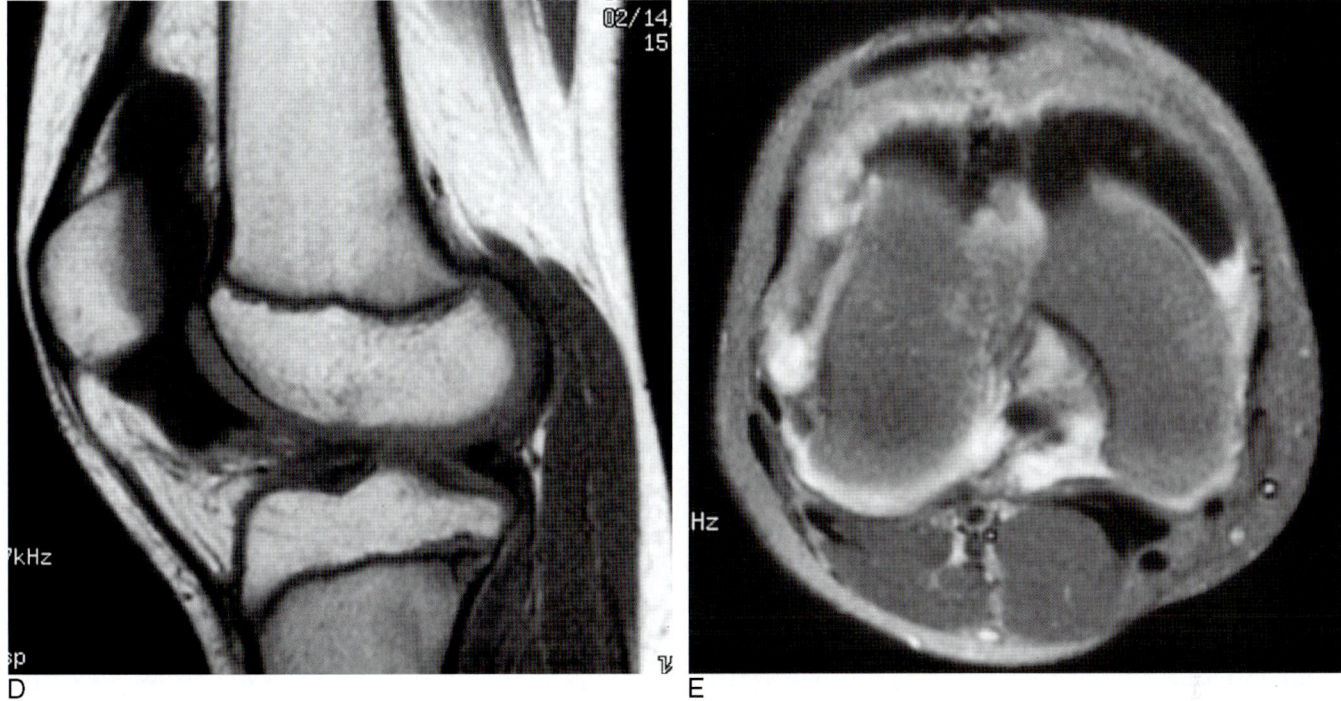

■ **FIGURE 68-34—Cont'd** Sagittal T1-weighted (TR 316, TE 16) (**D**), and axial T1-weighted with fat-saturation postcontrast (**E**) images of the same knee show a large joint effusion and moderate synovial enhancement (on **E**).

changes can also be observed (Fig. 68-35). One study on Lyme versus septic arthritis evaluated by MRI in children showed that the presence of subcutaneous edema significantly favors septic over Lyme arthritis.[1] Multifocal bone marrow abnormalities were reported in a middle-aged woman suffering from Lyme disease and presenting as acrodermatitis chronica atrophicans.[8]

Multidetector Computed Tomography

Joint effusions, periarticular soft tissue edema, and all other abnormalities that are seen in Lyme arthritis on radiographs can be better characterized by CT.[3]

Ultrasonography

Ultrasonography is reported to be utilized in the evaluation of joint effusion and articular and periarticular inflammation in patients with Lyme arthritis.[9,10]

Nuclear Medicine

Bone scintigraphy is nonspecific but can help in detecting multiple sites of inflammatory joint involvement by Lyme disease.[9-11] Gallium-67 shows increased radiotracer uptake in the affected muscle groups.[3]

Positron Emission Tomography/ Computed Tomography

Although MRI is the primary imaging modality for most suspected central nervous system pathology, the practical

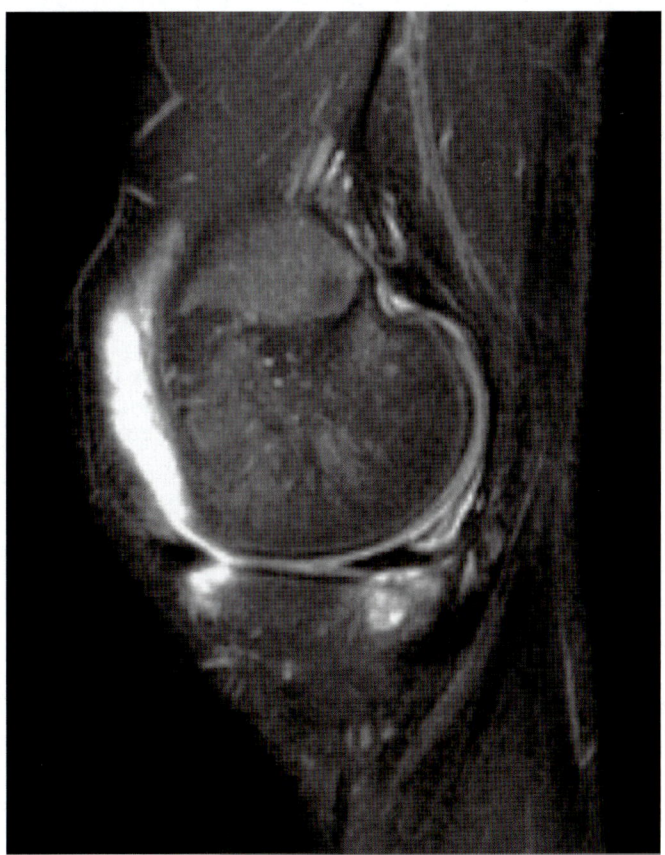

■ **FIGURE 68-35** Sagittal T2-weighted image with fat saturation in a patient with advanced Lyme arthritis shows a joint effusion and erosive changes in the proximal tibia. *(Courtesy of Sandra Moore, MD, NYU Medical Center, NY.)*

applications of PET continue to expand.[12] The role of PET in the diagnosis and evaluation of Lyme arthritis is to be determined.

DIFFERENTIAL DIAGNOSIS

With its numerous manifestations Lyme disease has become the latest great imitator in the spirochete family like syphilis.[6] Early differentiation of Lyme arthritis from septic arthritis is difficult and is particularly important because of the disparate therapeutic implications of each diagnosis. The differential diagnosis also includes inflammatory and degenerative arthritides as well as granulomatous infection such as tuberculosis.[1,3,4]

SYNOPSIS OF TREATMENT OPTIONS

Medical Treatment

Most patients can be cured with a few weeks of oral antibiotics. Antibiotics commonly used for oral treatment are doxycycline, amoxicillin, or cefuroxime axetil. Patients with certain neurologic or cardiac forms of disease may require intravenous treatment with drugs such as ceftriaxone or penicillin. A few patients, particularly those diagnosed with later stages of disease, may have persistent or recurrent symptoms. These patients may benefit from a second 4-week course of therapy.[1,13,14]

Ten to 20 percent of untreated patients with Lyme arthritis achieve spontaneous long-term remission yearly.[3]

Prior vaccination with the second-generation polyvalent outer-surface protein (OspC) vaccine preparation may reduce the risk of developing Lyme disease associated with tick bites. The development of the next generation of Lyme disease vaccine is in its infancy.[15]

Surgical Treatment

Surgery is generally not utilized in the treatment of Lyme disease. There was a case report of Lyme arthritis with advanced degenerative changes localized to the midcarpal joint treated with a limited wrist arthrodesis with relief of pain and improved function.[16] Malawista found that in persistent Lyme arthritis, arthroscopic synovectomy was often curative, although this statement is not accepted for all age groups.[17]

SUGGESTED READINGS

Ecklund K, Vargas S, Zurakowski D, Sundel RP. MRI features of Lyme arthritis in children. AJR Am J Roentgenol 2005; 184:1904–1909.
Lawson JP, Rahn DW. Lyme disease and radiologic findings in Lyme arthritis. AJR Am J Roentgenol 1992; 158:1065–1069.

REFERENCES

1. Ecklund K, Vargas S, Zurakowski D, Sundel RP. MRI features of Lyme arthritis in children. AJR Am J Roentgenol 2005; 184:1904–1909.
2. Centers for Disease Control and Prevention (CDC) and Jajosky RA, Hall PA, Adams DA, et al. Summary of notifiable diseases—United States, 2004. MMWR Morb Mortal Wkly Rep 2006; 53:1–79.
3. Lawson JP, Rahn DW. Lyme disease and radiologic findings in Lyme arthritis. AJR Am J Roentgenol 1992; 158:1065–1069.
4. Resnick D. Osteomyelitis, septic arthritis, and soft tissue infection: organisms. In Resnick D (ed). Diagnosis of Bone and Joint Disorders, 4th ed. Philadelphia, WB Saunders, 2002, pp 2510–2624.
5. Aguero-Rosenfeld ME, Wang G, Schwartz I, Wormser GP. Diagnosis of Lyme borreliosis. Clin Microbiol Rev 2005; 18:484–509.
6. Stechenberg BW. Lyme disease: the latest great imitator. Pediatr Infect Dis J 1988; 7:402–409.
7. Buchmann RF, Jaramillo D. Imaging of articular disorders in children. Radiol Clin North Am 2004; 42:151–68, vii.
8. Schmitz G, Vanhoenacker FM, Gielen J, et al. Unusual musculoskeletal manifestations of Lyme disease. JBR-BTR 2004; 87:224–228.
9. Ushakova MA, Anan'eva LP, Mach ES, et al. [The clinical instrumental characteristics of the locomotor involvement in patients who have had Lyme disease]. Ter Arkh 1995; 67:45–49. Russian.
10. Ushakova MA, Mach ES, Anan'eva LP, et al. [Methods for the instrumental diagnosis and verification of Lyme arthritis]. Ter Arkh 1997; 69:15–19. Russian.
11. Brown SJ, Dadparvar S, Slizofski WJ, et al. Triple-phase bone image abnormalities in Lyme arthritis. Clin Nucl Med 1989; 14:730–733.
12. Kalina P, Decker A, Kornel E, Halperin JJ. Lyme disease of the brainstem. Neuroradiology 2005; 47:903–907. Epub 2005 Sep 13.
13. Wormser GP, Nadelman RB, Dattwyler RJ, et al. Practice guidelines for the treatment of Lyme disease. The Infectious Diseases Society of America. Clin Infect Dis 2000; 31(Suppl 1):1–14.
14. Wormser GP, Ramanathan R, Nowakowski J, et al. Duration of antibiotic therapy for early Lyme disease: a randomized, double-blind, placebo-controlled trial. Ann Intern Med 2003; 138:697–704.
15. Hanson MS, Edelman R. Progress and controversy surrounding vaccines against Lyme disease. Expert Rev Vaccines 2003; 2:683–703.
16. Scerpella TA, Engber WD. Chronic Lyme disease arthritis: review of the literature and report of a case of wrist arthritis. J Hand Surg [Am] 1992; 17:571–575.
17. Malawista SE. Resolution of Lyme arthritis, acute or prolonged: a new look. Proceedings of the International Conference on Lyme Borreliosis, Brussels, November 16, 2001.

Syphilis

ETIOLOGY

Syphilis originates from ancient myth and was highlighted in 1530 in a poem "Syphilis, sive morbus Gallicus" by Girolamo Fracastoro.[1] It is caused by a spirochete *Treponema pallidum* that is transmitted by sexual and intimate contact (acquired syphilis). A fetus can be infected by transmission of the organism through the placenta (congenital syphilis).[2,3]

PREVALENCE AND EPIDEMIOLOGY

In some parts of the world, syphilis remains a common heterosexually transmitted disease. The World Health Organization estimated in 1999 that of a global total of 12 million adults with syphilis, 11 million were living in sub-Saharan Africa, Latin America, and south and southeast

Asia. In recent years there has been a striking increase in the number of cases of syphilis in Eastern Europe, especially in the former Soviet Union. In Western Europe and North America, although there are some cases reflecting international contacts, there has also been an increase in cases among homosexual men, which seems to reflect changing patterns of sexual behavior.

In 2000, the rate of primary and secondary syphilis in the United States was 2.1 cases per 100,000 population, the lowest since reporting began in 1941. From 2001 to 2004, the rate increased to 2.7, primarily as a result of increases in cases among homosexual men. The disparity between syphilis rates among blacks and whites in 2004 increased for the first time since 1993 and is associated with a substantial increase of syphilis among black men. After declining for 13 years, the rate of primary and secondary syphilis in 2004, compared with 2003, increased in the South and remained the same among women. The rate of infection among Hispanics also increased. A higher rate of syphilis might increase the transmissibility of human immunodeficiency virus (HIV) infection.[4]

PATHOPHYSIOLOGY

Congenital Syphilis

Congenital syphilis results from the transplacental migration of *T. pallidum,* which invades multiple organs, including perichondrium, cartilage, and bones, with active osteochondral ossification, such as metaphysis of the tubular bones. Depending on the severity of infection the fetus may be aborted or the infant can be stillborn, can die shortly after birth, or survive with early or late characteristics of congenital syphilis. Clinical manifestations of early congenital syphilis include rhinorrhea, rash, anemia, hepatosplenomegaly, ascites, and the nephrotic syndrome (Figs. 68-36 and 68-37). The characteristic stigmata of late congenital syphilis are interstitial keratitis, saber-shin

> ### KEY POINTS
>
> - Osteoarticular manifestations of syphilis can be seen with congenital, secondary, and tertiary syphilis.
> - Manifestations of congenital syphilis include osteochondritis, diaphyseal osteomyelitis (osteitis), periostitis, and miscellaneous changes.
> - The characteristic stigmata of late congenital syphilis are interstitial keratitis, saber-shin deformity of the tibia, and Hutchinson's teeth (peg-shaped, notched, and hypoplastic dental structures).
> - Clutton's joints represent a late manifestation of congenital syphilis.
> - Musculoskeletal manifestations of secondary syphilis are rare and include arthralgias, arthritis, back pain, sacroiliitis, spondylitis, osteitis, and periostitis.
> - Neuropathic arthropathy (Charcot joint), gummatous and nongummatous syphilitic periostitis, osteitis, and osteomyelitis represent musculoskeletal manifestations of tertiary syphilis.

deformity of the tibia, and Hutchinson's teeth (peg-shaped, notched, and hypoplastic dental structures).[2,3,5]

Acquired Syphilis

In acquired syphilis, *T. pallidum* penetrates mucous membranes and enters the lymphatics. The organism reaches the regional lymph nodes in a few hours. It may enter the bloodstream and cause spirochetemia. Three to 6 weeks after the initial infection a primary lesion, which represents a skin ulceration known as a chancre, develops at the inoculation site. This lesion heals spontaneously.[2,3,5]

Approximately 6 weeks later the patient develops secondary syphilis with various systemic manifestations, including skin eruption, arthritis, tenosynovitis, and a variety of visceral involvement. Secondary syphilis

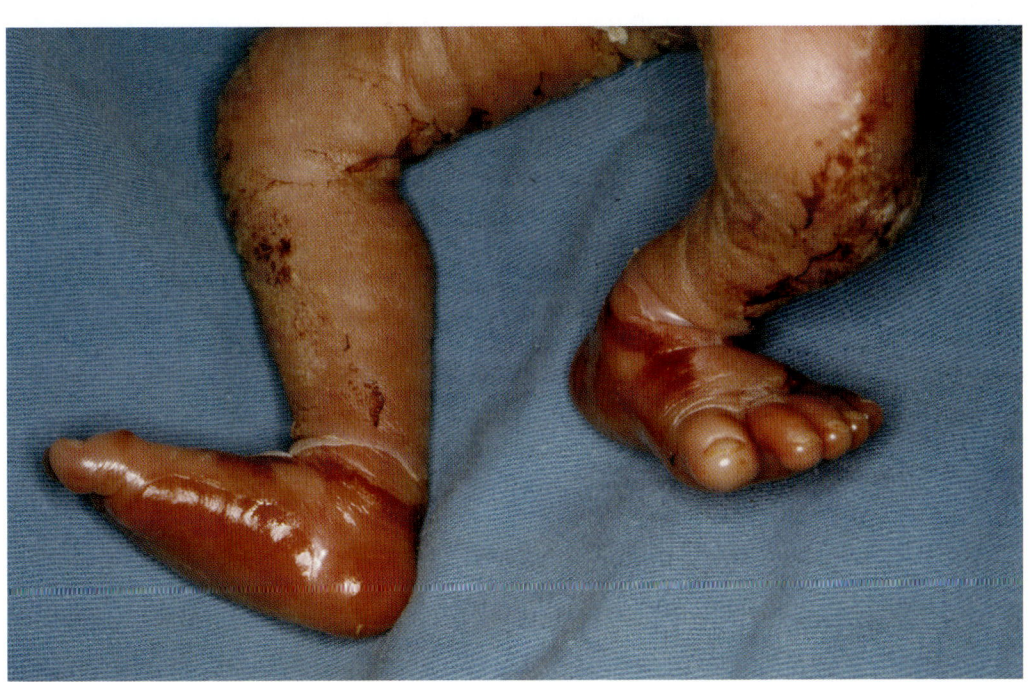

■ FIGURE 68-36 A 1-day-old newborn with congenital syphilis with characteristic skin lesions. *(Courtesy of G. Barnes, MD, Tucson, AZ.)*

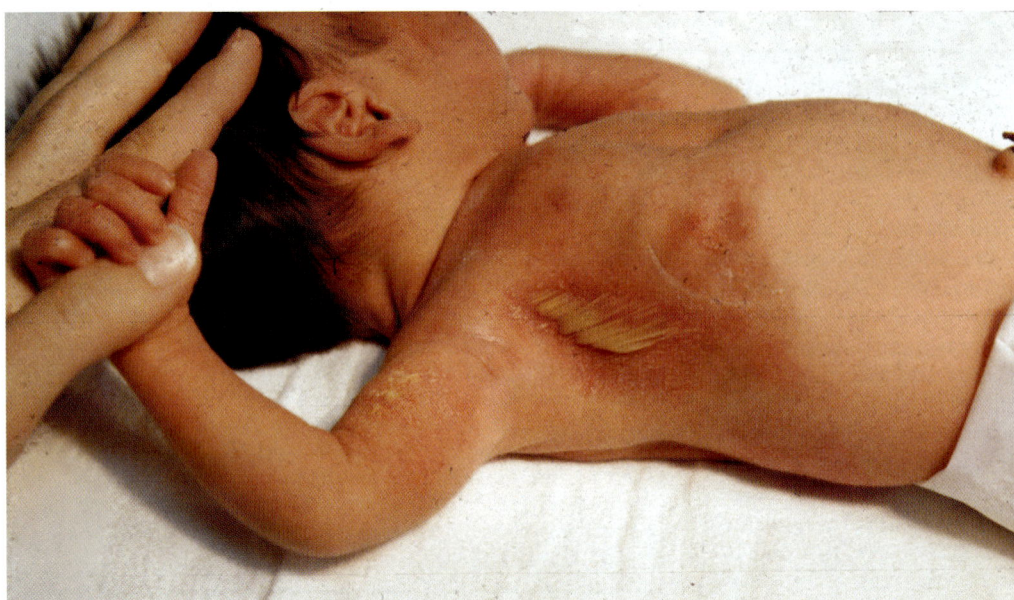

■ **FIGURE 68-37** Neonate with congenital syphilis with skin lesions. *(Courtesy of G. Barnes, MD, Tucson, AZ.)*

is observed in up to 20% of patients. Patients with HIV infection may have unusual clinical manifestation of syphilis, including prominent constitutional symptoms (lues maligna).[2,3,5,6]

Latent syphilis follows the primary and secondary disease. During this phase of the disease the patient may be without symptoms, although the disease may be progressing slowly in various organ systems.[2,3,5]

Syphilitic meningitis and meningovascular syphilis occur early, within the first few years of infection. General paresis and tabes dorsalis occur later, typically 5 to 30 years after infection. Tertiary syphilis, including cardiovascular and neurosyphilis, may occur in approximately 50% of infected patients. Late manifestations include large destructive lesions in any organ of the body, termed *gummas,* and neuropathic arthropathy.[2,3,5,7] In patients with coexisting HIV infection the course of disease may be modified.[2,3,8,9]

The diagnosis can be made by darkfield microscopic visualization of *T. pallidum* sampled from chancre. Under the microscope this organism has a distinctive spiral appearance. Two types of serologic testing are normally used to diagnose syphilis. Both tests detect antibodies, but neither is fully reliable in diagnosing the disease. The first type of test detects antibodies to lipids, called "reagin" antibodies. The Venereal Disease Research Laboratory (VDRL) test is used on serum or sometimes on cerebrospinal fluid taken from the spinal column by lumbar puncture. The rapid plasma reagin (RPR) test is used only on serum. These tests may be positive in patients with a range of other infections, including malaria and rheumatologic illnesses such as systemic lupus erythematosus or during pregnancy. Reagin antibody levels due to syphilis go down when syphilis is treated, so these tests can be used to monitor treatment. The treponemal-specific tests that are used to detect the antibodies to proteins made by *T. pallidum* are very specific but usually remain positive even after a patient has been cured of syphilis. These "treponemal" tests include *T. pallidum* hemagglutination assay (TPHA), *T. pallidum*

particle agglutination test (TPPA), and fluorescent treponemal antibody absorption test (FTA-ABS), along with a number of enzyme immunoassay (EIA) tests that are similar to antibody tests for HIV. It can take up to 90 days for the body to develop antibodies to the bacterium that causes syphilis, so a blood test immediately after exposure to syphilis may not detect infection. In HIV-infected patients the test result can be false negative.[2,3,10]

MANIFESTATIONS OF THE DISEASE

Osteoarticular manifestations of syphilis were recognized since the beginning of the 20th century and can be seen with congenital, secondary, and tertiary syphilis.[1,3,5]

Musculoskeletal manifestations of congenital syphilis in fetuses, neonates, and very young children include osteochondritis, diaphyseal osteomyelitis (osteitis), periostitis, and miscellaneous changes.[2,3,5]

Musculoskeletal manifestations of secondary syphilis are nonspecific. The diagnosis is usually suspected because of association with mucocutaneous findings, including an erythematous maculopapular rash involving the palms and soles, mucosal patches, condylomata lata, and generalized lymphadenopathy.[2,3,6]

Musculoskeletal manifestations of tertiary syphilis are rare, and the neuropathic or Charcot joint is the most characteristic finding. Gummatous involvement of the joints is an unusual manifestation.[2,3,5,7]

Radiography

Early Congenital Syphilis

Osteochondritis

Radiographic findings of syphilitic osteochondritis, which usually results in symmetric involvement of sites of enchondral ossification, are seen in approximately 60% of infants with congenital syphilis. This is seen during the first 3 to 6 weeks of life and rarely after 3 months.

The upper extremity is more commonly involved than the lower. The epiphyseal-metaphyseal junction of the long bones, the costochondral regions, and, in severe cases, the flat and the other bones are affected. Radiography demonstrates irregular epiphyseal lines, subchondral metaphyseal radiolucent bands, diaphyseal cupping, metaphyseal erosion at the growth plate junction, and periosteal thickening. Metaphyseal destruction may result in epiphyseal separation. Bone erosion at the surface of the proximal tibial shaft, usually sparing the most recently formed few millimeters of metaphysis (Laval-Jeantet collar), is considered characteristic and termed *Wimberger's sign*. Complete healing is usually achieved after penicillin therapy within 2 months. Residual osseous deformities and scars are not common but include saddle-nose, nasal septal perforation, Deformity of frontal bones, and saber shins (anterior bowing of the tibia) (Figs. 68-38 to 68-40).[2,3,5]

Osteitis (Diaphyseal Osteomyelitis)

Osteitis may occur in untreated infants or after inadequate antibiotic treatment. It affects the metaphysis and extends to the diaphysis of large tubular bones (Fig. 68-41). Osteolytic areas surrounded by dense bone, and periosteal new bone formation may be observed. Bone lesions are usually polyostotic. Nontubular bone is occasionally involved (Fig. 68-42).[2,3,5]

Periostitis

Periostitis may be seen as an isolating diffuse and symmetric finding or in combination with the other findings and usually affects the long tubular bones. It is less frequent than osteochondritis. Periostitis is associated with pain and decreased motion, which is termed *pseudoparalysis of Parrot*[2,3,5] (see Figs. 68-38, 68-41 and 68-42C).

Miscellaneous Findings

Gummas are rarely seen in congenital syphilis, usually in flat bones. Joint effusions may complicate epiphyseal destruction or separation.[2,3,5]

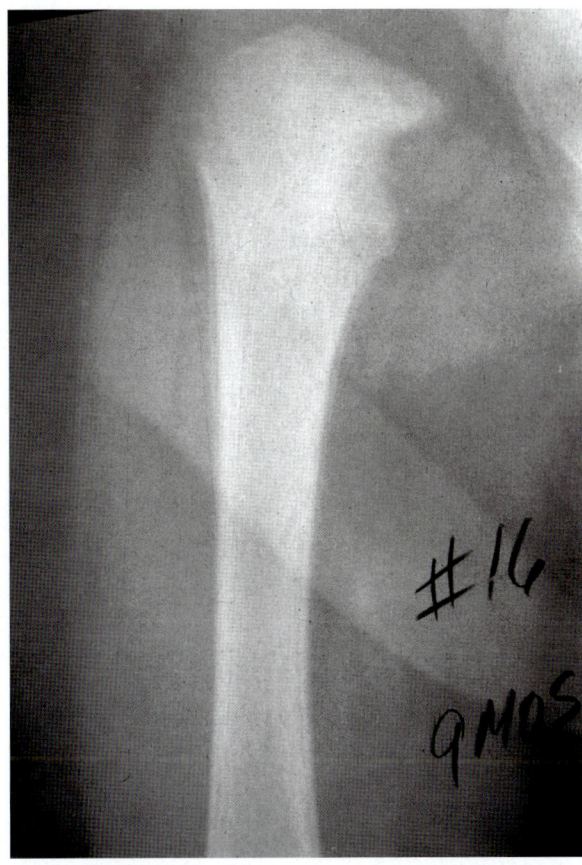

■ **FIGURE 68-38** A 9-month-old newborn was born with congenital syphilis. Radiograph of the right femur demonstrates an erosion at the medial aspect of the proximal metaphysis consistent with osteochondritis. There is associated periostitis along the femoral shaft. *(Courtesy of G. Barnes, MD, Tucson, AZ.)*

Late Congenital Syphilis

The late lesions of congenital syphilis correspond to the tertiary lesions of acquired syphilis. They occur after the age of 2 years and rarely after the third decade of life.[2,3,5]

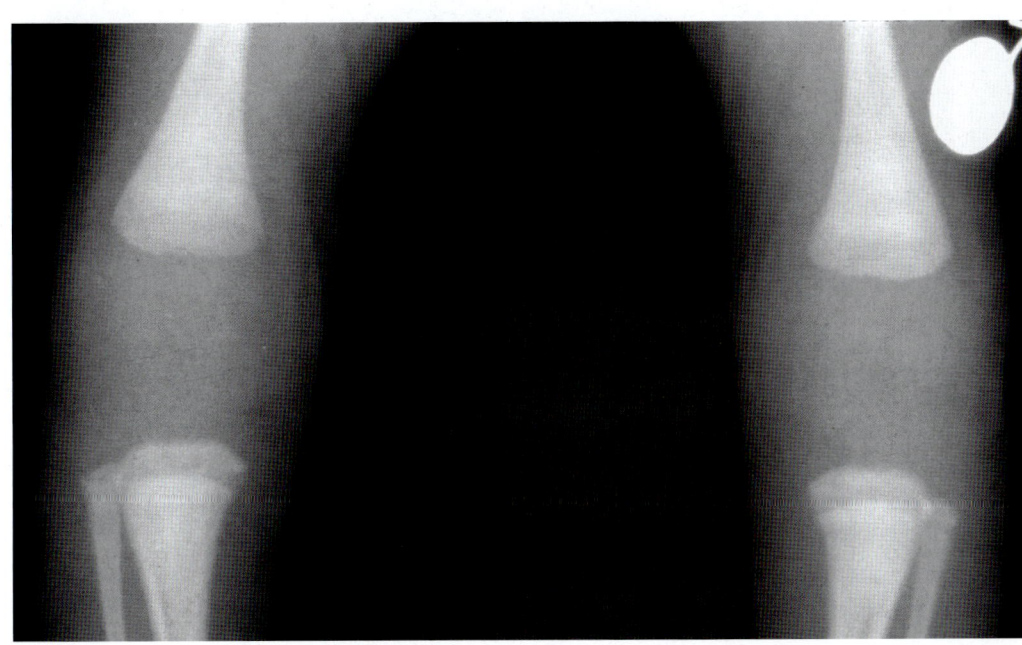

■ **FIGURE 68-39** Neonate with congenital syphilis. Frontal radiograph of both knees shows lucent metaphyseal lines. *(Courtesy G. Barnes M.D. Tucson, AZ.)*

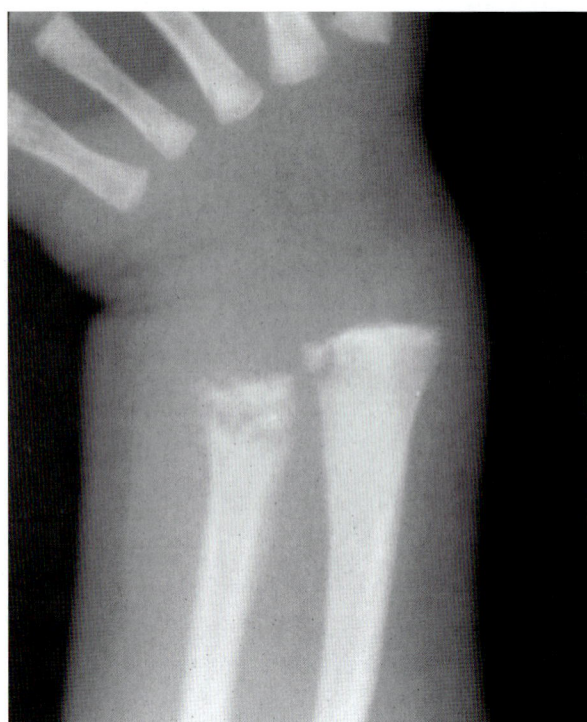

■ **FIGURE 68-40** Neonate with congenital syphilis. Radiograph of the wrist shows metaphyseal irregularities with associated pathologic fractures. *(Courtesy of G. Barnes, MD, Tucson, AZ.)*

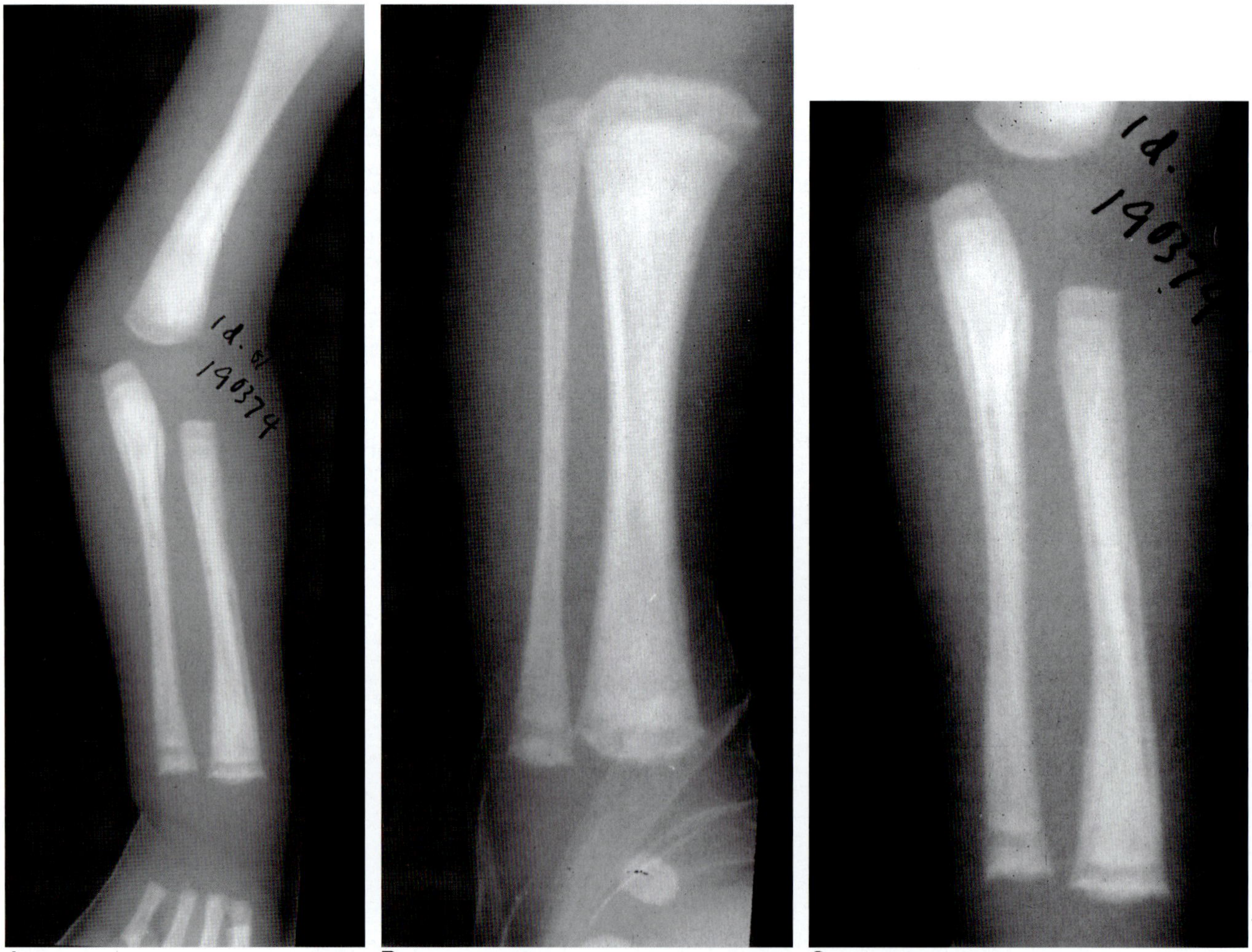

A

B

C

■ **FIGURE 68-41** A to C, Radiographs in neonates with congenital syphilis show osteomyelitis (osteitis), periostitis, and lucent metaphyseal lines involving the long tubular bones.

(Continued)

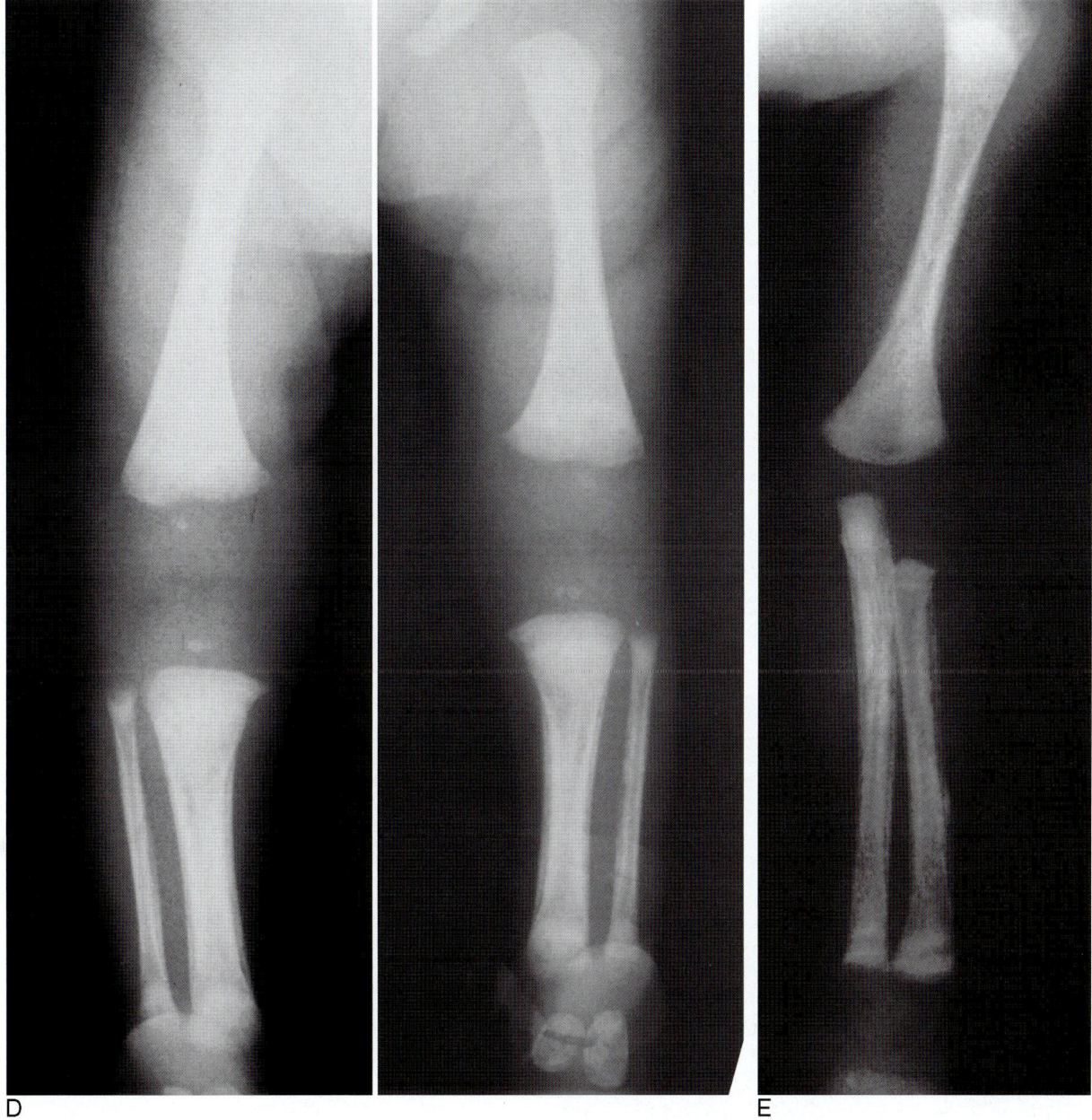

D   E

■ **FIGURE 68-41—Cont'd**   **D** and **E,** Radiographs in neonates with congenital syphilis show osteomyelitis (osteitis), periostitis, and lucent metaphyseal lines involving the long tubular bones. (Courtesy of G. Barnes, MD, Tucson, AZ.)

Both gummatous and nongummatous osteomyelitis result in diffuse hyperostosis of the involved bone. Endosteal proliferation narrows the medullary cavity, whereas the periosteal proliferation creates undulating, enlarged, and dense bone contour. Anterior bowing of the tibia can result, termed *saber shin*. The flat bones, including cranium, can be involved. Dactylitis can also occur (Fig. 68-43).[3,5]

Clutton's Joints

Clutton's joints represent late manifestation of congenital syphilis and manifests usually as symmetric oligoarthritis that involves predominantly the large joints. Joint effusion, periarticular soft tissue swelling, and synovitis are observed. The synovitis generally occurs between the ages of 8 and 15 years.[2,3,5]

Secondary Syphilis

Musculoskeletal manifestations of secondary syphilis are rare and were first described by Wile in 1914.[6] They include arthralgias, arthritis, back pain, sacroiliitis, spondylitis, osteitis, and periostitis.[2,3,5,6]

Tertiary Syphilis

Neuropathic arthropathy (Charcot joint) is observed in 5% to 10% of patients with tabes dorsalis. Lost of deep sensation and chronic trauma lead to extensive destructive changes

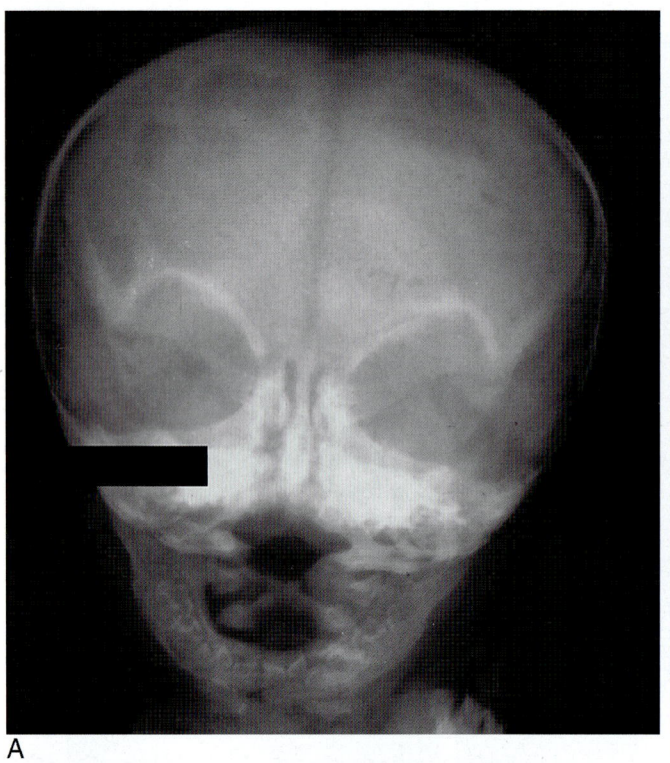

A

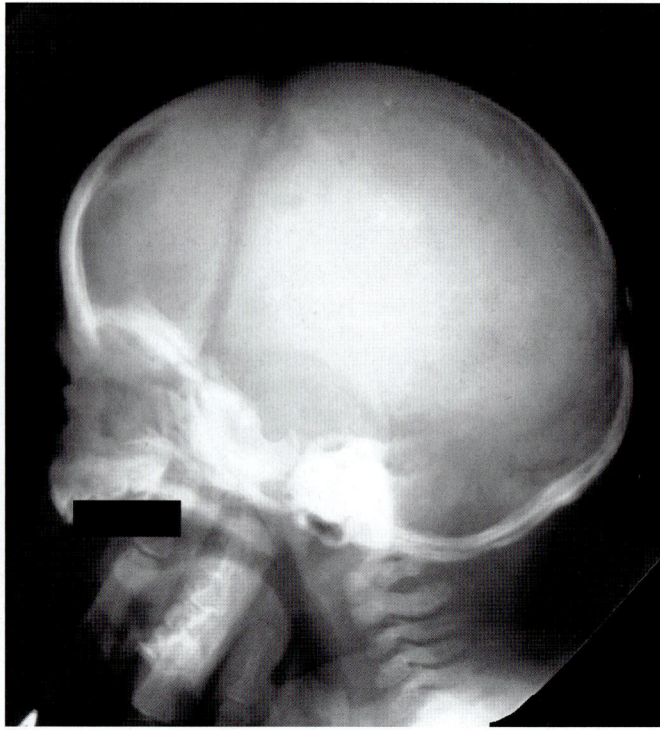

B

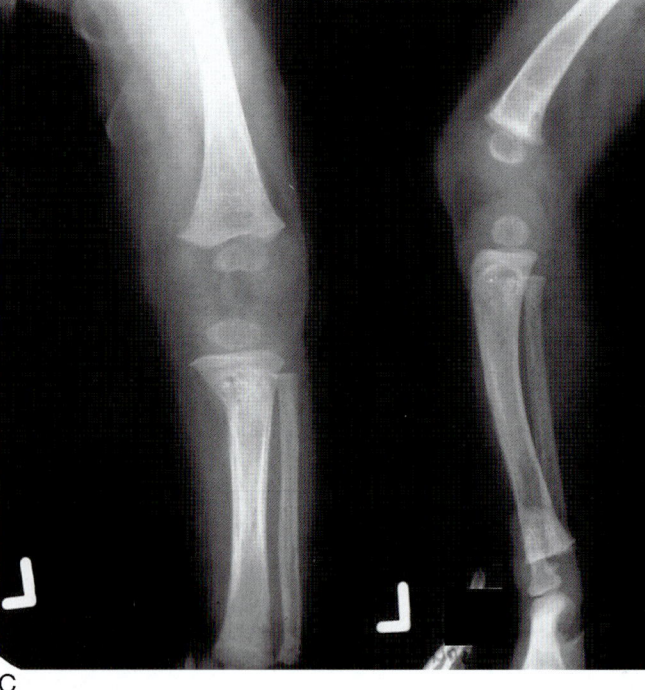

C

■ **FIGURE 68-42** **A** and **B,** Multiple lytic lesions in calvarial bones in an infant with congenital syphilis. **C,** In the same infant note the presence of osteomyelitis and periostitis involving the long bones. *(Courtesy of W. Martel, MD, Ann Arbor, MI.)*

in the affected bones. The most commonly affected joints are knees, hips, and those of the spine. Upper extremity joints and sacroiliac joints are affected less commonly. Radiography demonstrates extensive destructive changes, cupping of the articular surfaces, new bone formation, bone fragmentation, increased density, intra-articular loose bodies, and intra-articular and periarticular calcifications, with associated soft tissue swelling and joint effusion. Association between the Charcot joints due to tertiary syphilis and calcium pyrophosphate deposition disease arthropathy has been reported (Figs. 68-44 and 68-45).[2,7,11,12]

Gummatous involvement of joints and bones became rare after initiation of penicillin therapy. Radiographs show erosive changes of subchondral bone, areas of bone resorption, and reactive changes mimicking those in other chronic infections. A gumma is a discrete lesion of variable size that contains necrotic material. On microscopic examination it contains granulation tissue, and the

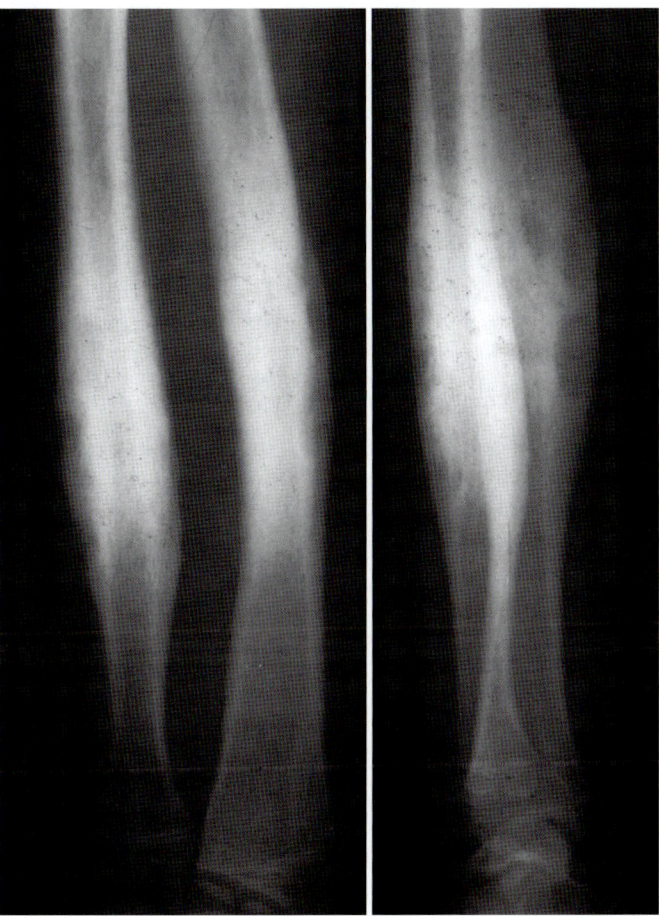

■ **FIGURE 68-43** Late congenital syphilis. Osteomyelitis is evident in the long bones of the leg. *(Courtesy of D. Resnick, MD, San Diego, CA.)*

organisms are usually not seen. Resorption of bone about the gumma is termed *caries sicca,* and detachment of necrotic bone caries necrotica. Radiography shows lytic and sclerotic lesions in bone of variable size. The lesions are frequently associated with periostitis. Pathologic fractures may be observed (Fig. 68-46).[2,3,5]

Nongummatous syphilitic periostitis, osteitis, or osteomyelitis can occur independently or in conjunction with gummas. Radiography reveals destructive and productive bone changes associated with periostitis.[2,3,5]

In gummatous and nongummatous acquired syphilis skeletal lesions can be seen in both the axial and the appendicular skeleton.[2,3]

Nuclear Medicine

Bone scintigraphy typically demonstrates increased radiotracer uptake in the regions of skeletal abnormality caused by syphilis.[13-15]

DIFFERENTIAL DIAGNOSIS

Musculoskeletal manifestations can be associated with congenital, secondary, and tertiary syphilis and can mimic a wide variety of rheumatic and systemic diseases. The differential diagnosis of skeletal syphilis includes yaws, an infection caused by *T. pertenue,* an organism morphologically indistinguishable from *T. pallidum.* Yaws occurs in tropical climates and has radiologic manifestations similar to those of syphilis. The correct diagnosis is made by the isolation of *T. pertenue* from a skin lesion. Other types of infections caused by bacteria, fungi, and mycobacteria are also included in the differential

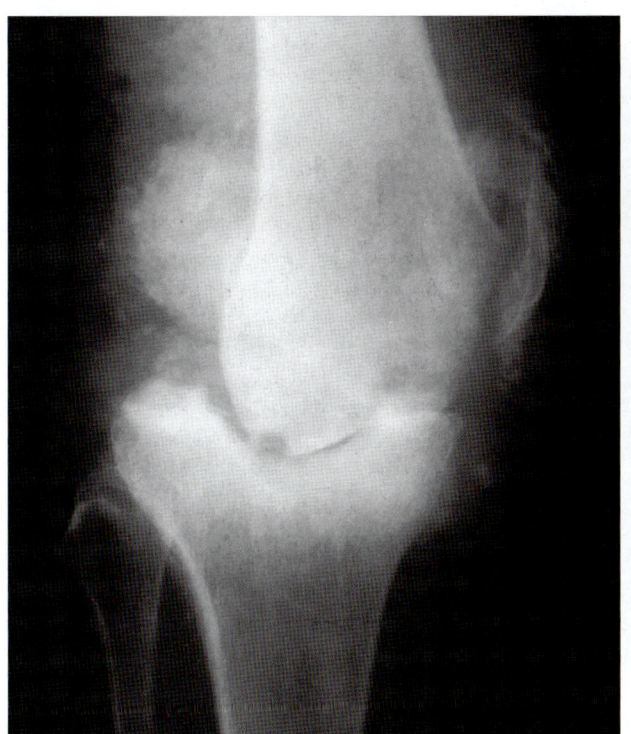

A

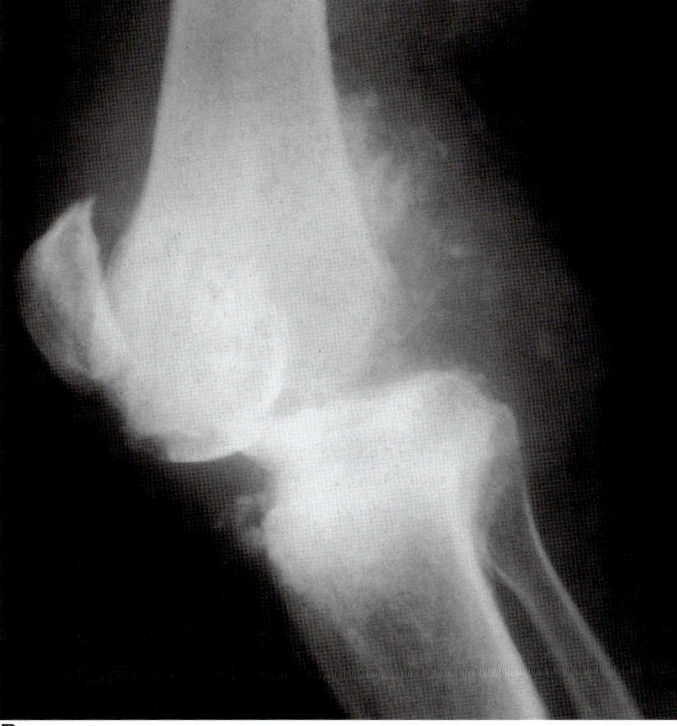

B

■ **FIGURE 68-44** Acquired tertiary syphilis. Frontal (**A**) and lateral (**B**) radiographs of the knee show marked destructive changes consistent with a neuropathic/Charcot joint. *(Courtesy of D. Resnick, MD, San Diego, CA.)*

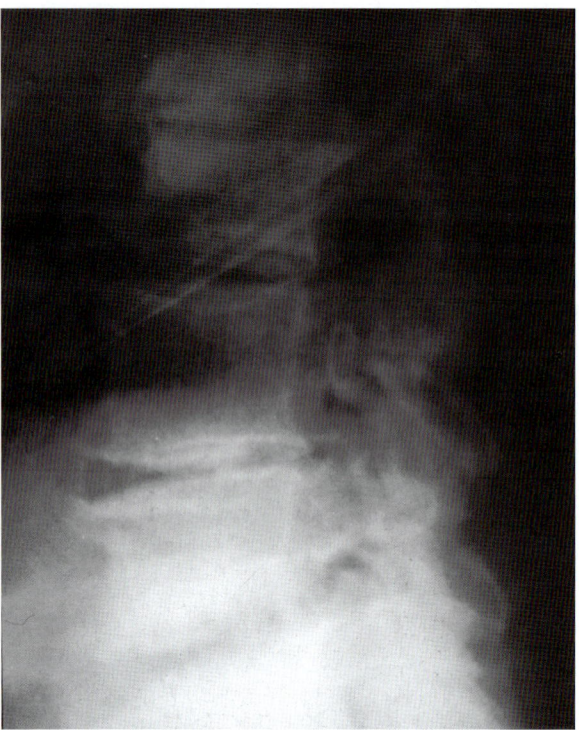

■ **FIGURE 68-45** Tertiary syphilis. Lateral radiograph of the lumbar spine shows changes compatible with a neuropathic/Charcot joint. *(Courtesy of D. Resnick, MD, San Diego, CA.)*

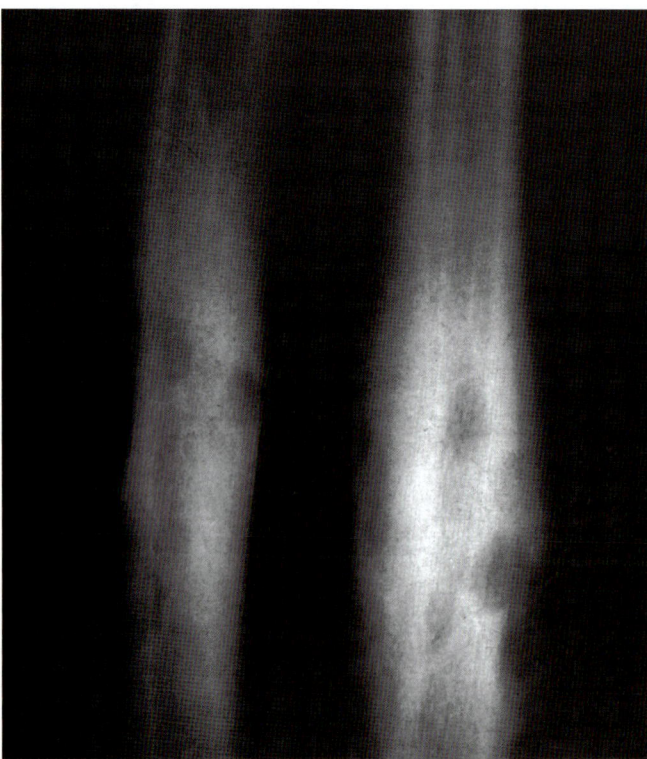

■ **FIGURE 68-46** Tertiary syphilis. Images of the long bones show findings of osteomyelitis with destructive lesions consistent with gummas. *(Courtesy of D. Resnick, MD, San Diego, CA.)*

diagnosis. Sometimes the lesion can resemble a tumor such as osteosarcoma.[3]

SYNOPSIS OF TREATMENT OPTIONS

Medical Treatment

Treponema pallidum remains exquisitely sensitive to penicillin. Patients allergic to penicillin should be treated with tetracycline or erythromycin. In HIV-positive patients, syphilis is usually treated with high doses of antibiotics such as penicillin, benzylpenicillin (Crystapen), or doxycycline (Vibramycin/Vibramycin D).[2,8,9,16]

Surgical Treatment

Surgery may be offered to those most impaired by forms of tabes arthropathy. Joint arthrodesis may be performed. Joint arthroplasty often resulted in loosening, although fair results have been reported in some cases.[2,11,17,18]

What the Referring Physician Needs to Know

■ Syphilis is transmitted by sexual and intimate contact.
■ Syphilis again has become a significant clinical problem, and clinicians must be familiar with the classic as well as the changing clinical manifestations, new diagnostic methods, interaction with HIV infections, and outcomes of therapy.
■ Musculoskeletal manifestations can be associated with congenital, secondary, and tertiary syphilis and can mimic a wide variety of rheumatic and systemic diseases.
■ Musculoskeletal manifestations due to congenital and secondary syphilis usually subside completely after accurate diagnosis and antibiotic therapy.

SUGGESTED READING

Reginato AJ. Syphilitic arthritis and osteitis. Rheum Dis Clin North Am 1993; 19:379–398.

REFERENCES

1. Lipozencic J, Marinovic B. 2005 centennial year marking the discovery of the spirochete treponema pallidum. Acta Dermatovenerol Croat 2006; 14:61.
2. Reginato AJ. Syphilitic arthritis and osteitis. Rheum Dis Clin North Am 1993; 19:379–398.
3. Resnick D. Osteomyelitis, septic arthritis, and soft tissue infection: organisms. In Resnick D (ed). Diagnosis of Bone and Joint Disorders, 4th ed. Philadelphia, WB Saunders, 2002, pp 2510–2624.
4. Centers for Disease Control and Prevention (CDC). Primary and secondary syphilis—United States, 2003–2004. MMWR Morb Mortal Wkly Rep 2006; 55:269–273.
5. Jeffe HL. Metabolic, Degenerative, and Inflammatory Diseases of Bones and Joints. Philadelphia, Lee & Febiger, 1972.
6. Wile UJ. Arthopathy in secondary syphilis. J Cutan Incl Syph 1914; 32:20–23; J Clin Microbiol 2006; 44:1335–1341.
7. Resnick D. Neuropathic osteoarthropathy. In Resnick D (ed). Diagnosis of Bone and Joint Disorders, 4th ed. Philadelphia, WB Saunders, 2002, pp 3564–3595.
8. From the MMWR. Recommendations for diagnosing and treating syphilis in HIV-infected patients. Arch Dermatol 1989; 125:15–16.

9. Recommendations for diagnosing and treating syphilis in HIV-infected patients. MMWR Morb Mortal Wkly Rep 1988; 37:600–602, 607–608.
10. Muller I, Brade V, Hagedorn HJ, et al. Is serological testing a reliable tool in laboratory diagnosis of syphilis? Meta-analysis of eight external quality control surveys performed by the German infection serology proficiency testing program.
11. Allali F, Rahmouni R, Hajjaj-Hassouni N. Tabetic arthropathy: a report of 43 cases. Clin Rheumatol 2006; 25:858–860.
12. Jones EA, Manaster BJ, May DA, Disler DG. Neuropathic osteoarthropathy: diagnostic dilemmas and differential diagnosis. RadioGraphics 2000; 20(Spec No):S279–S293.
13. Gomez Martinez MV, Gallardo FG, Cobo Soler J, et al. [Osteitis in secondary syphilis]. Rev Esp Med Nucl 2003; 22:424–426. Spanish.
14. Cronin EB, Williams WH, Tow DE. Radionuclide imaging in a case of tertiary syphilis involving the liver and bones. J Nucl Med 1987; 28:1047–1051.
15. Moreno AJ, Yedinak MA, Rahnema A, Fredericks P. Bone scintigraphy in latent congenital syphilis. Clin Nucl Med 1985; 10:824–825.
16. Lafond RE, Lukehart SA. Biological basis for syphilis. Clin Microbiol Rev 2006; 19:29–49.
17. Gualtieri G, Sudanese A, Toni A, Giunti A. Loosening of a hip prosthesis in a patient affected with tabetic disease. Chir Organi Mov 1991; 76:83–85.
18. Yoshino S, Fujimori J, Kajino A, et al. Total knee arthroplasty in Charcot's joint. J Arthroplasty 1993; 8:335–340.

Tuberculosis

Tuberculosis is still a common disease in underdeveloped parts of the world. The prevalence of this disease has significantly decreased after development of chemotherapy. In the 1940s and 1950s, skeletal tuberculosis occurred in 3% to 5% of patients with pulmonary tuberculosis and in approximately 30% of patients with extrapulmonary tuberculosis. In the 1960s and 1970s the prevalence of tuberculosis had decreased, but it started to rise again in the mid 1980s in the United States. The factors that have contributed to an increased rate of tuberculosis include an increased number of immunocompromised patients, the development of drug-resistant strains of mycobacteria, changing patterns of travel and immigration, and an increased number of health care workers exposed to the disease. Additionally, in rare occasions modern therapeutic techniques, including bacille Calmette-Guérin vaccination, can cause an iatrogenic infection.[1-3]

ETIOLOGY

Mycobacterium tuberculosis is the main causative organism of musculoskeletal tuberculosis. A few cases are attributable to *M. bovis*. Atypical mycobacteria such as *M. kansasii, M. marinum, M. sacrofulaceum,* and *M. avium* complex account for 1% to 4% of tuberculosis cases. These produce chronic infection, are of low virulence, and usually are more resistant to the standard drugs.[4]

PREVALENCE AND EPIDEMIOLOGY

The majority of cases are found in south and east Asia, sub-Saharan Africa, and Eastern Europe. In 1997, 1.9 billion people were infected with tuberculosis.[8]

During 2004, a total of 14,511 confirmed tuberculosis cases (4.9 cases per 100,000 population) were reported in the United States, representing a 3.3% decline in the rate from 2003. Slightly more than half (53.7%) of U.S. cases were in foreign-born persons. Findings indicate that although the 2004 tuberculosis rate was the lowest recorded in the United States since national reporting began in 1953, the declines in rates for 2003 (2.3%) and 2004 (3.3%) were the smallest since 1993. In addition, tuberculosis rates greater than the U.S. average continue to be reported in certain racial/ethnic populations; in 2004, Hispanics, blacks, and Asians had tuberculosis rates 7.5, 8.3, and 20.0 times higher than whites, respectively. Essential elements for controlling tuberculosis in the United States include sufficient local resources, interventions targeted to populations with the highest tuberculosis rates, and continued collaborative efforts with other nations to reduce tuberculosis globally.[9,10]

Bone and joint tuberculosis may account for up to 30% to 35% of cases of extrapulmonary tuberculosis. Skeletal tuberculosis most often involves the spine, followed by tuberculous arthritis in weight-bearing joints and extraspinal tuberculous osteomyelitis.[1,10] Skeletal tuberculosis equally affects males and females. Lesions in hands and feet are not uncommonly seen in children, immunocompromised patients, and the elderly. Extra-axial tuberculous arthritis is usually monarticular, and involvement of multiple joints is rare.[1,11]

CLINICAL PRESENTATION

Skeletal tuberculosis can be seen in any age group; it is rare in the first year of life. In the non-Hispanic white population the median age is about 60 years, and among the minority groups it is about 40 years. In the communities with a high prevalence the majority of patients are infected by the age of 20 years. Extrapulmonary tuberculosis is more common in children than in adults, with common involvement of lymph nodes (scrofulosis). The delay in diagnosis is common and is reported to be 16 to 19 months.[13]

The spine is most commonly affected, followed by the pelvis, hip, and knee joints. The joints of the lower extremity are more commonly involved than the joints of the upper extremity. Tuberculosis of the spine was first described by Sir Percival Pott in 1779.

The initial symptoms vary. The patients with tuberculous spondylitis present with an insidious onset of back pain, stiffness, local tenderness, neurologic abnormalities,

---

KEY POINTS

■ The disease has an indolent course.
■ There is commonly a delay in diagnosis.
■ Prompt diagnosis and treatment are important.

and possibly fever. Paralysis can occur as a result of spinal cord compression from abscesses, granulation tissue, bone fragments, arachnoiditis, ischemia of the cord from endarteritis, or intramedullary granulomas. This form of skeletal tuberculosis is most commonly associated with pulmonary disease.

Tuberculous arthritis can lead to pain, swelling, weakness, muscle wasting, and a draining sinus. A history of trauma may be obtained in 30% to 50% of cases.

Tuberculous dactylitis usually manifests as a painless swelling of the hand and foot.

Tuberculous tenosynovitis and bursitis can produce soft tissue swelling and tenderness. Very infrequently carpal tunnel syndrome results from tuberculous involvement of tendon sheaths and bursae in the wrist.

A positive tuberculin skin test is not reliable for the diagnosis of tuberculosis. Elderly patients who have never had any clinical manifestation of tuberculosis as well as those who have received the bacillus Calmette-Guérin vaccine have a high frequency of a positive skin test. However, a negative tuberculin skin test generally excludes the disease, except in immunocompromised and malnourished patients in whom the test can be false negative.

PATHOPHYSIOLOGY

Musculoskeletal tuberculosis mainly results from hematogenous dissemination or lymphangitic spread from a primary or reactivated infected focus. Rarely, this disease may be the result of direct inoculation. Injuries may result in reactivation of preexisting tuberculous infection. The contributing factors for the reactivation of disease include poor socioeconomic conditions, and immunodeficiency, mainly in the patients with HIV infection and AIDS.[4]

Mycobacteria reach the skeletal system through the vascular system, mainly arterial as a result of bacteremia, but may also reach the axial skeleton through the venous plexus of Batson.[4] Localization to the metaphyseal segments of the long bones is noted in this disease, like in pyogenic osteomyelitis, perhaps related to tuberculous infarcts from emboli within the nutrient vessels.[1] Tuberculous involvement of the joints may result from hematogenous dissemination through the subsynovial vessels, or indirectly form epiphyseal or metaphyseal lesions, which erode into the joint space. A tuberculous granuloma develops within the bone at the site of mycobacterial deposition. This lesion undergoes caseous necrosis and expands, causing trabecular destruction. Further expansion can cause cortical destruction, with subsequent development of a soft tissue mass.[4] The margins of the bony lytic lesions are usually distinct.[1,5] In children, the periosteal reaction can occur. Bone sclerosis and ankylosis occur only when the disease has chronically faded out.[5-7]

Tuberculosis is one among multiple many other diseases associated with formation of bone marrow granulomas. The typical response of tissue is the formation of sharply demarcated tubercles. In the central part of the tubercle are multinucleated giant cells and at the periphery is a mantle of lymphocytes. Around a central zone are clusters of epithelioid cells with elongated vascular nuclei. The tuberculin produced by the acid-fast bacilli causes the characteristic caseating necrosis. As necrosis

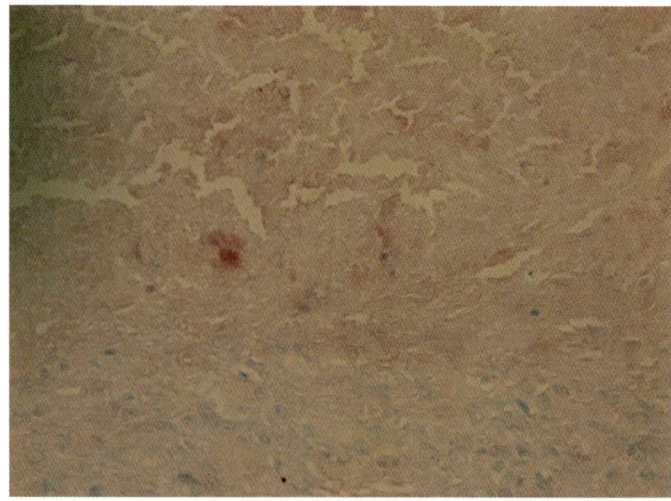

■ **FIGURE 68-47** *Mycobacterium tuberculosis.* Note a small number of slightly beaded, bright rose-pink bacilli. This paucity of organisms is the usual finding in an immunocompetent patient. (Acid-fast bacillus stain.) *(Courtesy of Anna Graham, MD, Tucson, AZ.)*

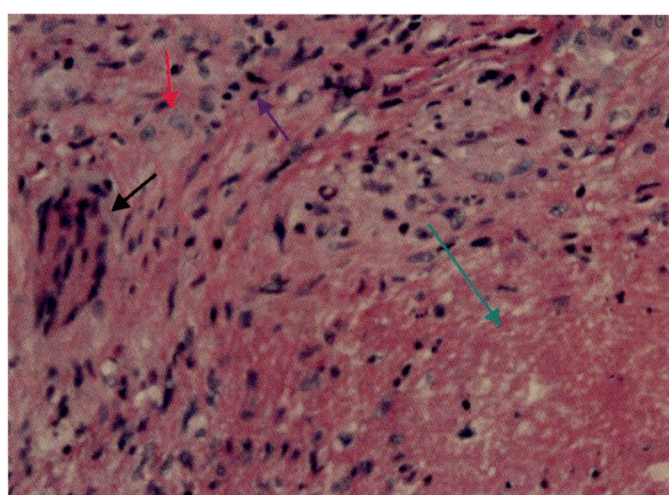

■ **FIGURE 68-48** *Mycobacterium tuberculosis.* Note the giant cell (*black arrow*), the epithelioid histiocyte cells (*pink arrow*), lymphocytes (*blue arrow*), and caseation necrosis (*green arrow*). These features characterize a well-formed granuloma, formed as a response to *M. tuberculosis* in an immunocompetent patient. (Hematoxylin and eosin stain.) *(Courtesy of Anna Graham, MD, Tucson, AZ.)*

progresses the epithelioid cells degenerate and become grouped into an amorphous mass. Peripheral growth of the tubercle relates to the influx of new mononuclear cells that mature into the epithelioid cells, as long as viable bacilli are present. Healing lesions are associated with the production of hyaline fibrous nodules and encapsulation, which leads to formation of a connective tissue scar. Calcifications and ossifications of caseating lesions may also occur (Figs. 68-47 and 68-48).[1,13]

IMAGING TECHNIQUES

Radiography should be always the initial imaging modality obtained in evaluation of skeletal tuberculosis.[13,38] Regardless of results of the radiographic study MRI should be performed for evaluation of local extent of disease. MRI has a superb contrast resolution and multiplanar imaging capability and is superb in evaluation of soft tissue and bone involvement.[1,13] CT with the better spatial resolution than MRI is superior in evaluation of cortical destruction especially in the posterior elements, and for depiction of soft tissue calcifications (within an intraspinal abscess).[13] Nuclear medicine studies including ^{99m}Tc-methylene diphosphonate (MDP) and ^{67}gallium citrate scans are of limited value but should be performed to evaluate for multicentricity of disease.[13] Ultrasonography is of limited value but can demonstrate abdominal paraspinal abscesses and soft tissue infection.[1]

MANIFESTATIONS OF THE DISEASE

The spine is involved in the majority of cases of musculoskeletal tuberculosis, followed by hips and knees. Other joints and soft tissues can also be involved. Tuberculosis can also affect any bone in the body as well as soft tissues including bursae, tendon sheaths, muscles, and other soft tissue structures.

Tuberculous spondylitis frequently affects the lower thoracic and upper lumbar spine in adults. Other sites in the spine are less frequently involved. Most frequently, tuberculous spondylitis begins in the anterior aspect of the vertebral body adjacent to the subchondral end plate. The lesion can be detected by radiography usually in 2 to 5 months. Infection can spread beneath the anterior or posterior longitudinal ligaments, allowing the osseous invasion at distant sites. The infection can violate the peripheral aspect of the intervertebral disc. The disease can penetrate the subchondral bone and involve the disc and cause decrease of disc height. The involvement of posterior elements is rare. Discovertebral destruction is similar as in pyogenic infection but usually more indolent. Long segments of the spine can be involved. Extension of tuberculous infection into the paraspinal, usually anterolateral and rarely posterior, soft tissues is common. Paraspinal abscesses can cause periosteal stripping and avascular necrosis. The infection can also penetrate the adjacent organs. Tuberculous psoas abscesses are prone to calcify. Destruction of vertebral bodies leads to kyphotic deformities that are more severe in thoracic than in cervical or lumbar region. Scoliosis and ankylosis of multiple vertebral bodies can be observed (Figs. 68-49 to 68-54).

Tuberculous osteomyelitis can involve any bone but is most common in femur and tibia and small bones of the hands and feet. Typically the metaphyses are involved. Transphyseal extension is more common in tuberculous than in pyogenic osteomyelitis. The cystic type of tuberculous osteomyelitis is more common in children than in adults. In children these lesions involve the metaphysis of long bones, whereas in adults the skull, shoulder, and axial skeleton are more commonly involved. Solitary involvement is predominant.

Tuberculous dactylitis is more common in children than in adults. Hands are affected more often than feet, with the proximal phalanges of the index and middle fingers and the metacarpals of the middle and ring fingers being the most frequent locations. Soft tissue swelling is

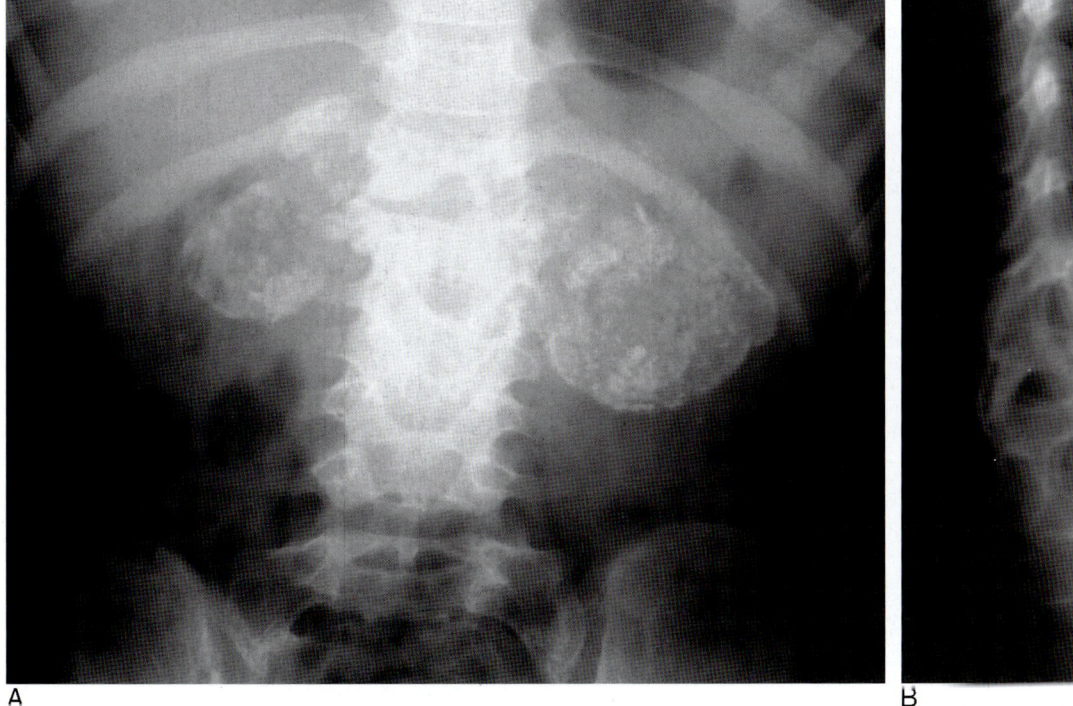
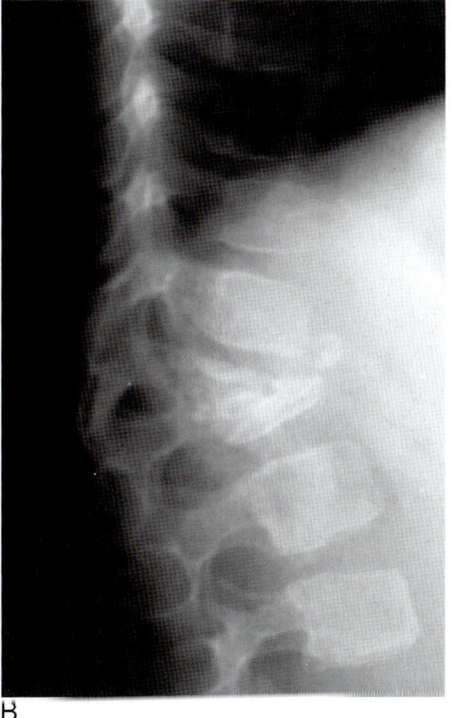

A   B

■ **FIGURE 68-49**   Tuberculous spondylitis. Frontal (**A**) and lateral (**B**) radiographs of the lumbar spine show tuberculous involvement of L1 vertebral body with loss of height, wedging, and kyphosis, and with associated calcified paraspinal abscess (cold abscess). *(Courtesy of G. Barnes, MD, Tucson, AZ.)*

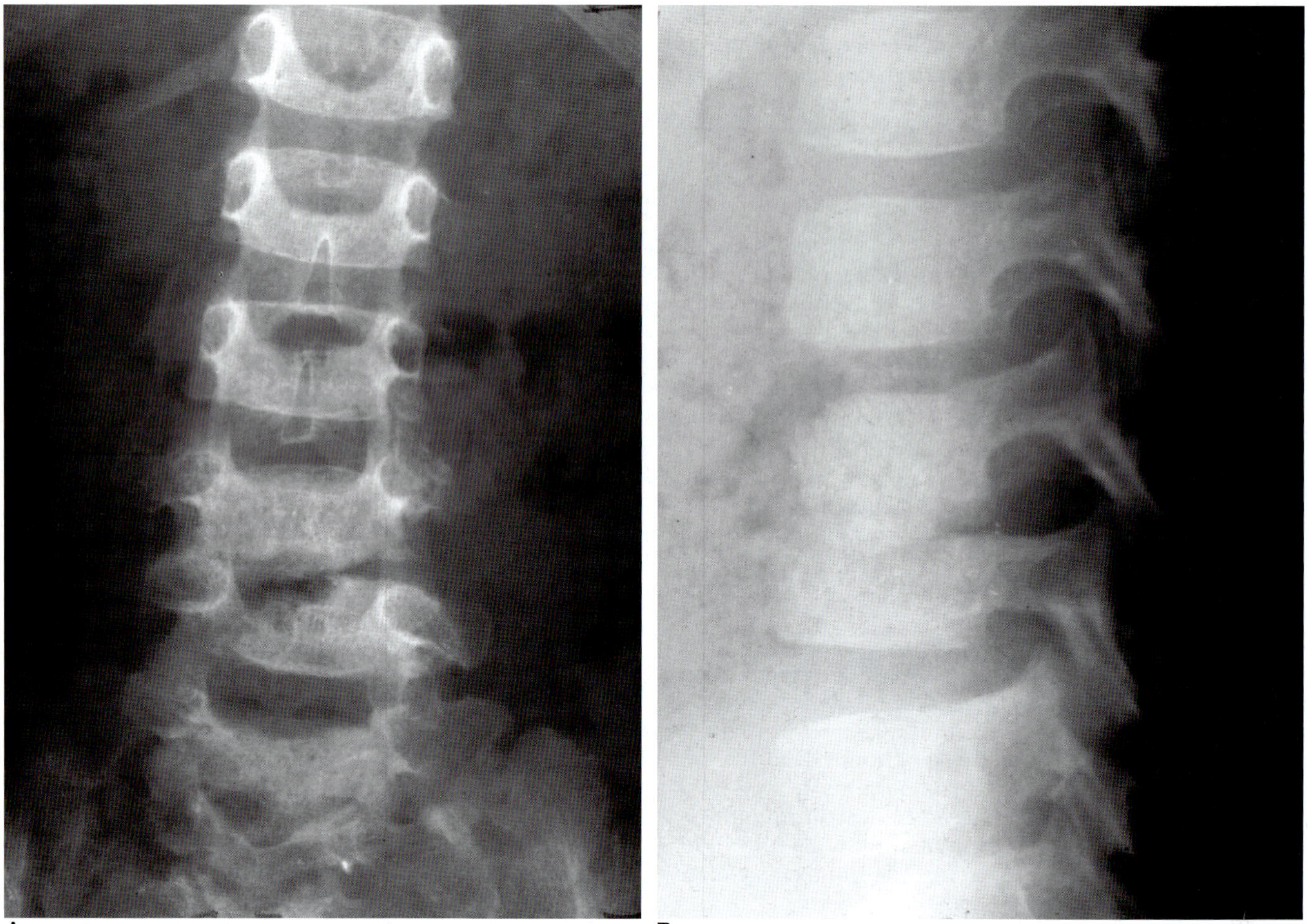

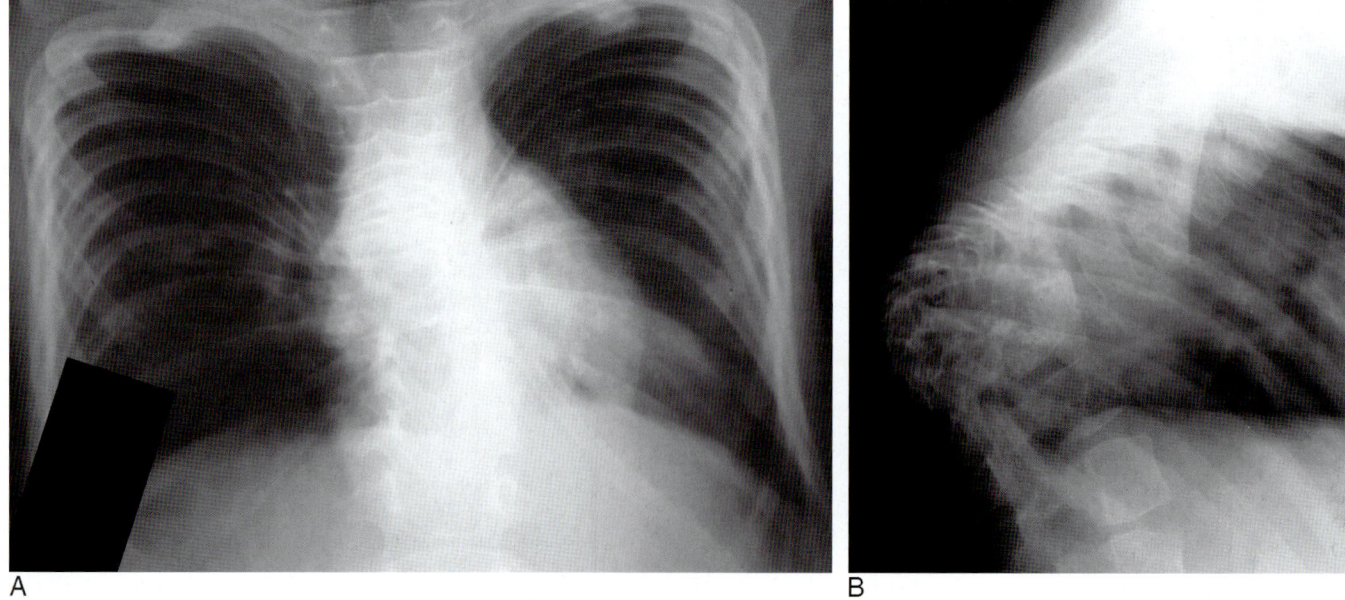

A   B

■ **FIGURE 68-50**   Tuberculous spondylitis. Frontal (**A**) and lateral (**B**) radiographs of the lumbar spine show disc space loss and end plate erosions at the L3-L4 level. *(Courtesy of G. Barnes, MD, Tucson, AZ.)*

A   B

■ **FIGURE 68-51**   Tuberculous spondylitis. Frontal (**A**) and lateral (**B**) radiographs of the chest/thoracic spine show gibbus deformity in the lower thoracic spine secondary to tuberculous infection. *(Courtesy of G. Barnes, MD, Tucson, AZ.)*

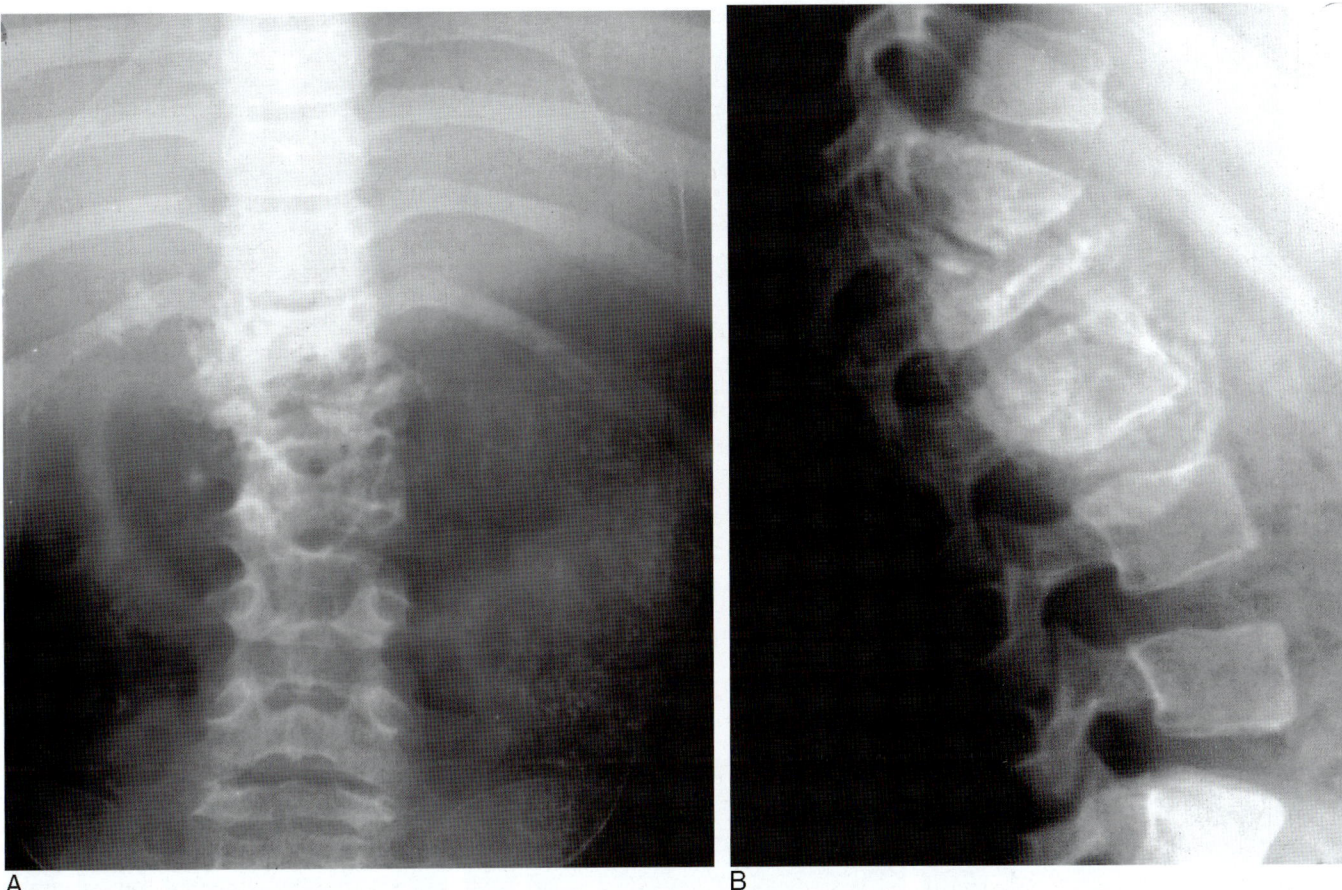

■ **FIGURE 68-52** Tuberculous spondylitis. Frontal (**A**) and lateral (**B**) radiographs of the thoracolumbar spine show marked loss of height of L1 and, to a lesser extent, of T12 vertebral bodies with erosive changes at the T12–L2 levels and associated kyphosis and calcified soft tissue abscess. *(Courtesy of G. Barnes, MD, Tucson, AZ.)*

the initial symptom in virtually all cases, whereas stiffness, pain, and finger numbness may be present in some (Fig. 68-55).[1,13]

Tuberculous arthritis most commonly involves hip and knee joints, but any joint can be involved. It is most commonly monarticular disease. The presenting symptoms are usually the insidious onset of joint pain and swelling. Other presenting symptoms include weakness, muscle wasting, and draining sinuses. Trauma, drug addiction, intra-articular corticosteroid injection, and systemic illness predispose to tuberculous arthritis (Figs. 68-56 and 68-57).

In tuberculous bursitis and tenosynovitis synovial membrane of bursae and tendon sheaths and tendons themselves are infected. Typical sites of infection include the radial and ulnar bursae of the hand, flexor tendon sheaths of the fingers, bursae about the ischial tuberosity, subacromial-subdeltoid bursa and subgluteal bursae. The other locations are affected less often.

Tuberculous myositis and soft tissue infection are frequently associated with underlying disease such as collagen vascular disease, immunosuppression therapy, or local trauma. Soft tissue abscesses are more frequent in patients with AIDS. Tuberculous myositis is rare.

Radiography

Early radiographic findings in tuberculous spondylitis are loss of end plate definition and only slight disc space narrowing. Later radiography shows vertebral end plate destruction with paucity of sclerosis or periosteal reaction, associated with paraspinal abscesses. Paraspinal abscesses may be detected as areas of fusiform soft tissue swelling around the spine. They frequently contain calcifications. Bone loss results in vertebral deformity. Multiple vertebral levels may be involved in noncontiguous fashion. In most severe cases, nearly an entire vertebral body is destroyed with progression to vertebra plana. Severe kyphosis (gibbus deformity) develops as the disease progresses (see Figs. 68-49 to 68-54).[1,14,28]

Radiographic findings of tuberculous osteomyelitis include osteopenia, osteolytic foci with poorly defined edges, and minimal surrounded sclerosis. Transphyseal extension of disease is common.

In tuberculous dactylitis, prominent fusiform soft tissue swelling and periostitis are the most common findings. Periostitis is the earliest sign of bone involvement, followed by gradual bone destruction and sequestrum formation. Destruction of underlying bone leads to cyst-like

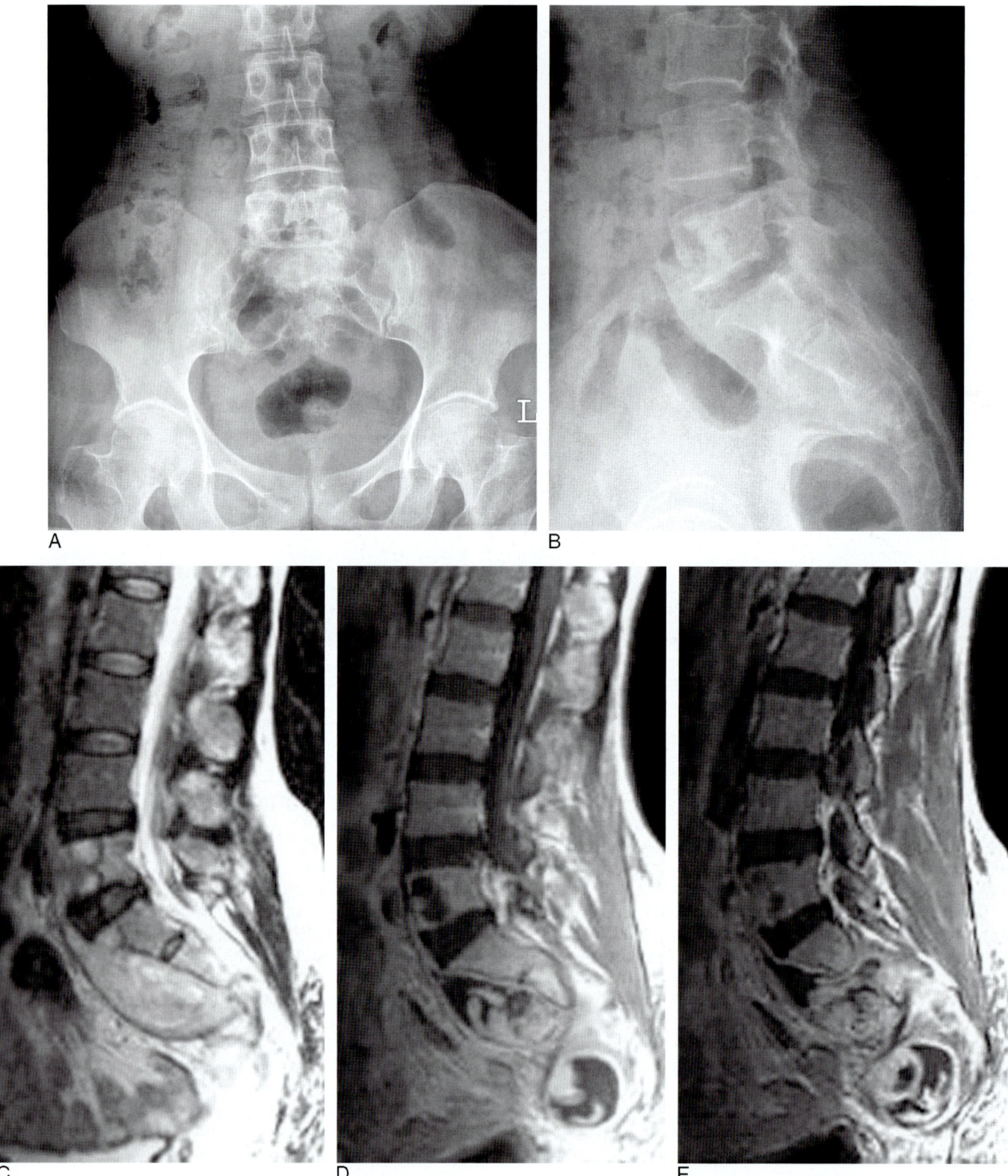

■ **FIGURE 68-53** Tuberculous spondylitis. Frontal (**A**) and lateral (**B**) radiographs of the lumbosacral spine show a lytic lesion involving the anterior aspect of the L5 vertebral body with associated cortical erosions of the anterior aspect of the L5 and S1 vertebrae and prevertebral soft tissue thickening/paraspinal abscess. **C,** T2-weighted sagittal MR image shows increased signal intensity in the regions of abnormality and associated paraspinal abscess. **D** and **E,** Sagittal T1-weighted images after intravenous administration of gadolinium-based contrast agent show heterogeneous enhancement in the regions of abnormality consistent with osteomyelitis and paraspinal abscess. Note sparing of the L5–S1 disc space. *(Courtesy of Hilary Umans, MD, Bronx, NY.)*

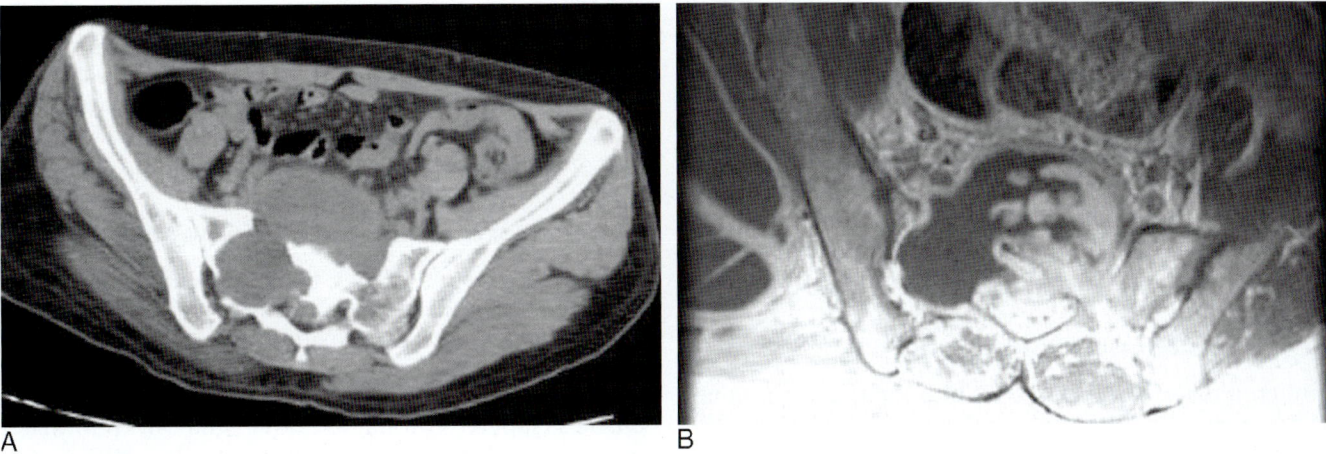

■ **FIGURE 68-54** Sacral tuberculous osteomyelitis. **A,** Axial CT image of the sacrum shows destructive lytic lesion involving the right sacral site with associated cortical discontinuity and parasacral mass/abscess anteriorly. **B,** Axial T1-weighted image after intravenous administration of gadolinium-based contrast agent heterogeneous enhancement in the region of abnormality consistent with osteomyelitis and abscess. *(Courtesy of Hilary Umans, MD, Bronx, NY.)*

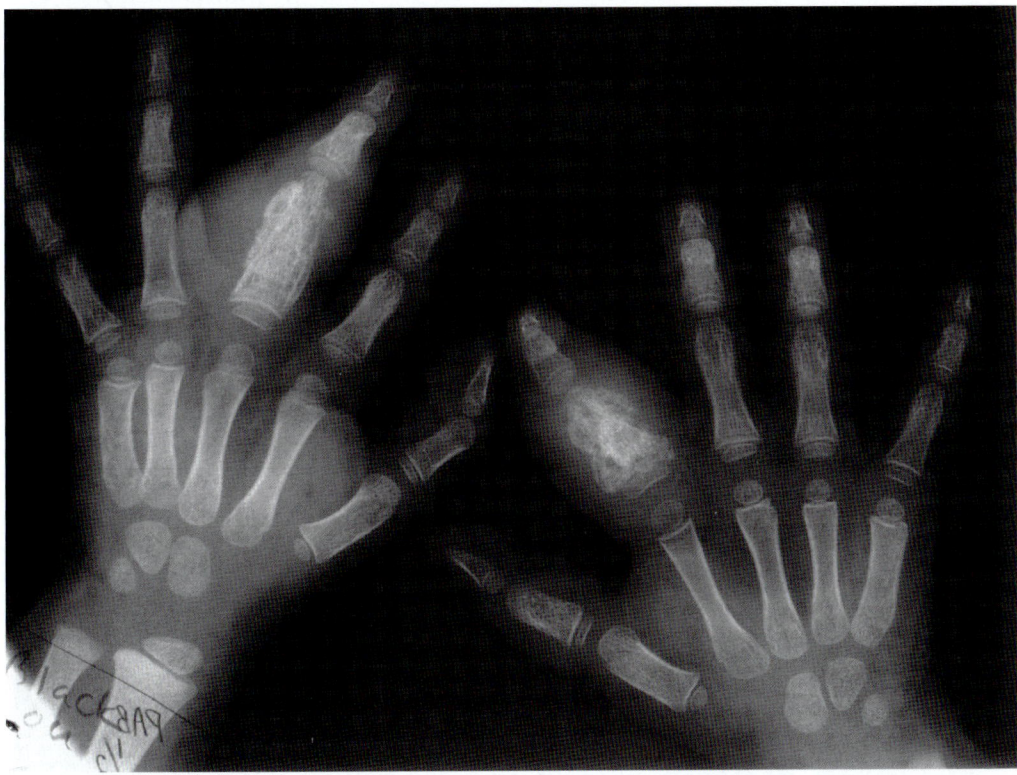

■ **FIGURE 68-55** Tuberculous dactylitis is evident as spina ventosa in this child. Radiograph shows expansion and destructive changes involving the proximal phalanges of the right index finger and left third finger. *(Courtesy of George Barnes, MD, Tucson, AZ.)*

cavity formation with the remaining bone ballooned out. This is most marked in the diaphyses of metacarpal and metatarsal bones in children and is termed *spina ventosa* ("wind-filled sail"). Other radiographic features include diffuse bone infiltration with a coarse trabecular pattern and localized destruction of the end of the phalanx with reactive sclerosis and bone involvement (see Fig. 68-55).[1,13]

In early stages, joint effusion and soft tissue edema may be the only signs of tuberculous arthritis. Classic radiographic signs of tuberculous arthritis include juxta-articular osteoporosis, peripheral osseous erosions, and gradual reduction of the joint space and are termed *Phemister's triad* (see Fig. 68-56). If the disease is left untreated, complete joint obliteration and fibrous ankylosis of the joint may result. Periostitis and bone proliferation are less common and less extensive than in pyogenic arthritis. When present, tuberculous periostitis is linear, paralleling the contour of the bone. In skeletally immature patients synovitis and chronic hyperemia can lead to epiphyseal overgrowth and premature physeal fusion.[13]

In tuberculous bursitis and tenosynovitis, soft tissue swelling and osteoporosis may be observed. Osseous involvement may develop in the region of the greater trochanter. In any bursal location dystrophic calcifications may appear.

Magnetic Resonance Imaging

In tuberculous spondylitis MRI is best for assessing signal change within the disc space and adjacent vertebral bodies, intraosseous abscess, skip lesions, subligamentous spread of infection and epidural extension. Characteristic changes in affected vertebral bodies are decreased signal intensity on the T1-weighted, increased signal on the T2-weighted and inversion recovery images, and enhancement after intravenous administration of gadolinium-based contrast. A thick enhancing rim is observed about the paraspinal abscesses.[1,13,14,28,29] Intraosseous abscesses also demonstrate rim enhancement. MRI is very sensitive in detection of early changes of tuberculous arthritis, but the appearances are nonspecific. MRI is useful in diagnosis of tuberculous tenosynovitis, bursitis, and myositis with similar signal abnormalities as with osseous infection (see Figs. 68-53C-E, 68-54-B, and 68-56C-E).

Multidetector Computed Tomography

In tuberculous spondylitis CT is sensitive in detecting early bone changes, paraspinal abscesses, and involvement of posterior elements. It provides superb visualization of bone fragmentation and calcifications within paraspinal abscesses. Multislice CT provides thin-cut imaging that enables superb coronal, sagittal, and 3D reformatted images (see Figs. 68-54-A and 68-57).[1,14,28] MRI is superior to CT in evaluation of soft tissue infection, including tenosynovitis, bursitis, and myositis.

Ultrasonography

Ultrasonography allows diagnosis of abdominal tubercular abscesses and can confirm clinical suspicion. It is

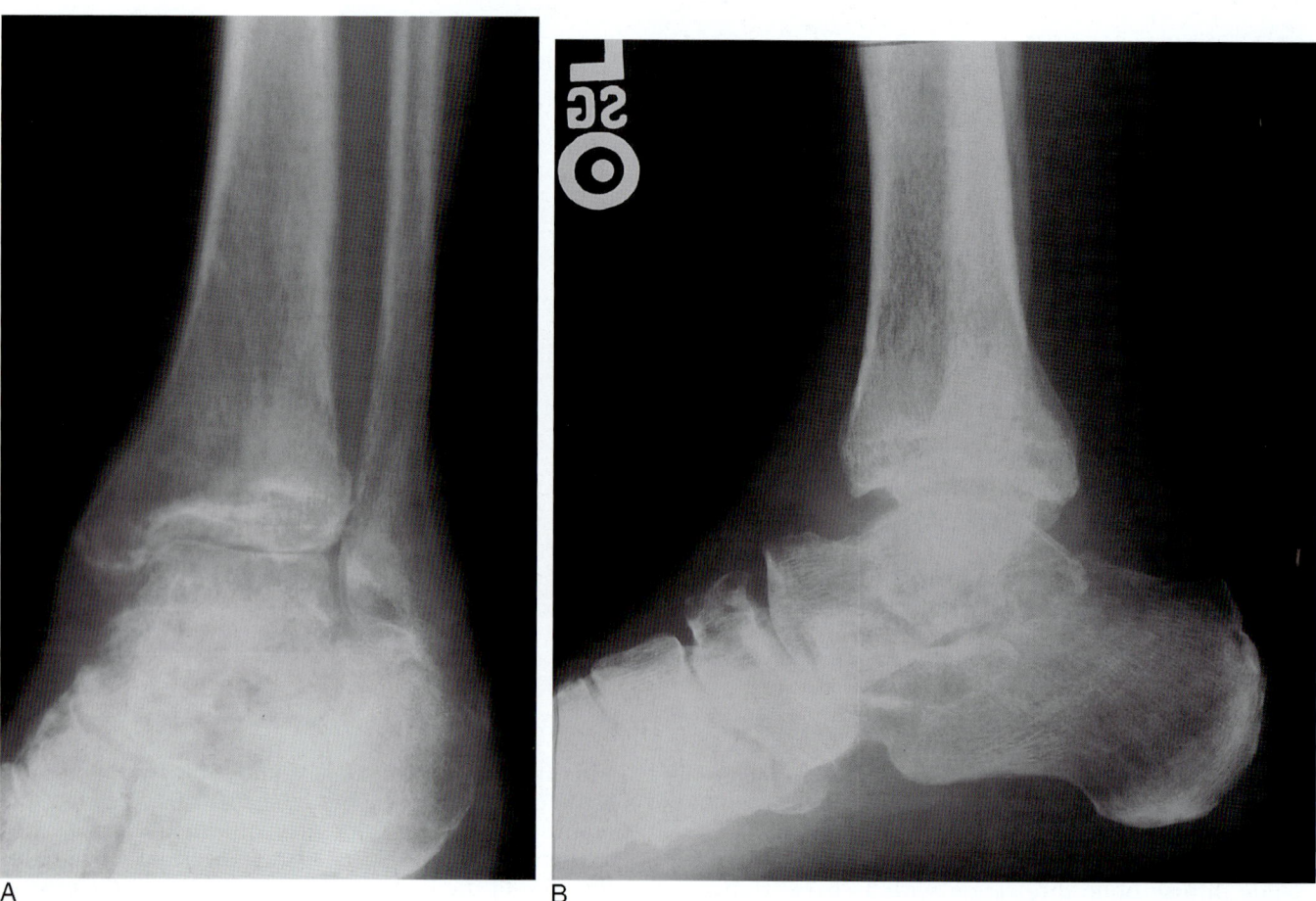

A   B

■ **FIGURE 68-56** Tuberculous arthritis in a 66-year-old man. Frontal (**A**) and lateral (**B**) radiographs of the ankle show osteopenia, small ankle effusion, narrowing of the subtalar joint, and probable erosive changes about the subtalar joint.

(Continued)

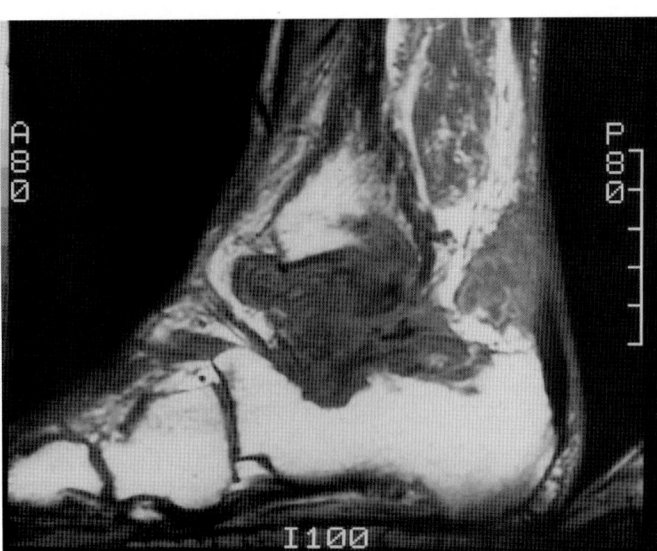

C

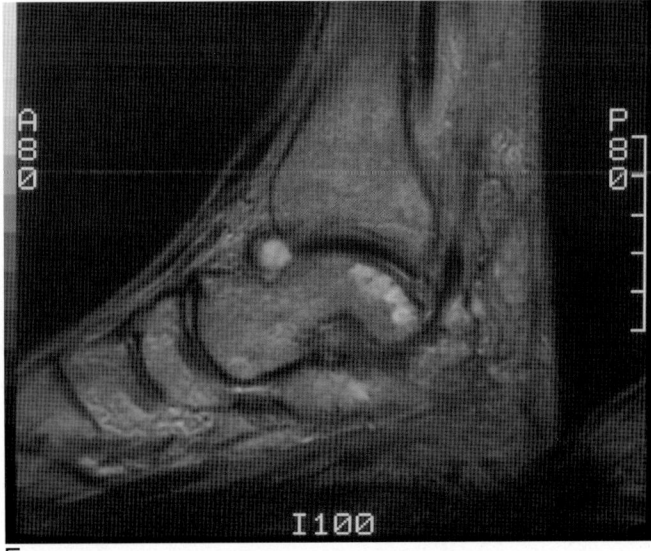

D

E

■ **FIGURE 68-56—Cont'd**   Sagittal (**C**) and coronal (**D**) T1-weighted images show abnormal low signal intensity of the talus and portion of calcaneus and distal tibia consistent with osteomyelitis and tuberculous arthritis. In **C**, note the abnormal intermediate signal intensity in the region of Kager's fat pad and erosion of the Achilles tendon compatible with soft tissue infection. Ankle joint effusion is present. **E**, The regions of abnormality show intermediate increased signal intensity on the fluid-sensitive sequence. *(Courtesy of E. Outwater, MD, Tucson, AZ.)*

also useful to guide percutaneous drainage and to follow the patients after drainage. However, MRI and CT remain methods of choice to depict vertebral involvement. Ultrasonography can be used in evaluation of tuberculous tenosynovitis, bursitis, and myositis.

Nuclear Medicine

Evaluation of spinal tuberculosis with scintigraphy early in the course of infection is limited by the indolent nature of skeletal tuberculosis. ^{99m}Tc-methylene diphosphonate and ^{67}gallium citrate scans may be negative initially despite the presence of active disease clinically and radiographically.[13] The complementary use of these two radionuclide agents is recommended by some investigators to improve accuracy (86%). As the infection progresses,

extensive osseous changes and attempts at healing result in increased bone metabolism, manifested as areas of increased radionuclide uptake on bone scans. Bone scintigraphy is helpful in evaluation of multifocal involvement and in monitoring the response to therapy.[1,14] ^{111}In-labeled white blood cells may show either increased or decreased radiotracer accumulation in the affected region, with reported accuracy for vertebral osteomyelitis of 63% to 66%.[1,14,30]

Positron Emission Tomography/ Computed Tomography

The value of PET in evaluation of skeletal tuberculosis is not determined. A preliminary study showed moderate uptake of fluorodeoxyglucose (FDG) in the capsule

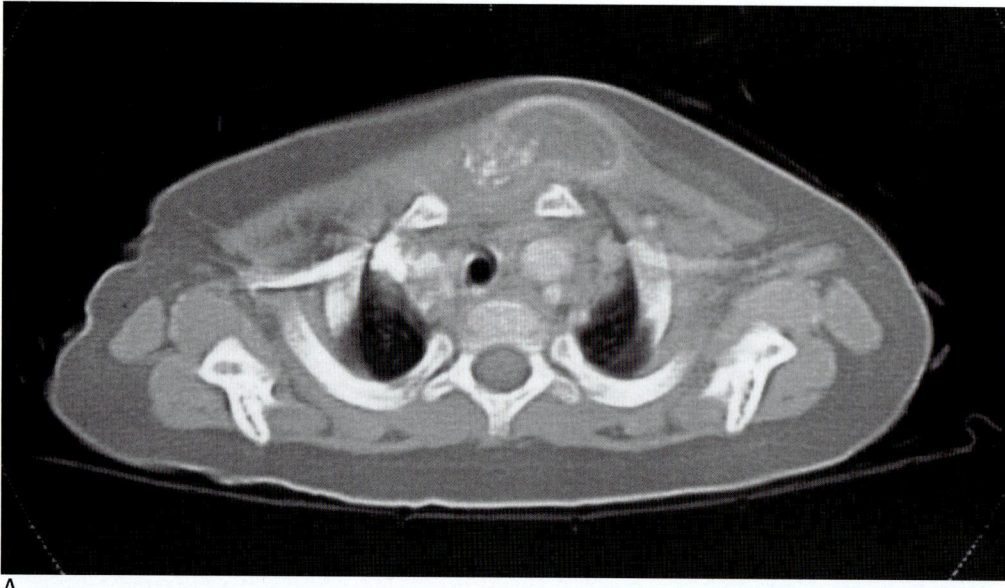

A

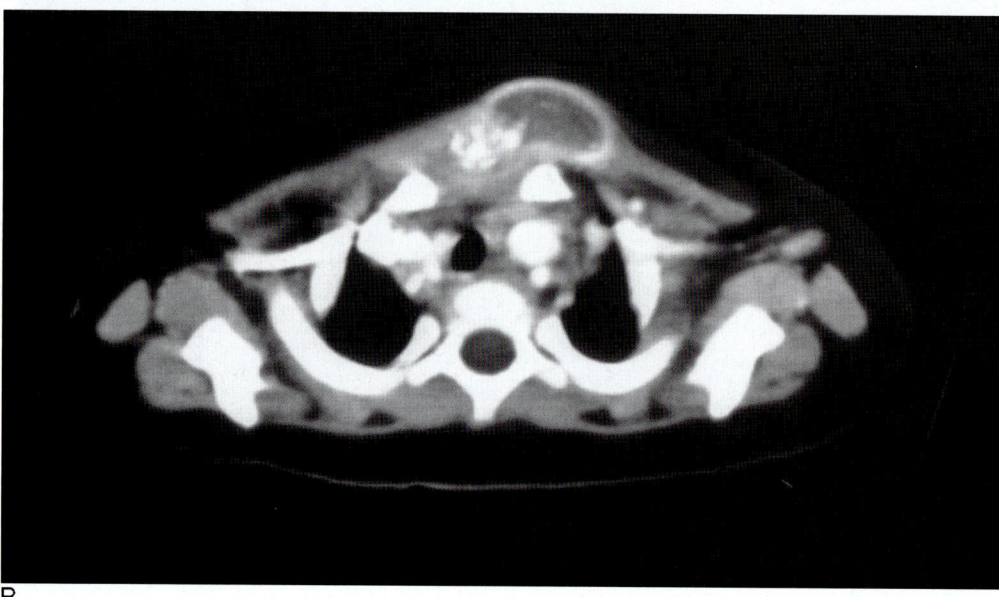

B

■ **FIGURE 68-57** Tuberculous arthritis in a 1-year-old child with pulmonary tuberculosis. **A** and **B,** Axial CT images of the upper thorax show destructive changes involving the left sternoclavicular joint with associated periarticular abscess and soft tissue calcifications. *(Courtesy of George Barnes, MD, Tucson, AZ.)*

and low uptake in the center of two tuberculous cold abscesses. These features are unique compared with nontuberculous abscess and typical tuberculosis lesions, which are characterized by high FDG uptake. Pathologically, a tuberculous cold abscess is not accompanied by active inflammatory reaction. These findings suggest that the FDG uptake by tuberculous lesions varies according to the grade of the inflammatory activity. This new diagnostic feature of a tuberculous cold abscess may be useful in the evaluation of such lesions by FDG PET.[41,42]

Classic Signs

- Late disc involvement
- Cold paraspinal abscess with calcifications
- Multiple vertebral levels may be involved in noncontiguous fashion
- Thick enhancing rim about paraspinal abscess
- Phemister's triad
- Transphyseal extension of metaphyseal infection
- Spina ventosa

DIFFERENTIAL DIAGNOSIS

Differential diagnosis for tuberculous spondylitis includes low-grade pyogenic infection such as brucellosis, fungal infections, tumors, and sarcoidosis. Clinical data favoring tuberculosis are an insidious onset of symptoms, presence of pulmonary tuberculosis, late onset of paraplegia, and a normal erythrocyte sedimentation rate.[1,13] Tuberculous osteomyelitis and arthritis have a more indolent course similar to fungal infection when compared with pyogenic infections.

None of the radiographic findings is pathognomonic for tuberculous spondylitis. However, delay in destruction of intervertebral disc, large calcified paravertebral abscesses with thick enhancing rim, subligamentous spread, and absence of sclerosis favor tuberculous infection.[1,13,28]

Differentiation of tuberculous and pyogenic osteomyelitis is difficult. Acute pyogenic osteomyelitis has a more rapid course and less frequent extent across the physis into the adjacent joint than tuberculous osteomyelitis. Tuberculous infection has a similar course as fungal skeletal infection.

Differential diagnosis for tuberculous dactylitis includes syphilitic dactylitis with bilateral and symmetric involvement, more prominent periostitis, and less prominent soft tissue swelling. Phalangeal, metacarpal, and metatarsal changes can be observed in various other diseases, including fibrous dysplasia, hyperparathyroidism, leukemia, sarcoidosis, and sickle cell anemia but radiographic abnormalities at other sites allow accurate diagnosis of these conditions. Dactylitis in coccidioidomycosis can have a similar appearance.

The differential diagnosis of tuberculous arthritis includes pyogenic and fungal arthritis, rheumatoid arthritis, gout, idiopathic chondrolysis, pigmented villonodular synovitis, and synovial osteochondromatosis. Slow progression of disease, significant osteoporosis, and mild sclerosis are typically seen in tuberculous and fungal disease.

SYNOPSIS OF TREATMENT OPTIONS

Medical Treatment

Chemotherapy for tuberculosis in general and osteoarticular tuberculosis in particular poses certain peculiar problems that include chronicity of infection, infection by resistant mycobacteria, persistent mycobacteria, possibility of concomitant human immunodeficiency virus infection, and drug toxicity during prolonged treatment. Although the success rate of chemotherapy is greater than 90% with optimum drug combination regimens currently used, there is a need for additional improvement.[4,36,37]

Of the commonly used first-line drugs against the large population of mycobacteria actively multiplying in the walls of a cavity, isoniazid, rifampicin, and streptomycin are bactericidal, pyrazinamide is inactive, whereas ethambutol is bacteriostatic. Against a small bacterial population multiplying slowly inside the microphage at acidic pH, pyrazinamide is the most effective drug, followed by isoniazid and rifampicin, with streptomycin being inactive. Against intermittently multiplying

bacilli in solid caseous lesions, only rifampicin is active. Therefore, rifampicin is effective in preventing relapse of disease.[4]

Second-line (reserve) drugs include capreomycin, kanamycin, fluoroquinolones (ciprofloxacin, ofloxacin, sparfloxacin), ethionamide, cycloserine, and para-aminosalicylic acid. In general, these drugs are less effective and more toxic than the standard drugs. The newer drugs include amikacin, fluoroqinolones, rifabutin, clarithromycin, and clofazimine. Glucocorticoids may be required during chemotherapy to counter a hypersensitivity reaction to standard antimycobacterial agents. Bacillus Calmette-Guérin vaccination has some role in prophylaxis of tuberculosis.[4]

On diagnosis, treatment is started immediately without waiting for the results of susceptibility test, which may take a long time. If required, the regimen can be modified after the results of susceptibility tests are available. From a bacteriostatic viewpoint, isoniazid and rifampicin is the most effective combination. To prevent primary and secondary drug resistance a combination of three rather than two bactericidal drugs should be used initially in an optimum regimen. Isoniazid usually always is present. The duration of treatment never must be less than 6 months.[4,36] Treatment of multidrug-resistant latent tuberculosis infection can represent a challenge.[37]

Surgical Treatment

Spinal tuberculosis is usually seen at an advanced anatomic and clinical stage with major destruction of several vertebrae. Significant instability and deformity of the spine can result, mandating prompt diagnosis and treatment to prevent permanent neurologic damage. Surgery allows assessment of the diagnosis, opportunity to treat a vertebral compression, evacuation of pus, and treatment or stabilization of spinal deformation.[13,39]

Anti-tuberculous therapy is beset by important factors that limit its efficacy, such as the emergence of drug toxicity and multiresistant mycobacterial strains. Surgical treatment may be indicated in selected cases where medical therapy alone is not sufficient to eradicate the problem. Chemotherapy should be commenced preferably before surgery to prevent miliary disease.[36,39]

What the Referring Physician Needs to Know

- The diagnosis of musculoskeletal tuberculous infection remains a challenge to clinicians and requires a high index of suspicion.
- The combination of indolent onset of symptoms, positive tuberculin skin test, and compatible radiographic findings strongly suggest the diagnosis.
- Tuberculosis, however, must be confirmed by positive culture or histologic proof from the aspiration of synovial fluid or biopsy of the bone or synovium.
- Prompt diagnosis and treatment of skeletal TB are important to prevent serious bone and joint destruction and severe neurologic sequelae in the case of spinal involvement.

SUGGESTED READINGS

Extrapulmonary tuberculosis: an overview. Am Fam Physician 2005;
72:1761–1768.
Moore SL, Rafii M. Advanced imaging of tuberculosis arthritis. Semin
Musculoskelet Radiol 2003; 7:143–153.

Moore SL, Rafii M. Imaging of musculoskeletal and spinal tuberculosis. Radiol Clin North Am 2001; 39:329–342.
Shembekar A, Babhulkar S. Chemotherapy for osteoarticular tuberculosis. Clin Orthop Relat Res 2002; (398):20–26.

REFERENCES

1. Resnick D. Osteomyelitis, septic arthritis, and soft tissue
infection: organisms. In Resnick D (ed). Diagnosis of Bone and
Joint Disorders, 4th ed. Philadelphia, WB Saunders, 2002, pp
2510–2624.
2. De Backer AI, Mortele KJ, Vanhoenacker FM, Parizel PM. Imaging
of extraspinal musculoskeletal tuberculosis. Eur J Radiol 2006;
57:119–130.
3. Moore SL, Rafii M. Imaging of musculoskeletal and spinal
tuberculosis. Radiol Clin North Am 2001; 39:329–342.
4. Shembekar A, Babhulkar S. Chemotherapy for osteoarticular
tuberculosis. Clin Orthop Relat Res 2002; (398):20–26.
5. De Vuyst D, Vanhoenacker F, Gielen J, et al. Imaging features of
musculoskeletal tuberculosis. Eur Radiol 2003; 13:1809–1819.
6. Morris BS, Varma R, Garg A, et al. Multifocal musculoskeletal
tuberculosis in children: appearances on computed tomography.
Skeletal Radiol 2002; 31:1–8.
7. Teo HE, Peh WC. Skeletal tuberculosis in children. Pediatr Radiol
2004; 34:853–860.
8. Moore SL, Rafii M. Advanced imaging of tuberculosis arthritis.
Semin Musculoskelet Radiol 2003; 7:143–153.
9. Centers for Disease Control. Trends in tuberculosis morbidity—
United States, 2004. MMWR Morb Mortal Wkly Rep 2005;
54:245–249.
10. Jensen PA, Lambert LA, Iademarco MF, Ridzon R and Centers
for Disease Control. Guidelines for preventing the transmission
of *Mycobacterium tuberculosis* in health-care settings, 2005.
MMWR Recomm Rep 2005; 54:1–141.
11. Extrapulmonary tuberculosis: an overview. Am Fam Physician
2005; 72:1761–1768.
12. Koh DM, Bell JR, Burkill GJ, et al. Mycobacterial infections:
still a millennium bug—the imaging features of mycobacterial
infections. Clin Radiol 2001; 56:535–544.
13. Yao DC, Sartoris DJ. Musculoskeletal tuberculosis. Radiol Clin
North Am 1995; 33:679–689.
14. Shanley DJ. Tuberculosis of the spine: imaging features. AJR Am
J Roentgenol 1995; 164:659–664.
15. Schultz E, Richterman I, Dorfman HD. Case report 739:
Tuberculous arthritis of knee. Skeletal Radiol 1992; 21:330–334.
16. Araki Y, Tsukaguchi I, Shino K, Nakamura H. Tuberculous arthritis
of the knee: MR findings. AJR Am J Roentgenol 1993; 160:664.
17. Merdina EV, Mitusova GM, Sovetova NA. [Ultrasound diagnosis
of retroperitoneal abscesses in spinal tuberculosis]. Probl Tuberk
2001; (4):19–21. Russian.
18. Gandolfo N, Serrato O, Sandrone C, Serafini G. [The role of
echography in osteolytic tubercular abscesses]. Radiol Med
(Torino) 1993; 85:574–578. Italian.
19. Babic M, Mihelic R. [Ultrasonic diagnosis of abscesses in tubercular
spondylitis of the vertebrae]. Reumatizam 1991; 38:39–43. Croatian.
20. Soler R, Rodriguez E, Remuinan C, Santos M. MRI of musculoskeletal
extraspinal tuberculosis. J Comput Assist Tomogr 2001; 25:177–183.
21. Cormican L, Hammal R, Messenger J, Milburn HJ. Current
difficulties in the diagnosis and management of spinal
tuberculosis. Postgrad Med J 2006; 82:46–51.
22. Li H, You C, Yang Y, et al. Intramedullary spinal tuberculoma: report
of three cases. Surg Neurol 2006; 65:185–188; discussion 188–189.

23. Almeida A. Tuberculosis of the spine and spinal cord. Eur J Radiol
2005; 55:193–201.
24. Narlawar RS, Shah JR, Pimple MK, et al. Isolated tuberculosis of
posterior elements of spine: magnetic resonance imaging findings
in 33 patients. Spine 2002; 27:275–281.
25. Yago Y, Yukihiro M, Kuroki H, et al. Cold tuberculous abscess
identified by FDG PET. Ann Nucl Med 2005; 19:515–518.
26. De Backer AI, Mortele KJ, Vanschoubroeck IJ, et al. Tuberculosis
of the spine: CT and MR imaging features. JBR-BTR 2005;
88:92–97.
27. Kalita J, Misra UK, Mandal SK, Srivastava M. Prognosis of
conservatively treated patients with Pott's paraplegia: logistic
regression analysis. J Neurol Neurosurg Psychiatry 2005;
76:866–868.
28. Joseffer SS, Cooper PR. Modern imaging of spinal tuberculosis.
J Neurosurg Spine 2005; 2:145–150.
29. Smith AS, Weinstein MA, Mizushima A, et al. MR imaging
characteristics of tuberculous spondylitis vs vertebral
osteomyelitis. AJR Am J Roentgenol 1989; 153:399–405.
30. Lisbona R, Derbekyan V, Novales-Diaz J, Veksler A. Gallium-
67 scintigraphy in tuberculous and nontuberculous infectious
spondylitis. J Nucl Med 1993; 34:853–859.
31. Chang DS, Rafii M, McGuinness G, Jagirdar JS. Primary multifocal
tuberculous osteomyelitis with involvement of the ribs. Skeletal
Radiol 1998; 27:641–645.
32. Evangelista E, Itti E, Malek Z, et al. Diagnostic value of 99mTc-
HMDP bone scan in atypical osseous tuberculosis mimicking
multiple secondary metastases. Spine 2004; 29:E85–E87.
33. Bakshi G, Satish R, Shetty SV, Anjana J. Primary skeletal muscle
tuberculosis. Orthopedics 2003; 26:327–328.
34. Ahmed J, Homans J. Tuberculosis pyomyositis of the soleus muscle
in a fifteen-year-old boy. Pediatr Infect Dis J 2002; 21:1169–1171.
35. Kapukaya A, Subasi M, Bukte Y, et al. Tuberculosis of the shoulder
joint. Joint Bone Spine 2006; 73:177–181.
36. Butorac R, Littlejohn GO, Hooper J. Mycobacterial disease in the
musculoskeletal system. Med J Aust 1987; 147:388–391.
37. Papastavros T, Dolovich LR, Holbrook A, et al. Adverse events
associated with pyrazinamide and levofloxacin in the treatment
of latent multidrug-resistant tuberculosis. Can Med Assoc J 2002;
167:131–136.
38. Taljanovic MS, Hunter TB, Fitzpatrick KA, et al. Musculoskeletal
magnetic resonance imaging: importance of radiography. Skeletal
Radiol 2003; 32:403–411.
39. Ghadouane M, Elmansari O, Bousalmame N, et al. [Role of surgery
in the treatment of Pott's disease in adults. Apropos of 29 cases].
Rev Chir Orthop Reparatrice Appar Mot 1996; 82:620–628.
French.
40. Paradisi F, Corti G. Skeletal tuberculosis and other granulomatous
infections. Baillieres Best Pract Res Clin Rheumatol 1999;
13:163–177.
41. Yago Y, Yukihiro M, Kuroki H, et al. Cold tuberculous abscess
identified by FDG PET. Ann Nucl Med 2005; 19:515–518.
42. Ichiya Y, Kuwabara Y, Sasaki M, et al. FDG-PET in infectious
lesions: The detection and assessment of lesion activity. Ann Nucl
Med 1996; 10:185–191.

Hematologic/ Vascular Disease

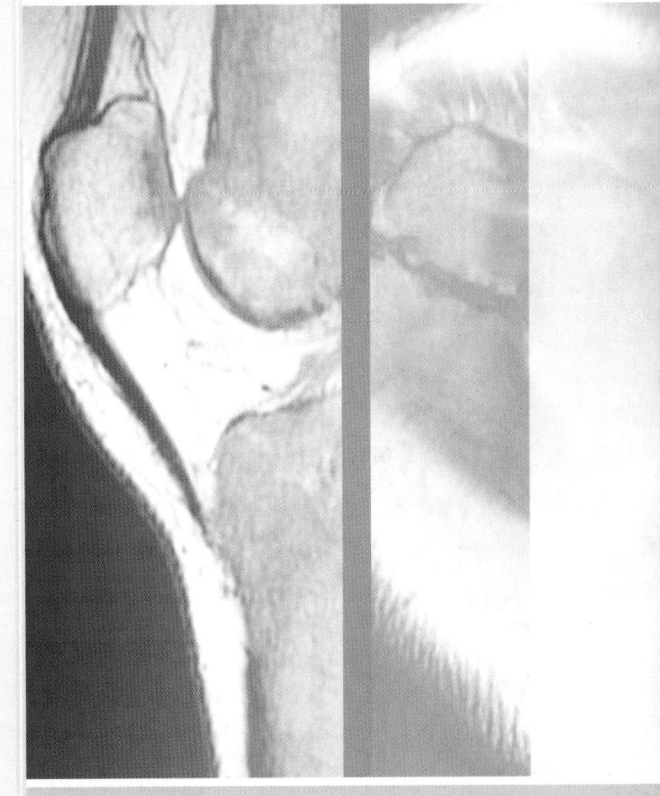

69

General Principles of Magnetic Resonance Imaging of the Bone Marrow

Bruno Vande Berg

The current chapter addresses general concepts on MRI of the bone marrow with emphasis on common normal and abnormal marrow patterns. MRI plays a key role in marrow imaging because of its high sensitivity for detecting focal or diffuse alterations in marrow content. MRI of the bone marrow is also performed for other purposes, including medullary lesion characterization, disease staging, prognosis, and monitoring of treatment response.

MRI of the skeleton yields information on the medullary content of the bones (Fig. 69-1). The calcified components of the skeleton—either cortical or cancellous—are best depicted by using ionizing imaging modalities (radiographs, CT, and bone scintigraphy). Therefore, it is not surprising that MR and CT images of the same lesion occasionally yield different information (Fig. 69-2).

ANATOMY AND PHYSIOLOGY OF NORMAL BONE MARROW

The medullary cavity of the adult human skeleton contains red and yellow marrow. In adults, red marrow occupies the cranial vault, the spine, the ribs, the sternum, the pelvic region, and the proximal aspects of the femur and humerus.[1,2] Red marrow contains about 50% of fat cells and 50% of hematopoietic cells embedded in a network of highly permeable sinusoids (Table 69-1). The relative proportion of fat and non-fat cells varies among individuals according to poorly understood parameters but also according to age and sex; it also depends on the bone considered and on the anatomic region of each individual bone (Fig. 69-3).

Yellow marrow almost exclusively contains fat cells and few capillaries. It is mainly found in the appendicular skeleton of the human adults. All long bones epiphyses, except the proximal humeral and femoral epiphyses, contain yellow marrow.

The possibility of red marrow to convert to yellow marrow and, conversely, of yellow marrow to transform into red marrow, is a unique feature of the marrow.[3] It occurs as a physiologic process during growth and until adulthood: at birth, red marrow occupies almost the entire skeleton. It progressively converts to yellow marrow, starting distally in the limbs and centrally in the long bones. In case of demand for more hematopoietic cells, expansion of red marrow occurs in a centripetal direction.

MAGNETIC RESONANCE IMAGING TECHNIQUES

T1-Weighted Spin-Echo Sequence

The T1-weighted spin-echo (SE) sequence is the most important sequence for bone marrow MRI. It is able to depict the wide changes in normal red marrow distribution and composition that occur with aging because the marrow signal intensity is directly proportional to the amount of fat-laden adipocytes of the marrow cavity. The rationale for its use as the main sequence for marrow imaging is that it is able to demonstrate the changes in the amount of fat cells that occur in almost any abnormal marrow condition (Fig. 69-4). Consequently, this sequence lacks specificity because it depicts the disappearance of fat and not the concomitant appearance of

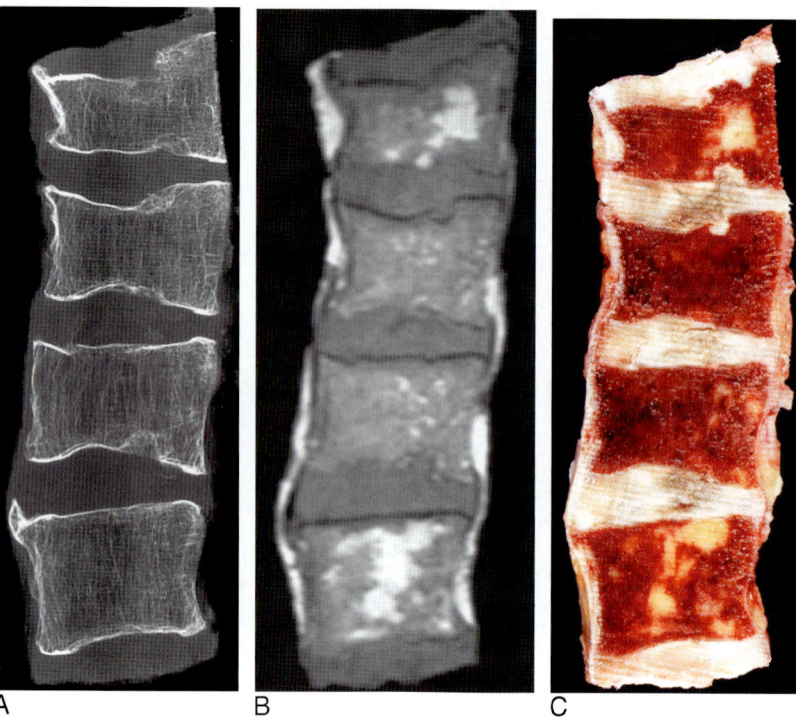

■ **FIGURE 69-1** Bone and marrow imaging. **A,** Radiograph of a spine specimen depicts the cortical and trabecular bone. **B,** The corresponding T1-weighted SE MR image depicts red and yellow marrow, as demonstrated on the specimen photograph (**C**). The bone pattern seen on the radiograph differs from that of the marrow seen on the T1-weighted SE MR image.

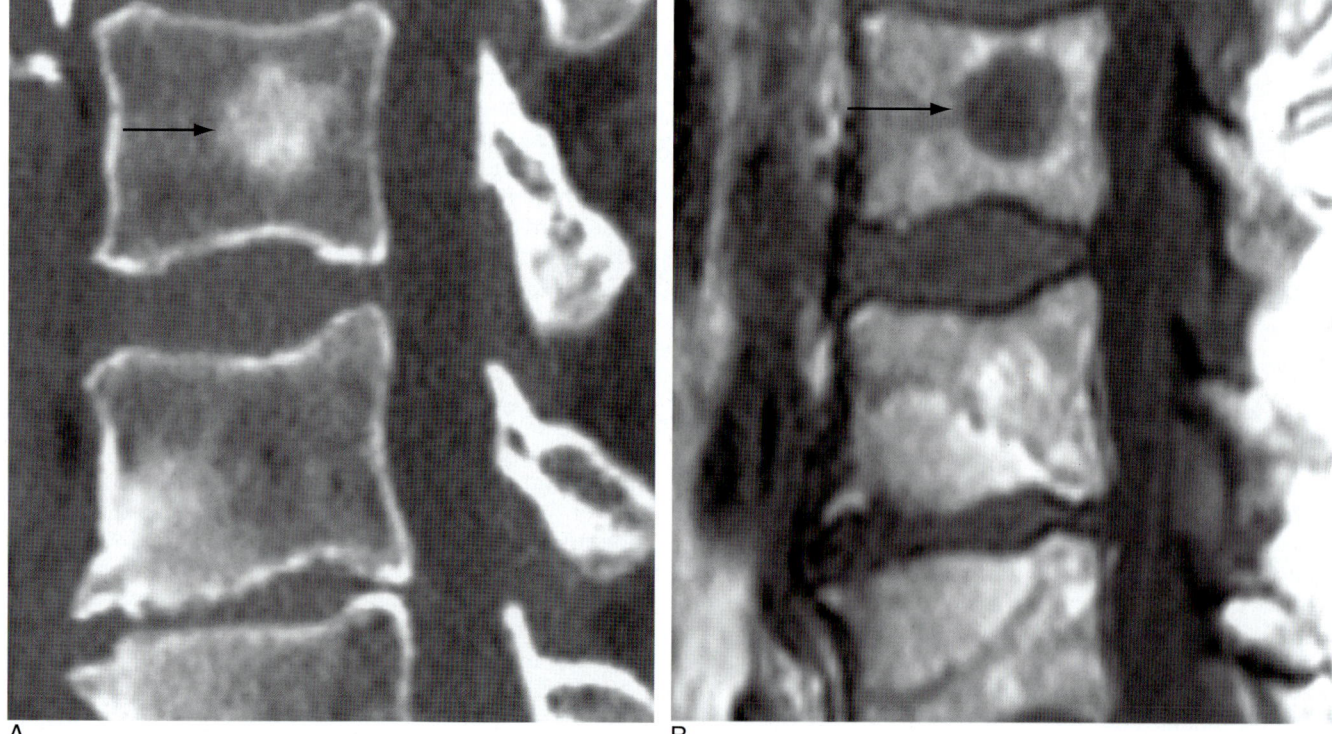

■ **FIGURE 69-2** **A,** Sagittal CT reformatted image of the lumbar spine shows multiple sclerotic bone lesions in L2 (*arrow*), L3, and L4. **B,** On the corresponding T1-weighted SE MR image, the signal pattern of these sclerotic lesions is variable: the L2 lesion shows low signal intensity (disappearance of fat?) (*arrow*); the L3 and L4 lesions show high signal intensity (presence of fat?). Similar bone patterns on the CT image can have variable MR appearance that depends on each marrow alteration.

TABLE 69-1 Anatomy of Red and Yellow Marrow

	Yellow Marrow	Red Marrow
Chemical Composition	80% lipids, 15% water	40% lipids, 40% water
Main Cellular Composition	Fat cells	Hematopoietic and fat cells
Vasculature	Few capillaries	Permeable sinusoids
Main Distribution	Appendicular skeleton	Axial skeleton

abnormal cells. In addition, the T1-weighted SE sequence is widely available and it is reproducible over time and among imaging centers.

Intermediate-Weighted Spin-Echo Sequence

The intermediate-weighted SE sequence without fat saturation has no role to play in marrow imaging because many marrow constituents show a similar intermediate signal intensity.

T2-Weighted Fast Spin-Echo Sequence

The T2-weighted fast SE sequence has a limited value for lesion detection but can contribute to lesion characterization. However, it is generally obtained mainly for the assessment of adjacent structures (see Fig. 69-4). Many marrow lesions do not significantly alter the amount of marrow water, and the lesion's signal intensity widely varies according to poorly understood parameters (Fig. 69-5).

Fat-Saturated Spin-Echo Sequences

Fat saturation plays an important role in bone marrow imaging.[4] Actually, fat protons so heavily contribute to the medullary signal on T1- and T2-weighted SE images that they occasionally decrease the MR sensitivity for the detection of abnormal marrow components. Therefore, the application of techniques that decreases the influence of fat protons on signal intensity is likely to facilitate lesion detection (Fig. 69-6). The STIR sequence, in which the inversion time is selected to suppress fat contribution, provides valuable information because the signal of fat is suppressed and T1 and T2 contrast are additive. Fat saturation can also be achieved by selective presaturation of hydrogen protons from fat molecules and can be followed by T1-, intermediate-, or T2-weighted sequences.[5] STIR sequence and fat-saturated intermediate-weighted sequences give similar results in the detection of subtle marrow alterations.[6]

As a significant drawback, the specificity of fat-saturated sequences is lower than that of T1- and T2-weighted SE sequences, partly because several tissue components that can be recognized on T1- or T2-weighted SE images will present a less specific signal intensity after fat saturation.

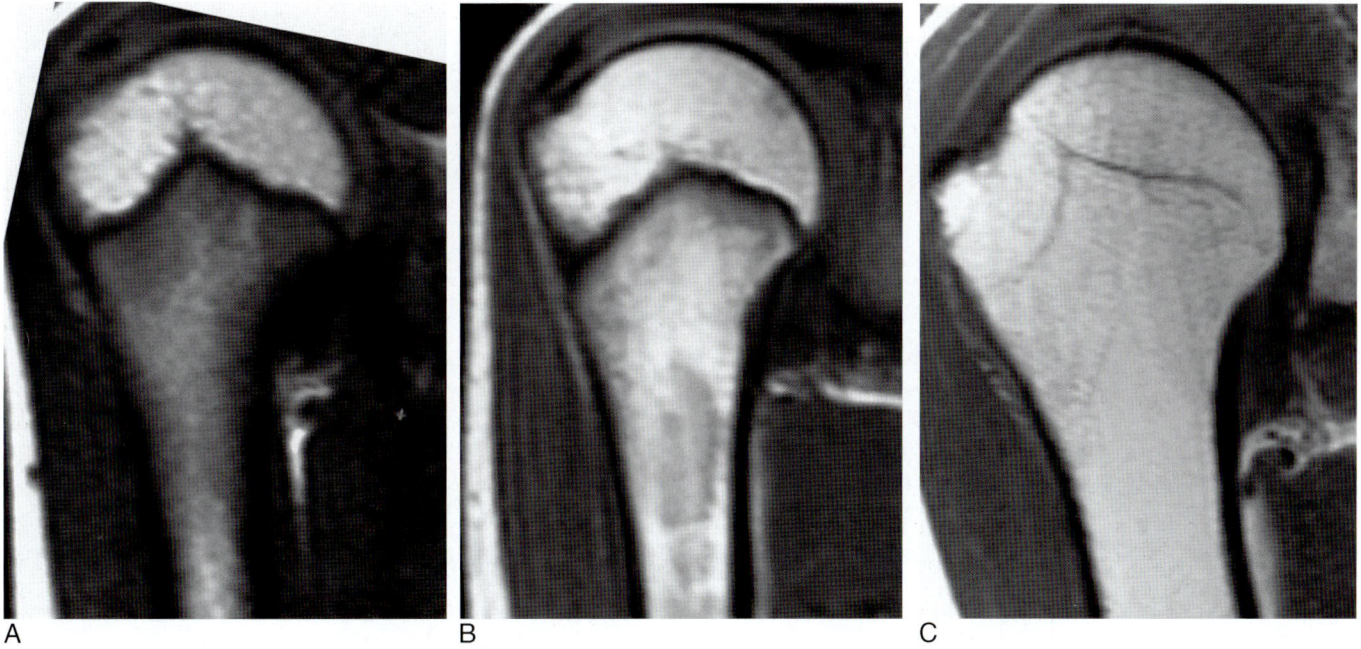

A   B   C

■ **FIGURE 69-3** **Variation in MR appearance of the bone marrow with age.** Coronal T1-weighted SE MR images of the proximal humeri of different patients age 4 years (**A**), 10 years (**B**), and 64 years (**C**). The metaphyseal cavity of the child contains red marrow, whereas that of the adult contains fatty marrow. Fatty marrow is consistently seen in the epiphyses.

■ **FIGURE 69-4** **A,** Sagittal T1-weighted SE MR image of the spine shows multiple marrow areas (*arrows*) of low signal intensity, indicating marrow replacement by metastases. **B,** On the corresponding T2-weighted SE image, marrow lesions are barely visible. Note spinal cord compression due to a posterior mass at C4 level and high signal in C5-C6 vertebral bodies due to fatty marrow as demonstrated in **A.**

Gradient-Echo Sequences

Gradient-echo sequences play a limited role in marrow imaging. The network of cancellous bone is responsible for local field inhomogeneities that account for a marked decrease in signal intensity of cancellous bone containing areas on T2*-weighted gradient-echo sequences. These sequences are occasionally used for the detection of purely lytic lesions and also for the selective evaluation of the cancellous bone network such as in osteoporosis.

Gadolinium-Enhanced Sequences

Gadolinium-enhanced sequences may contribute to bone marrow imaging in many ways. It may be used to demonstrate normal signal enhancement in questionable red marrow areas or abnormal enhancement for lesion characterization. Gadolinium-enhanced T1-weighted SE sequence is recommended for intradural lesion detection, but it is generally not necessary for bone marrow lesion detection, at least without fat saturation, because many lesions become invisible on this sequence. If fat saturation is applied, marrow lesions become more conspicuous. There is general agreement that fat-saturated gadolinium-enhanced T1-weighted SE images and fat-saturated intermediate-weighted SE images are equivalent for the detection of subtle marrow changes that are not obvious on T1- and T2-weighted SE images.[6]

Other Sequences

Several techniques including diffusion-weighted sequences, perfusion imaging, spectroscopy, and relaxation

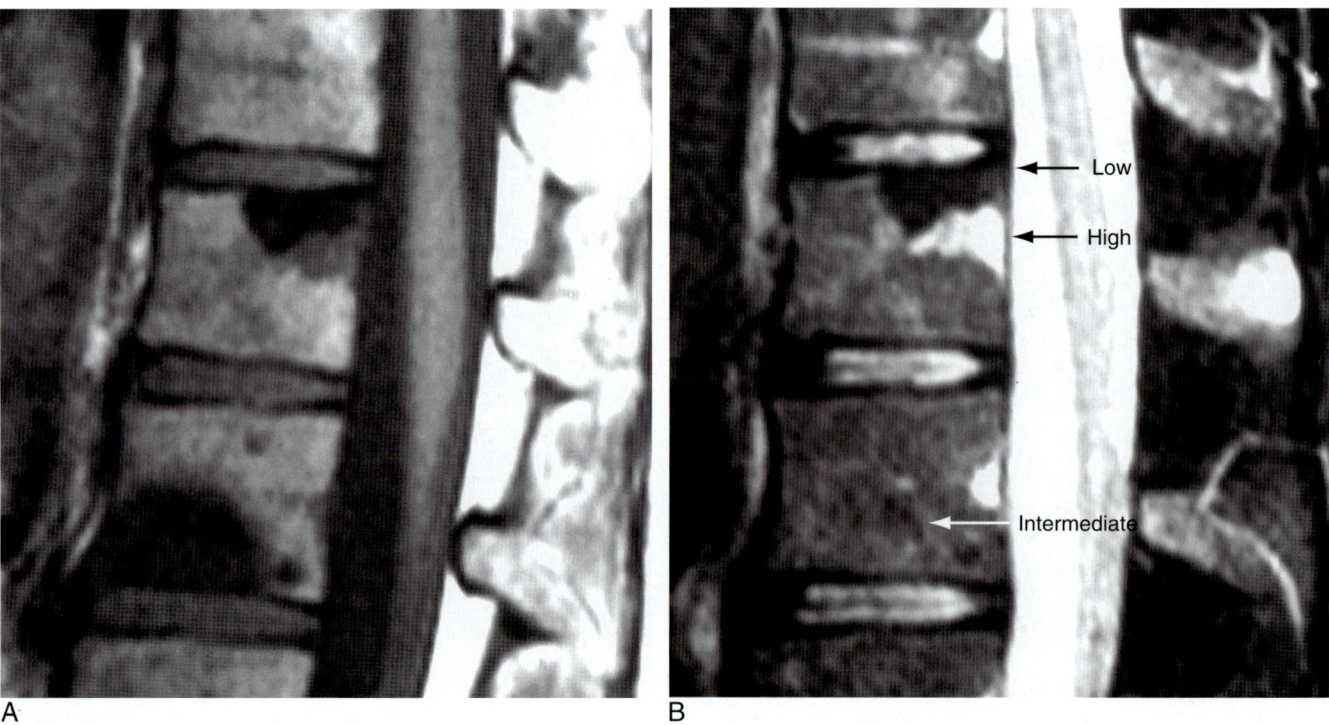

■ **FIGURE 69-5** Marrow replacement due to bone metastases on sagittal T1-weighted (**A**) and fat-saturated T2-weighted (**B**) SE MR images. The signal intensity is consistently low on the T1-weighted image, whereas it is variable on the T2-weighted SE MR image.

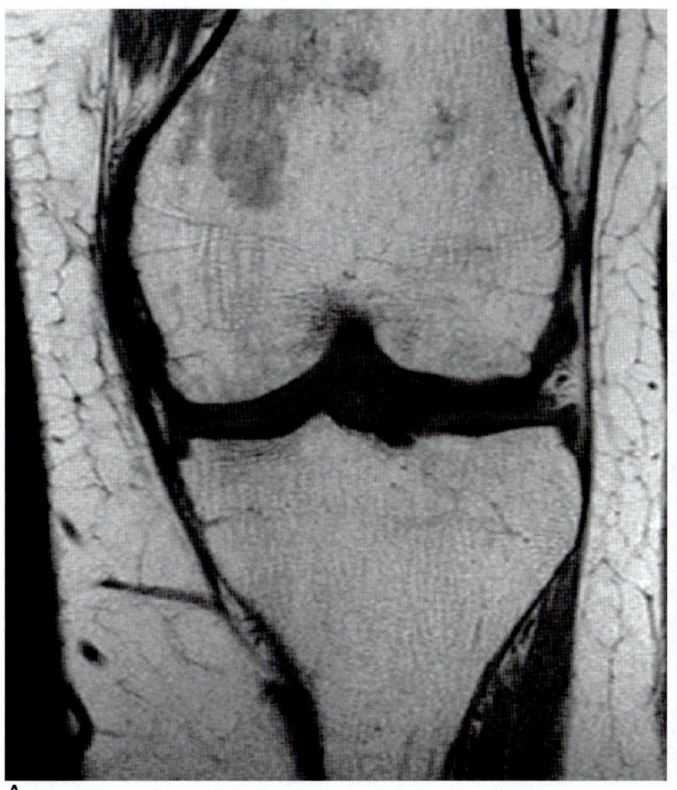
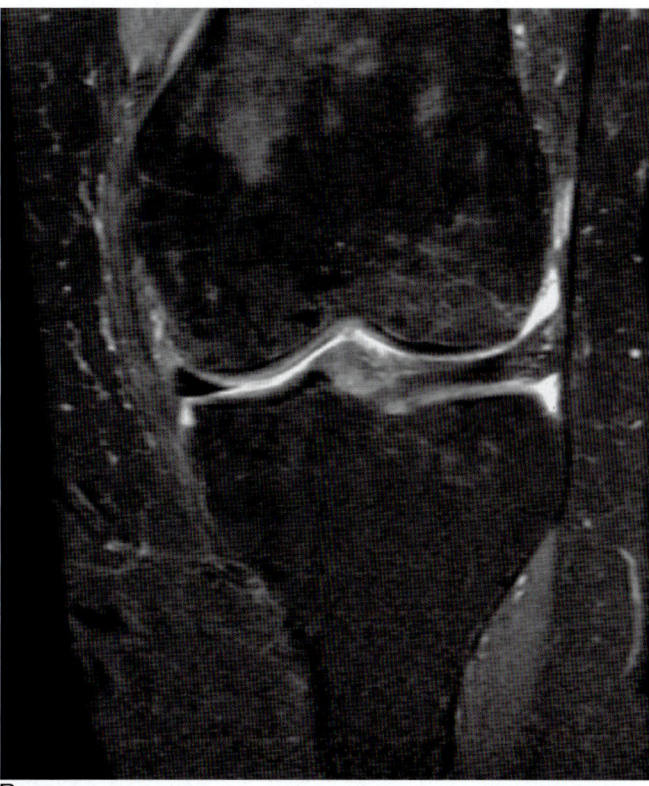

A   B

■ **FIGURE 69-6** **A,** Coronal T1-weighted image of the knee shows normal fatty marrow in the femoral condyles. Note the presence of normal red marrow in the femur metaphysis. **B,** The corresponding fat-saturated intermediate-weighted SE MR image shows abnormal increase in signal intensity in both femoral condyles. Subtle marrow alterations seen on fat-saturated images are occasionally occult on T1-weighted SE MR images, most likely due to the presence of fat.

times measurements are under evaluation for the detection of components of specific lesions. There is a need for better detection of specific cell components in two situations: (1) the amount of specific cells is limited (low tumor burden cancers, assessment of response to chemotherapy) and (2) the specific cells are hidden in a background of abnormal marrow (in edema-like changes around tumors or in spontaneous vertebral fractures, in hypercellular but normal red marrow). There is no general agreement on the added value of these sequences to resolve these two challenges. One should always keep in mind that even a normal looking T1-weighted SE image of the marrow does not enable one to exclude marrow infiltration by abnormal cells because a certain level of infiltration must be reached before the water/fat balance becomes sufficiently altered.

NORMAL ANATOMY

Magnetic Resonance Appearance of the Normal Marrow

Normal red marrow of the adult human shows intermediate signal intensity on both T1- and T2-weighted SE images (Table 69-2; Fig. 69-7).

On T1-weighted SE images, signal intensity of normal lumbar vertebral bodies must be higher than that of adja-

cent intervertebral disc in an adult patient.[7] In the thoracic spine, marrow signal intensity can be lower than that of disc because of the relatively high signal of thoracic discs. In the pelvis, normal marrow signal intensity should be higher than that of adjacent normal muscles on T1-weighted SE images.[8] It is unreliable to assess the marrow status on T2-weighted SE images because there is no internal standard with which marrow signal intensity can be compared. On fat-saturated T2- or intermediate-weighted fast SE images, vertebral marrow signal intensity normally ranges from intermediate to moderately elevated.

TABLE 69-2 Magnetic Resonance Imaging Characteristics of Red and Yellow Marrow

MR Sequence	Red Marrow	Yellow Marrow
T1-weighted SE	Intermediate	High
T2-weighted fast SE	Intermediate	Intermediate/high
STIR, fat-saturated intermediate SE	Moderately high	Low
Gradient-echo	Low	Intermediate
Contrast medium enhancement	Moderate	None

SE, spin-echo; STIR, short tau inversion recovery.

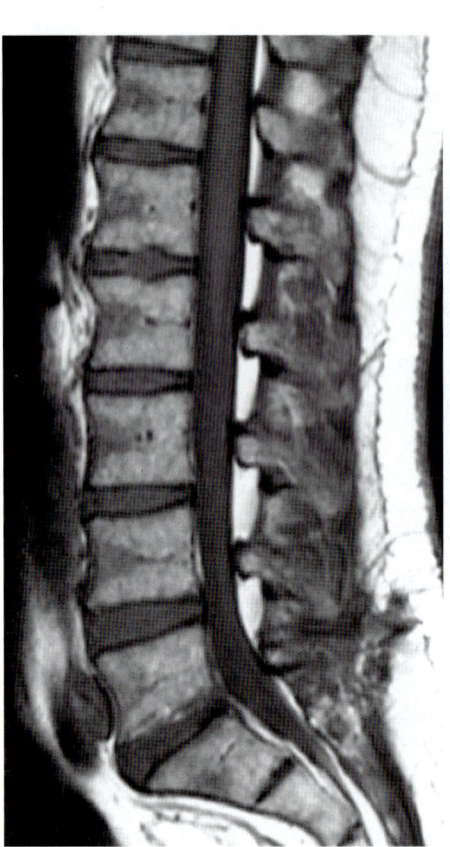 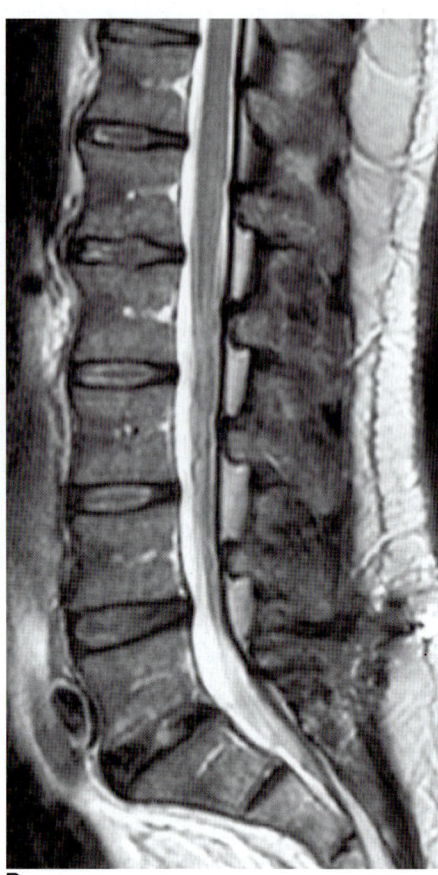 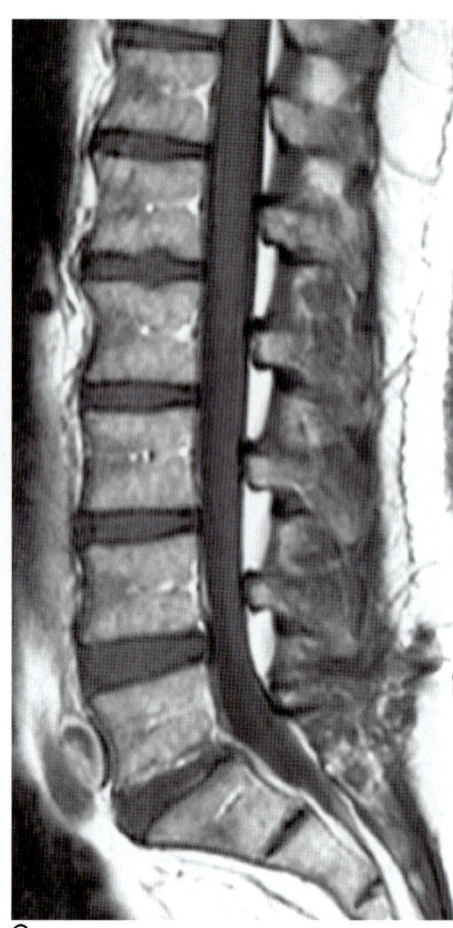

A   B   C

■ **FIGURE 69-7** Sagittal T1- (**A**), T2- (**B**), and enhanced T1- (**C**) weighted SE MR images of the lumbar spine show normal marrow pattern with low signal intensity red marrow and moderate signal intensity enhancement after injection of contrast material. Intramedullary and perivertebral veins normally enhance, which indicates that contrast material has been successfully injected.

After intravenous injection of gadolinium-containing contrast material, enhancement of marrow signal intensity is barely visible at visual inspection on T1-weighted SE images (see Fig. 69- 7) despite the important marrow vascularization. This observation can be partly explained as follows: on T1-weighted images, signal intensity enhancement of a given tissue parallels the gadolinium-induced shortening of the T1 relaxation time in that tissue. Because of the short T1 relaxation time of red marrow due to the presence of fat, the gadolinium-induced shortening in T1 relaxation time is small and, therefore, barely visible. Signal enhancement is more obvious on fat-saturated T1-weighted SE images or can be quantitatively assessed by performing dynamic MR studies. Usually, normal marrow signal intensity should not increase more than 35% in adults older than 35 years of age.[9] In normal fatty marrow, contrast-induced alteration of signal intensity is not visible.

There are important interindividual variations in marrow MR appearance among normal subjects of the same age range, partly because of variations in red marrow cellularity. However, there is limited variation in marrow MR appearance in the same subject, in the spine (between different vertebral bodies), and in the axial skeleton (between paired bones) (see Fig. 69-7). Several distribution patterns of red marrow can be recognized in each bone, which are systematically observed in the paired bones of the same subject.[8,10]

MAGNETIC RESONANCE IMAGING PATTERNS OF MARROW LESIONS

Bone marrow lesions can be classified into a small number of lesion categories based on their signal intensity on T1-weighted SE images (Table 69-3; Fig. 69-8).[2,11] These patterns are generally nonspecific and can be observed within the same lesion.

Marrow Depletion

Marrow depletion is a pattern characterized on T1-weighted images by an increase in signal intensity in comparison to adjacent red marrow (Figs. 69-9 and 69-10). This signal pattern reflects an increase in fat content and a concomitant decrease in the non-fat marrow content. Focal red marrow depletion occurs in the spine of normal

TABLE 69-3 Elementary Lesion Patterns on Magnetic Resonance Imaging

Lesion Patterns	Signal Intensity on T1 Weighting	Fat Amount
Depletion	High	Increased
Infiltration	Moderately low	Moderately reduced
Replacement	Low	Markedly reduced

subjects, with an increased frequency according to age[12]; it also occurs in bone lesions, including quiescent lesions, Paget's disease, and vertebral hemangioma. Regional red marrow depletion occurs after radiation therapy. Diffuse red marrow depletion can be induced by drugs, including corticosteroids and chemotherapeutic agents, and in aplastic anemia.

Marrow Infiltration

Marrow infiltration is a pattern characterized by a subtle to moderate decrease in marrow signal intensity on T1-weighted spin-echo images (see Fig. 69-10). Margins are generally indistinct with a gradual zone of transition toward normal bone marrow. The term *infiltration* suggests that the abnormal marrow component infiltrates or permeates the normal marrow constituents with some possible residual adipocytes in the lesion. The term *bone marrow edema* is frequently used to characterize marrow infiltration with high signal intensity on T2-weighted SE images and a return to normal signal intensity on gadolinium-enhanced T1-weighted images. The term *edema-like changes* could be more appropriate because numerous marrow changes can alter signal intensity in a similar manner, including interstitial hemorrhage, edema, necrosis, or fibrosis.

Focal marrow infiltration involves the periphery of many abnormal processes including fracture, tumor, infection, osteoarthritis, and so on. Diffuse marrow infiltration occurs in systemic disorders including anemia, chronic infection, the acquired immunodeficiency syndrome (AIDS), and bone marrow cancers. Marrow infiltration by neoplastic cells, interstitial fibrosis, or storage disorders can result in a similar MR abnormality.

Marrow Replacement

Marrow replacement is a pattern characterized by a marked decrease in signal intensity on T1-weighted SE

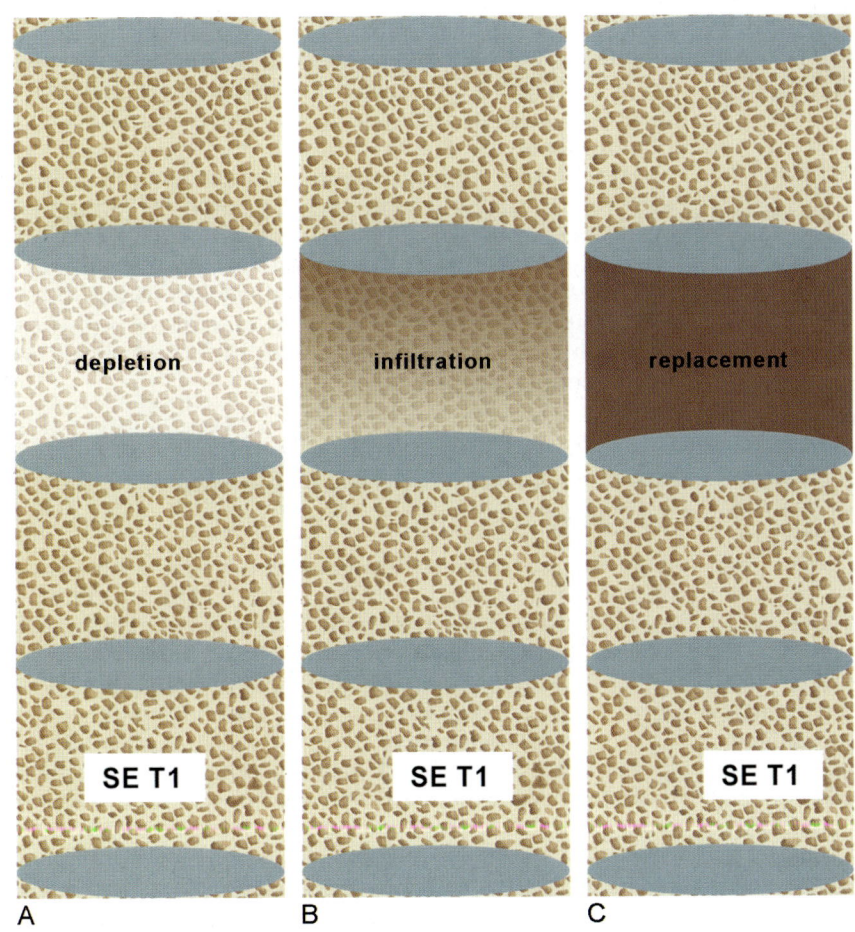

depletion

infiltration

replacement

SE T1   SE T1   SE T1

A   B   C

■ **FIGURE 69-8** Schematic drawings of three marrow lesion patterns on T1-weighted SE image including (**A**) marrow depletion (increased signal intensity), (**B**) marrow infiltration (slight decrease in signal intensity) and (**C**) marrow replacement (marked decrease in signal intensity).

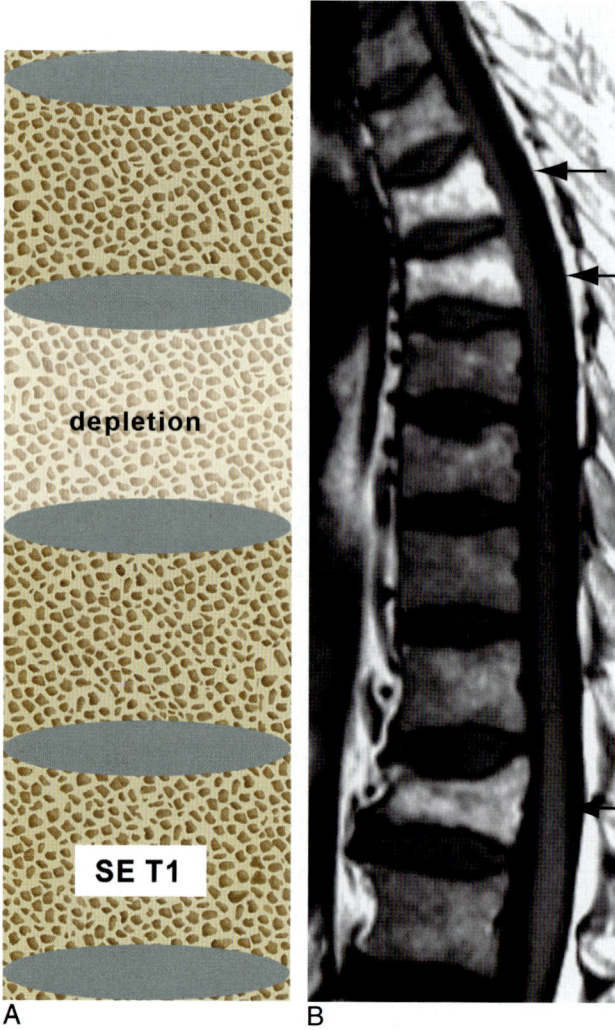

■ FIGURE 69-9 **A,** Marrow depletion. **B,** Several vertebral bodies show increased signal intensity with respect to adjacent vertebral bodies on a T1-weighted SE MR image. These lesions correspond to healed vertebral fractures in a young male patient with severe osteoporosis.

WHAT THE RADIOLOGIST NEEDS TO KNOW

How Does One Increase Sensitivity of Bone Marrow Magnetic Resonance Imaging?

Three fundamental options can be proposed to increase sensitivity for marrow lesion detection, including optimal sequence selection, utilization of gadolinium, and whole-body imaging.

The T1-weighted SE sequence generally enables accurate marrow lesion detection. Its value decreases in many situations in which the difference in amount of fat between the lesion and the adjacent marrow—or fat gradient—is reduced (Fig. 69-13). The fat gradient is decreased if the lesion still contains fat cells or if the adjacent marrow contains little fat. In those situations, fat-saturated intermediate or T2-weighted fast SE sequences or STIR sequences are superior to the T1-weighted SE image for lesion detection, probably because of the low signal intensity of the background marrow and the intermediate to high signal intensity of the abnormal marrow. Fat-saturated gadolinium enhanced T1-weighted SE images seem to provide similar results. Examples of situations in which the signal of normal marrow is low (and cause decreased fat gradient) include children (Fig. 69-14) and young adults, patients treated with drugs that induce marrow hypercellularity, and patients with chronic infection. In these situations, fat-saturated intermediate- or T2-weighted images or gadolinium-enhanced fat-saturated T1-weighted SE images are superior to the standard T1-weighted SE sequence for lesion detection. Several studies demonstrated the value of T2*-weighted gradient-echo images in patients with purely lytic bone lesions such as in multiple myeloma.

MRI of the spine generally enables accurate lesion detection in cancer patients. Adding coronal T1-weighted SE images of the pelvis enables assessment of a larger amount of the red marrow–containing space and increases the likelihood of lesion detection. Whole-body MRI enables to analyze the largest amount of body and should become more popular with the development of new technologies.[13]

How Does One Increase Specificity of Bone Marrow Magnetic Resonance Imaging?

As a rule, characterization of bone marrow lesions with MRI remains limited, mainly in the setting of multiple focal or diffuse marrow replacement for which biopsy may still be the most accurate diagnostic modality.

In the setting of an isolated bone lesion, analysis of several MR sequences, including gadolinium-enhanced images, may contribute to narrow the differential diagnosis list. Plain films and CT images also greatly contribute to lesion characterization by depicting several lesional components that are not easily recognized at MRI: cartilaginous, bony or fibrous matrices, calcium, sequestrum, and gas are all more specifically recognized on CT than on MR images. In addition, the patterns of adjacent

images (Fig. 69-11). The term *replacement* suggests that normal marrow components are completely replaced by abnormal marrow components without residual adipocytes. Margins can be either sharp or indistinct depending on the absence or presence of surrounding marrow infiltration. Signal intensity on other sequences and enhancement patterns vary greatly, probably reflecting the histopathologic changes of the abnormal marrow component. Marrow replacement can be diffuse or focal (Fig. 69-12).

Differentiating focal marrow "replacement" from "infiltration" is important: marrow infiltration is frequently reactional to adjacent lesions and its biopsy is unlikely to be diagnostic. Marrow replacement is nonspecific but can be a valuable target for a biopsy if necessary. In red marrow, the distinction between marrow replacement and infiltration can be difficult because, in red marrow, a slight increase in non-fat cells can rapidly induce complete marrow replacement.

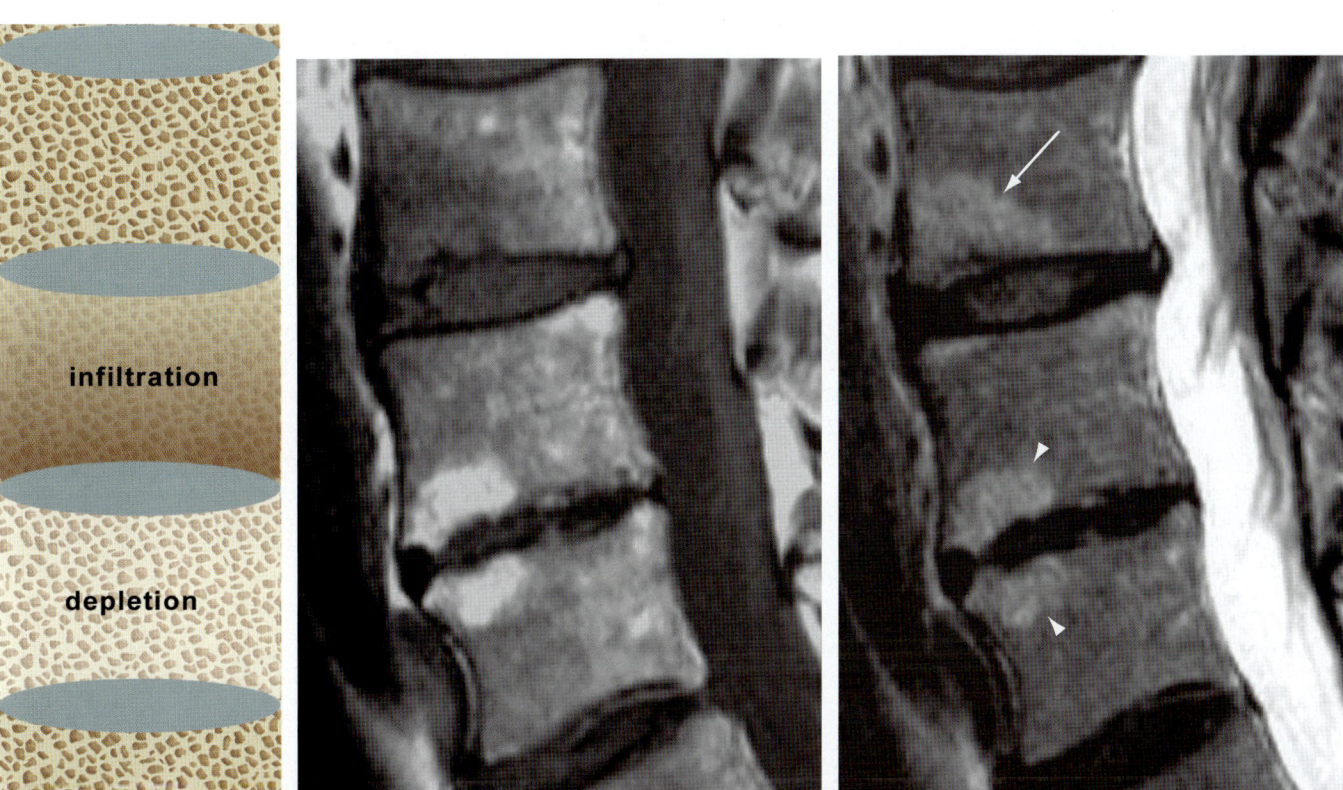

■ **FIGURE 69-10** **A,** Marrow infiltration and depletion. Sagittal T1- (**B**) and T2- (**C**) weighted SE MR images of the lumbar spine with focal marrow infiltration in L3 (**C**, *arrows*) and focal marrow depletion in L4 and L5 (**C**, *arrowheads*) adjacent to intervertebral disc disease. Marrow infiltration shows moderate decrease in signal intensity on the T1-weighted SE image and moderate increase in signal intensity on the T2-weighted image, consistent with marrow edema. The T2-weighted image cannot be used to discriminate between both lesions' patterns because they have similar signal intensities.

trabecular bone and periosteum changes can help in lesion characterization by indicating growth patterns. In a nutshell, combining bone and marrow analysis by looking at CT and MR images, respectively, often contribute to a specific diagnosis of an isolated lesion.

With or Without Fat Suppression?

The use of fat suppression with either T2- or enhanced T1-weighted images has gained general agreement mainly because it displays marrow lesions in a favorable way, that is, with high signal intensity on a low signal intensity background. The dynamic range of signal intensity is smaller on fat-saturated images than on T1- and T2-weighted SE images. Therefore, the use of fat saturation can induce loss in signal intensity information. At this stage of understanding of MRI, we consider that, in general, fat saturation should be used for optimal lesion detection but not for lesion characterization. This hypothesis remains to be validated.

Is This a Normal Variant?

Several marrow alterations are fortuitously discovered and should not be confused with significant marrow changes.

Islands of Fatty Marrow

During adulthood, foci of yellow marrow appear in the vertebral bodies.[12] Their signal intensity is high on T1-weighted SE images and low on fat-saturated images (see Fig. 69-11). On intermediate- or T2-weighted fast SE images, they also show high signal intensity and they should not be confused with clinically significant marrow lesions (see Fig. 69-4).

Vertebral Hemangioma

Vertebral hemangioma, a common asymptomatic vertebral lesion, contains dilated, blood-filled vascular spaces set in a stroma containing large amounts of adipose tissue without hematopoietic cells. On T1-weighted images, its

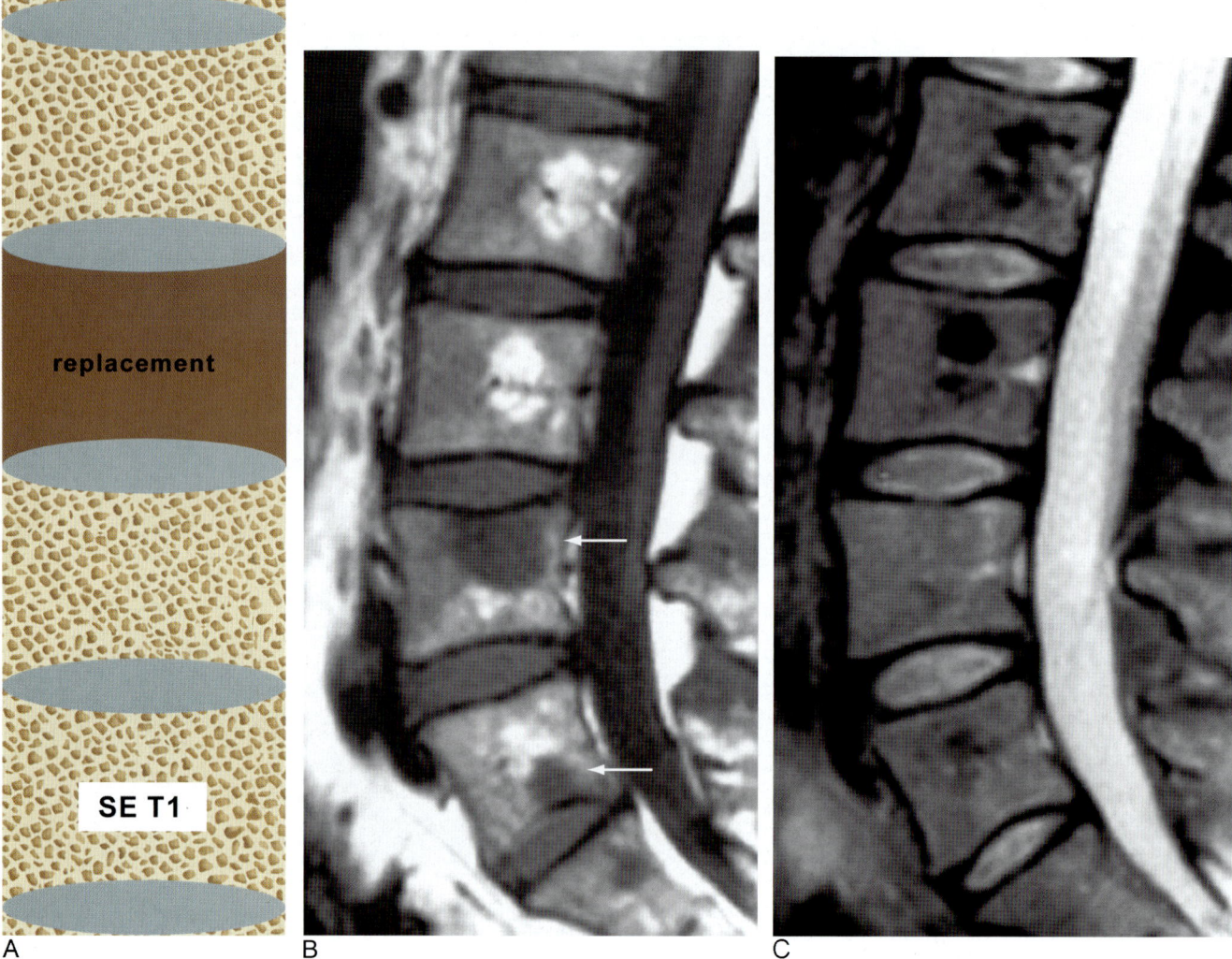

■ **FIGURE 69-11** **A,** Marrow replacement. **B,** A sagittal T1-weighted SE MR image shows marrow areas of decreased signal intensity consistent with marrow replacement (*arrows*). Areas of high signal intensity in L2 and L3 vertebral bodies are not clinically significant (fatty marrow). **C,** On the fat-saturated intermediate-weighted SE MR image, lesions are barely visible.

signal is generally higher than that of adjacent marrow, although it can also be equivalent and therefore not visible on T1-weighted images.[14] On T2-weighted SE images, their signal is consistently high (see Fig. 69-4). The presence of fat cells and dilated vessels with interstitial edema most likely accounts for its high signal intensity on T1-and T2-weighted images, respectively.[15] Punctuated or linear areas of low signal intensity are also seen on T1- and T2-weighted images, probably due to the presence of thickened trabeculae. Signal enhancement of hemangioma after gadolinium injection is variable, depending on its appearance on T1-weighted images and the type of sequence that is obtained after contrast medium injection.

Enostosis

Enostosis or a compact bone island consists of lamellar cortical bone embedded within cancellous bone. Its

signal intensity is very low on all sequences, its contours are spiculated, and adjacent marrow generally has a normal appearance.

Islands of Red Marrow

Random variations in red marrow cellularity occur and cause the presence of areas of more pronounced decrease in signal intensity than adjacent marrow on T1-weighted SE MR images (Fig. 69-15). The margins of these nodules are sharp if the marrow conversion process is advanced and fuzzier if the marrow conversion process is limited.[16] Occasionally, central areas of high signal intensity on T1-weighted images due to the persistence of fat cells are present, which are an additional argument in favor of a normal variant. Presence of low to intermediate signal intensity on T2-weighted, lack of evident signal enhancement on T1-weighted images after gadolinium injection,

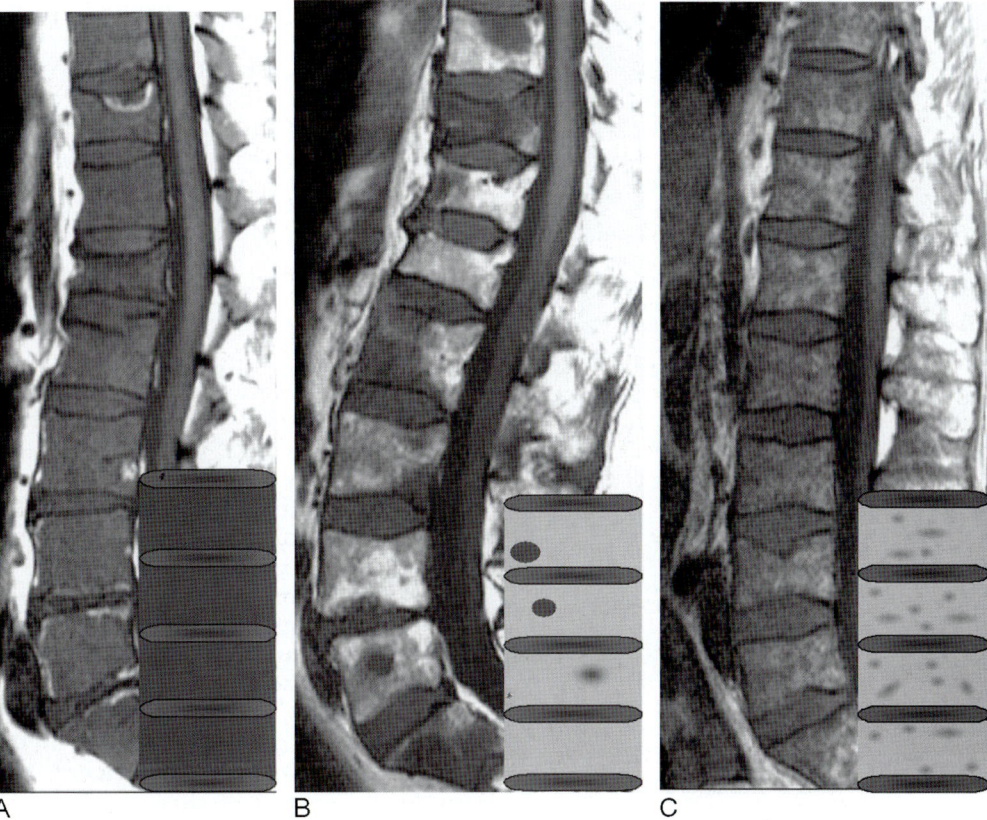

■ **FIGURE 69-12** Diffuse marrow replacement shows a homogeneous low signal intensity. Marrow replacement can be either diffuse (**A**) or focal (**B**). **C,** The variegated or pepper-and-salt pattern is defined by the presence of multiple tiny areas of decreased signal intensity on T1-weighted images.

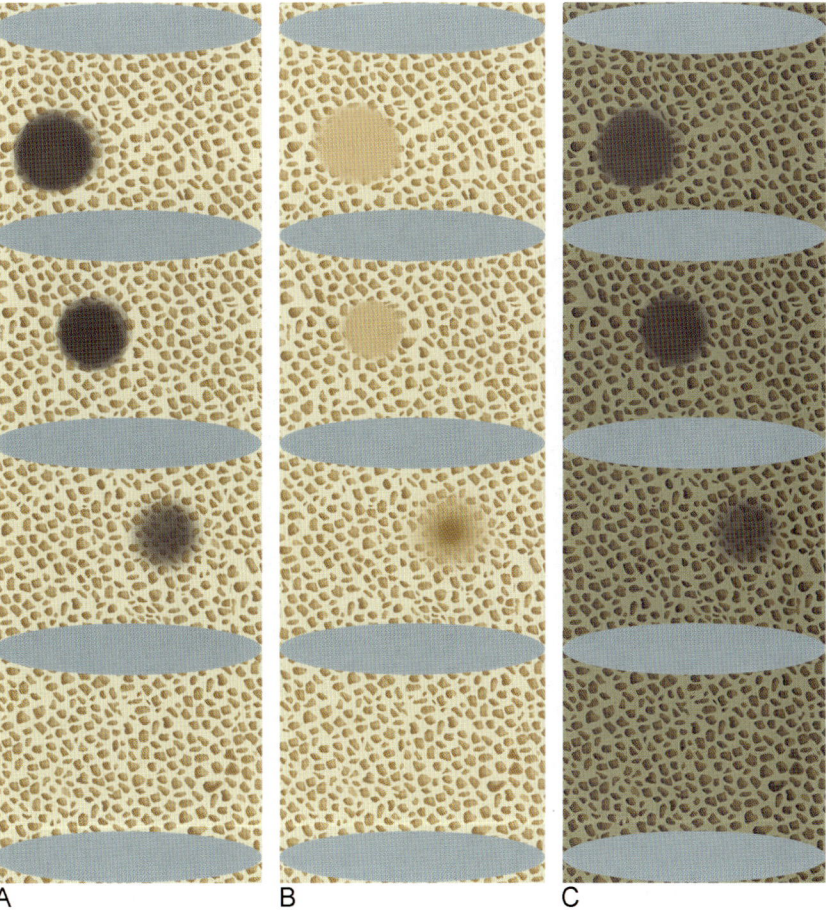

■ **FIGURE 69-13** Schematic drawings of situations in which the T1-weighted SE MR sequence shows limited value for lesion detection. **A,** In the normal situation, the intensity gradient is important between normal marrow and focal lesion. Decreased lesion conspicuity can occur if the lesion shows a relatively high signal intensity (**B**) or if the normal marrow shows decreased signal intensity on the T1-weighted SE MR image (**C**) (lower intensity gradient).

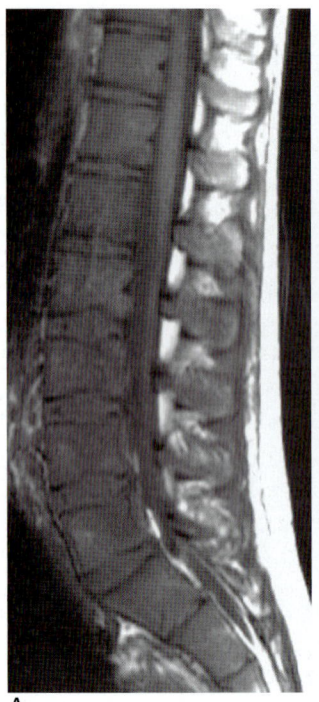
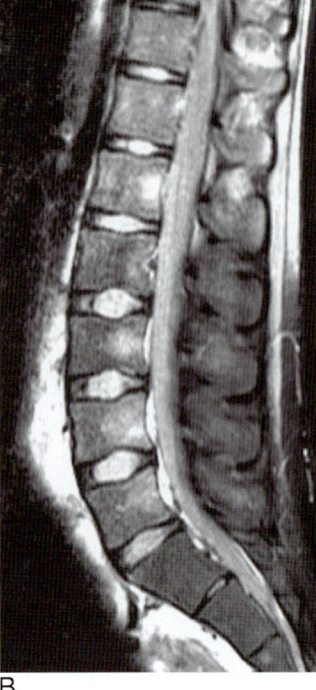

■ **FIGURE 69-14** A 15-year-old boy presented with Ewing's tumor of the iliac wing. **A,** The lumbar bone marrow shows diffuse low signal intensity on the T1-weighted SE MR image and focal lesions are barely visible. **B,** On the corresponding fat-saturated T2-weighted fast SE MR image, multiple focal lesions with intermediate to high signal intensity become visible.

and lack of trabecular bone changes on CT images and of changes at follow-up MR studies generally help to differentiate these benign heterogeneities from clinically relevant abnormalities. Experience with glucose-6-phosphate dehydrogenase (G6PD)- fluorodeoxyglucose (FDG)–labeled positron emission tomography is limited, but these areas may show slight increased hypermetabolic uptake in comparison with adjacent red marrow.[17]

Hematopoietic Marrow Hyperplasia

Diffuse hematopoietic marrow hyperplasia is defined by the presence of hypercellular hematopoietic marrow in the axial skeleton and by expansion of hematopoietic marrow in the appendicular skeleton (marrow reconversion).[18] It can be idiopathic, mainly in middle-aged obese woman (Fig. 69-16). It also occurs in heavy smokers and in subjects with intensive sports activities, mainly long distance runners.[19] It is similar to what occurs in patients in response to stimuli that trigger the production of red marrow cells, including administration of hematopoietic growth factors during chemotherapy, chronic infection, and any other cause of chronic anemia, such as hereditary hemoglobinopathies.

On T1-weighted SE images, hematopoietic marrow hyperplasia is associated with a marked decrease in signal intensity of vertebral marrow that becomes lower than that of adjacent disc (or gluteus muscles in the pelvis). Marrow signal intensity is low on T2-weighted SE images and intermediate on fat-saturated intermediate-weighted

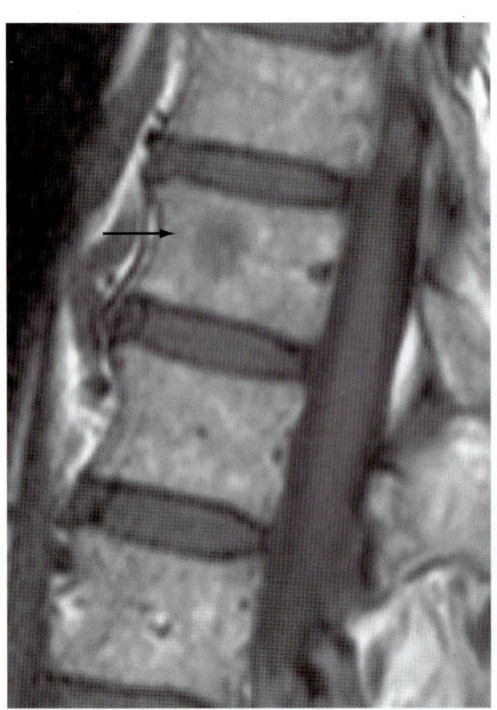
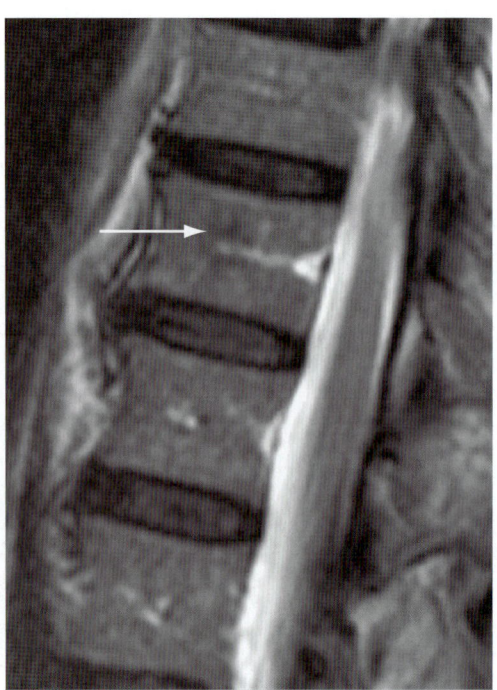

■ **FIGURE 69-15** Presumed island of red marrow. **A,** On the sagittal T1-weighted MR image, a small area of slight decrease in signal intensity is present in the center of the vertebral body (*arrow*). **B,** The lesion shows low signal intensity on the T2-weighted SE MR image. Note that the central vein of the body and its surrounding fat (*arrow*) is preserved, although they are within the lesion.

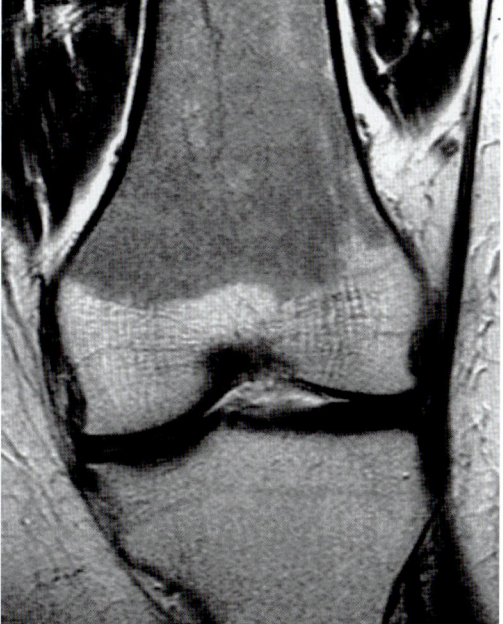

A   B

■ **FIGURE 69-16** On the coronal T1- (**A**) and T2- (**B**) weighted SE MR images of the right knee of a 64-year-old obese woman, the distal femur metaphysis shows low signal intensity, indicating the presence of red marrow, which is uncommon by that age and indicates red marrow hyperplasia. The signal intensity of red marrow is higher than that of muscles and there is no red marrow in the epiphyses.

images. After intravenous gadolinium injection, signal intensity enhancement is moderate but can increase up to 80% on dynamic T1-weighted SE images. In the appendicular skeleton, expansion of red marrow in distal limbs can be observed along with nodules of regenerating red marrow that can simulate bone metastasis.

Differentiation of hematopoietic marrow hyperplasia from diffuse marrow infiltration remains extremely difficult, and blind iliac crest biopsy could be the most accurate technique to definitely address this occasionally difficult problem. As a rule, normal marrow hyperplasia should have a signal intensity similar to that of red marrow on all sequences. In- and out-phase gradient-echo images, T1 relaxation time determination, hydrogen proton spectroscopy, dynamic contrast MR studies, and diffusion-weighted images have all been shown to be of some help, but none has demonstrated definite conclusive results. Preliminary observations with FDG-PET imaging also shown confusing overlapping findings because diffuse hypermetabolic marrow can be observed in both conditions.[20]

SUGGESTED READINGS

Steiner RM, Mitchell DG, Rao VM, et al. Magnetic resonance imaging of bone marrow: diagnostic value in diffuse hematologic disorders. Magn Reson Q 1990; 6:17–34.

Steiner RM, Mitchell DG, Rao VM, Schweitzer ME. Magnetic resonance imaging of diffuse bone marrow disease. Radiol Clin North Am 1993; 31:383–409.

Vande Berg BC, Galant C, Lecouvet FE, et al. The lumbar vertebral body and diskovertebral junction. Radiol Clin North Am 2000; 38:1153–1175.

Vande Berg BC, Malghem J, Lecouvet FE, Maldague BE. Magnetic resonance imaging of the normal bone marrow. Skeletal Radiol 1998; 27:471–483.

Vande Berg BC, Malghem J, Lecouvet FE, Maldague BE. Classification and detection of bone marrow lesions with magnetic resonance imaging. Skeletal Radiol 1998; 27:529–545.

Vogler JBI, Murphy WA. Bone marrow imaging. Radiology 1988; 168:679–693.

REFERENCES

1. Kricun ME. Red-yellow marrow conversion: its effect on the location of some solitary bone lesions. Skeletal Radiol 1985; 14:10–19.
2. Vogler JBI, Murphy WA. Bone marrow imaging. Radiology 1988; 168:679–693.
3. Cristy M. Active bone marrow distribution as a function of age in humans. Phys Med Biol 1981; 26:389–400.
4. Mirowitz SA. Fast scanning and fat-suppression MR imaging of musculoskeletal disorders. AJR Am J Roentgenol 1993; 161:1147–1157.
5. Delfaut EM, Beltran J, Johnson G, et al. Fat suppression in MR imaging: techniques and pitfalls. Radiographics 1999; 19:373–382.
6. Zanetti M, Bruder E, Romero J, Hodler J. Bone marrow edema pattern in osteoarthritic knees: correlation between MR imaging and histologic findings. Radiology 2000; 215:835–840.
7. Carroll KW, Feller JF, Tirman PF. Useful internal standards for distinguishing infiltrative marrow pathology from hematopoietic marrow at MRI. J Magn Reson Imaging 1997; 7:394–398.

8. Dawson KL, Moore SG, Rowland JM. Age-related marrow changes in the pelvis: MR and anatomic findings. Radiology 1992; 183:47–51.

9. Baur A, Stabler A, Bartl R, et al. MRI gadolinium enhancement of bone marrow: age-related changes in normals and in diffuse neoplastic infiltration. Skeletal Radiol 1997; 26:414–418.

10. Ricci C, Cova M, Kang YS, et al. Normal age-related patterns of cellular and fatty bone marrow distribution in the axial skeleton: MR imaging study [see comments]. Radiology 1990; 177:83–88.

11. Vande Berg BC, Malghem J, Lecouvet FE, Maldague BE. Classification and detection of bone marrow lesions with magnetic resonance imaging. Skeletal Radiol 1998; 27:529–545.

12. Hajek PC, Baker LL, Goobar JE, et al. Focal fat deposition in axial bone marrow: MR characteristics. Radiology 1987; 162(1 pt 1):245–249.

13. Eustace S, Tello R, DeCarvalho V, et al. A comparison of whole-body TurboSTIR MR imaging and planar ^{99m}Tc-methylene diphosphonate scintigraphy in the examination of patients with suspected skeletal metastases. AJR Am J Roentgenol 1997; 169:1655–1661.

14. Laredo JD, Assouline E, Gelbert F, et al. Vertebral hemangiomas: fat content as a sign of aggressiveness. Radiology 1990; 177:467–472.

15. Baudrez V, Galant C, Vande Berg BC. Benign vertebral hemangioma: MR-histological correlation. Skeletal Radiol 2001; 30:442–446.

16. Levine CD, Schweitzer ME, Ehrlich SM. Pelvic marrow in adults. Skeletal Radiol 1994; 23:343–347.

17. Bordalo-Rodrigues M, Galant C, Lonneux M, et al. Focal nodular hyperplasia of the hematopoietic marrow simulating vertebral metastasis on FDG positron emission tomography. AJR Am J Roentgenol 2003; 180:669–671.

18. Deutsch A, Resnick D, Niwayama G. Case report 145: bilateral, almost symmetrical skeletal metastases (both femora) from bronchogenic carcinoma. Skeletal Radiol 1981; 6:144–148.

19. Shellock FG, Morris E, Deutsch AL, et al. Hematopoietic bone marrow hyperplasia: high prevalence on MR images of the knee in asymptomatic marathon runners. AJR Am J Roentgenol 1992; 158:335–338.

20. Elmstrom RL, Tsai DE, Vergilio JA, et al. Enhanced marrow [18F]fluorodeoxyglucose uptake related to myeloid hyperplasia in Hodgkin's lymphoma can simulate lymphoma involvement in marrow. Clin Lymphoma 2004; 5:62–64.

70

Ischemic Bone Lesions

Bruno Vande Berg

Ischemic bone lesions cover a wide spectrum of conditions with variable clinical, imaging, and pathologic findings. In general, oxygen delivery to the bone and marrow cells is impaired at least in some areas of any ischemic bone lesion. Epiphyseal ischemic lesions have been more extensively investigated because of their clinical importance.[1] MRI has definitely contributed to their detection and staging.

ETIOLOGY

Ischemic bone lesions occur in several conditions, although they are frequently idiopathic. The etiologic factors that have been identified include joint fracture and dislocation, systemic corticosteroid use, Cushing's disease, alcohol abuse, sickle cell disease, other hemoglobinopathies, vasculitis, trauma, renal transplantation and osteodystrophy, radiation therapy, pancreatitis, gout, Gaucher's disease, connective tissue diseases (e.g., systemic lupus erythematosus), caisson disease, and cytotoxic agents (e.g., vinblastine, vincristine, cisplatin, cyclophosphamide, methotrexate, bleomycin, 5-fluorouracil).[1] Several diseases including the acquired immunodeficiency syndrome (AIDS) and severe acute respiratory syndrome (SARS) seem to be associated with an increased prevalence of ischemic bone lesions, although lesions could be related either to the diseases or to their treatments. A Japanese survey of femoral head osteonecrosis estimated that 34.7% were due to corticosteroid use, 21.8% to alcohol abuse, and 37.1% to idiopathic mechanisms.[2]

PREVALENCE AND EPIDEMIOLOGY

The prevalence of ischemic bone lesions is unknown, mainly because many lesions are clinically silent. The rate of symptomatic epiphyseal osteonecrosis of the hip is 2 to 4.5 cases per patient-year with approximately 15,000 new cases reported each year in the United States. Femoral head osteonecrosis accounts for more than 10% of total hip replacement surgeries performed in the United States. A Japanese survey estimated that 2500 to 3300 cases of epiphyseal osteonecrosis of the hip occur each year.[2]

Age at onset of epiphyseal osteonecrosis depends on the underlying cause. Idiopathic femoral head osteonecrosis most often develops in male subjects aged between 35 and 55 years and is bilateral in 40% to 80% of cases. On average, women present almost 10 years later than men.

The male-to-female ratio also depends on the underlying cause, although idiopathic epiphyseal osteonecrosis is more common in men, with an overall male-to-female ratio ranging from 4 to 8:1. There is no racial predilection, except for osteonecrosis associated with sickle cell disease and hemoglobin S and SC disease, which predominantly occurs in people of African and Mediterranean descent.

CLINICAL PRESENTATION

Clinical presentation ranges from fortuitous discovery at MRI in asymptomatic patients to deep excruciating bone pain in patients with sickle cell crisis. In post-traumatic and in corticosteroid-induced osteonecrosis, symptoms occur generally several months after the trauma or the onset of treatment, respectively. Joint pain develops spontaneously, and in the lower limbs pain is generally worsened by weight bearing.

PATHOPHYSIOLOGY

The pathophysiology of osteonecrosis remains poorly understood, and four different conditions are recognized (Table 70-1).

In *systemic osteonecrosis* (e.g., corticosteroid-induced osteonecrosis) impaired perfusion with subsequent necrosis of bone and marrow can be caused by several mechanisms, including thrombotic or embolic occlusion of blood vessel (e.g., fat embolism, sickle cell crisis, caisson disease), injury to vessel wall (e.g., vasculitis, connective tissue diseases such as systemic lupus erythematosus, radiation, infection), and increased pressure on the vessel wall (e.g., extravasated blood in marrow, inflammation caused by lipid accumulation in osteocytes, intraosseous hypertension from proliferating Gaucher cells in Gaucher's disease). Systemic osteonecrosis can involve any bone segment and yellow or red marrow.

TABLE 70-1   Post-traumatic, Systemic, and Overuse Osteonecrosis in Adults

	Post-traumatic Osteonecrosis	Systemic		Overuse Osteonecrosis
		*Yellow Marrow**	*Red Marrow*	
Likely Pathophysiology	Interrupted blood supply	Various causes of ischemia	Various causes	Trabecular bone fracture
Lesion Number	Unique	Multiple	Multiple	Unique
Age	Any	Any	Any	Elderly
Topography	Epiphysis	Epi-metaphysis	Any	Epiphysis
Background	Yellow	Yellow	Red	Yellow
MR Pattern	Segmental	Segmental	Edema	Edema
Lesion Model	Subcapital femoral neck fracture	Corticosteroid-induced osteonecrosis	Vaso-occlusive crisis in sickle cell disease	Spontaneous osteonecrosis of the knee

*The segmental pattern can also be idiopathic and unique in case of no risk factor.

In *post-traumatic osteonecrosis* anatomic disruption of the blood supply after bone fracture or joint dislocation can cause bone osteonecrosis, given the terminal blood supply of the involved area (an epiphysis or a cortical bone fragment).

In *overuse osteonecrosis* (e.g., "spontaneous osteonecrosis of the knee") subchondral trabecular bone fracture could impair perfusion with subsequent bone and marrow necrosis. Overuse osteonecrosis is confined to the epiphyses, mainly of the lower limbs.

Histopathology

At the microscopic level *cell necrosis* may take several patterns. but coagulation necrosis is the most common pattern of necrosis in bones. It results in complete absence of osteocytes within the bone trabeculae, loss of adipocyte nuclei with lipid cysts formation, and death of hematopoietic cells (Fig. 70-1).[3]

An *infarct* is a localized area of necrosis in *tissue* resulting from reduction from either its arterial supply or venous drainage.[4] The term *bone infarct* is generally

used to describe a metaphyseal or diaphyseal ischemic lesion but not an epiphyseal lesion rather for cultural than for medical reasons (Fig. 70-2). The histopathologic changes that occur in infarcts merely depend on the type of marrow vasculature. In yellow marrow, arterial occlusion produces a bloodless or white infarct because of the poor vasculature of yellow marrow. Marrow remains fatty and demonstrates normal signal intensity on MR images. The reactive interface of fibrovascular tissue that progressively appears and surrounds the ischemic lesion is the hallmark of yellow marrow infarct. In red marrow, hemorrhagic or red infarcts may develop because of the rich vascular network of red marrow.[4]

Collapsed epiphyseal osteonecrosis is characterized by the presence of an irreversible fracture of the subchondral bone plate and adjacent trabeculae that frequently runs parallel underneath the subchondral bone plate itself (Fig. 70-3). Collapsed *epiphyseal osteonecrosis* is a radio-clinical condition characterized by pain and functional disability of the joint considered as an *organ*, related to an irreversible spontaneous fracture of the epiphysis, generally associated with an epiphyseal infarct.

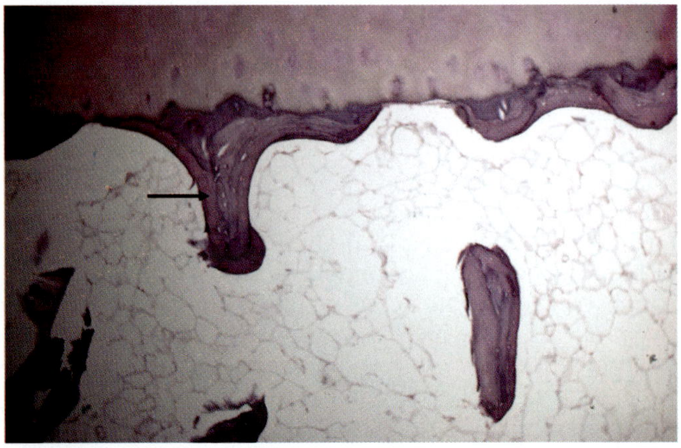

IMAGING TECHNIQUES

Radiographs are relatively insensitive for the detection of the early stages of ischemic bone lesions. However, they play a key role in the assessment of symptomatic joints because they may demonstrate the subchondral bone fracture and the epiphyseal collapse in case of epiphyseal osteonecrosis or they may indicate another condition. Multiple high-resolution radiographs including distraction views (frog-leg view of the hips) are often required to demonstrate the epiphyseal fracture.

MRI is the imaging modality of choice in the assessment of both symptomatic and asymptomatic joints because it is sensitive in the detection of marrow content alteration. Technical characteristics of the MR unit such as magnetic field strength do not influence its accuracy in the detection of bone lesions. Investigation of both sides of the body is advisable in patients with unilateral symptoms (mainly in the hips) because of the high frequency

■ **FIGURE 70-1   Necrosis.** Microscopic features of bone necrosis: bone trabeculae with empty lacunae (*arrow*) and marrow with preserved fatty content.

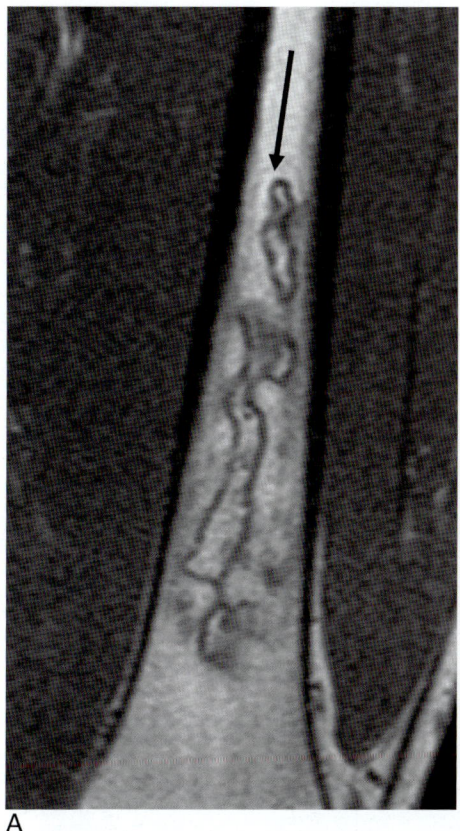 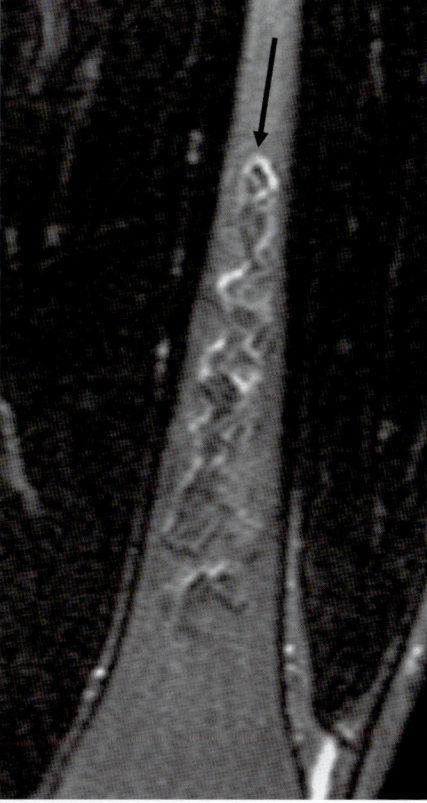

■ **FIGURE 70-2 Diaphyseal infarct.**
A, Coronal T1-weighted image of the femur shows a fat-containing lesion (*arrow*) with serpiginous contours located a few millimeters at a distance from the endosteal bone.
B, Corresponding T2-weighted image shows the double-line sign (*arrow*).

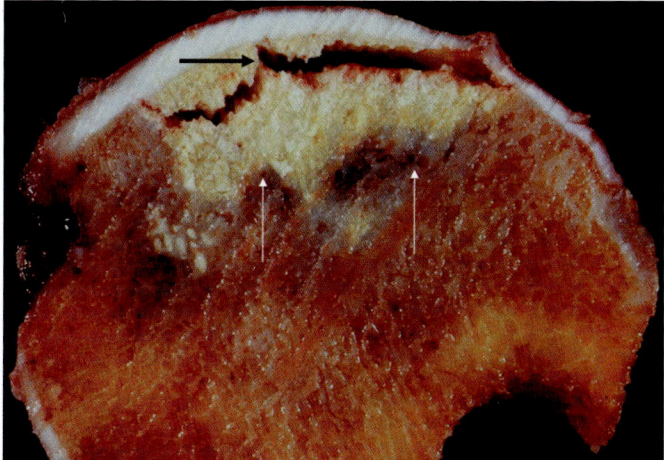

■ **FIGURE 70-3 Femoral head osteonecrosis.** Photograph of a resected femoral head with osteonecrosis shows the subchondral fracture (*black arrow*), the infarct (*thin arrows*), and surrounding marrow changes.

of bilateral involvement in systemic epiphyseal osteonecrosis (Fig. 70-4). T1-weighted spin-echo images should first be obtained because of their sensitivity to the presence of any marrow changes. Normal T1-weighted images may be sufficient to rule out ischemic marrow lesions in the vast majority of the cases. T2-weighted spin-echo or fat-saturated intermediate-weighted images are also necessary to accurately assess the articular cartilage and the subchondral bone plate. Contrast-enhanced MR images

generally do not contribute significantly to the assessment of ischemic bone lesions in the adult except in post-traumatic lesions in which the interface may be lacking at the early stage or when complications such as infection or tumor are suspected.

MANIFESTATIONS OF THE DISEASE

Radiography

Radiographs are insensitive to the detection of early infarcts because dead bone remains normal on radiographs and because the reactive interface that surrounds the infarct cannot be detected before it calcifies (see Fig. 70-4). With some nuances, post-traumatic, systemic, and overuse osteonecrosis show similar radiographic changes because they depict late reactive changes and subchondral bone plate fractures.

Bone sclerosis that delineates the ischemic lesion is an early radiographic sign, although it occurs late in the disease course. Bone resorption is generally limited, and cystic changes generally indicate collapsed epiphyseal osteonecrosis. Periosteal bone reactions adjacent to diaphyseal or metaphyseal lesions are rarely present.

The fracture of the subchondral bone plate is the hallmark of epiphyseal osteonecrosis. It can appear as frank and abrupt depression of the subchondral bone plate or as a crescentic radiolucent line parallel to the subchondral bone plate (Fig. 70-5; also see Fig. 70-4). These two features may coexist in the same epiphysis, although in different areas, probably owing to the joint biomechanics.

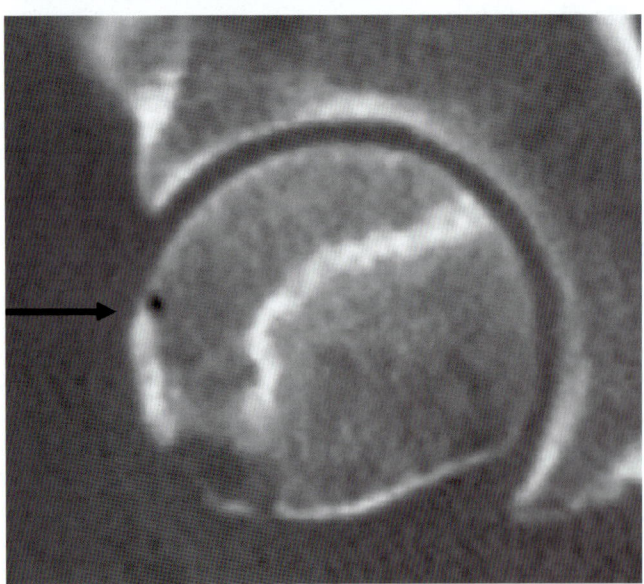

■ FIGURE 70-4 **Patient with right hip pain. A,** Coronal
T1-weighted image of the pelvis shows right hip joint effusion
and ischemic lesions in both femoral heads (*arrows*) with right
femoral neck marrow infiltration. The rim of low signal intensity is
specific for ischemic lesions. **B,** Oblique radiograph of the right hip
demonstrates fracture of the subchondral bone plate (*arrow*). **C,**
Sagittal CT reformatted image shows the sclerotic interface. Subtle
deformity of the anterior aspect of the femoral head with a small gas
bubble is depicted (*arrow*). **D,** Sagittal fat-saturated intermediate-
weighted MR image better displays the subchondral trabecular bone
fracture (*arrow*). The interface is no longer visible (well seen on the
T1-weighted image). **E,** Sagittal CT reformatted image of the left hip
shows the sclerotic interface but neither subchondral bone fracture
nor femoral head deformity.

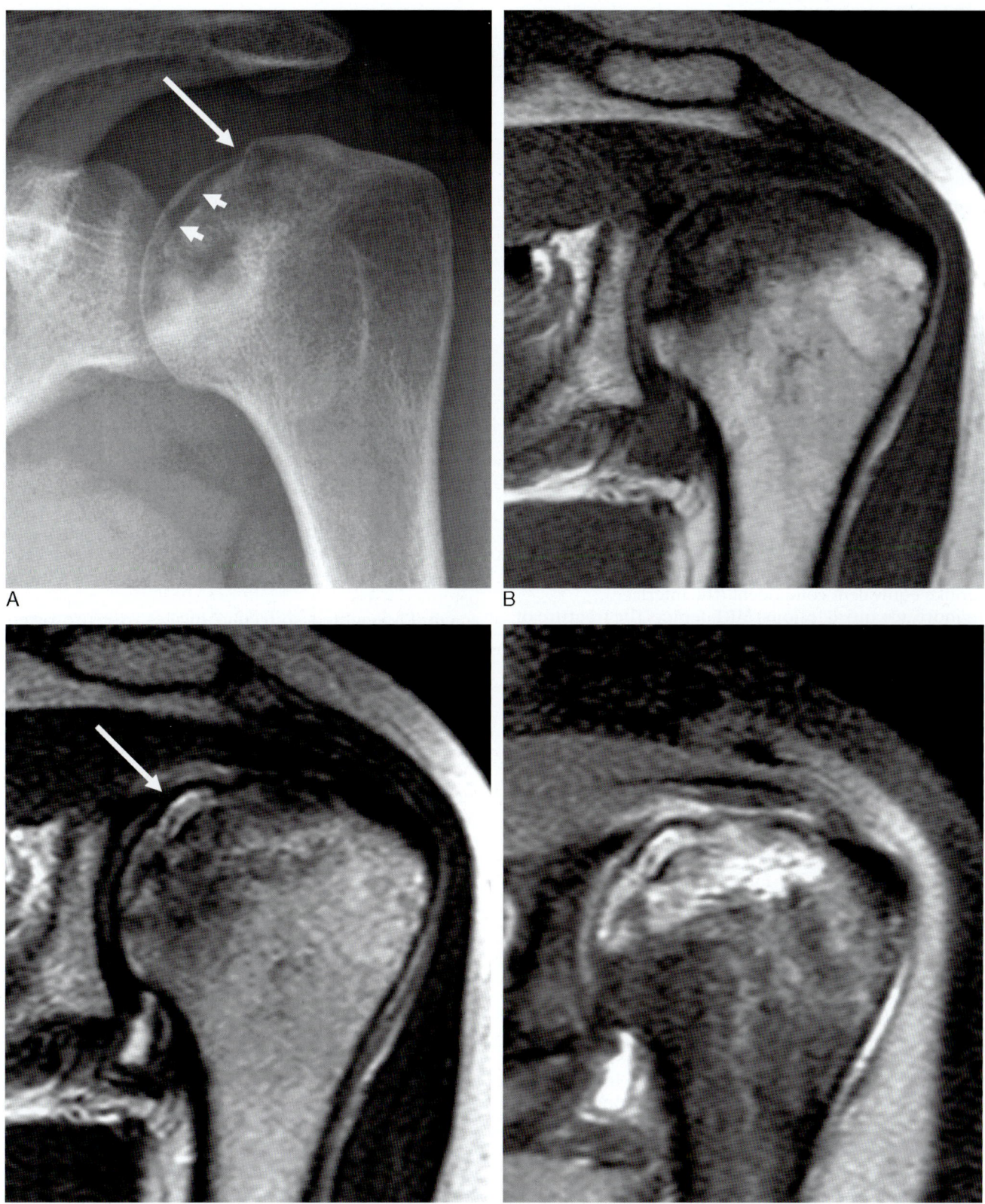

■ **FIGURE 70-5** **A,** Specific radiographic signs of osteonecrosis include epiphyseal collapse (*arrow*) and subchondral fracture (*arrowheads*). Note sclerosis of the trabecular bone within the humeral head. **B,** On a coronal T1-weighted spin-echo MR image, the entire lesion shows a homogeneous low signal intensity that lacks specificity. **C,** On the corresponding T2-weighted spin-echo MR image, the lesion shows low signal and the subchondral fracture (*arrow*) has high signal intensity. **D,** On the fat-saturated intermediate-weighted MR image, the lesion's signal is intermediate and nonspecific. Abnormal epiphyseal contour is better depicted on the fat-saturated intermediate-weighted image than on the T1- and T2-weighted images. MR images of advanced epiphyseal osteonecrosis are generally more complex and less specific than the corresponding radiographs.

Later on, radiographs accurately depict the abnormal epiphyseal shape and the altered bone structure (mixed bone sclerosis and resorption) of the involved epiphysis (see Fig. 70-5). Generally, the rate of development of secondary osteoarthritis parallels the degree of epiphyseal deformity: the more important the deformity, the more rapid the development of osteoarthritis.

Magnetic Resonance Imaging

The MR pattern of ischemic necrosis merely depends on the marrow in which it develops and therefore on its origin, its topography, and its stage.

The MR appearance of a yellow marrow infarct is that of an area of normal fatty signal intensity delineated by a rim of low signal intensity on T1-weighted images (see Fig. 70-4).[5] At the early stage, the signal of an ischemic yellow marrow lesion remains normal on T1- and T2-weighted spin-echo images because of the persistence of mummified lipid-containing cells.[5] Later, a rim of reactive tissue develops at the periphery of the lesions. On T2-weighted spin-echo images, the peripheral rim shows the double-line sign with an outer low and inner high signal intensity line, in 65% to 85% of ischemic lesions.[5] This double-line pattern probably results from chemical-shift misregistration artifact[6] related to the fact that there is fat on both sides of a water-like equivalent component (the interface).

In more advanced lesions, MRI depicts the fracture of the subchondral bone plate as a frank and abrupt depression of the subchondral bone plate or as a high signal intensity line on T2-weighted images extending under the subchondral bone plate (see Fig. 70-5). Occasionally, the fracture shows low signal intensity on T2-weighted images (Fig. 70-6). Contour depression usually occurs in the weight-bearing areas of the epiphysis (e.g., lateral aspect of femoral head) and subchondral cleft fracture usually appears in the non–weight-bearing areas (e.g., anterior aspect of the femoral head).

In late stages of the disease, with marked epiphyseal deformity (which can be more conspicuous on radiographs than on MR images), signal intensity changes within the lesion are prominent and complex (without residual fat) whereas surrounding marrow may appear normal (see Figs. 70-5 and 70-6).

Ischemic bone lesions developing in patients with marrow diseases including chronic anemia (sickle cell disease) or marrow infiltration (Gaucher's disease) frequently show a nonspecific pattern of low signal intensity on T1-weighted images and high signal intensity on T2-weighted images, in other words, the bone marrow edema pattern (Fig. 70-7). Because yellow marrow has been replaced by abnormal cells, all infarcts develop in red marrow equivalent areas and demonstrate bone marrow edema, whatever the topography.[7,8] After contrast injection, nonenhanced areas are visible within the lesion, the extent of which could depend on the chronicity of the lesion. The differential diagnosis between infected and noninfected marrow infarcts remains delicate, and the presence of soft tissue abscess could be the most important finding indicative of infection. At a later stage, several other MR patterns will develop that differ from those observed in yellow marrow infarcts.

Post-traumatic Osteonecrosis

Post-traumatic epiphyseal osteonecrosis also shows the segmental pattern because it involves a fat-containing epiphysis (Fig. 70-8). Early changes after the fracture or joint dislocation are absent or include marrow and soft tissue changes directly related with the trauma. Several weeks after the trauma, a reactive interface surrounding an ischemic area appears at some distance from the fracture level. Fat-suppressed enhanced T1-weighted sequences could enable early depiction of the infarcted area before the development of the interface, although it remains difficult to differentiate normal fatty marrow from avascular fatty marrow.

Overuse Epiphyseal Osteonecrosis

Overuse osteonecrosis generally involves a unique and subchondral area of a lower limb epiphysis. It is consistently symptomatic and is not associated with classic risk factors of systemic osteonecrosis. Additional infarcts at a distance from the involved joint are generally lacking. This pattern typically involves the medial femoral condyle of an elderly patient, but it can be observed in other lower limb epiphyses, including the femoral head, the medial tibial plateau, the talus, the metatarsal heads, as well as the lunate. In the femoral head, this pattern represents about 10% of symptomatic femoral head osteonecrosis.

On T1-weighted spin-echo images, overuse osteonecrosis shows decreased signal intensity in a subchondral area, with normal overlying cartilage (Fig. 70-9). The lesion lacks well-delimited margins, and there is no residual fat within the lesions (Fig. 70-10; also see Fig. 70-9). On T2-weighted spin-echo images, the lesion has low signal intensity in the subchondral area corresponding to necrotic, avascular tissue with adjacent edema-like marrow changes (see Figs. 70-9 and 70-10).[9] Subchondral bone plate fracture is usually present, but it usually appears as contour deformity without fluid-containing subchondral cleft, probably because the lesion involves a weight-bearing region of the joint. Spontaneous osteonecrosis of the knee is frequently associated with a medial meniscal lesion (frequently a radial tear or a root tear) and with subchondral impaction fractures.[10]

The demonstration with MRI of two different patterns of epiphyseal osteonecrosis—the systemic or segmental pattern and the edema-like pattern—suggests that epiphyseal osteonecrosis could represent a common end point of at least two different pathways.[11,12] In the segmental pattern of systemic or post-traumatic origin, vascular failure of the bone marrow is the triggering event and leads to marrow infarct with possible subsequent epiphyseal fracture. In the diffuse pattern of overuse origin, mechanical failure of bone (trabecular bone fracture) or cartilage abrasion could lead to fracture of the subchondral bone plate with subsequent development of necrosis at the interface between the broken osteocartilaginous plate and the epiphysis.[10,13]

Multidetector Computed Tomography

Multidetector computed tomography has not been widely used for the assessment of ischemic bone lesions.

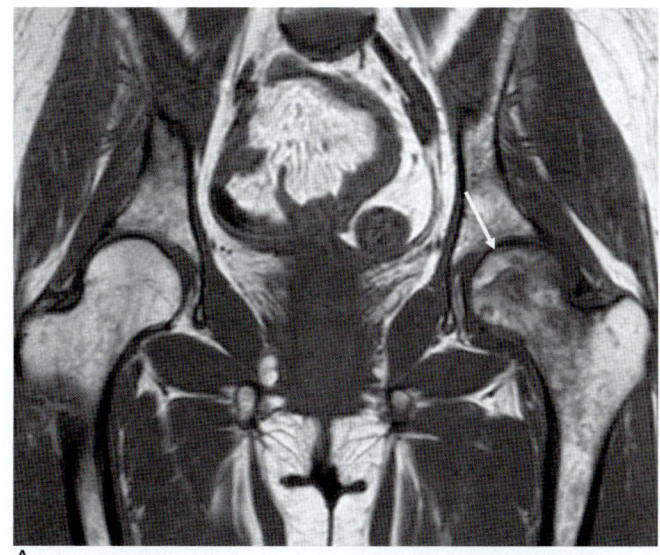

A

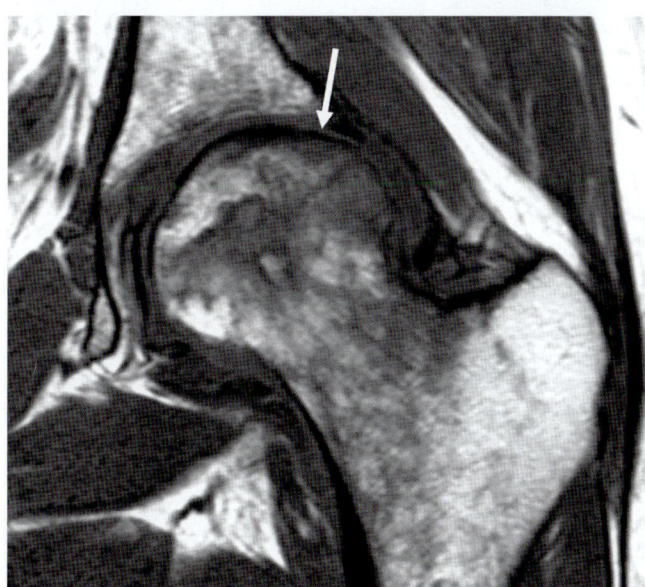

B

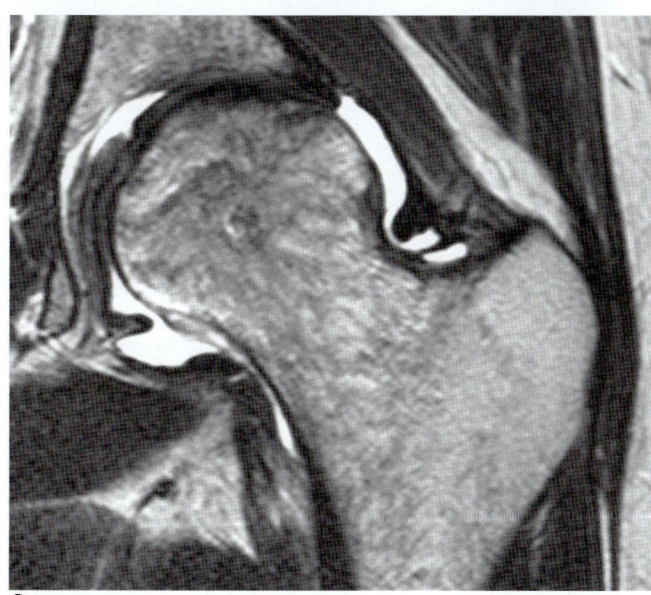

C

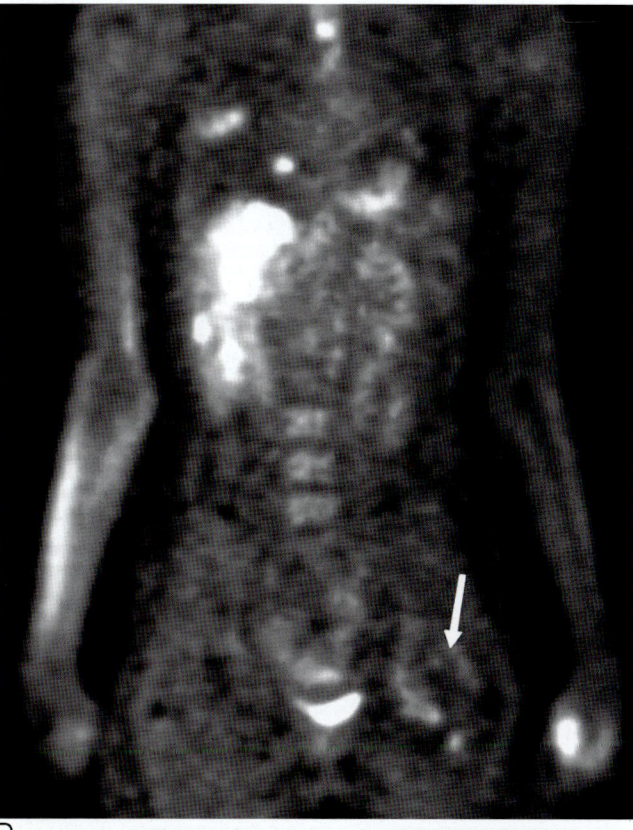

D

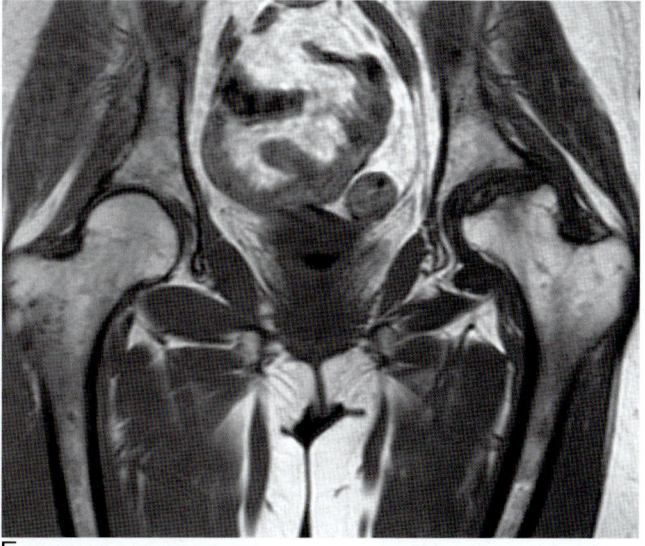

E

■ **FIGURE 70-6** **A,** Coronal T1-weighted MR image of the pelvis of a woman with treated non-Hodgkin's lymphoma and acute left hip pain demonstrates an ischemic lesion of the left femur (*arrow*). **B,** On a high-resolution coronal T1-weighted spin-echo MR image the subchondral lesion has both high and low signal intensity with subtle depression of the lateral aspect of the femoral head (*arrow*). The femoral neck marrow is infiltrated. **C,** On the corresponding T2-weighted spin-echo MR image, the ischemic lesion also shows variable signal intensity patterns. The interface is barely visible. Joint effusion is present. **D,** Coronal FDG-PET image shows mild hypermetabolic activity in the left capsule (*arrow*). **E,** Coronal T1-weighted MR image obtained several months later shows epiphyseal collapse. The lesion shows low signal intensity, and femoral neck marrow is normal.

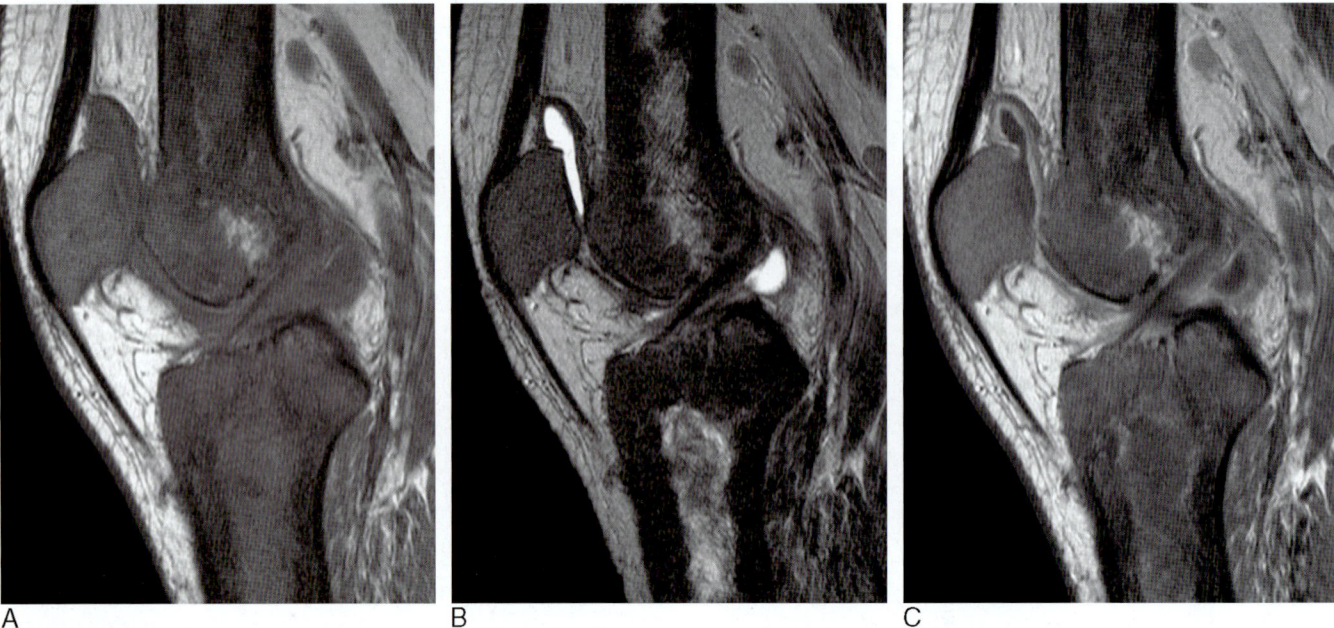

A   B   C

■ **FIGURE 70-7** **Systemic osteonecrosis in red marrow.** On the sagittal (**A**) T1- and (**B**) T2-weighted MR images of the knee of a patient with sickle cell disease the whole marrow shows an abnormal low signal intensity. High signal intensity areas involve the center of the medullary cavity. These focal marrow alterations are not specific but are compatible with marrow infarcts. **C,** On the enhanced T1-weighted image the focal lesions show peripheral enhancement. Note associated joint effusion.

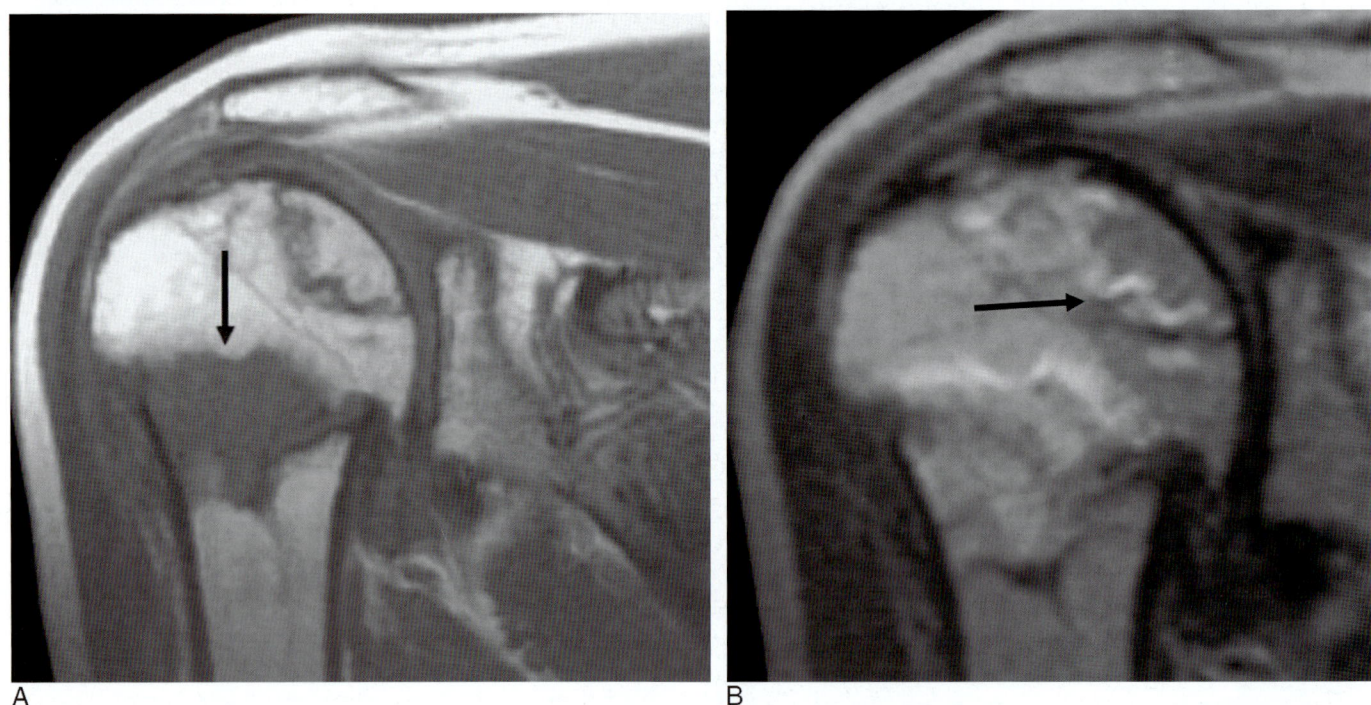

A   B

■ **FIGURE 70-8** **Post-traumatic osteonecrosis. A,** Coronal T1-weighted spin-echo MR image of the right shoulder shows a neck fracture (*arrow*) and a humeral head infarct. **B,** On the corresponding T2-weighted spin-echo MR image, the fracture converts to high signal intensity and a double-line sign is visible at the periphery of the subchondral infarct (*arrow*).

A preliminary study suggested that MDCT could be valuable in the detection of the subchondral bone plate fracture.[14] In our experience, MDCT could also contribute to the assessment of post-traumatic osteonecrosis treated with metallic hardware.

Nuclear Medicine

Bone scintigraphy using technetium diphosphonate has been used for decades in the assessment of articular pain, mainly because of the relatively high negative predictive

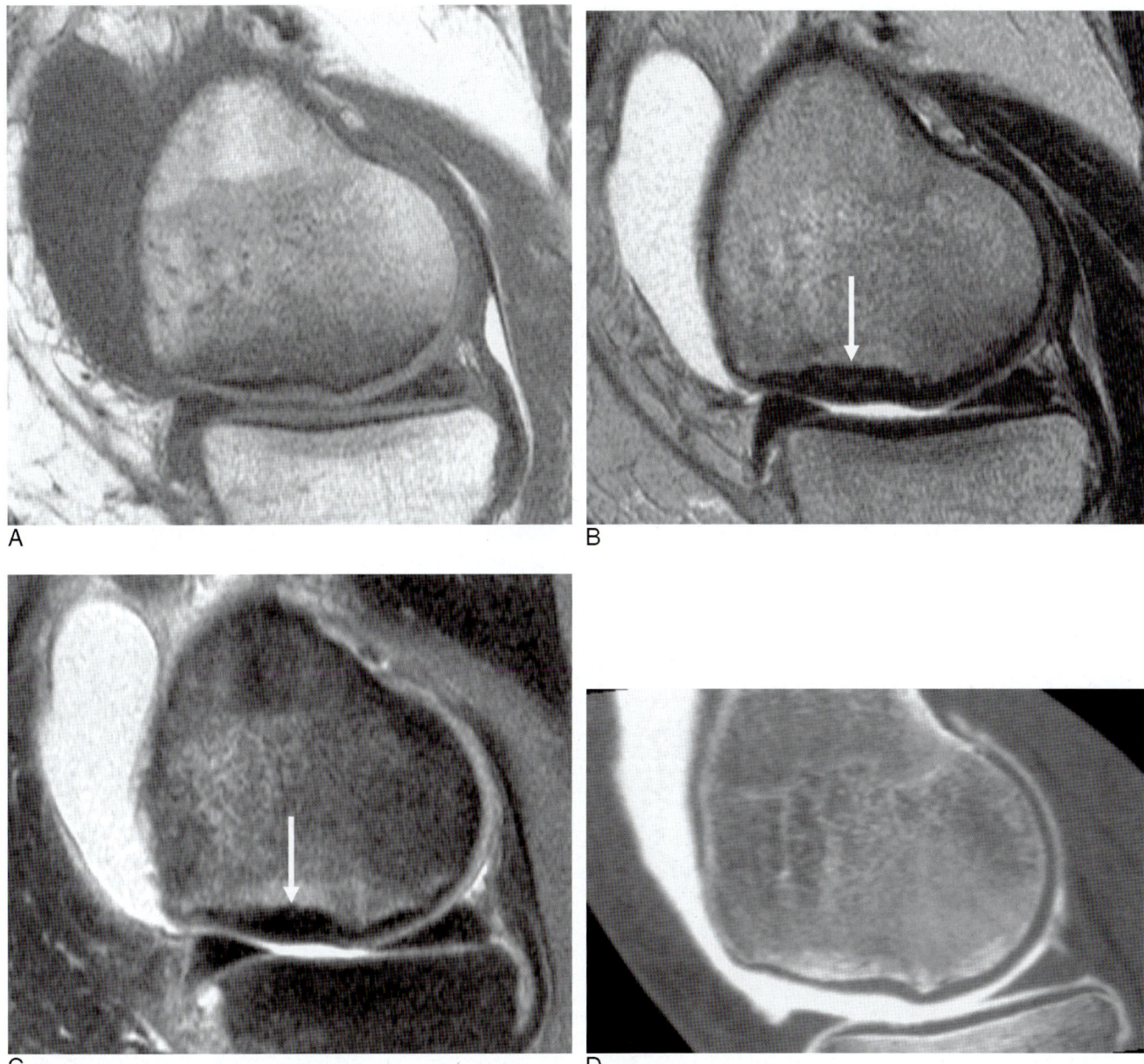

■ FIGURE 70-9   Spontaneous osteonecrosis of the knee. A, Sagittal T1-weighted MR image demonstrates ill-delimited infiltration of the subchondral marrow of the femoral condyle and deformity of the subchondral bone plate. B, Sagittal T2-weighted MR image shows a low signal intensity subchondral area (*arrow*). C, On the fat-saturated intermediate-weighted MR image, the lesion more clearly consists of a low signal subchondral area (*arrow*) and edema-like changes in the adjacent marrow. D, Sagittal reformatted image after CT arthrography also shows condyle deformity, subchondral sclerosis, and a normal overlying cartilage.

value in the setting of symptomatic epiphyseal osteonecrosis. Its use has progressively decreased because of the availability of MRI and the well-known limitations in the analysis of abnormal bone scans owing to its poor specificity and poor spatial resolution.

Positron Emission Tomography/ Computed Tomography

There are limited literature data on the value of PET in ischemic bone lesions. Ischemic bone lesions could remain occult on PET images except for slight marker accumulation in the joint capsule (see Fig. 70-6).

Classification Systems

Over the years, numerous different classification systems have been developed to stage the disease, mainly for femoral head osteonecrosis. Although there is no standard unified classification system used by all investigators, there is general agreement on the fact that the presence of subchondral bone fracture represents a pivotal

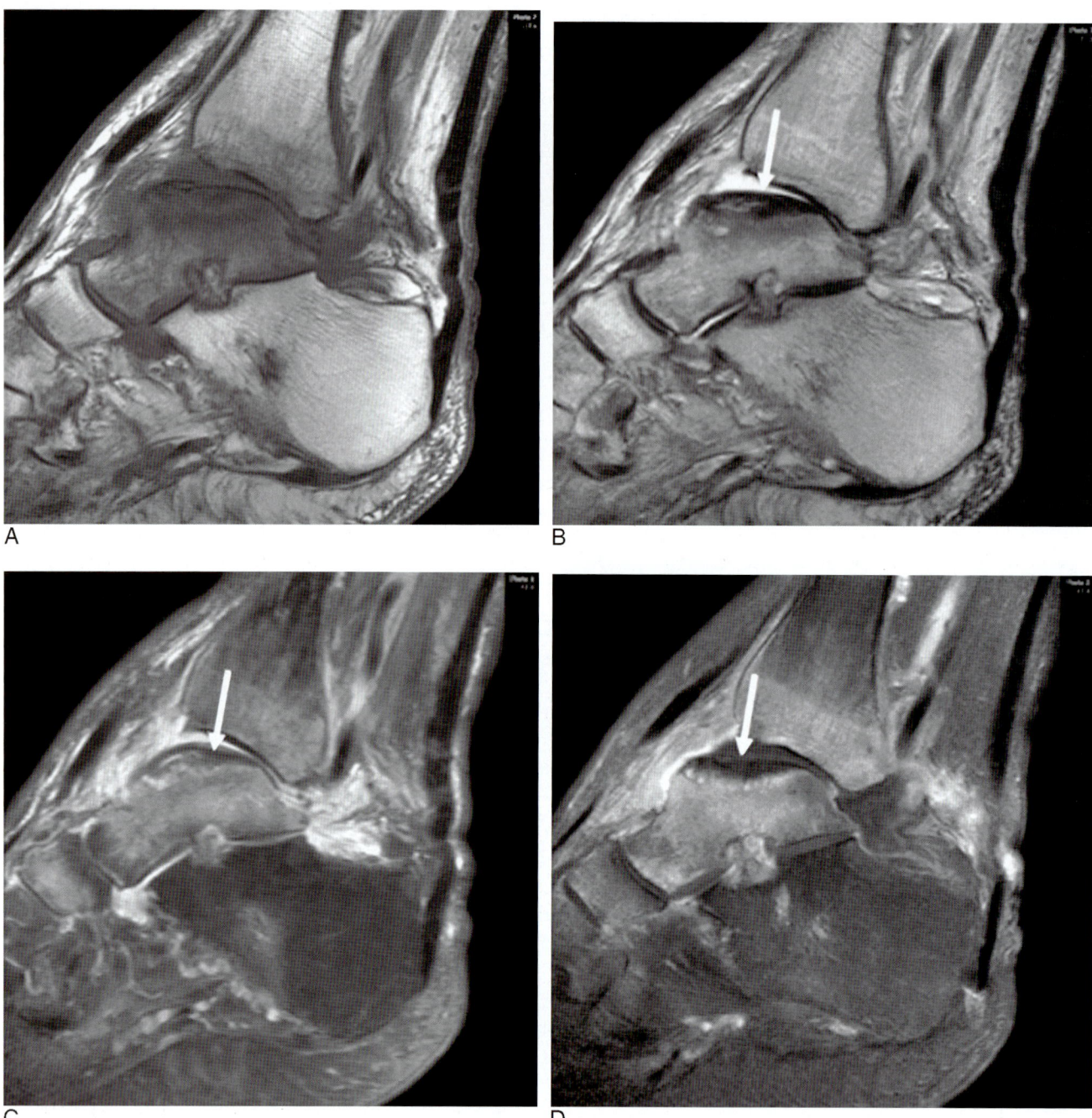

■ **FIGURE 70-10**   **Overuse osteonecrosis of the ankle. A,** Sagittal T1-weighted MR image of the ankle shows talar dome collapse and low signal in the talus. **B,** On the corresponding T2-weighted MR image, the subchondral area shows low signal intensity (*arrow*), suggestive of necrotic tissue. **C,** On the fat-saturated intermediate-weighted MR image the subchondral area (*arrow*) also shows low signal intensity. Adjacent marrow infiltration is better depicted. **D,** The enhanced T1-weighted MR image demonstrates marked enhancement in abnormal marrow except in the necrotic subchondral area (*arrow*).

position (generally at stage III, whatever the classification system). Ficat and Arlet originally developed a four-stage classification system based on radiographic changes and the functional exploration of bone (intraosseous phlebography and measurement of bone marrow pressure) (Table 70-2).[15] Steinberg's and Arco's classification systems included MRI evaluation, allowing for quantification and topography of the epiphyseal lesion (Table 70-3).[16] Mitchell's classification system[5] included signal pattern of

necrotic lesion (A: fat; B: blood; C: edema; D: fibrosis), but it showed limited utility because of the variability of signal intensity of the lesion within the same lesion.

Natural History of Ischemic Bone Lesions

Metaphyseal marrow infarcts remain stable for life and do not lead to bone fracture. Infection and malignant transformation are two rare complications.

TABLE 70-2   Ficat Staging System of Avascular Necrosis of the Hip

Stage	Clinical and Radiologic Findings
Stage I	Normal radiographs Decreased or increased uptake on bone scan No pain Increased medullary pressure
Stage II	Variable change in trabecular bone appearance (sclerosis, delimited area of sclerosis, cyst changes) but preserved femoral head shape Variable pain
Stage III	Specific changes on radiographs include collapse of subchondral bone and/or crescent sign due to subchondral bone fracture Pain
Stage IV	Marked collapse of subchondral bone with preserved joint space
Stage V	Secondary osteoarthritis

TABLE 70-3   Staging System Based on the Consensus of the Subcommittee of Nomenclature of the International Association on Bone Circulation and Bone Necrosis (ARCO)

Stage	Clinical and Laboratory Findings
Stage 0	No symptoms Normal radiographs and MR images Osteonecrosis at histology
Stage I	Presence or absence of symptoms Normal radiographs Abnormal MR images Osteonecrosis at histology
Stage II	Symptoms Trabecular bone changes on radiographs without subchondral bone changes Preserved joint space Diagnostic MR findings
Stage III	Symptoms Variable trabecular bone changes with subchondral bone fracture (crescent sign and/or subchondral bone collapse) Preserved shape of femoral head and preserved joint space Subclassification based on extent of crescent, as follows: Stage IIIa: Crescent is less than 15% of the articular surface. Stage IIIb: Crescent is 15%-30% of the articular surface. Stage IIIc: Crescent is more than 30% of the articular surface.
Stage IV	Symptoms Altered shape of femoral head with variable joint space Subclassification depends on the extent of collapsed surface, as follows: Stage IVa: Less than 15% of surface is collapsed. Stage IVb: Approximately 15%-30% of surface is collapsed. Stage IVc: More than 30% of surface is collapsed.

The natural history of epiphyseal infarcts is more controversial. Natural outcome of symptomatic femoral head osteonecrosis conservatively treated is usually poor, with a high frequency of irreversible collapse. Conversely, the natural history of asymptomatic femoral head lesions discovered fortuitously at systematic MRI performed in a patient with a high risk of necrosis showed a 15% to 20% risk of appearance of symptoms at 1-year follow-up, with the majority of lesions remaining silent at follow-up (see Fig. 70-11). Quantitative determination of the extent and location of uncollapsed femoral head infarcts on MR images enables one to estimate the fracture risk.[17-19] Femoral heads in which the infarct is either small or involves a limited proportion of the weight-bearing area are less likely to collapse than those with large lesions. Signal changes in lesions could also indicate impending fractures because infarcts with fat-like signal intensity show a collapse-free survival much longer than those with heterogeneous signal.[17]

DIFFERENTIAL DIAGNOSIS

The diagnosis of ischemic bone lesions heavily relies on medical imaging. The alert clinician may suspect the diagnosis when facing a patient with acute and spontaneous articular pain and risk factors for ischemic lesions. Clinical examination has little diagnostic value except for accurate localization of the involved area (knee pain due to femoral head osteonecrosis).

Blood tests generally do not contribute to the diagnosis of the ischemic lesions, but it is of importance in the recognition of eventual underlying disease (e.g., anemia, hyperuricemia, intoxication).

Magnetic Resonance Imaging

Metaphyseal infarcts should not be confused with enchondromas. On T1-weighted images, the signal of enchondromas is low with small fatty-like signal intensity septa trapped between cartilaginous nodules. Contours are lobulated and not serpiginous-like in infarcts.

A noncollapsed epiphyseal infarct has a typical MR appearance. Rarely, a chronic subchondral fracture can show a transient similar pattern with a subchondral low signal intensity line and adjacent fatty marrow. Generally, this line that represents the healed trabecular bone fracture does not completely circumscribe a subchondral marrow area and is located very near to the subchondral bone plate.

Collapsed epiphyseal osteonecrosis shows a more complex MR appearance and must be differentiated from other lesions, including subchondral cysts in osteoarthritis, sequelae of osteochondritis dissecans, fractures, and tumors. Analysis of the overlying cartilage is critical: cartilage adjacent to subchondral cysts is generally abnormal, whereas cartilage adjacent to recently collapsed osteonecrosis remains relatively preserved. In clinical practice, radiographs of advanced lesions are easier to understand than MR images.

Overuse epiphyseal osteonecrosis must be differentiated from numerous conditions showing the bone marrow edema pattern because of their considerable differences

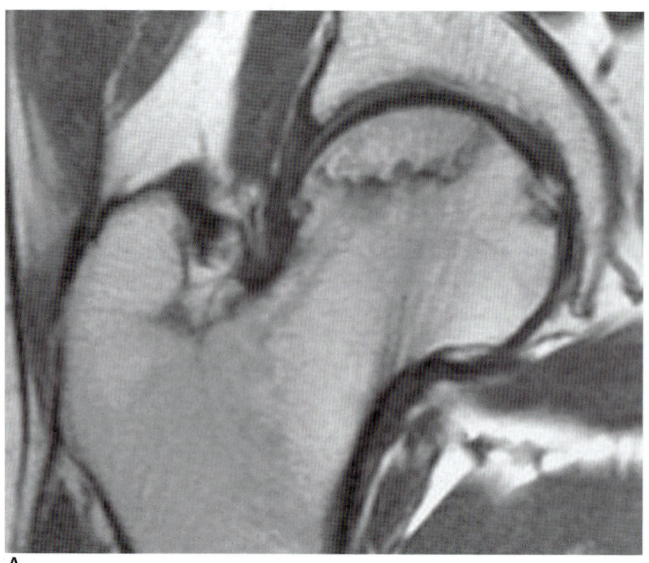
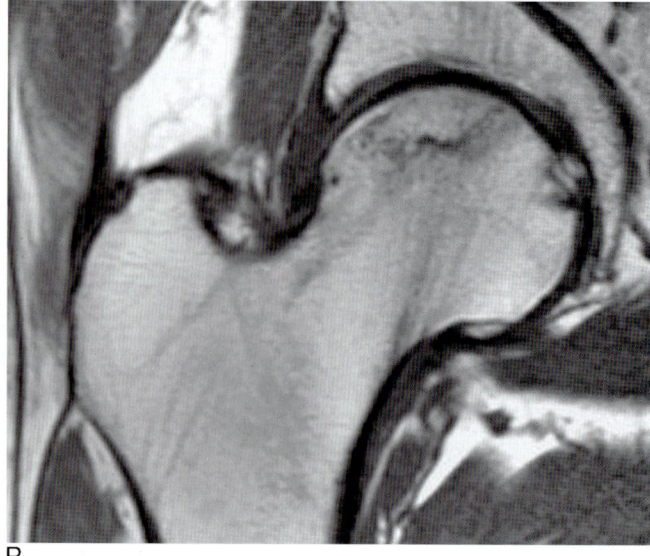

■ **FIGURE 70-11** **A** and **B**, Coronal T1-weighted spin-echo MR images of the right hip obtained in a patient 1 and 2 years after the onset of corticosteroid treatment show a femoral head infarct that does not collapse at follow-up.

in treatment and prognosis.[20] Transient osteoporosis, transient bone marrow edema, and epiphyseal stress fracture are generally self-limited.[6,10,21,22] On the contrary, osteoarthritis (Fig. 70-12)[23-25] and epiphyseal osteonecrosis[17-19,26-28] are not reversible.

Insufficiency stress fracture can be either reversible or irreversible. Careful analysis of the articular cartilage, the subchondral bone plate, and the subchondral marrow on high-resolution coronal and sagittal T2-weighted fast spin-echo images or fat-saturated intermediate-weighted fast spin-echo images is mandatory for this differential diagnosis. Several prognostic rules must be used: (1) abnormal cartilage indicates a clinically irreversible lesion, even if marrow edema resolves at follow-up MRI; (2) epiphyseal collapse indicates an irreversible lesion, whatever the marrow pattern at MRI; and (3) a fluid-like signal intensity line underneath the epiphyseal contour also suggests irreversibility. If the hyaline cartilage and the epiphyseal shape are preserved, and if there is no subchondral bone cleft, detection and determination of the size of low signal intensity subchondral areas help to differentiate osteonecrosis from transient lesions. In the hip and knee joints, a crescent-shaped low signal intensity area in the subchondral region with a thickness equal or superior to 4 mm on T2-weighted images suggests an irreversible lesion. In other situations, the outcome is uncertain, unless there are no other changes than edema, in which case the lesion is reversible.

SYNOPSIS OF TREATMENT OPTIONS

Medical Treatment

Treatment efficacy of ischemic epiphyseal lesions remains controversial for many reasons: the lack of generally accepted diagnostic gold standard (intraosseous pressure determination, histology, MRI), the difficulty in classifying

the patients and in detecting subchondral bone plate fracture, the coexistence of different lesion patterns in the same studies, and the limited knowledge on the natural history of ischemic bone lesions.

Despite the use of a large spectrum of drugs or conservative methods, medical management of symptomatic ischemic bone lesions has not proved to be effective in preventing or arresting the disease process.[29] Pain control is usually achieved by nonsteroidal analgesics, and patients should be advised to use crutches or other supports to avoid weight bearing. Several drugs or other therapeutic methods can be applied, including diphosphonates, hyperbaric oxygen therapy, and magnetic field strength appliance.

Surgical Treatment

Several surgical procedures have been tried with variable success, mainly in the femoral head. Core decompression of the hip with or without bone graft is the most common procedure currently used to treat the early stages of femoral head osteonecrosis, and it is effective in pain control. This procedure has been used for approximately three decades, but there are numerous publications analyzing its efficacy, and there is no consensus among investigators regarding either the indication for this procedure or its effect on the fate of the femoral head.[30] In late stages, characterized by collapse, femoral head deformity, and secondary osteoarthritis, total hip arthroplasty is the most appropriate treatment, although several osteotomy procedures have been tried with variable success.[1]

SUMMARY OF MAGNETIC RESONANCE IMAGING FINDINGS

Epiphyseal osteonecrosis may show two different patterns of involvement based on a T1-weighted spin-echo image, namely, the segmental and the diffuse patterns. The

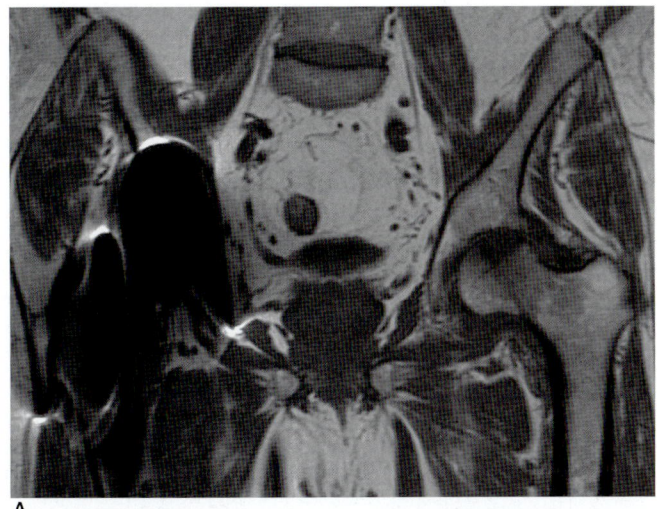

A

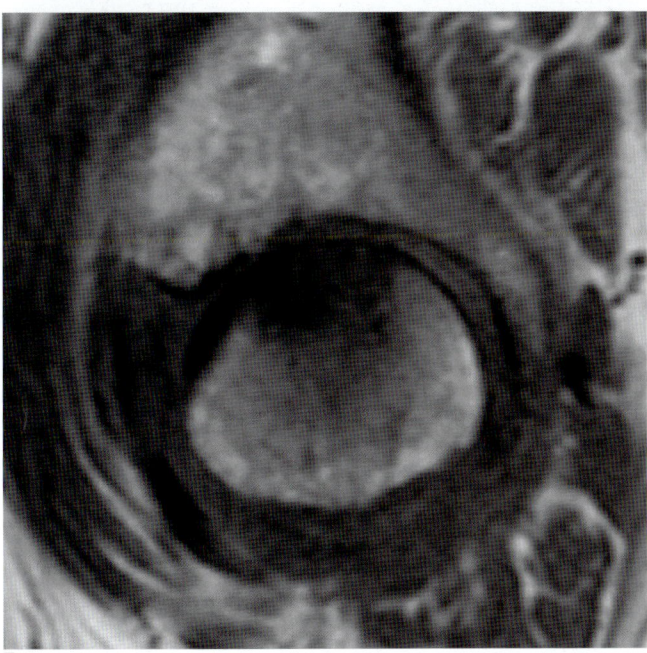

B

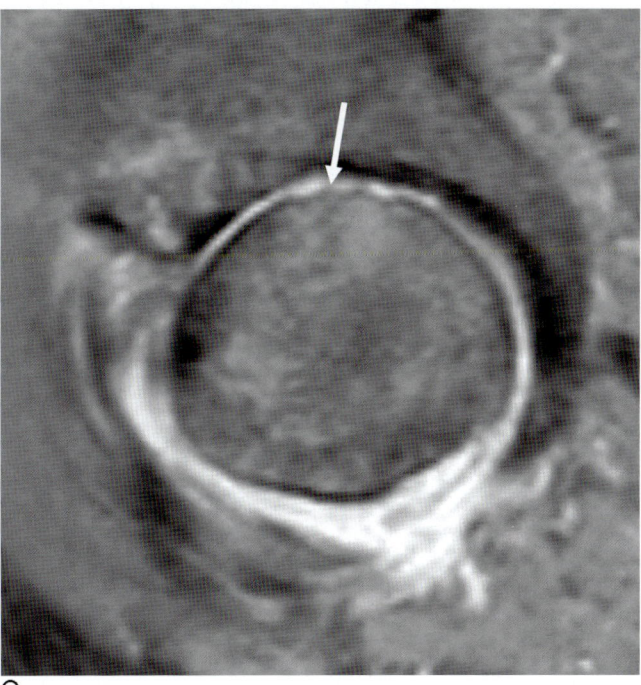

C

■ **FIGURE 70-12 A,** Coronal T1-weighted spin-echo MR image shows a low signal lesion in the left femoral head and neck. **B,** On the sagittal T1-weighted MR image, the subchondral marrow demonstrates low signal intensity, without clear margin. The sphericity of the femoral head is preserved. **C,** On the corresponding fat-saturated intermediate-weighted MR image, extensive cartilage abrasion (*arrow*) indicative of osteoarthritis is clearly demonstrated. In osteonecrosis, cartilage abrasion is secondary to epiphyseal deformity, which is lacking in the current case.

segmental pattern is observed in yellow marrow areas in patients with systemic osteonecrosis (with known risk factors for marrow infarcts) (see Fig. 70-5). On T1-weighted spin-echo images, the segmental pattern is defined by the presence of a well-demarcated lesion with necrotic tissue of variable signal intensity, generally including some high signal intensity areas in the subchondral lesion. Specific MRI features include the reactive interface and the subchondral bone fracture. The reactive interface shows the same MR appearance as in marrow infarcts, but it is frequently blurred by adjacent reactive changes.[31] The signal intensity of the necrotic tissue is either equivalent to that of fat or is low on T1-, T2-, and enhanced T1-weighted images, reflecting the presence of mummified fat or eosinophilic necrosis, respectively.[32-34] Reactive changes that surround the lesion show low signal intensity on T1-weighted images and intermediate to high signal intensity on T2-weighted images, depending on the balance among fibrous, sclerotic, edematous hemorrhagic and cellular components.[32,33,35-37] These surrounding changes that are more frequent in symptomatic than in asymptomatic lesions[35] probably indicate incipient epiphyseal fracture[14,35,36,38,39] rather than extension of ischemia.

Actually, in rapidly progressive and destructive osteoarthritis (see Fig. 70-11), in which cartilage destruction is the primary event, subchondral bone plate fracture and bone contusion could also lead to irreversible collapse of the epiphysis.[23,40]

What the Referring Physician Needs to Know

- Is there a bone lesion?
- Is it likely to be the cause of the pain?
- Is it an ischemic lesion or not?

- If thought to be an ischemic lesion:
  - Is there a fracture of the subchondral bone plate (staging)?
  - If there is no fracture, what is the risk for fracture (prognosis)?

REFERENCES

1. Mankin HJ. Nontraumatic necrosis of bone (osteonecrosis). N Engl J Med 1992; 326:1473-1479.
2. Ito H, Kaneda K, Matsuno T. Osteonecrosis of the femoral head. J Bone Joint Surg Br 1999; 81:969-974.
3. Glimcher MJ, Kenzora JE. Nicolas Andry award. The biology of osteonecrosis of the human femoral head and its clinical implications: 1. Tissue biology. Clin Orthop Relat Res 1979; (138):284-309.
4. Robbins SL, Cotran RS, Kumar V. Fluid and hemodynamic derangements. In Robbins SL, Cotran RS, Kumar V (eds). Pathologic Basis of Disease. Philadelphia, WB Saunders, 1984, pp 85-117.
5. Mitchell DG, Rao VM, Dalinka MK, et al. Femoral head avascular necrosis: correlation of MR imaging, radiographic staging, radionuclide imaging, and clinical findings. Radiology 1987; 162:709-715.
6. Vande Berg BC, Malghem J, Labaisse MA, et al. MR imaging of avascular necrosis and transient marrow edema of the femoral head. RadioGraphics 1993; 13:501-520.
7. Rao VM, Fishman M, Mitchell DG, et al. Painful sickle cell crisis: bone marrow patterns observed with MR imaging [published erratum appears in Radiology 1987;162(1 pt 1):289]. Radiology 1986; 161:211-215.
8. Vande Berg BC, Malghem J, Labaisse MA, et al. Apparent focal bone marrow ischemia in patients with marrow disorders: MR studies. J Comput Assist Tomogr 1993; 17:792-797.
9. Lecouvet FE, Vande Berg BC, Maldague BE, et al. Early irreversible osteonecrosis versus transient lesions of the femoral condyles: prognostic value of subchondral bone and marrow changes on MR imaging. AJR Am J Roentgenol 1998; 170:71-77.
10. Yamamoto T, Schneider R, Bullough PG. Subchondral insufficiency fracture of the femoral head: histopathologic correlation with MRI. Skeletal Radiol 2001; 30:247-254.
11. Mitchell DG. Using MR imaging to probe the pathophysiology of osteonecrosis. Radiology 1989; 171:25-26.
12. Vande Berg BC, Malghem J, Lecouvet FE, Maldague B. Magnetic resonance imaging and differential diagnosis of epiphyseal osteonecrosis. Semin Musculoskelet Radiol 2001; 5:57-67.
13. Glimcher MJ, Kenzora JE. The biology of osteonecrosis of the human femoral head and its clinical implications: III. Discussion of the etiology and genesis of the pathological sequelae; comments on treatment. Clin Orthop Relat Res 1979; (140):273-312.
14. Stevens K, Tao C, Lee SU, et al. Subchondral fractures in osteonecrosis of the femoral head: comparison of radiography, CT, and MR imaging. AJR Am J Roentgenol 2003; 180:363-368.
15. Ficat RP. Idiopathic bone necrosis of the femoral head. Early diagnosis and treatment. J Bone Joint Surg Br 1985; 67:3-9.
16. Steinberg ME, Hayken GD, Steinberg DR. A quantitative system for staging avascular necrosis. J Bone Joint Surg Br 1995; 77:34-41.
17. Shimizu K, Moriya H, Akita T, et al. Prediction of collapse with magnetic resonance imaging of avascular necrosis of the femoral head. J Bone Joint Surg Am 1994; 76:215-223.
18. Lafforgue P, Dahan E, Chagnaud C, et al. Early-stage avascular necrosis of the femoral head: MR imaging for prognosis in 31 cases with at least 2 years of follow-up. Radiology 1993; 187:199-204.
19. Takatori Y, Kokubo T, Ninomiya S, et al. Avascular necrosis of the femoral head: natural history and magnetic resonance imaging. J Bone Joint Surg Br 1993; 75:217-221.
20. Conway WF, Totty WG, McEnery KW. CT and MR imaging of the hip. Radiology 1996; 198:297-307.
21. Bloem JL. Transient osteoporosis of the hip: MR imaging. Radiology 1988; 167:753-755.
22. Wilson AJ, Murphy WA, Hardy DC, Totty WG. Transient osteoporosis: transient bone marrow edema? Radiology 1988; 167:757-760.
23. Boutry N, Paul C, Leroy X, et al. Rapidly destructive osteoarthritis of the hip: MR imaging findings. AJR Am J Roentgenol 2002; 179:657-663.
24. Sugano N, Ohzono K, Nishii T, et al. Early MRI findings of rapidly destructive coxopathy. Magn Reson Imaging 2001; 19:47-50.
25. Watanabe W, Itoi E, Yamada S. Early MRI findings of rapidly destructive coxarthrosis. Skeletal Radiol 2002; 31:35-38.
26. Turner DA, Templeton AC, Selzer PM, et al. Femoral capital osteonecrosis: MR finding of diffuse marrow abnormalities without focal lesions [see comments]. Radiology 1989; 171:135-140.
27. Mitchell DG, Kressel HY. MR imaging of early avascular necrosis [letter]. Radiology 1988; 169:281-282.
28. Thickman D, Axel L, Kressel HY, et al. Magnetic resonance imaging of avascular necrosis of the femoral head. Skeletal Radiol 1986; 15:133-140.
29. Lieberman JR, Berry DJ, Mont MA, et al. Osteonecrosis of the hip: management in the twenty-first century. J Bone Joint Surg Am 2002; 84:834-853.
30. Lieberman JR. Core decompression for osteonecrosis of the hip. Clin Orthop Relat Res 2004; (418):29-33.
31. Coleman BG, Kressel HY, Dalinka MK, et al. Radiographically negative avascular necrosis: detection with MR imaging. Radiology 1988; 168:525-528.
32. Lang P, Jergesen HE, Moseley ME, et al. Avascular necrosis of the femoral head: high-field-strength MR imaging with histologic correlation. Radiology 1988; 169:517-524.
33. Jergesen HE, Lang P, Moseley M, Genant HK. Histologic correlation in magnetic resonance imaging of femoral head osteonecrosis. Clin Orthop Relat Res 1990; (253):150-163.
34. Vande Berg BC, Malghem J, Labaisse MA, et al. Avascular necrosis of the hip: comparison of contrast-enhanced and nonenhanced MR imaging with histologic correlation. Work in progress. Radiology 1992; 182:445-450.
35. Koo KH, Ahn IO, Song HR, et al. Bone marrow edema and associated pain in early stage osteonecrosis of the femoral head: prospective study with serial MR images. Radiology 1999; 213:715-722.
36. Sakai T, Sugano N, Nishii T, et al. MR findings of necrotic lesions and the extralesional area of osteonecrosis of the femoral head. Skeletal Radiol 2000; 29:133-141.
37. Kubo T, Yamamoto T, Inoue S, et al. Histological findings of bone marrow edema pattern on MRI in osteonecrosis of the femoral head. J Orthop Sci 2000; 5:520-523.
38. Iida S, Harada Y, Shimizu K, et al. Correlation between bone marrow edema and collapse of the femoral head in steroid-induced osteonecrosis. AJR Am J Roentgenol 2000; 174:735-743.
39. Huang GS, Chan WP, Chang YC, et al. MR imaging of bone marrow edema and joint effusion in patients with osteonecrosis of the femoral head: relationship to pain. AJR Am J Roentgenol 2003; 181:545-549.
40. Ryu KN, Kim EJ, Yoo MC, et al. Ischemic necrosis of the entire femoral head and rapidly destructive hip disease: potential causative relationship. Skeletal Radiol 1997; 26:143-149.
41. Kopecky KK, Braunstein EM, Brandt KD, et al. Apparent avascular necrosis of the hip: appearance and spontaneous resolution of MR findings in renal allograft recipients. Radiology 1991; 179:523-527.

71

Hemophilia and Related Disorders

G. M. Allen, C. J. Fang, and D. J. Wilson

The term *hemophilia* is used to refer to a group of blood coagulation disorders that result from deficiencies in specific plasma clotting factors.

The earliest descriptions of what appears to be hemophilia date to the 11th and 12th centuries. Jewish writings describe rabbinical rulings exempting male boys from circumcision if two previous brothers had died of bleeding after the procedure, suggesting an appreciation of the hereditary nature of the condition. The first modern description of hemophilia is attributed to Dr. John Conrad Otto, a physician in Philadelphia, who clearly appreciated the cardinal feature of hemophilia: an inherited tendency of males to bleed. In 1803 he published a treatise entitled "An Account of a Hemorrhagic Disposition Existing in Certain Families." It is not until 1828 that the first use of the word "hemophilia" appears in an account of the condition written by Hopff ("Uber die Haemophilie oder die erbliche Anlage zu todlichen Blutungen").

Despite these historical descriptions of hemophilia dating back to ancient times and the early 19th and 20th century understanding of the symptoms and inheritance, the biochemical basis was only elucidated in the early 1950s. In the 19th century, the majority of physicians believed that bleeding in hemophilia was due to a structural abnormality in the blood vessels. The major breakthrough took place in 1937, when Patek and Taylor, at Harvard University, identified a fraction precipitated from normal plasma by dilution with mild acid. They showed this fraction would correct the clotting of hemophilic blood. In 1944, Pavlovsky, from Buenos Aires, described a case in which mutual correction of in-vitro clotting tests occurred when plasma from two different hemophiliacs was mixed. This finding was only explained in 1952 when Macfarlane and Biggs, at Oxford University, described the first case of hemophilia B, which they named Christmas disease after the surname of the 10-year-old boy they studied. They determined that the disease was due to deficiency of factor IX. It was subsequently appreciated

that many proteins were involved in the coagulation pathway. Names were assigned to the various coagulation factors by an International Committee in 1962: the factor missing in hemophilia A was subsequently termed *factor VIII*. A scheme for the interaction of the various factors in a coagulation pathway was independently devised by two groups shortly thereafter. Macfarlane called his scheme a "cascade" in an article in *Nature* in 1964, and Ratnoff used the term "waterfall" in a publication in the same year.

In the musculoskeletal system, these disorders manifest in a spectrum of abnormalities affecting joints and soft tissues. Imaging plays an important part in detecting, staging, and monitoring disease. The severe damage that may occur in joints is apparent on plain films, whereas cross-sectional techniques are ideal for judging the extent and progress of soft tissue hemorrhage. Imaging may assist in locating the source of chronic pain. This patient group is also afflicted by conventional diseases unrelated to their hemophilia, and imaging is useful in excluding other causes of symptoms.

ETIOLOGY

Of all causes of hemophilia, types A and B are most associated with intraosseous and intra-articular bleeding. Hemophilia A (classic hemophilia) results from a deficiency

---

KEY POINTS

- Hemophilia is a rare, sex-linked recessive but devastating disease.
- It can be treated by replacing the relevant blood-clotting factors VIII and IX.
- Radiologists can detect hemorrhage in joints and soft tissue
- Radiologists can detect the chronic diseases associated with the condition: arthropathy and pseudotumors.

of factor VIII. Hemophilia B (Christmas disease) is due to a functional deficiency of plasma thromboplastin component (factor IX). These disorders are both X linked and therefore manifest clinically in men but are carried by women.

PREVALENCE AND EPIDEMIOLOGY

Classic hemophilia occurs in 1 in 10,000 males in the United States. Christmas disease is rarer, affecting approximately 1 in 100,000 males. Although both forms are almost exclusive to males, reports exist of disease occurring in females. Twenty-five percent of hemophilia is due to spontaneous mutation. Acquired hemophilia due to antibodies to factor VIII is rare but severe and can affect women.

CLINICAL PRESENTATION

Acute Hemarthrosis

Between 75% to 90% of hemophilia patients will suffer from hemarthrosis. Adults are better able to protect their joints from trauma and, consequently, hemarthrosis is more common in young children and adolescents.

Acute intra-articular bleeding will present as pain and dysfunction. Swelling and effusion will be apparent in the more superficial joints. When it is already known that the patient has a coagulation disorder and the clinical findings are clearcut, imaging is of limited immediate value. Because these patients are often in severe pain and are prone to worsening of the hemorrhage it is unwise to perform even the least invasive examination. In the acute phase the priority is resuscitation and coagulation control with blood factor replacement not radiologic investigation. Once the patient is stabilized, radiographs and other imaging may be useful to exclude fracture and evaluate preexisting arthropathy.

Deep and impalpable joints such as the hip are difficult to examine, and ultrasonography is the best means of demonstrating or excluding intra-articular bleeding or effusion. This will also be the case in peripheral joints with small effusions or in obese patients. Joints related to the spine may require CT or MRI to detect involvement, although this would be an unusual occurrence.

Hemarthrosis may be first detected by imaging when patients present with less specific complaints, including pain, anemia, and limitation of movement. Therefore, the imaging criterion for the diagnosis of blood in a joint should be known for all the standard techniques.

Recurrent Hemarthrosis

Synovial thickening occurs as a result of repeated hemarthrosis. There seems to be a trigger that can turn reactive synovial thickening into an aggressive and progressively destructive synovitis leading to subsequent destruction of the articular surface. Repeated bleeding is the most potent cause, although the exact reason for its onset is not clear. Clinically the patient will suffer from progressive joint dysfunction, manifest by increased stiffness.

In this stage of disease, imaging may be misleading in distinguishing free fluid from synovial thickening, especially if too much reliance is placed on MRI. Synovial thick-

ening and fluid are indistinguishable on plain films. The synovial tissue will have a rich blood supply, and although bone scintigraphy may reflect this on blood pool images it cannot reliably differentiate between the low-grade synovial irritation seen in virtually all joint effusions and significant synovial proliferation. Ultrasonography is arguably the most useful test. Fluid has minimal echoes whereas synovial thickening is echogenic with blood flow seen on spectral Doppler imaging. CT with intravenous contrast medium enhancement can be used, whereas plain CT may confuse the two intra-articular substances. Regrettably, the MRI appearances of fluid and synovial thickening are the same on T1- and T2-weighted images. The blood supply to synovium will become apparent after intravenous administration of gadolinium-diethylenetetramine-pentaacetic acid (Gd-DTPA), especially if fat suppression is employed on postcontrast T1-weighted images. It is tempting but inaccurate to rely on conventional MR signal changes to "exclude" synovitis. Intra-articular contrast would work with either CT or MRI, but fortunately there is a better alternative. If ultrasonography is available this is a less expensive and faster means to diagnose synovial fluid and thickening than either CT or MRI contrast studies.

Chronic Joint Pain and Dysfunction

Whereas radiographs will give an overview of joint degeneration, showing a widened intercondylar notch, MRI is usually the investigation of choice when surgery is being contemplated. MRI will show hemorrhage at varying ages with hemosiderin deposition, which appears as a signal void (i.e., "black") on all sequences. The differential diagnosis of such a patient's arthropathy would be pigmented villonodular synovitis. Operating on a hemophilic patient is so hazardous and expensive that it would be wise to obtain as much data as possible by noninvasive techniques even when clinical circumstances may not warrant complex imaging in a similar patient with normal coagulation.

Acute Soft Tissue Hemorrhage

Patients present with acute pain, swelling, and dysfunction. There may be secondary complications resulting from the enlargement of a hematoma. For example, there may be compression of adjacent nerves or vascular structures. In this phase of disease, acute hematomas or soft tissue collections can cause severe compression of a nerve or vessel such that urgent surgery will be considered.

It may be argued that MRI should be the first and only investigation for the investigation of soft tissue hemorrhage and its complications. CT with ultrasonography should only be employed when MRI is not available (Fig. 71-1).

Recurrent Soft Tissue Hemorrhage

For the reasons listed earlier, ultrasonography or MRI is the best means of showing a recurrent soft tissue hemorrhage.

Chronic Mass Lesion/Pseudotumor

Pseudotumors are a rare complication of hemophilia, occurring in 1% to 2% of patients with severe hemophilia

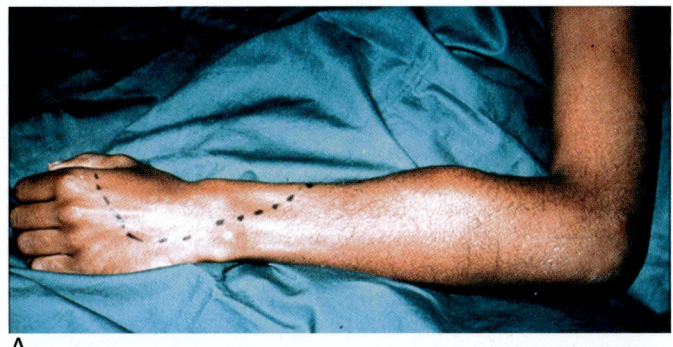

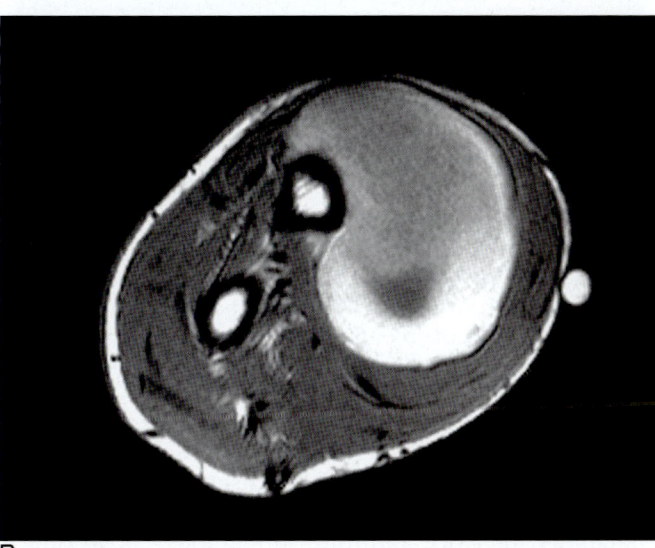

■ **FIGURE 71-1** Soft tissue hemorrhage. **A,** Clinical photograph depicting soft tissue swelling due to a hematoma compressing the radial nerve resulting in paresthesia (as demarcated by the ink markings). **B,** Axial T1-weighted MR image through the forearm shows an acute hematoma.

(clotting factor level <1% of normal). The pseudotumor grows as a chronic, slowly expanding, encapsulated cystic mass as a result of recurrent hemorrhage into extra-articular soft tissue sites and therefore presents as a slowly enlarging mass. Pseudotumors are categorized as osseous and soft tissue lesions, on the basis of anatomic location. The sites most frequently affected are, in order of descending frequency, the femur, pelvis, tibia, and small bones of the hand. Radiographic findings vary greatly with the extent, location, and different stages of hemorrhage and reflect the presence of medullary bone destruction, cortical changes, internal opacities, various types of periosteal reaction, and surrounding soft tissue abnormalities. With these variable radiographic appearances, osseous hemophilic pseudotumors can be confused with other tumorous or infectious conditions.[1]

MRI is unrivaled in the detection, staging, and follow up of soft tissue bleeding with mass effects.

Life-Threatening Blood Loss

Because transfusion factor replacement and immobilization are the emergency treatments for massive blood loss, imaging has little immediate role and probably should be avoided.

Exceptions to this rule would be in a penetrating injury or fracture when the same protocols that would be considered for those with normal coagulation should be applied.

Fracture

When the nature of the injury might have caused a fracture, then radiographs are always indicated. CT may be used to support the diagnosis and further characterize complex fractures if surgery is necessary.

PATHOPHYSIOLOGY

It is well recognized that repeated bleeding into the joint is responsible for synovial and cartilage changes.[2,3] Blood appears to have three effects that result in joint destruction: a direct effect on the cartilage and indirect effects of synovial proliferation and induction of inflammatory cells.

Blood appears to have a direct toxic effect on cartilage before and independent of its other effects. The direct effects of blood on cartilage precede synovial changes, and synovitis may be secondary to articular cartilage damage. Studies show that after exposure to blood there is inhibition of matrix formation and increased matrix breakdown, resulting in a loss of matrix.[4]

Iron deposition seems to be the mechanism by which bleeding into a joint exerts its indirect effects. Acute episodes of bleeding result in the formation of a dark clot containing fluid within the joint. After repeated episodes, resorption is incomplete, resulting in the synovial membrane taking on a brown tint caused by blood pigment absorption. This progressive accumulation of iron deposits in the synovium is an important characteristic and thought to be the trigger for synovial inflammation with proliferation in number and hypertrophy of the synovial villi. The hemosiderin deposits may attract lymphocytes. The inflammatory changes are mild in comparison with true inflammatory arthropathies such as rheumatoid arthritis. The presence of synovial iron deposits is also seen in other joint disorders such as pigmented villonodular synovitis, hemangiomas, and hemosiderotic synovitis. All of these disorders share a pattern of joint destruction that resembles hemophilic arthropathy, suggesting iron deposition is important. It is thus thought that the accumulation of iron within the joint is a stimulus for synovial proliferation[5-8] and an attractant for inflammatory cells that produce enzymes and cytokines that cause destruction of articular cartilage.[9]

Pseudotumors represent an uncommon complication of hemophilia and occur in 1% to 2% of patients with severe forms of the disease.[10] Pseudotumors represent chronic, slowly expanding hematomas. The lesions are encapsulated and often occur in the soft tissues but may arise in bone or subperiosteum. Pseudotumors that occur in muscles with broad tendon insertions progress to cause severe pressure erosion of adjacent bone.[11] The bones most commonly affected are the femur, pelvis, tibia, and bones of the hand.

Pathologically, pseudotumors consist of blood products in various stages of evolution with a fibrous capsule (Fig. 71-2). Hemosiderin-laden macrophages are seen within the

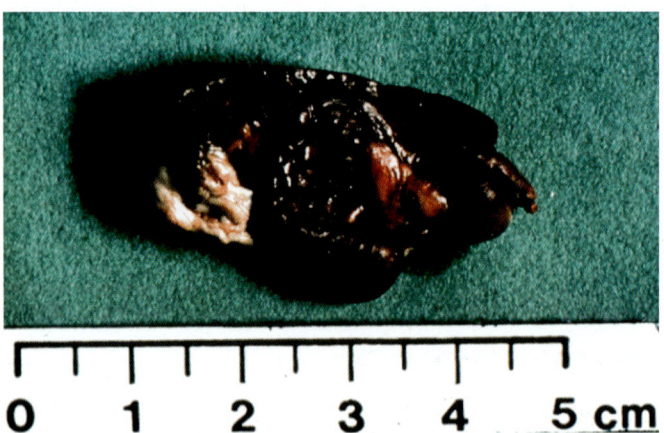

■ **FIGURE 71-2** Pseudotumor specimen. Note the predominant composition is dark material, indicative of hemosiderin deposition.

fibrous capsule.[12] As the pseudotumor enlarges there may be increasing pressure on adjacent structures that may undergo necrosis. The result can be destruction of adjacent bone or necrosis of muscle and skin. Compartment syndromes and joint contractures can also occur.[11] The tumors are usually painless, but there may be compression of adjacent nerves resulting in pain or neurologic dysfunction. Pain can also result from pathologic fractures. As pseudotumors progress, function of the extremity will be compromised. Rarely, pseudotumors have ruptured, resulting in exanguination.[11] These complications may develop suddenly in patients who previously exhibited no symptoms or appeared clinically stable.[10,13]

MANIFESTATIONS OF THE DISEASE

Acute Hemarthrosis

It is usually difficult on clinical and imaging grounds to determine if an effusion is composed of fresh blood as opposed to transudate or pus. It would normally be necessary to aspirate the joint to confirm hemarthrosis. This may be a hazardous procedure without factor replacement capability, and this will always occur when the coagulation disorder is not yet discovered. Those who aspirate joints must be aware of this risk. Imaging control or guidance is useful to ensure that the joint was punctured and not an adjacent vessel. Joint aspiration techniques are described elsewhere, but there are specific precautions to be taken when a coagulopathy is known or suspected. These include adequate cover with blood factor replacement, strict aseptic technique to minimize the risk of infection, and immobilization after the procedure in those with antibodies to injected coagulation factor. The risk of introducing infection or precipitating fresh hemorrhage should be balanced against the risk of failing to detect septic arthritis. A principal role of imaging is to avoid unnecessary joint puncture when there is no fluid present. CT, MRI, or ultrasonography can all be used to guide the needle placement. After the procedure, CT, ultrasonography, or MRI may be used to assess how much fluid remains. For practical and financial reasons, ultrasonography is the method of choice.

Radiography

If careful attention is paid to the soft tissue planes, radiographs may show joint effusion, but in practice these signs are of minimal value. When radiographic signs are apparent, joint distention is clinically obvious. In the early stages when the effusion is small and difficult to detect clinically the assessment of fat stripes next to joints may be very misleading and, with the exception of the elbow (Fig. 71-3), prone to overinterpretation.[14] The availability of other imaging methods means that the plain radiographic signs of acute disease are now largely of historic interest.

Magnetic Resonance Imaging

Magnetic resonance imaging is very sensitive to joint fluid, especially on T2-weighted images where fluid returns a high signal (Fig. 71-4). If a fat suppression technique is employed, the signal from fat cannot obscure the details of the joint effusion. Unenhanced MRI cannot determine the degree of synovitis. The swollen synovium has the same signal as fluid within the joint on most conventional images. Some would argue that magnetisation (or saturation) transfer contrast (MTC) in MRI is an improvement but there are still problems, and enhancement with intravenous Gd-DTPA is necessary for precision.

Multidetector Computed Tomography

Computed tomography may be used to demonstrate swelling and hemorrhage into joints. With the now wide availability of MRI and ultrasonography, however, it is less important in the acute phase of a hemarthrosis. As with ultrasonography, the presence of fluid in the joint

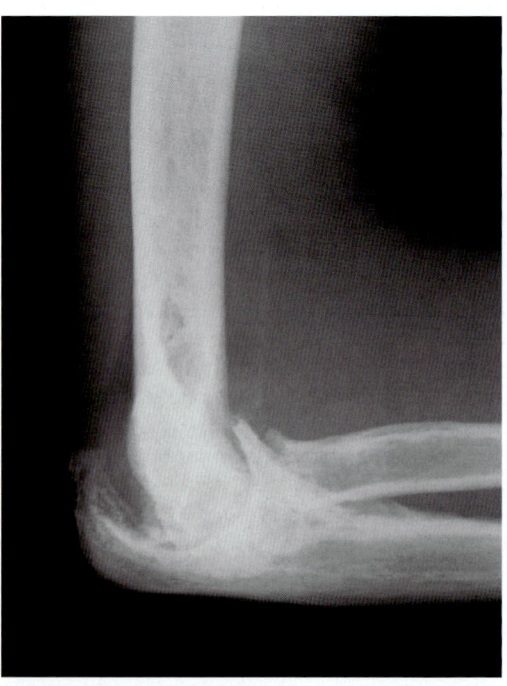

■ **FIGURE 71-3** Lateral radiograph of the elbow in a hemophiliac patient. There is elevation of the anterior and posterior fat pads indicating elbow joint effusion. Note also the accompanying degenerative changes.

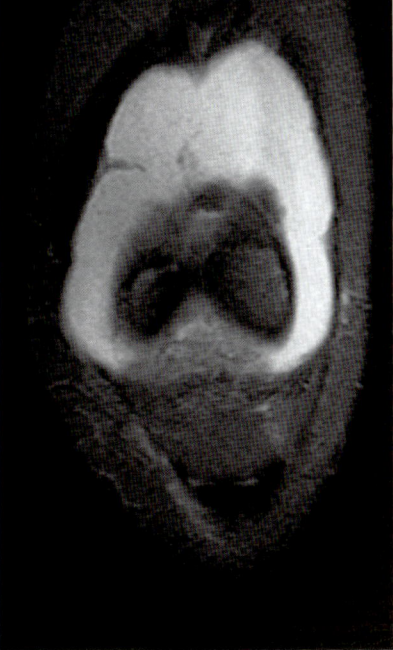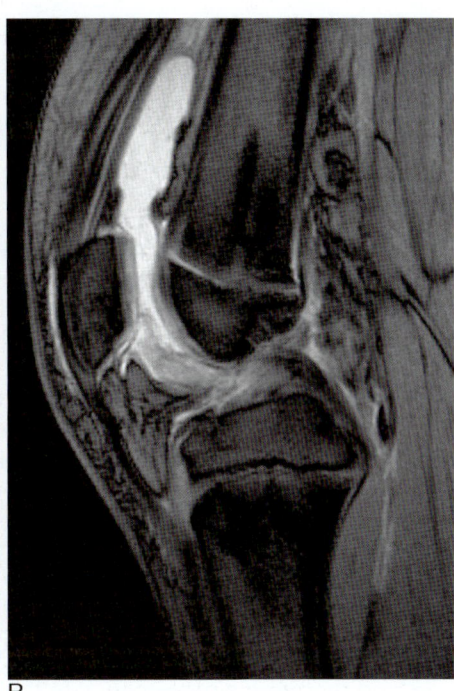

A   B

■ **FIGURE 71-4** Acute effusion. **A,** Coronal STIR MR image shows fluid in the suprapatellar pouch. **B,** Sagittal gradient-echo MR image depicts an acute hemarthrosis in a skeletally immature patient (note the unfused epiphysis).

is not specific to the type of fluid and the technique adds little to the simple detection of fluid. Differentiation of synovial thickening from joint fluid is sometimes possible but less reliable than with ultrasound evaluation. To be certain, intravenous administration of a contrast agent is required. The synovial blood supply will enhance the perfused tissues whereas only very late images will show attenuation change in the joint fluid.

Ultrasonography

Ultrasonography is the best means of detecting joint effusions.[15] Fluid, whether it is transudate, pus, or blood, is seen as an echo-free area adjacent to bone and within the capsule. Comparison with the normal side is useful. Effusions of as little as 1 mL can be detected (Fig. 71-5). Unfortunately, severe hemorrhages into the hip may cause the joint to sublux or dislocate. Fluid then falls into the gap and is less obvious on ultrasonography and may be very difficult to identify. Therefore, to avoid this diagnostic pitfall, any irritable hip that looks normal on ultrasonography should be examined by plain radiographs.[16] Synovial thickening is easily identified as echogenic layers on the inner aspect of the capsule. It may be that synovial hypertrophy predicts the onset of an aggressive arthropathy, but this hypothesis is not yet confirmed. Should further work confirm this, then ultrasonography will have an important role in deciding when to treat synovial hypertrophy aggressively.

Chronic Joint Changes

Five pathologic processes take place in joints subjected to recurrent chronic hemorrhage: hyperemia, synovial hypertrophy, hemosiderin deposition, articular surface destruction, and osseous cysts. Each produces its own radiologic

features, and only some or all of these may be present in the same joint. Appearances vary widely between joints in the same patient, making asymmetry the norm.

Although plain films will give an overview of joint degeneration, MRI is usually the investigation of choice when surgery is being contemplated. Operating on a hemophilic patient is so hazardous and expensive that it would be wise to obtain as much data as possible by

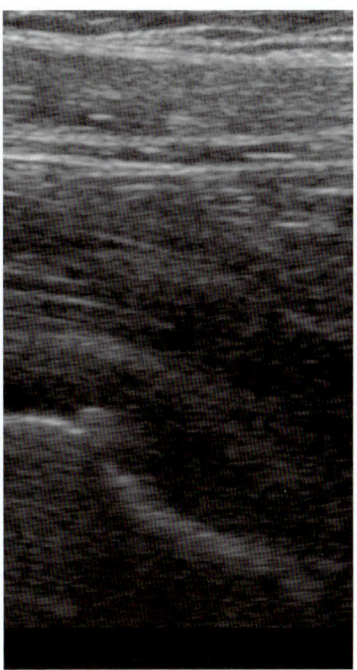

■ **FIGURE 71-5** Joint effusion in hip joint. The effusion is seen on an ultrasound image as a hypoechoic abnormality anterior to the femoral head and neck. A small osteophyte is present.

noninvasive techniques even when clinical circumstances may not warrant complex imaging in a similar patient with normal coagulation.

Radiography

Hyperemia

Hemarthrosis leads to immobility of a joint and disuse osteoporosis. Recurrent hemarthrosis results in increased blood supply to the joint. Apart from the direct imaging signs of this phenomenon (increased signal on short tau inversion recovery [STIR] sequences and increased activity on bone scintigraphy) there may be an effect on growth of the immature skeleton. This can lead to hypertrophy of the areas of growth, leading to some of the classic radiographic signs of hemophilia. For example, in the knee there is squaring of the patella (Fig. 71-6A) and enlargement of the femoral condyles (see Fig. 71-6B). At the ankle, overgrowth of the medial malleolus in relation to the lateral tibial epiphysis results in tibiotalar slant (see Fig. 71-6C). In the elbow, there is enlargement of the radial head. Hyperemia can lead to premature epiphyseal closure and therefore a discrepancy in limb size with apparent hemihypertrophy. Any bones adjacent to a recurrent hemarthrosis may be affected. Harris growth lines are also a prominent feature in growing bone due to interval stresses. These features are summarized in Table 71-1, but many are not exclusive to hemophilia and may be seen in chronic infection and some juvenile inflammatory arthropathies.

Synovial Hypertrophy

Although many hemarthroses settle with no residual sequelae, on occasion an aggressive synovial response may follow. This causes prolonged or chronic synovial hypertrophy and, in due course, invasion of the adjacent joint margins. There will be some evidence of joint space thickening with fat pad displacement followed by an erosive destruction reminiscent of rheumatoid arthritis. These changes are unpredictable and vary widely between joints that have been affected by similarly severe hemorrhages in the same patient. They may be rapid and disabling (Fig. 71-7). Erosion at the site of ligamentous attachments may account for some of the well-recognized features of hemophilia, such as widening of the intercondylar notch of the knee (Fig. 71-8).

Hemosiderin Deposition

Each time blood is present within the joint hemosiderin is deposited in the synovial lining. This gradually increases the density of the synovium and adjacent tissues on plain radiographs. Although the sign of a homogenous increase in density of the joint tissues is described as an "opaque effusion," strictly it is not the effusion that is dense but the soft tissues (Fig. 71-9).

Articular Surface Damage

After recurrent hemorrhage within a joint, synovial hypertrophy, and bony overgrowth there is likely to be premature and accelerated osteoarthritis. This has many of the usual and typical features of this condition, although there is often a paucity of osteophytes and subchondral cyst formation may be out of proportion to the joint space narrowing. Unlike degenerative osteoarthritis, arthritis that results from hemarthroses occurs asymmetrically (Fig. 71-10) and in young patients. Joint ankylosis is now rare in hemophilia, probably owing to better medical management of the acute hemarthrosis and its prevention.

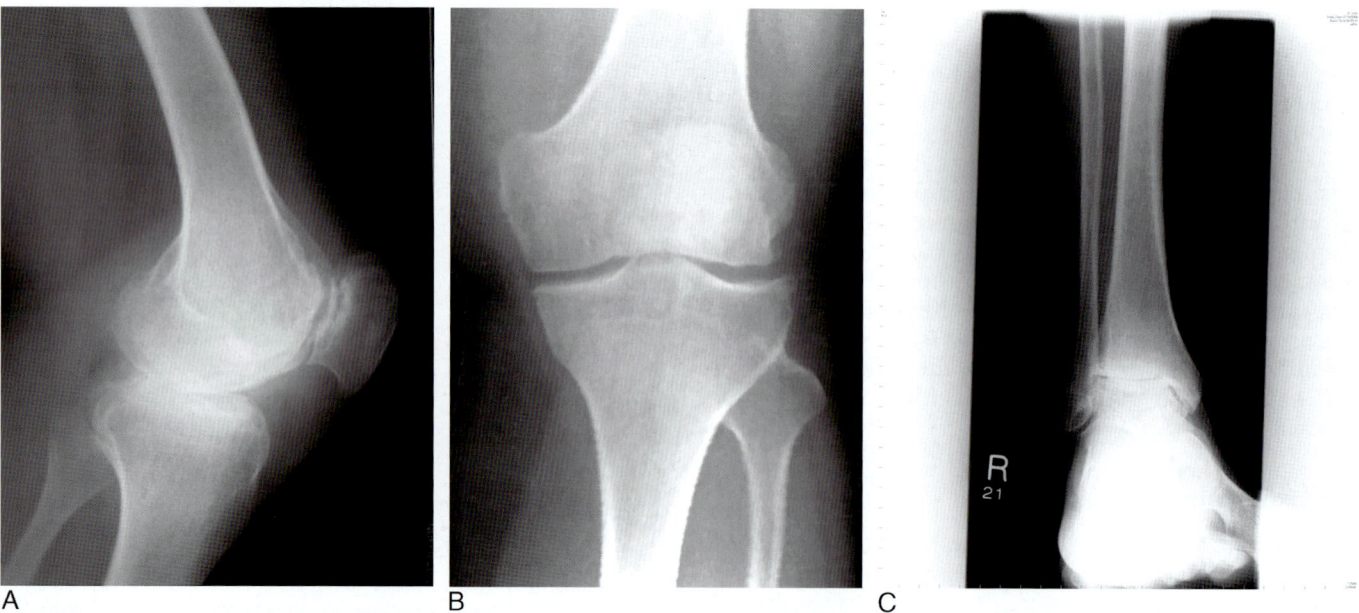

A   B   C

■ **FIGURE 71-6** Classic radiographic findings in hemophilia. **A,** Note squaring of inferior pole of patella. **B,** Enlarged femoral condyles. **C,** Tibiotalar slant.

TABLE 71-1 Manifestations of Hemophilia in Different Joints

Joint Affected (in order of frequency)	Typical Radiographic Changes
Knee	Enlarged femoral condyles, widened intercondylar notch, squared patella
Elbow	Radial head enlargement, cystic change at the radial notch of the ulna, olecranon fossa enlargement leading to a large olecranon foramen
Ankle	Tibiotalar slant
Shoulder	Osteophyte formation, cysts, small humeral head with a varus deformity
Wrist	Distal ulnar growth disturbance, subluxed distal radioulnar joint, carpal cysts
Hip	Avascular necrosis of the femoral head mimicking Legg-Calvé-Perthes disease thought to be due to occlusion of the epiphyseal vessels secondary to hemarthrosis; axial migration of the femoral head with protrusio acetabuli
Hand	Cysts
Foot	Talar collapse, mimicking a Charcot joint, plantarflexion, forefoot adduction

Intraosseous Cyst Formation

Subchondral cysts may be the result of osteoarthritis, but some intraosseous cysts seen in coagulopathy-induced joint disease occur in the metaphysis at a surprising distance from the affected joint surfaces. These are thought to be due to intraosseous bleeding or erosion from the hypertrophied synovium. Remote cysts may collapse, presenting as acute pain and mechanical derangement (Fig. 71-11).

Magnetic Resonance Imaging

Magnetic resonance imaging is the best method of judging the nature and extent of joint destruction and soft tissue change. Subchondral and distant cysts are obvious as areas of high signal intensity replacing bone on T2-weighted images. They will be of low signal compared with the bright marrow on T1-weighted images (Fig. 71-12). Synovial erosion and deformity are well demonstrated. Articular surface damage is seen best on MRI, although not with the accuracy of arthroscopy. Because it is unlikely that a patient with a coagulation disorder will be subjected to "routine" diagnostic arthroscopy, this limitation of MRI should be recognized. Synovial fibrosis and hemosiderin deposition will be demonstrated as areas of low signal intensity on all sequences (Fig. 71-13). Most important, MRI has the ability to exclude most other pathologic processes, such as infection, tears of the menisci, fracture, and tumor. A normal MRI study should be considered very reassuring.

Multidetector Computed Tomography

Hemosiderin deposition will increase the attenuation of the soft tissues around the joint. All the bony features of chronic arthropathies are well demonstrated on CT, with the possible exception of articular surface damage. Because the images are acquired in the supine position, even with the advent of 3D reconstruction and the modest soft tissue contrast provided by CT, radiographs especially when obtained with the patient bearing weight are more precise.

Ultrasonography

Other than in the detection of synovial thickening there is no obvious role for ultrasonography in patients with chronic hemophilic arthropathy.

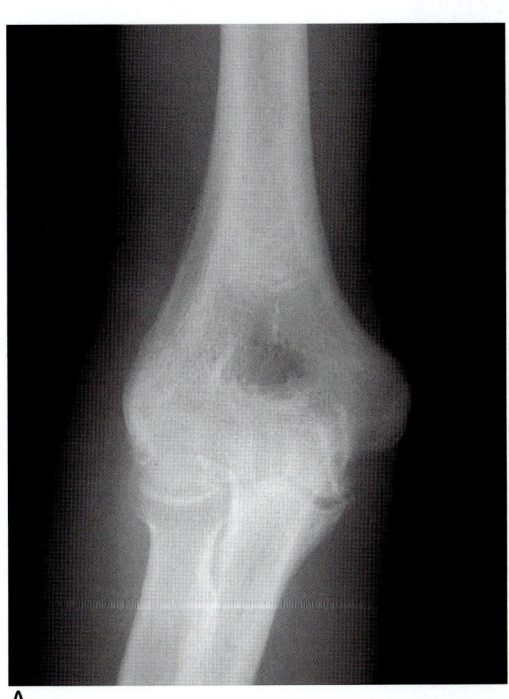
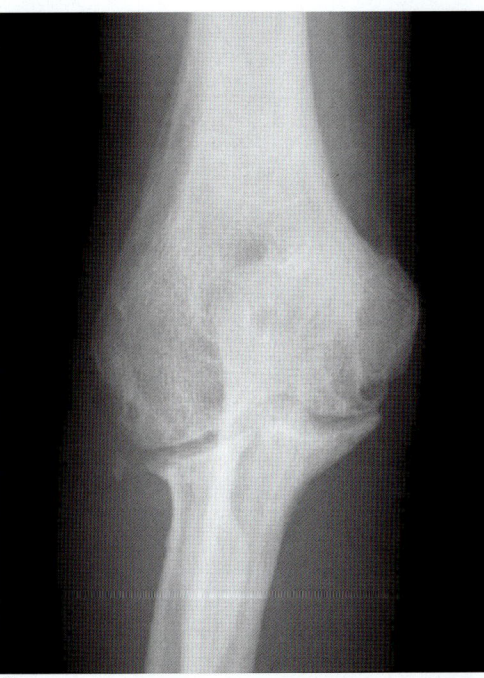

■ **FIGURE 71-7** A and B, Radiographs of elbow in the same patient 3 years apart. Note the rapid progress in degenerative changes over this time interval.

A

B

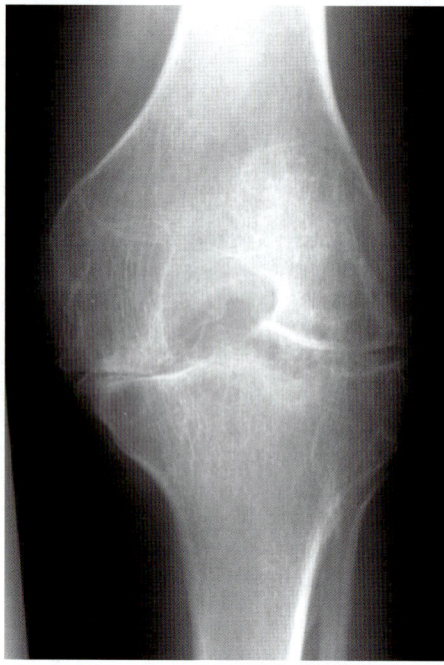

FIGURE 71-8 Widening of the intercondylar notch. This radiographic finding appears to be secondary to erosion at ligamentous attachments.

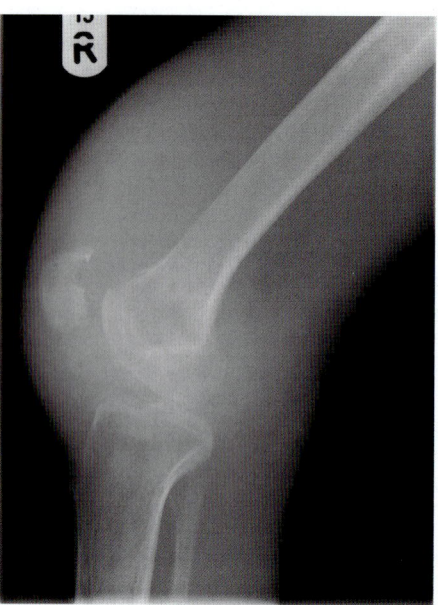

FIGURE 71-9 Radiograph of an opaque effusion. Note increased opacity in the suprapatellar pouch. This is not secondary to bleeding into the joint but indicates chronic synovitis and hemosiderin deposition.

Acute Soft Tissue Changes

Ultrasonography, CT, and MRI can all be used for detection of acute soft tissue hemorrhage. Ultrasound evaluation is not effective in showing the full extent of the hemorrhage and in this respect cannot act as a baseline investigation. In these cases, it should be regarded as a screening test and MRI relied on for precise diagnosis. It may be argued that MRI should be the first and only investigation.

Radiography

Plain radiographs are insensitive to soft tissue hemorrhage and have little value except when an associated fracture is suspected.

Magnetic Resonance Imaging

Magnetic resonance imaging is the best method of demonstrating the presence and extent of a soft tissue

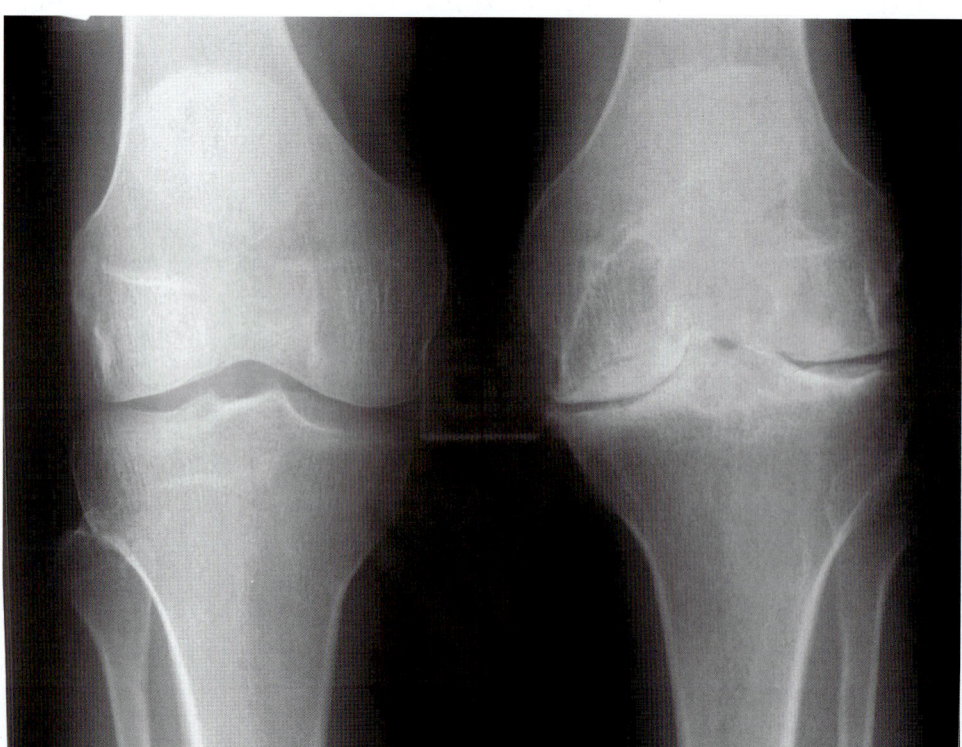

FIGURE 71-10 Radiography demonstrates the asymmetric distribution of disease at the knee joints in this patient with hemophilia.

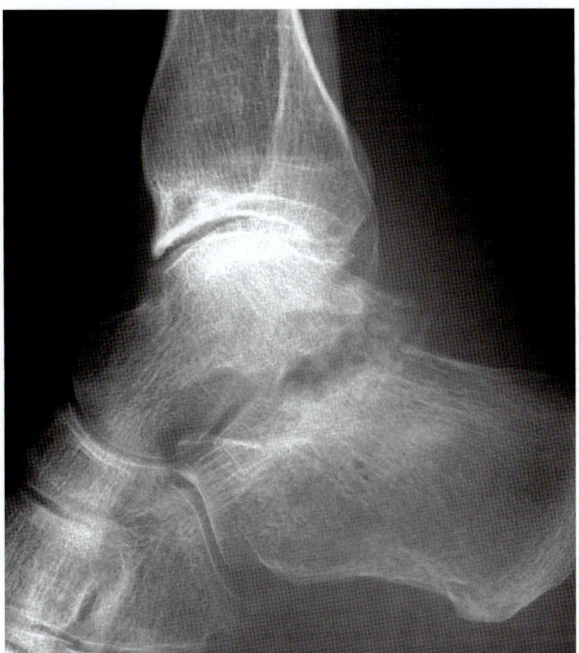

■ FIGURE 71-11 Anteroposterior and lateral view of ankle. There is loss of joint space with subchondral cyst formation.

hemorrhage. Fat-saturated or fast STIR techniques have the contrast that rivals ultrasonography. In early hemorrhages when ultrasound shows echogenic blood, MRI is probably more accurate in differentiation of a hemorrhage from normal muscle. MRI also has the advantage of being easily reproduced and of providing large

field-of-view multiplanar images that allow accurate follow-up and surgical planning (Figs. 71-14 and 71-15).

Multidetector Computed Tomography

Multidetector CT will show new soft tissue hemorrhage as a mass effect displacing other structures that appears of higher attenuation than muscle. As the form of the hematoma changes, the attenuation will diminish through patchy changes, to one with a thick wall and pseudocapsule. Further imaging will be necessary if there is pseudotumor formation. Comparison with the normal side is useful in detecting smaller hemorrhages. As an acute hematoma matures, CT shows less contrast between blood and muscle than does ultrasonography. In the subacute phase, blood becomes isodense to muscle on CT.

Ultrasonography

Hemorrhage into soft tissue is easily and reliably detected by ultrasonography, provided that the examiner understands the spectrum of appearances and their relationship to the age of the hemorrhage. In muscles, the hemorrhage can take two forms, either diffuse bleeding with dissociation of the muscle fibers and exaggeration of the "penniform" appearance or a discrete hematoma. An acute hemorrhage is seen as a low echo zone and can look like fluid, with posterior acoustic enhancement. Within 1 or 2 hours, areas of fibrin clot appear in the hemorrhage. These are highly echogenic. Note that most coagulopathies do not prevent the fibrin cascade and clots are expected in hemophilia. After 1 or 2 days the

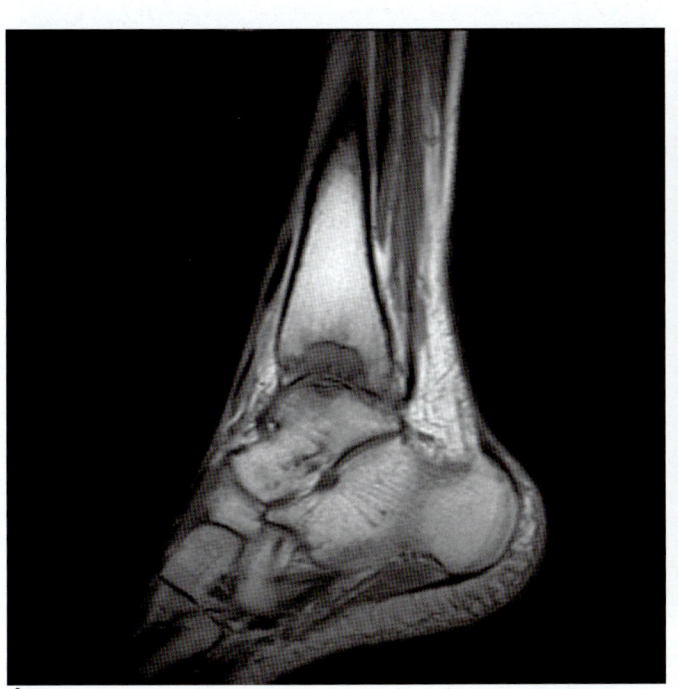

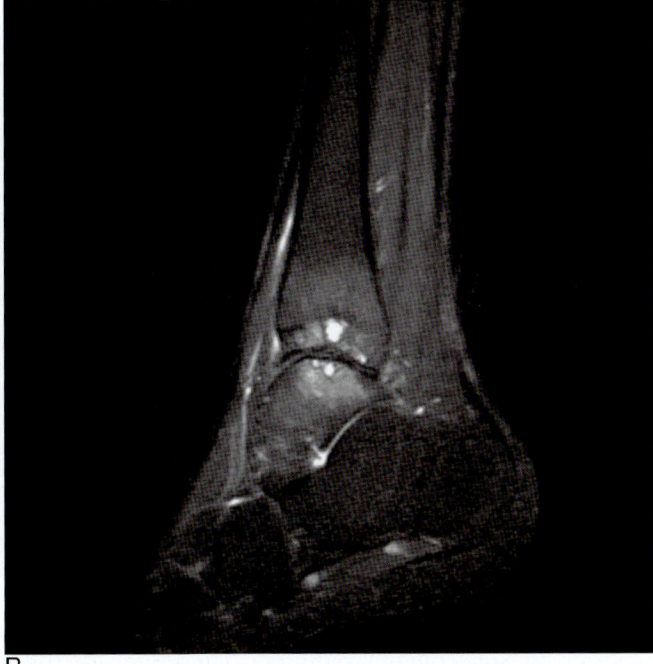

A   B

■ FIGURE 71-12 Subchondral cysts. MR images of ankle of the same patient as in Figure 71-11 show low signal intensity on T1-weighted imaging (**A**) and high signal intensity on T2-weighted imaging (**B**).

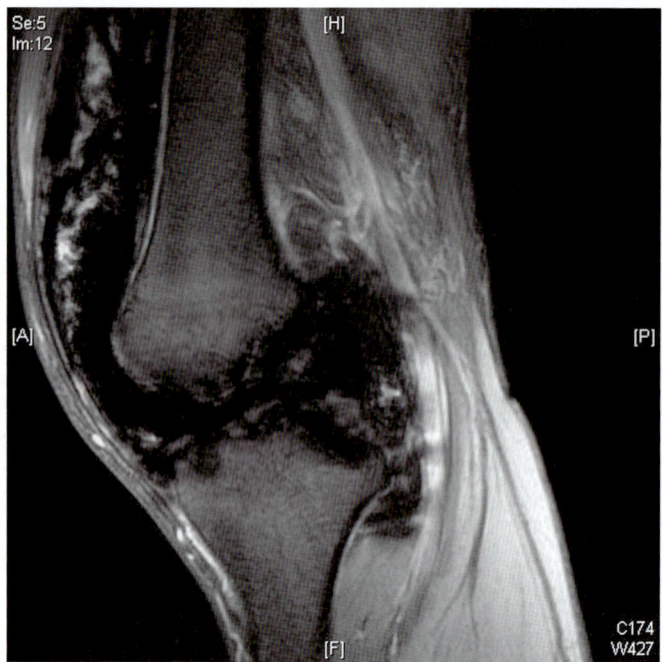

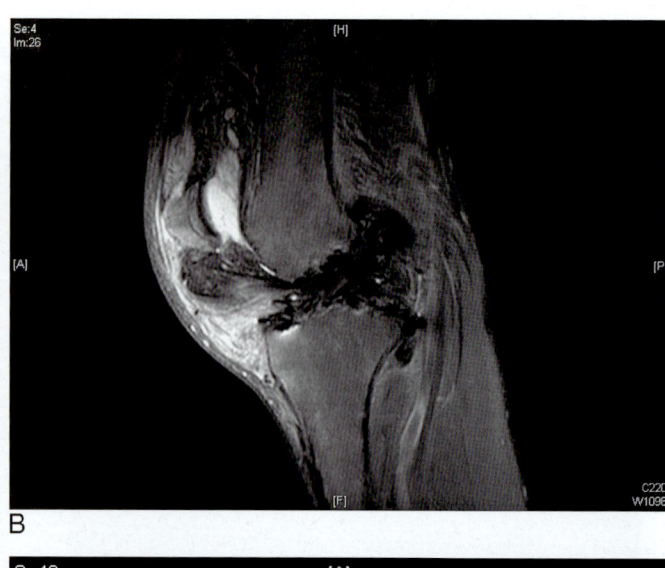

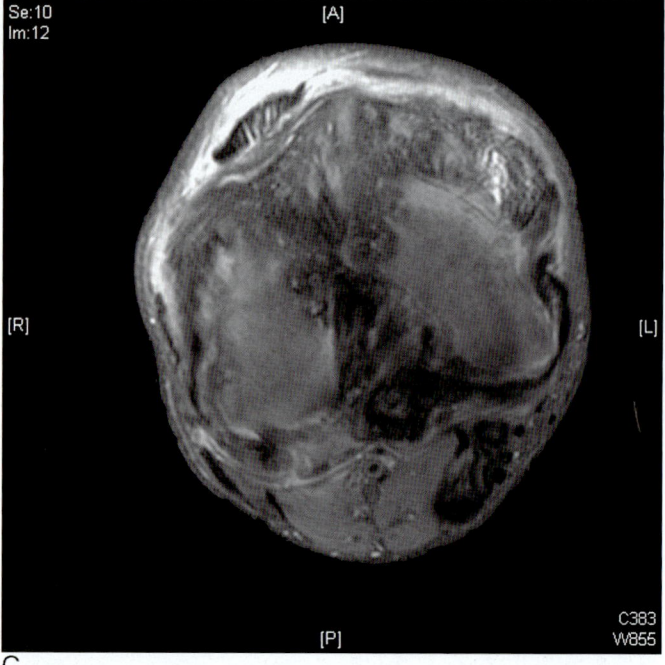

■ **FIGURE 71-13** **A** and **B,** Gradient-echo MR images of the knee of a patient with advanced hemophilia. There is low signal abnormality in the synovium, secondary to hemosiderin deposition. Gradient-echo images are most sensitive to susceptibility, and this can be seen in the marked "blooming" artifact. **C,** Proton density–weighted fat-suppressed MR image. Again, low signal is seen in the synovium. The degree of artifact is less than seen on the gradient-echo sequence. There is florid synovitis.

whole hematoma becomes echogenic. After a few more days and certainly by the end of a week the solid mass starts to liquefy and areas of hypoechogenicity appear. They coalesce to form an inspissated collection that is largely fluid. It can be months or even years before it fully resolves, but the hematoma may resorb fully at any stage and only the minority will still be present a year from the onset (Fig. 71-16). Unfortunately, ultrasonography is very observer dependent and it is difficult to record the spread of the hemorrhage in a way that can be interpreted and compared by subsequent examiners. Therefore, for this purpose MRI is preferred.

Chronic Soft Tissue Changes

Magnetic Resonance Imaging

Hemosiderin deposition will lead to susceptibility artifact exaggerated on gradient-echo images because they are more sensitive to the presence of metal than other sequences. Indeed, gradient-echo sequences may be chosen for their marked sensitivity to metal deposition. The hemosiderin will be seen as areas of low signal intensity on all MRI sequences; this is, however, not pathognomonic to hemophilia, and other conditions such as pigmented villonodular synovitis, synovial hemangioma, neuropathic

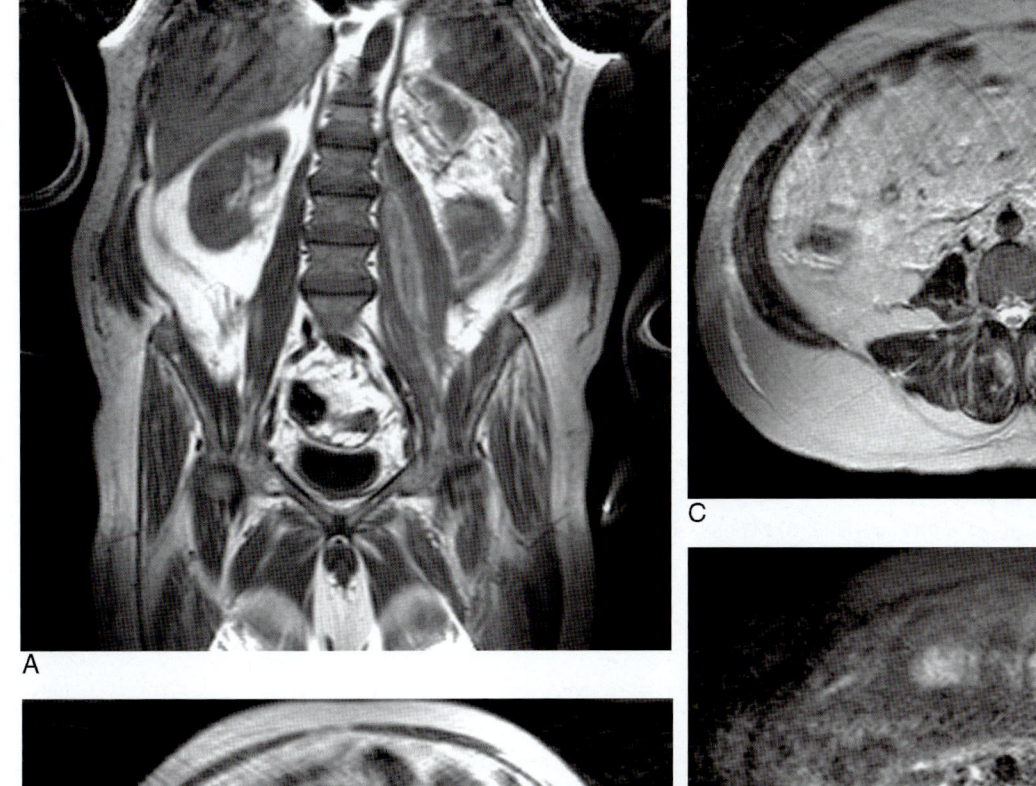

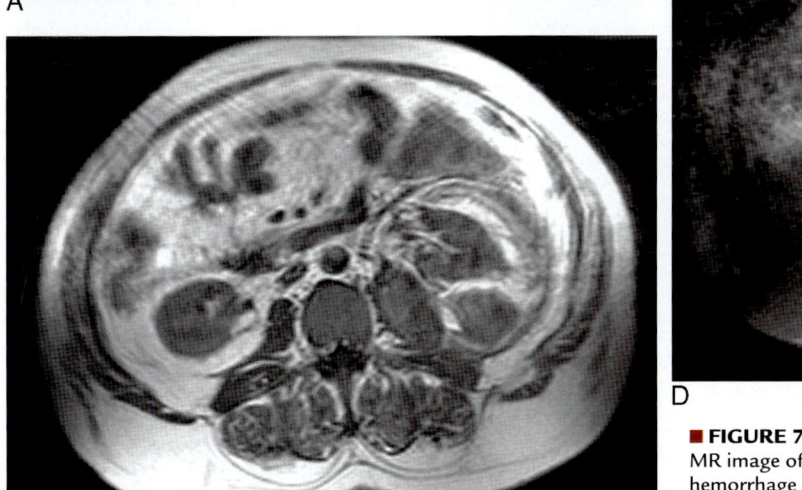

■ **FIGURE 71-14** Hemorrhage in the psoas muscle. **A,** Coronal MR image of the posterior abdominal wall showing an intramuscular hemorrhage into the left psoas muscle. **B** to **D,** Axial T1- and T2-weighted MR images of an acute intramuscular hemorrhage into the left psoas. Note that there is intermediate intensity on the T1-weighted sequences and brightness on the T2-weighted sequences, indicating acute hemorrhage.

osteoarthropathy, and amyloid deposition in chronic renal failure should also be considered. Calcification and ossification may be difficult to detect using MRI. They are seen as focal areas of reduced signal on all sequences, and they are easily overlooked because they have similar appearances to the fibrous septa between muscles.

Multidetector Computed Tomography

Hemosiderin deposition will increase the density of the soft tissues. Calcification and ossification will be readily seen on multidetector CT.

Ultrasonography

Old hematomas, scars, muscle atrophy, old areas of hemorrhage and calcification/ossification all may be observed using ultrasound. Ultrasound evaluation can be done under dynamic conditions because it is possible to ask the patient to reproduce the symptoms while watching the image in real time. By this means, partial muscle tears, tethered scars, and muscle herniation through fascial planes may uniquely be seen.

Recurrent Hemorrhage

Magnetic Resonance Imaging

The MRI signal from a hematoma changes with time. There is less knowledge regarding the timing of changes because MRI is a much newer technique than ultrasonography, but this will change with experience. Our studies suggest that MRI has the same or better potential for dating hemorrhages and in detecting recurrence of ongoing hemorrhage (Table 71-2).

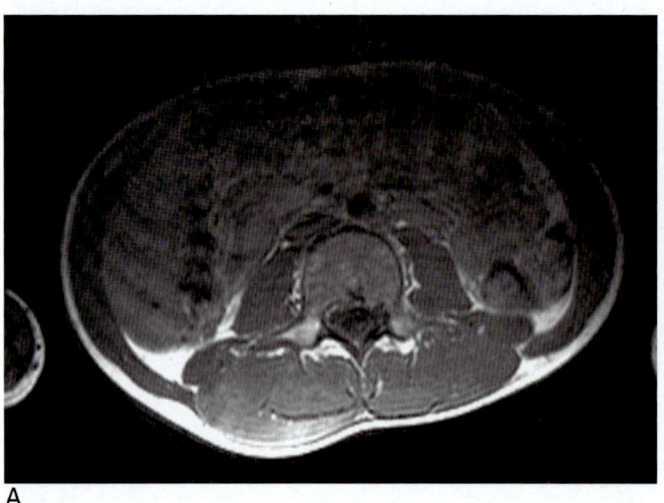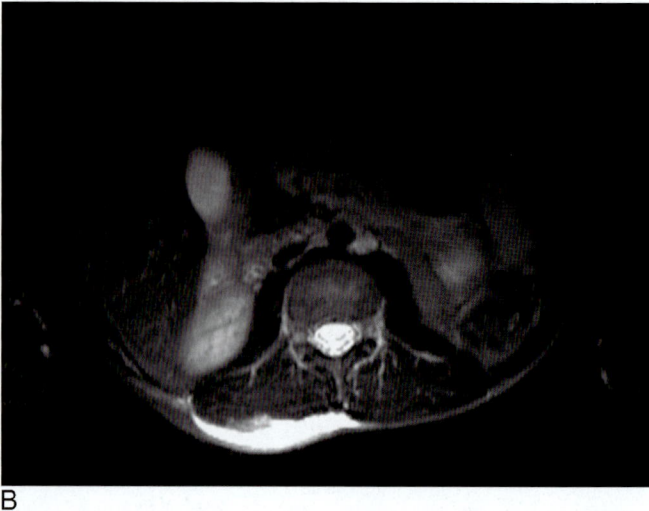

A   B

■ **FIGURE 71-15** Axial T1-weighted (**A**) and T2-weighted (**B**) MR images of an acute soft tissue hemorrhage, posterior to the right paraspinal muscle, enclosed within the fascial layer and deep to the fat layer. Note the high signal intensity on STIR imaging but intermediate signal intensity on T1-weighted imaging that characterizes a recent hemorrhage.

Multidetector Computed Tomography

Computed tomography will show the focal changes of a recurrent hemorrhage but with less contrast than on ultrasonography. In addition, the disadvantage of the radiation dose from repeated CT examinations should be considered if ultrasonography or MRI is available.

As the limb falls into disuse because of pain and mechanical dysfunction there will be muscle atrophy. This may be sufficiently rapid to mask the fact that the hematoma is enlarging. As the limb decreases in cross section on serial studies an enlarging hematoma may be overlooked.

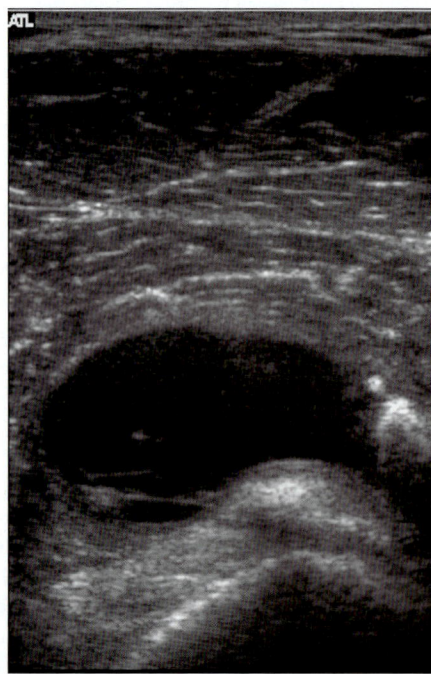

■ **FIGURE 71-16** Ultrasound image of recent and chronic hemorrhage.

Ultrasonography

Ultrasonography has a particular role in recurrent hemorrhage. A newly echogenic area within the echo-free semichronic collection is a strong indication of additional and recent hemorrhage.

Pseudotumor

Pseudotumors are categorized as osseous and soft tissue lesions on the basis of anatomic location. The sites most frequently affected, are, in order of descending frequency, the femur, pelvis, tibia, and small bones of the hand. Radiologic findings vary greatly across all modalities and with the extent, location, and different stages of hemorrhage. The variable radiographic appearances mean that osseous hemophilic pseudotumors can be confused with other tumors or infectious conditions.

Radiography

Pseudotumors have a variable radiographic appearance, although there are some common features. The lesions tend to be lytic, but usually with a well-defined margin. Pseudotumors can become extensive, replacing segments of bone.

They may be placed in an intramedullary or eccentric location within the bone. The lesions are expansile, and osseous trabeculae often traverse the lesion.

When bleeding occurs in the subperiosteal region the hematoma may exhibit aggressive bone destruction. This may mimic an invasive soft tissue neoplasm. In adults, extrinsic destruction of the bone is typical whereas in children there is more often intrinsic expansion of bone with little soft tissue enlargement. Clues that hemophilia is the cause of a destructive mass are the combination of aggressive destruction and reparative bone formation (Fig. 71-17). This is similar to chronic osteomyelitis in its complex pattern of bone changes.

TABLE 71-2	Magnetic Resonance Imaging Characteristics in Hemophilia		
Finding	**T1-Weighted Signal Intensity**	**T2-Weighted Signal Intensity**	**Gradient-Echo T2*-Weighted Signal Intensity**
Early hemorrhage	Low	High	High
Recent hemorrhage	Intermediate	Varied/low with bright margin	High
Established hemorrhage	High	High	High
Old hemorrhage	Low/high mixed	Low/high mixed	Susceptibility

Magnetic Resonance Imaging

Magnetic resonance imaging is the definitive technique for the same reasons as soft tissue staging. It is marginally less precise than CT in showing bony change but is probably better at showing the full extent of the bone involvement because it will pick up edema in the marrow at the margins of a lesion. The pseudotumor has a capsule whose peripheral margin is often of low signal intensity on T1- and T2-weighted spin-echo sequences owing to the hemosiderin with a less uniform signal in the interior. As for ultrasonography, the detection of mural nodules is important and straightforward to recognize.

Multidetector Computed Tomography

Computed tomography not only shows the soft tissue element of a pseudotumor, but it is the most precise way of showing the bone damage and destruction (Fig. 71-18).

Ultrasonography

Ultrasonography will detect and demonstrate the soft tissue elements of a pseudotumor. With extended field-of-view imaging it can now go some way to providing a permanent set of images for follow-up comparison or surgical planning (Fig. 71-19). This information is, however, not as good as MRI or CT. Ultrasonography is unable to demonstrate the full extent of bony destruction. It may demonstrate mural plaques on the inner wall of a low-echo pseudotumor cavity, which suggests the diagnosis of pseudotumor. It is a sign that gives a strong pointer to the diagnosis because it is not seen in the conditions that may mimic pseudotumor, such as infection or soft tissue tumor.

DIFFERENTIAL DIAGNOSIS

Imaging is not wholly specific for hemophilia. Other processes result in the deposition of hemosiderin besides hemophilia. These disorders include pigmented villonodular synovitis, neoplasm (e.g., synovial hemangioma), neuropathic osteoarthropathy, and chronic renal disease.

Patients with hemophilia also suffer from nonbleeding disease. Acute appendicitis may be confused with a retroperitoneal hemorrhage. The conventional protocols for imaging patients without a coagulation disorder should be employed. However, the power of MRI to exclude

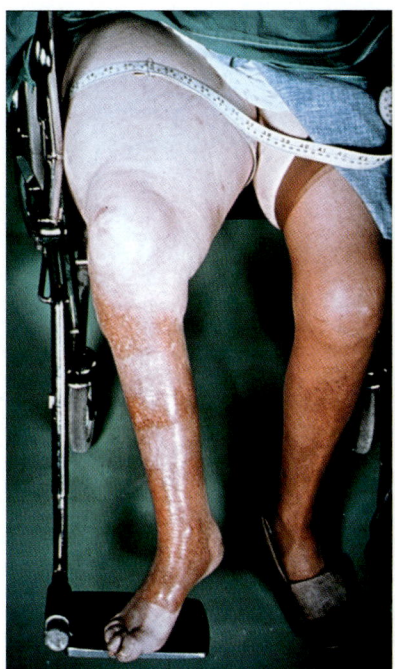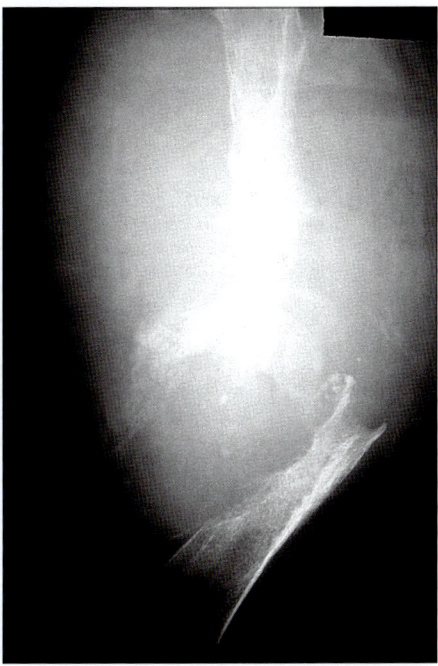

A   B

■ **FIGURE 71-17** Pseudotumors. **A,** Clinical photograph of hemophilia patient with large swelling of right thigh. **B,** Radiograph of femur of the same patient shows soft tissue swelling with underlying bone destruction.

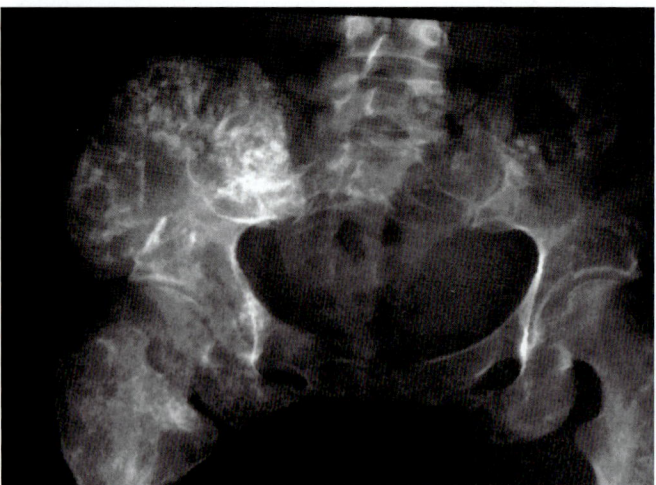

■ **FIGURE 71-18** Pseudotumor. Radiograph of pelvis shows destructive lesion in ileum.

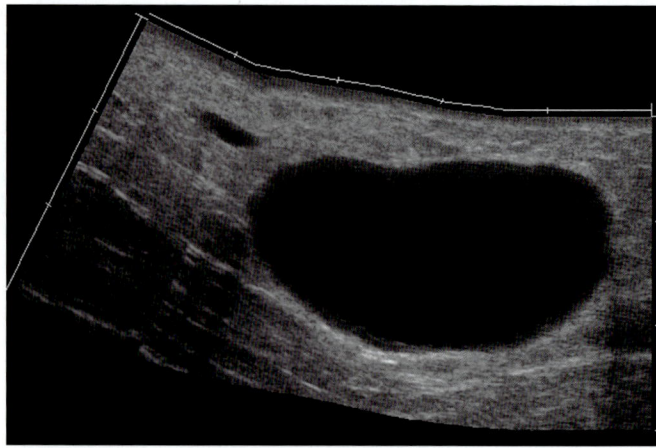

■ **FIGURE 71-19** Ultrasound image show how extended field-of-view imaging can provide an overview of a large area.

a wide range of conditions with its precision and low miss rate in acute hemorrhage suggests that it should be an early adjunct to diagnosis in patients known to have a coagulation disorder.

SYNOPSIS OF TREATMENT OPTIONS

The immediate infusion of factor VIII is the best way of limiting hemorrhage into joints and soft tissue and preventing the sequelae. Urgent access to this has been set up by units dealing with hemophiliacs as a 24-hour service. This has made significant impact in the progress of those afflicted with this disease.

Hematoma aspiration has been tried but can lead to sepsis. If it is attempted, it needs to be performed under ultrasound guidance and with factor VIII coverage.

Surgical treatment is hazardous unless absolutely necessary.

What the Referring Physician Needs to Know

- Could the patient have hemophilia?
- Is there a hemorrhage into the joint or soft tissue?
- How extensive is the hemorrhage, and is it resolving; acute on chronic hematomas are common.

- Has the patient developed chronic problems within joints?
- Has the patient developed a pseudotumor?

REFERENCES

1. Keller A, Terrier F, Schneider PA, et al. Pelvic haemophilic pseudotumor: management of a patient with high level of inhibitors. Skeletal Radiol 2002; 31:550-553.
2. Roy S, Ghadially FN. Pathology of experimental haemarthrosis. Ann Rheum Dis 1966; 25:402-415.
3. Mainardi CL, Levine PH, Werb Z, Harris ED Jr. Proliferative synovitis in hemophilia: biochemical and morphologic observations. Arthritis Rheum 1978; 21:137-144.
4. Roosendaal G, Vianen ME, Marx JJ, et al. Blood-induced joint damage: a human in vitro study. Arthritis Rheum 1999; 42:1025-1032.
5. Kerr R. Imaging of musculoskeletal complications of hemophilia. Semin Musculoskelet Radiol 2003; 7:127-136.
6. Hakobyan N, Kazarian T, Jabbar AA, et al. Pathobiology of hemophilic synovitis: I. Overexpression of *mdm2* oncogene. Blood 2004; 104:2060-2064.
7. Valentino LA, Hakobyan N, Kazarian T, et al. Experimental haemophilic synovitis: rationale and development of a murine model of human factor VIII deficiency. Haemophilia 2004; 10:280-287.
8. Hakobyan N, Kazarian T, Valentino LA. Synovitis in a murine model of human factor VIII deficiency. Haemophilia 2005; 11:227-232.
9. Blake DR, Gallagher PJ, Potter AR, et al. The effect of synovial iron on the progression of rheumatoid disease: a histologic assessment of patients with early rheumatoid synovitis. Arthritis Rheum 1984; 27:495-501.
10. Ahlberg AK. On the natural history of hemophilic pseudotumor. J Bone Joint Surg Am 1975; 57:1133-1136.
11. Jaovisidha S, Ryu KN, Hodler J, et al. Hemophilic pseudotumor: spectrum of MR findings. Skeletal Radiol 1997; 26:468-474.
12. Wilson DA, Prince JR. MR imaging of hemophilic pseudotumors. AJR Am J Roentgenol 1988; 150:349-350.
13. van Ommeren JW, Mooren DW, Veth RP, et al. Pseudotumor occurring in hemophilia. Arch Orthop Trauma Surg 2000; 120:476-478.
14. Royle SG. Investigation of the irritable hip. J Pediatr Orthop 1992; 12:396-397.
15. Wilson DJ, Green DJ, MacLarnon JC. Arthrosonography of the painful hip. Clin Radiol 1984; 35:17-19.
16. Mathie AG, Benson MK, Wilson DJ. Lessons in the investigation of irritable hip: failure of ultrasound to detect haemarthrosis. J Bone Joint Surg Br 1991; 73:518-519.

72

Sickle Cell Anemia

Hilary R. Umans and Thomas L. Pope

ETIOLOGY

Sickle cell anemia (SCA), first described in a 20-year-old dental student from Grenada by Herrick in 1910, is the most common single gene disorder in African-Americans.[1] Dr. Linus Pauling and his team identified the cause of SCA as a single substitution in the gene encoding of the β-hemoglobin chain (valine substituted for glutamic acid). An individual with two abnormal chromosomes was designated as Hg SS and manifested the major clinical features of SCA. The person with one normal and one sickle cell β-globin chain, designated as Hg SA, was a carrier of the gene and had the sickle cell trait.[2] This genetic mutation has survived in Africa by natural selection because affected individuals have resistance to malaria.

The overall designation of SCA refers to any patient with at least one Hg S chain and one other abnormal β-globin chain. If this is another sickle cell β-globin chain, the individual is homozygous for Hg SS and by definition has SCA, Hg SC, or one of the thalassemias (e.g., Hg S-thal). Hg SS accounts for 60% to 70% of the cases of the disease in the United States and these individuals have the most severe manifestations of the disease. Individuals with Hg SA (one abnormal sickle cell gene designated S and one normal hemoglobin gene designated A or the "sickle cell trait") generally have a more benign clinical course without the vaso-occlusive complications and have fewer musculoskeletal abnormalities. Hemoglobin S reduces in a dose-dependent manner the susceptibility to malaria (*Plasmodium falciparum* infection). Therefore, a patient with homozygous Hg SS is more resistant to the infection than a patient with heterozygous Hg SA.[3] However, individuals with sickle cell trait are at a higher risk for developing medullary carcinoma of the kidney. There are other rarer combinations of the sickle cell gene, but none of these has significant clinical sequelae.[3]

The second most common disorder in which hematopoietic cells assume a sickle cell shape is hemoglobin C disease. These patients have two normal α and two variant β chains. Because the amount of Hb S is generally less than 50%, these individuals have a relatively benign form of hemolytic anemia that clinically is manifested by sporadic joint pain, pigmented gallstones, retinopathy, and splenomegaly.[4]

The aberrant hemoglobin cells of a patient with sickle cell disease have a life span approximately one fifth of that of normal hemoglobin cells. Therefore, these sickle cells are continually removed from the circulation and destroyed at an increased rate, resulting in anemia. Therefore, SCA is characterized as one of the many hemolytic anemias. Furthermore, Hg S, when deoxygenated, exhibits decreased solubility and forms long aggregates with other hemoglobin molecules within the red blood cells (RBCs). These molecules distort the RBCs into the characteristic sickle-shaped cells, which have a tendency to adhere to the endothelial wall and impair blood flow. The resultant vascular occlusion in various organ systems is believed to be the etiology for the most identifiable manifestations of this disease.[4]

PREVALENCE AND EPIDEMIOLOGY

Affecting 1 in 375 blacks in the United States, SCA is present in about 0.15% of the black U.S. population. Approximately 1 in 12 Americans of African descent carries the heterozygous sickle cell trait. SCA, however, can also be seen in many ethnic groups, particularly those from the Mediterranean basin (Turkey, the Arabian peninsula) and the subcontinent of India. Because of migration the disease can also be found in the Caribbean and South and Central America.[4]

KEY POINTS

- The diagnosis of sickle cell is almost always known at the patient's presentation.
- Major manifestations of sickle cell anemia are from infarction or infection.
- It may be difficult to distinguish infection from infarction in many cases. Clinical follow-up is often necessary.

CLINICAL PRESENTATION

The most common clinical scenario seen in SCA is recurrent acute, painful vaso-occlusive crises thought to be secondary to microvascular occlusion with organ and tissue ischemia. Almost 40% of patients with SCA experience at least one crisis before 5 years of age. In young patients these episodes most commonly present as dactylitis of the hands, fingers, feet, and toes (so-called hand-foot syndrome).[5,6] Table 72-1 outlines the major clinical features of SCA. The five "In's" of this disease, listed in Table 72-2, represent the major consequences of this disorder.

IMAGING TECHNIQUES

As with many diseases of the musculoskeletal system, the initial imaging evaluation is radiography. The radiograph gives an overview of the osseous structures and can show areas of bone resorption or proliferation. If clarification of osseous findings suspected on the radiograph is required, CT can be used as the next imaging study because this technique shows cortical bone to advantage. The actual clinical setting determines which technique is most appropriate after the radiograph. For patients with a high clinical suspicion of pathology who have normal radiographs and CT, MRI or radionuclide bone scanning can be used. In suspected infarction, MRI or radionuclide bone scanning may be used. MRI, although more expensive, can identify the infarction at an earlier stage and has the spatial resolution to identify other possible causes of the patient's symptoms. If soft tissue or osseous infection (osteomyelitis) is suspected clinically, gadolinium-enhanced MRI is the most appropriate modality after radiography. If a survey of the osseous structures is required, radionuclide bone scanning is the most accepted modality at this time, although whole-body MRI, although not widely used, has been reported to show promise in this setting.[7]

MANIFESTATIONS OF THE DISEASE

The skeletal features of SCA are changes in bone and bone marrow caused by tissue hypoxia from the intermittent episodic occlusion of the microcirculation by the individual's sickled cells. The major imaging findings are compensatory bone marrow hyperplasia, infarction of bone and bone marrow, secondary osteomyelitis, and secondary growth aberrations.

Bone Marrow Changes (Marrow Hyperplasia)

Because the bone marrow is the primary source for hematologic cells it is rational to assume that any disease resulting in an increased turnover of these cells will have an effect on this organ. In normal patients there is a gradual conversion of red (hematopoietic) marrow to yellow (fatty) marrow, a process that begins at the distal appendicular skeleton in early childhood. This process is usually completed by the second decade of life and in adults this red marrow generally only remains in the sternum, pelvis, ribs, and vertebrae. The epiphyses remain as fat-containing structures throughout life in normal individuals.[8] The shortened survival of erythrocytes in patients with SCA (10–20 days) leads to the imaging findings outlined in Table 72-3.

Radiography

Radiographic changes include osteopenia, a coarsened or accentuated trabecular pattern, and widening of the medullary spaces with resultant cortical thinning and loss of the normal diaphyseal constriction in the long bones (Fig. 72-1). All patients with SCA do not necessarily manifest all of these features. However, all patients with SCA have, in general, one or two of these imaging findings, which are best seen on radiography. Rarely, patients with SCA may show diploic widening secondary to marrow hyperplasia in the calvaria (the "hair-on-end" appearance), but this calvarial finding is much more common and characteristic of thalassemia, a disease that is discussed under Differential Diagnosis.

Magnetic Resonance Imaging

Magnetic resonance imaging can demonstrate the replacement of fatty marrow with hematopoietic marrow, and the persistence of red marrow may make detection of

---

TABLE 72-1 Major Clinical Manifestations of Sickle Cell Anemia

Osteonecrosis (multiple sites)
Infarction
   Diaphyseal
   Medullary
   Epiphyseal
Infection
   Osteomyelitis
   Septic arthritis
Fractures
Crystal deposition
Splenic infarction (involution)
Splenic sequestration
Acute chest syndrome (lung infarction)
Papillary necrosis
Renal insufficiency
Stroke

TABLE 72-2 The Five "In's" of Sickle Cell Anemia

*In*sufficient ossification (marrow hyperplasia)
*In*farction
*In*fection
In failure (because of the anemia)
*In*volution (of spleen)

TABLE 72-3 Imaging Findings of Marrow Hyperplasia

Osteopenia
Coarsened or accentuated trabecular pattern
Increase in the size of vascular channels
Widened medullary spaces
Cortical thinning
Loss of the normal diaphyseal constriction

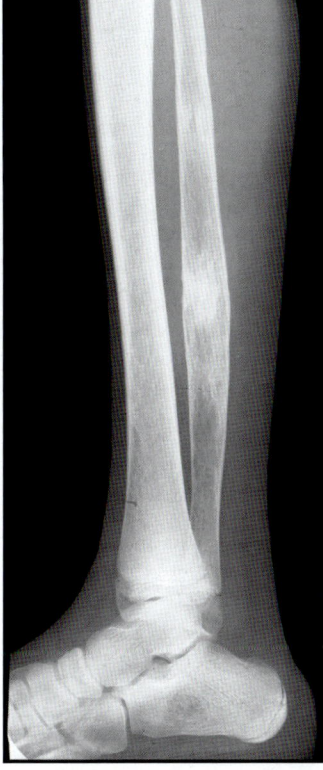

■ **FIGURE 72-1** Lateral tibia and fibula in child with sickle cell disease showing coarsened trabecular pattern and slight widening of the medullary spaces *(Courtesy of Dr. Mark Murphey, Armed Forces Institute of Pathology.)*

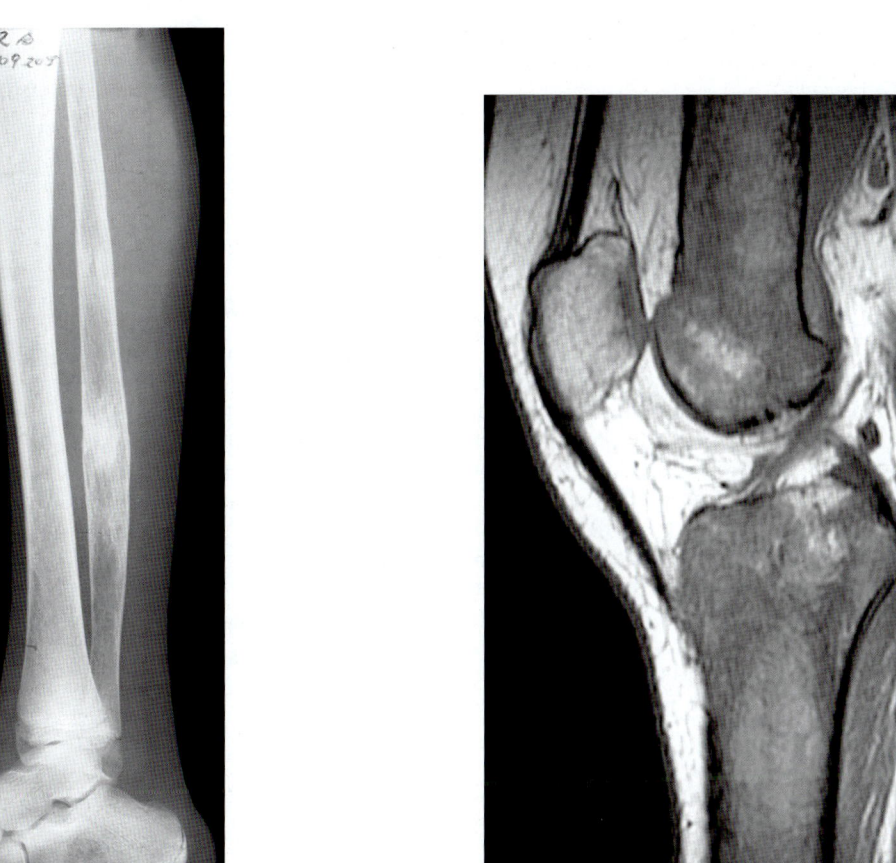

■ **FIGURE 72-2** Lateral knee in patient with long-standing sickle cell disease showing marked diffuse marrow replacement.

infarction or infection more difficult (Fig. 72-2).[7] Rarely, extramedullary hematopoiesis is encountered but is much more common in thalassemia.[8]

Multidetector Computed Tomography

Multidetector CT will confirm the findings of osteopenia, a coarsened or accentuated trabecular pattern, and widening of the medullary spaces with resultant cortical thinning and loss of the normal diaphyseal constriction in the long bones but is not needed for the detection of these features because the radiograph suffices.

Ultrasonography

There is no role for ultrasonography in the evaluation of bone marrow changes of SCA.

Nuclear Medicine

There is no role for nuclear medicine in the evaluation of bone marrow changes of SCA.

Positron Emission Tomography/Computed Tomography

Combined PET/CT plays no role in the evaluation of bone marrow changes of SCA.

Classic Signs

■ Marrow replacement with hematopoietic elements
■ Rarely, the "hair-on-end" appearance in the skull

Vascular Occlusion

Vascular occlusion, thought to be the underlying cause of the painful crises in SCA regardless of the location, is estimated to be 50 times more common than osteomyelitis.[9] Vascular compromise resulting in infarction produces some of the most recognizable musculoskeletal imaging features of this disease, which are listed in Table 72-4 and described in detail below.

Sickle Cell Dactylitis (Hand-Foot Syndrome, Aseptic Dactylitis)

Sickle cell dactylitis is one of the earliest manifestations of SCA and predominately involves children aged 6 months to 2 years. It is also one of the most commonly encountered clinical entities in this age group, occurring in up to 50% of patients with SCA. SCA patients with dactylitis

TABLE 72-4 Skeletal Manifestations of Vascular Occlusion in Sickle Cell Anemia

Dactylitis
Epiphyseal infarction and osteonecrosis (especially of the femoral head)
"H"-shaped (Lincoln log) vertebral bodies
Metaphyseal infarcts
Medullary infarction
Epiphyseal infarction
Growth disturbances

present with hand and foot pain, point tenderness, limitation of motion, soft tissue swelling, and fever. The cause of dactylitis is infarction of the bone marrow and cortex in the small bones of the hands and feet. The syndrome does not occur after 5 to 6 years of age because the red marrow in these bones is replaced by fibrous tissue, which requires less oxygenation. The major differential diagnosis in this setting is diffuse osteomyelitis and the clinical scenario and blood cultures help differentiate these two diseases.[5,6,8,9] With supportive therapy, patients usually recover from the acute episode, although the involved bones may show either deformity or complete repair from the vascular insult.

Radiography

The imaging findings of dactylitis are best appreciated by radiography, and the earliest manifestations are diffuse soft tissue swelling of the hands and the feet. Within 10 days to 2 weeks patients may develop relatively symmetric mixed osteosclerosis and osteolysis of the shafts of the involved bones with diffuse periostitis (Figs. 72-3 and 72-4).

Magnetic Resonance Imaging

Magnetic resonance imaging has no role in the evaluation of dactylitis.

Multidetector Computed Tomography

Multidetector CT has no role in the evaluation of dactylitis.

Ultrasonography

A combination of scintigraphy and ultrasonography has been advocated in the literature to help differentiate osteomyelitis from bone infarction in the patient suspected of having hand-foot syndrome. Scintigraphy will localize the site of increased activity, and ultrasonography can be used to identify subperiosteal fluid collections that can be aspirated for culture and sensitivity.[10]

Classic Signs

■ Mixed lucency and sclerosis in the hands and feet
■ Soft tissue swelling

Epiphyseal Infarction and Osteonecrosis

Diaphyseal Infarction

Infarction of cortical perforating vessels may lead to linear osteosclerosis that parallels the cortical margin

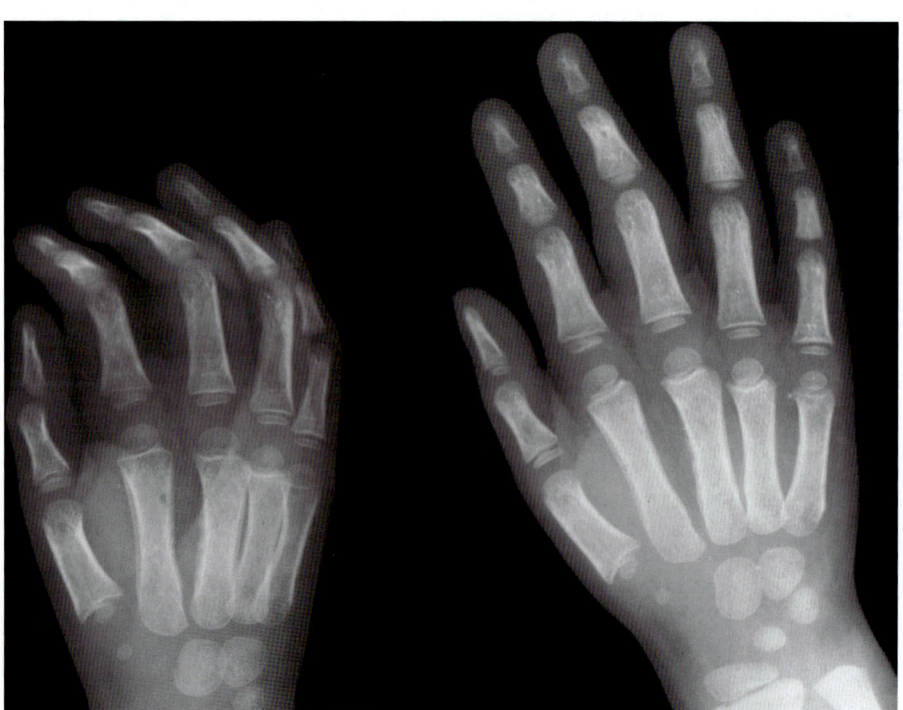

■ **FIGURE 72-3** Frontal and oblique views of the hands in a patient with hand-foot syndrome showing exuberant periosteal reaction.

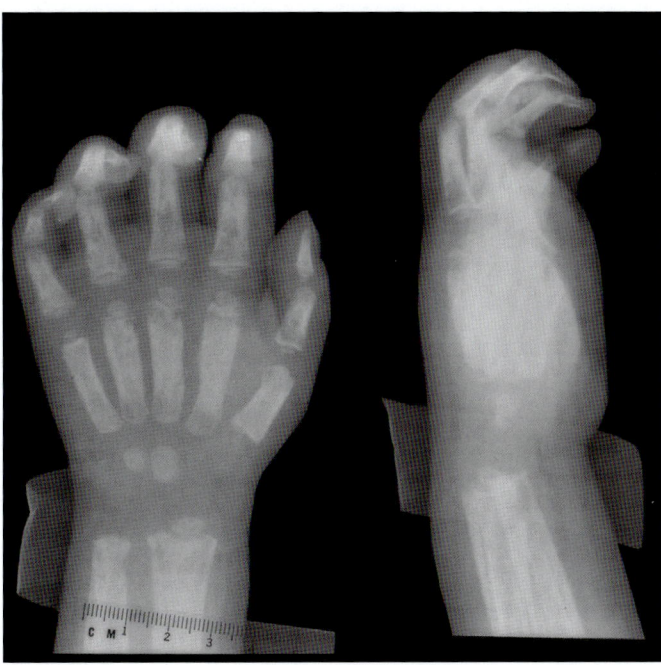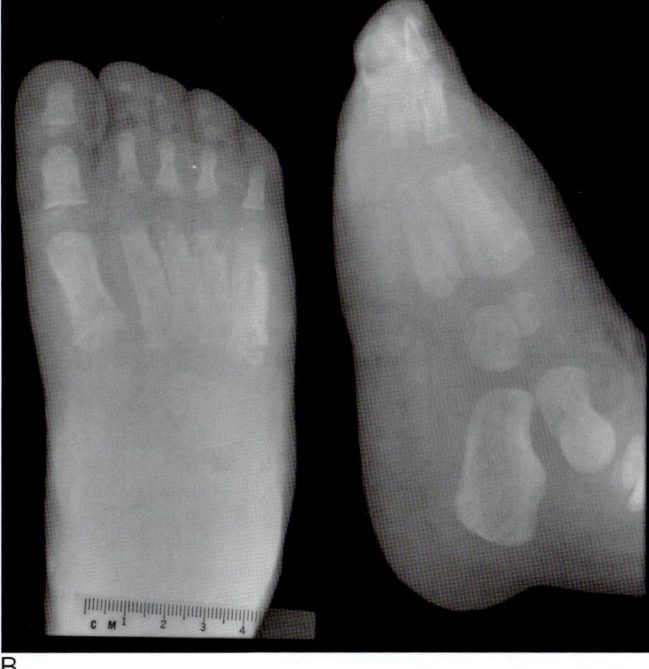

A   B

■ **FIGURE 72-4**   Hands (**A**) and feet (**B**) of a child with hand-foot syndrome showing marked periosteal reaction and diffuse osteolysis and osteosclerosis.

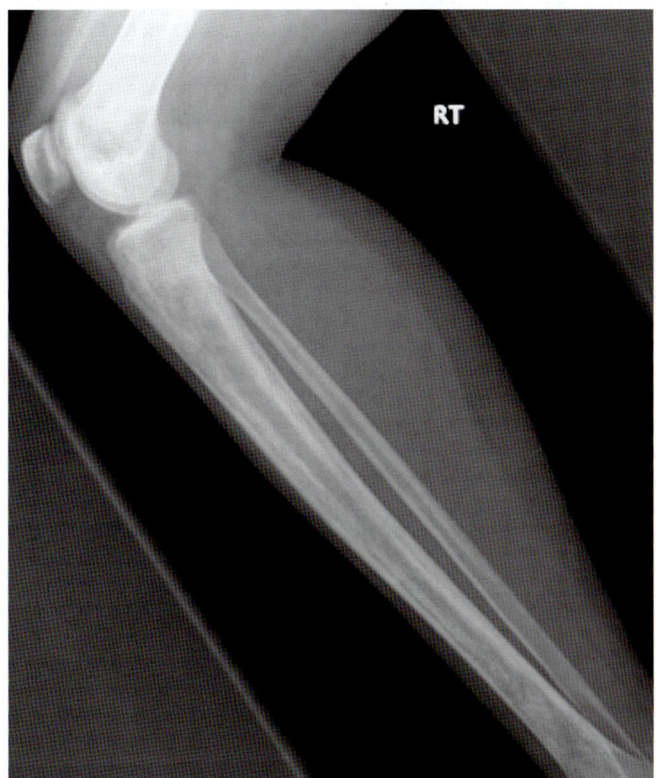

■ **FIGURE 72-5**   Lateral tibia and fibula in a child with sickle cell disease showing the "bone-within-bone" appearance.

of the involved bone. This finding is termed the "bone-within-bone" appearance (Fig. 72-5).

Miscellaneous Findings

There are a host of other miscellaneous findings that have been described in patients with SCA. These include crystal deposition, hemarthroses, joint effusions, synovitis, protrusion acetabuli, bony ankylosis of the spine and hip, growth disturbances, and fractures. However, these abnormalities are discussed elsewhere in the book and are not elucidated here because none of them is unique or pathognomonic of SCA.

Imaging Features

Epiphyseal infarction in SCA has a predilection for the proximal femora and humeri but can occur in any bone. SCA is the most common cause of femoral head osteonecrosis in children, and almost 50% of SCA patients will develop osteonecrosis by the age of 35.[7,11,12] In the younger patient epiphyseal infarction may mimic Legg-Calvé-Perthes disease (Figs. 72-6 and 72-7). (See Differential Diagnosis section.)

Another manifestation of infarction is the "H"-shaped or "Lincoln log" vertebral bodies. The normal vertebral body has vessels that perforate the cortex centrally and then curve to supply the superior and inferior end plates. Infarction of these perforating vessels may lead to resorption and loss of central subchondral bone. This "H"-shape with midline concavities is virtually pathognomonic of

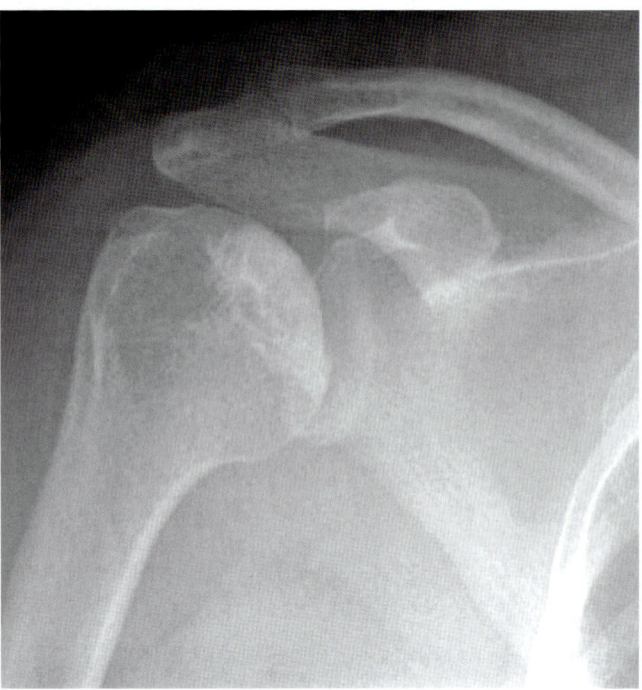

■ **FIGURE 72-6** Avascular necrosis (with collapse of the articular surface) of the proximal humerus ("snowcapping") in a patient with sickle cell disease.

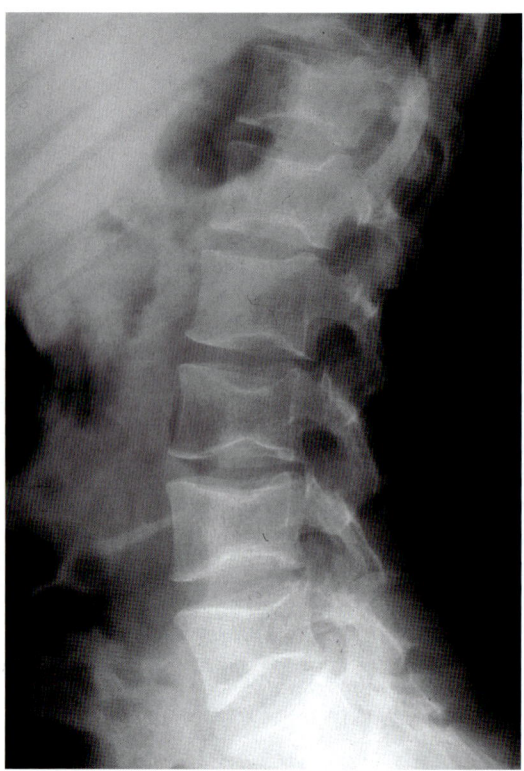

■ **FIGURE 72-8** Lateral lumbar spine showing the characteristic "H"-shaped vertebrae and biconcave end plates typical of sickle cell anemia. This is also a manifestation of infarction in these patients.

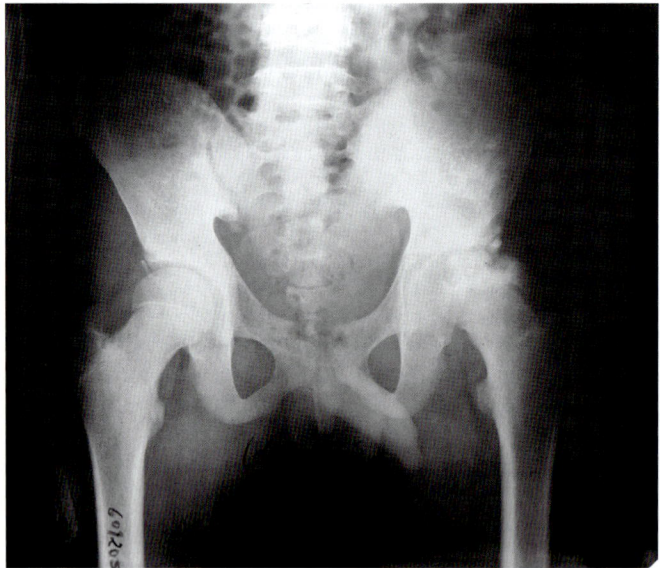

■ **FIGURE 72-7** Avascular necrosis of the left femoral head in a patient with sickle cell anemia.

SCA (Fig. 72-8).[13] The metaphyses of long bones are other sites of infarction and result from vascular sludging at the end arteriovenous anastomosis.

Radiography

Epiphyseal infarction (osteonecrosis) in the adult with SCA has no specific radiographic features to distinguish it from other causes of osteonecrosis. The femoral head

is the most common site for this finding, and MRI is the modality that will diagnose this complication at its earliest stages. In the later stages of osteonecrosis radiography may be used to follow the progression of fragmentation, collapse, and secondary osteoarthrosis that occurs in the weight-bearing bones (see Fig. 72-7). In the epiphyses of non–weight-bearing bones without (most notably the humeral head) osteonecrosis, sclerosis may occur without significant contour changes (see Fig. 72-8). Finally, in some patients with SCA massive infarction of bone may result in diffuse sclerosis that may mimic osteoblastic metastatic disease on radiography.[14]

Magnetic Resonance Imaging

Acute epiphyseal infarction is manifested by diffuse decreased signal intensity on short echo time (TE) (T1-weighted) images and increased signal intensity on fluid-sensitive (T2-weighted or inversion recovery) images. As the process matures and in the subacute setting, the involved area develops into a more focal region and the T1-weighted images will show a serpentine line of low signal intensity surrounding the hyperintense marrow. A double line of low signal intensity surrounding an inner rim of higher signal intensity ("the double-line" sign) is sometimes seen on the T2-weighted MR images.[8]

Acute medullary infarction is best demonstrated with MRI that shows areas of edema within the cancellous bone marrow and the periosteal soft tissues (Fig. 72-9). Some authors have concluded that osteomyelitis cannot be distinguished from infarction by imaging alone.[15-17]

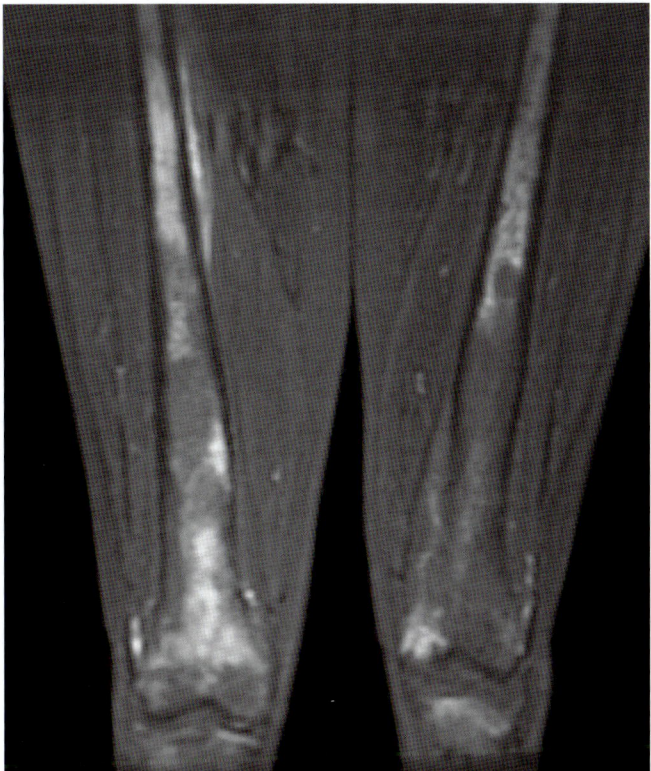

■ **FIGURE 72-9** Fat-suppressed T2-weighted coronal MR image of both mid and distal femora demonstrate multiple geographic foci of increased medullary signal intensity as a result of acute infarction. Note the associated parosteal soft tissue edema tracking along the medial shaft of the right femur.

However, in a small series of 11 patients, Umans and associates reported that MRI with contrast medium enhancement could distinguish infection from infarction. In their study, acute infarcts demonstrated thin, linear rim enhancement presumably reflecting nonenhancing central necrosis whereas osteomyelitis revealed more geographic and irregular marrow enhancement (Figs. 72-10 and 72-11).[17] Healed infarctions show areas of mixed osteolysis and sclerosis on radiography (Fig. 72-12).

Multidetector Computed Tomography

Multidetector CT, with its ability to generate high-resolution reformatted images in sagittal and coronal planes, can be used to evaluate the hip in patients with acute pain and suspected recent collapse of the articular surface. In general, however, CT has a limited role in evaluation of osteonecrosis in SCA compared with less expensive (radiography) and more specific (MRI) modalities.

Classic Signs

- Classic avascular necrosis (cannot be differentiated from avascular necrosis from other causes)
- Epiphyseal infarction of the proximal humerus ("snowcap" sign)
- "H"-shaped vertebral bodies
- Medullary infarction in long bones

Infection (Osteomyelitis and Septic Arthritis)

Infection in patients with SCA is much less common than infarction but SCA patients are 100 times more likely to develop infection than the normal population. The most serious infection is osteomyelitis, which is often encountered in the diaphyseal regions of the femur, tibia, and humerus.[9] The presenting clinical symptoms of patients with osteomyelitis include pain, fever, erythema at the site of involvement, and leukocytosis. The most common infecting organism in SCA patients is the *Salmonella* species (especially the nontypical serotypes), and the second most common organism is *Staphylococcus aureus*. Other organisms reported to cause osteomyelitis in this setting are gram-negative enteric bacilli.[15,16] The exact predisposing mechanism is unknown. It is suspected that ischemic bowel infarction allows *Salmonella* (and other enteric organisms) to enter the circulatory system. The resultant bacteremia leads to osteomyelitis. Other reported reasons for the SCA patients' susceptibility to *Salmonella* and other enteric pathogens are decreased clearance of portal bacteria by the liver, interference with bacterial phagocytosis of macrophages, and abnormalities of the complement system.[9,18] Another less common mechanism for the development of osteomyelitis is contiguous spread from a soft tissue infection.

Osteomyelitis is difficult to distinguish from infarction clinically or radiographically. Both entities may have similar clinical presentations and laboratory abnormalities.

Septic arthritis, although reported in SCA patients, is much less common than osteomyelitis. The exact cause of this complication is unknown, but intravascular sickling in synovial capillaries can cause hyperviscosity and plugging that can lead to increased susceptibility to joint infection. Also, hypoxia, acidosis, and hyperthermia from articular inflammation can cause sickling of red blood cells, which results in further stasis.[18]

Radiography

On radiographs, both infection and infarction may show soft tissue swelling, periostitis, and mixed areas of osteosclerosis and osteolysis (Fig. 72-13).

Magnetic Resonance Imaging

After the radiograph is performed, gadolinium-enhanced MRI is the next best imaging study to evaluate the patient suspected of having osteomyelitis. As mentioned earlier, acute infarcts usually show thin, linear rim enhancement after gadolinium administration whereas osteomyelitis often reveals a more geographic and irregular marrow enhancement pattern on post-contrast MRI (see Figs. 72-10B and 72-11).[16]

Multidetector Computed Tomography

Computed tomography may show subperiosteal abscesses and fluid collections thought more common in osteomyelitis. In general, soft tissue involvement, including soft tissue masses, is more common in the setting of osteomyelitis. Nevertheless, soft tissue extension of infection is an inconstant finding, making it an unreliable distinguishing feature between infection and infarction.[8,9]

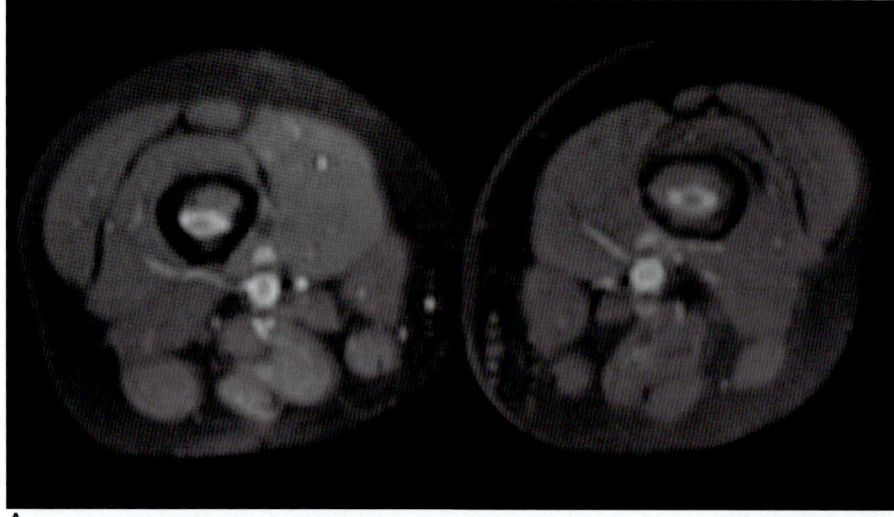

A

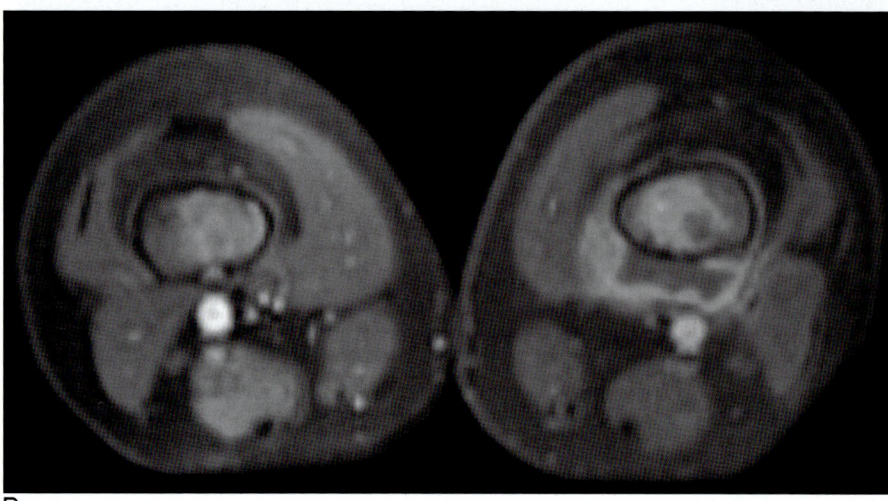

B

■ **FIGURE 72-10** Axial enhanced, fat-suppressed T1-weighted MR images of the midshaft and distal femora in a patient with medullary infarcts and osteomyelitis. **A,** Thin peripheral linear enhancement about infarcts. **B,** Superimposed osteomyelitis characterized by more geographic marrow enhancement in the left distal femoral shaft and a thick rim of enhancement of a posterior parosteal abscess.

Ultrasonography

Ultrasonography may show soft tissue fluid collections in an abscess and be a reasonable tool to guide aspiration of these fluid collections if needed and desired by the referring physician.

Nuclear Medicine

At radionuclide scintigraphy, both infection and infarction will be "hot." In general, soft tissue involvement (and, thus, soft tissue masses) is more prominent in osteomyelitis but soft tissue extension of the infection may not always be present to use this as a discriminator.

Classic Signs

■ Osteomyelitis in the setting of SCA is identical in its imaging findings to osteomyelitis in any other setting.

DIFFERENTIAL DIAGNOSIS

Sickle cell anemia is one of the hematologic diseases that may have similar clinical and imaging features. The differential diagnosis can be discussed as it relates to the major imaging findings of SCA.

Sickle cell-thalassemia is a disease caused by inheritance of one gene for Hb S and one for thalassemia. The clinical and imaging features of this disorder are variable and may range from no symptoms to full-blown sickle cell disease. These patients may develop any of the signs and symptoms of SCA, including infarction, septic arthritis, and osteomyelitis.[19]

Thalassemia, first described in 1925 by Cooley and Lee, is a group of diseases related to an inherited abnormality of globin production and not to a structural abnormality in the globin chain as is present with SCA.[20] Patients with thalassemia may have features similar to SCA. Marrow expansion is the most prominent imaging feature of the disease and is usually more pronounced than in SCA. In fact, the "hair-on-end" appearance of the skull is the most

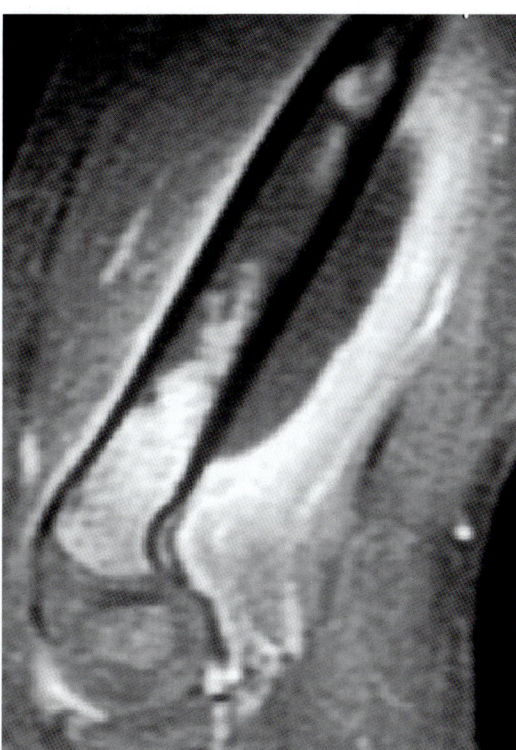

■ **FIGURE 72-11** Sagittal fat-suppressed T1-weighted MR image of the distal humerus and elbow after the administration of gadolinium demonstrates geographic marrow enhancement surrounding a segment of nonenhancement in the distal shaft indicative of osteomyelitis and intraosseous abscess. Note the large volar parosteal abscess with a thick rind of surrounding soft tissue enhancement.

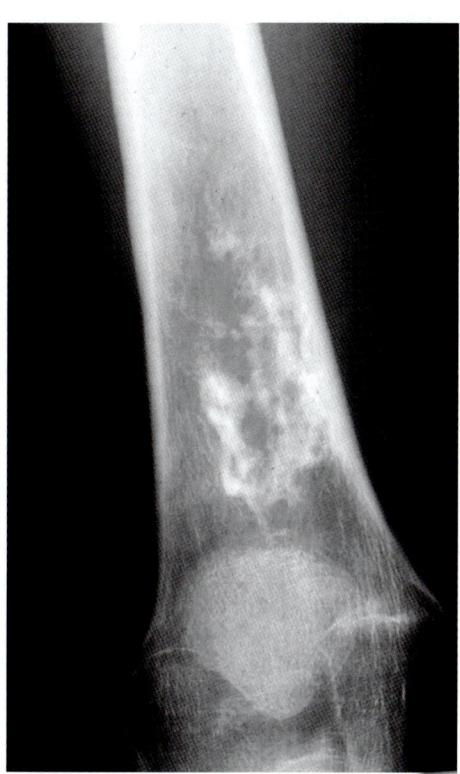

■ **FIGURE 72-12** Anteroposterior radiograph of the distal femur demonstrates peripheral sclerosis related to a chronic or healed medullary bone infarct.

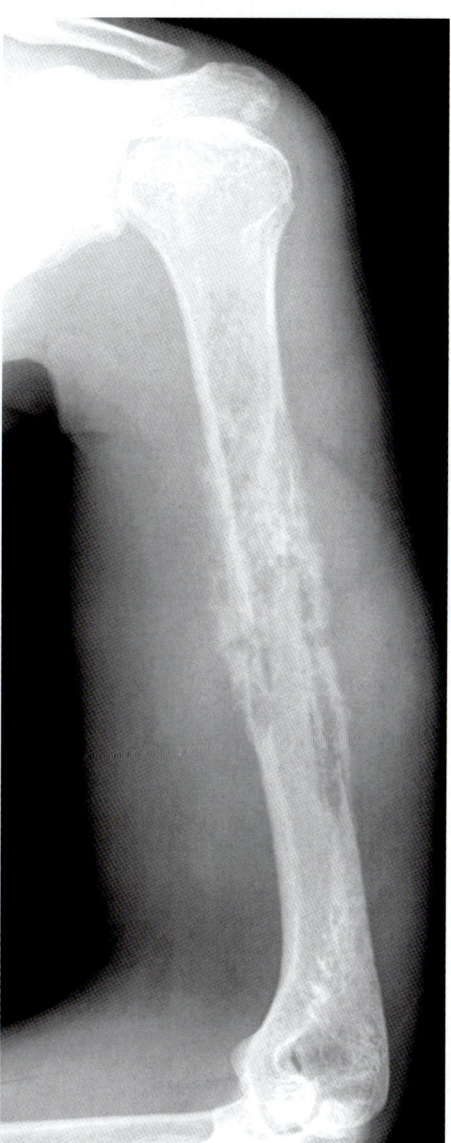

■ **FIGURE 72-13** Lateral radiograph of the humerus demonstrates mixed osteosclerosis and osteolysis with associated periostitis and surrounding soft tissue swelling in the midshaft related to subacute osteomyelitis.

characteristic feature of thalassemia, and this finding is rare in SCA patients (Fig. 72-14). Other radiographic manifestations of cortical thinning and a prominent trabecular pattern characterize thalassemia and are not seen as often with SCA. Growth disturbances, crystal deposition and fractures, and extramedullary hematopoiesis may also occur with thalassemia.[21]

Hip pain is a common presenting complaint in adolescents. The infarction of the femoral head that occurs in SCA may mimic Legg-Calvé-Perthes disease, an idiopathic avascular necrosis of the capital femoral epiphysis. However, Legg-Calvé-Perthes disease is most common in white children aged 3 to 12. Only about 15% of cases are bilateral. This is in contradistinction to the femoral head infarction seen in SCA in which the patient is usually of African descent, is often older at presentation,

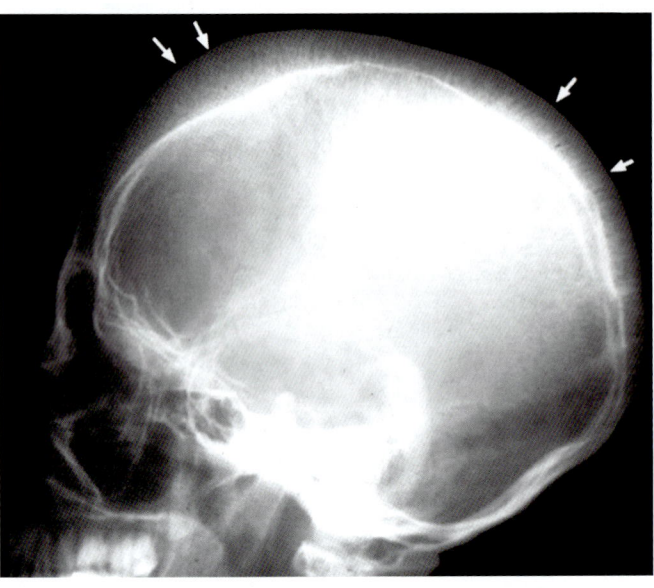

■ **FIGURE 72-14** Lateral skull radiograph demonstrates the "hair-on-end" appearance (*arrows*) with widening of the diploic space in an individual with thalassemia.

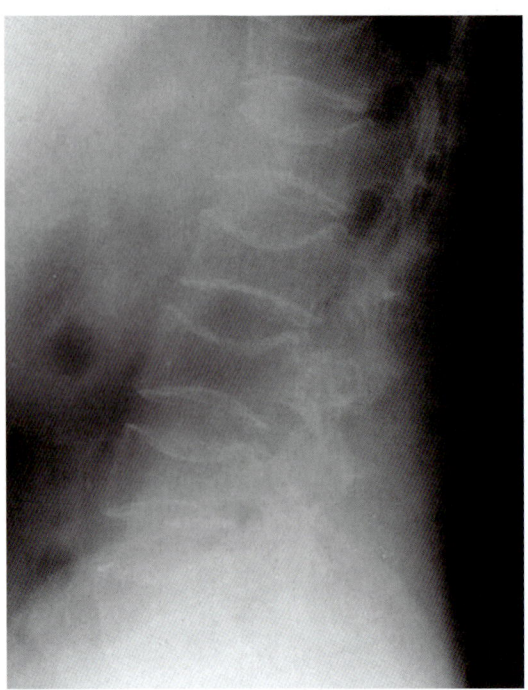

■ **FIGURE 72-15** Lateral lumbar spine radiograph of 72-year-old female shows "codfish" vertebral bodies associated with osteoporosis.

and in whom the symptoms and signs are often bilateral. Otherwise, infarction of the femoral head seen in any disease may mimic that seen in SCA.[22]

The structural changes to the vertebral bodies in SCA may mimic those caused by osteoporosis from any cause. However, in osteoporosis, the end-plate depressions are usually more rounded and do not have the "H" shape seen in SCA. The rounded depressions or "biconcave" appearance of the superior and inferior end plates have been referred to as "fish" vertebral bodies because of their resemblance to actual fish vertebrae or "fish mouth" spine, referring to the resultant ovoid appearance of the disc space (Fig. 72-15).[23] Note that the end plates are more rounded than in SCA.

SYNOPSIS OF TREATMENT OPTIONS

Medical Treatment

The current major therapies for SCA are geared toward replacing lost Hb SS cells by transfusion or by decreasing the number of Hb S cells that are produced. Transfusions are usually given as needed except in those patients with SCA who are at an increased risk of stroke. These individuals generally receive monthly maintenance transfusions aimed at keeping the total hemoglobin concentration at 12 g/dL and Hb SS concentration to under 30%. Ideally, this is accomplished by bone marrow and stem cell transplantation (from umbilical cord blood) before any major complications of SCA occur. These transfusions, however,

are not without risks themselves and can be associated with a variety of complications, including alloimmunization, transfusion reaction, infection (hepatitis C and human immunodeficiency virus infections), and total-body iron overload.[24,25]

Decreasing the amount of Hb SS cell production can be accomplished by two mechanisms. One way is to change the marrow cell population. This is accomplished by bone marrow and stem cell transplantation (from umbilical cord blood). Ideally this is done before any major complications of SCA occur. If successful, this procedure is essentially curative. Limited availability of marrow donor matches and umbilical cord blood donors for SCA patients curtails widespread use of this procedure.[26,27]

The second method of reducing the production of Hb SS-containing red blood cells is to induce fetal hemoglobin (Hb F) production in the native marrow, which can be accomplished by the administration of hydroxyurea, a cytotoxic agent, which increases the production of Hb F, replacing some of the abnormal β-globin chains and thereby lowering the relative amount of Hb SS in the blood. Hydroxyurea has also been shown to decrease the incidence of painful crises, hemolytic crises, days in hospital, and transfusions.[4,28-30]

Of course, SCA patients who present with suspected osseous infection are treated symptomatically until an organism is isolated. They are then administered the appropriate antibiotic, or the infection is drained surgically.

Surgical Treatment

Surgical treatment is not commonly employed in patients with SCA. The major surgical therapy is to perform hip replacements on patients with avascular necrosis and to drain soft tissue abscesses. Of these, the most common is hip replacement surgery.

What the Referring Physician Needs to Know

- Evidence of acute infarction
- Evidence of avascular necrosis
- Infection versus infarction if possible (difficult without gadolinium-enhanced MRI)
- Progression of disease in patients seen on ongoing basis

SUGGESTED READING

Lonergan GJ, Cline DB, Abbondanzo SL. Sickle cell anemia. RadioGraphics 2001; 21:971–994.

REFERENCES

1. Herrick JB. Peculiar elongated and sickle-shaped red blood corpuscles in a case of severe anemia. Arch Intern Med 1910; 6:517–521.
2. Pauling L, Itano HA, Singer SJ, Wells IE. Sickle-cell anemia: a molecular disease. Science 1949; 110:543–549.
3. Alouch JR. Higher resistance to *Plasmodium falciparum* infection in patients with homozygous sickle cell disease in western Kenya. N Engl J Med 1997; 317:781–787.
4. Bowman JE, Murray RFJ. Genetic Variation in Peoples of African Origin. Baltimore, Johns Hopkins University Press, 1990; 196–201.
5. Weinberg AG, Currarino G. Sickle cell dactylitis: histopathologic observations. Am J Clin Pathol 1972; 58:518–523.
6. Babhulkar SS, Pande K, Babhulkar S. The hand-foot syndrome in sickle-cell haemoglobinopathy. J Bone Joint Surg Br 1995; 77:310–312.
7. Deely DM, Schweitzer ME. MR imaging of bone marrow disorders. Radiol Clin North Am 1997; 35:193–212.
8. Gilkeson RC, Basile V, Sands MI, Hsu IT: Chest case of the day: extramedullary hemopoiesis (EHMH). AJR Am J Roentgenol 1997; 169:270–273.
9. Keeley K, Buchanan GR. Acute infarction of long bones in children with sickle cell anemia. J Pediatr 1982; 101:170–175.
10. Rafai A, Nyman R: Scintigraphy and ultrasonography in differentiating osteomyelitis from bone infarction in sickle cell disease. Acta Radiol 1997; 38:139–143.
11. Frush DP, Heyneman LE, Ware RE, Bissett GS. MR features of soft-tissue abnormalities due to acute marrow infarction in five children with sickle cell disease. AJR Am J Roentgenol 1999; 173:989–993.
12. Ware HE, Brooks AP, Toye R, Berney SI. Sickle cell disease and silent avascular necrosis of the hip. J Bone Joint Surg Br 1991; 73:947–949.
13. Cordner S, De Ceulaer K. Musculoskeletal manifestations of hemoglobinopathies. Curr Opin Rheumatol 2003; 15:44–47.
14. Munk P, Helms CA, Holt RG: Immature bone infarcts: findings on plain radiographs and MR scans. AJR Am J Roentgenol 1989; 152:547–549.
15. Skaggs DL, Kim SK, Greene NW, et al. Differentiation between bone infarction and acute osteomyelitis in children with sickle-cell disease with use of sequential radionuclide bone-marrow and bone scans. J Bone Joint Surg Am 2001; 83:1810–1813.
16. Atkins BL, Price EH, Tillyer L, et al. *Salmonella* osteomyelitis in sickle cell disease children in the east end of London. J Infect 1997; 34:133–138.
17. Umans H, Haramati N, Flusser G. The diagnostic role of gadolinium enhanced MRI in distinguishing between acute medullary bone infarct and osteomyelitis. Magn Reson Imaging 2000; 18:255–262.
18. Burnett MW, Bass JW, Cook BA. Etiology of osteomyelitis complicating sickle cell disease. Periatrics 1998; 101:296–297.
19. Reynolds J: Radiologic manifestations of sickle cell hemoglobinopathy. JAMA 1972; 38:247–250.
20. Cooley TB, Lee P: A series of cases of splenomegaly in children with anemia and peculiar bone changes. Trans Am Pediatr Soc 1925; 37:29–35.
21. Caffey J. Cooley's anemia: a review of the roentgenographic findings in the skeleton. AJR Am J Roentgenol 1957; 78:381–391.
22. Wenger DR, Ward WT, Herring JA. Current concepts review: Legg-Calvé-Perthes disease. J Bone Joint Surg Am 1991; 73:778–788.
23. Rexroad JT, Moser RP III, Georgia JD: "Fish" or "fish mouth" vertebrae? AJR Am J Roentgenol 2003; 181:886–887.
24. Adams RJ, McKie YC, Hsu L, et al. Prevention of a first stroke by transfusions in children with sickle cell anemia and abnormal results on transcranial Doppler ultrasonography. N Engl J Med 1998; 339:5–11.
25. Adams RJ. Stroke prevention in sickle cell disease. Curr Opin Hematol 2000; 7:101–105.
26. King KE, Ness PM. Treating anemia. Hematol Oncol Clin North Am 1996; 10:1305–1320.
27. Castro O. Management of sickle cell disease: recent advances and controversies. Br J Haematol 1999; 107:2–11.
28. Steinberg MH. Management of sickle cell disease. N Engl J Med 1999; 340:1021.
29. Charache S. Mechanism of action of hydroxyurea. Semin Hematol 1997; 34:15–21.
30. Koren A, Segal-Kupershmit D, Zalman L, et al. Effect of hydroxyurea in sickle cell anemia: a clinical trial in children and teenagers with severe sickle cell anemia and sickle cell beta-thalassemia. Pediatr Hematol Oncol 1999; 16:221–232.

CHAPTER 73

Thalassemia

Apostolos Karantanas

ETIOLOGY

In 1925, Cooley and Lee described a series of patients suffering from severe anemia associated with splenomegaly and bone abnormalities.[1] The name thalassemia, combining the Greek words *thalassa* meaning "sea" and *aima* meaning "blood," underlines the Mediterranean origin of the patients. Thalassemia is not a single disease but rather a group of diseases related to an inherited abnormality of globin production.[2] The defects in the rate of synthesis of one of the globin chains leads to impaired erythropoiesis, hemolysis, and a variable degree of anemia. The main groups of thalassemia consist of the α type and the β type, with α-globin chain and β-globin chain synthesis deficiency, respectively. Thalassemia major represents the homozygous form, whereas thalassemia minor is the heterozygous form of the disease. A poorly defined intermediate variety of the disease is called thalassemia intermedia. The disease is a single gene disorder inherited in a mendelian recessive manner that is indigenous in people of Mediterranean and Southeast Asian origin. Thalassemia is a severe anemia treated by regular blood transfusions throughout life and by systematic removal of excess iron. The recommended treatment for thalassemia major requires regular blood transfusions every 2 to 5 weeks to maintain the pretransfusion hemoglobin level above 9 to 10.5 g/dL. This transfusion regimen promotes normal growth, allows normal physical activities, suppresses bone marrow activity, and minimizes iron accumulation.[3]

PREVALENCE AND EPIDEMIOLOGY

Life expectancy in β-thalassemia is poor worldwide owing to lack of chances for efficient therapy. Nevertheless, life span has increased during past decades as a result of improvements in transfusion and iron chelation therapy in developed countries. It has been estimated that there are probably as many as 100,000 living patients with homozygous β-thalassemia. In this chapter the focus is on the more common and severe form, β-thalassemia major. The presence and severity of bone disease in β-thalassemia major patients depends on the optimization of the transfusion and iron chelation therapy.

CLINICAL PRESENTATION

The clinical presentation depends significantly on the regularity and efficiency of treatment. In untreated or undertreated patients, growth arrest, spontaneous fractures, and acute spinal cord compression are the most common musculoskeletal manifestations of the disease. In optimally treated patients, arthralgia, mainly of the knees, is the most common clinical presentation.

PATHOPHYSIOLOGY AND IMAGING TECHNIQUES

Bone Disease in Untreated or Undertreated Thalassemia Major

Untreated or inadequately transfused children with β-thalassemia major demonstrate an expansion of the bone marrow up to 15 to 30 times normal owing to ineffective erythropoiesis and anemia. Marrow hyperplasia, exhibiting decreased radiographic density, is responsible for

---

KEY POINTS

- Untreated or poorly treated β-thalassemia is demonstrated radiologically by medullary expansion and extramedullary hematopoiesis.
- Regular transfusion has resulted in the decrease of the classic radiologic signs of the disease.
- Iron chelation may be associated with skeletal dysplasia that mainly affects growth plates and epiphyses.
- MRI is the method of choice for imaging iron chelation–induced bone disease.
- Osteoporosis in thalassemia results from many causes, but bone mineral densitometry yields variable results, owing to the unpredictable pattern of bone marrow siderosis.

most of the radiographic features of the disease. Skeletal abnormalities in untreated β-thalassemia major are usually seen in children older than 1 year of age. Both the axial and appendicular skeletons are involved, but around puberty there is an increased predominance of the former. Extramedullary hematopoiesis represents the body's attempt to maintain a normal erythropoiesis level and is observed in a variety of disorders that alter the bone marrow composition. Extramedullary hematopoiesis is a well-recognized finding in β-thalassemia major patients in whom extraosseous extension of marrow tissue is observed. Endocrine diseases also contribute to bone abnormalities in β-thalassemia major, in particular hypoparathyroidism, hypothyroidism, and hypogonadism, as well as low concentrations of serum 1,25-dihydroxyvitamin D and osteocalcin.[4] It has been reported that by raising the baseline hemoglobin from 6.5 to 9.5 g/dL, most of the β-thalassemia major–related skeletal abnormalities could be avoided.[5]

Skull

Skull contains hematopoietic marrow, and therefore any alterations result from hyperactivity of the red marrow in response to anemia. Marrow hyperplasia widens the diploic space with thinning or virtual disappearance of the outer table, thickening of the inner table, reduction of the trabeculae, granular osteopenia, solitary or multiple circumscribed osteolytic areas, and widened and tortuous vascular channels (Figs. 73-1 and 73-2). The residual trabeculae are thickened and occasionally arranged perpendicular to the curvature of the cranial vault, producing the "hair-on-end" appearance on plain radiographs

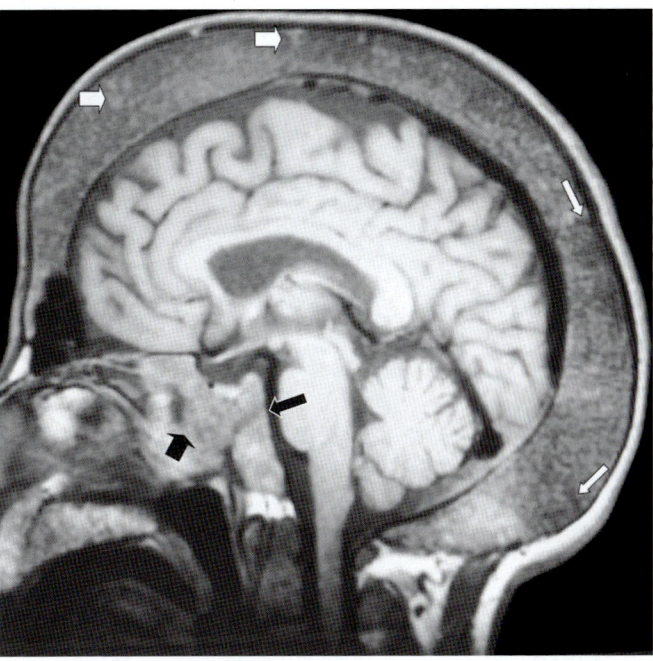

■ **FIGURE 73-2** Sagittal T1-weighted (TR ms/TE ms, 500/20) MR image in a 10-year-old boy with β-thalassemia major. There is marked widening of the diploic space containing hypointense trabeculae (*thin white arrows*) and hyperintense marrow (*thick white arrows*). The clivus is expanded (*thin black arrow*) and the sphenoidal sinuses obliterated (*thick black arrow*).

(see Fig. 73-1). The skull may obtain an elongated remodeling, also known as "tower" skull, with frontal and posterior bossing.[6] The marrow hyperplasia also involves the facial bones, resulting in osseous expansion with subsequent obliteration of the paranasal sinuses (see Figs. 73-1 and 73-2). Ethmoidal air cells are usually well pneumatized owing to absence of red marrow within the surrounding bones. Marrow hyperplasia in the maxilla causes lateral displacement of the orbits and ventral displacement of the incisors, giving rise to the typical appearance of a deformed face with widened nasal bridge. The radiologic findings associated with marrow hyperplasia are not pathognomonic of β-thalassemia major and are also found in iron-deficiency anemia, sickle cell disease, and spherocytosis.[7]

Thorax

The ribs contain hematopoietic marrow in all ages. As a result, overactive marrow results in osteopenia, expansion, localized lucencies, cortical erosions and thinning, and "rib-within-a-rib" appearance (Figs. 73-3 and 73-4). The latter is usually seen in the middle and anterior portions of the ribs and occurs when hypertrophied marrow perforates the cortex and extends longitudinally beneath the periosteum. Marrow extension anteriorly through the cortex of the rib is easier, compared with extension posteriorly, owing to firm muscular attachment in the latter. The type of rib abnormality has been reported to be related to the age at onset of the transfusion regimen.[8] In the same study, patients with abnormal but not expanded ribs started the low transfusion regimen earlier

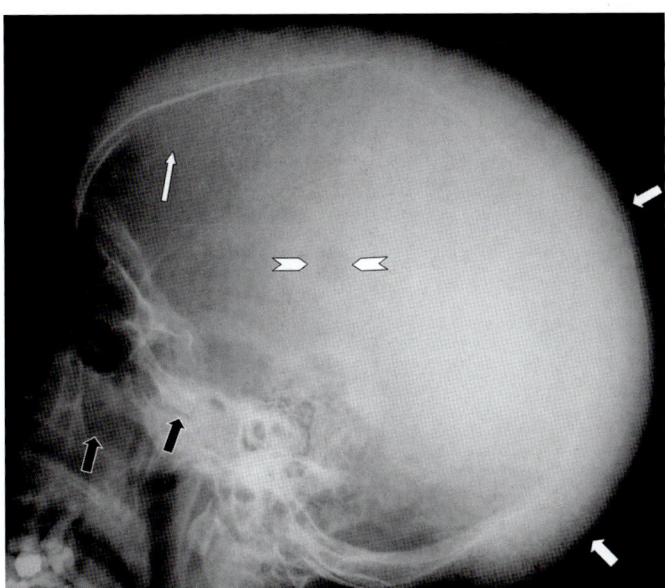

■ **FIGURE 73-1** Lateral skull radiograph in a patient with β-thalassemia major shows widening of the diploic space, granular osteopenia (*long white arrow*), and thinning of the outer table. The marked vertical striations give the appearance of the characteristic "hair-on-end" sign (*white arrows*). Absence of normal paranasal sinus pneumatization results from marrow overgrowth (*black arrows*). A solitary well-defined osteolytic area is also seen (*arrowheads*).

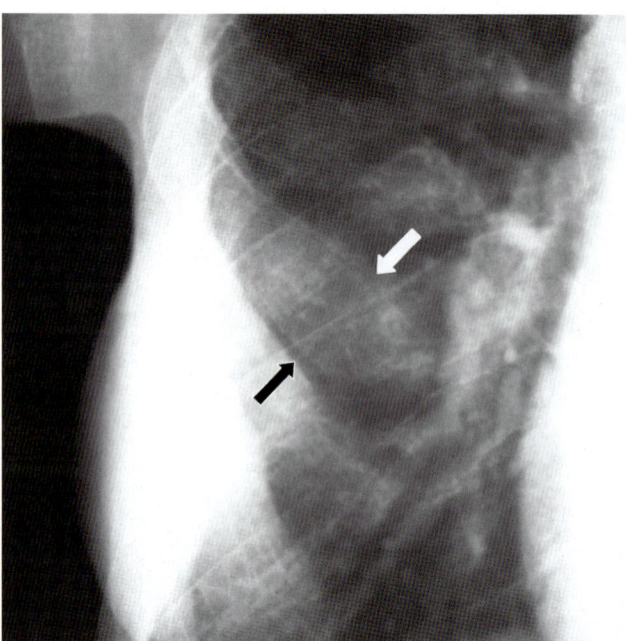

■ **FIGURE 73-3** Posteroanterior plain radiograph shows expansion of the anterior rib with localized lucencies, osteopenia, and cortical thinning in a patient with β-thalassemia major (*arrows*).

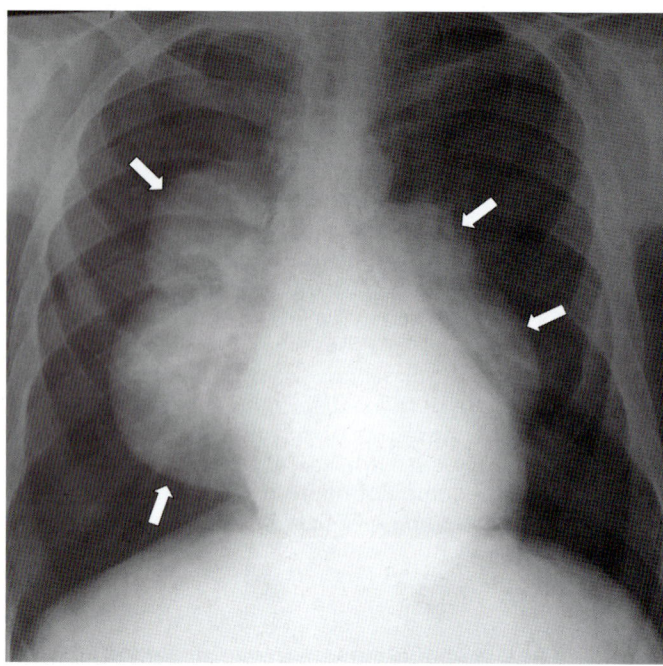

■ **FIGURE 73-5** Posteroanterior plain radiograph of a β-thalassemia major male patient shows posterior mediastinal masses corresponding to bilateral paravertebral extramedullary hematopoiesis.

than patients with expanded ribs, and approximately two thirds of the rib abnormalities did not regress even if a hypertransfusion regimen was applied.

Extramedullary hematopoiesis masses usually develop bilaterally in the thoracic paraspinal areas (Fig. 73-5).[9] These lesions are located either circumferentially around the vertebral bodies or appear as bilateral lobulated ones,

simulating "psoas muscles" into the thorax (Figs. 73-6 and 73-7). Extramedullary hematopoiesis appears on CT as well-defined, soft tissue lobular lesions, with density similar to muscles. On MRI the lesions are of intermediate signal intensity on T1-weighted images, variable signal intensity on T2-weighted images, and moderate enhancement after contrast medium administration (see Fig. 73-7).

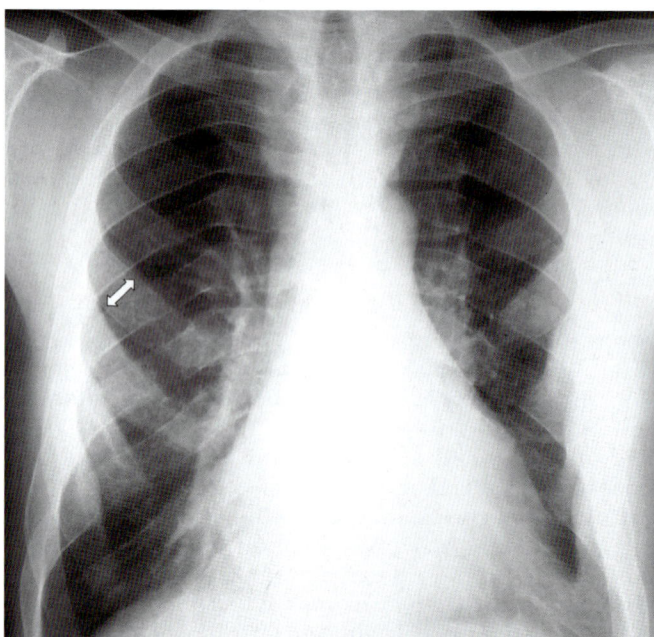

■ **FIGURE 73-4** Posteroanterior plain radiograph of a 42-year-old man with β-thalassemia major who had irregular transfusion and recent onset of desferrioxamine treatment. The "rib-in-rib" appearance is shown (*arrow*).

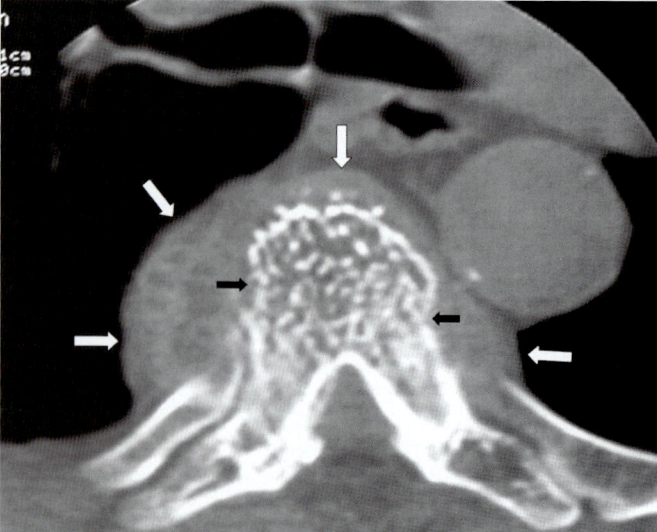

■ **FIGURE 73-6** Axial CT image in a 34-year-old β-thalassemia major patient shows reduction and unequally distributed thick trabeculae, as well as discontinuity along the very thin cortex (*black arrows*). Bilateral paraspinal soft tissue lesions represent extramedullary hematopoiesis (*white arrows*). A previous laminectomy was performed to alleviate symptoms from epidural extramedullary hematopoiesis with cord compression.

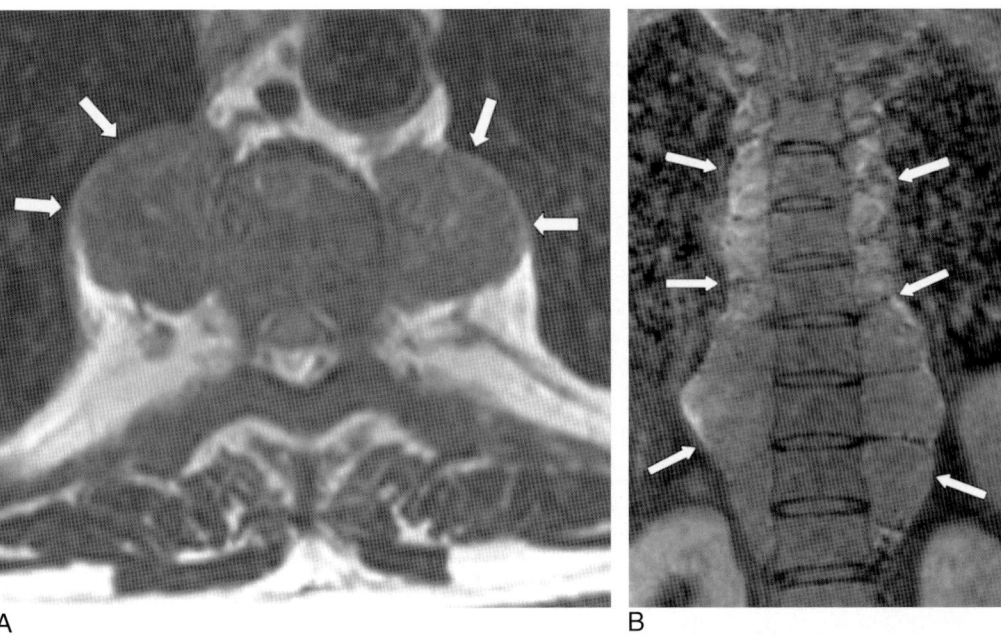

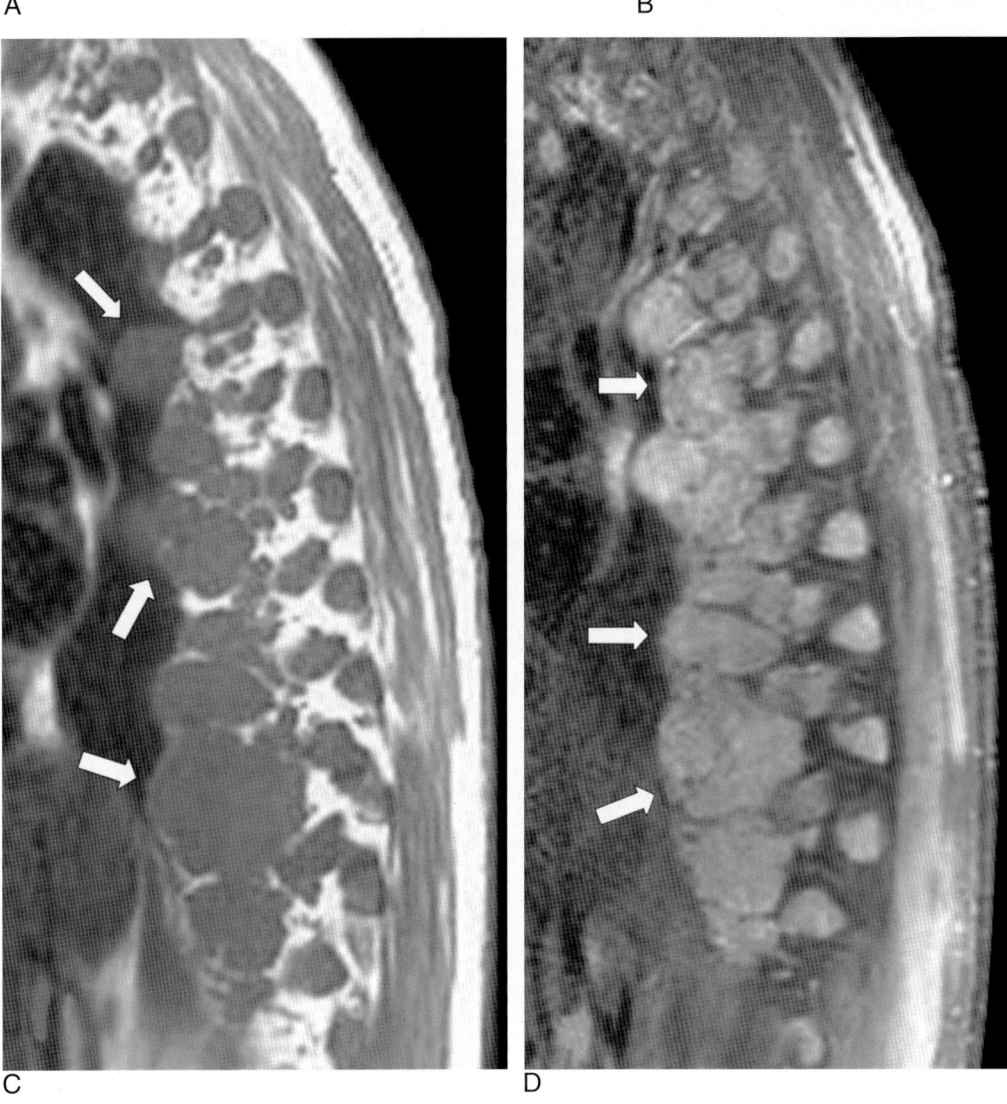

■ **FIGURE 73-7** A 44-year-old β-thalassemia major patient presented with irregular transfusion schema and extramedullary hematopoiesis. **A,** 2D Multi-echo gradient-recalled-echo MR image at the T10 level shows rounded paraspinal lesions (*arrows*) isointense to the vertebral bone marrow. **B,** Contrast medium–enhanced fat-suppressed T1-weighted spin-echo image shows multiple bilateral paravertebral lesions. The parasagittal T1-weighted spin-echo (**C**) and contrast medium–enhanced fat-suppressed T1-weighted spin-echo (**D**) images show the moderate and homogeneous enhancement of the lesions (*arrows*).

Spine

The spinal changes in untreated or poorly treated patients with β-thalassemia major result from bone marrow overgrowth and include deformities (scoliosis, kyphosis), vertebral collapse, osteoporosis, and extramedullary hematopoiesis.[10]

Radiologically, osteoporosis is evident in the vertebral bodies with diminished number and coarsening of trabeculae, thinning of the subchondral bone plates, and biconcave or wedge-shaped deformities (Figs. 73-8 and 73-9; see also Fig. 73-6). Rarely, H-shaped vertebrae of unclear pathogenesis, similar to changes of sickle cell anemia, can be observed. A "bone-within-bone" appearance may also be noted (see Fig. 73-8). Early degeneration of the intervertebral discs occurs in the lower thoracic and lumbar spine and are depicted promptly by MRI (see Fig. 73-9). Extramedullary hematopoiesis results from extraosseous extension of medullary tissue and develops in the paravertebral and presacral spaces, whereas epidural extension may cause cord compression (see Figs. 73-9 and 73-10).[9]

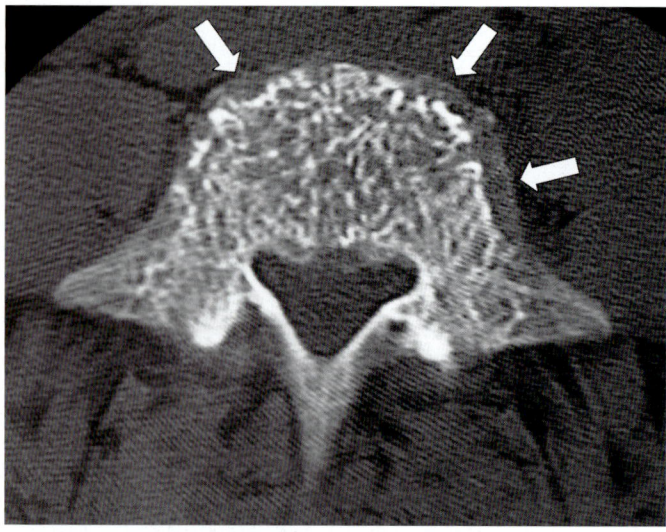

■ **FIGURE 73-8** Axial CT scan in a 13-year-old patient with β-thalassemia shows "bone-within-bone" appearance (*arrows*) and coarsening of the trabeculae.

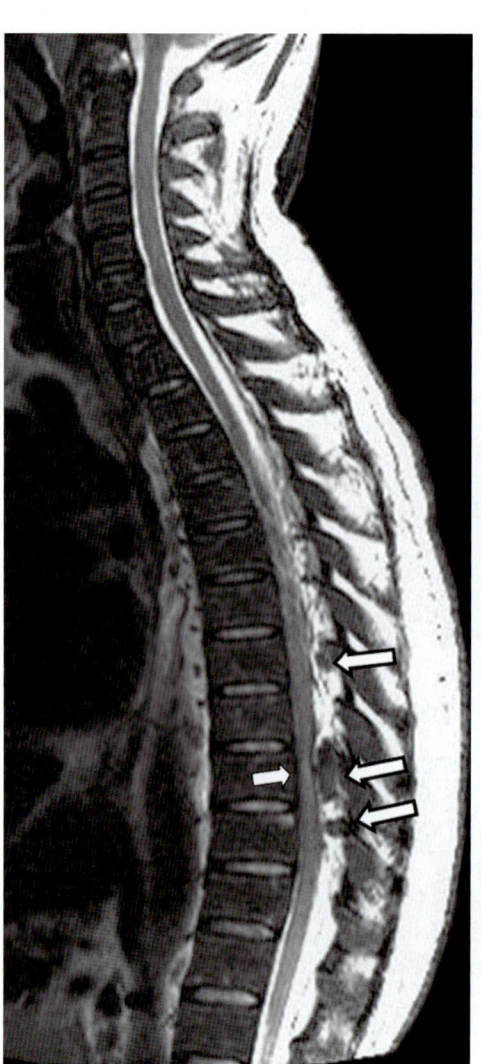

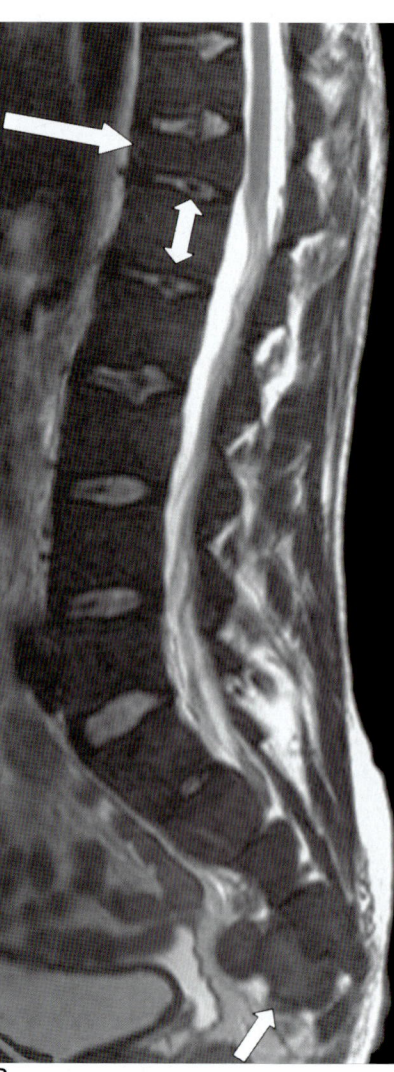

■ **FIGURE 73-9** **A,** A 44-year-old patient with β-thalassemia major presented with a 12-month history of pain in the midthoracic region and recent severe weakness in the lower extremities. The sagittal T2-weighted turbo spin-echo MR image shows extramedullary hematopoietic lesions in the posterior epidural space (*arrows*) compressing the cord, which exhibits high signal intensity (*short arrow*). **B,** A 33-year-old patient with β-thalassemia major presented with a recent history of lower limbs weakness. The sagittal T2-weighted turbo spin-echo MR image shows extramedullary hematopoietic lesions in the presacral area (*short arrow*), expansion of the S2 body, disc degeneration (*double-head arrow*), and an osteoporotic fracture of the T12 vertebral body (*long arrow*).

A

B

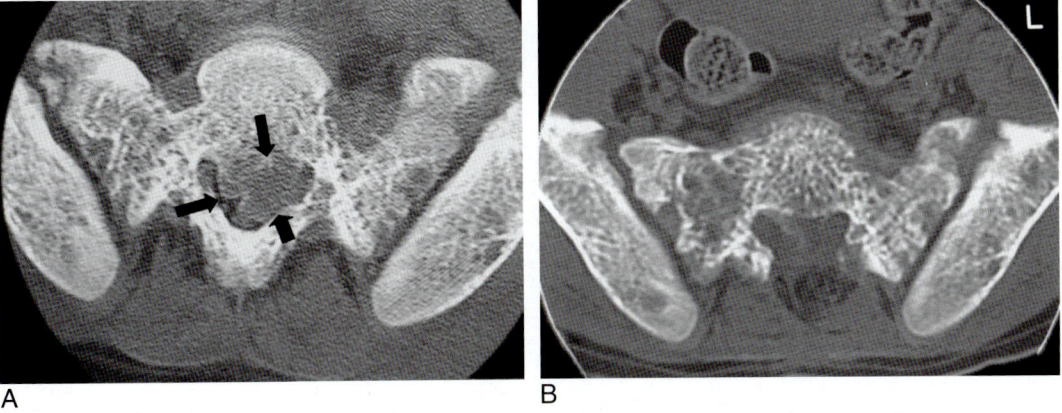

■ **FIGURE 73-10** Axial CT scan of a 12-year-old β-thalassemia major patient with acute paraparesis. **A,** Extramedullary hematopoiesis in the spinal canal causes severe central spinal canal stenosis (*arrows*). Laminectomy was performed within 6 hours of the onset of symptoms and the patient showed complete recovery. **B,** Follow-up CT scan 6 months postoperatively.

MRI is the method of choice for demonstrating epidural disease, owing to its multiplanar and superb soft tissue contrast capability. Various treatment options have been proposed for acute myelopathy due to epidural hematopoiesis, including laminectomy, hypertransfusion, and administration of cytotoxic drugs. Low dose radiation therapy alone has been efficient in prompt resolution of neurologic deficiencies.

Tubular Bones

Bone marrow overgrowth results in widened marrow cavities, cortical thinning, and a coarse appearance of the trabeculae (Fig. 73-11). The osseous contour may be altered with loss of the normal concave outline. The associated widening of the metaphyses and epiphyses resembles the appearance of a flask (see Fig. 73-11). Irregular transverse radiodense lines may be seen close to the ends of the long bones, representing growth arrest and recovery lines in untreated or poorly treated patients (Fig. 73-12). Premature fusion of the growth plates in the tubular bones is found in 10% to 15% of children with β-thalassemia major, usually after the age of 10.[11] Growth arrest mainly involves proximal humeri and distal femora. A discrepancy in leg length might be observed, in which case surgical correction may be required.[11] Premature femoral

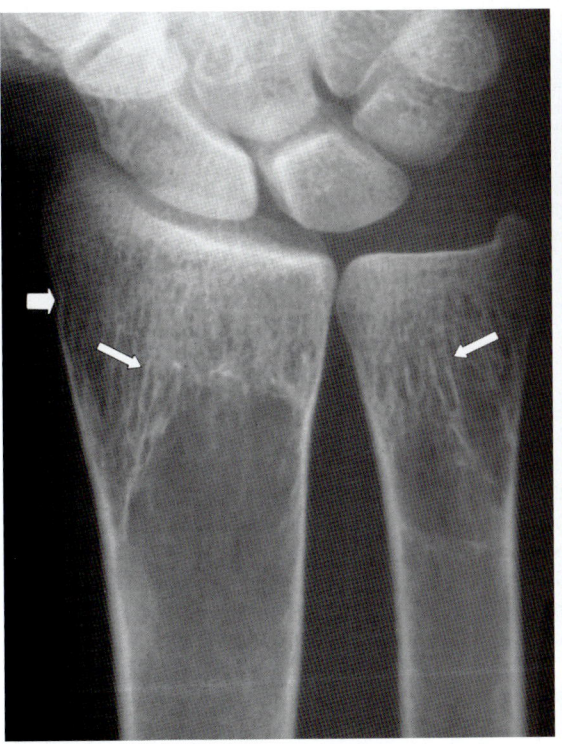

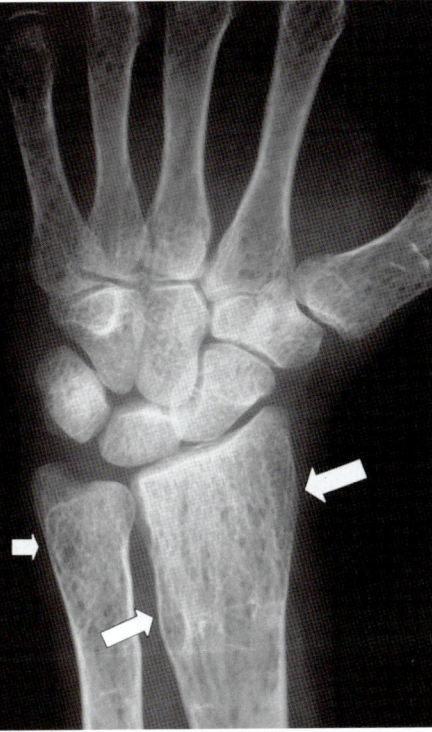

■ **FIGURE 73-11** A and B, Radiographs in two different β-thalassemia major patients show coarse trabeculation (*thin arrows*), thinned cortices (*thick short arrows*), and widened flask-like shafts from medullary expansion (*thick arrows*).

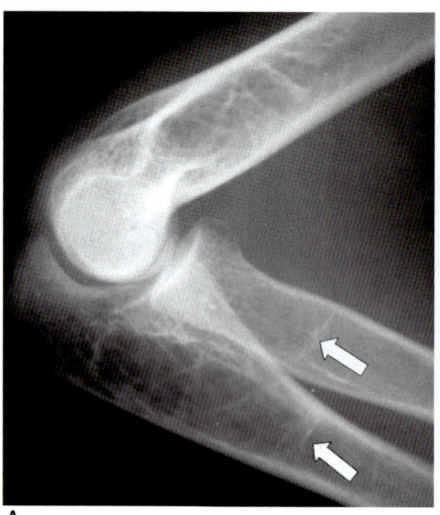
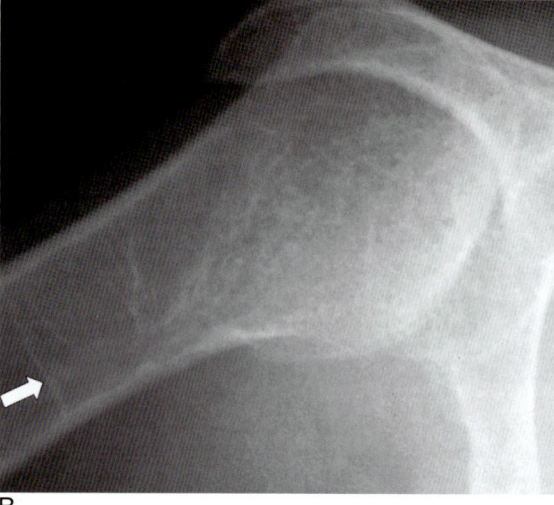

A   B

■ **FIGURE 73-12** Irregular transverse radiodense lines (*arrows*) represent growth arrest and recovery lines in poorly treated patients. **A,** A 35-year-old β-thalassemia major patient who had irregular transfusion. **B,** Same patient as in Figure 73-4.

and humeral fusion is in contrast to the delayed fusion that is frequently seen in superior iliac crest secondary ossification centers. Enlargement of nutrient foramina in the phalanges of the hand may occur secondary to increased blood supply to the highly vascular proliferated hematopoietic marrow.[6] Increased foraminal size usually does not regress regardless of the transfusion treatment.

Spontaneous fractures in untreated or undertreated patients with β-thalassemia major occur in about one third of the patients and may be multiple or recurrent; they occur more ofter in the long bones of the lower extremity and less often in the forearm. A multicenter study on transfused patients reported a fracture prevalence of 19.7%, suggesting that the risk for fractures exists even when hemoglobin levels are over 9 g/dL and serum ferritin levels less than 1000 ng/mL.[12] Marrow ischemic infarcts and osteonecrosis have been reported to occur more commonly in patients with β-thalassemia major than in the general population (Fig. 73-13).[13] Rarely, spontaneous subperiosteal hematoma may occur (Fig. 73-14).

Bone and Joint Disease after Optimal Transfusion and Iron Chelation

Radiologic abnormalities caused by medullary expansion have become less frequent with the introduction of optimal transfusion treatment strategies. In 1989, Scutellari and associates observed a decrease in the classic radiographic findings of medullary expansion among the high-transfusion group of β-thalassemia major compared with the low-transfusion group.[14] This was further confirmed by others, who showed that only 2 of 41 patients with β-thalassemia major had radiographic evidence of medullary expansion.[15] Both studies indicated the effectiveness of blood transfusion treatment, which is able to preserve excellent health and increase life expectancy.

Before the introduction of iron-chelation therapy, hypertransfused patients were prone to develop joint disease, possibly caused by hemosiderosis, epiphyseal

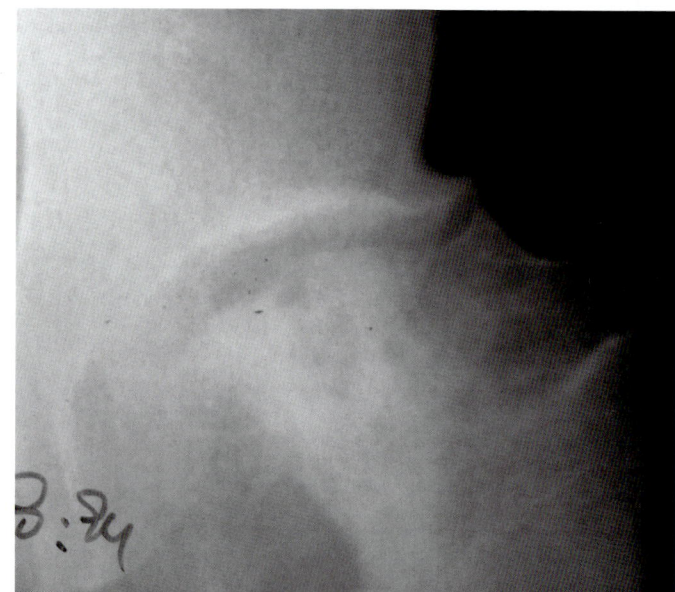

■ **FIGURE 73-13** Plain radiograph of left hip shows osteonecrosis with femoral head collapse and early secondary osteoarthritis in a 19-year-old man with β-thalassemia major.

osteonecrosis, growth disturbances, infection, crystal deposition, hemarthrosis, synovial membrane microvascular obstruction, and localized consequences due to marrow expansion.[16] Hyperuricemia may also appear secondary to repeated blood transfusions; gout is rarely seen, but when it occurs it affects small joints and unusual sites such as the sacroiliac joints. High serum iron levels may cause synovial and articular cartilage abnormalities, usually in the large joints. Radiologic findings of β-thalassemia major–related joint disease include joint space loss, cystic lesions, flattening of the subchondral bone, and osteophyte formation. MRI may show bone iron deposition in the bone marrow and the synovium (Fig. 73-15).

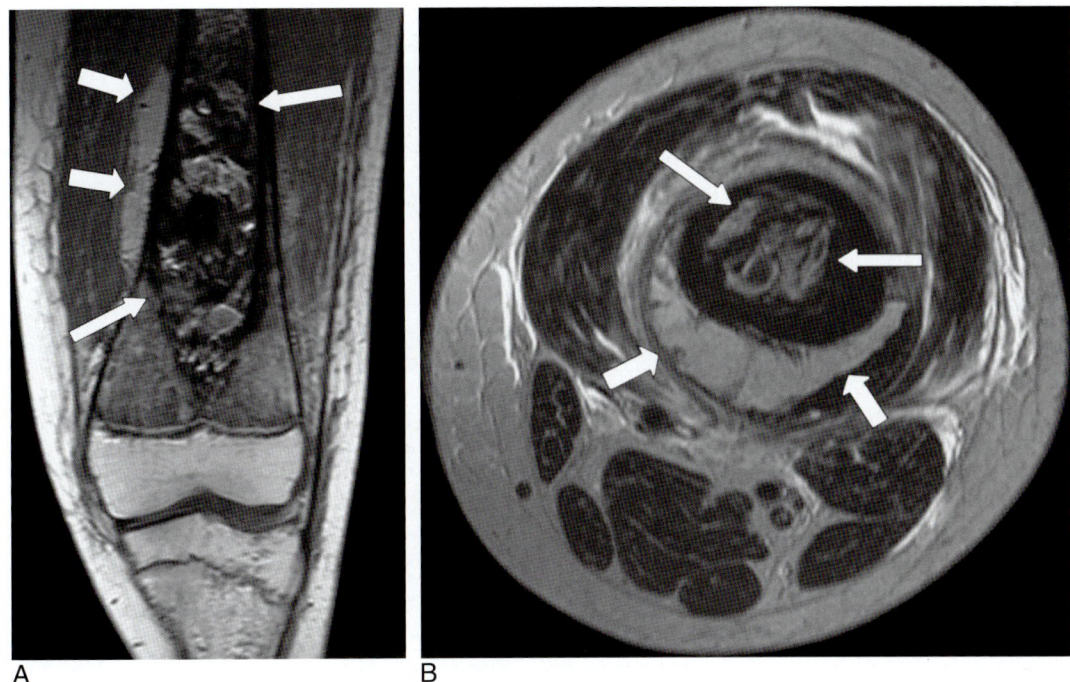

■ **FIGURE 73-14** MR images from a male patient with β-thalassemia major with diaphyseal femoral bone infarcts (*thin arrows*) and spontaneous subperiosteal hematoma presenting with high signal intensity on both T1-weighted spin-echo (**A**) and T2-weighted turbo spin-echo (**B**) sequences (*thick arrows*).

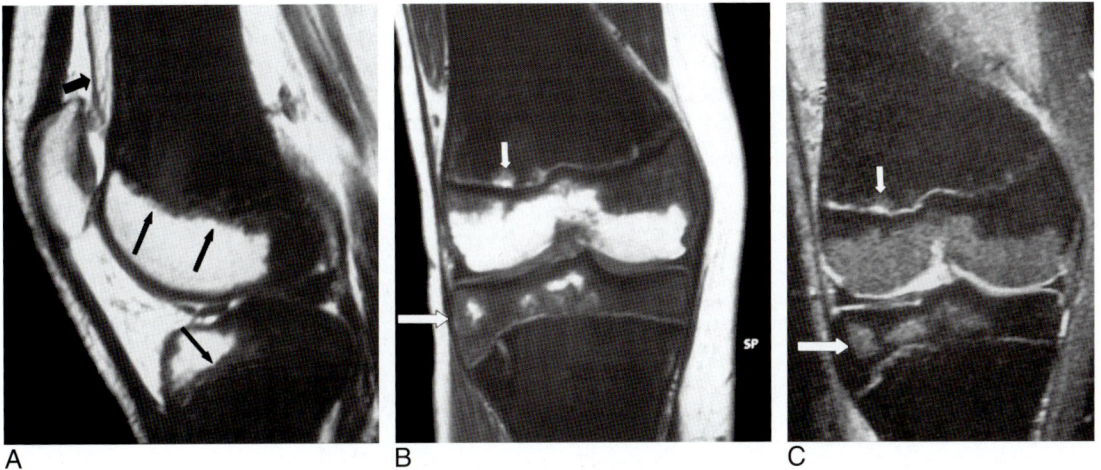

■ **FIGURE 73-15** MR images from a 23-year-old man with β-thalassemia major. **A,** The T2-weighted turbo spin-echo image in the sagittal plane shows diffusely low signal intensity bone marrow (*thin black arrows*) and a low signal intensity synovium (*small black arrow*) consistent with iron deposition. The T1-weighted spin-echo (**B**) and turbo short tau inversion recovery (**C**) images in the coronal plane show juxtaphyseal lesions in the metaphyses (*small white arrows*) and epiphyseal areas of intermediate signal intensity (*white arrows*) that may be attributed to desferrioxamine-induced changes.

Chondrocalcinosis and subchondral erosions may occasionally be seen; they usually do not dissolve after iron-chelation treatment (Fig. 73-16).

Prevention of iron overload can be achieved by optimum chelation therapy. In this case, two agents, namely, desferrioxamine (DFO) and deferiprone, are given parenterally and orally, respectively. Therapeutic agents may cause changes related to toxicity. Prompt imaging recognition of the iron-chelator toxicity may guide treatment with regard to dose reduction or change to another chelator.

DFO is a safe drug administered to β-thalassemia major patients from early childhood throughout life. Patients who receive high doses of DFO, particularly when the iron burden is low, complain frequently of pain in the hips and lower back. A dose of DFO of less than

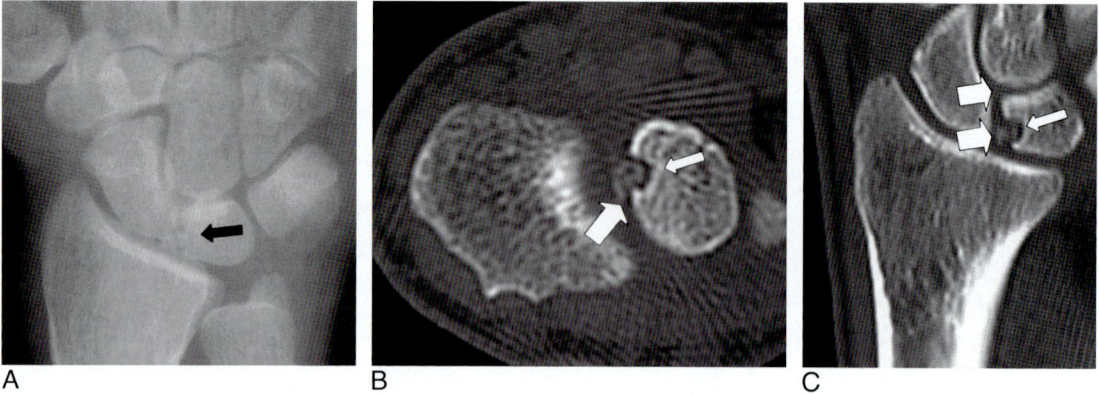

A B C

■ **FIGURE 73-16** A 30-year-old male β-thalassemia major patient was transfused twice a month and presented with a history of 24 years of desferrioxamine therapy and 3 years of deferiprone therapy. Plain anteroposterior radiograph (**A**), axial multidetector CT scan (**B**), and coronal multidetector CT reconstruction (**C**) show secondary hemochromatosis with chondrocalcinosis (*thick arrows*) and subchondral erosion in the lunate (*arrows*). Minus ulnar variant may have occurred secondary to iron-chelated–related growth arrest.

50 mg/kg/day appears to be safe in hypertransfused patients older than the age of 3. DFO administration appears to interfere with enchondral ossification and can result in growth retardation and reduction of growth velocity. The exact mechanism by which DFO interferes with normal bone growth is not known. Inhibition of osteoblast proliferation and chelation of zinc, related to binding of iron, have been shown to play a role.[17] Bone dysplasia occurs in about one third of β-thalassemia major patients who receive DFO iron-chelation therapy. These patients may have a short trunk with discrepancy between the upper and lower limbs. However, it has not been clarified yet whether the altered bone growth is related to drug dose or age at onset of chelation.[17] The balance between DFO and the amount of iron available for chelation may be more important than the age of treatment onset. Bone biopsy in β-thalassemia major patients treated with DFO showed that osseous lesions correspond to areas with a paucity of mineralization. Radiologic changes of the DFO-related bone disease consist of flattening of the thoracic and lumbar vertebral bodies that resemble spondylometaphyseal dysplasia, metaphyseal abnormalities, and growth retardation (Figs. 73-17 to 73-19). Metaphyseal abnormalities include widening, sclerotic longitudinal trabeculations, irregularity of the metaphyseal zone with sclerotic and radiolucent cystic areas, and widened growth

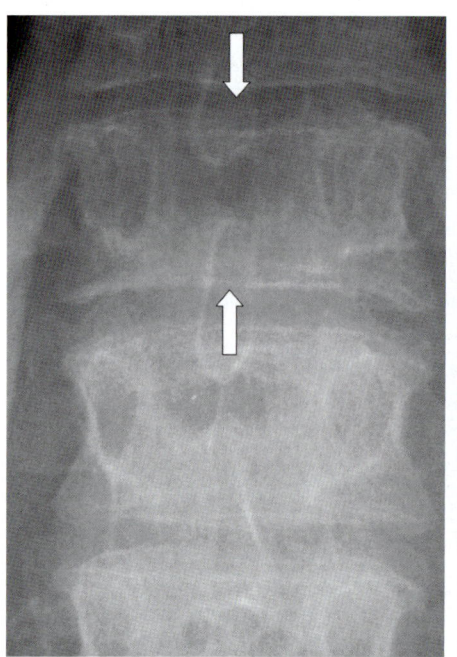

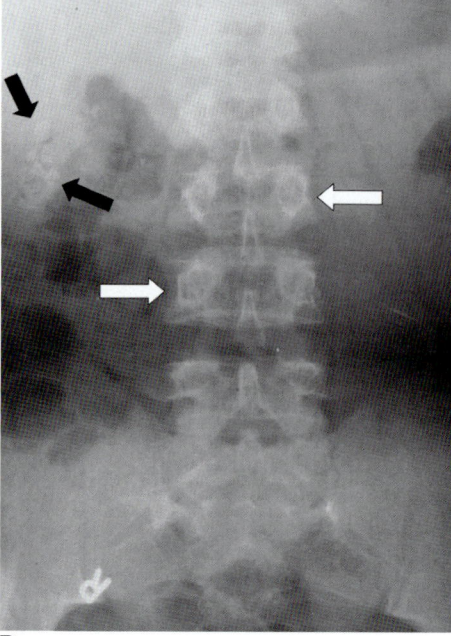

A B

■ **FIGURE 73-17** Plain radiographs of the spine in a 28-year-old woman (**A**) and a 31-year-old man (**B**) with β-thalassemia on desferrioxamine treatment show platyspondyly (*white arrows*). Gallstones are seen on the second patient (*black arrows*).

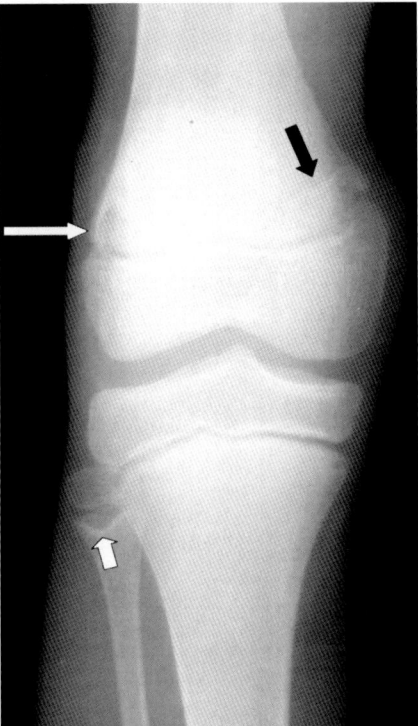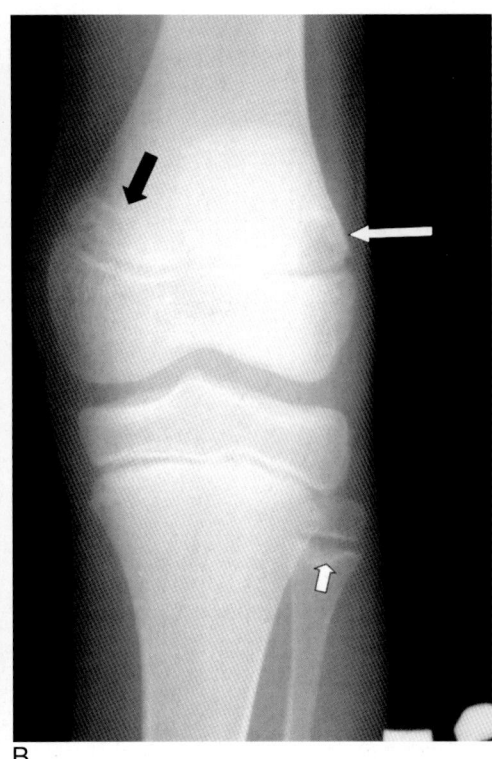

■ **FIGURE 73-18** Radiographs from a 13-year-old boy with β-thalassemia major who had been transfused since 2½ years of age and chelated with desferrioxamine since 5 years of age. The knee region shows mild genu valgum, distal femoral metaphyseal sclerosis (*black arrows*), juxta-metaphyseal lucencies (*white arrows*), and widened growth plates (*small arrows*).

A B

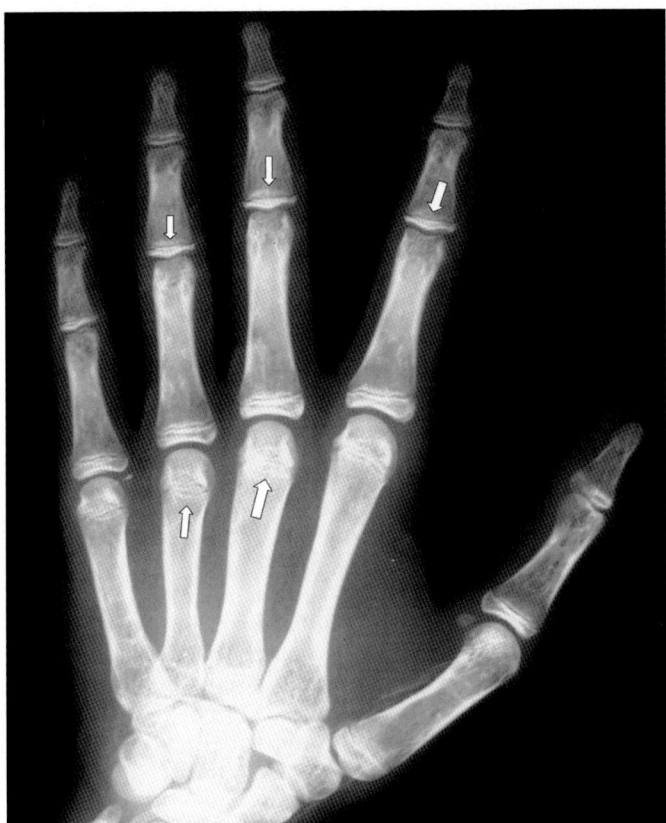

■ **FIGURE 73-19** Radiograph from a 19-year-old male β-thalassemia major patient who was begun on transfusion therapy at 1 year of age and chelation therapy at 5 years of age. Plain radiograph of the left hand reveals metaphyseal sclerosis at the distal metacarpal and proximal phalangeal metaphyses (*arrows*). Growth plates are still open due to retardation.

plate.[17] Radiologic findings are usually bilateral and more prominent in the metaphyses of the knees and wrists, characteristically starting to appear at about the age of 3 and possibly associated with a genu valgum deformity. In one study, all of 12 β-thalassemia major patients with evidence of long-bone changes due to DFO administration had distal ulna involvement.[18] Only one study addressed the MRI findings in a series of patients treated with DFO.[19] In this study, epiphyseal involvement occurred in 45% of patients exhibiting lateral distal physeal widening and blurring of the physeal-metaphyseal junction of the femur. In addition, metaphyseal lesions that are hypointense on T1-weighted images and hyperintense on T2-weighted images seem to match the well-known DFO-induced dysplastic changes seen on plain radiographs. Patients with MRI evidence of bone dysplasia have a significantly lower body height compared with patients without evidence of bone dysplasia.[19] Reduction of the DFO dose has a positive influence on healing of the metaphyseal abnormalities with partial or complete obliteration of the cystic defects and increased bone sclerosis.[17]

Deferiprone has been introduced in clinical use as an iron chelator rather recently and is administered orally. Toxic side effects of this therapy result in an arthropathy involving mainly the knees that is manifested clinically with stiffness, joint pain, swelling, and effusion.[20] Previous reports have suggested that this arthropathy is more frequent in patients who are more heavily iron loaded and who receive larger doses of the drug (100 mg/kg/day).[21] The exact cause of the deferiprone-related arthropathy is not well understood.[20] It has been suggested that this disorder could have resulted from a toxic effect of the deferiprone-mediated free radicals.[20] Iron deposits in

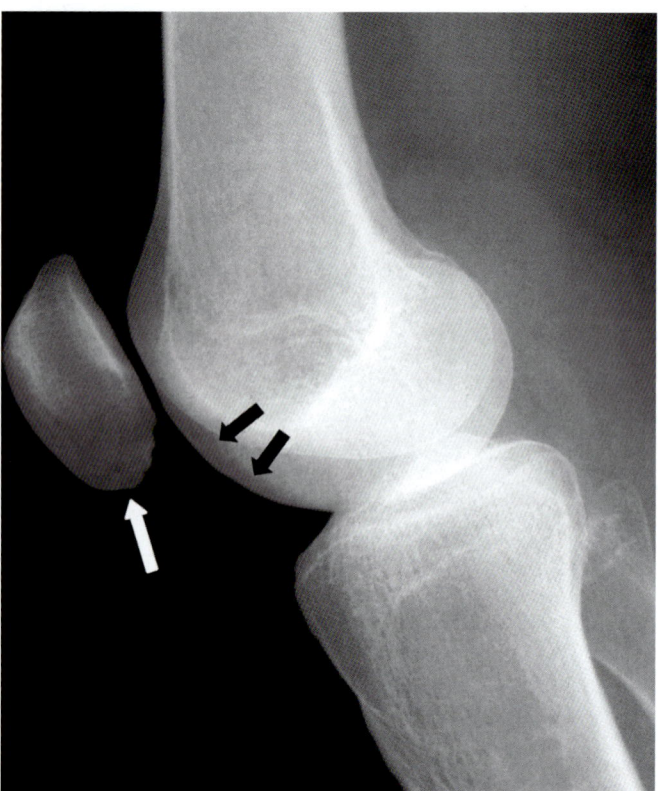

■ **FIGURE 73-20** A 33-year-old woman with β-thalassemia major who was treated with transfusion for 29 years and with chelation with both desferrioxamine and deferiprone. Plain lateral radiograph shows subcortical erosions of the lower pole of the patella (*white arrow*) and subchondral cortical irregularity and subcortical lesions of the femoral condyle (*black arrows*).

synovium have been confirmed with biopsy.[22] The reason why deferiprone predominantly affects epiphyseal cartilage, as opposed to DFO which affects the growth plate, has not been clarified. The radiographic findings of deferiprone-related arthropathy have not been well described in the literature. In one study, 64% of patients complained of arthralgia whereas abnormal imaging findings were present in 86% of the patients and included irregular flattening of the subchondral femoral condyles, the tibial plateau and the patella, and a broad beak of the superior patellar pole (Fig. 73-20).[22] In the same study, MRI findings on contrast enhanced T1-weighted images included diffuse thickening and intense enhancement of the synovium; and on T2-weighted images, hypointense bands were most conspicuous in the region of the infrapatellar fat pad and high signal intensity lesions were evident in the articular cartilage extending into defects of the subchondral bone.

Osteoporosis-Bone Mineral Densitometry

Osteoporosis is characterized by low bone mass, resulting in reduced bone strength and increased risk of fractures of the vertebral bodies, distal forearm, and proximal femur. Osteoporosis may become a major cause of morbidity in β-thalassemia major patients who, if optimally

treated, will have a longer life expectancy. Factors contributing to the development of osteoporosis include failure to achieve a peak bone density during skeletal growth, anemia with chronic disease-related reduced activity, hypogonadism, excessive bone resorption, DFO toxicity, and calcium/vitamin D deficiency.[23] Bone formation is not impaired although bone resorption is grossly increased in β-thalassemia major patients, and its severity appears to depend on the levels of hemoglobin.[24]

Various quantitative studies with dual-energy x-ray absorptiometry (DXA) have addressed the degree of osteoporosis in β-thalassemia major patients. In a series of 82 optimally treated β-thalassemia major patients, osteoporosis was present in 42%, with a pattern of spinal involvement in females and one of spinal and femoral involvement in males.[25] Similar results were reported by others on 50 patients, who also proved that hormonal replacement therapy is important and successful in increasing the bone mineral density.[26]

A discrepancy, was found by others, between DXA and quantitative computed tomography (QCT), the mean Z score of the spine by DXA being −2.46 whereas by QCT it was −1.25.[26] In another similar study on 48 patients, it was shown that the overall prevalence of spinal osteoporosis was 44% with DXA and only 6% with QCT.[27] In the same study, the 10-year follow-up showed that in spite of the high percentage of osteoporosis, as defined with DXA, a low number of patients had been complaining of symptoms as backache, and only 4 have suffered fractures of the peripheral skeleton. On the island of Crete, data from the two thalassemia units showed that none of the 75 optimally transfused and iron-chelation treated patients suffered any osteoporotic fracture (personal communication). Another study with single-energy QCT in thalassemic patients and controls found statistically significant difference between mean bone mineral density values (173.4 and 158.2 mg/cm³, respectively).[28] This discrepancy between the two methods may be related to differential involvement of cortical and trabecular bone, considering that DXA measures bone density across the whole vertebrae whereas QCT measures trabecular density and cortical density separately. A possible explanation for the increased bone mineral density values in QCT is the transfusion-related iron deposition in the marrow.[29,30] Single-energy QCT thus may overestimate the real mineral vertebral content, and the same phenomenon occurs using DXA but to a lesser degree owing to the two x-ray energies employed. In conclusion, with regard to the presence of osteopenia or osteoporosis in β-thalassemia major patients, it seems that estimation of bone mineral density yields variable results depending highly on the technique used and the underlying status of the disease. Most of the patients should be classified as osteopenic and/or osteoporotic with DXA, but this is not in accordance with the absence of osteoporotic fractures in optimally treated patients.

Bone Marrow and Magnetic Resonance Imaging

The MRI appearance of bone marrow reflects the patient's transfusion and chelation history. In optimally transfused patients there is little marrow expansion.

Hypertransfused, but not optimally chelated patients with raised serum ferritin levels demonstrate iron deposition in the central and peripheral skeleton, resulting in marrow that is of low signal intensity on all pulse sequences (see Figs 74-9 and 74-15). Iron deposition is greatest in areas of high red marrow concentration. Patients with optimal transfusion and chelation therapy may still demonstrate some iron deposition in the skeleton. The long-term effects of this clinically undetectable level of iron deposition are unknown. It has been shown with quantitative signal intensity correlation that bone marrow hypointensity on MRI, due to iron deposition, is a frequent finding in β-thalassemia major patients.[30] The degree of marrow siderosis, expressed as a marrow to paraspinal muscles ratio, correlates with splenic siderosis and serum ferritin levels, which is a serum marker of iron overload, but does not correlate with liver siderosis, possibly implying differences in the mechanisms of iron deposition between bone marrow and liver.[30]

DIFFERENTIAL DIAGNOSIS

The clinical differential diagnosis depends on the status of the treatment. The "hair-on-end" and the marrow hyperplasia-associated radiologic findings are also found in iron-deficiency anemia, sickle cell disease, and spherocytosis. Growth arrest and osteoporosis can be found in any chronic disease and in many congenital disorders.

Patients who are undertreated may show a bone-within-bone appearance in the spine that might resemble osteopetrosis or renal osteodystrophy. H-shaped vertebrae are quite similar to the changes of sickle cell anemia. Patients taking DFO may show flattening of the thoracic and lumbar vertebral bodies that resemble spondylometaphyseal dysplasia.

SYNOPSIS OF TREATMENT OPTIONS

Medical Treatment

A defect in globin chain synthesis in homozygous β-thalassemia major results in diminished red blood cell life span and severe hypochromic anemia. Untreated or undertreated patients suffer from marked red marrow hyperplasia, resulting in characteristic radiographic features of medullary expansion. Extramedullary hematopoiesis may occur in the paravertebral or epidural anatomic spaces. The introduction of regular blood transfusion to maintain high levels of pretransfusion hemoglobin and of chelation therapy to reduce iron overload has improved the clinical status and life span of these patients.

Surgical Treatment

Acute spinal cord compression due to extramedullary hematopoiesis needs urgent surgical decompression with or without adjuvant radiotherapy.

What the Referring Physician Needs to Know

- The classic radiologic signs due to marrow expansion or extramedullary hematopoiesis are now rare.
- Well-transfused patients present with iron deposition- or iron chelation-related bone disease and osteoporosis.
- Plain radiographs, MRI, and bone mineral densitometry are currently used in assessing bone disease in β-thalassemia major patients.
- Accurate interpretation of imaging findings of β-thalassemia major patients requires exact knowledge of transfusion schema and iron chelation.
- Bone mineral studies should be applied and interpreted with caution because the underlying variable degree of marrow siderosis might interfere with the measurements.

SUGGESTED READINGS

Low LC. Growth, puberty and endocrine function in beta-thalassaemia major. J Pediatr Endocrinol Metab. 1997;10:175–184.

Wonke B. Bone disease in beta-thalassaemia major. Br J Haematol. 1998;103:897–901.

Tunaci M, Tunaci A, Engin G, et. al. Imaging features of thalassemia. Eur Radiol 1999;9:1804–1809.

Rund D, Rachmilewitz E. Beta-thalassemia. N Engl J Med. 2005;353:1135–1146.

Tyler PA, Madani G, Chaudhuri R, Wilson LF, Dick EA. The radiological appearances of thalassaemia. Clin Radiol. 2006;61:40–52.

REFERENCES

1. Cooley TB, Lee P. A series of cases of splenomegaly in children with anemia and peculiar bone change. Transact Am Pediatr Soc 1925; 37:29.
2. Spritz RA, Forget BG. The thalassemias: molecular mechanisms of human genetic disease. Am J Hum Genet 1983; 35:333–361.
3. Cazzola M, Borgna-Pignatti C, Locatelli F, et al. A moderate transfusion regimen may reduce iron loading in beta-thalassemia major without producing excessive expansion of erythropoiesis. Transfusion 1997; 37:135–140.
4. Mahachoklertwattana P, Sirikulchayanonta V, Chuansumrit A, et al. Bone histomorphometry in children and adolescents with beta-thalassemia disease: iron-associated focal osteomalacia. J Clin Endocrinol Metab 2003; 88:3966–3972.
5. Piomelli S, Danoff SJ, Becker MH, et al. Prevention of bone malformations and cardiomegaly in Cooley's anemia by early hypertransfusion regimen. Ann N Y Acad Sci 1969; 165:427–436.
6. Lawson JP, Ablow RC, Pearson HA. Colonial and phalangeal vascular impressions in thalassemia. AJR Am J Roentgenol 1984; 143:641–645.
7. Moseley JE. Skeletal changes in the anemias. Semin Roentgenol 1974; 3:169–184.

8. Lawson JP, Ablow RC, Pearson HA. The ribs in thalassemia: I. The relationship to therapy. Radiology 1981; 140:663–672.

9. Loh CK, Alcorta C, McElhinney AJ. Extramedullary hematopoiesis simulating posterior mediastinal tumors. Ann Thorac Surg 1996; 61:1003–1005.

10. Korovessis PG, Papanastasiou D, Tiniakou M, Beratis NG. Prevalence of scoliosis in beta-thalassemia. J Spinal Disord 1996; 9:170–173.

11. Currarino G, Erlandson ME. Premature fusion of the epiphyses in Cooley's anemia. Radiology 1964; 83:656–664.

12. Ruggiero L, De Sanctis V. Multicentre study of prevalence of fractures in transfusion-dependent thalassaemic patients. J Pediatr Endocrinol Metab 1998; 11(Suppl 3):773–778.

13. Orzincolo C, Castaldi G, Scutellari PN, et al. Aseptic necrosis of femoral head complicating thalassemia. Skeletal Radiol 1986; 15:541–544.

14. Scutellari PN, Orzincolo C, Franceschini F, et al. The radiographic appearances following adequate transfusion in beta-thalassaemia. Skeletal Radiol 1989; 17:545–550.

15. Chan YL, Li CK, Pang LM, Chik KW. Desferrioxamine-induced long bone changes in thalassaemic patients—radiographic features, prevalence and relations with growth. Clin Radiol 2000; 55:610–614.

16. Gratwick GM, Bullough PG, Bohne WH, et al. Thalassemic osteoarthropathy. Ann Intern Med 1978; 88:494–501.

17. Brill PW, Winchester P, Giardina PJ, Cunningham-Rundles S. Deferoxamine-induced bone dysplasia in patients with thalassemia major. AJR Am J Roentgenol 1991; 156:561–565.

18. Orzincolo C, Scutellari PN, Castaldi G. Growth plate injury of the long bones in treated beta-thalassemia. Skeletal Radiol 1992; 21:39–44.

19. Chan YL, Li CK, Chu WCW, et al. Deferoxamine-induced bone dysplasia in the distal femur and patella of pediatric patients and young adults: MR imaging appearance. AJR Am J Roentgenol 2000; 175:1561–1566.

20. Diav-Citrin O, Koren G. Oral iron chelation with deferiprone. Pediatr Clin North Am 1997; 44:235–247.

21. Agarwal MB. Oral iron chelation: a review with special emphasis on Indian work on deferiprone (L1). Indian J Pediatr 1993; 60:509–516.

22. Kellenberger CJ, Schmugge M, Saurenmann T, et al. Radiographic and MRI features of deferiprone-related arthropathy of the knees in patients with beta-thalassemia. AJR Am J Roentgenol 2004; 183:989–994.

23. Jensen CE, Tuck SM, Agnew JE, et al. High prevalence of low bone mass in thalassaemia major. Br J Haematol 1998; 103:911–915.

24. Voskaridou E, Kyrtsonis MC, Terpos E, et al. Bone resorption is increased in young adults with thalassaemia major. Br J Haematol 2001; 112:36–41.

25. Molyvda-Athanassopoulou E, Sioundas A, Karatzas N, et al. Bone mineral density of patients with thalassemia major: four-year follow-up. Calcif Tissue Int 1999; 64:481–484.

26. Danesi L, Cherubini R, Ciceri L, et al. Evaluation of spine and hip bone density by DXA and QCT in thalassemic patients. J Pediatr Endocrinol Metab 1998; 11:961–962.

27. Mylona M, Leotsinides M, Alexandrides T, et al. Comparison of DXA, QCT and trabecular structure in beta-thalassemia. Eur J Haematol 2005; 74:430–437.

28. Akpek S, Canatan D, Arac M, Ilgit ET. Evaluation of osteoporosis in thalassemia by quantitative computed tomography: is it reliable? Pediatr Hematol Oncol 2001; 18:111–116.

29. Kalef-Ezra J, Zibis A, Chaliassos N, et al. Body composition in homozygous beta-thalassemia. Ann N Y Acad Sci 2000; 904:621–624.

30. Drakonaki EE, Maris T, Papadakis A, Karantanas AH. Bone marrow changes in beta-thalassemia major: quantitative MR imaging findings and correlation with iron stores. Eur Radiol 2006 Dec 16; Epub.

74

Myelofibrosis

Eoin Carl Kavanagh

ETIOLOGY

Myelofibrosis is a chronic myeloproliferative disorder characterized by bone marrow fibrosis and the development of extramedullary hematopoiesis. Myelofibrosis can occur as a primary disease entity (also termed *idiopathic myelofibrosis* or *agnogenic myeloid metaplasia*) or can occur secondary to diffuse bony metastatic disease, infections (e.g., tuberculosis and fungal infections), sarcoidosis, myeloma, and lymphoma. The etiology of primary myelofibrosis is unknown, but an increased incidence of this disease is seen after exposure to radiation and to bone marrow toxins such as benzene. Primary myelofibrosis occurs as a result of a clonal proliferation of myeloid cells with variable maturity and hematopoietic efficiency.

The marrow fibrosis that occurs is a reactive process of nonclonal fibroblasts, mediated by cytokines such as platelet-derived growth factor (PGDF) and transforming growth factor (TGF)-β, shed from clonally expanded megakaryocytes. A variety of genetic factors have been implicated in the development of primary myelofibrosis, including the *JAK2* tyrosine kinase mutation that has been described in a variety of myeloproliferative disorders.[1]

PREVALENCE AND EPIDEMIOLOGY

Primary myelofibrosis is a rare disorder with reported incidence figures that range from 0.5 to 1.5 in 100,000. The male-to-female ratio has been reported as 1.2 to 1.6:1. The median age at diagnosis is 60 years, with rare cases reported in young adults and children. Cases of primary myelofibrosis in children often have a more indolent course than those in adults.

CLINICAL PRESENTATION

Myelofibrosis is typically insidious in onset, and many patients are asymptomatic at the time of diagnosis. The most common presenting symptoms are fatigue due to anemia or abdominal fullness related to splenomegaly (a site of extramedullary hematopoiesis). Less common presenting symptoms include bleeding and bone pain.

On examination there is splenomegaly in virtually all patients, which can be massive. Hepatomegaly is seen in 50% of patients, and lymphadenopathy is seen in 10%. As the disease progresses the associated anemia becomes more severe and may require repeated transfusions. Splenic infarction can occur, leading to episodes of abdominal pain. Extramedullary hematopoiesis in the epidural space can lead to cord compression late in the course of the disease.

PATHOPHYSIOLOGY

Myelofibrosis is characterized by the replacement of normal marrow with fibrous material (reticulin and collagen) and by the presence of extramedullary hematopoiesis. The fibrotic changes that occur in bone are due to a process of nonclonal fibroblasts, mediated by cytokines that are shed from clonal megakaryocytes. The major cytokines implicated are PGDF and TGF-β. PGDF stimulates fibroblasts to proliferate and secrete collagen whereas TGF-β enhances the secretion of extracellular matrix proteins. The degree of bone marrow cellularity seen is variable and depends on the degree of fibrosis present. In acute cases the bones may appear osteopenic on radiographs with marrow infiltration seen on scintigraphy and MRI. As the disease progresses, the marrow becomes hypocellular and fibrotic. In more chronic cases, bone marrow fibrosis is then seen as areas of osteosclerosis on radiographs and as areas of T1 and T2 hypointensity on MRI.

KEY POINTS

- Myelofibrosis can occur as a primary disease entity or secondary to infiltrative disorders of bone marrow.
- Bone marrow fibrosis and splenomegaly are key imaging features of myelofibrosis.
- MRI is the investigation of choice for bone marrow assessment.
- Myelofibrosis is a progressive disorder with no specific medical treatments showing any overall benefit.

Almost all cases of myelofibrosis have splenomegaly, and splenic histology shows extramedullary hematopoiesis. Foci of extramedullary hematopoiesis can also be seen in the liver, kidneys, lymph nodes, adrenal glands, lungs, and the epidural space. At these sites, mesenchymal cells responsible for fetal hematopoiesis can be activated. The mechanisms responsible for extramedullary hematopoiesis are not fully understood. Sites of extramedullary hematopoiesis may enlarge significantly after splenectomy.

IMAGING TECHNIQUES

Techniques and Relevant Aspects

A variety of imaging techniques can be used in the investigation of myelofibrosis. Typically, radiographs will show osteosclerosis in 30% to 70% of patients. Abdominal radiographs can also show splenomegaly. MRI is the investigation of choice for evaluation of the bone marrow due to its superior soft tissue resolution. CT can show osteosclerosis and sites of extramedullary hematopoiesis.

Pros and Cons

The advantages of MRI over CT for evaluation of marrow pathology include its superior ability to evaluate soft tissues and the fact that it does not employ ionizing radiation.

MANIFESTATIONS OF THE DISEASE

The most frequently encountered radiographic manifestations of myelofibrosis are diffuse bone marrow fibrosis and sites of extramedullary hematopoiesis. Although all these findings can be seen on radiographs, MRI is the investigation of choice to evaluate the fibrotic marrow changes seen in myelofibrosis.

Radiography

Osteosclerosis is seen in 30% to 70% of patients, particularly in the axial skeleton and proximal long bones. Abdominal radiographs may show the classic combination of axial osteosclerosis and splenomegaly. Radiographs can also show areas of patchy demineralization in more acute cases of myelofibrosis. The cortical thickening seen in long bones is secondary to endosteal sclerosis. This results in obliteration of the normal interface between cortical and medullary bone.

Magnetic Resonance Imaging

The bone marrow in myelofibrosis shows low signal intensity on T1- and T2-weighted sequences, reflecting fibrotic marrow change (Fig. 74-1). Focal areas with reconversion of fatty marrow to red marrow are typically seen in the shafts of long bones. Areas of hyperintensity on inversion recovery images within the bone marrow have been described in myelofibrosis, and spectroscopic studies have shown a large resonance of water in such cases.[2] Typically, heterogeneous marrow enhancement is seen after administration of gadolinium. Areas of ischemic bone marrow will not enhance, and therefore the enhancement patterns can be variable. MRI has not been demonstrated to be of use in distinguishing between primary and secondary myelofibrosis because the marrow changes seen in both entities are identical. MRI may also be of value in planning

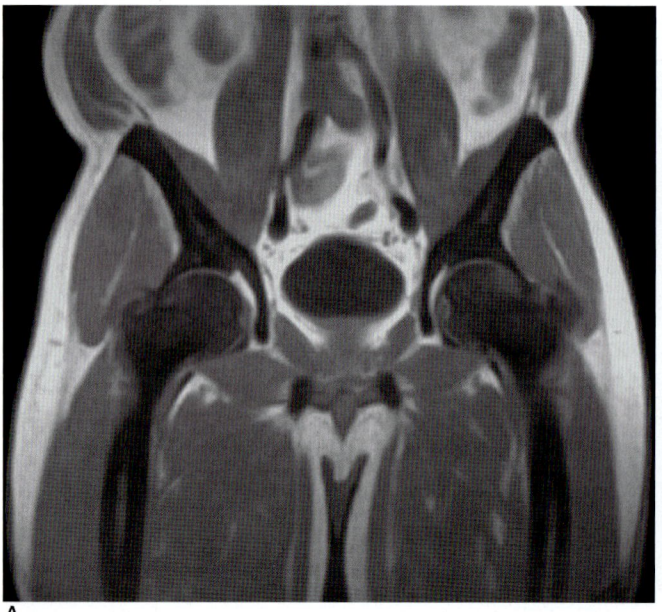
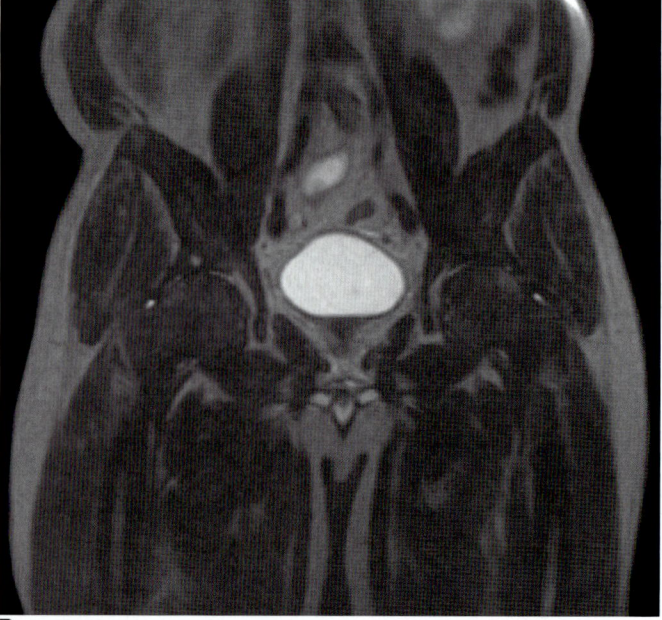

A   B

■ **FIGURE 74-1**   **A,** Coronal T1-weighted image of the pelvis in a 67-year-old man with myelofibrosis shows extensive areas of T1 hypointensity throughout the pelvis and proximal femora. **B,** Coronal T2-weighted image of the pelvis in a 67-year-old man with myelofibrosis shows extensive areas of T2 hypointensity throughout the pelvis and proximal femora.

site-specific bone biopsy. The MRI findings of marrow fibrosis will vary depending on the severity and stage of the disease.[3] MRI is also very useful for the assessment of sites of extramedullary hematopoiesis (Fig. 74-2).[4]

Multidetector Computed Tomography

Multidetector CT shows areas of osteosclerosis throughout the axial skeleton and proximal long bones (Fig. 74-3). MDCT can also show sites of extramedullary hematopoiesis such as splenomegaly, hepatomegaly, lymphadenopathy, and soft tissue masses (Fig. 74-4).[5]

Ultrasonography

Abdominal ultrasonography can demonstrate splenomegaly and hepatomegaly in patients with myelofibrosis.

Nuclear Medicine

Diffusely increased uptake is typically shown on routine bone scintigraphy, secondary to osteosclerosis. Markedly increased uptake can be seen throughout the spleen and liver on technetium-99m colloid scans and on indium-111 chloride scans.

Positron Emission Tomography/Computed Tomography

Combined PET/CT can show markedly increased uptake throughout the spleen and liver and diffusely throughout the bone marrow.[6]

Dual-Energy X-ray Absorptiometry

Elevated bone densitometry measurements have been reported in cases of myelofibrosis.[7]

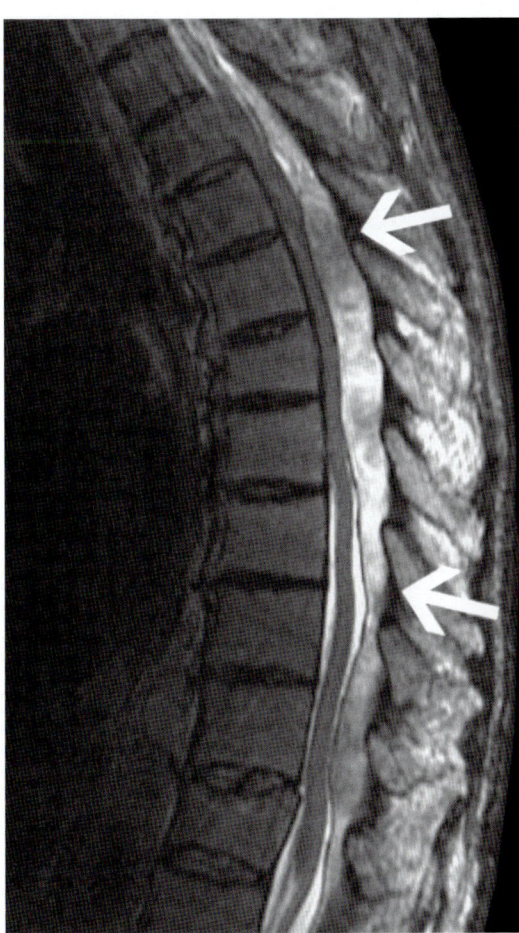

■ **FIGURE 74-2** Sagittal T2-weighted image of the thoracic spine in a 65-year-old woman with a history of myelofibrosis and bilateral lower limb neurologic signs. A lobulated hyperintense mass is present in the posterior epidural space (*arrows*). Surgical decompression was performed, and intraoperative biopsy revealed extramedullary hematopoiesis.

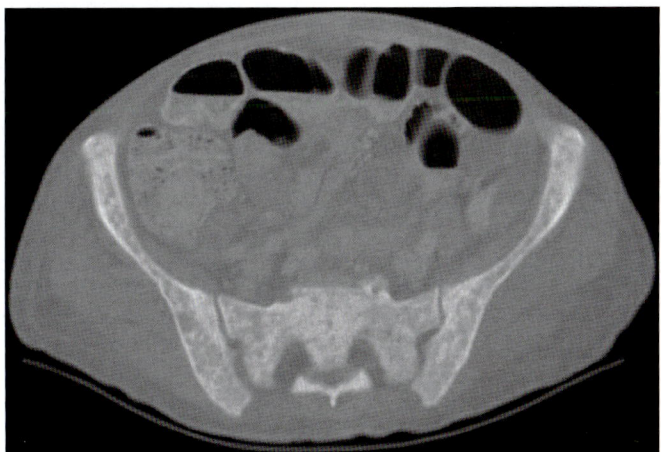

■ **FIGURE 74-3** Axial noncontrast CT scan in a 70-year-old man with myelofibrosis shows diffuse osteosclerosis in the iliac bones and sacrum.

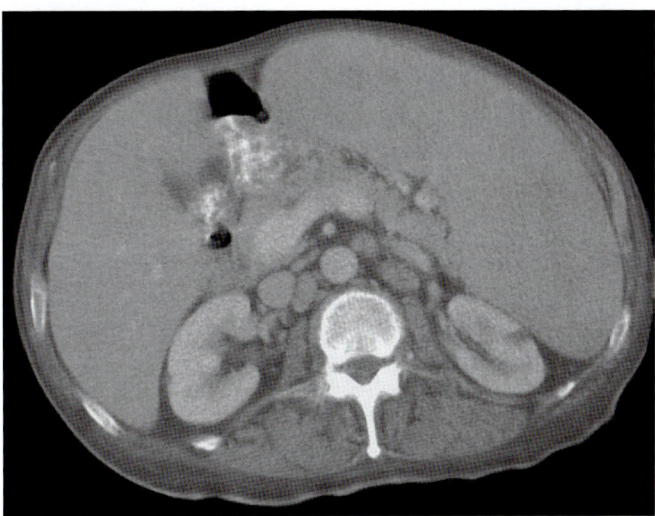

■ **FIGURE 74-4** Axial postcontrast CT image of the upper abdomen in a 55-year-old man with myelofibrosis shows massive splenomegaly.

Classic Signs

- Osteosclerosis
- Bone marrow fibrosis
- Splenomegaly

DIFFERENTIAL DIAGNOSIS

The differential diagnosis for such a clinical presentation is broad. Any potential cause of chronic anemia should be considered in the differential diagnosis. Consideration should be given to other myeloproliferative disorders such as chronic myelogenous leukemia, essential thrombocytosis, and polycythemia vera. Any potential secondary causes for myelofibrosis should be considered in the differential diagnosis, such as diffuse bony metastatic disease, infections (e.g., tuberculosis and fungal infections), sarcoidosis, myeloma, and lymphoma.

A mild anemia is seen in more than 50% of patients at the time of diagnosis. The anemia is typically progressive and is eventually seen in all patients with myelofibrosis. Typically, the peripheral blood smear shows poikilocytosis and numerous teardrop forms in the red cell line. Often the platelet morphology is bizarre with megakaryocytes evident. Leukocytosis is noted in approximately 30% of patients at presentation, with a leukoerythroblastic blood picture in greater than 90% of cases. A leukoerythroblastic blood picture can also be seen in association with severe infection, inflammation, or other marrow infiltrative processes. A triad of teardrop poikilocytosis, leukoerythroblastic blood, and giant abnormal platelets is highly suggestive of myelofibrosis. Bone marrow biopsy typically shows fibrosis, using a silver stain to show increased reticulin fibers. In contradistinction to chronic myelogenous leukemia, there are no specific associated chromosomal abnormalities in myelofibrosis.

SYNOPSIS OF TREATMENT OPTIONS

Medical Treatment

In general, no specific drug therapy has been shown to alter the natural history of the disease. The asymptomatic patient with myelofibrosis requires no specific therapy. Therapy is therefore typically supportive and palliative. Anemia is treated with transfusion therapy, and corticosteroids are used in patients with a hemolytic component of the disease. Thalidomide has been shown to produce favorable responses in some patients with minimal toxicity. Lenalidomide may have equivalent efficacy with less toxicity. Hydroxyurea is useful for control of splenomegaly, thrombocytosis, and leukocytosis. Radiotherapy can be performed for symptomatic extramedullary hematopoietic tumors and splenomegaly.

Surgical Treatment

Allogenic bone marrow transplantation has been performed in younger patients with the disease with 50% long-term survival. Splenectomy is not routinely performed because it has no impact on outcome, but it is indicated for recurrent painful episodes related to splenic enlargement.

What the Referring Physician Needs to Know

- The extent of bone marrow infiltration
- The degree of splenomegaly
- Sites of extramedullary hematopoiesis and their potential to cause significant complications (e.g., spinal cord compression from extramedullary hematopoiesis in the epidural space)

SUGGESTED READING

Guermazi A, de Kerviler E, Cazals-Hatem D, et al. Imaging findings in patients with myelofibrosis. Eur Radiol 1999; 9:1366–1375.

REFERENCES

1. Tefferi A. New insights into the pathogenesis and drug treatment of myelofibrosis. Curr Opin Hematol 2006; 13:87–92.
2. Amano Y, Onda M, Amano M, Kumazaki T. Magnetic resonance imaging of myelofibrosis. Clin Imaging 1997; 21:264–268.
3. Olipitz W, Beham-Schmid C, Aigner R, et al. Acute myelofibrosis: multifocal bone marrow infiltration detected by scintigraphy and magnetic resonance imaging. Ann Hematol 2000; 79:275–278.
4. Guermazi A, Miaux Y, Chiras J. Imaging of spinal cord compression due to thoracic extramedullary haematopoiesis in myelofibrosis. Neuroradiology 1997; 39:733–736.
5. Georgiades CS, Neyman EG, Francis IR, et al. Typical and atypical presentations of extramedullary hemopoiesis. AJR Am J Roentgenol 2002; 179:1239–1243.
6. Burrell SC, Fischman AJ. Myelofibrosis on F-18 FDG PET imaging. Clin Nucl Med 2005; 30:674.
7. Diamond T, Smith A, Schnier R, Manoharan A. Syndrome of myelofibrosis and osteosclerosis: a series of case reports and review of the literature. Bone 2002; 30:498–501.

Metabolic/ Hormonal/ Systemic Disease

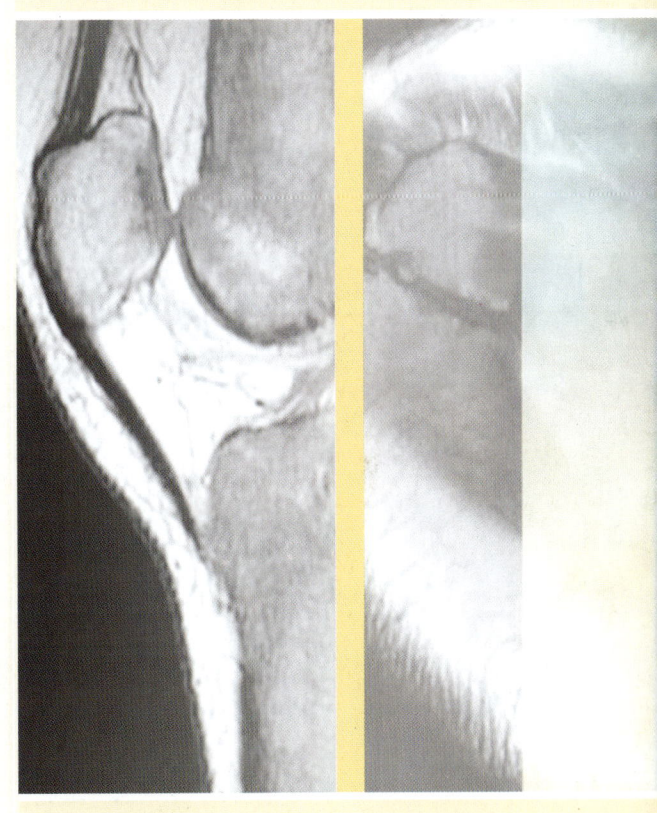

CHAPTER 75

Osteoporosis

Judith Adams

Metabolic disorders of the skeleton affect bone as a tissue, so that all bones are involved histologically, although radiologic features are not always evident. Such diseases can be caused by genetic, endocrine, nutritional, or biochemical disorders.[1]

Osteoporosis is the most common metabolic bone disease. It is a *quantitative* abnormality of bone ("too little bone"), in contrast to rickets/osteomalacia, which are *qualitative* abnormalities of bone (reduced mineral-to-osteoid ratio). In osteoporosis there is reduction in bone mass and altered trabecular structure. Bones become brittle and fracture with little, or no, trauma (insufficiency fractures). Osteoporosis is now defined as a systemic skeletal disease characterized by low bone mass and microarchitectural deterioration of bone tissue, with a consequent increase in bone fragility and susceptibility to fracture. Not only is the amount of bone tissue reduced, the structural integrity and biomechanical strength of bone are compromised by destruction of trabeculae, resulting in loss of continuity and interconnectivity of these bone struts.[2] The latter has been the drive for striving to develop noninvasive methods to image trabecular structure.[3]

ETIOLOGY

All bones contain both outer cortical (compact) and inner trabecular (net-like) bone tissue; the relative amounts of each type vary in different skeletal sites, and both contribute to bone strength. Bone is a specialized tissue made up of a matrix of collagen fibers, mucopolysaccharides, and inorganic crystalline mineral matrix (calcium hydroxyapatite) that is distributed along the length of the collagen fibers. Despite its hardness, bone remains metabolically active throughout life (bone turnover), with bone being constantly resorbed (by osteoclasts) and accreted (by osteoblasts), the activity of which can be modified by many factors. As a consequence, bones remodel from birth to maturity, maintaining their basic shape, repairing after fracture and responding to physical forces (i.e., mechanical stresses related to bone deformity) throughout life. The strength of a bone is related not only to its hardness and other physical properties but also to its size, shape, and architectural arrangement of the compact and trabecular bone.[2]

Bone Turnover

Bone formation (osteoblastic activity) and bone resorption (osteoclastic activity) constitutes *bone turnover,* a process that takes place on bone surfaces and continues throughout life. Trabecular bone has a greater surface-to-volume ratio than compact bone and is consequently some eight times more metabolically active. Bone formation and bone resorption are linked in a consistent sequence under normal circumstances. Precursor bone cells are activated at a particular skeletal site to form osteoclasts, which erode a fairly constant amount of bone. After a period of time the bone resorption ceases and osteoblasts are recruited to fill the eroded space with new bone tissue. This coupling of osteoblastic and osteoclastic activity constitutes the basal multicellular unit (BMU) of bone and is normally in balance, with the amount of bone eroded being replaced with the same amount of new bone and the cycle lasting 3 to 4 months. At any one time there are numerous BMUs throughout the skeleton at different stages of this cycle. The amount of bone in the skeleton at any moment in time depends on peak bone mass attained during puberty and adolescence and on the balance between bone resorption and formation. If the process of

---

KEY POINTS

- Radiographic features include osteopenia, thinned cortex, and reduced trabeculae; DXA bone densitometry should be suggested to confirm the diagnosis.
- The presence of vertebral fracture should be clearly and accurately reported by radiologists and should stimulate further investigation/management.
- Other imaging techniques (radionuclide imaging, CT, MRI) are helpful in differentiating whether fractures are acute/chronic or due to other pathologic processes.

bone turnover becomes uncoupled, excessive osteoclastic resorption or defective osteoblastic function result in a net loss of bone (osteoporosis). Increased activation frequency of resorption units also results in high bone turnover states (hyperparathyroidism, postmenopausal bone loss). Bisphosphonate therapy reduces the activation of resorption units by inhibiting osteoclastic function, and reversal in the mineral deficit with such treatment contributes to an increase in bone mineral density (BMD).

Osteoporosis should not be considered as a single disease entity but rather an end result of many disease processes.[4] It may result from defective skeletal accretion during bone growth and development. Alternatively, it can result from disease processes in which bone resorption exceeds new bone formation, resulting in a net loss of bone mass and consequent compromise to skeletal strength.

Osteoporosis may be broadly classified as being (1) generalized (involving the entire skeleton), which may be primary (Table 75-1) or secondary in adults and children (Tables 75-2 and 75-3), or (2) regional (involving a segment of the skeleton) (Table 75-4), for which there are several causes.

TABLE 75-1	Causes of Primary Osteoporosis

Idiopathic juvenile
Postmenopausal
Senile
Osteogenesis imperfecta

TABLE 75-2	Causes of Osteoporosis in Children

Systemic long-term glucocorticoid therapy
Chronic inflammatory disease (e.g., juvenile inflammatory arthritis)
Hypogonadism—primary or secondary
Prolonged immobilization
Osteogenesis imperfecta
Idiopathic juvenile osteoporosis

TABLE 75-3	Causes of Secondary Osteoporosis

Endocrine
Glucocorticoid excess
Estrogen/testosterone deficiency
Hyperthyroidism
Hyperparathyroidism
Growth hormone deficiency (childhood onset)
Nutritional
Intestinal malabsorption
Chronic alcoholism
Chronic liver disease
Partial gastrectomy
Vitamin C deficiency (scurvy)
Hereditary
Homocystinuria
Marfan syndrome
Ehlers-Danlos syndrome
Hematologic
Sickle cell disease
Thalassemia
Gaucher's disease
Others
Rheumatoid arthritis
Hemachromatosis
Long-term heparin therapy

TABLE 75-4	Causes of Regional Osteopenia

Disuse osteoporosis
Reflex sympathetic osteodystrophy (Sudeck's atrophy)
Regional migratory osteoporosis
Periarticular osteoporosis (of inflammatory arthritis)

Generalized Osteoporosis

Generalized osteoporosis may be primary (see Table 75-1) or secondary (see Table 75-3) in origin, and there may be many causes that fall into four categories:

1. Factors that reduce peak adult bone mass
2. Age-related bone loss
3. Bone loss associated with the menopause or hypogonadal state
4. Bone loss that is secondary to other medical conditions and drugs

Primary Osteoporosis

Idiopathic juvenile osteoporosis is a self-limiting form of osteoporosis that occurs in prepubertal children.[5] It is a rare disorder, occurring in children aged 8 to 14 years who have previously been healthy. The disease runs an acute course over a period of 2 to 4 years, during which there is growth arrest and fractures. There is a wide spectrum of severity, and both cortical and trabecular bone are affected. In the mild form only one or two vertebral fractures may be present, but in more severe cases deformity involves all the vertebrae and the extremities, particularly the metaphyseal region of the distal tibia. A few affected patients may develop severe kyphoscoliosis, deformities of the extremities, and even death from respiratory failure due to deformity of the thorax. The disease is reversible and remits spontaneously, and affected patients may be left with only a mild or moderate kyphosis, short stature, and some bone deformity after fractures. Investigations indicate uncoupling of the two components of bone turnover due to both increase in resorption and decrease in formation. The condition has to be differentiated from osteogenesis imperfecta and other forms of juvenile osteoporosis. Affected patients do not have the blue sclerae characteristic of osteogenesis imperfecta. The other important differential diagnoses in children with vertebral fractures are hypercortisolism and leukemia.

Osteoporosis of young adults is a heterogeneous condition that occurs equally in young men and women. The disease generally runs a mild course, with multiple vertebral fractures occurring over a decade or more and associated loss in height. Fractures of metatarsals and ribs are also common, and hip fractures may occur. The cause of the condition is uncertain, and in some individuals it may simply be that inadequate bone mass has been formed during skeletal growth. Some affected individuals may have a mild variant of osteogenesis imperfecta. Exceptionally, osteoporosis may present during pregnancy, but whether this is a causal or coincidental association is unknown.

Postmenopausal (type I) osteoporosis occurs at the time of menopause when reduction in levels of estrogen results in all women losing bone; some lose trabecular bone at a rate three times greater than is usual (2%–10% per year). The bone loss is greatest during the first 4 years after the menopause. The condition characteristically becomes clinically evident in women 15 to 20 years after the menopause. Fractures occur in sites of the skeleton rich in trabecular bone, including the vertebral bodies and distal forearm (Colles' fracture). In premature menopause bone loss can be prevented by hormone replacement therapy up to the age of natural menopause (approximately 50 years of age). However, hormone replacement therapy should not be used long term after this age for the purpose of bone protective therapy because there are other more specific and effective bone agents now available[6] and because of the increased risk of breast cancer and cardiovascular events with long-term use of hormone replacement therapy in elderly women.

Senile (type II) osteoporosis occurs in both men and women 75 years or older and is due to age-related bone loss. This occurs as a result of age-related impaired bone formation associated with secondary hyperparathyroidism. The latter is a consequence of reduced calcium absorption from the intestine secondary to decreased production of the active metabolite of vitamin D (1,25-dihydroxyvitamin D) in the kidney of the elderly population. There is reduction in both cortical and trabecular bone. The syndrome manifests mainly as hip fractures and wedge fractures of the vertebrae, but fractures may also occur in the proximal tibia, proximal humerus, and pelvis.

Osteogenesis Imperfecta

A number of inherited disorders of connective tissue can result in osteoporosis.[4] Osteogenesis imperfecta, or "brittle bone" syndrome, results from mutations affecting either the *COL1A1* or *COL1A2* genes of type I collagen.[7,8] Although the disease is usually apparent at birth or in childhood, more mild forms of the disease may not become apparent until adulthood, when affected individuals present with insufficiency fractures and osteopenia.

The classification (types I-IV) of osteogenesis imperfecta is that devised by Sillence and coworkers.[7] The important characteristics in this classification include blue sclerae, the severity of the disorder, and the mode of inheritance (dominant, recessive, sporadic/new mutation), although accurate classification is difficult because of phenotypic overlap. Affected subjects who do not have dental involvement are designated in group "A." Subjects with dentinogenesis imperfecta are designated as group "B."

Other causes of osteoporosis in children are given in Table 75-2.

Secondary Osteoporosis

A large number of conditions may lead to osteoporosis and may be of endocrine, nutritional, hereditary, hematologic, or other origin. Radiologically, these may be indistinguishable from involutional (senile) osteoporosis.[9] However, some may have specific and diagnostic radiologic features (i.e., subperiosteal erosions of the phalanges in primary hyperparathyroidism). In glucocorticoid excess[10] (endogenous and exogenous) there is reduced bone formation due to a direct effect on the osteoblast, with increased osteoclastic activity, probably mediated through secondary hyperparathyroidism, stimulated by reduced gastrointestinal absorption of calcium. There is also evidence that glucocorticoids induce premature apoptosis of both osteoblasts and osteoclasts. The adverse effect is primarily on trabecular bone. Fractures occur particularly in the vertebral bodies and ribs; the latter may heal with profuse callus formation. Thyrotoxicosis stimulates catabolic activity and increases osteoclastic bone resorption and may occasionally be severe enough to cause recognizable osteoporosis. Long-term heparin therapy has also been reported to cause osteoporosis, possibly due to release of collagenase from lysosomes. Formation of osseous matrix also requires other substances such as protein and vitamin C (for the formation of collagen). Hence, osteoporosis may develop in deficiency states involving lack of proteins (e.g., in starvation or severe malnutrition) or in scurvy. Finally, a number of other disorders, including hepatic disease and chronic alcoholism, may cause osteoporosis by various mechanisms, many of which are still not clearly understood.

Regional Osteopenia

The growth and development of the skeleton, and maintenance of bone health throughout life, depends on normal activity and loading of the skeleton. If, for any reason, there is inactivity (e.g., stroke, polio, cord transsection) there will be localized (disuse) osteopenia involving the affected part of the skeleton. Such a process may be acute (e.g., after a fracture) or chronic (e.g., after a stroke).

Reflex sympathetic dystrophy (Sudeck's atrophy) is a more severe form of localized osteopenia that can occur in children or adults and can be precipitated by a variety of pathologic processes. Fracture is a common cause, but other causes include infection, peripheral neuropathy, tumor, or central nervous system abnormality. In approximately 25% of cases, no predisposing cause is found. The causative mechanism is not clearly understood, but it is thought that the precipitating factor results in abnormal neural reflexes traveling along the peripheral nerves and giving rise to localized symptoms. There are, consequently, sympathetic nervous system influences through increased sensitivity to catecholamines and other neuropeptides that result in pain, soft tissue swelling, and hyperemia.[11] There is excessive bone resorption (probably stimulated by cytokines), which occurs particularly in a periarticular distribution and may simulate malignant disease. Any joint may be affected, with involvement of the shoulder and hand being most common. Multiple joints may rarely be affected. Reflex sympathetic dystrophy tends to be progressive, and atrophic changes may eventually be evident in the skin, which has a smooth and glistening appearance.

Regional migratory osteoporosis, also known as migratory osteolysis, is an uncommon and self-limiting condition presenting as arthralgia and migrating between weight-bearing joints of the lower limb.[12,13] The condition is often associated with generalized osteoporosis and may be the result of microinsufficiency fractures in the subarticular region of the affected joint. Transient osteoporosis of the hip is the most common site and was originally described in pregnant women.[12] However, it is now known to be just as common in middle-aged men. Clinically, there is hip pain with no history of injury. The pain may progress and be severe enough to cause a limp and restrict movement in the affected joint. There may be an effusion due to a mild chronic synovitis. Joint aspirations are often performed to exclude infection as a cause of the symptoms and signs and are sterile. Recovery usually occurs spontaneously in 6 to 12 months without late sequelae. Symptoms may develop rapidly and then resolve, only to recur again in some other joint. The joint adjacent to the diseased one is usually the next to be affected, but there may be two or more joints that are symptomatic simultaneously.

Periarticular osteoporosis occurs in inflammatory (e.g., rheumatoid arthritis) or some infective arthropathies and results in juxta-articular focal osteopenia (Fig. 75-1).

PREVALENCE AND EPIDEMIOLOGY

Osteoporosis is a serious public health problem in which, over the past 20 years, there have been significant advances in knowledge of its epidemiology, pathophysiology, and

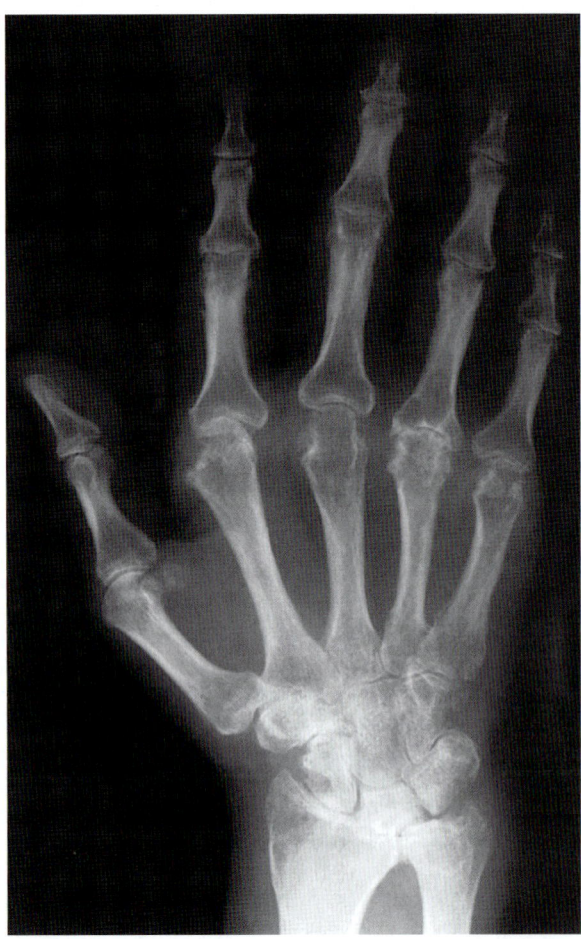

■ **FIGURE 75-1** Regional osteoporosis. Radiograph of the hand in a patient with early rheumatoid arthritis shows periarticular osteopenia at the metacarpophalangeal and interphalangeal joints, with joint space narrowing and juxta-articular erosions. Periarticular osteopenia is the earliest radiographic feature of rheumatoid arthritis and is related to hyperemia, inflammation, and cytokines, which stimulate osteoclastic bone resorption.

treatment. In the Western world osteoporosis is reported to affect 1 in 2 women and 1 in 5 men older than the age of 50 years in their lifetime.[14] The risk of fracture increases with advancing age and progressive loss of bone mass and varies with the population being considered. In the United Kingdom each year 60,000 hip, 50,000 wrist, and 120,000 vertebral fractures occur. These fractures result in considerable morbidity and mortality for those affected, and they incur considerable social and health care costs (£2 billion). The age-adjusted incidence of fragility fractures in both sexes is 25% higher in the United States than in Britain and other areas of Europe, and the financial burden of managing osteoporotic fractures in the United States was estimated to be $17 billion in 2001. The incidence of hip fracture has doubled over the past 3 decades and is predicted to continue to rise beyond what one would predict from increased longevity, particularly in the Far East.

After hip or vertebral fracture, mortality at 5 years is about 20% greater than that expected. The mortality rate is highest in men older than 75 years with other comorbidities. Most of the excess deaths occur in the first 6 months after hip fracture. At 1 year after hip fracture 40% of patients are unable to walk independently, 60% have difficulty with one essential activity of daily living, 80% are restricted in other living activities (e.g., driving, shopping), and 27% will be admitted to a nursing home for the first time.[14]

Vertebral fractures are the most common type of osteoporotic fracture. They may occur in the absence of trauma or after only minimal trauma. In the United States it is estimated that 25% of women older than age 50 years will have a vertebral fracture, and this will rise to 33% in those older than 75.[15] In Europe, there is a similar prevalence of 20% in women over 50 and a strong age dependency.[14] A prevalence of 20% is found in men older than the age of 50, but because more of these cases were present at an earlier age, traumatic events are presumed to be the cause.[16]

CLINICAL PRESENTATION

Generalized osteoporosis is a chronic disease with late clinical consequences (low trauma, insufficiency fractures) and so might only come to clinical diagnosis when such fractures occur. For this reason it is sometimes referred to as the "silent epidemic." Acute fractures will be associated with pain and may later cause deformity (e.g., wrist fractures).

Vertebral fractures are the most commonly occurring osteoporotic fracture. They occur as an acute event related to minor trauma and can be accompanied by pain, which generally resolves spontaneously over 6 to 8 weeks. This resolution of symptoms serves to distinguish osteoporotic vertebral fractures from similar events due to more sinister pathology, such as metastases, in which the symptoms are more protracted. However, 30% of vertebral fractures can be present in asymptomatic patients. The clinical symptoms include back pain, loss of height, spinal kyphotic deformity (dowager's hump), and ribs that may override the iliac crest. These fractures may be associated with respiratory compromise and gastrointestinal symptoms (esophageal reflux) and lead to depression and reduced quality of life for those affected. Vertebral fractures cause disability and limited spinal mobility and are associated with increased mortality. They are powerful predictors of future fracture; if a single vertebral fracture is present, then there is a 12% increased risk of a future vertebral fracture within 12 months; if multiple vertebral fractures are present, this risk rises to 22%. Patients with vertebral fracture are at fivefold increased risk of further vertebral fractures and at twofold increased risk of hip fracture. Consequently, the accurate identification and clear reporting of vertebral fracture by radiologists have a vital role to play in the diagnosis and appropriate management of patients with, or at risk of, osteoporosis. There is evidence that vertebral fractures are underreported.[17,18] As a consequence there has been a joint vertebral fracture initiative between the European Society of Skeletal Radiology (Osteoporosis Group) and the International Osteoporosis Foundation to raise the profile of osteoporosis and its diagnosis among radiologists, particularly emphasizing the importance of accurate reporting of the presence of vertebral fractures. An educational compact disk can be obtained from www.osteofound. org. A patient with the combination of vertebral fracture and low bone density has a 25-fold increased risk for subsequent vertebral fracture than does a patient with no fracture and high bone density.

PATHOPHYSIOLOGY

Anatomy

Changes of osteoporosis are often most prominent in areas of the skeleton rich in trabecular bone, particularly in the axial skeleton (vertebrae, pelvis, ribs, and sternum).[9] This is because trabecular bone is some eight times more metabolically active than cortical bone. Eventually, changes may be evident in the bones of the appendicular skeleton also. Trabeculae become thin and may disappear completely; they may be sparse, but those that remain may become thickened due to stresses to which the skeleton is exposed. The cortex becomes reduced in width through endosteal bone resorption, and in states of increased bone turnover there will be intracortical tunneling and porosity.

Pathology

Regional Osteoporosis

Chronic disuse is characterized by a uniform pattern of bone loss; acute immobilization causes more focal and irregular bone formation and resorption. This results in different patterns of bone loss, which include diffuse osteopenia, linear translucent bands, speckled radiolucent areas, and cortical bone resorption.[9]

Reflex sympathetic dystrophy (Sudeck's atrophy) can be diagnosed by radionuclide scanning, especially if no radiographic abnormality is present; this modality is reported to have a sensitivity and specificity of over 80%.[9] The predominant feature is intense and diffuse isotope uptake in the affected bones in the blood flow, blood pool, and static images. MRI may be normal or may show nonspecific soft tissue edema, soft tissue atrophy, or marrow edema.

Regional osteoporosis is most common in the hip. Radiographically there is reduction in density of the proximal femur. There may be an underlying abnormality of perfusion of the marrow, which is edematous. Radionuclide scan shows nonspecific increased uptake of isotope in the affected hip. MRI is sensitive to demonstrating the edematous marrow, before any radiographic abnormality is present.[12,13] There may be increased joint fluid, with diffuse decreased T1-weighted and increased T2-weighted signal changes in the femoral head and intracapsular portion of the femoral neck. The use of chemical shift, fat suppression, and short tau inversion recovery (STIR) imaging is effective in accentuating the signal changes and improves the detection of marrow edema.[9] Focal bone loss and marrow edema can also occur with tumor, arthritis, or infection, which must be excluded before the diagnosis of transient osteoporosis of the hip can be made.

Periarticular osteoporosis is probably the most common form of regional osteoporosis encountered in clinical practice and is related to hyperemia of the inflamed joint and the presence of local cytokines that stimulate osteoclastic bone resorption. Periarticular osteoporosis is a characteristic early feature of rheumatoid arthritis (see Fig. 75-1), but a generalized reduction in bone mass can also occur, which involves both compact and trabecular bone. There is generally increased bone resorption, with normal or reduced bone formation. The causes of these changes are complex. Immobilization and glucocorticoid therapy contribute to the osteoporosis.

Generalized Osteoporosis

In osteogenesis imperfecta radiographic features vary according to the type of disease and its severity[1] and include osteopenia and fractures, which may heal with florid callus formation, mimicking osteosarcoma. Bones are thin and undertubulated (gracile) and are normal in length or shortened, thickened, and deformed by multiple fractures (Fig. 75-2). Intrasutural (wormian) bones can be identified on skull radiographs. In severe forms of osteogenesis imperfecta the diagnosed may be made before birth by detailed ultrasound scanning in the second trimester. Diagnostic features include cranial enlargement, reduced echogenicity of bone, and deformity and shortening of limb bones as a result of intrauterine fractures.

Type I is the mildest and most common form of the disease and may only become apparent in adulthood. There is a history of fractures, generally dating back to childhood. In children the fractures may become radiographically and clinically apparent as the child becomes more active (5+ years) and may take the form of overt fractures or microfractures involving the metaphyses. In infancy these features may resemble those found in nonaccidental injury. The differential diagnosis can usually be resolved by the presence of associated extraskeletal manifestations (blue sclera, dentigenesis imperfecta), or evidence of a family history of the condition, so that bone biopsy for diagnosis is infrequently required. Affected patients are short in stature, with only 10% being of normal height, and have joint laxity, blue sclerae, and presenile hearing loss. Transmission is by autosomal dominant trait. Radiologically, the bones are usually reduced in density, although some patients may have normal bone

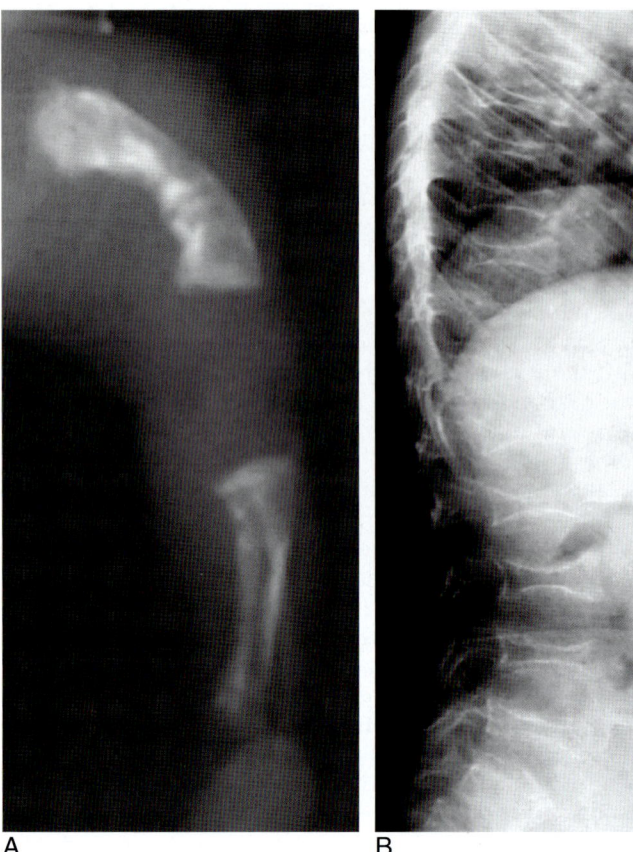

A   B

■ **FIGURE 75-2** Osteogenesis imperfecta ("brittle bone" disease) results from mutations affecting the genes of type I collagen. Affected individuals present with fractures and osteopenia and the presentation and severity vary. The fractures cause deformity, as seen on radiographs of the femur of this neonate (**A**) and in the spine (**B**) where there are grade 3 (severe) fractures involving all vertebrae. A differential diagnosis for the latter appearance in children is leukemia. *(Courtesy of Dr. A. Offiah, Great Ormond Street, London, UK.)*

density. Bones may be thin and undertubulated (gracile) or normally modeled. Vertebral fractures occur in the fourth decade. When scoliosis is present, it is mild.

Type II (lethal, perinatal)–affected infants are small for dates, with deep blue sclerae and shortened and deformed limbs due to multiple fractures. Fractures involve the ribs, and death is usually the result of pulmonary insufficiency. Survival is rare beyond the first 3 months. Other complications include brain and spinal cord injury. Radiologically, multiple fractures are present with a characteristic "concertina" deformity of the lower limbs. The ribs can appear "beaded" due to multiple rib fractures, which may occur in utero. The cranial vault is severely undermineralized and may be distorted by molding, with wormian (sutural) bones in the occipital and parietal region and with platyspondyly. Histology reveals defective enchondral ossification at the epiphyses, which appear disorganized with persistent islands of calcified cartilage and undermineralized bone. There is defective transformation of woven bone to lamellar bone, in both the cortical and trabecular skeletal components. Formation of membrane bone is also deficient, accounting for the marked calvarial thinning.

Type III (severe progressive) is inherited as an autosomal recessive trait. Fractures are usually present at birth

and involve the long bones, clavicles, ribs, and cranium, leading to deformity. Although size at birth is normal, growth retardation is evident in the first year of life, and many affected patients reach only 3 to 4 feet in height. As growth proceeds, increasing deformity of the calvaria occurs, with associated facial distortion, malocclusion, and mild prognathism, basilar invagination, and progressive hearing loss. Sclerae are blue at birth, but this diminishes with age, and sclerae are white in adults. Vertebral fractures occur at an early age and contribute to the progressive and severe kyphoscoliosis that develops during childhood. Affected patients tend to be wheelchair bound because of progressive deformities as a consequence of fractures. Complications include progressive pulmonary insufficiency through distortion of the thorax. Radiologically, the bones may be slender or broad due to recurrent fractures. Epiphyses are abnormal, with expansion and islands of calcified ("popcorn") cartilage. As with other forms of osteogenesis imperfecta, the incidence of fracture declines after puberty.

Type IV (moderately severe) is inherited as an autosomal dominant trait and can vary in severity and is sometimes confused with either type I or type III. There is generally more severe osteopenia and bone deformity than in type I. The sclerae are blue in children, and although this may persist into adulthood, they may also fade to white. Subjects are short in stature, with abnormal molding of the calvaria and basilar invagination in a high proportion of patients. Bones of the axial and appendicular skeleton are osteopenic and dysplastic, resulting in scoliosis and deformity, particularly of the pelvis. Joint laxity can result in dislocation, particularly of the ankle or knee.

In primary and secondary osteoporosis the radiologic appearances of osteoporosis are essentially the same, irrespective of the cause. Despite the advent of newer imaging methods (CT, MRI), osteoporosis is still most commonly, and probably best, diagnosed on radiographs. However, radiography is relatively insensitive in detecting early bone loss (less than 30% to 40% loss of bone tissue), bone density will be affected by patient size and the radiographic factors used, and visual judgment of bone density is subjective, hence the importance of quantitative bone densitometry techniques. The main radiographic features of generalized osteoporosis are decreased bone density and cortical thinning (Fig. 75-3).

Decrease in radiographic bone density, in the absence of fractures, is termed *osteopenia*. It is due to resorption and thinning of trabeculae, some of which may be lost completely. The process initially affects secondary trabeculae, and the primary trabeculae may appear more prominent as they are affected at a later stage. In the proximal femur the principal compressive and tensile trabeculae are accentuated, with loss of trabeculae in the area (Ward's) between them, which appears more radiolucent.

Cortical thinning occurs as a result of endosteal, periosteal, or intracortical (cortical tunneling) bone resorption or a combination of all these sites of resorption. Endosteal resorption is the least specific radiographic finding because it may be evident in many metabolic disorders, including osteoporosis. Intracortical tunneling is slightly more specific, occurring mainly in disorders with rapid bone turnover such as disuse osteoporosis and reflex sympathetic

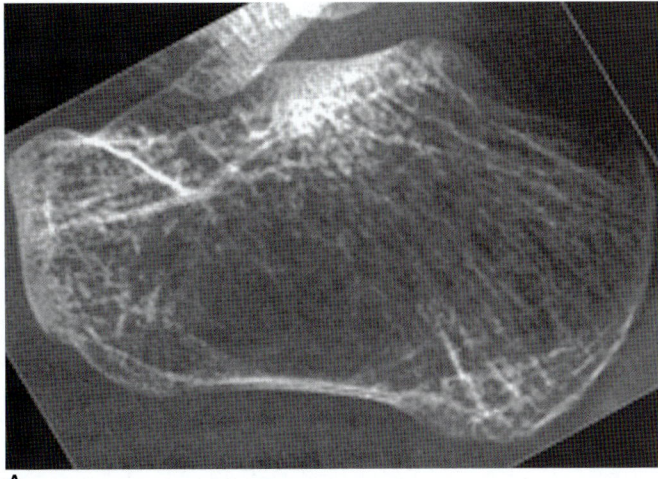

A

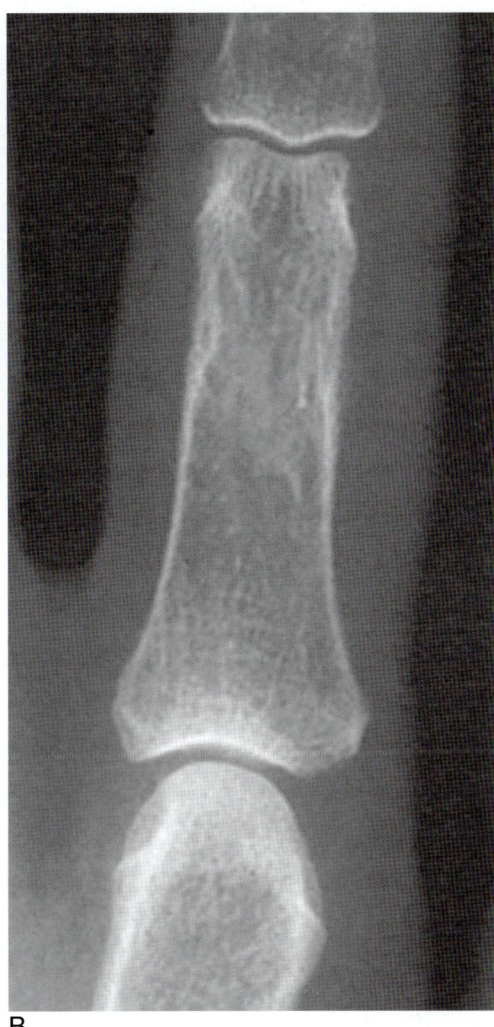

B

■ **FIGURE 75-3** General osteoporosis. There is reduced radiographic density (osteopenia), with reduction in the number of trabeculae, which may be destroyed completely, and the bone cortex becomes thinned, as evident in the lateral radiograph of the calcaneus (**A**) and radiograph of the phalanx (**B**).

dystrophy. Subperiosteal resorption is the most specific finding, being diagnostic of hyperparathyroidism.[1,19]

The radiographic features of generalized osteoporosis predominate in the axial skeleton and proximal long bones, which are rich in trabecular bone. In some sites the presence of multiple microfractures and callus formation can cause osteosclerosis on radiographs, which must be distinguished from other more sinister malignant pathologies (metastases). Such insufficiency fractures occur in particular anatomic sites, including the symphysis pubis, the sacrum, pubic rami, and calcaneus.[20,21] Other sites involved are the sternum, supra-acetabular area and elsewhere in the pelvis, femoral neck, and proximal and distal tibia. Some of these fractures may be accompanied by considerable osteolysis, particularly those involving the symphysis pubis, and may be erroneously diagnosed on radiographs as due to malignant tumor. Other imaging techniques (radionuclide scan, CT, and MRI) may help to differentiate insufficiency fractures from other pathologic processes (Fig. 75-4). On radionuclide scans there is increased uptake in regions of acute insufficiency fractures. When the sacrum is involved. this often gives a characteristic H pattern ("Honda" sign) of radionuclide uptake.[22] CT is particularly helpful in defining the fracture lines of insufficiency fractures involving the sacrum (fractures are usually parallel to the sacroiliac

joint) and in the calcaneus. In these sites, fractures may not be identified on radiographs because of complex anatomy and superimposition of other anatomic structures. MRI is particularly sensitive at identifying insufficiency fractures in the femoral neck before they are evident radiographically, as is radionuclide scanning.[21,22]

Vertebral fractures (Fig. 75-5) are perhaps related to biomechanical forces through the spine; as trabeculae are lost, the process particularly involves the horizontally orientated secondary trabeculae. The vertical trabeculae actually become more prominent and thickened.[1,9] This results in a vertical "striated" appearance to the vertebral body on lateral spinal radiographs (see Fig. 75-5B). This feature is generally seen in several, or all, of the vertebrae when it is related to osteoporosis, a feature that serves to distinguish a similar appearance in a single vertebral body when it is related to hemangioma. In contrast to fractures of long bones, osteoporotic vertebral fractures are rarely associated with a demonstrable break in the cortex or accompanied by significant callus formation. The exception to this is in Cushing's syndrome in which exuberant callus may be seen due to calcification of incompletely formed osteoid. This results in the characteristic marginal vertebral condensation.[9]

Vertebral fractures are the most common of osteoporotic fractures (see Fig.75-5C). The anterior and cen-

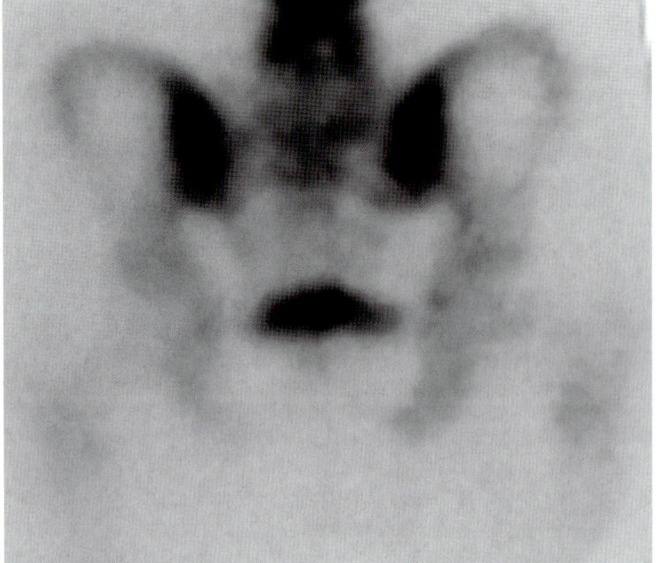

A

■ **FIGURE 75-4** Radionuclide imaging may be a more sensitive method of imaging acute fractures before they are evident on radiographs, especially insufficiency fractures in the sacral ala (**A**) in which there is increased uptake of isotope, giving a "Honda" sign. Acute vertebral fractures in the thoracic and lumbar spine (**B**) show increased uptake of isotope. Radionuclide imaging can be used to differentiate between acute and chronic vertebral fractures.

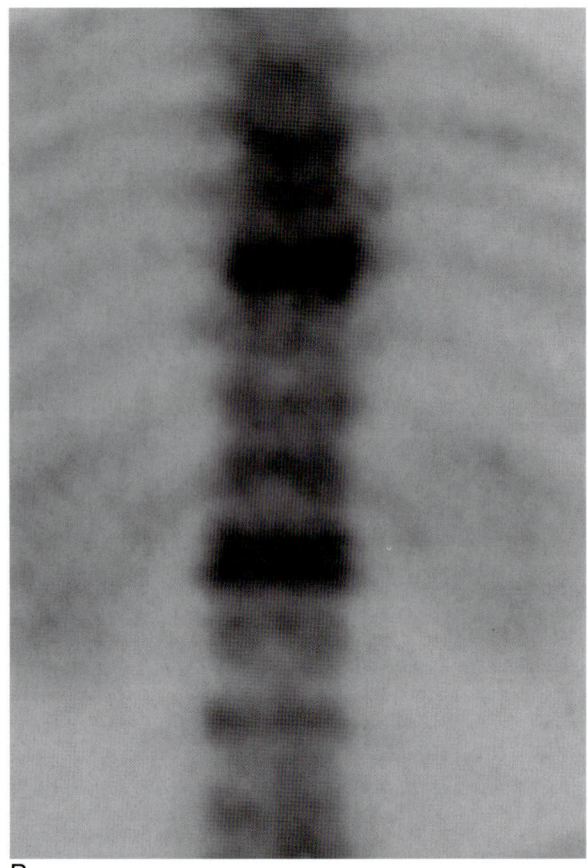

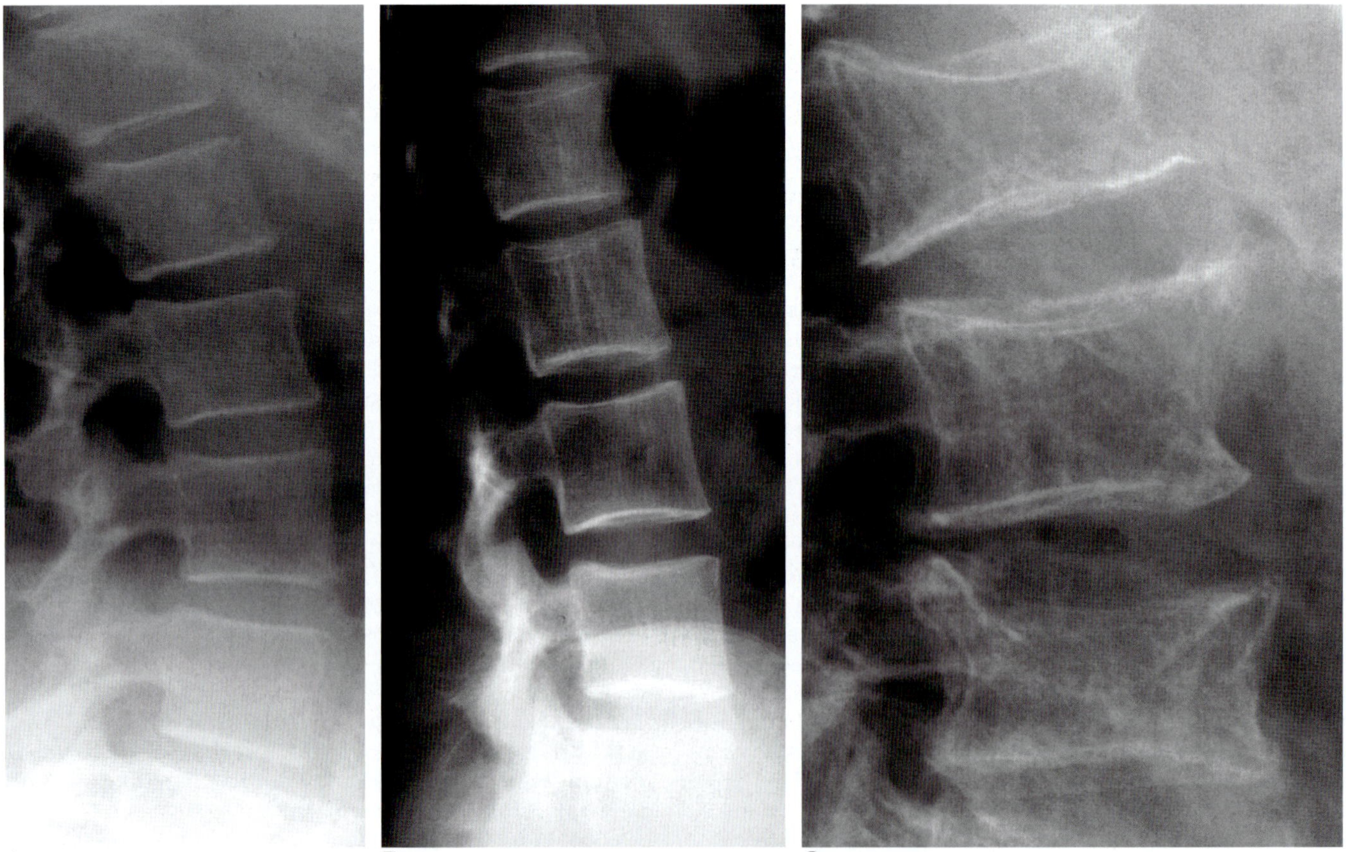

B

A   B   C

■ **FIGURE 75-5** Vertebral fractures are the most common osteoporotic fracture, and their presence is a powerful predictor of future fracture (vertebral fracture, 5×; hip fracture, 2×). **A,** Lateral lumbar spine radiograph shows normal vertebrae. **B,** The earliest feature of spinal osteoporosis is prominent vertical striations due to loss of secondary horizontal trabeculae. **C,** Multiple vertebral fractures in the lumbar spine of varying types and grades (top vertebra: grade 2 [moderate] wedge fracture; mid vertebra: grade 1 [mild] upper end plate fracture; lower vertebra: grade 3 [severe] crush fracture).

tral midportion of the vertebrae withstand compression forces less well than the posterior and outer ring elements of the vertebrae, resulting in wedge or end plate fractures or, less commonly, crush fractures.[23,24] Vertebral fractures can be graded[25]: the semi-quantitative grading method is the one currently most frequently applied to define the prevalence and incidence of vertebral fractures in epidemiology studies and pharmaceutical trials of the efficacy of new osteoporosis therapies. The more severe the grade of vertebral fracture, the greater the risk of future fracture. Although vertebral fractures are generally associated with change in shape of the vertebrae, this is not always so; and it is important to observe subtle density changes adjacent and inferior to the vertebral end plate that indicate fracture of just the middle portion of the end plate.

Good radiographic techniques are required when imaging the spine, particularly in the lateral projection. The spine must be parallel to the radiographic table to prevent the vertebrae appearing to have an apparent biconcave end plate, which is caused as an artifact due to tilting of the vertebrae or the divergence of the x-ray beam ("beam can" effect) (Fig. 75-6A). Other pathologic processes (trauma, myeloma, metastases, Scheuermann's disease, Schmorl's nodes, infection, degenerative disease, and congenital anomalies) and normal variants ("Cupid's bow") (see Fig. 75-6B) may cause deformities of the vertebra and have to be differentiated from osteoporotic vertebral fracture (see Fig. 75-6B and C).[23-26] Scheuermann's disease causes end plate irregularity, most commonly in the thoracic spine, and involves several adjacent vertebrae. With spondylosis there may be change in modeling of the vertebrae, which appear slightly wedged and elongated in an anteroposterior diameter. Other imaging methods such as CT (particularly the midsagittal reformatted image from 3D volume imaging now feasible on multidetector spiral CT scanners) (see Fig. 75-6C), MRI (see Fig 75-6D), and radionuclide scanning (see Fig 75-4B) can be helpful in this differentiation.[26] MRI is particularly useful in differentiating acute from chronic vertebral fractures, because in the former there is marrow edema and the fracture may fill with fluid and show high signal intensity on T1-weighted images (Fig. 75-7A), which are useful differentiating features from other infiltrating causes of vertebral fracture (e.g., metastases). Old vertebral fractures regain the high signal intensity of marrow fat.

IMAGING TECHNIQUES

Quantitative measurements used in any field require ideally to have good accuracy and precision. *Accuracy* expresses how close the measurement made is to the actual chemical composition (e.g., how close BMD measured relates to the chemical analysis of bone). *Precision* assesses the reproducibility of the measurement technique and is usually expressed as a percentage of coefficient of variation (CV%). A high precision (low CV%—about 1%) is essential in any longitudinal studies to detect small changes over reasonable periods of time. A statistically significant change in measurement is 2.77 × precision.

Radiographic Morphometry

Methods have been used to standardize skeletal measurements of cortical thickness (radiogrammetry), trabecular pattern (Singh index), and vertebral deformity (morphometry) from radiographs.

Radiogrammetry involves the measurement of cortical thickness of various long bones on radiographs. The most frequently used bone for this measure is the second metacarpal of the nondominant hand. The method also has been applied to other bones (clavicle, radius, humerus, femur, and tibia) in the past. In the metacarpal the mid-diaphyseal diameter of the bone (from each periosteal surface) and the medullary cavity (distance between endosteal surface) are measured using calipers.[27] A variety of indices have been described, including bone width (BW), cortical thickness (CT), metacarpal index (MCI), and parameters of "areal" cortical density (g/cm^2) . The technique is simple to perform, uses a low radiation dose, and was widely applied. However, the reproducibility is limited (CV% up to 11%), because the endosteal surface becomes irregular and more difficult to identify with bone resorption that occurs with age and in osteoporosis. Consequently, longitudinal studies had to extend over a decade or more to assess change with time. This established technique has been rejuvenated by the application to it of modern computer vision methods (active shape models [ASM]) to make it automated, with great improvement in precision to better than 1% (digital x-ray radiogrammetry [DXR])[27] (Fig. 75-8A).

The *Singh index* assesses the two principal arches of trabeculae in the proximal femur: the compressive group lies in the medial portion of the femoral neck and the tensile group is in the lateral aspect in the femoral neck. The number, thickness, and arrangement of trabeculae in the femoral neck change with age, owing to resorption and altered stresses. On radiographs this change in trabecular pattern can be graded as an index of osteopenia. Six grades were described by Singh and colleagues, ranging from grade 6 (normal) to grade 1 (severe osteoporosis).[28] The subjectivity of the Singh grading scale limits its reproducibility. However, computer analysis has the potential to make the measurement more rapid and accurate.[28]

Various methods of *vertebral morphometry* have been proposed to standardize the subjective visual assessment of vertebral fracture and to quantitate alterations in vertebral height and shape.[25] These developments have been stimulated by the need for comparable methods to be applied in epidemiologic studies and by the prevalence and incidence of vertebral fractures being used as inclusion criteria and treatment outcome measures in therapeutic trials assessing the efficacy of new treatments for osteoporosis.

When performing vertebral morphometry the protocol for spinal radiography must be standardized, with a fixed film focus distance (FFD), and the spine must be parallel to the radiographic table. Any scoliosis or tilting of the spine due to poor positioning will cause apparent, but false, biconcavity of the end plates ("bean can effect") (see Fig. 75-6A). The x-ray beam is centered at the T7 spinous process for the lateral thoracic spine and at the L3 spinous process for the lateral lumbar spine projections. Assessments for vertebral fractures are usually made from T4 to L4 on the lateral spinal projections. Vertebral fractures are defined as end

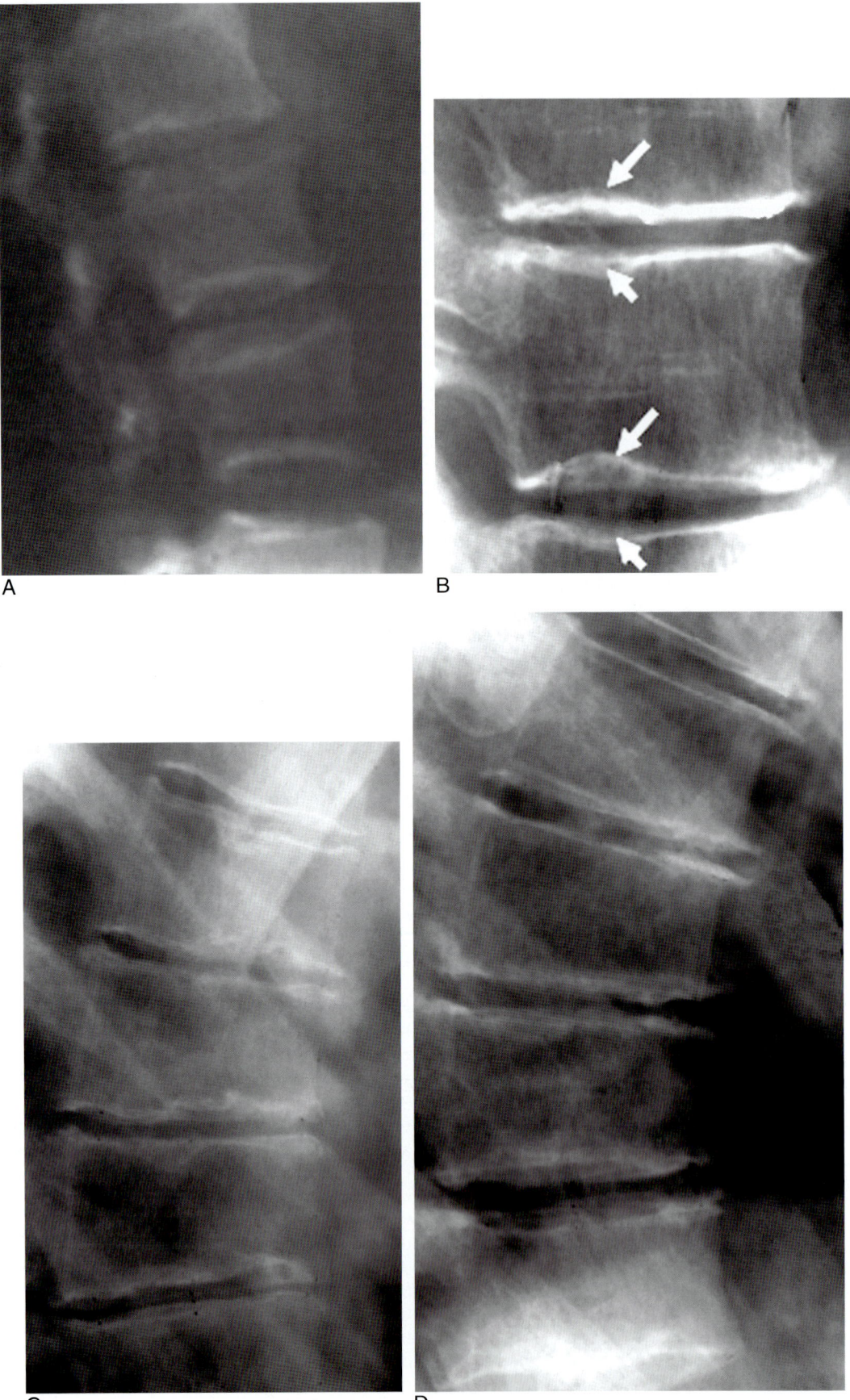

■ **FIGURE 75-6** Some differential diagnoses of vertebral fractures. **A,** Technical in origin ("bean can" effect) due to tilting of the vertebrae, either from scoliosis of the spine or divergence of the x-ray beam, which results in artifact of apparent biconcave vertebral end plate. **B,** Normal variant with prominent posterior biconcavities of end plates (*arrows*) ("Cupid's bow"). These can be differentiated form vertebral fractures by their posterior position and distinct end plate cortical margin. **C,** Scheuermann's disease involves several adjacent vertebrae and causes some mild wedging of the affected vertebrae, the end plates of which are irregular. **D,** Spondylosis is associated with some change in modeling of the vertebrae, which can be mildly wedged and elongated in their anteroposterior diameter, with osteophytes.

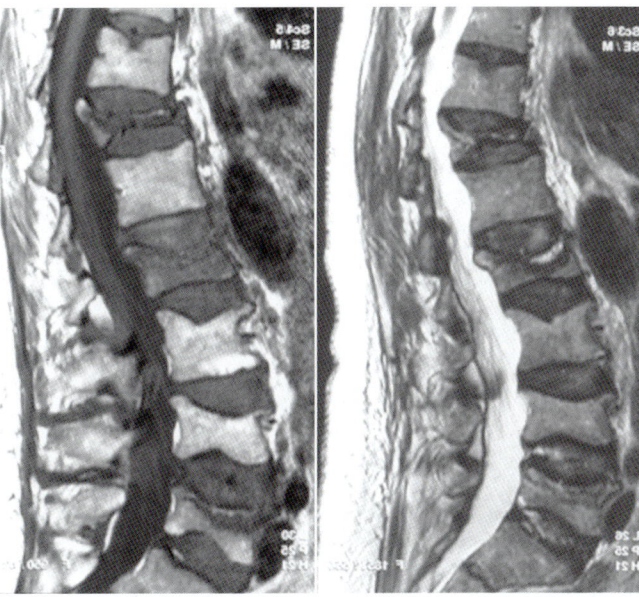

A

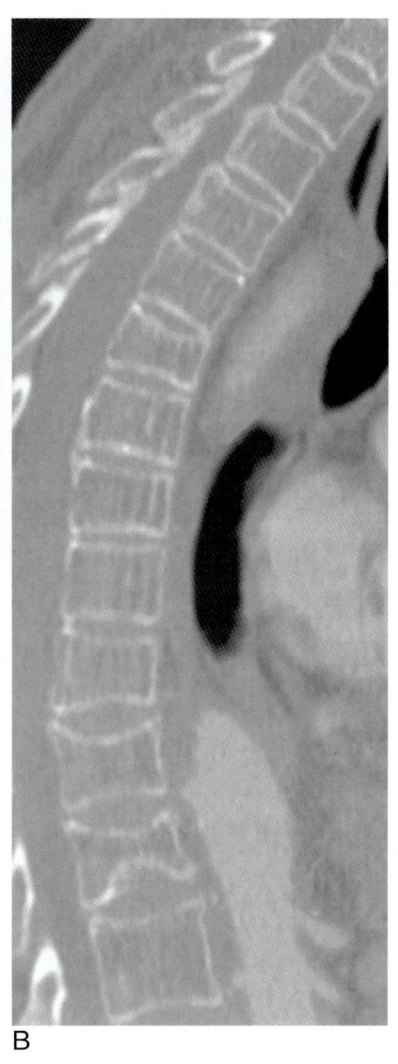

B

■ **FIGURE 75-7** Other imaging methods for diagnosing vertebral fractures. **A,** Sagittal MR images: *left,* T1-weighted; *right,* T2-weighted. There is a severe grade 3 fracture of T12: in L3 there is an acute grade 3 severe upper end plate fracture with high signal intensity fluid in the fracture line on the T1-weighted image, which helps to confirm that this is an acute osteoporotic fracture and excludes it from being due to an infiltrating process (tumor). There are also fractures of L3, L4, and L5 of varying types, grades, and ages. **B,** Midsagittal reformatted image from a 3D volume MDCT scan showing prominent vertical striations indicating loss of horizontal trabeculae and osteoporosis. There are also fractures of several vertebrae in the mid and lower thoracic spine and in the upper lumbar spine. Because the middle is the weakest portion of the vertebral end plate, such sagittal CT sections may make end plate fractures more obvious than on lateral spinal radiographs. (*A courtesy of Dr. Richard Whitehouse, Manchester Royal Infirmary, UK.*)

plate, wedge, or crush (see Fig 75-8B). Changes in shape of the vertebrae (deforming events) are generally defined by the six-point method, in which the anterior, mid, and posterior points of the superior and inferior end plates of the vertebral body are identified, to measure anterior, mid, and posterior heights. These points can be placed directly on a radiograph or, more usually, the radiograph is digitized and the points placed using a translucent cursor on a digitizing tablet. The change in shape can be graded (see Fig 75-8C): grade 0 = normal; grade 1 (mild) = 20% to 25% reduction in anterior, middle, and/or posterior height and 10% to 20% reduction of the projected vertebral area; grade 2 (moderate) = 25% to 40% reduction in anterior, middle and/or posterior height and 20% to 40% reduction in projected vertebral area; grade 3 (severe) = 40% or greater reduction in anterior, middle, and/or posterior height and in the projected area.[25]

The introduction of fan beam technology in dual-energy x-ray absorptiometry (DXA) has enabled good quality (dual- and single-energy modes) images (posteroanterior and lateral projections) of the thoracic and lumbar spine, from which instant vertebral assessment (IVA) and morphometric measurements can be made (MXA).[29,30] It may be feasible for this process to be automated by computer techniques.[31] The advantage of MXA over conventional spinal radiography is a lower radiation dose (1/100th), less end plate distortion, because the x-ray beam is parallel to the end plate at each vertebral level, and visualization of the entire spine on a single image (Fig. 75-9).

Bone Densitometry

Whether a fracture occurs depends on a variety of factors, including the patient's age, propensity to fall and response to the fall; however, BMD is an important determinant of fracture, accounting for approximately 70% of bone strength. Reduced BMD is a useful predictor of increased fracture risk. The lower the peak bone density, the higher the risk of fracture in later life. Methods of measuring bone density are therefore relevant to the study of skeletal development, the detection of osteopenia, and the assessment of efficacy of treatment of osteoporosis. Such methods for measuring BMD should be accurate, precise (reproducible), sensitive both to small changes with time and to differences in patient groups (i.e., fracture compared with nonfracture), inexpensive, and involve a minimal exposure to ionizing radiation. Some of the techniques now available come close to these ideal requirements.[1]

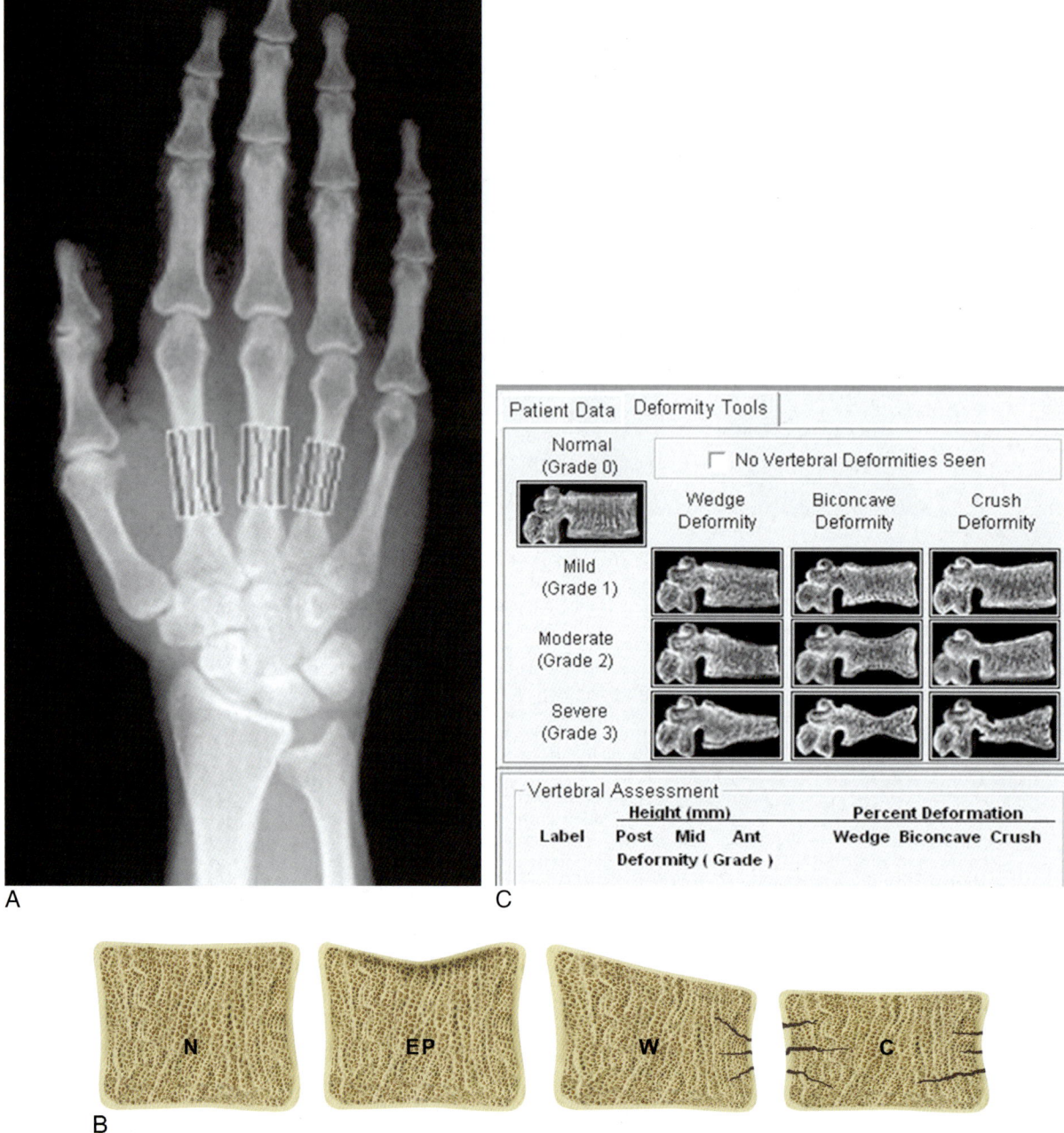

■ **FIGURE 75-8** Quantitative assessment of the skeleton. Radiogrammetry is a long-established technique to measure cortical thickness in the midshaft of the second metacarpal of the nondominant hand (metacarpal index) using calipers. **A,** More recently there has been application of computer vision methods (active shape models [ASM]) to automate this measurement to the second to fourth metacarpals, which improves precision (digital x-ray radiogrammetry [DXR]). **B,** Vertebral fractures can be described as end plate (EP), wedge (W), or crush (C), depending on the change in shape in relation to normal vertebral shape (N). **C,** The change in shape can be graded as indicated from the Instant Vertebral Assessment (IVA) tool of the Hologic QDR 4500 Discovery DXA scanner (Hologic Inc, Bedford, MA, USA): Grade 0 = normal; grade 1 (mild) = 20%–25% reduction in anterior, middle, and/or posterior height and 10%–20% reduction of the projected vertebral area; grade 2 (moderate) = 25%–40% reduction in anterior, middle and/or posterior height and 20%–40% reduction in projected vertebral area; grade 3 (severe) = 40% or greater reduction in anterior, middle, and/or posterior height and in the projected area.

Dual-Energy X-ray Absorptiometry

Dual-energy x-ray absorptiometry (DXA)[32] has now become the most widely available bone density technique since its introduction in 1987. X-ray beams of two peak energies are produced by a variety of techniques (k-edged filtration, energy switching) by different scanner manufacturers. The energies used are selected to optimize the separation of the mineralized and soft tissue components of the areas scanned. Original scanners had a pencil beam and coupled detector and scanned in a rectilinear fashion. Now scanners have a fan-beam x-ray source and banks of detectors. These allow rapid scanning with improved spatial resolution. The higher photon flux enables lateral imaging of the entire spine (single or dual

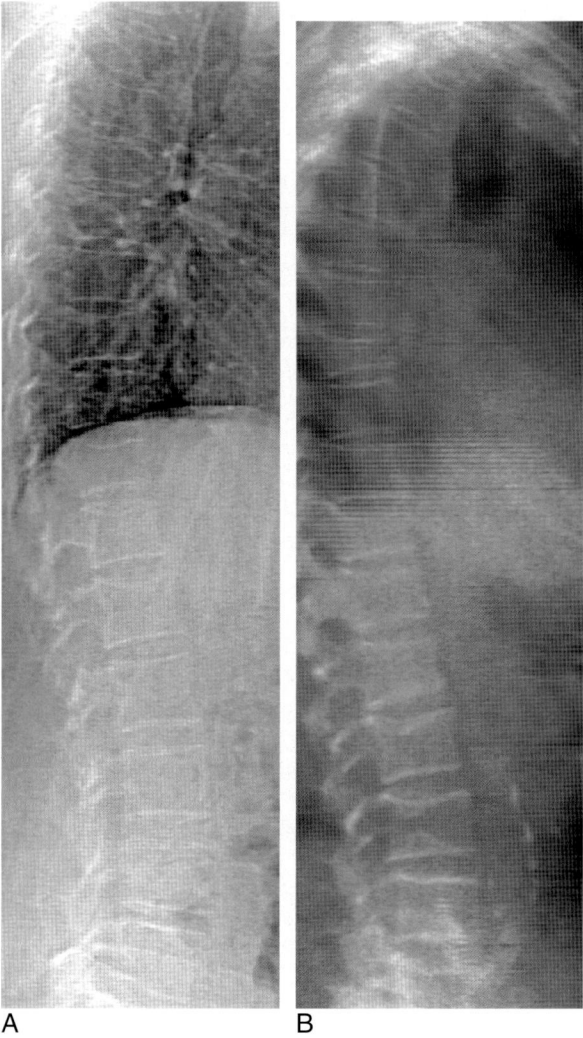

■ FIGURE 75-9 Spinal imaging using DXA scanner. **A,** The introduction of fan beam technology in DXA has enabled posteroanterior and lateral images of the spine to be obtained in single (**A**) and dual (**B**) energy; the thoracic spine is better visualized on the dual-energy image. The single-energy images are obtained at 1/100th of the radiation dose of conventional spinal radiographs; the entire spine is on a single image and does not have the problems of parallax of the divergent beam of radiographs. **A,** Normal appearances. **B,** Vertebral fractures at T8, L2, L3, and L4 and aortic calcification are present; linear artifact over the thoracolumbar junction is caused by diaphragmatic movement during acquisition of the image. The exact clinical role of DXA in the identification of vertebral fractures is still to be determined.

energy) from which morphometric x-ray absorptiometry analysis (MXA) of vertebral fractures can be made (see Figs. 75-8C and 75-9).[29,30] In clinical diagnosis, DXA is applied to the lumbar spine (L1-L4), the proximal femur (regions of analysis include the femoral neck, trochanter, and Ward's area), and total hip (Fig. 75-10A to C). Whole-body DXA with regional analysis gives information not only on bone density but also on body composition (lean muscle mass and fat mass) (see Fig. 75-10D). DXA measures integral (trabecular + cortical) BMD; different skeletal sites have variable cortical/trabecular ratios (50/50 in the lumbar spine (posteroanterior), 10/90 in the lateral projection of the lumbar spine, 60/40 in the proximal femur, and 80/20 in the whole body). The accuracy of DXA is between 3%

and 8%, with good precision (CV%); better than 1% in the posteroanterior spine and total femur, and 1% to 2% in the femoral neck. The advantages of DXA are the rapid scanning (<1 minute) and precise results if performed with meticulous care and extremely low doses of radiation (1-6 µSv per site scanned).[33] There are some limitations. Measurements are of integral bone and projected "areal" (g/cm^2), rather than true volumetric (g/cm^3), density. DXA measurements are therefore size dependent, a particular problem in children, in whom the bones are growing in size and changing in shape.[34,35] Additionally, all calcium within the path of the photon beam contributes to the BMD and can cause errors in BMD measures by DXA in the lumbar spine (Table 75-5).

Extraneous calcification (wall of aorta, vertebral fractures, and particularly degenerative and hyperostotic changes consequent to disc and apophyseal joint disease) will cause inaccuracies and overestimation of BMD (Fig. 75-11). This limits the usefulness and sensitivity of spinal DXA in elderly patients in whom such degenerative changes are commonly present (60% in those aged 70 years or more). Such artifacts require the results from affected individual vertebral bodies to be excluded from analysis; a minimum of two vertebrae must be available for analysis. Treatment with strontium ranelate causes artifactual increase in BMD, with approximately 50% of the increase being due to the high atomic number strontium being in the bones. DXA body scanners can now be used for scanning of peripheral sites (forearm) and to study regional bone density around a prosthesis after hip arthroplasty. Small, less-expensive, and more-mobile DXA scanners are manufactured for specific application to the forearm and the calcaneus.

To interpret BMD results in an individual patient it is essential to have appropriate race- and sex-matched BMD reference ranges, because there are ethnic differences in BMD and fracture prevalence. The patient's results can then be expressed as a standard deviation (SD) Z score, the percentage of expected or percentile of mean for age and sex, or as an SD T score, the percentage of expected or percentile of sex-matched young normal individuals (peak bone mass). The Z and T score methods are most commonly applied currently. In terms of bone densitometry the World Health Organization (WHO) has defined osteoporosis as a T score of below −2.5 using DXA in the proximal femur (neck, total) and lumbar spine (L1-L4).[32] Although there is consensus on this diagnostic definition from bone density, there is as yet no similar consensus on how these diagnostic definitions might most appropriately be applied consistently to therapeutic intervention. It is anticipated that in the near future the WHO will revise how patients are identified for cost-effective therapeutic interventions by calculating 5- and 10-year risk of fracture using age (>65 years), prior low trauma fracture, parental hip fracture, use of systemic glucocorticoids, excess alcohol intake, smoking, and rheumatoid arthritis.[36] This might separate patients into low risk (reassure), high risk (treat), and intermediate risk, in whom DXA BMD will be performed to recategorize a patient's risk as high or low.

In longitudinal studies the absolute BMD is used to calculate change with time or treatment in an individual patient. The interval of time between measurements will

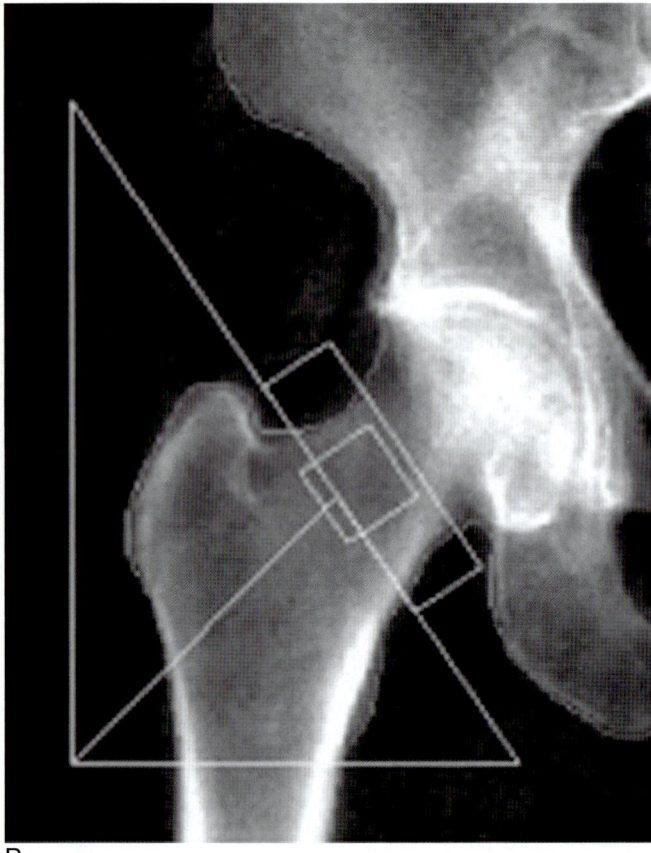

A

B

■ **FIGURE 75-10** Dual-energy X-ray absorptiometry (DXA) provides "areal" BMD (g/cm²) and is currently the gold standard method for diagnosis of osteoporosis by bone densitometry (WHO definition T score −2.5 or below in posteroanterior lumbar spine (L1-4) **(A)** or (femoral neck or total hip) acquired on GE Lunar Prodigy **(B)**

(Continued)

depend on the site of measurement (axial or appendicular skeleton), the type of bone measured (trabecular, cortical or integral), the expected rate of change in BMD, the measuring technique used, and its precision. The preferred measurement site for assessing change is the lumbar spine by DXA (high precision of better than 1%). In individual patients a minimal period of 1, but preferably 2, years should elapse between measurements to ensure change in BMD is significant (2.77 × precision error).

Quantitative Computed Tomography

Quantitative computed tomography (QCT)[37] uniquely allows for the separate estimation of trabecular and cortical BMD and provides a true volumetric density in grams per liter (milligrams per milliliter), rather than the "areal" (grams per square centimeter) density of DXA. QCT is therefore not size dependent, which is of particular relevance in children and in patients with diseases that result in small stature (Turner's syndrome, growth hormone deficiency, ill health). The technique is generally applied to the lumbar spine. A lateral projection radiograph is obtained, and for 2D QCT a scanning plane is selected (10-mm slice) through the middle of each vertebra, generally L1-L3, parallel to the end plates (Fig. 75-12A). If vertebral fractures are present, thinner (5-mm) sections may be required to avoid including the vertebral end plate in the section scanned, which will cause overestimation of BMD. A low-dose scanning technique (80 kV, 70 mA, 2 s) can be used to reduce patient radiation dose.[33] The entry of the basivertebral vein on the transverse axial section confirms the section to be in the midplane of the vertebral body. An oval region of interest to include as much of the vertebral trabecular bone as possible, without including the cortical rim or basivertebral vein, is selected for analysis (see Fig. 75-12B). QCT is performed with a calibration reference phantom to transform Hounsfield units into bone mineral equivalents. These phantoms were initially fluid (K_2HPO_4) but are now made of solid hydroxyapatite material. The results from different types of calibration phantoms are not interchangeable, unless a cross-calibration calculation can be made. In longitudinal studies it is preferable that the same reference phantom be used.

Original CT scanners used rotate-translate technology that permitted only single 2D sections. The recent

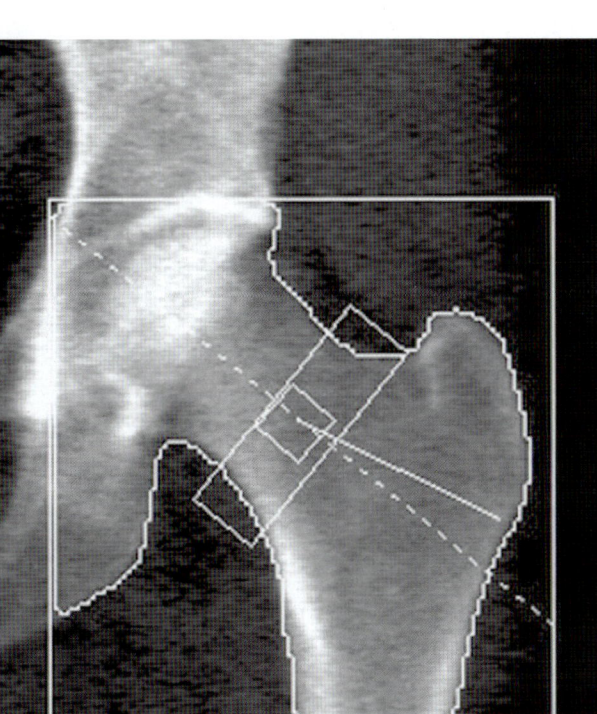

C

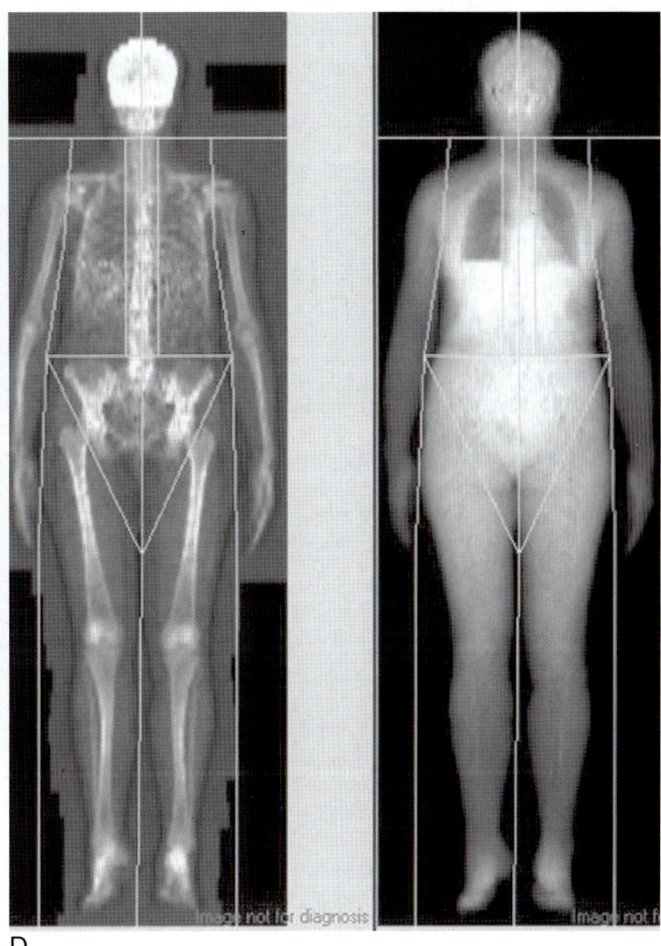

D

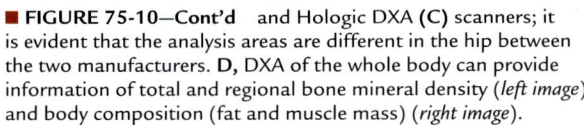

■ FIGURE 75-10—Cont'd and Hologic DXA **(C)** scanners; it is evident that the analysis areas are different in the hip between the two manufacturers. **D,** DXA of the whole body can provide information of total and regional bone mineral density (*left image*) and body composition (fat and muscle mass) (*right image*).

TABLE 75-5 Causes of Erroneous Bone Mineral Density Measures by DXA in the Lumbar Spine

Overestimation of Bone Mineral Density
Extraneous calcification (lymph nodes, aorta)
Degenerative disc and spine disease (osteophytes)
Ankylosing spondylitis
Vertebral fracture
Sclerotic metastases
Vertebral hemangioma
Overlying metal artifacts (navel rings)
Surgical interventions (metallic rods, spinal fusion)
Vertebroplasty
Paget's disease
Treatment with strontium ranelate
Underestimation of Bone Mineral Density
Laminectomy

---

technical developments in CT of continuous spiral rotation of the x-ray tube and multiple rows of detectors enable rapid 3D volume scanning (see Fig. 75-12A and B). As a consequence, precision has improved (better than CV = 1%) and the method is applicable to measure bone size and density in the hip. The WHO definition of osteoporosis (T score below −2.5) is *not* applicable to QCT; a Z score of −2.0 and below is abnormal. Some use the definition of a QCT of 100 mg/cm³ or below as "osteopenia" and 80 mg/cm³ or below as "osteoporosis."

Although usually applied to the vertebral trabecular bone, more recently dedicated, small CT scanners (peripheral pQCT) have been developed that allow separate analysis of cortical and trabecular bone in the nondominant forearm (see Fig. 75-12C and D) and in other sites of the skeleton, including the tibia. Measurement of cross-sectional bone and muscle area, and certain biomechanical parameters, can also be made from these scans.[34,35] These dedicated pQCT scanners use older CT technology (rotate and translate), and each section consequently takes about 1 minute to obtain.

Radiation Dose in Bone Densitometry (Table 75-6)

DXA scans (and pQCT) have extremely low radiation doses at between 1 to 6 μSV per site scanned, which is equivalent to about 3 hours of background equivalent radiation (BER, 2400-7200 μSv, depending on geographic area).[33] This makes it possible to gain ethical approval for application in normal children to study growth and development of the skeleton. The radiation dose from QCT is higher but still compares favorably with conventional radiographic exposures. With a low kV, the dose

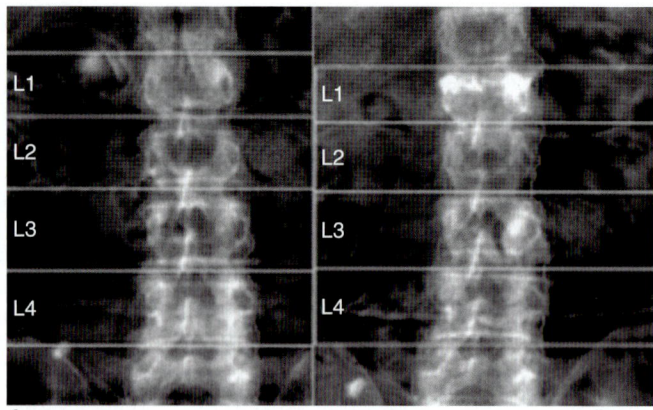

A

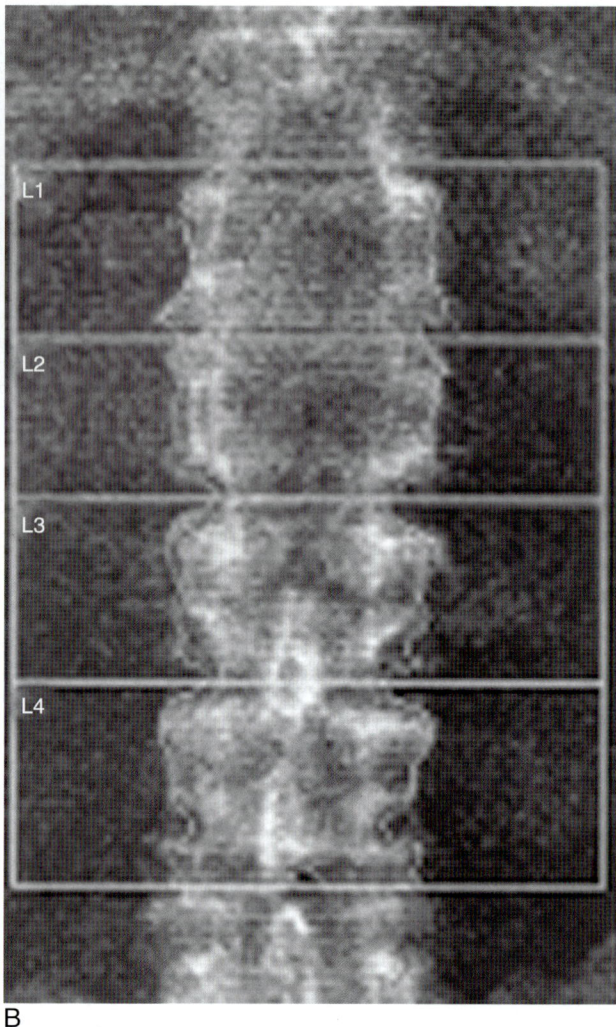

B

■ **FIGURE 75-11** Causes of artifacts on DXA images and measurements. **A,** A vertebral fracture of L1 has occurred between the first scan (*left image*) and the follow-up scan (*right image*); the fractured vertebra will have the same amount of calcium in a smaller area and so the bone mineral density measurement will be falsely elevated; to calculate accurately the change in bone mineral density L1 must be excluded from both scans. **B,** There have been laminectomies at L1 and L2; the DXA bone mineral density measurement will be falsely reduced at these levels and must be excluded from analysis to avoid an erroneous classification of osteoporosis being made. A minimum of two vertebrae must be available for analysis.

for QCT (including the initial scout view) will be approximately 90 μSV.

Other Research Methods

Quantitative ultrasonography (QUS) measures broadband ultrasound attenuation (BUA) and speed of sound (SOS). It is predominantly applied to the calcaneus, where it predicts fracture risk in elderly females. However, it cannot be used to diagnose osteoporosis as defined by the WHO, is temperature sensitive, is a poor monitoring tool, and has been applied to numerous other skeletal sites (e.g., phalanges); and it is not clear how it should be used in clinical practice in other patient groups (men, young women, and children). Quantitative magnetic resonance imaging (QMRI) has been applied in research to assessing bone density and trabecular bone structure.[38] The diameters of bone trabeculae range from 50 to 200 μm. Trabecular structure can be demonstrated on conventional radiographs, particularly in the appendicular skeleton (hands), where visualization can be enhanced by magnification techniques. More recently, there has been increase in the research application of high-resolution CT and high-resolution MRI to examining trabecular structure in vivo.

MicroCT systems are under development with increased spatial resolution, but these are generally only applicable to examine small tissue samples in vitro.[38]

DIFFERENTIAL DIAGNOSIS

The main differential clinical diagnosis of generalized osteoporosis includes multiple myeloma and acute leukemia. There are many causes of secondary osteoporosis (see Table 75-3), which can present as a wide variety of clinical symptoms and signs. However, their discussion is beyond the scope of this chapter.

Vertebral fractures with more persistence pain (over 6 to 8 weeks), and those occurring above T7, should raise the possibility of a malignant etiology (e.g., metastasis, myeloma) rather than due to osteoporosis. Clinical features of bruising, bleeding, and recurrent infections can be features of acute leukemia. Localized lytic bone destruction at the site of a pathologic fracture on radiographs also indicates a malignant cause. Specific clinical features may direct diagnosis to a cause of secondary osteoporosis; for instance, "moon" facies, increase in weight, abdominal obesity and striae, hypertension, and hair loss indicate Cushing's syndrome.

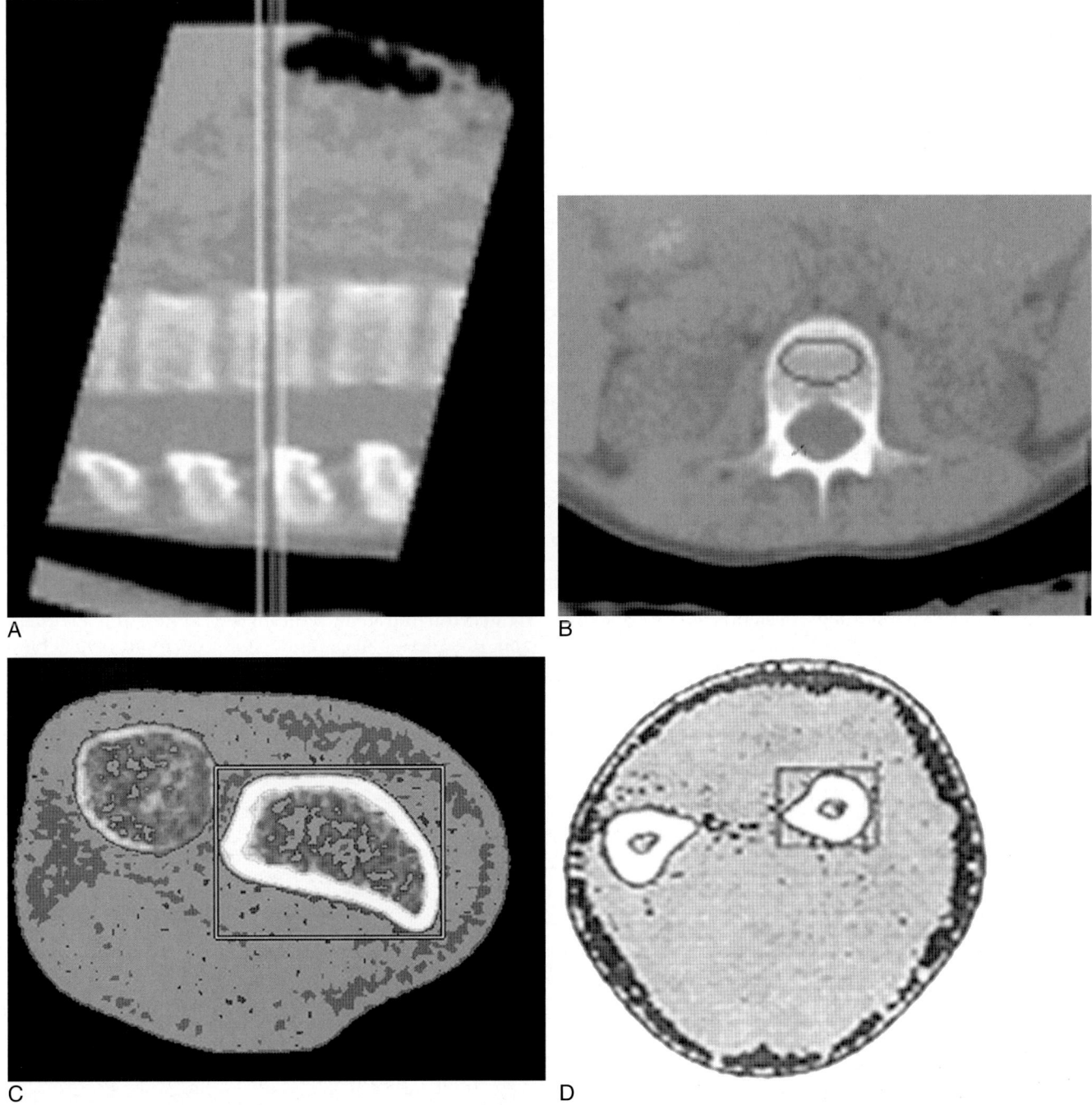

■ **FIGURE 75-12** Quantitative computed tomography (QCT) uniquely provides separate measures of cortical and trabecular bone mineral density as true volumetric density (mg/cm³) and is applied to the spine (**A** and **B**) and peripheral sites (forearm and tibia) (**C** and **D**). With technical developments in CT (spiral, multislice), 3D volume imaging (**A**) of L1-L3 improves precision to CV = 1% and the appropriate section can be selected for analysis of an oval region in the trabecular bone (**B**). A bone mineral phantom (solid hydroxyapatite) enables Hounsfield unit numbers to be transformed into bone mineral equivalents. Peripheral QCT, using dedicated peripheral CT scanners, is generally performed in the distal radius (4% site) (**C**) to provide volumetric bone mineral density of the cortical and trabecular bone and at the midshaft (50% site) (**D**) from which can be measured cortical thickness and density and endosteal and periosteal cross-sectional area from which biomechanical parameters (moment of inertia and stress strain index) can be extracted, together with cross-sectional muscle and fat area.

In the primary causes of osteoporosis there are no blood or urine tests that are diagnostic, because measures all are usually normal. There may be evidence of increased bone turnover with raised levels of collagen degradation products in the urine (pyridinium cross-links). In leukemia there will be an abnormal blood cell count and marrow aspirate. In multiple myeloma (plasma cell cancer) there will be abnormal marrow that is infiltrated with plasma cells, hypercalcemia, and Bence Jones (light chain) protein in the urine. In hyperparathyroidism there is a raised calcium concentration, normal or reduced phosphate level, normal or raised alkaline phosphatase value, and calciuria and phosphaturia.

TABLE 75-6 Radiation Doses in Bone Densitometry Methods with Some Comparators

Technique	Site	EDE (μSv)	NBR	Fatal Cancer Risk
DXA	Spine	2.4–4.0	13 hours	<1 in a few million
	Femur	2.4–5.4	20 hours	<1 in a few million
	Total body	1.0–3.4	11 hours	<1 in a few million
Quantitative CT	Spine	55–100	10 days	1 in 200,000
Peripheral quantitative QCT	Radius/tibia	0.43/slice	1.7 hours	<1 in a few million
Radiographs	Hand	<1	<1 hour	<1 in a few million
	Chest	20–40	3–6 days	1 in a million
	Lumbar spine	700–1,000	7 months	1 in 200,000
CT	Abdomen/pelvis	10,000	4.5 years	1 in 2,000
Trans-Atlantic flight (return)		80	12 days	
Background radiation (NBR)		7–21 per day		
		2400–7300 pa		

EDE, effective dose equivalent; NBR, natural background radiation.

SYNOPSIS OF TREATMENT OPTIONS

Medical Treatment

Adequate analgesia should be given to manage pain during the episode of an acute fracture or appropriately as improves the quality of life thereafter for those severely affected by osteoporosis; physiotherapy may also be helpful.

Pharmaceutical intervention of established osteoporosis was, in the past, limited and unsatisfactory. However, over the past decade there has been the introduction of effective therapies. These include bisphosphonates, selective estrogen receptor modulators (SERMs), teriparatide (parathyroid hormone), and strontium ranelate, which have been shown to increase bone mineral density by varying degrees (by between 4% to 12%) but more importantly significantly reduce future vertebral fracture (by between 30% to 70%). Treatment strategies have generally favored prevention of osteoporosis by maximizing peak bone mass, minimizing age-related and postmenopausal bone loss (hormone replacement therapy in premature menopause), avoidance of risk factors (e.g., smoking, excessive alcohol consumption) with

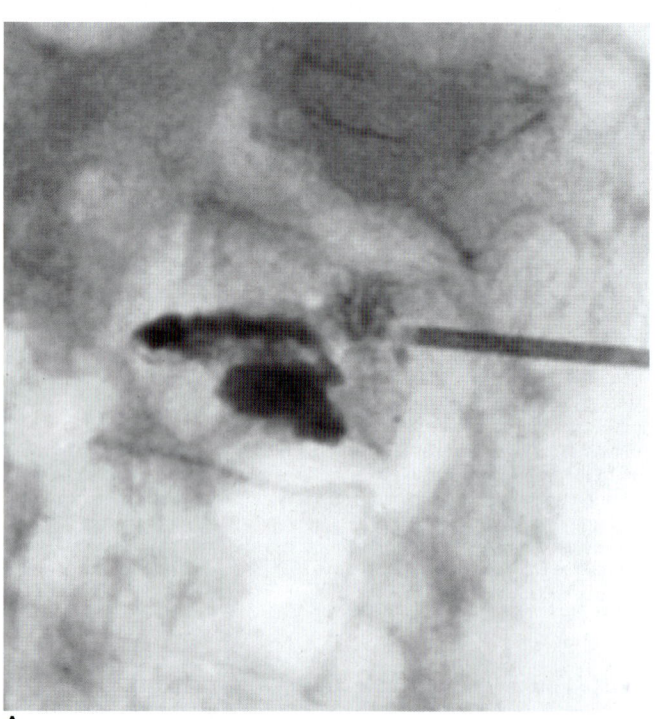
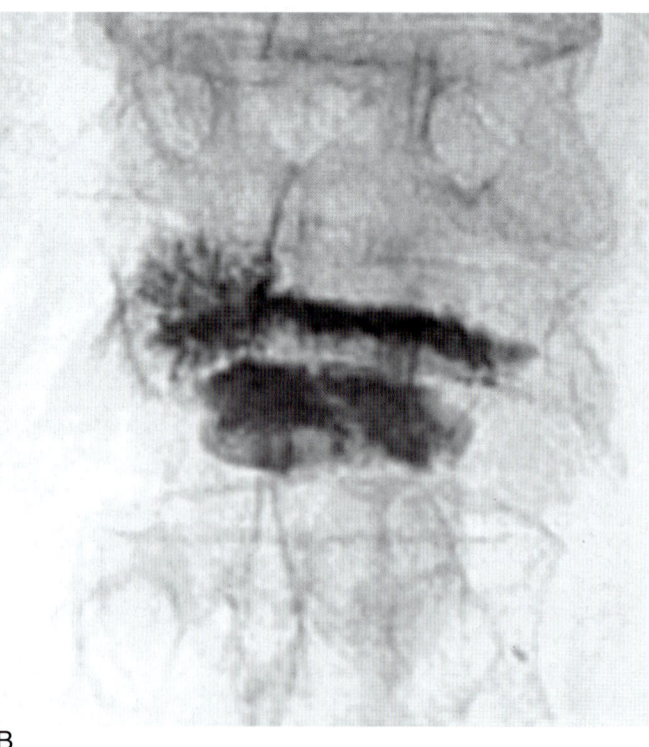

A   B

■ **FIGURE 75-13** Vertebroplasty. In selected cases, pain from osteoporotic vertebral fractures that have not responded to conservative and bisphosphonate therapy may be treated by injection of cement (methylmethacrylate) into the vertebral body. Lateral **(A)** and frontal **(B)** projections show opaque cement entering the fracture line and marrow space of the vertebra of the patient whose MR image is illustrated in Figure 76-7A. Vertebroplasty in the lumbar region will cause false elevation on bone mineral density as measured by DXA, and the specific vertebra would have to be excluded from analysis. *(Courtesy of Dr. R. W. Whitehouse, Manchester Royal Infirmary, UK.)*

adequate dietary intake of calcium and vitamin D (1 g elemental calcium and 800 units vitamin D), and physical activity. Compliance and persistence with oral bone protective therapies taken daily is relatively poor, being approximately 50% at 1 year. This situation has been improved with the introduction of monthly dosing for some bisphosphonates. Some bisphosphonates are given intravenously; it is with these, rather than with oral preparations, and when they are being given for hypercalcemia in patients with metastatic cancer, that there has been reported the uncommon complication of osteonecrosis of the jaw.

Surgical Treatment

Vertebroplasty (see Procedures on CD) has selected application in patients with osteoporotic vertebral fractures that are persistently painful.[39,40] Although performed by several medical specialists, radiologists are probably the most appropriate group to perform this image-guided interventional technique, particularly because imaging (radiographs, radionuclide scans, CT, and MRI) plays a role in selecting patients appropriate for the procedure. Vertebroplasty is the injection of cement (methylmethacrylate) into a fractured vertebral body as a means of treating pain (Fig. 75-13). Kyphoplasty is the injection of cement into the fractured vertebral body after a balloon has been used to decompress the fracture and correct some of the deformity, although the latter is limited (<15 degrees).[40] Both

techniques are intended to relieve pain in patients who have not responded to conservative measures and time. There is no clear evidence as to how long to wait before treating with vertebroplasty, but the current consensus is that a minimum of 4 weeks should pass with adequate medical treatment; some will delay the procedure 6 to 8 weeks. Adequate medical treatment should include analgesia, and many believe there should be a trial of bisphosphonates. Patient selection is crucial to success. The pain should arise from vertebral fractures that are temporally related to the onset of symptoms. MRI with water-sensitive sequences and fat suppression (fast STIR) will show edema and hemorrhage in a fracture of recent onset. As yet there are no randomized controlled trials that compare medical management with vertebroplasty, and which compare vertebroplasty with kyphoplasty, although some such studies are underway. The chance of successful pain relief for osteoporotic fracture is between 70% and 95%. There are fewer data on the efficacy of kyphoplasty and none to show that this relatively complex and more expensive procedure has advantage in outcome when compared with vertebroplasty. Overall complication rates from reports suggest that symptom-inducing or potentially serious complications occur in approximately 2% of patients treated for osteoporotic fracture. All patients treated by vertebroplasty or kyphoplasty for osteoporotic compression fractures should be under the care of a clinician with special interest in osteoporosis management and on appropriate medical therapy to reduce future fracture risk.

What the Referring Physician Needs to Know

- Osteoporosis is a common problem (1 in 2 women; 1 in 5 men affected over 50 years).
- Fractures are associated with considerable morbidity, mortality, and health care costs.
- Effective therapies are available to reduce future fracture risk.
- Radiographic features may be present before fractures occur.
- Thirty percent of vertebral fractures may be present without symptoms.

- Vertebral fractures are powerful predictors of future fracture (vertebral 5×; hip 2×).
- Dual-energy x-ray absorptiometry (DXA) (hip, spine) is the quantitative method for confirming the diagnosis of osteoporosis in terms of bone densitometry.

SUGGESTED READINGS

Adams JE, Shaw N (eds). A Practical Guide to Bone Densitometry in Children. Bath, England, National Osteoporosis Society, 2004.

Blake GM, Wahner HW, Fogelman I. The Evaluation of Osteoporosis: Dual Energy X-ray Absorptiometry and Ultrasound in Clinical Practice, 2nd ed. London, Martin Dunitz, 1999.

Favus MJ (ed). Primer on the Metabolic Bone Diseases and Disorders of Mineral Metabolism, 6th ed. American Society of Bone and Mineral Research, Washington, DC., 2006.

Genant HK, Guglielmi G, M. Jergas M (eds). Bone Densitometry and Osteoporosis. Berlin, Springer-Verlag, 1999.

Genant HK, Jergas M, van Kuijk C (eds). Vertebral Fracture in Osteoporosis. San Francisco, CA, Osteoporosis Research Group, University of San Francisco, 1995.

Grampp S (ed). Radiology of Osteoporosis. Berlin, Springer, 2003.

Mathis JM, Deramond H, Belkoff SM (eds). Percutaneous Vertebroplasty. New York, Springer-Verlag, 2002.

Njeh CF, Hans D, Fuerst T, et al (eds). Quantitative Ultrasound: Assessment of Osteoporosis and Bone Status. London, Martin Dunitz, 1999.

Orwoll E (ed). Osteoporosis in Men Elsevier, Academic Press, 1999.

Sawyer AJ, Bachrach LK, Fung EB (eds). Bone Densitometry in Growing Patients: Guidelines for Clinical Practice. Totowa, NJ, Humana Press, 2006.

REFERENCES

1. Adams JE. Metabolic and endocrine skeletal disease. In Grainger RG, Allison DJ, Dixon AK (eds). Grainger and Allison's Diagnostic Radiology: A Textbook of Medical Imaging, 5th ed. Philadelphia, Churchill Livingstone, 2008, pp 1043-1113.
2. Bouxsein ML, Karasik D. Bone geometry and skeletal fragility. Curr Osteoporos Rep 2006; 4:49-56.
3. Link T, Majumdar S. Osteoporosis imaging. Radiol Clin North Am 2003; 41:813-839.
4. Marcus R, Feldman, Kelsey J (eds). Osteoporosis, 2nd ed. San Diego, CA, Academic Press, 2001.
5. Kauffman RP, Overton TH, Shiflett M, Jennings JC. Osteoporosis in children and adolescent girls: case report of idiopathic juvenile osteoporosis and review of the literature. Obstet Gynecol Surg 2001; 56:492-504.
6. Meunier PJ, Delmas PD, Eastell R, et al. Diagnosis and management of osteoporosis in postmenopausal women: clinical guidelines. International Committee for Osteoporosis Clinical Guidelines. Clin Ther 1999; 21:1025-1044.
7. Sillence D. Osteogenesis imperfecta: an expanding panorama of variants. Clin Orthop Rel Res 1981; 59:11-25.
8. Rauch F, Glorieux FH. Osteogenesis imperfecta. Lancet 2004; 363;1377-1385.
9. Quek ST, Peh WC. Radiology of osteoporosis. Semin Musculoskelet Radiol 2002; 6:197-206.
10. van Staa TP, Leufkens HG, Cooper C. The epidemiology of corticosteroid induced osteoporosis: a meta-analysis. Osteoporos Int 2002; 13:777-787.
11. Pham T, Lafforgue P. Reflex sympathetic dystrophy and neuromediators. Joint Bone Spine 2003; 70:12-17.
12. Toms AP, Marshall TJ, Becker E, et al. Regional migratory osteoporosis: a review illustrated by five cases. Clin Radiol 2005; 60:425-438.
13. van de Berg BC, Lecouvet FE, Maldague B, Malghem J. Osteonecrosis and transient osteoporosis of the femoral head. In Davies AM, Johnson K, Whitehouse RW (eds). Imaging of the Hip and Bony Pelvis—Techniques and Applications. Heidelberg, Springer, 2006, pp 195-216.
14. Sambrook P, Cooper C. Osteoporosis. Lancet 2006; 367:2010-2018.
15. Melton LJ, Lane AW, Cooper C, et al. Prevalence and incidence of vertebral fracture. Osteoporos Int 1993; 3:113-119.
16. O'Neill T, Felsenberg D, Varlow J, et al. The prevalence of vertebral fracture in European men and women: the European Vertebral Osteoporosis Study. J Bone Miner Res 1996; 11:1010-1018.
17. Gehlbach SH, Bigelow C, Heimisdottir M, et al. Recognition of vertebral fractures in a clinical setting. Osteoporos Int 2000; 11:577-582.
18. Delmas PD, van de Langerijt L, Watts NB, et al. Underdiagnosis of vertebral fractures is a worldwide problem: the IMPACT study. J Bone Miner Res 2005; 20:557-563.
19. Adams JE. Radiology of rickets and osteomalacia. In Feldman D, Pike JW, Glorieux FH (eds). Vitamin D, 2nd ed. San Diego, Elsevier, 2005, pp 967-994.
20. Peh W. Imaging of pelvic insufficiency fracture. RadioGraphics 1996; 16:335-348.
21. Peh W, Davies AM. Bone trauma: stress fractures. In Davies AM, Johnson K, Whitehouse RW (eds). Imaging of the Hip and Bony Pelvis—Techniques and Applications. Heidelberg, Springer, 2006, pp 247-266.
22. Hain SF, Fogelman I. Nuclear medicine studies in metabolic bone disease. Semin Musculoskelet Radiol 2002; 6:323-329.
23. Jiang G, Eastell R, Barrington NA, Ferrar L. Comparison of methods for the visualisation of prevalent vertebral fracture in osteoporosis. Osteoporos Int 2004; 15:887-896.
24. Ferrar L, Jiang G, Adams J, Eastell R. Identification of vertebral fractures: an update. Osteoporos Int 2005; 16:717-728.
25. Guermazi A, Mohr A, Grogorian M, et al. Identification of vertebral fractures in osteoporosis. Semin Musculoskelet Radiol 2002; 6:241-252.
26. Link TM, Guglielmi G, van Kuijk C, Adams JE. Radiologic assessment of osteoporotic fracture: diagnostic and prognostic implications. Eur Radiol 2005; 15:1521-1532.
27. Nielsen SP. The metacarpal index revisited: a brief overview. J Clin Densitom 2001; 4:199-207.
28. Smyth PP, Adams JE, Whitehouse RW, Taylor CJ. Application of computer texture analysis to the Singh Index. Br J Radiol 1997; 70:242-247.
29. Blake GM, Rea JA, Fogelman I. Vertebral morphometry studies using dual-energy X-ray absorptiometry. Semin Nucl Med 1997; 27:276-290.
30. Duboeuf F, Bauer DC, Chapurlat RD, et al. Assessment of vertebral fracture using densitometric morphometry. J Clin Densitom 2005; 8:362-368.
31. Roberts M, Cootes T, Adams JE. Vertebral morphometry: semi-automated determination of detailed vertebral shape from dual-energy X-ray absorptiometry images using Active Appearance Models. Invest Radiol 2006; 41:849-859.
32. Blake GM, Fogelman I. Role of dual-energy X-ray absorptiometry in the diagnosis and treatment of osteoporosis. J Clin Densitom 2007; 10:102-110.
33. Kalender WA. Effective dose values in bone mineral measurements by photon absorptiometry and computed tomography. Osteoporos Int 1992; 2:82-87.
34. Mughal M, Ward K Adams J. Assessment of bone status in children by densitometric and quantitative ultrasound techniques. In Carty H, Brunelle F, Stringer DA, Kao S (eds). Imaging Children, 2nd ed. London, Churchill Livingstone, 2005, pp 477-486.
35. van Rijn RR, van der Sluis IM, Link TM, et al. Bone densitometry in children: a critical appraisal. Eur Radiol 2003; 13:700-710.
36. Kanis JA, Borgstrom F, De Laet C, et al. Assessment of fracture risk. Osteoporos Int 2005; 16:581-589.
37. Guglielmi G, Lang TF. Quantitative computed tomography. Semin Musculoskelet Radiol 2002; 6:219-227.
38. Link TM, Bauer JS. Imaging of trabecular bone structure. Semin Musculoskelet Radiol 2002; 6:253-261.
39. Peh WC, Gilula LA. Percutaneous vertebroplasty: an update. Semin Ultrasound CT MR 2005; 26:52-64.
40. Deramond H, Saliou G, Aveillan M, et al. Retrospective contributions of vertebroplasty and kyphoplasty to the management of osteoporotic vertebral fractures. Joint Bone Spine 2006; 73:610-613.

76

Hyperparathyroidism, Renal Osteodystrophy, Osteomalacia and Rickets

Murali Sundaram and Jean Schils

Hyperparathyroidism

ETIOLOGY

A review of more than 20,000 cases of primary hyperparathyroidism found that in 89% of patients the cause was a solitary adenoma in the parathyroid gland and that 10% had multiglandular hyperplasia. Parathyroid carcinoma and cysts causing primary hyperparathyroidism are very unusual, occurring in less than 1% of cases.[1]

PREVALENCE AND EPIDEMIOLOGY

In the United States, primary hyperparathyroidism is said to affect 10 to 30 people per 100,000 population. The prevalence is higher in Italy and Sweden where up to 2% of women older than 55 years will be affected by the disease. Women are affected three times more frequently than men.[2] The disease appears ancient in view of a recent report describing pathognomonic lesions of primary hyperparathyroidism in a skeleton from 7000 years ago.[3]

CLINICAL PRESENTATION

The clinical syndrome can be remembered as "stones, bones, abdominal groans, and psychic overtones." Some medical abnormalities that may be encountered are renal stones, osteoporosis, and pancreatitis.

PATHOPHYSIOLOGY

Parathyroid hormone (PTH) acts on kidney and bone. It decreases tubular absorption of phosphorus, resulting in increased urinary phosphorus excretion and reduced serum phosphorus levels. A second action on the kidney is increasing the active form of vitamin D (25-dihydroxyvitamin D), which increases calcium and phosphorus absorption from the gastrointestinal tract.

PTH stimulates bone resorption, with a resultant increase of calcium and phosphorus in the blood. Consequently, there is an increase in serum concentrations of calcium.

IMAGING TECHNIQUES

The classic and earliest radiographic sign of primary hyperparathyroidism is subperiosteal phalangeal resorption along the radial aspects of the index, long, and ring

---

KEY POINTS

- The classic radiographic changes of hyperparathyroidism in primary hyperparathyroidism are largely historical because diagnosis and treatment are based on serum calcium and PTH levels.
- DEXA scanning to monitor osteoporosis in nonsurgical candidates with primary hyperparathyroidism is currently approved practice.
- Chondrocalcinosis may be the presenting radiographic finding in patients with primary hyperparathyroidism.

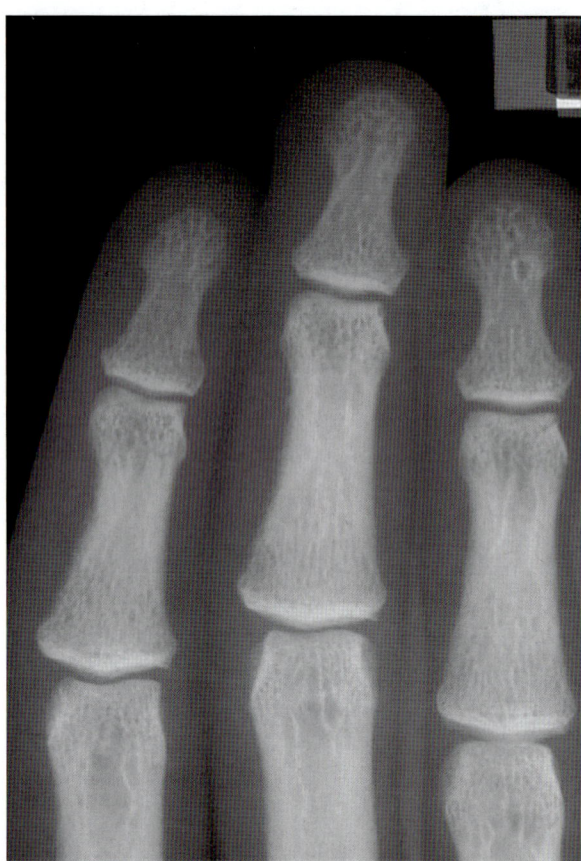

■ **FIGURE 76-1** Early but unequivocal radiographic signs of hyperparathyroidism. The radial aspects of the middle phalanges of the index and long fingers show cortical resorption (compared with ring finger) and fine spiculation, constituting the classic subperiosteal resorption of hyperparathyroidism. This appearance may represent primary, secondary, or tertiary hyperparathyroidism.

fingers (Fig. 76-1). This finding is now hardly encountered in the Western Hemisphere because of the widespread availability and use of routine serum chemistry panels. The well-described classic changes of primary hyperparathyroidism in textbooks of radiology are today, in adults, largely of historical interest. Because routine serum chemistry panels are not performed in children, advanced radiographic changes of hyperparathyroidism due to primary hyperparathyroidism may still be encountered.[4]

MANIFESTATIONS OF THE DISEASE

The imaging that tends to be performed for patients with biochemical evidence of primary hyperparathyroidism is outside the realm of musculoskeletal radiology. Because the cause is usually an adenoma and, less frequently, multiglandular parathyroid hyperplasia, technetium-99m sestamibi imaging and ultrasonography may be performed. These imaging studies are usually reserved for failed parathyroidectomy or in planning minimally invasive parathyroid surgery.

The majority of patients with primary hyperparathyroidism are asymptomatic, because the disease is detected biochemically. About 5% of women with renal stones have primary hyperparathyroidism.

Radiography

As previously mentioned, the classic signs of primary hyperparathyroidism are now rarely encountered. These patients, however, are osteoporotic. Bone densitometry is considered an important tool for detecting and monitoring osteoporosis due to hyperparathyroidism to identify those patients at future fracture risk. Bone loss in hyperparathyroidism involves the outer compact bone whereas in postmenopausal osteoporosis the loss of bone is cancellous/trabecular. Hence, dual-energy x-ray absorption (DEXA) may be normal in the spine in patients with mild primary hyperparathyroidism because it is rich in cancellous bone. The bone density of the femoral neck will be intermediate in degree of abnormality because bone at this location is composed of both cancellous and cortical bone. The most reliable site for measuring bone loss in primary hyperparathyroidism is the distal part of the forearm, which contains proportionately a large amount of cortical bone.

Chondrocalcinosis typically in the knees and, less commonly, in the triangular ligament of the ulna in patients younger than 50 years of age should raise the possibility of a hypercalcemic state. The most common hypercalcemic state is primary hyperparathyroidism, and it should be considered in the absence of joint space narrowing or other signs of degenerative arthritis. It would also be reasonable to raise this consideration in older patients if there are no accompanying signs of degenerative joint disease in the presence of chondrocalcinosis. Although it has been mentioned that primary hyperparathyroidism is now usually diagnosed biochemically, radiologists need to be aware that routine biochemical laboratory evaluations are not always done in the outpatient setting, which makes the observation of chondrocalcinosis and its possible relationship to hypercalcemia important (Fig. 76-2).

DIFFERENTIAL DIAGNOSIS

There are numerous other causes for hypercalcemia besides primary hyperparathyroidism. A partial list includes familial hypocalciuric hypercalcemia; idiopathic hypercalcemia; familial hyperparathyroidism; multiple endocrine neoplasia (MEN) type 1; neoplasia from breast, lung, colon, prostate, and kidney; and multiple myeloma. Sarcoidosis and histoplasmosis may also present as hypercalcemia.

The critical breakthrough permitting primary hyperparathyroidism to be distinguished from tumor-induced hypercalcemia was estimating serum PTH levels. The diagnosis of primary hyperparathyroidism requires both elevated serum calcium and PTH levels.

SYNOPSIS OF TREATMENT OPTIONS
Medical Treatment

A normal diet is prescribed with normal intake of calcium but without calcium supplementation. Thirty to 50 mg per day of cinacalcet, which is a calcium emetic, reduces serum concentrations of PTH and calcium.[5]

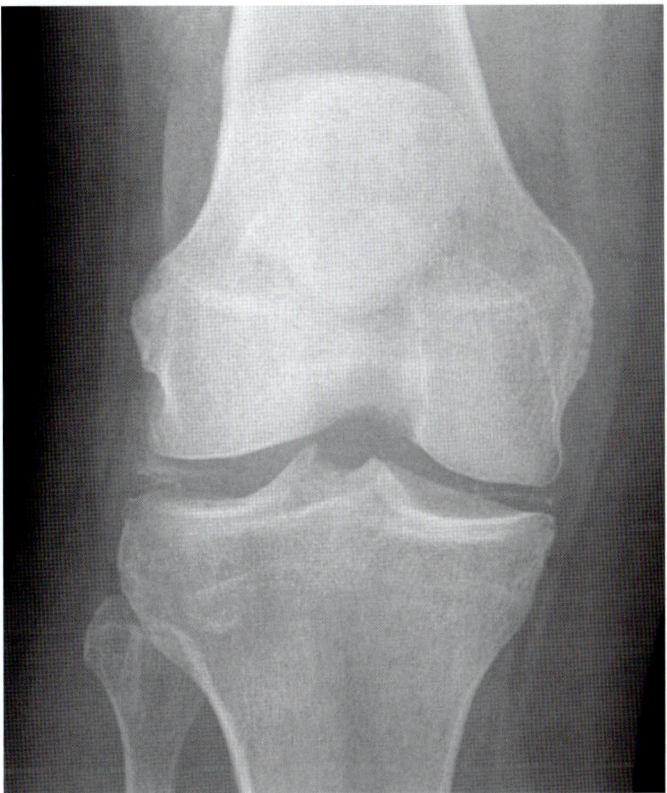

■ **FIGURE 76-2** Chondrocalcinosis in a patient with primary hyperparathyroidism showing well preserved femorotibial joint space and without signs of degenerative joint disease.

What the Referring Physician Needs to Know

- A skeletal survey or hand radiographs to demonstrate signs of primary hyperparathyroidism is redundant.
- A skeletal survey or a technetium bone scan would be appropriate if malignancy is a consideration for hypercalcemia.

SUGGESTED READING

Levine MA. Primary hyperparathyroidism: 7,000 years of progress. Cleve Clin J Med 2005; 72:1084–1097.

REFERENCES

1. Ruda JM, Hollenbeaker CS, Stach BC Jr. A Systematic review of the diagnosis and treatment of primary hyperparathyroidism, 1995–2003. Otolaryngol Head Neck Surg 2005; 132:259–372.
2. Levine MA. Primary hyperparathyroidism: 7,000 years of progress. Cleve Clin J Med 2005; 72:1084–1097.
3. Zink AR, Panzer S, Fesq-Martin M, et al. Evidence for a 7,000 year old case of primary hyperparathyroidism [Letter]. JAMA 2005; 293:40–42.
4. Kollaris J, Zarroug AE, van Hwerden J, et al. Primary hyperparathyroidism in pediatric patients. Pediatrics 2005; 115:974–980.
5. Peacock M, Bilezikiang P, Klassen PS, et al. Cinacalcet hydrochloride maintains long term normal calcemia in patients with primary hyperparathyroidism. J Clin Endocrinol Metab 2005; 90:135–141.

Renal Osteodystrophy

ETIOLOGY

The connection between chronic impairment of renal glomerular function and bone disease was made a little over a hundred years ago.[1] The term *renal osteodystrophy* to describe the musculoskeletal manifestations of chronic renal failure was described in 1943 by Liu and Chu.[2] The traditional view has been that renal osteodystrophy encompasses hyperparathyroidism, osteomalacia, osteoporosis, and soft tissue calcification. In fact, renal osteodystrophy is the result of two major pathologic processes occurring in varying severity and proportion; hyperparathyroidism from an excess of parathyroid hormone and rickets or osteomalacia from a deficiency of 1,25-dihydroxycholecalciferol (1,25-DHCC, the renal hormone of vitamin D).[3] The natural history of renal osteodystrophy, that is, hyperparathyroidism and osteomalacia, has been modified by dialysis and renal transplantation.

PREVALENCE AND EPIDEMIOLOGY

Worldwide there are over 1 million patients on maintenance hemodialysis.[4] Because it is held that even in undialyzed uremic patients that hyperparathyroidism is almost universal, it can be assumed that all of these patients, irrespective of findings on imaging, have renal osteodystrophy.

CLINICAL PRESENTATION

The clinical presentation of chronic renal failure includes sodium and water retention, hypercalcemia, and metabolic acidosis. These manifestations may be associated with cardiovascular, pulmonary, hematologic, endocrine, or neuromuscular abnormalities.

PATHOPHYSIOLOGY

The underlying etiologic causes leading to chronic renal failure include diabetes mellitus (28%), hypertension (25%), glomerulonephritis (21%), polycystic kidney disease (4%), and others (23%), such as obstruction, infection, and so on.[5] A patient is considered azotemic with a glomerular filtration rate of 30% to 35% and uremic when excretion is less than 20% of normal excretory capacity.

KEY POINTS

- Hyperparathyridism is universal in chronic renal failure.
- Maintenance hemodialysis for 15 years results in amyloid deposition in almost 100% of patients.
- Soft tissue calcification in renal osteodystrophy should be reversed medically and not surgically.
- Short T2 on MRI of a destructive vertebral or discovertebral lesion suggests amyloid.

MANIFESTATIONS OF THE DISEASE

Because of the advances in understanding the underlying mechanisms that result in hyperparathyroidism and osteomalacia, the routine performance of skeletal surveys, which was once prevalent, is not utilized.[6] The radiographic signs of hyperparathyroidism that may be manifest in patients with chronic renal failure are phalangeal resorption in the hands (Fig. 76-3)[7] and/or exclusive phalangeal tuft resorption (Fig. 76-4).[8] The hands are the earliest and most sensitive site for the detection of hyperparathyroidism. Depending on the extent and severity of disease, resorption may be encountered in the heads of the clavicles (Fig. 76-5), sacroiliac joints (Fig. 76-6), and other

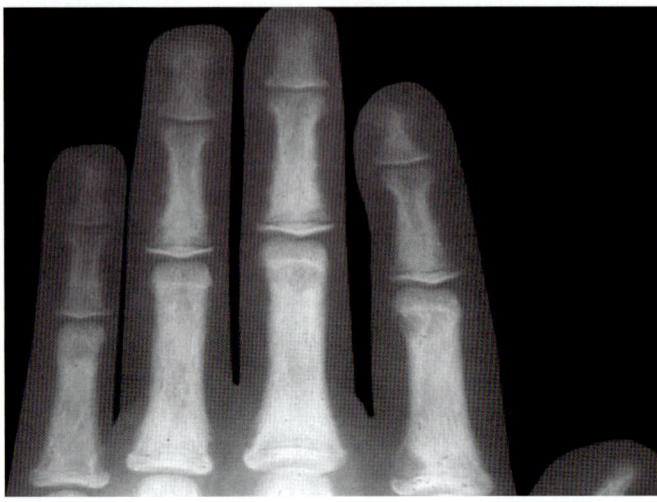

■ **FIGURE 76-3** Extensive phalangeal and tuftal cortical resorption of secondary hyperparathyroidism in a young patient with open growth plates. Presumed brown tumor at base of ulna aspect of proximal phalanx.

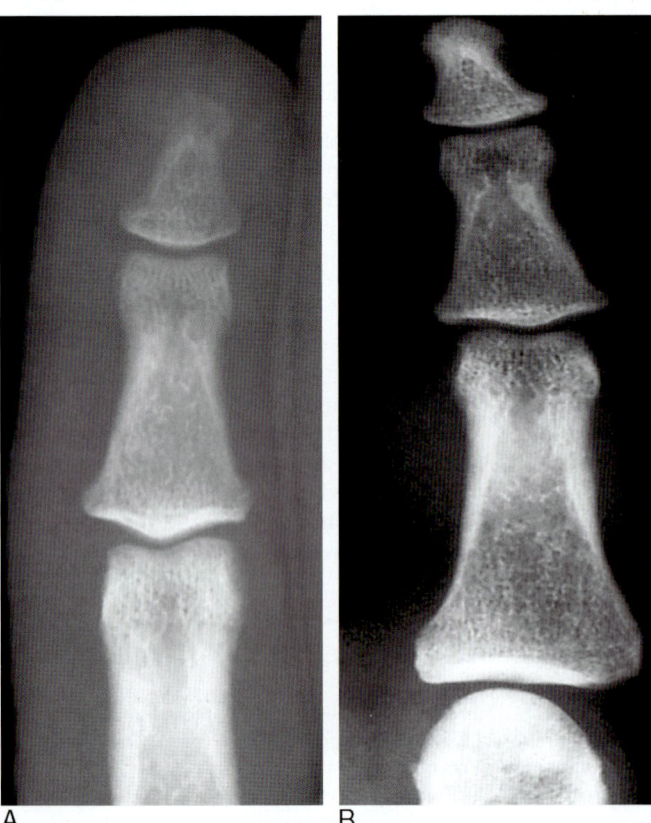

■ **FIGURE 76-4** **A,** Tuft resorption preceding midphalangeal changes in renal osteodystrophy. **B,** Reconstitution of tuft, reflecting improvement of renal osteodystrophy on medical management alone.

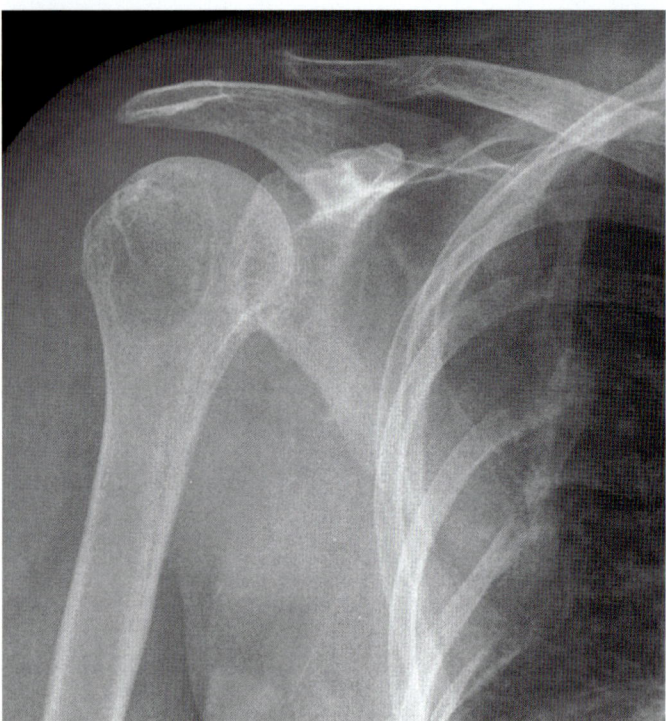

■ **FIGURE 76-5** Resorbed head of clavicle in poorly controlled patient with renal osteodystrophy. Note brown tumor and multiple rib fractures. As in Figure 76-4B, this will reconstitute after improved medical management or successful renal transplantation and does not represent irreversible destruction.

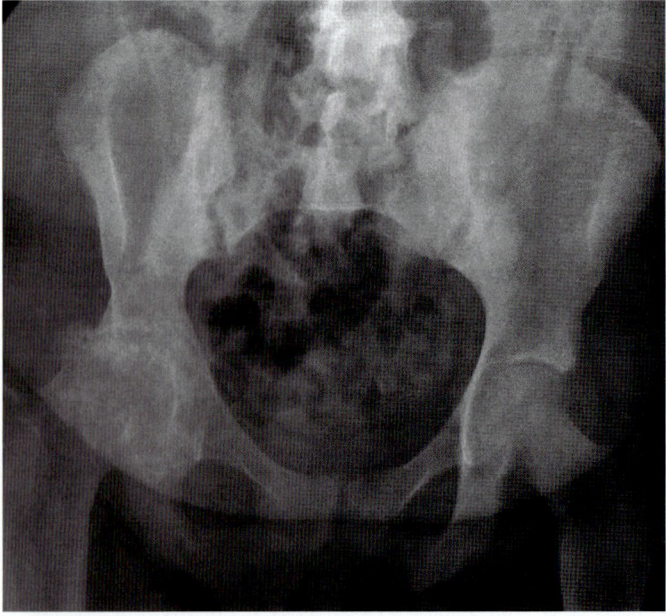

■ **FIGURE 76-6** Widened sacroiliac joints and sclerotic bones are characteristic of advanced renal osteodystrophy.

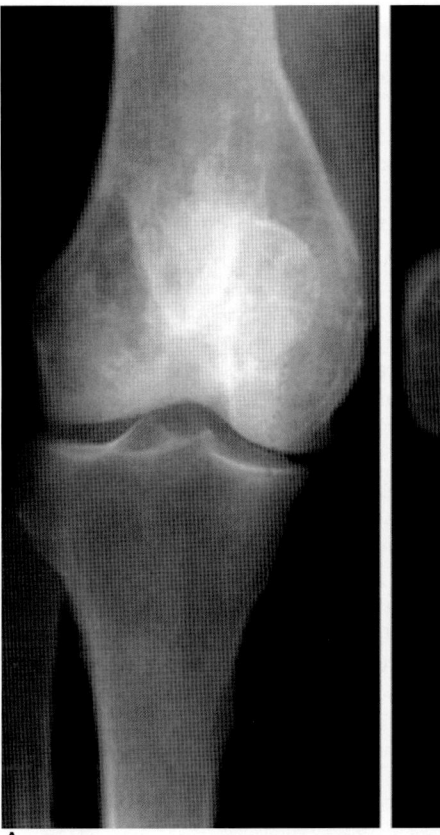
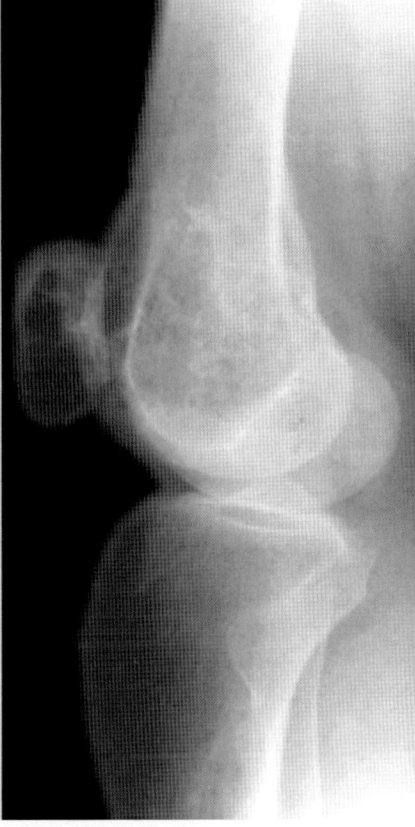
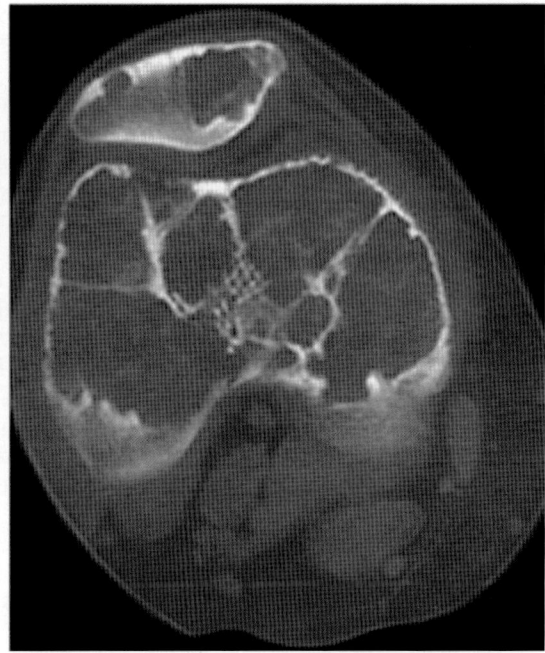

A

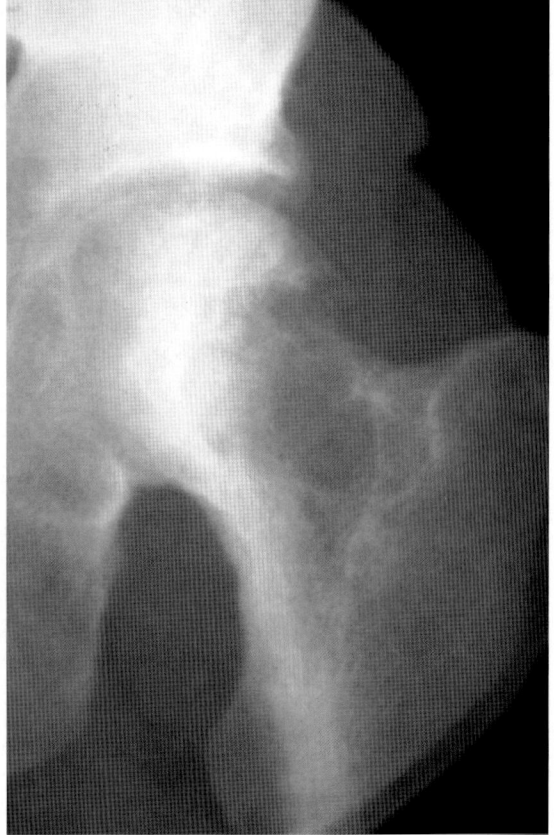

B

■ **FIGURE 76-7** **A,** Radiographs and CT scan of a 30-year-old patient show multilocular brown tumor in the femur and two discrete brown tumors in the patella, raising the differential diagnosis of multicentric giant cell tumor if unaware of the patient's medical background. **B,** Brown tumor in femoral neck. Osteolytic lesion in the femoral neck of a 50-year-old woman indistinguishable from a metastasis. Brown tumor or amyloidoma would reasonably only be considered if there was a known history of chronic renal failure.

periosteal surfaces, such as the proximal humeri or proximal femora. Periostitis may be an accompanying finding. Osteoclastomas or brown tumors occur in renal osteodystrophy (Fig. 76-7) and, in fact, will be encountered more frequently than in primary hyperparathyroidism because of the large numbers of patients with renal failure being kept alive by dialysis and the early diagnosis of primary hyperparathyroidism now routinely being made by serum biochemistry. In the presence of brown tumors there will almost always be phalangeal signs of hyperparathyroidism. Osteosclerosis, despite osteoclasis being the primary pathophysiologic action on the skeleton, may be encountered in renal osteodystrophy and is most commonly appreciated in vertebrae, pelvis ribs, and long bones. In vertebrae, sclerosis may affect the entire body but is frequently confined to the end plates, producing a characteristic appearance of alternating bands of different density that Dent called "the rugger jersey spine" (Fig. 76-8).[9]

Erosions in the peripheral and axial skeleton have been reported with incidences of approximately 30% and 25%, respectively.[10,11] These erosions are usually minor and progress slowly, but in some instances destruction especially in the axial skeleton could be extensive (Figs. 76-9 and 76-10).[11,12]

Soft Tissue Calcification

There are five main locations for soft tissue calcification: (1) ocular, (2) arterial, (3) cartilaginous, (4) periarticular or soft tissues, and (5) visceral. In some instances, the calcification may be massive, appearing tumor-like. When massive, there is little merit in referring to them as tumoral calcinosis (which is an entity in itself and a diagnosis of exclusion) but merely recognize them as a manifestation of poorly controlled renal osteodystrophy (Fig. 76-11). Surgery is not curative for massive calcification because it is a manifestation of the medical disease. The presence of calcification correlates with elevated levels of serum phosphorus. When the level of serum phosphorus is lowered, the calcium amount will decrease and could disappear.

In the United States, osteomalacia is usually a minor component of untreated renal osteodystrophy. The only reliable radiographic evidence for osteomalacia in patients with renal failure is the presence of Looser zones. Looser zones are wide, straight bands of radiolucency perpendicular to and abutting the bony cortex. They are usually symmetric and may have a narrow surrounding region of sclerosis.[13]

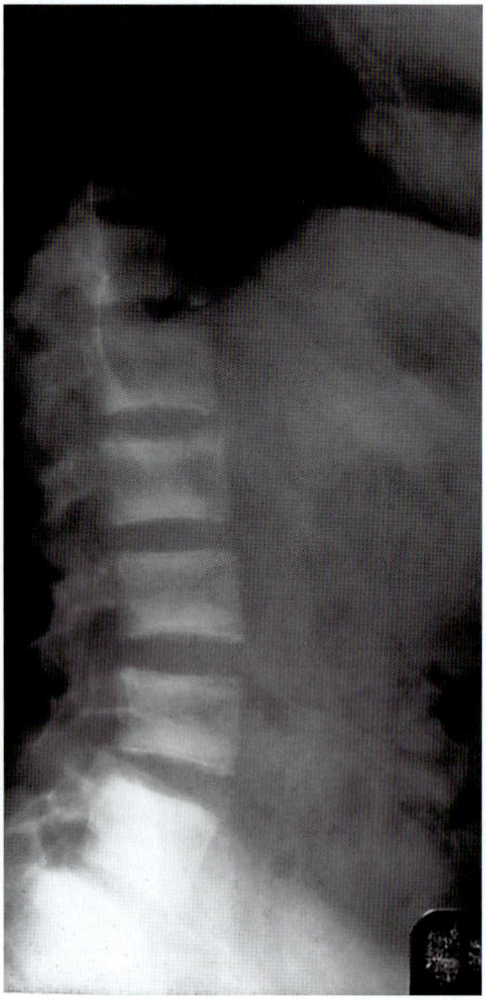

■ **FIGURE 76-8** Characteristic "rugger jersey" spine with sclerosis of the end plates and normal lucency in the midvertebral bodies.

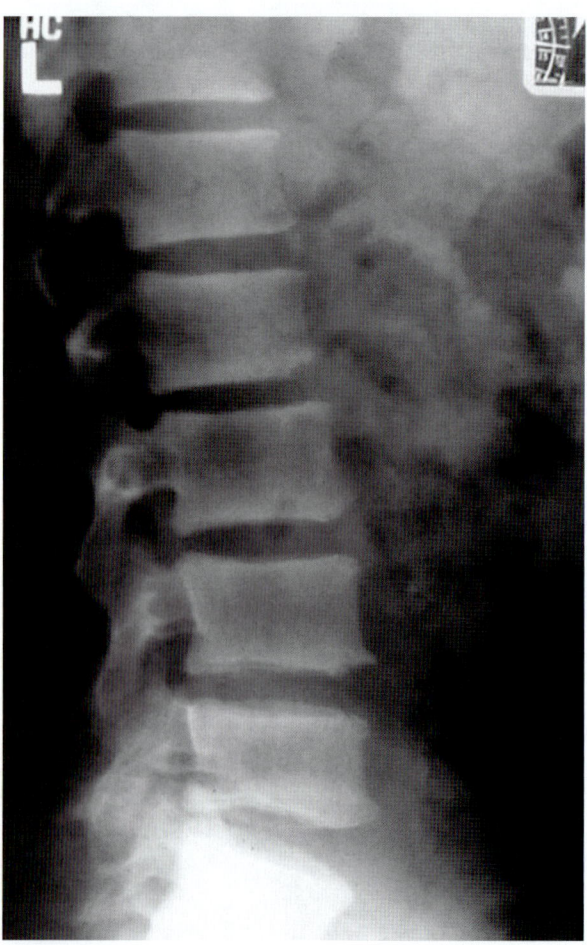

■ **FIGURE 76-9** Renal spondyloarthropathy. Associated with faint vertebral sclerosis are erosions at the anterior inferior corners of L2 to L4 reminiscent of the Romanus or discovertebral erosions of ankylosing spondylitis.

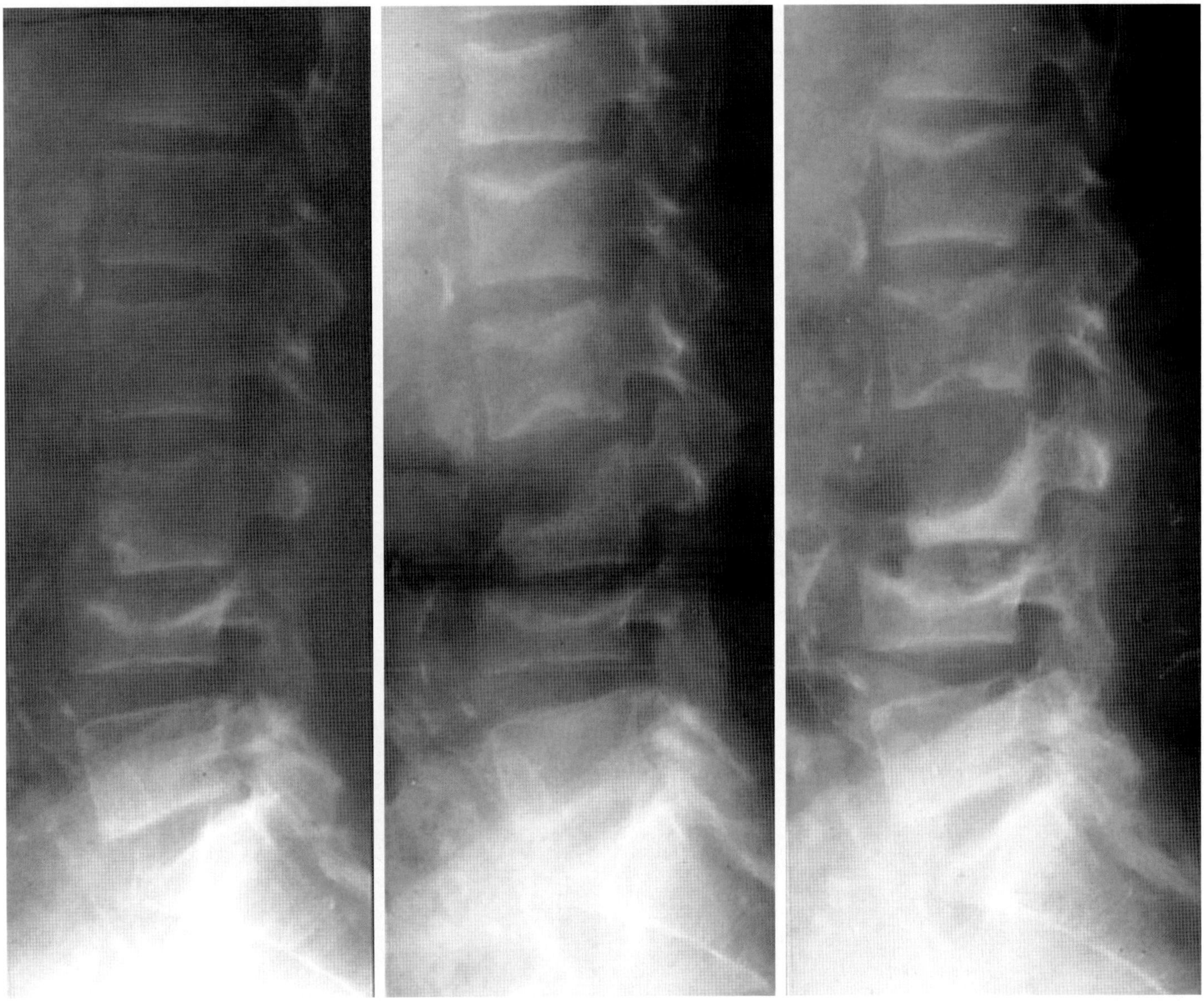

■ **FIGURE 76-10** Radiographs of spine of a female patient who was on dialysis for more than 12 years. Note the progressive dissolution of L3 over 12 months and end plate deformities of the other vertebrae. Deformed L4 was secondary to remote trauma. The patient declined any surgical intervention and died suddenly of other causes.

In Children

Osteosclerosis is a feature more frequently encountered in uremic children than in adults. Children usually have a lower incidence of soft tissue and arterial calcification. Rickets-like lesions are seen in renal osteodystrophy and, because of the similarity to nutritional rickets, have led to what many believe is the unfortunate term of "renal rickets" used to describe this appearance. The skeletal changes that are seen in patients with chronic renal failure are due to hyperparathyroidism rather than rickets (Fig. 76-12). This observation made almost 60 years ago holds true today.[14]

Osteoarticular Manifestations and Chronic Dialysis

A complication unknown to medicine before the introduction of dialysis was the development of a completely new condition, amyloidosis, occurring as a direct consequence of the use of dialysis. The problem of amyloid deposition in patients on long-term dialysis is unresolved and has been referred to as "the rise and rise" of dialysis amyloidosis.[15]

Amyloid deposition is a consequence of β_2-microglobulin, which is elevated 30 to 50 times normal in renal failure patients. The complications of amyloidosis tend to become evident about 8 years after the beginning of dialysis and are almost universal in patients who have been on dialysis for 15 years or longer. The most common symptomatic location for these deposits is the carpal tunnel. Because of the relative frequency of this association and a fairly straightforward clinical diagnosis of carpal tunnel disease, confirmatory imaging is rarely sought or required. Amyloid deposits have also been considered responsible for cystic lesions in bone and tendon thickening.

Spontaneous tendon ruptures have been a well-recognized complication of renal osteodystrophy since

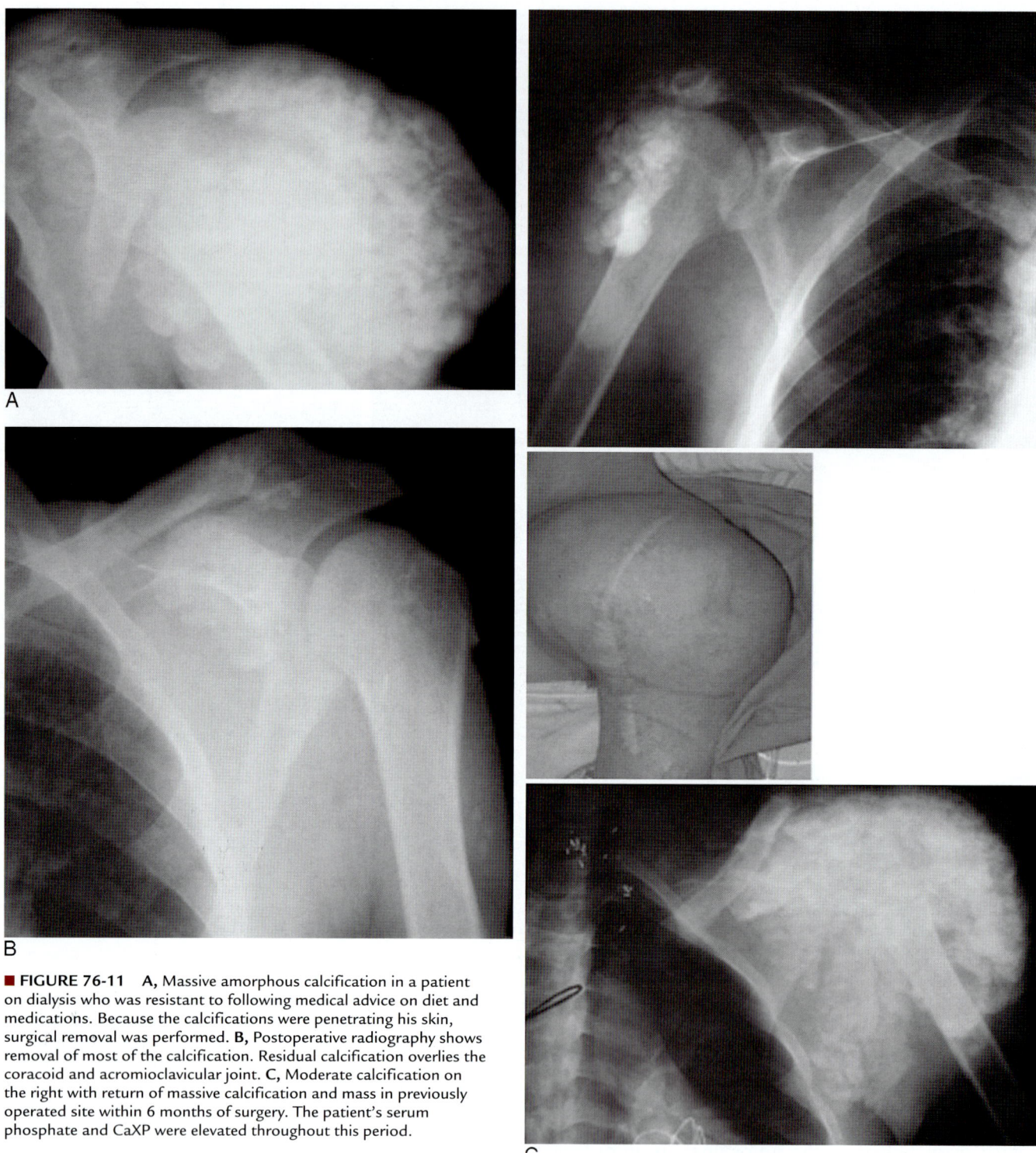

■ **FIGURE 76-11** **A,** Massive amorphous calcification in a patient on dialysis who was resistant to following medical advice on diet and medications. Because the calcifications were penetrating his skin, surgical removal was performed. **B,** Postoperative radiography shows removal of most of the calcification. Residual calcification overlies the coracoid and acromioclavicular joint. **C,** Moderate calcification on the right with return of massive calcification and mass in previously operated site within 6 months of surgery. The patient's serum phosphate and CaXP were elevated throughout this period.

the predialysis era and have been attributed to the sustained levels of elevated parahormone. Tendon ruptures are not considered a direct complication of amyloidosis. Amyloid deposits may be found in the synovium, and when large in bone they appear aggressive and osteolytic (Fig. 76-13). Aluminum toxicity is not discussed because this devastating disease has virtually disappeared since the recognition of its dual causes of aluminum contamination in the dialysate and excessive ingestion of phosphate binders.

Magnetic Resonance Imaging

Magnetic resonance imaging can be of help in suggesting the diagnosis of amyloidosis in patients on maintenance

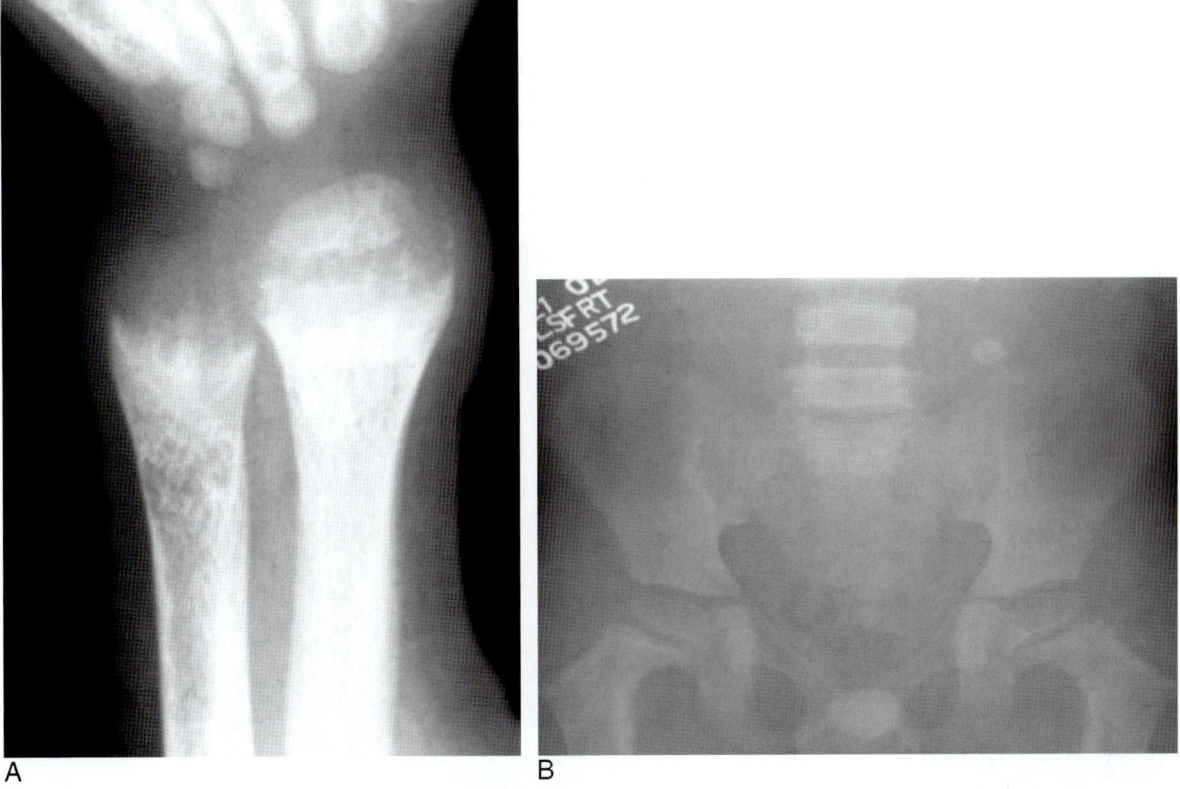

A   B

■ **FIGURE 76-12** **A,** Adolescent with renal osteodystrophy. Note dense bones and widened growth plates (radius) and metaphyseal cupping and fraying (ulna) with periostitis along with distal radius. The combination of sclerotic bones and a rickets-like appearance should primarily suggest renal osteodystrophy. **B,** Adolescent with renal osteodystrophy. Densely sclerotic lumbar vertebrae, widened sacroiliac joint spaces, and widened femoral growth plates are virtually diagnostic of renal osteodystrophy.

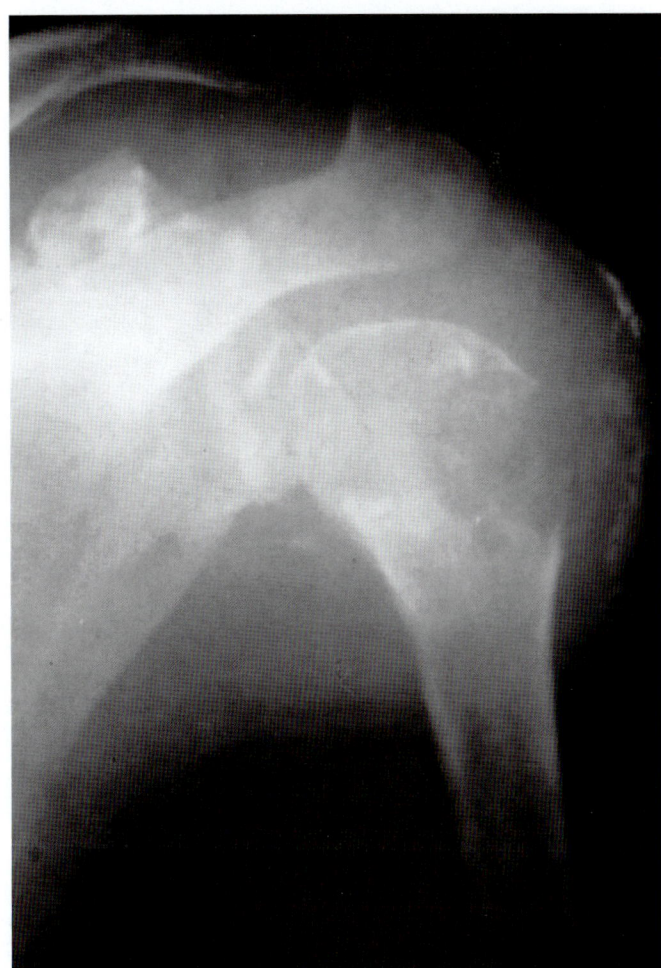

■ **FIGURE 76-13** Amyloidoma of the humerus. Destructive osteolytic lesion is indistinguishable from a malignant disease process. There is minimal soft tissue calcification and a large soft tissue mass.

hemodialysis when a destructive lesion of a vertebra is associated with a lesion that has low signal intensity on T2-weighted images (Fig. 76-14). The deposition of amyloid in synovial tissue is recognizable in patients with chronic renal failure because its low signal intensity on T2-weighted images would be indistinguishable from pigmented villonodular synovitis. Low signal intensity on T2-weighted images would in essence exclude discitis (Fig. 76-15).

Tendon ruptures, a complication of renal osteodystrophy, can readily be detected on MRI (Fig. 76-16).

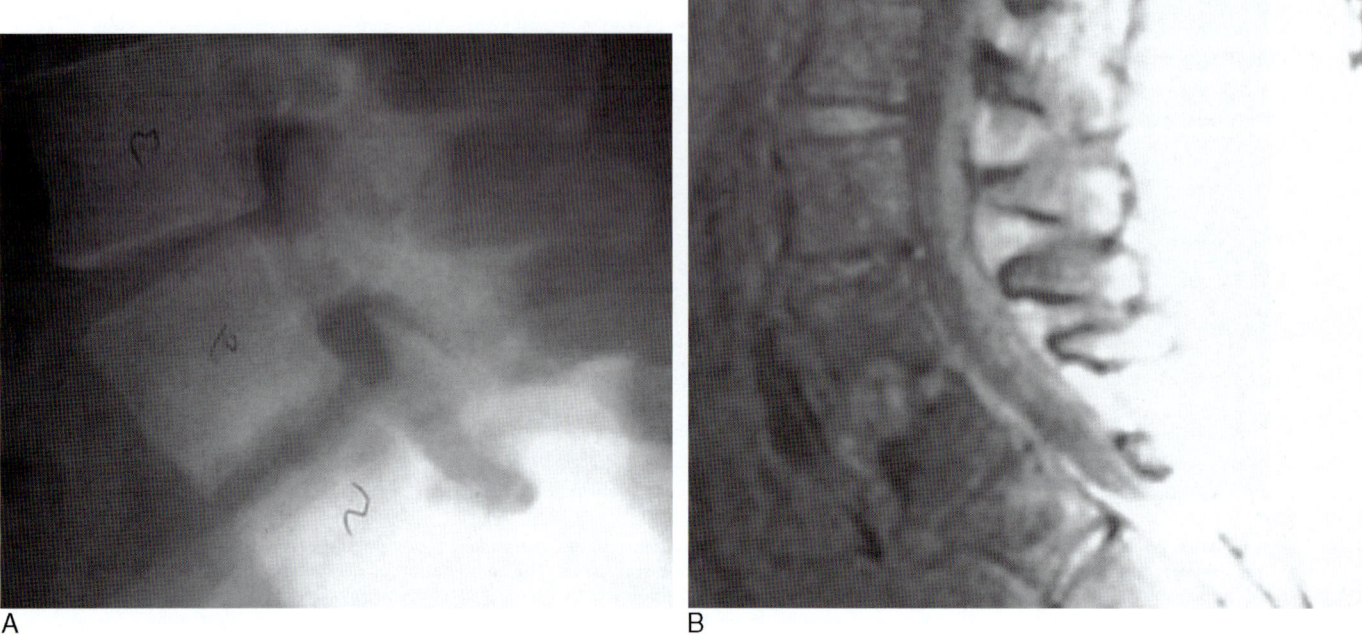

A   B

■ **FIGURE 76-14** On the radiograph there was concern for discitis at L4-L5 in this patient on long-term hemodialysis who presented to the emergency department with a fever and back pain. T2-weighted sagittal MR image shows low signal intensity at L4-L5. Resorptive changes are present at L3-L4 with intermediate signal. A biopsy was not performed, and an infected graft was later identified as the cause for fever and signs of infection.

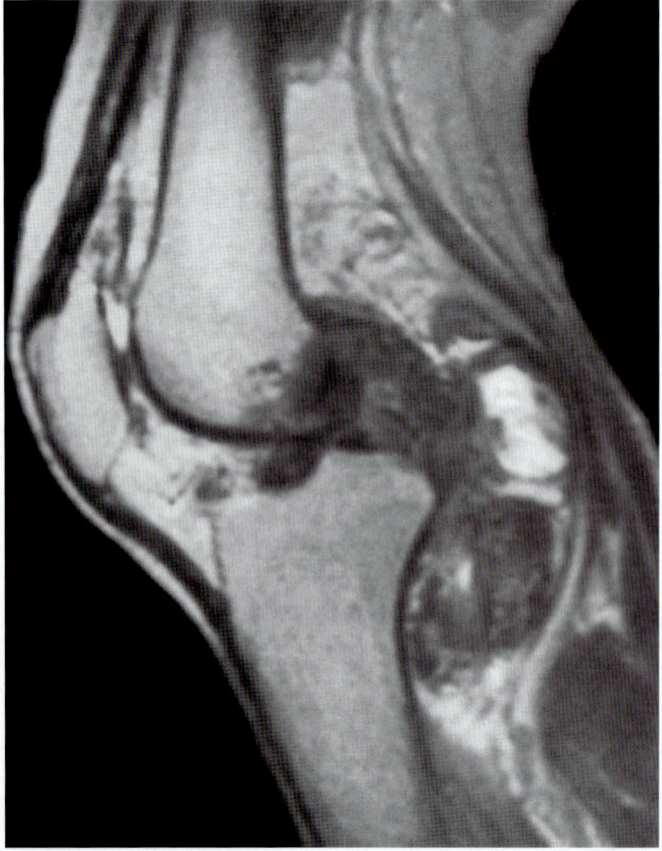

■ **FIGURE 76-15** Low signal intensity synovial-based mass (on T1- and T2-weighted images) would quite correctly suggest pigmented villonodular synovitis in everyday clinical practice. In patients on dialysis this appearance may be secondary to amyloid deposition.

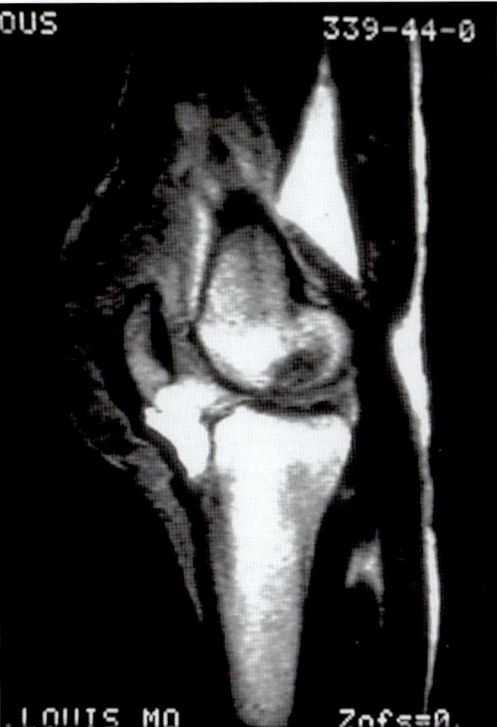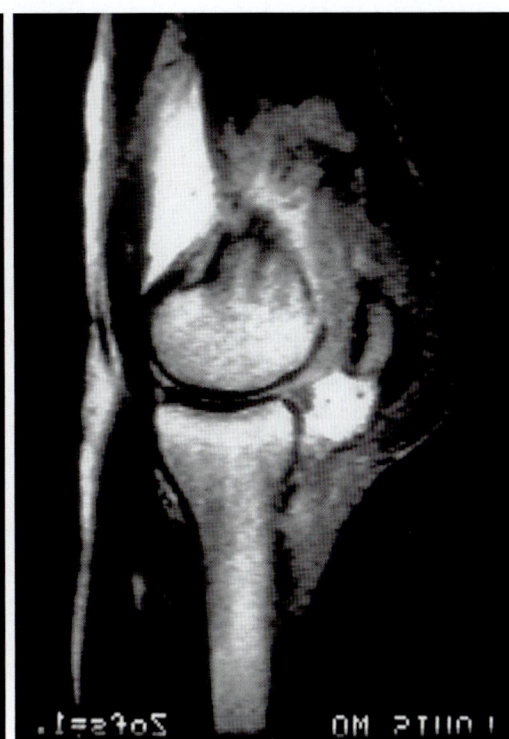

■ **FIGURE 76-16** Bilateral quadriceps tendon ruptures in a patient on long-term hemodialysis. This patient also had bilateral triceps tendon ruptures.

DIFFERENTIAL DIAGNOSIS

When radiographic abnormalities are identified in a patient known to be on maintenance hemodialysis, the appearances are usually not a diagnostic challenge. However, when the spectrum of abnormalities that encompass renal osteodystrophy are encountered without knowing the clinical background, the differential diagnosis would depend on the location of the abnormalities. Subperiosteal resorption of the radial aspects of the phalanges is virtually pathognomonic of hyperparathyroidism. However, selective loss of bone tufts of the phalanges could be seen in other entities such as scleroderma, systemic lupus, and thermal injury. Similarly, soft tissue calcification in the hands may be encountered in systemic lupus erythematosus and scleroderma. The presence of midphalangeal cortical resorption would separate renal osteodystrophy from the aforementioned conditions.

Diffusely dense bones in the pelvis and vertebral bodies would generate a differential diagnosis dependent on the patient's age. As a rule, in the United States, the prime differential diagnosis in a male patient younger than the age of 30 would be sickle cell disease. Other causes of dense bones such as myeloproliferative disease, osteopetrosis, or sclerosing dysplasias are rarer considerations. In a young female, disseminated sclerotic metastatic disease from breast carcinoma could have an appearance similar to that seen in renal osteodystrophy. Dense bones in men older than the age of 50 need to be distinguished from prostatic metastasis and, in women, from breast metastasis.

Sacroiliac resorption could mimic the seronegative spondyloarthropathies, which, however, are not associated with dense pelvis or vertebrae or resorptive changes in the femoral cortices.

SYNOPSIS OF TREATMENT OPTIONS

Medical Treatment

An appropriate diet should be maintained along with maintenance hemodialysis.

Surgical Treatment

With the exception of dense bones, most of the imaging findings of renal osteodystrophy are reversed by successful renal transplantation.

What the Referring Physician Needs to Know

- Soft tissue calcification deposition in renal osteodystrophy is not a surgical disease.
- Soft tissue calcification will disappear on medical treatment and dialysis if the serum phosphate level is successfully lowered.
- If the serum phosphate level remains elevated and calcific masses are surgically removed, they are almost certain to recur.
- Brown tumors and amyloid of bone can coexist and be indistinguishable on imaging.
- Destructive spondyloarthropathy with a short T2 on MRI favors amyloid deposition and would speak against an infection.

SUGGESTED READING

Sundaram M. Renal osteodystrophy. Skeletal Radiol 1989; 18:415–426.

REFERENCES

1. Lucas RC. A form of late rickets associated with albuminuria: Rickets of adolescents. Lancet 1883; 1:993.
2. Liu SH, Chu HI. Studies of calcium and phosphorous metabolism with special reference to pathogenesis and effects of dihydrotachysterol and iron. Medicine 1946; 22:103.
3. Parfitt AM. The actions of parathyroid hormone on bone: relation to bone remodeling and turnover, calcium homeostasis and metabolic bone disease. Metabolism 1976; 25:1157.
4. Cameron JS. Dialysis Today and Tomorrow: History of the Treatment of Renal Failure by Dialysis. Oxford, Oxford University Press, 2002, p 336.
5. Lingappa VR. Renal disease: chronic renal failure—pathophysiology of disease. In McPhee SJ, Lingappa VR, Ganong WF, Lange JD: Pathophysiology of Disease: An Introduction to Clinical Medicine, 3rd ed. New York, Lang, 2000, pp 394–398.
6. Sundaram M, Wolverson MK. The prevalence of skeletal surveys of patients in maintenance hemodialysis. Ann Intern Med 1982; 97:780.
7. Pugh D. Subperiosteal resorption of bone. AJR 1951; 66:577.
8. Sundaram M, Joyce PF, Shields JB, et al. Terminal phalangeal tufts: earliest site of renal osteodystrophy findings in hemodialysis patients. AJR Am J Roentgenol 1979; 133:25.
9. Dent CE. Clinical section. Proc R Soc Med 1955; 48:530.
10. Sundaram M, Wolverson MK, Heiberg EH, Grider RD. Erosive azotemic osteodystrophy. AJR Am J Roentgenol 1981; 1936:363.
11. Sundaram M, Seelig R, Pohl D. Vertebral erosions in patients undergoing maintenance hemodialysis for chronic renal failure. AJR Am J Roentgenol 1987; 149:323.
12. Kaplan P, Resnick D, Murphey M, et al. Destructive non-infectious spondyloarthropathy in hemodialysis patients: a report of four cases. Radiology 1987; 162:241.
13. Looser E. Late rachitis osteomalacia: clinical, roentgenologic and pathological-anatomic investigations. J Dtsch Xlschr Chir 1920; 152: 210.
14. Albright F, Reifenstein C. The Parathyroid Glands and Metabolic Bone Disease: Selected Studies. Baltimore, Williams & Wilkins, 1948, p 115.
15. Cameron JS. The Rise and Rise of Dialysis Amyloidosis: A History of the Treatment of Renal Failure by Dialysis. Oxford, Oxford University Press, 2002, p 263.

Rickets and Osteomalacia

The terms *rickets* and *osteomalacia* respectively refer to the same pathophysiologic processes manifesting in different age groups. The disease, before the closure of growth plates, is conventionally termed *rickets,* and when encountered after closure of the growth plates it is referred to as *osteomalacia*. Irrespective of the underlying disease that leads to rickets/osteomalacia, the radiographic signs are the same.[1,2] Therefore, the recognition of rickets or osteomalacia by the radiologist requires clinical and biochemical evaluation to determine the causative disease.

KEY POINTS

- Adults: Looser zones
- Children: widened growth plates, metaphyseal cupping and fraying

---

ETIOLOGY

The etiologic causes include malnourishment (vitamin D deficiency), genetic causes, inadequate sunshine, gastrointestinal malabsorption, liver disease, anticonvulsant therapy, renal glomerular and tubular diseases, and tumor-induced osteomalacia.

PREVALENCE AND EPIDEMIOLOGY

The epidemiology and prevalence is uncertain because the nutritional states and diseases that lead to rickets or osteomalacia are varied and multifactorial. In countries where the population is at risk from nutritional rickets the ready availability of sunlight would appear to protect from overt clinically apparent rickets. However, X-linked hypophosphatemia occurs in approximately 1 in 25,000 and is the most common form of genetically induced rickets.[3]

CLINICAL PRESENTATION

Common presenting symptoms are failure to thrive in children and dull, aching bone pain and generalized weakness in adults. Usually, however, the symptoms associated with the disease states leading to rickets/osteomalacia would represent the dominant clinical features at presentation.

PATHOPHYSIOLOGY

Although for some years it has been established that vitamin D is not a vitamin but acts more like a hormone, the term *vitamin* continues to be used because of the historical association of the term with its associated disease states. The physiologically active form of vitamin D is 1,25-dihydroxyvitamin D. The presence of this vitamin with normal calcium, phosphorus, pH, and alkaline phosphates is required for normal mineralization of bone matrix. Vitamin D_3 is produced by the interaction of ultraviolet B radiation from sunlight with the skin. Small amounts of vitamin D_3 will be obtained from dietary sources such as dairy products and fish liver oil. Vitamin D_2 is prepared artificially and found in food supplements. These prohormones need to be hydroxylated twice to reach its active state of 1,25-dihydroxyvitamin D_3. The first hydroxylation is in the liver and again in the mitochondria of the kidney, resulting in the biologically active form of vitamin D. The active form of vitamin D is required for calcium absorption in all segments of the small intestine. Because the liver, kidney, and intestines all play an important part in vitamin D metabolism, disease states affecting any of these organs can potentially lead to rickets or osteomalacia. Rickets and osteomalacia are generally associated with a low serum calcium level, which, in turn, results in secondary hyperparathyroidism, which is always present histologically but, rarely, radiographically, and accompanying brown tumors are rare.[4,5]

Not widely recognized is that a low phosphate level with a relatively normal calcium level can also result in rickets/osteomalacia. These findings are usually associated with renal tubular defects (de Toni-Fanconi syndrome, cystinosis, X-linked hypophosphatemia) or the condition of tumor-induced ostemalacia (oncogenic osteomalacia/rickets). Two of these conditions that will be discussed further are X-linked hypophosphatemia and tumor-induced osteomalacia.[6,7] In X-linked hypophosphatemia the syndrome is genetically transmitted as an X-linked dominant trait, and in tumor-induced osteomalacia the cause of phosphate loss is an occult tumor. In these patients 1,25-dihydroxyvitamin D may be undetectable to very low. Fifty percent of these tumors occur in bone, and 50% occur in soft tissues. Some of these lesions are reactive in origin, and few are malignant. Fibroblast growth factor-23 is elevated in these patients, and the tumor is believed to elaborate this product.[8] Removal of the tumor results in dramatic improvement in symptoms of weakness and reversal of biochemical abnormalities and disappearance of radiographic abnormalities if they were present in the first place.

IMAGING TECHNIQUES

The radiographic signs of rickets and osteomalacia are constant in their appearances irrespective of the cause. The identification of rickets or osteomalacia should be considered a manifestation of any one of several disease processes rather than being considered the manifestation of a single disease process.

The classic signs of rickets are a widened physeal growth plate and metaphyseal cupping and fraying best identified at rapidly growing ends of bones such as the wrists, knees, anterior ends of ribs, and proximal femoral growth plates (Fig. 76-17).[9,10] The only reliable sign for the diagnosis of osteomalacia is the presence of the Looser zone. A Looser

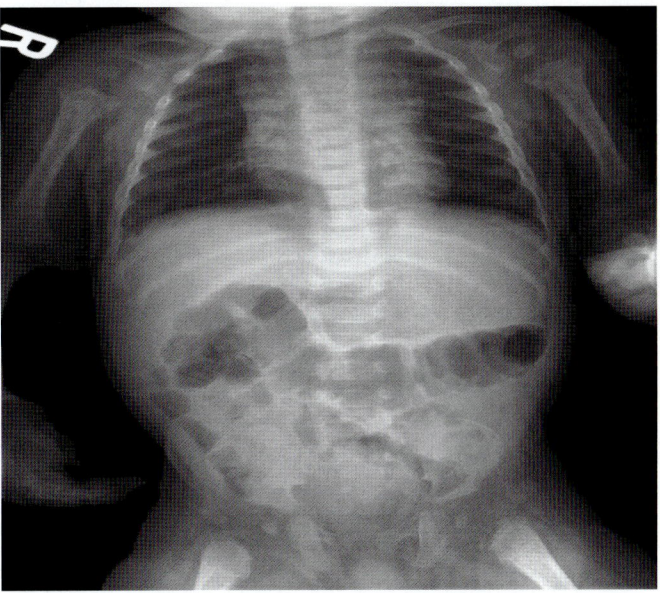

■ **FIGURE 76-17** Manifestations of rickets in the proximal humeri and femora with widened growth plates and splayed humeral metaphyses. This child from a recent immigrant family had been breast fed for about 2 years. Note the widened anterior ends of ribs, the so-called rachitic rosary.

zone is a radiolucency that runs perpendicular to the cortex of the bone and may have a sclerotic margin and be indistinguishable from the now frequently encountered stress fracture. The lucency in osteomalacia represents unmineralized osteoid (Fig. 76-18).

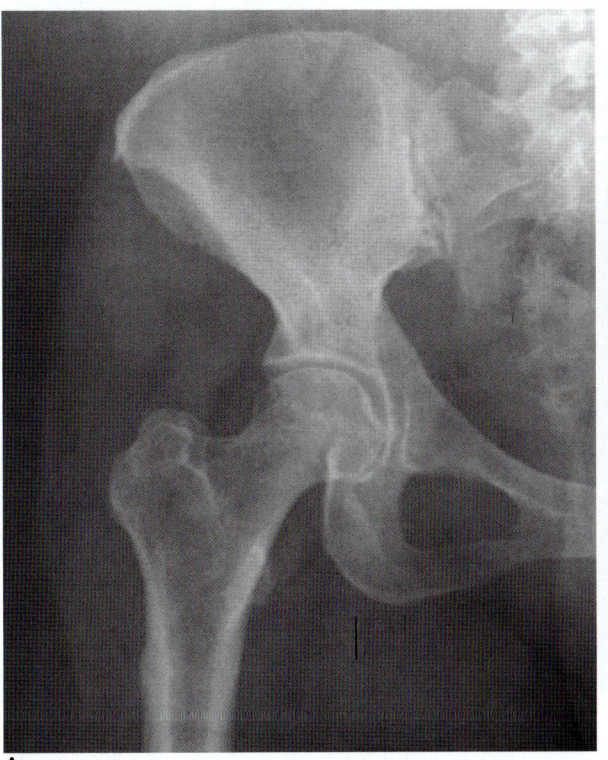
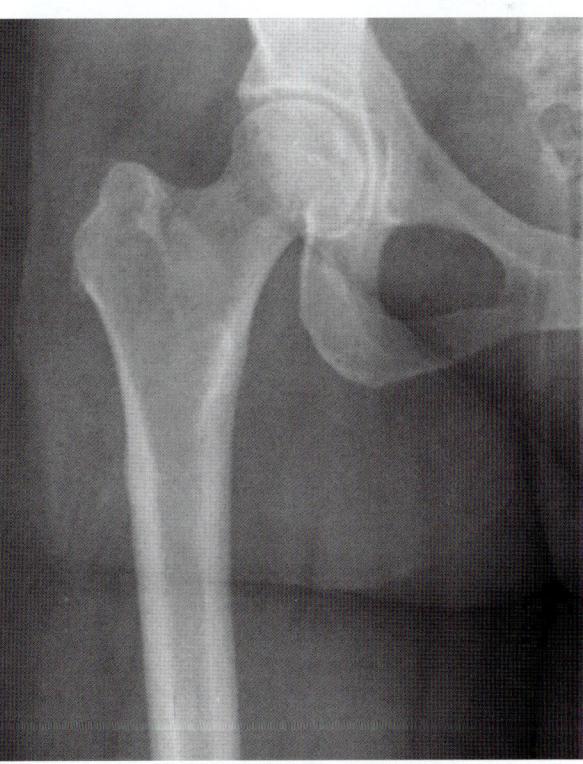

A   B

■ **FIGURE 76-18** **A,** Looser zone of osteomalacia in the outer aspect of the proximal femur. **B,** Healing of Looser zone after treatment.

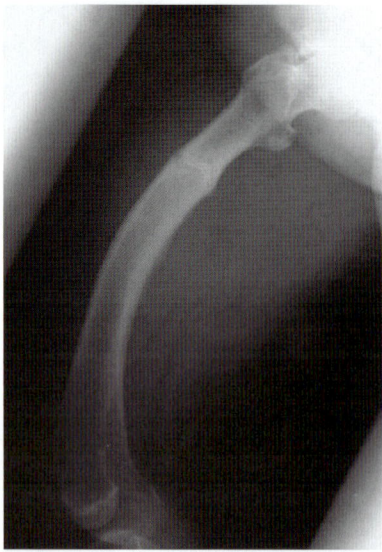

A

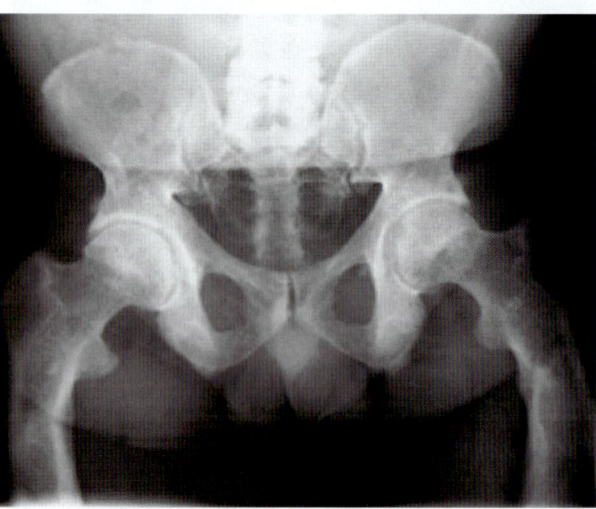

B

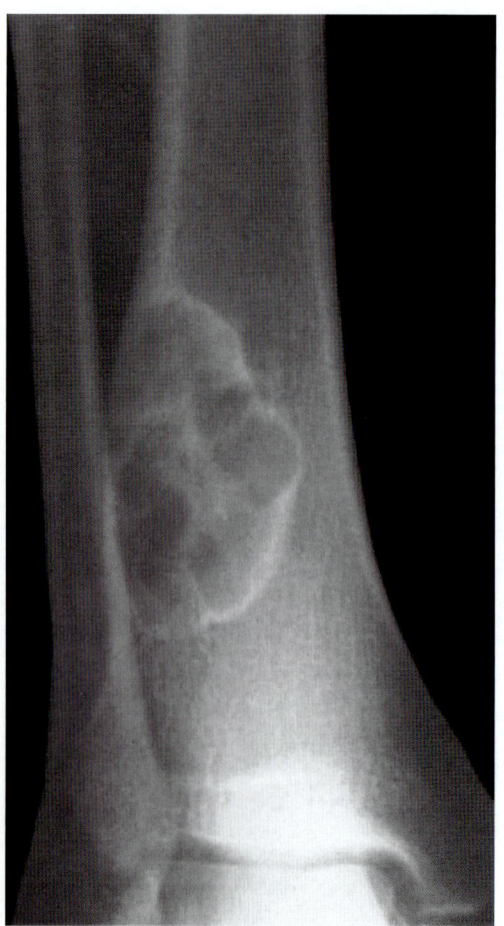

C

X-linked hypophosphatemic rickets/osteomalacia produces a somewhat paradoxical imaging appearance in that in this condition of abnormal bone mineralization, in addition to the well-established signs of rickets/osteomalacia the bones are dense and there may be extraskeletal ossification and even fusion of the entire spine (ankylosis) mimicking a seronegative spondylitis or fluorosis.[11] Intraspinal ossification may be encountered.[12] The long bones are often shorter than usual, widened, and bowed (Fig. 76-19).

In the condition of oncogenic osteomalacia no bone or soft tissue abnormality should be considered innocuous (Fig. 76-20). Many of these patients with a low serum phosphate tend to be evaluated by either whole-body MRI or radionuclide octreotide scanning. Sometimes, it is the patient who, in following the advice of the physician, discovers a tiny mass or lump in the performance of a routine whole-body self-examination.

DIFFERENTIAL DIAGNOSIS

For the classic signs of rickets/osteomalacia the cause needs to be determined. X-linked hypophosphatemia can mimic ankylosing spondylitis and fluorosis. However, the sacroiliac joints are not affected in X-linked hypophosphatemia.

■ **FIGURE 76-19** **A,** X-linked hypophosphatemic osteomalacia. Chronic Looser zone. Note the marked bowing of the femur due to chronic "soft" bone and reactive periostitis along the medial shaft. **B,** Small enthesophytes at both the lesser trochanters and left greater trochanter, bowed femora, and partially healed Looser zones. **C,** Patent sacroiliac joints, dense bones, and bowed femora in X-linked hypophosphatemic osteomalacia. *(Courtesy of Professor J. E. Adams, FRCR, Manchester University, England.)*

■ **FIGURE 76-20** After removal of this nonossifying fibroma the patient shown here with oncogenic rickets/osteomalacia was rapidly restored to a feeling of normal health. The serum phosphate level returned to normal levels in a few weeks.

Serum calcium, phosphorus, parathyroid hormone, and 1,25-dihydroxyvitamin D levels should be evaluated.

SYNOPSIS OF TREATMENT OPTIONS

The appropriate therapy depends on the cause. However, adequate nutrition and treatment of any significant underlying disease are imperative to avoid developing the sequelae of the disease.

What the Referring Physician Needs to Know

- In oncogenic osteomalacia no lesion of bone or soft tissue should be considered innocuous.
- A search for these lesions can be performed by whole-body MRI or radionuclide octreotide scanning.

SUGGESTED READINGS

Pitt MJ. Rickets and osteomalacia are still around. Radiol Clin North Am 1991; 29:97–118.

Sundaram M, McCarthy EF. Oncogenic osteomalacia. Skeletal Radiol 2000; 29:117–124.

Weissman Y, Hochberg Z. Genetic rickets and osteomalacia. Curr Ther Endocrinol 1994; 5:492–495.

REFERENCES

1. Harrison HE, Harrison HC. Rickets then and now. J Pediatr 1995; 87:1144.
2. Pitt MJ. Rickets and osteomalacia are still around. Radiol Clin North Am 1991, 29.97–118.
3. Weissman Y, Hochberg Z. Genetic rickets and osteomalacia. Curr Ther Endocrinol Metab 1994; 5:492–495.
4. Davies DR, Dent CE, Willcox A. Hyperparathyroidism and steatorrhoea. BMJ 1956; 2:1133–1137.
5. Bereket A, Casur Y, Driat P, Yordam N. Brown tumor as a complication of secondary hyperparathyroidism in severe long lasting vitamin D deficiency rickets. Eur J Paediatr 2000; 159:170–173.
6. Clarke BL, Wynne AG, Wilson D, Fitzpatrick LA. Osteomalacia associated with adult Fanconi's syndrome: clinical and diagnostic features. Clin Endocrinol 1995; 43:479–490.
7. Sundaram M, McCarthy EF. Oncogenic osteomalacia. Skeletal Radiol 2000; 29:117–124.
8. Wilkins GE, et al. Oncogenic osteomalacia: evidence for a humoral phosphatic factor. J Clin Endocrinol Metab 1995; 80:1628–1634.
9. Wharton B, Bishop N. Rickets. Lancet 2003; 362:1389–1400.
10. Oestevich AE, Ahmad BS. The periphysis and its effect on the metaphysic: II. Application to rickets and other abnormalities. Skeletal Radiol 2003; 22:115–119.
11. Polisson RP, et al. Calcification of entheses associated with X-linked hypophosphatemic osteomalacia. N Engl J Med 1985; 313:1–6.
12. Adams JE, Davies M. Intraspinal new bone formation and spinal cord compression in familial hypophosphatemic vitamin D resistant osteomalacia. Am J Med 1986; 61:1117–1129.

CHAPTER 77

Amyloidosis

Bryan T. Jennings, Michael S. Gibson, Mark D. Murphey, and Rogerich T. Paylor

ETIOLOGY

Amyloidosis is not a single disease but a heterogeneous group of diseases characterized by abnormal extracellular deposition of insoluble proteins in bone and soft tissue. The word *amyloid* means "starch" in Greek and was first used to describe this condition by Virchow in 1854.[1] Previously, amyloid was categorized as primary or secondary. These categories were further divided into systemic or localized forms. This classification became cumbersome with the progressive description of many types of amyloidosis. To date, 21 types of amyloidosis each with distinct precursor proteins have been identified. Differences in presentation reflect the targeted organ or organs of the produced amyloid protein. The World Health Organization (WHO) classifies amyloid on the basis of its precursor fibril protein. The initial letter of the WHO classification is A (for amyloid) followed by the initial for the specific precursor protein fibril.[2,3] WHO nomenclature has been suggested to replace the previous categorization of systemic amyloidosis as primary (WHO AL amyloidosis), secondary (WHO AA amyloidosis), familial and senile (WHO ATTR amyloidosis), dialysis-related (WHO ABeta2M amyloidosis), and so on.[3] Identifying the type of amyloidosis is critical because of the vastly different treatments and prognoses. Musculoskeletal manifestations of amyloidosis are common and are the focus of this chapter.

PREVALENCE AND EPIDEMIOLOGY

The epidemiology of amyloidosis is confounded by underdiagnosis in the community setting and by the selection bias inherent in studies performed at tertiary referral centers. It is estimated that AL amyloidosis has an incidence of 8 per million people per year and that it affects 10% to 15% of patients with multiple myeloma.[4] Referral centers have estimated cases of ATTR amyloidosis as representing 10% to 20% of the number of AL amyloidosis cases per year.[5] ABeta2M amyloidosis is estimated to occur in up to 80% of patients on dialysis for 10 years or more.[6,7] AA amyloidosis is present in 5% to 25% of patients with rheumatoid arthritis.[7]

CLINICAL PRESENTATION

Clinical presentations of amyloidosis have a moderate degree of overlap between subtypes. Clinical distinctions may be difficult and often rely on biopsy for confirmation and subtyping. Characterization of the subtype is important because treatment and prognosis vary dramatically. Amyloid arthropathy is present most commonly in AL amyloidosis and ABeta2 amyloidosis, and the musculoskeletal findings of these two subtypes are identical.[6]

AA amyloidosis can present at any age as a result of an acute-phase protein released in response to inflammation. Any long-standing inflammatory process could potentially result in AA amyloidosis, although it is present in less than 1% of patients with chronic inflammatory conditions.[6] A common association is with rheumatoid arthritis in which between 5% to 25% of patients may be affected, and 75% of patients with AA amyloidosis have rheumatoid arthritis.[6,7] AA amyloidosis usually occurs at least 2 years after the onset of rheumatoid arthritis.[7] Amyloid arthropathy is rare in AA amyloidosis, in which many of the articular abnormalities are due to the underlying rheumatoid arthritis.[6] Other associations with AA amyloidosis include inflammatory bowel disease and familial Mediterranean fever.[5] Renal dysfunction (which ranges from proteinuria to renal failure and is present in 90% of affected patients), hepatomegaly, autonomic neuropathy, and cardiomyopathy are less frequent manifestations.[8] The median survival in patients with AA amyloidosis is 4.5 years.[9]

AL amyloidosis is rare before the age of 40 and thereafter demonstrates increasing incidence with age.[10] It is often related to a plasma cell dyscrasia, and 30% of these patients eventually progress to multiple myeloma. AL amyloidosis occurs in 10% to 15% of patients with multiple myeloma.[9] The prognosis of systemic AL amyloidosis with or without myeloma is worse than that of myeloma alone, with a median survival time of 13.2 months after diagnosis.[8,11] AL amyloidosis may present initially as a solitary plasmacytoma, but typically it progresses to systemic disease over time.[12] The typical delay in progression ranges from 3 months to 9 years.[12] Clinical manifestations depend on the degree of the individual organ affected but include nephrotic syndrome, rapid and progressive congestive heart failure, sensory and autonomic nervous system involvement, hepatomegaly, macroglossia, and endocrine system involvement (e.g., hypoadrenalism and hypothyroidism).[5,8] Progressive renal failure is rare.[5] Although amyloid arthropathy is a rare manifestation involving only 3% of patients with AL amyloidosis, carpal tunnel syndrome is present in 10% to 30% of patients.[7,13]

ATTR amyloidosis is caused by mutations in the protein transthyretin. The inheritance pattern is autosomal dominant. Patients with this form of amyloidosis present with clinical manifestations that overlap with those of AL amyloidosis. However, unlike in AL amyloidosis, heart failure is uncommon and macroglossia is not present.[5,8] Median survival time is 10 to 15 years.[8]

ABeta2 amyloidosis is associated with long-term dialysis. Previous studies report development of amyloidosis in up to 80% of patients on dialysis for longer than 5 to 10 years. However, this figure is likely decreasing with newer dialysis filters.[14] Unlike the other systemic amyloidoses, visceral organ involvement occurs less frequently and late in the disease. Juxta-articular, articular, and intraosseous deposition of amyloid is common, with shoulders, knees, hips, wrists, and spine frequently affected.[14,15] Destructive spondyloarthropathy, carpal tunnel syndrome, and osseous and synovial involvement are common.[14]

PATHOPHYSIOLOGY

Amyloid fibrils have a three-dimensional structure known as the beta-pleated sheet regardless of their precursor protein. This structure accounts for their resistance to proteolysis and their apple-green birefringence under polarized light when stained with Congo red. At gross pathologic evaluation amyloid appears as a mass with a pink-yellow or white-yellow waxy surface. Amorphic eosinophilic material is demonstrated on microscopic examination. Histiocytes and multinucleated giant cells surround the amyloid deposits, which may be seen to thicken the interspersed vessel walls.[16]

MANIFESTATIONS OF THE DISEASE

Musculoskeletal manifestations of amyloidosis include carpal tunnel syndrome, neuropathic appearance, intraosseous and/or articular deposition, and destructive spondyloarthropathy. Frequently affected sites are the shoulder, hip, spine, and wrist. Sequelae may include pathologic fracture, joint destruction, joint contractures, or carpal tunnel syndrome.[5,8,14] Of note, carpal tunnel syndrome in amyloidosis has no sex predilection and no preference for the dominant hand (as seen with the idiopathic disease). Spinal involvement, in which the thoracic spine is the most common location, may demonstrate osteopenia with pathologic fracture.[7]

Radiography

Radiographs are often the initial imaging modality in amyloidosis. One classic clinical presentation is a juxta-articular mass that involves the shoulder girdle resulting in disproportionate prominence of the musculature in an elderly patient. Some authors have described this appearance as the "shoulder pad sign" because its appearance mimics the shoulder pad worn by American football players.[7,9] Other radiographic signs include osseous erosions, joint destruction, or dislocation and pathologic fractures, especially of the hip or spine. Well-defined lytic lesions may be present within cortical bone or the intramedullary canal and may occasionally be expansile.[17] These lytic lesions commonly affect the acetabulum, proximal femur, humerus, or carpal bones (Figs. 77-1 and 77-2). The appearance in the carpus may simulate subchondral cysts, and these findings have traditionally been referred to as dialysis cysts.[6] Fine sclerotic margins are characteristic.[9] Spinal involvement (destructive spondyloarthropathy) is usually centered at the disc space and mimics infectious spondylodiscitis on radiography. The disc space narrowing and end-plate destruction can be rapid and occur at multiple levels. Calcifications have been reported but are very uncommon and are almost always associated with multiple myeloma (AL amyloidosis). Occasionally, calcified lesions may mimic chondrosarcoma or osteosarcoma on radiographs.[17]

Magnetic Resonance Imaging

Magnetic resonance imaging is well suited for evaluating the extent and distribution of amyloidosis because it can simultaneously access the bones, joints, and soft tissue structures.[14] A common clinical presentation is diffuse synovial thickening around the joint. Amyloid-affected tissue is similar to or slightly lower in signal intensity than muscle on T1-weighted MR images.[7,15] T2-weighted MR images demonstrate low to intermediate signal intensity within the amyloid deposition, although high signal intensity may be present if there is a focal fluid collection (Fig. 77-3). This MR appearance helps differentiate amyloid from other articular processes and spinal processes (e.g., infectious spondylodiscitis), which typically have increased signal intensity on T2-weighted images (Fig. 77-4). This low signal intensity may be related to the fibrillar, collagen-like composition of amyloid and when present can obviate the need for biopsy. Bursitis may result from amyloid deposition in the bursa surrounding the shoulder or hips. Contrast agent administration results in mild to moderate diffuse enhancement.[7,15]

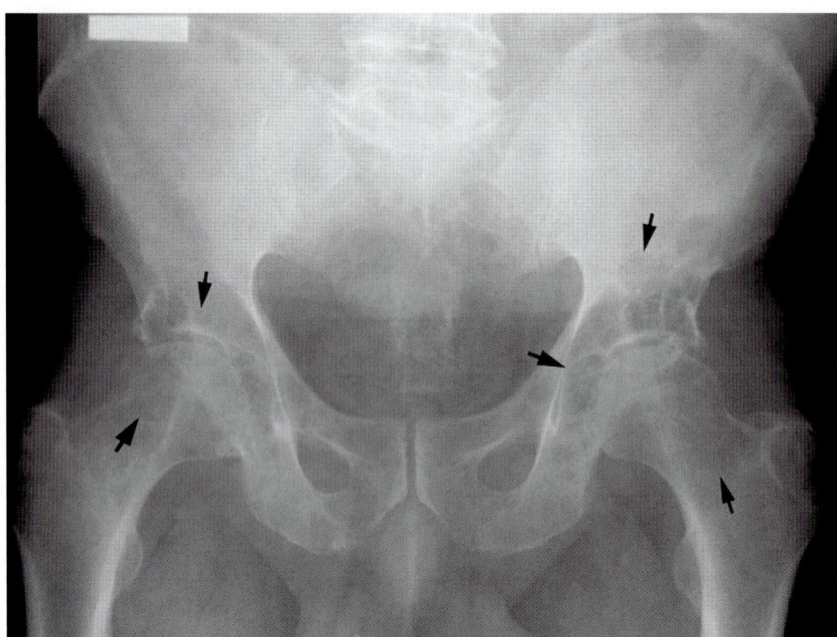

■ **FIGURE 77-1** Anteroposterior view of the pelvis demonstrates multiple lytic lesions on both sides of the joint space affecting the hips bilaterally (*arrows*).

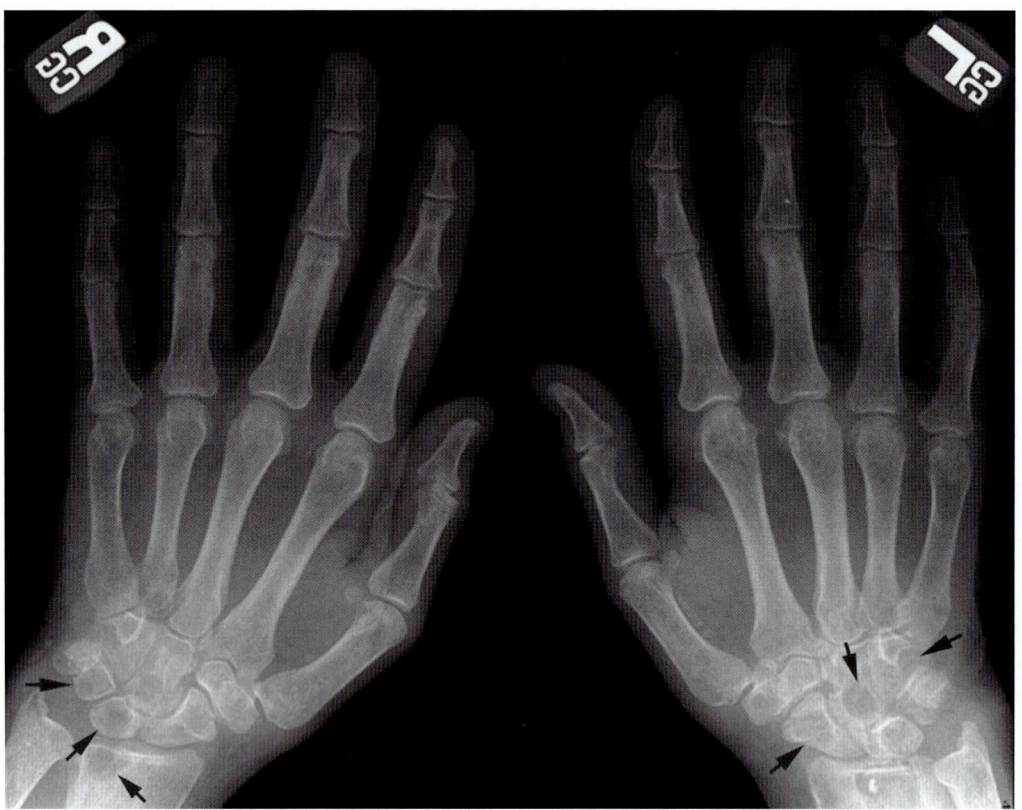

■ **FIGURE 77-2** Anteroposterior radiographs of the hands demonstrate multiple lytic lesions involving the carpal bones bilaterally (*arrows*). Relative preservation of bone mineralization and lack of distal erosions help to differentiate this pattern from inflammatory arthropathies, although the appearance can simulate gout.

Multidetector Computed Tomography

On CT, amyloid demonstrates diffuse joint thickening as a result of synovial amyloid deposition. Osseous erosions may be extrinsic or eccentric with a "punched out" appearance (Fig. 77-5). Soft tissue deposits are typically isodense to muscle and exhibit mild diffuse enhancement.[15]

Ultrasonography

The typical ultrasound appearance is that of hyperechoic material (amyloid deposition) in and around the joints.[15,18,19] Factors evaluated in patients with an appropriate clinical presentation and history, such as long-term dialysis with shoulder symptoms, sensitivities of 72% to

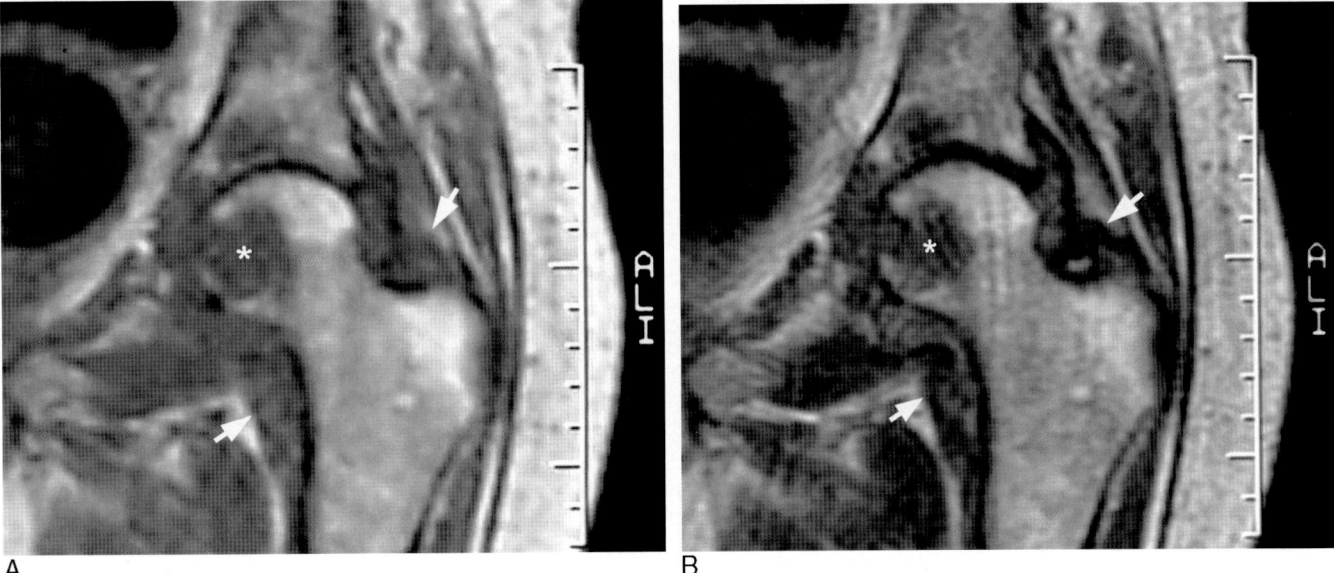

A   B

■ **FIGURE 77-3** T1-weighted (**A**) and T2-weighted (**B**) coronal MR images of the left hip demonstrate amyloid deposits filling the joint space (*arrows*) and eroding the left femoral head and acetabulum. Note that the deposits remain low on both sequences (*asterisks*).

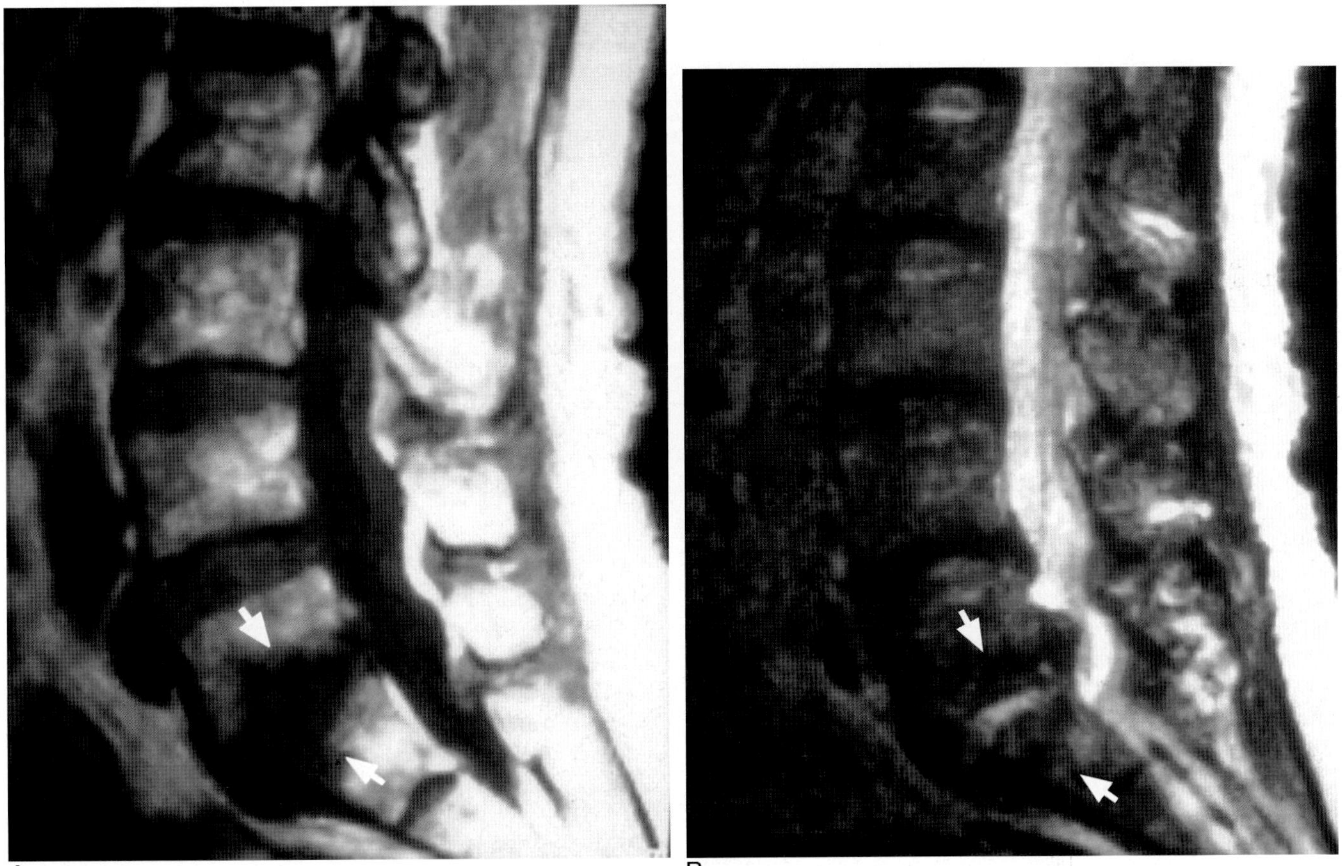

A   B

■ **FIGURE 77-4** T1-weighted (**A**) and T2-weighted fat-saturated (**B**) MR images of the lumbar spine in a long-term dialysis patient demonstrate a lesion centered at the L5/S1 disc space that is predominantly low in signal intensity on both sequences. This appearance is typical of amyloid deposition and helps to differentiate amyloidosis from infectious spondylodiscitis.

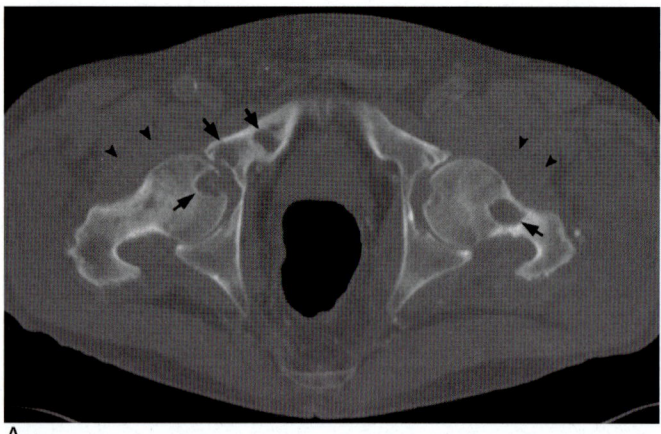
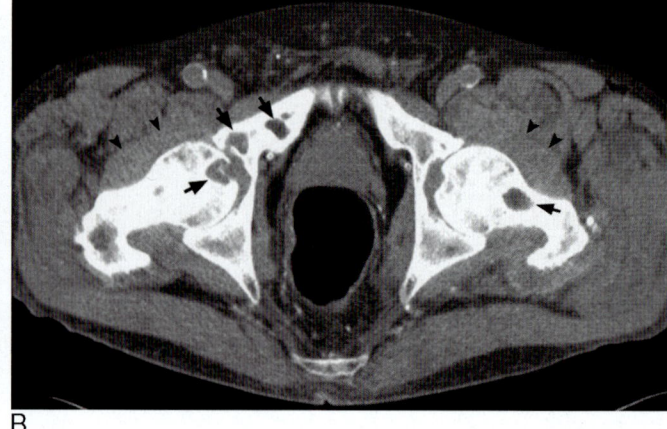

■ **FIGURE 77-5** **A** and **B,** Noncontrast CT images of the hips demonstrate multiple punched-out lesions with a thin sclerotic rim on both sides of the joint (*arrows*). Soft tissue density is present within the joint space representing synovial deposition (*arrowheads*) and within the punched-out lesions.

79% and specificities of 79% to 100% for identification of amyloid involvement that have been reported, included presence of an echogenic pad overlying the rotator cuff, biceps tendon thickening (4 mm), supraspinatous thickening (8 mm), and/or a rotator cuff tear. Tenosynovitis can result in similar abnormalities, limiting both the sensitivity and specificity of these measurements in painful shoulders.[15,18]

Nuclear Medicine

Uptake within amyloid deposits on bone scintigraphy using technetium-99m–labeled methylene diphosphonate is variable, and thus this technique's utility is limited. However, antibody studies using iodine-123–labeled serum amyloid P can show the extent of disease. The serum amyloid P binds to amyloid independently of its precursor protein, thus accumulating in amyloid-laden tissues. However, this is used more often as a quantitative method to follow efficacy of treatment.[8]

DIFFERENTIAL DIAGNOSIS

The differential diagnosis includes pigmented villonodular synovitis, gout, and rheumatoid arthritis. Noncalcified synovial chondromatosis may mimic amyloid on radiography. Unlike amyloidosis, however, synovial chondromatosis has increased signal intensity on T2-weighted MR images. Pigmented villonodular synovitis appears similar to amyloidosis on CT and MRI. However, it is typically monarticular, whereas amyloidosis is almost invariably polyarticular. Amyloid arthropathy and rheumatoid arthritis may both involve the wrist, but osteopenia, commonly seen in rheumatoid arthritis, is not a typical feature of amyloidosis.[6] Gout may be very difficult to differentiate because both diseases may occur in dialysis patients and appear as intermediate to low signal intensity on T2-weighted images. The distribution of the processes may aid in the radiographic distinction. Both gout and amyloidosis may affect large joints and the carpal bones. However, gout often involves the more distal joints of the hands and feet. Also, rheumatoid arthritis tends to have

increased signal intensity on T2-weighted MR images and involves other joints (e.g., metacarpophalangeal joints) in the hand. Appropriate clinical workup and biopsy may be needed to confirm the diagnosis.

SYNOPSIS OF TREATMENT OPTIONS

Treatment options depend on the type of amyloidosis. The basic approach relies on the tenet that if the synthesis of the amyloid precursor protein can be disrupted then the affected organs can reabsorb accumulated deposits and organ function can be restored. However, if the deposits are sufficiently advanced the underlying organ dysfunction may be irreversible.

Autologous stem cell bone marrow transplant after chemotherapy with melphalan in high doses is the preferred treatment for AL amyloidosis in appropriate candidates.[4] Clinical control of the underlying inflammatory process is the preferred treatment for AA amyloidosis. Liver transplantation is used to treat ATTR amyloidosis because it is the predominant site of transthyretin (TTR) production.[5] Treatment of ABeta2M amyloidosis has focused on improved hemofiltration, high-flux dialysis methods, and renal transplantation.[15]

What the Referring Physician Needs to Know

- *Amyloidosis* is a broad term used to describe a group of diseases whose prognosis and treatments can be quite variable.
- Amyloid should be considered in the differential diagnosis of multiple lytic lesions on both sides of the joint and in all lesions that are low in signal intensity on both T1-weighted and T2-weighted MR images.
- Biopsy plays an important role in the confirmation of amyloidosis and identification of the subtype in those amyloidoses in which clinical presentation may overlap.

ACKNOWLEDGMENT

The views expressed in this chapter are those of the authors and do not necessarily reflect the official policy or position of the Department of the Navy, Department of Defense, or the U.S. Government.

SUGGESTED READINGS

Falk RH, Comenzo RL, Skinner M. The systemic amyloidoses. N Engl J Med 1997; 337:898–909.

Hazenberg BP, van Gameren I, Bijzet J, et al. Diagnostic and therapeutic approach of systemic amyloidosis. Neth J Med 2004; 62:121–128.

Kiss E, Keusch G, Zanetti M, et al. Dialysis related amyloidosis revisited. AJR Am J Roentgenol 2005; 185:1460–1467.

Sheldon PJ, Forrester DM. Imaging of amyloid arthropathy. Semin Musculoskelet Radiol 2003; 7:195–203.

REFERENCES

1. Virchow VR. Ueber einem Gehirn and Rueckenmark des Menschen. Virchows Arch 1854; 6:135–138.
2. WHOIUIS Nomenclature Sub-Committee. Nomenclature of amyloid and amyloidosis. Bull WHO 1993; 71:105–112.
3. Westermark P, Benson MD, Buxbaum JN, et al. Amyloid fibril protein nomenclature—2002. Amyloid J Protein Folding Disord 2002; 9:197–200.
4. Gertz MA, Merlini G, Treon SP. Amyloidosis and Waldenström's macroglobulinemia. Hematology Am Soc Hematol Educ Program 2004; 257–282. Review.
5. Falk RH, Comenzo RL, Skinner M. The systemic amyloidoses. N Engl J Med 1997; 337:898–909.
6. Sheldon PJ, Forrester DM. Imaging of amyloid arthropathy. Semin Musculoskeletal Radiol 2003; 7:195–203.
7. Resnick D. Diagnosis of Bone and Joint Disorders, 4th ed. Philadelphia, WB Saunders, 2002, pp 2087–2111.
8. Hazenberg BP, van Gameren I, Bijzet J, et al. Diagnostic and therapeutic approach of systemic amyloidosis. Neth J Med 2004; 62:121–128.
9. Georgiades CS, Neyman EG, Barish MA, et al. Amyloidosis: Review and CT manifestations. RadioGraphics 2004; 24:405–416.
10. Kyle RA, Linos A, Beard CM, et al. Incidence and natural history of primary systemic amyloidosis in Olmsted County, Minnesota, 1950 through 1989. Blood 1992; 79:1817–1822.
11. Comenzo RL, Gertz MA. Autologous stem cell transplantation for primary systemic amyloidosis. Blood 2002; 99:4276–4282.
12. Flores M, Nadarajan P, Mangham D. Soft-tissue amyloidoma: A case report. J Bone Joint Surg Br 1998; 80:654–656.
13. Skinner M, Anderson JJ, Simms R, et al. Treatment of 100 patients with primary amyloidosis: A randomized trial of melphalan, prednisone, and colchicine versus colchicine only. Am J Med 1996; 100:290–298.
14. Cobby M, et al. Dialysis-related amyloid arthropathy: MR findings in four patients. AJR Am J Roentgenol 1991; 157.
15. Kiss E, Keusch G, Zanetti M, et al. Dialysis-related amyloidosis revisited. AJR Am J Roentgenol 2005; 185:1460–1467.
16. Enzinger FM, Weiss SW: Soft Tissue Tumors, 4th ed. St. Louis, Mosby, 2001.
17. Remus WR, Kyriakos M, Gilula LA, et al. Plasma cell tumors with calcified amyloid deposition mistaken for chondrosarcoma. Radiology 1993; 189:505–509.
18. Sommer R, Valen GJ, Ori Y, et al. Sonographic features of dialysis-related amyloidosis of the shoulder. J Ultrasound Med 2000; 19:765–770.
19. Cloft HJ, Quint DJ, Markert JM, et al. Primary osseous amyloidoma causing spinal cord compression. AJNR Am J Neuroradiol 1995; 16:1152–1154.

CHAPTER 78

Pituitary and Thyroid Disorders

Calvin Ma, Paul Marten, and Rodrigo Dominguez

Acromegaly and Pituitary Gigantism

ETIOLOGY

Acromegaly and pituitary gigantism are conditions resulting from hypersecretion of growth hormone (GH) from the pituitary gland. The onset of GH hypersecretion in adults after the growth plates have fused results in acromegaly. The onset of GH hypersecretion in children and adolescents before fusion of the growth plates results in pituitary gigantism.

The most common cause of GH hypersecretion is a benign pituitary tumor composed of somatotrophs (GH-secreting cells) or mammosomatotrophs (GH-secreting and prolactin-secreting cells). Most are confined to the anterior pituitary gland. Other less common causes include diffuse pituitary hyperplasia, pituitary somatotroph carcinoma, a hypothalamic tumor secreting growth hormone-releasing hormone (GHRH), a nonendocrine tumor secreting GHRH, and ectopic secretion of GH by a nonendocrine tumor.[1]

PREVALENCE AND EPIDEMIOLOGY

Acromegaly has an incidence of 3 to 4 cases per million people per year and a prevalence of 50 to 70 cases per million population.[1] Pituitary gigantism is extremely rare, with approximately 100 reported cases to date. There is no known gender or racial predilection.

CLINICAL PRESENTATION

Acromegaly typically has its onset in the third or fourth decade of life and is insidious, resulting in a delay in diagnosis by an average of 12 years. The mean age at diagnosis is 40 to 45 years.[1] In contrast, pituitary gigantism may occur at any age before epiphyseal fusion. Symptoms of GH hypersecretion have been observed as early as 6 months of life. Pituitary gigantism typically has dramatic linear growth acceleration that prompts early investigation and diagnosis.

Acromegaly and pituitary gigantism share many similar clinical manifestations because of the universal effect of

---

KEY POINTS

- Onset of GH hypersecretion in children or adolescents before the growth plates have fused results in pituitary gigantism. Onset of GH hypersecretion in adults after epiphyseal fusion results in acromegaly.
- In pituitary gigantism, skeletal growth is usually proportional. In acromegaly, skeletal growth is mainly in bone width.
- The most common etiology of GH hypersecretion is a pituitary adenoma.
- Clinical presentations include coarse facial features, macroglossia, prognathic mandible, enlarged hands and feet, hyperhidrosis, organomegaly, arthritis, back pain and spinal stenosis, obstructive sleep apnea, cardiovascular diseases, other pituitary endocrine dysfunctions, fatigue, and lethargy. In addition, pituitary gigantism is characterized by tall stature.
- Radiographic findings include enlarged pituitary gland on MRI, prognathic mandible, hyperostosis of calvaria, enlarged distal phalangeal tufts, widened joint spaces, soft tissue hypertrophy, thickened heel pad, widened atlantoaxial and intervertebral disk spaces, increased anteroposterior and transverse diameter of vertebral bodies, and scalloped posterior vertebral bodies.
- Diagnostic workup includes measuring IGF-1 level (highly sensitive), followed by GH level after a glucose load (highly specific). Laboratory confirmation should be followed with MRI of sella turcica to detect for pituitary tumors and if MRI is negative, CT of the body should be done to evaluate for ectopic GH/GHRH secretions by tumors.

growth hormones. The main difference in their clinical features is a growth in bone width seen in the acromegaly and a longitudinal or proportional bone growth seen in the pituitary gigantism. Patients with pituitary gigantism may eventually develop many of the clinical manifestations of acromegaly (Table 78-1) if they live long enough and are not adequately treated.

The characteristic features of acromegaly, many of which may also be seen in pituitary gigantism, include enlarged and protruded mandible; poor dental closure with separation of the teeth; coarse facial features with prominent forehead, supraorbital ridge, and zygomatic arch; and enlarged hands and feet.

Patients develop thickened skin and skin tags as a result of soft tissue hypertrophy. They often experience hyperhidrosis, which makes them malodorous. Hypertrophy of the tongue, pharynx, and larynx may result in macroglossia, deepened voice, and obstructive sleep apnea. Hypertrophy of muscles and connective tissues in the extremities may cause nerve compression and result in peripheral neuropathy such as carpal tunnel syndrome.

The visceral organs are enlarged, including the liver, spleen, pancreas, kidneys, heart, and thyroid. There is also increased incidence of benign tumors such as uterine myomas, prostatic hypertrophy, and colon polyps.

Cardiovascular diseases are common. The cardiac abnormalities include hypertension, left ventricular hypertrophy, cardiomyopathy, heart failure, and valvular heart disease.

Cartilage and synovial hypertrophy eventually lead to arthropathy commonly affecting the large joints such as the hips, knees, and shoulders, as well as more peripheral joints such as the elbows, wrists, and ankles.

Back pain is a common complaint due to degenerative disc disease in the lower back and painful kyphosis in the thoracic spine. Spinal cord compression from soft tissue and osseous hypertrophy in the spinal column resulting in spinal stenosis are present in some patients.

Headaches and visual changes are common symptoms resulting from local mass effect of the tumor.

The pituitary adenoma can also diminish secretion of other pituitary hormones, most commonly gonadotropins. Women may experience menstrual dysfunction such as amenorrhea or oligomenorrhea, vaginal atrophy, and hot flashes. Men may experience erectile dysfunction, testicular atrophy, and diminished libido. Both sexes may show decreased bone mineral density secondary to a hypogonadal state. Fatigue and lethargy are common complaints. They probably result from sleep apnea, cardiovascular dysfunction, hyperglycemia, hypogonadism, or other associated clinical conditions of GH hypersecretion.

Although typically occurring as an isolated disorder, gigantism may occasionally present as a feature of other conditions, such as McCune-Albright syndrome, multiple endocrine neoplasia type 1, neurofibromatosis, tuberous sclerosis, or Carney complex.

PATHOPHYSIOLOGY

Anatomy

The pituitary gland (hypophysis) lies in the sella turcica and is suspended from the hypothalamus by the infundibular stalk. It is regulated by the hypothalamus and is divided into two sections. The posterior section is the neurohypophysis, which is an extension of the hypothalamus and releases vasopressin and oxytocin into the blood. The anterior section is the adenohypophysis, which is a pharyngeal derivative that secretes six trophic hormones, including GH, lactogenic hormone, adrenocorticotropic hormone, thyroid-stimulating hormone, follicle-stimulating hormone, and luteinizing hormone.

Pathology

Secretion of GH from the anterior pituitary somatotrophs is usually controlled by GHRH synthesized in the hypothalamus and transported via the pituitary stalk to the somatotrophs in the anterior pituitary gland. Once released into circulation, GH stimulates the liver to produce insulin-like growth factor 1 (IGF-1). IGF-1 is the primary mediator of many of the growth-promoting effects of GH and is therefore responsible for most of the clinical manifestations of acromegaly and gigantism.[1]

In the immature skeleton, in which the growth plates are still open, GH hypersecretion stimulates endochondral bone formation at the physeal growth plates, leading to excessive bone growth in both length and width and thus resulting in the very tall but normally proportioned person seen in gigantism.

Once the physeal growth plates have fused, GH hypersecretion reactivates endochondral bone formation at various cartilage-bone junctions and stimulates periosteal bone formation, leading to mainly growth in bone width. The osseous as well as soft tissue hypertrophy, particularly in the acral parts of the body such as the hands, feet, and mandible, results in the characteristic appearance of acromegaly.

Stimulation of endochondral bone formation in acromegaly at various cartilage-bone junctions results in deposition of new cartilage on preexisting cartilage and enlargement of the joint. Excessive GH stimulates articular chondrocyte proliferation and increased matrix production, leading to thickening of the articular cartilage and widening of the joint spaces. The growth hormone also stimulates hypertrophy of periarticular tissues, resulting in

TABLE 78-1	Clinical Presentation of Acromegaly

Coarse facial features with enlarged, protruded mandible and prominent supraorbital ridges
Poor dental closure with wide separation of teeth
Macroglossia
Deepened voice
Obstructive sleep apnea
Thickened skin and skin tags
Enlarged hands and feet
Hyperhidrosis
Organomegaly
Peripheral neuropathy
Arthropathy
Back pain, kyphosis, degenerative back disease
Hypertension, cardiomyopathy, and heart failure
Headaches and visual changes
Fatigue and lethargy
Menstrual dysfunction, vaginal atrophy, and hot flashes in women
Erectile dysfunction, testicular atrophy, and diminished libido in men

ligamentous laxity and joint instability. Eventually, these processes lead to wear and fissuring of the cartilage. The repair mechanisms are impaired, owing to excessive GH, and consequently allow overproliferation of regenerating fibrocartilages, which may subsequently become calcified and result in osteophyte formation. Eventual destruction and thinning of the articular cartilage lead to joint space narrowing.

Stimulation of periosteal bone formation results in many characteristic findings of acromegaly. In the skull, periosteal bone deposition leads to thickening of the calvaria, enlargement and forward protrusion of the mandible, prominence of the supraorbital ridges and facial bones, and deepening of the alveolar sockets of the teeth with separation of the teeth. In the long bones, subperiosteal and subligamentous bone formation result in thickening and irregularity of the cortex, prominence of the bony tuberosities, and osteophytosis. One characteristic finding is enlargement of the distal phalangeal tufts. In the vertebral column, there is increase in anteroposterior and transverse diameters of the vertebral bodies without proportional increase in height, giving the vertebral bodies a short appearance. There is associated increase in the size of the intervertebral disc, which is produced by marginal subperiosteal formation of cartilage. Osteophytes of the spine may be extensive.

Stimulation of soft tissue hypertrophy by excessive GH leads to thickening of the skin, enlargement of the hands and feet, organomegaly, muscular hypertrophy, and other connective tissue overgrowth that contribute to many of the clinical manifestations of acromegaly and pituitary gigantism.

IMAGING TECHNIQUES

Techniques and Relevant Aspects

Radiographs and MRI are the most commonly used imaging modalities in the evaluation and workup of acromegaly and pituitary gigantism. Radiographs can demonstrate characteristic features that are often sufficient to suggest the diagnosis and prompt further evaluation.

After confirmation of GH hypersecretion by laboratory studies, MRI of the sella turcica is often used to detect for pituitary adenoma because it is the most common etiology. If MRI is contraindicated, CT of the sella turcica is performed.

If MRI or CT findings of the sella turcica are negative, CT of the chest, abdomen, and pelvis is useful in the evaluation for rare ectopic secretion of GH/GHRH by tumors in the lung, pancreas, adrenal, or ovaries.

Ultrasonography is occasionally used instead of radiography to observe for response to treatments. Colao and colleagues reported the use of ultrasonography in evaluating soft tissue thickness and joint space widening for reversibility in response to treatment.[2]

Pros and Cons

Magnetic resonance imaging has several advantages over CT, including the ability to display pathologic lesions in three orthogonal planes without loss of information and the ability to demonstrate the relationship of the pituitary lesions to the optic chiasm and cavernous sinuses. MRI provides more detailed information of the surrounding structures that may be affected by the GH- or GHRH-secreting tumors.

CT has the advantage of providing better visualization of the bony septa in the sphenoidal sinus, which may be important if a transsphenoidal surgical approach is being considered.

MANIFESTATIONS OF THE DISEASE

Radiography

Soft Tissue

Skin thickening may be observed as a result of collagen tissue response to excessive growth hormone. Many articles have documented the utility of measuring heel pad thickness as a diagnostic aid for acromegaly.[3-5] The shortest distance between the calcaneus and the plantar skin surface is usually measured. Although there are variations in heel pad thickness related to body weight, gender, and race, values greater than 25 mm in men and 23 mm in women are highly suggestive of the disease in the absence of other local causes of skin thickening, such as infection, injury, or edema.

Muscular and connective tissue hypertrophy in the extremities may cause peripheral neuropathy due to nerve compression, and this can be seen on MRI as edema around the nerve along with soft tissue hypertrophy.

Skull

The calvaria is usually thickened, but uncommonly it can be thinned. The sella turcica may be enlarged or destroyed. The paranasal sinuses are prominent, and there is increased pneumatization of mastoid air cells. The supraorbital ridges and zygomatic arches are prominent as well. There is enlargement of the mandible and widening of the mandibular angle, resulting in forward protrusion of the mandible, giving the "lantern jaw" appearance. Consequently, there is poor dental closure and inability to properly incise food. Anterior tilting of the teeth and interdental separation may be observed, as well as hypercementosis of the teeth and macroglossia (Fig. 78-1).

Hand

The hand contains many diagnostic clues in a patient with acromegaly. Some characteristic findings include enlarged distal phalangeal tufts, widened articular spaces of the metacarpophalangeal joints, squared phalanges and metacarpal bones, thickened soft tissues of the fingers, enlarged sesamoid bone, beak-like osteophytosis at the metacarpal heads, and bone formation at insertion sites of tendons and ligaments. A distal phalangeal tuft width of more than 12 mm in men and over 10 mm in women is virtually diagnostic of acromegaly.[6] A metacarpophalangeal joint space width of more than 2.5 mm in both men and women is suggestive of acromegaly. A soft tissue thickness measured at the proximal midphalanges

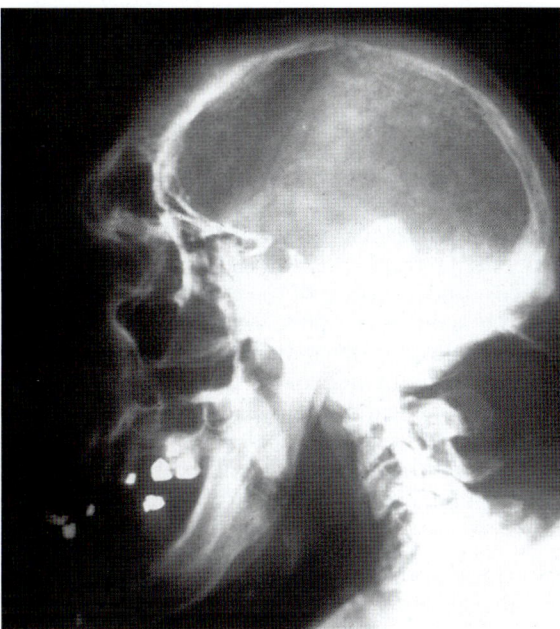

■ FIGURE 78-1 Skull radiograph of a patient with acromegaly. The mandible is elongated and protruded with an associated wide mandibular angle. The paranasal sinuses are prominent. Hypercementosis of the teeth with interdental separation can be seen. *(Courtesy of Javier Beltran, MD.)*

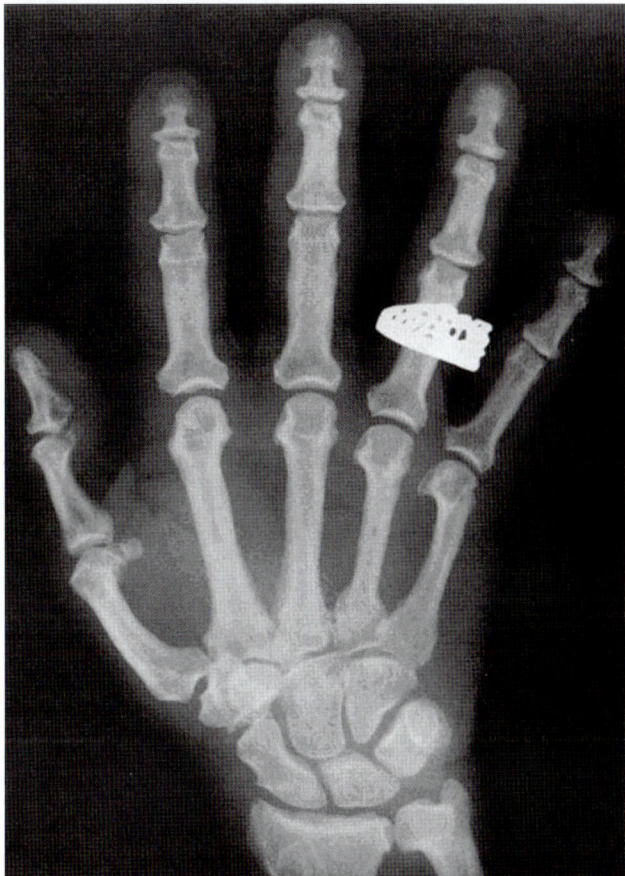

■ FIGURE 78-2 Hand radiograph in a patient with acromegaly. Note the enlarged distal phalangeal tufts, squared proximal phalanges, beak-like osteophytosis at the metacarpal heads, widened metacarpophalangeal joint spaces, and thickened soft tissues. *(From Littlejohn GO, Urowitz MB, et al. Radiographic features of the hand in diffuse idiopathic skeletal hyperostosis [DISH]: comparison with normal subjects and acromegalic patients. Radiology 1981; 140:626, with permission.)*

of more than 27 mm in men and 26 mm in women is also suggestive of acromegaly (Fig. 78-2).[7,8]

Some studies have been done using the sesamoid index as a diagnostic aid for acromegaly.[6,9] To determine the sesamoid index, the medial sesamoid of the first metacarpophalangeal joint is measured on a nonmagnified radiograph with a 36-inch focus-film distance. The greatest diameter of this sesamoid bone in millimeters is multiplied by the greatest diameter of the same sesamoid image perpendicular to the first measurement. The reliability of this sesamoid index approach has been challenged owing to variations in measurement in normal men and women, but generally values greater than 40 in men and 32 in women are suggestive of acromegaly.[6,9] The sesamoid index from normal men and women is generally around 20, with a range from 12 to 29.[9] Acromegaly is less likely, with values less than 30, but cannot be excluded. In addition to increased size of sesamoid bones, an increased number of sesamoids may also be seen.

Foot

Radiographic findings in the foot are similar to those in the hands and include soft tissue thickening; widening of the distal phalangeal tufts; widening of the articular joint space, particularly the metatarsophalangeal joint spaces; prominence of metatarsal heads; beak-like osteophytes at the metatarsal heads; metatarsal penciling; increased size and number of sesamoid bones; and bone proliferation at sites of tendon and ligament attachments.

Spine

In the spine there is increased anteroposterior and transverse diameters of vertebral bodies secondary to anterior

and lateral appositional bone growth. There is no change in the vertebral body height, resulting in the appearance of a short vertebral body. These findings are more often seen in the thoracic and lumbar spine and are less common in the cervical spine. There is also increased height of the intervertebral disc space, which may account for the increased spinal mobility. This is particularly evident in the lumbar region. The anterior and lateral osteophytes in the thoracic and lumbar spine may be extensive, perhaps due to excessive spinal mobility from lax paraspinal ligaments and thickened intervertebral discs. In the cervical spine, widening of the atlantoaxial joint space may be observed. Commonly, there is an increase in kyphotic curvature of the thoracic spine and lordotic curvature of the lumbar spine.

A few studies have reported the incidence of spinal stenosis in patients with acromegaly and pituitary gigantism, resulting from hypertrophy of bones and ligaments, widening of vertebral bodies, and developmental narrowing of the spinal canal.[10]

Scalloping of the posterior margins of the vertebral bodies may be observed (Fig. 78-3), and the etiology is unclear. There is a predilection for the lumbar spine. This

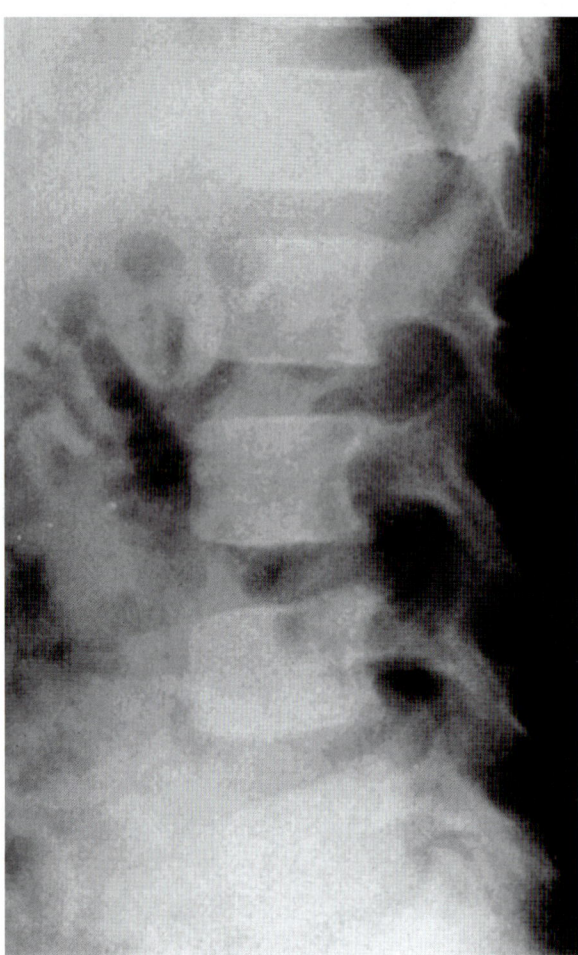

■ **FIGURE 78-3** Acromegaly with scalloping of the posterior vertebral bodies in the lumbar spine. *(From Kumar R, et al. The vertebral body: Radiographic configurations in various congenital and acquired disorders. RadioGraphics 1988; 8:469, with permission.)*

finding is not specific for acromegaly and can be found in a number of other conditions.[11] (See discussion under Differential Diagnosis.)

Peripheral Joints

Patients with acromegaly and pituitary gigantism eventually develop arthropathies that commonly affect the hip, knee, and shoulder, as well as at more distant sites such as the elbow, wrist, hand, ankle, and foot.[12] Early changes include widening of joint spaces from hypertrophy of the cartilage, osseous surface, soft tissue, and synovium. In advanced stages when cartilaginous and osseous degeneration predominate[13] there is joint space narrowing, subchondral cyst formation, sclerosis, and osteophytosis resembling degenerative disease. However, involvement at sites not commonly affected by degenerative disease and the presence of prominent osteophytes and bony excrescences should suggest acromegaly. Acromegalic arthropathy has been found to be noninflammatory and osteoarthritic. Synovial effusions are not common, but when they are present synovial fluid analyses revealed color, cell count, and mucin clot characteristics to be similar to those seen in joint effusions of degenerative

disease.[12] Rheumatoid factors and crystal analyses were negative. The most common abnormalities detected radiographically were osteophytosis and joint space narrowing in late stages.

Bony Excrescences

Bony excrescences may be observed in many locations, including sites of tendon and ligament attachments, posterior and inferior aspect of the calcaneus, anterior margin of the patella, trochanters of the femur, tuberosities of the humerus, undersurface of the distal clavicles, superior aspect of the symphysis pubis, and numerous other locations. Beak-like osteophytes on the inferior aspect of the humeral head, lateral aspect of the acetabulum, medial portion of the femoral head, superior surface of the symphysis pubis, medial aspect of the metacarpals, and metatarsals can be prominent in acromegaly and pituitary gigantism.

Bone Mineral Density

The results of bone mineral density measurements in patients with acromegaly from studies to date have been conflicting. The inconsistent results may be due to difference in sites of bone mineral density measurement, the duration and severity of acromegaly, and the gonadal status. Several studies suggest an important relationship between the bone mineral density with the gonadal status, with some studies finding normal or increased bone mineral density in eugonadal acromegalic patients and other studies finding preserved or decreased bone mineral density in hypogonadal patients (Table 78-2).

TABLE 78-2　Radiographic Findings of Acromegaly
Skull
Thickened calvaria
Prognathic mandible, wide mandibular angle
Prominent paranasal sinuses
Hypercementosis of teeth, wide interdental separation
Hand and Foot
Enlarged distal phalangeal tufts >12 mm in men and > 10 mm in women
Widened metacarpophalangeal joint space >2.5 mm
Thickened soft tissue thickness at midphalanges >27 mm in men and >26 mm in women
Sesamoid index >40 in men and >32 in women
Heel pad thickness >25 mm in men and >23 mm in women
Spine
Increased anteroposterior and transverse diameter without corresponding increase in height
Increased height of intervertebral disc space in lumbar spine
Extensive anterior and lateral osteophytes
Thoracic kyphosis
Scalloping of posterior vertebral bodies in lumbar spine
Peripheral Joints
Early changes include widening of joint spaces
Advanced stage manifested by joint space narrowing, subchondral cyst formation, sclerosis, and osteophytosis resembling degenerative disease
Distinguished from degenerative disease by involvement of sites not commonly affected by degenerative disease and presence of prominent bony excrescences
Bony Excrescences
At sites of tendon and ligament attachments

DIFFERENTIAL DIAGNOSIS

Acromegaly

A combination of radiographic findings would be sufficient to suggest a diagnosis of acromegaly. Some of these radiographic findings when viewed individually are not specific to acromegaly and may be seen in other disorders. For example, widened phalangeal tufts are seen in patients working in heavy manual labor.[14] Scalloped vertebral bodies can result from increased intraspinal pressure from intraspinal neoplasm, cyst, or syringomyelia or from dural weakness predisposing vertebral bodies to deformity, as may be seen in Marfan syndrome, neurofibromatosis, and Ehlers-Danlos syndrome.[15] The joint space narrowing, osteophytosis, cyst formation, and sclerosis seen in late stages of acromegalic arthropathy resemble those in degenerative disease. Soft tissue enlargement and peripheral neuropathy such as carpal tunnel syndrome may be seen in hypothyroidism secondary to myxedematous tissue. A prognathic jaw can also be seen in hypopituitarism.

One disorder that has been reported to have similar clinical and radiographic findings to acromegaly is familial pachydermoperiostosis, characterized by abundant periosteal new bone formation, enlargement of the distal extremities with spade-like hands, squaring of the phalanges, thickening of the skin, coarsening of facial features, and prominent paranasal sinuses.[16] However, unlike acromegaly, there are no signs of endochondral bone formation. The sella turcica is normal, the phalangeal tufts are not widened, the mandibular size and angle are normal, and the articular joint spaces are preserved. In pachydermoperiostosis, the growth hormone level is normal.

Another condition that can mimic acromegaly is long-term therapy with phenytoin (Dilantin), which can lead to development of thickened calvaria, thickened heel pad, and coarse facies.[13,17]

Pituitary Gigantism

Most children who present with gigantism do not have pituitary gigantism. There are many causes of tall stature that should be excluded, including chromosomal causes of tall structure (Sotos, Weaver, Marshall-Smith, and XYY syndromes), precocious puberty, hyperthyroidism, Marfan syndrome, and Beckwith-Wiedemann syndrome. Other associated disorders should be considered as well, such as McCune-Albright syndrome, multiple endocrine neoplasia type 1, neurofibromatosis, tuberous sclerosis, and Carney complex.

SYNOPSIS OF TREATMENT OPTIONS

Medical Treatment

Surgery is usually the first-line therapy for most patients because pituitary adenoma is the most common cause of GH hypersecretion and often can be resected. If surgery fails to sufficiently reduce the GH and IGF-1 levels to normal, medical treatment is usually the first choice for secondary treatment for residual disease. Medical treatment can also be considered as a primary therapy in patients who are not surgical candidates due to unacceptable risks, patients who refuse surgery, and patients with adenomas that are surgically inaccessible. The medical treatments available include pharmacologic agents such as somatostatin analogues, dopamine agonists, and GH receptor antagonists.

The somatostatin analogues commonly used are octreotide and lanreotide.[18] The somatostatin analogues are effective in lowering the serum GH level, reducing the tumor size, and improving the clinical manifestations of acromegaly.

The dopamine agonists have limited effectiveness in the treatment of acromegaly. They are generally less effective than the somatostatin analogues. An exception is with tumors that co-secrete prolactin, which have a better response rate to dopamine agonists than to the somatostatin analogues. The dopamine agonists include bromocriptine and cabergoline, with the latter being somewhat more effective. These dopamine agonist agents have the advantage over other treatments in that they are taken orally.

A novel pharmacologic option when there is no response to the just-listed medical treatments is a GH receptor antagonist such as pegvisomant. This mutated GH molecule blocks the native hormone from binding and is reported to be very effective in lowering the IGF-1 level. Long-term studies are still needed, and this antagonist has not been tested in children.

Surgical Treatment

Surgery is the first-line therapy for acromegaly in most patients. The treatment of choice is transsphenoidal surgical resection if the pituitary adenoma is small or large but still resectable. If the adenoma is very large and not completely resectable or if it is not entirely accessible surgically, as much tissue should be surgically removed as possible to facilitate other treatment options. A remission rate of 80% to 85% can be expected for microadenomas, with a rate of 50% to 65% for macroadenomas. Surgery is

---

What the Referring Physician Needs to Know

- Combination of radiographic findings would be sufficient to suggest diagnosis of acromegaly; however, some findings when viewed individually are not specific to acromegaly and may be seen in other disorders.
- Most gigantism is not pituitary gigantism. One must exclude other causes of tall stature.
- After laboratory confirmation, MRI of the sella turcica should be performed to evaluate for pituitary tumor. If MRI is negative, CT of the chest, abdomen, and pelvis is done to look for ectopic GH/GHRH secretion by tumors in the lung, adrenal, pancreas, and ovaries.
- Transsphenoidal surgical resection of pituitary adenoma is the first choice of treatment. Medical treatments are available if surgery fails to induce complete remission or if surgery is contraindicated. Radiation treatment is generally reserved for refractory cases.

as safe in children as it is for adults. The major morbidity of surgery is permanent diabetes insipidus.

Radiation treatment is generally reserved for refractory cases or used as an adjuvant when surgery is contraindicated. Adenoma growth is arrested, but the decline in GH secretion and the clinical improvement is very slow. More than half of the patients eventually develop panhypopituitarism. And cranial irradiation in children may cause learning disabilities and emotional changes.

SUGGESTED READINGS

Colao A, Marzullo P, Vallone G, et al. Reversibility of joint thickening in acromegalic patients: An ultrasonography study. J Clin Endocrinol Metab 1998; 83:2121-2125.
Melmed S. Acromegaly. N Engl J Med 1990; 322:966-977.
Molitch ME. Clinical manifestations of acromegaly. Endocrinol Metab Clin North Am 1992; 21:597-614.

REFERENCES

1. Melmed S. Acromegaly. N Engl J Med 1990; 322:966-977.
2. Colao A, Marzullo P, Vallone G, et al. Reversibility of joint thickening in acromegalic patients: An ultrasonography study. J Clin Endocrinol Metab 1998; 83:2121-2125.
3. Gonticas SK, Ikkos DG, Stergiou LH. Evaluation of the diagnostic value of heel-pad thickness in acromegaly. Radiology 1969; 92:304-307.
4. Steinbach HL, Russell W. Measurement of the heel pad as an aid to diagnosis of acromegaly. Radiology 1964; 82:418-423.
5. Kho KM, Wright AD, Doyle FH. Heel pad thickness in acromegaly. Br J Radiol 1970; 43:119-125.
6. Anton HC. Hand measurements in acromegaly. Clin Radiol 1972; 23:445-450.
7. Lin SR, Lee KF. Relative value of some radiographic measurements of the hand in the diagnosis of acromegaly. Invest Radiol 1971; 6:426-431.
8. Littlejohn GO, Urowitz MB, Smythe HA, Keystone EC. Radiographic features of the hand in diffuse idiopathic skeletal hyperostosis (DISH): comparison with normal subjects and acromegalic patients. Radiology 1981; 140:623-629.
9. Kleinberg DL, Young IS, Kuperman HS. The sesamoid index: an aid in the diagnosis of acromegaly. Ann Intern Med 1966; 64:1075-1078.
10. Epstein N, Whelan M, Benjamin V. Acromegaly and spinal stenosis. J Neurosurg 1982; 56:145-147.
11. Kumar R. The vertebral body: radiographic configurations in various congenital and acquired disorders. RadioGraphics 1988; 8:469-484.
12. Detenbeck LC, Tressler HA, O'Duffy JD, Randall RV. Peripheral joint manifestations of acromegaly. Clin Orthop Relat Res 1973; 91:119-127.
13. Kattan KR. Thickening of the heel-pad associated with long-term Dilantin therapy. AJR Am J Roentgenol 1975; 124:52-56.
14. Poznanski AK. The Hand in Radiologic Diagnosis. Philadelphia, WB Saunders, 1974, pp 510-513.
15. Mitchell GE, Lourie H, Berne AS. The various causes of scalloped vertebrae with notes on their pathogenesis. Radiology 1967; 89:67-74.
16. Harbison JB, Nice CM Jr. Familial pachydermoperiostosis presenting as an acromegaly-like syndrome. AJR Am J Roentgenol 1971; 112:532-536.
17. Lefebvre EB, Haining RG, Labbe RF. Coarse facies, calvarial thickening and hyperphosphatasia associated with long-term anticonvulsant therapy. N Engl J Med 1972; 286:1301-1302.
18. Drange M, Melmed S. Long-acting lanreotide induces clinical and biochemical remission of acromegaly caused by disseminated growth hormone-releasing hormone-secreting carcinoid. J Clin Endocrinol Metab 1998; 83:3104-3109.

Hypopituitarism

ETIOLOGY

Hypopituitarism refers to a condition in which there is partial or complete insufficiency of pituitary hormone secretion. The most common pituitary hormone deficiency, growth hormone deficiency (GHD), is the main focus of this section.

The cause of hypopituitarism in pediatric patients can be divided into two categories: congenital and acquired. Congenital causes include central nervous system tumors (e.g., craniopharyngioma, metastatic carcinoma, pituitary adenoma, pituitary carcinoma, meningioma), central nervous system malformations, septo-optic dysplasia, pituitary hypoplasia or aplasia, and empty sella syndrome. Acquired causes include cranial irradiation, infection (e.g., tuberculosis, fungal, abscess), infiltrative diseases (e.g., sarcoidosis, histiocytosis X, hemochromatosis, lymphocytic hypophysitis, and leukemia), trauma, and hypoxic insult.[1]

In adults, most patients have pituitary disease caused by a pituitary tumor, surgery, or radiation therapy for the tumor. Other causes include trauma and infiltrative diseases (e.g., sarcoidosis, tuberculosis, histiocytosis X, hemochromatosis, and lymphocytic hypophysitis).

PREVALENCE AND EPIDEMIOLOGY

In the United States, the incidence of hypopituitarism with multiple pituitary hormone deficiency is very rare in childhood, with possibly less than 3 cases per million people per year. However, GHD is more frequent and has a prevalence of approximately 1 in 4000 children.[2] The prevalence of adult-onset GHD in the United States is not known.

CLINICAL PRESENTATION

Clinical manifestations of GHD in children are summarized in Table 78-3.[1-4]

PATHOPHYSIOLOGY

Anatomy

The pituitary gland (hypophysis) lies in the sella turcica, where it is suspended from the hypothalamus by the

---

KEY POINTS

- The radiographic manifestation for hypopituitarism is nonspecific.
- The skeletal findings in children include delayed skeletal growth and maturation, delayed appearance and growth of ossification centers as well as delayed fusion and disappearance of the ossification center, delayed dental eruptions, and osteopenia.
- The skeletal findings in adults are nonspecific and mainly consist of osteoporosis with increased incidence of fracture.

TABLE 78-3 Clinical Presentation of Growth Hormone Deficiency

GHD in Children	Adult-Onset GHD
Short stature	Reduced bone mineral density
Low growth velocity	Increased risk of osteoporotic bone fractures
Characteristic facies with frontal bossing, flattened nasal bridge, and prominent forehead	Reduced muscle strength
Delayed dental eruption	Altered body composition with increased fat and central obesity and decreased muscle volume
Delayed skeletal maturation and bone age	Impaired cardiac function
Increased weight-to-height ratio	High-risk cardiovascular profile (elevated low density lipoprotein cholesterol levels, high body fat, insulin resistance)
Abnormal distribution of fat with excess subcutaneous fat and central obesity	Impaired renal functions
Poor hair and nail growth	Decreased exercise capacity
Delayed puberty and sexual maturity	Emotional and psychosocial disturbances

infundibular stalk. It is regulated by neuropeptide-releasing and release-inhibiting hormones produced in the hypothalamus and delivered via the infundibular stalk. The pituitary gland comprises two regions. The posterior gland is the neurohypophysis, which is an extension of the hypothalamus and releases vasopressin and oxytocin into the blood. The anterior gland is the adenohypophysis, which is a pharyngeal derivative that secretes six trophic hormones, including GH, prolactin, adrenocorticotropic hormone, thyroid-stimulating hormone, follicle-stimulating hormone, and luteinizing hormone.

Pathology

Any disease process affecting the pituitary gland or infundibular stalk can affect the pituitary's secretion of growth hormones along with other pituitary hormones. Trauma causing transection of the infundibular stalk will prevent GH-releasing hormone and other neuropeptide-releasing hormones produced in the hypothalamus from reaching the pituitary gland. Cranial irradiation can lead to panhypopituitarism. Infiltrative diseases, brain tumors affecting the pituitary gland, and pituitary aplasia or hypoplasia can all lead to hypopituitarism.

IMAGING TECHNIQUES

Techniques and Relevant Aspects

Radiography is helpful in determining bone age. Skeletal maturation is a useful diagnostic tool to determine the status of GH secretion because it more accurately reflects an individual's growth and development. Weight and height are less reliable because they vary with familial characteristics, nutritional state, and fluctuations in health. Anteroposterior radiographs of the left hand and wrist, or knee or ankle in children younger than 1 year old, are used to evaluate the progress of epiphyseal ossification by comparing the results with age- and sex-matched reference ranges.

A lateral skull radiograph is occasionally obtained to evaluate the sella turcica. However, with the high false-negative rate of plain skull radiographic findings, MRI is the procedure of choice to exclude an intracranial mass or developmental abnormalities arising from the pituitary gland. In cases in which MRI of the pituitary gland cannot be done, CT should be performed.

Pros and Cons

Magnetic resonance imaging has several advantages over CT in the evaluation of the pituitary gland, including the ability to display pathologic lesions in multiple planes and the ability to provide more detailed information on the structures surrounding the pituitary gland, such as the optic chiasm and cavernous sinuses.

On the other hand, CT has the advantage of providing better visualization of the bony septa in the sphenoidal sinus, which may be important if a transsphenoidal surgical approach is being considered for treatment of a tumor.

MANIFESTATIONS OF THE DISEASE

Radiography

The skeletal manifestation of GHD is delayed skeletal growth and maturation. Hypopituitarism has been reported to affect the linear growth and stature of the bones more than the skeletal maturation.[5] There is a delay in the appearance and growth of ossification centers. Their fusion and disappearance are also delayed. Absence of growth lines in tubular bones may be observed. The bones may be osteoporotic if GHD is not treated. There is also an increased incidence of slipped capital femoral epiphysis.[6]

The findings on the skull radiograph may include a small pituitary fossa or empty sella turcica. Alternatively, an enlarged or eroded sella turcica may be seen, suggesting the possible presence of a tumor. Suprasellar calcifications may suggest a craniopharyngioma. Other findings on the skull radiograph that may be noted include delayed closure of sutures and delayed dental eruptions.

The skeletal finding in adult-onset GHD is nonspecific and mainly characterized by osteoporosis due to reduced bone mineral density with an increased rate of fracture.[3] Spine radiographs may demonstrate reduced vertebral body height due to vertebral compression fracture and osteoporosis (Table 78-4).

DIFFERENTIAL DIAGNOSIS

Pituitary dwarfism accounts for less than 10% of short stature. Other conditions to consider in the differential diagnosis are listed in Table 78-5.

TABLE 78-4 Radiographic Findings of Growth Hormone Deficiency

GHD in Children	Adult-Onset GHD
Delayed skeletal growth and maturation	Nonspecific, mainly characterized by osteopenia with increased incidence of fracture
Delay in appearance and growth of ossification centers	Reduced vertebral body height due to vertebral compression fractures and osteopenia
Delay in fusion and disappearance of ossification centers	
Delayed closure of sutures and dental eruptions	
Osteopenia	

TABLE 78-5 Differential Diagnosis of Short Stature

Familial short stature
Hypothyroidism
Turner syndrome
Noonan syndrome
Laron syndrome
Prader-Willi syndrome
Osteochondrodysplasia
Intrauterine infection causing growth retardation
Child abuse and neglect with failure to thrive or psychosocial dwarfism
Malabsorption
Inflammatory bowel disease
Hypercortisolism
Diabetes
Renal tubular acidosis
Short stature accompanying systemic disease

SYNOPSIS OF TREATMENT OPTIONS

Medical Treatment

Growth hormone deficiency can be effectively treated with GH replacement therapy. GH replacement therapy can reverse many of the clinical manifestations of GHD, such as stimulating linear growth and skeletal maturation in children if treated promptly, increasing the bone mineral density, improving muscle strength, improving exercise capacity, and improving the psychological well-being in adults. For GH replacement to be effective, other pituitary deficiencies should be detected and treated as

What the Referring Physician Needs to Know

■ There is a broad differential diagnosis for short stature. Pituitary etiology accounts for less than 10% of short stature. Other causes must be excluded.

■ Many of the clinical manifestations of GHD can be reversed with GH replacement therapy if treated promptly.

■ In order for GH replacement to be effective, other pituitary deficiencies should be detected and treated.

well. Response to GH therapy should be monitored every 3 to 6 months by height measurements and occasionally by bone age determination.

Surgical Treatment

Surgery may be needed if a brain tumor or congenital abnormality is detected.

SUGGESTED READINGS

Carroll PV, Christ ER, Bengtsson BA, et al. Growth hormone deficiency in adulthood and the effects of growth hormone replacement: a review. Growth Hormone Research Society Scientific Committee. J Clin Endocrinol Metab 1998; 83:382–395.
Preece MA. Diagnosis and treatment of children with growth hormone deficiency. Clin Endocrinol Metab 1982; 11:1–24.

REFERENCES

1. Edeiken J, Murray D, Karasick D (eds). Edeiken's Roentgen Diagnosis of Diseases of Bone, 4th ed. Baltimore, Williams & Wilkins, 1990, vol 1, pp 1431–1460.
2. Preece MA. Diagnosis and treatment of children with growth hormone deficiency. Clin Endocrinol Metab 1982; 11:1–24.
3. Carroll PV, Christ ER, Bengtsson BA, et al. Growth hormone deficiency in adulthood and the effects of growth hormone replacement: a review. Growth Hormone Research Society Scientific Committee. J Clin Endocrinol Metab 1998; 83:382–395.
4. Shalet SM, Toogood A, Rahim A. The diagnosis of growth hormone deficiency in children and adults. Endocr Rev 1998; 19:202–223.
5. Hernandez RJ, Poznanski AW, Hopwood NJ. Size and skeletal maturation of the hand in children with hypothyroidism and hypopituitarism. AJR Am J Roentgenol 1979; 133:405–408.
6. Rappaport EB, Fife D. Slipped capital femoral epiphysis in growth hormone-deficient patients. Am J Dis Child 1985; 139:396–399.

Hyperthyroidism

ETIOLOGY

Hyperthyroidism refers to a condition in which the thyroid hormones, specifically free thyroxine (T_4) and triiodothyronine (T_3), are elevated and lead to a clinical state of thyrotoxicosis. The most common causes of hyperthyroidism are toxic diffuse goiter (Graves disease), toxic multinodular goiter (Plummer disease), and solitary toxic adenoma. Less common causes include thyroiditis, pituitary neoplasm with hypersecretion of thyroid-stimulating hormone, and thyroid carcinoma.[1,2]

PREVALENCE AND EPIDEMIOLOGY

Because Graves disease is the most common cause of hyperthyroidism in the United States, the prevalence of hyperthyroidism can be approximated to the prevalence of Graves disease. In adults, Graves disease contributes to

KEY POINTS

- Musculoskeletal abnormalities of hyperthyroidism:
  - Accelerated skeletal maturation
  - Osteopenia from increased bone turnover
  - Myopathy
  - Thyroid acropachy
- Clinical and radiographic features of thyroid acropachy:
  - Exophthalmos
  - Soft tissue swelling
  - Pretibial myxedema
  - Clubbing
  - Periostitis—usually seen involving the metacarpal or metatarsal bones and proximal phalanges bilaterally, predominantly on the radial sides

TABLE 78-6   Clinical Presentation of Hyperthyroidism
Heat intolerance
Tachycardia, palpitations, atrial fibrillation
Weight loss
Muscle weakness (proximal > distal) and cramps
Insomnia
Inability to concentrate
Fine resting finger tremors
Fine hair, warm and smooth skin
Stare and lid lag
Hyperreflexia
Arthralgia
Palpable enlarged thyroid

60% to 80% of hyperthyroidism and occurs in up to 2% of women but it is about one tenth as frequent in men.[3,4]

In children, Graves disease accounts for more than 95% of hyperthyroidism. The prevalence of hyperthyroidism in children is 0.02%, which is less than 5% of all cases of hyperthyroidism.

Hyperthyroidism is quite rare in infancy and is usually seen when the mother is hyperthyroid at the time of delivery. If the mother has had medical treatment or surgical thyroidectomy during gestation, the infant may be born hyperthyroid, even if the mother reverts back to a euthyroid state during the remainder of the pregnancy.

CLINICAL PRESENTATION

The clinical symptoms of hyperthyroidism include weight loss, heat intolerance, tachycardia with episodes of palpitations, diarrhea, arthralgias, muscle weakness, muscle cramps, anxiety, insomnia, and inability to concentrate.[1,5]

Physical examination may demonstrate an enlarged thyroid; moist, warm, and smooth skin; onycholysis; fine hair; stare and lid lag, tachycardia or atrial fibrillation; fine resting finger tremors; hyperreflexia; and proximal greater than distal muscle weakness (Table 78-6).

Hyperthyroidism is also associated with syndromes such as polyostotic fibrous dysplasia (McCune-Albright syndrome) and ovarian dermoids.

PATHOPHYSIOLOGY

Anatomy

The thyroid gland is located in the neck anterior to the trachea and between the cricoid cartilage and suprasternal notch. It usually consists of two lobes, with the left and right lobes extending around the trachea and esophagus to as far as the carotid sheath on each side in the neck. The isthmus connects the left and right thyroid lobes and lies just anterior to the trachea. A pyramidal lobe is occasionally seen extending superiorly from the middle of the isthmus. This important endocrine gland contains follicular cells that produce thyroxine, which regulates metabolism, and parafollicular cells, that produce calcitonin, which regulates calcium balance. The thyroid gland is part of the hypo-thalamus-pituitary-thyroid axis and is closely regulated by thyrotropin-releasing hormone from the hypothalamus and thyroid-stimulating hormone from the pituitary gland.

Pathology

In hyperthyroid patients, the laboratory findings of hyperphosphatemia, hypercalcemia, elevated alkaline phosphatase, and hypercalciuria suggest increased bone turnover with a negative calcium balance.

The increased bone turnover and bone loss can be seen radiographically as osteoporosis with increased spontaneous fracture rates in the spine, pelvis, femoral neck, long bones, hands, and feet. In the spine, osteoporosis causes rarefaction of the midportion of the vertebral body with exaggerated biconcave deformity of the anterior and posterior margins, giving a "fish" vertebrae appearance. The spine can also be characterized by vertebral compression fractures and kyphosis. In the hands and feet, cortical striations have been observed in the phalanges due to hyperosteoclastosis in the cortical bone that results in longitudinal splitting of the cortex, giving it a striated appearance.[6] Interestingly, the cancellous bone is relatively spared. Osteoblastic foci are also seen more prominent in the cortical bone than the trabecular bone, suggesting the presence of both increased bone resorption and bone formation in the cortex. However, in the setting of osteoporosis and reduced bone mass, osteoclastic activity is more dominant.

Hyperthyroidism is rare in children, and its course is usually rapid without any bone abnormality. In long-standing hyperthyroidism, the most notable effect on the bones is acceleration of skeletal maturation, premature craniosynostosis, and decreased bone mass.[7] In the hand, the second metacarpal bone is the most sensitive to bone loss.

In addition to osseous changes in hyperthyroid patients, the muscles are commonly affected in hyperthyroidism. Muscle weakness, cramps, tenderness, and wasting have been observed, more commonly involving the proximal muscles of the extremities than the distal muscles.[8]

IMAGING TECHNIQUES

Whereas ultrasonography and nuclear medicine thyroid scan can be used to evaluate the thyroid gland, skeletal manifestations of hyperthyroidism are often adequately evaluated with radiography.

MANIFESTATIONS OF THE DISEASE

Radiography

The main radiographic findings of hyperthyroidism include accelerated skeletal maturation, osteoporosis from increased bone turnover, and thyroid acropachy.

The degree of acceleration of skeletal maturation depends on the timing and degree of the hormonal imbalance. Long exposures lead to faster linear growth and maturation. Neonatal and infantile forms manifest as premature craniosynostosis and brachydactyly. Older children can develop myopathy with cardiomegaly seen on chest radiography from cardiomyopathy. Because of marked acceleration of maturation, there is early epiphyseal fusion and premature calcification of costochondral cartilage in adolescents. Mothers with severe thyrotoxicosis, particularly in the third trimester, can also affect their children with these changes.

Acceleration of bone turnover from stimulation of osteoblastic and osteoclastic activity can result in net osteoporosis, which is radiographically more detectable if the patient is hyperthyroid for more than 5 years. Skeletal changes are less apparent in patients younger than age 50 and more common in older men and postmenopausal women. The accelerated osteoporosis transcends that which is expected after menopause. Hyperthyroidism can demonstrate intracortical striations of tubular bones, showing evidence of rapid bone turnover, most pronounced in the metacarpals. Cortical striations can also be seen in acromegaly and hyperparathyroidism. Hyperthyroid osteoporosis is best observed at the distal femurs and shows a more diffuse distribution, including the extremities, cranium, and pelvis. Like other forms of osteoporosis, spinous changes include loss of vertebral body height due to vertebral compression fractures and biconcave "fish mouth" vertebrae, which are more pronounced in the thoracic and lumbar vertebrae. Focal rarefaction of bone may be seen throughout the skeleton and may be confused with multiple myeloma, especially when it is seen in the skull (Fig. 78-4).

Thyroid acropachy (hyperthyroid osteoarthropathy) is detected in approximately 1% of patients with Graves disease, although the incidence is likely higher because it is asymptomatic and therefore underdiagnosed.[9] Although the etiology is unknown, it is usually seen in patients after treatment for hyperthyroidism who had radioactive iodine ablation or thyroidectomy. The patient may be euthyroid, hypothyroid, or hyperthyroid at the time of radiographic presentation. Although thyroid acropachy can occur at any age, it is more common in adults and is relatively rare in children. The clinical symptoms include soft tissue swelling of the extremities, clubbing of the fingers (Fig. 78-5) and toes, pretibial myxedema, and exophthalmos.[10] Erythema of fingers and toes may also accompany the soft tissue swelling. There is no associated pain.

Radiographically, thyroid acropachy is characterized by diaphyseal periosteal reaction that is most pronounced in the metacarpal, metatarsal, proximal, and middle phalanges and less common in other long tubular bones. Periostitis is noted beginning as early as 18 months after treatment

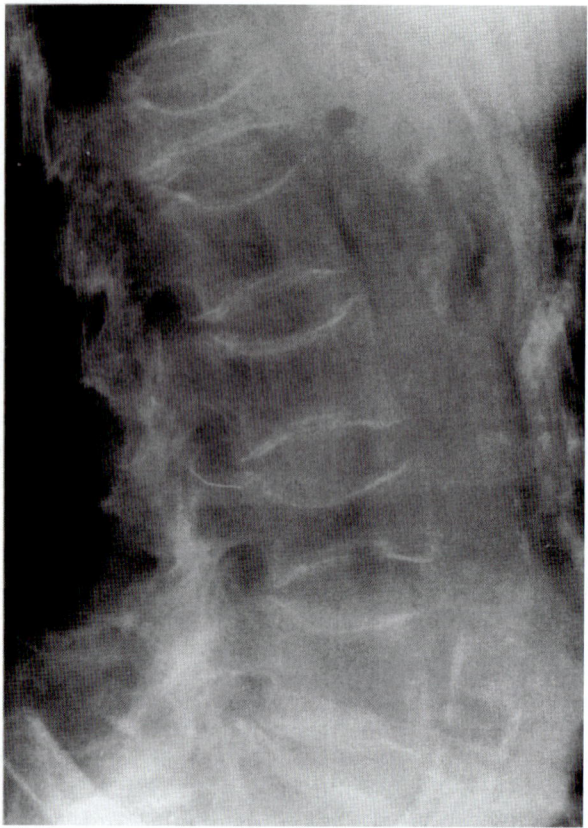

■ **FIGURE 78-4** Hyperthyroid osteoporosis in the spine. There are biconcave "fish mouth" deformities of the lumbar vertebral bodies in this osteoporotic patient. *(From Kumar R. The vertebral body: radiographic configurations in various congenital and acquired disorders. RadioGraphics 1988; 8:472.)*

and does not depend on the current thyroid state of the patient. Periostitis of the bone initially results in a solid and dense appearance with lacy and feathery margins. In later stages, a thick, smooth, periosteal cloaking is formed. The periostitis in thyroid acropachy is usually asymmetric and more prominent in the radial sides of the bones. Acropachy is seen only with patients with a history of Graves disease treated with thyroidectomy and radioactive iodine and is not noted in patients treated with antithyroid drugs (e.g., propylthiouracil) alone.[11]

DIFFERENTIAL DIAGNOSIS

The differential diagnosis for periostitis involving multiple bones is long (Table 78-7). The periostitis seen in hypertrophic pulmonary osteoarthropathy (HPO) is most commonly seen symmetrically in the tibia, fibula, radius, and ulna. Periostitis involving the hands and feet as in thyroid acropachy is very unusual for HPO. In addition, the feathery pattern of periostitis seen in thyroid acropachy is not seen in HPO. Pachydermoperiostitis, also known as primary hypertrophic osteoarthropathy, also has periosteal bone formation that is generally seen symmetrically in the tibia, fibula, radius, and ulna. Fluorosis affects the axial skeleton and long bones to a greater extent than thyroid acropachy. Phalangeal

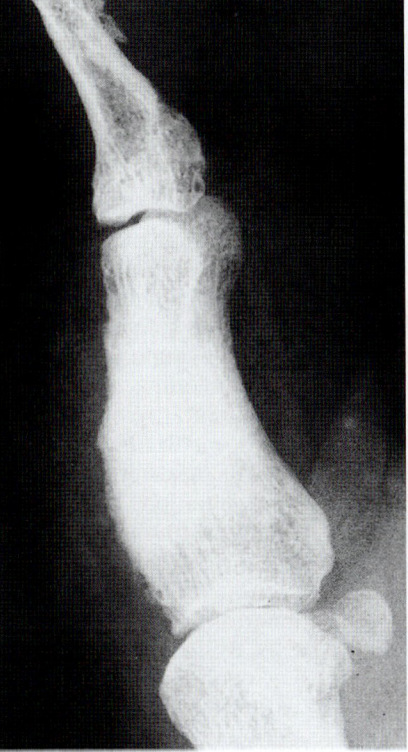

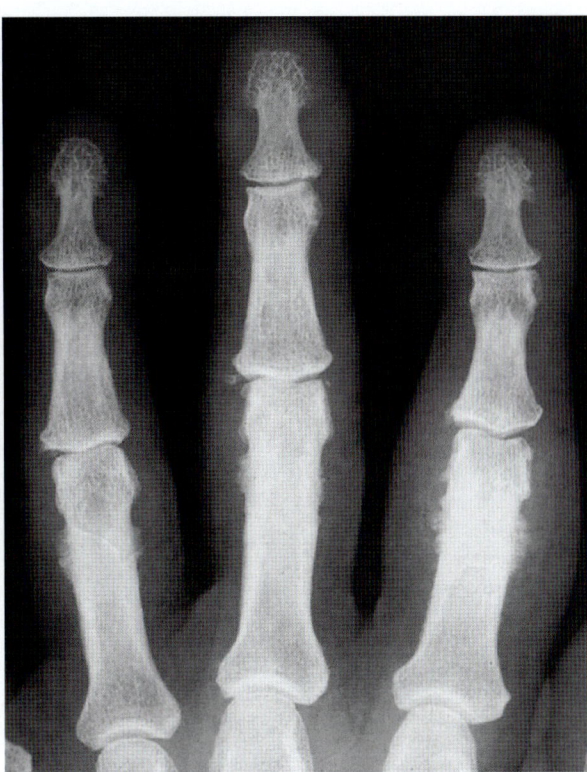

A

B

■ **FIGURE 78-5** Thyroid acropachy in the hand. Fluffy diaphyseal periosteal reaction is most pronounced in the metacarpal bones in the hand and more prominent on the radial sides of the bones. Soft tissue swelling and clubbing of the fingers are also present (*arrows*). *(From Resnick D. Thyroid disorders. In Resnick D. Diagnosis of Bone and Joint Disorders, 4th ed. Philadelphia, WB Saunders, 2002, vol 3, p 2031.)*

TABLE 78-7   Differential Diagnosis of Hyperthyroidism
Differential Diagnosis of Periosteal Reaction of Multiple Bones
Thyroid acropachy
Hypertrophic pulmonary osteoarthropathy
Venous stasis/varicose veins
Vascular insufficiency
Pachydermoperiostosis
Hypervitaminosis A
Fluorosis
Leukemia
Infection
Trauma
Differential Diagnosis of Accelerated Skeletal Age
Hyperthyroidism (maternal or acquired)
Polyostotic fibrous dysplasia (McCune-Albright syndrome)
Idiopathic isosexual precocious puberty
Premature thelarche
Premature adrenarche
Hypothalamic tumors
Pinealoma
Liver tumors (choriocarcinoma, hepatoma)
Adrenocortical tumor or hyperplasia
Gonadal tumors (androgen or estrogen secreting)
Exogenous steroids
Acrodysostosis
Cerebral gigantism (Soto syndrome)
Pseudohypoparathyroidism
Lipodystrophy
Weaver syndrome

involvement of leukemic acropachy is different from that of thyroid acropachy in that it is most pronounced in the terminal phalanges.[12] Clinical correlation can often distinguish periostitis found in venous stasis, hypervitaminosis A, infection, and trauma.

SYNOPSIS OF TREATMENT OPTIONS

Medical Treatment

The medical therapies available for hyperthyroidism include pharmacologic agents and radioactive iodine ablation of the thyroid gland. The pharmacologic agents available include thiourea drugs such as propylthiouracil and methimazole, iodinated contrast agents, and propranolol for symptomatic relief.

Use of radioactive iodine (^{131}I) is an excellent way of destroying overactive thyroid tissue. It causes damage to the thyroid cells that concentrate it without increasing the risk of subsequent thyroid cancers, leukemia, or other malignancies. It is contraindicated in pregnant or breast-feeding patients.

Surgical Treatment

Thyroid surgery is performed less frequently as radioactive iodine ablation has become more widely accepted.

It is usually performed in pregnant patients who cannot undergo radioactive iodine ablation, in patients with very large goiters, or in patients who have a high chance of malignancy.

In children with total craniosynostosis, surgery may be needed to relieve the increased intracranial pressure.

The methods used to treat hyperthyroidism will depend on the etiology, severity, patient's age, clinical situation, and patient's preference.

What the Referring Physician Needs to Know

- The presence of thyroid acropachy on radiograph is virtually diagnostic of thyrotoxicosis.
- Treating hyperthyroidism can reverse some of the clinical manifestations of the condition, such as myopathy and osteoporosis.
- Radioactive iodine (^{131}I) is contraindicated in pregnant or breast-feeding women.

SUGGESTED READINGS

Chew FS. Radiologic manifestations in the musculoskeletal system of miscellaneous endocrine disorders. Radiol Clin North Am 1991; 29:135–147.

Kinsella RA Jr, Back DK. Thyroid acropachy. Med Clin North Am 1968; 52:393–398.

McKeown NJ, Tews MC, Gossain VV, Shah SM. Hyperthyroidism. Emerg Med Clin N Am 2005; 23:669-685.

REFERENCES

1. McKeown NJ, Tews MC, Gossain VV, Shah SM. Hyperthyroidism. Emerg Med Clin N Am 2005; 23:669-685.
2. Reid JR, Wheeler SF. Hyperthyroidism: diagnosis and treatment. Am Fam Physician 2005; 72:623-630.
3. Turnbridge WM, Evered DC, Hall R, et al. The spectrum of thyroid disease in a community: the Whickham survey. Clin Endrocrin (Oxf) 1977; 7:481-493.
4. Weetman AP. Graves disease. N Engl J Med 2000; 343:1236-1248.
5. American Association of Clinical Endocrinologists Medical Guidelines for Clinical Practice for Evaluation and Treatment of Hyperthyroidism and Hypothyroidism (AACE Thyroid Guidelines). Endocr Pract 2002; 8:457-467.
6. Meunier PJ, Bianchi CS, Edouard CM, et al. Bony manifestation of thyrotoxicosis. Orthop Clin North Am 1972; 3:745-774.
7. Riggs W Jr, Wilroy RS Jr, Etteldorf JN. Neonatal hyperthyroidism with accelerated skeletal maturation, craniosynostosis, and brachydactyly. Radiology 1972; 105:621-625.
8. Segal AM, Sheeler LR, Wilke WS. Myalgia as the primary manifestation of spontaneously resolving hyperthyroidism. J Rheumatol 1982; 9:459-461.
9. Gimlette TMD. Thyroid acropachy. Lancet 1960; 1:22-24.
10. Vanhoenacker FM, Pelckmans MC, De Beuckeleer LH, et al. Thyroid acropachy: correlation of imaging and pathology. Eur Radiol 2001; 11:1058-1062.
11. Kinsella RA Jr, Back DK. Thyroid acropachy. Med Clin North Am 1968; 52:393-398.
12. Glatt W, Weinstein A. Acropachy in lymphatic leukemia. Radiology 1969; 92:125-126.
13. Fisher DA. Thyroid disease in the neonate and in childhood. In DeGroot LJ, editor. Endocrinology. 2nd ed. Philadelphia, WB Saunders, 1989, pp 733-745.

Hypothyroidism

ETIOLOGY

Hypothyroidism refers to a clinical condition in which there is inadequate production of thyroid hormone. Primary hypothyroidism is the most common cause of hypothyroidism, and it is characterized by an abnormality in the thyroid gland that results in deficient production of thyroid hormone. Causes include treatment of Graves disease (thyroidectomy or radioiodine ablation), autoimmune thyroiditis such as Hashimoto thyroiditis, iodine deficiency, poor iodine metabolism, medications (e.g., lithium), and infiltrative processes such as metastatic disease, lymphoma, and amyloidosis.[1]

Congenital hypothyroidism, which is characterized by hypothyroidism present since birth and previously known as cretinism, may result from in utero iodine deficiency, inborn error of thyroid hormone metabolism, or anatomic defect in the thyroid gland (e.g., thyroid agenesis, dysgenesis, or ectopia).

Secondary hypothyroidism is less common and results from an abnormality in the pituitary gland, resulting in deficient thyroid-stimulating hormone (TSH), or from an abnormality in the hypothalamus, resulting in inadequate thyrotropin-releasing hormone.

PREVALENCE AND EPIDEMIOLOGY

The incidence of thyroid disorders in North America is approximately 2% in women and 0.2% in men. The prevalence of overt hypothyroidism is around 0.1% to 2% and subclinical hypothyroidism is around 4%[1]. There are no known racial differences.

For congenital hypothyroidism, the incidence is 1 in 4000 newborns.[2] It is observed in all racial and ethnic groups. Any observed racial difference is most likely related to geographic and socioeconomic status rather than to any specific racial predilection. Congenital hypothyroidism caused by iodine deficiency has all but been eliminated in the developed world. The populations of areas of the world with underiodinated or noniodinated salt, and with less seafood consumption such as Africa and land-locked regions of Asia and Indonesia, still suffer.

KEY POINTS

- The key radiographic finding for congenital hypothyroidism is retarded skeletal maturation and epiphyseal dysplasia with secondary articular degeneration.
- There is no diagnostic radiographic finding for adult-onset hypothyroidism, although dystrophic calcification and arthropathy may be seen.
- Many clinical manifestations are reversible with thyroid hormone replacement.

CLINICAL PRESENTATION

The extent of clinical findings generally depends on the etiology, severity, and duration of hypothyroidism.

Infants with in utero thyroid hormone deficiency during the critical period of development of the central nervous system often develop cerebral diplegia, severe mental retardation, and deaf-mutism. If thyroid hormone deficiency is perpetrated after birth, diffuse edema, severe growth retardation, and delayed skeletal maturation ensue. There is reported interaction between thyroid hormone levels affecting the amount of growth and sex hormones excreted.

At birth, congenital hypothyroid neonates may demonstrate prolonged jaundice, large fontanelles, umbilical hernia, hypotonia, or hoarse cry or may subtly present as a "good baby" who sleeps most of the time and rarely cries. Newborns can initially appear normal in size. The child will progressively fall off the growth chart over several months, as slow skeletal growth and delayed ossification centers manifest. Closure of the fontanelles is also delayed and accompanies delayed ossification.

Thyroid deficiency occurring in children results in juvenile myxedema with mental retardation and developmental delays.

The symptoms and signs of infantile and childhood hypothyroidism, depending on the age of onset, are presented in Table 78-8.[2,3]

PATHOPHYSIOLOGY

Anatomy

The thyroid gland develops from the buccopharyngeal cavity between the 4th and 10th weeks of gestation. It arises from the fourth brachial pouches and develops into a bilobed gland that is located in the neck just anterior to the trachea between the cricoid cartilage and suprasternal notch. Both thyroid lobes normally extend from the side to the level of the carotid sheath. The two lobes are connected by the isthmus, which lies anterior to the trachea. Occasionally, a pyramidal lobe can be seen arising superiorly from the middle of the isthmus. Errors in the formation or migration of thyroid tissue can result in thyroid aplasia, dysplasia, or ectopy (lingual or sublingual location). The thyroid gland is regulated by TSH from the pituitary gland, which in turn is regulated by thyrotropin-releasing hormone from the hypothalamus.

Pathology

Thyroid hormones are vital to skeletal growth because they stimulate differentiation and maturation of the chondrocytes at the growth plate cartilage. They also stimulate osteoblast and osteoclast activities for bone remodeling. They are required for the expression of many of the skeletal actions of growth hormone.[4]

The consequences of hypothyroidism include delayed skeletal maturation and growth in infants and children, delayed closure of growth plates, and delayed appearance of secondary ossification centers. Whereas skeletal retardation can be seen in other conditions, it is usually more severe in hypothyroidism. Although children with hypothyroidism commonly have low levels of growth hormone as well, treatment with growth hormone alone does not restore normal development. The degree and progress of skeletal maturation strongly correlate with thyroid function. Lack of thyroid hormone stimulation prevents normal growth and maturation at the cartilaginous growth plate. It also prevents expression of the growth hormones.

Delayed closure of the growth plates can be seen into adulthood secondary to delayed appearance of secondary ossification centers. Histologic examination of the persisting growth plate does not show any evidence of cellular proliferation in the cartilage.[5] The bony tissue of the metaphysis apposed to the cartilage growth zone eventually closes off the growth plate and subsequently impedes longitudinal growth of the bone even though there is persistence of the growth plate.

Delayed, fragmented, and irregular ossification centers are commonly seen, most often described in the femoral heads and knees. Unlike normal focal growth and enlargement, hypothyroid children can have numerous ossification centers that grow and coalesce to form an irregular epiphysis with uneven density called hypothyroid epiphyseal dysgenesis. Epiphyseal dysgenesis classically occurs in the hips and less commonly in the hands and feet. The irregular ossifications are less pronounced than those from Down syndrome or osteochondrodystophy. Chronic irregular epiphysis in the femoral head can lead to flattened femoral heads, widening of the femoral neck, and coxa vara deformity. Abnormal epiphyseal development may also be a risk factor for slipped capital femoral epiphysis reported in a few hypothyroid children, but such association is rare.[6] Epiphyseal dysgenesis may be explained by an imbalance in thyroid function between the stimulatory mitogenic effect of elevated TSH and the lack of differentiation by thyroid hormones, which are deficient.[7]

In addition to epiphyseal dysgenesis, hypothyroidism may manifest as destructive joint arthropathies. Joint pain,

TABLE 78-8 Clinical Presentation of Hypothyroidism	
Infantile and Childhood Hypothyroidism	**Adult-Onset Hypothyroidism**
Prolonged jaundice	Fatigue, lethargy, weakness
Large fontanelles	Mental or physical slowness
Umbilical hernia	Dry waxy skin
Hypotonia	Coarse brittle hair, alopecia
Mottled, cool, and dry skin	Diffuse nonpitting edema, periorbital edema
Hoarse cry	
Hypersomnia and minimal crying	Pallor
Decreased activity	Cold intolerance, hypothermia
Constipation	Hoarseness
Poor feeding and weight gain	Constipation
Small stature or poor growth	Weight gain
Developmental delay, mental retardation	Macroglossia
	Bradycardia
Coarse facial features	Menstrual disturbance
Macroglossia	Depression
Pallor	Prolonged deep tendon reflex relaxation phase
Myxedema	
Prolonged deep tendon reflex relaxation phase	Myalgia, arthralgia, paresthesias
Goiter	
Myalgia, arthralgia, paresthesias	

effusion, and stiffness are common complaints in patients with hypothyroidism. Arthropathic changes commonly involve the hands and knees in adults, whereas the hips and epiphysis of the femoral heads are more often involved in children. The joints may be enlarged and painful secondary to thickening of the synovium, joint effusion, or both. The joint effusion is cloudy and viscous but noninflammatory.[8] It has a high hyaluronic acid content and may be explained by the presence of a TSH-responsive adenylate cyclase in the synovial membrane and the stimulation of hyaluronic acid production as well as synovial thickening by elevated TSH in hypothyroidism.[8] Destructive arthropathy of the proximal interphalangeal and metacarpal joints presenting similarly to rheumatoid arthritis has been described.[9,10] A destructive lesion in the tibial plateau suggesting compression has also been reported in literature.[6] Avascular necrosis has been described in the femoral head and carpal lunate.[11] The association of hypothyroidism with calcium pyrophosphate dihydrate crystal deposition, although suggested, remains uncertain because results to date have been conflicting.

Hypothyroid myopathy may also manifest as diffuse muscular hypertrophy and muscle weakness that is predominantly proximal. Diffuse muscle hypertrophy, stiffness, weakness, and cramps are known as Hoffman's syndrome.[12] Symmetric proximal muscle weakness with marked serum muscle enzyme elevations clinically resemble polymyositis and has been misdiagnosed as such.[13] Generalized myalgias when accompanied by trigger point tenderness may suggest fibromyalgia and may be the initial presentation of hypothyroidism.[14]

Myxedema can cause entrapment neuropathy such as carpal tunnel syndrome, which is seen in 7% of hypothyroid patients.

IMAGING TECHNIQUES

Although ultrasonography and nuclear medicine thyroid scan are the most commonly used modalities to evaluate the thyroid gland, plain radiographs are sufficient to evaluate most of the musculoskeletal changes of hypothyroidism. The radiographs can be supplemented with CT or MRI in evaluating joint complaints for signs of joint destruction, effusion, or avascular necrosis. MRI is also helpful in evaluating extremities for suspicion of neuropathy caused by nerve compression by myxedema (e.g., carpal tunnel syndrome).

MANIFESTATIONS OF THE DISEASE

Radiography

Retardation of skeletal maturation is a key radiographic finding in hypothyroidism. Delayed skeletal maturation is radiographically detected by observing a delay in appearance and growth of epiphyseal ossification centers, which is best seen in the infant by examining the knees or feet.[15]

Prompt appearance of the ossifications (best evaluated at the knees) followed by normal osseous development after thyroid hormone replacement can confirm the diagnosis of juvenile hypothyroidism if laboratory and clinical findings suggest the diagnosis. The distal femoral epiphysis is usually ossified at 36 weeks' gestation, and the proximal tibial epiphysis is ossified at 38 weeks' gestation. Epiphyseal plates may stay open well into adulthood if untreated. Delayed areas of synchondrosis in the sacrum or sternum parallel areas of delayed ossification (Figs. 78-6 to 78-8 and Table 78-9.

In the epiphyses, irregular epiphyseal appearance may result from ossification occurring from multiple centers rather than from a single site. The fragmented appearance of the epiphysis can simulate other conditions and can be mistaken for Legg-Calvé-Perthes disease. Chronic epiphyseal dysgenesis and delayed or inadequate treatment can lead to irregular epiphysis with eventual articular degeneration and intra-articular loose osseous and cartilaginous bodies. In the hips this can lead to the trifecta of coxa plana, coxa magna, and coxa vara.

In the skull, plain radiographs or CT may show delayed closure of fontanelles, prominent sutures with accessory (wormian) bones developing within the sutures, hypoplastic paranasal sinuses and mastoid air cells, delayed dentition, protruding mandible, and brachycephaly resulting from decreased growth of the spheno-occipital synchondrosis. The sella turcica may be enlarged secondary to hyperplasia of the pituitary gland as a result of feedback from low thyroid hormone level on the hypothalamus and pituitary gland (Figs. 78-9 and 78-10).[16]

In the spine, one to three of the vertebral bodies at the thoracolumbar junction may demonstrate a short, bullet-shaped appearance with beak-like anterior margin or anterosuperior vertebral body notching.[17] Exaggerated kyphosis at the thoracolumbar junction may be observed, resulting in a gibbus deformity that may improve with thyroid hormone replacement. These findings are nonspecific and may be seen in a number of other conditions, such as Hurler disease, Morquio disease, and achondroplasia.

In the hands, delayed skeletal maturation can be seen as it can be seen elsewhere. Hypothyroidism affects the linear

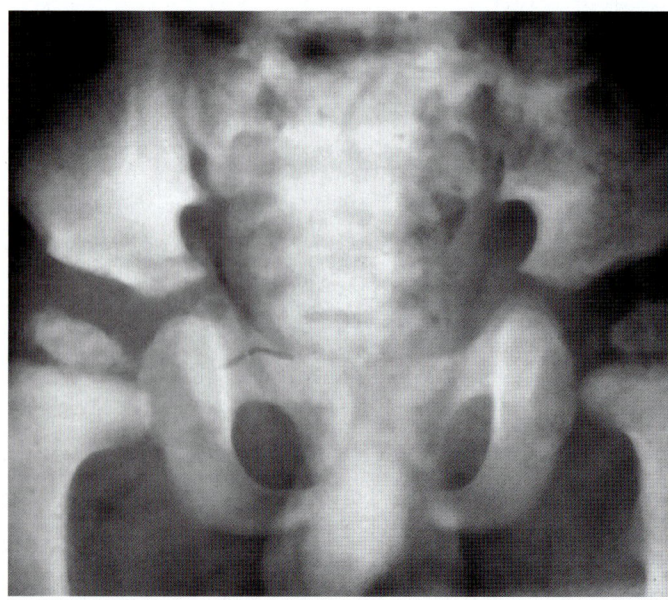

■ **FIGURE 78-6** Bilateral femoral epiphyseal dysgenesis. *(Courtesy of Javier Beltran, MD.)*

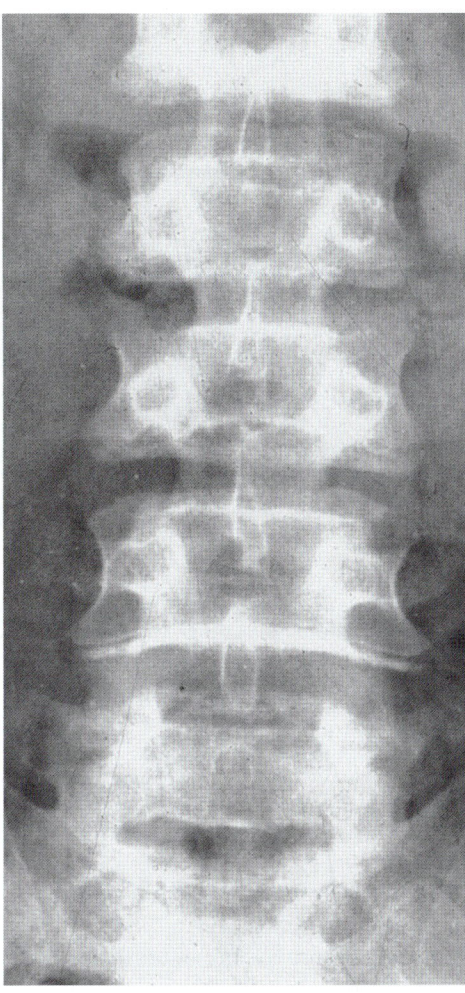

■ **FIGURE 78-7** The epiphyseal end plates of the vertebral bodies remain open in this 23-year-old patient. *(Courtesy of Javier Beltran, MD.)*

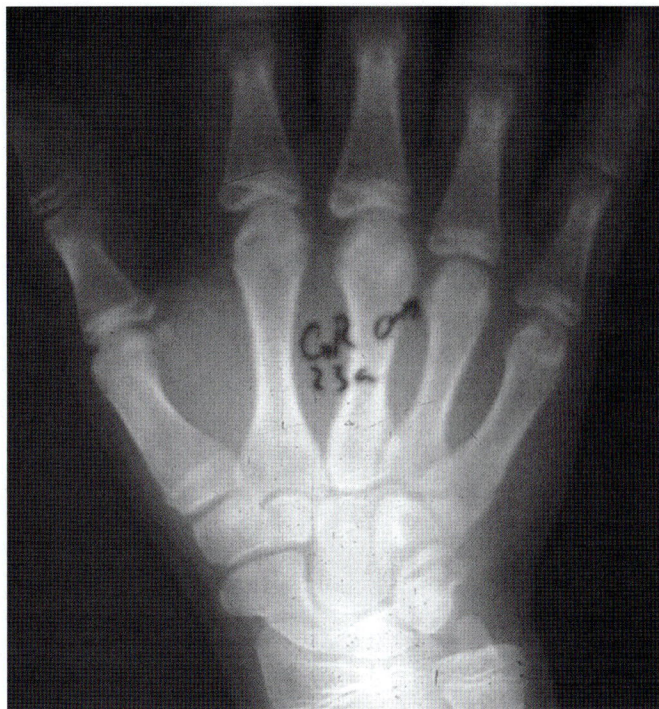

■ **FIGURE 78-8** The epiphyses in the hand are still open in this 23-year-old patient. *(Courtesy of Javier Beltran, MD.)*

growth less than it affects skeletal maturation, whereas in hypopituitarism, linear growth is affected more than skeletal maturation.[18] In addition to delayed skeletal maturation, a radiographic finding of the hand specific to untreated primary hypothyroidism is osseous projections from the midportion of the metaphyses of the distal phalanges into the epiphyseal plate, which is noted in 80% of the cases.[19] Its presence along with delayed skeletal maturation suggests the diagnosis of hypothyroidism.

In adult-onset hypothyroidism, the skeletal changes are mild and may include slightly increased bone density and joint arthropathies. Destructive changes in the proximal interphalangeal joints and metacarpal joints simulating rheumatoid arthritis should include hypothyroid arthropathy on the differential diagnosis. Sclerosis in the femoral heads and neck should also raise the suspicion for avascular necrosis. In the knees, destructive lesions in the tibial plateau suggest compression.

Abnormal soft tissue calcification and increased bone sclerosis may be seen on imaging studies. Increased bony eburnation of the periorbital region results in the "lunette" sign of hypothyroidism.[20] Parotid calcification, premature atherosclerosis, nephrocalcinosis, and dystrophic calcifications in various soft tissues may all be evident.

TABLE 78-9 Reported Musculoskeletal Abnormalities in Hypothyroidism
Retarded skeletal maturation
Accessory sutural bones
Epiphyseal dysplasia
Epiphyseal deformity with secondary degenerative joint disease
Gibbus deformity
Dystrophic calcification
Carpal tunnel syndrome
Synovial effusion, tenosynovitis
Myopathy
Neuropathy
Soft tissue edema
Osteoporosis
Slipped capital femoral epiphysis
Ligamentous laxity
Calcium pyrophosphate dihydrate crystal deposition
Erosive arthritis

Reprinted from Resnick D. Thyroid disorders. In Resnick D. Diagnosis of Bone and Joint Disorders, 4th ed. Philadelphia, WB Saunders, vol 3, p 2034.

Magnetic Resonance Imaging

A hyperplastic pituitary with a relatively enlarged pituitary fossa can be seen with a chronically hypofunctioning thyroid and should not be mistaken for a pituitary tumor.

DIFFERENTIAL DIAGNOSIS

The differential diagnosis of hypothyroidism is presented in Table 78-10.[21]

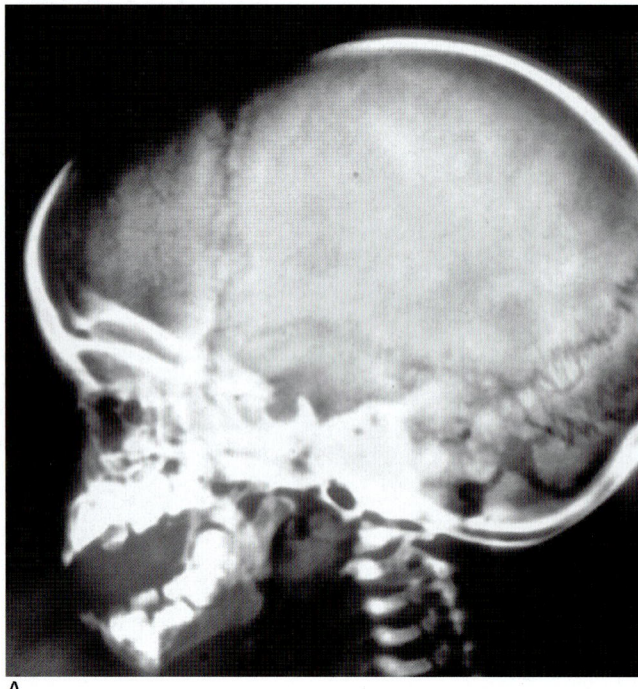

A

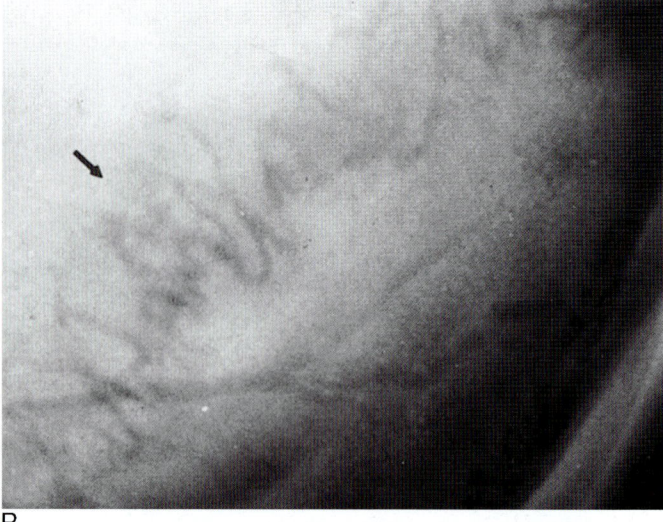

B

■ **FIGURE 78-9   A,** Note the prominent sutures and accessory (wormian) bones. The paranasal sinuses are hypoplastic. **B,** Wormian bones (*arrow*). (***B*** *from Resnick D. Thyroid disorders. In Resnick D. Diagnosis of Bone and Joint Disorders, 4th ed. Philadelphia, WB Saunders, 2002, vol 3, p 2036.*)

TABLE 78-10 Differential Diagnosis of Hypothyroidism		
Generalized Delayed Skeletal Age	**Stippling of Epiphyseal Ossification Centers**	**Wormian Bones**
Hypothyroidism	Congenital hypothyroidism	Pyknodysostosis
Chronic severe anemia (e.g., sickle cell anemia, thalassemia)	Spondyloepiphyseal dysplasia	Pachydermoperiostosis
Constitutional	Multiple epiphyseal dysplasia (Fairbank disease)	Osteogenesis imperfecta
Addison disease	Legg-Calvé-Perthes disease	Rickets—hypophosphatasia
Cushing syndrome	Aseptic necrosis	Kinky hair syndrome
Corticosteroid therapy	Normal variant	Cleidocranial dysostosis
Hypogonadism (e.g., Turner syndrome)	Endemic cretinism	Hypothyroidism, cretinism
Panhypopituitarism	Down syndrome	Primary acro-osteolysis (Hadju-Cheney)
Growth hormone deficiency	Mucopolysaccharidosis (Morquio syndrome)	Down syndrome
Chromosomal disorders (e.g., trisomy 21, trisomy 18)	Stickler syndrome (hereditary arthro-ophthalmopathy)	Normal variant
Skeletal dysplasia	Osteopoikilosis	Congenital hypophosphatasia
Congenital malformation syndrome	Osteopathia striata	Chromosomal abnormalities
Congenital heart disease (especially cyanotic)	Dysplasia epiphysialis hemimelica (Trevor disease)	Major central nervous system abnormalities
Juvenile diabetes mellitus		
Chronic illness		
Inflammatory bowel disease		
Intrauterine growth retardation		
Legg-Calvé-Perthes disease		
Malnutrition		
Malabsorption (e.g., celiac disease)		
Neurogenic disorders		
Chronic renal disease		
Rickets		
Idiopathic		

Reprinted from Kottamasu SR. Bone changes in endocrinopathies. In Kuhn JP, Slovis TL, Haller JO (eds). Caffey's Pediatric Diagnostic Imaging, 10th ed. St. Louis, Mosby, 2004, vol 2, p 2436-2437.

SYNOPSIS OF TREATMENT OPTIONS

Levothyroxine (thyroxine, T_4), also known as Synthroid, is the treatment of choice. It is taken daily orally, and the dose is adjusted every 3 weeks until the patient is euthyroid.

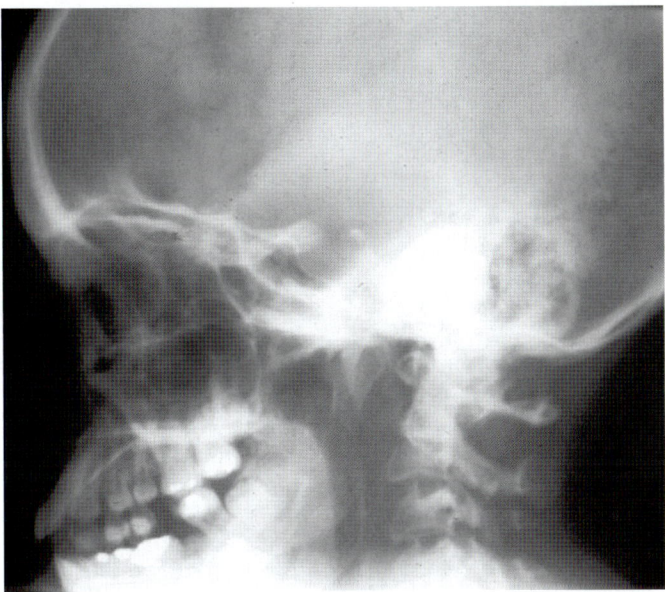

■ **FIGURE 78-10** Enlarged sella turcica suggesting pituitary hyperplasia secondary to chronic hypothyroidism. *(Courtesy of Javier Beltran, MD.)*

What the Referring Physician Needs to Know

- Although the key radiographic manifestation of hypothyroidism is delayed skeletal maturation, the diagnosis of hypothyroidism is based on clinical findings.
- In infants, absence of the distal femoral and proximal tibial epiphyses is an important radiographic clue for hypothyroidism.
- Unexplained delay in closure of the fontanelles or sutures in children should raise the suspicion of hypothyroidism and prompt investigation.
- Hypothyroidism can initially present in children or adults with unexplained joint pain or effusion, local or generalized muscle pain, or paresthesias.
- Hypothyroid myopathy may simulate polymyositis clinically.
- Hypothyroidism in adults can present like rheumatoid arthritis of the hand as pain and swelling in the metacarpophalangeal and proximal interphalangeal joints.
- Hypothyroidism can lead to life-threatening myxedema coma with a mortality rate of up to 100% if it is not treated.
- Many of the clinical manifestations of hypothyroidism can be at least partially reversed if it is treated promptly with thyroid hormone replacement.

SUGGESTED READINGS

Chew FS. Radiologic manifestations in the musculoskeletal system of miscellaneous endocrine disorders. Radiol Clin North Am 1991; 29:135-147.

McLean RM, Podell DN. Bone and joint manifestations of hypothyroidism. Semin Arthritis Rheum 1995; 24:282-290.

REFERENCES

1. Devdhar M, Ousman YH, Burman KD. Hypothyroidism. Endocrinol Clin N Am 2007; 36:595-615.
2. Delange F. Neonatal screening for congenital hypothyroidism: results and perspectives. Horm Res 1997; 48:51-61.
3. American Association of Clinical Endocrinologists Medical Guidelines for Clinical Practice for Evaluation and Treatment of Hyperthyroidism and Hypothyroidism. Endocr Pract 2002; 8:457-467 (AACE Thyroid Guidelines).
4. Lewinson D, Harel Z, Shenzer P, et al. Effect of thyroid hormone and growth hormone on recovery from hypogonadism of epiphyseal growth plate cartilage and its adjacent bone. Endocrinology 1989; 124:937-945.
5. Jaffe HL. Metabolic, Degenerative and Inflammatory Diseases of Bones and Joints. Philadelphia, Lea & Febiger, 1972, p 346.
6. Crawford AH, MacEwen GD, Fonte D. Slipped capital femoral epiphysis co-existent with hypothyroidism. Clin Orthop Relat Res 1977; 122:135-140.
7. McLean RM, Podell DN. Bone and joint manifestations of hypothyroidism. Semin Arthritis Rheum 1995; 24:282-290.
8. Dorwart BB, Schumacher HR. Joint effusions, chondrocalcinosis and other rheumatic manifestations in hypothyroidism: a clinicopathologic study. Am J Med 1975; 59:780-790.
9. Neeck G, Riedel W, Schmidt KL. Neuropathy, myopathy and destructive arthropathy in primary hypothyroidism. J Rheumatol 1990, 17.1697-1700.
10. Gerster JC, Valceschini P. Destructive arthropathy of fingers in primary hypothyroidism without chondrocalcinosis. J Rheumatol 1992; 19:637-641.
11. Rubinstein HM, Brooks MH. Aseptic necrosis of bone in myxedema. Ann Intern Med 1977; 87:580-581.
12. Klein I, Parker M, Sherbert R, et al. Hypothyroidism presenting as muscle stiffness and pseudohypertrophy: Hoffmann's syndrome. Am J Med 1981; 70:891-894.
13. Madariaga MG. Polymyositis-like syndrome in hypothyroidism: review of cases reported over the past twenty-five years. Thyroid 2002; 12:331-336.
14. Wilke WS, Sheeler LR, Makarowski WS. Hypothyroidism with presenting symptoms of fibrositis. J Rheumatol 1981; 8:626-631.
15. Resnick D. Thyroid disorders. In Resnick D (ed). Diagnosis of Bone and Joint Disorders, 4th ed. Philadelphia, WB Saunders, 2002, vol 3, pp 2026-2042.
16. Swischuk LE, Sarwar M. The sella in childhood hypothyroidism. Pediatr Radiol 1977; 6:1-3.
17. Swischuk LE. The beaked, notched, or hooked vertebra: its significance in infants and young children. Radiology 1970; 95:661-664.
18. Hernandez RJ, Poznanski AW, Hopwood NJ. Size and skeletal maturation of the hand in children with primary hypothyroidism. AJR Am J Roentgenol 1979; 133:405-408.
19. Hernandez RJ, Poznanski AK. Distinctive appearance of the distal phalanges in children with hypothyroidism and hypopituitarism. Radiology 1979; 132:83-84.
20. Borg SA, Fitzer PM, Young LW. Roentgenologic aspects of adult cretinism: two case reports and review of the literature. Am J Roentgenol Radium Ther Nucl Med 1975; 123:820-828.
21. Kottamasu SR. Bone changes in endocrinopathies. In Kuhn JP, Slovis TL, Haller JO (eds). Caffey's Pediatric Diagnostic Imaging, 10th ed. Philadelphia, Elsevier, 2004, pp 2436-2439.

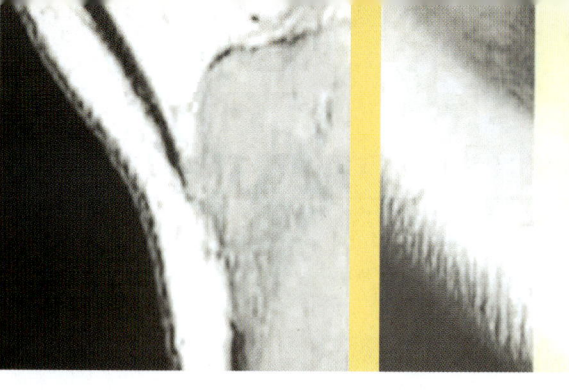

79

Gaucher Disease

Daniel Rosenthal

ETIOLOGY

Gaucher disease bears the name of Philippe Gaucher, a French dermatologist who first described the clinical syndrome. Understanding of the condition was greatly enhanced in 1965 when it was recognized that the disease was due to a functional deficiency of the enzyme β-glucosidase. This deficiency results in accumulation of glucosylceramide, a cell membrane metabolite, in lysosomes of cells of the monocyte/macrophage lineage.[1]

PREVALENCE AND EPIDEMIOLOGY

There are several thousand individuals in the United States with Gaucher disease. It is particularly prevalent among the Ashkenazi Jewish population, among whom as many as 1 in 14 may be carriers. More than 300 mutations that may result in clinical disease have been identified; 7 of these account for the majority of nucleotide substitutions. Four alleles account for approximately 90% of cases: *N370S, 84GG, L444P,* and *IVS2+1.* Inheritance is autosomal recessive.

CLINICAL PRESENTATION

The clinical features result from the accumulation of glucosylceramide in cells of the reticuloendothelial system. Apoptosis is inhibited in these cells. Their relative immortality leads to progressive accumulation of characteristic Gaucher cells, which replace normal marrow elements and cause hepatosplenomegaly.

Although the severity of disease is variable, the most prevalent forms of Gaucher disease are associated with a normal or near-normal life expectancy. The presence and degree of central nervous system involvement has been used to delineate three more-or-less distinct forms of the disease.[2]

The most prevalent form of Gaucher disease is known as the type 1 variant. It does not affect the central nervous system. Although this has been referred to as the "adult type," 66% of individuals with type 1 Gaucher disease develop some manifestations of the disease in childhood. Onset early in childhood is usually predictive of a severe, rapidly progressive phenotype, and young children with type 1 Gaucher disease are at high risk for morbid complications.

Type 2 Gaucher disease is characterized by onset in infancy with severe central nervous system involvement and death in early childhood. Severely affected individuals have been identified as early as the second trimester of pregnancy, exhibiting polyhydramnios, hydrops fetalis with bilateral hydrothorax, hepatosplenomegaly, arthrogryposis, absent fetal movements, and thickened skin. Patients with type 3 Gaucher disease demonstrate milder central nervous system involvement with onset in adolescence or early adulthood and a more indolent course.

Diagnosis of Gaucher disease is typically confirmed by enzyme assay, DNA analysis, bone marrow biopsy, spleen or liver biopsy, or some combination of these four methods. Of these, assay for glucocerebrosidase activity of peripheral blood leukocytes is considered to be the most efficient and reliable means of diagnosis.

KEY POINTS

- MRI is the best modality to identify the major sites of organ involvement and areas of infarction in Gaucher disease.
- CT is an alternative modality that is useful but exposes the patient to radiation.
- Gaucher disease is due to functional deficiency of β-glucosidase, leading to accumulation of abnormal metabolites in the reticuloendothelial system.
- The most severe types produce visceral and hematologic disorders in infancy. Skeletal disorders predominate in less severely affected individuals.
- Skeletal imaging is dominated by marrow replacement, osteopenia, focal lytic lesions, osteonecrosis, fracture, and osteomyelitis.
- Erlenmeyer flask deformity is a highly characteristic, but inconstant and not pathognomonic, feature of the disease.

Portions of this chapter appear in the author's own discussion on this topic in the textbook Weissman B: Imaging of Arthritis and Metabolic Bone Disease. Philadelphia: Mosby, 2009.

PATHOPHYSIOLOGY

Anatomy

Nonskeletal

The accumulation of glucocerebroside in the lysosomes of visceral macrophages gives rise to multiple manifestations, including hepatosplenomegaly, anemia, thrombocytopenia, growth retardation, and skeletal disease. The most severe variants of Gaucher disease may cause death at an early age from visceral and hematologic manifestations.

Pulmonary infiltrates and thoracic lymph node enlargement can be the predominant imaging findings of some of the severe forms.[1] Even patients with type 1 disease may occasionally develop pulmonary involvement. Interlobular septal and intralobular interstitial thickening may result in a reticulated pattern, irregular interfaces at the pleural surfaces, and ground-glass appearance as seen on radiographs and high-resolution CT.

Cardiac involvement in Gaucher disease has been reported in only a few patients, mostly adults with pericardial changes. However, thickened, relatively immobile mitral and aortic valves have been seen, resulting in significant mitral regurgitation. Therefore, echocardiographic investigation of patients with suspected cardiac involvement with Gaucher disease is recommended.

Brain involvement occurs in the severe, neuronopathic forms. The severity of neurologic abnormalities has been shown to correlate with multifocal areas of cerebral hypoperfusion. Extensive hypoperfusion foretells clinical deterioration, and progressive cerebral atrophy has been demonstrated in the frontal and temporal lobes.

Enlargement of the liver and spleen is almost universal in patients with Gaucher disease (Fig. 79-1A). In addition, about 5% of patients have focal splenic or hepatic lesions. These presumably represent areas of infarction or fibrosis related to previous infarction, but focal defects can also be caused by other conditions such as metastatic carcinoma.

Hypersplenism leading to thrombocytopenia and moderate immunocompromise is a frequent complication of Gaucher disease, often requiring splenectomy. Partial splenic embolization may be performed to avoid the increased risk of serious infectious complications.[4] Complete removal of the spleen is thought to cause deterioration of the disease in other organs (especially the bones) possibly by removal of an important reservoir for the Gaucher cells. After institution of enzyme replacement therapy, there is usually an initial dramatic decline and then sustained decreases in organ size, especially in pediatric patients (see Fig. 79-1B).

Skeletal Features

In general, skeletal complications require time to develop; therefore, skeletal manifestations are less characteristic of the more fulminant forms of the disease. However, when present, the fundamental features of skeletal involvement are the same in all clinical forms of the disease.[3]

In some affected individuals there may be no clinical, radiographic, scintigraphic, or histologic evidence of bone involvement, but in others the skeleton can be completely devastated. Findings from the International Collaborative Gaucher Group Registry, an international database of more than 2600 patients, show that nearly all patients with Gaucher disease have radiologic evidence of skeletal involvement and the majority have a history of serious skeletal complications. For most patients with type 1 disease, the skeletal manifestations are probably its most disabling aspect.

The skeleton is not affected uniformly. With the exception of generalized osteopenia and marrow replacement, most manifestations are multiple and localized.

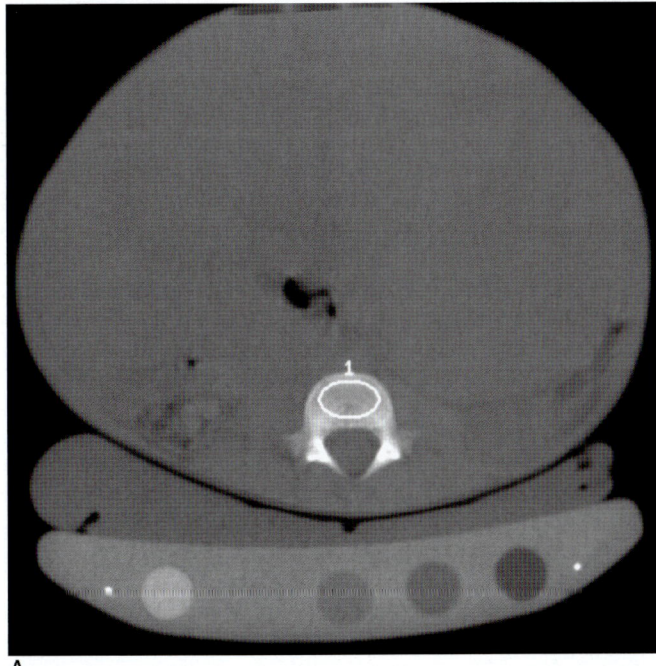

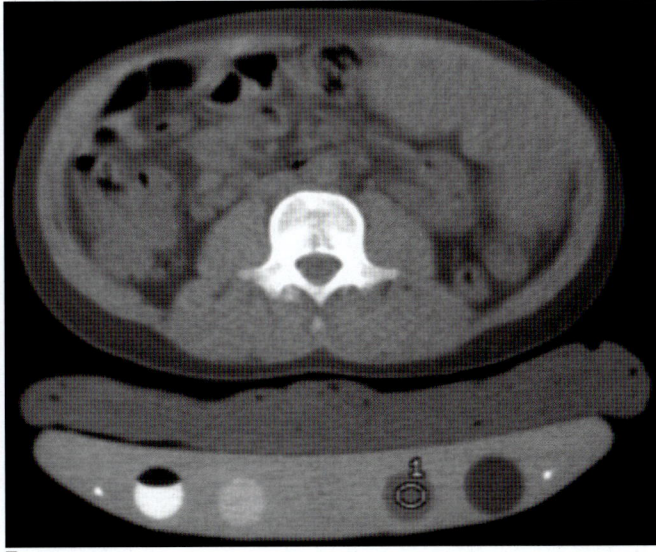

■ FIGURE 79-1   **A,** Abdominal CT scan reveals massive hepatosplenomegaly in this untreated child with Gaucher disease. **B,** After 3 years of enzyme replacement therapy there is no longer organ enlargement.

Sometimes much of the skeleton is preserved. These observations suggest that bone is affected by scattered, focal collections of Gaucher cells. It is possible that local effects may be the result of a toxic process around these foci. Alternatively, the storage of glucocerebroside in tissue macrophages may disturb the generation of competent osteoclasts and thus result in a failure to maintain a healthy skeleton.[5]

Patients commonly experience nonspecific bone pain, and some suffer from intermittent episodes of severe pain (bone crises) similar to those seen in sickle cell disease. Up to 20% have impaired mobility.

Radiographically demonstrable involvement results from five basic processes:

1. Marrow replacement
2. Generalized osteopenia
3. Skeletal resorption due to adjacent heavily involved marrow leading to focal lytic lesions
4. Acute focal bone disease including
   a. Osteonecrosis, especially collapse of the femoral head
   b. Osteomyelitis and "pseudo-osteomyelitis"
   c. Fractures
5. The Erlenmeyer flask deformity, a characteristic (but not universally present) modeling abnormality of the distal femur

Pathology

The histologic hallmark of Gaucher disease is the presence of lipid-laden histiocytes. These are widely distributed among the organs of the reticuloendothelial system and are particularly prominent in the liver, spleen, bone marrow, and lymph nodes but may also be found in other connective tissues. Accumulation of glucocerebroside within the macrophages imparts a characteristic foamy or "wrinkled cigarette paper" appearance to the cytoplasm (Fig. 79-2).

IMAGING TECHNIQUES

Techniques and Relevant Aspects

Because it affects multiple organ systems, virtually every imaging modality has a role to play in evaluation of patients with Gaucher disease. Some are used to evaluate the sever-

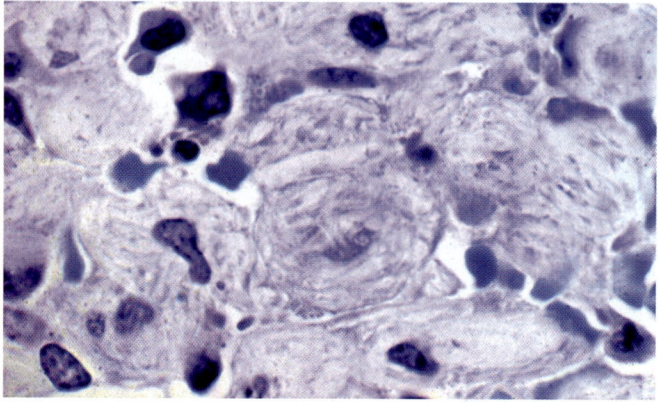

■ **FIGURE 79-2** Toluidine blue stain shows a Gaucher cell with the so-called wrinkled cigarette paper appearance of the cytoplasm.

ity of the disease itself, whereas others find their use in evaluation of the complications of the disease. In many instances, the evaluation of specific complications is not different when they occur in patients with Gaucher disease than when they occur in the general public. Thus, for example, fractures and osteomyelitis are evaluated no differently, although they are treated somewhat differently because of the bleeding tendencies and immune deficiencies often present in this population. For purposes of this discussion, we will focus on imaging aspects that are specific to Gaucher disease.

Pros and Cons

A number of quantitative and semiquantitative techniques have been applied to the investigation of Gaucher disease. These have been used to evaluate the severity of marrow replacement and the extent of organomegaly. Although these have been important in understanding the natural history of the disease, and in evaluating the effectiveness of therapy, they are probably too laborious and imprecise to be applied to individual patients. Furthermore, the effects of therapy are now largely known (see later) and therefore in most instances investigational techniques are not required.

MANIFESTATIONS OF THE DISEASE

Radiography

Radiography is the standard approach to detection and evaluation of fractures. Fractures are relatively common in patients with Gaucher disease. They may occur due to generalized osteopenia or to focal bone replacement, resulting in weakened skeletal areas at sites of osteolysis (Fig. 79-3A).

Radiography is also the best means to detect the presence of an Erlenmeyer flask deformity. This is a well-known and characteristic feature of Gaucher disease. It represents undertubulation of the distal femur due to failure of bone resorption in the "cut-back" zone of the metaphysis (Fig. 79-4). The Erlenmeyer flask deformity is not unique for Gaucher disease. It may also be seen in disorders associated with osteoclast failure (e.g., osteopetrosis) and may be associated with certain other rare marrow-packing diseases such as mannosidosis, a glycoprotein storage disease of lysosomes due to specific absence of α-D-mannosidase.[6] The Erlenmeyer flask deformity can be strikingly obvious or extremely subtle in patients with Gaucher disease. In our experience, its presence does not invariably reflect either the severity of disease or the local marrow involvement.

Notching of the medial aspect of the proximal humeral metaphysis, in some cases contributing to pathologic fracture, has also been reported as a manifestation of Gaucher disease and certain other infiltrative marrow processes such as leukemia, Niemann-Pick disease, Hurler syndrome, and metastatic neuroblastoma, but controversy remains as to whether this represents a normal variant.[7]

Focal accumulation of Gaucher cells may result in lytic lesions. These are typically not symptomatic unless

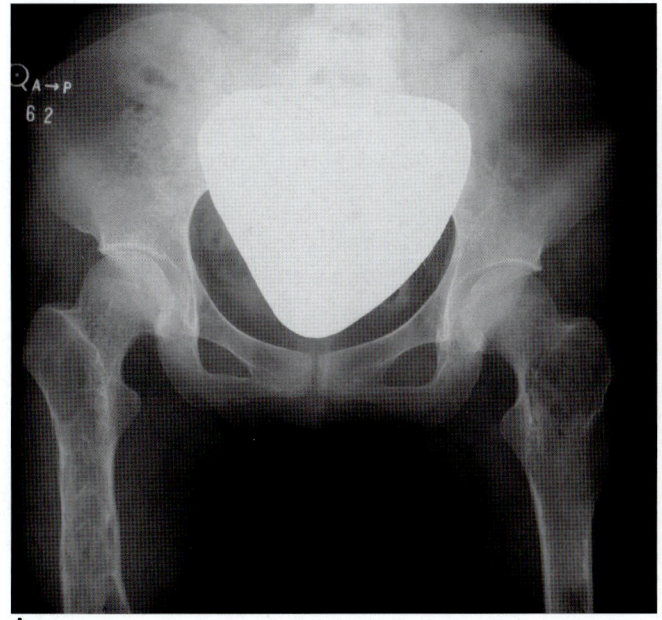

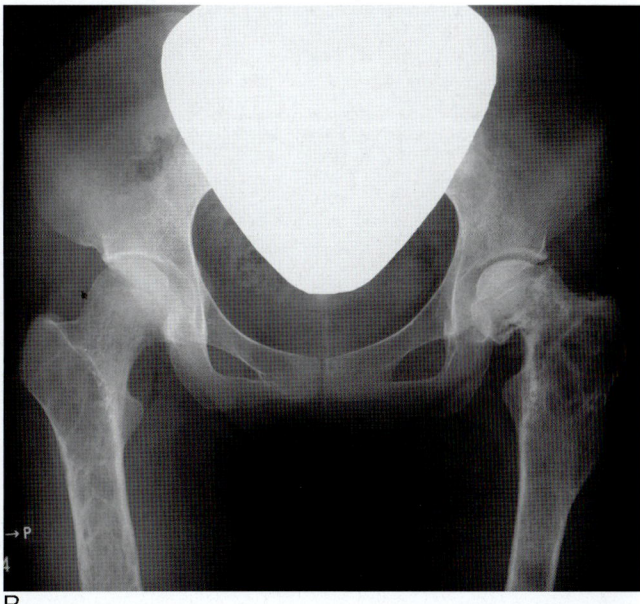

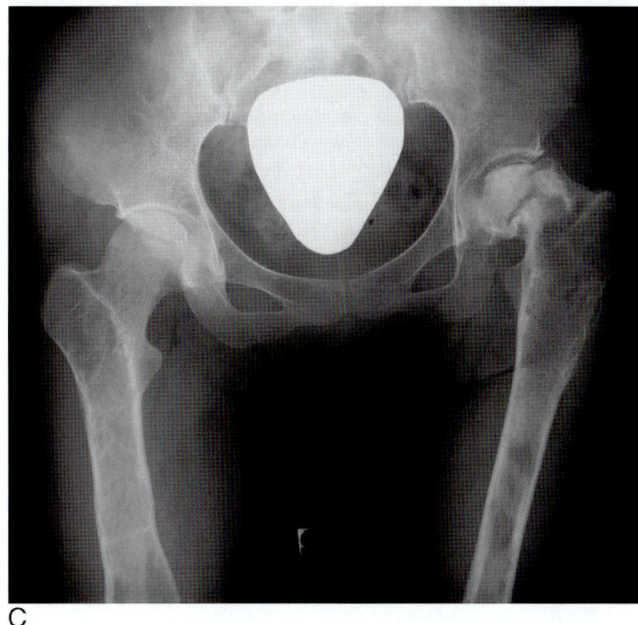

■ **FIGURE 79-3** **A,** Plain radiograph of the pelvis demonstrates severe osteopenia and bilateral large focal lytic lesions of the proximal femora. This is a common location for these lesions, which are typically bilaterally symmetric. **B,** Radiograph of the pelvis obtained on the same patient 7 months later shows a fracture through the lytic lesion of the left femur. Note that the trabecular bone of the femoral head appears somewhat dense, indicating osteonecrosis. **C,** Slightly less than a year later, a radiograph demonstrates nonunion of the femoral fracture and a subchondral "crescent sign" indicating subarticular fracture and impending collapse of the femoral head.

infarction or fracture supervenes (see Fig. 79-3B). When focal marrow deposits become so large that the cortex is violated, then extraosseous extension of Gaucher disease may occur (Fig. 79-5). Commonly referred to as a "gaucheroma," such focal deposits might simulate malignancy. This differential diagnosis may occasionally become problematic in view of the increased risk of multiple myeloma in patients with Gaucher disease. In one rare instance, an extraosseous Gaucher cell accumulation even produced a monoclonal IgG kappa gammopathy, further simulating a myeloma.[8] Gaucheromas tend to be very slowly progressive.[9] In some instances the connection to the bone (although always present) may be subtle, giving the incorrect impression of a soft tissue mass.[10]

Radiographs may also demonstrate the effects of bone infarction, although they are not useful for early diagnosis of this condition. Macroscopic infarction takes the form of a medullary zone demarcated from adjacent bone by a serpiginous sclerotic boundary. Occasionally, this may result in a "bone-within-bone" appearance (Fig. 79-6A). If the end of a bone is affected, osteoarticular necrosis may be followed by collapse of the surface and the need for total joint arthroplasty (see Fig. 79-3B and C). In the spine, collapse of the vertebral end plates with vertical or square sides may be seen, similar to sickle cell anemia. As in the latter condition, microscopic bone infarction may result in diffuse medullary sclerosis (see Fig. 79-6B). Complete replacement of the vertebral marrow with collapse may result in the findings of vertebra plana (see Fig. 79-6C).

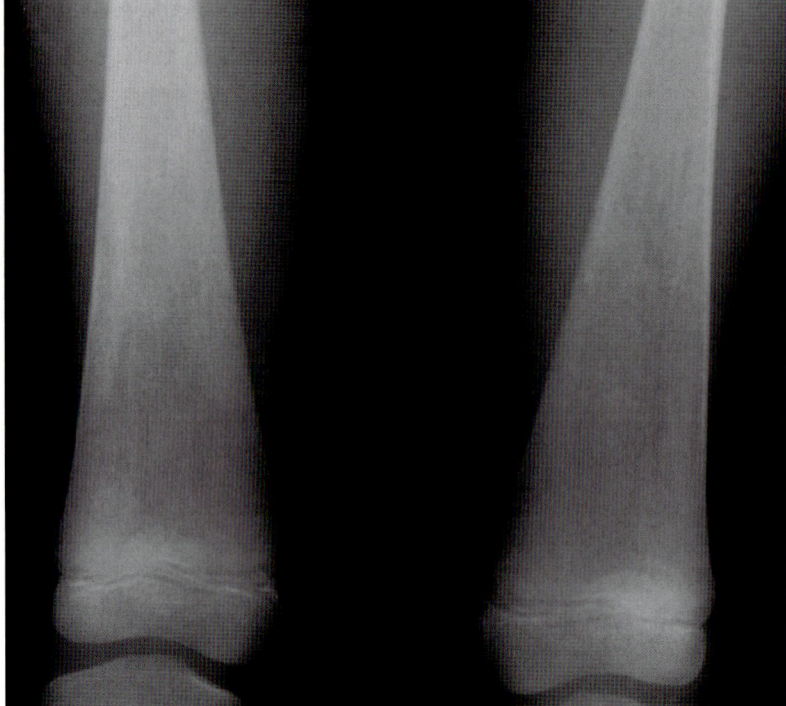

A

■ **FIGURE 79-4** **A,** Anteroposterior radiograph of both distal femora demonstrates striking widening of the distal metaphyses. In normal individuals, the distal metaphyses abruptly widen into the femoral condyles. In patients with an Erlenmeyer flask deformity, the femur takes on a conical shape due to dysfunction of the "cut-back" zone. **B,** After 3 years of treatment with enzyme replacement, the femur has taken on a more normal shape. This type of improvement may be observed in children who undergo therapy but is rare in adults.

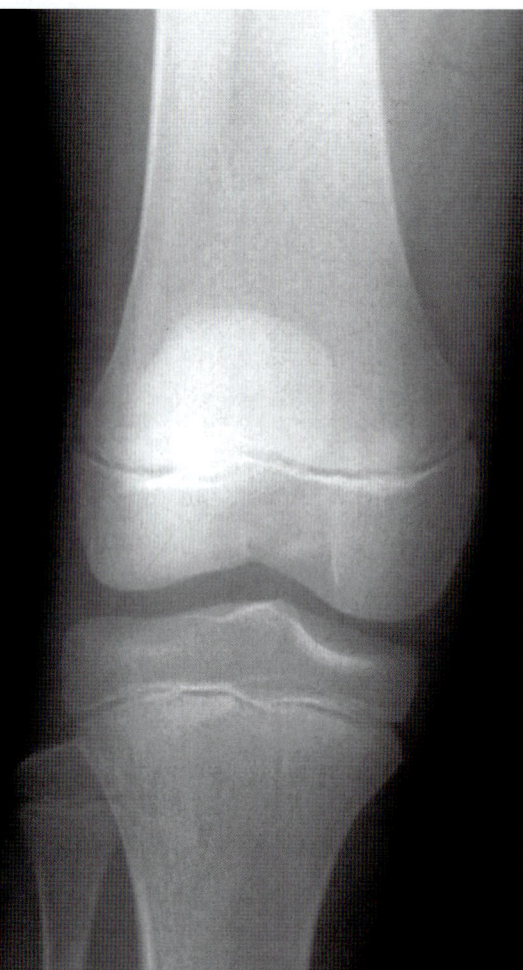

B

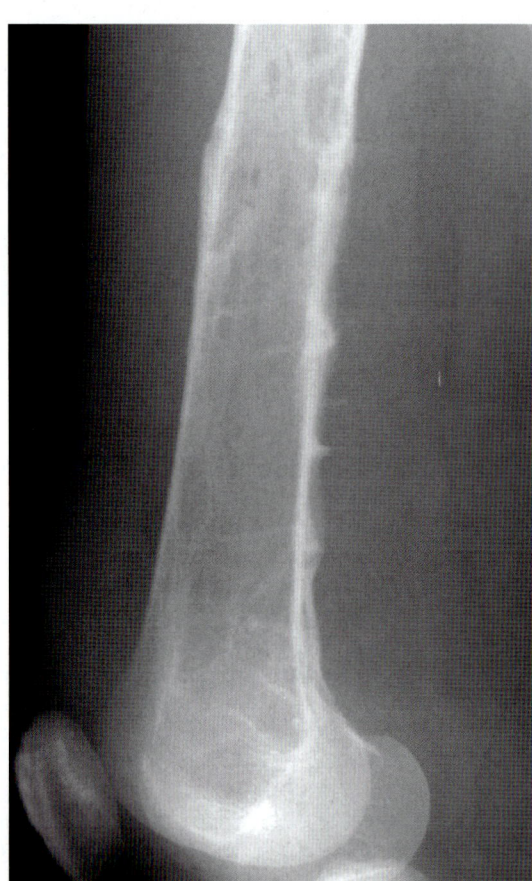

■ **FIGURE 79-5** Lateral radiograph of the distal femur demonstrates osteopenia, multiple lytic lesions, and a "hair-on-end" pattern of periosteal new bone formation due to extraosseous spread of Gaucher disease.

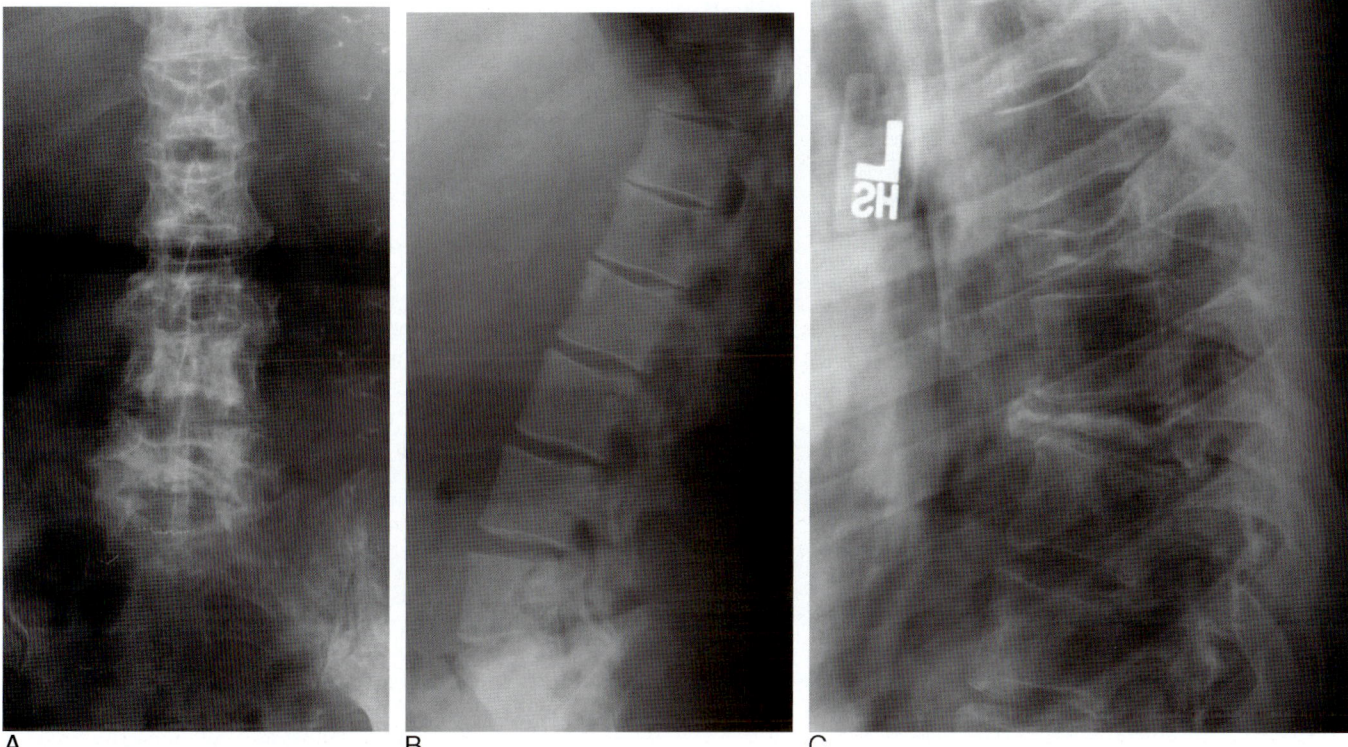

■ FIGURE 79-6 **A,** Anteroposterior spine radiograph (different patient from Fig. 79-3A) shows a "bone-within-bone" appearance due to multiple vertebral body infarctions. This is a relatively rare manifestation. **B,** Lateral radiograph of the spine demonstrates diffuse medullary sclerosis, a pattern that may also be observed in sickle cell disease. Presumably this represents the skeletal response to small vessel occlusion, without a discrete infarcted territory. **C,** Vertebra plana. As in other diseases that cause marrow replacement, vertebral fractures may result in vertebra plana.

Bone Densitometry

Low levels of bone density in Gaucher disease are associated with serum markers of accelerated bone turnover and breakdown, suggesting that the osteopenia associated with type 1 Gaucher disease is due to increased bone resorption.[11]

Patients with Gaucher disease are usually found to have osteopenia at all sites. The severity of osteopenia is related to overall disease severity and is correlated with genotype; the more severely affected individuals with the *N370S/84GG* mutation have lower density than those with the milder *N370S/N370S* mutation. As in individuals without Gaucher disease, density declines as a function of age. Bone densitometry (dual-energy x-ray absorptiometry [DEXA]) has been advocated for following the response to therapy for children with Gaucher disease, although absolute measurements do not correlate with severity of disease.[12] It is interesting that DEXA measurements are more consistently abnormal in patients than quantitative CT scans, an order of sensitivity that is opposite from that seen with osteoporosis. Because quantitative CT scans measure trabecular bone only, perhaps this indicates that in Gaucher disease the osteopenia has an important component of cortical bone loss.

Magnetic Resonance Imaging

Magnetic resonance imaging can also be used to evaluate the visceral and soft tissue manifestations of Gaucher disease. Like CT and ultrasonography, it can be used to accurately measure the volume of the liver and spleen. It is more expensive than ultrasonography, but more reproducible, and it does not involve radiation exposure like CT, something that is probably important in affected children who may require serial measurements. MRI of the brain may demonstrate progressive cerebral atrophy in the frontal and temporal lobes.

MRI is the most useful method for evaluation of bone marrow replacement, which is the most universally present skeletal manifestation of Gaucher disease. Normal bone marrow becomes infiltrated by cellular elements containing foam cells (macrophages packed with glucocerebroside). This feature is impossible to recognize on radiographs and is extremely subtle on CT scans but is quite obvious on MRI. Marrow affected by Gaucher disease characteristically demonstrates either homogeneous or patchy low signal intensity on both T1- and T2-weighted imaging sequences (Fig. 79-7). These signal alterations presumably reflect the combined effects of replacement of marrow fat and the highly structured microtubular arrays in which the glucocerebroside accumulates.

Gaucher disease extends into the marrow in a more-or-less predictable pattern. This pattern reverses the sequence of marrow conversion that normally occurs during childhood. During normal development, the maximal extent of red marrow occurs at the ninth month in utero. Subsequently, the red marrow is replaced by much less cellular yellow or fatty marrow, beginning in the distal parts of the appendicular skeleton and proceeding

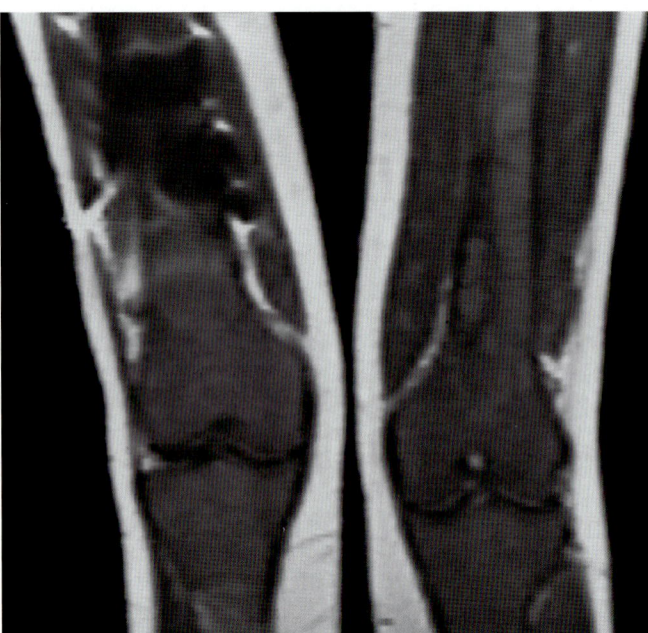

■ **FIGURE 79-7** T1-weighted coronal MR image of the knees. The bright marrow signal that is normally due to the presence of fat is absent because of infiltration of the marrow.

proximally. These changes cause progressive increase in the marrow signal on T1-weighted images. By age 10, adult degrees of signal intensity are achieved in most pelvic sites, although fatty replacement remains ongoing throughout life. Even by age 6, adult levels of fat content (40% to 45%) are reached in the posterior ilium; therefore, marrow with homogeneous low signal on T1-weighted images in these areas is abnormal. Most epiphyseal centers have fatty marrow throughout life. We believe that this is because the secondary centers are cartilaginous during early childhood and ossification occurs when physiologic requirement for red marrow is declining. Therefore, the normal pattern of marrow conversion is centripetal, except for the fact that the secondary centers do not participate.

In Gaucher disease the process is reversed, with accumulation of Gaucher-affected tissue beginning in the axial skeleton and proceeding into the proximal and then the distal long bones. The epiphyses are relatively spared, although with advanced disease they, too, are affected.[13]

This pattern is thought to reflect the availability of the macrophages that serve as reservoirs for the glucocerebroside accumulation. Such macrophages are primarily found in red marrow, and therefore areas of residual red marrow tend to be affected first. Replacement of the proximal marrow causes areas of red marrow to develop further peripherally, and Gaucher cell accumulation follows. This reverse process is known as "reconversion" and may also be seen in other marrow-replacing disorders.[14]

A number of different approaches have been devised to quantify the extent of marrow replacement. Simple scales based on the known pattern of disease progression and visual determination of the presence of disease have been developed by Rosenthal and Hermann.[15,16]

Since the vertebral marrow appears darker than expected on T1 images due to absence of fat, a "semiquantitative" approach has been devised to compare vertebral body signal intensity to disk brightness. If the normalized vertebra to disk ratio (NVDR) is taken to be 1.0 (95% confidence limits, 0.70 to 1.30), for untreated patients with Gaucher disease the ratio is below 0.7.[17]

It is also possible to calculate a numerical value for the volume percent of fat (fat fraction). This is generally done using the technique of quantitative chemical shift imaging. The fat fraction is decreased severalfold in patients with Gaucher disease compared with normal individuals.[18]

These approaches are valuable because the extent of marrow replacement indicates the probability of skeletal symptoms. There is a significant positive correlation between liver size, the risk of avascular necrosis, and the marrow scale used by Hermann. The spleen size does not seem to be related to these factors.[19]

A correlation has been demonstrated between fat fraction of axial bone marrow as calculated by Dixon quantitative chemical shift imaging (Dixon QCSI) and bone complications, with an 85% increase in risk of bone complication for every decrease of 0.1 in the fat fraction. Fat fractions are significantly lower in patients with Gaucher disease than in normal patients, and lower in Gaucher disease patients who have undergone splenectomy than in those who have not. The latter observation supports the clinical impression that removal of the splenic "reservoir" may worsen the skeletal disease.[20] Other studies have also demonstrated a relationship between fat fraction and clinical disease severity, although not always with bone complications.[15]

Computed Tomography

Like ultrasonography and MRI, CT can be used to demonstrate changes in the size of the liver and spleen. CT is faster to perform than MRI and can for that reason usually be done in children without the need for sedation. As with the other imaging techniques, focal changes due to infarction and infiltration can also be demonstrated by CT scans.

As mentioned earlier, CT can be used to measure bone density (quantitative CT [QCT]). In patients with osteoporosis this is advantageous because of its specific sensitivity to loss of trabecular bone, which makes it highly sensitive to early bone loss in the spine. However, in Gaucher disease, the reduction in trabecular bone mass as demonstrated by QCT has been only moderate. DEXA demonstrates greater degrees of loss. Presumably this is a reflection of the fact that cortical bone loss predominates. In addition, when performed using conventional single-energy QCT methods, replacement of normal marrow fat with Gaucher cells tends to artifactually elevate the apparent bone mass. Although rarely performed because of technical complexity, dual-energy measurements more accurately reflect the degree of bone loss.

Ultrasonography

Ultrasonography may be used to assess volume changes in the liver and spleen. As is the case for MRI, this is of particular interest in children because of the lack of exposure to ionizing radiation. Focal splenic or hepatic lesions can be hypoechoic, hyperechoic, or mixed. These lesions presumably represent areas of infarction or fibrosis related to previous infarction. After institution of enzyme replacement therapy, ultrasound has been used to demonstrate an initial dramatic decline and then sustained decrease in organ size. Ultrasonography can also be used to demonstrate suspected cardiac involvement.

Nuclear Medicine

Liver scintigraphy has been used to demonstrate both enlargement and inhomogeneous uptake. Focal defects may represent liver involvement with Gaucher disease; but as is the case in individuals without Gaucher disease, focal defects can also be caused by other conditions such as metastatic carcinoma. Like ultrasonography, scintigraphy can be useful in detecting splenic infarction and in following enlargement of the spleen after partial splenectomy.

Brain scans with technetium-99m hexamethylpropylene-amine-oxime and SPECT imaging have been used to demonstrate brain involvement in the severe, neuronopathic forms. Multifocal hypoperfusion of the brain has been shown to correlate with neurologic abnormalities, and extensive hypoperfusion foretells clinical deterioration.

Radioisotope scans have also been used to evaluate the marrow changes of Gaucher disease. As determined by ^{99m}Tc sulfur colloid, the extent of marrow involvement correlated well with the clinical and radiologic changes of the skeleton, but a normal pattern was found in the early stages of the disease. Bone scanning after inhalation of xenon gas has also been shown to correlate with disease activity.[15] Initially attempted in the belief that the Gaucher deposits would have xenon uptake characteristics similar to those of fat, it is now believed that the observed uptake is more likely due to increased blood flow in the affected marrow. ^{99m}Tc sestamibi (MIBI) has also been utilized to demonstrate glycolipid deposits in the bone marrow. Although MIBI scanning is a sensitive technique for detecting bone marrow deposits, it is unclear whether the observed uptake correlates well with clinical disease. Some studies suggest that MIBI scans are inadequate for early identification of patients at high risk for skeletal complications or for the follow-up of patients treated with enzyme replacement. Others, however, have found that a semiquantitative scintigraphic score was highly correlated with an overall clinical severity score index (SSI) and with various parameters contributing to the SSI, either positively or negatively. Scintigraphic score is most highly correlated with measurements of serum chitotriosidase, an overall biochemical marker of disease severity. Enzyme replacement therapy–naive patients showed high correlation of the scintigraphic score with the clinical SSI, with a radiographically based score, and with serum chitotriosidase. In patients receiving enzyme-replacement therapy the scintigraphic score was correlated with the clinical SSI, with hepatomegaly, and with hemoglobin.[21]

SYNOPSIS OF TREATMENT OPTIONS

Medical Treatment

Enzyme Replacement

Before the development of enzyme replacement therapy, treatment of Gaucher disease was mainly focused on symptomatic relief. However, enzyme replacement therapy makes it possible to reverse the manifestations of the disease itself. Alglucerase (Ceredase, Genzyme Corporation, Cambridge, MA) is a mannose-terminated form of glucocerebrosidase derived from human placentae and developed to treat patients with Gaucher disease. The first objective evidence (1992) that enzyme replacement therapy with alglucerase might be effective for treatment of bone disease was the report of one child treated for 2 years. Bone biopsies showed a progressive return to normal marrow and cortical thickness.[22] Since then, in vitro methods of protein production have led to creation of imiglucerase (Cerezyme, Genzyme Corporation, Cambridge MA), a synthetic enzyme with a more predictable composition.[2]

Enzyme replacement allows removal of the lipid metabolite whose accumulation causes the pathology. After implementation of therapy, improvements became evident within 6 months. Patients have increased hemoglobin levels and platelet counts and decreased incidence of epistaxis and bruising. Spleen and liver size are reduced, and skeletal symptoms improve. Children gain height, and most patients are able to resume work and daily activities. Enzyme replacement therapy is well tolerated, with few mild adverse reactions reported.[23]

Enzyme Replacement Therapy in Children

It appears clear that symptomatic children treated with enzyme replacement therapy will experience significant increases in skeletal growth and bone mineral density (BMD). Enzyme replacement therapy therefore has the potential to prevent serious and irreversible skeletal complications such as fractures and vertebral compression later in life.[24] Because early disease onset frequently heralds a poor prognosis, and because optimal doses of enzyme therapy can ensure adequate, potentially normal, development through childhood and adolescence, very few children diagnosed by signs and symptoms should go untreated.

Monitoring the Effects of Treatment

Imaging can be used to track the progress of improvement with enzyme replacement therapy. MRI demonstrates return of marrow fat in treated individuals.[18] Subsequently, response to enzyme replacement therapy has been repeatedly observed as a quantitative increase in signal intensity on T1-weighted images, even when it is not perceptible as a change in the pattern of marrow involvement.[25]

In our own work, the lipid composition of bone marrow, determined by direct chemical analysis, began to improve after 6 months of treatment at a time when noninvasive imaging studies showed no significant changes.

By 42 months, improvement in marrow composition was demonstrable on all noninvasive, quantitative imaging modalities (magnetic resonance score, quantitative xenon scintigraphy, and quantitative chemical shift imaging). Quantitative chemical shift imaging, the most sensitive technique, demonstrated a dramatic normalization of the marrow fat content in all patients. Net increases in either cortical or trabecular bone mass, as assessed by combined cortical thickness measurements and dual-energy quantitative CT, respectively, also occurred.[26] Other studies have also demonstrated modest improvement in patients treated for 2 years or more, and there have been a number of anecdotal reports of improvement.

Changes in the skeleton in response to enzyme replacement therapy have been most striking in children. In adults, the marrow response (increase in fat fraction) is similar. However, whether enzyme replacement produces demonstrable changes in the bone mass of adult skeletons has been controversial. In some reports there was little benefit, possibly because of the splenectomized state.[27]

Costs

Enzyme replacement therapy for Gaucher disease is among the most expensive of all drug regimens. Alternative approaches to lowering the cost of treatment include the use of lower dosages[28] and alternatives to this type of therapy.

It is unclear when in the course of the disease that enzyme replacement therapy should be implemented. In the opinion of some experts, it is important that patients be monitored closely and that enzyme replacement should be initiated before development of irreversible skeletal complications such as infarction and fibrosis.[29] Some evidence indicates that the vulnerable period is during childhood, adolescence, or early adulthood when there is the greatest risk of progression. There is a marked tendency for stabilization thereafter. This observation suggests that Gaucher disease is not necessarily a relentlessly progressive disorder but may become stable during adulthood.

There has been an effort to reach consensus recommendations for a comprehensive schedule of monitoring of all relevant aspects to confirm the achievement, maintenance, and continuity of the therapeutic response.[30] The current recommendations for enzyme replacement therapy suggest that adults at increased risk of complications and all affected children should begin therapy with an intravenous infusion of 60 units/kg every 2 weeks. Adults at lower risk may begin at a dose of 30 to 45 units/kg every 2 weeks. After clinical improvement, dose decreases may be considered in 15% to 25% increments every 3 to 6 months in higher-risk adults and children, with a minimum recommended maintenance dose of 30 units/kg

every 2 weeks; adults at lower risk can be maintained at a minimum of 20 units/kg every 2 weeks.[31]

Surgical Treatment

Surgical interventions continue to be required in the era of enzyme replacement therapy. Osteonecrosis of the joints—particularly the hips but also the knees and shoulders—and pathologic fractures of the long bones including the ribs, as well as episodic "crises" of bone pain in children and young adults, are common manifestations. Surgical interventions such as joint arthroplasties are important adjuvant treatments in this population. Surgical treatment may be complicated because of problems related to marrow insufficiency and increased risk of infection. Therefore, presurgical hematologic profiling plus antibiotic coverage are important.[32]

Because many patients are young, aseptic loosening of total hip arthroplasty may occur soon after operation. Osteotomy may be an alternative to arthroplasty for such individuals.[33]

Hypersplenism leading to thrombocytopenia and moderate immune compromise is a frequent complication of Gaucher disease, often requiring splenectomy. Partial splenic embolization may be performed to avoid the increased risk of serious infectious complications and deterioration of the disease associated with operative splenectomy.[4]

Efforts continue to be made to find a more "biologic" cure. Bone marrow transplantation has been successful in a small number of patients (although attended with the usual problems), suggesting that in advanced Gaucher disease bone marrow transplant may be an option if a human leukocyte antigen–identical related or unrelated donor is available.[34]

What the Referring Physician Needs to Know

- Sites and degrees of organ involvement
- Monitoring of changes in organ involvement to plan and monitor therapy
- Quantitative imaging techniques (other than dual-energy x-ray absorptiometry) have produced advances in understanding the disease but are probably not necessary for the management of the individual patient.
- Enzyme replacement therapy has been highly effective in suppressing the manifestations of Gaucher disease. For visceral disease, treatment can be withheld until symptoms warrant it. However, skeletal disease is difficult to reverse; therefore, prevention should be the goal.

SUGGESTED READINGS

Mankin HJ, Rosenthal DI, Xavier R. Gaucher disease. Curr Concepts Rev 2001; 83A:748-762.

Pastores GM, Weinreb NJ, Aerts H, et al. Therapeutic goals in the treatment of Gaucher disease. Semin Hematol 2004; 41(4 Suppl 5):4-14.

REFERENCES

1. Brady RO, Kanfer JN, Shapiro D. Metabolism of glucocerebrosides: II. Evidence of an enzymatic deficiency: Gaucher disease. Biochem Biophys Res Commun 1965; 18:221-225.
2. Mankin HJ, Rosenthal DI, Xavier R. Gaucher disease. Curr Concepts Rev 2001; 83A:748-762.
3. Hill SC, Damaska BM, Tsokos M, et al. Radiographic findings in type 3b Gaucher disease. Pediatr Radiol 1996; 26:852-860.
4. Thanopoulos BD, Frimas CA, Mantagos SP, Beratis NG. Gaucher disease: treatment of hypersplenism with splenic embolization. Acta Paediatr Scand 1987; 76:1003-1007.
5. Stowens DW, Teitelbaum SL, Kahn AJ, Barranger JA. Skeletal complications of Gaucher disease. Medicine (Baltimore) 1985; 64:310-322.
6. DeFriend DE, Brown AEM, Hutton CW, Hughes PM. Mannosidosis: an unusual cause of a deforming arthropathy. Skeletal Radiol 2000; 29:358-361.
7. Li JK, Birch PD, Davies AM. Proximal humeral defects in Gaucher disease. Br J Radiol 1988; 61:579-583.
8. Kaloterakis A, Cholongitas E, Pantelis E, et al. Type I Gaucher disease with severe skeletal destruction, extraosseous extension, and monoclonal gammopathy. Am J Hematol 2004; 77:377-380.
9. Hermann G, Shapiro R, Abdelwahab IF, et al. Extraosseous extension of Gaucher cell deposits mimicking malignancy. Skeletal Radiol 1994; 23:253-256.
10. Poll LW, Koch J-A, et al. Type I Gaucher disease: extraosseous extension of skeletal disease. Skeletal Radiol 2000; 29:15-21.
11. Fiore CE, Barone R, Pennisi P, et al. Bone ultrasonometry, bone density, and turnover markers in type 1 Gaucher disease. J Bone Miner Metab 2002; 20:34-38.
12. Charrow J, Andersson HC, Kaplan P, et al. Enzyme replacement therapy and monitoring for children with type 1 Gaucher disease: consensus recommendations. J Pediatr 2004; 144:112-120.
13. Rosenthal DI, Scott JA, Barranger J, et al. Evaluation of Gaucher disease using magnetic resonance imaging. J Bone Joint Surg Am 1986; 68:802-808.
14. Baur A, Stabler A, Lamerz R, et al. Light chain deposition disease in multiple myeloma: MR imaging features correlated with histopathological findings. Skeletal Radiol 1998; 27:173-176.
15. Rosenthal DI, Barton NW, McKusick KA, et al. Quantitative imaging of Gaucher disease. Radiology 1992; 185:841-845.
16. Hermann G, Shapiro RS, Abdelwahab IF, Grabowski G. MR imaging in adults with Gaucher disease type I: evaluation of marrow involvement and disease activity. Skeletal Radiol 1993; 22:247-251.
17. Vlieger EJP, Maas M, Akkerman EM, et al. The application of the vertebra-disc ratio in a population of patients with Gaucher disease [Abstract]. Proc Intl Soc Magn Reson Med 2000; 8:2131.
18. Johnson L, Hoppel B, Gerard E, et al. Quantitative chemical shift imaging of vertebral bone marrow in patients with Gaucher disease. Radiology 1992; 182:451-455.
19. Terk MR, Esplin J, Lee K, et al. MR imaging of patients with type I Gaucher disease: relationship between bone and visceral changes. AJR Am J Roentgenol 1995; 165:599-604.
20. Maas M, Hollak CEM, Akkerman EM, et al. Quantification of skeletal involvement in adults with type I Gaucher disease: fat fraction measured by Dixon quantitative chemical shift imaging as a valid parameter. AJR Am J Roentgenol 2002; 179:961-965.
21. Mariani G, Filocamo M, Giona F, et al. Severity of bone marrow involvement in patients with Gaucher disease evaluated by scintigraphy with ^{99m}Tc-sestamibi. J Nucl Med 2003; 44:1253-1262.
22. Barton NW, Brady RO, Dambrosia JM, et al. Dose-dependent responses to macrophage-targeted glucocerebrosidase in a child with Gaucher disease. J Pediatr 1992; 120(2 pt 1):277-280.
23. Whittington R, Goa KL. Alglucerase: a review of its therapeutic use in Gaucher disease. Drugs 1992; 44:72-93.
24. Bembi B, Ciana G, Mengel E, et al. Bone complications in children with Gaucher disease. Br J Radiol 2002; 75(Suppl 1): A37-A44.
25. Poll LW, Koch J-A, vom Dahl S, et al. Magnetic resonance imaging of bone marrow changers in Gaucher disease during enzyme replacement therapy: first German long-term results. Skeletal Radiol 2001; 30:496-503.
26. Rosenthal DI, Doppelt SH, Mankin HJ, et al. Enzyme replacement therapy for Gaucher disease: skeletal responses to macrophage-targeted glucocerebrosidase. Pediatrics 1995; 96(4 pt 1):629-637.
27. Schiffmann R, Mankin H, Dambrosia JM, et al. Decreased bone density in splenectomized Gaucher patients receiving enzyme replacement therapy. Blood Cells Mol Dis 2002; 28:288-296.
28. Figueroa ML, Rosenbloom BE, Kay AC, et al. A less costly regimen of alglucerase to treat Gaucher disease. N Engl J Med 1992; 327:1632-1636.
29. Pastores GM, Patel MJ, Firooznia H. Bone and joint complications related to Gaucher disease. Curr Rheumatol Rep 2000; 2:175-180.
30. Pastores GM, Weinreb NJ, Aerts H, et al. Therapeutic goals in the treatment of Gaucher disease. Semin Hematol 2004; 41(4 Suppl 5):4-14.
31. Andersson HC, Charrow J, Kaplan P, et al. Individualization of long-term enzyme replacement therapy for Gaucher disease.[erratum appears in Genet Med 2005 Jul-Aug;7(6):460]. Genet Med 2005; 7:105-110.
32. Itzchaki M, Lebel E, Dweck A, et al. Orthopedic considerations in Gaucher disease since the advent of enzyme replacement therapy. Acta Orthop Scand 2004; 75:641-653.
33. Iwase T, Hasegawa Y, Iwata H. Transtrochanteric anterior rotational osteotomy for Gaucher disease: a case report. Clin Orthop Relat Res 1995; (317):122-125.
34. Ringden O, Groth CG, Erikson A, et al. Ten years' experience of bone marrow transplantation for Gaucher disease. Transplantation 1995; 59:864-870.

CHAPTER 80

Storage Diseases (Mucopolysaccharidoses/ Glycogenoses)

Calvin Ma and Rodrigo Dominguez

Lysosomal storage diseases are a group of inborn errors of metabolic disorders characterized by accumulation of incompletely metabolized substrates inside lysosomes due to deficiency in one of the numerous enzymes required for substrate degradation. They comprise more than 30 different syndromes and are generally divided into lipidoses, glycogenoses, and mucopolysaccharidoses. Most of these disorders are severely debilitating and lead to premature death. The focus of this chapter is on mucopolysaccharidoses and glycogenoses. Only the clinical and radiographic findings are discussed. Detailed biochemical and pathophysiologic aspects of each disorder are extensively covered in many articles and textbooks, some of which are listed in the suggested readings and references at the end of this chapter.

ETIOLOGY

Mucopolysaccharidoses

Mucopolysaccharidoses (MPS) result from the absence or defect of enzymes required for the breakdown of glycosaminoglycan (GAG), also formerly known as mucopolysaccharide. GAGs are long-chain carbohydrates that contribute to the formation of bones, cartilage, tendons, corneas, skin, and connective tissues. A deficiency in one of the enzymes that break down GAG will result in intracellular substrate accumulation, leading to structural and functional abnormalities at the cellular and tissue level. The specific enzyme deficiencies that lead to a specific substrate accumulation and their corresponding syndromes are listed in Table 80-1.[1] The mucopolysaccharidoses are inherited in an autosomal recessive pattern, with the exception of MPS II (Hunter syndrome), which is inherited in an X-linked recessive mode.

Glycogenoses

The glycogenoses (glycogen storage diseases, GSD) are another group of lysosomal storage disorders that result from deficiency in enzymes required for the breakdown of glycogen. Failure to completely metabolize glycogen results in accumulation and storage of glycogen substrates in lysosomes of hepatic and muscle tissues where glycogen is most abundant. These tissues are therefore most commonly and severely affected by the glycogen storage disorders. The specific enzyme deficiency and its associated syndromes are summarized in Table 80-2.[2-4] The glycogenoses are inherited in an autosomal recessive pattern, with the exception of type IX in which several subtypes are inherited as an X-linked pattern.

PREVALENCE AND EPIDEMIOLOGY

The incidence for all types of mucopolysaccharidoses is estimated to be 1 in 25,000 births.[5] There is no known racial or gender predilection for any of these disorders

KEY POINTS

- Mucopolysaccharidoses are progressive disorders involving multiple organs, including the brain, liver, spleen, heart, and blood vessels; and many are associated with coarse facial features, clouding of the cornea, and mental retardation.
- Glycogenoses are also progressive disorders involving multiple organs, but the liver and skeletal muscles are most commonly and severely affected. Most types of glycogenoses are associated with some degree of hepatomegaly or muscle weakness.

TABLE 80-1   Mucopolysaccharidoses

Type	Enzyme Deficiency	Substrate Accumulated
MPS I H-Hurler	α-L-Iduronidase	Heparan sulfate
MPS I H/S-Hurler-Scheie		Dermatan sulfate
MPS I S-Scheie		
MPS II-Hunter	Iduronidate sulfatase	Heparan sulfate
		Dermatan sulfate
MPS IIIA-Sanfilippo A	Heparan-N-sulfatase	Heparan sulfate
MPS IIIB-Sanfilippo B	N-Acetyl-α-glucosaminidase	
MPS IIIC-Sanfilippo C	α-Glucosaminidase	
MPS IIID-Sanfilippo D	N-Acetylglucosamine-6-sulfate	
MPS IV-Morquio	N-Acetylgalactosamine-6-sulfatase	Keratan sulfate, chondroitin sulfate
MPS VI-Maroteaux-Lamy	Arylsulfatase B	Dermatan sulfate
MPS VII-Sly	β-Glucuronidase	Heparan sulfate
		Dermatan sulfate
MPS IX-Natowicz	Hyaluronidase	Chondroitin sulfate

Data from Neufeld EF, Muenzer J. The mucopolysaccharidoses. In Scriver C, Beaudet AL, Valle D, Sly W (eds). The Metabolic and Molecular Bases of Inherited Disease, 8th ed. New York, McGraw-Hill, 2001, vol 3, pp 3421–3452.

TABLE 80-2   Glycogen Storage Diseases

Type	Enzyme Deficiency	Target Organ	Key Clinical Findings
I: von Gierke, hepatorenal glycogenosis	Ia: Glucose-6-phosphatase Ib: Glucose-6-phosphate translocase	Liver, spleen, kidney, intestines, leukocytes	Hypoglycemia, hyperuricemia, hyperlipidemia, lactic acidosis, hepatosplenomegaly, nephromegaly
II: Pompe, acid maltase deficiency	α-1,4-Glucosidase (acid maltase)	Heart, skeletal muscles	Hypotonia, cardiomyopathy
III: Forbes-Cori, limit dextrinosis	Amylo-1,6-glucosidase (debrancher)	Liver, heart, muscle, leukocytes	Hypotonia, hepatomegaly, cirrhosis, fasting ketosis
IV: Andersen, amylopectinosis	Amylo-1,4-1,6-transglucosidase (debrancher)	Liver	Hepatomegaly, cirrhosis
V: McArdle	Muscle phosphorylase	Skeletal muscles	Exercise intolerance, rhabdomyolysis, renal failure
VI: Hers	Liver phosphorylase	Liver, leukocytes	Hepatomegaly, mild hypoglycemia
VII: Tarui	Phosphofructokinase	Skeletal muscles, erythrocytes	Exercise intolerance, rhabdomyolysis, renal failure
IX	Liver phosphorylase kinase	Liver, skeletal muscles, heart, erythrocytes	Hepatomegaly, hyperlipidemia, fasting ketosis

Data from references 2 to 4.

except for Hunter syndrome (MPS II), which is inherited as X-linked recessive and thus predominantly affects males.

The cumulative incidence of glycogen storage diseases is estimated to be around 1:20,000 to 1:25,000 births.[4] There are no racial differences for most of the glycogen storage diseases. However, the highest incidence for GSD III has been recorded in non-Ashkenazi Jews in northern Africa, and GSD VI has been most commonly reported in Japanese and Ashkenazi Jews. There is no gender preference except for subtypes of GSD IX that are inherited in an X-linked pattern in which mostly male patients are affected.

CLINICAL PRESENTATION

Mucopolysaccharidoses[6-11]

Hurler Syndrome (MPS I H)

Hurler syndrome is the most severe form and one of the most commonly encountered mucopolysaccharidoses. Infants with Hurler syndrome usually appear normal at birth and are not diagnosed until early in their second year of life. Clinical features begin to develop after 6 to 12 months with coarsening of facial features. The head is enlarged with widely spaced eyes, corneal clouding, frontal bossing, flattened nasal bridge, everted lips, protruded tongue, and widely separated and hypoplastic teeth. Umbilical or inguinal hernias may be present. Hepatosplenomegaly results in a protuberant abdomen. Lumbar gibbus leads to a stooped posture accentuated by flexion contractures of the hip and knee joints. Flexion contracture of the hand leads to claw hand deformity, stiff joints, and carpal tunnel syndrome. Mucopolysaccharide deposition in the trachea, nasopharynx, and esophagus leads to aerodigestive tract obstruction with persistent rhinitis, adenotonsillar hypertrophy, sleep apnea, recurrent upper respiratory tract infection, and feeding difficulties.[12] Deposition in cardiac valves and coronary arteries eventually results in valvular dysfunction, coronary artery disease, and ischemic cardiomyopathy.[13] Deposition in the leptomeninges leads to communicating hydrocephalus and an enlarged cranium with sutural diastasis. Growth disturbance results in severe dwarfism. There is progressive mental deterioration. These children eventually die between 10 and 15 years of age from pneumonia or cardiac failure. Many of the other mucopolysaccharidoses, with the exception of MPS IV or Morquio syndrome, have clinical and radiographic findings similar to Hurler syndrome, although with different degrees of severity (Fig. 80-1).

Scheie Syndrome (MPS I S)

Scheie syndrome is the least severe form of the MPS I group. There is nearly normal height, intellect, and life span, although the life span may be somewhat shortened by the presence of aortic valve disease, which is seen in almost all cases. Somatic presentations include corneal clouding, joint stiffness, and carpal tunnel syndrome. Psychosis is common.

Hurler-Scheie Syndrome (MPS I H/S)

Hurler-Scheie syndrome is intermediate in severity between Hurler syndrome and Scheie syndrome. The clinical and skeletal features more closely resemble those of Hurler syndrome, but the patients survive slightly longer into their 20s and the psychomotor retardation and dwarfism are less severe.

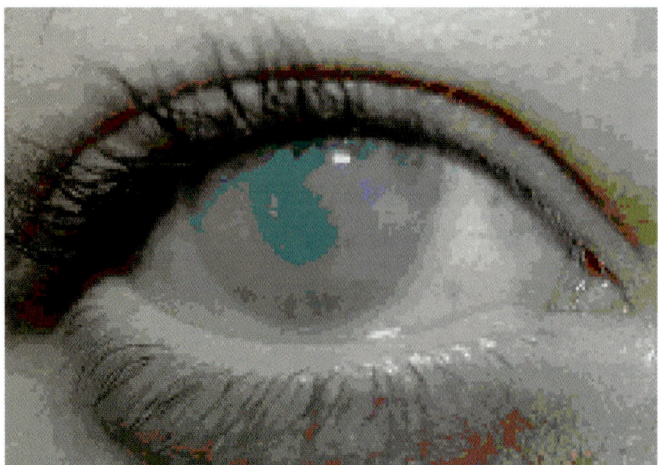

■ **FIGURE 80-1** Corneal clouding in Hurler syndrome. *(From Ashworth JL, Biswas S, Wraith E, Lloyd IC. Mucopolysaccharidoses and the eye. Surv Ophthalmol 2006; 51:7. Copyright 2006 by Elsevier, with permission.)*

Hunter Syndrome (MPS II)

Hunter syndrome is the only mucopolysaccharidosis that is X-linked recessive. The clinical features are similar to those of Hurler syndrome but less severe. Coarse facies, hepatosplenomegaly, growth failure, and joint stiffness occur later than in Hurler syndrome. Psychomotor retardation is less severe. Seizures are common. Corneal clouding is not apparent but can be detected on slit-lamp examination. Half of the children become deaf. Cutaneous nodules over the scapula and upper back are uniquely seen with Hunter syndrome. The patients are typically diagnosed around 2½ to 5 years old. Patients with the severe form of Hunter syndrome usually die in 10 to 15 years secondary to cardiac causes, and those with the mild form may survive to the fourth decade or later.

Sanfilippo Syndrome (MPS III)

The Sanfilippo syndrome can result from four different enzyme deficiencies (see Table 80-1) that lead to accumulation of the same substrate—heparan sulfate—and result in clinically indistinguishable features. The patients appear normal until 3 to 5 years old when there is progressive and profound mental deterioration, which is the most striking feature in this mucopolysaccharide group. There are learning difficulties and behavioral disturbances characterized by severe hyperactivity and aggression. Seizures are common. The patients do not have dwarfism and do not have cardiac disease. Corneal clouding is minimal and detected on slit-lamp examination. Joint stiffness is mild. Other clinical and skeletal changes are similar to those of Hurler syndrome and Hunter syndrome but milder. Most patients die between 10 and 30 years of age.

Morquio Syndrome (MPS IV)

Previously, Morquio syndrome was divided into types A and B, with both types thought to occur from defects in separate enzymes. However, MPS IVB is now considered a variant of GM_1-gangliosidosis. Morquio syndrome does not closely resemble other mucopolysaccharide disorders; it has distinctive skeletal manifestations that are usually diagnostic. Morquio syndrome is usually not apparent at birth but can be diagnosed by 1 year old. There is striking dwarfism, with height rarely exceeding 4 feet in adult life. Intelligence is normal; mental retardation is rare. The cornea is slightly clouded and only detectable on slit-lamp examination. The head is of normal size. Morquio syndrome is one of the most commonly encountered mucopolysaccharidoses, along with Hurler syndrome.

Maroteaux-Lamy Syndrome (MPS VI)

The striking clinical features of this syndrome are dwarfism and corneal clouding without mental impairment. The somatic and skeletal changes are very similar to those of Hurler syndrome. Patients have coarse facial features, hepatosplenomegaly, inguinal hernias, severe cardiac abnormalities, hydrocephalus, and hearing defects. Growth slows down at 4 years old and stops completely by 8 years of age, resulting in severe dwarfism.

Sly Syndrome (MPS VII)

The clinical and radiographic findings of Sly syndrome are similar to those of Hurler syndrome, but there is great variation in severity. In general, there is restricted growth and mental development. Sly syndrome often presents as nonimmune hydrops fetalis, and the patients rarely survive more than a few months.

Natowicz Syndrome (MPS IX)

There has only been one patient reported to date with this syndrome. Mild short stature and periarticular soft tissue masses were noted, but there were no neurologic or ocular findings.[14]

Glycogenoses

Glycogen is most abundantly found in the liver and skeletal muscles. Consequently, these organs are most commonly and seriously affected by the glycogen storage diseases.[2,3,4,9,15,16] A disorder in hepatic glycogen metabolism results in fasting hypoglycemia, seizures, hepatomegaly, and, in some types, cirrhosis of the liver. A disorder in muscle glycogen metabolism results in muscle weakness, cramps, and exercise intolerance. A summary of the enzyme deficiency of each specific glycogen storage disease and the target organs with key clinical findings is provided in Table 80-2.

von Gierke Disease (GSD I)

Type I glycogenosis, also called von Gierke disease, presents early in infancy with hypoglycemia, lactic acidosis, and marked hepatomegaly. Severe hypoglycemia results in seizures. Hepatomegaly results in a protuberant abdomen and may be the first sign noted by the mother. Splenomegaly and nephromegaly may be seen. Hyperuricemia also develops and predisposes to gouty arthritis, which is found later in life around puberty along with uric acid renal stones. Hyperlipidemia is also present and manifests as skin xanthomas in the extremities and predisposes to pancreatitis. Easy bruising and epistaxis are common as a result of impaired platelet aggregation and adhesion. Hepatic adenomas develop in most patients by their second or third decades of life. Growth retardation results in short stature, and puberty is delayed. Osteoporosis is present, with frequent fractures reported. Other late complications include renal disease, renal stones, and hypertension. A variant of GSD I known as type Ib is caused by a deficiency in glucose-6-phosphate translocase. In addition to these clinical findings, von Gierke disease is further characterized by neutropenia and presents as recurrent bacterial infections and chronic inflammatory diseases such as inflammatory bowel disease with oral lesions and intestinal ulcers.

Pompe Disease (GSD II)

Type II glycogenosis, or Pompe disease, has three different clinical phenotypes: classic or infantile form (type IIa), juvenile form (type IIb), and adult form (type IIc). The classic or infantile form presents early in infancy as profound hypotonia and muscle weakness manifesting as respiratory and feeding difficulties. Cardiomegaly, cardio-

myopathy, and heart failure are prominent. Macroglossia and hepatomegaly may be noted. These patients typically die in the first year of life. Despite the hypotonia and flaccidity, the muscles in these patients are actually firm and even hypertrophic. The juvenile form presents later in infancy after age 6 to 12 months and may have both cardiac enlargement and muscle weakness or muscle involvement only without cardiomegaly. Muscle weakness is predominantly proximal. Patients may have recurrent pneumonia due to respiratory muscle weakness. Death is usually in the first decade of life. In the adult form, the disease course is milder and more slowly progressive, with symptoms beginning from the second to sixth decades. There is progressive myopathy in striated muscles that may eventually lead to paralysis of diaphragmatic muscles and death. The heart is not affected in the adult form.

Forbes-Cori Disease (GSD III)

Type III glycogenosis, also known as Forbes-Cori disease or limit dextrinosis, results from a deficiency of glycogen debranching enzyme activity, resulting in impaired release of glucose from glycogen. GSD III shares many similar clinical features with GSD I, but the symptoms are milder and most patients with type III disease survive longer. During infancy and childhood, GSD III may be clinically indistinguishable from GSD I, with hypoglycemia, hepatomegaly, hyperlipidemia, and growth retardation as the predominant clinical findings. Splenomegaly may be seen, but the kidneys are not enlarged in type III disease. Unlike type I disease, lactic acid and uric acid levels are normal in GSD III. On the other hand, elevated levels of liver transaminases are prominent and progressive liver cirrhosis and failure may occur. In adults, progressive muscle weakness and distal muscle wasting can become severe after the third or fourth decade. Fasting ketosis is a common finding in this type of glycogenosis.

Andersen Disease (GSD IV)

Type IV glycogenosis, also called Andersen disease or amylopectinosis, is another disease resulting from deficiency of a debranching enzyme. It is very rare and typically presents in the first few months of life as hepatomegaly, splenomegaly, and failure to thrive. The infant develops progressive hepatic cirrhosis and subsequently portal hypertension, ascites, and esophageal varices. Most patients die before 5 years of age.

McArdle Disease (GSD V)

Type V glycogenosis, known as McArdle disease, exclusively involves skeletal muscles and restricts physical activity. Clinical symptoms typically present in young adulthood with complaints of muscle cramps and exercise intolerance. These patients may report lack of endurance and weakness since childhood. They are unable to sustain brief intense activities such as sprinting or carrying heavy loads and less intense but sustained activities such as climbing stairs or walking up a hill. However, they are able to sustain exercises that are moderate in intensity at their own pace. Rhabdomyolysis with myoglobinuria and even acute renal failure may develop after vigorous exercise.

Hers Disease (GSD VI)

Type VI glycogenosis, or Hers disease, shares many features with type I but is milder and has a benign course. The patients present with hepatomegaly and growth retardation early in childhood. They may have mild hypoglycemia, hyperlipidemia, and hyperketosis. Unlike GSD I, lactic acid and uric acid are normal. The heart and skeletal muscles are not affected in Hers disease. The hepatomegaly usually regresses by puberty.

Tarui Disease (GSD VII)

Type VII glycogenosis, also known as Tarui disease, is clinically similar to GSD V but results from a deficiency in a different enzyme. The patients present with fatigue and pain with exercise. Vigorous activities will result in muscle cramps and rhabdomyolysis. However, compared with McArdle disease, the exercise intolerance is seen at a younger age in childhood and is more severe. A compensated hemolytic anemia also occurs in this disease. Hyperuricemia is often seen and exaggerated by exercise.

GSD IX

Type IX glycogenosis has many subtypes, but the most common form of type IX is liver phosphorylase kinase deficiency, which accounts for 75% of all cases and is X-linked, unlike the rest of the GSD types. Patients present with growth retardation, hepatomegaly, mild hyperlipidemia, and fasting ketosis. These clinical findings disappear with time, and most adults are asymptomatic. Although initially presenting with growth retardation, most patients reach a final normal adult height.

PATHOPHYSIOLOGY

Briefly, the lysosomal storage diseases result from a deficiency in one of the many enzymes required for substrate degradation. Absence of any one of the enzymes in the sequence of substrate metabolism results in an incompletely digested product that accumulates within lysosomes, cells, and tissues, altering the structural and biomechanical properties of the affected tissue.

MANIFESTATIONS OF THE DISEASE: MUCOPOLYSACCHARIDOSES

With the exception of Morquio syndrome, the skeletal abnormalities of the mucopolysaccharidoses are qualitatively similar and referred to as dysostosis multiplex.[6–10,17–22] They have varying degrees of dysostosis multiplex. Radiographic abnormalities are not present at birth but generally can be seen by 2 years of age. The mucopolysaccharidoses that have significant skeletal manifestations include MPS I, II, IV, VI, and VII.

Radiography

Hurler Syndrome (MPS I H)

Skull

The skull is normal at birth with the earliest changes noted after 6 months. The skull will usually enlarge due

to communicating hydrocephalus or arachnoid cysts. Diastasis of the coronal sutures may be observed. There is usually a scaphocephalic configuration due to premature fusion of the sagittal and lambdoid sutures. There is frontal bossing and calvarial thickening. Deepening of the optic chiasm recess results in a J-shaped sella turcica. The mandible is thickened and short, the mandibular angle is widened, the rami are short, and the condyles are flat or concave secondary to hypoplasia. The teeth are hypoplastic and widely spaced (Fig. 80-2).

Chest

The ribs are oar-shaped and wider than the intercostal spaces but become narrower in the paravertebral region. The clavicles are short and thick medially and hook-shaped laterally. The scapulas are small and irregular. The glenoid fossa may be hypoplastic. Tracheal narrowing may be observed on the chest radiograph (Fig. 80-3).

Spine

A thoracolumbar gibbus deformity usually develops by age 18 months due to hypoplasia of the anterosuperior aspect of the vertebral body at the thoracolumbar junction, which gives an anteroinferior beaking appearance. The other vertebral bodies have short anteroposterior diameter with concave anterior and posterior surfaces. The vertebral bodies are ovoid with convex superior and inferior end plates. The spinous process is dysplastic (Fig. 80-4). Odontoid hypoplasia, a characteristic feature of Morquio syndrome, has been described in Hurler syndrome and a few other mucopolysaccharidoses.[23] Under fluoroscopy, dynamic craniovertebral junction instability may be observed secondary to odontoid hypoplasia and ligamentous laxity (see Fig. 80-8).

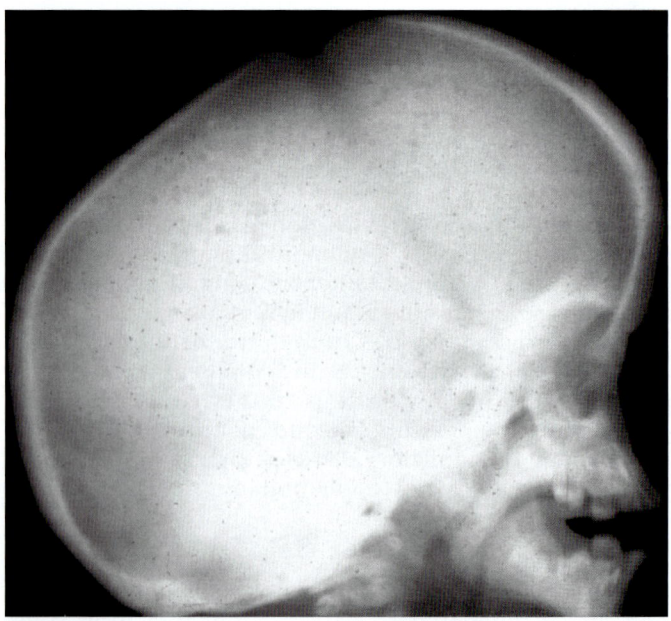

■ **FIGURE 80-2** Hurler syndrome. The cranium is enlarged with premature fusion of the sagittal and lambdoid sutures, resulting in a scaphocephalic configuration. The sella turcica is J shaped. The mandibular rami are short, and the mandibular angle is widened. The teeth are hypoplastic and widely spaced.

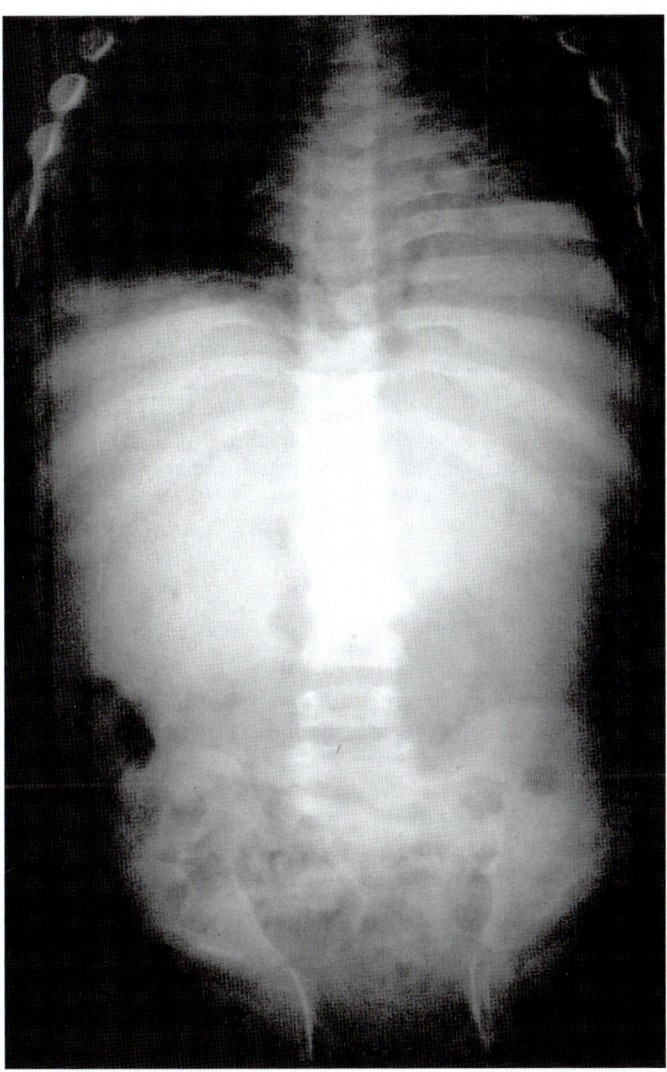

■ **FIGURE 80-3**   Hurler syndrome. The ribs are oar-shaped and wider than the intercostal spaces but become narrower in the paravertebral region. The iliac wings of the pelvis are flared, and the iliac body is constricted inferiorly.

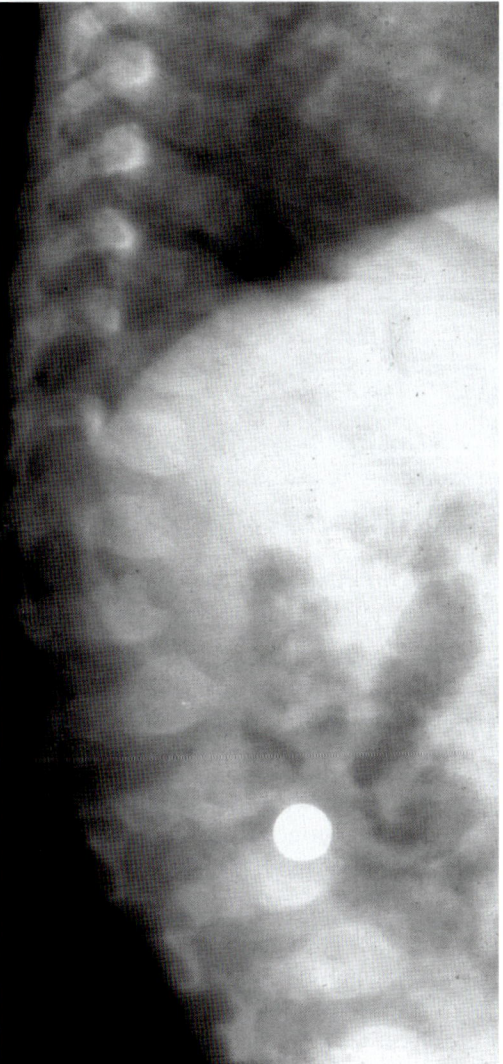

■ **FIGURE 80-4**   Hurler syndrome. There is hypoplasia of the anterosuperior aspect of the vertebral body at the thoracolumbar junction resulting in an anteroinferior beaking appearance. The other vertebral bodies have a short anteroposterior dimension and are ovoid with concave anterior and posterior margins and convex superior and inferior end plates. Thoracolumbar gibbus deformity is typically present in Hurler syndrome.

Pelvis

The iliac wings are flared, and the iliac body is constricted inferiorly. The acetabula are oblique (Figs. 80-3, 80-5). Coxa valga is frequently seen, but dislocation of the hip is uncommon (see Fig. 80-5).

Hand

The carpal bones are small and irregular. The metacarpals and proximal and middle phalanges are short and wide without normal diaphyseal constrictions. The second to fifth metacarpal bones are tapered and pointed proximally. The distal phalanges are hypoplastic (Fig. 80-6). There is coarse bony trabeculation. Flexion contracture of the hand results in a claw hand deformity.

Long Bones

There is defective modeling in the long bones with diaphyseal widening. The upper extremities are generally affected more than the lower extremities. Proximal

humeral constriction leads to varus configuration of humeral heads. The long tubular bones are short and poorly modeled. The diaphyses are wide, whereas the metaphyses are concomitantly constricted. The humeral neck is in varus configuration. The distal radius and ulna are tilted toward each other (see Fig. 80-6).

The Other Mucopolysaccharidoses (Except Morquio Syndrome)

In Scheie syndrome, the radiographic findings are minimal. The skeleton and stature are almost normal. There are mild hypoplastic and cystic deformities of the carpal bones and base of the metacarpophalangeal bones. There is a claw hand deformity. In Hurler-Scheie syndrome the dysostosis multiplex is moderate. In Hunter syndrome there is moderate dysostosis multiplex in the classic form and mild dys-

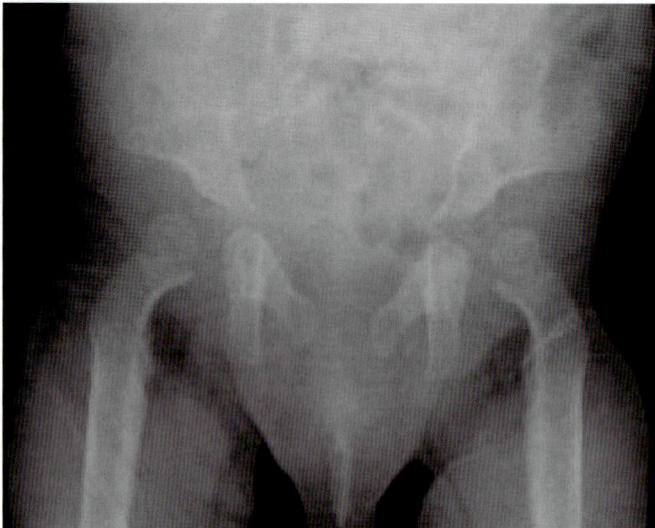

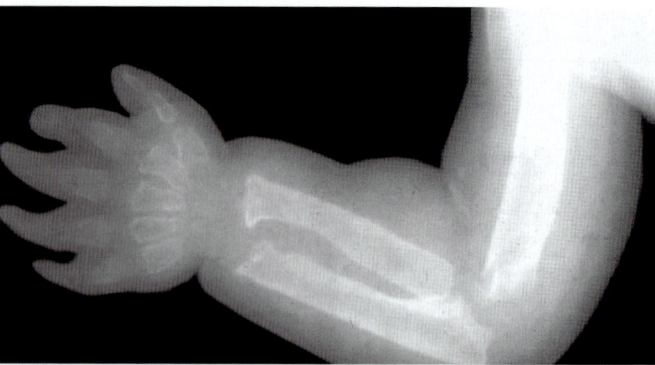

■ **FIGURE 80-6** Hurler syndrome. The metacarpal bones are tapered and pointed proximally. The distal phalanges and carpal bones are hypoplastic. There is defective modeling of the long bones with diaphyseal widening, with the upper extremities generally affected more than the lower extremities. The distal radius and ulna are tilted toward each other.

■ **FIGURE 80-5** Hurler syndrome. The iliac wings are flared with constriction of the iliac body inferiorly. The acetabula are oblique. Coxa valga is observed.

ostosis in the mild form of the disease. However, unlike in Hurler syndrome, gibbus deformity and coxa valga are not usually seen. The calvaria is normal, and the sella turcica is also normal. In Sanfilippo syndrome, the dysostosis multiplex may be mild. However, marked hyperostosis of the parietal and occipital bones, normal sella turcica, and sclerotic nonpneumatized mastoids are commonly observed. Morquio syndrome has distinctive skeletal findings (see later). Maroteaux-Lamy syndrome has skeletal changes that are very similar to those of Hurler syndrome but with varying severity. There is characteristic deficient ossification of the superior portion of femoral capital epiphyses in most children, and this may be misdiagnosed as Legg-Calvé-Perthes disease or cretinism. In later stages of the disorder, the femoral heads are flat and wide (coxa plana, coxa magna). Coxa valga is observed. Joint restriction at the hips, knees, and elbows is common. Pectus carinatum is also observed. In Sly syndrome there is great variability in the radiographic findings.

Morquio Syndrome (MPS IV)

Unlike the other mucopolysaccharidoses, Morquio syndrome has distinctive skeletal findings. In the spine there is universal vertebra plana or platyspondyly, which can be distinguished from the oval vertebral bodies of Hurler and other mucopolysaccharidoses. In addition, the anterior beaking in Morquio is central, compared with the inferior beaking in Hurler syndrome (Fig. 80-7). Odontoid hypoplasia is characteristic of Morquio syndrome, with associated ligamentous laxity potentially resulting in atlantoaxial subluxation and spinal cord compression (Fig. 80-8). Cervical cord compression from atlantoaxial instability was a major cause of death in Morquio syndrome, but nowadays patients often undergo elective cervical fusion so they can survive to their third or fourth decades, where they often die of respiratory complication. Another characteristic finding is a fixed pectus carinatum deformity with restriction of chest wall motion. In the upper extremities, ulnar deviation may

be seen secondary to shortening of the ulna. The articular surfaces of the distal radius and ulna are angled toward each other. The carpal bones are small and irregular, the scaphoid does not ossify, and the metacarpal bones are short. The metaphyseal ends of the bones are widened and the epiphyseal ends are irregular. There is brachydactyly. In the pelvis, there is flaring of the iliac wings with sloping acetabular roofs beginning at 1 year old. The body of the iliac bones becomes very constricted inferiorly. The developing femoral capital epiphyses show early compression. The epiphyses initially appear fragmented and eventually disappear. The femoral necks become progressively wider and are eroded. Coxa valga increases. The lower limbs also include prominent features such as pes planus and genu valgum, with the latter resulting from hypoplasia of the lateral portions of the proximal tibial epiphyses. There are flexion deformities of both knees and hips, resulting in a semicrouching stance. The long bones are characterized by diaphyseal constriction with abrupt metaphyseal widening (Figs. 80-7 and 80-8).

Although certain types of mucopolysaccharidoses may have prominent features that suggest one type over another, urinary testing for excretion of mucopolysaccharides should be performed when the disorder is suspected. Confirmation is made by demonstration of specific enzyme deficiency in peripheral blood leukocytes or fibroblast cells.

Magnetic Resonance Imaging

Magnetic resonance imaging is usually obtained of the brain and cervical spine, with particular attention made to the craniocervical junction. The odontoid may be hypoplastic, predisposing the patient to atlantoaxial instability. In addition, thickening of the dura mater can result in cord compression. On T1-weighted images, there is hypointense to isointense periodontoid soft tissue mass and hypointense thickened dura. On T2-weighted images, the hypoplastic dens, periodontoid soft tissue mass, and thickened dura are hypointense. If cord compression is present, there is hyperintense signal within the cord.

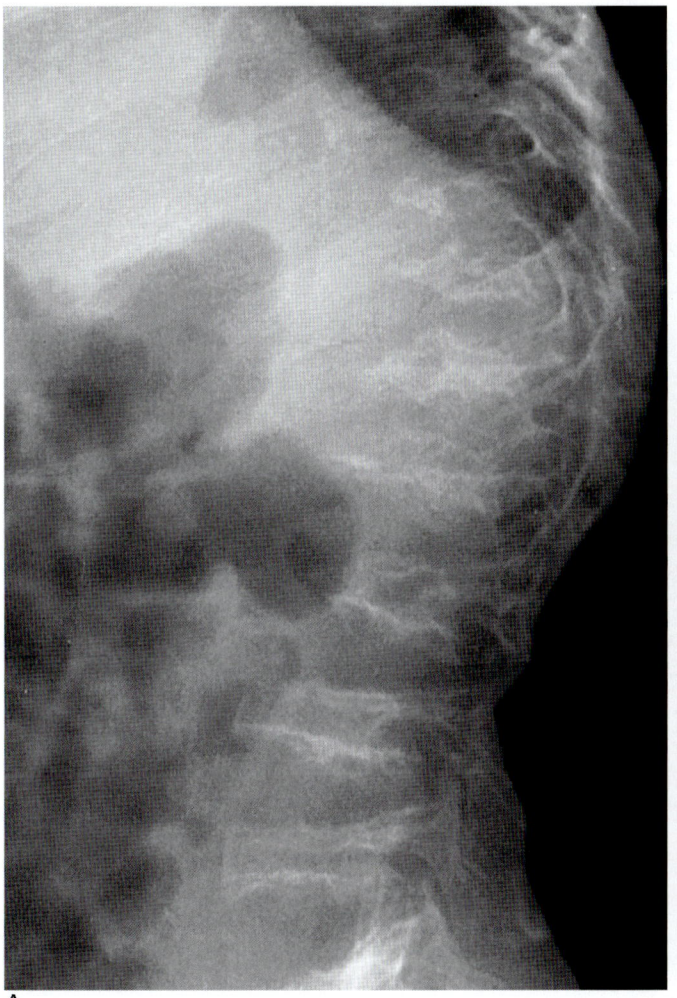
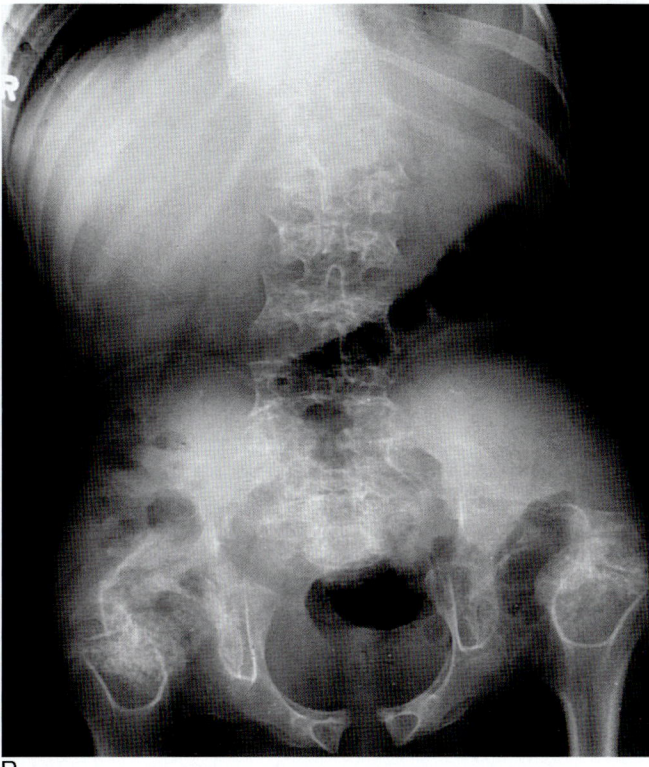

A B

■ **FIGURE 80-7** Morquio syndrome. **A,** There is universal vertebra plana, or flattened vertebral bodies. This can be distinguished from the ovoid vertebral bodies of Hurler syndrome and other mucopolysaccharidoses. The central anterior beaking of Morquio syndrome also differs from the anteroinferior beaking of Hurler syndrome and other mucopolysaccharidoses. **B,** Note again the platyspondyly of the vertebral bodies and the severe changes in the hip. *(From Resnick D. Osteochondrodysplasias, dysostoses, chromosomal aberrations, mucopolysaccharidoses, and mucolipidoses. In Resnick D, Kransdorf MJ [eds]. Bone and Joint Imaging, 3rd ed. Philadelphia, Elsevier, 2005, pp 1321, 1323.)*

On contrast-enhanced T1-weighted images, no abnormal enhancement is seen (Fig. 80-9).

Multidetector Computed Tomography

On CT images of the cervical spine, central and foraminal narrowing may be observed at the craniovertebral junction. In severe cases, compression on the cord may be observed. On contrast-enhanced CT, there is marked dural thickening without or with only mild enhancement.[24] Abnormal dens ossification may also be noted (Fig. 80-10).

MANIFESTATONS OF THE DISEASE: GLYCOGENOSES

Unlike mucopolysaccharidoses, glycogenoses do not involve many skeletal changes. The bone changes are nonspecific.[2,9,25]

Radiography

The radiograph may demonstrate osteopenia, as evidenced by thinned cortices, expansion of medullary cavities, and loss of trabeculation. Fractures are frequently seen as a result of osteopenia and hypoglycemic seizures. Bone maturation is retarded. Multiple growth arrest lines may be seen. Scalloping of the anterior surface of the thoracolumbar vertebral bodies (T11-L2) has been reported in several types of glycogenoses. Exaggerated lumbosacral lordosis or scoliosis may be seen. Nutrient foramina may be prominent in the middle phalanx of the third finger. Failure of constriction of the metaphysis of tubular bones has been described in some cases. In other cases there is overconstriction of the long bones. Spiculation of the physeal plate was seen in all types except GSD II. Patients with type I disease may develop gouty arthritis secondary to long-standing hyperuricemia.

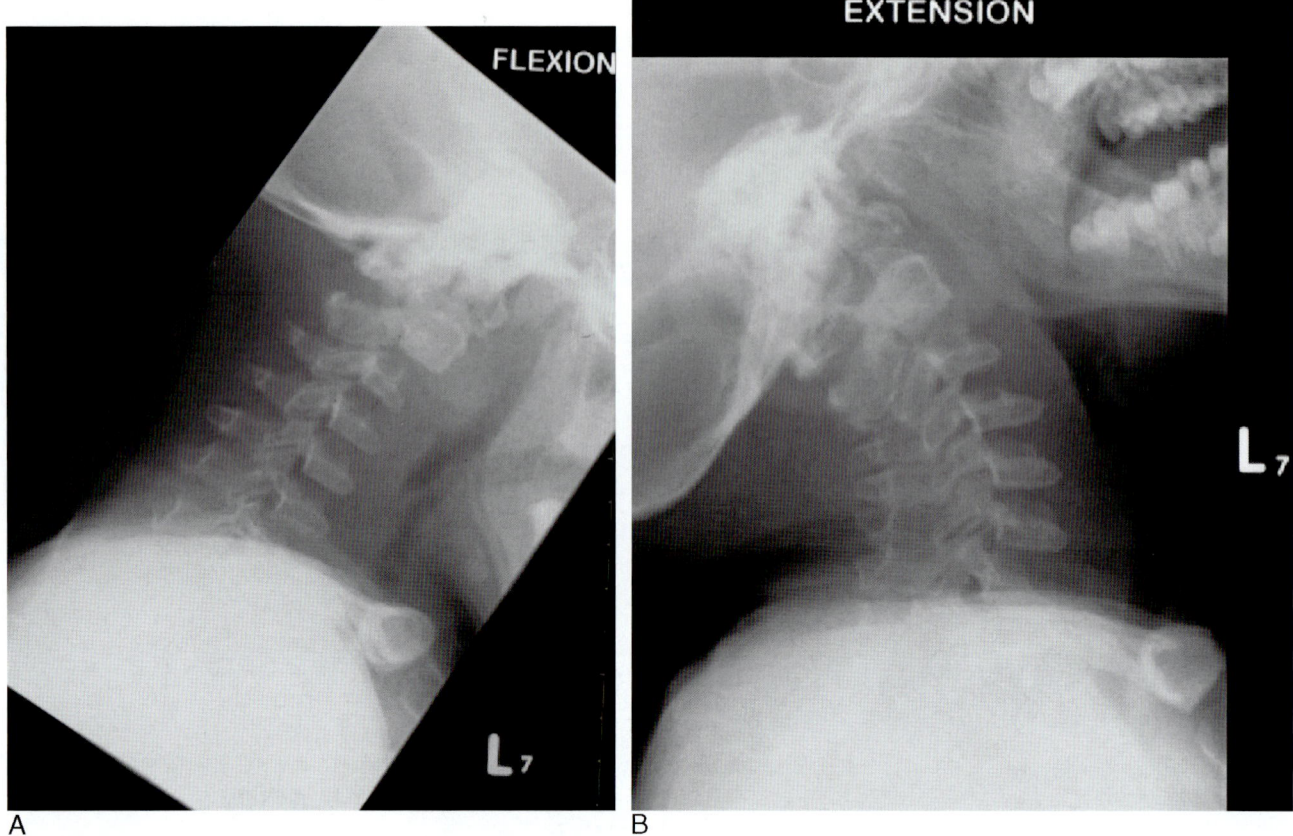

■ **FIGURE 80-8**   Flexion (**A**) and extension (**B**) views of the cervical spine from a patient with Morquio syndrome. There is hypoplasia of the odontoid that predisposes to atlantoaxial subluxation and spinal cord compression. Also observed is platyspondyly of the vertebral bodies. *(Courtesy of Martin Williams, MD.)*

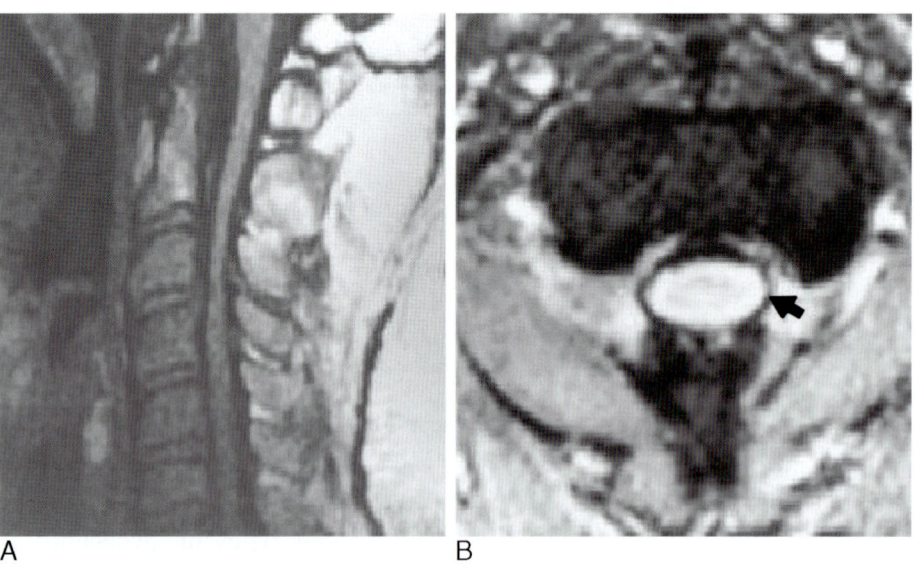

■ **FIGURE 80-9**   MR images of the cervical spine in a patient with Hunter syndrome. **A,** Sagittal T1-weighted image demonstrates marked cord compression at the level of C2 and C3 by hypointense thickened dura. **B,** Axial T2-weighted gradient-echo MR image demonstrates thinned spinal cord surrounded by a hypointense thickened dura (*arrow*). *(From Vinchon M, Cotten A, Clarisse J, et al. Cervical myelopathy secondary to Hunter syndrome in an adult. AJNR Am J Neuroradiol 1995; 16:1403. Copyright 1995 by American Society of Neuroradiology, with permission.)*

Magnetic Resonance Imaging

Magnetic resonance imaging may demonstrate pseudohypertrophy of skeletal muscles. In GSD type 1b, MRI of the extremities may demonstrate hematopoietic marrow in regions in which normal fatty conversion is expected, reflecting bone marrow hypercellularity accompanying the neutropenia.[26]

Multidetector Computed Tomography

Computed tomography may demonstrate atrophy of the posterior paraspinal and psoas muscles.[27] The psoas muscles were observed to be spared in McArdle disease.

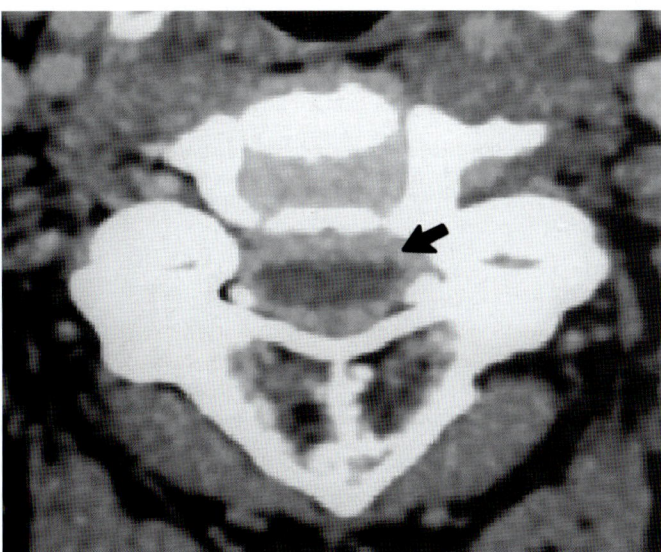

■ **FIGURE 80-10** Axial nonenhanced CT image of the cervical spine in a patient with Hunter syndrome demonstrates markedly thickened dura mater with cord compression (*arrow*). *(From Vinchon M, Cotten A, Clarisse J, et al. Cervical myelopathy secondary to Hunter syndrome in an adult. AJNR Am J Neuroradiol 1995; 16:1403. Copyright 1995 by American Society of Neuroradiology, with permission.)*

DIFFERENTIAL DIAGNOSIS

The differential diagnosis of the mucopolysaccharidoses and glycogen storage diseases is presented in Table 80-3.

SYNOPSIS OF TREATMENT OPTIONS

Managing the systemic involvement of lysosomal storage disorder patients requires a multidisciplinary team effort coordinated by the patient's pediatrician or internist.

Medical Treatment

In mucopolysaccharidoses, the main therapeutic options include bone marrow transplantation and enzyme replacement therapy.[1,7] Bone marrow transplantation may result in improvement of airway disease, cardiomyopathy, and abdominal organ enlargement. Neurologic conditions may stabilize. Skeletal changes unfortunately do not respond to treatment, and patients continue to need orthopedic intervention. Laronidase treatment in MPS I patients has been reported to decrease storage of GAG and improve respiratory function, sleep apnea, and overall functional capacity.

In glycogenoses, the current treatment includes nocturnal nasogastric infusion of glucose or oral administration of uncooked cornstarch for GSD I, high-protein diet and supportive therapies in GSD II, symptomatic treatment in GSD III, oral administration of glucose or fructose during exercise for GSD V and GSD VII, and high-carbohydrate diet and frequent feedings in GSD VI.[4,15] Enzyme replacement therapy has been reported to improve cardiac function and structure, increase overall muscle strength, and improve survival in patients with Pompe disease.[28]

Surgical Treatment

Surgical management of mucopolysaccharidoses may include elective occipital-cervical fusion to avoid compromising the cord from atlantoaxial instability and surgery to relieve compression on the cord from thickened dura mater, surgery for hip dislocation, bracing for thoracolumbar kyphosis, epiphyseal stapling, and tibial osteotomy for knee deformity. Other possible procedures include valve replacements, angioplasty, hernia repair, carpal tunnel release, and ventriculoperitoneal shunting for hydrocephalus.

In the glycogenoses, surgical treatment may include liver transplantation and renal transplantation.

TABLE 80-3 Differential Diagnosis of Mucopolysaccharidoses and Glycogen Storage Diseases	
Mucopolysaccharidoses	**Glycogen Storage Diseases**
Achondroplasia	Duchenne muscular dystrophy
Spondyloepiphyseal dysplasia	Limb girdle dystrophy
Other skeletal dysplasias	Polymyositis
Down syndrome	Danon disease
Klinefelter syndrome	Other myopathies or neuromuscular disorders
	Other storage disorders
Mucolipidoses such as Gaucher disease, Fabry disease	
Other storage disorders	

What the Referring Physician Needs to Know

- Diagnosis of mucopolysaccharidosis can often be made by examination of urine for excretion of GAG fragments.
- Prenatal screening for mucopolysaccharidosis is possible with sampling of amniotic fluid or chorionic villus.
- Patients with odontoid hypoplasia should undergo elective cervical spine fusion to avoid cord compression from atlantoaxial subluxation.
- In glycogenosis, abdominal ultrasonography should be performed to detect for hepatic adenomas in the liver and rare but possible malignant degeneration.
- Echocardiography should be performed to detect for cardiac involvement in glycogenosis.

SUGGESTED READINGS

Ashworth JL, Biswas S, Wraith E, Lloyd IC. Mucopolysaccharidoses and the eye. Surv Ophthalmol 2006; 51:1–17.

Eggli KD, Dorst JP. The mucopolysaccharidoses and related conditions. Semin Roentgenol 1986; 21:275–294.

Kachur E, Del Maestro R. Mucopolysaccharidoses and spinal cord compression: case report and review of the literature with implications of bone marrow transplantation. Neurosurgery 2000; 47:223–228.

Mikles M, Stanton RP. A review of Morquio syndrome. Am J Orthop 1997; 26:533–540.

Muenzer J. Mucopolysaccharidoses. Adv Pediatr 1986; 33:269–302.

Northover H, Cowie RA, Wraith JE. Mucopolysaccharidosis type IVA (Morquio syndrome): a clinical review. J Inherit Metab Dis 1996; 19:357–365.

REFERENCES

1. Neufeld EF, Muenzer J. The mucopolysaccharidoses. In Scriver C, Beaudet AL, Valle D, Sly W (eds). The Metabolic and Molecular Bases of Inherited Disease, 8th ed. New York, McGraw-Hill, 2001, vol 3, pp 3421–3452.
2. Miller JH, Stanley P, Gates GF. Radiography of glycogen storage diseases. AJR Am J Roentgenol 1979; 132:379–387.
3. Kishnani PS, Howell RR. Pompe disease in infants and children. J Pediatr 2004; 144:S35-S43.
4. Chen YT. Glycogen storage diseases. In Scriver CR, Beaudet AL, Sly WS, Valle D (eds). The Metabolic and Molecular Bases of Inherited Diseases, 8th ed. New York, McGraw-Hill, 2001, vol 1, pp 1521–1551.
5. Mucopolysaccharidoses Fact Sheet. National Institute of Neurological Disorders and Strokes. Available at: http://www.ninds.nih.gov/disorders/mucopolysaccharidoses/detail_mucopolysaccharidoses.htm. Accessed 3/20/06.
6. Edeiken J, Dalinka M, Karasick D (eds). Edeiken Roentgen Diagnosis of Diseases of Bone, 4th ed. Baltimore, Williams & Wilkins, 1990, vol 2, pp 1745–1764.
7. Eggli KD, Dorst JP. The mucopolysaccharidoses and related conditions. Semin Roentgenol 1986; 21:275–294.
8. Murray RO, Jacobson HG, Stoker DJ. The Radiology of Skeletal Disorders, Exercises in Diagnosis, 3rd ed. Edinburgh, Churchill Livingstone, 1990, vol 2, pp 930–945.
9. Taybi H, Lachman RS. Radiology of Syndromes, Metabolic Disorders, and Skeletal Dysplasias, 4th ed. St. Louis, Mosby, 1996, pp 593–598, 669–681.
10. Resnick D, Kransdorf MJ. Bone and Joint Imaging, 3rd ed. Philadelphia, Elsevier Saunders, 2005, pp 1318–1325.
11. Ashworth JL, Biswas S, Wraith E, Lloyd IC. Mucopolysaccharidoses and the eye. Surv Ophthalmol 2006; 51:1–17.
12. Sharpiro J, Strome M, Crocker AC. Airway obstruction and sleep apnea in Hurler and Hunter syndromes. Ann Otol Rhinol Laryngol 1985; 94:458–461.
13. Schieken RM, Kerber RE, Ionasescu VV, et al. Cardiac manifestations of the mucopolysaccharidoses. Circulation 1975; 52:700–705.
14. Natowicz MR, Short MP, Wang Y, et al. Clinical and biochemical manifestations of hyaluronidase deficiency. N Engl J Med 1996; 335:1029–1033.
15. Hirschhorn R, Reuser AJ. Glycogen storage disease type II: Acid α1,4-glucosidase (acid maltase) deficiency. In Scriver CR, Beaudet AL, Sly WS, Valle D (eds). The Metabolic and Molecular Bases of Inherited Diseases, 8th ed. New York, McGraw-Hill, 2001, vol 3, pp 3389–3420.
16. Kannourakis G. Glycogen storage disease. Semin Hematol 2002; 39:103–106.
17. Ross JS, Brant-Zawadzki M, Moore KR, et al (eds). Diagnostic Imaging, Spine. Amirsys, 2004, pp 156–159.
18. Steinbach HL, Gold RH, Preger L (eds). Roentgen Appearance of the Hand in Diffuse Disease. Chicago, Year Book Medical Publishers, 1975, pp 158–165.
19. Kulkarni MV, Williams JC, Yeakley JW, et al. Magnetic resonance imaging in the diagnosis of the cranio-cervical manifestations of mucopolysaccharidoses. Magn Reson Imaging 1987; 5:317–323.
20. Vinchon M, Cotten A, Clarisse J, et al. Cervical myelopathy secondary to Hunter syndrome in an adult. AJNR Am J Neuroradiol 1995; 16:1402–1403.
21. Kachur E, Del Maestro R. Mucopolysaccharidoses and spinal cord compression: case report and review of the literature with implications of bone marrow transplantation. Neurosurgery 2000; 47:223–229.
22. Schmidt H, Ullrich K, von Lengerke HJ. Radiological findings in patients with mucopolysaccharidosis I H/S (Hurler-Scheie syndrome). Pediatr Radiol 1987; 17:409–414.
23. Thomas SL, Childress MH, Quinton B. Hypoplasia of the odontoid with atlanto-axial subluxation in Hurler syndrome. Pediatr Radiol 1985; 15:353–354.
24. Taccone A, Tortori Donati P, Marzoli A, et al. Mucopolysaccharidosis: thickening of dura mater at the craniocervical junction and other CT/MRI findings. Pediatr Radiol 1993; 23:349–352.
25. Preger L, Sanders GW, Gold RH, et al. Roentgenographic skeletal changes in the glycogen storage diseases. Am J Roentgenol Radium Ther Nucl Med 1969; 107:840–847.
26. Schrerer A, Engelbrecht V, Neises G, et al. MR imaging of bone marrow in glycogen storage disease type 1b in children and young adults. AJR Am J Roentgenol 2001; 177:421–425.
27. Cinnamon J, Slonim AE, Black KS, et al. Evaluation of the lumbar spine in patients with glycogen storage disease: CT demonstration of patterns of paraspinal muscle atrophy. Am J Neuroradiol 1991; 12:1099–1103.
28. Schiffmann R, Brady RO. New prospects for the treatment of lysosomal storage diseases. Drugs 2002; 62:733–742.

81

Osteogenesis Imperfecta

James Teh and Roger Smith

Osteogenesis imperfecta (OI), also known as brittle bone syndrome, is an uncommon heritable disorder of collagen synthesis that results in defective, weak bony matrix, leading to bone fragility with fractures and deformity. A wide range of clinical manifestations may be seen, ranging from perinatal death to premature osteoporosis presenting in middle-aged adults. Important secondary clinical features are growth impairment, resulting in a rhizomelic dwarfism, hearing loss, blue sclerae, dentinogenesis imperfecta, cardiopulmonary complications, and neurologic compromise due to basilar invagination.

The radiologic findings play a key role in diagnosing the condition. The multiple fractures encountered in OI often raise suspicion of nonaccidental injury, and radiologists must therefore have an understanding of the clinical manifestations of OI, the range of its genetic variability, and its imaging findings.

ETIOLOGY

Osteogenesis imperfecta may be inherited (autosomal dominant) or result from a sporadic mutation. Autosomal recessive cases are possible but rare. The main pathologic process in OI is a disturbance in the synthesis of type I collagen, which is the predominant protein of the extracellular matrix of most tissues. Type I collagen fibers are found in bones, ligaments, sclera, dentin, tendons, meninges, and skin. In bone, the defective extracellular matrix causes osteoporosis, which leads to bone fragility.

The collagen molecule is synthesized from procollagen, which is secreted into the extracellular compartment. These molecules then assemble into an ordered fibril. Gene mutations that interfere with the expression of the collagen gene, formation of the triple helix, or procollagen secretion affect the structure and function of collagen fibrils, resulting in OI.[1]

Most forms of OI arise from mutations in one of two genes that encode the synthesis and/or structure of type I collagen: the *COL1A1* gene on chromosome 17 and the *COL1A2* gene on chromosome 7. Mutations in these genes may result in abnormal collagen or decreased production of normal collagen, or a combination, resulting in the different phenotypic expressions of OI.[2] Milder forms of OI are caused primarily by the decreased production of normal collagen, whereas more severe forms are caused primarily by the production of abnormal collagen. A wide variation in clinical severity may occur between family members with the same genetic mutation.[3]

PREVALENCE AND EPIDEMIOLOGY

The frequency of OI is based primarily on data from Sillence and associates in Australia.[4] OI is reported to occur in around 1 in 20,000 births, but this is likely to be an underestimate because milder forms may remain undiagnosed.[1] Males and females are equally affected.

Over the 30-year period between 1950 and 1979 it was estimated that there were 10,000 individuals with skeletal dysplasia in the United Kingdom (excluding stillbirths, perinatal deaths, and patients with chromosome anomalies and metabolic bone disease).[5] About 6000 required substantial orthopedic care, and half of these were severely physically handicapped throughout life. In this group OI was the most common diagnosis.

CLINICAL PRESENTATION AND PATHOPHYSIOLOGY

The Sillence classification is the most widely recognized.[4] This classification is based on both clinical and radiographic features. Four main types of OI were initially

---

KEY POINTS

- Osteogenesis imperfecta is an uncommon heritable disorder caused by abnormal collagen synthesis.
- There is a very wide range of clinical presentation.
- Four main types are described in the original Sillence classification, and several additional types have been described subsequently.
- Diagnosis relies on clinical and radiologic features.
- Treatment requires a multidisciplinary approach.

described, but over the years several subsequent types have been added.

Previously, OI was divided into two forms: "congenita" and "tarda," depending on the severity of disease, but this classification has been superceded because it fails to encompass the wide range of clinical presentation. In OI congenita the fractures occur in utero, whereas in OI tarda the fractures occur at birth or later. OI tarda can be further subdivided into "gravis," with fractures first occurring at the time of birth or during the first year of life, and "levis," with fractures first occurring after the first year.

Type I

Type I OI is the most common form of disease, comprising up to 60% of people with OI.[4] It is generally associated with the best prognosis. This condition is transmitted as an autosomal dominant trait, although new mutations may occur. The most frequent genetic mutation causing type I OI results in a decreased production of normal collagen. Type I OI is divided into A and B subtypes based on the absence or presence of dentinogenesis imperfecta, respectively. Individuals with type IB have more severe disease, with a greater fracture rate and a greater likelihood of growth impairment.[6] Life expectancy of patients with type IA OI is normal. In type 1B OI, mortality is slightly increased compared with that of the general population.

Type I OI is usually not detected at birth. Clinically, its distinguishing features are blue sclerae and presenile conductive hearing loss.[4] Patients may have their first fracture when learning to walk. In the prepubertal years mild trauma may lead to a series of fractures. The incidence of fractures tends to decrease significantly after puberty. In some cases exuberant callus formation may occur with healing. Patients may be of small or normal stature. Ligamentous laxity, resulting in joint hypermobility or subluxation, is common. Cardiovascular problems, particularly aortic valve disease, can occur. In some patients postmenopausal vertebral compression fractures may be the first presentation.[7]

Type II

In type II OI collagen is improperly formed. Type II OI is the most severe form, characterized by extreme bone fragility, leading to intrauterine or early infant death.[8] Clinically, distinguishing features include intrauterine growth retardation, thin and beaded ribs, crumpled long bones, and poor craniofacial bone ossification. The affected infants tend to have flat triangular facies with a small beaked nose. The sclerae are blue and occasionally almost black. Unexplained widespread arterial calcification occurs in some infants.[1]

Type III

Type III OI, also known as the progressive deforming type, is the most severe form of OI compatible with survival beyond infancy. In this form, collagen is improperly formed. Its hallmark feature is severe bone fragility. Abnormalities are present at birth in more than 50% of patients. Postnatal growth failure is often severe, and fractures are frequent in the first 2 years of life. Children with type III OI tend to have severe dwarfism due to vertebral compression fractures, limb deformities, and disruption of growth plates. Individuals are frequently wheelchair bound, although some are able to walk with aids. The sclerae are normal. The midface is flat with frontal bossing. Patients with type III OI can have a full life span, but many succumb to cardiorespiratory or neurologic complications, either during childhood or in early adulthood.[9]

Type IV

Type IV OI is rare.[4] Although type IV OI may be considered as intermediate in severity between types I and III, this is a heterogeneous group, with a wide spectrum of disease. The mode of inheritance is autosomal dominant. Type IV OI is classified into two groups according to the absence (type IVA) or presence (type IVB) of dentinogenesis imperfecta.

Type IV OI is clinically distinguished from type I OI by the increased severity of bone fragility and by the presence of white sclerae. Furthermore, in type IV OI the first fracture occurs more commonly at birth, dentinogenesis imperfecta is more frequent, and bruising is less common. Differentiation between these two types may be difficult, however.[10]

Other Forms of Osteogenesis Imperfecta

Some cases of OI do not fit neatly into the four main types described by Sillence. Types V and VI OI fall within the phenotypic range of type IV OI but are primarily distinguished from patients with type IV OI by iliac crest histology and histomorphometry.

Type V OI includes individuals with osteoporosis, dense metaphyseal bands, interosseous membrane ossification of the forearms and legs, and a high frequency of hypertrophic callus formation.[11] Inheritance is autosomal dominant. Qualitative histology of iliac biopsy shows that lamellae are arranged in an irregular fashion or have a mesh-like appearance. Quantitative histomorphometry reveals decreased amounts of cortical and cancellous bone. The type I collagen of these patients has normal electrophoretic mobility, and no mutations have been detected at the gene level.

The proposed type VI OI is phenotypically similar to type IV but is distinguished on histologic criteria. Inheritance is autosomal dominant. Patients with this type of OI are moderately to severely affected. Qualitative histology of iliac crest bone biopsy specimens shows an absence of the birefringent pattern of normal lamellar bone under polarized light, often with a "fish-scale" pattern. Quantitative histomorphometry reveals thin cortices and hyperosteoidosis.

The proposed type VII phenotype is characterized by fractures at birth, bluish sclerae, early deformity of the lower extremities, coxa vara, and osteopenia.[12] Rhizomelia is a prominent feature. Inheritance is autosomal recessive. Histomorphometric analyses of iliac crest bone reveals findings similar to OI type I, with decreased cortical width and trabecular number, increased bone turnover, and preservation of the birefringent pattern of lamellar bone.

There are also unusual forms of OI that are not classified into the numerical system described by Sillence. Bruck syndrome is a recessively inherited phenotypic disorder featuring the combination of skeletal changes resembling OI with congenital arthrogryposis multiplex (contractures of the large joints).[13] In the Cole-Carpenter syndrome there are bone deformities and multiple fractures reminiscent of osteogenesis imperfecta but also ocular proptosis with craniosynostosis and hydrocephalus.[14]

IMAGING FINDINGS

Type I

Many imaging features are shared with other types of OI, particularly type IV.

The radiographic hallmark is osteopenia, which is manifest by decreased bone density and cortical thinning, particularly of the metaphyses. "Feathering" and coarsening of trabeculae may also be seen.[15] Harris growth arrest lines are often present, corresponding to transient periods of epiphyseal disturbance and growth arrest (Fig. 81-1). Apart from osteopenia, bowing and healing fractures may be evident. The long bones may appear overtubulated and gracile.

In mild forms of OI, radiographs of the skull may be normal. With more severe forms of OI the skull demon-strates poor mineralization and multiple wormian, or intrasutural, bones.[16] Wormian bones are considered significant when there are more than 10 and they measure more than 6 by 4 mm and are arranged in a general mosaic pattern (Fig. 81-2; Table 81-1).[16]

Basilar invagination may be demonstrated on radiographs of the cervical spine or skull (see Fig. 81-2).[17] Although seen in all types of OI, it is more commonly associated with type IV, in which it may eventually lead to brain-stem compression.[18] Although numerous radiographic criteria have been described for assessing basilar invagination (e.g., Clark, Chamberlain, McGregor), no single criterion is completely accurate and a combination of criteria may be required for a definitive diagnosis.[17] Basilar invagination combined with a large, thin skull vault may lead to the "tam-o'-shanter" skull on the anteroposterior view, with flattening in the vertical axis and widening in the transverse axis (Fig. 81-3). On the lateral view the skull shape has also been described as resembling Darth Vader's helmet (Fig. 81-4). If basilar invagination is suspected, the patient should be further assessed for brain-stem compression or syringohydromyelia by MRI (Fig. 81-5).

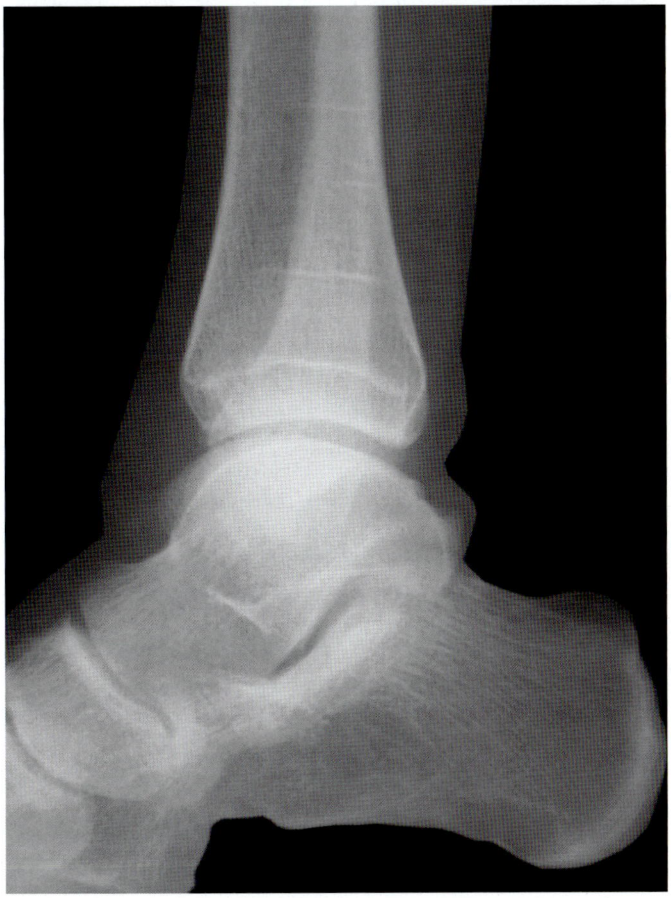

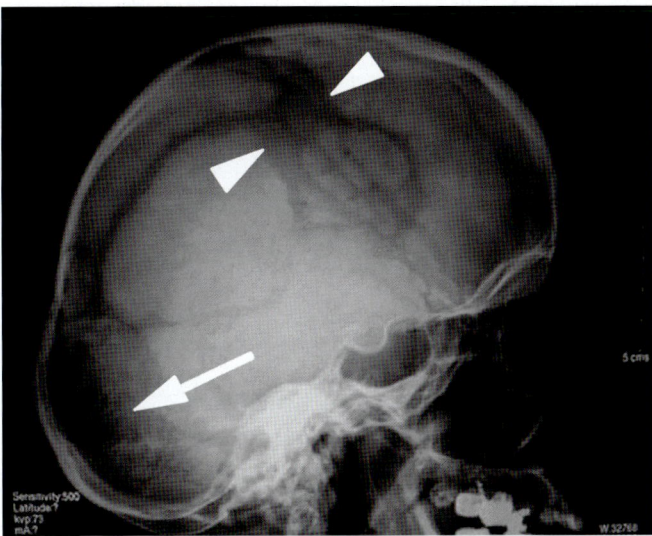

■ **FIGURE 81-2** Lateral radiograph of the skull demonstrating decreased enchondral ossification of the skull (*arrowheads*) leading to the appearance of very large intrasutural bones. Multiple small wormian bones are also seen (*long arrow*). There is basilar invagination.

TABLE 81-1 Differential Diagnosis of Wormian Bones
Osteogenesis imperfecta
Pyknodysostosis
Rickets in healing phase
Menkes kinky hair syndrome
Cleidocranial dysostosis
Hypothyroidism
Hypophosphatasia
Otopalatodigital syndrome
Primary acro-osteolysis (Hajdu-Cheney syndrome)
Pachydermoperiostosis
Progeria
Down syndrome

■ **FIGURE 81-1** Lateral radiograph of the ankle demonstrating osteopenia with prominent Harris growth arrest lines.

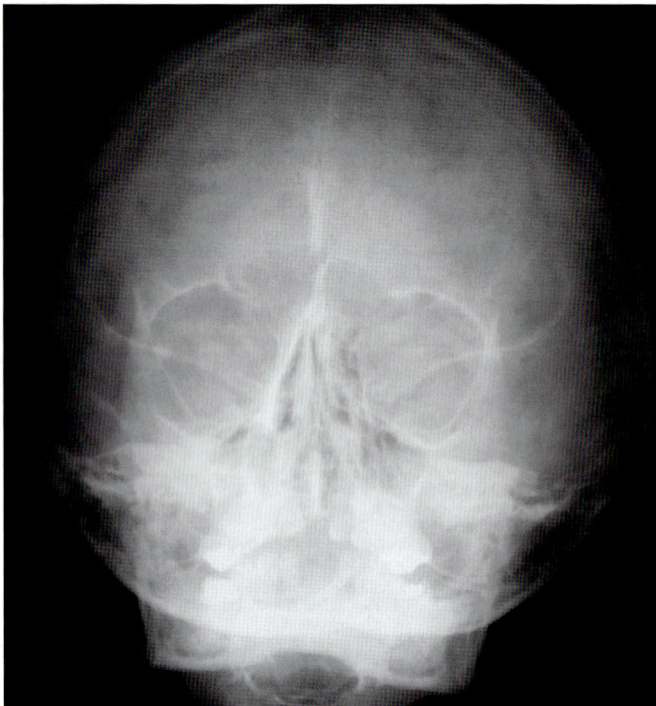

■ **FIGURE 81-3** Anteroposterior radiograph of the skull showing widened biparietal diameter with superior flattening giving the "tam-o'-shanter" appearance.

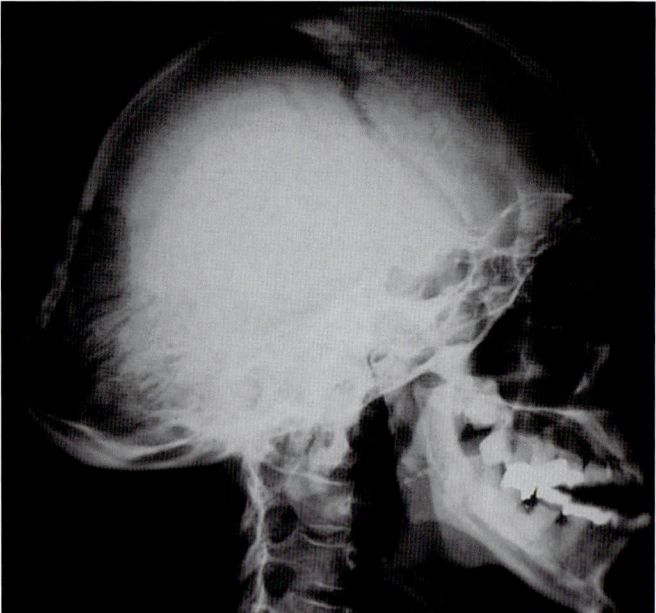

■ **FIGURE 81-4** Lateral radiograph of the skull demonstrating basilar invagination and wormian bones. The skull shape resembles Darth Vader's helmet.

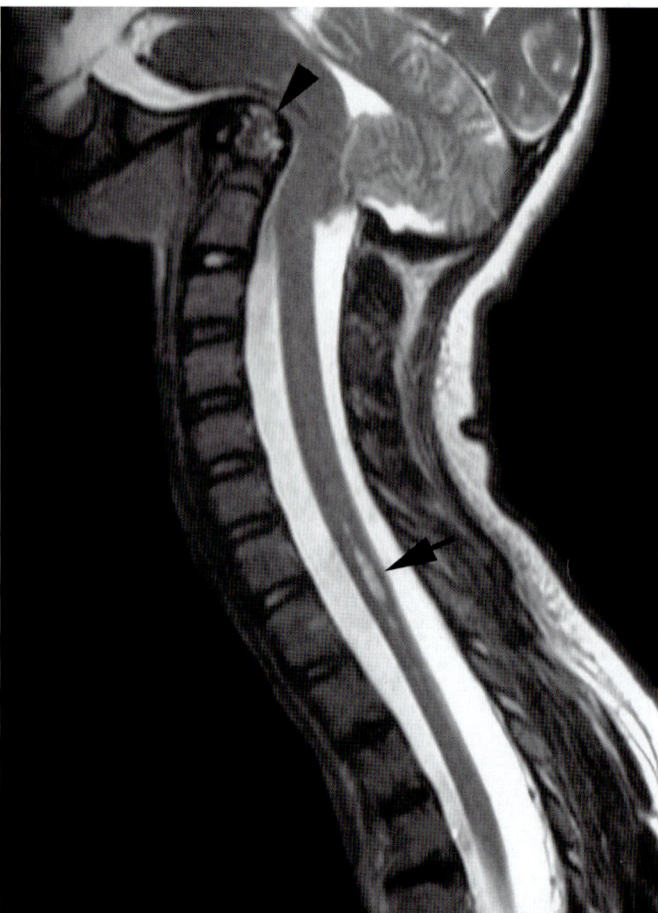

■ **FIGURE 81-5** Sagittal T2-weighted MRI demonstrating basilar invagination with brain stem compression (*arrowhead*) and a small syringohydromyelia (*arrow*). Projection of the tip of the dens above McGregor line (which is defined as a straight line between the upper surface of the posterior edge of the hard palate to the most caudal point of the occiput) suggests basilar invagination.

OI is sometimes associated with either relative or absolute macrocephaly.[19] Between the ages of 2 to 3 years, the child's head circumference may rapidly increase. Communicating hydrocephalus may occur, with prominence of sulci and ventricular enlargement seen on CT or MRI.[19]

The association of OI with hearing impairment is known as Van der Hoeve-de Kleyn syndrome.[20] The CT findings of temporal bone involvement in OI include proliferation of undermineralized bone involving the otic capsule, proliferation of the bony labyrinthine capsule just anterior to the oval window, and envelopment of the stapes footplate. The osteosclerotic foci may be single or multiple. The bone changes may extend to the upper margin of the superior semicircular canal.[21] Eventually, the cochlea may become completely surrounded by a ring of hypodense bone. The changes seen in OI are identical to those seen in patients with otosclerosis. (Fig. 81-6). The differential diagnosis includes Paget disease, syphilis, and Camurati-Engelmann disease.

The incidence of scoliosis in OI has been documented as between 39% and 80% with a greater incidence in the more severe forms.[22] There is often severe platyspondyly with vertebral compression fractures giving the appearance of codfish vertebrae (Fig. 81-7). Vertebral compression fractures after menopause may be the first presentation of OI.[7]

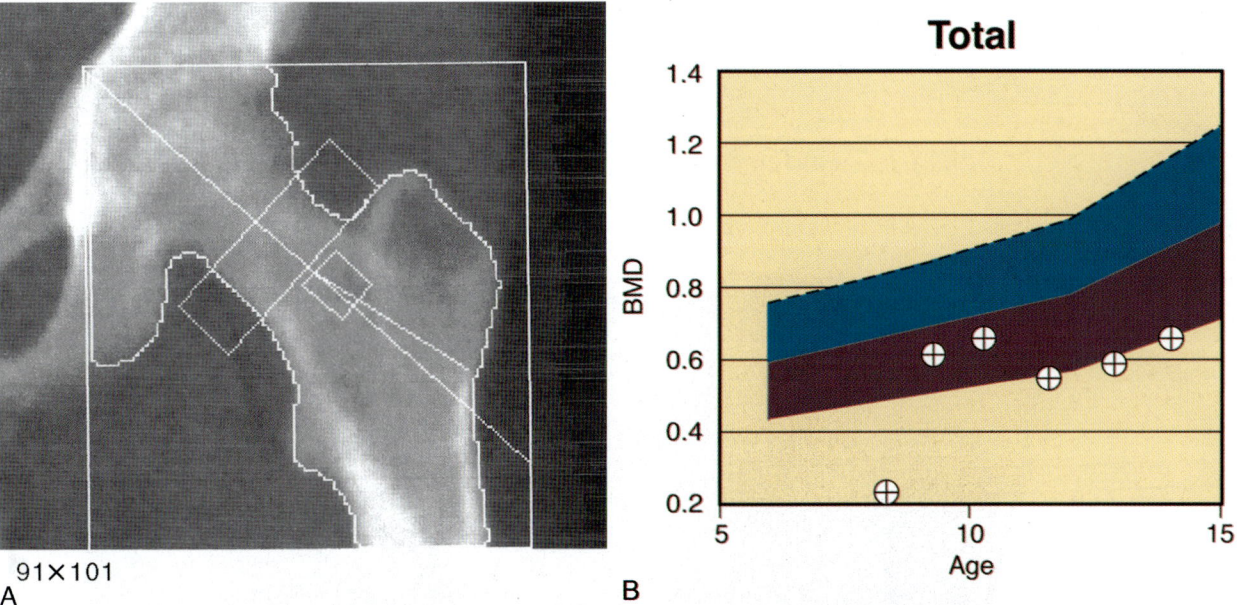

Total

■ **FIGURE 81-6** DEXA scan demonstrating the dramatic improvement in bone mineral density (BMD) after bisphosphonate treatment at the age of 8. Scan Information: Scan Type: xLeft hip; Analysis: 13:44 version 12.4 left hip; Operator: MW; Model: Discovery A (s/N 80379); Comment: NOC 4303E.

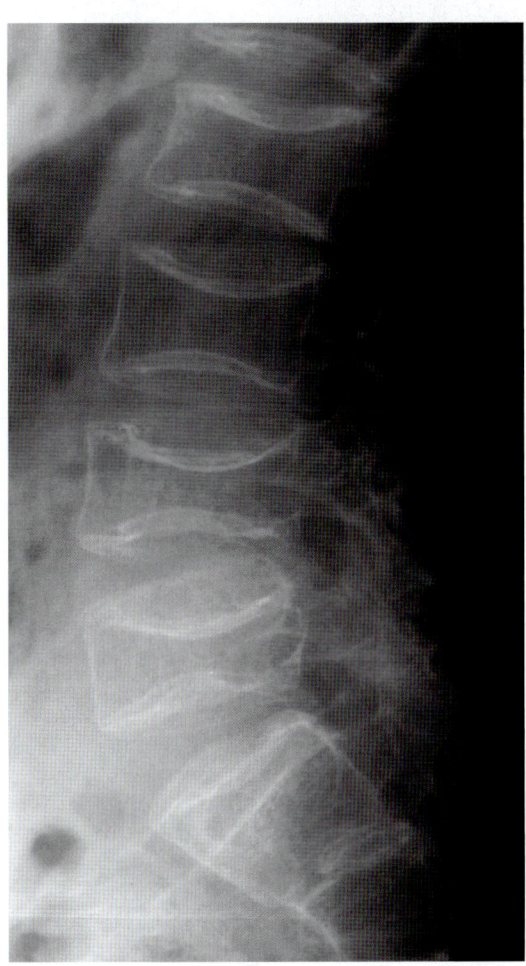

■ **FIGURE 81-7** Lateral radiograph of the lumbar spine demonstrating multiple osteoporotic collapses with the appearance of "codfish" vertebrae.

Type II

Radiographic examination reveals multiple in utero fractures at various stages of healing.[23] The long bones are extremely osteoporotic with very thin cortices. The morphology of the long bones in the upper extremities is better maintained than in the lower extremities. There is severe rhizomelic dwarfism with short, curved, and angulated long bones (Fig. 81-8). The legs are often abducted into a frog-leg position. Relative macrocephaly with enlargement of the anterior and posterior fontanelles invariably occurs. Only the lateral plates of the skull may be ossified due to the enlarged fontanelles.

Type II OI can be further subdivided into types IIA, IIB, and IIC on the basis of the radiographic features of the long bones and ribs.[8] Individuals with type IIA demonstrate short, broad, "crumpled" long bones, angulation of tibiae, and continuously beaded ribs. With type IIB there are short, broad, crumpled femora, angulation of tibiae, but normal ribs (or ribs with incomplete beading). With type IIC there are long, thin, inadequately modeled, undertubulated long bones with multiple fractures and thin beaded ribs.

Type III

The imaging findings in type III OI overlap with other types. The bones are soft as well as fragile. Bowing deformities of up to 90 degrees may be present, caused either by the tension of normal muscle deforming the bone or by previous fractures.[24] In the upper limb bowing deformity most commonly affects the humerus, followed by the ulna and radius. With bowing deformity the bone may become buttressed, usually on the concavity of the curve (Fig. 81-9).[15] In the lower limb the femur

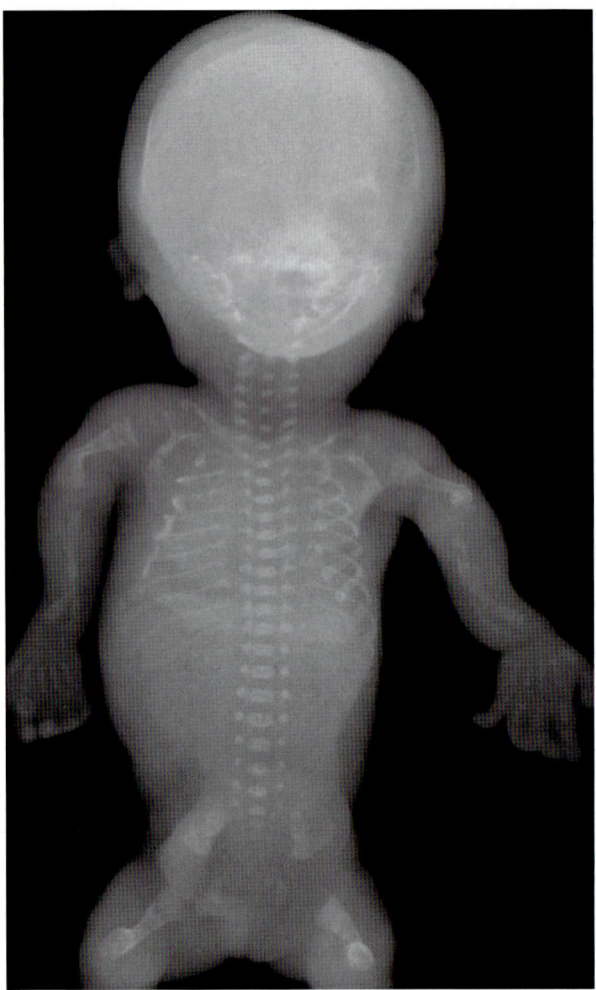

■ **FIGURE 81-8**   Type IIB osteogenesis imperfecta. Postmortem radiograph. There is relative macrocephaly with severe shortening of the long bones and multiple fractures. The ribs are thin but not crumpled.

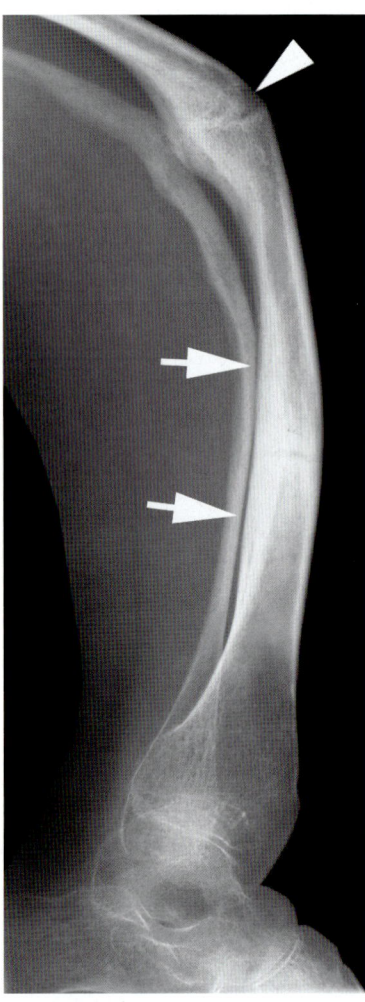

■ **FIGURE 81-9**   Lateral radiograph of the tibia demonstrating marked bowing deformity with buttressing of the cortex in the concavity (*arrows*). There is an old malunited fracture (*arrowhead*).

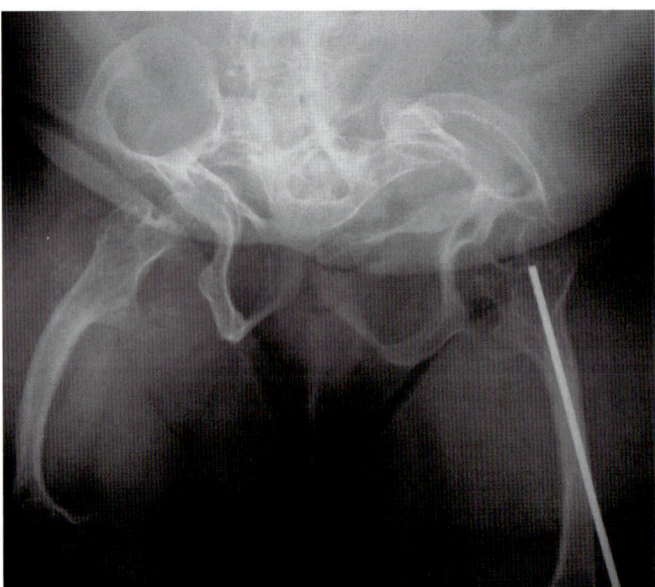

■ **FIGURE 81-10**   Radiograph of the pelvis showing marked osteopenia with severe bilateral protrusio acetabuli and modeling deformity of the pelvis with marked bowing of the femora. A nonexpandable rod has been inserted into the left femoral shaft.

is most commonly involved. In the pelvis, protrusio acetabuli is a common finding in association with coxa vara (Fig. 81-10).[25] As the child develops, there may be undertubulation of the long bones with development of an Erlenmeyer flask deformity. Alternatively, there may be overtubulation with exaggerated metaphyseal flaring accompanied by a slender diaphysis resulting in a trumpet-shaped deformity (Fig. 81-11). The extreme slenderness of the diaphysis combined with bone fragility may result in pseudarthrosis of the fibula (Fig. 81-12; Table 81-2).

The cyclical treatment of OI with bisphosphonates can result in distinctive imaging findings, with bands of sclerotic growth arrest lines (also known as "Harris lines") seen at the metaphyses of the long bones. There is no evidence that these iatrogenic changes have any clinical implications, but their appearance should be recognized to prevent unnecessary further investigation (Fig. 81-13).

A characteristic but inconstant finding is the presence of "popcorn" calcifications in the metaphyses or epiphyses of the long bones, usually at the knee or ankle. This is thought to result from repeated microfractures at the growth plate, leading to spread of cartilaginous islands into the adjacent metaphysis or epiphysis (Fig. 81-14).[1,15]

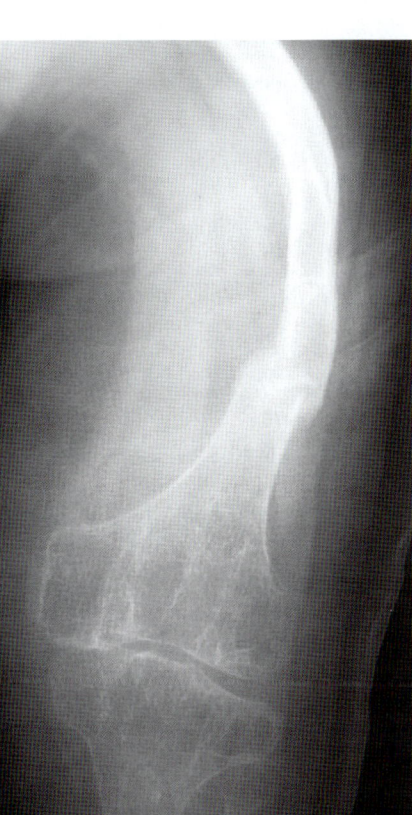

■ **FIGURE 81-11** Radiograph of the left lower limb demonstrating severe osteopenia with "trumpet-shaped" long bones with metaphyseal flaring and slender diaphyses.

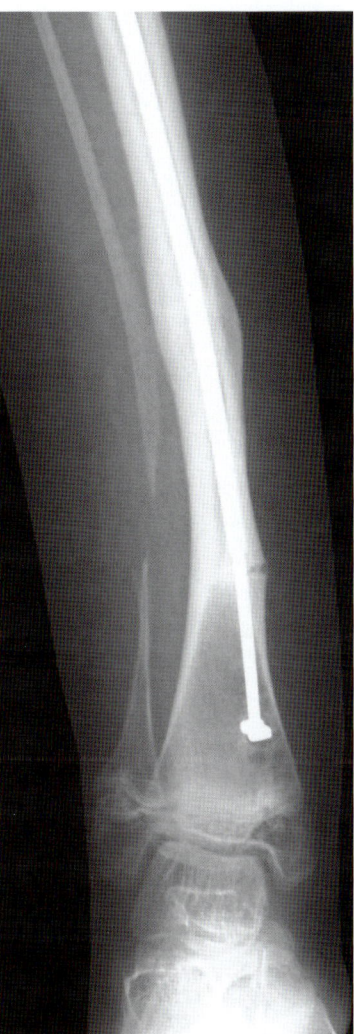

■ **FIGURE 81-12** Radiograph of the fibula demonstrating an extreme thinning of the fibula diaphysis leading to a fibular pseudoarthrosis. There is an expandable rod across the tibia.

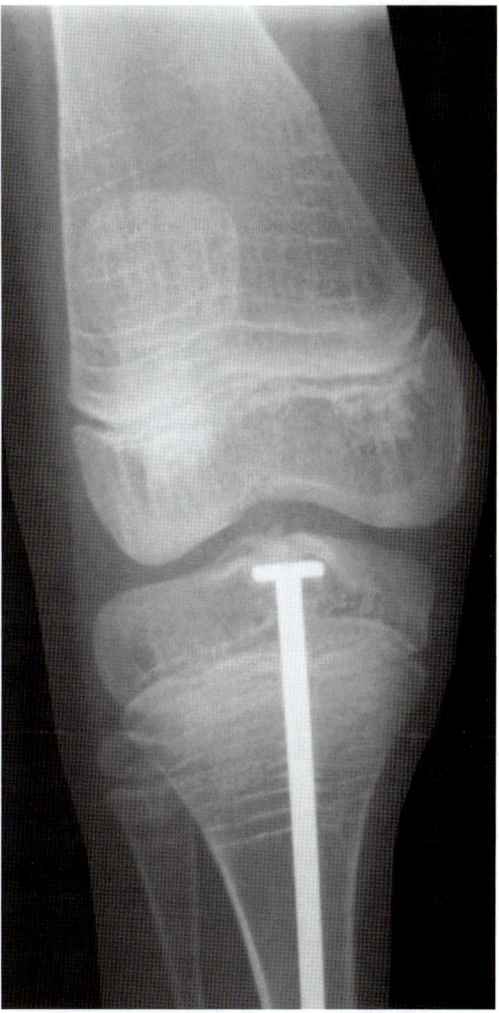

■ **FIGURE 81-13** Radiograph of the knee demonstrating alternating dense metaphyseal bands in a patient who had undergone cyclical bisphosphonate therapy. There is an expandable rod across the tibia.

Virtually all individuals with OI type III develop significant kyphoscoliosis (Fig. 81-15).[26] Patients with type III osteogenesis imperfecta demonstrate elongation of the pedicles, which may be very thin, a deformity that is not seen in other types of OI (Fig. 81-16).[27] Pars defects are common, which may result in spondylolisthesis (Fig. 81-17).

Spinal deformity combined with rib fractures and remodeling result in a very high incidence of chest wall abnormalities.[28] Pectus carinatum occurs more frequently than pectus excavatum (Fig. 81-18). Restrictive lung dis-

ease due to chest wall deformity, as well as decreased mobility, predisposes the patients to recurrent pneumonias, which are a major cause of morbidity and mortality.

As with other forms, in the skull there is relative macrocephaly, often with basilar invagination; and wormian bones are usually present.[29]

Type IV

There is a wide overlap between the imaging findings in type IV and type I, and, to a lesser degree, type III OI (see earlier).

Hyperplastic callus formation can occur after fractures or surgical intervention in all types of OI but is particularly associated with types IV and V.[11] Patients present with a painful vascular mass. The femur is most often affected, with the callus appearing as a dense, irregular mass arising from the cortex of bone. The appearances may mimic osteosarcoma, myositis ossificans, chronic osteomyelitis, or osteochondroma. CT may demonstrate a well-defined

TABLE 81-2 Differential Diagnosis of Pseudarthrosis of the Fibula
Osteogenesis imperfecta
Neurofibromatosis
Fibrous dysplasia
Osteofibrous dysplasia

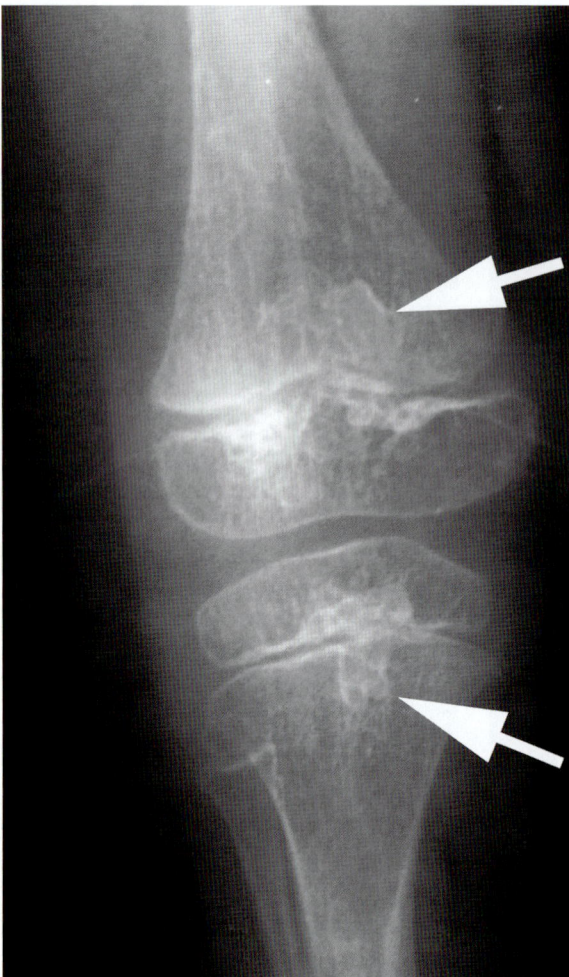

■ FIGURE 81-14 Radiograph of the knee showing "popcorn" calcifications of the diametaphyseal regions (*arrows*), thought to result from spread of cartilaginous islands from the growth plate.

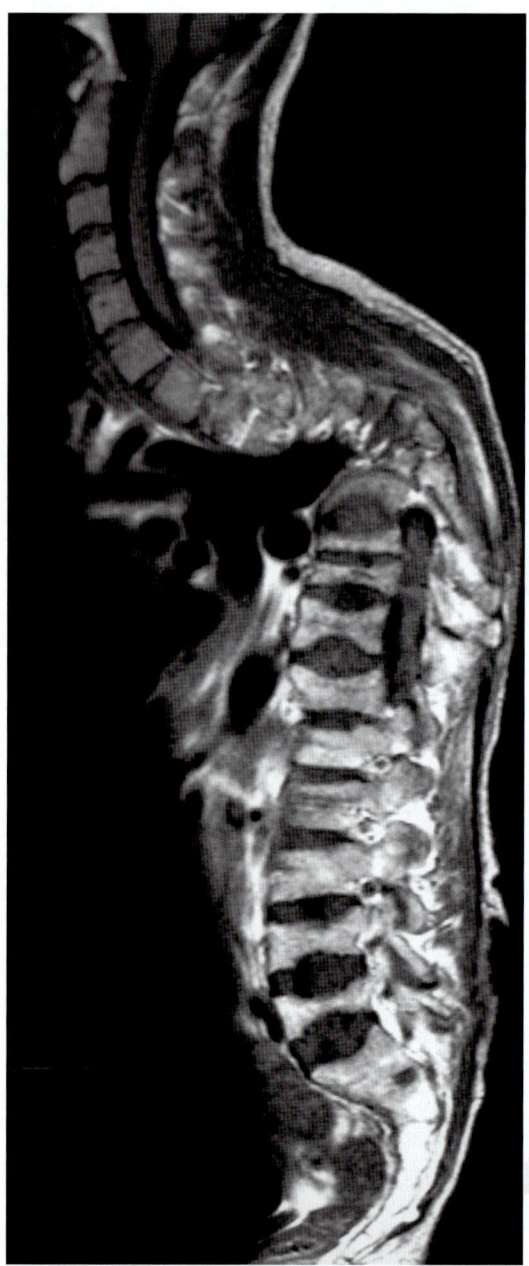

■ FIGURE 81-15 Sagittal T1-weighted MR image demonstrating a severe thoracic kyphoscoliosis.

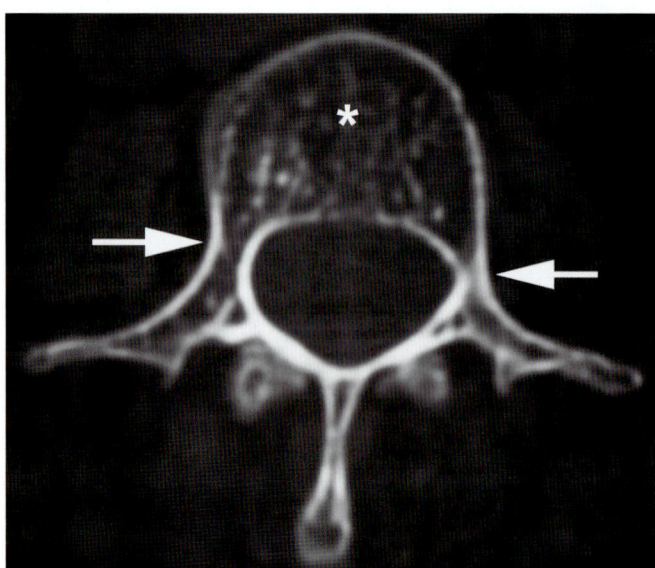

■ FIGURE 81-16 Axial CT scan through the lumbar region demonstrating severe osteopenia with prominence of the trabeculae (*asterisk*). The pedicles are thin and elongated (*arrows*).

calcified rim, allowing differentiation of hyperplastic callus from more aggressive lesions such as osteosarcoma. The plasma alkaline phosphatase level may be elevated.

MANIFESTATIONS OF THE DISEASE

Radiography

In cases of suspected OI, a selective skeletal survey should be performed. Views of the long bones, skull, chest, pelvis, and thoracolumbar spine should be obtained. The radiographic features are dependent on the type of OI and on the severity of disease. The radiographic findings may be nonspecific because some findings may be seen across

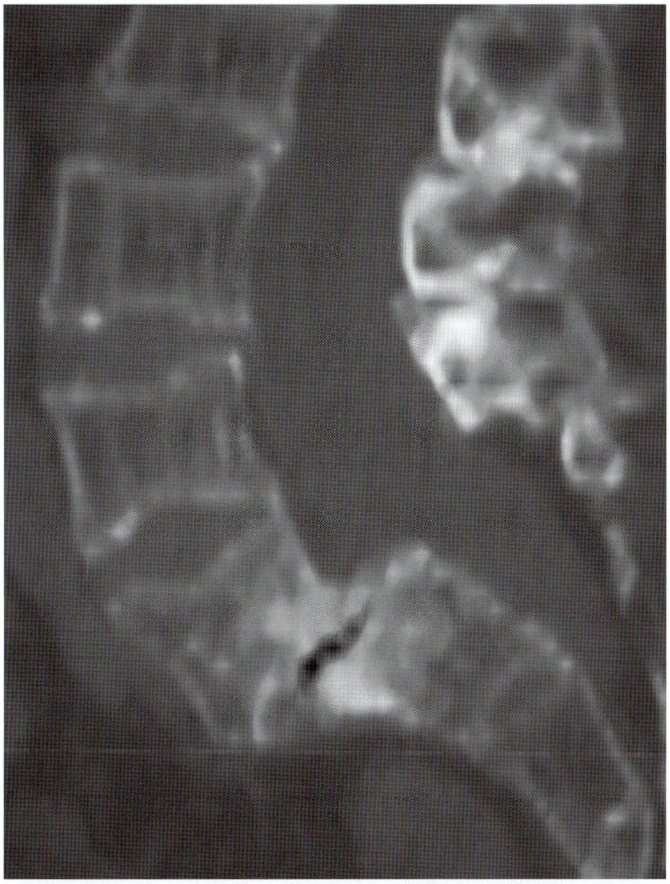

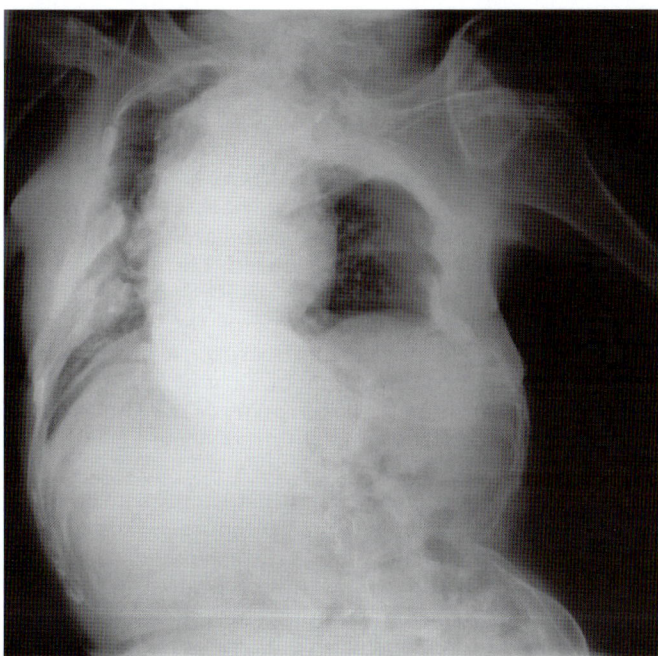

■ **FIGURE 81-17** Sagittal CT reformatted image of the lumbar spine demonstrating severe osteopenia with a 40% spondylolisthesis.

all subtypes. In the more severe forms of OI (i.e., type II) the radiographic findings are considered diagnostic.

Magnetic Resonance Imaging

Magnetic resonance imaging is particularly useful for assessment of neurologic impairment in OI. In patients with basilar invagination, MRI has the advantage over radiographs and CT of detecting associated cord compression or syringohydromyelia.

Classic Signs

TYPE I

- Most frequent and mildest type of OI
- Most fractures occur before puberty
- Normal or near-normal stature
- Joint laxity
- Sclerae usually blue
- Bone deformity absent or minimal
- Dentinogenesis imperfecta may occur
- Hearing loss possible
- Collagen structure normal, but amount of collagen less than normal

TYPE II

- Most severe form
- Frequently lethal at or shortly after birth, often due to respiratory compromise
- Multiple fractures and severe bone deformity
- Triangular facies
- Small stature with hypoplastic lungs
- Collagen structure abnormal

TYPE III

- Bones fracture easily
- Fractures often present at birth
- Short stature
- Sclerae usually blue
- Joint laxity and poor muscle development
- Chest deformity
- Triangular face
- Kyphoscoliosis
- Bone deformity often severe
- Dentinogenesis imperfecta may occur
- Hearing loss possible
- Collagen improperly formed

TYPE IV

- Between type I and type III in severity
- Bones fracture easily, mostly before puberty
- Short stature
- Normal sclerae
- Mild to moderate bone deformity
- Scoliosis common
- Barrel-shaped rib cage and chest wall deformities
- Dentinogenesis imperfecta may occur
- Hearing loss possible
- Collagen structure abnormal

■ **FIGURE 81-18** Chest radiograph demonstrating chest wall deformity due to a combination of kyphoscoliosis and rib remodeling.

In patients who develop scoliosis, MRI is the modality of choice for evaluating neurologic symptoms or for excluding congenital anomalies such as a tethered cord or Arnold-Chiari malformation before surgery.[30]

MRI is the investigation of choice for back pain and should be used in lieu of radiographs. Both sagittal T1-weighted and short tau inversion recovery images should be obtained to allow the differentiation of acute from chronic vertebral fractures.

Multidetector Computed Tomography

Computed tomography has an important role in evaluating neurologic symptoms and hearing impairment. CT with 2D and 3D reformatted images can also be used to assess the vertebral column anatomy in cases of scoliosis or spondylolisthesis before surgery. CT also has a role in the detection of occult fractures.

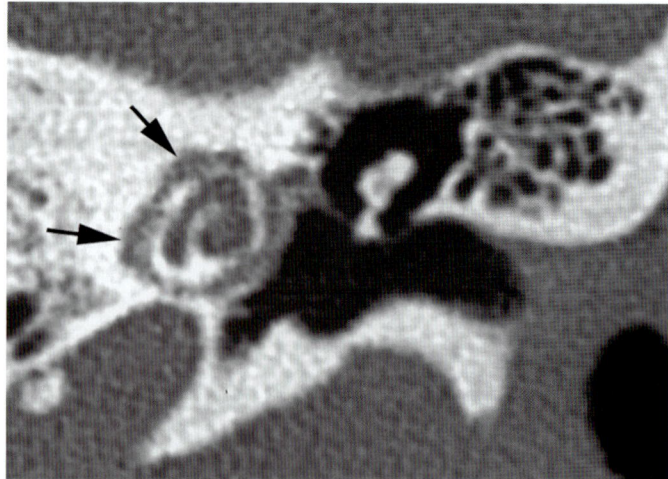

■ **FIGURE 81-19** CT scan of the temporal bone demonstrating low density mineralization around the cochlea (*arrows*).

Ultrasonography

Ultrasonography plays a key role in the prenatal diagnosis of OI, which is one of the more commonly encountered skeletal dysplasias in utero. In the more severe types of OI (types II and III), ultrasonography during the second trimester may reveal hypoechogenicity of the calvaria owing to decreased mineralization, with supervisualization of the intracranial structures.[31] Compression of the skull vault by the ultrasound probe should raise the suspicion of skeletal dysplasia but is not diagnostic for OI. Bowing and fractures of the long bones may be present, along with shortening of the long bones. Multiple rib fractures may also be seen. Increased nuchal translucency has also been described. The diagnosis of OI may be confirmed by DNA analysis of chorionic villus cells obtained by ultrasound-guided chorionic villus sampling.

Bone Mineral Densitometry

Measurements of bone mineral density can be used to help establish the diagnosis, assess prognosis, and monitor the response to treatment in patients with OI.[32] In recent years, dual-energy x-ray absorptiometry (DEXA) has become the most widely accepted technique for bone mineral density measurements in children, superceding single-photon absorptiometry and quantitative CT of the lumbar spine (Fig. 81-19).

A clear relationship between bone mineral density and clinical severity in patients with OI is not always present, but bone mineral density may predict long-term functional outcome.[33] Serial DEXA scanning is now routinely used as an objective assessment of response to bisphosphonate therapy, but there are considerable difficulties in interpretation, particularly if there are bone deformities in the spine and/or hip (see Fig. 81-6).

DIFFERENTIAL DIAGNOSIS

The differential diagnosis of OI varies according to the age of the patient. On prenatal ultrasonography, severe OI may be confused with thanatophoric dysplasia, achondrogenesis type I, or campomelic dysplasia, all of which demonstrate relative macrocephaly and limb shortening.

Type III OI may appear similar to infantile hypophosphatasia, which presents as severe osteoporosis and micromelia. Serum biochemistry in hypophosphatasia demonstrates low serum alkaline phosphatase and increased inorganic pyrophosphate, whereas in OI the serum alkaline phosphatase level is normal or increased.

After infancy, OI may be confused with primary juvenile osteoporosis or other secondary causes of osteoporosis in childhood, such as hypogonadism or chronic steroid use.

An important consideration in early childhood is non-accidental injury (NAI).

In middle-aged women, OI may be mistaken for post-menopausal osteoporosis.[7]

Differentiation from Nonaccidental Injury

Osteogenesis imperfecta type IVA is the form most likely to be confused with NAI.[34] The diagnosis of NAI can be reached in the majority of cases by assessment of the social circumstances combined with careful clinical and imaging evaluation by experienced clinicians. When diagnostic uncertainty persists in cases of suspected NAI, such as when the supposed force of the injury seems insufficient to have caused the fracture, when fractures occur in a protected environment, or when there are no external signs of abuse, collagen analysis may be useful.[35] However, routine biopsy for children suspected to have been abused is unwarranted.

Some authors have suggested that there is a self-limiting variant of OI, referred to as temporary brittle bone disease.[36] It is postulated that a transient defect in collagen formation results in multiple fractures in children younger than the age of 6 months. The condition is highly controversial because the main radiologic and clinical features described for this variant are very similar to those seen in NAI.[35] Unless further research establishes the exis-

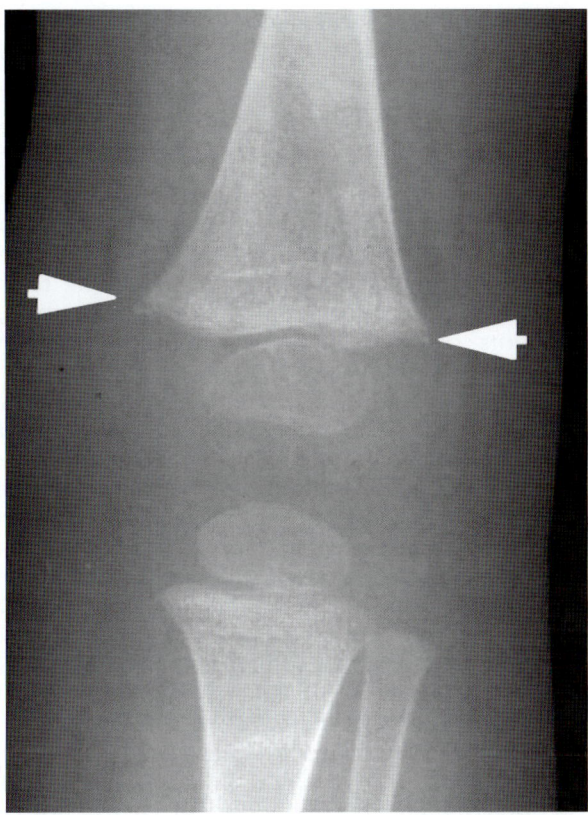

■ **FIGURE 81-20** Radiograph of the knee in a child showing small corner metaphyseal fractures (*arrowheads*) typical for nonaccidental injury.

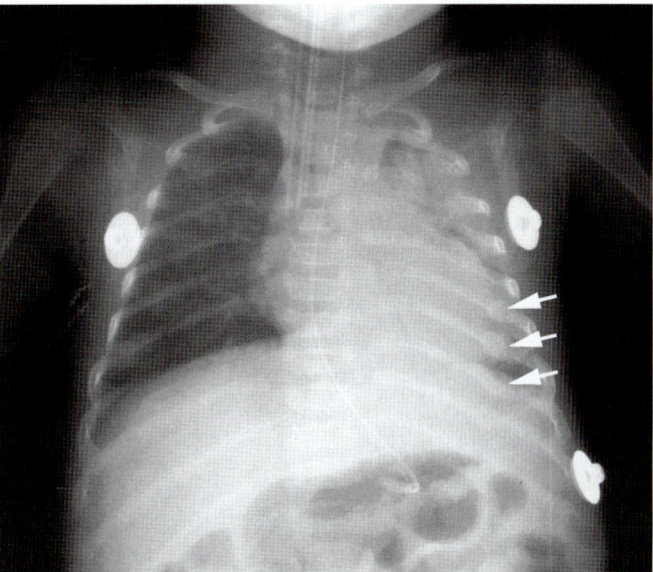

■ **FIGURE 81-21** Chest radiograph showing multiple posterior rib fractures (*arrows*) in a child suffering from nonaccidental injury. The endotracheal tube lies in the right main bronchus with collapse of the left lung.

tence of temporary brittle bone disease, it should only be considered a hypothetical entity.

It should always be remembered that OI and NAI can coexist; however, there are specific features that help differentiate these two conditions. Metaphyseal corner fractures, which are common in child abuse, are very rare in OI (Fig. 81-20).[35] If metaphyseal corner fractures are present in OI, they are usually associated with thin cortices and osteopenia.[37] In addition, bucket-handle fractures and fractures of the sternum, scapula, and skull vault are rare in OI. Certain fractures in infants, such as hand fractures in the nonambulatory child, fractures of the outer end of the clavicle, and spinal and posterior rib fractures are strongly suggestive of NAI (Fig. 81-21).[35] In children subject to NAI, serial radiographs should show normal healing and remineralization. In children with OI, fractures continue to occur even with the child in protective custody. NAI can also be differentiated from OI on the basis of nonskeletal manifestations, such as intracranial hemorrhages and visceral trauma.[35]

DNA Testing

DNA testing can be performed on blood samples to determine the presence of a genetic mutation causing OI. There is a false-negative rate of around 5%.

Collagen Analysis

Collagen synthesis analysis can be performed to determine the quantity or quality of type I collagen by culturing dermal fibroblasts obtained from skin biopsy. This may be useful for prenatal screening, genetic counseling, and differentiating OI from child abuse, but the process takes around 3 months or longer.[38] Furthermore, there is a consensus that the routine use of collagen analysis is unnecessary because in most cases comprehensive clinical evaluation by an experienced clinician is adequate for diagnosis. There is a false-negative rate of approximately 15%.

SYNOPSIS OF TREATMENT OPTIONS

The prevention and management of fractures in individuals with OI require a multidisciplinary approach. Treatment should be tailored to the individual needs of the patient, taking into account the age and severity of disease. The long-term goal for children with OI is independence in the daily functions of life, including self-care, mobility, and recreation. Regular exercise and a good diet should be encouraged in all patients. Individuals with OI should avoid smoking, excessive alcohol or caffeine consumption, and corticosteroids, which may affect bone density. In patients with severe disease, bisphosphonates are being routinely used for improving bone density.

Medical Treatment

Cyclical intravenous bisphosphonates have been shown to reduce bone pain and fracture incidence and to increase bone density and mobility, with minimal side effects.[39] Most clinical trials have involved treatment of children with severe forms of OI. At present, there is insufficient evidence to recommend bisphosphonates for all children with mild OI. A number of issues regarding the use of bisphosphonate therapy in children and adolescents remain to be resolved, including the optimal dose, frequency, and duration of administration. Bisphosphonate therapy should, therefore, only be administered by specialist physicians. Other drugs, such as the parathyroid hormone–like protein teriparatide are also being studied as treatments for patients with OI.

Future therapeutic options for OI may include allogeneic bone marrow transplantation to engraft functional mesenchymal progenitor cells and thus help increase the production of normal bone.

Surgical Treatment

Surgical intervention is indicated for recurrent fractures or deformity that impairs function.

In many circumstances it may be preferable to treat fractures with short-term immobilization in lightweight casts, splints, or braces to allow mobilization as soon as possible.

Surgery is often undertaken in children with OI in which metal rods are inserted into the long bones to control fractures and improve bowing deformities.[40] Fractures may still occur after rodding, but the rod provides an internal splint that can maintain bony alignment. There are two basic types of rods. Nonexpandable rods are more versatile but may need replacement as the child grows (see Fig. 81-9). Expandable rods have a telescopic design and can change in length as the bone grows. Due to their thickness they can only be used in larger bones, such as the femur and tibia. These rods need to be firmly anchored at both ends (Fig. 81-22; see also Figs. 81-12 and 81-13).

Percutaneous vertebroplasty is an effective technique for relieving painful vertebral compression fractures in osteoporosis, but its routine use in OI has not been established.

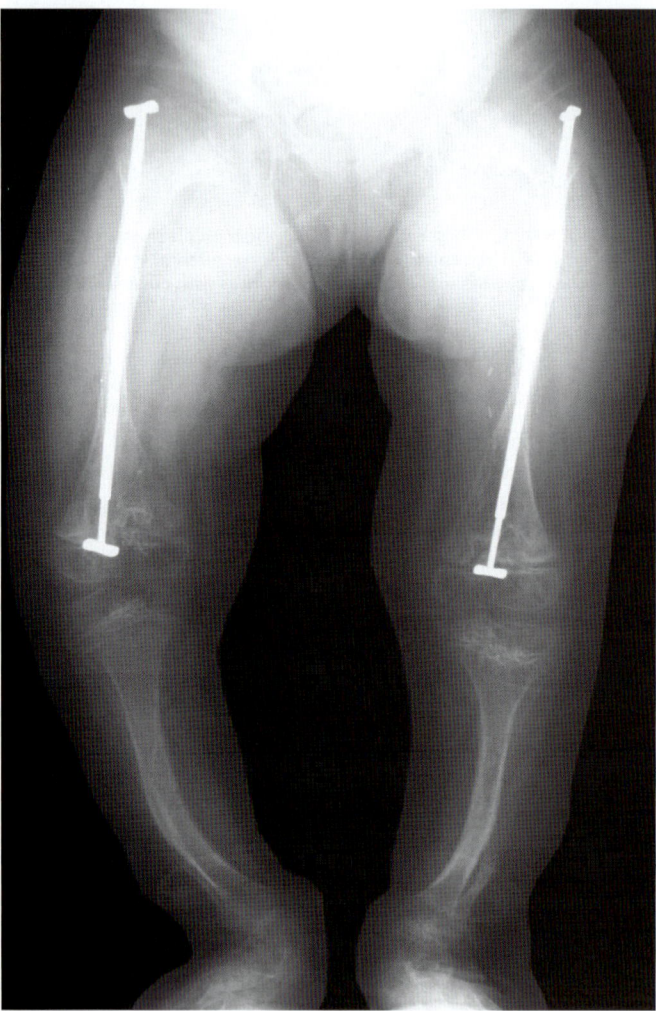

■ **FIGURE 81-22** Radiograph of both lower limbs demonstrating extendable rods in situ within both femoral shafts in a child with OI type III. Note that the rods are anchored at both ends.

What the Referring Physician Needs to Know

- The diagnosis of OI is based on clinical and radiologic features.
- Many radiologic findings are nonspecific and may be seen across all subtypes.
- The differential diagnosis of OI is based on the age at presentation.
- The cornerstone of imaging is radiography.
- CT is useful for evaluating neurologic complications and for investigating hearing loss.
- MRI is useful for evaluating neurologic complications and for differentiating acute from chronic vertebral fractures.
- DEXA can sometimes help to establish the diagnosis, assess prognosis, and monitor response to treatment.

SUGGESTED READINGS

Chapman S, Hall CM. Non-accidental injury or brittle bones. Pediatr Radiol 1997; 27:106–110.

Smith R. Osteogenesis imperfecta, non-accidental injury, and temporary brittle bone disease. Arch Dis Child 1995; 72:169–171; discussion 171–176.

Smith R, Wordsworth P. Osteogenesis Imperfecta: Clinical and Biochemical Disorders of the Skeleton. Oxford, Oxford University Press, 2005.

REFERENCES

1. Smith R, Wordsworth P. Osteogenesis Imperfecta: Clinical and Biochemical Disorders of the Skeleton. Oxford, Oxford University Press, 2005.
2. Byers PH. Inherited disorders of collagen gene structure and expression. Am J Med Genet 1989; 34:72-80.
3. Smith R. Osteogenesis imperfecta: from phenotype to genotype and back again. Int J Exp Pathol 1994;75:233-241.
4. Sillence DO, Senn A, Danks DM. Genetic heterogeneity in osteogenesis imperfecta. J Med Genet 1979; 16:101-116.
5. Wynne-Davies R, Gormley J. The prevalence of skeletal dysplasias: an estimate of their minimum frequency and the number of patients requiring orthopaedic care. J Bone Joint Surg Br 1985; 67:133-137.
6. Paterson CR, McAllion S, Miller R. Heterogeneity of osteogenesis imperfecta type I. J Med Genet 1983; 20:203-205.
7. Paterson CR, McAllion S, Stellman JL. Osteogenesis imperfecta after the menopause. N Engl J Med 1984; 310:1694-1696.
8. Bauze RJ, Smith R, Francis MJ. A new look at osteogenesis imperfecta: a clinical, radiological and biochemical study of forty-two patients. J Bone Joint Surg Br 1975; 57:2-12.
9. Cremin B, et al. Wormian bones in osteogenesis imperfecta and other disorders. Skeletal Radiol 1982; 8:35-38.
10. Riew KD, et al. Diagnosing basilar invagination in the rheumatoid patient: the reliability of radiographic criteria. J Bone Joint Surg Am 2001; 83:194-200.
11. Hayes M, et al. Basilar impression complicating osteogenesis imperfecta type IV: the clinical and neuroradiological findings in four cases. J Neurol Neurosurg Psychiatry 1999; 66:357-364.
12. Charnas LR, Marini JC. Communicating hydrocephalus, basilar invagination, and other neurologic features in osteogenesis imperfecta. Neurology 1993; 43:2603-2608.
13. Ross UH, et al. Osteogenesis imperfecta: clinical symptoms and update findings in computed tomography and tympanocochlear scintigraphy. Acta Otolaryngol 1993; 113:620-624.
14. Mafee MF, et al. Use of CT in the evaluation of cochlear otosclerosis. Radiology 1985; 156:703-708.
15. Benson DR, Donaldson DH, Millar EA. The spine in osteogenesis imperfecta. J Bone Joint Surg Am 1978; 60:925-929.
16. Sillence DO, et al. Osteogenesis imperfecta type II: delineation of the phenotype with reference to genetic heterogeneity. Am J Med Genet 1984; 17:407-423.
17. Spranger J, Cremin B, Beighton P. Osteogenesis imperfecta congenita: features and prognosis of a heterogenous condition. Pediatr Radiol 1982; 12:21-27.
18. McAllion SJ, Paterson CR. Causes of death in osteogenesis imperfecta. J Clin Pathol 1996; 49:627-630.
19. Amako M, et al. Functional analysis of upper limb deformities in osteogenesis imperfecta. J Pediatr Orthop 2004; 24:689-694.
20. Aarabi M, et al. High prevalence of coxa vara in patients with severe osteogenesis imperfecta. J Pediatr Orthop 2006; 26:24-28.
21. Engelbert RH, et al. Spinal complications in osteogenesis imperfecta: 47 patients 1-16 years of age. Acta Orthop Scand 1998; 69:283-286.
22. Versfeld GA, et al. Costovertebral anomalies in osteogenesis imperfecta. J Bone Joint Surg Br 1985; 67:602-604.
23. Widmann RF, et al. Spinal deformity, pulmonary compromise, and quality of life in osteogenesis imperfecta. Spine 1999; 24:1673-1678.
24. Sillence DO, et al. Osteogenesis imperfecta type III: delineation of the phenotype with reference to genetic heterogeneity. Am J Med Genet 1986; 23:821-832.
25. Paterson CR, McAllion S, Miller R. Osteogenesis imperfecta with dominant inheritance and normal sclerae. J Bone Joint Surg Br 1983; 65:35-39.
26. Glorieux FH, et al. Type V osteogenesis imperfecta: a new form of brittle bone disease. J Bone Miner Res 2000; 15:1650-1658.
27. Ward LM, et al. Osteogenesis imperfecta type VII: an autosomal recessive form of brittle bone disease. Bone 2002; 31:12-18.
28. Viljoen D, Versfeld G, Beighton P. Osteogenesis imperfecta with congenital joint contractures (Bruck syndrome). Clin Genet 1989; 36:122-126.
29. Cole DE, Carpenter TO. Bone fragility, craniosynostosis, ocular proptosis, hydrocephalus, and distinctive facial features: a newly recognized type of osteogenesis imperfecta. J Pediatr 1987; 110:76-80.
30. Alam A, Teh J. MRI assessment of scoliosis. Imaging 2005; 17:226-235.
31. Constantine G, et al. Prenatal diagnosis of severe osteogenesis imperfecta. Prenat Diagn 1991; 11:103-110.
32. Astrom E, Soderhall S. Beneficial effect of bisphosphonate during five years of treatment of severe osteogenesis imperfecta. Acta Paediatr 1998; 87:64-68.
33. Huang RP, et al. Functional significance of bone density measurements in children with osteogenesis imperfecta. J Bone Joint Surg Am 2006; 88:1324-1330.
34. Smith R. Osteogenesis imperfecta, non-accidental injury, and temporary brittle bone disease. Arch Dis Child 1995; 72:169-171; discussion 171-176.
35. Chapman S, Hall CM. Non-accidental injury or brittle bones. Pediatr Radiol 1997; 27:106-110.
36. Paterson CR, Burns J, McAllion SJ. Osteogenesis imperfecta: the distinction from child abuse and the recognition of a variant form. Am J Med Genet 1993; 45:187-192.
37. Astley R. Metaphyseal fractures in osteogenesis imperfecta. Br J Radiol 1979; 52:441-443.
38. Gahagan S, Rimsza ME. Child abuse or osteogenesis imperfecta: how can we tell? Pediatrics 1991; 88:987-992.
39. Glorieux FH, et al. Cyclic administration of pamidronate in children with severe osteogenesis imperfecta. N Engl J Med 1998; 339:947-952.
40. Cole WG. Orthopaedic treatment of osteogenesis imperfecta. Ann N Y Acad Sci 1988; 543:157-166.

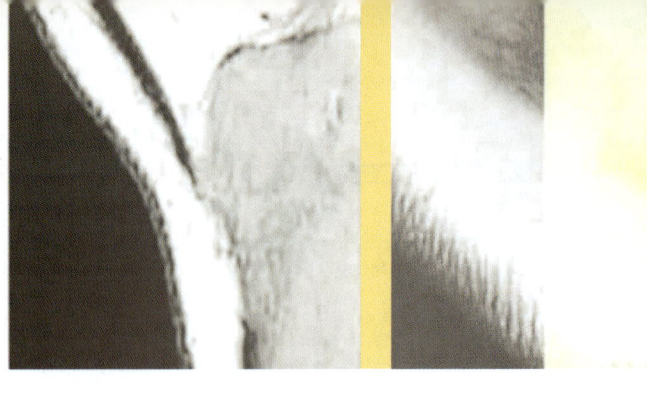

82

Marfan Syndrome

Filip M. Vanhoenacker, A. Snoeckx, and M. Biervliet

ETIOLOGY

Marfan syndrome is an autosomal dominant disorder.

PREVALENCE AND EPIDEMIOLOGY

The incidence in the general population is estimated as 1 in 5,000 to 10,000.[1] The majority of patients will have familial incidence, although approximately 15% of cases occur sporadically, representing new mutations.

CLINICAL PRESENTATION

Marfan syndrome is a disorder of connective tissue, involving the cardiovascular, ocular, and skeletal systems, as well as the lungs, dura, and skin.[1,2]

PATHOPHYSIOLOGY

Abnormalities in synthesis, secretion, or matrix incorporation of the glycoprotein fibrillin-1 are responsible for the clinical manifestations. The genetic defect has been linked to the *FBN1* gene on chromosome 15q21.1. More than 135 mutations have been described so far.[2,3] At present, it is possible to identify mutations in 70% of affected people.[4] Prenatal and preimplantation diagnosis is currently possible for families with known mutations.[5,6]

IMAGING TECHNIQUES

Plain radiography still plays a pivotal role in the initial imaging evaluation of Marfan syndrome. For evaluation of spinal manifestations (dural ectasia), CT and/or MRI are more appropriate techniques.

MANIFESTATIONS OF THE DISEASE

The phenotypic features of Marfan syndrome are highly variable, but most patients can be diagnosed clinically. The major clinical findings involve three major organ systems: ocular, cardiovascular, and skeletal.[2] Ocular signs are myopia, increased axial globe length, corneal flatness, and lens subluxation. Cardiovascular manifestations (Fig. 82-1A) include mitral valve prolapse, aortic root dilatation, mitral and/or aortic valve regurgitation, and aortic dissection and rupture. Cardiovascular complications, which begin in the first or second decade of life, are responsible for a reduction of the life expectancy.[7,8]

Clinical musculoskeletal findings include increased height and arm span, chest and vertebral column deformity, joint hypermobility, arachnodactyly, pes planus, and a narrow, highly arched palate and a narrow jaw, resulting in crowded and poor dentition.[2] Skeletal symptoms are predominant in childhood.[9]

Other clinical features include spontaneous pneumothorax, recurrent inguinal hernia, and striae atrophicae.[2]

The diagnostic criteria (including major and minor criteria for various organ systems) for Marfan syndrome have been described in detail by De Paepe and colleagues.[10] These clinical criteria, regarding the musculoskeletal system, are summarized in Table 82-1. Further discussion of diagnostic criteria of other organ systems is, however, beyond the scope of this chapter.

In the absence of family history, an affected person should display major criteria in at least two organ systems and involvement of a third organ system. In the presence of a positive family history, only one major criterion of an

---

KEY POINTS

- Chest deformity including pectus excavatum or pectus carinatum is encountered in 66% of patients.
- Severe scoliosis with a curve of more than 20 degrees or midthoracic lordosis and thoracolumbar kyphosis occurs in about two thirds of patients.
- Dural ectasia occurs in up to 63% of patients and is best assessed by MRI.
- Acetabular protrusion is seen in nearly 50% of patients.
- The value of the metacarpal index for assessment of arachnodactyly has been questioned.

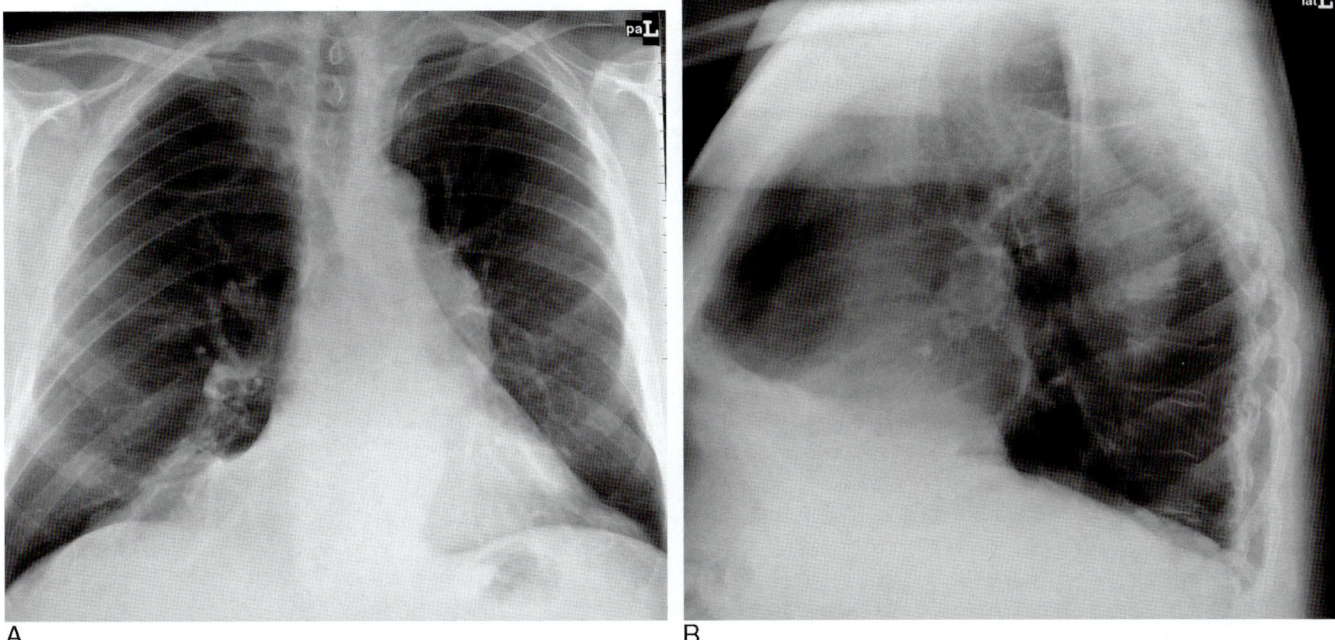

■ **FIGURE 82-1** Posteroanterior (**A**) and lateral (**B**) chest radiographs of a patient with Marfan syndrome. There is dilatation of the descending aorta. Note also a localized bulla in the right upper lung.

TABLE 82-1 Major and Minor Diagnostic Skeletal Criteria for Marfan Syndrome

Major Criteria
Presence of at least four of the following manifestations:
Pectus carinatum
Pectus excavatum requiring surgery
Reduced upper to lower segment ratio or arm span to height ratio
   greater than 1.05
Wrist and thumb signs
Scoliosis of more than 20 degrees or spondylolisthesis
Reduced extension at the elbows (<170 degrees)
Medial displacement of the medial malleolus causing pes planus
Acetabular protrusion
Minor Criteria
Pectus excavatum of moderate severity
Joint hypermobility
Highly arched palate with crowding of teeth
Facial appearance (dolichocephaly, malar hypoplasia, enophthalmos,
   retrognathia, down-slanting palpebral fissures)

Note: The skeletal system is considered to be involved if at least two major
   criteria or one major criterion and two minor criteria are present.

organ system and involvement of a second organ system are required.

In this chapter, the discussion of imaging abnormalities of Marfan syndrome is focused solely on musculoskeletal involvement.

Chest Deformity

In approximately 66% of patients, a pectus excavatum or pectus carinatum (pigeon chest) is encountered (Fig. 82-2). Elongated ribs are responsible for the pectus deformity. Thoracic lordosis and scoliosis (Fig. 82-3) may be associated and may further aggravate chest deformity,

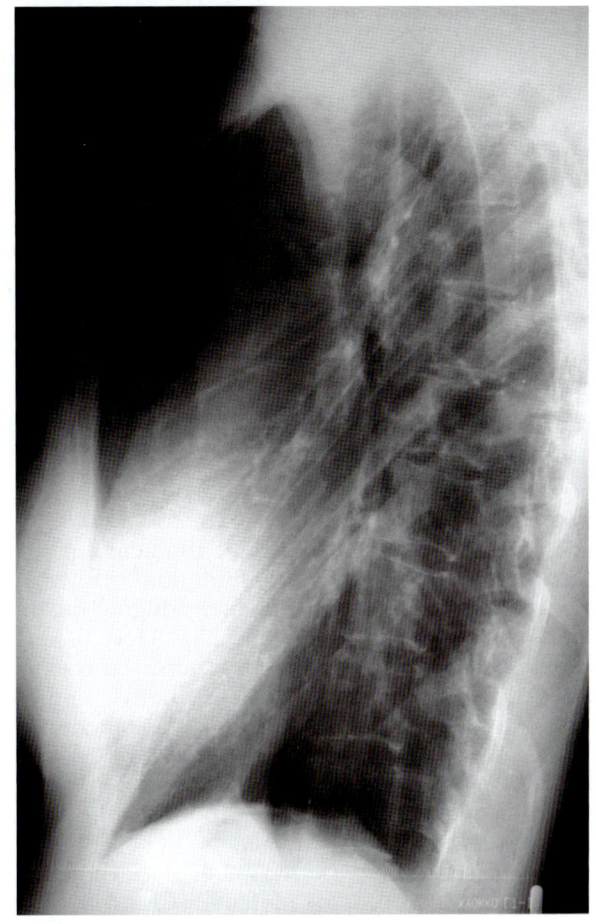

■ **FIGURE 82-2** Lateral chest radiograph demonstrating a pigeon chest deformity.

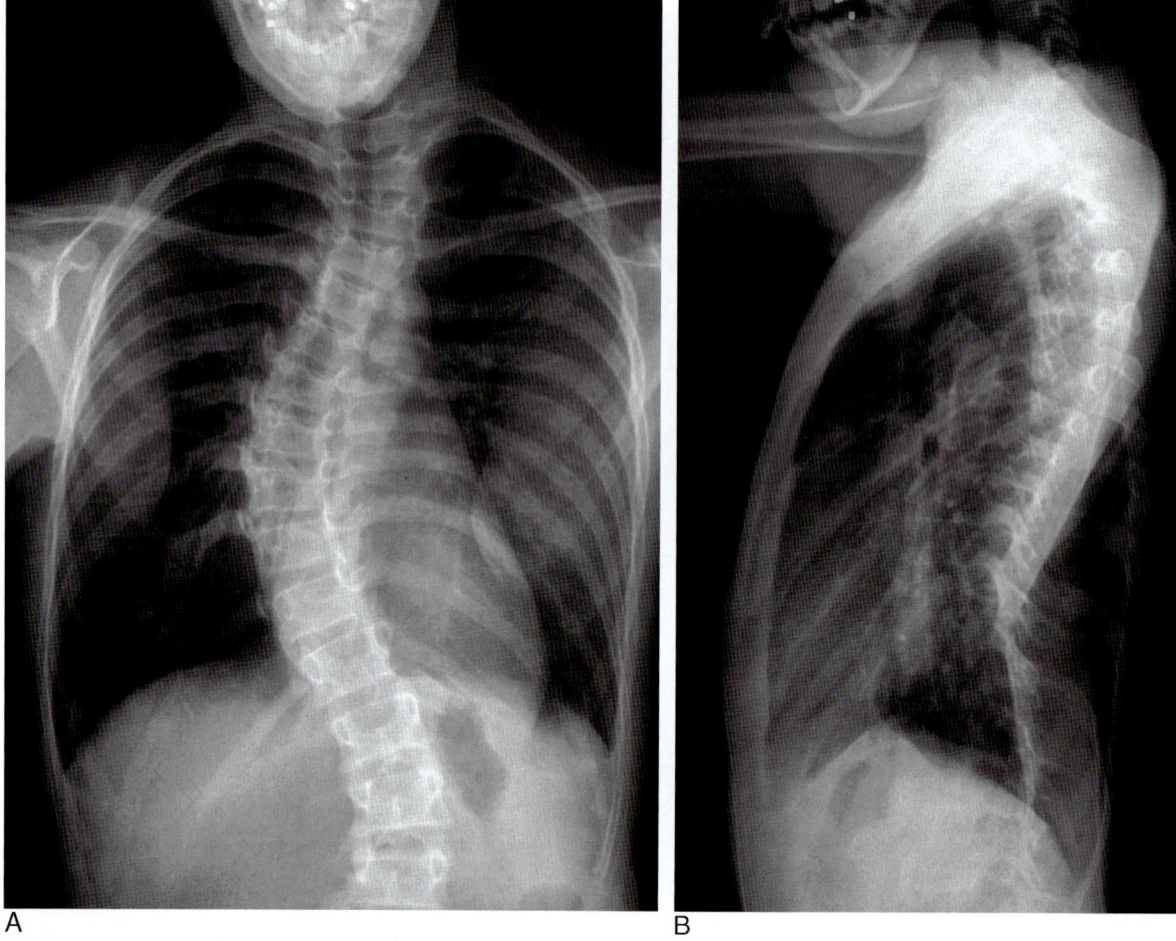

A   B

■ **FIGURE 82-3**   Posteroanterior (**A**) and lateral (**B**) chest radiographs. Severe chest deformity due to scoliosis and thoracic lordosis. Note also the presence of elongated ribs on the posteroanterior view.

compromising pulmonary function.[2] Apical bullae (see Fig. 82-1B) and spontaneous pneumothorax may further complicate the respiratory status of the patient.

Spine

A variety of abnormalities may be seen in the spine. Severe scoliosis with a curve of more than 20 degrees or midthoracic lordosis and thoracolumbar kyphosis occurs in about two thirds of patients.[11] The scoliosis is frequently a double major or right thoracic curve (see Fig. 82-3A), developing early in childhood.[12] Other manifestations of the lumbar spine include a higher incidence of spondylolisthesis, tall vertebrae (Fig. 82-4), biconcave vertebrae, transition vertebrae and increased transverse process distances, smaller pedicle widths, and laminar thickness.[2,13,14] The interpedicular distance may be widened.[15]

In the cervical spine, increased atlantoaxial translation, basilar impression, increased odontoid height, and focal kyphosis have been reported.[16]

Dural ectasia is a major criterion of Marfan syndrome, occurring in up to 63% of patients.[2] Clinically, it may be associated with back pain and headaches. The neural symptoms are thought to be related to stretching

and traction mechanisms. Dural ectasia may result in bony erosion with posterior scalloping of the vertebral bodies (Fig. 82-5) and thinning of the pedicles and lamina. Additionally, anterior meningoceles may develop (Fig. 82-6).

Radiography

Conventional radiography can be used to assess dural ectasia in adult patients.[17] At least one of the following criteria is required: an interpediculate distance at L4 greater than or equal to 38 mm, scalloping value at L5 greater than or equal to 5.5 mm, or sagittal diameter at S1 greater than or equal to 18 mm. Although conventional radiography has a high specificity of 91.7%, it has a low sensitivity of only 57.1%.[17]

Magnetic Resonance Imaging and Multidetector Computed Tomography

Because of the low sensitivity of standard radiography, guidelines for assessment of dural ectasia on CT and MRI have been developed by measuring the sagittal width of the dural sac and the dural sac ratio.[18,19] The dural sac ratio consists of the anteroposterior dural sac diameter (DSD) divided by the anteroposterior vertebral body diameter

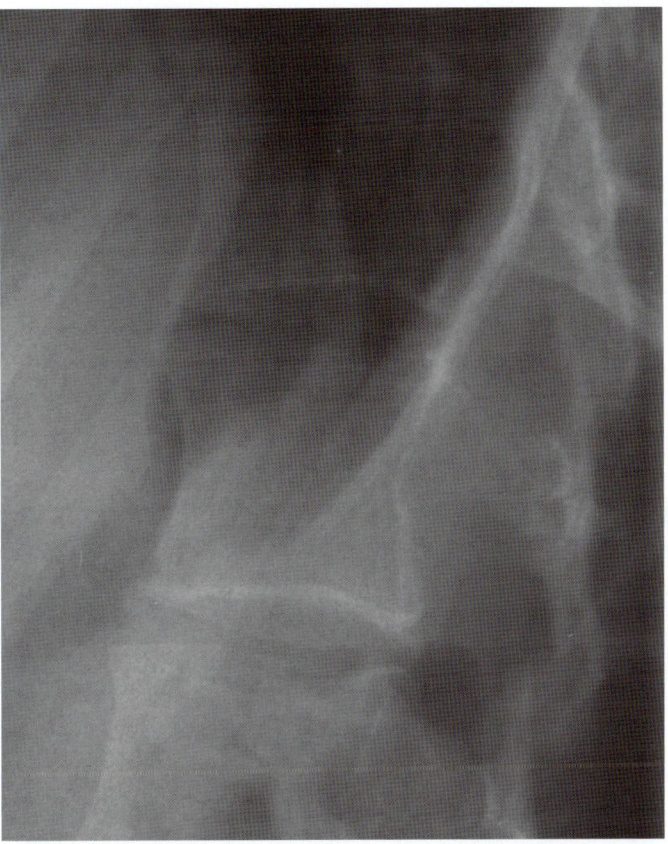

■ FIGURE 82-4 Lateral spot view of the thoracolumbar spine, showing tall vertebrae, which have a slightly biconcave morphology. Note the slight posterior scalloping.

(VBD). According to recent data, only the dural sac ratio at L5 and S1 and a sagittal dural width at S1 greater than that at L4 are statistically significant criteria (Fig. 82-7) for assessment of dural ectasia in children, adolescents, and young adults.[20] A dural sac ratio greater than 0.57 at S1 is sufficient for diagnosing Marfan syndrome.

Pelvis

Unilateral or bilateral acetabular protrusion (Fig. 82-8) is another frequent finding in Marfan syndrome, occurring in nearly 50% of patients.[21] Developmental dysplasia of the hip may occur due to increased joint mobility.[2]

Radiography

Radiographically, acetabular protrusion may be evaluated by the acetabular teardrop crossing the ilioischial line or by crossing of the acetabular and iliopectineal lines.[2]

Bone Mineral Density

A decreased bone mineral density has been reported, but the etiology and clinical significance in relation to fracture risk remain uncertain.[22]

Elongation of the Extremities and Arachnodactyly

Elongation of the extremities without an increase in width is classic (Fig. 82-9). The lower extremity exhibits greater overgrowth than the upper. Leg-length discrepancy may be associated with increased structural scoliosis.[23]

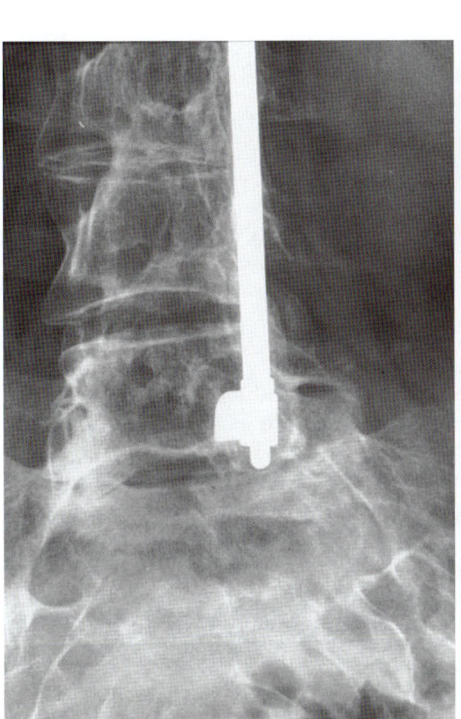
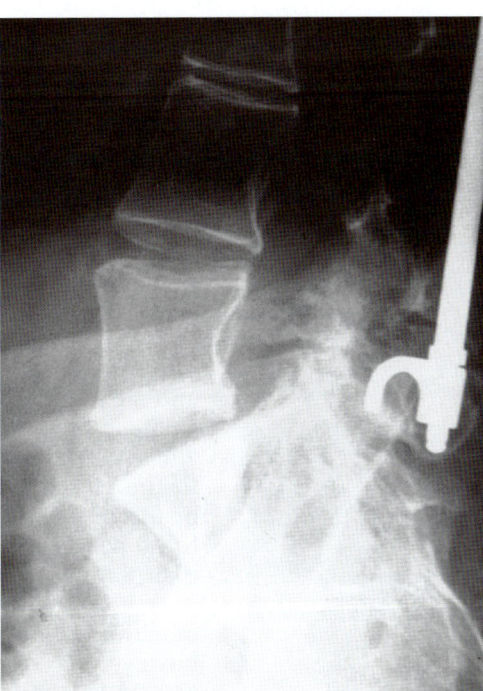

■ FIGURE 82-5 Radiograph of the lumbar spine, showing more severe posterior scalloping. Note also the presence of scoliosis, for which a surgical correction was performed (rod).

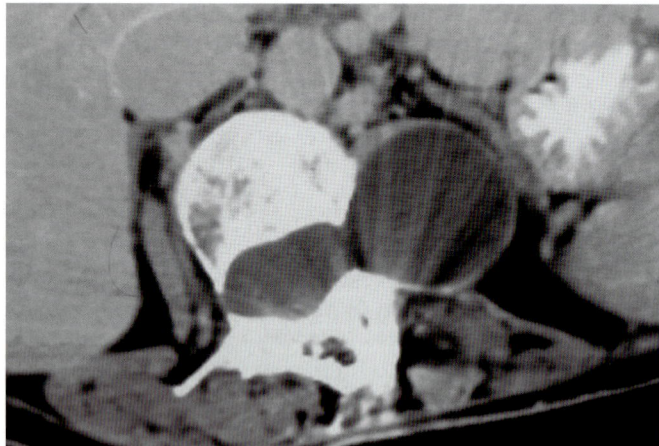

■ **FIGURE 82-6** CT scan of the upper abdomen. Note anterolateral meningocele on the left side of the spine.

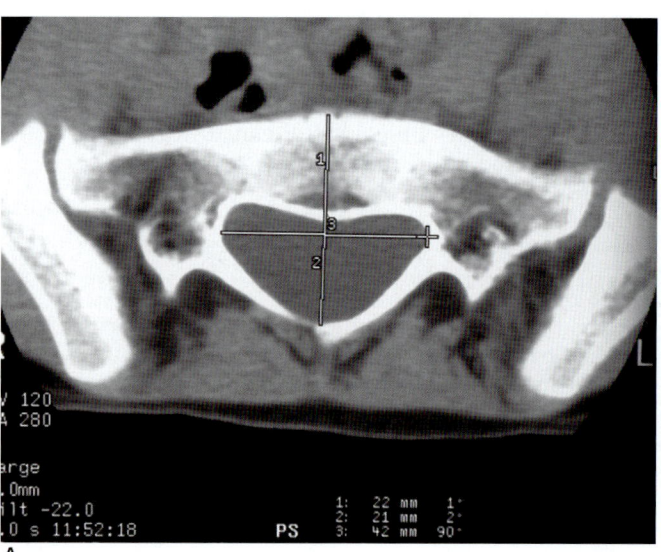

A

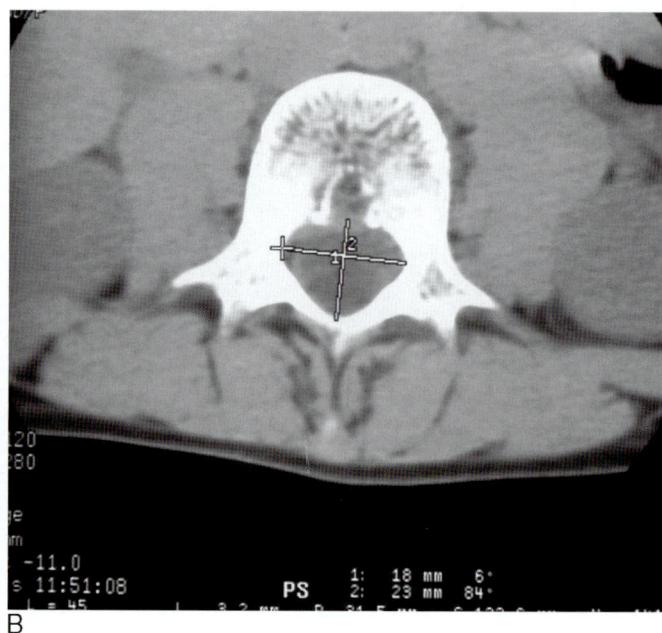

B

■ **FIGURE 82-7** CT scan of the lumbar spine. The anteroposterior dural sac diameter (DSD) at S1 (**A**) exceeds the DSD at L4 (**B**), which is indicative of dural ectasia.

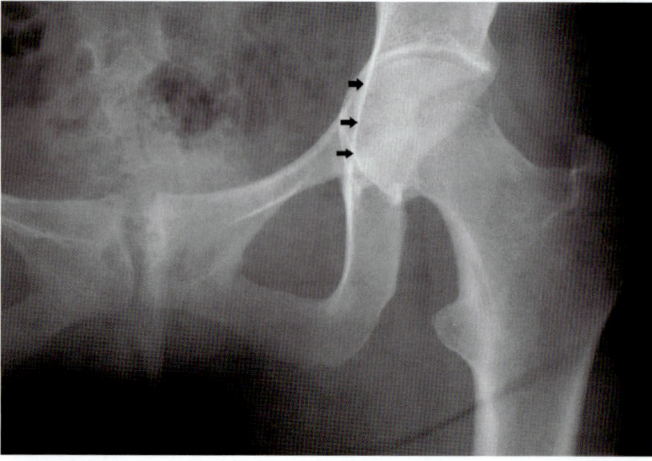

■ **FIGURE 82-8** Radiograph of the left hip. The acetabular teardrop crosses the ilioischial line, which indicates the presence of protrusio acetabuli (*arrows*).

Radiography

The tubular bones of the hands and feet are gracile, long, and slender ("spider-like"), which is designated by the term *arachnodactyly* (Fig. 82-10). The cortices are generally thinned, and the trabecular pattern is often delicate. In the past, the metacarpal index (MCI) was calculated by measuring the ratio of the average length and width of the second through fourth metacarpals. A ratio of more than 8.8 in males and 9.9 in females was believed to be indicative of arachnodactyly. The diagnostic value of this radiation-dependent and time-consuming measurement, however, has been questioned. According to Thomas and associates, the MCI does not have a role in assessment of

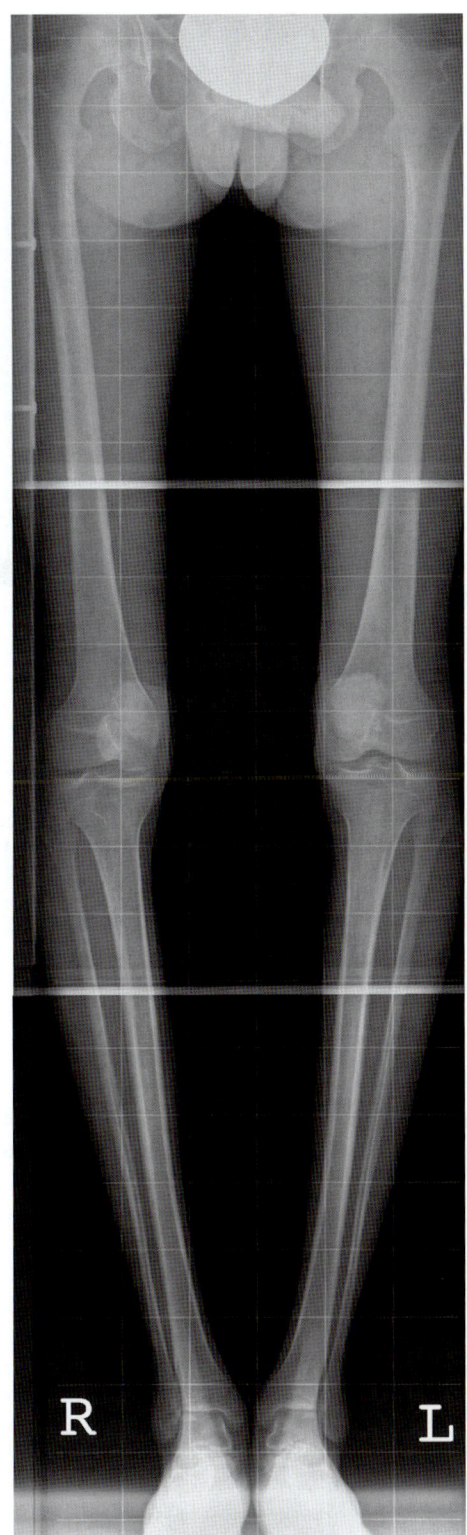

■ **FIGURE 82-9** Full-leg radiograph demonstrating elongation of the femoral, tibial, and fibular bones.

Marfan syndrome except possibly in two specific circumstances: (1) when the diagnosis is suspected but all other skeletal criteria are normal and (2) when there is clinical doubt and sophisticated tests are not available, as may occur in parts of the developing world.[24]

Feet

Radiography

Foot radiographs (anteroposterior and lateral weight-bearing views) may demonstrate pes planovalgus secondary to ligamentous laxity.

Skull

Radiography

Compared with the normal skull, the Marfan skull is found to be longer, taller, and thicker and to have an increased frontal sinus area. A high-arched palate may be present as well.[25]

DIFFERENTIAL DIAGNOSIS

Several disorders are included in the differential diagnosis of Marfan syndrome on the basis of similar skeletal, cardiac, and ophthalmologic manifestations. Many individuals referred for possible Marfan syndrome are shown to have evidence of a systemic disorder of the connective tissue, including long limbs, deformity of the thoracic cage, striae atrophicae, mitral valve prolapse, and mild and nonprogressive dilatation of the aortic root but do not meet diagnostic criteria for the disorder. This constellation of features is referred to by the acronym MASS phenotype (Mitral valve, Aorta, Skeleton, and Skin).

Marfan syndrome should be distinguished from other syndromes with cardiac and vascular involvement as well as musculoskeletal manifestations. This includes Ehlers-Danlos syndrome, homocystinuria, Loeys-Dietz syndrome, and Shprintzen-Goldberg syndrome. Differential diagnosis for cardiovascular and ocular involvement without musculoskeletal manifestations includes familial thoracic aortic aneurysm syndrome, bicommissural aortic valve, and ascending aortic aneurysm and familial ectopia lentis.

In a patient with prominent arachnodactyly, disorders such as congenital contractural arachnodactyly and acromegaly should be included in the differential diagnosis.[26]

SYNOPSIS OF TREATMENT OPTIONS

Medical Treatment

Treatment options for Marfan syndrome vary, depending on the organ system affected. Medical treatment by β-adrenergic receptor blockade is directed to prevent aortic dissection, which is the most fearful complication of Marfan syndrome.[26] Currently, a cure for Marfan syndrome does not exist. Because Marfan syndrome is an autosomal dominant disorder, genetic counseling is highly recommended.

Surgical Treatment

Main surgical treatment options include cardiovascular surgery for aortic dissection and aortic aneurysm, ocular surgery, and scoliosis surgery. In the early-onset

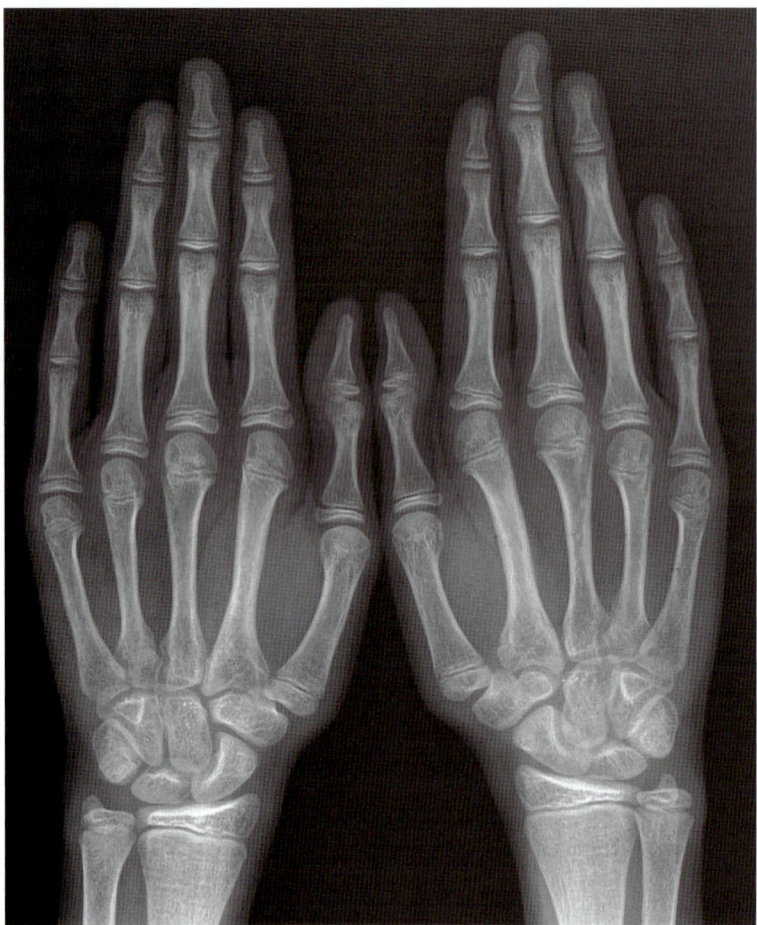
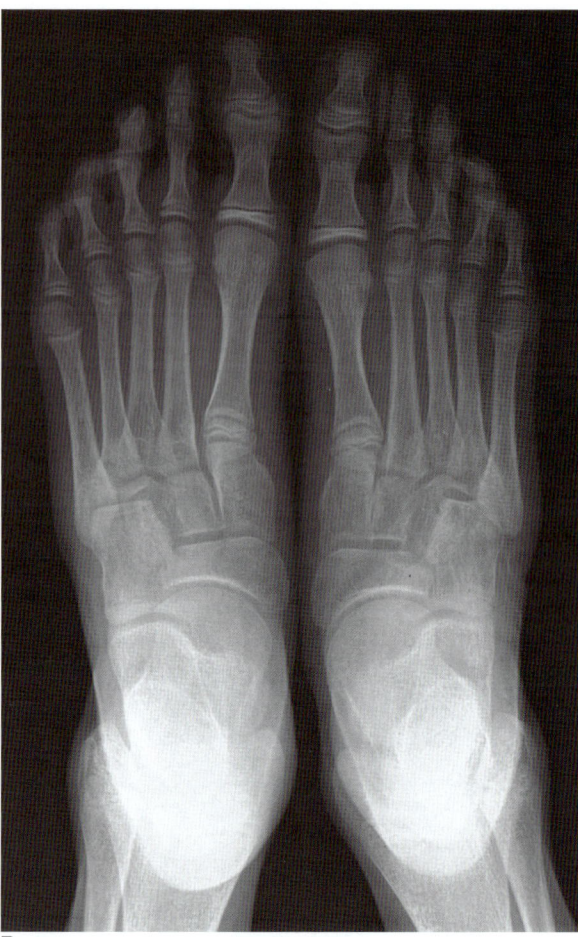

■ **FIGURE 82-10** Radiographs of the hands (**A**) and feet (**B**) showing slender and gracile metacarpals, metatarsals, and phalanges.

scoliosis or "infantile scoliosis" in Marfan syndrome, bracing is not recommended for halting progression of curves greater than 40 degrees. Moreover, surgery should not be performed on children younger than 4 years of age because many patients with large curves before this age will succumb spontaneously to cardiac complications.[12]

What the Referring Physician Needs to Know

- Phenotypic features of Marfan syndrome are highly variable.
- Diagnostic criteria include major and minor criteria.
- Because Marfan syndrome is an autosomal dominant disorder, genetic counseling is highly recommended.
- Curative treatment for Marfan syndrome does not exist.
- Surgery for scoliosis should not be performed on children younger than 4 years of age.

SUGGESTED READINGS

Aburawi EH, O'Sullivan J, Hasan A. Marfan's syndrome: a review. Hosp Med 2001; 62:153–157.

Giampietro PF, Raggio C, Davis J. Marfan syndrome: orthopedic and genetic review. Curr Opin Pediatr 2002; 14:35–41.

Magid D, Pyeritz RE, Fishman EK: Musculoskeletal manifestations of the Marfan syndrome: Radiologic features. AJR Am J Roentgenol 1990; 155:99.

REFERENCES

1. Pyeritz RE, McKusick VA: The Marfan syndrome: diagnosis and management. N Engl J Med 1979; 300:772-777.
2. Giampietro PF, Raggio C, Davis JG. Marfan syndrome: orthopedic and genetic review. Curr Opin Pediatr 2002; 14:35-41.
3. Toudjarska I, Kilpatrick MW, Lembessis P, et al. Novel approach to the molecular diagnosis of Marfan syndrome: application to sporadic case and in prenatal diagnosis. Am J Med Genet 2001; 99:294.
4. Nijbroek G, Sood S, McIntosh I, et al. Fifteen novel FBN1 mutations causing Marfan syndrome detected by heteroduplex analysis of genomic amplicons. Am J Hum Genet 1995; 57:8-21.
5. Rantamaki T, Raghunath M, Karttunen L, et al. Prenatal diagnosis of Marfan syndrome: identification of a fibrillin-1 mutation in chorionic villus sample. Prenat Diagn 1995; 15:1176-1181.
6. Harton GL, Tsipouras P, Sisson MD, et al. Preimplantation genetic testing for Marfan syndrome. Mol Hum Reprod 1996; 2:713-715.
7. Roseborough GS, William GM. Marfan and other connective tissue disorders: Conservative and surgical considerations. Semin Vasc Surg 2000; 13:272.
8. Murdoch JL, Walker BA, Halpren BI, et al. Life expectancy and causes of death in Marfan syndrome. N Engl J Med 1972; 286:804.
9. Lipscomb KJ, Clayton-Smith J, Harris R. Evolving phenotype of Marfan's syndrome. Arch Dis Child 1997; 76:41-46.
10. De Paepe A, Devereux RB, Dietz HC, et al. Revised diagnostic criteria for Marfan syndrome. Am J Med Genet 1996; 62:417-426.
11. Sponseller PD, Hobbs W, Riley LH, et al. The thoracolumbar spine in Marfan syndrome. J Bone Joint Surg Am 1995; 77:867-876.
12. Sponseller PD, Sethi N, Cameron DE, et al. Infantile scoliosis in Marfan syndrome. Spine 1997; 22:509-516.
13. Tallroth K, Malmivaara A, Laitinin ML, et al. Lumbar spine in Marfan syndrome. Skeletal Radiol 1995; 24:337-340.
14. Sponseller PD, Ahn NU, Ahn UM, et al. Osseous anatomy of the lumbosacral spine in Marfan syndrome. Spine 2000; 25:2797-2802.
15. Ahn NU, Ahn UM, Nallamshetty L, et al. The lumbar interpediculate distance is widened in adults with the Marfan syndrome. Acta Orthop Scand 2001; 72:67-71.
16. Hobb WR, Sponseller PD, Weiss AC, Pyeritz RE. The cervical spine in Marfan syndrome. Spine 1997; 22:983-989.
17. Ahn NU, Nallamshetty L, Buchowski JM, et al. Dural ectasia and conventional radiography in the Marfan lumbosacral spine. Skeletal Radiol 2001; 30:338-345.
18. Ahn NU, Sponseller PD, Ahn UM, at al. Dural ectasia in the Marfan syndrome: MR and CT findings and criteria. Genet Med 2000; 2:173-179.
19. Oosterhof T, Groenink M, Hulsmans F, et al. Quantitative assessment of dural ectasia as a marker for Marfan syndrome. Radiology 2001; 220:514-518.
20. Habermann CR, Weis F, Schoder V, et al. MR evaluation of dural ectasia in Marfan syndrome: reassessment of the established criteria in children, adolescents, and young adults. Radiology 2005; 234:535-541.
21. Yule SR, Hobson EE, Dean JC, Gibert FJ. Protrusio acetabuli in Marfan's syndrome. Clin Radiol 1999; 54:95-97.
22. Giampietro PF, Person M, Schneider R, et al. Assessment of bone mineral density in adults and children with Marfan syndrome. Osteopor Int 2003; 14:559-563.
23. Jones KB, Sponseller PD, Hobbs W, et al: Leg-length discrepancy and scoliosis in Marfan syndrome. J Pediatr Orthop 2002; 22:807.
24. Thomas SM, Younger KA, Child A, Wilson AG. Is the metacarpal index useful in the diagnosis of Marfan syndrome? Clin Radiol 1006; 51:570-574.
25. Beals RK, Mason L. The Marfan skull. Radiology 1981; 140:723-725.
26. Judge DP, Dietz HC. Marfan's syndrome. Lancet 2005; 366:1965-1976.

Paget's Disease

Iain Watt

Paget's disease, or osteitis deformans, was described by Sir James Paget when he presented his series of five cases on November 14, 1886, to the Medical and Chirurgical Society of London. He described a slowly progressive disorder leading to enlargement and deformity of bones, notably the patient's head, and increased risk of fracture. The following year, a detailed report was published of one of these patients, whom Paget had observed for approximately 20 years, as well as a brief summary of several other persons with the same disorder.[1]

PREVALENCE

The worldwide prevalence of Paget's disease varies appreciably. The rate is highest in the United Kingdom (the original site of description)[2] and countries settled from the United Kingdom, including Australia, New Zealand, and the United States. The disease is much rarer in continental Europe and is very rare in Asia and Africa. Even within the United Kingdom prevalence rates vary considerably, with the highest grouped in the northwest of England (Fig. 83-1).[2] Currently, the disease affects 3% to 4% of adults older than 40 years of age in the United Kingdom and as many as 10% of those 80 years of age or older. The peak age at presentation is 60 to 69 years.[3] Although unusual, patients younger than the age of 40 can be affected.

ETIOLOGY

The exact etiology is unknown. A possible infectious cause has been suggested. Giant osteoclasts with numerous nuclei characterize active Paget's disease. Probable viral intracellular inclusion bodies have been shown in these osteoclasts that contain organized groups of microcylinders in the nuclei and cytoplasm, as found in other paramyxovirus infections such as measles. Other possible infective organisms have been suggested, including canine distemper virus.[4] In some populations, Paget's disease is rare, or apparently new. For example, Paget's disease was described first in Japan in 1921 but may have increased since then. This may reflect better detection, a spreading slow virus infection, or other unknown causes. Higher prevalences in association with HLA-DR2 antigen have been recorded in Ashkenazi Jews. This and reports of cases affecting several members of a family in various generations as well as affliction of identical twins suggest a genetic basis. The most important cause of classic Paget's disease is sequestosome 1, which is a scaffold protein in the NF-κB signaling pathway; mutations affecting the ubiquitin-associated domain of this protein occur in 20% to 50% of familial and 10% to 20% of sporadic cases.[5] Debate persists with regard to the balance between the influences of environmental versus familial factors. However, the high prevalence of familial disease supports the importance of heritable factors.[6] Whatever the underlying etiology, recent clinical, biochemical, and paleopathologic data from the United Kingdom and New Zealand suggest that the prevalence of Paget's disease is falling, as well as the severity of skeletal involvement (Figs. 83-2 and 83-3).[7-10]

PATHOPHYSIOLOGY

The major finding is an excessive and abnormal remodeling of bone with active and quiescent phases (Figs. 83-4 and 83-5). Three such phases are described but in reality represent a continuum. Individual sites progress at different rates, resulting in a thickened, disorganized trabecular and cortical pattern. The first phase corresponds to the radiographic lytic stage, when highly active osteoclasts dominate, resulting in osteolysis of bone as in osteoporosis circumscripta (Fig. 83-6) and the advancing resorption, or flame-shaped V front (Fig. 83-7). The second phase represents a mixed picture of osteoblastic repair coupled with ongoing bone resorption. This produces both trabecular and cortical thickening consisting of primitive or woven bone with increased vascularity and a pronounced connective tissue reaction. The final phase is osteoblast dominant and hence is dominantly sclerotic. Multiple cement lines are seen, each representing an episode of bone resorption and subsequent re-formation. The re-formed trabeculae lack normal orientation, and hence the bone is weaker and unable to shed load normally. As a consequence,

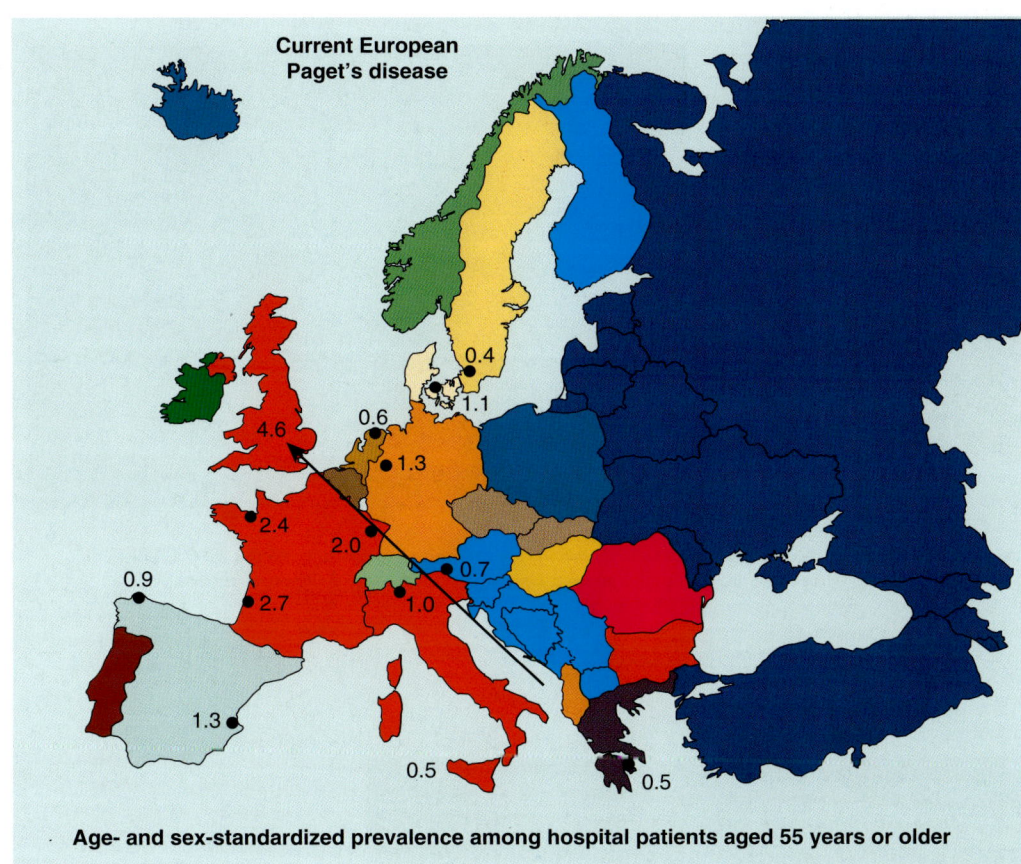

■ FIGURE 83-1 The prevalence of Paget's disease varies across Europe, being lowest in the southeast and greatest in the northwest (figures noted are percentages).

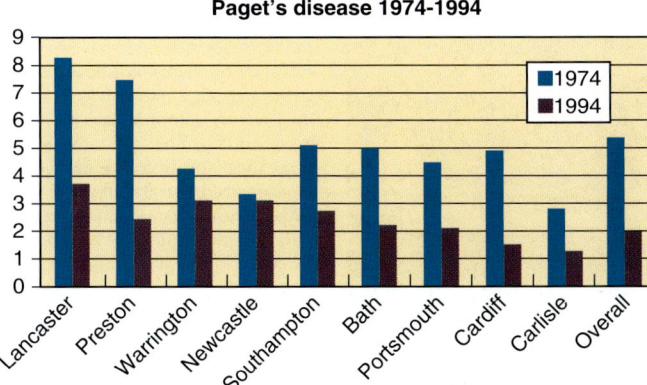

■ FIGURE 83-2 The regional prevalence of Paget's disease may be declining. These data show a reduction has occurred in the same British towns between 1974 and 1994. Note how the levels vary even within the United Kingdom and that the greatest prevalence is in the northwest (Lancaster and Preston). *(From Cooper C, Schafheutle K, Dennison E, et al. The epidemiology of Paget's disease in Britain: is the prevalence decreasing? J Bone Miner Res 1999; 14:192–197. Reproduced with permission of the American Society for Bone and Mineral Research.)*

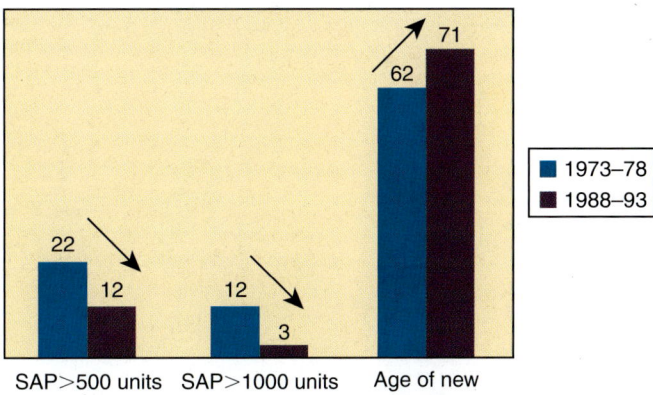

■ FIGURE 83-3 The severity of Paget's disease also may be declining. The age at onset in new cases is increasing while the severity, as measured by serum alkaline phosphatase (SAP), is less. *(From Cundy HR, Gamble G, Wattie D, et al. Paget's disease of bone in New Zealand: continued decline in disease severity. Calcif Tissue Int 2004; 75:358–364. Reprinted with kind permission from Springer Science and Business Media.)*

bone is softer, bows under load, and fractures more easily. Furthermore, pagetic bone does not form haversian systems or organize around blood vessels as normal bone does. The cortex is the site of the most active turnover, with hypervascularity typified by small-caliber vessels. In the bone marrow, fibrovascular replacement of normal fat occurs, especially in the lytic phase, but returns to fatty marrow again in the late mixed phase. Eventually, marrow fat is greater than normal. The coarse-fibered pagetic bone is avid for both calcium and phosphorus, as can be shown in isotopic studies. Pagetic bones may be ivory hard, difficult to cut, and heavier than normal.

An increase in regional blood flow is classic, shown clinically as a rise in skin temperature, and related to the

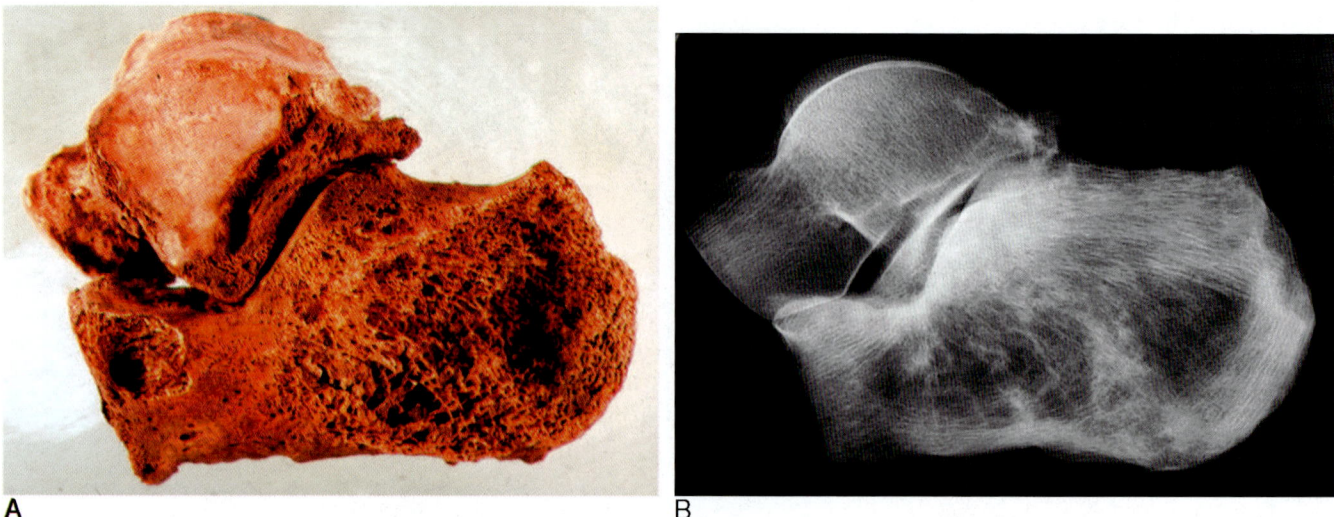

■ **FIGURE 83-4   A,** The macroscopic appearance of established Paget's disease is shown in this dry bone specimen. Note the cortical thickening; the "picture frame"–like outline; the disruption of normal trabeculation, especially the load-bearing trabeculae; and the expansion of bone. **B,** Radiograph of specimen.

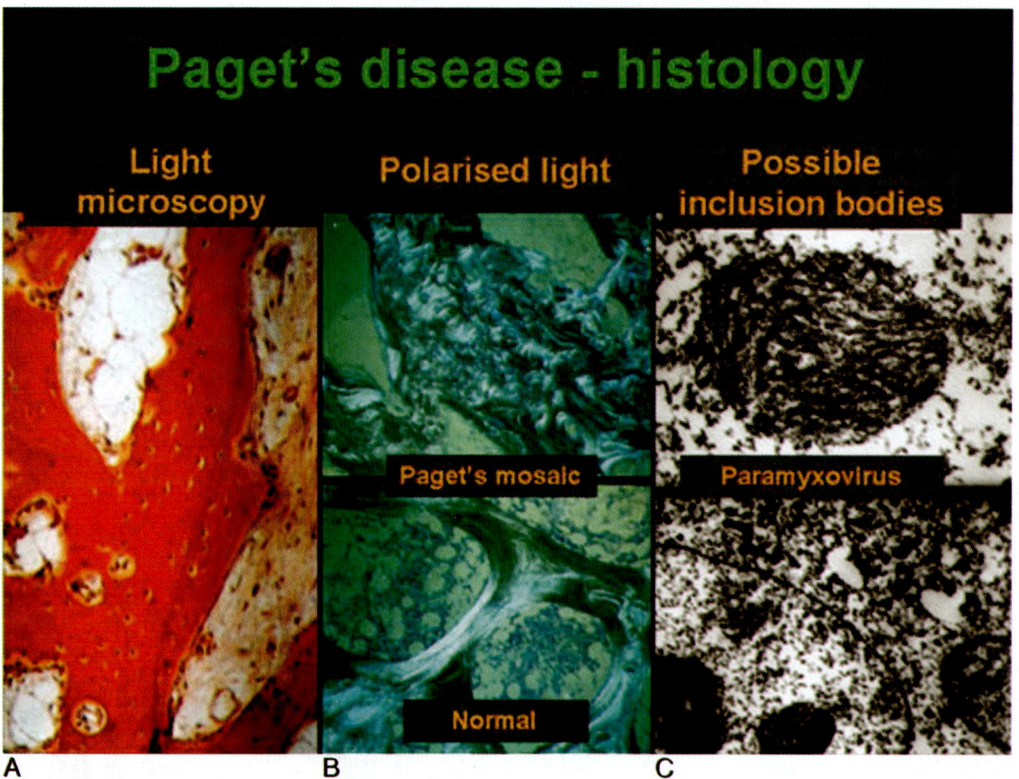

■ **FIGURE 83-5   A,** Histologically the normal trabeculae have been replaced by thickened, disorganized structures. **B,** Polarizing light microscopy demonstrates the replacement of normal lamellar bone (*below*) with a mosaic, disorganized pattern (stained with toluidine blue). **C,** Electron microscopy of nuclei of affected osteoclasts shows inclusion bodies resembling paramyxovirus-like structures.

hypervascularity of pagetic bone. As indicated, pagetic bone contains an increased number of capillaries, dilated arterioles, and large venous sinuses. This, coupled with a decrease in peripheral resistance, results in an increased cardiac output, particularly when involvement of the skeleton is extensive.

CLINICAL PRESENTATION

According to Paget, "the most frequent seats of the osteitis have been the tibiae, femora, clavicles, spine, and vault of the skull." Little has changed since this description in 1889; currently, the most commonly involved sites include

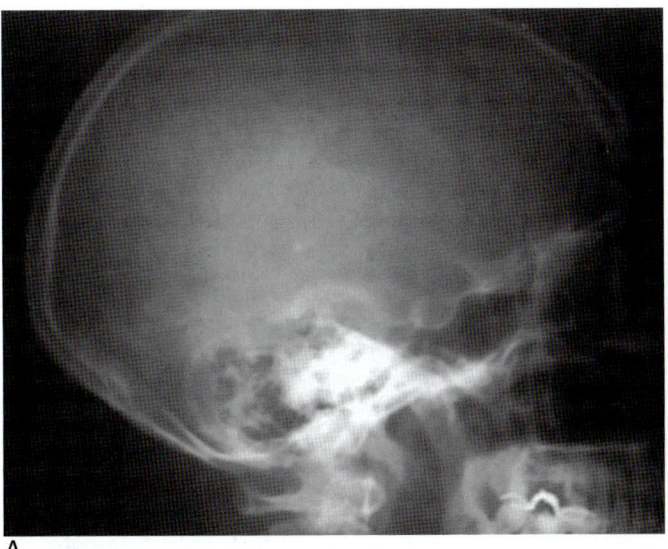

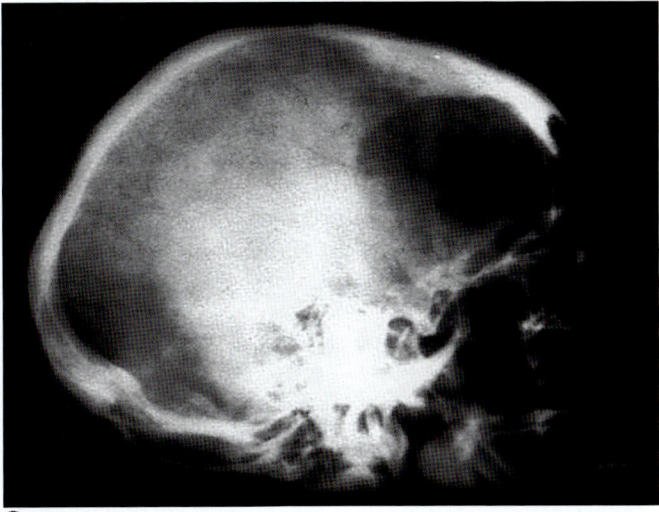

A

C

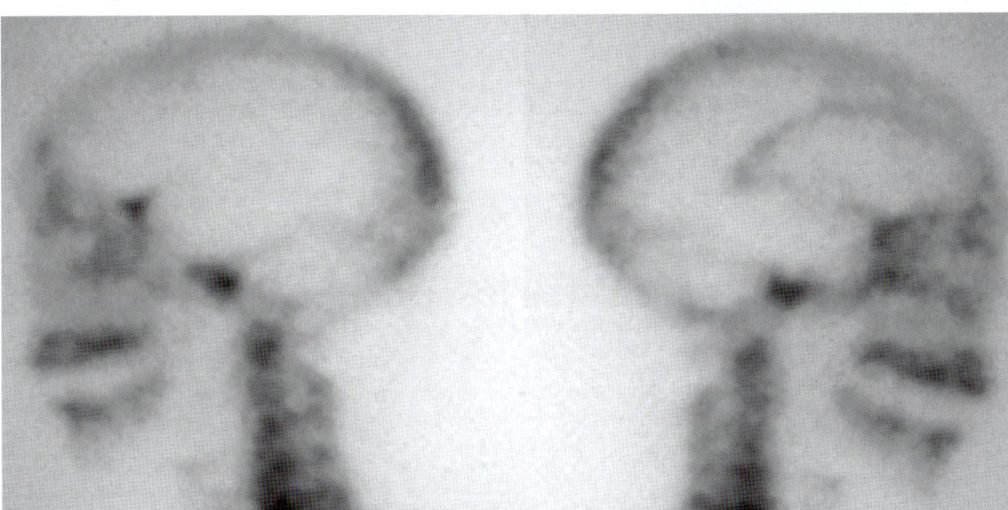

B

■ **FIGURE 83-6** Osteoporosis circumscripta in the skull. A rather subtle reduction in frontal bone density on the radiograph (**A**) is outlined by a margin of increased activity on a late-phase scintigram (**B**). In another patient, with more advanced disease, a classic, geographic area of frontal bone lucency is shown (**C**).

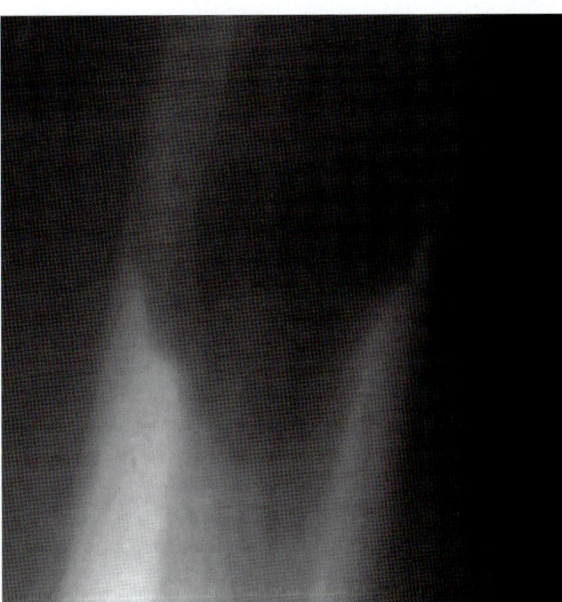

■ **FIGURE 83-7** A localized view of the femur demonstrates a classic V-shaped front between active lytic Paget's disease and normal bone.

the skull (25%–65%), spine (30%–75%), pelvis (30%–75%), and proximal long bones (25%–30%), whereas the shoulder girdle and arm are less involved (humerus, 31%; scapula, 24%; clavicle, 11%). Any bone may be affected, but pagetic changes in the ribs, fibulae, and small bones in the hand and foot are infrequent (Fig. 83-8). Although most commonly presenting as a polyostotic disease, Paget's disease may be monostotic (10%–35%), occurring most often in the spine. Polyostotic disease tends to be asymmetric in distribution and often predominantly right sided (Fig. 83-9).

Within an individual bone, Paget's disease almost always begins in the subarticular zone and spreads progressively along the shaft to the diaphysis. The rate of progression in active disease is about 1 mm per month. A particular exception is the tibial tubercle, where disease may begin and spread distally, leaving the subarticular zone of the knee uninvolved (Fig. 83-10). Occasionally the same process may be seen in the radius.

At least one patient in five is totally asymptomatic, with Paget's disease being an incidental finding during an investigation for other problems. This may include the finding of a raised serum alkaline phosphatase value on examination of the blood (see later). Hence,

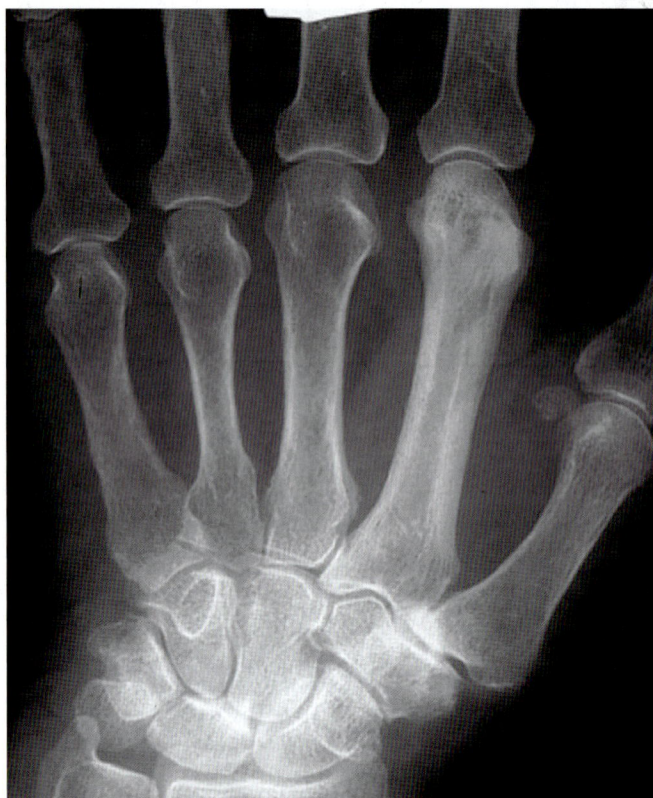

■ **FIGURE 83-8** Paget's disease may involve the small bones of the hand or foot as in this case of typical pagetic involvement of the index finger metacarpal.

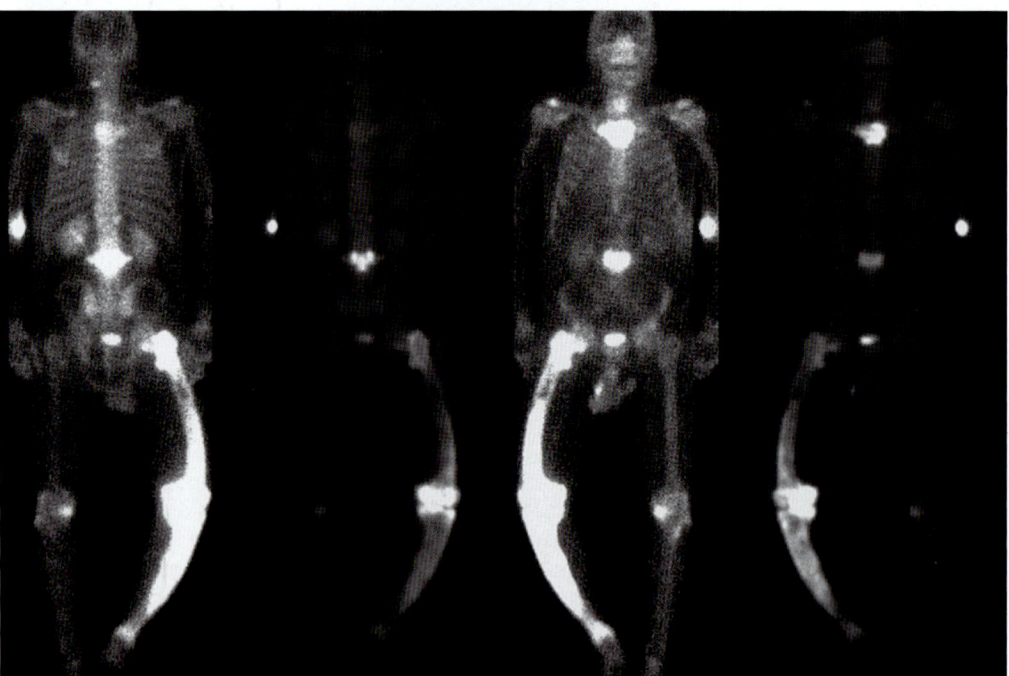

■ **FIGURE 83-9** A whole-body radionuclide scintiscan (late phase using ⁹⁹ᵐTc-labeled diphosphonate) shows a predominantly right-sided distribution of disease but also the apparently random sites of involvement. Note, however, the area of photon deficiency in the right femur. This should raise the possibility of a sarcoma, which was confirmed histologically.

the exact prevalence and true incidence of the disease is difficult to assess. On the other hand, the disease may present as severe symptoms and signs, including skeletal, neuromuscular, and cardiovascular complications. Typically, Paget's disease begins in middle age, progresses slowly, and gives no problems apart from those that are due to changes of shape, size, and angulation of affected bones. The major clinical features are shown in Box 83-1.

MANIFESTATIONS OF THE DISEASE

Laboratory Investigations

The classic findings are a raised serum alkaline phosphatase value and raised serum and urine levels of hydroxyproline, particularly in the active, lytic phase. Serum calcium and phosphate levels are usually normal, but less than 10% of patients may get secondary hyperparathyroidism due to hypercalcemia secondary to severe bone remodeling.

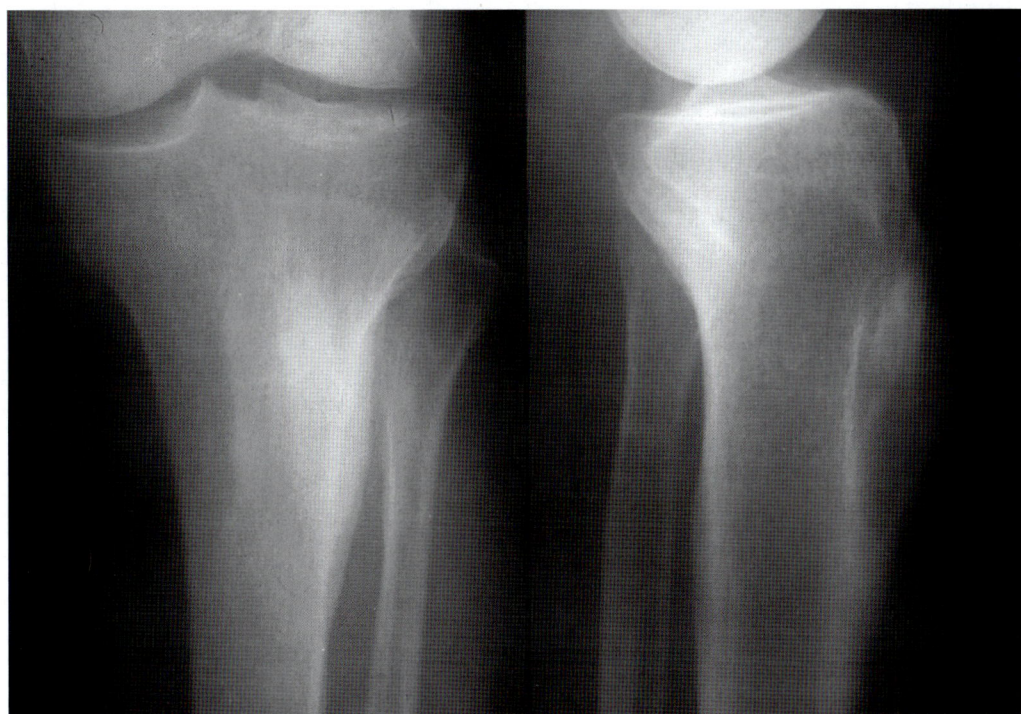

■ **FIGURE 83-10** Acute, lytic Paget's disease extending down the tibial shaft from the tibial tubercle and not the usual subarticular zone.

BOX 83-1   Clinical Features of Paget's Disease

SKELETAL

- Localized pain, often worse at night and unrelated to exercise
- Bony tenderness
- Increased skin temperature reflecting the hypervascularity of the underlying active disease
- Increasing bone size such as enlarging head, and therefore hat size
- Softening and remolding of bone, for example, bowing of the legs or an increasing kyphosis of the spine
- Fracture with minimal trauma

NEUROLOGIC

- Cranial nerve symptoms due to encroachment into foramina, for example, deafness and visual field defects
- Symptoms related to spinal cord compression or ischemia, including motor weakness or paralysis, sciatic claudication due to spinal stenosis, or incontinence

CARDIOVASCULAR

- The highly vascular bone of Paget's disease is associated with the need for a higher cardiac output. If severe, or associated with ischemic heart disease in an older patient, the result may be high-output congestive cardiac failure.
- Sudden acute heart failure may result from injudicious treatment of Paget's disease, when a sudden reduction in disease activity results in a dramatic increase in blood volume.
- Recent publications have reported a higher prevalence of aortic stenosis, complete heart block, and right bundle branch block in Paget's disease.

The raised levels of alkaline phosphatase may be related to an increased rate of bone formation, whereas the elevated urinary levels of hydroxyproline may indicate an increased rate of bone resorption. Urinary hydroxylysine (and hydroxylysine glycoside) excretion also increases in patients with Paget's disease. These abnormalities vary with the distribution and activity of disease and may be normal when the disease is inactive.

Radiography

For most indications, including diagnosis, staging, and surveillance, radiographs are usually sufficient. Paget's disease represents a continuum of pathology, but for convenience the features may be divided into three stages:

In the lytic phase, when excessive bone resorption dominates, the classic finding is of bone resorption and radiolucency. In the skull, large geographic areas of lucency develop that are often frontal or occipital, the so-called osteoporosis circumscripta. Both tables are involved, especially the inner table, in contradistinction to fibrous dysplasia, which usually involves the outer table particularly. Facial bone involvement is infrequent compared with the classic changes of fibrous dysplasia (Fig. 83-11). In the active, lytic phase, osteoblastic activity is absent or greatly reduced and thus sclerosis is not a feature. In long bones, the advancing edge of radiolucency presents a sharply defined margin that is V or wedge shaped, sometimes likened to a blade of grass or a flame. As indicated earlier, rare cases may start at the tibial tubercle; very rarely, the radius is the second most common site of diaphyseal Paget's disease. Paget's disease may present acutely and painfully after recent skeletal

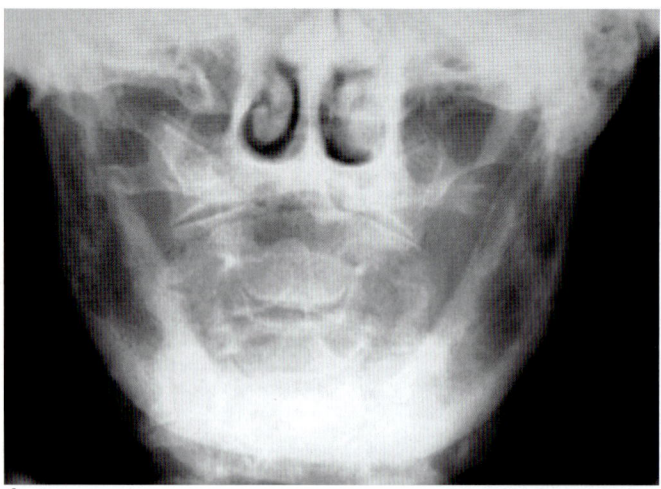

A

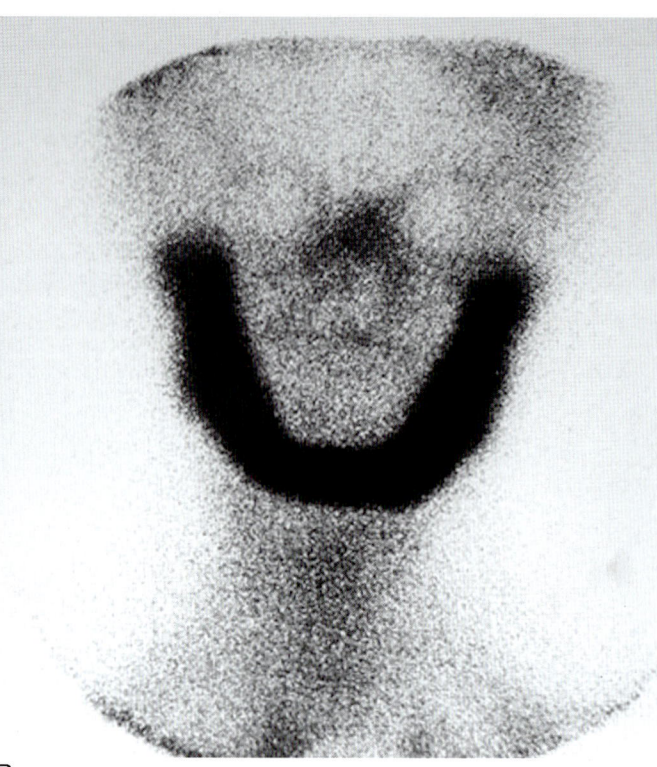

B

■ **FIGURE 83-11** It is unusual for the facial bones to be involved with Paget's disease. In this case, however, typical features are shown both on a radiograph (**A**) and the late phase of a scintiscan (**B**) in the mandible.

trauma that also may induce reactivation of an existing lesion (Fig. 83-12).

During the mixed phase, when secondary reparative, osteoblastic changes occur, the obvious feature is of coarsening and thickening of both trabeculae and cortex. The thickening is most obvious along lines of stress. In the pelvis, the iliopectineal and ischiopubic lines thicken in particular (Fig. 83-13) and the iliac wings often appear asymmetric in size, shape, and consistency. The combination of bone resorption and haphazard deposition results in abnormal molding of bone, and as bone enlarges in the pelvis this is most obvious at the pubic rami and ischium. In the spine, the combination of cortical thickening and coarsening trabeculation results in the so-called picture frame appearance. Paget's disease may be distinguished from other causes of sclerotic vertebrae, such as osteodystrophy, because it involves all four margins of the vertebra as opposed to the predominantly superior and inferior end-plate changes in the latter. Furthermore, the mainly vertical thickening is coarser than that seen in a hemangioma. Hemangiomas do not usually cause the end plate changes typical of Paget's disease.

In the later *blastic phase*, the individual lesions of Paget's disease progress variably and independently. In long bones, extensive sclerosis may develop that may obscure the underlying trabecular changes. Bony enlargement is common and may be considered a hallmark of Paget's disease. In the skull, patchy, ill-defined areas of sclerosis develop that may, at first sight, suggest metastasis. However, they are typically fluffy, are likened to cotton wool, and may cross over cranial sutures (Fig. 83-14). Marked thickening of the diploic space occurs, especially involving the inner table. Softening of bone, especially the skull base, results

in basilar invagination, causing the so-called tam-o'-shanter skull. The blastic phase in the spine is associated with diffuse sclerosis, resulting in marked sclerosis, often involving multiple levels. The sclerotic vertebrae are one of the causes of an "ivory vertebra" (Table 83-1; Fig. 83-15).

Skeletal Scintigraphy

Scintigrams using technetium-99m (^{99m}Tc)–labeled diphosphonates accurately reflect the marked increase in bone turnover in active Paget's disease. Increased activity is shown in all three phases of the disease, indicating the underlying pathologic process. Increased activity occurs in the early, blood pool phase, reflecting hypervascularity as well as the later, and osteoblastic, bone-forming image (Fig. 83-16). Scintigraphy may be used to show the polyostotic distribution of the disease and thereby assist staging before therapy. The scintigrams may be abnormal before any radiographic change and may give a so-called false-positive finding when a patient has been scanned for potential metastasis or other indications. However, Paget's disease is typified in long bones by the presence of elongated scintigraphic lesions beginning from an articular surface, unlike the rounded foci of metastasis.

The extent of increased activity recorded on scintiscans varies according to the underlying disease activity. So, for example, in one review scintigrams and corresponding radiographs were both abnormal in 56% to 86% of lesions, radiographs were only abnormal in 11% to 20%, and scintiscans were only abnormal in 2% to 23%.[11] This spectrum is important when assessing the presence of disease, when staging the disease, or when monitoring therapy.

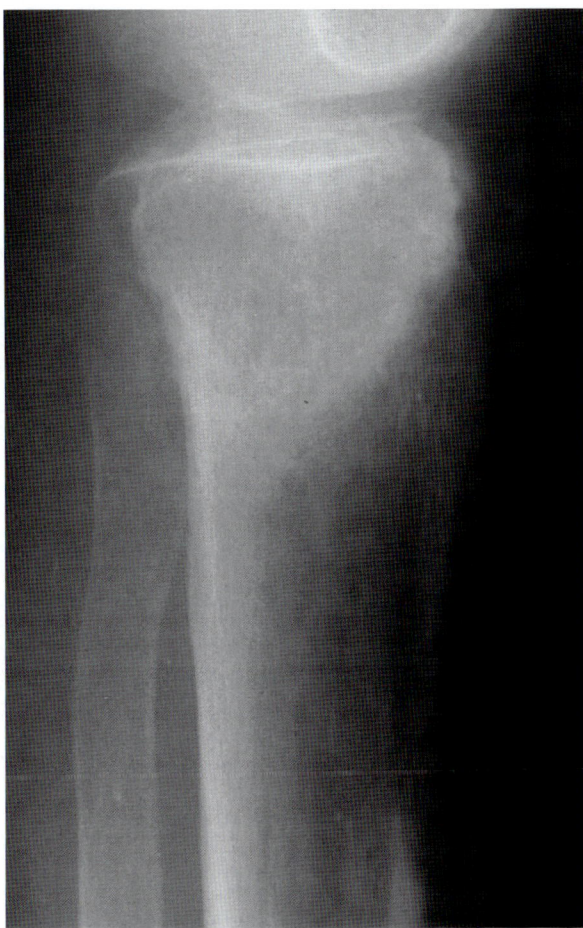

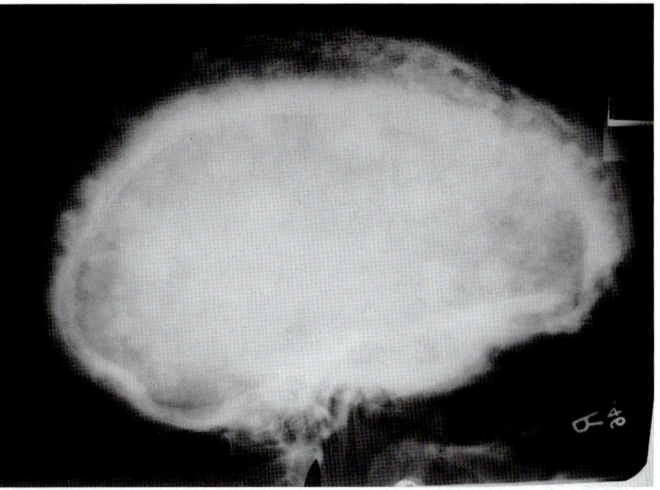

■ **FIGURE 83-14** Gross Paget's disease of the skull. Note the marked thickening of the vault, the multiple "cotton wool" opacities, and the extensive involvement of the base of the skull.

■ **FIGURE 83-12** Acute, lytic Paget's disease is present in the upper anterior tibia of this elderly woman. She had sustained an undisplaced, proximal tibial fracture 4 weeks before this radiograph (note the band of sclerosis running obliquely to the Paget's disease representing callus). This case illustrates how acute Paget's disease may occur after trauma and explained the ongoing severe pain that the patient felt in this limb.

TABLE 83-1 Most Common Differential Diagnosis to Paget's Disease in a Vertebra	
Diffuse Vertebral Body Sclerosis	**Focal Vertebral Body Sclerosis**
Hemangioma	Osteoblastic metastasis
Osteoblastic metastasis	(breast/prostate)
(breast/prostate)	Lymphoma
Myelosclerosis	Mastocytosis
Lymphoma	Osteoid osteoma
Mastocytosis	Osteoblastoma
Renal osteodystrophy	Chordoma
Fluorosis	
Sickle cell disease	
Chronic osteomyelitis	

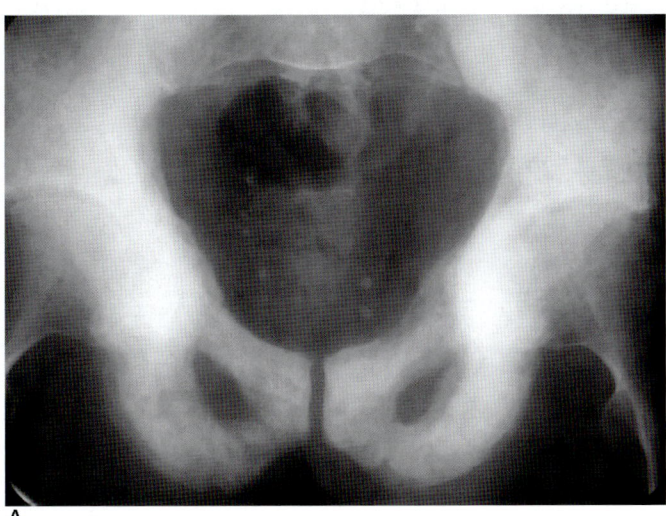

A

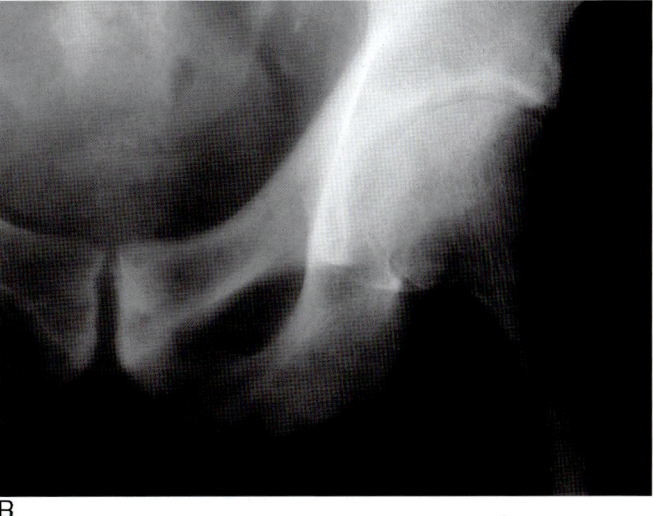

B

■ **FIGURE 83-13** Typical sclerotic Paget's disease of the pelvis. **A,** Extensive involvement should create no diagnostic difficulty, particularly the expansile disorganized nature of the bone. **B,** More subtle changes are shown in the left pubic ring of another patient.

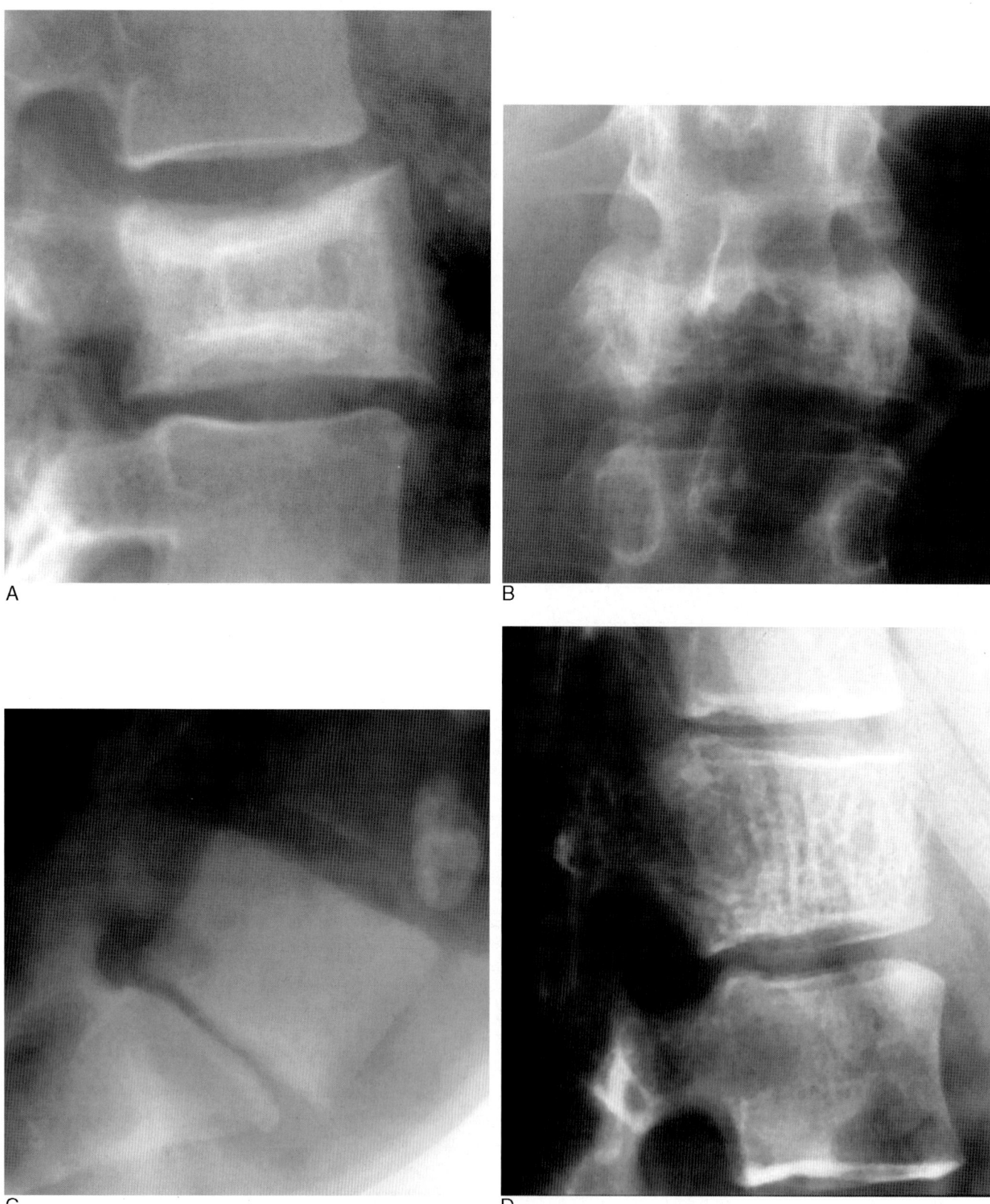

A

B

C

D

■ **FIGURE 83-15** Paget's disease of the lumbar spine. **A** and **B,** Typical features include expansion of bone, the "picture frame" appearance, obvious softening of bone, plasticity, and posterior element involvement. **C,** The denser, blastic phase is marked also by bone expansion. **D,** Note the important differences from a classic vertebral hemangioma.

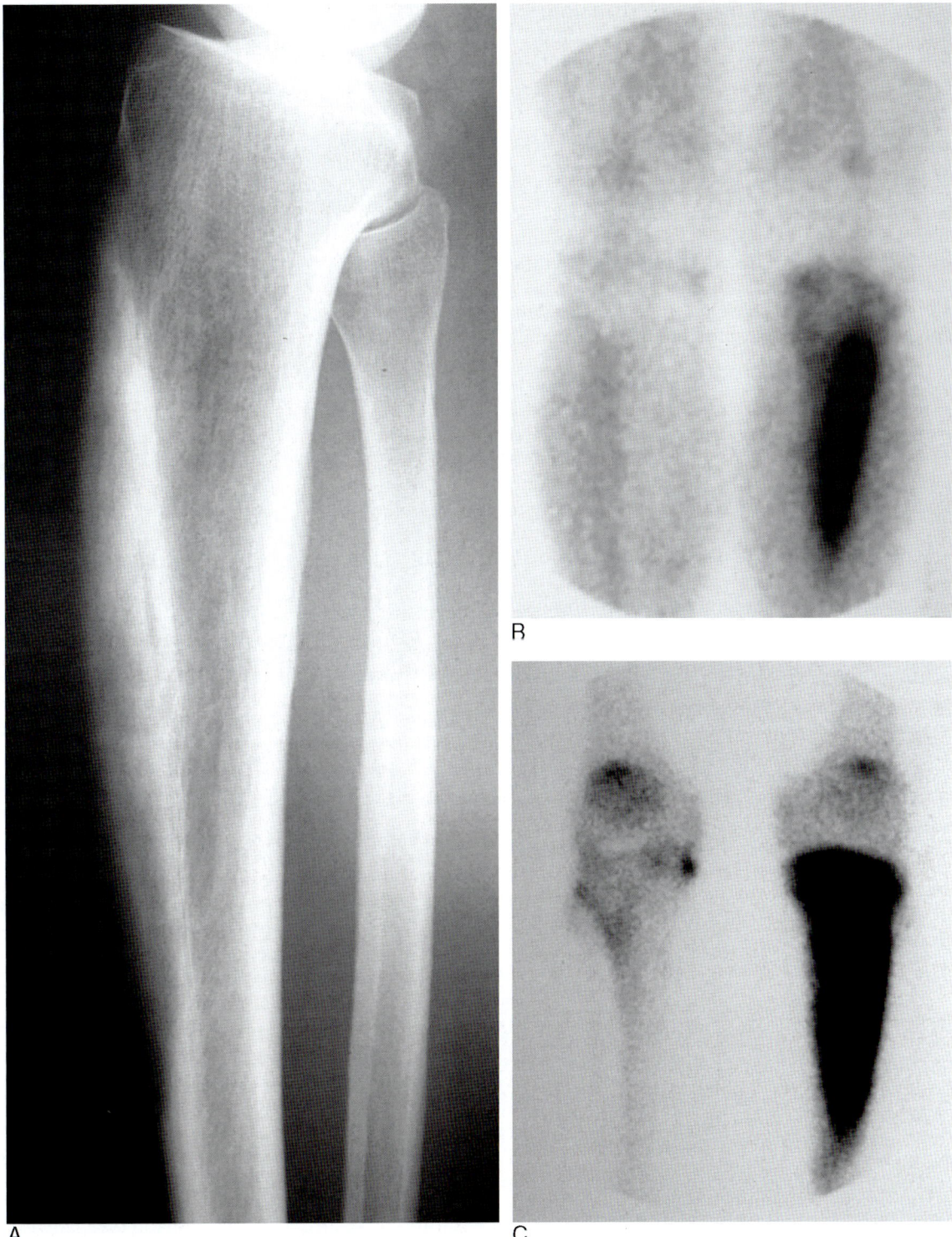

A   C

■ **FIGURE 83-16** **A,** ^{99m}Tc-labeled diphosphonate scintigraphy in active, lytic Paget's disease. Note the marked increase in activity on the early, blood pool image (**B**) as well as the grossly increased activity on the late phase (**C**). Although the radiograph suggests that the disease is confined to the anterior tibia, and confirmed largely by the blood pool image, the late phase suggests rather greater involvement.

Scintigraphy does not assist in the differentiation of the various complications of Paget's disease. Other radiopharmaceuticals have been employed, for example, gallium-67 citrate, but the results have not proved useful overall.

Computed Tomography and Magnetic Resonance Imaging

Both CT and MRI have questionable roles in most cases of Paget's disease. CT typically shows a reduced number of coarsened trabeculae as well as cortical and trabecular thickening. Patchy sclerosis may be more obvious, as is bony enlargement. Although these features are shown to better advantage on CT, radiographic changes are usually obvious.

MRI shows the same structural changes but with the added benefit of visualizing marrow fat. Cortical destruction and/or soft tissue masses are absent in uncomplicated Paget's disease. However, different phases of appearances are described in bone marrow. Usually yellow, fatty marrow signal is maintained regardless of pathologic phase, often more fat than usual.[12,13] Furthermore, the volume of the medullary canal may be reduced, owing to cortical encroachment. In the lytic to early mixed phase, bone marrow may show heterogeneous signal intensity on T1- and T2-weighted images. The T1-weighted signal intensity is decreased to that of muscle but still has fatty deposits within it. On T2-weighted images bone marrow shows heterogeneous high signal, accentuated on water-sensitive sequences due to fibrovascular replacement. Lastly, in late phase Paget's disease increasing low signal intensity is shown on all pulse sequences, corresponding to bony sclerosis. At all stages of disease the increased blood flow of Paget's disease is mirrored by gadolinium enhancement of involved bone. This is typically patchy or speckled and is most marked in active disease.

COMPLICATIONS

Benign

Paget's disease is heir to many multisystem complications. The major skeletal problems relate to bone softening and abnormal molding and bending, leading to deformity and fracture. Adjacent joints may develop an arthropathy, and bony expansion results in neurologic compromise.

Bone Softening

The most obvious complication is bowing of long bones, especially anteriorly or laterally in tibiae or femora. In the spine, an increasing scoliosis or kyphosis may occur; and in the pelvis, acquired protrusio acetabuli may be very marked, resulting in an almost triangular pelvic configuration.

Fracture

Fractures are of two types, either a horizontal cortical fracture or a complete, usually transverse pathologic fracture. The cortical fracture is a stress fracture usually at right angles to the cortex of a long bone (Figs. 83-17 and 83-18). Often one or two in number they are particularly common

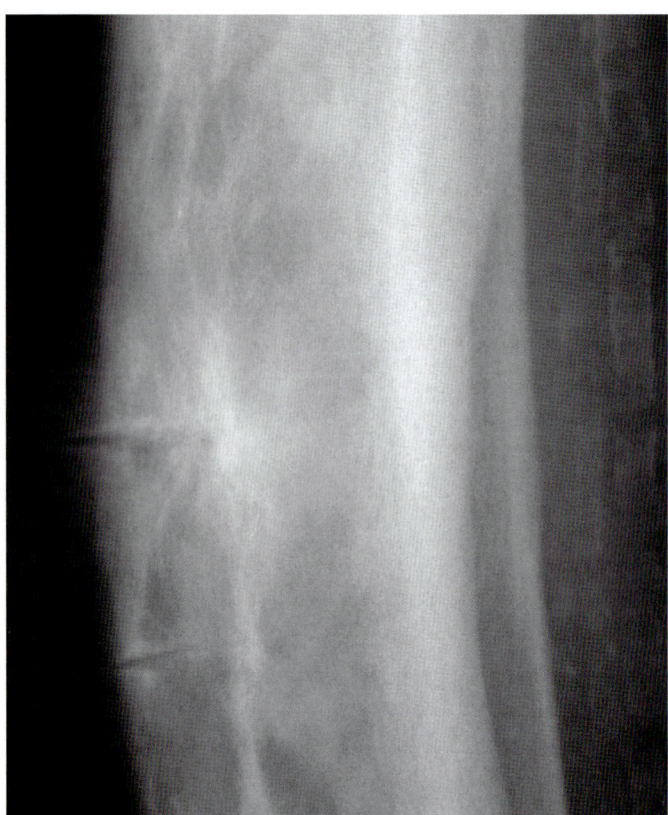

■ **FIGURE 83-17** Cortical fractures in active lytic Paget's disease. Note that they are aligned at right angles to the cortex and are on the convexity of this curved bone (tibia).

in the lower extremities, especially in the femur and the tibia. The femoral fractures are often subtrochanteric. They occur most frequently in patients with long-standing (often inactive) disease, are more common in women, and are found typically on the convexity of a curved bone. This is in contradistinction to Looser's zones, which occur on the concavity. These stress fractures are due to an excess of immature callus as opposed to unmineralized osteoid in Looser's zones. Other common sites include the humeri, pelvis, and spine. These lesions may remain static or progress to a typical transverse pathologic fracture that has a high prevalence of nonunion (Fig. 83-19). Careful examination of the fracture margins is necessary under these circumstances because it is possible a fracture may have occurred as the result of Paget's sarcoma. Any evidence of ill-defined bone resorption at the fracture site should be regarded with suspicion (see later).

Associated Arthritis

Associated arthritis is a common problem. It may fall into one of two types. First, an aggressive osteoarthritis is associated with joint collapse and deformity secondary to Paget's disease in adjacent bone or bones, most commonly the hip or knee, although any joint with adjacent pagetic bone may be affected (Fig. 83-20). The second, more subtle form of joint disease occurs in the hip, often referred to as Paget's coxopathy.[14] Best thought of as a secondary form of osteoarthritis, the typical appearances may be confused

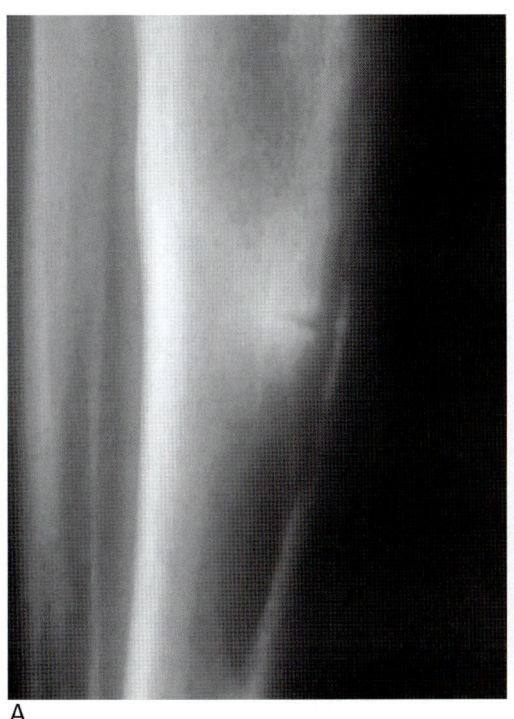

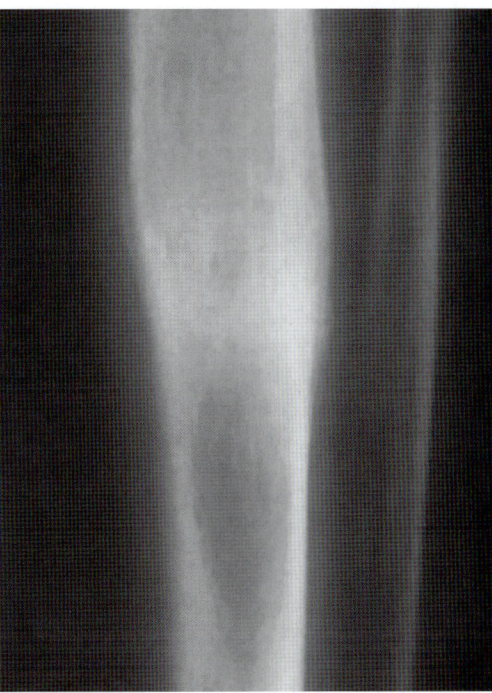

A   B

■ **FIGURE 83-18** Cortical fractures in a more lytic, active phase of Paget's disease, again typically placed in this acutely softened bone.

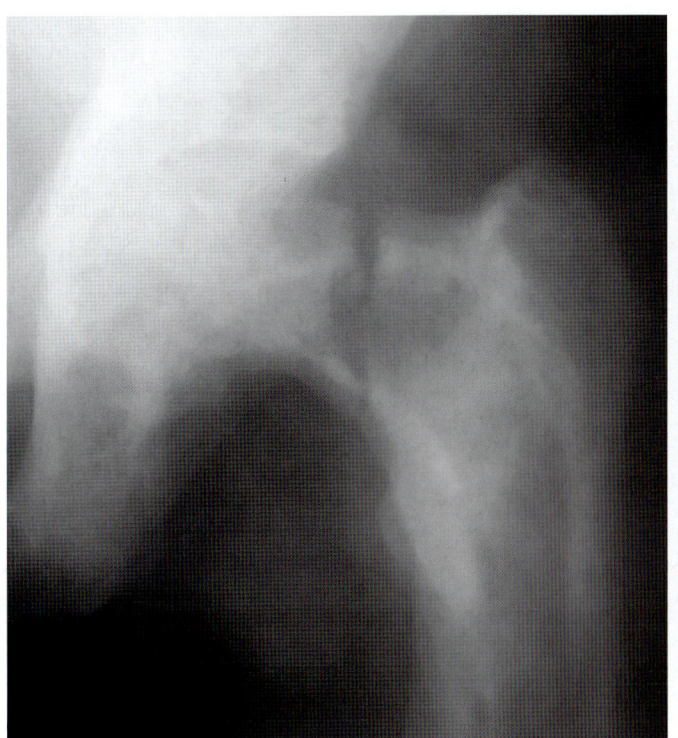

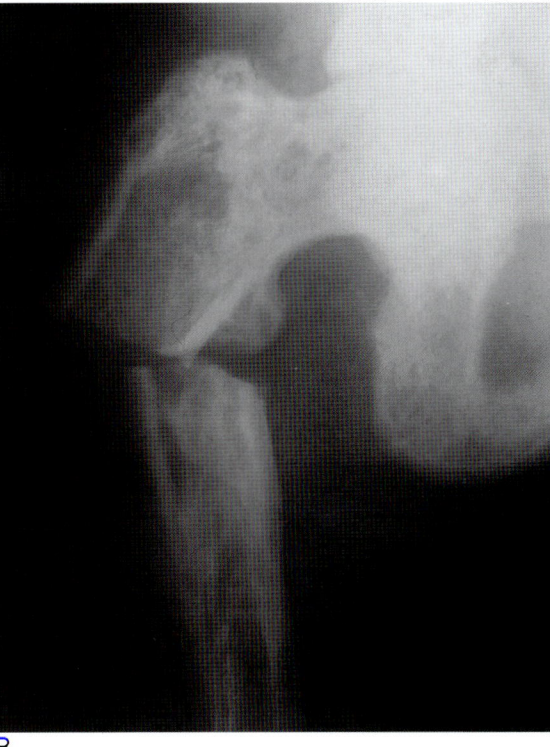

A   B

■ **FIGURE 83-19** Complete transverse fractures in established Paget's disease. Both are in the upper femur. Both are sharply defined and at right angles across the shaft of these bowed bones. The clarity of the margins militates against a malignant pathology underlying these typical pathologic fractures.

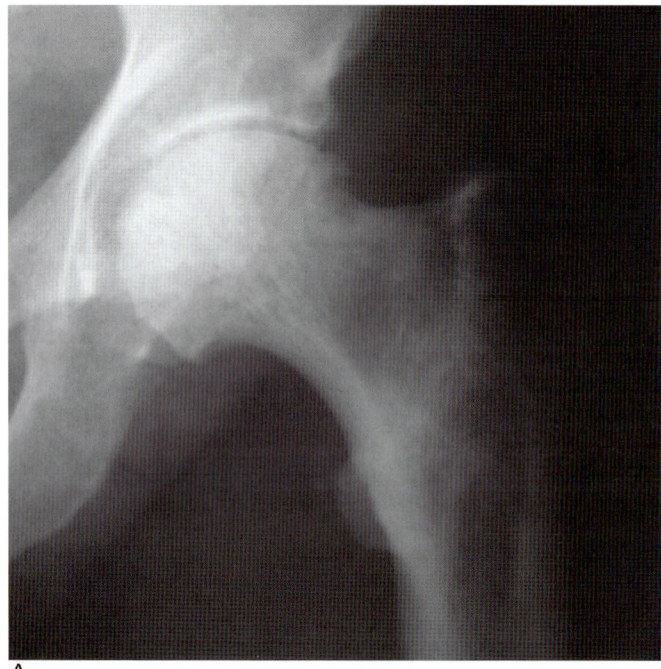

A

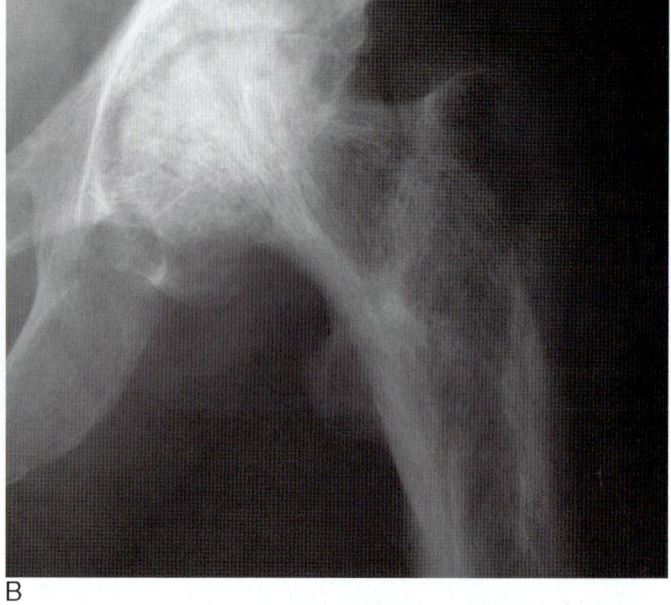

B

■ **FIGURE 83-20** Progressive, destructive osteoarthritis in Paget's disease. Initially (**A**) only modest, symmetric hyaline cartilage thinning is shown. One year later (**B**), obvious subchondral changes have occurred, particularly in the femoral head. Finally, 3 years after presentation (**C**) the hip shows gross destructive osteoarthritis.

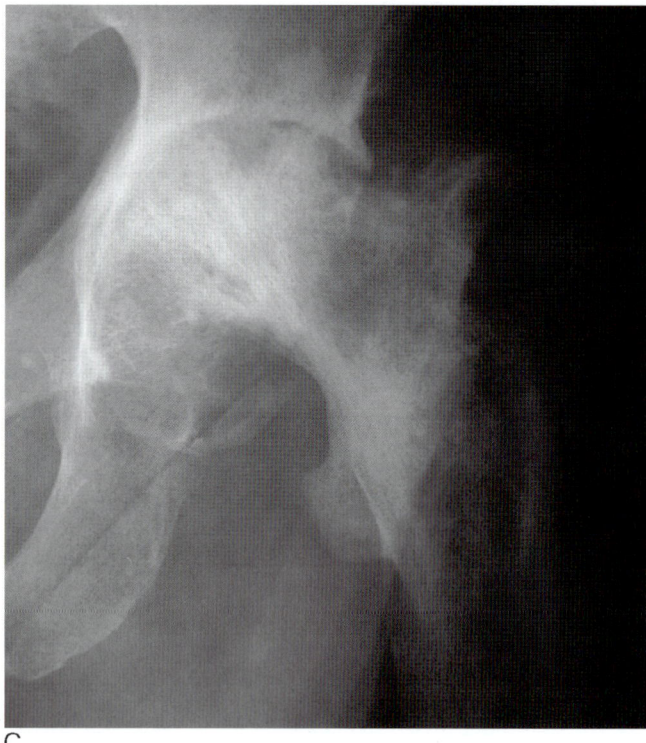

C

with an inflammatory arthropathy. The major feature is concentric joint space narrowing with very little secondary bone response in the form of osteophytes, cysts, or sclerosis. Furthermore, because protrusio acetabuli also may be present, a misdiagnosis of an inflammatory arthropathy is understandable. Indeed, on occasion, joints adjacent to pagetic bone may undergo spontaneous bony fusion, especially the sacroiliac joint, such that a spondyloarthropathy becomes considered. Lastly, hyperuricemia

is reported in about 40% of patients with Paget's disease secondary to high cell turnover. However, prevalence of overt acute or tophaceous gout is low.

Neurologic Complications

Paget's disease frequently involves the vertebral column, particularly the lumbar spine and the sacrum (Fig. 83-21).[15] Thoracic and cervical involvement is less

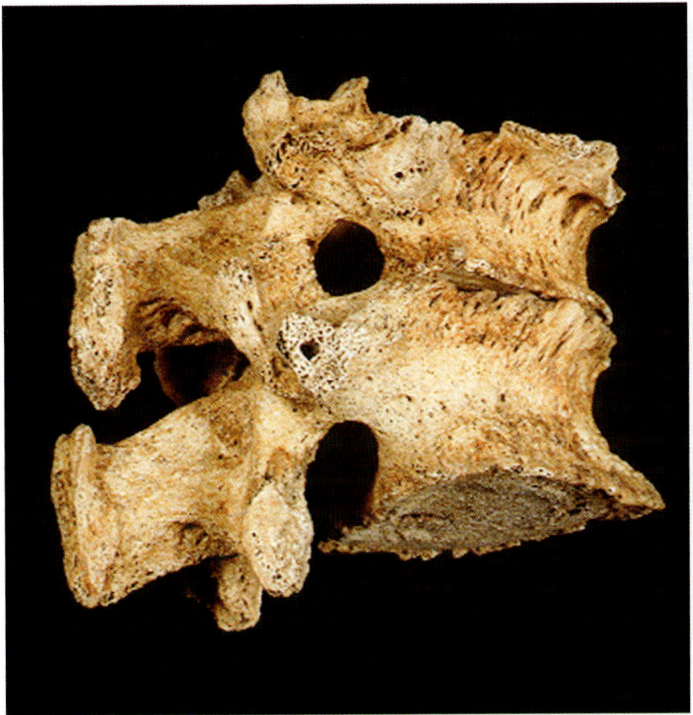

A

■ **FIGURE 83-21** Paget's disease of a lumbar vertebra (paleopathologic specimen from the United Kingdom, circa AD 1550). Note the expansion of bone and involvement of the posterior elements. In this case no spinal stenosis is present.

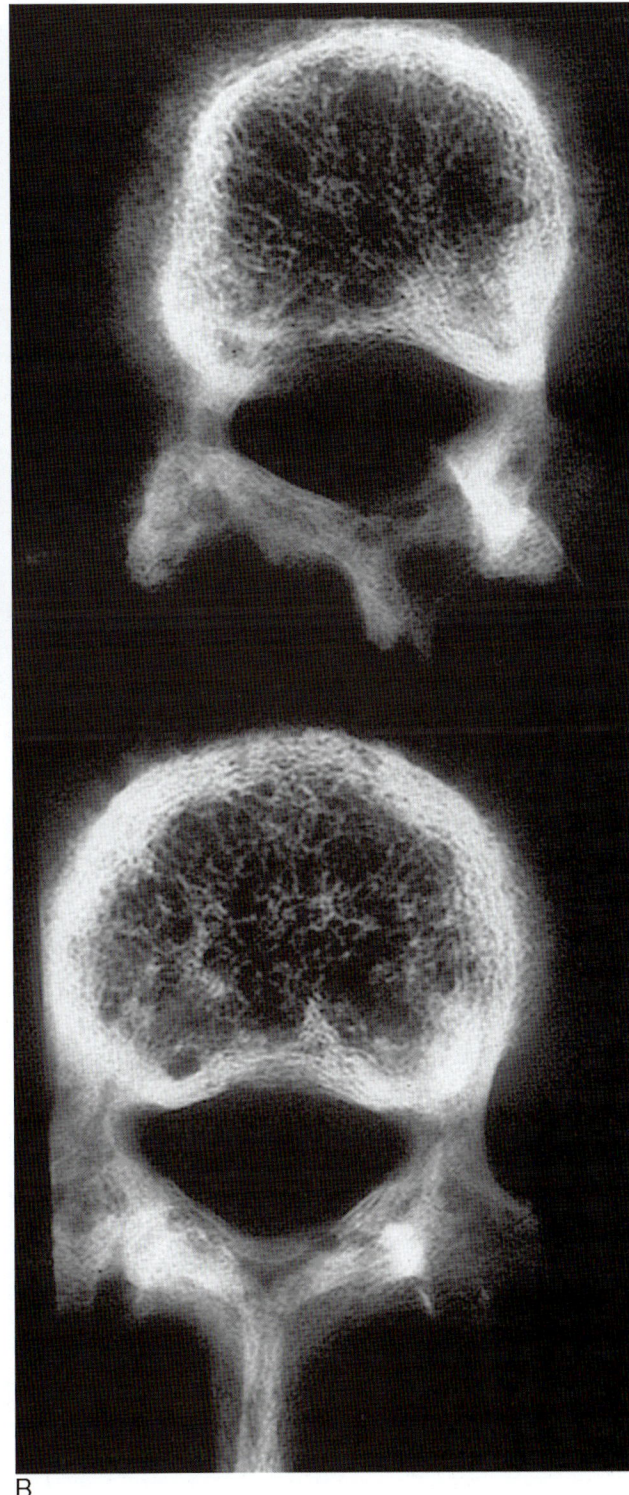

B

common. Monostotic disease may cause difficulty in diagnosis because of a potentially wide differential diagnosis (see Table 83-1). The key features are vertebral enlargement, involvement of the posterior elements, and changes in all four cortices on any view. Simple bony enlargement may create spinal canal stenosis or foraminal encroachment. This may be exaggerated by rapid degenerative disease in disks and facet joints. The neural canal is narrowest in the upper thoracic region and hence is the site at greatest risk of cord compression. Fractures, including vertebra plana, may occur (Fig. 83-22). Spinal cord hypoxia may be difficult to diagnose and is thought to be secondary to hyperemic pagetic bone stealing flow. Neurogenic (sciatic) claudication results from lumbar canal stenosis. Less common complications include extramedullary hematopoiesis,

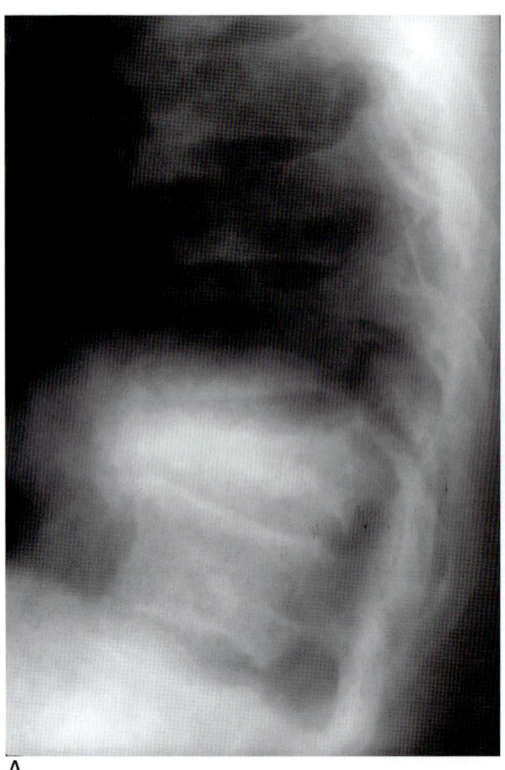
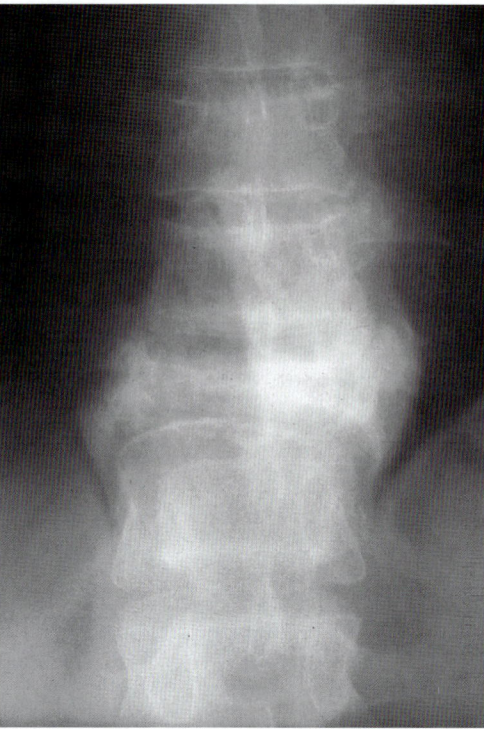

A   B

■ **FIGURE 83-22** Paget's disease in the thoracic spine. This patient complained of severe midthoracic pain and had some long tract signs. Note the collapse reminiscent of vertebra plana, the local kyphosis, and the retropulsion of the middle column.

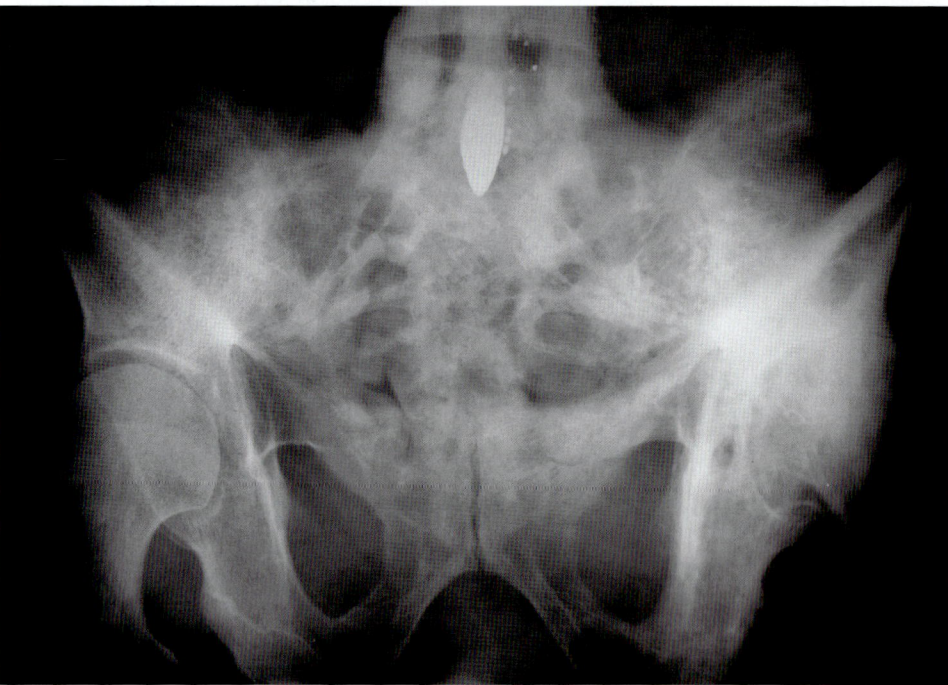

■ **FIGURE 83-23** Paget's disease and previous ankylosing spondylitis. Note how the pagetic bone has spread to cross the already fused sacroiliac joints and is spreading up the spine in the paraspinal bone of the ankylosing spondylitis. The softening of bone is also obvious with a triangular shape of the pelvis. Previously injected Myodil is noted.

which may cause spinal cord compression, and osseous bridging between vertebral bodies. The latter may resemble a congenital fusion, be mistaken for a spondyloarthropathy, or develop typical features of Paget's disease in the fusion bone (Fig. 83-23). Indeed, Paget's disease may develop at a site of bone grafting when pagetic bone has been used.[16]

Calvarial enlargement associated with foraminal stenosis compresses individual cranial nerves causing anosmia, absent papillary reflexes, blindness, ptosis, facial pain, tinnitus, dysphagia, trigeminal neuralgia, deafness, and ocular muscle palsies (Fig. 83-24). Bone softening with basilar invagination occurs in as many as 30% of patients with cranial involvement and results in secondary stenosis of the foramen magnum. As with other complications, these features are worse in women and increase in frequency with progressive disease severity. Stretching or occlusion of the vertebral and/or basilar arteries, internal

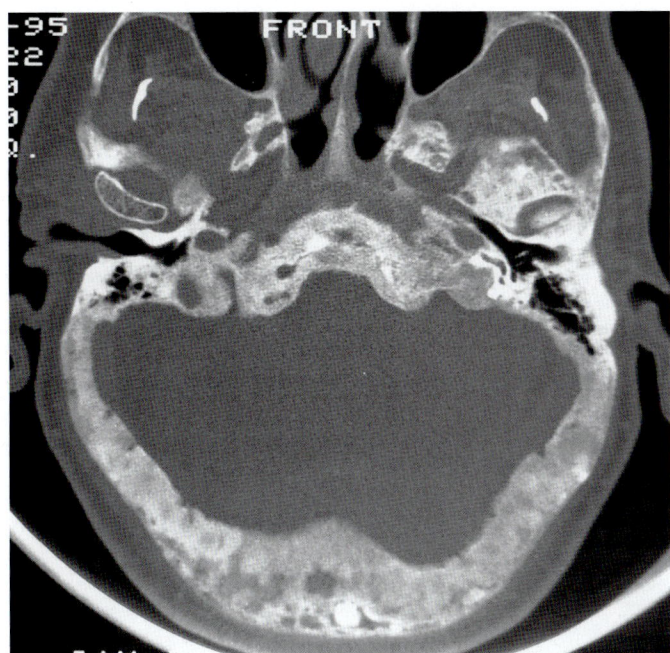

■ **FIGURE 83-24** Compression and distortion of the internal auditory meatuses and middle ears is shown on CT secondary to Paget's disease of the skull.

hydrocephalus from obstruction of cerebrospinal fluid flow, and syringomyelia may be associated features.

Evaluation of neurologic complications requires CT to best assess the bony changes, but MRI is mandatory for the neural complications.

Neoplastic

Neoplasms, although rare, are a complication of Paget's disease. The malignant lesion is a high-grade sarcoma often called Paget's sarcoma. Giant cell tumors (GCTs) also occur, and a debate exists as to whether or not metastatic disease may be more frequent in the hypervascularized pagetic bone.

Paget's sarcoma occurs in about 1% of patients with long-standing disease, the risk being greater with polyostotic disease (5%–10%). It is of interest to note that this was a complication in some of Paget's original five patients. The sarcoma most frequently involves men (2:1) in the 55- to 80-year age group. Clinical symptoms include new local pain, swelling, and fracture most commonly of the femur, the pelvis, and, disproportionately so, the proximal humerus. Histologically, this high-grade sarcoma may differentiate into several types, mainly osteosarcoma (50%–60%), malignant fibrous histiocytoma or fibrosarcoma (20%–25%), and chondrosarcoma (10%). Prognosis is poor, with a survival rate of 14% at about 2.5 years reflecting a high degree of anaplasia (Fig. 83-25).[17] Metastasis is frequent.

Radiographs demonstrate an aggressive ill-defined area of bone destruction, cortical lysis, and a soft tissue mass. A periosteal reaction is unusual, in contradistinction to conventional osteosarcomas, reflecting the rapidly progressive nature of the tumor. Comparison with results of previous examinations is very helpful because it may alert one to the development of a zone of bone resorption not present previously. Skeletal scintigraphy usually demonstrates an area of focal photopenia in the otherwise increased activity of pagetic bone. Gallium-67 has been used to confirm a sarcoma by showing increased activity in the zone of osteopenia. CT and MRI produce nonspecific findings with intermediate signal intensity on T1-weighted sequences and high signal intensity on T2-weighted sequences, usually with patchy postgadolinium enhancement. Central necrosis may be seen on both CT and MRI. Paget's sarcoma requires that a high index of suspicion be maintained when a focus of bone destruction occurs in pagetic bone.

GCTs arise in pagetic bone and may be solitary or multiple. However, they are very much rarer in Paget's disease than in the general population and often involve unusual sites such as skull or facial bones. Almost by definition, they occur in patients older than usual and are associated with long-standing polyostotic Paget's disease.

The radiographic appearance usually is typical of GCT but with obvious Paget's disease in the underlying bone (Fig. 83-26). CT or MRI may demonstrate a mass-like lesion in bone, which is difficult to differentiate from a sarcoma except that a GCT is better defined and more localized. The soft tissue component is prominent with intermediate signal intensity on T1-weighted images and foci of increased signal intensity on T2-weighted images. Cystic and hemorrhagic areas may be present with florid contrast enhancement.

Metastasis

Debate exists as to whether Paget's disease, with an inherent high blood flow, is or is not susceptible to the implantation of hematogenous metastasis. Personal experience suggests that a metastasis arising in pagetic bone is very rare (Fig. 83-27).

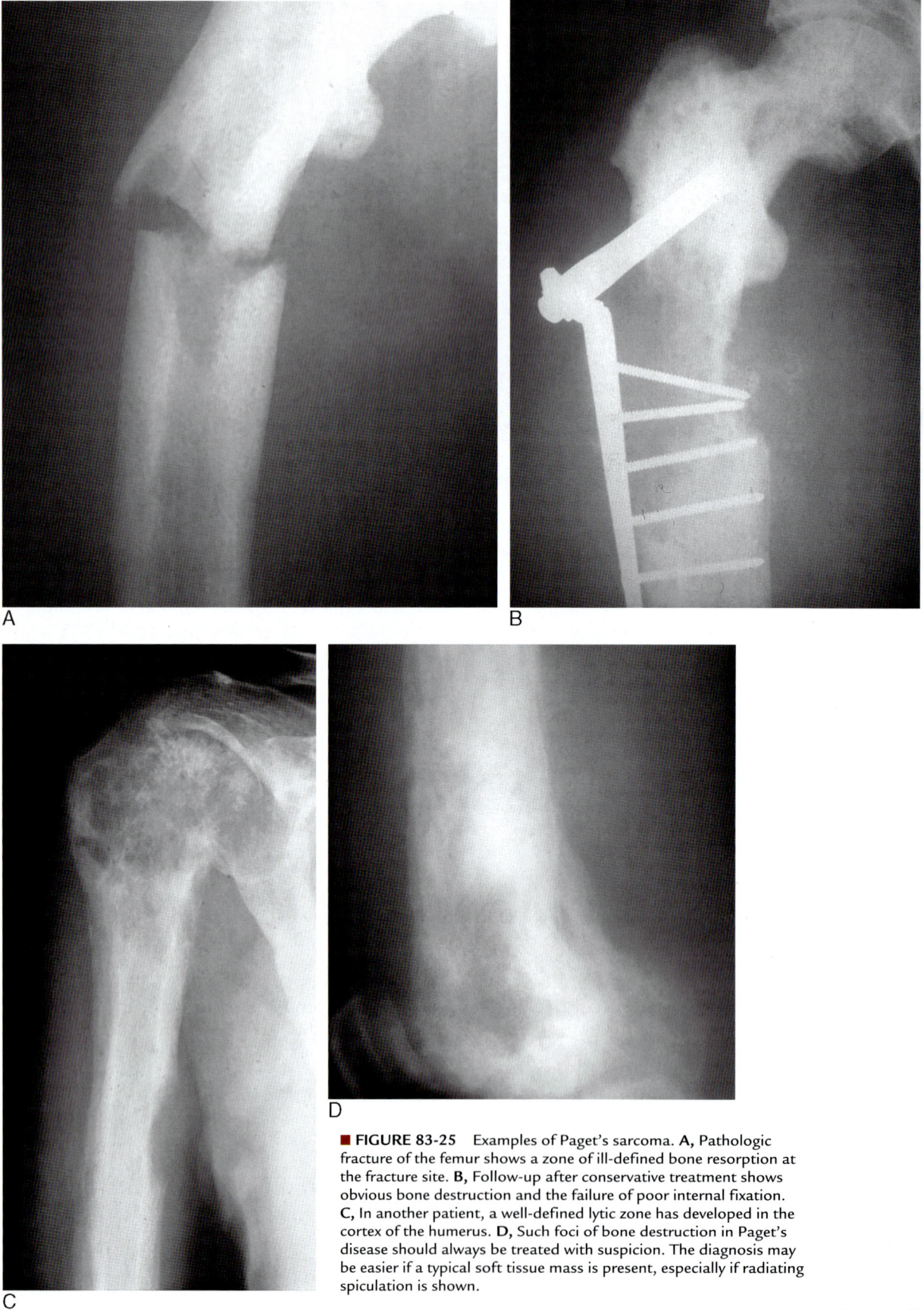

■ **FIGURE 83-25** Examples of Paget's sarcoma. **A,** Pathologic fracture of the femur shows a zone of ill-defined bone resorption at the fracture site. **B,** Follow-up after conservative treatment shows obvious bone destruction and the failure of poor internal fixation. **C,** In another patient, a well-defined lytic zone has developed in the cortex of the humerus. **D,** Such foci of bone destruction in Paget's disease should always be treated with suspicion. The diagnosis may be easier if a typical soft tissue mass is present, especially if radiating spiculation is shown.

(Continued)

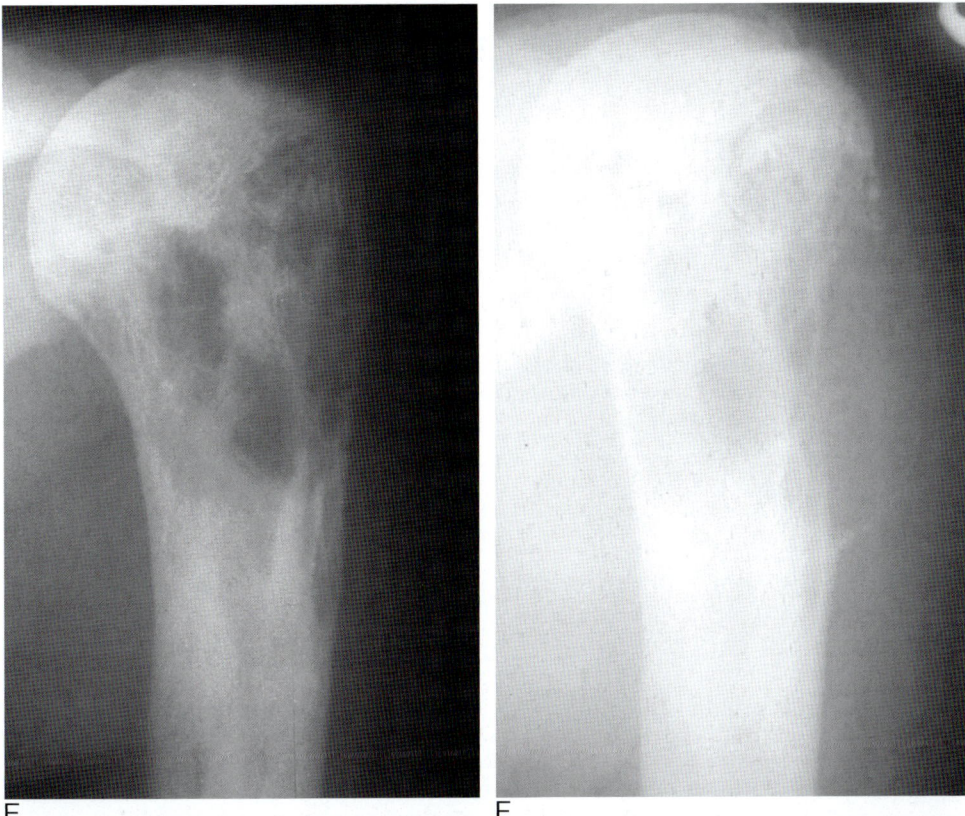

E

F

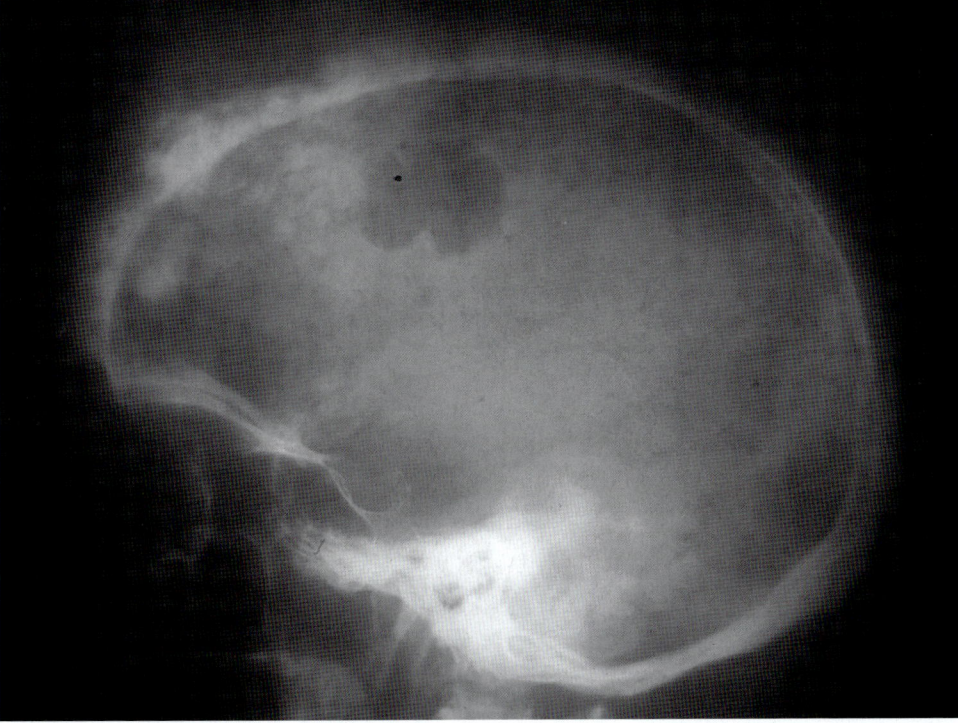

G

■ **FIGURE 83-25—Cont'd** **E** and **F,** The combination of bone destruction and a soft tissue mass should present no difficulty in diagnosis in this humerus. **G,** Paget's sarcoma can arise in any pagetic bone, as in this skull.

Soft Tissue Masses

Several reports have been made of soft tissue masses arising from pagetic bone (Fig. 83-28).[18] These rare pseudo-tumors are usually solitary, presenting as local pain and swelling and a periosteal-based soft tissue mass. The underlying cortex may be eroded. Periosteal new bone formation is present, sometimes with a "pumice-like" appearance. Distinction from a sarcoma is difficult and may require biopsy for differentiation, but preservation of fatty marrow signal on MRI is reassuring.[19]

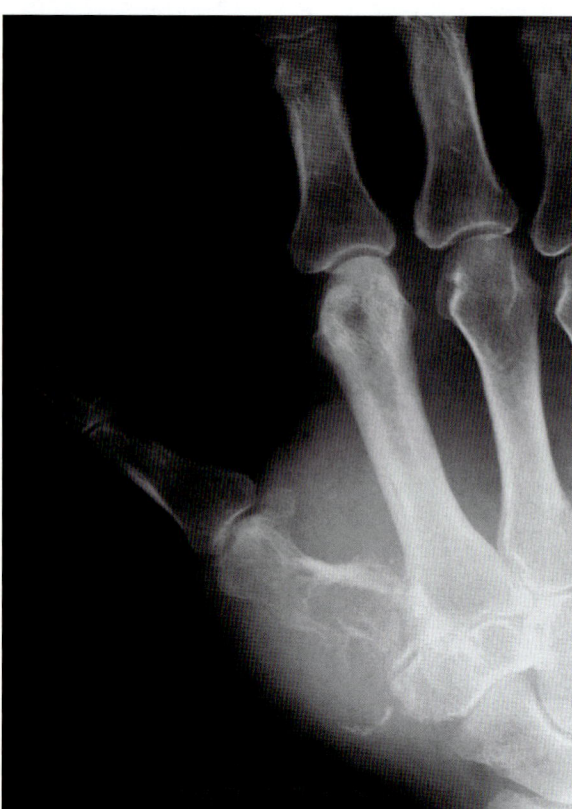

■ **FIGURE 83-26** Giant cell tumor arising in pagetic bone. Note also the involvement of the index finger metacarpal. The lesion is large, lytic, and expansile with an apparent soft tissue mass. The histology was benign.

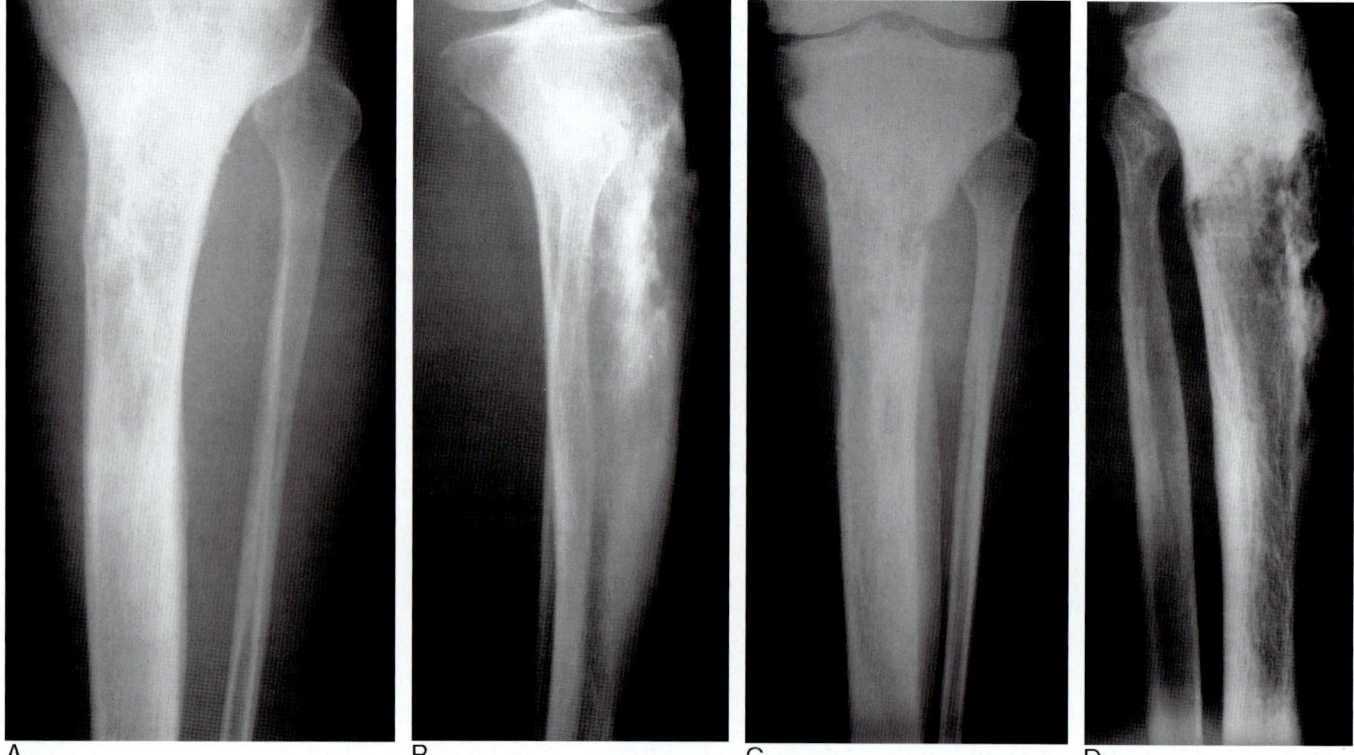

A   B   C   D

■ **FIGURE 83-27** Metastasis arising in active, lytic Paget's disease. **A** and **B,** Patchy, ill-defined sclerosis deep to Paget's disease is unusual in lytic disease. A possible soft tissue component is also present. **C** and **D,** Subsequent images a month later reveal an obvious malignant process with frank bone destruction. Histology revealed a metastasis from carcinoma of the prostate superimposed on active Paget's disease.

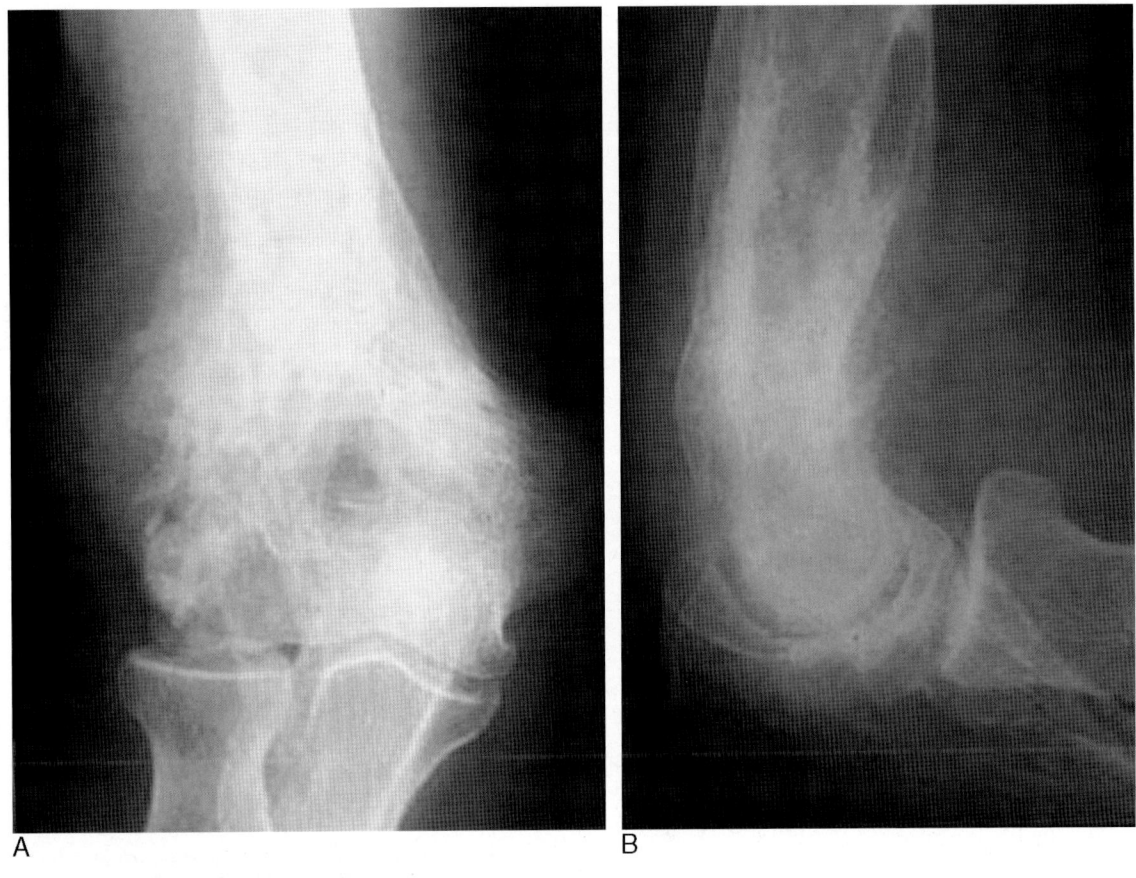

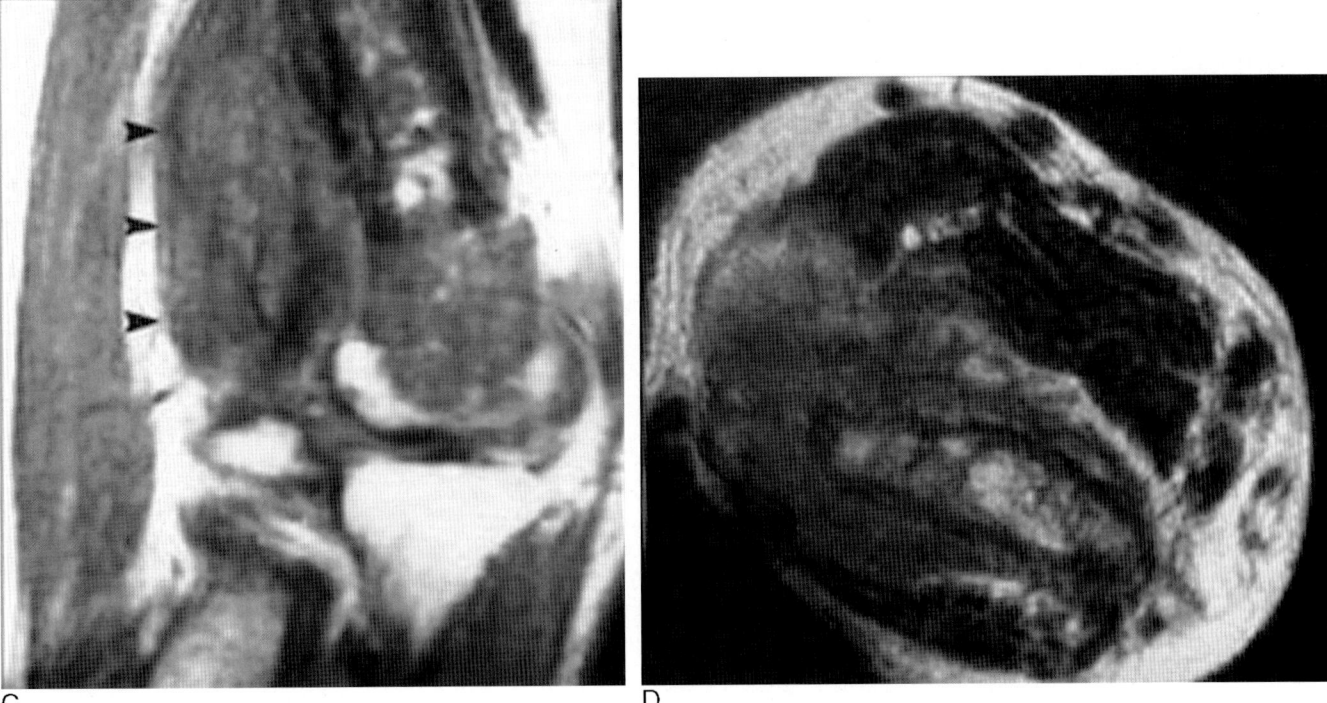

■ FIGURE 83-28 **A** and **B,** A pseudotumor is shown arising from the distal humerus. An apparent soft tissue mass and amorphous bone formation suggest a sarcoma on the radiographs. **C,** The T1-weighted image shows low signal in the mass and in the medullary canal. **D,** The T2-weighted image also reveals a low signal intensity, but relatively well-defined lesion. The useful and helpful sign may be the presence of fat within the soft tissue mass suggesting that it is a pseudotumor. *(From Tins BJ, Davies AM, Mangham DC. MR imaging of pseudosarcoma in Paget's disease of bone: a report of two cases. Skeletal Radiol 2001; 30:161–165, with permission.)*

SUGGESTED READING

Smith SE, Murphey MD, Motamedi K, et al. Radiologic spectrum of Paget disease of bone and its complications with pathologic correlation. Radiographics 2002; 22:1191–1216.

REFERENCES

1. Paget J. On a form of chronic inflammation of bones (osteitis deformans). Med Chir Trans 1887; 60:37.
2. Cooper C, Dennison K, Schafheutle K, et al. Epidemiology of Paget's disease of bone. Bone 1999; 24(Suppl):3S–5S.
3. Davie M, Davies M, Francis R, et al. Paget's disease of bone: a review of 889 patients. Bone 1999; 24(Suppl):11S–12S.
4. Mee AP, Sharpe PT. Dogs, distemper and Paget's disease. Bioessays 1993; 15:783–789.
5. Daroszewska A, Ralston SH. Genetics of Paget's disease of bone. Clin Sci 2005; 109:257–263.
6. New England Registry for Paget's Disease of Bone. Analysis of environmental factors in familial versus sporadic Paget's disease of bone. J Bone Miner Res 2003; 18:1519–1524.
7. Cooper C, Schafheutle K, Dennison E, et al. The epidemiology of Paget's disease in Britain: is the prevalence decreasing? J Bone Miner Res 1999; 14:192–197.
8. Morales-Piga AA, Bachiller-Corral FJ, Abraira V, et al. Is the clinical expressiveness of Paget's disease of bone decreasing? Bone 2002; 30:399–403.
9. Rogers J, Jeffrey DR, Watt I. Paget's disease in an archaeological population. J Bone Miner Res 2002; 17:1127–1134.
10. Cundy HR, Gamble G, Wattie D, et al. Paget's disease of bone in New Zealand: continued decline in disease severity. Calcif Tissue Int 2004; 75:358–364.
11. Lavender JP, Evans IM, Arnot R, et al. A comparison of radiography and radioisotope scanning in the detection of Paget's disease and in the assessment of response to human calcitonin. Br J Radiol 1977; 50:243–250.
12. Kaufmann GA, Sundaram M, McDonald DJ. Magnetic resonance imaging in symptomatic Paget's disease. Skeletal Radiol 1991; 20:413–418.
13. Vande Berg BC, Malghem J, Lecouvet FE, Maldague B. Magnetic resonance appearance of uncomplicated Paget's disease of bone. Semin Musculoskelet Radiol 2001; 5:69–77.
14. Helliwell PS, Porter G. Controlled study of the prevalence of radiological osteoarthritis in clinically unrecognised juxta-articular Paget's disease. Ann Rheum Dis 1999; 58:762–765.
15. Saifuddin A, Hassan A. Paget's disease of the spine: unusual features and complications. Clin Radiol 2003; 58:102–111.
16. Hamadouche M, Mathieu M, Topouchian V, et al. Transfer of Paget's disease from one part of the skeleton to another as a result of autogenous bone-grafting. J Bone Joint Surg Am 2002; 84:2056–2061.
17. Mankin HJ, Hornicek FJ. Paget's sarcoma. Clin Orthop Relat Res 2005; 438:97–102.
18. Tins BJ, Davies AM, Mangham DC. MR imaging of pseudo sarcoma in Paget's disease of bone: a report of two cases. Skeletal Radiol 2001; 30:161–165.
19. McNairn JDK, Damron TA, Landas SK, Ambrose JL. Benign tumefactive soft tissue extension from Paget's disease of bone simulating malignancy. Skeletal Radiol 2001; 30:157–160.

CHAPTER 84

Hypertrophic Osteoarthropathy

Michael S. Gibson, Bryan T. Jennings, and Mark D. Murphey

ETIOLOGY

Hypertrophic osteoarthropathy (HOA), formerly known as hypertrophic pulmonary osteoarthropathy, is characterized by digital clubbing and periosteal proliferation along tubular bones. It was first described in 1890 by Pierre Marie in patients with chronic lung disease.[1] Multiple nonpulmonary causes of HOA have now been described, accounting for the change in nomenclature. HOA can be classified as either primary or secondary. The primary form of the disease, also known as pachydermoperiostosis, is a familial disorder with variable degrees of expression. The secondary form is related to any one of a large number of underlying conditions, of which primary bronchogenic carcinoma is the most common.[2] A summary of the diseases associated with secondary HOA is presented in Box 84-1.

PREVALENCE AND EPIDEMIOLOGY

Primary HOA is a rare disorder that most commonly presents in males by a ratio of 9:1.[3] The onset of disease has a bimodal distribution, with one peak during the first year of life and a second peak around the age of puberty. Secondary HOA related to lung cancer is relatively common. One study found evidence of HOA in 17% of staging bone scintigrams performed on patients with lung cancer.[4] On clinical examination, up to 30% of patients with lung cancer have evidence of digital clubbing.[5] The presence of secondary HOA has no prognostic significance in patients with lung cancer.[4] The age and sex distribution of secondary HOA follow that of the underlying condition.

CLINICAL PRESENTATION

Hypertrophic osteoarthropathy commonly presents as painful swelling and tenderness of the distal extremities, associated with digital clubbing. Arthralgias and joint effusions may occur, typically in a large joint such as the knee.

Primary HOA is characterized by diffuse skin and soft tissue thickening. In the lower extremity, soft tissue swelling and bone enlargement can lead to a cylindrical appearance, with disruption of the normal extremity contours. Dramatic skin thickening in the face and scalp can result in deep furrows and transverse folds known as cutis verticis gyrata. Additional characteristic features of primary HOA include hyperhidrosis of the extremities and seborrhea of the face, nose, and scalp.[6]

Secondary HOA may be the initial presentation of bronchogenic carcinoma. The presence of bilaterally symmetric periostosis and digital clubbing should alert the clinician to the possibility of underlying malignancy.

PATHOPHYSIOLOGY

The pathogenesis of HOA remains uncertain. Localized vascular proliferation and endothelial cell hyperplasia have been demonstrated histologically in the soft tissues of patients with HOA.[7] These histologic findings are believed to be related to the presence of one or more growth factors in the systemic circulation that are normally inactivated in the lungs. Megakaryocytes and platelet clumps that are normally fragmented in the lungs reach the distal extremities and are thought to cause a local tissue reaction via release of cytokines.[8] Platelet-derived growth factor (PDGF) and vascular endothelial growth factor (VEGF) have been proposed as having a role in clubbing and HOA.[9]

KEY POINTS

- HOA is manifested by digital clubbing and periostosis of tubular bones.
- The diagnosis of primary HOA only can be made after exclusion of all potential causes of secondary HOA.

BOX 84-1 Diseas Associated with Secondary Hypertrophic Osteoarthropathy

PULMONARY

- Bronchogenic carcinoma
- Metastases
- Pulmonary abscess
- Tuberculosis
- Bronchiectasis
- Cystic fibrosis
- Arteriovenous malformation
- Mesothelioma
- Pulmonary fibrosis

CARDIAC

- Cyanotic congenital heart disease
- Bacterial endocarditis

GASTROINTESTINAL

- Inflammatory bowel disease
- Cirrhosis
- Biliary atresia
- Esophageal carcinoma
- Esophagitis
- Polyposis

MISCELLANEOUS

- Nasopharyngeal carcinoma
- Hodgkin's lymphoma
- Vascular graft infection
- Prostaglandin therapy
- AIDS

MANIFESTATIONS OF THE DISEASE

Radiography

Periosteal proliferation in the tubular bones is the radiographic hallmark of HOA (Fig. 84-1).

The morphology of the periostosis evolves with increasing degrees of disease severity.[10] In mild cases, a monolayer of periosteal reaction is present. Multilayer periostosis represents moderate disease, and irregular periostosis indicates severe disease. Ossification of the interosseous membrane is seen in the most severe cases. The longitudinal extent of periostosis within a given bone also changes over time.[10] Diaphyseal involvement is the earliest finding. With long-standing disease, the

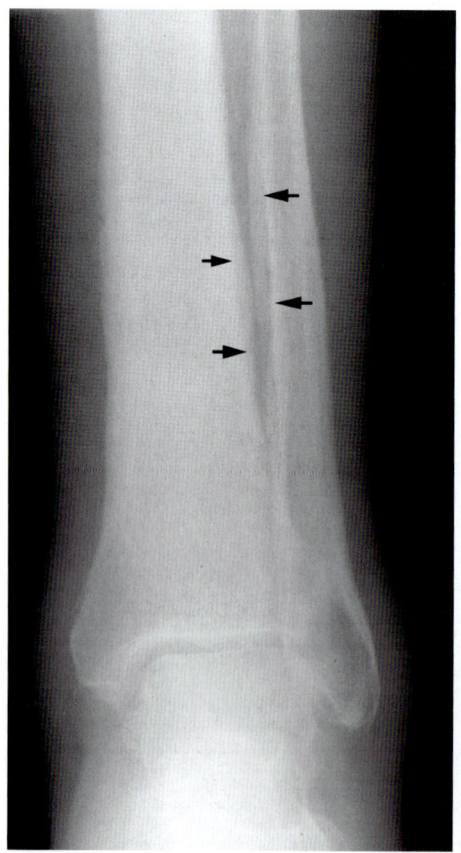
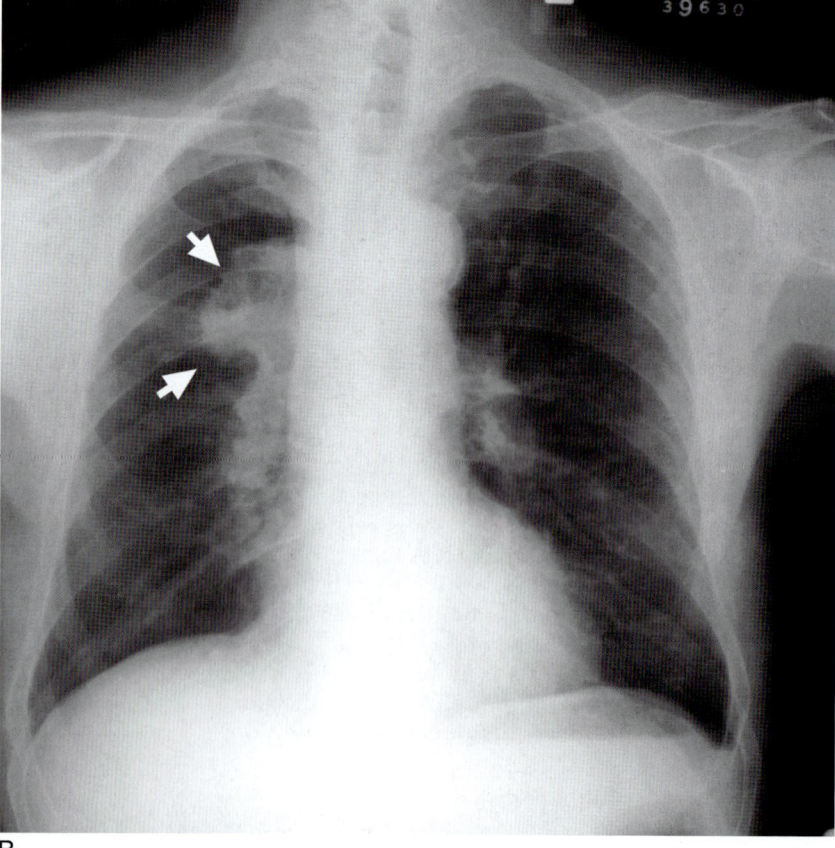

A   B

■ **FIGURE 84-1** **A,** A 54-year-old man presented with secondary hypertrophic osteoarthropathy from lung cancer. Anteroposterior radiograph of the left ankle demonstrates smooth, thick monolayer periosteal reaction (*arrows*) involving the distal tibia and fibula. **B,** Posteroanterior chest radiograph in the same patient reveals a primary bronchogenic carcinoma in the right suprahilar region (*arrows*).

periostosis can extend to involve the metaphyses and epiphyses. Epiphyseal involvement suggests primary HOA, because secondary HOA often allows only a short survival time. There is a direct relationship between the duration of disease and the number of bones involved.[10] The tibia and fibula are the most common bones affected, followed by the femur, metacarpals, carpus, radius, ulna, metatarsals, and humerus.[11] Skeletal changes are typically bilateral and symmetric. Unilateral involvement has been reported in cases of HOA distal to sites of vascular graft infection.

Bone remodeling can occur in the distal phalanges of patients with long-standing clubbing.[12] The remodeling may be hypertrophic, with "mushroom-like" overgrowth of the tuft, or it may be osteolytic. The age at onset determines which type of remodeling occurs. Clubbing that appears during childhood is associated with osteolysis, whereas clubbing that develops after puberty is associated with hypertrophy.[13]

Joint swelling is a common manifestation of HOA. Effusions may be seen on radiographs, typically at the knee or ankle. The effusions are not inflammatory; therefore, joint space narrowing, juxta-articular osteoporosis, and erosions are not characteristic of HOA. The presence of erosions in a patient with HOA should suggest a concomitant inflammatory arthropathy.[13]

Nuclear Medicine

Radionuclide bone scintigraphy is highly sensitive for detection of periosteal proliferation. Abnormalities may be seen on scintigraphy before they are radiographically apparent. The classic appearance of HOA is diffuse, symmetric, increased linear uptake along the diaphyseal cortical margins of tubular bones, known as the "parallel tract" or "double stripe" sign.[11] Scintigraphy is useful in delineating the extent of skeletal involvement and in assessing disease progression or response to therapy (Fig. 84-2).

DIFFERENTIAL DIAGNOSIS

The differentiation of primary from secondary HOA is based on clinical exclusion of underlying conditions associated with secondary HOA. A positive family history is present in many cases of primary HOA.[3] The differential diagnosis of symmetric bilateral periostosis includes shin splints, venous stasis, thyroid acropachy, hypervitaminosis A, infantile cortical hyperostosis, diffuse idiopathic skeletal hyperostosis, fluorosis, and diaphyseal dysplasia (Camurati-Engelmann disease).

SYNOPSIS OF TREATMENT OPTIONS

Medical Treatment

Digital clubbing is typically painless and does not require therapy. Treatment of HOA is directed toward identification and management of the underlying condition. Symptomatic HOA is typically treated with nonsteroidal anti-inflammatory drugs or oral corticosteroids. Successful

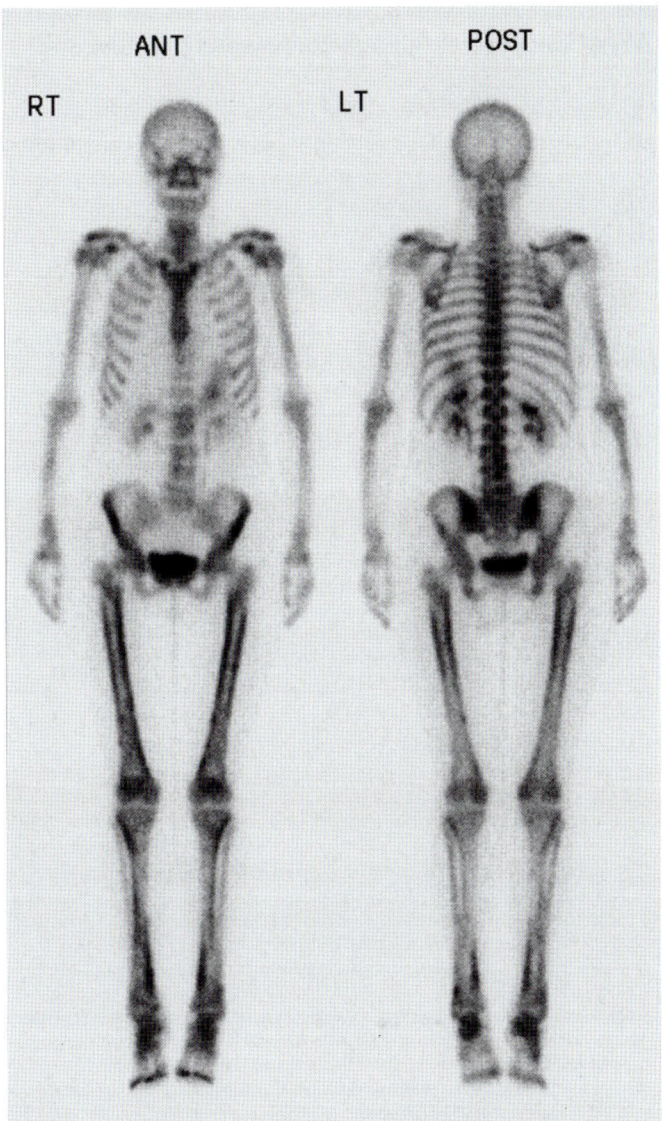

■ **FIGURE 84-2** A 63-year-old woman presented with secondary hypertrophic osteoarthropathy from lung cancer. Whole-body bone scintigram demonstrates increased radionuclide uptake with the "parallel tract" sign in the femora. Linear cortical uptake is also present in both tibiae.

treatment of refractory cases has been reported with intravenous bisphosphonates[14] as well as with subcutaneous octreotide.[15] Various chemotherapeutic agents used in the treatment of underlying malignancies have resulted in symptomatic and radiographic improvement in patients with secondary HOA.

Surgical Treatment

The skeletal manifestations of secondary HOA typically regress after thoracotomy for treatment of primary lung cancer. There is no role for direct surgical intervention on bones affected by HOA.

What the Referring Physician Needs to Know

■ The presence of HOA should raise the question of underlying disease, particularly bronchogenic carcinoma.
■ Radiographs of the chest should be obtained in the appropriate clinical setting.

ACKNOWLEDGMENT

The views expressed in this chapter are those of the authors and do not necessarily reflect the official policy or position of the Department of the Navy, Department of Defense, nor the U.S. Government.

SUGGESTED READINGS

Dickinson CJ. The aetiology of clubbing and hypertrophic osteoarthropathy. Eur J Clin Invest 1993; 23:330–338.
Martinez-Lavin M, Pineda C, Valdez T, et al. Primary hypertrophic osteoarthropathy. Semin Arthritis Rheum 1988; 17:156–162.
Pineda C. Diagnostic imaging in hypertrophic osteoarthropathy. Clin Exp Rheum 1992; 10(Suppl 7):27–33.

REFERENCES

1. Marie P. De l'osteoarthropathie hypertrophiante pneumonique. Rev Med (Paris) 1890; 10:1–36.
2. Martinez-Lavin M, Matucci-Cerinic M, Jajic I, Pineda C. Hypertrophic osteoarthropathy: consensus on its definition, classification, assessment and diagnostic criteria. J Rheumatol 1993; 20:1386–1387.
3. Martinez-Lavin M, Pineda C, Valdez T, et al. Primary hypertrophic osteoarthropathy. Semin Arthritis Rheum 1988; 17:156–162.
4. Morgan B, Coakley F, Finlay DB, Belton I. Hypertrophic osteoarthropathy in staging skeletal scintigraphy for lung cancer. Clin Radiol 1996; 51:694–697.
5. Baughman RP, Gunther KL, Buchsbaum JA, Lower EE. Prevalence of digital clubbing in bronchogenic carcinoma by a new digital index. Clin Exp Rheumatol 1998; 16:21–26.
6. Jajic Z, Jajic I, Nemcic T. Primary hypertrophic osteoarthropathy: clinical, radiologic, and scintigraphic characteristics. Arch Med Res 2001; 32:136–142.
7. Silveira LH, Martinez-Lavin M, Pineda C, et al. Vascular endothelial growth factor in hypertrophic osteoarthropathy. Clin Exp Rheumatol 2000; 18:57–62.
8. Dickinson CJ, Martin JF. Megakaryocytes and platelet clumps as the cause of finger clubbing. Lancet 1987; 2:1434–1435.
9. Atkinson S, Fox SB. Vascular endothelial growth factor (VEGF)-A and platelet-derived growth factor (PDGF) play a central role in the pathogenesis of digital clubbing. J Pathol 2004; 203:721–728.
10. Pineda CJ, Martinez-Lavin M, Goobar JE, et al. Periostitis in hypertrophic osteoarthropathy: relationship to disease duration. AJR Am J Roentgenol 1987; 148:773–778.
11. Ali A, Tetalman MR, Fordham EW, et al. Distribution of hypertrophic pulmonary osteoarthropathy. AJR Am J Roentgenol 1980; 134:771–780.
12. Pineda CJ, Guerra J Jr, Weisman MH, et al. The skeletal manifestations of clubbing: a study in patients with cyanotic congenital heart disease and hypertrophic osteoarthropathy. Semin Arthritis Rheum 1985; 14:263–273.
13. Pineda C, Fonseca C, Martinez-Lavin M. The spectrum of soft tissue and skeletal abnormalities of hypertrophic osteoarthropathy. J Rheumatol 1990; 17:773–778.
14. Speden D, Nicklason F, Francis H, Ward J. The use of pamidronate in hypertrophic pulmonary osteoarthropathy (HPOA). Aust NZ J Med 1997; 27:307–310.
15. Johnson SA, Spiller PA, Faull CM. Treatment of resistant pain in hypertrophic pulmonary osteoarthropathy with subcutaneous octreotide. Thorax 1997; 52:298–299.

85

Sarcoidosis

Hakan Ilaslan and Murali Sundaram

ETIOLOGY

Sarcoidosis is a systemic disorder characterized by the accumulation of non-necrotizing granulomas in affected organs, with varying degrees of associated inflammation or fibrosis. Its exact etiology is not known. The pattern of organ involvement and disease progression is variable and often difficult to predict at presentation.

PREVALENCE AND EPIDEMIOLOGY

Epidemiologic characterization of sarcoidosis is problematic owing to variability in disease course, ascertainment bias, and lack of precise diagnostic methods. Results of population-based radiographic screening studies in Scandinavia and the United Kingdom have suggested that there are a significant number of asymptomatic patients whose disease never becomes overt. Based on these studies, prevalence rates have ranged from less than 1 per 100,000 population in the United Kingdom to 102 per 100,000 in Sweden.[1]

In the United States, the incidence of sarcoidosis in African Americans is 3.8-fold higher than whites, conferring an overall lifetime risk of 2.4% versus 0.85%.[2]

Musculoskeletal involvement by sarcoidosis is rare, and a bone incidence is difficult to determine. Based on a worldwide review of the pre-MRI era, Perry and coworkers[3] identified 98 patients with bone lesions from 2483 patients with sarcoidosis, making for an incidence of 4%. A recent prospective MRI series found 17 of 40 patients with sarcoidosis to have intramedullary lesions.[4] Muscle and subcutaneous lesions were uncommon.

CLINICAL PRESENTATION

Arthralgia with overt synovitis tends to occur early in the course of the disease and may be the presenting feature. It is usually oligoarticular but occasionally polyarticular and rarely monoarticular.[5] The most commonly involved joints are the ankles. It may also involve the knees, wrists, and elbows. Symmetric ankle arthritis at onset has been shown to have a high degree of sensitivity (95%) and specificity (92%) for acute sarcoid arthritis.[5] Other joints such as the small joints of the hands and feet, hips, and sternoclavicular and sacroiliac joints are less frequently involved.[6,7] Enthesitis is present in up to 33% of the patients, with acute sarcoid arthritis involving mainly the Achilles tendon.[5]

Acute sarcoid arthritis is usually self-limited, and recurrences are uncommon. Destructive changes are absent, and the symptoms are present from just a few weeks to more than 3 months.[7,8] The triad of acute arthritis, bilateral hilar adenopathy, and erythema nodosum is known as Löfgren syndrome. Chronic arthritis is uncommon and is almost always associated with multiorgan disease. In the chronic form, the shoulders, knees, wrists, ankles, and hands are affected most frequently and response to treatment is poor.

Osseous sarcoidosis is often clinically occult; pain and swelling (dactylitis) may occur, but overt bony disease is uncommon overall (<5%). Any bony structure may be involved, but the middle and distal phalanges of the hands and feet are the most frequent sites.[9] Significant osseous involvement is associated with multisystemic disease and indicates a poor prognosis.

Muscle involvement may cause weakness, elevated muscle enzyme levels, and pain; the diagnosis is supported by electromyographic abnormalities and enhancement on gadolinium-enhanced MRI or nuclear gallium scan. The proximal muscles are most commonly affected. Although the incidence of symptomatic sarcoid myositis is reportedly less than 5%, muscle biopsy in asymptomatic

KEY POINTS

- Hands and feet are the most frequent sites of involvement.
- Phalangeal findings (honeycomb or latticework pattern and cystic changes) are typical.
- Imaging findings on MRI are usually nonspecific and similar to those of other marrow-infiltrating lesions.
- Destructive lesions are rare.

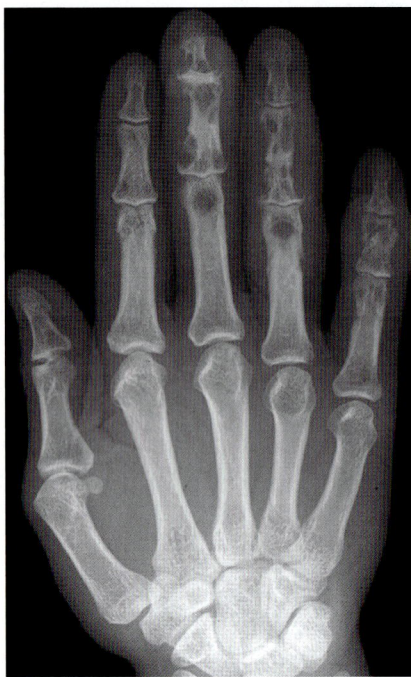

■ FIGURE 85-1 Anteroposterior radiograph of right hand demonstrates a lace-like pattern in the third, fourth, and fifth digits with associated soft tissue swelling and a nondisplaced fracture of the fifth distal phalanx.

patients will reveal granulomas in 50% to 80% of patients.[10] Unrecognized myositis may be an important contributor to generalized fatigue and limitation in exercise in these patients.

MANIFESTATIONS OF THE DISEASE

Radiography

Because of the infrequent occurrence of musculoskeletal sarcoid and the lack of large series, neither clear-cut sites of predilection nor imaging patterns have emerged. Yet, there are circumstances when the disease might be considered. The best-known radiographic sign of osseous sarcoid is the lace-like or honeycomb pattern described in the phalanges of the hands. (Fig. 85-1). These phalangeal changes are usually seen in the presence of cutaneous sarcoid and, in that clinical setting, rare as the finding is, would appear to be pathognomonic. The lack of cortical destruction with lesions of the large bones might explain why these lesions could be occult radiographically (Fig. 85-2C). Sclerotic lesions of sarcoid are most commonly seen in spine, pelvis, skull, and ribs and can be focal or diffuse.

Magnetic Resonance Imaging

On MRI, focal areas of marrow infiltration may be seen (see Fig. 85-2A). These areas may show increased uptake

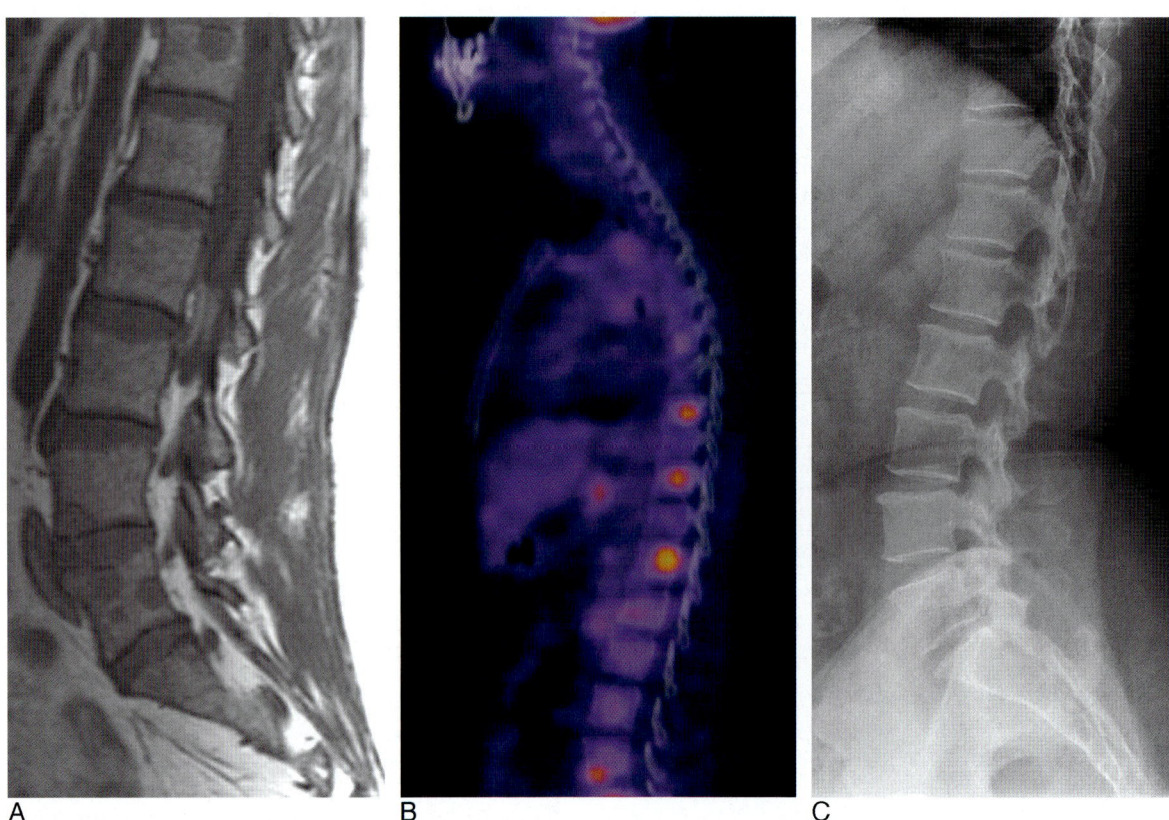

A   B   C

■ FIGURE 85-2 **A,** Sagittal T1-weighted (TR 450/TE 14) MR image of lumbar spine shows several focal areas of marrow-infiltrating lesions. Biopsy revealed non-necrotizing granulomas consistent with sarcoidosis. **B,** Sagittal PET/CT fusion image demonstrates increased uptake in these lesions. **C,** Lateral radiograph of the lumbar spine is unremarkable without lytic or sclerotic lesions. *(From Cohen AA. Rheumatologic manifestations of sarcoidosis. Curr Opin Rheumatol 2004; 16:51–55.)*

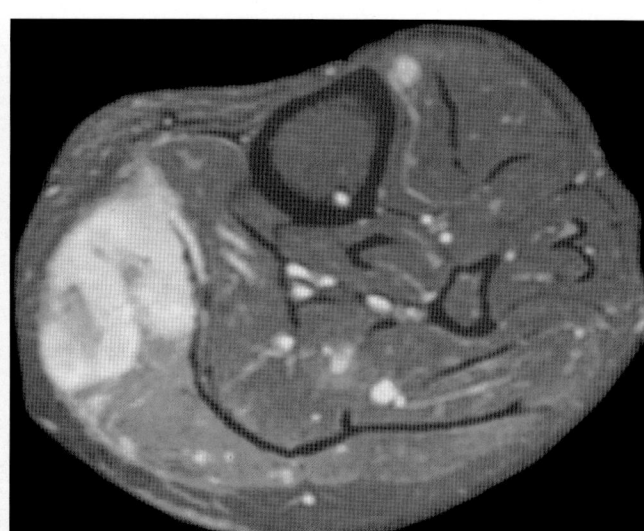

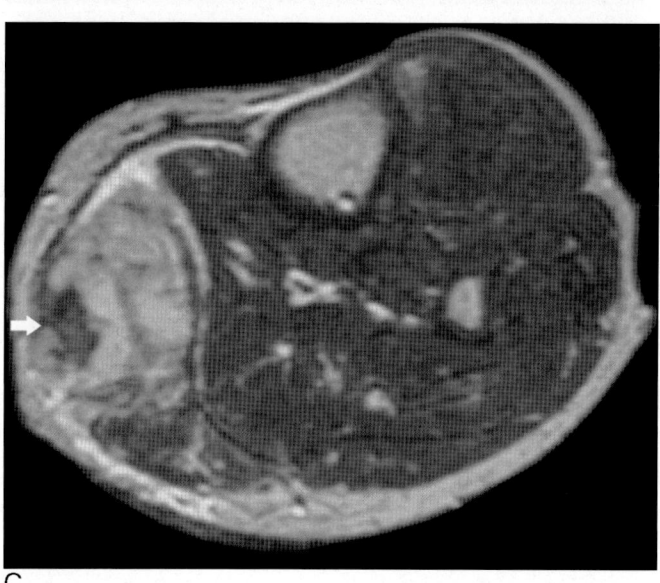

■ **FIGURE 85-3** Axial MR image through the left calf. T1-weighted precontrast (TR 340/TE 17) (**A**) and T1-weighted fat-suppressed postcontrast (TR 500/TE 17) (**B**) MR images show mass-like nodular involvement of the medial head of the gastrocnemius muscle with diffuse enhancement in the periphery. A central nodule of low signal intensity is seen on a T2-weighted image (TR 2000/TE 90) (**C**). *(Courtesy of Shigeru Ehara, Iwate Medical University School of Medicine Morioka, Japan.)*

on PET/CT (see Fig. 85-2B). In a recent study, MRI revealed more axial skeleton and disease of large bones than had been recognized on radiographs.[4] However, large appendicular and axial bone lesions are usually confined to the medullary cavity,[4] although cortical disruption and extraosseous extension is rarely reported.[11]

The occurrence of muscle sarcoid on MRI may result in two quite different patterns[12]: (1) a nodule of low signal intensity (on all pulse sequences) with radiating strands and surrounding high signal intensity and (2) an edema-like pattern in muscle suggestive of a myositis.

The nodular pattern of muscle involvement by sarcoidosis is considered on MRI as a relatively specific appearance. The characteristic feature on axial imaging is a nodular mass with distinctive signal features. The periphery of the nodule has increased signal intensity on all sequences and enhances after intravenous administration of gadolinium contrast medium (Fig. 85-3A and B). Centrally within the nodular mass is a smaller nodule that is dark on all sequences (described as "a dark star") (see Fig. 85-3C). On coronal and sagittal planes the nodule has an orientation following the muscle fibers and the just-described signal features are seen as a low-signal central stripe with outer or peripheral stripes of increased signal intensity.[4] The pattern of myositis is less specific and would warrant biopsy for a diagnosis of sarcoidosis to be established.[3] The MRI finding of fatty atrophy of the muscles can be seen with sarcoidosis in the later stages (Fig. 85-4).

Although arthralgia is a common symptom, joint involvement is infrequently documented in sarcoidosis. MRI can demonstrate nonspecific synovitis (Fig. 85-5) reminiscent of an inflammatory arthritis.

The MRI findings of musculoskeletal sarcoidosis lesions may indicate systemic involvement and a greater burden

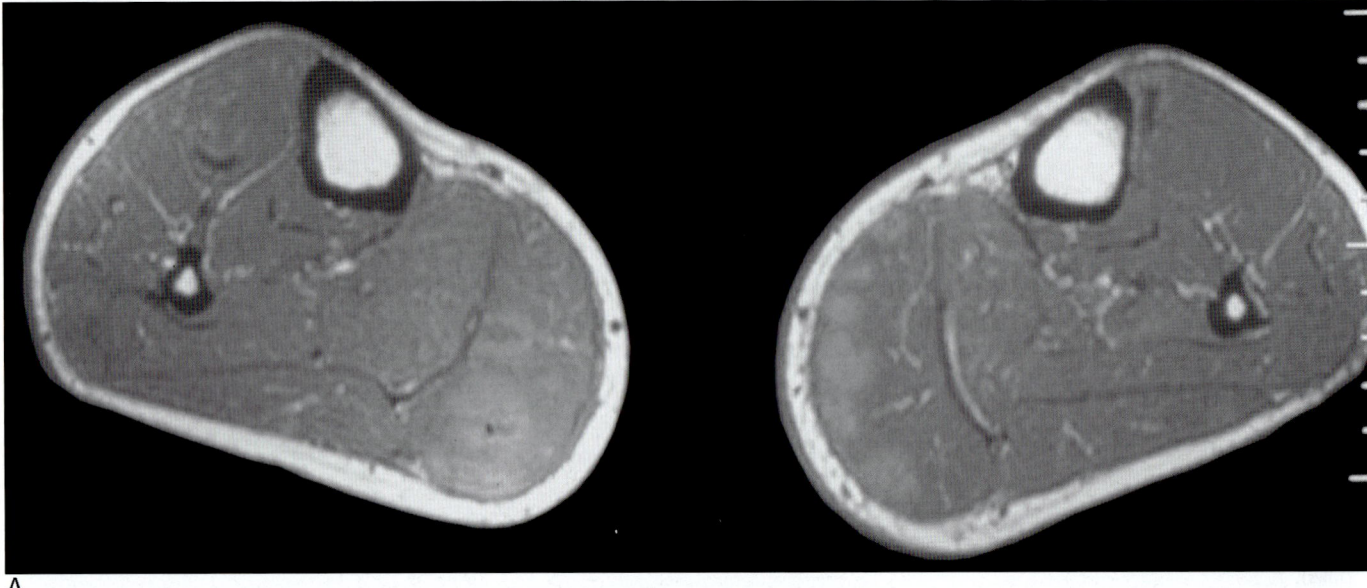

A

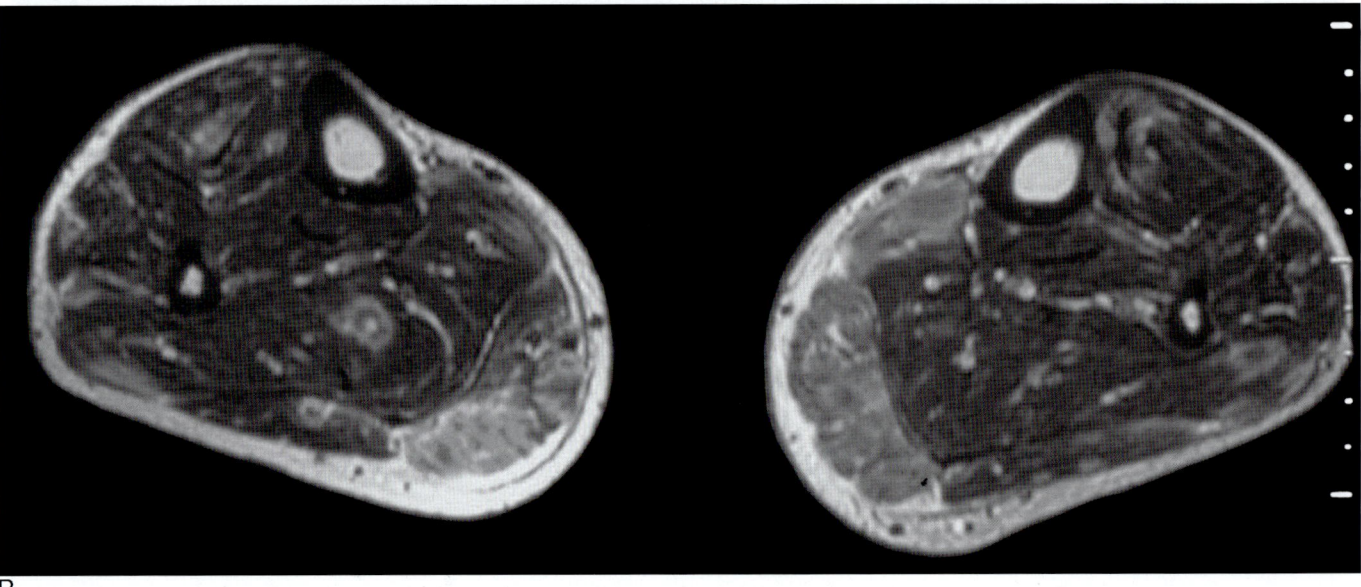

B

■ **FIGURE 85-4** Axial MRI through the bilateral calves. T1-weighted (TR 460/TE 8) (**A**) and T2-weighted (TR 3200/TE 112) (**B**) MR images show diffuse myositis pattern involving several different muscle groups, most marked in the medial head of gastrocnemius muscles. *(Courtesy of Shigeru Ehara, Iwate Medical University School of Medicine Morioka, Japan.)*

of granulomas, which may have therapeutic and prognostic significance.[4] In addition, when musculoskeletal manifestations are demonstrated, MRI can also guide biopsy in patients with suspected sarcoidosis and can be used to follow response to treatment.

Nuclear Medicine

Bone scintigraphy has been used to delineate the extent of skeletal involvement in patients with sarcoidosis. Appearance on the scintigram is usually more extensive when compared with that on radiographs.

Positron Emission Tomography/ Computed Tomography

Sarcoid is PET avid, and PET/CT may be helpful to assess activity and extent of disease in patients with known sarcoidosis.

DIFFERENTIAL DIAGNOSIS

The characteristic phalangeal lesions, albeit rare, do not usually require differential diagnosis. The MRI appearance of osseous sarcoid is not specific and should be dif-

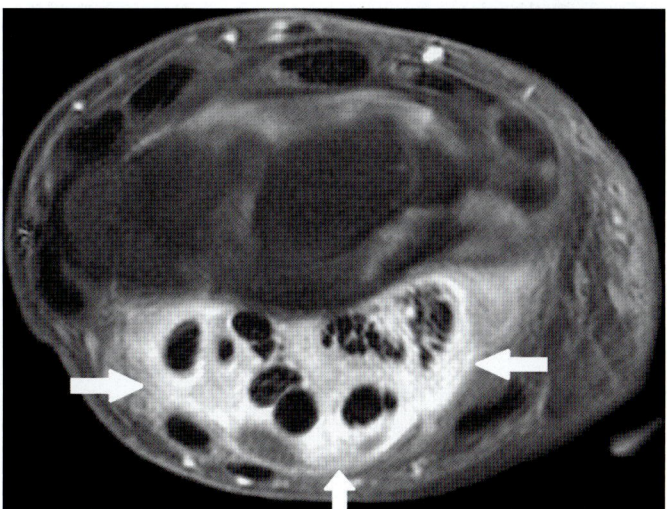

■ **FIGURE 85-5** Axial T1-weighted postcontrast (TR 663/TE 16) MR image through the wrist demonstrates marked synovitis of flexor tendons (*arrows*). *(Courtesy of Mark Kransdorf, MD, Mayo Clinic, Jacksonville, FL.)*

ferentiated from metastatic disease, multiple myeloma, lymphoma, and disseminated granulomatous infection Also, multifocal fibrous dysplasia and tuberous sclerosis may be considered in the differential diagnosis for sclerotic lesions.

Differentiation of sarcoidosis myopathy from other muscle disorders, including corticosteroid myopathy, sequel of trauma, chronic disuse, and/or chronic denervation myopathies requires correlation with electromyography, which shows greater muscle irritability with sarcoidal myopathy than corticosteroid myopathy. Creatine kinase levels are often elevated in muscle sarcoidosis but not in corticosteroid myopathy. MRI does not differentiate

between these causes but can be used to assess the degree of atrophy and guide the selection of a muscle biopsy site, obviating a biopsy of fatty-replaced muscle.

Patients with active pulmonary sarcoidosis have elevated angiotensin-converting enzyme (ACE) levels, which become negative after treatment with corticosteroids or when the disease is inactive, and it may be useful to monitor disease activity and response to therapy. ACE is produced within the sarcoid granulomas by epithelioid cells and alveolar macrophages through the release of an ACE-inducing factor. Elevated ACE levels are present in 40% to 90% of patients; however, this test is not specific for sarcoidosis and may be present in other granulomatous conditions.

SYNOPSIS OF TREATMENT OPTIONS

Nonsteroidal anti-inflammatory drugs are used as initial therapy for patients with acute arthritis due to sarcoid. Patients with refractory disease, myopathy, or widespread organ involvement may require corticosteroids. Patients with chronic arthritis often require corticosteroids as well, because it is usually associated with organ involvement.

What the Referring Physician Needs to Know

■ Osseous sarcoidosis is often clinically occult.
■ Acute arthritis may be the presenting symptom.
■ Chronic arthritis is uncommon and is almost always associated with multiorgan disease.
■ Muscle sarcoidosis may take the form of nodular involvement or diffuse myositis.

SUGGESTED READINGS

Cohen AA. Rheumatologic manifestations of sarcoidosis. Curr Opin Rheumatol 2004; 16:51-55.

Wilcox A, Bharadwaj P, Sharma OP. Bone sarcoidosis. Curr Opin Rheumatol 2000; 12:321-330.

REFERENCES

1. James DG. Epidemiology of sarcoidosis. Sarcoidosis 1992; 9:79-87.
2. Rybicki BA, Major M, Popovich J Jr, et al. Racial differences in sarcoidosis incidence: a 5-year study in a health maintenance organization. Am J Epidemiol 1997; 145:234-241.
3. Perry LT, et al. Sarcoidosis. Br J Hosp Med 1994; 5:293-295.
4. Moore SL, Terrstein A, Golimbu C. MRI of sarcoidosis patients with musculoskeletal symptoms. AJR Am J Roentgenol 2005; 185:154-159.
5. Visser H, Vos K, Zanelli E, et al. Sarcoid arthritis: clinical characteristics, diagnostic aspects, and risk factors. Ann Rheum Dis 2002; 61:499-504.
6. Perruquet JL, Harrington TM, Davis DE, et al: Sarcoid arthritis in a North American Caucasian population. J Rheumatol 1984; 11:521-525.
7. Gran JT, Bøhmer E: Acute sarcoid arthritis: a favourable outcome? Scand J Rheumatol 1996; 25:70-73.
8. Pettersson T: Rheumatic features of sarcoidosis. Curr Opin Rheumatol 1998; 10:73-78.
9. Neville E, Carstairs LS, James DG. Sarcoidosis of bone. Q J Med 1977; 46:215-227.
10. Silverstein A, Siltzbach LE. Muscle involvement in sarcoidosis: asymptomatic, myositis, and myopathy. Arch Neurol 1969; 21:235-241.
11. Sundaram M, Place H, Shaffer WO, Martin DS. Progressive destructive vertebral sarcoid leading to surgical fusion. Skeletal Radiol 1999; 28:717-722.
12. Otake S, Ishigaki T. Muscular sarcoidosis. Semin Musculoskelet Radiol 2001; 5:167-170.

86

Tuberous Sclerosis

Luis Beltran

Tuberous sclerosis (Bourneville syndrome, Bourneville-Pringle syndrome, Bourneville-Brissaud disease, Pringle disease, phakomatosis, epiloia) is a neurocutaneous syndrome that is classically characterized by a clinical triad of epileptic seizures, mental retardation, and adenoma sebaceum (dermal angiofibroma). Despite the classic triad, tuberous sclerosis can manifest in a wide variety of clinical, pathologic, and radiologic features, including the presence of hamartomas (benign neoplasms composed of cellular elements normally present in tissue) in multiple organ systems. These lesions may include renal angiomyolipomas, cerebral and paraventricular hamartomas, and cardiac rhabdomyomas. Various skin abnormalities such as hypomelanotic macules, shagreen patches, and periungual fibromas may be noted, and pulmonary involvement may include lymphangioleiomyomatosis and the development of pneumothorax.

Two thirds of patients with tuberous sclerosis additionally present with musculoskeletal involvement, including sclerotic lesions in the calvaria, ribs, pelvis, vertebrae, and long bones as well as bone lucencies in the phalanges of the hands and feet. There is also evidence of an association between tuberous sclerosis and fibrous dysplasia[1-10] (disorder of progressive replacement of normal bone elements by fibrous tissue) and an association between tuberous sclerosis and congenital macrodactyly.[11-18]

ETIOLOGY

The etiology of tuberous sclerosis has been linked to mutations in two separate genes, *TSC1* and *TSC2*.[1] The *TSC1* gene, which maps to chromosome 9q34, encodes a protein termed *hamartin,* which is widely expressed in normal tissues. Although the precise function of hamartin in normal tissues is unknown, it forms a complex with the tuberin protein that is encoded by the *TSC2* gene, and the complex is thought to function in part as a negative regulator of the cell cycle. Several different types of *TSC1* mutations have been identified, most of which result in a truncated protein with loss of function. The *TSC2* gene, which maps to chromosome 16p13.3, is ubiquitously expressed in all adult normal tissues and encodes the tuberin protein. Although the exact function of the tuberin protein is unknown, it

appears to participate in normal brain development and in withdrawal of the normal cardiomyocyte from the cell cycle during terminal differentiation.

PREVALENCE AND EPIDEMIOLOGY

Tuberous sclerosis is a hereditary autosomal dominant disorder with an incidence of 1 in 10,000 live births but is sporadic and without family history in 50% to 84% of cases.[1]

CLINICAL PRESENTATION

The result of mutations in *TSC1* and *TSC2* is abnormal benign cell growth in the tissues involved, leading to the hamartomatous lesions in multiple organ systems. Although the malignant potential of these lesions is very low, the tumors can significantly compromise the function of the organs involved, leading to the multiple clinical manifestations of tuberous sclerosis: seizures, mental retardation, symptoms of obstructive hydrocephalus, or focal neurologic deficits. Common presenting signs and symptoms include headaches, vomiting, or neurologic deficits, including vision loss with cerebral and periventricular hamartomas; renal failure and hemorrhage in renal angiomyolipomas; flow abnormalities, arrhythmias, and heart failure in cardiac rhabdomyomas; and dyspnea and pneumothorax in lymphangioleiomyomatosis.

IMAGING TECHNIQUES

The use of CT, MRI, and ultrasonography in the detection of cerebral and paraventricular hamartomas, renal angiomyolipomas, and cardiac rhabdomyomas has been extensively

---

KEY POINTS

■ Skeletal manifestations of tuberous sclerosis are rare and nonspecific and include cystic lesions in the short tubular bones and sclerotic lesions in the spine.
■ Tuberous sclerosis and fibrous dysplasia may coexist.

documented in the literature on tuberous sclerosis, playing a primary role in the diagnosis of this protean disease.[1] The use of plain films, CT, and MRI in the evaluation of musculoskeletal lesions in tuberous sclerosis, on the other hand, is less extensive and plays a more complementary role. Despite the lack of documented cases, musculoskeletal involvement is frequent (45% to 66%) in patients with tuberous sclerosis[2]; therefore, further radiologic investigation of such lesions is warranted and could aid the treating physician in diagnosing, treating, and following the progression of tuberous sclerosis. Reported cases of CT and MRI evaluation of hamartomatous lesions in tuberous sclerosis have provided more detailed and specific information that may aid the treating physician in diagnosing this disease.

MANIFESTATIONS OF THE DISEASE

Radiography

Plain radiographic evidence of musculoskeletal lesions in tuberous sclerosis is more documented in the literature than are CT or MRI findings, but they are nonspecific and not noted early enough to have a significant role in the diagnosis of tuberous sclerosis.

The classic lesions of tuberous sclerosis described on plain films include the following:

- Sclerotic bone lesions in the vertebral bodies and neural arches[2] and in the iliac bones of the pelvis (Figs. 86-1 to 86-3).[3]
- Fibrous dysplasia. A rare but early thoracic radiographic finding of tuberous sclerosis is an unusual but characteristic, expanded rib deformity due to diffuse sclerosis.[2] In 1988, Breningstall and colleagues reported a case of tuberous sclerosis and radiographic abnormalities, including marked sclerosis and thickening of the left wing of the sphenoid and osteosclerotic areas in the left acetabulum.[4] Biopsy specimens of these lesions were characteristic of fibrous dysplasia. Fibrous dysplasia is a sporadic skeletal abnormality, typically seen in adolescents and young adults, in which normal bone

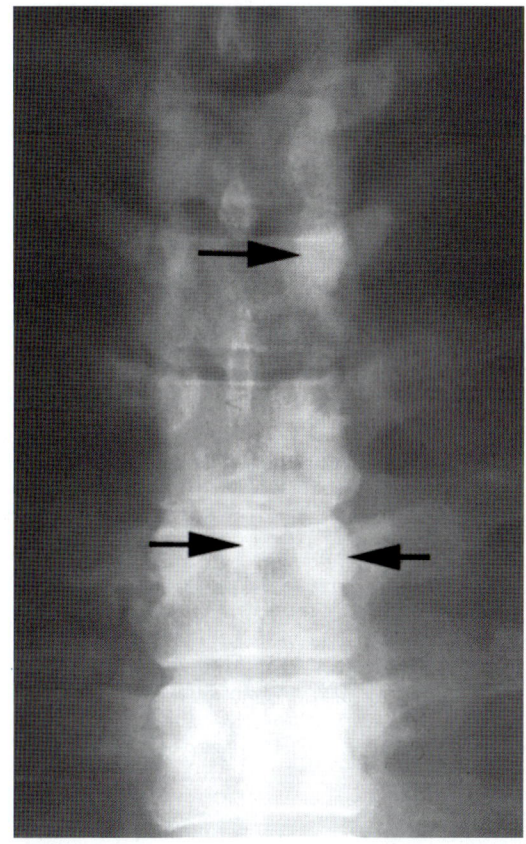

■ **FIGURE 86-2** Anteroposterior view of the thoracic spine showing focal areas of sclerosis involving the neural arch (*arrows*).

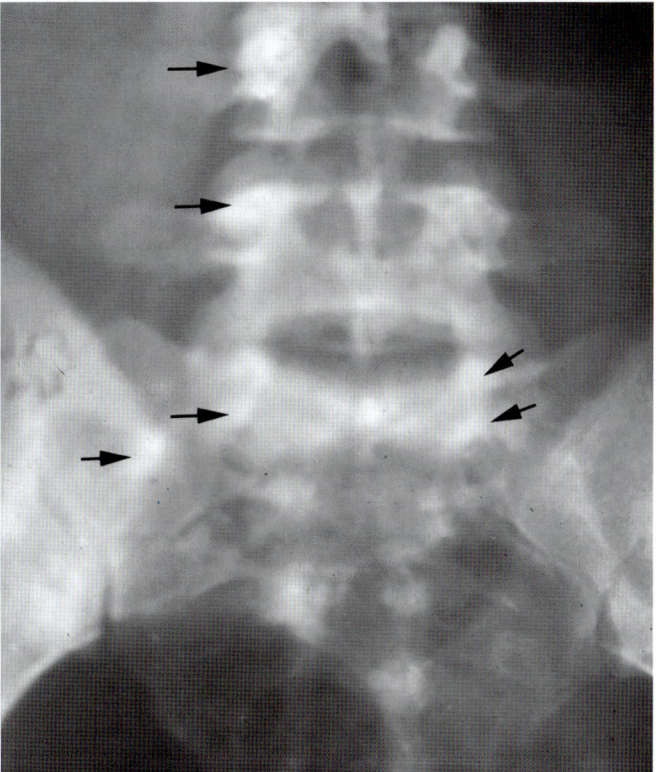

■ **FIGURE 86-3** Anteroposterior view of the lumbosacral area demonstrating multiple focal sclerotic lesions (*arrows*).

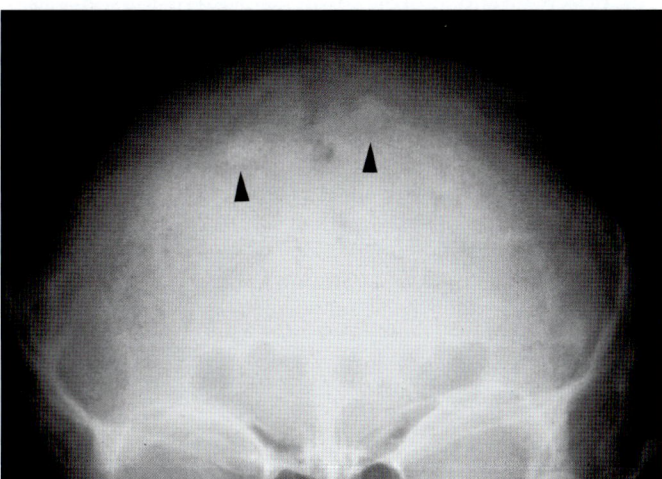

■ **FIGURE 86-1** Anteroposterior view of the skull demonstrates focal areas of sclerosis (*arrowheads*).

marrow is replaced by fibro-osseous tissue. It may be associated with either solitary or multiple lesions in one or more bones. The histologic features of fibrous dysplasia include a background of whorled bundles of spindle cells and multiple trabeculae that vary in both size and shape. These trabeculae are composed of immature woven bones that presumably result from osseous metaplasia. Scattered osteoclasts are also seen but are not a dominant histologic feature.[5] Several other reported cases of associated tuberous sclerosis and fibrous dysplasia show similar findings.[5-10]

● Cyst-like radiolucencies in the hands and feet (Fig. 86-4)[2]
● Periosteal new bone in the metatarsals
● Congenital macrodactyly. Multiple reports of an association between tuberous sclerosis and congenital macrodactyly involving hypertrophy of the phalanges of the hands and feet have also been made.[11-18]

Magnetic Resonance Imaging

Patients with tuberous sclerosis do not routinely undergo MRI of the musculoskeletal system; thus, MRI data in the literature are limited. In 2005, Stosic-Opincal and coworkers described a case of a patient with tuberous sclerosis

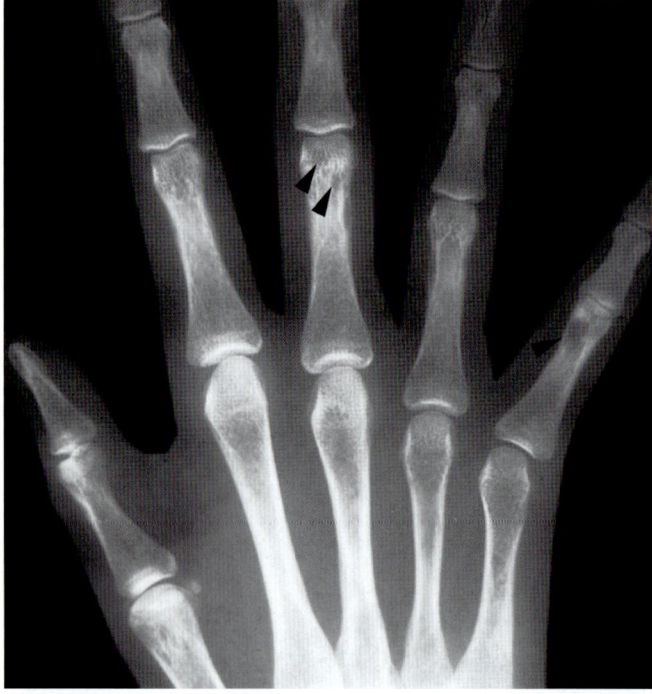

■ FIGURE 86-4 Small cystic lesions in the short tubular bones of the hand (*arrowheads*).

in which multiple focal lesions (up to 2 cm in diameter) of the vertebral bodies, pedicles, and laminae were detected using spine MRI.[19] All the lesions showed the same MRI features: low signal intensity on both T1-weighted and T2-weighted images and no contrast enhancement after intravenous administration of gadolinium. Similar lesions were present in the same patient in the iliac bones and femur. These findings are consistent with multiple hamartomatous lesions in several locations of the axial and peripheral skeleton.

Multidetector Computed Tomography

Computed tomographic evaluation of hamartomatous lesions has provided more detailed and specific information that may aid the treating physician in the diagnosis of tuberous sclerosis. A case of associated tuberous sclerosis and fibrous dysplasia was reported in 2003 by Gasparetto and colleagues in which an 11-year-old girl with tuberous sclerosis who presented with a right nasal mass had a CT examination revealing fibrous dysplasia involving the frontal, ethmoid, sphenoid, and vomer bones. These findings were confirmed with biopsy, and follow-up revealed marked expansion of these lesions.[5]

In 2004, Abel and associates reported a case of a 6-year old girl with tuberous sclerosis who had a mass involving the right inferior orbital rim.[3] The mass was examined with CT of the head and orbits that showed a bony mass arising from the upper portion of the right maxillary bone just below the orbital rim. There was no evidence of bony erosion or excavation, and the mass was described as a bony exostosis. The lesion was surgically excised, and histologic examination revealed medullary bone surrounded by dense fibrosis with numerous interconnecting bony trabeculae present within the normal bone marrow. Osteoblasts were present on the surface of the trabeculae. The diagnosis of a bony hamartoma of the inferior orbital rim was made based on these findings.

DIFFERENTIAL DIAGNOSIS

The differential diagnosis of the skeletal lesions on radiographs can be diverse:

● Sclerotic lesions can be mistaken for osteomas, osteoblastic metastases, or Paget disease.
● Cystic lesions in the hands and feet may also be seen in sarcoidosis or enchondromatosis.
● Periosteal new bone in the metatarsals may also be found in hyperparathyroidism.
● Destructive lesions in the flat bones may also be found in lytic metastases and osteomyelitis.

SUGGESTED READINGS

Aughenbaugh GL. Thoracic manifestations of neurocutaneous diseases. Radiol Clin North Am 1984; 22:741–756.

Hoffman A. Imaging of tuberous sclerosis lesions outside of the central nervous system. Ann N Y Acad Sci 1991; 615:94–111.

REFERENCES

1. Lendvay TS, Marshall FF. The tuberous sclerosis complex and its highly variable manifestations. J Urol 2003; 160:1635–1642.
2. Bernauer TA, Mirowski GW, Caldemeyer KS. Tuberous sclerosis: II. Musculoskeletal and visceral findings. J Am Acad Dermatol 2001; 45:450–452.
3. Abel A, Brockbank DT, Farber M, Meyer DR. Bony hamartoma of the inferior orbital rim in a patient with tuberous sclerosis. Arch Opthalmol 2004; 122:780–782.
4. Breningstall GN, Faerber EN, Kolanu R. Fibrous dysplasia in a patient with tuberous sclerosis. J Child Neurol 1988; 3:131–134.
5. Gasparetto EL, de Carvalho Neto A, Bruck I, Antoniuk S. Tuberous sclerosis and fibrous dysplasia. AJNR Am J Neuroradiol 2003; 24:836–837.
6. Chong VF, Khoo JB, Fan YF. Fibrous dysplasia involving the base of the skull. AJR Am J Roentgenol 2002; 178:717–720.
7. Jee WH, Choi KH, Choe BY, et al. Fibrous dysplasia: MR imaging characteristics with radiopathologic correlation. AJR Am J Roentgenol 1996; 167:1523–1527.
8. Terada T, Nakai R, Moriwaki H, et al. Tuberous sclerosis with an atypical radiological skull change: case report. Neurosurgery 1985; 16:804–807.
9. Moore AT, Buncic JR, Munro IR. Fibrous dysplasia of the orbit in childhood: clinical features and management. Ophthalmology 1985; 92:12–20.
10. Brown EW, Megerian CA, McKenna MJ, Weber A. Fibrous dysplasia of the temporal bone: imaging findings. AJR Am J Roentgenol 1995; 164:679–682.
11. Zaremba J. Tuberous sclerosis: a clinical and genetic investigation. J Ment Defic Res 1968; 12:63–80.
12. Ortonne JP, Jeune R, Fulton R, Thivolet J. Primary localized gigantism and tuberous sclerosis. Arch Dermatol 1982; 118:877–878.
13. Colamaria V, Zambelli L, Tinazzi P, Bernardina BD. Tuberous sclerosis associated with partial gigantism in a child. Brain Dev 1988; 10:78–181.
14. Wallis CE, Beighton PH. Tuberous sclerosis with macrodactyly: further phenotypic overlap within the phakomatoses. Dysmorph Clin Genet 1989; 3:2–4.
15. Kousseff BG. Tuberous sclerosis and macrodactyly. Dysmorph Clin Genet 1989; 3:5–7.
16. Norman-Taylor F, Mayou BJ. Macrodactyly in tuberous sclerosis. J R Soc Med 1994; 87:419–420.
17. Shin AY, Garay AA. Unilateral insensate macrodactyly secondary to tuberous sclerosis in a child. Am J Orthop 1997; 26:30–32.
18. Lustberg H, Gagliardi J, Lawson J. Digital enlargement in tuberous sclerosis. Skeletal Radiol 1999; 28:116–118.
19. Stosic-Opincal T, Peric V, Lilic G, et al. Spine MRI findings in a patient with tuberous sclerosis: a case report: part I. Spine 2005; 30:844.

87

Drug-Related Bone and Soft Tissue Disorders

Natalie Zelenko, Romulo Baltazar, and Javier Beltran

Numerous pharmacologic agents may affect the musculoskeletal system. Often radiographic manifestations of these effects are apparent before or despite the lack of clinical symptomatology. As such, the radiologist may at times be the first physician to make the appropriate findings. The scope of drug-related disorders with radiographic abnormalities involving the musculoskeletal system is reviewed in this chapter.

CORTICOSTEROIDS

The spectrum of bone and joint abnormalities that may arise in patients on long-term corticosteroid therapy is wide and includes osteoporosis, pathologic fractures, osteonecrosis, neuropathic-like articular destruction, osteomyelitis, septic arthritis, tendinous and soft tissue injury, periarticular and capsular calcification, and abnormalities in the distribution of fat.

Osteoporosis and Pathologic Fractures

The precise mechanism by which osteoporosis results from corticosteroid treatment is not known. However, the two most probable mechanisms are (1) direct inhibition of bone formation and (2) indirect activation of bone resorption related to diminished intestinal calcium absorption and parathyroid hormone upregulation.[1-3] Women, the elderly, and patients on high-dose therapy may be particularly susceptible to corticosteroid-induced osteoporosis (Fig. 87-1). The process is at least partially reversible upon termination of treatment.[4,5]

Osteonecrosis

As in the case of osteoporosis, the mechanism by which osteonecrosis results from corticosteroid use is not definitively known. Although an association between osteonecrosis and corticosteroid use is well accepted, a causal relationship has not always been directly established. The

two most commonly cited mechanisms in the pathogenesis of corticosteroid-induced osteonecrosis are (1) mechanical microfractures resulting in osseous collapse[6] and (2) vascular compromise due to marrow accumulation of fat cells, fat embolization, vasculitis, and hyperviscosity.[7,8] Findings related to osteonecrosis typically appear at least 2 or 3 years

---

KEY POINTS

- Numerous pharmacologic agents may cause disturbances in bone metabolism and therefore affect radiographic appearance of numerous osseous structures.
- The radiologist can often be the first to suggest the diagnosis by recognizing the radiographic changes in bones.
- Corticosteroids may lead to osteoporosis, osteonecrosis, neuropathic-like arthropathy, and osteomyelitis/septic arthritis.
- Phenytoin, phenobarbital, deferoxamine, aluminum, and ifosfamide are the main pharmacologic agents that may result in various forms of osteomalacia and rickets-like appearance of bones.
- Vitamin A and retinoids have different manifestations in the pediatric and adult populations; both involve acceleration in the process of bone maturation.
- Vitamin D toxicity may cause soft tissue calcifications in adults and metaphyseal bands in children.
- Fluorosis leads to increased bone production, including osteosclerosis, osteophytosis, periostitis, and ligamentous calcification.
- Prostaglandin E is associated with periostitis.
- Polyvinyl chloride has been implicated in acro-osteolysis.
- Methotrexate toxicity is associated with osseous radiographic findings most similar to scurvy (vitamin C deficiency).
- Vitamin A, retinoids, alcohol, cocaine, thalidomide, and warfarin all have teratogenic effects, particularly musculoskeletal abnormalities.

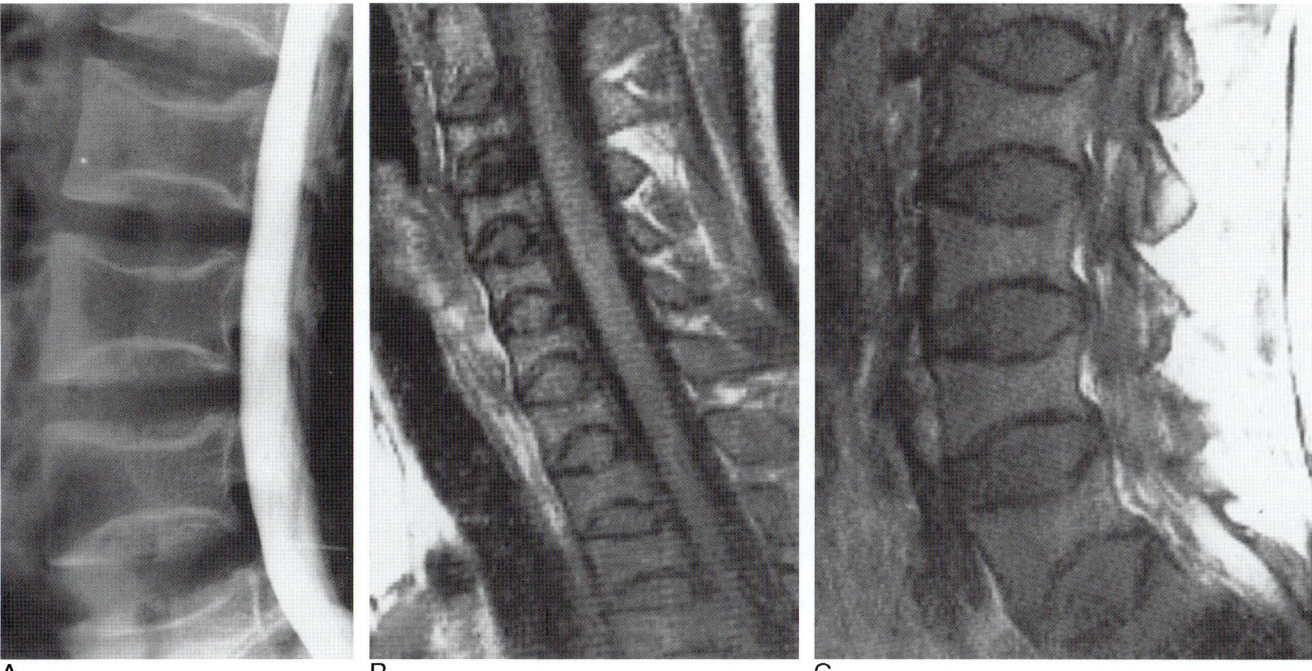

A   B   C

■ **FIGURE 87-1   Corticosteroid-induced osteoporosis.** This 22-year-old woman had received systemic corticosteroid therapy for many months as a child. She subsequently developed cushingoid features. Lateral radiograph (**A**) obtained during a lumbar myelogram (performed for investigation of low back pain) reveals osteopenia, biconcave deformities of multiple vertebral bodies, and well-defined subchondral bone plates. Sagittal T1-weighted (TR/TE, 200/26) spin-echo MR images of the cervical spine (**B**) and lumbar spine (**C**) show the biconcave deformities to good advantage. The signal intensity of the bone marrow reflects the presence of hematopoietic tissue and is within normal limits. *(Courtesy of G. Greenway, MD, Dallas, TX. From Resnick D [ed]: Diagnosis of Bone and Joint Disorders, 4th ed. Philadelphia, WB Saunders, 2002.)*

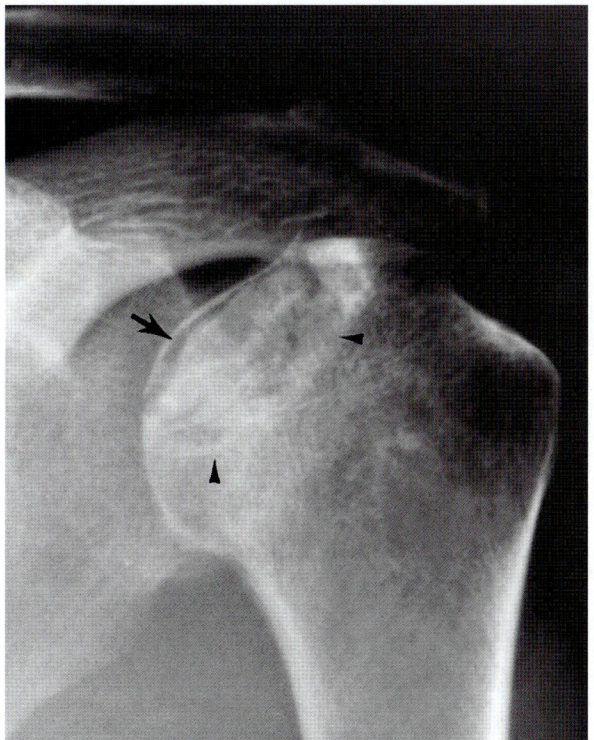

■ **FIGURE 87-2   Corticosteroid-induced osteonecrosis.** Proximal end of the humerus. Abnormalities consist of flattening of the humeral head with a subchondral radiolucent line (crescent sign) (*arrow*), surrounding osteolysis and osteosclerosis (*arrowheads*), and relative preservation of joint space. *(From Resnick D [ed]: Diagnosis of Bone and Joint Disorders, 4th ed. Philadelphia, WB Saunders, 2002.)*

after the initiation of treatment. Reports on the incidence of these findings have been highly variable and contingent on the underlying disease, dose, and duration of treatment (Figs. 87-2 to 87-7).[9]

Neuropathic-Like Articular Destruction

Intra-articular corticosteroid administration is believed by many, but not all,[10] to be a cause of joint disease that mimics the neuropathic joint. This entity is most frequently seen in the hip and the knee. As in cases of neuropathic joint, recurrent trauma in the context of diminished pain sensation results in joint space narrowing, fracture, and fragmentation, leading eventually to severe osseous and cartilaginous collapse (Figs. 87-8 and 87-9).

Osteomyelitis and Septic Arthritis

Rarely, corticosteroid administration may predispose a patient to bone and joint infections owing to immunosuppression.[11,12] The most commonly involved joint is the knee, but any joint is susceptible and multiple joints may be simultaneously affected. Bacteria, particularly *Staphylococcus aureus,* are typically the causative organisms.

Other Disorders

Tendon rupture may occur in the setting of systemic corticosteroid therapy or local injection. Corticosteroids

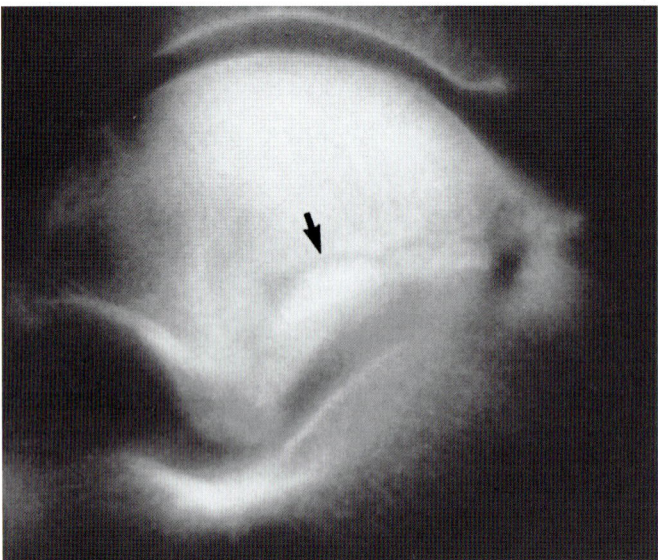

■ **FIGURE 87-3   Corticosteroid-induced osteonecrosis: talus.**
A conventional tomogram in the lateral projection shows sclerosis, mainly in the proximal portion of the bone, and a subchondral radiolucent line (*arrow*). (*From Resnick D [ed]: Diagnosis of Bone and Joint Disorders, 4th ed. Philadelphia, WB Saunders, 2002.*)

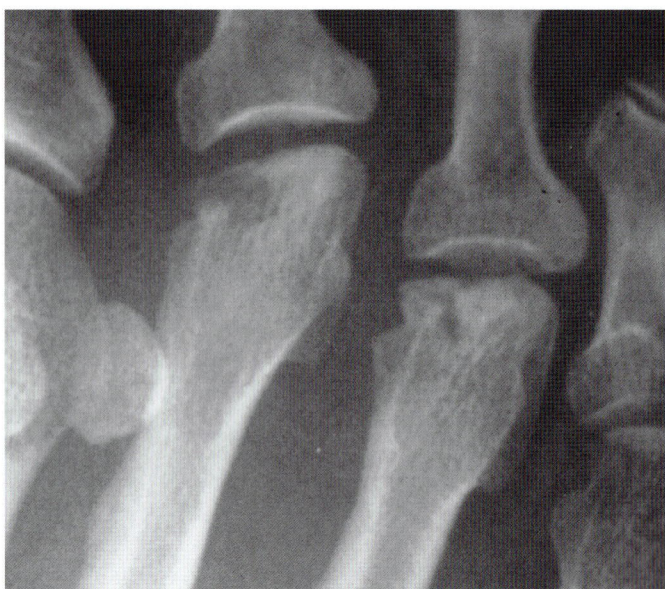

■ **FIGURE 87-4   Corticosteroid-induced osteonecrosis: metatarsal heads.** Note sclerosis, radiolucent zones, and collapse of the second and third metatarsal heads. (*Courtesy of M. Murphey, MD, Washington, DC. From Resnick D [ed]: Diagnosis of Bone and Joint Disorders, 4th ed. Philadelphia, WB Saunders, 2002.*)

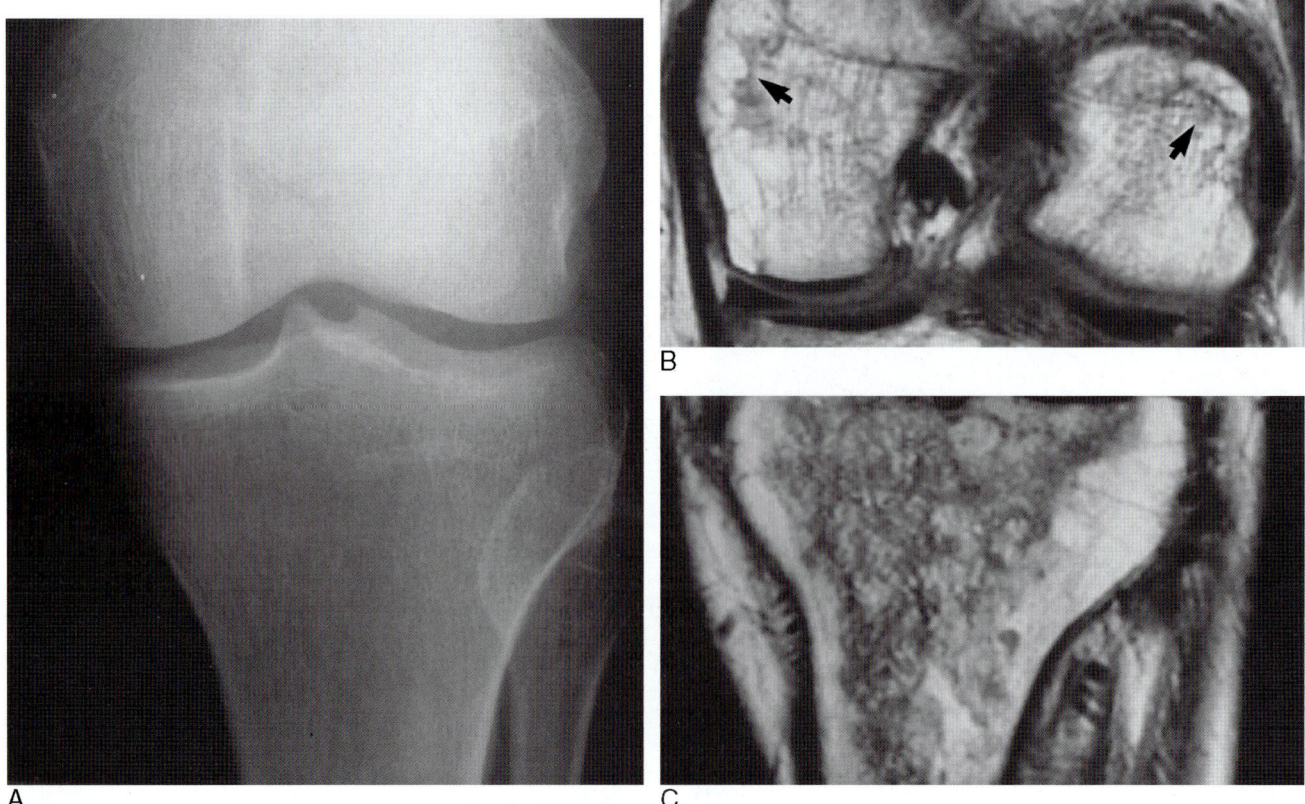

■ **FIGURE 87-5   Corticosteroid-induced osteonecrosis: distal end of the femur and proximal portion of the tibia. A,** The routine radiograph is normal. **B** and **C,** Two coronal T1-weighted (TR/TE, 750/20) spin-echo MR images show characteristic findings of osteonecrosis involving both femoral condyles (*arrows*) and tibia. (*From Resnick D [ed]: Diagnosis of Bone and Joint Disorders, 4th ed. Philadelphia, WB Saunders, 2002.*)

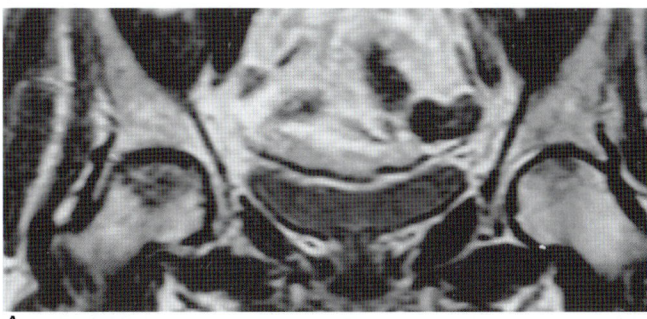

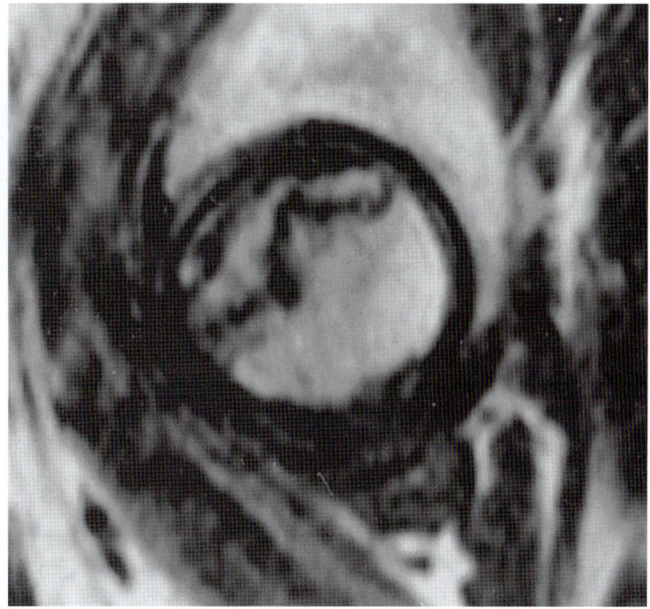

■ **FIGURE 87-6 Corticosteroid-induced osteonecrosis: femoral heads.** This 62-year-old woman had received intraocular corticosteroids for glaucoma. Coronal (**A**) intermediate-weighted (TR/TE, 2000/30) and sagittal (**B**) T1-weighted (TR/TE, 600/12) spin-echo MR images reveal bilateral osteonecrosis of the femoral heads. The sagittal image in **B** is of the right femoral head. Note the serpentine regions of low signal intensity. *(From Resnick D [ed]: Diagnosis of Bone and Joint Disorders, 4th ed. Philadelphia, WB Saunders, 2002.)*

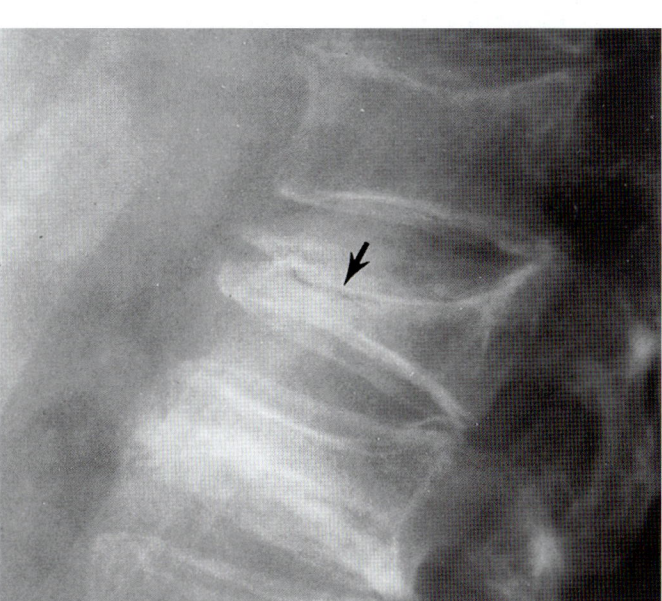

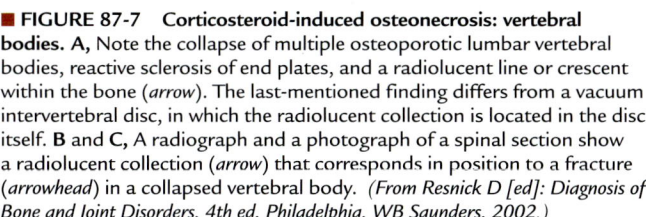

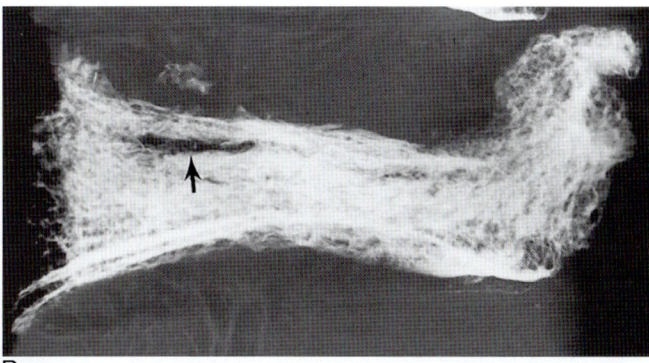

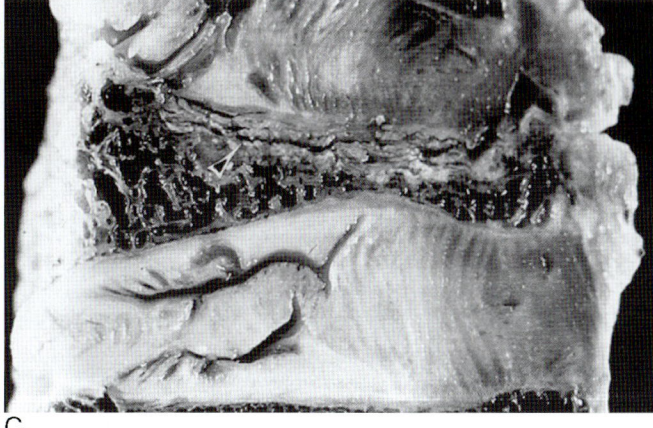

■ **FIGURE 87-7 Corticosteroid-induced osteonecrosis: vertebral bodies. A,** Note the collapse of multiple osteoporotic lumbar vertebral bodies, reactive sclerosis of end plates, and a radiolucent line or crescent within the bone (*arrow*). The last-mentioned finding differs from a vacuum intervertebral disc, in which the radiolucent collection is located in the disc itself. **B** and **C,** A radiograph and a photograph of a spinal section show a radiolucent collection (*arrow*) that corresponds in position to a fracture (*arrowhead*) in a collapsed vertebral body. *(From Resnick D [ed]: Diagnosis of Bone and Joint Disorders, 4th ed. Philadelphia, WB Saunders, 2002.)*

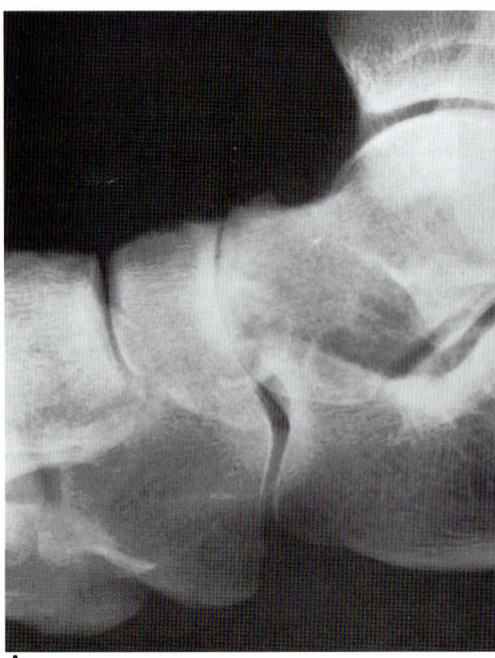

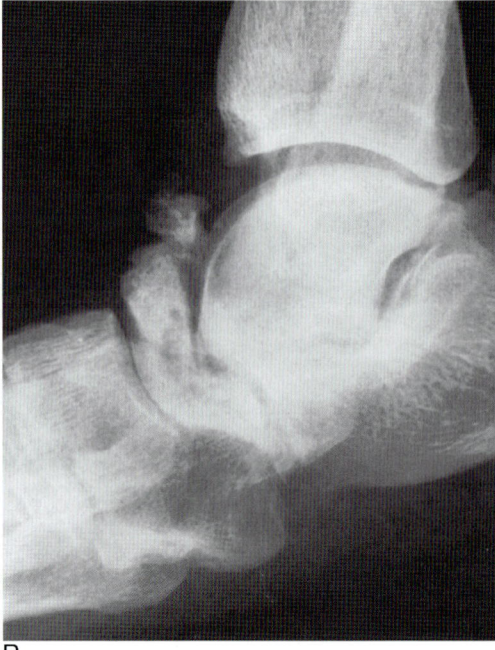

A   B

■ **FIGURE 87-8** Corticosteroid-induced neuropathic-like arthropathy. This patient with rheumatoid arthritis had had repeated injections of corticosteroids into the talonavicular space. Radiographs obtained 2 years apart indicate progressive abnormalities. The initial film (**A**) demonstrates joint space narrowing, sclerosis, and subchondral cyst formation, whereas the later film (**B**) reveals fragmentation of the talus and navicular bone. The findings are unlike those of uncomplicated rheumatoid arthritis and resemble neuropathic changes. *(From Resnick D [ed]: Diagnosis of Bone and Joint Disorders, 4th ed. Philadelphia, WB Saunders, 2002.)*

are believed to induce changes in healthy tendons and inhibit normal healing of diseased tendons. Subcutaneous tissue atrophy and calcification may also be present in the region of local application of corticosteroids.[13-16] Calcification due to hydroxyapatite deposition has been reported in synovial membranes, joint capsules, periarticular tissues, and cartilage (Fig. 87-10). Finally, systemic

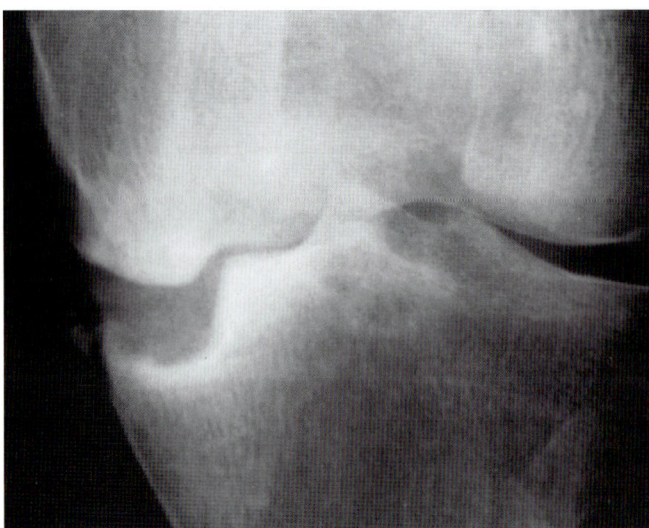

■ **FIGURE 87-9** Corticosteroid-induced neuropathic-like arthropathy. In this 70-year-old woman with rheumatoid arthritis, multiple corticosteroid injections into the knee were associated with significant bone abnormalities. Note the gouged-out area of destruction in the medial tibial plateau. *(From Resnick D [ed]: Diagnosis of Bone and Joint Disorders, 4th ed. Philadelphia, WB Saunders, 2002.)*

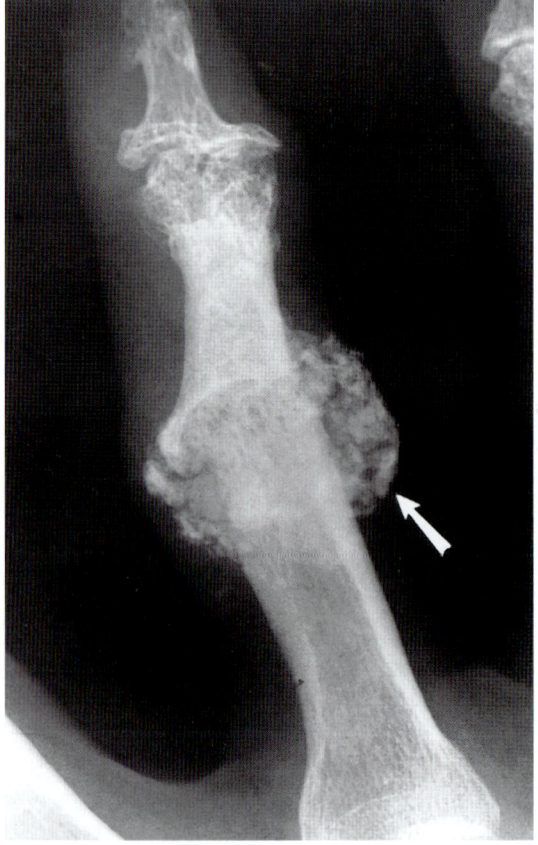

■ **FIGURE 87-10** Corticosteroid-induced intra-articular and periarticular calcification. In a 57-year-old woman with osteoarthritis of the interphalangeal joints of both hands, multiple intra-articular injections of triamcinolone hexacetonide were followed by the development of intra-articular and periarticular calcifications (*arrow*), presumably related to calcium hydroxyapatite crystal deposition. *(Courtesy of M. Dalinka, MD, Philadelphia, PA. From Resnick D [ed]: Diagnosis of Bone and Joint Disorders, 4th ed. Philadelphia, WB Saunders, 2002.)*

corticosteroid treatment, as in Cushing disease, may result in abnormal accumulation of fat. This may manifest in the mediastinum,[17-19] paraspinal region,[20,21] and epidural spine. Epidural lipomatosis may have neurologic manifestations.

OTHER DRUGS ASSOCIATED WITH OSTEOPOROSIS

Gonadotropin-releasing hormone used in the treatment of endometriosis, premenopausal breast cancer, male breast cancer, and prostatic cancer is associated with loss of trabecular bone in lumbar vertebrae. Heparin, in large doses, is associated with osteoporosis that may be complicated by rib fractures and vertebral collapse.[22] These findings are attributed to a collagenolytic property of heparin.

PHENYTOIN AND PHENOBARBITAL

Phenytoin and phenobarbital are commonly prescribed antiepileptics that may result in generalized abnormalities of bone formation indistinguishable from rickets and osteomalacia. The associated radiographic changes were present in 20% of patients on long-term anticonvulsant treatment in one study. The biochemical basis of these changes is reflected in an elevation in serum alkaline phosphatase level present in an even larger fraction of patients early in the course of therapy. Although the mechanism underlying the altered bone metabolism remains unclear, the most compelling implicated pathway involves the induction of hepatic microsomal hydroxylase activity and consequential inactivation of vitamin D and 25-hydroxyvitamin D. Phenytoin has also been demonstrated to impair intestinal absorption of calcium.[23] Data attempting to define the dose and treatment duration necessary to enact bony changes are inconclusive.

Radiographic changes, first described in 1968, include diffuse osteopenia, joint space widening, and the development of "Looser zones"[24] (Fig. 87-11). These findings are nonspecific and indistinguishable from other causes of osteomalacia and rickets.

Other findings that have been reported in association with phenytoin include diffuse calvarial thickening; dental root abnormalities; gross enlargement of the lips, nose, and soft tissues of the face and scalp; and heel pad thickening. Finally, phenytoin is a known teratogen and is implicated in the formation of cleft palate deformity and syndactyly.

ALUMINUM

Although aluminum is usually efficiently eliminated from the body by renal filtration, it may accumulate in the serum of patients with chronic renal failure, patients on dialysis, and patients receiving total parenteral nutrition.[24] Aluminum toxicity most dramatically involves the brain and the skeletal system, although deposits may occur in multiple organs, including liver, muscles, and gonads. In adults, aluminum intoxication manifests itself in the skel-

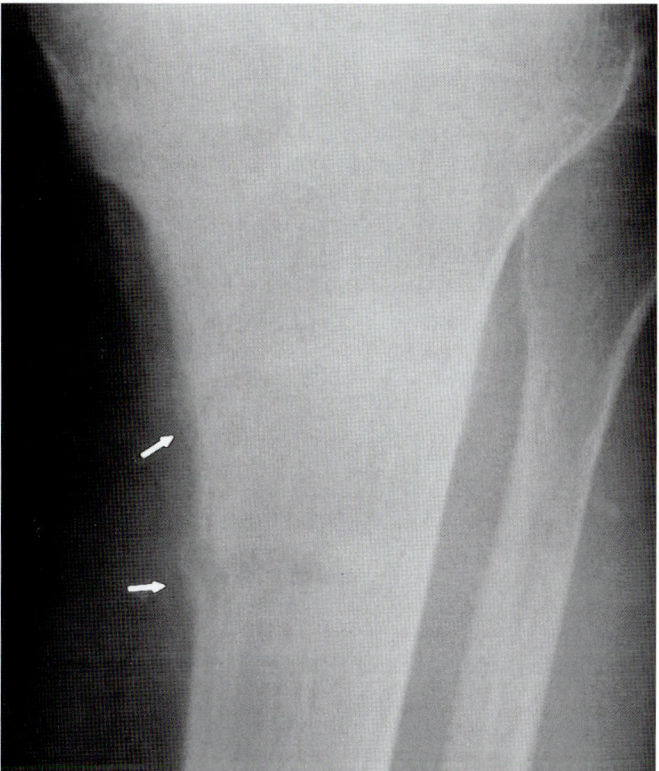

■ **FIGURE 87-11   Phenytoin (Dilantin)-induced osteomalacia.** In this adult with a seizure disorder, long-term phenytoin therapy has resulted in osteomalacia with Looser zones, or insufficiency fractures (*arrows*). *(From Resnick D [ed]: Diagnosis of Bone and Joint Disorders, 4th ed. Philadelphia, WB Saunders, 2002.)*

etal system as an osteomalacia resistant to vitamin D therapy. Radiographs may show evidence of osteomalacia and spontaneous fractures. Healing of these fractures results in only minimal callus formation. The radiographic features of aluminum toxicity are similar to those seen with renal osteodystrophy. The distinguishing clinical triad that accompanies aluminum intoxication consists of skeletal pain, proximal muscle weakness, and pathologic fractures. The pathologic basis for these effects of aluminum is probably the formation of insoluble complexes with phosphates and the inhibition of the deposition of calcium apatite.[25]

Children with impaired renal function can develop aluminum toxicity from oral intake of aluminum alone, as well as from aluminum contents of vaccines. Radiographically, the effects of aluminum intoxication in these infants result in osteopenia with pathologic fractures, fraying of the metaphyses of the long bones, and widening of the physes.[26]

DEFEROXAMINE

Deferoxamine is administered for long-term chelation therapy in combination with the hyperperfusion regimen in the treatment of thalassemia. It has been demonstrated that subcutaneous administration of high doses of deferoxamine in children younger than 3 years of age is associated with a decrease in mean body length, joint stiffness, and a rickets-like syndrome.[27] Short trunk, prominent sternum, genu valgum, and enlargement of the distal fibula and distal radius and ulna have been noted. Humerus, femur, and tibia may also be affected. Radiographs reveal widening of the metaphyses, followed by cupping, fraying, and eventually irregular mineralization with a jagged and thickened metaphyseal line. Genu valgum deformity occurs secondary to involvement of the proximal tibial metaphysis. Changes in the axial skeleton consist of loss of height in the thoracic and lumbar vertebrae.[27,28]

DIPHOSPHONATES

Sodium etidronate, which is used in the treatment of Paget disease, may result in development of osteomalacia. Radiolucency may develop in the bones affected by Paget disease. Pathologic fractures at these sites may occur as a result.[29] Effects of sodium etidronate have also been described in children with myositis ossificans progressiva, whereby it may cause widening/irregularity of the physis, generalized demineralization, and irregular sclerosis.[30] There have also been reports of the development of pseudogout in patients treated with cyclical etidronate for osteoporosis.[31]

IFOSFAMIDE

As a derivative of cyclophosphamide, ifosfamide is used in oncologic therapy, specifically in the treatment of Ewing sarcoma. There are several associated side effects, of which the most relevant to this discussion is the tox-icity to the renal glomeruli and tubules.[32] As a result of the nephrotoxicity, excess phosphate excretion may occur that leads to the development of hypophosphatemic rickets. The abnormalities reverse after cessation of therapy with ifosfamide and supplementation with oral phosphate.[33]

OTHER DRUGS ASSOCIATED WITH RICKETS AND OSTEOMALACIA

Isolated accounts of osteomalacia have been reported in relation to administration of rifampicin in the treatment of tuberculosis[34] and of cholestyramine in the treatment of hypercholesterolemia,[35] laxative abuse,[36] excessive magnesium and aluminum intake,[37] glutethimide therapy,[38] furosemide therapy,[39] and intravenous hyperalimentation in premature neonates. A child born to a mother taking long-term intravenous magnesium for tocolysis exhibited clinical and radiographic findings of osteomalacia.[40]

VITAMIN A

Chronic toxicity from excessive intake of vitamin A usually occurs in the pediatric population as a result of overzealous vitamin supplementation by the parents.[41] Signs and symptoms of vitamin A intoxication include anorexia, itching, low-grade fevers, and irritability. The hallmark of bony change is cortical hyperostosis in the long bones, particularly the ulna and the metatarsal bones, producing a wavy diaphyseal contour (Fig. 87-12). Clinically this may manifest as painful bony swelling over the site of

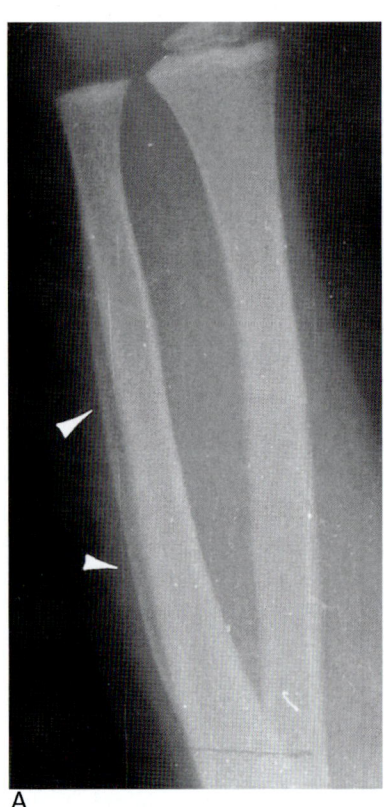
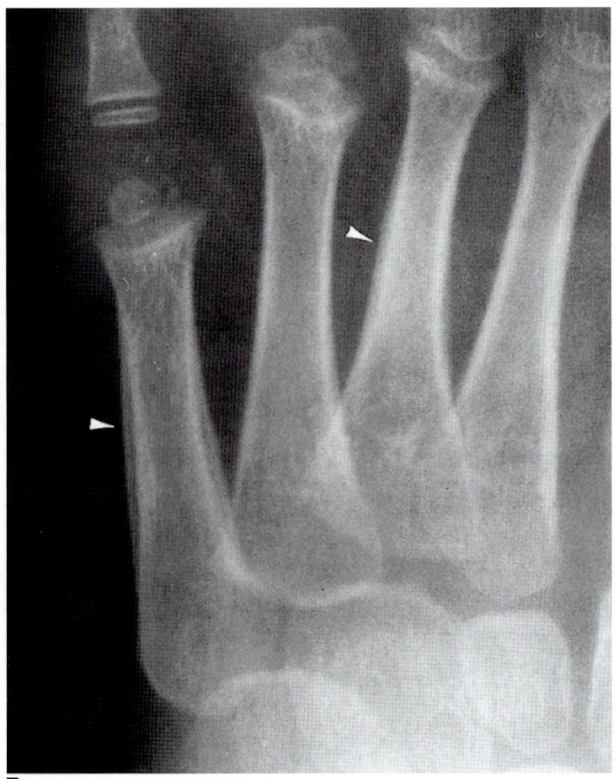

■ **FIGURE 87-12 Hypervitaminosis A: periostitis and cortical hyperostosis. A,** Note periosteal bone formation in the diaphysis of the ulna (*arrowheads*). **B,** In a different child, periosteal proliferation is evident in the diaphyses of multiple metatarsals (*arrowheads*). (*A courtesy of F. Silverman, MD, Stanford, CA. A and B from Resnick D [ed]: Diagnosis of Bone and Joint Disorders, 4th ed. Philadelphia, WB Saunders, 2002.*)

A

B

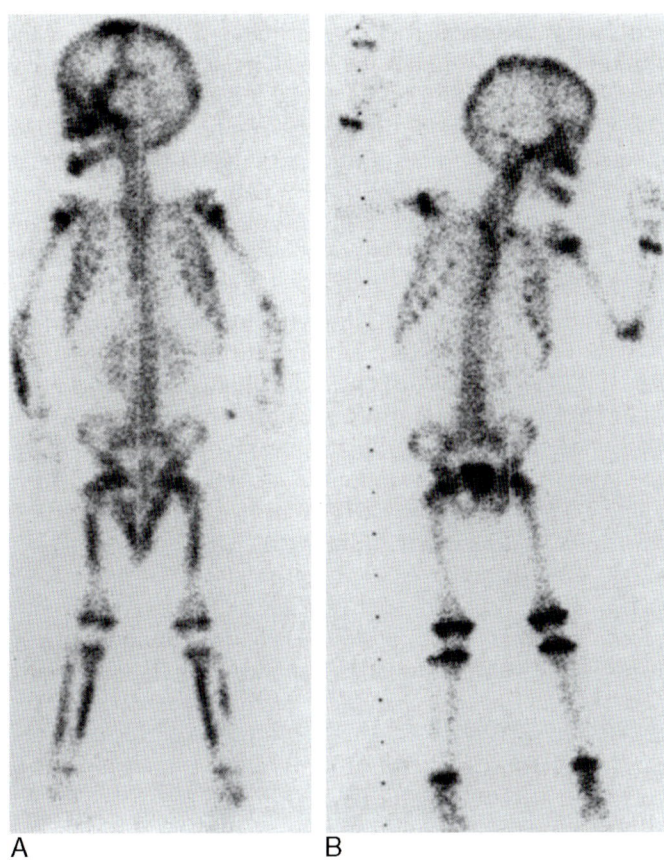

A   B

■ **FIGURE 87-13** **Hypervitaminosis A: scintigraphic abnormalities.** A 3-year-old boy, who had been eating a high-protein, low-carbohydrate diet supplemented with vitamins A, D, E, and K, developed discomfort on standing, muscle spasm, and abdominal pain. Physical examination documented desquamation of the skin and loss of hair. Radiographs (not shown) revealed diastasis of the cranial sutures without evidence of periostitis in the tubular bones. There was evidence of marked elevation of serum vitamin A levels. **A,** An initial bone scan, using ^{99m}Tc-methylene diphosphonate, shows an abnormally increased accumulation of the radionuclide in the diaphyseal regions of the ulnae, femora, tibiae, and fibulae and along the sutures of the calvaria. The megavitamin therapy was discontinued. Five weeks later periostitis became visible in the shafts of the tibiae and fibulae. **B,** A repeat bone scan using the same radiopharmaceutical agent obtained 4 months after **A** is normal. *(From Miller JH, Hayon II: Bone scintigraphy in hypervitaminosis A. AJR Am J Roentgenol 1985; 144:767. © 1985, American Roentgen Ray Society. Reprinted with permission from the American Journal of Roentgenology.)*

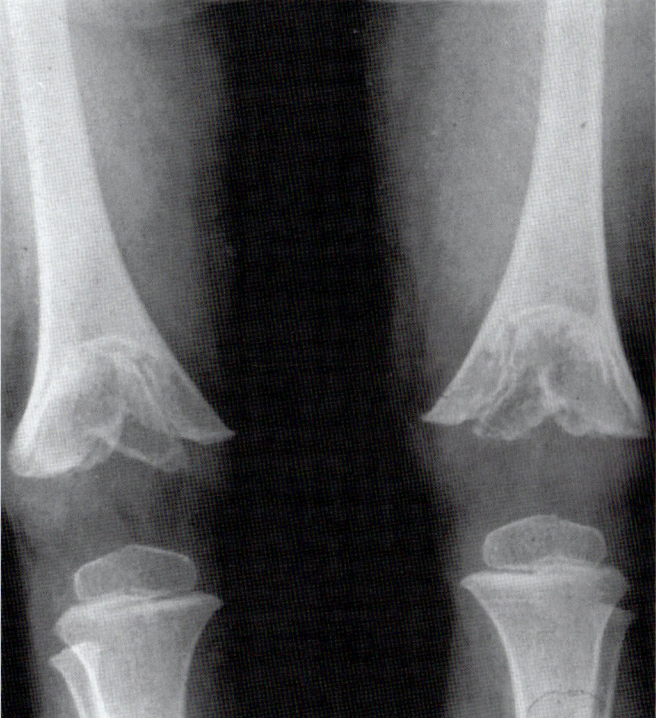

■ **FIGURE 87-14** **Hypervitaminosis A: metaphyseal and epiphyseal changes.** Observe the striking splaying and cupping of the distal femoral metaphyses, with narrowing of the cartilaginous growth plates and hypertrophy and invagination of the epiphyses. *(From Resnick D [ed]: Diagnosis of Bone and Joint Disorders, 4th ed. Philadelphia, WB Saunders, 2002.)*

the hyperostosis and appearance of hard, tender soft tissue nodules.[42] Another characteristic finding often seen with vitamin A toxicity is thickening of the shafts of the affected bones due to subperiosteal new bone formation. In addition to the ulna and metatarsal distribution of findings, the clavicles, tibiae, and fibulae are often affected, whereas the femoral bones, humeri, metacarpals, and ribs are less commonly involved. Nuclear medicine bone scintigraphy can be used to demonstrate the characteristic distribution of abnormalities[43] (Fig. 87-13). Late sequelae of vitamin A toxicity may occur in a subset of patients and include enlargement of the epiphysis with splaying and cupping of the metaphysis in the affected long bones, as well as shortening of the affected long bones secondary to premature fusion of the physes (Fig. 87-14). The cartilaginous growth plates may appear irregular and

narrowed, and there may be hypertrophy and premature fusion of the epiphyseal ossification centers that may lead to crippling deformities.[44] Unlike the cortical hyperostosis, the damage to the epiphyseal cartilage may be irreversible if the exposure to vitamin A has been prolonged. Although it is rare to see these just-described osseous changes in an adult, proliferative enthesopathies involving the long bones and flaval ligaments of the spine have been described in adults with vitamin A toxicity. After discontinuation of vitamin A intake the signs and symptoms clinically subside, whereas radiographic findings regress more gradually over a course of weeks to months in both the adult and pediatric populations.

RETINOIDS

Retinoids are synthetic derivates of vitamin A that are currently being used in standard medical practice to treat a number of dermatologic conditions such as acne and psoriasis. In addition, retinoids are sometimes used in the prevention of certain skin, bladder, and cervical cancers.[25] Bony changes associated with long-term retinoid administration occur in a spectrum of findings that appear to be irreversible.[45-47] Retinoids, like vitamin A, appear to accelerate the process of bone maturation, and manifestations include increased endochondral bone formation, rapid remodeling, premature fusion of the physes, as well as subperiosteal appositional growth of the cortex (Figs. 87-15 and 87-16). In adults, again similar to manifestation of vitamin A toxicity,

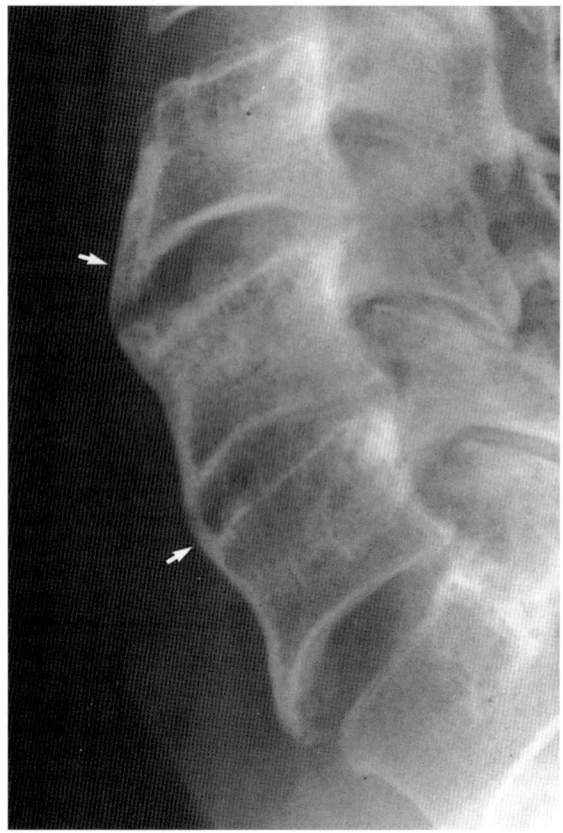

A

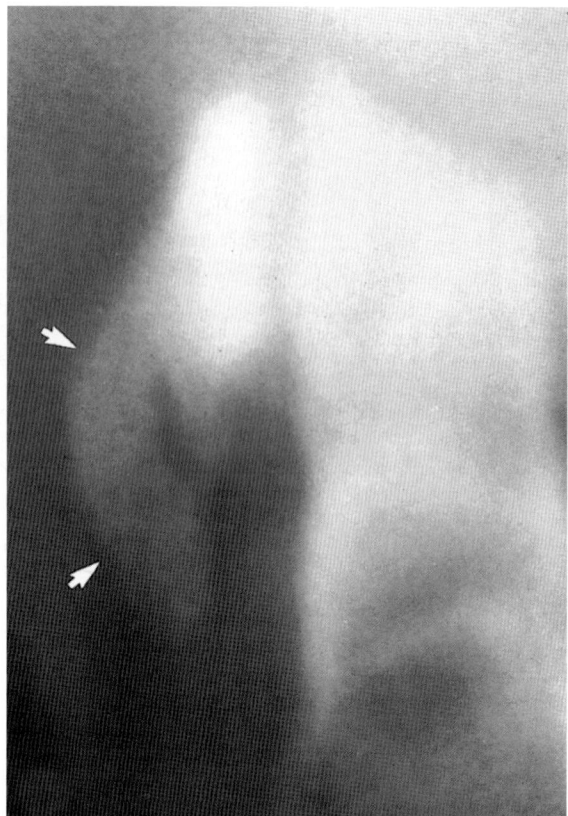

B

■ **FIGURE 87-15**   **Isotretinoin hyperostosis.** In three different patients, prominent ligamentous ossification is apparent (*arrows*) in the midcervical spine (**A**) and about the anterior arch of the atlas (**B** and **C**). *(A courtesy of J. Mink, MD, Los Angeles, CA; **B** courtesy of J. Lawson, MD, New Haven, CT; **A** and **B** from Resnick D [ed]: Diagnosis of Bone and Joint Disorders, 4th ed. Philadelphia, WB Saunders, 2002.)*

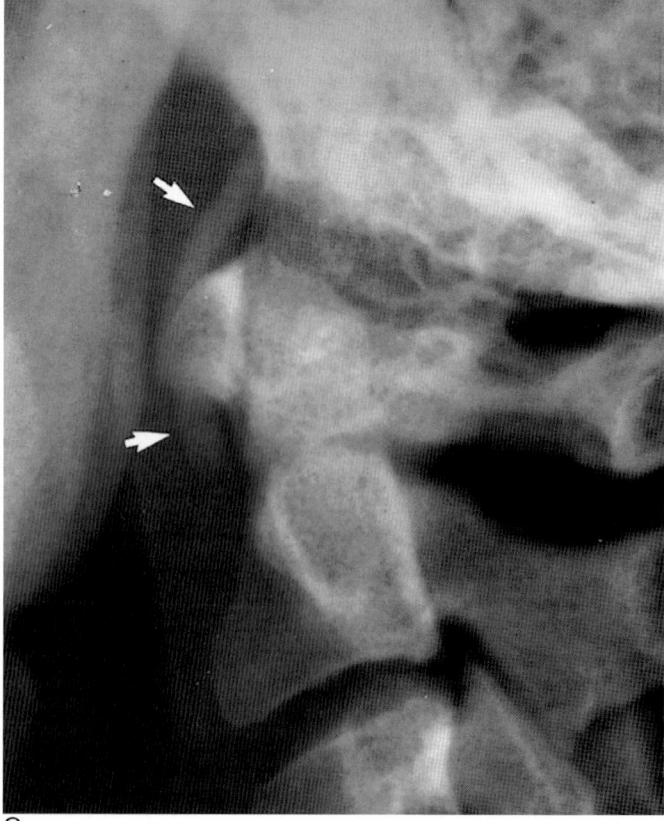

C

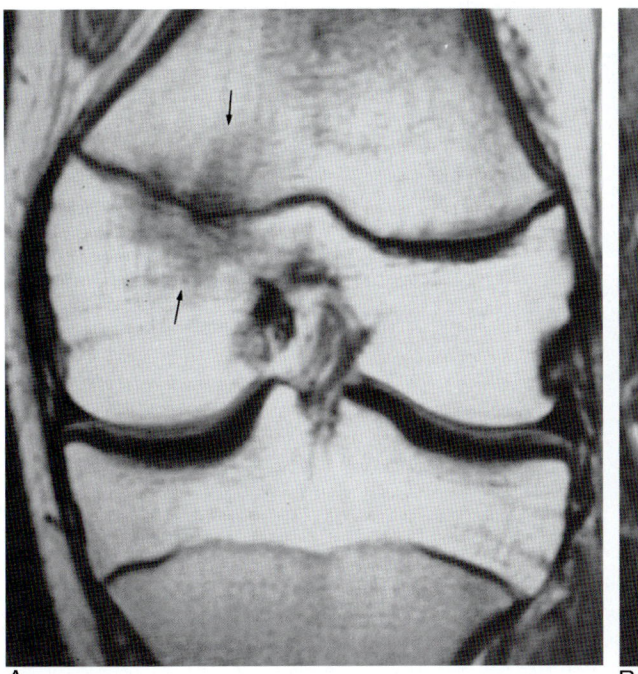
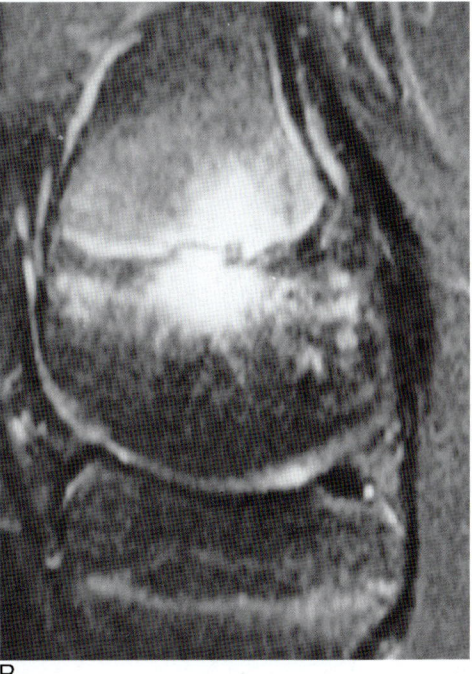

A   B

■ **FIGURE 87-16**   **Premature physeal fusion related to isotretinoin.** This 16-year-old patient had received isotretinoin therapy for acne. Subsequently, he developed knee pain unrelated to physical activity. **A,** Coronal T1-weighted (TR/TE, 722/20) spin-echo MR image shows fusion of a portion of the growth plate in the distal aspect of the femur with surrounding edema (*arrows*). **B,** The edema is more apparent in a sagittal STIR (TR/TE, 5300/30; inversion time, 150 ms) MR image. *(From Resnick D [ed]: Diagnosis of Bone and Joint Disorders, 4th ed. Philadelphia, WB Saunders, 2002.)*

proliferative enthesopathies are often observed. Long-term use of retinoids may produce findings that bear radiographic resemblance to diffuse idiopathic skeletal hyperostosis (see Fig. 87-15). Additional findings described in the axial skeleton include ossification of the atlantoaxial ligament and premature calcification of the atlanto-occipital and stylohyoid ligaments. Findings in the appendicular skeleton may consist of calcification or ossification in the tendons and ligaments around the pelvis, hips, knees, ankles, as well as in the coracoclavicular ligament. Of particular note is a case report describing development of a parosteal osteosarcoma in a patient after long-term etretinate therapy.[48] There are no other reports of an association between any malignancy and long-term retinoid use.

VITAMIN D

Initial reports of vitamin D toxicity were described in patients taking excessive amounts of vitamin D for treatment of rickets and later Paget disease or rheumatoid arthritis.[49,50] Clinical signs and symptoms of vitamin D intoxication include nausea, anorexia, dehydration, thirst, and urinary frequency. Vomiting, diarrhea, and abdominal pain often manifest in later stages. Patients with preexisting renal or gastrointestinal conditions may be especially susceptible to high amounts of vitamin D.[51] In adults, musculoskeletal manifestations of excess vitamin D intake include focal or diffuse osteoporosis and soft tissue calcification with smooth, lobulated deposition of calcium in synovial bursae and periarticular soft tissues[51,52] (Fig. 87-17). In the pediatric population the hallmarks of vitamin D toxicity are heavy calcifications of the proliferating cartilaginous matrix, man-

ifested on radiographs as increased density bands in the metaphyseal regions.[53] Cortical thickening may be seen at some sites, whereas cortical thinning with osteoporosis can be seen at others. Calcification of periarticular structures, laryngeal and tracheal cartilage, and muscles has also been described.[54]

FLUOROSIS

Chronic fluorine intoxication arises in patients drinking water with high fluorine concentrations, in persons with industrial or laboratory exposure to fluorine over a period of years, as well as in individuals who drink large quantities of fluorine-containing wine. Fluorosis has also been described in patients receiving a prolonged treatment of niflumic acid, a nonsteroidal anti-inflammatory drug that contains fluorine.[55] Skeletal changes seen in fluorine intoxication are characteristic and consist of osteosclerosis, increased thickness of bony trabeculae, vertebral osteophyte formation, and ligamentous calcification.[56-58] These changes are usually most pronounced in the spine, pelvis, and ribs, with relative sparing of the skull and appendicular skeleton (Figs. 87-18 and 87-19). When present in the appendicular skeleton, there may be calcification or ossification at the site of ligamentous or tendinous insertions, as well as osteophyte formation around the joints that may result in pain in limited range of motion. Osteophyte formation in the spine can at times be large enough to compromise the spinal canal and neural foramina. Calcification may also occur in the paraspinal ligaments. Soft tissue ossification resembling myositis ossificans has likewise been described.[59]

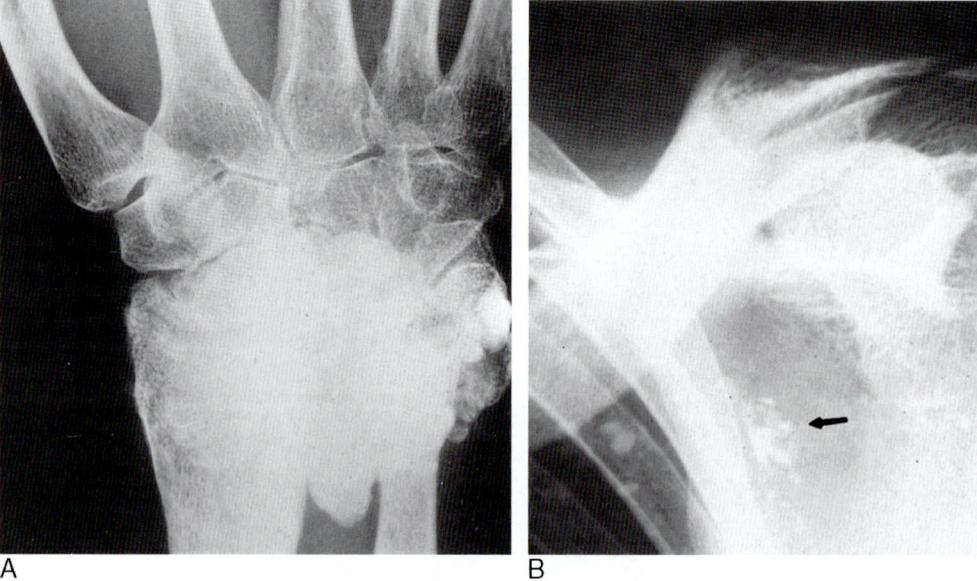

■ FIGURE 87-17
Hypervitaminosis D: soft tissue abnormalities. A, In a patient with rheumatoid arthritis who was treated with vitamin D, note massive soft tissue calcification about the wrist. **B,** In a different patient without articular disease, small calcific deposits in the soft tissue are evident (*arrow*). (*From Resnick D [ed]: Diagnosis of Bone and Joint Disorders, 4th ed. Philadelphia, WB Saunders, 2002.*)

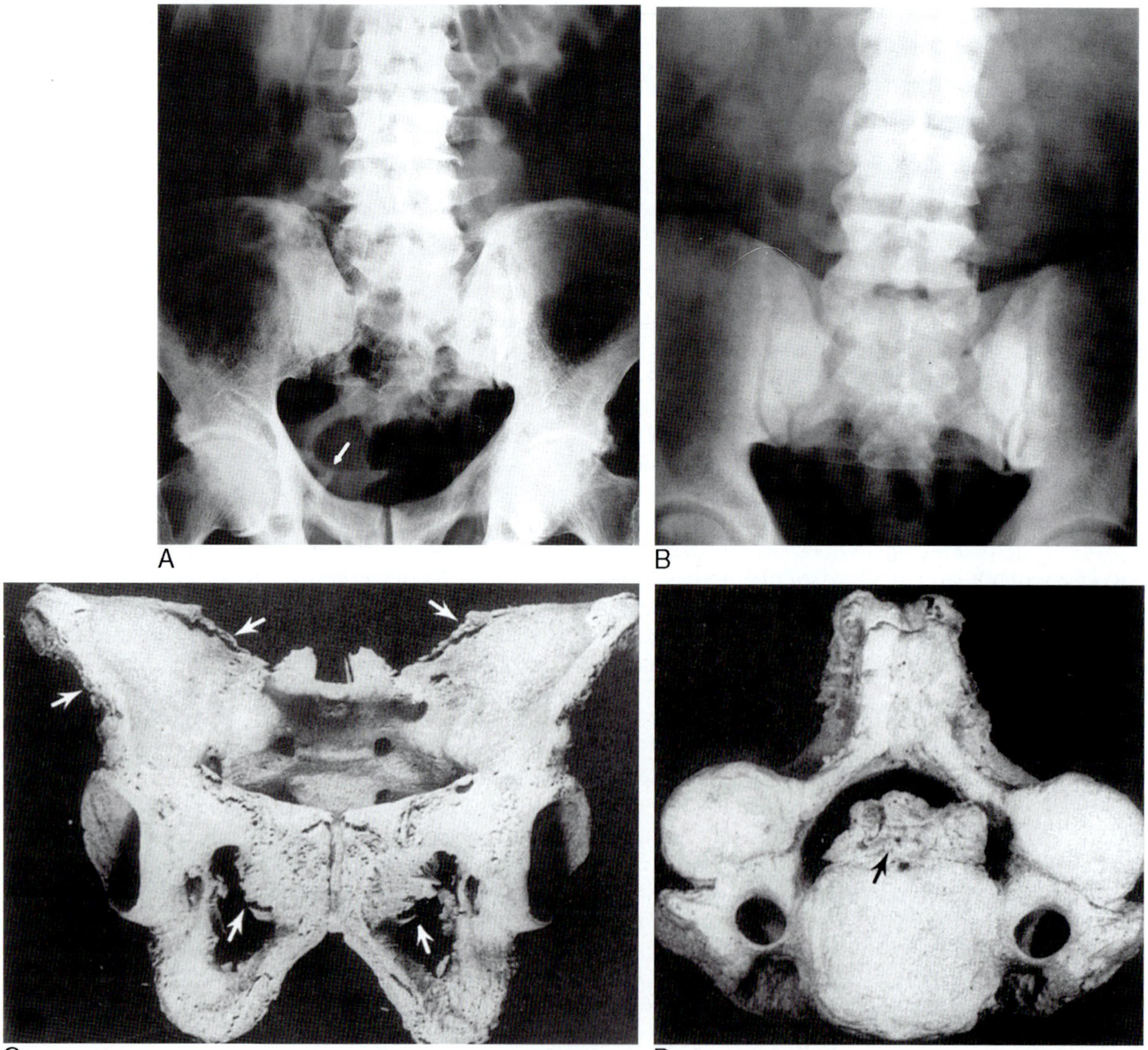

■ **FIGURE 87-18   Fluorosis: axial skeletal abnormalities. A,** Osteosclerosis with a coarsened trabecular pattern, vertebral osteophytosis, and sacrotuberous ligament ossification (*arrow*) are the observed radiographic changes. **B,** Osteosclerosis and vertebral osteophytosis are evident in a different patient with fluorosis. Note the bony eburnation about the sacroiliac joints. **C,** A macerated pelvis of a 45-year-old farmer from India with fluorosis reveals proliferation at ligamentous attachments, especially about the iliac crests and the ischial and pubic rami (*arrows*). **D,** In the same patient as in **C,** a photograph of the inferior surface of the third cervical vertebra reveals calcification and ossification of the posterior longitudinal ligament (*arrow*) and osseous overgrowth about the spinous processes and articular pillars. (*A and B from Resnick D [ed]: Diagnosis of Bone and Joint Disorders, 4th ed. Philadelphia, WB Saunders, 2002; C and D from Singh A, Dass R, Hayreh SS, Jolly SS. Skeletal changes in endemic fluorosis. J Bone Joint Surg Br 1962; 44:806. Copyright © of the British Editorial Society of Bone and Joint Surgery.*)

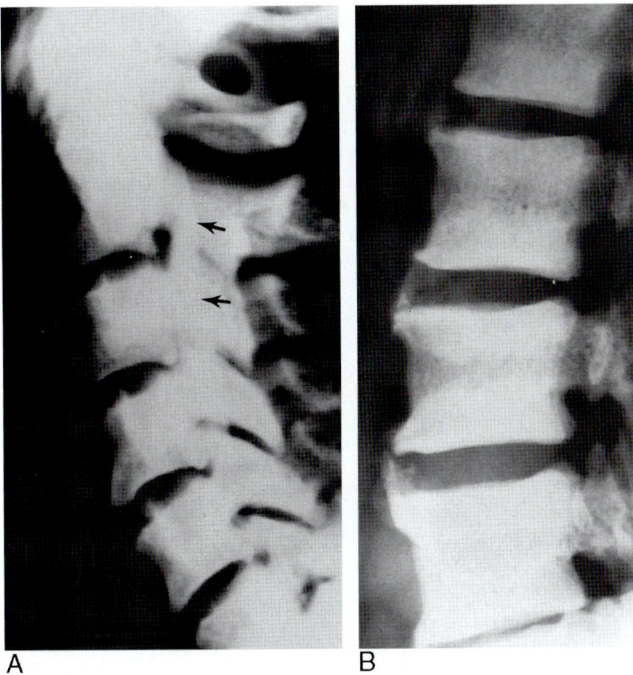

■ FIGURE 87-19   Fluorosis: axial skeletal abnormalities. In this 47-year-old woman, an extreme increase in radiodensity of the cervical and lumbar spine is observed. Note spinal osteophytes and ossification of the posterior longitudinal ligament (*arrows*). *(Courtesy of G. Beauregard, MD, Montreal, Quebec, Canada; from Resnick D [ed]: Diagnosis of Bone and Joint Disorders, 4th ed. Philadelphia, WB Saunders, 2002.)*

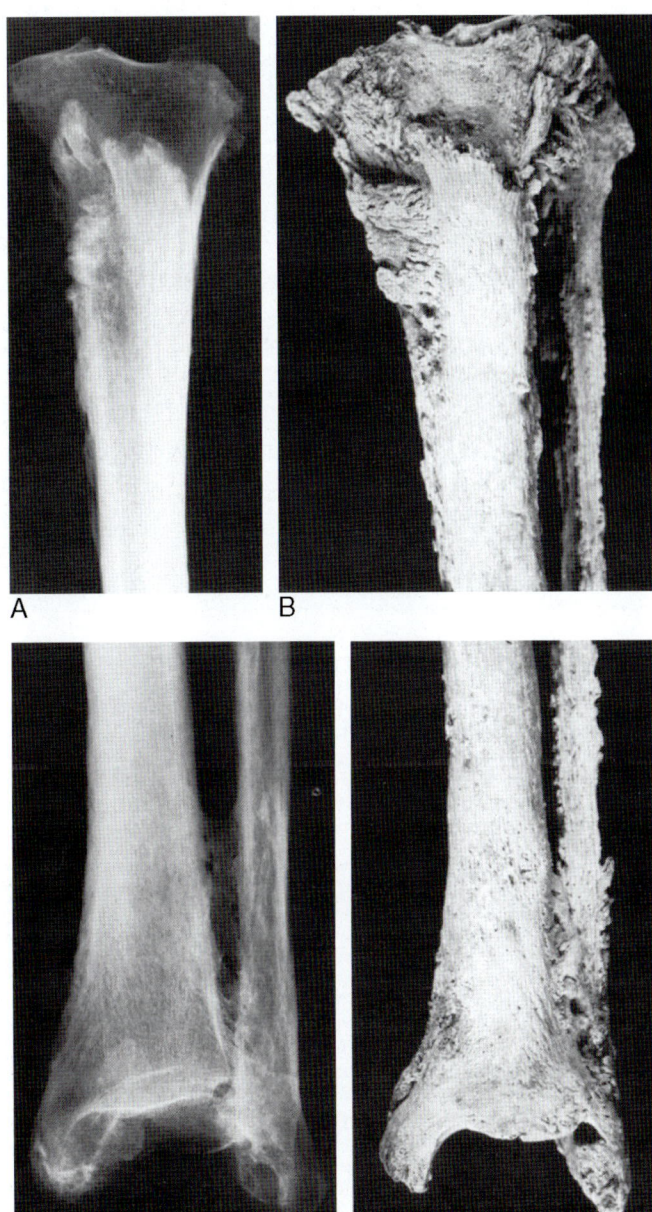

■ FIGURE 87-20   Fluorosis: appendicular skeletal abnormalities. A and B, Changes in the proximal portions of the tibia and fibula include exuberant periosteal proliferation, especially in the area of the tibial tuberosity. **C and D,** In the same cadaver, similar alterations affect the distal portions of the bones, particularly in the region of the interosseous membrane. *(From Resnick D [ed]: Diagnosis of Bone and Joint Disorders, 4th ed. Philadelphia, WB Saunders, 2002.)*

Periostitis can also occur in fluorosis and in some cases can take a very extreme form termed *periostitis deformans,* in which cloaks of heaving periosteal bone can be seen surrounding the shafts of the involved bones with associated encroachment on the medullary canal and extensive periarticular excrescences that can extend into tendons and muscles, especially around the hip, knee, or elbow[59] (Fig. 87-20).

In advanced stages, fluorosis can lead to crippling deformities, including kyphosis, limitation of movement, and contractures of the hips and knees. Neurologic complications have also been described and consist of paresthesias, muscle weakness, sensory disturbances, and paralysis.[56] Secondary hyperparathyroidism has been described in patients with endemic fluorosis,[60] possibly due to resistance of bone to the circulating parathyroid hormone, decreased availability of calcium in the bones, or a combination of both factors.

PROSTAGLANDIN E

Prostaglandin E is used to maintain a patent ductus arteriosus in patients with congenital heart disease resulting in a right-to-left shunt.[61] In most cases the treatment is short term in those who are awaiting definitive surgical repair. However, in some situations, prolonged prostaglandin E therapy may be needed. Cortical hyperostosis is the primary osseous abnormality that has been observed in patients receiving a protracted course of treatment with prostaglandin E.[62] Findings are typically noted after 30 to 40 days of medication but may occur as early as after 9 days. Characteristically, the periosteal reaction involves the diaphyses of the ribs, clavi-cles, and ulnae, usually in a symmetric fashion. Subsequent to discontinuation of therapy the periosteal reaction undergoes remodeling and consolidates with the bony cortex (Figs. 87-21 and 87-22).

VASOCONSTRICTORS, CALCIUM GLUCONATE, AND MILK-ALKALI SYNDROME

Vasoconstrictive drugs including dopamine (in high doses), ergotamines, vasopressin, and epinephrine are

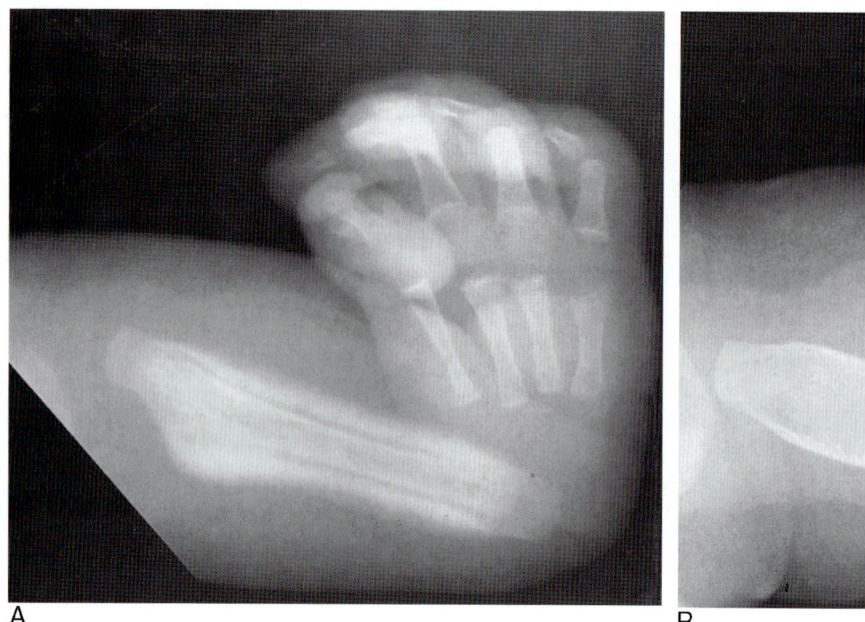
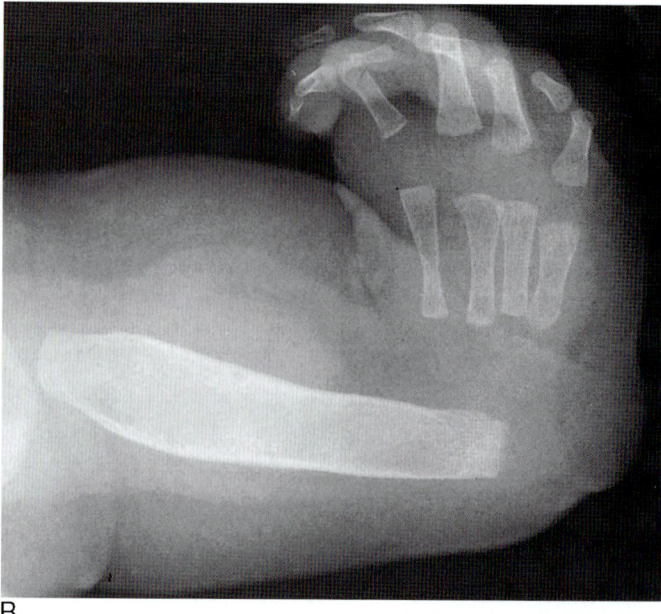

A   B

■ **FIGURE 87-21** **Prostaglandin periostitis.** This male infant was noted to have multiple congenital abnormalities at birth. A cardiac catheterization confirmed the presence of a severe tetralogy of Fallot. An infusion of prostaglandin E was begun when the patient was 3 weeks old and maintained for 7 weeks, after which it was discontinued. Bone changes were observed initially in the ribs and clavicle after 20 days of therapy. **A,** Radiograph of the forearm, obtained when the infant was 43 days old, reveals extensive periosteal elevation in the ulna. Note the absence of the radius, a finding of the VATER syndrome. **B,** At 6 months of age, the periosteal bone has been incorporated into the diaphysis of the ulna. *(From Poznanski AK, Fernbach SK, Berry TE. Bone changes from prostaglandin therapy. Skeletal Radiol 1985; 14:20.)*

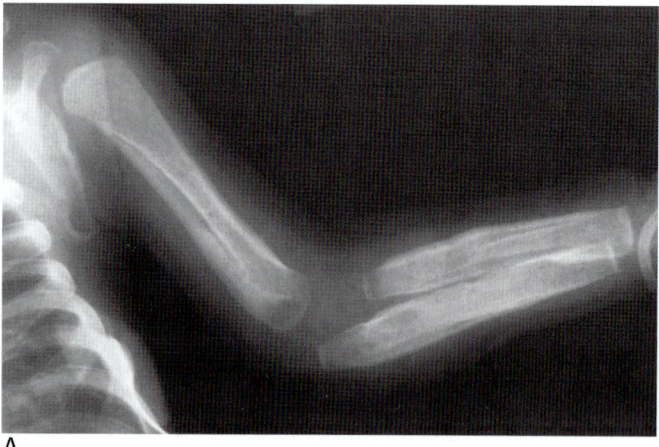

A

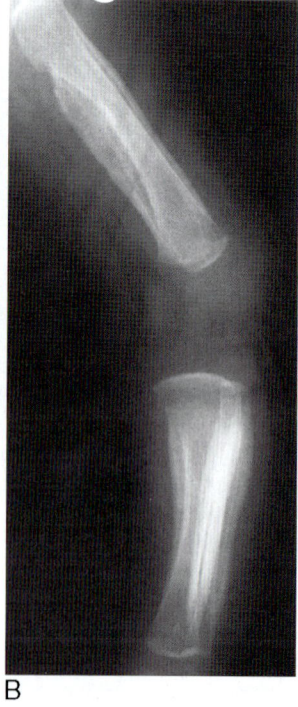

B

■ **FIGURE 87-22** **Prostaglandin periostitis.** In a 3-month-old infant receiving prostaglandin E_1 infusions, exuberant periosteal new bone is observed in the ribs, humerus, radius, ulna, femur, tibia, and fibula. *(Courtesy of T. Broderick, MD, Orange, CA; from Resnick D [ed]: Diagnosis of Bone and Joint Disorders, 4th ed. Philadelphia, WB Saunders, 2002.)*

associated with ischemic tissue necrosis, gangrene, and calcification. Soft tissue calcification related to tissue necrosis is also seen within injection sites after intravenous administration of calcium gluconate (Fig. 87-23). Calcification in these cases is characteristically amorphous and may be localized or distributed along fascial planes.[63]

In the chronic form of milk-alkali syndrome, excessive intake of calcium carbonate by middle-aged men suffering from heartburn is implicated as the cause of metastatic soft tissue calcification.[64] Renal failure with hyperphosphatemia, alkalosis, and hypercalcemia ultimately results in diffuse calcium deposition. Radiologic findings may include widespread calcification in the kidneys, vessels,

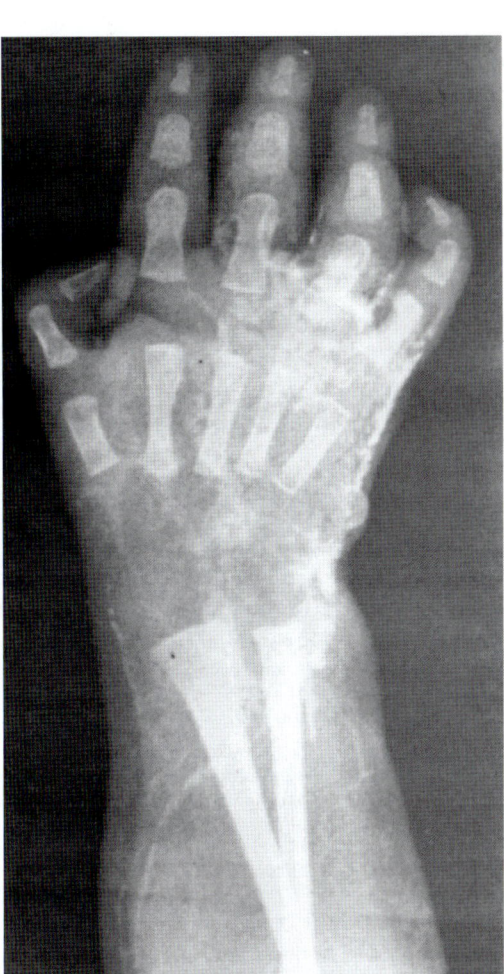

■ **FIGURE 87-23** **Calcium gluconate extravasation.** This 3-lb, 6-oz infant received an infusion of calcium gluconate into a vein in the dorsum of the hand that subsequently infiltrated into the soft tissues. A radiograph taken approximately 1 week later reveals extensive linear and plate-like subcutaneous deposits with vascular calcification. *(From Berger PE, Heidelberger KP, Poznanski AK. Extravasation of calcium gluconate as a cause of soft tissue calcification in infancy. AJR Am J Roentgenol 1974; 121:109. © American Roentgen Ray Society. Reprinted with permission from the American Journal of Roentgenology.)*

and ligaments and amorphous periarticular deposits of varying size (Fig. 87-24).

POLYVINYL CHLORIDE

Exposure to polyvinyl chloride is implicated in the development of acro-osteolysis in certain types of industrial plant workers. As many as 1% to 2% of such workers exhibited these findings in a study published in 1978.[65] The incidence in recent times has dramatically decreased owing to the implementation of preventative measures. Clinical manifestations include fatigue, asthenia, nervousness, and insomnia.[65] Nonspecific systemic symptoms early on are followed by a Raynaud phenomenon—like disorder. Exposure is also linked to the development of liver fibrosis and tumors (most notably angiosarcomas), splenomegaly, portal hypertension, thrombocytopenia, and pulmonary changes.[66]

On radiography, band-like radiolucency is present across the waist of several terminal phalanges of the hand or, less often, the foot. The tufts are resorbed, often resulting in beveling and osseous fragmentation. The findings are identical in appearance to the acro-osteolysis seen in hyperparathyroidism, reaction to abnormal stress, and after exposure to snake or scorpion venom.

BISMUTH POISONING

Children born to mothers who are being treated with bismuth for syphilis have demonstrated a bone disease with radiographic findings similar to those of lead or phosphorus poisoning (Fig. 87-25).[67] As adults, these individuals have also demonstrated radiographic findings comparable to osteonecrosis.[68,69]

METHOTREXATE

Methotrexate is a folic acid antagonist that interferes with DNA synthesis and has thus found use in the treatment of malignant diseases such as acute lymphoblastic leukemia and inflammatory disorders such as psoriasis. After 2 to 24 months of treatment, children may experience bone pain, joint swelling, and fractures favoring the lower extremities. Radiographic findings are most similar to those of scurvy. They include osteoporosis with a band of mineralization in the metaphysis (early) and prominent zone of provisional calcification and ring-like epiphyses (late). Metaphyseal and diaphyseal fractures often in the lower extremities may occur even in the absence of osteoporosis (Fig. 87-26). Healing is impaired, as evidenced by poor callus formation with delayed union or nonunion. Resolution of bony abnormalities can be expected on withdrawal.[70]

TERATOGENS
Vitamin A and Retinoids

Teratogenic effects have been associated with large doses of vitamin A and its synthetic derivatives isotretinoin (Accutane) and etretinate (Tegison). Estimates for the possibility of fetal malformations range in the area of 25%. The main documented abnormalities include hydrocephalus and microcephalus. Other described anomalies include those of the external ear, cardiovascular system, facial dysmorphism, cerebellar malformation, microphthalmia, and abnormalities of the thymus.[71]

Alcohol

Alcohol may cause numerous congenital abnormalities, together comprising what is known as fetal alcohol syndrome. The spectrum of findings is very broad and includes craniofacial anomalies, distorted motor function, cardiac and genitourinary anomalies, and capillary hemangiomas. Musculoskeletal abnormalities have been described in one third of patients with fetal alcohol syndrome. These include congenital hip dislocation, phalangeal abnormalities (clinodactyly and camptodactyly), radioulnar synostosis, scoliosis, vertebral fusion, and general limitation of

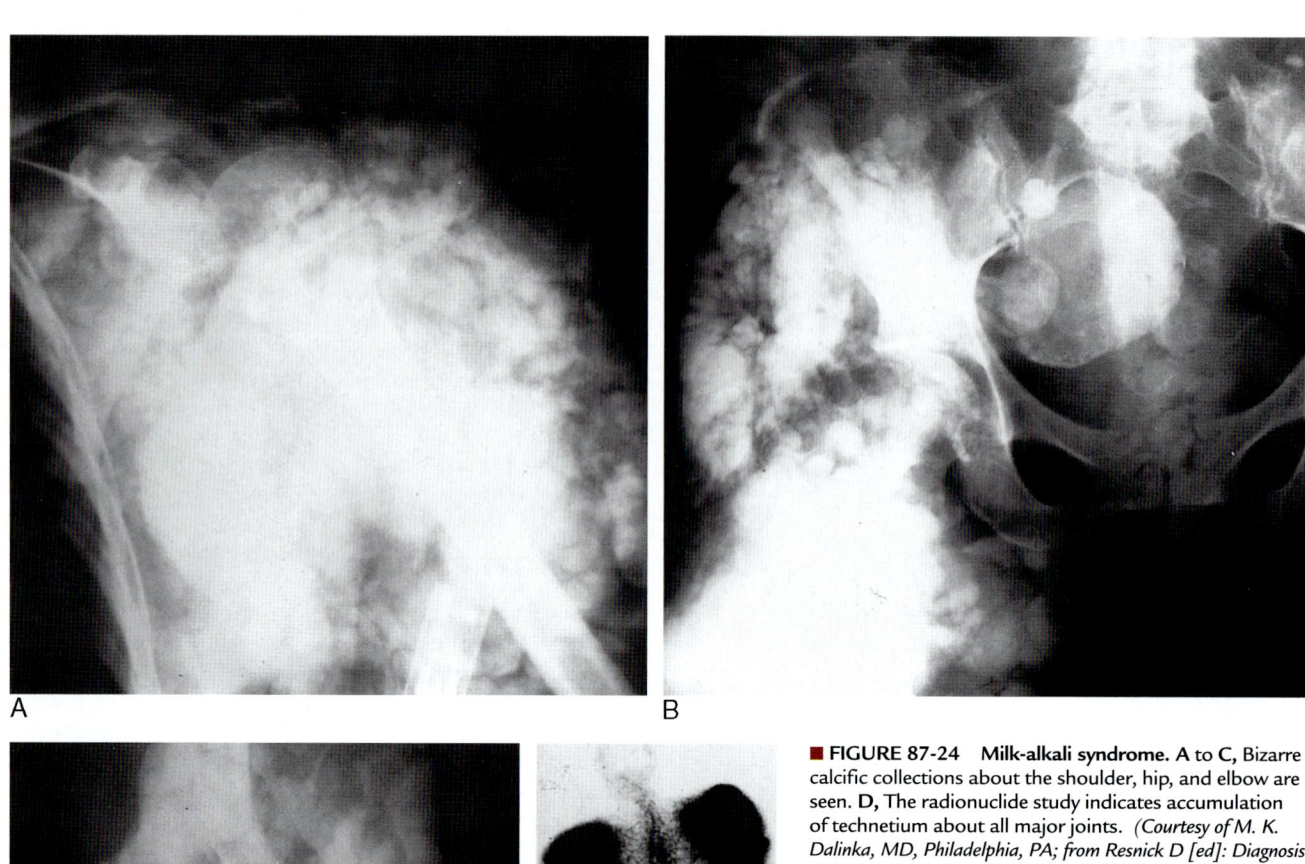

■ **FIGURE 87-24**   **Milk-alkali syndrome. A to C,** Bizarre calcific collections about the shoulder, hip, and elbow are seen. **D,** The radionuclide study indicates accumulation of technetium about all major joints. *(Courtesy of M. K. Dalinka, MD, Philadelphia, PA; from Resnick D [ed]: Diagnosis of Bone and Joint Disorders, 4th ed. Philadelphia, WB Saunders, 2002.)*

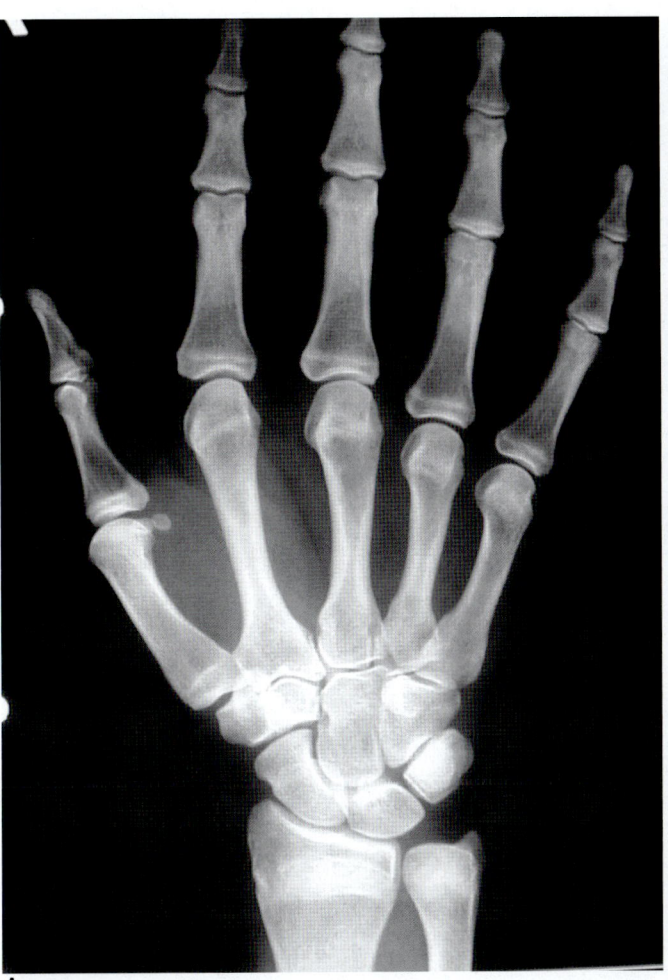

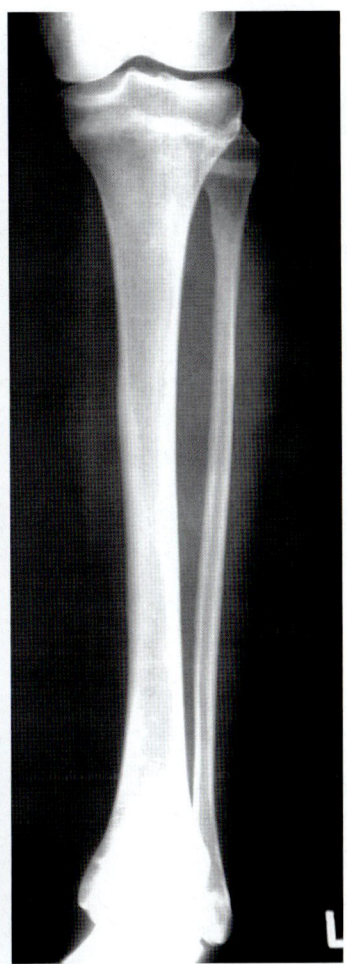

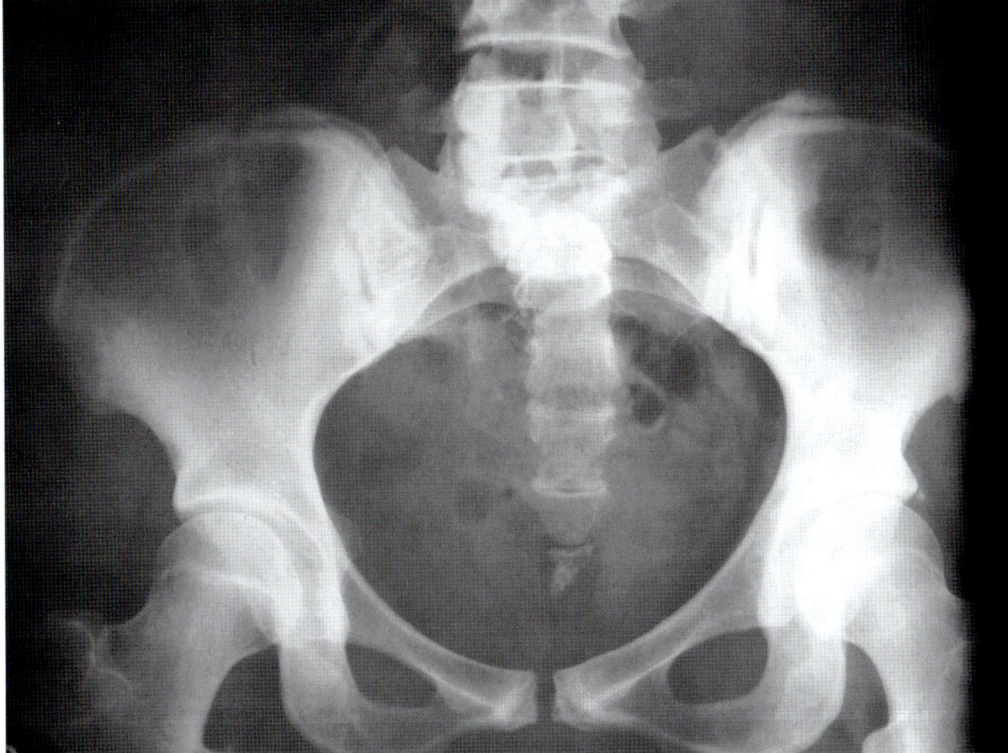

■ **FIGURE 87-25 Phosphorus poisoning.** A to C, Note the metaphyseal bands in the hand, leg, and pelvis of a young girl with phosphorus toxicity. Lead and bismuth poisoning would have a similar appearance. *(Courtesy of Dr. Sajid Butt, RNOH, Radiology Library.)*

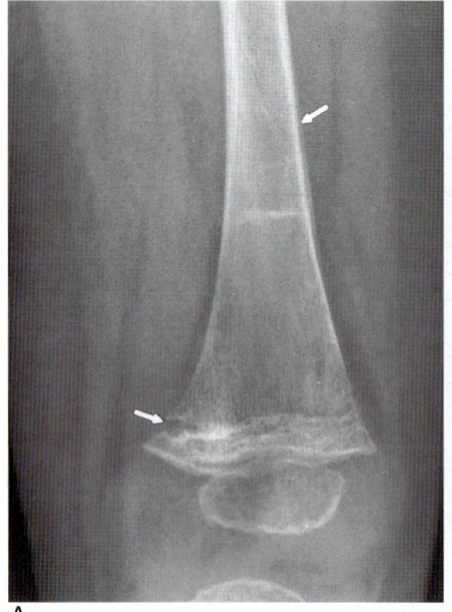

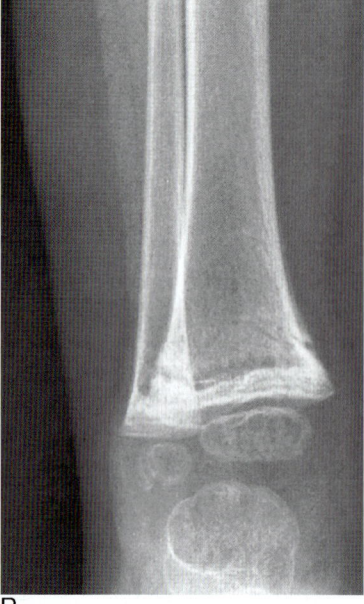

A   B

■ **FIGURE 87-26   Methotrexate osteopathy.** An 18-month-old boy with acute lymphocytic leukemia was treated with a variety of drugs, including methotrexate. Approximately 2 years later, these radiographs were obtained because the patient had pain and weakness in the legs. Findings in **A** include osteopenia, periostitis, and fractures both in the diaphysis and in the metaphysis of the left femur (*arrows*). A growth recovery line is seen. In **B,** note osteopenia, growth recovery lines, and a fracture of the metaphysis of the right tibia. Although these fractures healed well, additional ones occurred subsequently. (*From Schwartz AM, Leonidas JC: Methotrexate osteopathy. Skeletal Radiol 1984; 11:13.*)

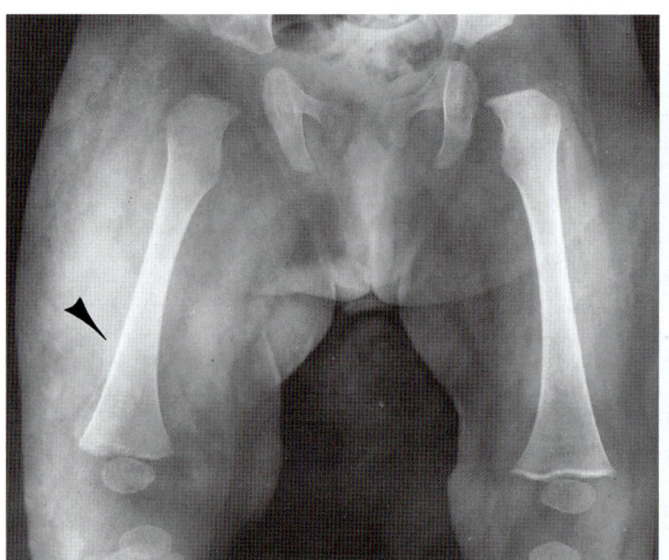

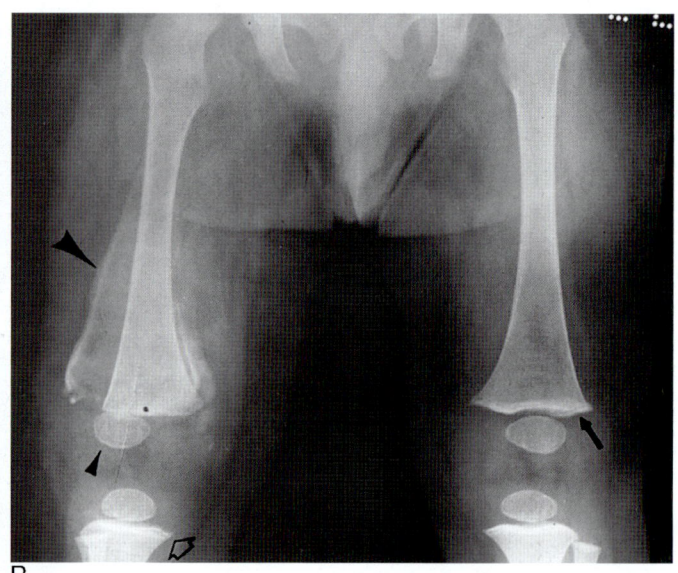

A   B

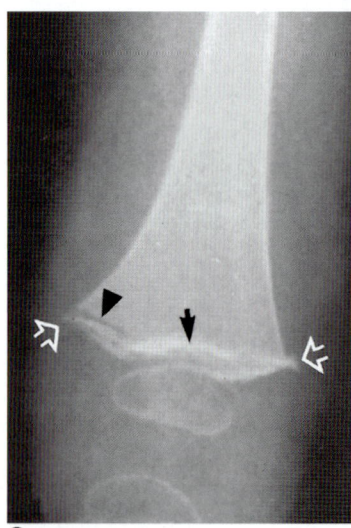

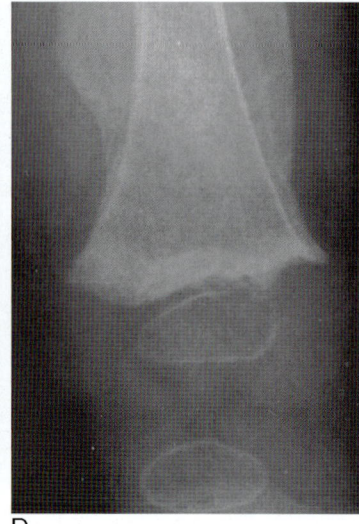

C   D

■ **FIGURE 87-27   Hypovitaminosis C: radiographic abnormalities. A** and **B,** At the ends of tubular bones, osteoporosis, a thick sclerotic metaphyseal line beneath which is a radiolucent line ("scurvy line") (*solid arrow*), small beak-like excrescences (*open arrow*), epiphyseal displacement (*small arrowhead*), and subperiosteal hemorrhage with periostitis (*large arrowheads*) can be noted. **C** and **D,** Radiographs obtained 1 month apart show initially a sclerotic metaphyseal line (**C,** *arrow*), beak-like excrescences (**C,** *open arrows*), and a metaphyseal radiolucent line (**C,** *arrowhead*). Subsequently (**D**), a thicker band of metaphyseal sclerosis and periostitis is seen. A sclerotic line about the epiphysis is also seen both in **C** and **D.** (*A and B courtesy of F. Silverman, MD, Stanford, CA; A to D from Resnick D [ed]: Diagnosis of Bone and Joint Disorders, 4th ed. Philadelphia, WB Saunders, 2002.*)

joint movement.[72] One report cited seven cases of chondrodysplasia punctata in infants of alcoholic mothers: the lower extremities, the sacrum, and the dorsal spine were affected, whereas the upper extremities were spared in all seven cases.[73]

Thalidomide

Teratogenic effects attributable to thalidomide mainly involve two organ systems: the skeletal system and skin. The most severe cases described included amelia and phocomelia with the absence or shortening/underdevelopment of the extremity, respectively. The mechanism responsible for the anomalies is thought today to be secondary to injury to the embryo's developing nervous system or neural crest. As a consequence, an embryonic neuropathy develops that results in failure of formation of tissue, not unlike sensory neuropathy in adults results in destruction of formed tissues.[25]

Cocaine

Evidence of teratogenic effects of cocaine is limited, and the topic remains somewhat controversial. So-called limb-body wall complex (a fetal malformation in which limb anomalies occur with disruption of the body wall) has been detected by ultrasound and described in two cases in which the mothers smoked a large amount of cocaine during the first trimester of pregnancy.[74] Disruption of uteroplacental blood supply to the fetus has been suggested as the mechanism responsible for the teratogenic effects of cocaine. Teratogenicity due to maternal cocaine intake should be considered in the differential diagnosis of congenital limb defects and/or amputations.

Warfarin

Stippling of ossification centers in bones and nasal hypoplasia is characteristic of fetal exposure to warfarin therapy in the mother during the first trimester of pregnancy. The involved bones primarily include, but are not limited to, the spine, femora, tarsal, and carpal bones. Past the age of 1 year the stippling may no longer be identifiable on radiographs.[75] Variable degree of hypoplasia of the extremities with normal growth and development may occur.[25]

DISORDERS ASSOCIATED WITH NUTRITIONAL DEFICIENCIES

Hypovitaminosis C (Scurvy)

Long-term deficiency of vitamin C has different manifestations in the pediatric and adult populations. Subsequently, this discussion will be divided into infantile and adult types of scurvy.

Infantile Scurvy

Because the process of heating milk leads to disruption of vitamin C, the pediatric form of this disorder usually occurs in infants who are fed pasteurized or boiled milk. The disease becomes clinically apparent after the deficiency of vitamin C has existed for 4 to 10 months. Clinical hallmarks of infantile scurvy are the hemorrhagic manifestations of the deficiency: petechial hemorrhages, swelling and ulceration of gums, hematuria, hematemesis, melena, and secondary infections.

Radiographically, this pediatric disorder includes changes in the metaphyses, epiphyses, and diaphyses of bony structures, resulting from decrease in normal cellular activity.[76] Depressed osteoblast activity leads to decreased formation of bony matrix, which is most pronounced in areas of active endochondral bone growth. There is likewise a reduction in the number of proliferating cartilage cells at the cartilaginous growth plate. Overall, the pathologic abnormalities in the ends of long bones have a characteristic radiologic appearance (Fig. 87-27). A sclerotic radiodense line is seen at the border of the physis, representing a prominent provisional zone of calcification. On the side of the metaphysis a transverse radiolucent band (scurvy line) is observed, which is so often described in cases of infantile scurvy. Metaphyseal beak-like excrescences may also occur, representing lateral extension of the heavy provisional zone calcification.[77] Other distinctive features of infantile scurvy include (1) subepiphyseal infarctions, known as the "corner sign" or "angle sign," (2) periosteal elevation secondary to periosteal hemorrhage, and (3) a radiodense shell around the ossification center at the epiphysis with central lucency.

Despite the severity of epiphyseal separation, long-term disturbances in bone growth after infantile scurvy are not common. Apparent early fusion of the physes may occur as a result of epiphyseal intrusion into the exaggerated metaphyseal concavity ("metaphyseal cupping").[77] However, the degree of limb shortening, when it occurs, is usually minimal.

Patients being treated for infantile vitamin C deficiency may exhibit characteristic radiographic signs. These include thickening of the cortex and increased density of the radiolucent zone of the metaphysis. Burying of the thickened provisional zone in the shaft of the long bone may appear as transverse densities within the shaft during treatment. Other signs that may appear during treatment are extensive subperiosteal bone formation and increased epiphyseal density.[76]

Adult Scurvy

Hemarthrosis, bleeding at the synchondroses, and osteoporosis are the main features of adult vitamin C deficiency.[78] Associated findings can include collapse of the subchondral bone in a joint with hemarthrosis, most commonly the femoral head. The possible etiology of the collapse may be ischemic necrosis secondary to the vascular compromise produced by the hemarthrosis. Osteoporosis in scurvy is most prominent in the axial skeleton and in the tubular bones and is essentially indistinguishable from osteoporosis from other causes.[77] Because clinical manifestations of scurvy require a long-standing deficiency of vitamin C, adult scurvy is a very rare diagnosis.

Deficiencies of Zinc and Other Elements

Deficiencies of zinc and trace elements such as magnesium, cobalt, molybdenum, chromium, and manganese are difficult to analyze precisely because they usually occur concurrently with other nutritional deficiencies.

Zinc, as a heavy metal, is in some form responsible for normal bone metabolism, and it is reasonable to suppose that its deficiency could lead to osteopenia and growth disturbances.[79] Deficiency in magnesium is associated with abnormal bone mineral formation.[80]

SUGGESTED READINGS

Lawson J. Drug induced metabolic bone disorders. Semin Musculoskel Radiol 2002; 4:285–297.

Resnick D. Disorders due to medications and other chemical agents. In Resnick D (ed). Diagnosis of Bone and Joint Disorders, 4th ed. Philadelphia, WB Saunders, 2002.

Resnick D. Heavy metal poisoning and deficiency. In Resnick D (ed). Diagnosis of Bone and Joint Disorders, 4th ed. Philadelphia, WB Saunders, 2002.

Resnick D. Hypervitaminosis and hypovitaminosis. In Resnick D (ed). Diagnosis of Bone and Joint Disorders, 4th ed. Philadelphia, WB Saunders, 2002.

REFERENCES

1. Gluck OS, Murphy WA, Hahn TJ, Hahn B. Bone loss in adults receiving alternate day glucocorticoid therapy: a comparison with daily therapy. Arthritis Rheum 1981; 24:892–898.
2. Hahn TJ, Halstead LR, Teitelbaum SL, Hahn BH. Altered mineral metabolism in glucocorticoid-induced osteopenia: effect of 25-hydroxyvitamin D administration. J Clin Invest 1979; 64:655–665.
3. Hahn TJ. Drug-induced disorders of vitamin D and mineral metabolism. Clin Endocrinol Metab 1980; 9:107–127.
4. Riggs BL, Jowsey J, Kelly PJ. Quantitative microradiographic study of bone remodeling in Cushing's syndrome. Metabolism 1966; 15:773–780.
5. Litvin Y, Hage S, Catane R, Horne T. Reversibility of glucocorticoid-induced osteopenia: a case report. Clin Nucl Med 1982; 7:269–271.
6. Frost HM. The etiodynamics of aseptic necrosis of the femoral head. In Proceedings of the Conference on Aseptic Necrosis of the Femoral Head. St. Louis, National Institute of Health, 1964, p 393.
7. Boettcher WG, Bonfiglio M, Hamilton HH, et al. Non-traumatic necrosis of the femoral head: I. Relation of altered hemostasis to etiology. J Bone Joint Surg Am 1970; 52:312–321.
8. Cosgriff SW. Thromboembolic complications associated with ACTH and cortisone therapy. JAMA 1951; 147:924–926.
9. Richards JM, Santiago SM, Klaustermeyer WB. Aseptic necrosis of the femoral head in corticosteroid-treated pulmonary disease. Arch Intern Med 1980; 140:1473–1475.
10. Gibson T, Burry HC, Poswillo D, Glass J. Effect of intra-articular corticosteroid injections on primate cartilage. Ann Rheum Dis 1977; 36:74–79.
11. Mills LC, Boylston BF, Greene JA, Moyer JH. Septic arthritis as a complication of orally given steroid therapy. JAMA 1957; 164:1310–1314.
12. Tondreau RL, Hodes PJ, Schmidt ER Jr. Joint infections following steroid therapy: roentgen manifestations. Am J Roentgenol Radium Ther Nucl Med 1959; 82:258–270.
13. Goldman L. Reactions following intralesional and sublesional injections of corticosteroids. JAMA 1962; 182:613–616.
14. Fisherman EW, Feinberg AR, Feinberg SM. Local subcutaneous atrophy. JAMA 1962; 179:971–972.
15. Schetman D, Hambrick GW Jr, Wilson CE. Cutaneous changes following local injection of triamcinolone. Arch Dermatol 1963; 88:820–828.
16. Rostron PK, Calver RF. Subcutaneous atrophy following methylprednisolone injection in Osgood-Schlatter epiphysitis. J Bone Joint Surg Am 1979; 61:627–628.
17. Koerner HJ, Sun DI. Mediastinal lipomatosis secondary to steroid therapy. Am J Roentgenol Radium Ther Nucl Med 1966; 98:461–464.
18. Price JE Jr, Rigler LG. Widening of the mediastinum resulting from fat accumulation. Radiology 1970; 96:497–500.
19. van de Putte LB, Wagenaar JP, San KH. Paracardiac lipomatosis in exogenous Cushing's syndrome. Thorax 1973; 28:653–656.
20. Streiter ML, Schneider HJ, Proto AV. Steroid-induced thoracic lipomatosis: paraspinal involvement. AJR Am J Roentgenol 1982; 139:679–681.
21. Bein ME, Mancuso AA, Mink JH, Hansen GC. Computed tomography in the evaluation of mediastinal lipomatosis. J Comput Assist Tomogr 1978; 2:379–383.
22. Jaffe MD, Willis PW. Multiple fractures associated with long term sodium heparin therapy. JAMA 1965; 193:152–154.
23. Caspary WF, Hesch RD, Matte R, et al. Intestinal calcium absorption in epileptics under anticonvulsant therapy. In Vitamin D and Problems Related to Uremic Bone Disease. Proceedings of the Second Workshop on Vitamin D. Weisbaden, West Germany, 1974, p 737. New York, Walter de Gruyter, 1975.
24. Kruse R. Osteopathien bei antiepileptisher. Lang-zeittherapie (Borlaufiege Mitteilung). Monatsschr Kinderheilkd 1968; 116:378–381.
25. Lawson J. Drug induced metabolic bone disorders. Semin Musculoskel Radiol 2002; 4:285–297.
26. Andreoli SP, Smith JA, Bergstein JM. Aluminum bone disease in children: radiographic features from diagnosis to resolution. Radiology 1985; 156:663–667.
27. De Virgiliis S, Congria M, Frau F, et al. Deferoxamine-induced growth retardation in patients with thalassemia major. J Pediatr 1988; 113:666–669.
28. Brill PW, Winchester P, Giardina PJ, Cunningham-Rundles S. Deferoxamine-induced bone dysplasia in patients with thalassemia major. AJR Am J Roentgenol 1991; 156:561–565.
29. Stamp TCB. Drug and chemical-induced rickets (and osteomalacia). In Preger L (ed). Induced Disease: Drug, Irradiation, Occupation. New York, Grune & Stratton, 1980, pp 27–43.
30. Wood BJ, Robinson GC. Drug induced changes in myositis ossificans progressiva. Pediatr Radiol 1976; 5:40–43.
31. Gallacher SJ, Boyle IT, Capell HA. Pseudogout associated with the use of cyclical etidronate therapy. Scott Med J 1991; 36:49.
32. Van Dyke JJ, Falkson HC, van der Merve AM, et al. Unexpected toxicity in patients treated with ifosfamide. Cancer Res 1972; 32:921–924.
33. Sweeney LE. Hypophosphatemic rickets after ifosfamide treatment in children. Clin Radiol 1993; 47:345–347.
34. Brodie MJ, Boobis AR, Dollery CT, et al. Rifampicin and vitamin D metabolism. Clin Pharmacol Ther 1980; 27:810–814.
35. Heaton KW, Lever JV, Barnard D. Osteomalacia associated with cholestyramine therapy for postiliectomy diarrhoea. Gastroenterology 1972; 62:642–646.
36. Frame B, Guing HL, Frost HM, Reynolds WA. Osteomalacia induced by laxative (phenolphthalein) ingestion. Arch Intern Med 1971; 128:794–796.
37. Neumann L, Jenson BG. Osteomalacia from aluminium and magnesium antacids: report of a case of bilateral hip fracture. Acta Orthop Scand 1989; 60:361–362.

38. Greenwood RH, Prunty FTG, Silver J. Osteomalacia after prolonged glutethimide administration. BMJ 1973; 1:643–645.
39. Chudney AE, Brown DR, Holzman IR, Sang OK. Nutritional rickets in two very low birth weight infants with chronic lung disease. Arch Dis Child 1980; 55:687–690.
40. Lamm CI, Norton KI, Murphy RJ, et al. Congenital rickets associated with magnesium sulfate administration for tocolysis. J Pediatr 1988; 113:1078–1082.
41. Caffey J. Chronic poisoning due to excess of vitamin A. AJR Am J Roentgenol 1951; 65:12–26.
42. Toomey JA, Morissette RA. Hypervitaminosis A. Am J Dis Child 1947; 73:473.
43. Miller JH, Haon II. Bone scintigraphy in hypervitaminosis A. AJR Am J Roentgenol 1985; 144:767.
44. Pease CN. Focal retardation and arrestment of growth due to vitamin A intoxication. JAMA 1962; 182:980.
45. Pittsley RA, Yoder FW. Retinoid hyperostosis: skeletal toxicity associated with long-term administration of 13-*cis*-retinoic acid for refractory ichthyosis. N Engl J Med 1983; 308:1012–1014.
46. Lawson JP, McGuire J. The spectrum of skeletal changes associated with long-term administration of 13-*cis*-retinoic acid. Skeletal Radiol 1987; 16:91–97.
47. Di Giovanna JJ, Helffgott RK, Gerber LH, Peck GL. Extraspinal tendon and ligament calcification associated with long-term therapy with etretinate. N Engl J Med 1986; 315:1177–1182.
48. Vilon P, Fiche M, Maugars Y, et al. Sarcome parosteal du radius apparu lors d'un traitement par etretinate. Rev Rhum 1991; 58:825–827.
49. Thatcher L. Hypervitaminosis D with report of a fatal case in a child. Edinburgh Med J 1931; 38:457.
50. Danowski TS, Winkler AW, Peters JP. Tissue calcification and renal failure produced by massive dose vitamin D therapy of arthritis. Ann Intern Med 1945; 23:22.
51. Jaffe HL. Metabolic, Degenerative and Inflammatory Diseases of Bones and Joints. Philadelphia, Lea & Febiger, 1972, p 448.
52. Butler WJ, Dieppe PA, Keat ASC. Calcinosis of joints and periarticular tissues associated with vitamin D intoxication. Ann Rheum Dis 1985; 44:494.
53. Ross SG. Vitamin D intoxication in infancy: a report of four cases. J Pediatr 1952; 41:815.
54. Debre R. Toxic effects of overdosage of vitamin D in children. Am J Dis Child 1948; 75:787.
55. Bregeon C, Bernat M, Renier J-C, et al. Osteose fluorée après 11 ans de traitment interuptée par l'acide niflumique. Nouv Presse Med 1980; 9:1446–1447.
56. Singh A, Jolly SS, Bansal BC, Mathur CC. Endemic fluorosis: epidemiological, clinical and biochemical study of chronic fluorine intoxication in Panjab (India). Medicine 1963; 42:229.
57. Singh A, Dass R, Hayreh SS, Jolly SS. Skeletal changes in endemic fluorosis. J Bone Joint Surg Br 1962; 44:806.
58. Stevenson CA, Watson AR: Roentgenologic findings in fluoride osteosclerosis. Arch Indust Health 1960; 21:340.
59. Soriano M, Manchon F. Radiological aspects of a new type of bone fluorosis, periostitis deformans. Radiology 1966; 87:1089.
60. Teotia SP, Teotia M. Secondary hyperparathyroidism in patients with endemic fluorosis. BMJ 1973; 1:637–640.
61. Elliott RB, Starling MB, Neutze JM. Medical manipulation of the ductus arteriosus. Lancet 1975; 1:140–142.
62. Ueda K, Saito A, Nakano H, et al. Cortical hyperostosis following long-term administration of prostaglandin E$_1$ in infants with cyanotic congenital heart disease. J Pediatr 1980; 97:834–836.
63. Resnick D. Disorders due to medications and other chemical agents. In Resnick D (ed). Diagnosis of Bone and Joint Disorders, 4th ed. Philadelphia, WB Saunders, 2002.
64. Orwoll ES. The milk-alkali syndrome: current concepts. Ann Intern Med 1982; 97:242–248.
65. Gama C, Meira JB. Occupational acro-osteolysis. J Bone Joint Surg Am 1978; 60:86–90.
66. Binns CH. Vinyl chloride: a review. J Soc Occup Med 1979; 29:134–141.
67. Russin LA, Stadler HE, Jeans PC: The bismuth lines in the long bones in relation to linear growth. J Pediatr 1942; 21:211.
68. Gaucher A, Netter P, Faure G, et al. Les osteoarthropathies "bismuthiques": Intérêt du dosage du bismuth osseux. Rev Rhum Mal Osteoartic 1980; 47:31.
69. Mabille JP, Gaudet M, Charpin JF. Osteonecrose de la tête humerale au cours de l'encephalopathie bismuthique. Ann Radiol 1980; 23:515.
70. Ragab AH, Frech RS, Vietti TJ. Osteoporotic fractures secondary to methotrexate therapy of acute leukemia in remission. Cancer 1970; 25:580–585.
71. Lammer EJ, Chen DT. Retinoic acid embryopathy. N Engl J Med 1985; 313:837–841.
72. Jones KL, Smith DW, Ulleland CN. Patterns of malformation in offspring of alcoholic mothers. Lancet 1973; 1:1267–1269.
73. Marateaux P, Lavollay B, Bomsell F, et al. Chondrodysplasia punctata and maternal alcohol intoxication. Arch Fr Pediatr 1984; 41:547–550.
74. Viscarello RR, Ferguson DD, Nores J, Hobbins JC. Limb-body wall complex associated with cocaine abuse: further evidence of cocaine's teratogenicity. Obstet Gynecol 1992; 80:523–526.
75. Fourie DT, Hay IT. Warfarin as a possible teratogen. S Afr Med J 1975; 49:2081–2083.
76. Caffey J: Pediatric X-ray Diagnosis, 7th ed. Chicago, Year Book Medical Publishers, 1978, p 1466.
77. Resnick D. Hypervitaminosis and hypovitaminosis. In Resnick D (ed). Diagnosis of Bone and Joint Disorders, 4th ed. Philadelphia, WB Saunders, 2002.
78. Bevelaqua FA, Hasselbacher P, Schumacher HR. Scurvy and hemarthrosis. JAMA 1976; 235:1874.
79. Gordon EF, Gordon RC, Passal DB. Zinc metabolism: basic, clinical and behavioral aspects. J Pediatr 1981; 99:3414.
80. Boskey AL, Rimnac CM, Bansal M, et al. Effects of short term hypomagnesemia on the chemical and mechanical properties of rat bone. J Orthop Res 1992; 10:774.

Musculo-skeletal Tumors and Tumor-like Lesions

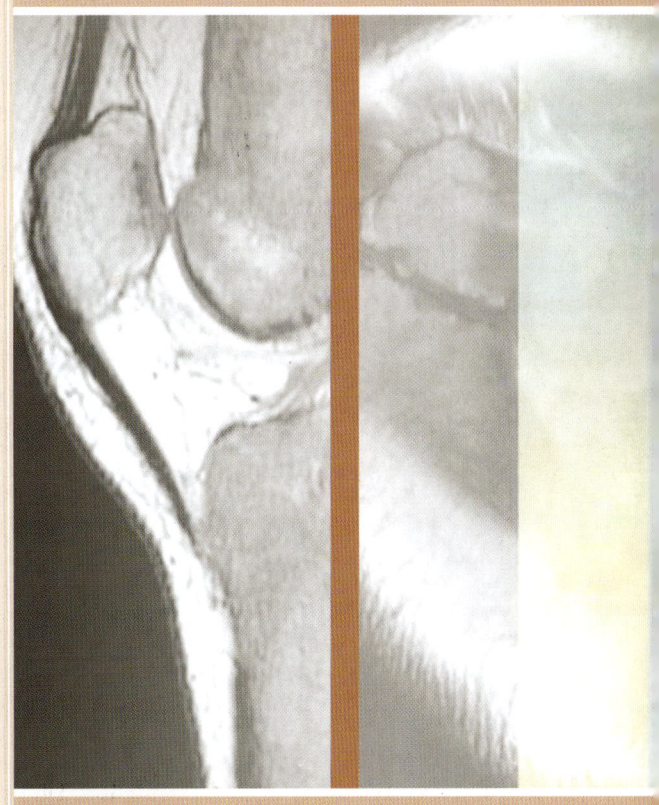

88

The Patient with a Tumor or Tumor-like Lesion of Bone

Hans L. Bloem and Herman M. Kroon

Tumors are typically detected on radiographs. A tumor is a space-occupying lesion. It may be neoplastic or non-neoplastic. The non-neoplastic tumor is also referred to as a tumor-like lesion. The group of tumor-like lesions is very heterogeneous and contains normal variants, fibrous dysplasia, osteomyelitis, and so on. The tumor or tumor-like lesion may be detected easily, with difficulty, or even not at all depending on the quality of radiographic examination, level of suspicion, location, presence of radiographically detectable tumor matrix such as ossification or calcification, amount of cancellous and/or cortical bone destroyed, and other host reactions such as reactive bone formation and periosteal reaction. Tumors are rare. Diagnosis is therefore challenging and requires a systematic as well as a multidisciplinary approach. It is a well-accepted axiom that the center of this approach is the collaboration between pathologist, orthopedic surgeon, and radiologist. This ensures that all available information is used when diagnosing and treating these rare conditions.

The first task of the radiologist is to identify any potential lesion. Many patients will not have a lesion, and most patients with an abnormality on the radiograph will not have a tumor. Because this setting decreases the level of suspicion, the radiologist should be aggressive in his or her diagnostic approach and should also be aware of the hazard of an undetected malignant tumor that is allowed to continue to grow and metastasize (Fig. 88-1).

The first question that needs to be addressed when an observation is made is are we dealing with a true lesion or is the observation a normal finding or normal variant (Table 88-1). Apparent lucencies representing paucity of bone mass are seen at typical locations such as in the humeral head, calcaneus (Fig. 88-2), and the neurocranium (impressions of venous lakes or pacchionian depressions).

Variants in the growing skeleton are of particular importance because primary osseous neoplasms are mainly found in this age group. Irregular chondral ossification with fragmentation and sclerosis at the side of a synchondrosis developing in a synostosis, for instance at the interface of the inferior pubic ramus and ischial bone, is frequently mistaken for a neoplasm. The clue to this diagnosis is the location in relation to the age of the patient (Fig. 88-3).

Another normal variant that can be mistaken for a neoplasm is an irregularity at the insertion or origin of a muscle observed in an adolescent (Figs. 88-4 to 88-6). The location in combination with the appearance of a small, well-demarcated scalloped periosteal defect allows a confident diagnosis to be made.

The second category consists of the non-neoplastic or tumor-like lesions. The most important lesions in this category are fibrous dysplasia, hemangioma, cysts, nonossifying fibroma, osteomyelitis, and post-traumatic sequelae such as old avulsion injuries and stress fractures (Fig. 88-7).[1] This category is included in the differential diagnosis when appropriate. The final category consists of true benign or malignant neoplasms.

KEY POINTS

- Osseous primary tumors occur mainly in the second decade of life.
- Metastases and myeloma occur mainly in patients older than 40 years of age.
- Detection of bone tumors requires a high level of suspicion.
- When a potential bone tumor is found, consultation of an experienced team consisting of a radiologist, pathologist, and orthopedic surgeon is required.
- Radiographs supported by epidemiologic data remain the mainstay in diagnosis.

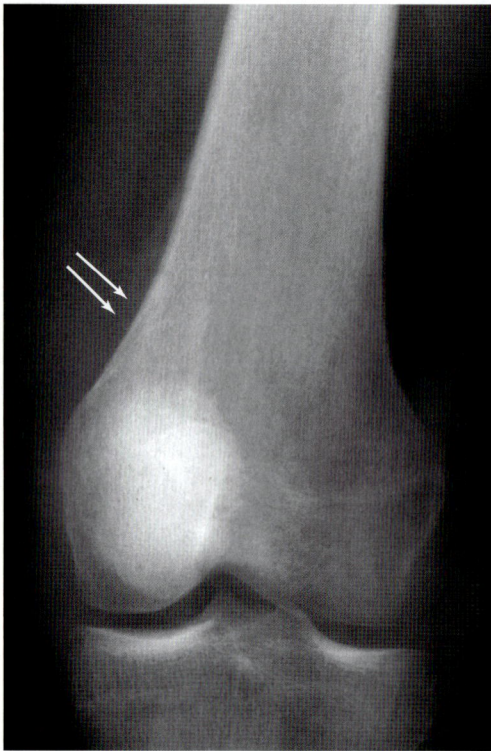
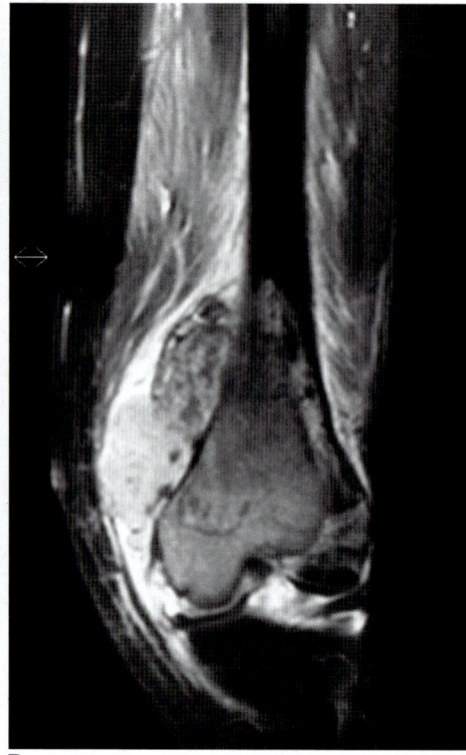

A   B

■ FIGURE 88-1   **A,** Subtle presentation of an osteosarcoma. Note the irregularity of metadiaphyseal cortex (*arrows*) on the medial site, displaying osteolysis and sclerosis. **B,** The tumor is easily detected on this fat-suppressed Gd-DTPA enhanced T1-weighted MR image.

TABLE 88-1	Anatomic Variants That May Mimic Tumor
Location	**Appearance and Explanation**
Distal posteromedial femoral metaphysis	Irregularity at origin of gastrocnemius muscle
Proximal diaphysis of humerus	Irregularity at insertion of deltoid muscle
Proximal radius	Irregularity at insertion of biceps muscle
Ischial-pubic synchondrosis	Irregularity, fragmentation at synchondrosis
Anterior ribs	Irregular ossification of cartilage
Parietal, occipital bone	Lucency because of thin neurocranium
Squamosal part temporal bone	Lucency because of thin neurocranium
Iliac bones	Lucency because of thin bone
Iliac bones	Apparent lucency because of gas in bowel
Scapula	Lucency because of thin bone
Calcaneus lateral view	Lucency because of paucity of cancellous bone
Humeral head	Lucency because of paucity of cancellous bone
Distal humerus anterior	Supracondylar process (see Fig. 88-6)
Radial tuberosity	Lucency because of paucity of cancellous bone
Femoral neck (Ward's triangle)	Lucency because of paucity of cancellous bone
Neurocranium	Small lucencies because of vascular impressions
Anterior clinoid process	Lucency because of pneumatization
Petrous bone	Lucency because of pneumatization
Vertebral body	Apparent osteochondroma due to elongated transverse process

The required systematic approach should include the analysis of not only radiographs but also other imaging studies.[2] A biopsy specimen should only be taken after all imaging studies, that are thought to be necessary based on initial clinical and radiographic findings, have been completed and analyzed. If malignancy is included in the radiographic differential diagnosis, MRI should routinely be performed as the next diagnostic step. The systematic approach should follow the steps listed in Table 88-2, and these issues are addressed in more detail later in this chapter. The final

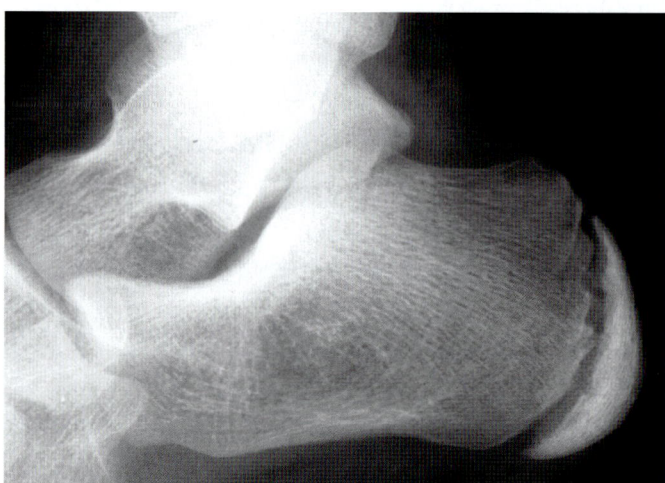

■ FIGURE 88-2   Normal calcaneus with central lucency representing normal paucity of trabecular bone.

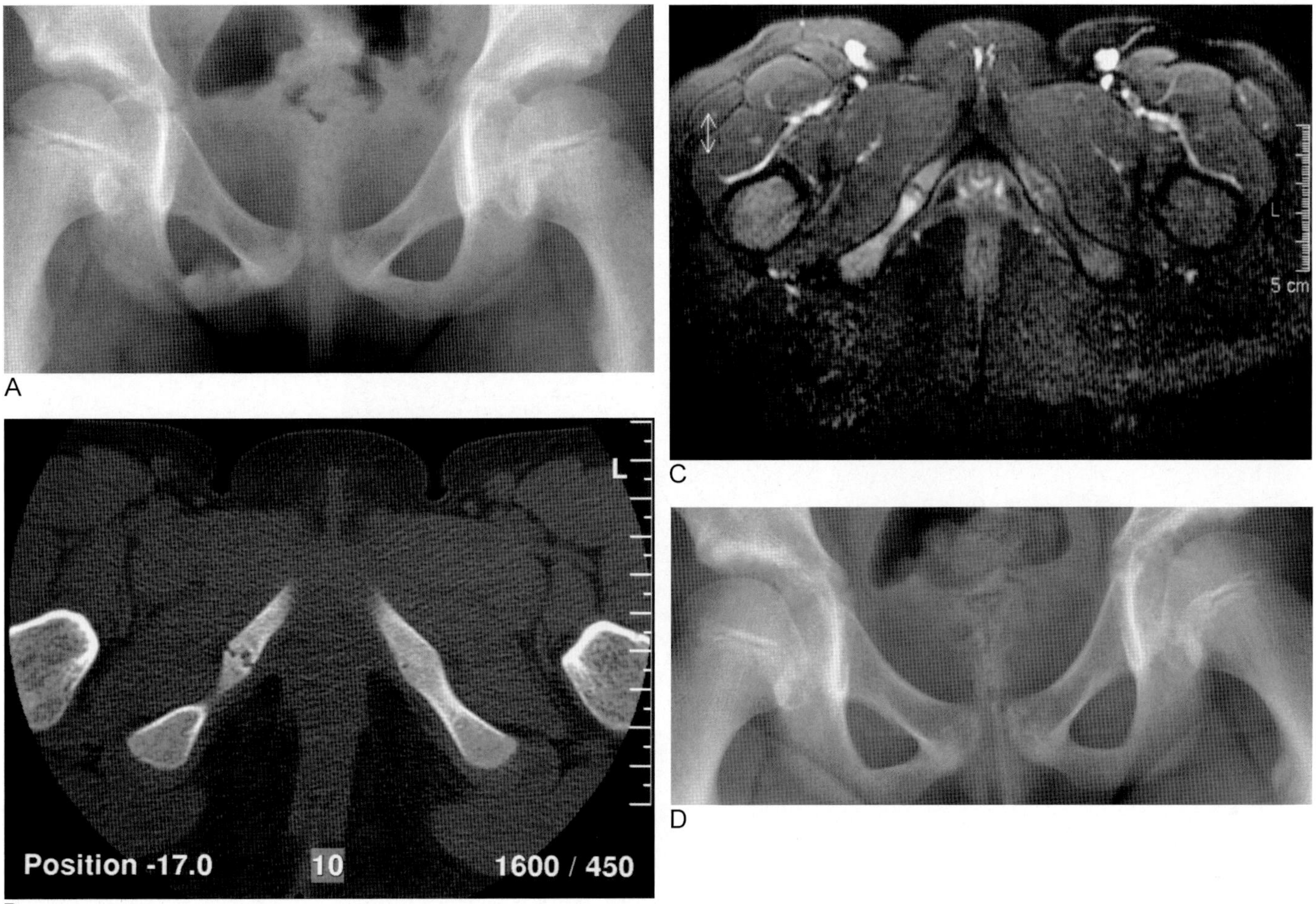

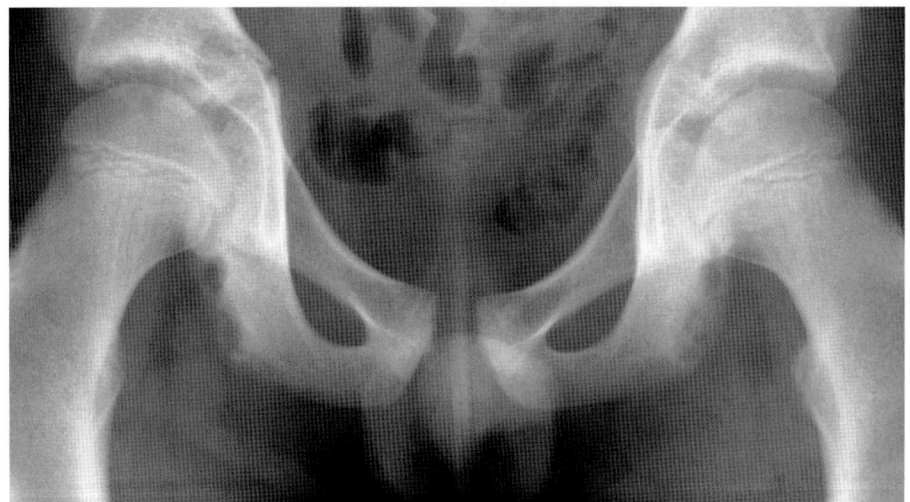

■ **FIGURE 88-3** Normal synchondrosis developing into a synostosis. **A,** The radiograph shows a pseudotumor on the right side where the inferior pubic ramus meets the ischial bone. **B,** CT shows the synchondrosis. **C,** High signal intensity is seen surrounding the synchondrosis on this T2-weighted MR image. **D,** One year later the synchondrosis matured into a normal synostosis.

■ **FIGURE 88-4** Bilateral scalloping at the origin of the rotator muscles of the hip (in particular the quadratus femoris muscle).

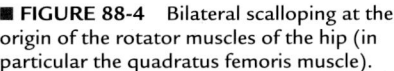

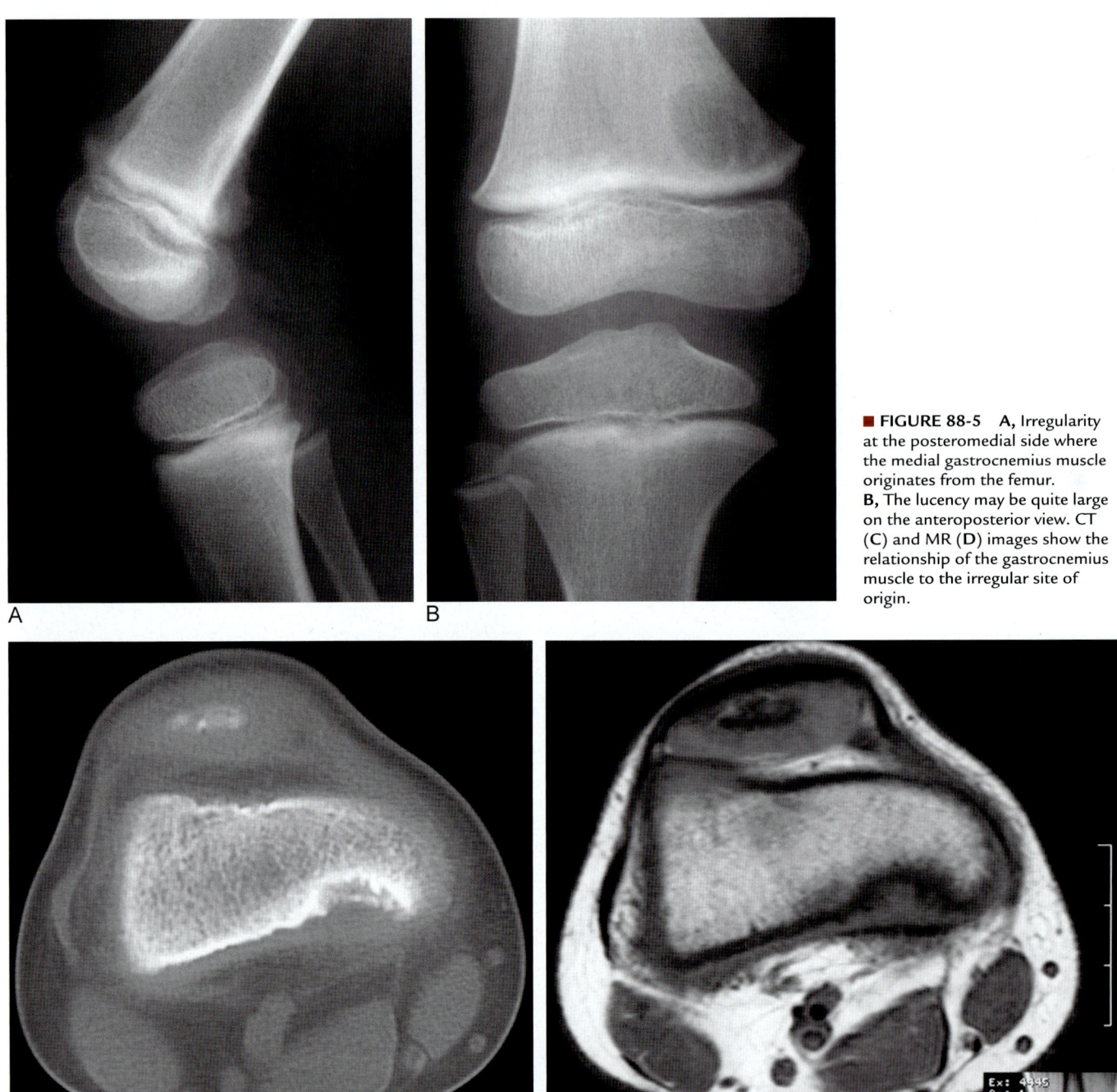

■ FIGURE 88-5   A, Irregularity at the posteromedial side where the medial gastrocnemius muscle originates from the femur. **B,** The lucency may be quite large on the anteroposterior view. CT **(C)** and MR **(D)** images show the relationship of the gastrocnemius muscle to the irregular site of origin.

diagnostic step before treatment is started frequently is an image-guided biopsy (see Biopsy: Bone in the Procedure Section on the CD).

PREVALENCE AND EPIDEMIOLOGY

Prevalence and epidemiologic data, such as location and age of the patient, are important parameters in the analysis of a patient presenting with a possible osseous tumor (see Table 88-2). However, specific tumors do occur outside their preferred locations, or age ranges. Although primary osseous neoplasm is rare in the general population, the incidence is significant in subpopulations. The incidence of primary osseous benign and malignant neoplasm is 2 to 3 cases per 100,000 population per year. The incidences of lung cancer and breast cancer are approximately 60 times higher than that of bone sarcoma. Bone sarcoma comprises only approximately 0.3% of newly diagnosed malignancies. Malignant primary bone tumors occur mainly in children and adolescents and have an annual incidence of 5 to 6 cases per 100,000 population of children younger than 15 years of age. Malignant lymphoma,

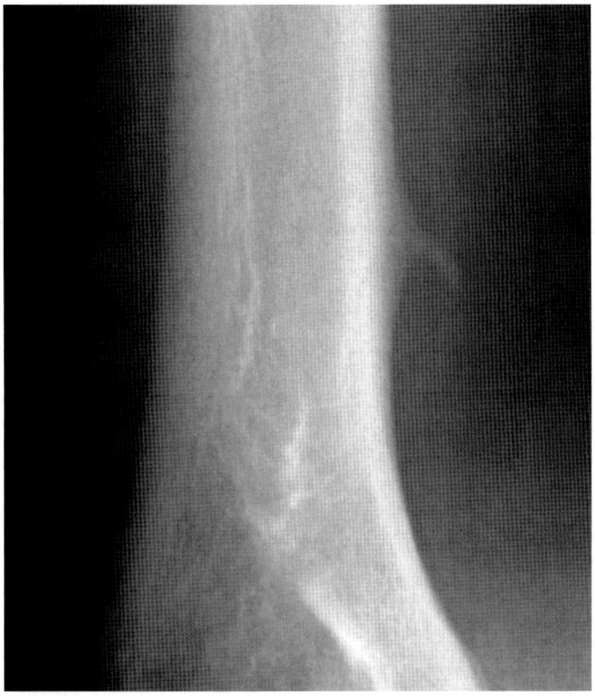

■ **FIGURE 88-6** Detail of a lateral view of the distal humerus shows the anteriorly located supracondylar process pointing toward the joint.

including the more common extraskeletal lymphoma, is the most common and bone sarcoma is the second most common solid malignant neoplasm in adolescence.

Myeloma is by far the most frequent osseous malignancy in adults, accounting for 45% of all malignant osseous tumors. Lymphoma is the other nonsarcomatous malignancy found in bone, accounting for 8% of malignant osseous tumors. These entities are discussed respectively in Chapters 91 and 92. The most frequently encountered sarcomas, benign osseous tumors, and tumor-like osseous lesions are listed in Table 88-3. Many benign lesions that are frequently asymptomatic, such as nonossifying fibroma, hemangioma, enchondroma, and fibrous dysplasia are underreported and therefore much more frequently encountered as an incidental finding.

Many lesions present within a specific age range, and age is therefore an important parameter to consider when a lesion that may be a primary bone tumor is analyzed. Myeloma and metastases are much more frequent than primary bone sarcoma when a patient is older than 40 years of age. Multiple osseous lesions are frequently found in children with neuroblastoma (see Chapter 96).[3] Bone sarcoma and benign osseous tumors typically present in the second decade of life. There is a second smaller peak late in the sixth decade. Age distribution of the more common lesions is presented in Tables 88-4 and 88-5.

In the next step of the analysis the location within the body is considered. As shown in Table 88-6, some tumors have a preference for certain locations within the body. Based on frequency distribution only, a tumorous lesion in the hand, and more specifically in the phalanges, is almost always an enchondroma because of the preference for this location in combination with the relatively high prevalence of enchondroma in general.[4] Adamantinoma is almost exclusively found in the tibia. However, a tumor in the tibia is more likely to be an osteosarcoma or nonossifying fibroma than adamantinoma, based on frequency distribution only. The reason is that osteosarcoma and especially nonossifying fibroma are relatively common and have a much higher prevalence than the extremely rare adamantinoma. Relatively common lesions are found

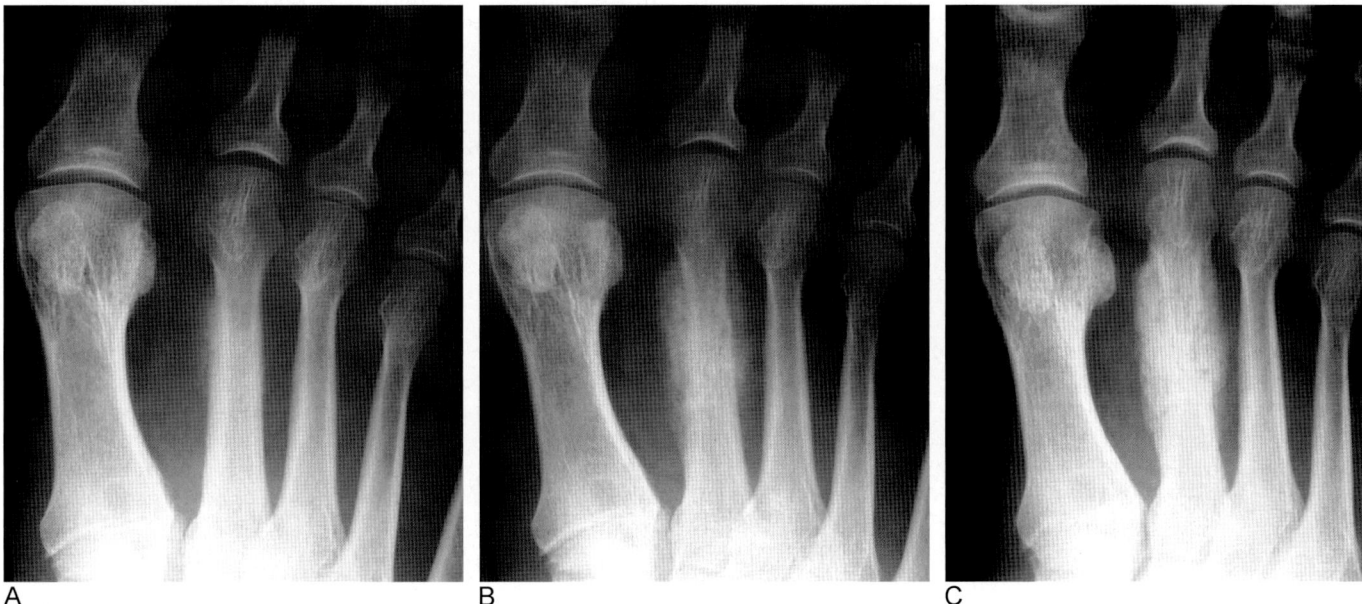

A   B   C

■ **FIGURE 88-7** **A,** The transversely oriented stress fracture is hard to appreciate, but callus formation is visible. Callus formation has an appearance that may raise concern because of its resemblance to tumor osteoid formation. **B,** Several weeks later, bone resorption and maturation of callus reflect fracture healing. At this stage the irregularity of callus may still raise suspicion. **C,** Two months later the fracture has healed and mature, solid callus allows a confident diagnosis of fracture healing; thus tumor is excluded.

TABLE 88-2 Systemic Approach in Diagnosing Osseous Tumors or Tumor-like Lesions

1. Categorize the radiograph (normal, variant, tumor-like lesion, tumor).
2. Determine prevalence of lesions in relation to the age of the patient.
3. Determine prevalence of lesions in affected bone.
4. Is the lesion solitary, or are there multiple lesions?
5. Determine prevalence of osseous lesions in affected part of the bone.
6. Analyze radiograph in detail.
7. Analyze additional information (MR, CT, clinical and laboratory data, etc.).
8. Perform biopsy, if needed, based on comprehensive imaging findings.

TABLE 88-3 Incidence, in Decreasing Order, of Lesions That May Present as a Primary Bone Tumor

Lesion	Incidence in % of All Tumors
Osteosarcoma	17%
Chondrosarcoma	11%
Enchondroma*	6%
Fibrous dysplasia*	6%
Giant cell tumor	6%
Nonossifying fibroma/fibrous cortical defect*	5%
Ewing's sarcoma	5%
Malignant fibrous histiocytoma/fibrosarcoma	5%
Osteochondroma*	4%
Aneurysmal bone cyst	4%
Metastasis	4%
Osteomyelitis	4%
Solitary bone cyst	3%
Osteoid osteoma	3%
Langerhans cell histiocytosis (eosinophilic granuloma)	3%
Chondroblastoma	2%
Others	12%

Note: Benign tumors and tumor-like lesions are in general underreported in these frequency distributions. * These lesions are often asymptomatic and therefore much more frequent than suggested in this table.
Data based on 6873 tumors on file in the Netherlands Committee on Bone Tumors.

much more frequently in aspecific or even uncommon locations than rare lesions are found in their preferential locations.

In the final step of analyzing epidemiologic data, one has to determine whether the lesion is solitary or multifocal. This may be apparent from the beginning, for instance when multiple lesions are seen on bone scintigraphy, on large field-of-view MRI, or on radiographs taken from symptomatic parts of the skeleton. It may also be necessary to start a search for other lesions using MRI, bone scintigraphy, or positron emission tomography. The most important lesions that are typically, but not always, multifocal are myeloma and metastasis. If we combine this with age, it is fairly straightforward to suggest a differential diagnosis, without even analyzing the images, of myeloma or metastases in a patient older than 40 years of age with multiple osseous lesions. Other lesions that may be multifocal are listed in Tables 88-7 and 88-8.

Although some tumors have a higher incidence in males, gender does not play a critical role in diagnosing bone tumors. There are some exceptions to this. Multiple myeloma and osteoid osteoma occur two to three times more frequently in males than in females. Examples of conditions that occur slightly more often in females than in males are hemangioma and giant cell tumor.

CLINICAL PRESENTATION

Radiographs, displaying findings that may reflect the presence of a tumor, are typically made because of local clinical symptoms such as pain, dysfunction, and/or swelling. These clinical signs may be misleading in children because of referred pain. The patient may for instance present with pain in the knee with or without a limp (dysfunction) secondary to a lesion in the hip region. The radiographic finding of a tumor may also be incidental or not related to the patient's symptoms.

Pain and/or local swelling are the most common, albeit nonspecific symptoms. Typically, pain has been present for several weeks or months. The onset is often gradual, and the patient may not recall when the pain started. Sudden onset of pain without adequate trauma occurs in pathologic fractures. In malignant tumors, pain may be rapidly progressive and may also be aggravating. When the tumor or tumor-like lesion is not fractured, pain is not related to physical activity and may be continuous or intermittent. Pain may be worse during the night. This is typically seen in osteoid osteoma in combination with good response to treatment with salicylates. When the tumor is located close to a joint, or when it is extending into a joint, the symptoms may erroneously be attributed to joint disease. Post-traumatic sequelae in and around joints are obviously much more frequently encountered in this young age group. This may even tempt the clinician to choose arthroscopy rather than radiography as a first diagnostic test, for instance when reactive synovitis is found at clinical examination.

Fever and general malaise may be present in high-grade malignancies, especially in Ewing's sarcoma. Because Ewing's sarcoma may look radiographically like osteomyelitis it is important to realize that also clinically the differentiation between infection and high-grade sarcoma may be challenging (Fig. 88-8). Temperature, sedimentation rate, and blood cultures may be normal in patients with osteomyelitis and may, with the exception of blood cultures, be abnormal in patients with Ewing's sarcoma.

At physical examination the soft tissue swelling typically is firm; it may be warm, but there is no discoloration of the skin. Specific skin abnormalities are seen at inspection in various syndromes such as neurofibromatosis. Dysfunction of joints or muscles may be observed.

PATHOPHYSIOLOGY

Imaging techniques may visualize the tumor, the host's response to the tumor, or both. Radiographs typically visualize the host's response. Parts of the tumor are only directly depicted using radiographs when there are

TABLE 88-4 Median Age in Increasing Order and 95% and 75% Prevalence of Malignant Tumors

Tumor	Median Age	90% Prevalence Age	75% Prevalence Age
Neuroblastoma	2	0–6	0–10
Ewing's sarcoma	14	5–30	5–20
Osteosarcoma conventional	17	5–55	5–25
Telangiectatic osteosarcoma	17	6–45	10–40
Adamantinoma	25	10–60	10–40
Synovial sarcoma	25	5–60	10–55
Chondrosarcoma central, grade III	26	10–60	10–55
Juxtacortical osteosarcoma	27	10–60	10–40
Chondrosarcoma peripheral, grade I, II	32	15–55	20–55
Non-Hodgkin's lymphoma	35	10–70	20–70
Malignant fibrous histiocytoma, fibrosarcoma	44	10–80	10–75
Chondrosarcoma central, grade I	44	15–75	20–70
Hemangioendothelioma	47	20–80	35–75
Chondrosarcoma central, grade II	55	25–80	30–80
Chordoma	58	30–80	40–75
Metastatic carcinoma	*	>40	40–80
Myeloma	60	40–80	45–75

*Absence of accurate data.
Data based on 6873 tumors on file in the Netherlands Committee on Bone Tumors.

TABLE 88-5 Median Age in Increasing Order and 90% and 75% Prevalence of Benign Osseous Tumors and Tumor-like Lesions

Lesion	Median Age	90% Prevalence	75% Prevalence
Langerhans cell histiocytosis	10	1–35	1–20
Solitary bone cyst	11	1–30	1–15
Chondroma, multiple	12	1–60	10–45
Aneurysmal bone cyst	14	1–25	1–20
Fibrous cortical defect, nonossifying fibroma	14	5–20	10–20
Osteoblastoma	15	1–30	5–25
Chondromyxoid fibroma	17	1–40	1–25
Osteoid osteoma	17	5–35	5–30
Chondroblastoma	17	10–30	10–20
Osteochondroma	20	1–50	5–30
Fibrous dysplasia	21	1–50	1–35
Myositis ossificans*	22	1–45	5–40
Giant cell granuloma	24	1–55	1–40
Chondroma juxtacortical	26	1–60	10–45
Fibromatosis*	29	1–70	1–45
Giant cell tumor	30	10–55	15–45
Pigmented villonodular synovitis*	32	15–60	15–50
Hemangioma	33	10–65	10–60
Desmoplastic fibroma	34	10–60	10–50
Chondroma solitary	35	6–65	10–60
Ganglion, cyst	38	10–70	30–60
Epidermoid cyst	42	25–60	30–55
Brown tumor (hyperparathyroidism)	52	40–70	45–70

*Includes soft tissue tumors invading bone.
NOF, nonossifying fibroma.
Data based on 6873 tumors on file in the Netherlands Committee on Bone Tumors.

calcifications within the tumor (e.g., in cartilaginous tumors), when tumor matrix is ossified (e.g., in osteosarcoma), or when there is a substantial soft tissue extension. Often more obvious is the host's response, including osteoclast activity (osteolysis), osteoblast activity (sclerosis), and periosteal reaction. Of these, osteolysis is the hardest to detect, especially in the diaphysis where there is a paucity of trabecular bone. Osteolysis becomes visible only when there is marked destruction of cortical bone and/or when more than 40% to 50% of trabecular bone is destroyed.[5] There is a complex and only partially understood interaction between tumor and host, using multiple signaling pathways, that initiates and maintains this dynamic process. The ensuing growth rate of the tumor has an important impact on the radiographic appearance (see Manifestations of the Disease).

In addition to these radiographically detectable reactions, angiogenesis is an important part of this interaction between tumor and host that can only be visualized using MRI, ultrasonography, and (early phase) bone scintigraphy.

TABLE 88-6 Frequency Distribution of Osseous Tumors and Tumor-like Lesions*

	Skull	Sternum	Clavicle	Rib	Spine/ Sacrum	Pelvis	Scapula	Humerus	Radius	Ulna	Hand	Femur	Patella	Tibia	Fibula	Foot
Osteosarcoma	17	7	3	9	5	9	2	17	5	9	1	30	0	23	17	2
Chondrosarcoma	8	57	4	27	10	24	8	8	5	11	9	8	0	5	1	8
Ewing's sarcoma	1	4	3	14	6	15	3	6	6	8	0	3	0	3	16	4
Malignant fibrous histiocytoma	7	2	6	2	2	5	2	5	2	0	0	8	0	3	2	0
Adamantinoma	0	0	0	0	0	0	0	0	1	0	0	0	0	2	0	0
Chordoma	2	0	0	0	12	0	0	0	0	0	0	0	0	0	0	0
Other malignancies	9	7	14	4	9	8	2	4	3	3	0	5	15	4	2	9
Osteoid osteoma	0	0	0	0	7	1	0	3	6	3	5	3	0	4	3	8
Osteoblastoma	1	0	1	1	10	1	1	1	0	1	2	1	0	1	1	8
Enchondroma	0	2	4	5	1	1	0	4	6	8	42	3	0	2	3	6
Osteochondroma	0	0	0	2	3	3	8	7	3	3	4	3	0	3	5	5
Chondroblastoma	0	2	0	1	0	1	0	6	0	1	1	3	23	3	1	10
Giant cell tumor	1	0	1	1	13	3	0	5	24	18	4	7	8	11	11	6
Other benign tumors	3	0	1	4	6	3	0	1	2	2	10	3	8	3	0	5
Aneurysmal bone cyst	2	0	20	2	9	4	3	3	8	10	4	2	15	4	10	7
Solitary bone cyst	0	0	1	0	0	3	0	17	2	1	1	3	15	0	2	4
Fibrous dysplasia	22	0	3	16	1	4	1	4	4	7	1	5	0	5	2	1
Nonossifying fibroma	0	0	0	0	0	0	0	1	1	1	0	6	0	14	11	1
Eosinophilic granuloma	7	0	9	5	4	5	3	2	2	0	0	2	0	1	0	0
Other tumor-like lesions	20	7	27	5	7	8	6	7	16	13	15	9	15	2	6	14

*For each location the distribution of the various histologic diagnoses is given in percent. Data based on 6873 tumors on file in the Netherlands Committee on Bone Tumors.

TABLE 88-7 Malignant Osseous Tumors That May Be Multifocal

Metastases
Myeloma
Angiosarcoma
Leukemia
Neuroblastoma
Ewing's sarcoma
Osteosarcomatosis
Lymphoma

TABLE 88-8 Benign Tumors and Tumor-like Conditions That May Be Multifocal

Fibrous dysplasia
Enchondromatosis
Osteochondromatosis
Synovial cysts
Brown tumors in hyperparathyroidism
Langerhans cell histiocytosis (eosinophilic granuloma)
Hemangiomatosis
Bone islands, osteoma (Gardner's syndrome)
Fibrous cortical defect, nonossifying fibroma
Giant cell tumor
Neurofibromatosis
Amyloidosis
Mastocytosis
SAPHO, chronic multifocal osteomyelitis

SAPHO, synovitis, acne, pustulosis, hyperostosis, osteitis.

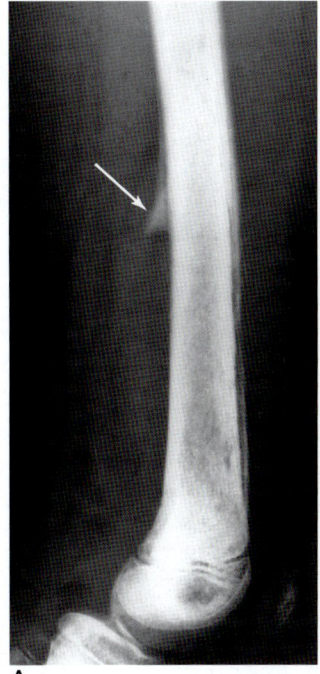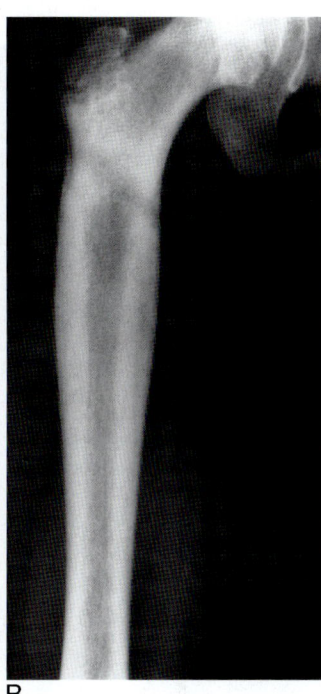

A   B

■ **FIGURE 88-8**   **A,** Atypical presentation of osteomyelitis in a child. The periosteal reaction (*arrow*) consisting of Codman's triangle and interrupted lamellar periosteal reaction is far more commonly seen in sarcoma. Because of this periosteal reaction, the predominantly diaphyseal location, the pattern of bone destruction, and the age of the patient, Ewing's sarcoma should be included in the differential diagnosis. **B,** Ewing's sarcoma in a young adolescent presenting with fever, high sedimentation rate, and elevated white cell count. Although this radiograph should raise the suspicion of Ewing's sarcoma, the periosteal reaction in Ewing's sarcoma usually is less solid than in this patient. Osteomyelitis should be included in the differential diagnosis because of this periosteal reaction and the absence of visible soft tissue mass.

Altered hemodynamics in the vicinity of the tumor, and even in large parts of the affected extremity, cause increased tracer uptake, seen on technetium-99m bone scintigraphy. Early cellular proliferation in the cambium layer of the periosteum that is not yet ossified can be observed on MRI and not on radiographs (Fig. 88-9). Inflammatory response and edema surrounding the tumor may be best seen on MRI, but the intraosseous component of this may be seen as rarefaction on radiographs. Periosteal reaction and inflammatory reaction are usually found close to the tumor but may be quite extensive, resulting in periosteal reaction seen away from the tumor, for instance in chondroblastoma. Extensive inflammatory reaction, as seen in osteoid osteoma and Langerhans cell histiocytosis, may even obscure the original lesion.

IMAGING TECHNIQUES

Clinical findings and symptoms, or a finding on another imaging study such as technetium-99m bone scintigraphy or MRI, are reasons to take radiographs. Good-quality radiographs taken in two orthogonal directions can, with important exceptions (Table 88-9), be used to confidently diagnose, or exclude the presence of a tumor. The cause of symptoms may also not be identified on radiographs when symptoms are secondary to pathology other than bone tumor, such as early osteomyelitis, intra-articular lesions, or soft tissue tumor.

The main reason to perform MRI in osseous lesions is local staging and monitoring of chemotherapy. In addition, dynamic Gd-chelate–enhanced MR can be used to differentiate benign from malignant cartilaginous tumors and to localize recurrent disease. These issues are addressed in the specific chapters.

Techniques and Relevant Aspects

With the advent of digital (DR) and computed (CR) radiography the quality of radiographs is excellent, but especially conventional film-screen radiographs may suffer from overpenetration or underpenetration. Because subtle findings may be easily hidden with suboptimal exposure, no compromise in quality should be accepted (Fig. 88-10).

Likewise, a small, or even large tumor may be missed if local anatomy is complex and/or if superimposing structures obscure the view (see Table 88-9). The best example is that of fairly large tumors located in the pelvis or sacrum that are being missed because of subtle abnormalities of curved cortical lines that are obscured by overlying bowel or superimposing anatomic structures. The second important point is visualizing the entire region of interest. A consequence of this is that no protection of the genitalia should be used when taking radiographs of the pelvis (Fig. 88-11).

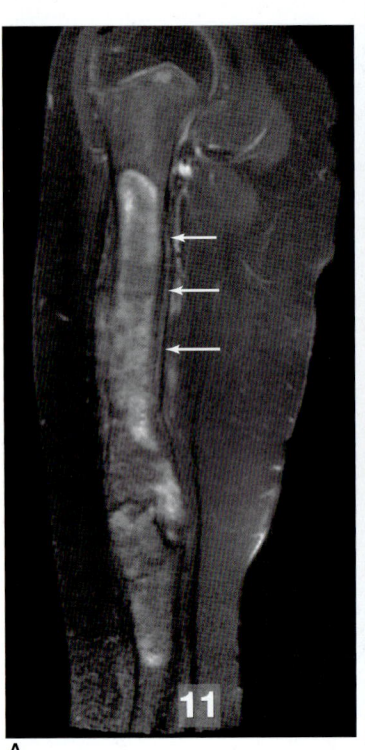

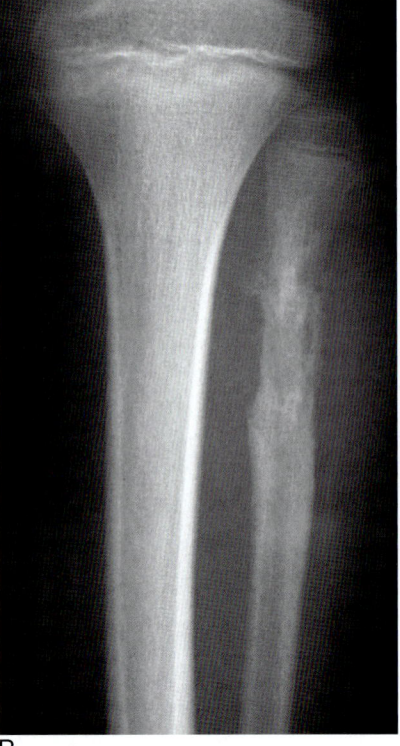

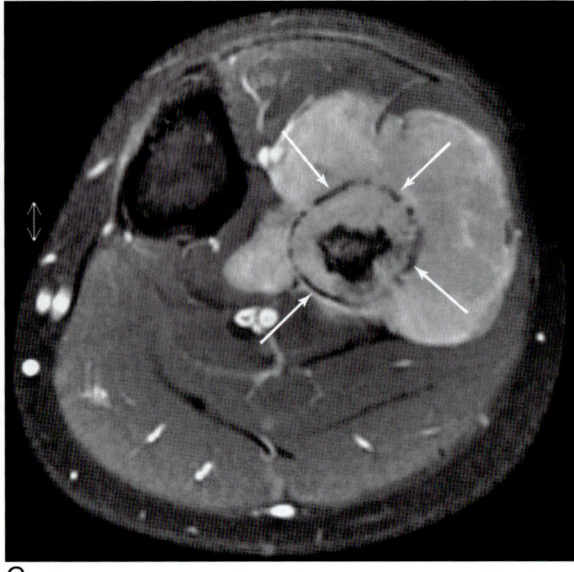

A   B   C

■ **FIGURE 88-9** **A,** Sagittal Gd-DTPA, fat-suppressed MR image of Ewing' sarcoma in the humerus. The high signal intensity line (*arrows*) represents the cellular layer of the periosteum. **B,** Destruction of bone, including cortex, is seen on this radiograph of Ewing's sarcoma in the proximal fibula. Ossification of periosteal reaction is very limited and is therefore not well appreciated on this radiograph. The tumor is shown originating in the fibula. **C,** Note the soft tissue extension and the low signal intensity of the fibrous component of the periosteum. The periosteum is interrupted at multiple sites. Axial Gd-DTPA enhanced MR image showing the tumor (*arrows*).

TABLE 88-9	Causes of a Missed Tumor on Radiographs
Cause	**Solution**
Referred pain	Radiography of adjacent body parts, technetium (Tc) bone scintigraphy
Poor quality radiograph	Repeat exposure
Lesion not included in field of view	Larger field of view, Tc bone scintigraphy
Superimposing structures in pelvis	Oblique views, CT, MRI
Complex anatomy in axial skeleton	Oblique views, CT, MRI
Cortical bone not involved	MRI
Paucity of cancellous bone (diaphysis, osteoporosis)	MRI
Small size of lesion (osteoid osteoma)	Tc bone scintigraphy, CT, or MRI
Growth pattern of myeloma	MRI

In the extremities at least one of the joints should be included in the radiographs. As mentioned earlier, special attention is needed to avoid mistakes in young children because of referred pain.

The same geometric requirements of radiography apply to MRI. A large field of view is needed, and at least one of the joints has to be included in the image when imaging lesions located in extremities. Also two orthogonal planes are required. The axial plane should always be used. The second plane may be sagittal for the spine, knee, and ankle or coronal for the shoulder and hip. A combination of T1- and T2-weighted contrast is needed. For these conventional spin-echo (SE) or turbo spin-echo (TSE), or fast spin-echo (FSE) with a small echo train length (3 to 5) for T1-weighted images can be used. Gradient-echo images should be avoided because contrast is generally poor. Whenever possible fat suppression should be used for the T2-weighted sequences. Short tau inversion recovery (STIR) sequences are basically T1-weighted sequences to which T2 contrast is added if the echo time is not too short. STIR sequences can be used if frequency selective fat suppression is suboptimal because of field inhomogeneity, secondary to large field of views (entire spine), bulk susceptibility (foot), or the presence of orthopedic hardware.

Contrast-enhanced MRI using gadolinium chelates is useful in the initial examination because it produces high-contrast, high spatial resolution images. T1-weighted SE or FSE images after contrast agent injection should be combined with frequency-selective fat suppression. STIR should be avoided because this nonselective suppression may decrease the signal intensity of enhancing tissue. When dynamic MRI is used these extracellular, interstitial contrast agents offer the possibility to reflect parameters such as vascular density, capillary leak, interstitial space, and pressure. These parameters in osseous tumors are of importance in monitoring therapy (see Chapter 99).

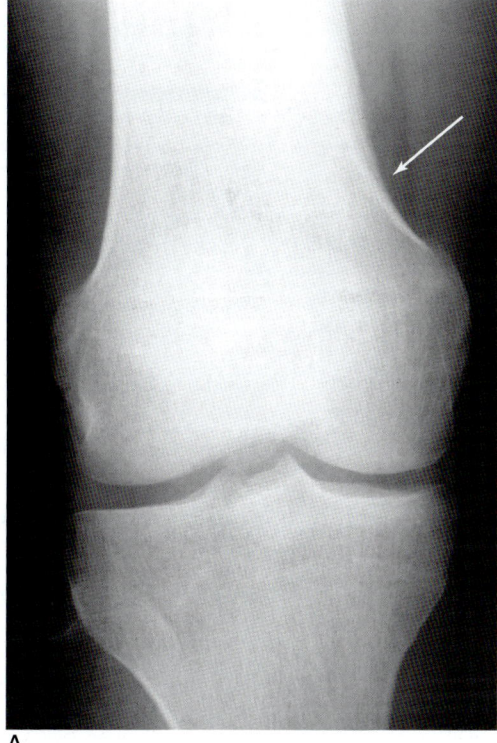
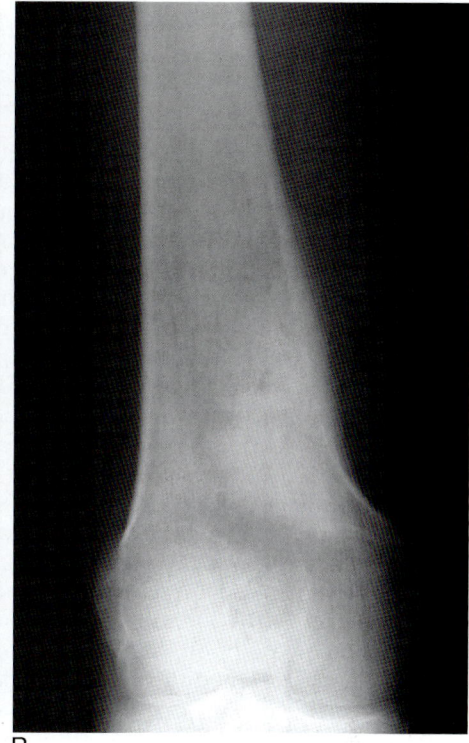

■ **FIGURE 88-10**   **A,** This analog, conventional radiograph is underexposed and does not allow analysis of osseous structure in the femur. The ossified lesion is therefore difficult to depict. Periosteal reaction on the medial side is depicted (*arrow*) but is incompletely visualized. **B,** With proper field of view and exposure, the osteoid matrix of the osteosarcoma in the medial femoral metaphysis is easily diagnosed.

A

B

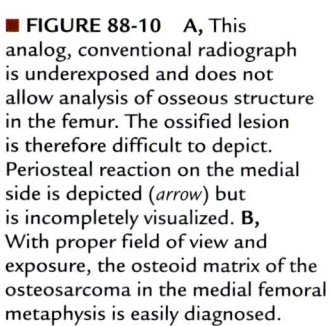

A

■ **FIGURE 88-11**   **A,** In this male adolescent, complaining of pain in the right hip, lead protection of the genitalia was used during radiography. **B,** The radiograph, repeated 2 months later because of persistent symptoms, taken with the proper technique clearly shows destruction of pubic bone caused by Ewing's sarcoma. **C,** The soft tissue extension is found to be huge on coronal T1-weighted MRI. This patient also illustrates the issue of referred pain.

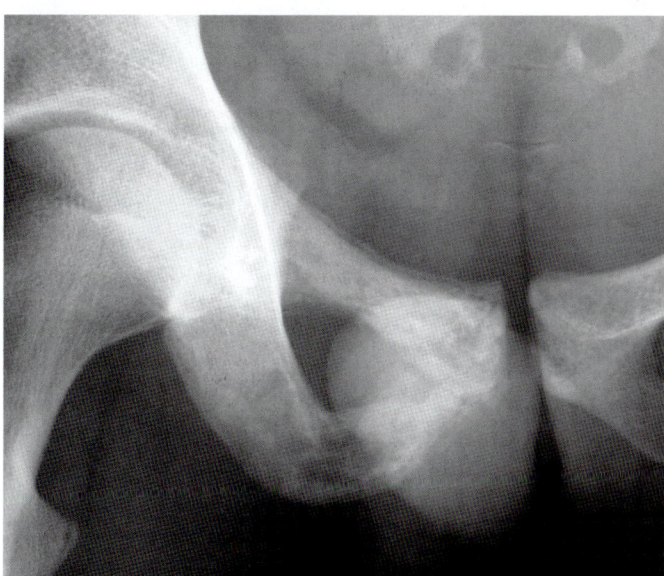

B

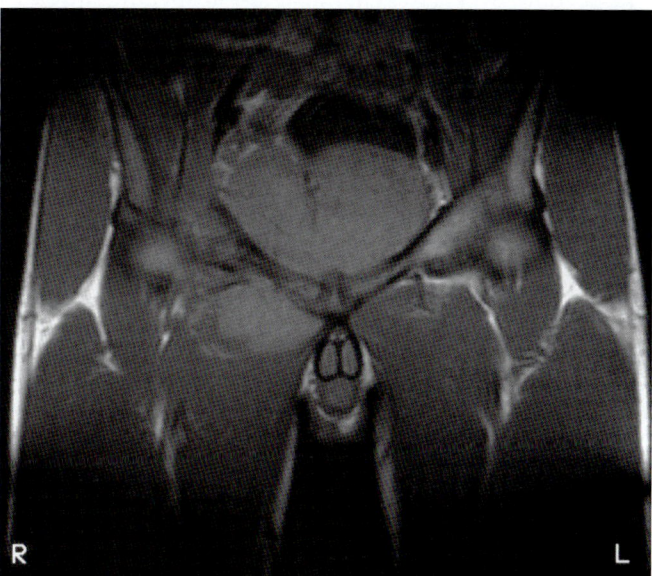

C

MANIFESTATIONS OF THE DISEASE

In Tables 88-10 to 88-15 the most frequently diagnosed tumors and tumor-like lesions are listed for the various anatomic areas within long bones. The general incidence of these tumors is taken into account. As a result, lesions with a relatively high incidence such as osteosarcoma are high on these lists irrespective of location. Lesions that are rare, such as adamantinoma, which has a preference for the diaphysis of the tibia, are, even if including their preferential site, relatively low on the list. The preferential sites for each bone tumor irrespective of general incidence are given in Chapters 90 and 92. A rule of thumb in the spine is that tumors arising in the vertebral body are often metastases whereas lesions arising in the posterior elements are usually benign. There are, however, exceptions such as hemangioma, osteomyelitis/spondylodiscitis, and Langerhans cell histiocytosis that arise in the vertebral body.[1]

In addition to the location of the tumor in the longitudinal axis of the bone, the location in the axial plane also is important in differential diagnosis. The lesion may be central, eccentric, cortical, or parosteal in origin (Fig. 88-12). When the hosting bone is small, or when the tumor is large, this differentiation in position of the tumor relative to the axis of the long bone often cannot be used.

Radiography

The radiographic analysis should, in combination with information on prevalence in relation to age and location, result in a differential diagnosis. The first level in the differential diagnosis is the classification of the lesion as follows:

A: definitely benign, no further action needed
B: benign with high level of confidence, clinical or radiographic follow-up, or treatment of specific condition needed
C: potentially malignant, biopsy in oncologic center needed
D: definitely malignant, biopsy and treatment in oncologic center needed.

The second level is to generate a lesion-specific differential diagnosis. This is important because a specific diagnosis may allow a confident diagnosis at the first level.

TABLE 88-11   Epi-metaphyseal Location of Lesions in Decreasing Order of Frequency

Giant cell tumor
Osteosarcoma
Chondroblastoma
Chondrosarcoma
Fibrosarcoma/malignant fibrous histiocytoma
Enchondroma

Frequency includes the general incidence of tumors (i.e., a common tumor that has a preference for another location may still have a higher prevalence in this specific location than a tumor with a general low prevalence that has a preference for this specific location).

TABLE 88-12   Epi-metadiaphyseal Location of Lesions in Decreasing Order of Frequency

Osteosarcoma
Giant cell tumor
Enchondroma
Fibrosarcoma/malignant fibrous histiocytoma
Chondrosarcoma
Aneurysmal bone cyst

Frequency includes the general incidence of tumors (i.e., a common tumor that has a preference for another location may still have a higher prevalence in this specific location than a tumor with a general low prevalence that has a preference for this specific location).

TABLE 88-13   Metaphyseal Location of Lesions in Decreasing Order of Frequency

Osteosarcoma
Fibrosarcoma/malignant fibrous histiocytoma
Enchondroma
Chondrosarcoma
Nonossifying fibroma/fibrous cortical defect
Osteochondroma
Solitary bone cyst
Giant cell tumor
Osteoid osteoma

Frequency includes the general incidence of tumors (i.e., a common tumor that has a preference for another location may still have a higher prevalence in this specific location than a tumor with a general low prevalence that has a preference for this specific location).

TABLE 88-10   Epiphyseal Location of Lesions in Decreasing Order of Frequency

Subchondral cyst
Chondroblastoma
Osteoid osteoma
Pigmented villonodular synovitis
Osteomyelitis (children)
Non-Hodgkin's lymphoma
Osteoblastoma
Langerhans cell histiocytosis (eosinophilic granuloma)
Dysplasia epiphysealis hemimelica (Trevor's disease)

Frequency includes the general incidence of tumors (i.e., a common tumor that has a preference for another location may still have a higher prevalence in this specific location than a tumor with a general low prevalence that has a preference for this specific location).

TABLE 88-14   Metadiaphyseal Location of Lesions in Decreasing Order of Frequency

Osteosarcoma
Enchondroma
Aneurysmal bone cyst
Fibrous dysplasia
Solitary bone cyst
Nonossifying fibroma/fibrous cortical defect
Ewing's sarcoma
Fibrosarcoma/malignant fibrous histiocytoma
Chondrosarcoma

Frequency includes the general incidence of tumors (i.e., a common tumor that has a preference for another location may still have a higher prevalence in this specific location than a tumor with a general low prevalence that has a preference for this specific location).

TABLE 88-15 Diaphyseal Location of Lesions in Decreasing Order of Frequency

Osteosarcoma
Nonossifying fibroma/fibrous cortical defect
Ewing's sarcoma
Osteochondroma
Enchondroma
Chondrosarcoma
Osteoid osteoma
Fibrous dysplasia
Fibrosarcoma/malignant fibrous histiocytoma
Solitary bone cyst
Aneurysmal bone cyst
Adamantinoma

Frequency includes the general incidence of tumors (i.e., a common tumor that has a preference for another location may still have a higher prevalence in this specific location than a tumor with a general low prevalence that has a preference for this specific location).

The appearance of a nonossifying fibroma (Fig. 88-13) is, in its location and morphology, very typical and allows a confident diagnosis to be made.

The differential diagnosis may also have an impact on clinical management. Especially in tumor-like lesions an unexpected radiologic diagnosis may initiate the start of a new diagnostic pathway, for instance when a brown tumor in association with signs of hyperparathyroidism is found. An unanticipated radiologic diagnosis may also initiate treatment for instance in infection or traumatic sequelae. The differential diagnosis also serves as a control mechanism when a histologic diagnosis is made. There are pitfalls in making a histologic diagnosis, such as sample errors, and it is essential that both the histologic and radiologic diagnosis are in accordance when a definitive diagnosis is made (Table 88-16; Fig. 88-14).

The morphology of a tumor or tumor-like lesion visualized on the radiograph reflects activity or aggressiveness. Malignant tumors are often, but not always, more biologically active than benign lesions. Lesion activity as depicted on radiographs is related to, but not identical to, malignancy. The morphologic criteria can be categorized as pattern of bone destruction, zone of transition, tumor matrix, cortical involvement, periosteal reaction, and soft tissue extension.

The three patterns of bone destruction are geographic, moth-eaten, and permeative. Combinations of these patterns are commonly seen in tumors. The most active pattern is the most significant one and should be used primarily in the analysis.

The geographic pattern (Fig. 88-15) of bone destruction reflects slow growth. The lesion is well circumscribed, and there is a narrow zone of transition from normal to abnormal bone. The margin is often, but not always, sclerotic. The presence and thickness of the sclerotic margin reflects slow growth or even absence of growth. Most lesions with this pattern of destruction are benign. A lesion showing geographic destruction with fading margins, or even cortical destruction, is more likely to be malignant.

The moth-eaten pattern of destruction is characterized by the presence of multiple, small, coalescing osteolytic areas (Fig. 88-16). Normal residual trabecular bone may be

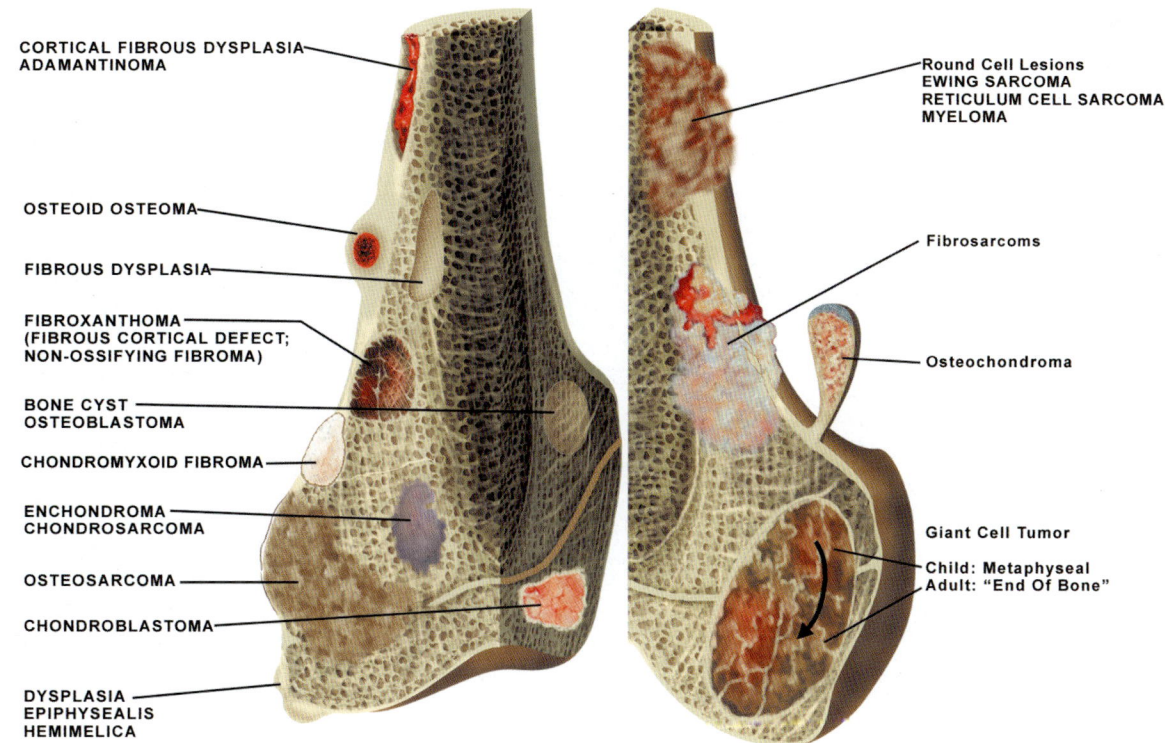

■ FIGURE 88-12 Diagram showing preferential locations of common tumors and tumor-like lesions within long bone. *(Adapted from Madewell JE, Ragsdale BD, Sweet DE: Radiologic and pathologic analysis of solitary bone lesions. Radiol Clin North Am 1981; 19:715–748.)*

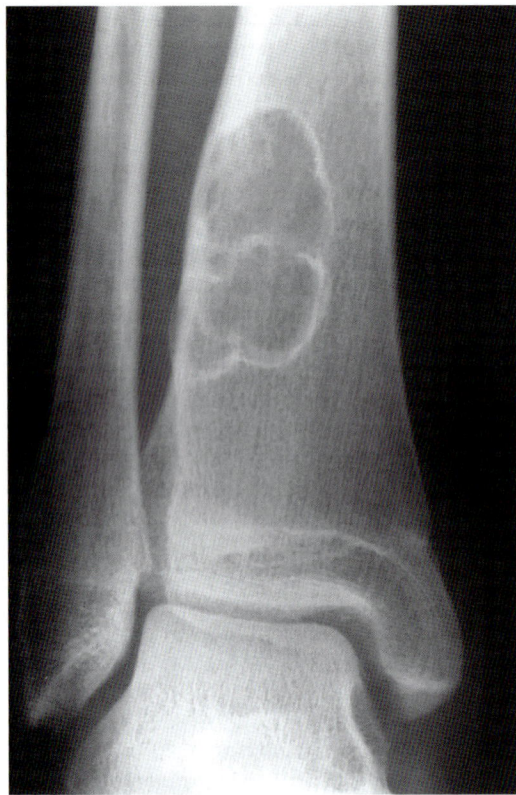

■ **FIGURE 88-13** Nonossifying fibroma in a young adolescent. The eccentric location relative to the axis of the long bone in combination with the lobulated sclerotic margin, intact cortical bone, solid new bone formation, and location in the region of the metadiaphysis are typical for the diagnosis. No biopsy is needed.

TABLE 88-16 Definitely Benign: No Further Action or Symptomatic Treatment Needed
Nonossifying fibroma/fibrous cortical defect
Normal variants
Post-traumatic sequelae
Bone island
Lipoma in calcaneus (see Fig. 88-14)
Osteochondroma (uncomplicated)
Dysplasia epiphysealis hemimelica
Hemangioma of the vertebral body
Enchondroma of the phalanges
Periosteal desmoid (irregularity in femur at origin of gastrocnemius muscle)
Bone infarction

seen within the lesion. Cortex may be partially destroyed. The margin is typically ill defined, and the zone of transition is fairly wide. This pattern reflects intermediate or even rapid growth and is a sign in favor of malignancy. Rapidly growing benign tumors such as giant cell tumor of bone may, however, also exhibit this type of destruction. Growth is too rapid for the host to be successful in containing the lesion. The permeative type of destruction is similar to the moth-eaten type, and distinction between the two serves no practical purpose (Fig. 88-17). The lucencies are larger, more confluent, and also more longitudinal. The margin is ill defined, and the zone of transition is wide. The true extent of the lesion often cannot be defined. These active or aggressive lesions are also characteristically malignant. Osteomyelitis is an example of a benign lesion that may be biologically very active and that may, as a consequence, display malignant features, including a moth-eaten or permeative type of bone destruction.

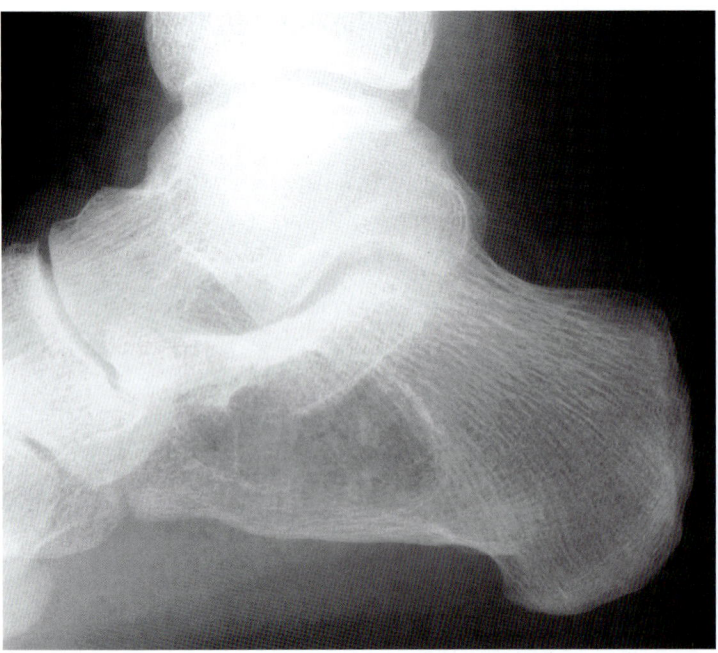

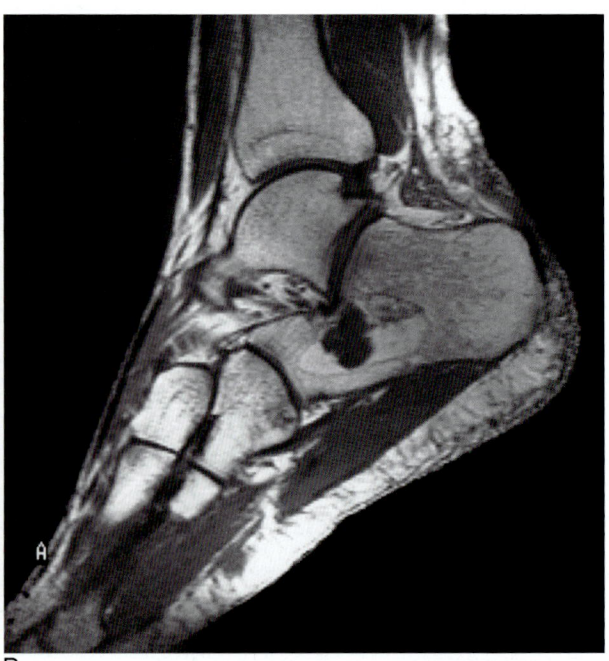

A   B

■ **FIGURE 88-14** **A,** This presentation of an oval osteolytic lesion with some calcifications along with a well-defined sclerotic margin located in the anterior part of the calcaneus is typical for an intraosseous lipoma. This is thought to be related to the location of the artery entering the calcaneus at this site. **B,** On the T1-weighted MR image the central cystic component has a low signal intensity whereas the peripheral fatty component has a high signal intensity.

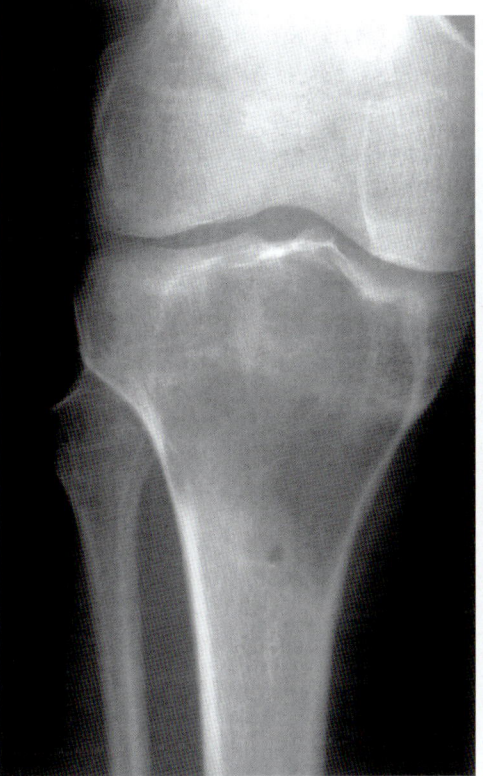
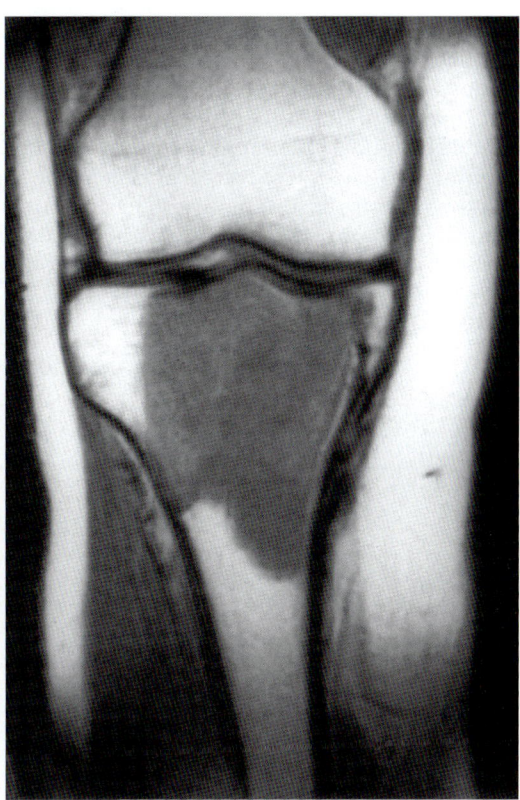

■ **FIGURE 88-15** **A,** Geographic pattern of bone destruction in giant cell tumor. The distal margin is not sclerotic but is well defined. The distal lucency is the biopsy tract. **B,** On the T1-weighted MR image the location of the margin is identical to that exhibited on the radiograph.

A

B

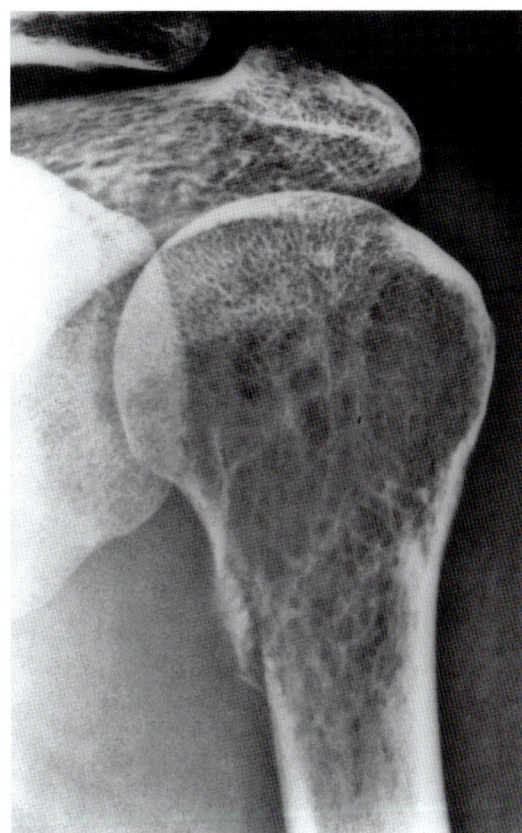

■ **FIGURE 88-16** Moth-eaten pattern of bone destruction with pathologic fracture in a giant cell tumor.

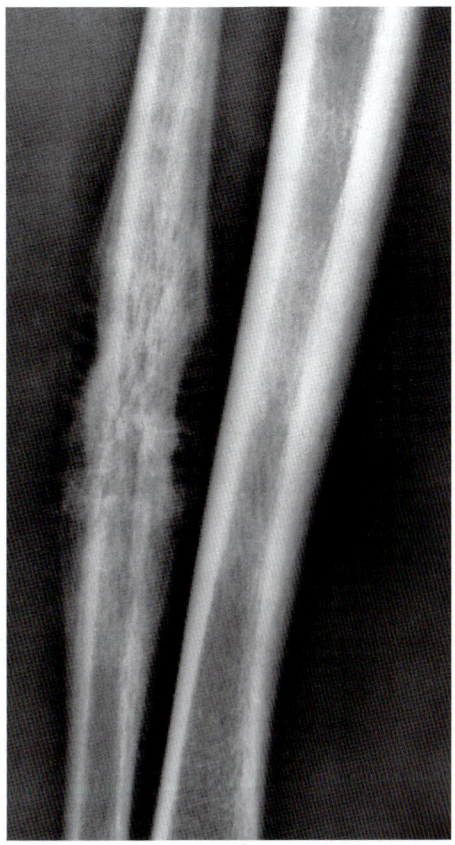

■ **FIGURE 88-17** Permeative pattern of bone destruction in a non-Hodgkin's lymphoma. Note also the spiculated interrupted periosteal reaction.

The periosteum consists of an outer fibrous layer and an inner cellular layer also called the cambium. When periosteum is thickened (cellular layer) or elevated from the cortical bone, it is visible on MRI as a separate structure. It is only visible on radiographs when elevated periosteum is ossified. Because of this delay of approximately 10 days, MRI is more sensitive to early periosteal reaction than radiography. Increased intramedullary pressure and cortical destruction initiate the formation of periosteal reaction in an attempt to contain the tumor or tumor-like lesion (e.g., infection) and to seal off the compartment in which the tumor originates. There are three types of periosteal reaction: continuous, interrupted, and complex (Fig. 88-18).[6]

When the tumor grows slowly the periosteum is successful in its attempt to contain the tumor. Cortex is (partially) destroyed, and an intact single or lamellar pattern of periosteal reaction is observed and forms the new cortex

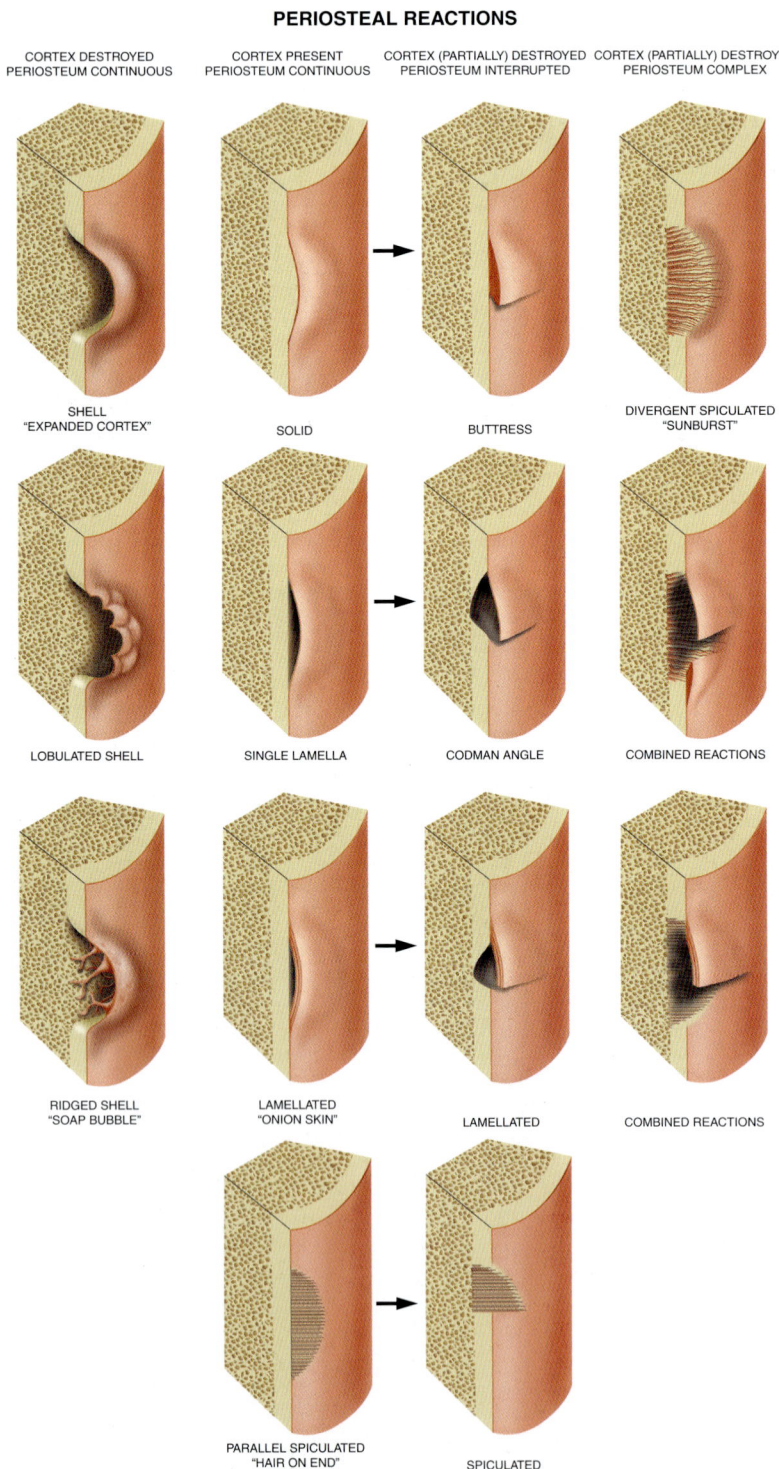

PERIOSTEAL REACTIONS

CORTEX DESTROYED PERIOSTEUM CONTINUOUS — SHELL "EXPANDED CORTEX", LOBULATED SHELL, RIDGED SHELL "SOAP BUBBLE"

CORTEX PRESENT PERIOSTEUM CONTINUOUS — SOLID, SINGLE LAMELLA, LAMELLATED "ONION SKIN", PARALLEL SPICULATED "HAIR ON END"

CORTEX (PARTIALLY) DESTROYED PERIOSTEUM INTERRUPTED — BUTTRESS, CODMAN ANGLE, LAMELLATED, SPICULATED

CORTEX (PARTIALLY) DESTROYED PERIOSTEUM COMPLEX — DIVERGENT SPICULATED "SUNBURST", COMBINED REACTIONS, COMBINED REACTIONS

■ **FIGURE 88-18** Diagram of the various types of periosteal reaction. *(Reprinted with permission from Ragsdale BD, Madewell JE, Sweet DE. Radiologic and pathologic analysis of solitary bone lesions: II. Periosteal reaction. Radiol Clin North Am 1981; 19:749–783.)*

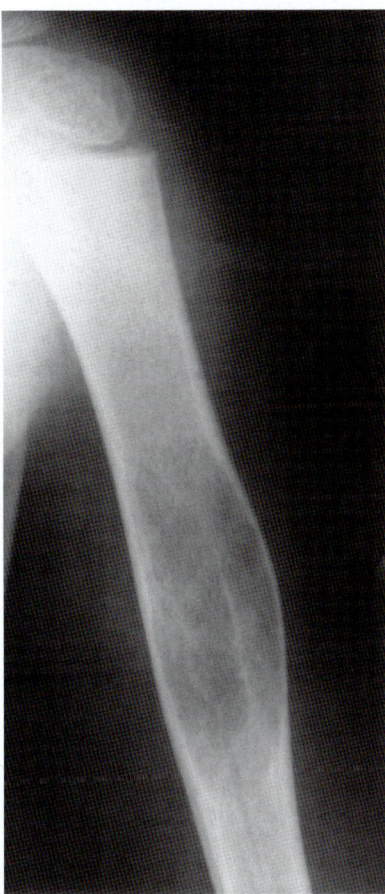

■ **FIGURE 88-19** A thin, but intact new cortex has developed that contains the intraosseous lesion (fibrous dysplasia).

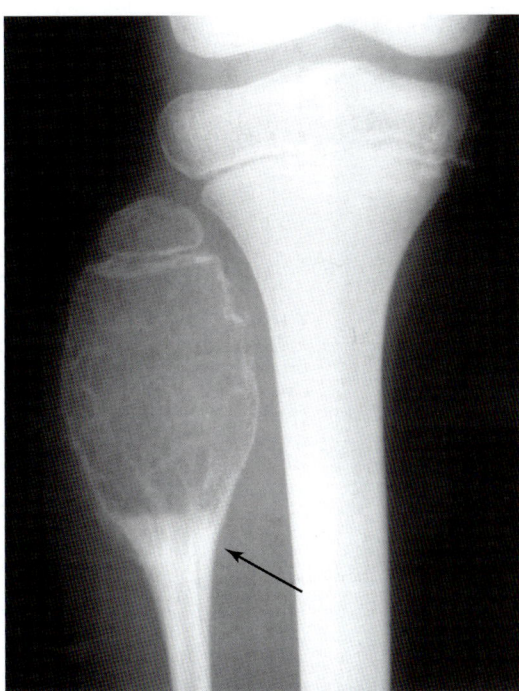

■ FIGURE 88-20 The new cortex is as thin as an eggshell in this aneurysmal bone cyst. This is also referred to as ballooning. Note the thickened sclerotic triangle of periosteal bone distally, also referred to as buttressing, or reactive triangle (*arrow*).

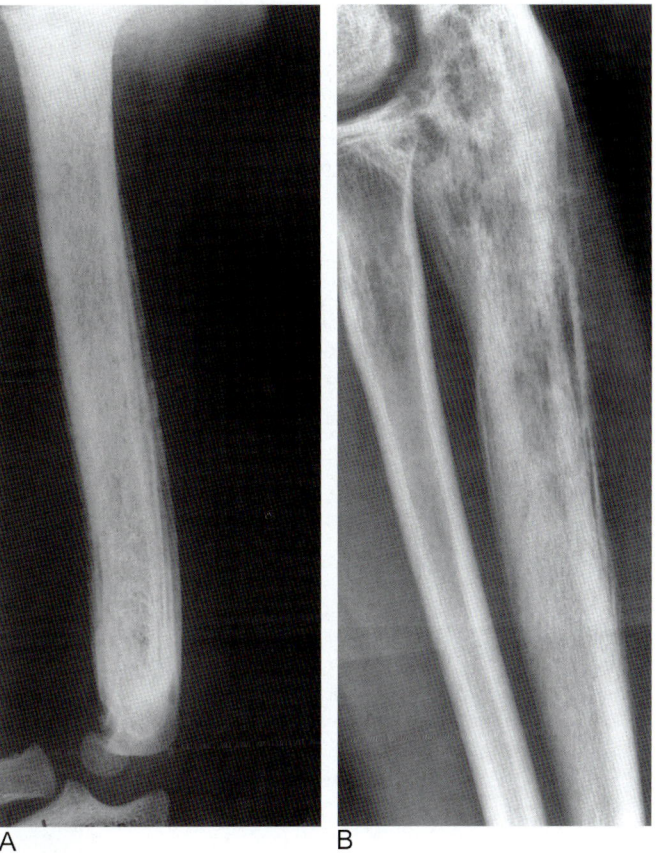

A   B

■ **FIGURE 88-21** **A,** Lamellated periosteal reaction in neuroblastoma. Proximally the periosteal reaction is interrupted. More distally the lamellated periosteal bone is intact. **B,** The lamellated periosteal reaction is clearly interrupted in this patient with osteomyelitis.

(Figs. 88-19 and 88-20). It is a single layer in slowly growing tumors. This is also referred to as ballooning when the new cortex is thin. Thin shells are seen in benign lesions such as aneurysmal bone cyst and giant cell tumor but also in vascular metastases. The periosteal new bone may be so thin (e.g., aneurysmal bone cyst) that it can only be appreciated as being continuous on CT. A solid buttress may accompany an intact shell in active benign conditions. The slower the growth, the thicker the continuous layer, which may even be completely merged with underlying cortex. Continuous periosteal reaction is seen not only in benign lesions but also in low-grade malignancies such as chondrosarcoma. There are multiple layers (lamellated, onion skin) when growth of the tumor is discontinuous. This pattern is also frequently seen in osteomyelitis.

When periosteum is not successful in containing the tumor, the single or multiple layers are interrupted (Fig. 88-21). This is a sign of rapid growth and is often seen in malignancy. When the tumor grows rapidly, the elevated periosteum is usually interrupted and linear ossifications are seen bridging the gap between original bone and elevated periosteum. This is also referred to as spiculation or "hair on end" (Fig. 88-22). The spiculated type of periosteal reaction is, especially in the cranial vault, also commonly seen in thalassemia or sickle cell anemia.

Codman's triangle is also seen in very rapidly growing malignant tumors (Fig. 88-23). Tumor grows on both sites

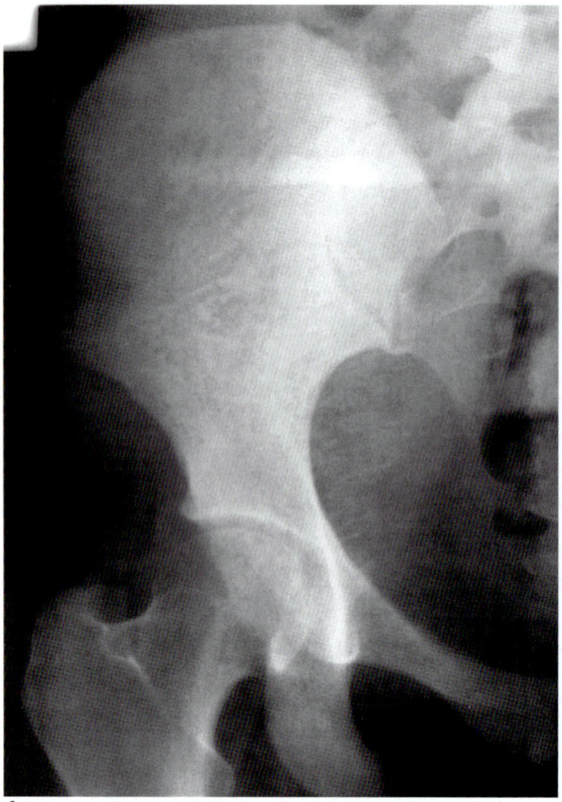

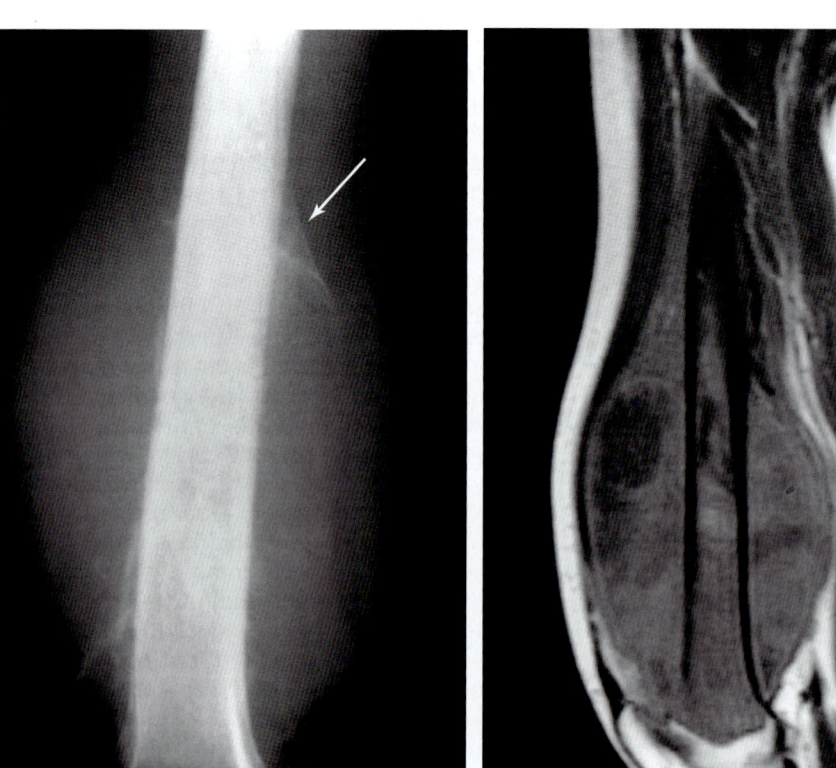

■ **FIGURE 88-22** Spiculated periosteal reaction in an osteosarcoma of the iliac bone is well seen on the radiograph (**A**) and CT (**B**) and MR (**C**) images.

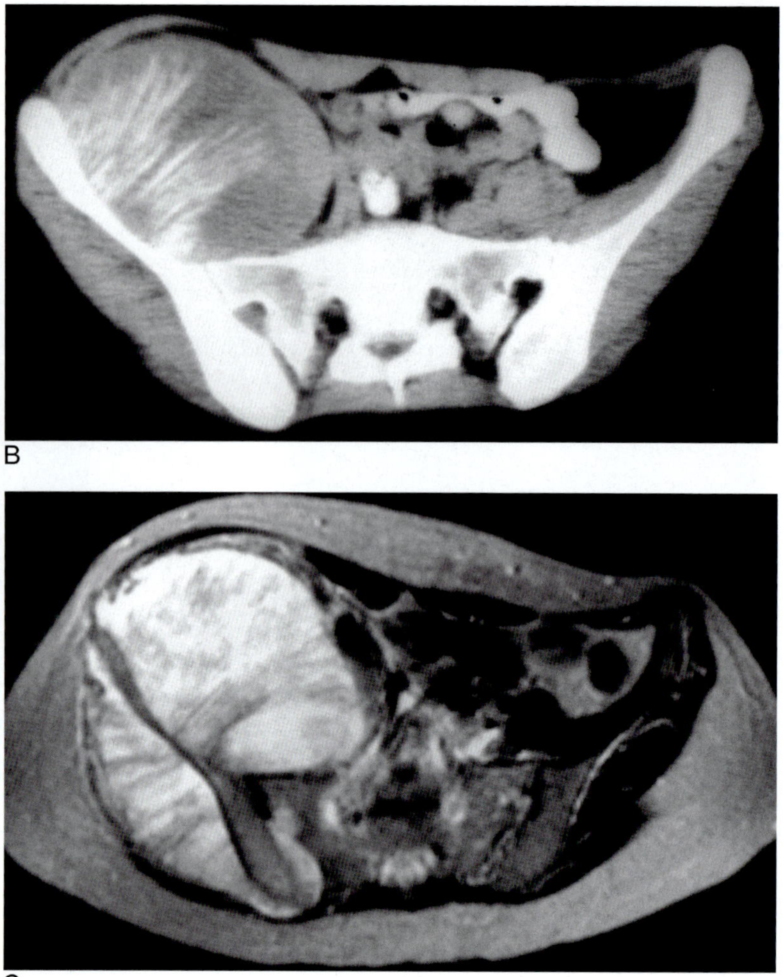

A

B

C

■ **FIGURE 88-23** Interrupted, irregular periosteal reaction is seen in this osteosarcoma. Note the elevated periosteal new bone at the proximal dorsal side forming Codman's triangle (*arrow*). This can be appreciated on the radiograph (**A**) and on the sagittal T1-weighted MR image (**B**).

A

B

of the cortex, and periosteum is elevated and interrupted. A cuff of ossified periosteum remains where the periosteum is lifted of the cortex. The complex types of periosteal reaction are a combination of various interrupted periosteal reactions and are indicative of malignancy.

Tumors may contain intercellular matrix formed by mesenchymal cells; this is referred to as tumor matrix. Osteoblasts create osteoid, chondroblasts create chondroid and myxoid, and fibroblasts create collagen. Mineralization of osteoid in osteosarcoma looks more like bone on radiographs than calcification in the chondroid matrix of cartilaginous tumors (Figs. 88-24 and 88-25). The appearance of matrix is addressed in other chapters, and these patterns may assist in making a specific diagnosis.

Extracompartmental extension of tumor is a sign of rapid growth that indicates the presence of malignancy. The presence of soft tissue extension can often be diagnosed on radiographs. MRI is used to identify and localize soft tissue extension (see Chapter 98) and to visualize invasion of other compartments such as muscular compartments and other structures.

Multiplicity is used in making a differential diagnosis. Multiplicity in combination with radiographic appearance may further narrow the differential diagnosis (Tables 88-17 and 88-18).

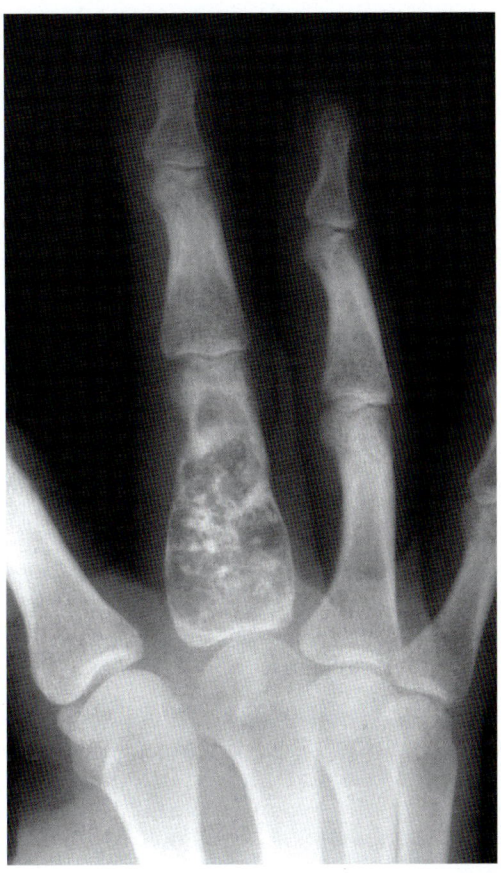

■ FIGURE 88-25   Linear and popcorn calcifications in chondroid tumor matrix are seen in this enchondroma of the proximal phalanx.

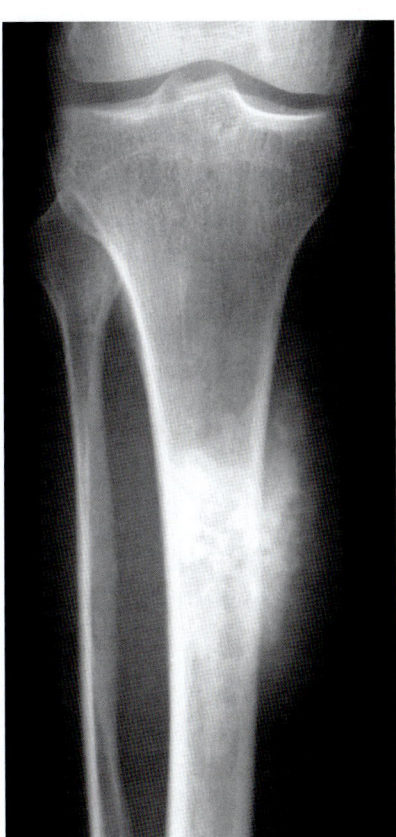

A   B

■ FIGURE 88-24   **A,** Osteoid matrix is seen in bone and soft tissue extension of this osteosarcoma. **B,** Because osteoid formation implies osteoblast activity, osteoid is seen on technetium-99 m bone scintigraphy because of increased tracer uptake. Metastases forming osteoid are therefore also depicted on bone scintigraphy.

TABLE 88-17   Common Multiple Osteolytic Benign Lesions
Cystic lesions in joint disease
Amyloidosis
Brown tumors in hyperparathyroidism
Enchondromatosis
Fibrous dysplasia
Osteomyelitis (including tuberculosis, hydatid, sarcoid, etc.)
Massive osteolysis (Gorham)
Mastocytosis
Neurofibromatosis
Langerhans cell histiocytosis (histiocytosis X)

TABLE 88-18   Common Multiple Osteosclerotic Benign Lesions
Bone infarcts
Bone islands
Callus
Osteomyelitis (chronic, multifocal)
Paget's disease
Fibrous dysplasia
Enchondromatosis
Mastocytosis
Matured benign lesions (e.g., nonossifying fibromas)
Osteomas (Gardner's syndrome)
Osteopathia striata
Osteopoikilosis

Magnetic Resonance Imaging

Cellularity, interstitial pressure, liquefaction, necrosis, hemorrhage, and specific components such as presence of osteoid, mature fat, collagen, or melanin are important in understanding the MRI appearance of the tumor itself. Characteristically, the tumor has prolonged T1 and T2 relaxation times, resulting in low signal intensity on T1-weighted and high signal intensity on T2-weighted MR images. Details and exceptions to this rule of thumb are discussed in the chapters dedicated to specific tumor types. The most important exceptions are listed in Tables 88-19 and 88-20 (Figs. 88-26 and 88-27).

Fluid-fluid levels are not very helpful in narrowing the differential diagnosis because they may occur not only in aneurysmal bone cyst but also in giant cell tumor, fibrous dysplasia, chondroblastoma, simple bone cyst, intraosseous lipoma, osteosarcoma, malignant fibrous histiocytoma, spindle cell sarcoma, and even osteomyelitis.[7] Most tumors are fairly well defined on MRI because of the presence of a pseudocapsule. An ill-defined reactive tissue zone, consisting of inflammatory tissue and edema, is frequently seen outside the pseudocapsule of sarcoma. Such a reactive tissue zone, however, is no sign of malignancy. It actually is more frequently found in benign conditions, especially in osteoid osteoma, chondroblastoma, Langerhans cell histiocytosis (eosinophilic granuloma), and osteomyelitis.[8] In stress fractures the MRI appearance may, erroneously, suggest the diagnosis of malignancy owing to the overwhelming reactive changes.

Appearance of enhancement patterns on dynamic and static MRI are determined by cardiac output, vessel density or total surface area, vessel leakage (tumor vessels lack a muscular wall and contain large endothelial gaps), interstitial pressure, and volume of interstitial space. Although the impact of these factors can be manipulated by the type and especially the size of contrast agents used, the commonly used extracellular-interstitial Gd-chelates reflect all these functions. Although most soft tissue sarcomas enhance fast (see Chapter 93), this is not the case in osseous tumors.[9] In bone, dynamic enhancement patterns play a role in cartilaginous tumors and giant cell tumor (see chapters on specific tumors), in monitoring response to therapy (see Chapter 99), and sometimes in staging (see Chapter 98).

Multidetector Computed Tomography

Magnetic resonance imaging has limited the role of CT to specific, but important, situations. The spatial resolution of MDCT is superior to that of MRI. As a consequence, CT may be used to visualize small tumors or anatomic structures that are not well visualized on MRI. The best example is visualizing osteoid osteoma. The nidus may be obscured by the vast reactive changes consisting of inflammatory tissue, edema, and reactive bone formation. A dedicated CT of the area with reactive changes as visualized by either MRI or technetium-99 m bone scintigraphy may be the only way to visualize the nidus of osteoid osteoma. The spatial resolution may also be used to visualize benign lesions to allow for surgical planning.

CT may also be used to visualize bone in detail in areas of complex anatomy such as in the spine and pelvis.

Finally, CT is commonly use to provide image guidance when osseous lesions are sampled.

Nuclear Medicine

Bone scintigraphy uses technetium-99 m–labeled phosphate compounds to visualize osteoblast activity on measurements taken 2 to 3 hours after intravenous injection of the tracer. The tracer interacts with hydroxyapatite crystals that are deposited on osteoid by osteoblasts. Bone scintigraphy is much more sensitive than radiographic techniques to this process because only small amounts of tracer are needed in the crystals, whereas a large volume of calcium in the newly formed osteoid is needed to be visualized by radiography or CT. In addition, earlier measurements, for instance taken 5 minutes after intravenous administration of the tracer, reflect blood flow.

TABLE 88-20 Lesions with High MR Signal Intensity on T1-Weighted Images	
Type of Lesion	**Histologic Reason**
Lipoma	Mature fat
Well-differentiated liposarcoma	Well-differentiated fat
Periphery in subacute hemorrhage	Methemoglobin
Hemangioma (mature)	Fatty marrow
Melanoma	Melanin

TABLE 88-19 Lesions with Low MR Signal Intensity on T2-Weighted Images	
Type of Lesion	**Histologic Reason**
Aggressive fibromatosis	Collagen
Osteosarcoma	Ossified, low cellularity osteoid
Old hemorrhage	Hemosiderin
Calcifications in various tumors	Dystrophic calcifications
Bone islands, osteoma	Osteoid
Mature nonossifying fibroma	Fibrous tissue, collagen

Classic Signs: Signs in Favor of Malignancy

- Multifocal disease
- Age older than 40 years
- Moth-eaten or permeative type of bone destruction
- Wide zone of transition
- Osteoid formation
- Cortical interruption with or without periosteal reaction
- Interrupted periosteal reaction
- Codman's triangle
- Spiculated periosteal reaction
- Lamellated periosteal reaction (onion skin)
- Extracompartmental extension

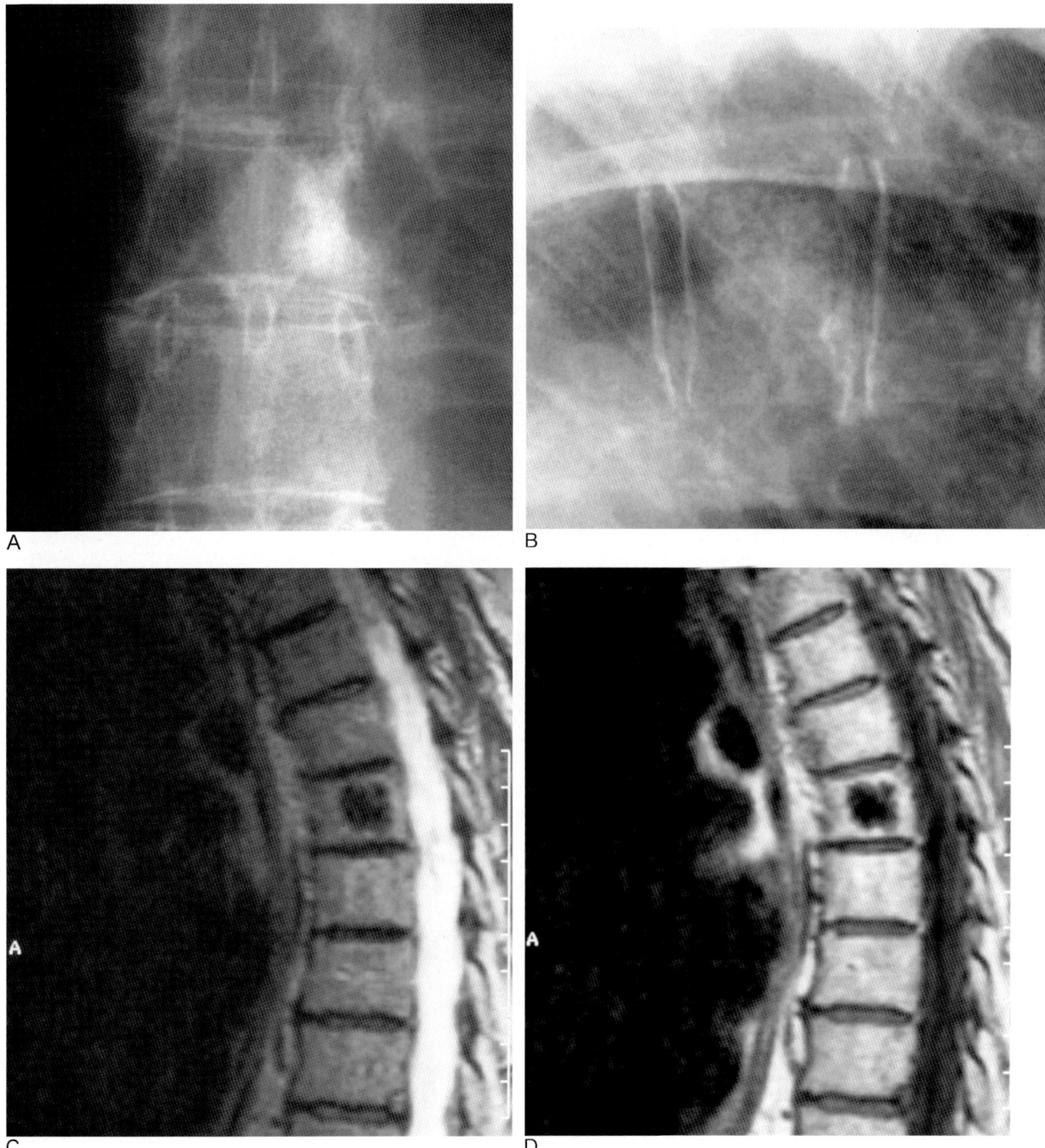

■ **FIGURE 88-26** **A** and **B,** Osteoma is seen as a sclerotic lesion on radiographs. It has a low signal intensity on T2-weighted (**C**) and T1-weighted (**D**) MR images.

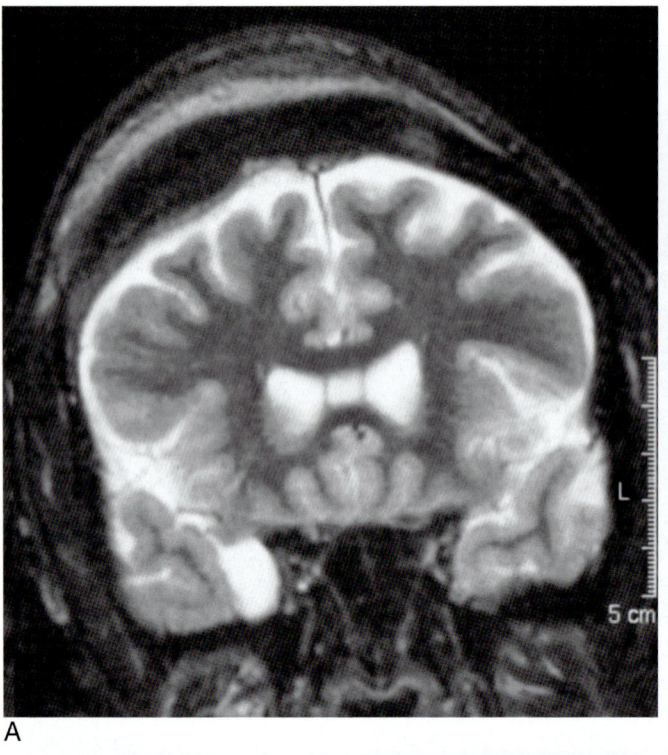

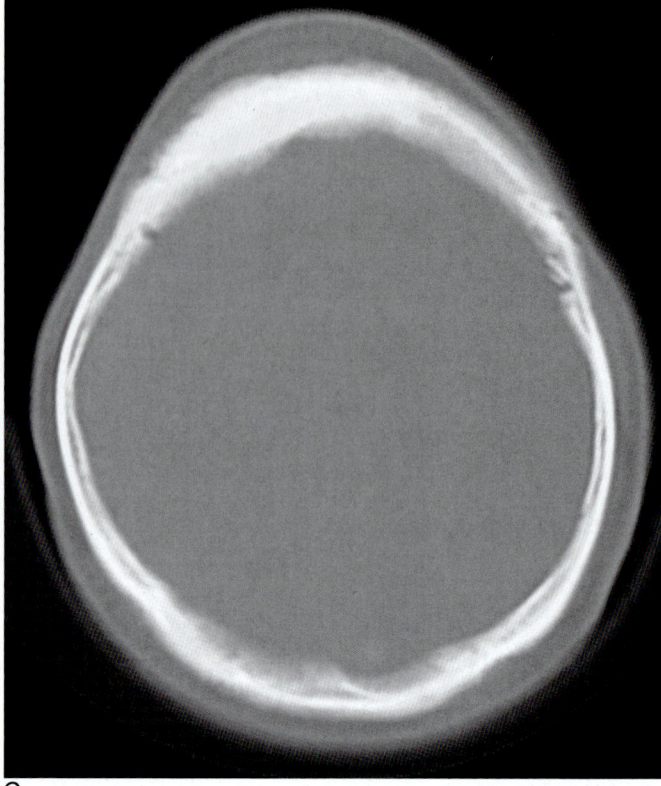

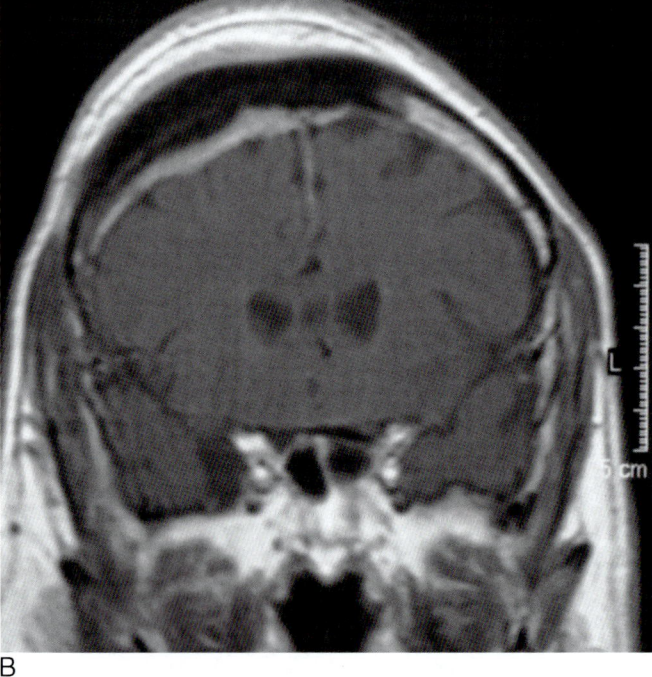

■ **FIGURE 88-27** **A,** On this T2-weighted MR image reactive bone is seen thickening the calvaria. The solid bone formation, which is reactive to meningioma en plaque, has low signal intensity. **B,** The signal intensity remains low on the Gd-DTPA enhanced image. Meningioma is enhancing. **C,** Solid reactive bone is also well seen on CT.

Because of the described mechanism, bone scintigraphy is a very sensitive method to detect primary and secondary osseous tumors. Bone scintigraphy has a poor sensitivity when osteoblast activity is insufficient, as in myeloma, metastases of renal cell, and thyroid cancer, or in general when the tumor grows too fast.

The main advantage of bone scintigraphy is its high sensitivity while imaging the entire body. It is thus mainly used to identify multifocal or diffuse disease (see Chapter 96) or to increase sensitivity of images, usually radiographs, when these are thought to be falsely negative. The main disadvantages are lack of anatomic resolution, low specificity, and dependency on osteoblast activity. For these reasons, positron emission tomography and MRI are also used for the traditional bone scintigraphy indications mentioned earlier. The expanding role of MRI is described in Chapters 91 and 96.

DIFFERENTIAL DIAGNOSIS

Laboratory tests have, with some exceptions, little to contribute to diagnosing bone tumors. There may be nonspecific abnormalities, such as elevated erythrocyte sedimentation rates, that reflect the inflammatory host's response to the presence of disease. Serum calcium levels increase secondary to destruction of bone. Beta-crosslaps are components of type 1 collagen of which increased serum concentrations can be measured secondary to increased osteoclast activity and ensuing increase of bone resorption. When there is marked bone turnover and osteoblast activity, alkaline phosphatase levels are increased. P1NP is a peptide of which increased serum concentrations can be measured secondary to increased osteoblast activity. An osteolytic lesion may be associated with increased alkaline phosphatase when other lesions (metastases, Paget's disease) are present or when growth of tumor is too rapid to allow the formation of reactive bone. Specific abnormalities may be found in multiple myeloma and in various metastases such as metastases from prostate cancer. Also in tumor-like lesions such as brown tumors in patients with hyperparathyroidism, elevated calcium and phosphorus levels are important in making a diagnosis and in differentiating brown tumor from giant cell tumor.

SYNOPSIS OF TREATMENT OPTIONS

As described in detail in Chapters 97 and 98, distinction has to be made between the various goals of treatment. This may be curative or palliative. Ablative surgery is the core of treatment. The importance of local staging is illustrated by the fact that limb salvage is preferred over amputation. Surgery can be supported by presurgical (neoadjuvant), or postsurgical (adjuvant) chemotherapy. Radiotherapy also is an important line of treatment that can be used in combination with surgery and chemotherapy, or it may be the only form of treatment.

What the Referring Physician Needs to Know

■ In what category (definitely benign/possibly benign/possibly malignant/definitely malignant) does the lesion belong?
■ What is the differential diagnosis?
■ Is there discordance between radiologic and histologic diagnosis?
■ Is a subsequent radiologic procedure required?

SUGGESTED READINGS

Bloem JL, van der Woude HJ, Geirnaerdt MJ, et al. Bone tumors. Eur Radiol 2000; 10:207-212.

Lodwick GS. A probabilistic approach to the diagnosis of bone tumors. Radiol Clin North Am 1965; 3:487-497.

Madewell JE, Ragsdale BD, Sweet DE. Radiologic and pathologic analysis of solitary bone lesions: I. Internal margins. Radiol Clin North Am 1981; 19:715-748.

Morrison WB, Dalinka MK, Daffner RH, et al. ACR appropriateness criteria: Bone tumors. Available at http://www.acr.org/s_acr/bin.asp?CID=1206(DID=11778(DOC=FILE.PDF.

Mulder JD, Schutte HE, Kroon HM, Taconis WK. Radiologic Atlas of Bone Tumors. Amsterdam, Elsevier, 1993.

Peterson JJ, Bancroft LW, Kransdorf MJ. Principles of tumor imaging. Eur J Radiol 2005; 56:319-330.

Ragsdale BD, Madewell JE, Sweet DE. Radiologic and pathologic analysis of solitary bone lesions: II. Periosteal reactions. Radiol Clin North Am 1981; 19:749-783.

Sweet DE, Madewell JE, Ragsdale BD. Radiologic and pathologic analysis of solitary bone lesions: III. Matrix patterns 1981; 19:785-814.

REFERENCES

1. Haddad MC, Sharif HS, Aideyan OA, et al. Infection versus neoplasm in the spine: differentiation by MRI and diagnostic pitfalls. Eur Radiol 1993; 3:439-446.

2. Moser RP, Madewell JE. An approach to primary bone tumors. Radiol Clin North Am 1987; 25:1049-1093.

3. Lonergan GJ, Schwab CM, Suarez ES, Carlson CL. From the archives of the AFIP: neuroblastoma, ganglioneuroblastoma, and ganglioneuroma: radiologic-pathologic correlation. RadioGraphics 2002; 22:911-934.

4. Oudenhoven LF, Dhondt E, Kahn S, et al. Accuracy of radiography in grading and tissue-specific diagnosis—a study of 200 consecutive bone tumors of the hand. Skeletal Radiol. 2006; 35:78-87.

5. Edelstyn GA, Gillespie PJ, Grebbel FS. The radiological demonstration of osseous metastases: experimental observations. Clin Radiol 1967; 18:158-162.

6. Ragsdale BD, Madewell JE, Sweet DE. Radiologic and pathologic analysis of solitary bone lesions: II. Periosteal reaction. Radiol Clin North Am 1981; 19:749-783.

7. Van Dyck P, Vanhoenacker FM, Vogel J, et al. Prevalence, extension and characteristics of fluid-fluid levels in bone and soft tissue tumors. Eur Radiol 2006; 16(12):2644-2651.

8. Kroon HM, Bloem JL, Holscher HC, et al. MR imaging of edema accompanying benign and malignant bone tumours. Skeletal Radiol 1994; 23:261-269.

9. van der Woude HJ, Verstraete KL, Hogendoorn PC, et al. Musculoskeletal tumors: does fast dynamic contrast-enhanced subtraction MR imaging contribute to the characterization? Radiology 1998; 208:821-828.

89

The Patient with a Soft Tissue Lump

Gina Allen

When someone notices a soft tissue lump it is inevitable that he or she will be worried and fearful until it is known what it is. The patient may have discovered the lump, or it may have been felt or noticed by a relative. Masses may be incidental findings during a physical examination by a medical practitioner who was performing an evaluation for an unrelated problem. Lumps that are painful, either because they are stretching sensitive tissues or because they are compressing nerves, are usually detected by the patient much earlier than the more common painless masses.

The clinical assessment of a soft tissue swelling can be very inaccurate. The history is important; if the lump has been present for a long period of time this would suggest that it is a benign lesion. A lump that is rapidly growing is of more concern to both patient and clinician and should be imaged urgently. Fortunately, malignant lesions are rare and, therefore, most soft tissue lesions are usually benign.[1]

The family physician is usually the first person to see a patient with a lump and may be able to reassure the patient that the lesion is benign on the basis of history, palpation, transillumination, and auscultation. The percentage of soft tissue lumps that are sent for imaging in the United Kingdom is not known, and the number of soft tissue lumps that are seen by family physicians when the patient is reassured has not been documented. Experience suggests that there are many mass lesions that are never seen by imagers or else we would spend a lot more time scanning lumps!

The important questions to pose when diagnosing the cause of a soft tissue lump are:

- Does the patient have a lesion rather than asymmetry or a normal variant (recognition)?
- What is the lesion composed of (define shape and structure)?
- What does it arise from?
- How big is it?
- Has it spread?
- Should a biopsy be done?

IMAGING TECHNIQUES

Recognition

The first role of imaging is to decide whether the patient does have a lump. Some lesions are due to normal asymmetry of the patient. This can be due to the patient having a strong right or left side dominance, resulting in muscle enlargement on the dominant side that can cause asymmetry, which is sometimes misinterpreted as a lesion. There can be asymmetry of tissue due to the presence of an asymmetric normal variant, such as an accessory muscle (see also Chapter 100).

Radiographs have little to offer in the diagnosis of a soft tissue lesion. They may show some calcification within the lesion. They may identify whether it is arising from bone, or they may suggest that it is of long standing because there is some erosion of adjacent bone. The majority of palpable swellings are due to soft tissue abnormality, and radiographs do not directly image the true abnormality. Sometimes if the lesion is due to fatty tissue and is large there may be some hyperlucency within the soft tissue on the radiograph, but often there is little to see, because small fat-containing lesions will be obscured on a two-dimensional image. Note that most liposarcomas do not have enough fat to demonstrate this sign.

Ultrasonography

Ultrasonography is the ideal means of screening soft tissue mass lesions.[2] It is very patient friendly, being neither painful nor frightening. The examiner must spend time with the patient, and the nature of the examination allows the patient to show the examiner the location of the swelling. This means that the examination can be directed exactly at the site of the patient's concern.

Ultrasonography is particularly useful in children; ionizing radiation is avoided and there is no need for the prolonged immobility needed for MRI. In many children, MRI may be possible only with the use of sedation or anesthesia. With ultrasonography the trust of both the child and the parent can be gained, and the experience of an ultrasound examination is usually far less psychologically traumatic than other forms of imaging. The greatest strength of ultrasonography is its ability to distinguish a cystic from a solid lesion (Table 89-1). An anechoic lesion with acoustic enhancement seen behind the lesion is a cystic lesion (Fig. 89-1).

Sometimes the use of ultrasound allows the examiner to fully reassure the patient that the lump is a benign lesion that needs no further investigation, for example, a small subcutaneous lipoma or a ganglion cyst in the popliteal fossa.

TABLE 89-1 Ultrasound Appearance of Cystic versus Solid Lesion

	Solid	Cystic
Echogenicity	Either hypoechoic, isoechoic, or hyperechoic	Anechoic
Acoustic enhancement behind lesion	Not usually; some nerve tumors may have	Present unless a very small lesion
Movement of contents on bouncing the probe on the skin	Never	Commonly present
Vascularity	May be within the lesion or absent	Never seen centrally unless artifact from movement of contents

Other benign lesions that can be excluded are muscle hernias (Fig. 89-2),[3] which are rarely visible using other imaging techniques, small foreign bodies (Fig. 89-3),[4] which have a characteristic appearance on ultrasonography, the presence of asymmetry of fatty tissue, or the presence of a normal variant. Ultrasound examination is an especially useful imaging technique because the patient can be shown the images during the study, thus enabling much more effective reassurance.

Ultrasonography is particularly useful for lumps less than 5 cm in diameter in the first 10 cm below the skin because high-resolution linear array probes can be used. Larger and deeper lumps can be seen by ultrasound using curvilinear array probes or on more modern apparatuses by using extended field-of-view technology, which builds up a composite picture along the length of a lesion (Fig. 89-4).

The presence of early calcification can be identified owing to the presence of acoustic shadowing behind the lesion. Ultrasonography is probably much more sensitive than radiography in the detection of calcium. The presence of vascularity within a lesion will not determine whether the lump is benign or malignant.

A vascular malformation can be identified on ultrasonography by the presence of serpiginous low signal intensity surrounded by high echogenicity, which is due to the presence of fat around the vessels. Some vascular malformations may have a predominance of slow flowing blood within them because they are mainly venous. In these lesions the use of compression of the lesion with the ultrasound probe while using color Doppler imaging can confirm the diagnosis because flow will be seen to fill all the serpiginous areas on releasing the pressure. These areas will not show flow within them using static color flow Doppler imaging or with conventional angiography or MR angiography. It may be possible to occlude the vessels in small lesions by the use of compression, a sign that will also be visible when using color Doppler imaging. This is a technique that sonographers also use for the detection of deep vein thrombosis.

Magnetic Resonance Imaging

Magnetic resonance imaging is the next best imaging technique for the screening of soft tissue abnormality and the best for staging its spread (see Chapter 98). It will show the extent of the lesion in detail and will also show bone marrow involvement. The lesion can be marked by the technician/radiographer who is performing the examination by a water/oil capsule to aid localization of the abnormality. Some lesions can be diagnosed confidently with MRI, for example, uniform areas of fat, which show absence of signal intensity using spectral fat suppression (see Chapters 93 and 94). One of the potential pitfalls when using MRI is the recognition of fluid versus a solid lesion. Sometimes a solid lesion with high water content can be misinterpreted as cystic. The use of intravenous contrast agents may confirm that the lesion is solid when enhancement is seen.[5] Alternatively, ultrasound can be used to further characterize a lesion found on non–contrast-enhanced MRI. The main advantage of MRI over ultrasonography is its ability to display

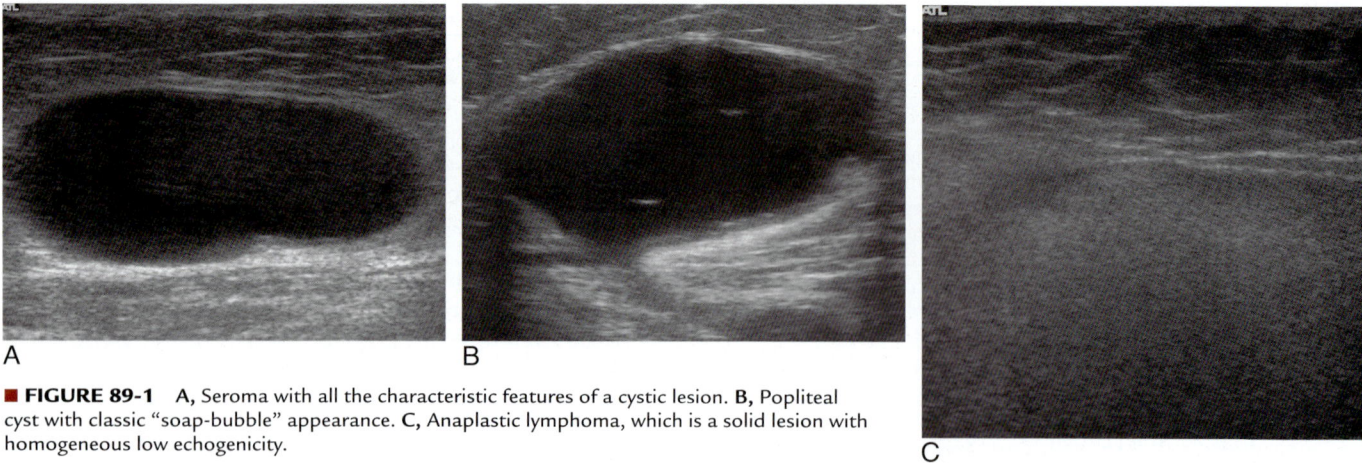

■ **FIGURE 89-1** **A,** Seroma with all the characteristic features of a cystic lesion. **B,** Popliteal cyst with classic "soap-bubble" appearance. **C,** Anaplastic lymphoma, which is a solid lesion with homogeneous low echogenicity.

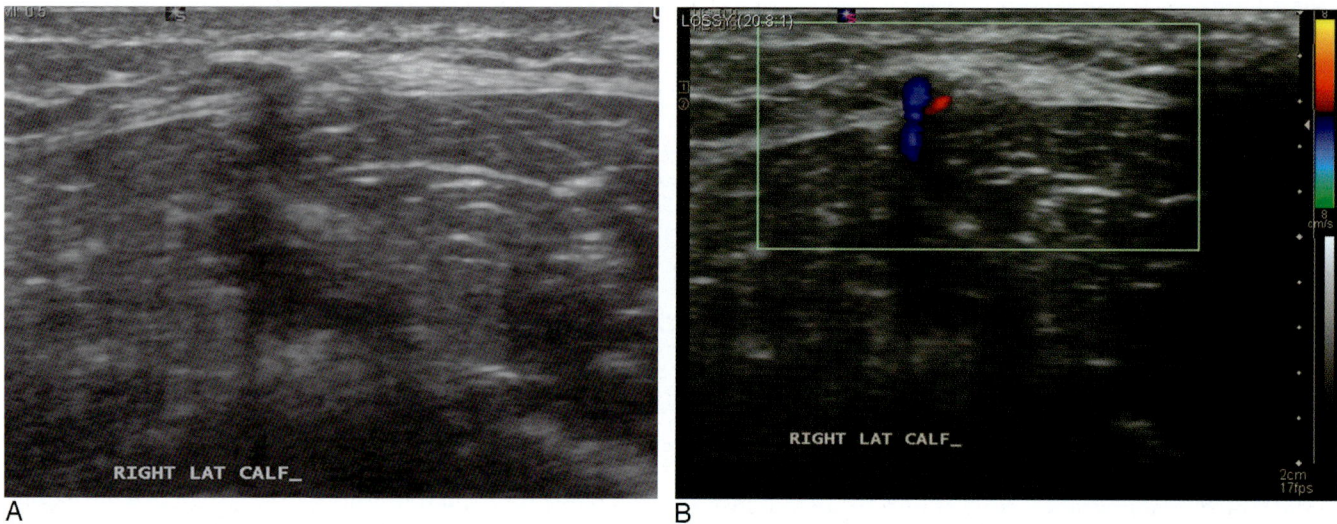

■ **FIGURE 89-2** **A,** Muscle hernia through a fascial plane of the peroneal muscles. **B,** Color Doppler image shows perforating vessels at the same site.

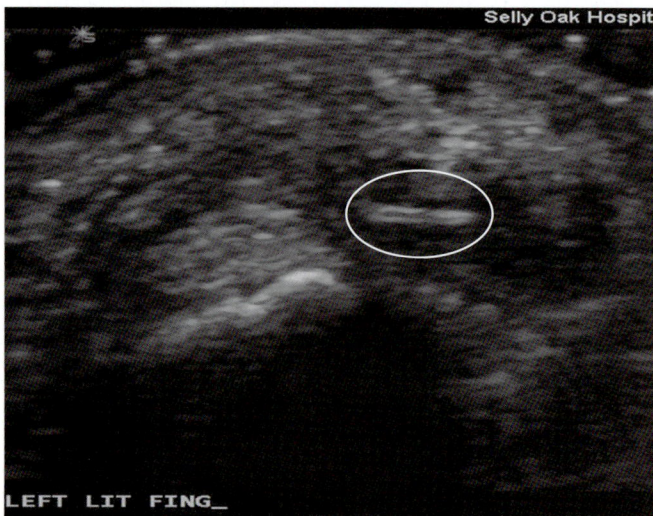

■ **FIGURE 89-3** Foreign body is seen next to flexor tendon. An oval surrounds the foreign body.

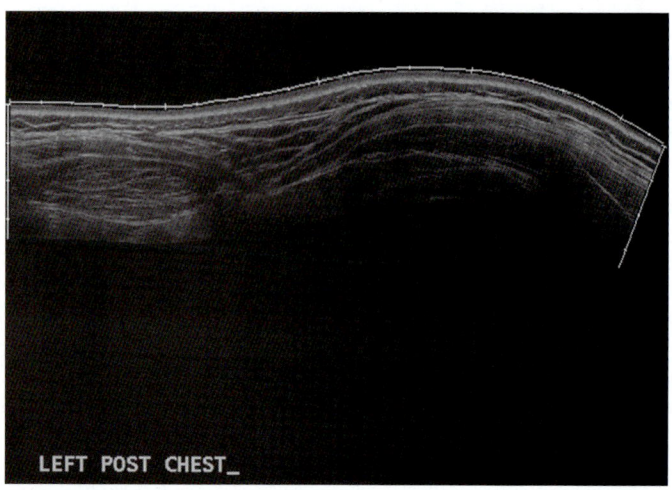

■ **FIGURE 89-4** Extended field-of-view sonogram of lipoma within the left erector spinae muscle; the right side is normal.

the lesion in relation to its surroundings, including bone (staging), but disadvantages include a patient's claustrophobia and the inability to safely examine patients who have intracranial aneurysm clips and pacemakers. With the growing obesity of the world's population a number of patients will not be able to have an MRI in a conventional MR scanner because they are too big to fit into the bore of the magnet!

Computed Tomography

Computed tomography is at best a modest means of imaging soft tissue. It has the same positive and negative attributes of radiographs, although reconstruction will allow a three-dimensional appearance. It may identify calcification in the presence of a lesion such as myositis ossificans, and it will demonstrate the pattern of calcium distribution. It will also show destruction of bone.[6] Unfortunately, CT cannot reliably show the true extent of the soft tissue lesion and, indeed, occasionally soft tissue lesions may be missed using CT. If circumstances mean that CT is the only way of imaging in cross section, then the use of an intravenous contrast agent can help improve the conspicuity of the lesion. CT will, as with radiographs, show fat as a low-attenuation lesion, which sometimes can be diagnostic (Fig. 89-5).

MANIFESTATIONS OF THE DISEASE

Defining the Shape and Structure of a Lesion

Ultrasonography can be confidently used to determine whether a lesion is cystic or solid (see Table 89-1). Ultrasonography gives a specific appearance of a low echogenic lesion with acoustic enhancement behind it. The use of compression in the assessment of a fluid filled lesion can also be helpful where swirling of the contents can be observed.

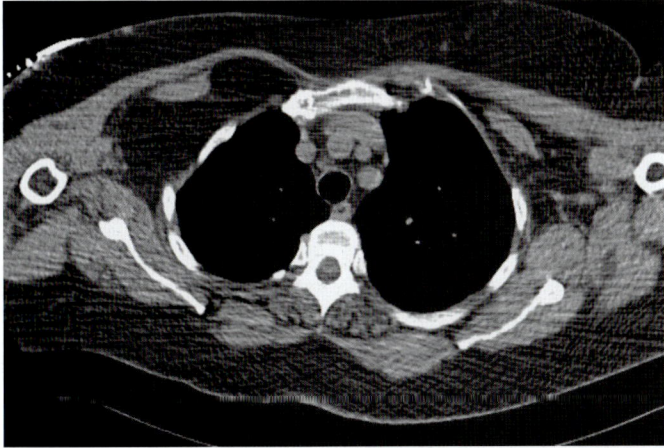

■ FIGURE 89-5 CT scan of a lipomatous tumor in the right axillary region. In this case no reliable differentiation between benign and malignant can be made on CT only.

The only pitfall is that some nerve-related tumors and homogeneous lymphatic tissue can give a similar appearance; for example, schwannomas can show hypoechogenicity and acoustic enhancement in approximately 50% of cases. This problem is overcome simply by careful attention to technique. If the gain (amplification) of the machine is set appropriately, then the solid but hypoechoic lesion will not be completely dark; there will be some echoes within it. If there is any doubt about the gain setting on an ultrasound machine, then an adjacent vessel should be examined and the gain setting adjusted so that the echoes within the vessel just disappear.[7]

Some common lesions can be very easily excluded or diagnosed using ultrasound, for example, ganglion cysts around the wrist and fingers and popliteal cysts in the knee. Fat-containing lesions are well seen by CT and MRI, but ultrasonography is also a useful technique. Fat-containing masses will be hyperechoic. If they are less than 5 cm, have no features of neovascularity, and are superficial with no extension through the deep fascia, they are likely to be benign (Fig. 89-6). However, well-differentiated liposarcomas may look very similar, and after a review of practice in one hospital, there has been some concern that low-grade liposarcomas may be overlooked. The tumor shown in Figure 89-6B is not very likely to be benign because of its size and homogeneous texture. Absence of flow does not exclude malignancy. Experienced examiners remain confident that ultrasonography may be used to determine which fatty masses should be referred for further investigation. Depending on the clinical circumstances, the certainty of diagnosis, and the experience or confidence of the operator, ultrasonography may be used as a test that predicts the safe postponement of other imaging. However, if there are any concerns that this may not be truly a fat containing lesion, then the performance of more sophisticated imaging such as MRI is indicated.

Vascularity

The vascularity of a lesion can be assessed by ultrasonography using either color or power Doppler imaging (Fig. 89-7). Conventional angiography and MR angiography can also be useful when assessing vascularity, especially in arteriovenous malformations when the possibility of treatment can also be included. Note that some low-flow arteriovenous lesions may be difficult to detect using contrast studies via an arterial route and retrograde examination by venography may show a much more extensive lesion. Ultrasonography and MRI will not miss slow-flowing regions.

Ultrasonography is effective as a first-line study in vascular lesions (Fig. 89-8). This can give an idea as to where the vascular supply originates and also whether there is a predominance of arterial and venous flow. The use of compression can also be invaluable. Some slow-flowing arteriovenous malformations are best seen by using color or pulsed Doppler imaging and applying pressure via the probe on the tissue and then gently releasing the pressure. If this is done, then a slow-flowing arteriovenous malformation will show flow.

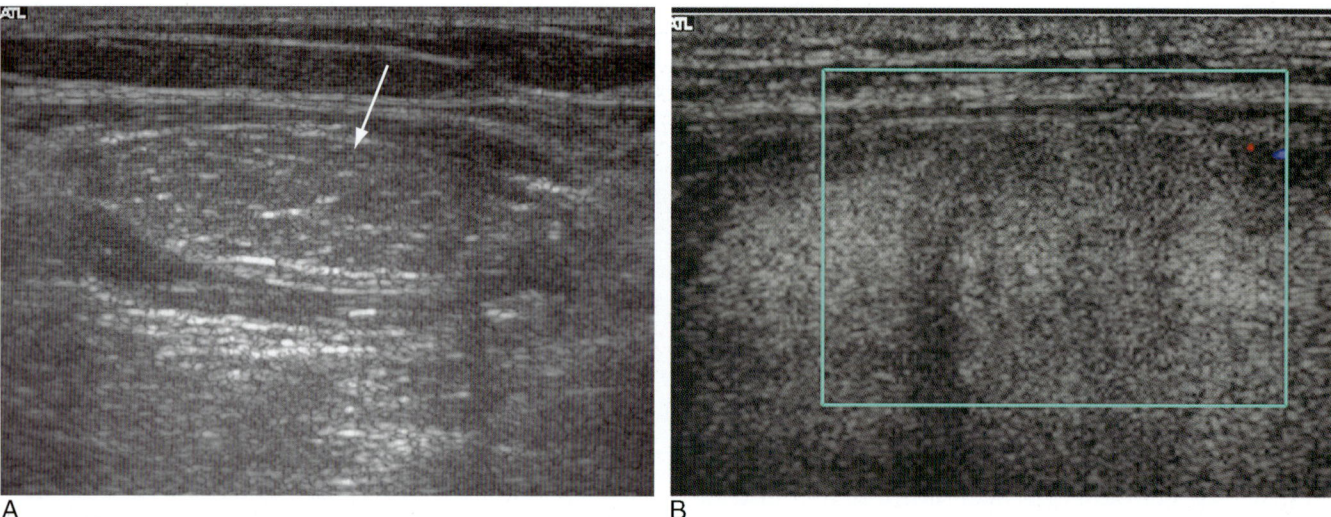

A   B

■ **FIGURE 89-6**   **A,** Sonogram of a lipoma (*arrow*). **B,** Sonogram of a liposarcoma. Color Doppler image shows homogeneous image of the large lesion with no flow.

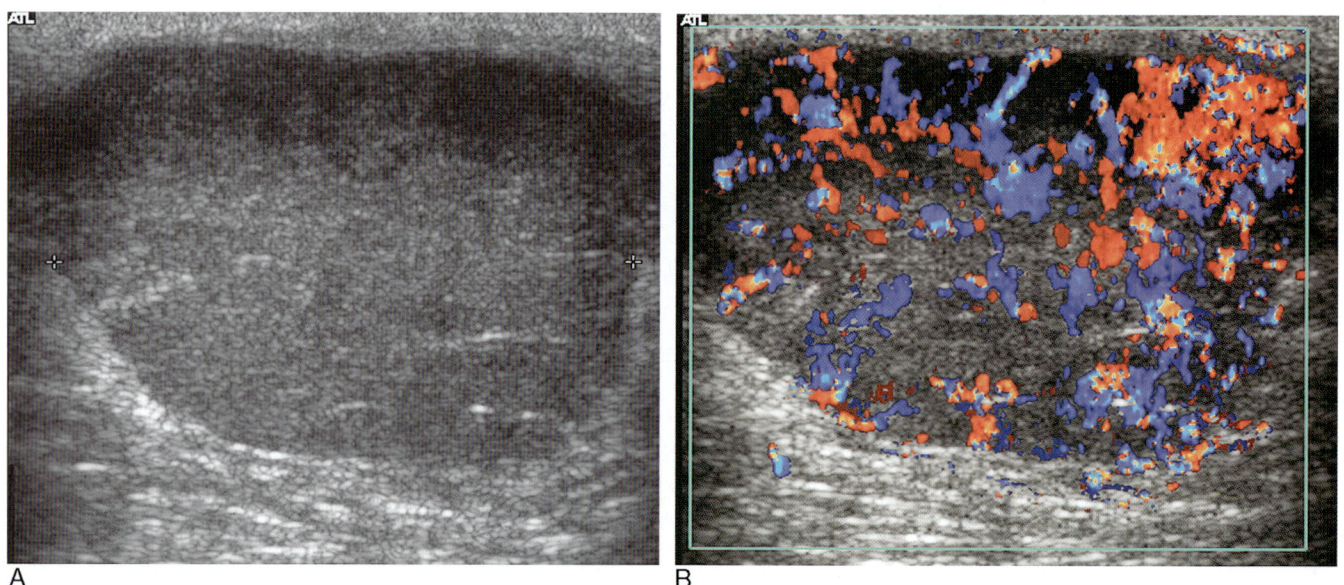

A   B

■ **FIGURE 89-7**   Sonogram of a Merkel cell tumor in the left buttock with (*right*) and without (*left*) color Doppler imaging.

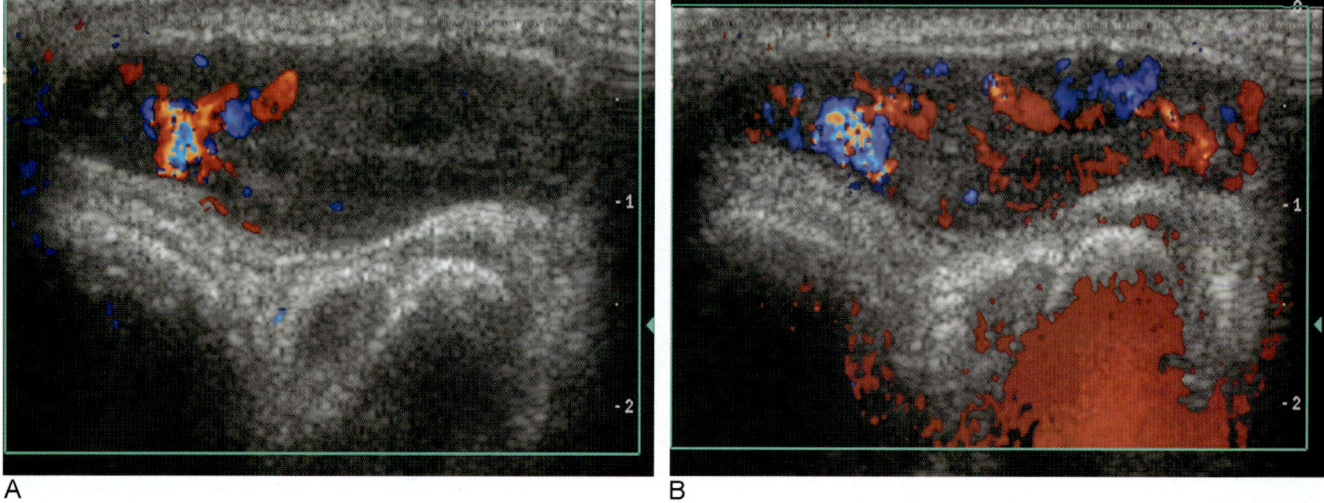

A   B

■ **FIGURE 89-8**   **A,** Color Doppler ultrasound image of a vascular malformation without compression. **B,** Compression has been applied, and on release of the probe pressure, more vessels can be seen.

Calcification

Calcification is best seen on plain films and CT. Early calcification can also be clearly identified using ultrasound where it causes acoustic shadowing behind the calcified region (Fig. 89-9). This is a specific finding in larger lesions, but in small lesions it can be absent. When large areas of calcification are present, the sonographer may not be able to see behind the initial calcification and therefore may underestimate its extent.

MRI is a poor means of assessing small areas of calcification. These areas have low signal intensity and are often overlooked, because the presence of low signal intensity can also be encountered in flow from a vessel or, indeed, fibrosis. If the amount of calcification present within a lesion needs to be analyzed, then CT is the best imaging method to use.

Mature fibrosis is of low signal intensity on all MR sequences and is of high echogenicity on ultrasonography (immature fibrosis may be rather cellular and may have fairly high signal intensity on T2-weighted MR images). The region behind the fibrosis will not have acoustic enhancement or shadowing. It is often easily detected in areas of previous injury to muscles and tendons, where it is often seen in association with the loss of the normal fibrillary structure. Some patients admit no history of injury, but on imaging a lump there is the presence of a partial muscle tear or a myofascial hernia that determines that it is from a previous but forgotten injury.

Muscle Injury

Scarring is common in muscles, and this can be seen with ultrasonography. The site of some lumps increases the chance that they are secondary to trauma. The rectus femoris muscle is a frequently injured muscle. The location of the lesion along the aponeurosis of the two muscle bellies is the most common area of injury.

At this site, hematoma, loss of the normal fibrillary pattern, calcification due to myositis ossificans, and scarring may all be seen.

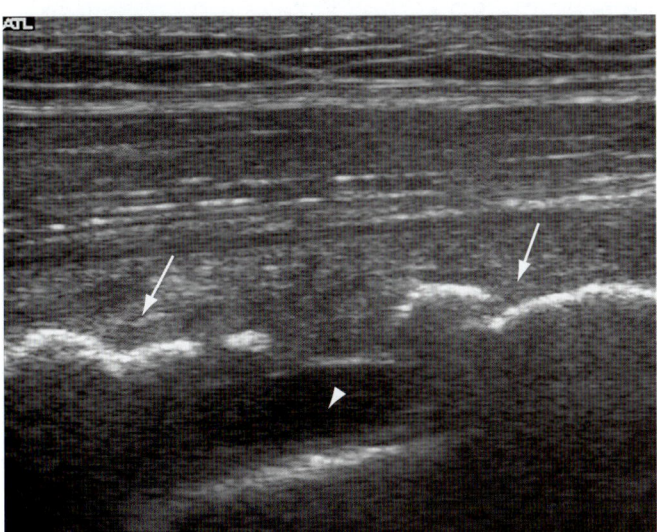

■ **FIGURE 89-9** Sonogram of myositis ossificans. Calcifications are marked by *arrows*. Posterior to the calcifications a liquefying hematoma can be seen (*arrowhead*).

Muscle hernias can be invisible because they may only be present when the patient is standing or straining. This means that when a supine MRI is performed it may appear completely normal. The use of dynamic ultrasound scanning can be invaluable in these patients. The patient can be imaged standing and after running. It is on stressing these muscles that muscle hernias can become obvious.

Ultrasonography of Muscle Trauma

Hematomas

When there has been an injury and hematoma forms it is initially of high echogenicity. After approximately 6 hours the hematoma starts to liquefy and becomes gradually anechoic (Fig. 89-10). This liquefaction can take up to 6 months to complete. A completely liquefied hematoma can therefore look like a cyst.

These lesions will present as lumps either with a clear history of trauma or no history (see also Chapter 94). The problem then is whether there is an underlying tumor that has bled. If the lesion is clearly anechoic with no echoes, then a liquefied hematoma can be confidently diagnosed. If there are echoes within the lesion, then the hematoma must be followed to resolution and liquefaction (Fig. 89-11). Alternatively, MRI and even biopsy may be indicated when suspicion for tumor is high.

Nerve-Related Lesions

The presence of a tail within a lesion, if it arises in the region of a neurovascular bundle, can suggest that it is a nerve-related lesion (see also Chapter 93).

On MRI, nerve lesions can show a central low signal intensity. On ultrasonography there is usually a central high signal intensity with a ring shadow, called a target lesion, within a neuroma. Schwannomas, if they become large, can become necrotic and cavitating. Nerve lesions can also show acoustic enhancement behind, which might suggest a more fluid-containing lesion. The importance of setting the machine appropriately cannot be overstated. Modern ultrasonography can effectively identify small nerves clearly down to the level of the digital nerves. The nerve fibers can be seen, and therefore small neuromas can be detected. The extent of disease within the nerve can also be assessed; for example, a portion of the nerve may be spared by the tumor, or it may only affect a branch of the nerve (Fig. 89-12). Ultrasonography can be used to answer these questions with its superior line pair resolution in the superficial regions when compared with MRI.

A pitfall of MRI is interpreting a neuroma as a ganglion when it does not have a tail because it often appears as a "fluid"-containing lesion with high signal intensity. Again, contrast-enhanced MRI is useful in differentiating these two conditions.

Lesions According to Site

Some lesions can be identified according to their site. In the hand, for example, the ganglion is the most common soft tissue swelling to be identified, followed by other rarer lesions, such as nerve tumors, giant cell tumors of tendon sheath, and lipomas. In the foot and ankle,

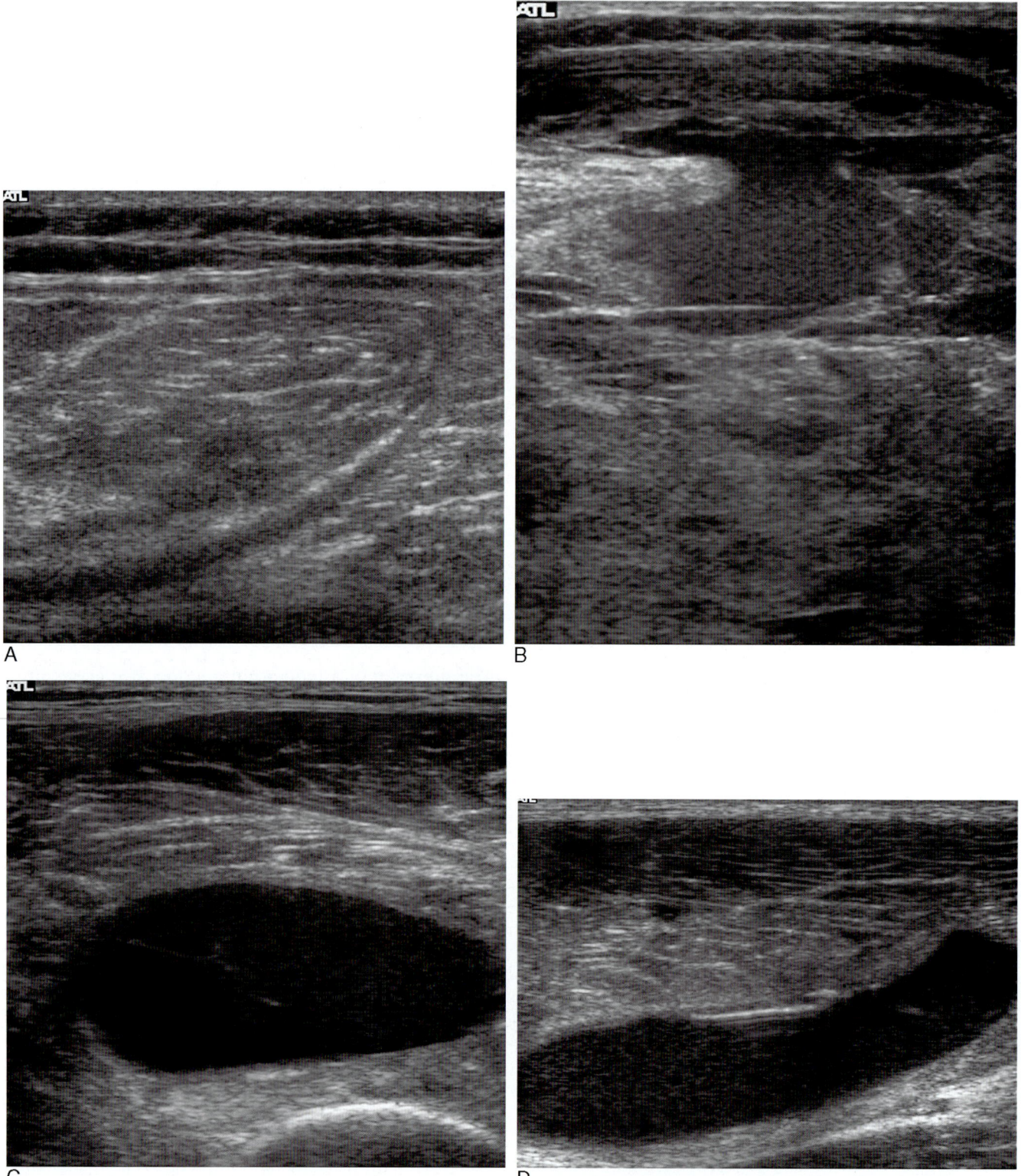

■ **FIGURE 89-10** **A,** Sonogram of liquefying hematoma in rectus femoris muscle. **B,** Liquefying hematoma with a mixture of cystic and solid components. **C,** Liquefied hematoma. **D,** Liquefied hematoma, injury seen behind the muscle belly (fascial plane injury).

ganglions are the most common lesions, followed by plantar fibromas and osteophytes. Tendinopathy around the ankle and wrist can also cause swelling. Around the knee the most common soft tissue swelling is the popliteal cyst. When this ruptures it is a great mimicker of a deep vein thrombosis. Here, ultrasonography is very useful because the assessment of the deep veins can be followed by an assessment of the presence of a popliteal cyst. Note that popliteal cyst rupture may lead to deep vein thrombosis, and both diagnoses may be made using ultrasonography.

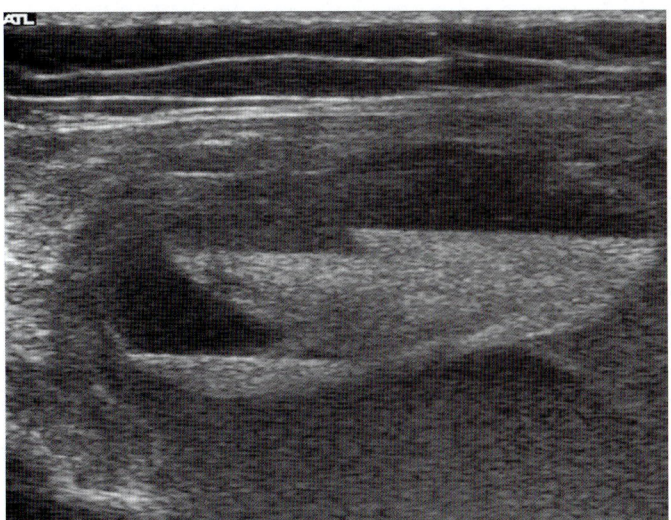

■ **FIGURE 89-11** Sonogram of telangiectatic osteosarcoma. Patient was originally thought to have a liquefying hematoma because he had a clear history of trauma. Note the fluid layers of acute (highly echogenic) hemorrhage and liquefied hemorrhage (low echogenicity).

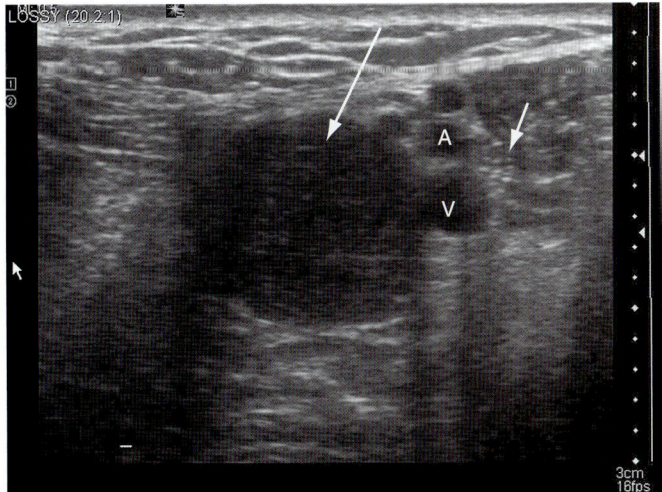

■ **FIGURE 89-12** Schwannoma (*long arrow*) arising from the medial calcaneal branch of the tibialis posterior nerve, with the main nerve trunk seen separately (*short arrow*). A, artery, V, vein.

Locating Spread

The presence and significance of spread will depend on the histology of the lesion. Local spread can be assessed by ultrasound initially, but MRI will be needed to assess extent in detail. MRI will then ascertain whether the lesion is arising from bone or whether indeed the soft tissue lesion is affecting bone by erosion or indentation. Local staging and diagnosis or exclusion of distant spread is addressed in Chapter 98.

The Decision to Biopsy

As indicated earlier, some lesions are very easily assessed and dismissed by the use of an ultrasound examination. The most common lesions that are imaged that are benign are ganglions and popliteal cysts (Fig. 89-13), followed by muscle

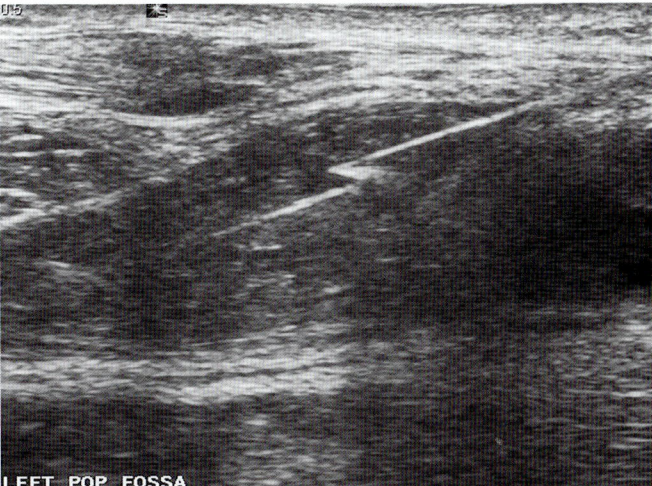

■ **FIGURE 89-13** Sonogram of a biopsy specimen of a complex popliteal cyst with synovitis.

hernia, fibrosis, and myositis ossificans after trauma and also foreign bodies, especially within the fingers and feet. There may be no history of foreign body inclusion even though one is clearly seen on imaging. The presence of a foreign body within the hand is very common and may be related to an injury after gardening or as a result of the patient's occupation, for example, metal working. Sometimes there has been a history of foreign body inclusion many years previously. It is not uncommon to see foreign bodies that relate to an injury over 20 years prior to the examination. The rate of growth of a lesion is very important. The size of a lesion is a major risk factor; for example, if a lipoma is greater than 5 cm and is deep, the likelihood of malignancy is much greater and these lesions should always be sampled after local staging with MRI.[8] Small lesions may be excised, or they could be followed up by ultrasound imaging to assess for an increase in growth. Lesions of less than 1 cm are difficult to biopsy. It can be attempted under ultrasound guidance, but if a diagnosis is vital, then sometimes an excision biopsy will need to be performed anyway (Table 89-2 and Figure 89-14).

SUMMARY

Imaging of soft tissue masses is of considerable value in showing which lesions are real and require investigation. Initial screening with ultrasound allows the examiner to take a specific history and to exclude patients with no mass, a cyst, a ganglion, and some of the sequelae of injury from further investigation. MRI is the best method of local staging and surgical planning and is mandatory in unexplained solid mass lesions. CT is an aid to diagnosis in some selected cases.

What the Referring Physician Needs to Know

■ Is the lesion a "leave me alone" lesion such as a ganglion or cyst?
■ Is malignancy excluded?
■ Is additional imaging needed?

TABLE 89-2   Comparison of Imaging Methods for Soft Tissue Lesions

	Radiography	CT	MRI	Ultrasound
Uses radiation	Yes	Yes	No	No
Show calcification	Excellent	Excellent	Low signal may be calcium	Good
Show bone involvement	Yes	Excellent	Excellent	Sometimes if accessible cortex eroded
Show soft tissue	Poorly	Sometimes	Excellent	Excellent, especially in extremities
Patient tolerance	Excellent	Good	May need sedation or general anesthesia in children	Excellent
Cross-sectional view	No	Good	Excellent	Limited (extended field-of-view imaging)
Contraindications	No	No	Pacemakers, aneurysm clips	No
Assessment of vascularity	No	With intravenous contrast	With intravenous contrast	Excellent

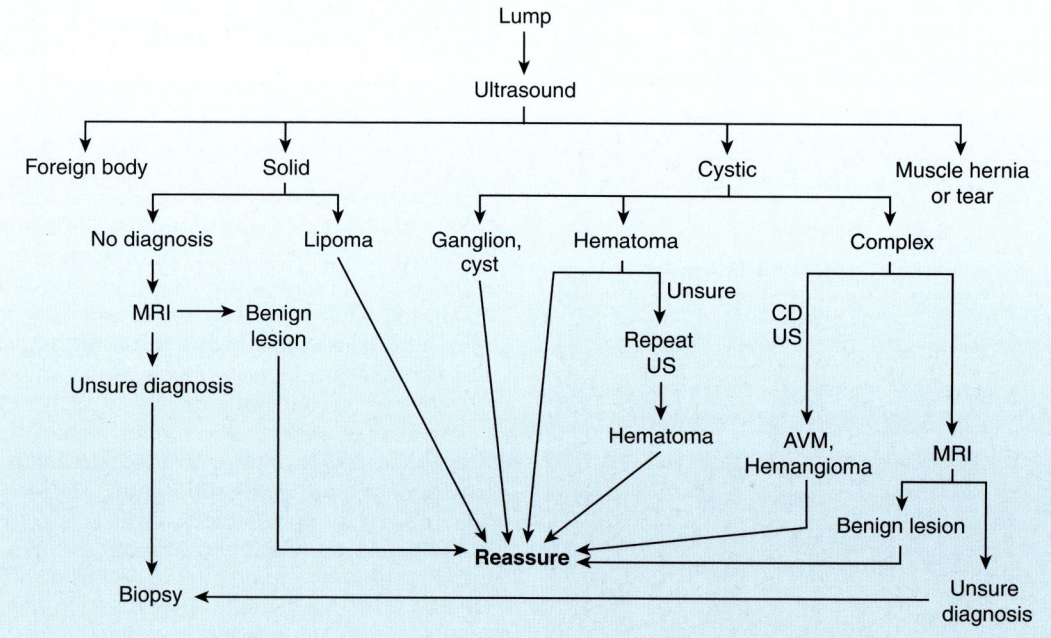

■ **FIGURE 89-14**   Algorithm for imaging soft tissue lesions. CT and radiographs have not been included here because they add little in the initial diagnosis and should be reserved for those lesions in which the assessment of calcification is needed or when the patient cannot undergo MRI. Advantages and disadvantages of the various imaging techniques are listed in Table 89-2.

REFERENCES

1. Siegel MJ. Magnetic resonance imaging of musculoskeletal soft tissue masses. Radiol Clin North Am 2001; 39:701–720.
2. Hwang S, Adler RS. Sonographic evaluation of the musculoskeletal soft tissue masses. Ultrasound Q 2005; 21:259–270.
3. Beggs I. Sonography of muscle hernias. AJR Am J Roentgenol 2003; 180:395–399.
4. Soudack M, Nachtigal A, Gaitini D. Clinically unsuspected foreign bodies: the importance of sonography. J Ultrasound Med 2003; 22:1381–1385.
5. Kransdorf MJ, Murphey MD. The use of gadolinium in the MR evaluation of soft tissue tumors. Semin Ultrasound CT MR 1997; 18:251–268.
6. Knapp EL, Kransdorf MJ, Letson GD. Diagnostic imaging update: soft tissue sarcomas. Cancer Control 2005; 12:22–26.
7. Hughes DG, Wilson DJ. Ultrasound appearances of peripheral nerve tumours. Br J Radiol 1986; 59:1041–1043.
8. Liu JC, et al. Sonographically guided core needle biopsy of soft tissue neoplasms. J Clin Ultrasound 2004; 32:294–298.

90

Primary Bone Tumors

A. Mark Davies

Primary bone tumors are rare and, unlike osseous metastases and myeloma, tend to occur in otherwise fit children, adolescents, and young adults. Patients typically present with either pain or swelling that may be initially mild or intermittent but in time becomes more severe and nonmechanical, particularly if the tumor is malignant. A pathologic fracture may be the initial presenting feature in a minority of cases, and small benign bone tumors can be incidental findings on radiographs obtained for other purposes. The vast majority of bone tumors will be first detected on radiographs, with only a minority of occult lesions being identified on other imaging, such as bone scintigraphy and MRI. This situation is unlikely to change significantly in the near future, because the radiograph remains relatively inexpensive and readily available. There is, however, an increasing tendency, particularly in younger patients, to go straight to noninvasive imaging such as MRI. Should a bone tumor be suspected on MRI then it is important to correlate the findings with contemporary radiographs as, arguably, of all the imaging techniques, the radiographs reveal the most diagnostic information in terms of pattern of bone destruction, periosteal new bone formation, and matrix mineralization. It can be a daunting task for the physician unfamiliar with bone tumors to understand the bewildering spectrum of bone tumors. The easiest way to comprehend primary bone tumors is to apply a pathologic classification according to their predominant tissue production and then the benign and malignant subtypes (Table 90-1). We, therefore, have both benign and malignant osteoid-producing/osteogenic tumors, cartilage-producing/chondrogenic tumors, round cell tumors, and so on. Both benign and malignant bone tumors may recur locally after surgical treatment, but only malignant tumors have the propensity to metastasize to distant organs. The likelihood of developing metastases depends on the histologic grade of the malignant tumor as well as the efficacy of the treatment. Some benign bone tumors have the ability to undergo malignant change, and some malignant tumors can dedifferentiate into a higher-grade sarcoma. The purpose of this chapter is to review the different types of primary bone tumors and provide a description of the principal imaging features. A number of non-neoplastic conditions are frequently included with bone tumors because of their tumor-like clinical and imaging features. These include simple bone cyst, aneurysmal bone cyst, and fibrous dysplasia and are covered in Chapter 92.

MANIFESTATIONS OF DISEASE

Osteoid-Producing Tumors

Osteoid-producing/osteogenic tumors are defined as neoplasms that produce an osteoid or bony matrix. According to their biologic behavior they are divided into benign and malignant lesions (see Table 90-1).

Osteoma

Osteoma is a slow-growing benign lesion surface lesion comprising well-differentiated mature bone. It classically occurs in the frontal and ethmoidal sinuses, the so-called ivory osteoma, and less commonly on the outer skull vault and the mandible (Fig. 90-1). In Gardner's syndrome, an autosomal-dominant disorder, osteomas particularly of the mandible are associated with cutaneous/subcutaneous lesions and colonic polyposis with a propensity for malignant change. Radiographs show an ivory dense mass with sharply defined margins firmly attached to the outer surface of bone. Osteomas rarely arise on the long bones, but if large they can mimic a parosteal osteosarcoma or melorheostosis. With the exception of Gardner's syndrome the identification of an osteoma is usually of little clinical significance. Large paranasal osteomas, however, may cause compressive and obstructive symptoms and erode into the anterior cranial fossa. Excision of large vault or mandibular lesions may be required for cosmetic reasons.

A lesion histologically identical to an osteoma but arising within trabecular bone is the bone island or enostosis. These are a common incidental finding on radiographic examinations and are typically small, oval or rounded, with a streaky or brush border that blends with the host trabeculae. Multiple bone islands crowded in the epimetaphyseal regions are a feature of the sclerosing bone

KEY POINTS

- The histologic grade of a bone tumor is a measure of its biologic aggressiveness and therefore indicates the risk of local recurrence after treatment and development of metastases.
- Peritumoral edema on MRI is more florid in benign conditions such as osteoid osteoma and chondroblastoma than sarcomas.
- A painful scoliosis in an adolescent may be the presenting feature of an osteoid osteoma or osteoblastoma.
- A tumor arising in the epiphysis before skeletal fusion is most commonly a chondroblastoma with sarcoma extremely unlikely.
- Malignant transformation of enchondroma and osteochondroma to central and peripheral chondrosarcoma is rare. The incidence is greater in Ollier's disease (20%) and hereditary multiple exostoses (<5%).
- Malignant spindle cell tumors of bone (fibrosarcoma, malignant fibrous histiocytoma, leiomyosarcoma, and pleomorphic sarcoma) have identical imaging features.
- Bone malignancies of vascular origin may present with multifocal disease affecting one limb.

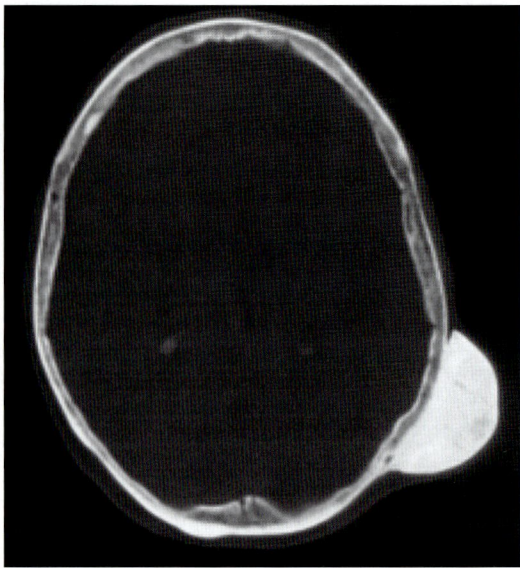

■ **FIGURE 90-1** CT image of head shows a vault osteoma.

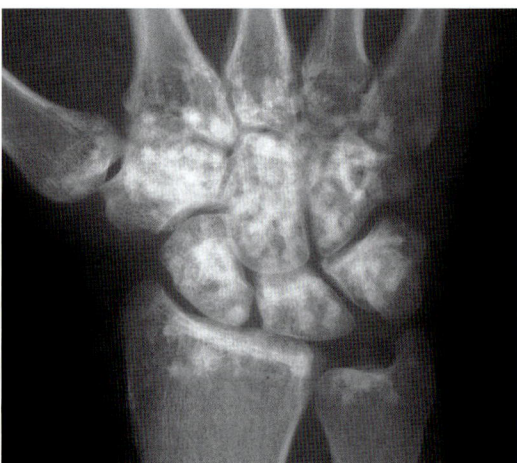

■ **FIGURE 90-2** Osteopoikilosis. Posteroanterior radiograph of wrist showing multiple bone islands.

TABLE 90-1 Classification of Primary Bone Tumors

	Benign	Malignant
Osteogenic tumors	Osteoma Osteoid osteoma Osteoblastoma	Osteosarcoma
Chondrogenic tumors	Osteochondroma Chondroma Chondroblastoma Chondromyxoid fibroma	Chondrosarcoma
Fibrogenic and fibrohistiocytic tumors	Desmoplastic fibroma Benign fibrous histiocytoma	Fibrosarcoma Malignant fibrous histiocytoma
Round cell tumor		Ewing's sarcoma
Hematopoietic (myeloproliferative) tumors		Plasmacytoma/ myeloma Lymphoma
Giant cell tumor	Giant cell tumor	Malignant giant cell tumor
Notochordal tumors	Chordoma	
Vascular tumors	Hemangioma	Hemangioendothelioma Angiosarcoma
Smooth muscle tumors	Leiomyoma	Leiomyosarcoma
Lipogenic tumors	Lipoma	Liposarcoma
Miscellaneous tumors	Adamantinoma	

Tumor-like lesions of bone, such as simple bone cyst and aneurysmal bone cyst, are frequently included in classifications of bone tumors but in this book are covered in Chapter 92.

dysplasia, osteopoikilosis (Fig. 90-2). Occasionally, bone islands grow to several centimeters in diameter showing increased activity on bone scintigraphy. These so-called giant bone islands need to be distinguished from other more significant causes of focal osseous sclerosis. The brush border on radiographs or CT can be a helpful diagnostic feature favoring a bone island.

Osteoid Osteoma and Osteoblastoma

Osteoid osteoma is one of the more common benign bone tumors arising in children, adolescents, and adults up to the age of 35 years. The classic clinical description is of night pain relieved by aspirin. It comprises a central lucent lesion (the nidus) that is usually less than or equal to 2 cm in diameter, with a varying degree of surrounding reactive sclerosis. The nidus consists of cellular highly vascularized tissue producing osteoid. It may be radiolucent or contain matrix mineralization depending on the degree of osteoid production. The most common locations are the femoral and tibial diaphyses, the femoral neck, and the posterior vertebral arch (Fig. 90-3). The most common variety is cortically based and arises in the tubular bone, stimulating florid, surrounding sclerosis, which may be sufficiently dense to obscure the nidus on radiographs. In this situation, osteoid osteoma may mimic a healing stress fracture or cortically based abscess. If the lesion arises

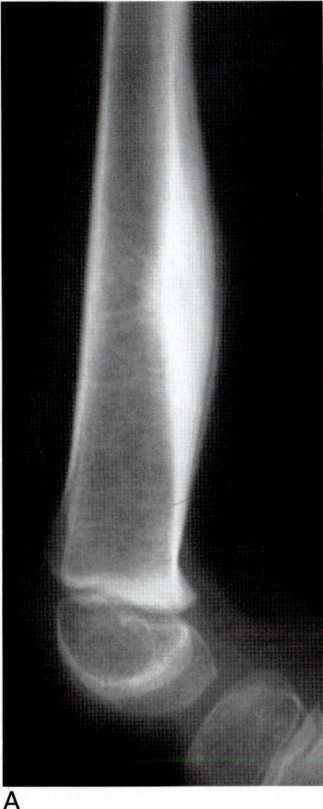

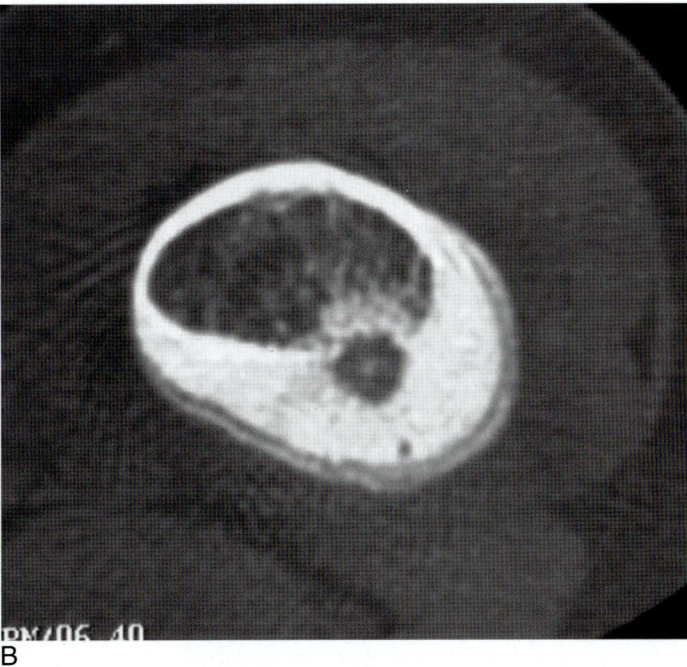

■ **FIGURE 90-3** Osteoid osteoma. **A,** Lateral radiograph showing hyperostosis along the posterior aspect of the femoral diaphysis. **B,** CT image of femur reveals the nidus.

in an intracapsular location, such as the femoral neck, the lack of periosteum means that the reactive sclerosis can be minimal or even absent. In this situation the florid inflammatory response typical of osteoid osteoma causes a reactive synovitis in the adjacent joint with a joint effusion and both marrow and juxtacortical edema. On MRI the bone, joint, and soft tissue inflammatory response may be the predominant feature with the nidus difficult to identify, particularly if a large field-of-view has been employed.[1] Dynamic gadolinium-enhanced MRI may be used to increase the conspicuity of the nidus.[2] CT is the imaging technique of choice in suspected osteoid osteoma (see Fig. 90-3B), first to identify the nidus and second to guide biopsy and thermal ablation, which is the currently preferred management for the majority of cases.[3] Osteoid osteoma may uncommonly arise in a subperiosteal location such as in the hindfoot and extremely rarely in an epiphysis. One classic presentation worth stressing is the painful scoliosis in the adolescent with an osteoid osteoma arising at the apex of the concavity. In a suspected case, in which spinal radiographs are frequently initially considered normal, bone scintigraphy is the technique of choice, followed by CT, to localize the nidus if a focus of abnormal activity is identified.

Osteoblastoma is approximately four times less common than osteoid osteoma. It has close histologic similarities to osteoid osteoma, so that some authorities consider the two conditions as part of the spectrum of the same entity. Both occur at similar ages and similar locations, with a painful scoliosis being a well-recognized presentation

of spinal lesions. Others, however, suggest that osteoid osteoma and osteoblastoma are two separate entities if only because the latter tends to be progressive and there is a rare incidence of malignant change. The radiographic appearances are variable with a well-defined lytic central lesion of greater than 2 cm in diameter containing matrix mineralization in a third of cases and with surrounding nonaggressive medullary sclerosis and periosteal new bone formation (Fig. 90-4).[4] MRI of spinal lesions will again show the adjacent inflammatory component with bone and soft tissue edema and, in long-standing cases, muscle wasting in the concavity of the scoliosis.

Osteosarcoma

Osteosarcoma is the most common primary malignant bone tumor in children and adolescents, and it is second in frequency to myeloma if all age groups are considered. High-grade intramedullary osteosarcoma, also known as conventional osteosarcoma, is the most common, but there are a number of other subtypes of osteosarcoma that differ in histologic grade, age at presentation, and site of origin (Table 90-2). Osteosarcoma may be secondary to malignant transformation of a preexisting bone lesion and can rarely be extraskeletal in origin. In addition, there is a group of rare congenital syndromes, now recognized to be due to inherited genetic aberrations, which are associated with an increased predisposition to osteosarcoma. These include Li-Fraumeni syndrome, congenital retinoblastoma, and Rothmund-Thomson syndrome.

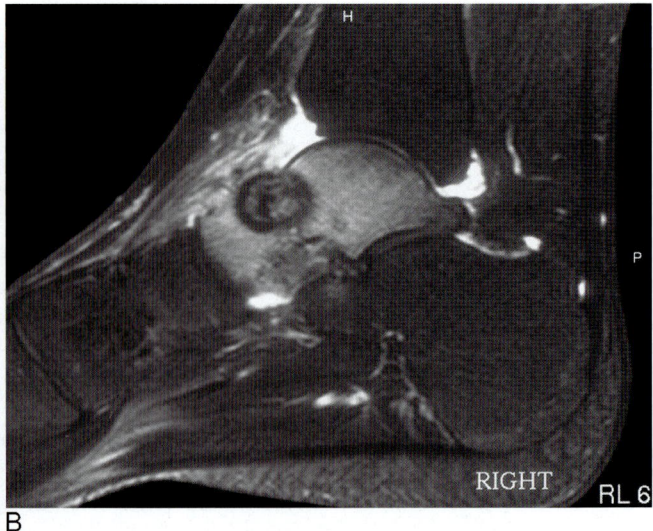

■ **FIGURE 90-4**   Osteoblastoma. **A,** CT image showing bone-forming lesion in the dome of the talus. **B,** Sagittal, T2-weighted, fat-suppressed MR image showing the low signal intensity osteoblastoma with florid surrounding hyperintense edema and inflammation.

TABLE 90-2	Osteosarcoma of Bone and Its Subtypes
Primary	**Secondary**
Conventional (85%)	Malignant transformation in
Osteoblastic	Paget's disease
Chondroblastic	Bone infarction
Fibroblastic	Fibrous dysplasia
Multicentric (1.5%)	Radiation-induced
Synchronous	Chronic osteomyelitis
Metachronous	Dedifferentiation of chondrosarcoma
Telangiectatic (4%)	
Small cell (1%)	
Low-grade central (<1%)	
Surface	
Parosteal (5%)	
Periosteal (<2%)	
High-grade surface (<1%)	

The percentages indicate approximate incidence in primary osteosarcomas.

Conventional (High-Grade Intramedullary) Osteosarcoma

Conventional osteosarcoma is the most common primary bone sarcoma in the adolescent age group, accounting for approximately 85% of all cases of osteosarcoma. Seventy-five percent of cases occur in patients younger than the age of 25 years. It most often arises in the long bones of the appendicular skeleton, particularly the distal femur, proximal tibia, and proximal humerus. Ninety percent are metaphyseal or metadiaphyseal, with only 10% diaphyseal. They are clearly highly aggressive tumors with permeative bone destruction, irregular cortical destruction, and complex periosteal reactions. The degree of malignant osteoid production can vary with a spectrum of radiographic appearances from purely lytic to densely osteoblastic, although most show a mixed pattern (Fig. 90-5). Textbooks understandably choose examples of osteosarcoma that tend to illustrate many or all of the typical features in a single case (Fig. 90-6). In clinical practice, however, cases may only show one or two of the classic signs. The radiologist needs to be alert to the diagnostic possibility of a sarcoma and recognize the significance of a single sign such as a Codman angle or subtle permeative bone destruction.[5] Indeed, if the matrix mineralization is minimal, the osteosarcoma may be radiographically indistinguishable from other sarcomas such as malignant round cell tumors. Failure to differentiate, for example, between an osteosarcoma and Ewing's sarcoma at presentation is of little consequence because the protocol for the staging studies and approach for the biopsy are identical for both tumors. Whether a high-grade intramedullary osteosarcoma is principally lytic or sclerotic has little influence on either management or prognosis. Similarly, pathologic subdivision into osteoblastic (50%), chondroblastic (25%), and fibroblastic (25%) types is of limited significance.

The diagnosis of an osteosarcoma is usually made after analysis of the radiographs with MRI largely utilized for staging purposes (see Chapter 98). Tumor infiltration of bone, irrespective of the precise histology, will show a T1-weighted signal that is isointense with surrounding muscle and is inhomogeneous but hyperintense on T2-weighted and STIR images (Fig. 90-7A). Low signal intensity areas in osteosarcoma correlate well with matrix mineralization. The identification of cortical destruction and soft tissue extension with a solid soft tissue mass are cardinal signs of a malignancy. Evidence of tumor on MRI beyond the confines of the host cortex is frequently taken to indicate soft tissue extension. In many cases the

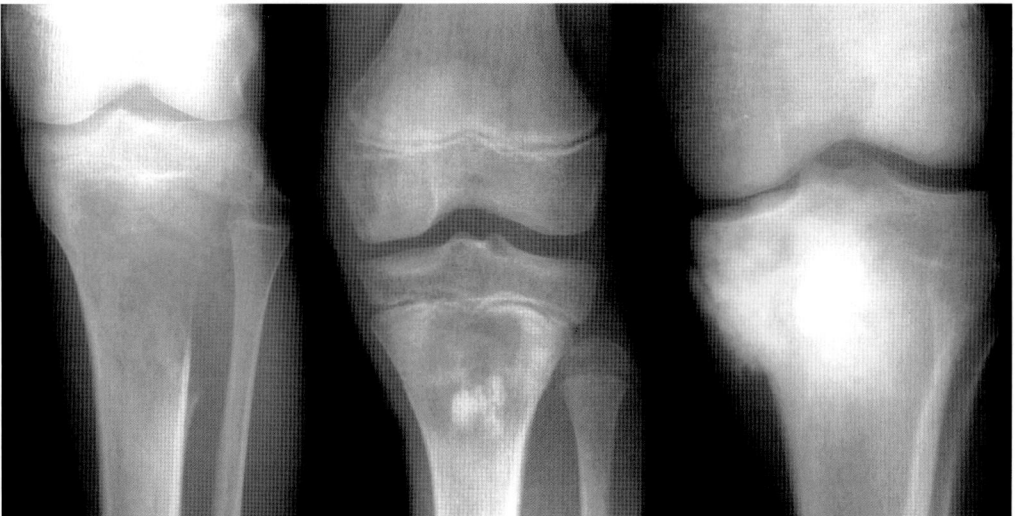

■ **FIGURE 90-5** Three cases of high-grade intramedullary osteosarcoma of the proximal tibia ranging (*left to right*) from purely lytic, mixed lytic with minor malignant osteoid production, to purely sclerotic.

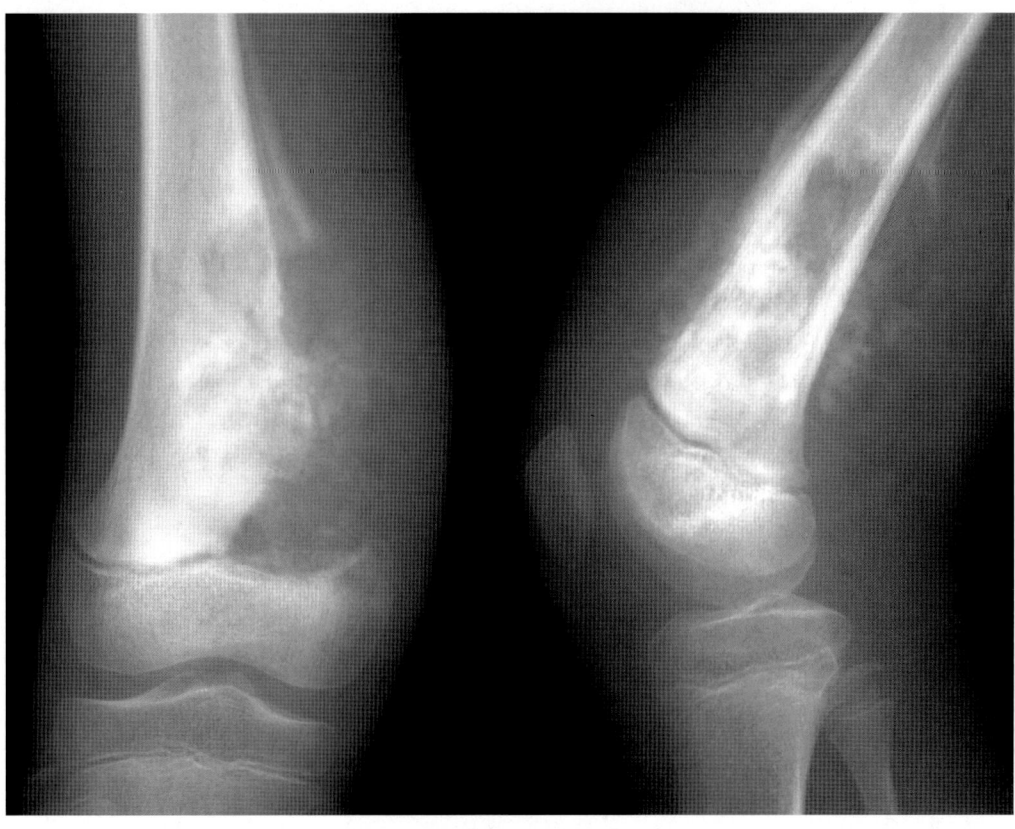

■ **FIGURE 90-6** Classic high-grade intramedullary osteosarcoma of distal femur. Radiograph shows lysis, malignant osteoid formation, complex periosteal new bone formation, and soft tissue extension.

tumor is displacing the periosteum rather than penetrating it and so remains "intraosseous," albeit with considerably greater dimensions than the parent bone. This can explain why there can be a discrepancy between the MRI findings and the pathologist's assessment of the extent of the excised tumor. Peritumoral edema, both medullary and soft tissue, may be seen with osteosarcoma and typically reduces after adjuvant chemotherapy. The degree of edema is significantly less florid than that seen in benign conditions such as osteoid osteoma and chondroblastoma. The use of dynamic contrast-enhanced MRI

may be useful in revealing viable areas of tumor before biopsy and as a baseline measurement for subsequent assessment of tumor response to chemotherapy. The significance of identifying growth plate, joint, and neurovascular involvement in osteosarcoma and other primary sarcomas of bone is discussed in Chapter 98. Bone scintigraphy will typically show marked increased activity over an osteosarcoma but again is largely reserved for staging purposes, that is, for confirming or excluding multifocal osteosarcomas or bone metastases (see Figs. 90-7B and 90-8).

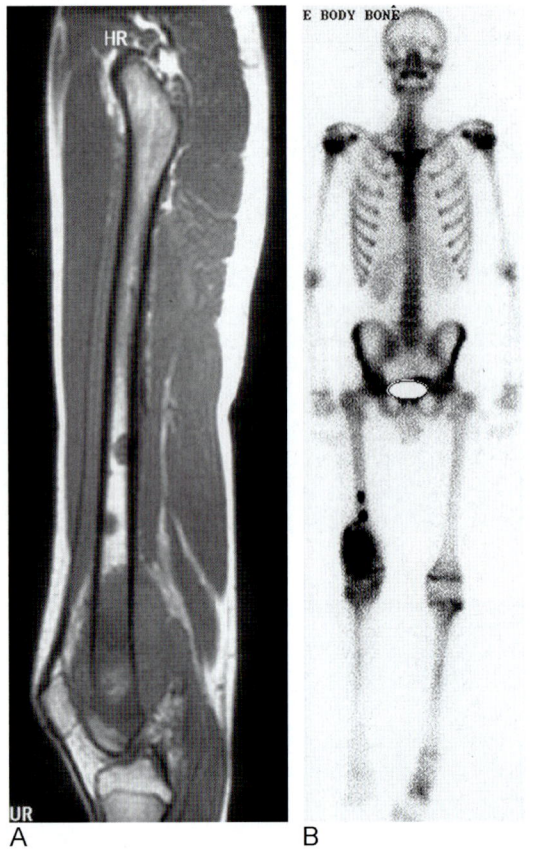

■ FIGURE 90-7 High-grade intramedullary osteosarcoma. Sagittal, T1-weighted MR image and whole-body bone scintiscan show the distal femoral osteosarcoma with two proximal skip metastases.

In less than 5% of cases noncontiguous intramedullary growth within the parent bone or across adjacent joints may occur. It is important that these so-called skip metastases are confirmed or excluded on the initial staging studies because this will influence subsequent surgical options (see Fig. 90-7B). High-grade intramedullary osteosarcoma has a high metastatic potential particularly via hematogenous spread to the lungs. Five to 10 percent of cases will have pulmonary metastases at initial presentation. After initial treatment with limb-salvage surgery (if practicable) and chemotherapy, disease relapse may arise due to local recurrence or the development of distant metastases, which typically are pulmonary. Because of the high-grade nature of these tumors this usually occurs within 2 to 3 years. The use of chemotherapy (particularly adjuvant) has greatly improved the prognosis for patients with a high-grade intramedullary osteosarcoma over surgery alone. The 5-year survival rate for most series of patients without evidence of metastatic disease at presentation is approximately 65%. Chemotherapy has modified the natural history of the disease, not just in terms of long-term survival but also in site of metastases. Approximately 15% of patients who subsequently develop metastases do so in the bones in the absence of imaging evidence of pulmonary disease.

Pathologists recognize a small cell variant of osteosarcoma that histologically resembles Ewing's sarcoma. It is of only passing interest to radiologists because the clinical and imaging features are indistinguishable from those of high-grade intramedullary osteosarcoma.

■ FIGURE 90-8 Multifocal osteosarcoma. **A,** Anteroposterior radiograph of the pelvis showing a large left iliac osteosarcoma. **B,** Whole-body bone scintigraphy shows further foci of osteosarcoma in the sacrum, right ilium, spine, and left proximal humerus. The chest CT in this case was clear of metastases.

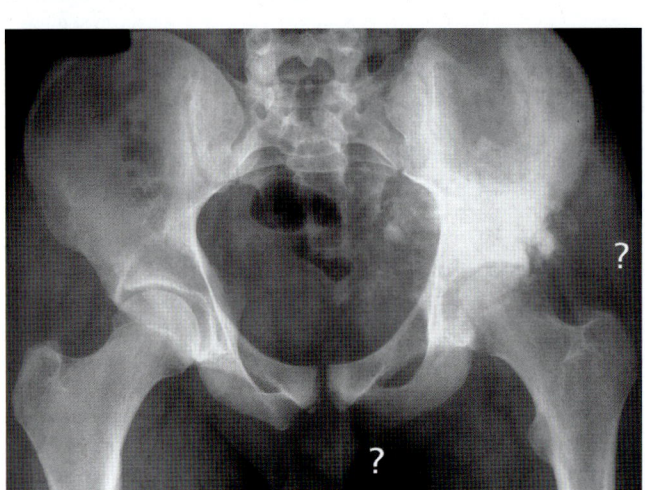

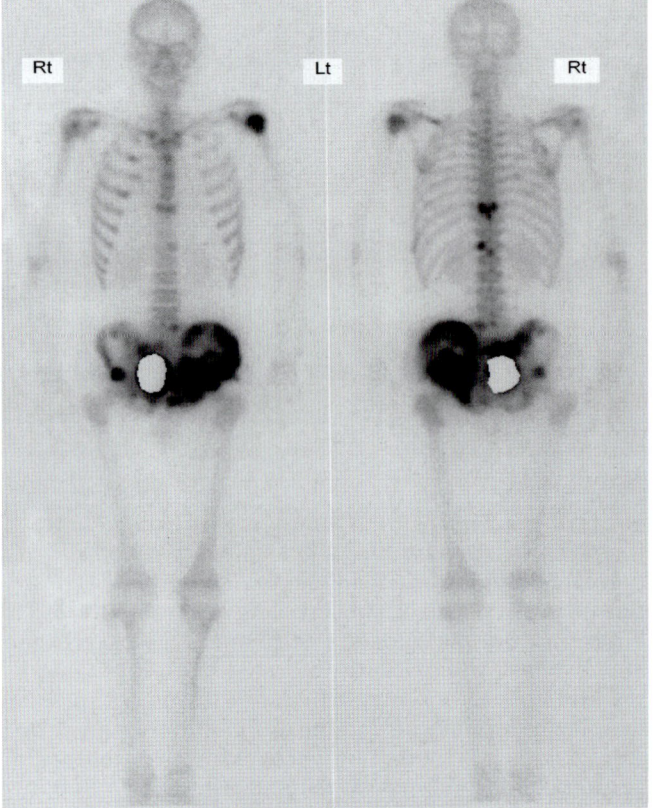

Multicentric Osteosarcoma

Approximately 1.5% of cases of osteosarcoma are classified as multicentric (multifocal). These tumors can be synchronous or metachronous in presentation, that is, multiple tumors identified at initial presentation or delayed over time (Fig. 90-8). For the diagnosis to be made, multiple bones are involved in the absence of pulmonary metastases. Whole-body bone scintigraphy or MRI will show the full extent of bone involvement with usually the index lesion being somewhat larger than the other lesions (see Fig. 90-8). This does beg the question as to whether multicentric osteosarcoma is a separate entity or a different manifestation of metastatic disease. It is likely that this is a diagnosis made less frequently than in the past because multislice CT is more sensitive in the detection of small lung nodules.

Telangiectatic Osteosarcoma

Telangiectatic osteosarcoma accounts for approximately 4% of all cases of osteosarcomas and has a minor male preponderance. It is a high-grade tumor that is most common in the second decade and affects the femur and tibia. It is predominantly lytic with aggressive features on radiographs (Fig. 90-9).[6] Histologically, it comprises multiple hemorrhagic spaces separated by thin septa. For this reason it may mimic both radiologically and histologically an aneurysmal bone cyst with fluid-fluid levels frequently identified on MRI. Clearly, it is of paramount importance to distinguish the two entities because the management and prognosis differ significantly.

Low-Grade Central Osteosarcoma

Low-grade central osteosarcoma accounts for less than 1% of all osteosarcomas. Typical sites include the femur and tibia (Fig. 90-10).[7] It is, as the name indicates, entirely intramedullary in location with nonaggressive radiographic features that frequently mimic either fibrous dysplasia or a cartilage lesion. For this reason, diagnosis is often delayed. Because of its rarity the author is reluctant to advise including it in the routine differential diagnosis of benign bone lesions. However, it is worth keeping the diagnosis in mind if biopsy of an otherwise innocuous bone lesion appears to show subtle malignant osteoid.

Surface Osteosarcoma

There are three types of surface or juxtacortical osteosarcoma that make up less than 7% of all osteosarcomas. These are the parosteal, periosteal, and high-grade surface variants.

Parosteal Osteosarcoma

Parosteal osteosarcoma is the second most common type of osteosarcoma and accounts for approximately 5% of cases. It is seen in a slightly older age group than high-grade intramedullary osteosarcoma, typically presenting in the third and fourth decades. Because it is a low-grade malignancy the prognosis is better, with a greater than 95% 5-year-survival after surgical excision, with chemotherapy only used in cases associated with dedifferentiation. Over 50% of cases arise on the posterior aspect of the distal femoral metaphysis (Fig. 90-11). Other sites include the proximal tibia and proximal humerus. The tumor is slow growing and is usually relatively large at presentation with particularly dense sclerosis due to mature osteoid, as compared with the immature osteoid typical of most high-grade osteosarcomas. The tumor is lobulated and wraps around the outer cortex of the underlying bone. Although it may be in contact with the cortex some areas will show a plane of cleavage readily visible on CT. On MRI up to 50% of cases will show evidence of cortical destruction with medullary invasion (see Fig. 90-11B). Up to 20% of cases

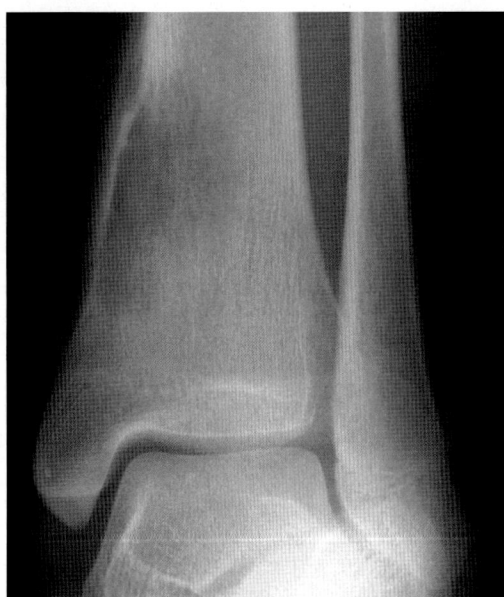
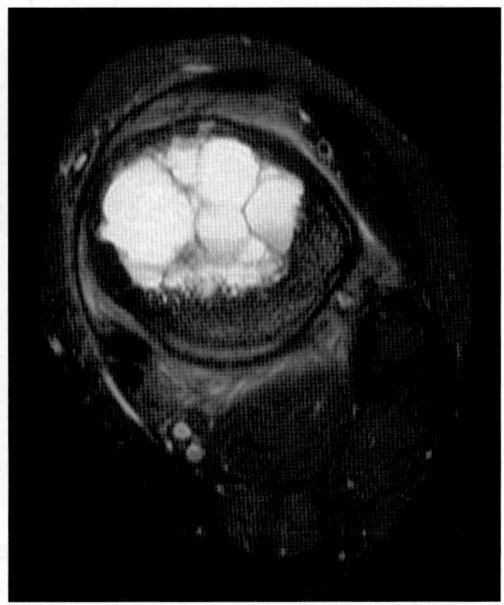

■ **FIGURE 90-9** Telangiectatic osteosarcoma. **A,** Anteroposterior radiograph showing an aggressive lytic lesion in the distal tibial metadiaphysis with overlying lamellar periosteal reaction. **B,** Axial, T2-weighted, fat-suppressed MR image shows a principally multilocular cystic lesion with several fluid-fluid levels mimicking an aneurysmal bone cyst.

A

B

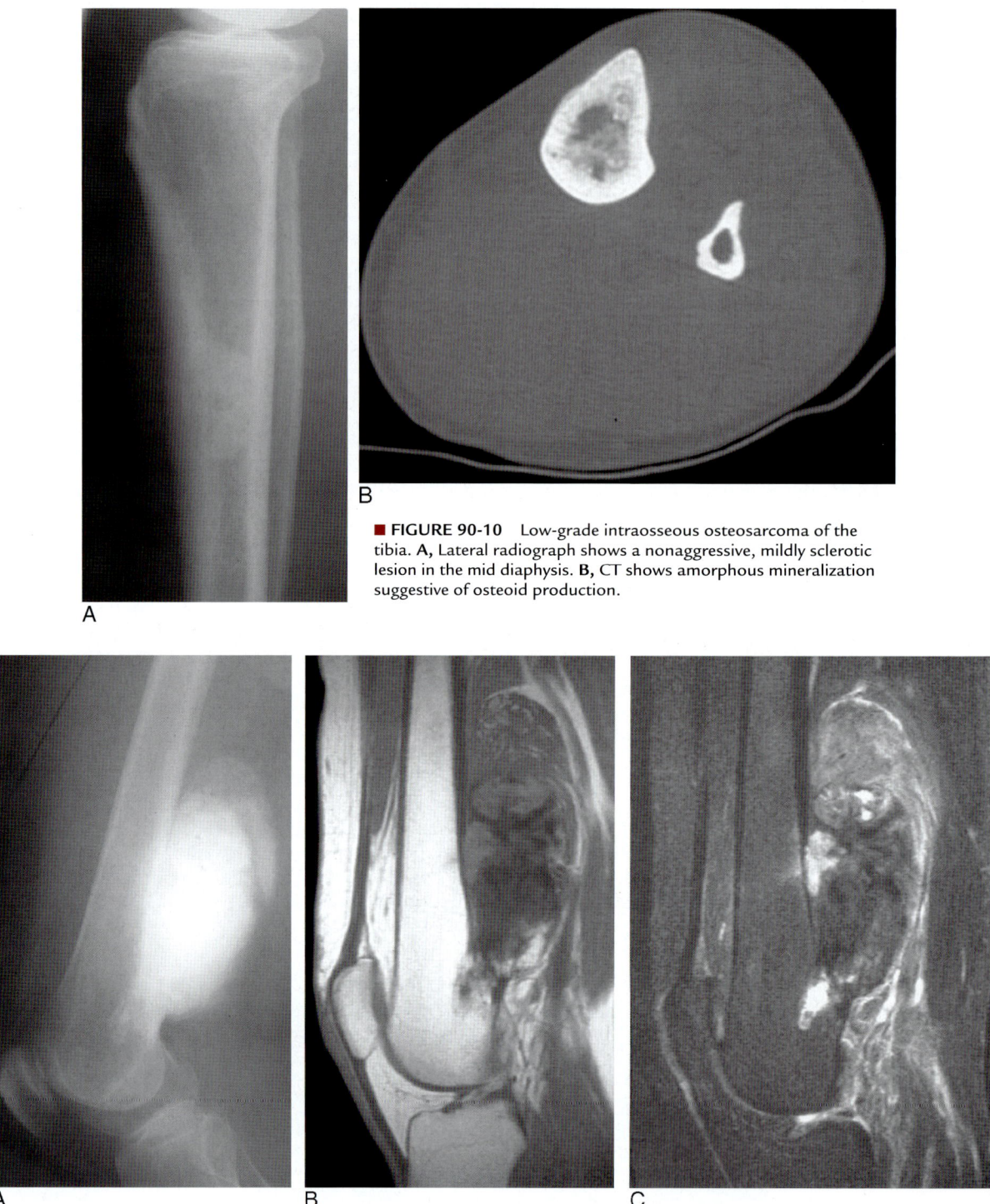

■ **FIGURE 90-10** Low-grade intraosseous osteosarcoma of the tibia. **A,** Lateral radiograph shows a nonaggressive, mildly sclerotic lesion in the mid diaphysis. **B,** CT shows amorphous mineralization suggestive of osteoid production.

■ **FIGURE 90-11** Dedifferentiated parosteal osteosarcoma. Lateral radiograph (**A**), sagittal T1-weighted (**B**), and STIR (**C**) MR images show a densely mineralized tumor arising on the posterior aspect of the distal femoral metadiaphysis. There is early medullary invasion distally and the lower density area proximally was shown to be due to dedifferentiation to high-grade osteosarcoma.

either at presentation or on recurrence will show dedifferentiation to a high-grade osteosarcoma. This should be suspected if there is a significant soft tissue component to the tumor. Biopsy should be directed to any suspected high-grade areas of the tumor because this will influence management. The differential diagnosis for parosteal osteosarcoma includes other mineralizing surface lesions, such as surface osteoma and myositis ossificans as well as

osteochondroma. The surface form of myositis ossificans (periostitis ossificans) can be diagnosed by identification of the zoning phenomenon whereby calcification and subsequent ossification first develops in the periphery of the lesion. This is in contrast to parosteal osteosarcoma, in which the matrix is densest centrally and may be less mature or absent peripherally. Parosteal osteosarcoma differs from osteochondroma in that the latter shows flaring of the cortex continuous with the cortex of the underlying bone and a trabecular component merging with the medulla of the host bone. Because it is a low-grade tumor, local recurrence may occur many years after presentation and initial surgical management.

Periosteal Osteosarcoma

Periosteal osteosarcoma accounts for less than 2% of cases of osteosarcoma. It tends to occur in adolescents and young adults and arises most often from the surface of the diaphyses of the tibia and femur (Fig. 90-12). It is a low- to intermediate-grade tumor with prominent chondrogenic components. There is a spectrum of imaging appearances ranging from features suggestive of a periosteal chondroma (due to the chondrogenic elements) with scalloping of the outer cortex to a patently more aggressive lesion with Codman angles and a spiculated/sunburst periosteal reaction (see Fig. 90-12).[8] The latter appearances resemble a high-grade surface osteosarcoma (see later). MRI confirms the surface nature of the tumor with intramedullary invasion uncommon.

High-Grade Surface Osteosarcoma

High-grade surface osteosarcoma is, as the name implies, a high-grade malignancy indistinguishable histologically from the intramedullary counterpart—the only difference being the surface origin. It is the rarest of the surface osteosarcomas, accounting for less than 1% of all osteosarcomas. The most frequent sites are the femur, tibia, and humerus (Fig. 90-13). Radiographically, these tumors resemble the more aggressive end of the spectrum of periosteal osteosarcoma, with prominent spiculated periosteal new bone formation and intramedullary invasion more common.[9]

Secondary Osteosarcoma

Secondary osteosarcoma develops in a preexisting bone lesion that may or may not be neoplastic (see Table 90-2). One distinctive feature of these secondary lesions is that they tend to occur in an older age group than primary osteosarcoma (e.g., Paget's osteosarcoma). This can have major implications on management because many affected patients are too old to undergo chemotherapy. This adversely affects the prognosis and ultimately the long-term survival of these patients. Dedifferentiated chondrosarcoma is discussed later under cartilage-producing tumors.

Paget's disease of bone, named after the 19th century British surgeon Sir James Paget, is a localized or multifocal disorder of bone characterized by abnormal bone turnover with increased osteoclastic activity and compensatory increased osteoblastic activity. The prevalence of Paget's disease increases with age, with significant geographic/ethnic variations. It is relatively common in the white races of northern Europe and yet rare in blacks and Asians. Recent studies, however, have shown that the disease is slowly disappearing. Of all the skeletal complications seen in Paget's disease malignant transformation is by far the most serious, with an incidence quoted as ranging from 0.7% to 6% affected cases. Paget's sarcoma is twice as common in men than women, is more common in patients with multifocal disease, and typically presents in the sixth and seventh decades of life. The most commonly affected bones, in descending order of frequency, are the femur, pelvis, and humerus (Fig. 90-14). By far and away the most frequent histology of Paget's sarcoma is osteosarcoma. In those regions where Paget's disease is common, 20% of patients with osteosarcoma who are older than 40 years of age and as high as 50% of patients with osteosarcoma older than the age of 60 have Paget's disease as the predisposing condition. In the older literature, the second most common histology in Paget's sarcoma was fibrosarcoma. More recent pathologic redefinition of spindle cell sarcomas means that other diagnoses such as malignant fibrous histiocytoma and leiomyosarcoma tend to be favored over fibrosarcoma. The majority of Paget's sarcomas will show rapidly progressive ill-defined bone destruction developing within an area of preexisting Paget's disease. Cortical destruction and a soft tissue mass are common features, whereas periosteal new bone formation is seen in less than 20% of cases. Despite the fact that most are secondary osteosarcomas, radiographically apparent malignant osteoid is not common. Unlike most sarcomas of bone, Paget's sarcoma frequently appears relatively photopenic against the background of increased activity of Paget's disease on bone scintigraphy. In uncomplicated Paget's disease the fat signal (hyperintense on both T1- and T2-weighted images) is typically

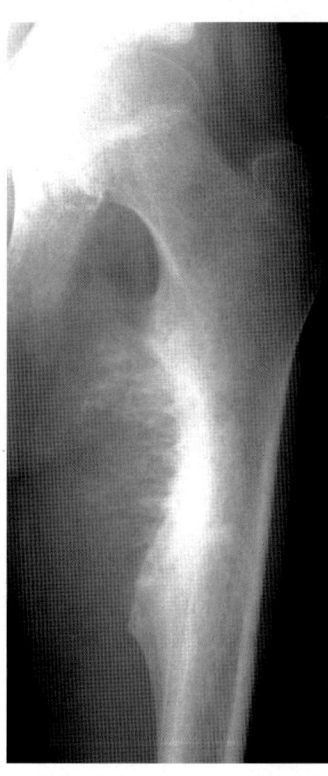

■ **FIGURE 90-12** Periosteal osteosarcoma. The radiograph shows typical spiculated periosteal reaction arising from the femur.

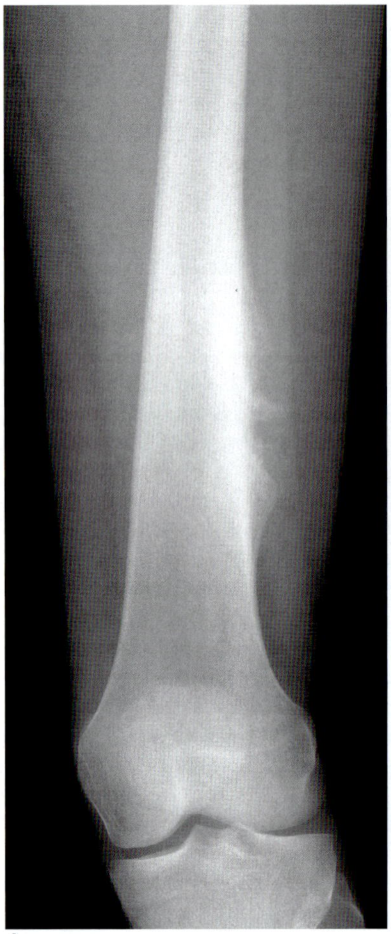

■ **FIGURE 90-13** High-grade surface osteosarcoma. Anteroposterior radiograph (**A**) axial T1-weighted (**B**), and axial, T2-weighted, fat-suppressed (**C**) MR images showing a surface lesion arising on the femur with early cortical involvement.

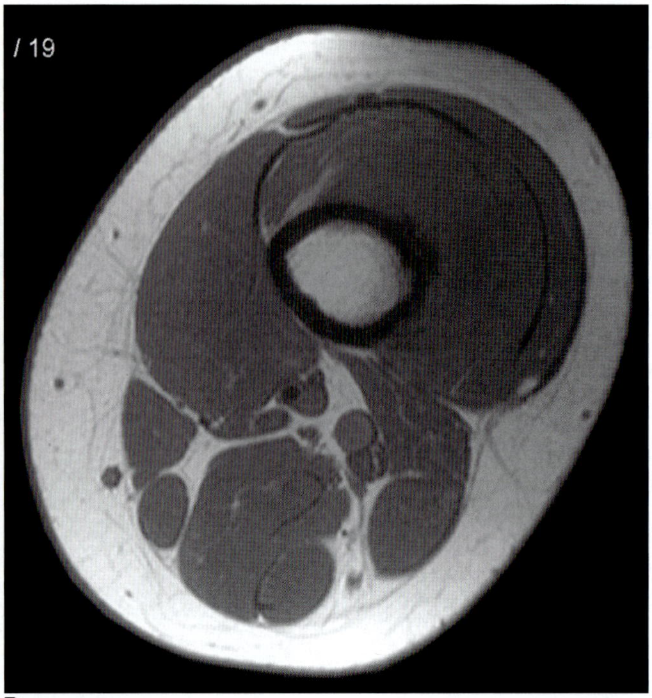

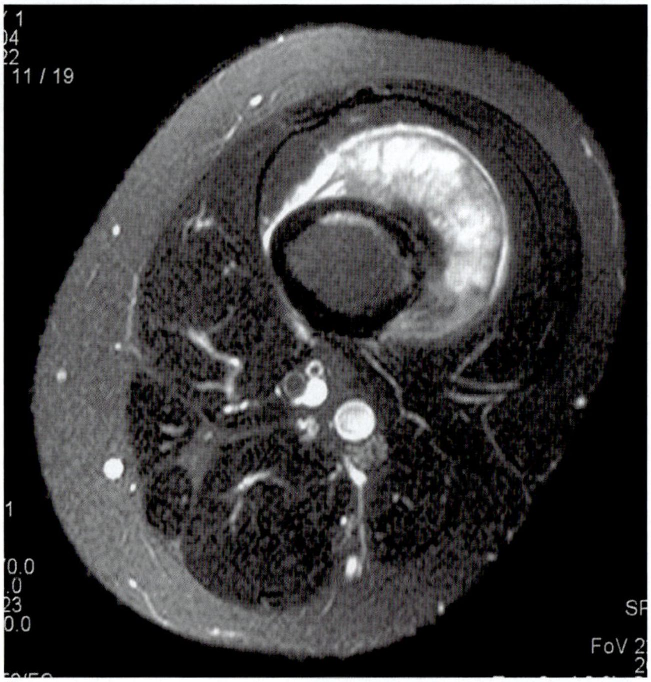

preserved in all phases of the disease. Paget's sarcoma, unless densely mineralized, typically shows intermediate- to low-signal-intensity tumor tissue on T1-weighted images with corresponding high signal intensity on T2-weighted or short tau inversion recovery (STIR) images. Most cases will show cortical destruction with a soft tissue mass. It is important to recognize that not all tumors arising in Paget's disease are sarcomas. There is a recognized association between Paget's disease and giant cell

tumors of bone. Also, in the elderly population, metastases, myeloma, and lymphoma may all develop in pagetic bone. Tumor-like conditions that may mimic Paget's sarcoma include pseudosarcoma due to the development of florid periosteal pagetic bone, accelerated disuse osteoporosis usually following immobilization, and drug-induced osteomalacia.

Radiation-induced sarcomas of bone are rare, accounting for approximately 1.5% of all bone sarcomas. The overall

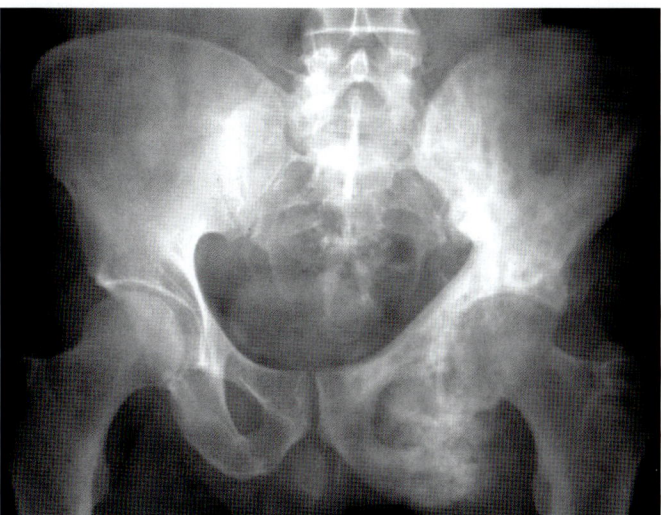

■ **FIGURE 90-14** Paget's sarcoma. The radiograph shows extensive Paget's disease involving the left hemipelvis. There is an osteosarcoma arising in the left ischium with malignant osteoid formation.

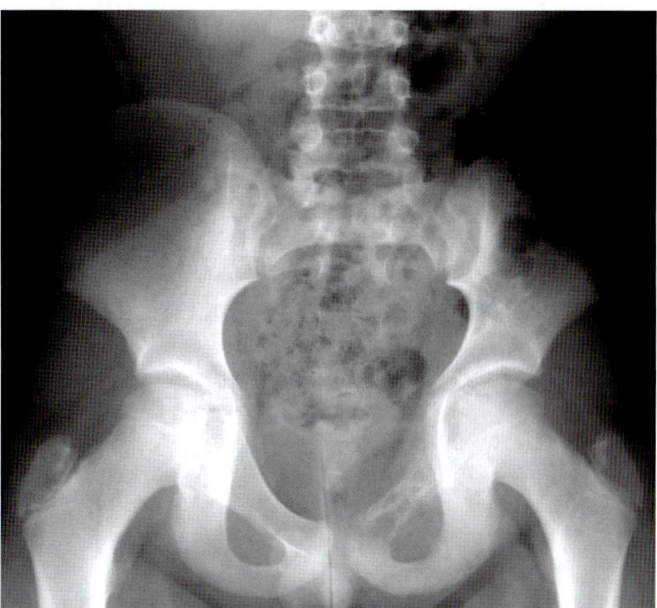

■ **FIGURE 90-15** Radiation sarcoma. The radiograph shows an aggressive lesion arising in the left superior pubic ramus due to an osteosarcoma. There is hypoplasia of the left hemipelvis also secondary due to radiotherapy administered as a child in the treatment of Wilms' tumor.

incidence ranges between 0.03% (of patients who receive radiation) to 0.2% (of patients who received radiation and survived 5 years). Sarcomas can develop in any bone exposed to either internal or external radiation sources. They may arise at the site of preexisting bone lesions or in bones that were normal at the time of irradiation, such as when radiation has been used to treat malignancy in adjacent soft tissue tumors without bony involvement. Approximately one third of post-irradiation sarcomas arise in preexisting lesions such as giant cell tumor, bone lymphoma, osteosarcoma, or round cell tumors such as Ewing's sarcoma. There was a vogue in the mid-20th century, long since ceased, to treat fibrous dysplasia with radiotherapy. As a result, radiation sarcomas were seen in association with fibrous dysplasia. Osteosarcoma and spindle cell sarcoma (fibrosarcoma, malignant fibrous histiocytoma) account for over 90% of radiation-induced sarcomas. Chondrosarcomas comprise less than 10% of the total. Established diagnostic criteria for the diagnosis of post-irradiation sarcoma are (1) malignancy arising within the irradiated field, (2) histologic proof of sarcoma, distinct from any original lesion, (3) and a long latent period of at least 4 years after irradiation. The latent period ranges from 4 to 55 years (mean, 11-14 years). It does not differ between children and adults, but in children a higher prevalence of radiation-induced sarcoma can be expected because the immature skeleton is more susceptible to radiation-induced induction of malignancy and because they have a longer period over which they are at risk and therefore have the potential to develop malignancy. Latency may be inversely proportional to radiation dose, with shorter latent periods often seen after administration of higher doses. Radiographically, an aggressive lytic lesion is present often with soft tissue extension (Fig. 90-15). Malignant osteoid formation with dense sclerosis is a feature of radiation-induced osteosarcoma. Coexisting radiation

bone changes are seen in up to 50% of patients. The cardinal features of cortical destruction and soft tissue extension are optimally demonstrated with MRI, but CT can also be used. Radiation-induced insufficiency fractures may mimic sarcoma or metastases, particularly on bone scintigraphy. These tend to occur at classic sites, for example, the sacrum in women who have undergone pelvic radiotherapy for a gynecologic malignancy.

Other conditions that rarely may be associated with the development of a secondary osteosarcoma as well as spindle cell sarcoma (malignant fibrous histiocytoma) are fibrous dysplasia, medullary infarction (Fig. 90-16), and chronic osteomyelitis. Increasing pain, medullary lysis, cortical breaching, and the development of a soft tissue mass, often without obvious radiographic evidence of malignant osteoid formation, should suggest the possibility of malignant transformation and prompt further investigation with MRI. Bone sarcomas have been rarely described arising adjacent to orthopedic implants, raising speculation as to an association. As yet, no convincing causal relationship has been proven in these cases.

Cartilage-Producing Tumors

Chondroid-producing/chondrogenic tumors are defined as neoplasms that produce a cartilaginous matrix. According to their biologic behavior they are subdivided into benign and malignant lesions (see Table 90-1) and further subdivided by intramedullary (central) and surface

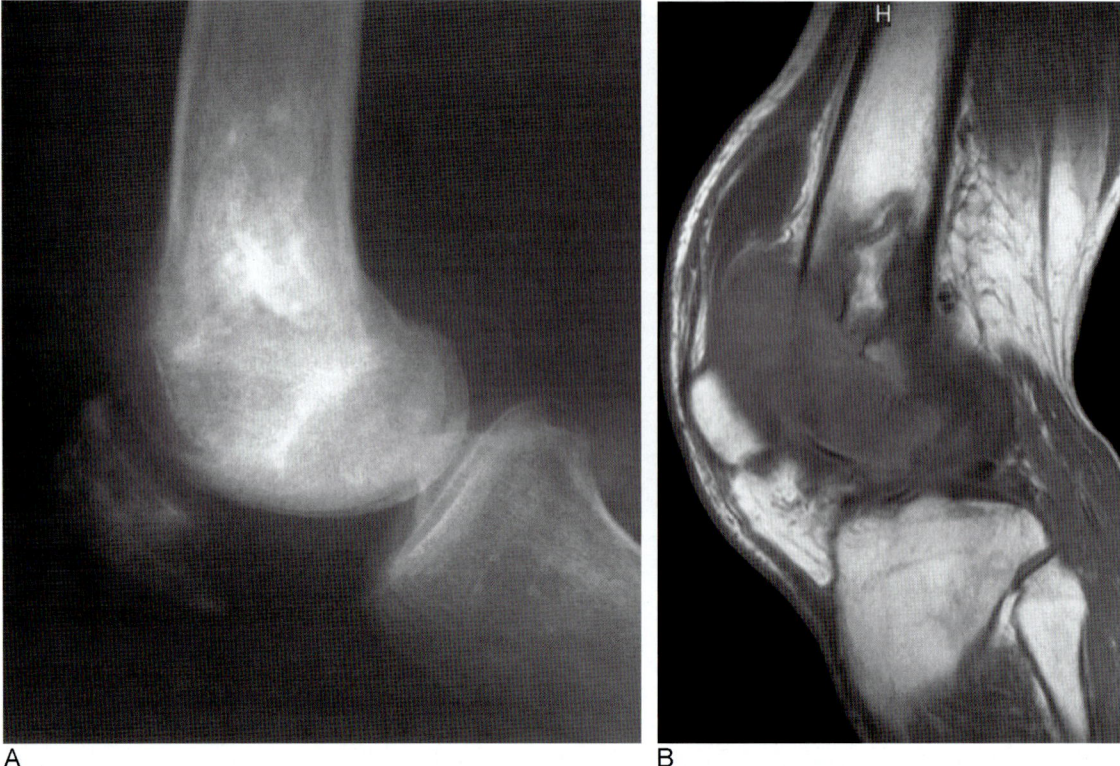

■ **FIGURE 90-16** Osteosarcoma associated with bone infarct. Lateral radiograph (**A**) and sagittal, T1-weighted MR image (**B**) showing a typical medullary infarct in the femoral metaphysis with a tumor distally invading the knee joint.

(peripheral) locations. The radiographic identification of cartilaginous matrix as annular, popcorn, or comma shaped is usually straightforward. Difficulties can occur in distinguishing between benign cartilaginous tumors with prominent cellular activity and low-grade chondrosarcoma both on imaging and histology.

Osteochondroma

Osteochondroma is a benign, cartilage-capped osseous projection arising on the outer surface of bone. The term *exostosis* is frequently used interchangeably with osteochondroma but, strictly speaking, an exostosis is a bony projection and can therefore be used loosely for any other calcifying/ossifying surface lesions of bone, such as surface osteoma and bizarre parosteal osteochondromatous proliferation. Osteochondroma is the most common bone tumor, comprising an estimated 35% of benign bone tumors and 10% of all bone tumors. As indicated in Table 88-3, the reported incidence of osteochondroma is too low because many osteochondromas are not detected or are not registered. They may present as an incidental finding on radiographs, owing to swelling and deformity around a joint or to one of the complications, including fracture, pressure on adjacent neurovascular structures, overlying bursal inflammation, and malignant transformation. They arise in childhood, although they may not present until adult life if at all, owing to an aberration/herniation originating at the growth plate (physis). There are three histologic

components. An outer fibrous perichondrium is present over a cartilage cap that, in turn, covers the bony base. Over 90% cases arise in the long bones of the extremities with 33% around the knee. They tend to be metaphyseal or diametaphyseal, projecting away from the adjacent joint, and can vary considerably in size.

The radiographic appearances of osteochondromas are distinctive with two typical forms: sessile (broad-based) and pedunculated (slender stalk or pedicle) with variable chondrogenic matrix in the cartilage cap that, if extensive, can resemble cauliflower (Figs. 90-17 and 90-18). The cortex and medulla of the underlying host bone is continuous with that of the osteochondroma, which helps to differentiate it from other surface lesions, such as parosteal osteosarcoma. Multiple osteochondromas, also known as diaphyseal aclasis, hereditary multiple exostoses, and osteochondromatosis, occur in approximately 1 in 50,000 persons in the general population. Apart from multiplicity it differs from the solitary type by the fact that the growth plate abnormalities tend to be circumferential rather than focal. This gives rise to sessile osteochondromas with greater modeling deformity and reduced longitudinal bone growth. The degree of skeletal involvement can vary significantly between patients even in the same family. Severely affected cases will show large juxta-articular bony lumps with reduced stature and bowing deformities. In the upper limb this can cause a Madelung-type deformity at the wrist and progressive dislocation of the radial head at the elbow.

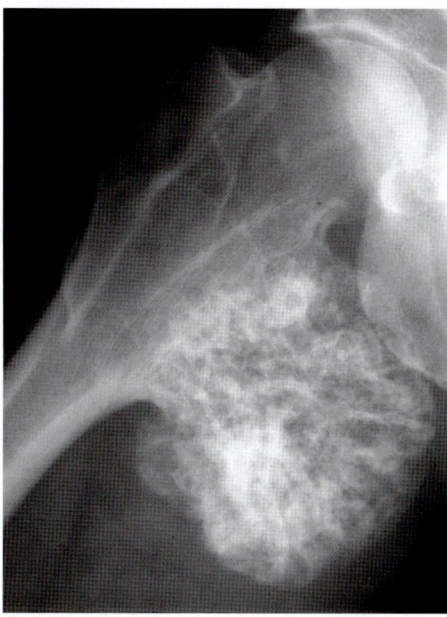

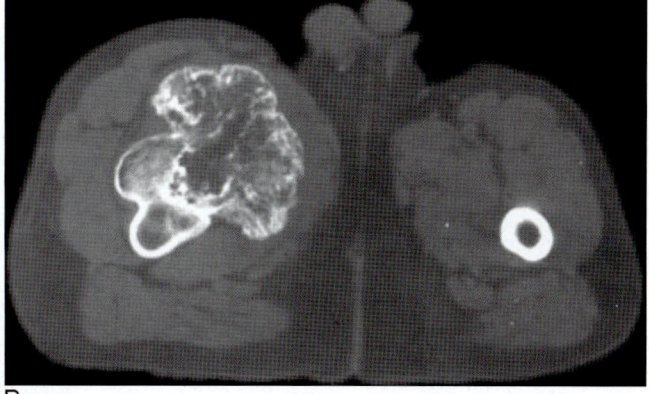

■ **FIGURE 90-17** Sessile osteochondroma. Anteroposterior radiograph (**A**) and CT image (**B**) showing a broad-based osteochondroma arising from the proximal femur.

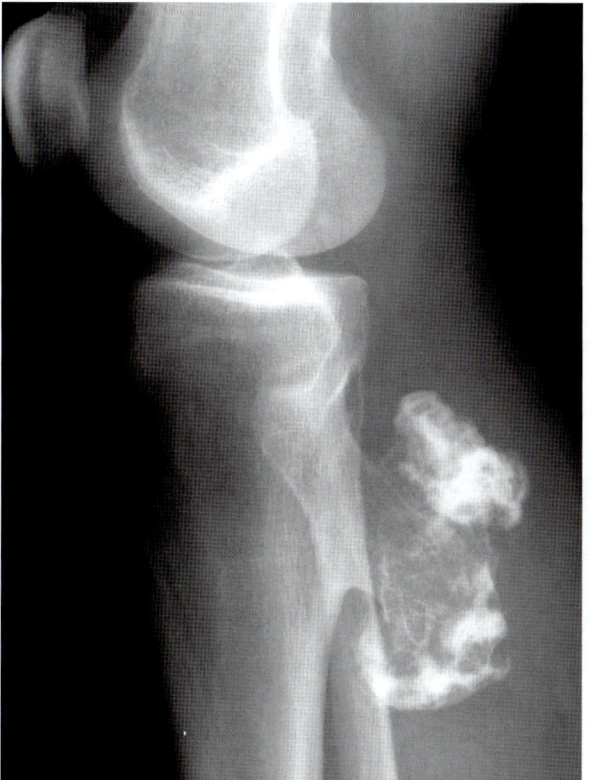

■ **FIGURE 90-18** Radiograph of pedunculated osteochondroma arising from the proximal tibia.

Most osteochondromas cease to grow at skeletal maturity. Growth in adult life can be due to persistent enchondral ossification or the most significant of all the complications of osteochondromas—malignant transformation to a low-grade peripheral chondrosarcoma. The latter complication occurs in less than 1% of solitary and in 3% to 5% of cases of hereditary multiple exostoses. Evidence clinically of pain and increasing size and with dispersal of the peripheral calcifications on review of serial radiographs suggests the possibility of malignant transformation (Fig. 90-19). Bone scintigraphy will show increased activity in the presence of both persistent enchondral ossification and malignant change. Normal background skeletal activity over a symptomatic osteochondroma would tend to exclude malignancy. The thickness of the cartilage cap can be readily measured using CT, MRI, or ultrasonography. If the cartilage cap is less than 2 cm in thickness, the possibility of malignancy is remote. If it is greater than 2 cm, the likelihood of malignancy increases (Fig. 90-20). Cross-sectional imaging is also useful in excluding other complications that may be associated with the development of an overlying soft tissue mass, including bursa and pseudoaneurysm formation (Fig. 90-21).

Radiation-induced osteochondroma is a recognized complication of radiotherapy, with an incidence of 5% to 10% of skeletally immature patients undergoing radiotherapy. Most reports are in children who received radiotherapy for Wilms' tumor or neuroblastoma, the majority of whom would have been treated before 6 years of age. However, they do occur after radiotherapy later than this. Lesions may be multiple, and development is reported between 3 and 18 years after radiotherapy. The time interval is extremely variable and largely dependent on the site of the lesion, any associated pressure, or mass effects, or if it is discovered incidentally on follow-up imaging. The imaging and pathologic features, surgical treatment, and prognosis are identical to those for a spontaneous osteochondroma.

Chondroma

Chondromas are benign tumors comprising abundant mature hyaline cartilage matrix that are relatively avascular. They are called enchondromas if they arise within

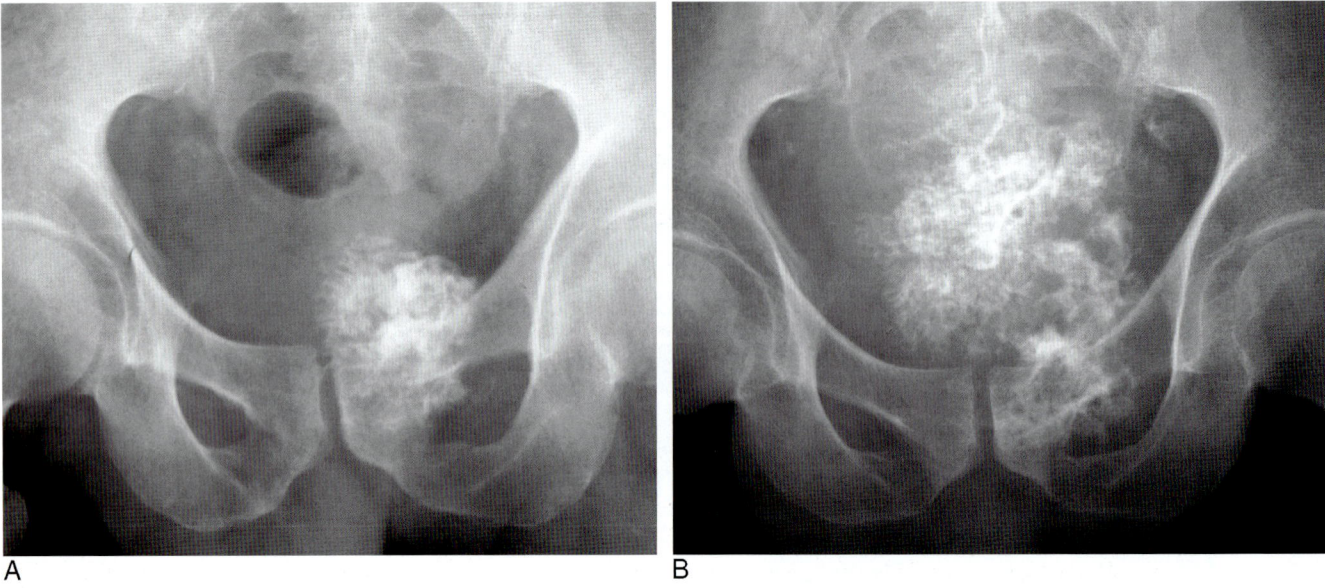

■ **FIGURE 90-19** Peripheral chondrosarcoma. **A** and **B,** Anteroposterior radiographs 4 years apart. In **B,** there is obvious increase in size of the lesion arising from the pubis with dispersal of the calcifications typical of a chondrosarcoma.

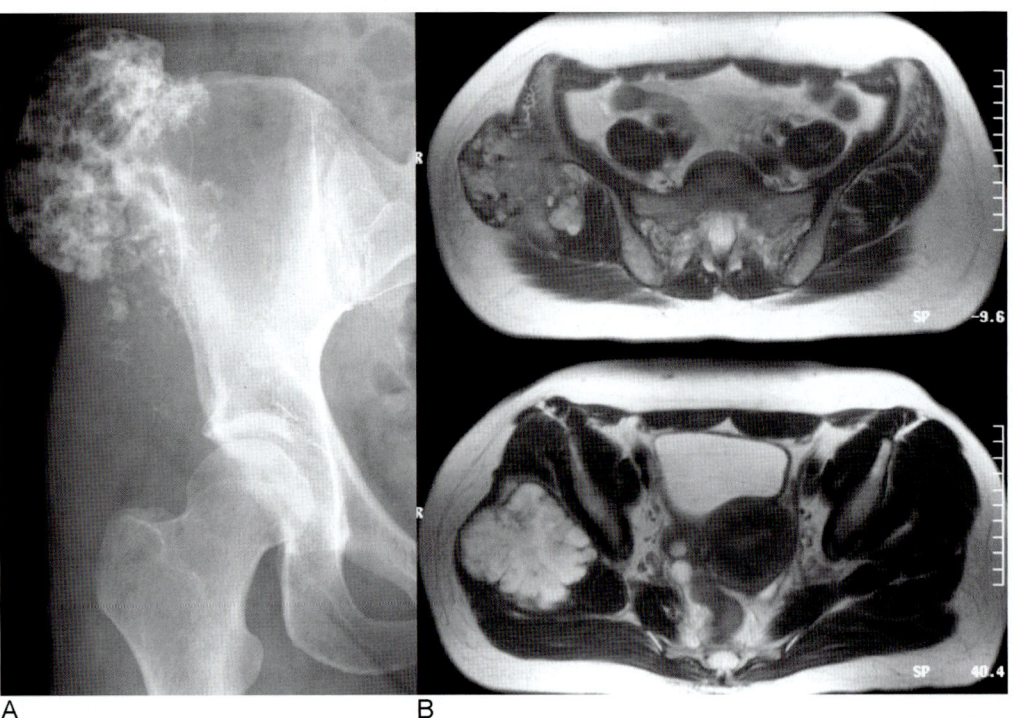

■ **FIGURE 90-20** Peripheral chondrosarcoma. Anteroposterior radiograph (**A**) and axial, T2-weighted MR images (**B**) of the pelvis showing the benign portion of the lesion arising from the superior aspect of the ilium. Distally there is dispersal of the calcifications in a soft tissue mass corresponding to the hyperintense lobules typical of low-grade chondrosarcoma.

the medulla and periosteal (juxtacortical) chondromas if they arise on the surface of bone. Enchondroma is the second most common benign bone tumor, accounting for up to 15% of cases. Like osteochondroma, the true incidence is higher than the registered incidence (see Table 88-3), as many are not detected. This explains the wide age range of presentation from 5 to 80 years, although most symptomatic cases present in the second to fourth decades. Fifty percent of cases arise in the tubular bones of the hands and feet; it is the most common

bone tumor of the distal extremities. The next most common sites are the metaphyses of the long bones, notably the distal femur and proximal humerus (Fig. 90-22). With the increasing use of MRI many more occult cases are being identified at these two sites, which then tends to initiate a series of further imaging tests, including bone scintigraphy before biopsy of the larger lesions to exclude a low-grade chondrosarcoma. Enchondromas are uncommon in the flat bones, such as the pelvis and ribs. Larger lesions relative to the underlying bone may

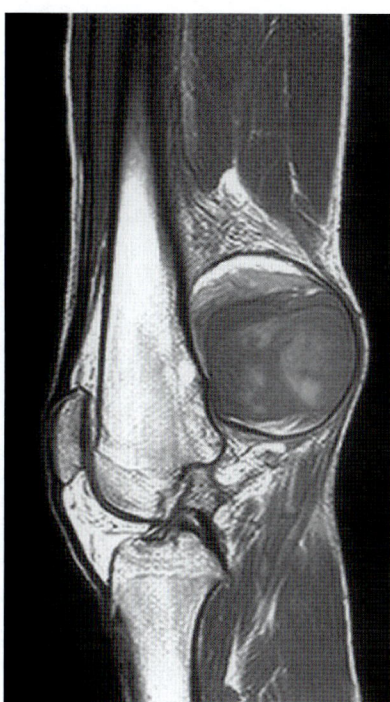

■ **FIGURE 90-21** Pseudoaneurysm of distal femoral artery. Sagittal T1-weighted MR image shows a rounded mass with hyperintense areas due to methemoglobin. The pseudoaneurysm is caused by mechanical friction on the artery from the sessile osteochondroma arising on the posterior aspect of the distal femur.

present as a pathologic fracture after only minor trauma. This is frequently the case with enchondromas of the fingers.

The typical radiographic features of an enchondroma are those of a lytic lesion arising within the medulla. The lesion is well defined to give a geographic pattern of bone destruction (Fig. 90-23). In relatively narrow bones, such as the hands and feet, bony expansion with cortical thinning is common. In the larger bones the tumor usually arises centrally within the metaphysis or metadiaphysis such that endosteal resorption/scalloping is only seen in the bigger lesions. Most tumors are less than 3 cm in length. If they are larger than 5 cm, the possibility of a low-grade chondrosarcoma is questioned.[10] Enchondromas may be purely lytic, particularly in the hands and feet. Identification of the classic mineralization variously called "ring-and-arc," "stippled," "punctate," and "popcorn" indicates the cartilaginous nature of the tumor but does not help distinguish benign from malignant lesions. In the adult, up to 30% of cases may show some increase in activity on bone scintigraphy owing to persistent enchondral ossification and so, again, cannot be used to distinguish benign from malignant cartilaginous tumors reliably. On MRI the hyperintense lobules of cartilage can be clearly identified on T2-weighted and STIR images, with the calcifications, if present, showing signal voids or low-signal foci. The high water content of the extracellular matrix explains the hyperintensity and may also cause some chemical shift artifact at the tumor/marrow fat interface.

Enchondromas are relatively avascular, so enhancement with gadolinium typically only shows a peripheral and septal pattern accentuating the lobular appearance of the tumor on T1-weighted images.

Periosteal (juxtacortical) chondroma is a benign hyaline cartilage tumor arising from the periosteum on the surface of bone. It is an uncommon lesion, comprising less than 2% of chondromas. They occur on the metaphyses of long bones, particularly the proximal humerus and around the knee (Fig. 90-24). On radiographs it shows as a surface lesion with saucerization of the outer cortex and peripheral buttress formation. The lesion may or may not show cartilaginous mineralization. The differential diagnosis on imaging includes periosteal osteosarcoma (because of its chondroblastic nature) and periosteal ganglion because of the erosion of the outer surface of the cortex adjacent to a joint. Larger lesions will show cartilaginous lobules on MRI and may simulate a sessile osteochondroma.

Multiple enchondromas, also known as enchondromatosis or Ollier's disease, is an uncommon bone dysplasia caused by failure of normal enchondral ossification. There is no hereditary or familial tendency, unlike hereditary multiple exostoses. The severity as well as extent of skeletal involvement can vary from just a few lesions in a single limb (monomelic), one side of the body (hemimelic), or bilateral involvement to very extensive disease with deformity and limb-length inequality. Typical radiographic features of severe disease include radiolucent columns of cartilage extending from the growth plate down to the metaphyses and variable quantities of cartilage calcification, with some lesions protruding into the soft tissues (Fig. 90-25). Disturbances at the growth plate lead to modeling deformities and shortening. Malignant transformation to a central low-grade chondrosarcoma occurs in approximately 20% cases. Multiple enchondromas in conjunction with soft tissue angiomas and, rarely, visceral angiomas is termed Maffucci's syndrome. It is also a developmental nonhereditary disorder. Identification of phleboliths within the soft tissues together with enchondromas clinches the diagnosis. However, the phleboliths may not calcify until adolescence or adulthood and thus until then the syndrome can be radiographically indistinguishable from multiple enchondromas. The angiomas may be detected on MRI, originally performed to assess the chondromas, if the soft tissue abnormality is within the scan field. The significance of Maffucci's syndrome is that the risk of malignant transformation is said to be even higher than multiple enchondromas, at approximately 30% to 35% of cases.

Chondroblastoma

Chondroblastoma is a benign cartilaginous tumor arising in the epiphyses and, less commonly, the apophyses, in the skeletally immature individual. It comprises less than 1% of all tumors and approximately 6% of benign bone tumors. Seventy-five percent of cases arise in the epiphyses around the knee and the proximal humerus (Fig. 90-26). It is one of the more common tumors, arising in the talus and patella after giant cell tumor of bone. Radiographically, it appears

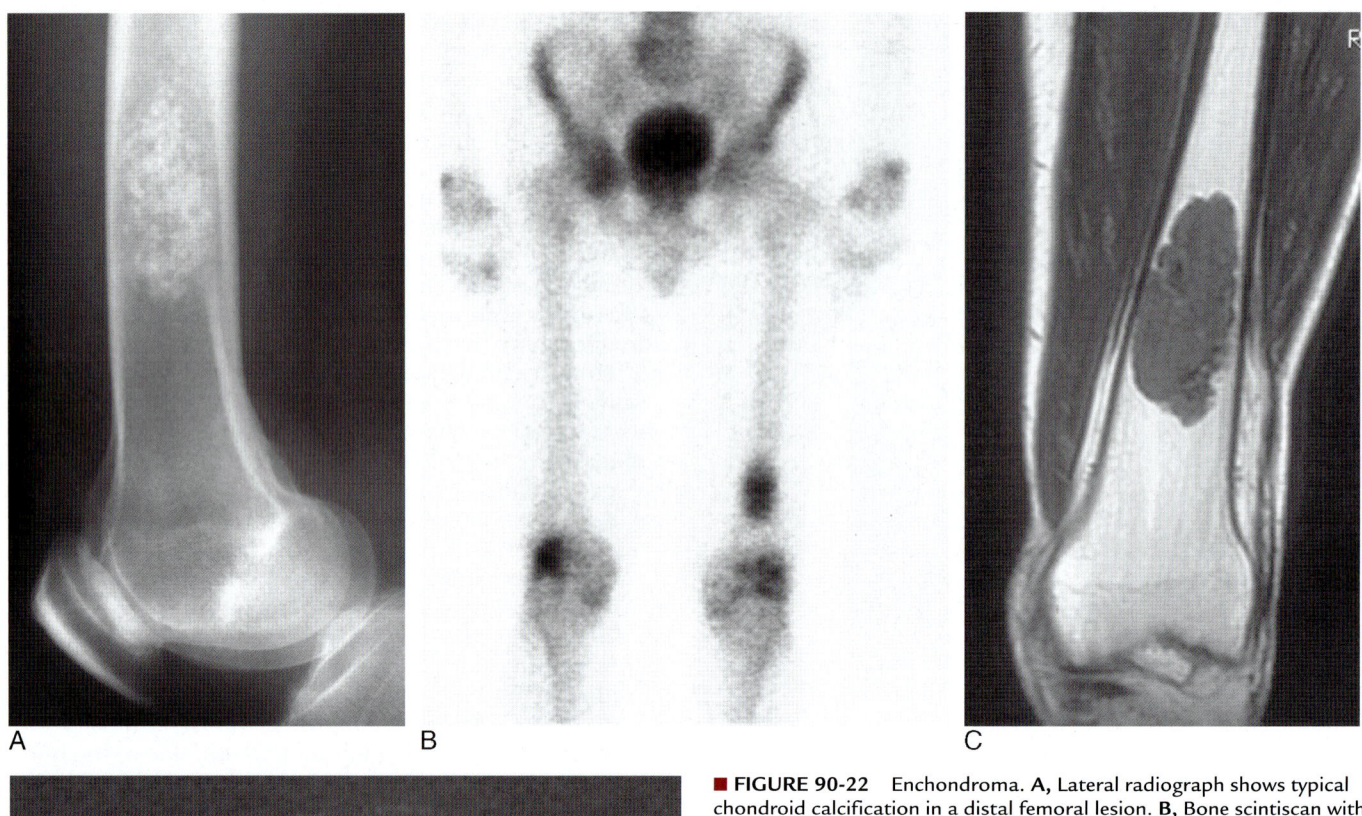

A   B   C

■ **FIGURE 90-22** Enchondroma. **A,** Lateral radiograph shows typical chondroid calcification in a distal femoral lesion. **B,** Bone scintiscan with moderately increased activity in the femoral lesion. There is also minor increased activity due to degenerative joint disease of the knees and right hip. Coronal T1-weighted (**C**) and axial T2-weighted, fat-suppressed (**D**) MR images showing the lobulated appearance of a cartilage tumor.

D

as a well-defined lytic lesion of variable size (depending on duration of symptoms) arising in an epiphysis (see Fig. 90-26A). Up to one third will show internal cartilage calcification on radiographs increasing to over half if CT is used. Large lesions may develop periosteal reaction along the metaphysis with involvement of the growth plate, simulating an aggressive lesion. The important factor to determine is the site of origin or epicenter of the lesion. Primary sarcoma arising in an epiphysis is remarkably rare. Most subarticular lytic lesions that might mimic chondroblastoma, such as clear cell chondrosarcoma and intraosseous ganglion, tend to occur in adulthood. In the child, the differential diagnosis includes an epiphyseal abscess. MRI will show an epiphyseal- or apophyseal-based lesion

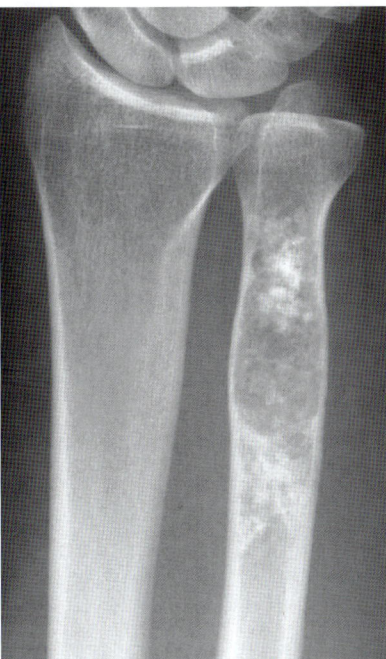

■ **FIGURE 90-23** Enchondroma. Posteroanterior radiograph of the forearm showing a lesion in the distal ulna with geographic bone destruction, chondroid matrix mineralization, endosteal resorption, and minor bony expansion.

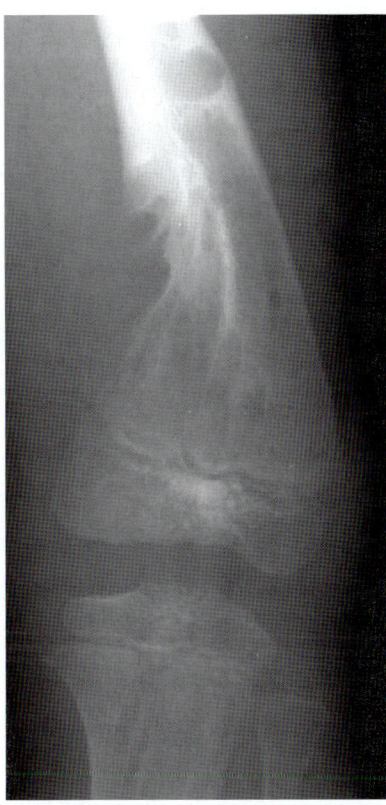

■ **FIGURE 90-25** Ollier's disease. Anteroposterior radiograph of the knee showing longitudinal radiolucent columns of cartilage involving the distal femoral and proximal tibial diaphyses. Differential growth has resulted in a varus deformity of the distal femur.

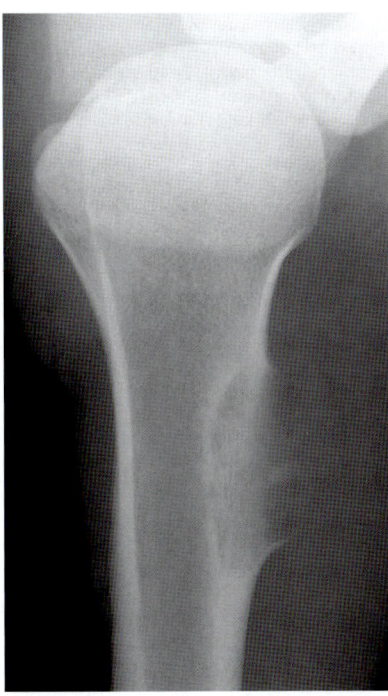

■ **FIGURE 90-24** Periosteal chondroma. Axial radiograph of shoulder showing a surface lesion with erosion of the outer cortex, a peripheral periosteal buttress, and absence of matrix mineralization.

ablation. Recurrence may be seen in 10% to 15% of cases. The presence of persistent marrow edema around the lesion on follow-up MRI is suggestive of recurrent disease. Malignant transformation has been described in a few cases of chondroblastoma.

Chondromyxoid Fibroma

Chondromyxoid fibroma is a rare benign cartilaginous tumor consisting of lobulated areas of spindle-shaped or stellate cells with abundant myxoid or chondroid intracellular matrix. It comprises less than 2% of benign bone tumors, occurs predominantly in the second and third decades, and has a predilection for the long bones of the lower limb, particularly the proximal tibia. The radiographic appearances are those of a well-defined oval or round lytic lesion arising eccentrically within the metaphysis of a long bone (Fig. 90-27). Matrix calcification is uncommon. MRI will reveal a typical lobulated pattern suggestive of a cartilage tumor. The differential diagnosis includes aneurysmal bone cyst and nonossifying fibroma.

Chondrosarcoma

Chondrosarcoma is a malignant tumor with hyaline cartilage differentiation with varying degrees of myxoid change and mineralization. It may be a central (medullary) or surface (peripheral) tumor as well as

with florid, surrounding reactive marrow edema and a joint effusion (see Figs. 90-26B and C).[11] Cystic spaces with fluid-fluid levels suggest secondary aneurysmal bone cyst formation (see Fig. 90-26C). Treatment usually involves curettage, although some centers are now trying thermal

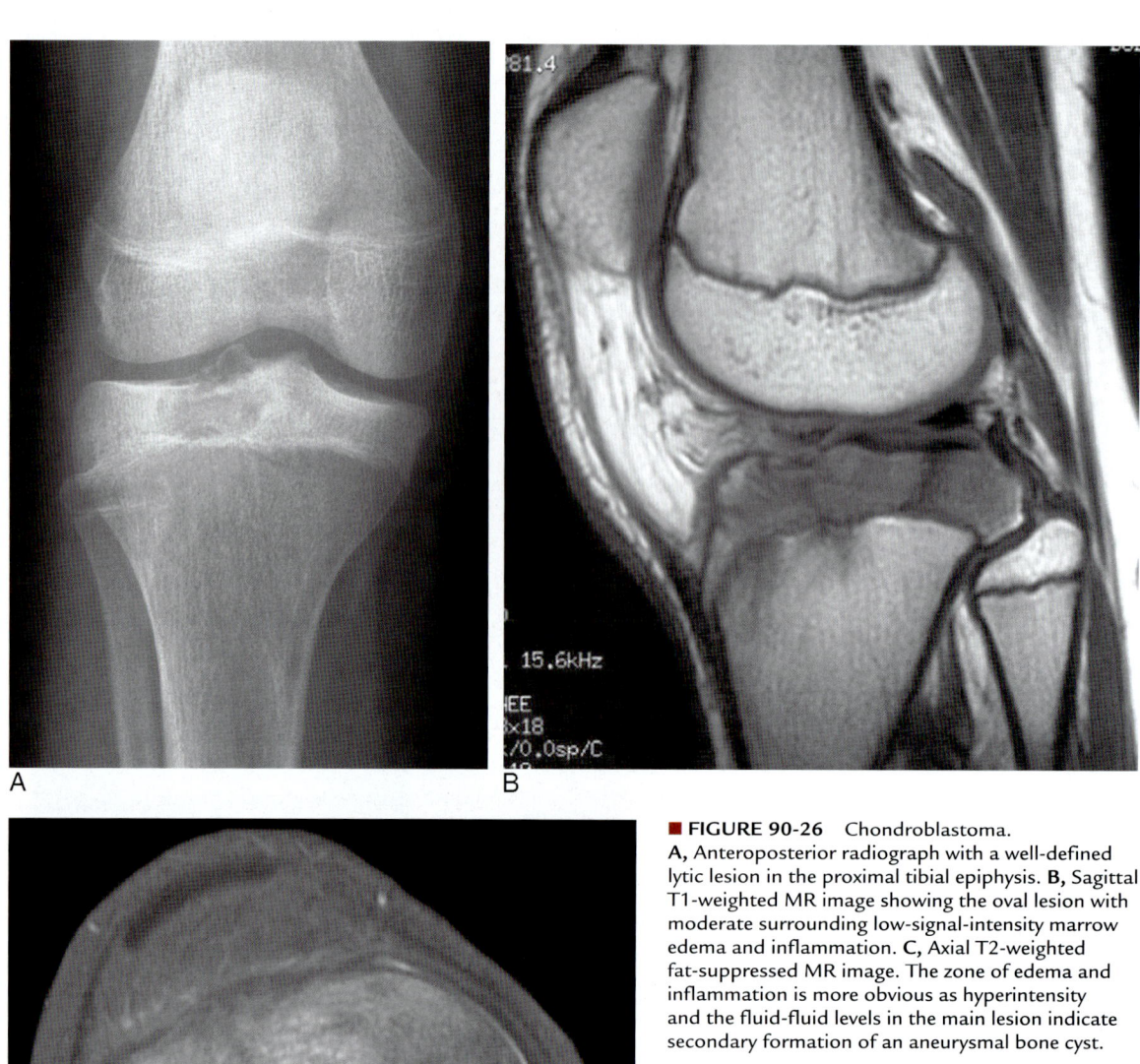

■ **FIGURE 90-26** Chondroblastoma.
A, Anteroposterior radiograph with a well-defined lytic lesion in the proximal tibial epiphysis. **B,** Sagittal T1-weighted MR image showing the oval lesion with moderate surrounding low-signal-intensity marrow edema and inflammation. **C,** Axial T2-weighted fat-suppressed MR image. The zone of edema and inflammation is more obvious as hyperintensity and the fluid-fluid levels in the main lesion indicate secondary formation of an aneurysmal bone cyst.

primary (arising de novo in normal bone) or secondary (arising in a preexisting benign cartilage tumor). It is the third most common primary malignant tumor of bone after myeloma and osteosarcoma. It is a disease of the middle-aged and elderly and more common in men than women. The diagnosis should be questioned if the patient is a child or adolescent. Chondosarcomas are graded pathologically on a scale of 1 to 3, otherwise known as of low, intermediate, and high grade. This is important because grading influences management and prognosis. As might be expected, high-grade tumors have an increased propensity to recur locally after surgery and develop distant metastases, which are typically pulmonary.

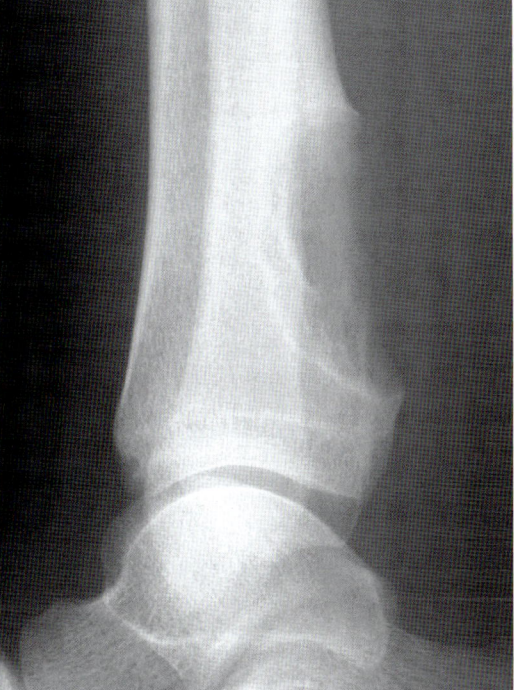
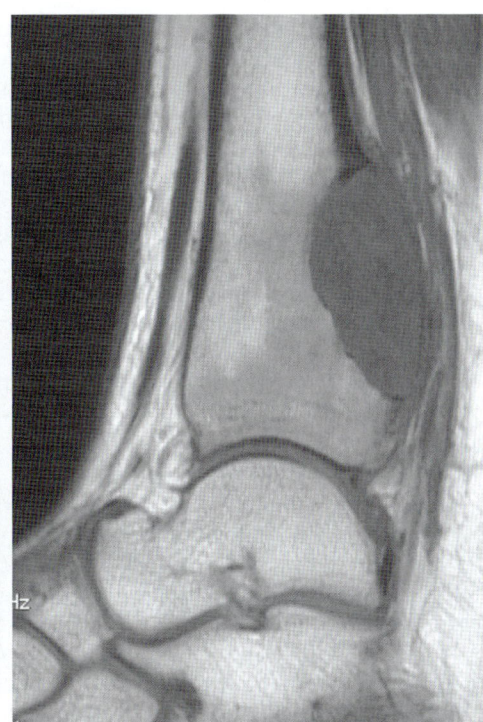

■ **FIGURE 90-27** Chondromyxoid fibroma. Lateral radiograph (**A**) and sagittal, T1-weighted MR image (**B**) of ankle show a well-defined, eccentric lytic lesion arising eccentrically within the distal tibial metaphysis.

Central Chondrosarcoma

Central chondrosarcoma arises centrally within the metaphyses or metadiaphyses of the long bones or flat bones of the pelvis and scapula. Approximately 90% are a primary malignancy, with a similar percentage histologically low grade. The lesions radiographically appear well defined with geographic bone destruction without a sclerotic margin. Cartilage mineralization is variable. These lesions are typically slow growing, with endosteal resorption resulting in scalloping and periosteal new bone formation causing cortical thickening (Fig. 90-28). This combination produces apparent bony expansion with an intact thickened cortex. In high-grade lesions the lysis appears more ill defined and there can be cortical destruction with soft tissue extension, both cardinal signs of a bone malignancy. Where problems arise is in distinguishing a low-grade chondrosarcoma from an active enchondroma that shows moderate cellularity. This applies to both the imaging and histologic assessment of the lesion. It is not unusual to see cartilage lesions in the bones of the hands and feet diagnosed pathologically as a chondrosarcoma and yet the metastatic potential at this site is almost negligible. Many of the imaging features described can at best be considered soft criteria, that is, suggestive but not specific for malignancy. These include tumor length exceeding 5 cm and increased activity on bone scintigraphy, which is seen in approximately 30% of enchondromas and 80% of chondrosarcomas.[10] MRI will show the typical lobules of cartilage that alone do not distinguish benign from malignant disease. Clearly, cortical destruction and soft tissue extension, which is not a feature of low-grade chondrosarcoma, are easily identified on MRI. Static contrast-enhanced MRI is also of little value because it will show peripheral and septal enhancement in both benign and malignant central cartilage tumors. Current

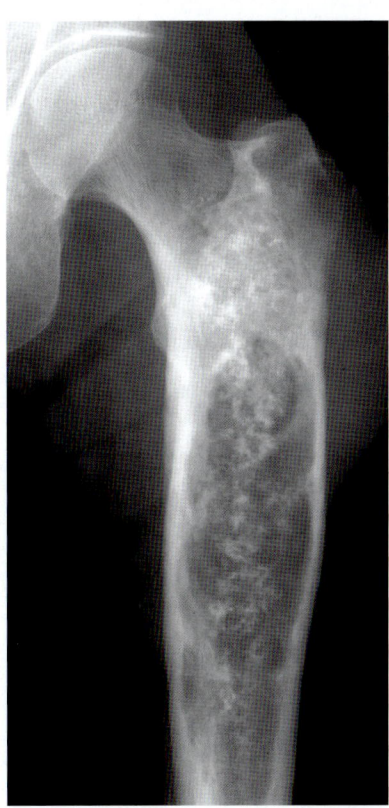

■ **FIGURE 90-28** Central chondrosarcoma. Anteroposterior radiograph shows an extensive lesion of the proximal femoral diaphysis with lysis, bony expansion, and chondroid matrix mineralization.

research is concentrating on the dynamic-enhancement characteristics of cartilage tumors, suggesting that chondrosarcomas tend to show more rapid enhancement than enchondromas.[12] Although the results of these studies are promising it should be noted that tumor vascularity is not a criterion used histologically to differentiate benign from malignant cartilage tumors. Similarly, some have claimed that positron emission tomography can be used in this respect, but it is difficult to envisage a sensitive and specific imaging test when the histologic diagnosis at least in low-grade lesions remains somewhat subjective. The distinction may in time become less important. Because chondrosarcoma is typically not responsive to either chemotherapy or radiotherapy it was always considered that wide surgical excision was the optimal treatment. There is now an increasing tendency with these borderline malignancies to treat them in a similar manner to an enchondroma with curettage but to ensure long-term follow-up to exclude local recurrence.

Surface Chondrosarcoma

Surface chondrosarcoma, as the name implies, arises on the outer surface of bone. There are two types. The first, the peripheral type, develops in the cartilage cap of a preexisting osteochondroma. The second, the periosteal (juxtacortical) chondrosarcoma, is a rare tumor typified by a cartilaginous mass usually greater than 5 cm in length closely applied to the external cortex of a bone without continuity with the underlying bone. The incidence of peripheral chondrosarcoma, association with hereditary multiple exostoses and distinction from benign osteochondroma were discussed in the section on osteochondroma (see Fig. 90-20).

Dedifferentiated Chondrosarcoma

Approximately 10% of cases of all chondrosarcomas show evidence of dedifferentiation. These tumors have a combination of a preexisting cartilage tumor, usually a low-grade chondrosarcoma, with areas of high-grade noncartilaginous sarcoma.[13] The histology of the high-grade component may be malignant fibrous histiocytoma, osteosarcoma, or, less commonly, fibrosarcoma and rhabdomyosarcoma. The imaging appearances are those of a cartilage tumor with superadded features of a more aggressive lesion, as shown by marked cortical destruction, soft tissue extension, periosteal new bone formation, malignant osteoid formation, and loss of the lobulated cartilaginous appearance on MRI (Fig. 90-29). Biopsy should be directed to the areas of the tumor with the highest grade because the treatment of chondrosarcoma relies largely on surgery alone whereas dedifferentiation may require chemotherapy and/or radiotherapy. As might be expected the prognosis for a patient with a dedifferentiated chondrosarcoma is poor, with a less than 20% five-year survival.

Clear Cell Chondrosarcoma

Clear cell chondrosarcoma comprises approximately 2% of all chondrosarcomas. It is more common in men than women; there is a large age range, but most arise in persons between 25 and 45 years of age. It appears as a well-defined lytic lesion arising in the epiphysis or subarticular portion of a long bone, particularly the humeral and femoral heads (Fig. 90-30).[14] The radiographic appearances overlap with those of chondroblastoma, although the age group tends to be older. Matrix calcification is uncommon. In can behave in a fairly indolent manner, showing slow progression on serial radiographs and thereby mimicking an intraosseous ganglion in the adult. Excision is required because there is a high recurrence rate with curettage alone.

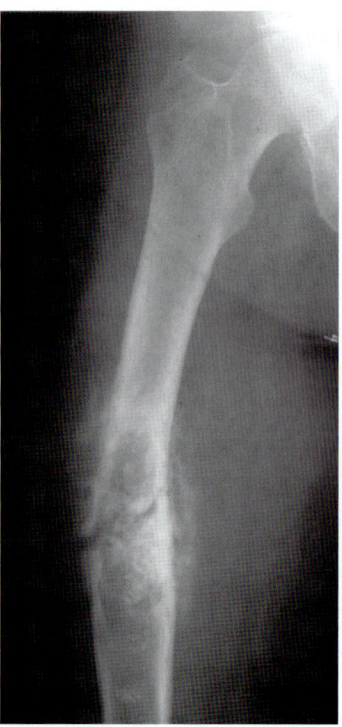

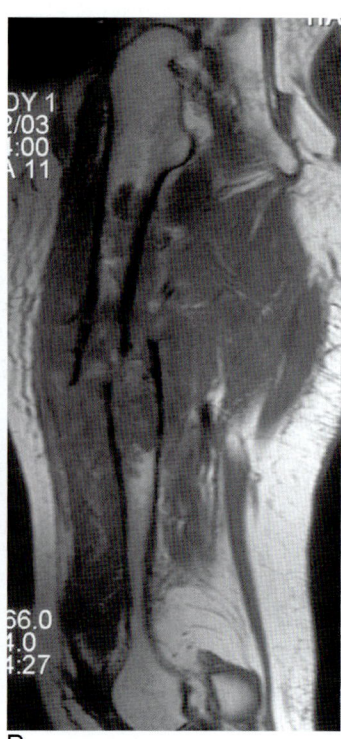

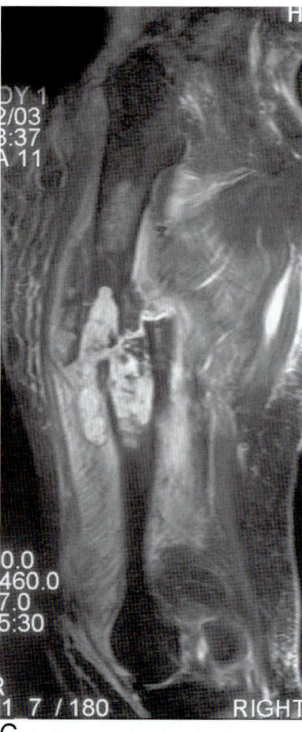

■ **FIGURE 90-29** Dedifferentiated chondrosarcoma. Anteroposterior radiograph (**A**) and coronal T1-weighted (**B**) and coronal STIR (**C**) MR images show a pathologic fracture of the midfemoral diaphysis through a cartilage tumor. The amorphous periosteal and juxtacortical mineralization suggests malignant osteoid consistent with malignant transformation to an osteosarcoma.

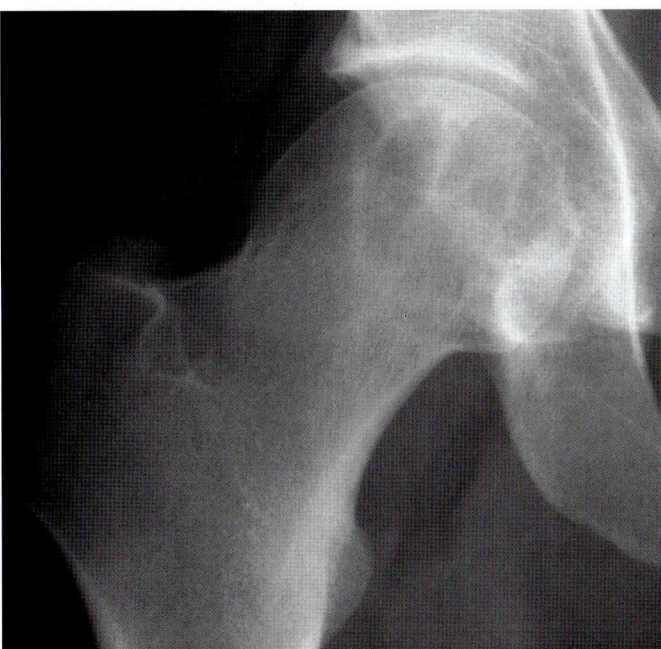

■ **FIGURE 90-30** Clear cell chondrosarcoma. Anteroposterior radiograph shows a well-defined subarticular lytic lesion in the femoral head. In the adult this mimics an intraosseous ganglion or giant cell tumor, and in the child, a chondroblastoma.

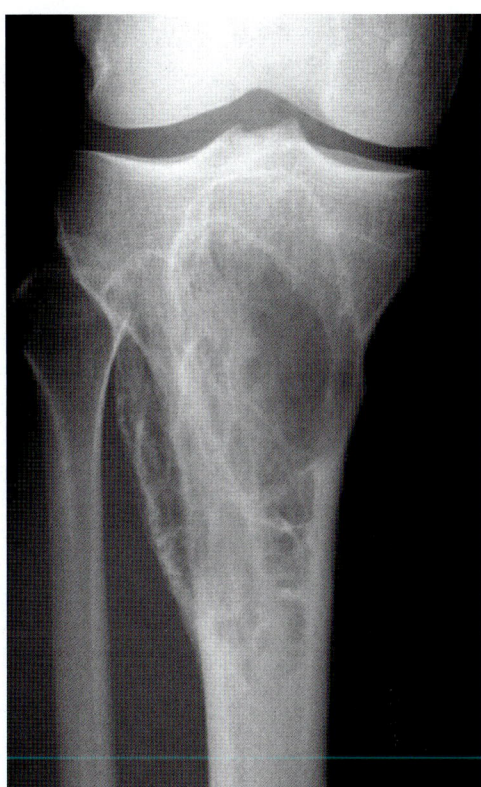

■ **FIGURE 90-31** Desmoplastic fibroma. Anteroposterior radiograph shows a lytic, expansile, trabeculated lesion in the proximal tibial metadiaphysis.

Mesenchymal Chondrosarcoma

Mesenchymal chondrosarcoma is a high-grade malignant tumor consisting of undifferentiated round cells and islands of well-differentiated hyaline cartilage. It comprises approximately 5% of all chondrosarcomas, with a predilection for the craniofacial bones, flat bones, and vertebrae. One third are extraskeletal, that is, they arise in the soft tissues. Unlike the other chondrosarcoma variants mesenchymal chondrosarcoma tends to occur at a younger age group, being most common in the second and third decades. The radiographic features are those of an aggressive bone lesion with varying degrees of chondroid matrix.

Fibrogenic and Fibrohistiocytic Tumors

This category of bone tumors consists of both benign and malignant lesions. Fibrogenic tumors are composed of spindle cells and produce a collagenous matrix, whereas fibrohistiocytic tumors are also composed of spindle cells but may or may not produce a collagenous matrix. Fibrous cortical defect, nonossifying fibroma, and fibrous dysplasia are common fibrous lesions of bone but are not considered true neoplasms and so are covered in Chapter 92.

Desmoplastic Fibroma

Desmoplastic fibroma is an extremely rare benign, but locally aggressive fibrogenic tumor comprising less than 0.1% of all primary bone tumors. It occurs in the second decade with the long bones, pelvis, and mandible the most commonly affected bones. Radiographically it appears as a central lytic lesion with geographic bone destruction and cortical expansion.[15] The majority of lesions show a degree of trabeculation to give a honeycomb appearance (Fig. 90-31). Radiographically, the differential diagnosis includes simple bone cyst, aneurysmal bone cyst, chondromyxoid fibroma, giant cell tumor, and fibrous dysplasia. More aggressive lesions can mimic a primary sarcoma. Clearly, all these conditions are more common and therefore would appear higher up on any list of differential diagnoses. Radiologic-pathologic correlation is important to identify the osseous origin of the tumor because the histology of desmoplastic fibroma is similar to that of periosteal desmoid and soft tissue desmoid tumor.

Benign Fibrous Histiocytoma

Benign fibrous histiocytoma is a rare, benign fibrohistiocytic tumor arising in bone with a large age range. Histologically, it resembles a nonossifying fibroma but differs on imaging in that it can arise centrally as well as eccentrically within the metaphyses of long bones. Geographic bone destruction with trabeculation and bony expansion are typical (Fig. 90-32).

Fibrosarcoma and Malignant Fibrous Histiocytoma

Fibrosarcoma and malignant fibrous histiocytoma are fibrogenic and fibrohistiocytic malignancies of bone, respectively. Although, distinct histologic entities, the imaging features are indistinguishable and the management is identical. For this reason they are frequently discussed together. Most occur in the middle aged and elderly,

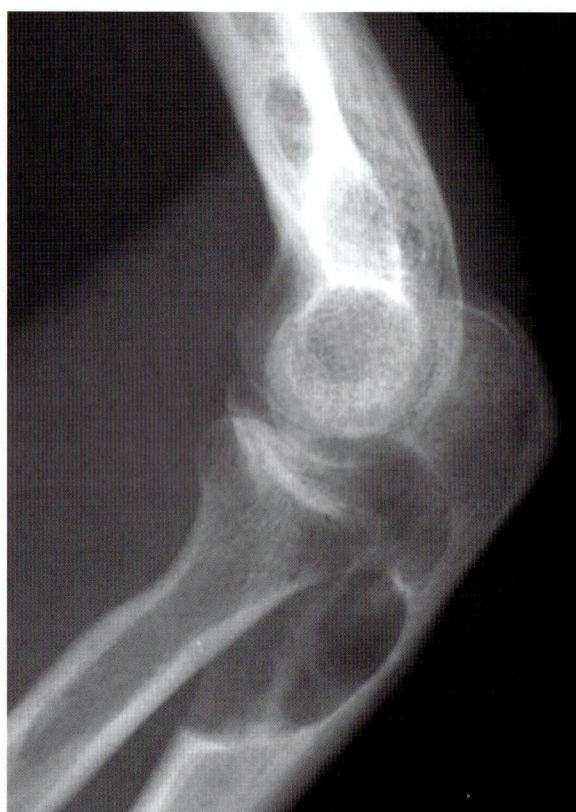

■ **FIGURE 90-32** Benign fibrous histiocytoma. Lateral radiograph shows geographic bone destruction in the proximal ulna.

comprising approximately 10% of all cases of malignant bone tumors. The most common sites are the metaphyses of the femur, humerus, and tibia. Radiographically, the tumors appear lytic and frequently eccentric, with a wide zone of transition, cortical breaching, minimal periosteal new bone formation, and no matrix mineralization (Fig. 90-33).[16] The tumors, therefore, mimic metastases and lymphoma of bone both in age of occurrence and imaging. The MRI features are nonspecific, showing the marrow infiltration, cortical destruction, and soft issue extension typical of malignancy, be it primary or metastatic. Both fibrosarcoma and malignant fibrous histiocytoma may be secondary, arising in association with a preexisting bone lesion such as Paget's disease, bone infarction, or fibrous dysplasia as well as irradiated bone. The incidence of secondary malignant fibrous histiocytoma is said to be approximately 25%, although this is somewhat higher than in my experience.

Round Cell Tumors

There are no benign round cell tumors. The malignancies in this category are Ewing's sarcoma and primitive neuroectodermal tumor (PNET), both considered part of a spectrum of round cell sarcomas with differing degrees of neuroectodermal differentiation. The clinical and imaging features of both conditions are similar and are covered in this text together. Malignant lymphoma of bone may be classified as either a round cell tumor or a myeloproliferative disorder (see later). A notable feature of the

Ewing family of tumors is the presence of a recurrent chromosomal translocation, identified in approximately 85% cases. Ewing's sarcoma is the most common primary malignant bone tumor in the first decade of life and second only to osteosarcoma in the second decade of life. Ninety percent of cases present in individuals younger than 20 years of age; there is a minor male predominance, and it is rarely seen in blacks. The long bones are the most commonly involved in the younger patients and the flat bones of the pelvis and scapula in older patients. The tumors may present as any primary malignancy with pain and swelling or uncommonly as a pathologic fracture. A minority of tumors, however, are well recognized to present as systemic symptoms, including pyrexia, anemia, and a raised white blood cell count and sedimentation rate, all suggestive of osteomyelitis, which is also one of the main differential diagnoses on imaging studies. The radiographic features are those of a highly aggressive lesion with permeative or moth-eaten bone destruction, cortical permeation or destruction, prominent soft tissue extension, and periosteal new bone formation that may be lamellar (onionskin), spiculated, and/or interrupted (Codman angle) (Fig. 90-34). The classic appearance of a Ewing sarcoma frequently illustrated in many textbooks is a diaphyseal lesion with onionskin periosteal reaction and Codman angles. However, in my experience many cases are similar in location to other primary sarcomas (i.e., diametaphyseal). In the absence of significant periosteal reaction or cortical destruction, particularly in complex anatomic areas such as the pelvis, the permeative bone destruction may be easily overlooked on the initial radiograph obtained at presentation. There is no tumor matrix, but up to 25% of cases will show mild to moderate sclerosis due to reactive bone changes (Fig. 90-35). This sclerosis, together with the periosteal reaction and a diametaphyseal location, may give appearances very similar to that of an osteosarcoma. The differential diagnosis in the younger patients includes acute osteomyelitis, Langerhans cell histiocytosis, neuroblastoma metastasis, and a leukemic deposit. In the older age group the differential diagnosis includes again other primary sarcomas and acute osteomyelitis as well as lymphoma of bone. The MRI appearances are relatively nonspecific, showing typical features of an aggressive tumor. However, the identification of a prominent solid soft tissue component helps to distinguish tumor from infection (Fig. 90-36). In my experience, less than 5% of cases of Ewing's sarcoma fail to show evidence of soft tissue extension on MRI. Ewing's sarcoma is a highly malignant sarcoma, with approximately 15% showing evidence of disseminated disease with lung and/or bone metastases at presentation. For this reason the prognosis for Ewing's sarcoma remains poorer than osteosarcoma, with a 5-year survival rate of approximately 55%. Central lesions, such as the pelvis, tend to have a poor prognosis because they present later and are consequently larger and it is also more difficult to undertake curative limb salvage surgery. A variant of Ewing's sarcoma is the periosteal type that arises on the surface of bone and presents as a soft tissue mass producing thickening and external erosion (saucerization).[17] In all other respects the imaging studies and management are as per conventional Ewing's sarcoma.

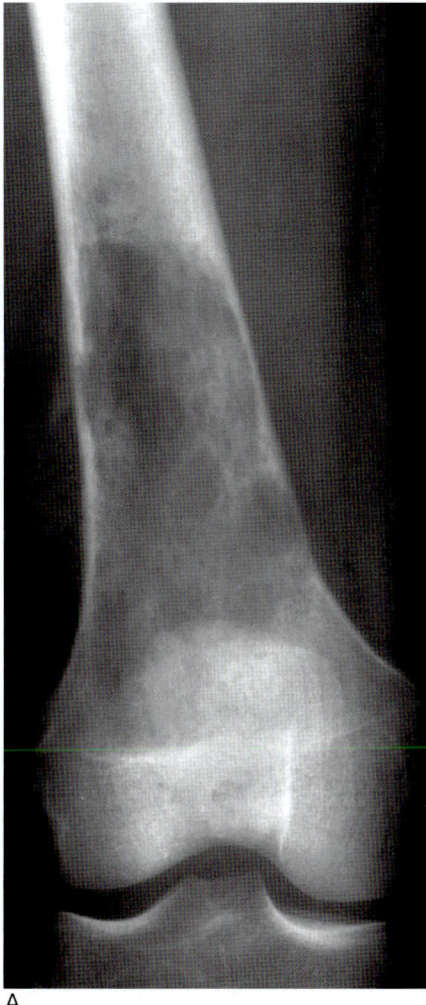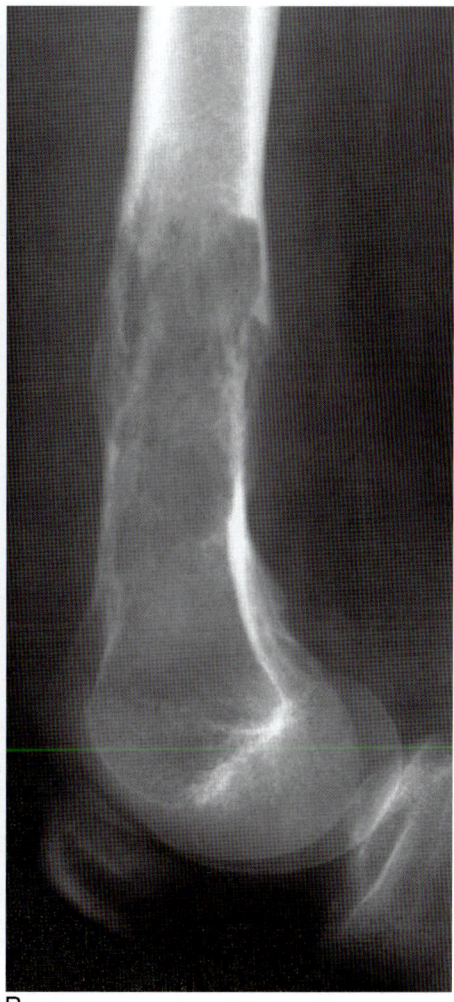

A   B

■ **FIGURE 90-33** Malignant fibrous histiocytoma. Anteroposterior (**A**) and lateral (**B**) radiographs show an aggressive lytic lesion of the distal femoral diaphysis with absent mineralization and periosteal new bone formation.

Hematopoietic (Myeloproliferative) Tumors

There are no benign tumors of hematopoietic derivation in the bone. The malignant tumors can be divided basically into two categories: plasmacytoma/myeloma and lymphoma. Myeloma is the most common primary malignancy of bone and is covered in Chapter 91. It should be stressed that in its solitary form, plasmacytoma, the typical radiographic appearances of an expansile, lytic, trabeculated lesion with geographic bone destruction can mimic an expansile metastasis, such as from renal or thyroid primary tumors, giant cell tumor, and intraosseous ganglion.

Lymphoma

Primary osseous lymphoma is defined as lymphoma with no evidence of systemic disease at the time of presentation or within 6 months of discovery of the original lesion. In a recent large series of lymphoma, 1% of cases had primary lymphoma of bone and 9% had secondary lymphoma.[10] It occurs in adults in the fourth to sixth decades. It typically arises at sites of persistent bone marrow, with the primary form showing a predilection for the femur, pelvis, and spine and the secondary form,

the spine. Radiographically, primary lymphoma appears highly aggressive with permeative bone destruction both of the medullary bone and the cortex, limited periosteal new bone formation, absent matrix mineralization, and frequently a very large soft tissue mass (Fig. 90-37). Sequestrum formation has been reported in up to 15% of cases, although my experience would suggest a lower percentage. The differential diagnosis includes other malignant round cell tumors such as Ewing's sarcoma/PNET as well as metastasis, malignant fibrous histiocytoma, and osteomyelitis. An uncommon but well-recognized radiographic appearance of lymphoma is dense sclerosis. In the spine, lymphoma can be one of the causes of the ivory vertebra sign. The MRI appearances of lymphoma are nonspecific, but malignancy can be inferred by the presence of a sizeable soft tissue mass. The sclerotic variant may not be associated with a significant mass, and the sclerosis will show decreased signal intensity on all sequences.

Giant Cell Tumor

Giant cell tumor (osteoclastoma) of bone is a benign, locally aggressive tumor comprising sheets of neoplastic

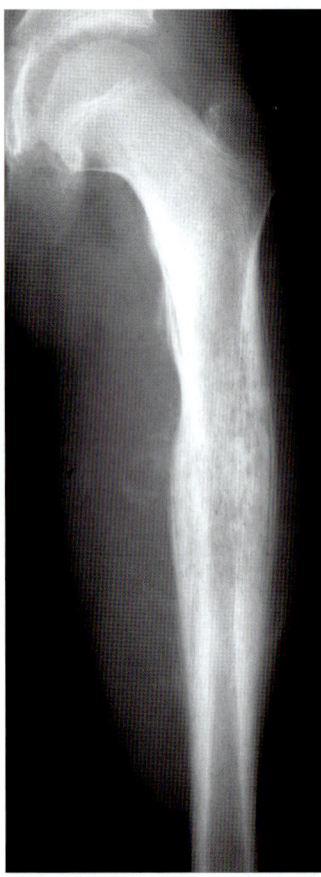

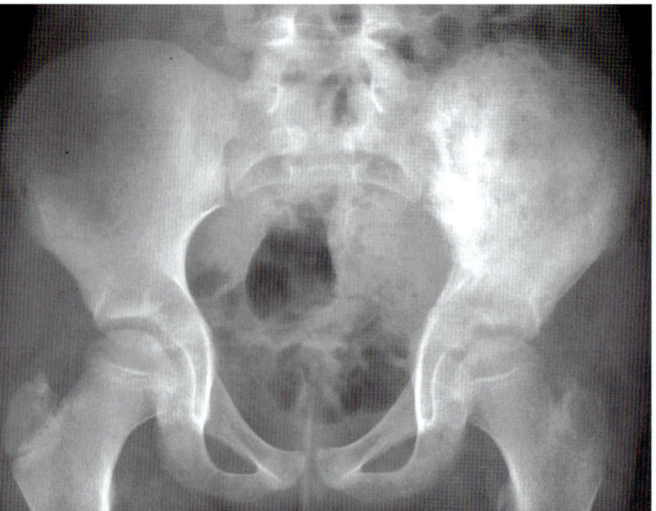

■ **FIGURE 90-35** Ewing's sarcoma. Anteroposterior radiograph shows permeative destruction of the left ilium with increased density due to a combination of reactive bone changes and periosteal new bone formation seen en face.

■ **FIGURE 90-34** Ewing's sarcoma. Anteroposterior radiograph of a classic diaphyseal Ewing's sarcoma in a child. There is permeative bone destruction and lamellar periosteal reaction and Codman angles.

ovoid mononuclear cells interspersed with uniformly distributed large, multinucleated, osteoclast-like giant cells. It is relatively common, representing approximately 5% of primary bone tumors and 20% of benign primary bone tumors. It is typically seen in the third to fifth decades inclusive, with less than 5% occurring before skeletal fusion. Common sites include the ends of the long bones, namely, the distal femur, proxi-mal tibia, and distal radius (Figs. 90-38 and 90-39). In the spine, the sacrum is the most common site. Less than 1% of cases of the tumors are multifocal, with most associated with Paget's disease of bone. The majority of solitary cases arise eccentrically in the metaphysis of a long bone and extend to a subarticular margin. Tumors in small tubular bones may appear central owing to the small volume of the parent bone. Occasionally, giant cell tumor may arise in an apophysis such as the greater trochanter. Textbooks frequently cite a radiographic grading system.[19] Type 1 is a *quiescent* lesion with geographic bone destruction and little or no cortical involvement. Type 2 is an *active* lesion that is still well defined but with no reactive sclerosis and now thinning and expansion of the cortex. Type 3 is an *aggressive* lesion, with a wide zone of transition, cortical breaching, and soft tissue extension. Periosteal new bone formation (in the absence of a pathologic fracture) and matrix mineralization are usually minimal. Although the grading

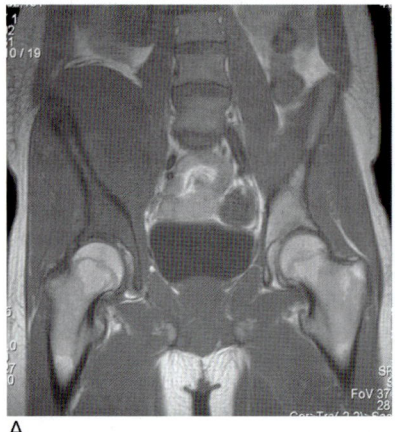

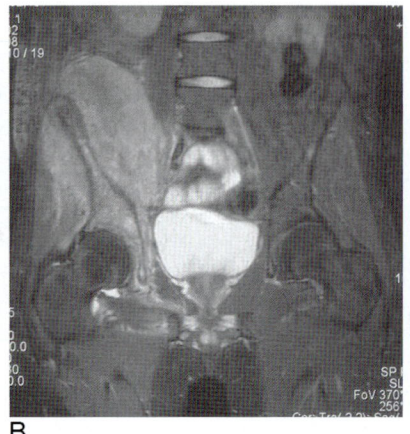

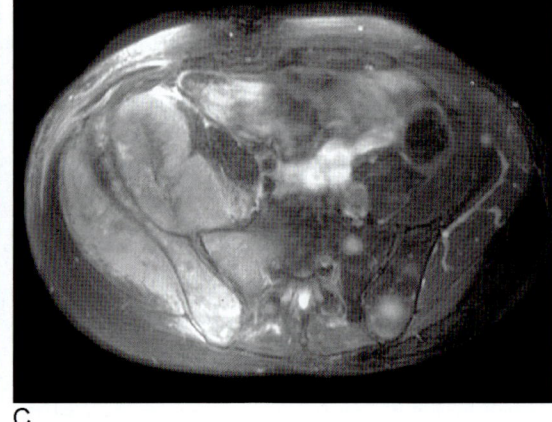

A   B   C

■ **FIGURE 90-36** Ewing's sarcoma. Coronal T1-weighted (**A**), coronal STIR (**B**), and axial T2-weighted, fat-suppressed (**C**) MR images show an extensive tumor infiltrating the right ilium and acetabulum with a large soft tissue mass. The foci of signal change in the sacrum and posterior aspect of the left ilium on the axial image indicates there is disseminated disease present even at presentation.

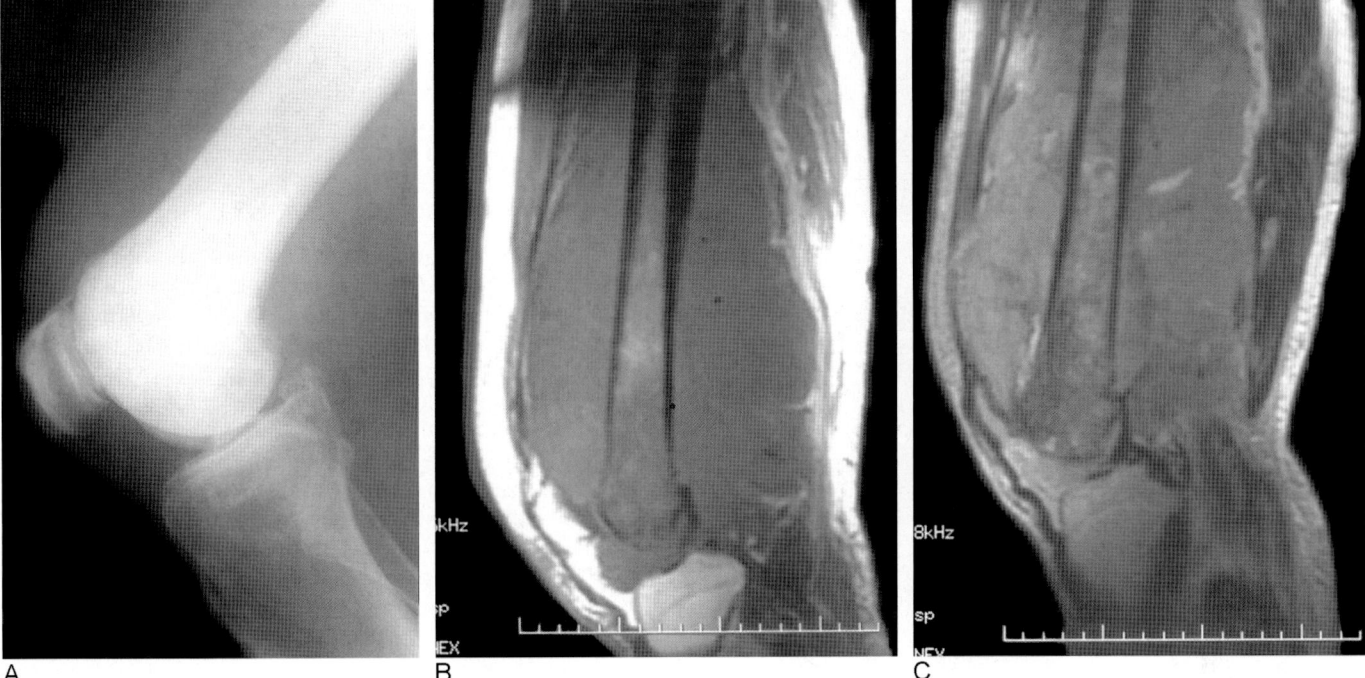

■ **FIGURE 90-37** Lymphoma. **A,** Anteroposterior radiograph shows generalized sclerosis of the distal femur. Sagittal T1-weighted (**B**) and sagittal T2-weighted (**C**) MR images show infiltration of the distal femur with massive soft tissue extension anteriorly, posteriorly, and into the knee joint.

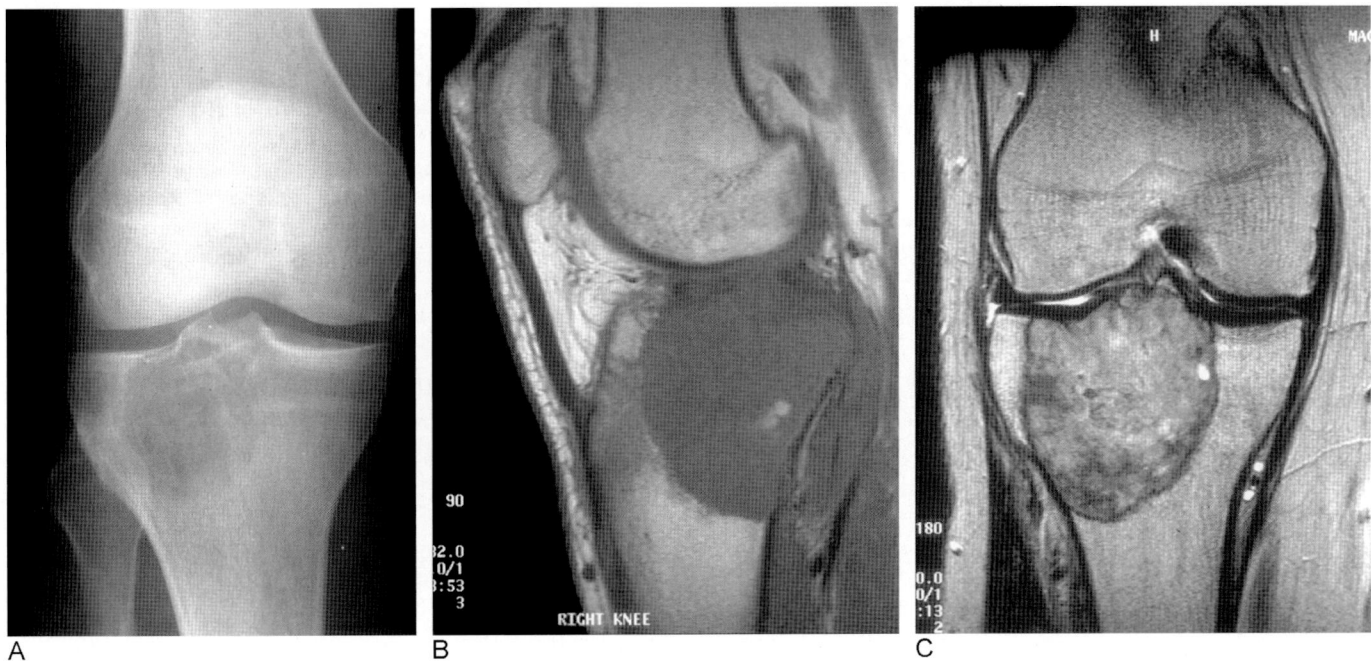

■ **FIGURE 90-38** Giant cell tumor. Anteroposterior radiograph (**A**), sagittal T1-weighted (**B**), and coronal T2-weighted (**C**) MR images show a lytic, eccentric, subarticular lesion that is solid on MRI.

system describes the spectrum of radiographic appearances of giant cell tumor from relatively indolent to locally highly aggressive it does not correlate well with the histologic findings and is therefore of limited value. Clearly, a type 3 lesion may well require more extensive surgery than a type 1 lesion to minimize the risks of local recurrence. The MRI features are nonspecific,

although some reports have highlighted the presence of low signal intensity areas on all sequences owing to large quantities of intratumoral hemosiderin. Fluid-fluid levels suggest coexistent secondary aneurysmal bone cyst formation. Dynamic contrast-enhanced MRI shows a rapid wash-in and a slower progressive wash-out time-intensity curve. Treatment of giant cell tumor largely

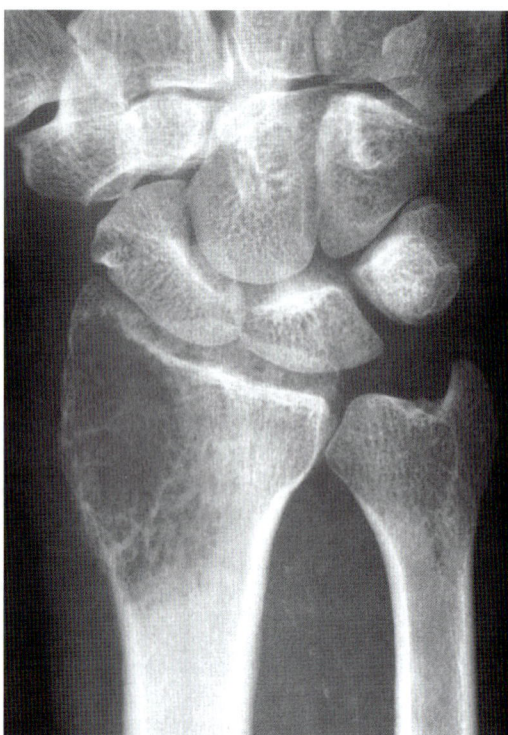

■ FIGURE 90-39 Giant cell tumor. Posteroanterior radiograph of the wrist shows a classic example comprising a subarticular, lytic, mildly trabeculated tumor eccentrically located in the distal radius.

relies on curettage. If the resultant bony defect is particularly large, the structural integrity of the bone may be aided by bone grafting or the insertion of bone cement (cementoplasty). Because of the aggressive nature of the tumor, local recurrence is seen in approximately 30% of cases. The distortion of the anatomy at the surgical site and healing response may make early detection of local recurrence difficult. Increasing lysis of the parent bone suggests recurrence. Lysis of bone graft material may be due to recurrence or just resorption as part of the healing process. When there is doubt, MRI with a dynamic contrast-enhanced sequence is advocated. Recurrent tumor will show a similar wash-in/wash-out time intensity curve to the primary tumor whereas postsurgical granulation tissue will show a slower more progressive wash-in curve and no rapid wash-out. Approximately 5% of cases of giant cell tumor will develop pulmonary metastases that, although histologically similar to the primary tumor, tend to behave in a fairly indolent manner with a moderate to good long-term prognosis. In distinction, approximately 1% of cases of giant cell tumor are truly malignant and may arise de novo, after surgical treatment with a variable latent period, or be secondary due to malignant transformation after previous radiation therapy. The management and prognosis in these situations is similar to other high-grade sarcomas of bone. It should be stressed that many different bone lesions can also contain giant cells. These include telangiectatic osteosarcoma and aneurysmal bone cyst. Therefore, close radiologic-pathologic correlation is important before the diagnosis of a giant cell tumor is

confirmed. This should include review of the serum calcium level because the brown tumor of hyperparathyroidism can be identical radiographically and histologically to a giant cell tumor. In the middle aged and elderly, metastasis and intraosseous ganglion may radiographically mimic a giant cell tumor.

Notochordal Tumors

Chordoma is a low-grade malignancy thought to arise from the embryonic remnants of the notochord. It is therefore a midline lesion with 50% arising in the sacrum, 35% from the clivus, and 15% in the rest of the spine (usually lumbar). It accounts for less than 4% of all primary malignant bone tumors presenting in the fourth to sixth decades. Sacrococcygeal tumors tend to present late with relatively subtle changes on radiographs frequently overlooked (Fig. 90-40). MRI reveals a midline destructive lesion with an anteriorly projecting soft tissue mass displacing rather than invading the pelvic organs. The tumor is frequently often lobulated, simulating a cartilaginous lesion; one recognized histologic variant of chordoma contains considerable chondroid matrix. CT may show marginal calcification and sparse matrix mineralization. The latter is thought to be due to intratumoral necrosis rather than cartilaginous differentiation. The differential diagnosis includes giant cell tumor, metastasis, chondrosarcoma, and lymphoma, although these are rarely midline in origin. The tumor is relatively nonresponsive to either chemotherapy or radiotherapy. Therefore, surgery is the mainstay of treatment, but it can be difficult to achieve a wide excision margin without major morbidity. Because of the desire to minimize bladder and bowel dysfunction, surgery may fail to remove the whole tumor and there is a high risk of local recurrence, albeit slowly progressive. Parachordoma is an extra-axial soft tissue and, rarely, bone lesion with some histologic similarities to chordoma, but the two entities are probably not related.

Vascular Tumors

Tumors arising from the vascular elements of bone may be benign (hemangioma), of an intermediate grade (hemangioendothelioma), or high-grade malignancy (angiosarcoma).

Hemangioma

Hemangioma of bone is a benign vascular malformation of endothelial origin. Depending on the predominant vessel type it may be classified as capillary, cavernous, venous, arteriovenous, or mixed. Hemangioma is a common lesion in the spine, with 10% of adults affected on one autopsy study. The next most commonly affected sites include the skull vault and craniofacial bones (Fig. 90-41). Involvement of the rest of the skeleton is relatively rare. In the spine, hemangioma affects the vertebral body and shows a coarsened vertical trabecular/corduroy pattern, giving a "polka dot" appearance on cross-sectional imaging. A distinctive MR feature is the relatively hyperintense signal on both T1- and T2-weighted images owing to the prominent fatty stroma. In the absence of gadolinium enhancement it is remarkably uncommon for any significant infiltra-

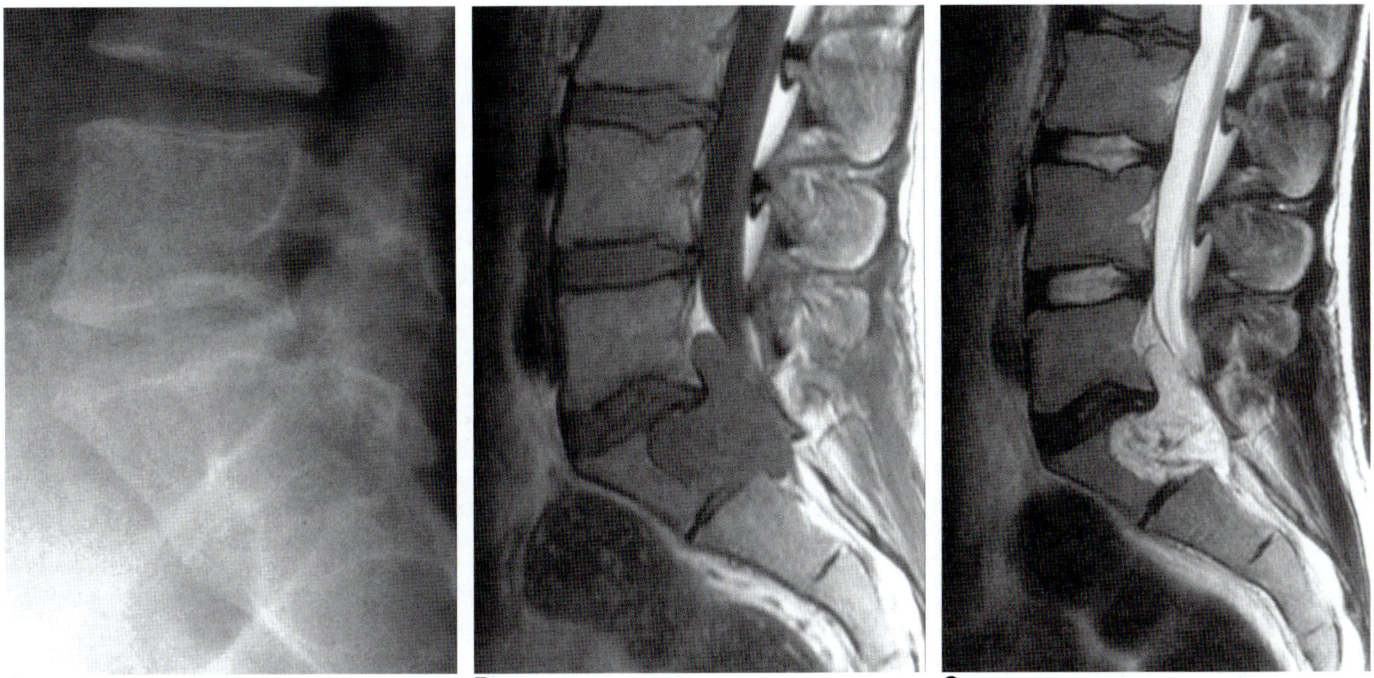

■ FIGURE 90-40   Chordoma. Lateral radiograph (**A**) and sagittal T1-weighted (**B**) and sagittal T2-weighted (**C**) MR images. The tumor is barely visible on the radiograph whereas the MR images reveal a heterogeneous tumor extending out of the posterior aspect of the body of S1 with extradural extension into the lumbar spinal canal.

tive lesion of the spine to exhibit hyperintensity on T1-weighted images. The vast majority of spinal hemangiomas are an incidental finding. On occasion, larger lesions may become symptomatic owing to a compression fracture or compromise of the spinal canal. Hemangiomas in which the fatty component is small, or even invisible relative to the vascular component, are more likely to compromise the vertebral canal and become symptomatic. Skull vault lesions show an area of lysis, with radiating thickened trabeculae likened to spokewheel or web patterns (see Fig. 90-41). In the long bones the hemangioma may give a lacelike or honeycomb pattern. Periosteal hemangioma is relatively rare but can be diagnosed by the association of focal reactive periosteal new bone formation on radiographs and adjacent serpiginous vessels with a fatty stroma on MRI.

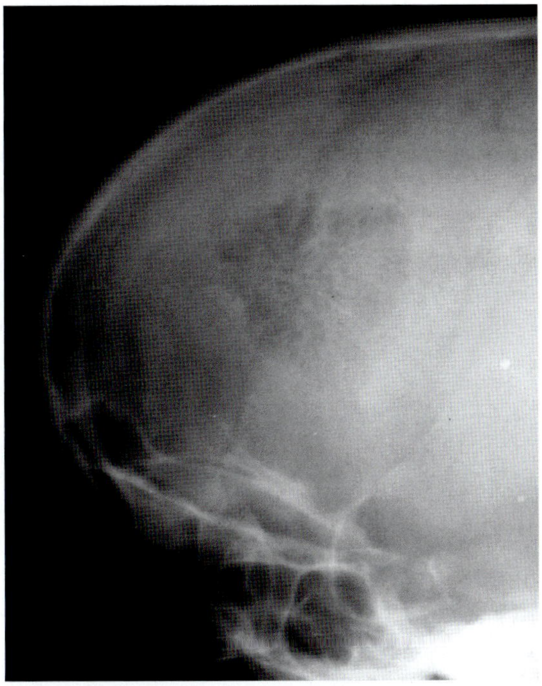

Glomus Tumor

The glomus tumor and its rarer variants, glomangioma and glomangiomyoma, arise from the neuromyoarterial glomus classically in the subungual portion of the fingers. The majority arise within the soft tissues and produce erosion of the terminal phalanx. Less common is the intraosseous type that produces lytic expansion of the terminal phalanx, simulating an epidermoid inclusion cyst (Fig. 90-42). A helpful distinguishing clinical feature is the localized pain and exquisite point tenderness typical of a glomus tumor.

Cystic Angiomatosis, Lymphangiomatosis, and Gorham's Disease

Cystic angiomatosis, lymphangiomatosis, and Gorham's disease (massive osteolysis or disappearing bone disease) are a spectrum of rare disorders typified by multiple lytic lesions in bone and usually presenting in children or young adults. Arguably, the importance of knowing about these interrelated conditions is in recognizing that they come far down in the differential diagnosis of multiple

■ FIGURE 90-41   Hemangioma. Lateral radiograph shows the web- or spoke-like appearance of a vault hemangioma.

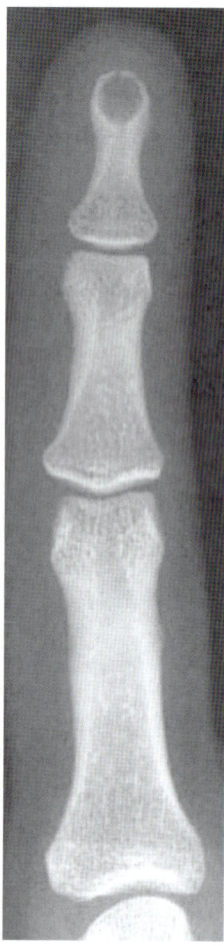

■ **FIGURE 90-42** Glomus tumor. Posteroanterior radiograph shows a well-defined, rounded lytic lesion in the terminal phalanx. The differential diagnosis would include an epidermal inclusion cyst.

lytic lesions in children, which includes Langerhans cell histiocytosis, polyostotic fibrous dysplasia, leukemic deposits, and neuroblastoma metastases. Bone-related symptoms are usually secondary to pathologic fractures through the lytic lesions.

Angiosarcoma and Hemangioendothelioma

There is a spectrum of malignant vascular tumors of bone with endothelial differentiation. The existing nomenclature varies and frequently leads to confusion. *Angiosarcoma* is the preferred term used for malignant vascular tumors in the World Health Organization classification. The term (epithelioid) hemangioendothelioma is still used for the more-differentiated, lower-grade malignancies. Radiographically, hemangioendothelioma produces geographic bone destruction (Fig. 90-43). Angiosarcoma is a high-grade malignancy that produces a permeative pattern of bone destruction with no matrix mineralization mimicking other malignancies such as metastases and lymphoma. As a group these tumors are rare, comprising less than 1% of primary malignant bone tumors. There is also a wide age distribution. These two facts mean that they are rarely considered high in a list of differential diagnoses of a bone lesion. One distinctive feature, however, is the tendency for multicentric presentation frequently involving a single (usually the lower) limb (see Fig. 90-43).

Smooth Muscle Tumors

Smooth muscle tumors of bone are rare. Leiomyoma of bone, in particular, is exceedingly rare. It is a benign spindle cell tumor with smooth muscle differentiation. It most commonly arises in the facial bones, showing a geographic pattern of bone destruction with a sclerotic border. Leiomyosarcoma of bone is also rare, being a relatively recently described entity. There has been a trend in the pathology community to subdivide malignant spindle cell tumors as knowledge increases. A generation ago the predominant diagnosis for these lesions was fibrosarcoma. Then malignant fibrous histiocytoma became the preferred diagnosis in the majority of cases. Today, many of these tumors are simply diagnosed as a pleomorphic spindle cell sarcoma with a small subset identified as leiomyosarcoma. The imaging features of leiomyosarcoma are indistinguishable from those of fibrosarcoma or malignant fibrous histiocytoma, namely, a permeative lytic lesion principally affecting the long bones with little or no periosteal new bone formation and no matrix miner-

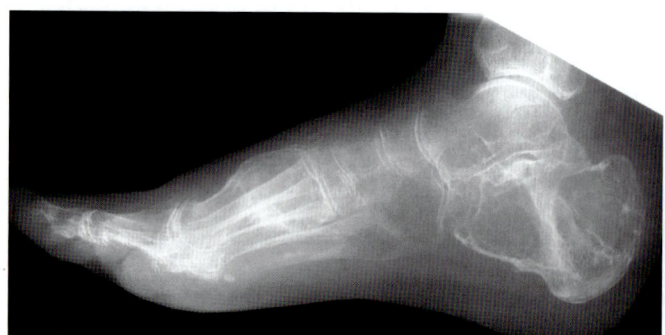

A

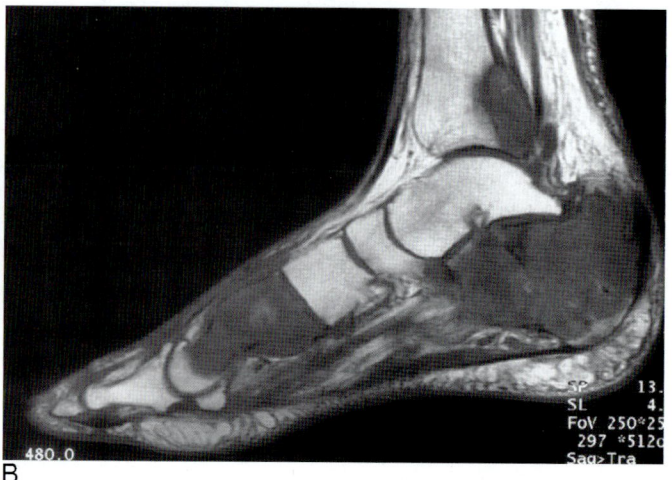

B

■ **FIGURE 90-43** Multiple hemangioendotheliomas. Lateral radiograph (**A**) and sagittal T1-weighted MR image (**B**) show lytic, mildly expansile lesions arising in the first metatarsal, calcaneus, and distal tibia. A multifocal monomelic distribution is typical of vascular tumors of bone.

alization. In this respect it can mimic a lytic osteosarcoma, although, like both fibrosarcoma and malignant fibrous histiocytoma, it tends to occur at a slightly older age group with a mean age of presentation of 45 years.

Lipogenic Tumors

Soft tissue lipomas are common. The intraosseous counterpart is a rare, entirely benign tumor classically arising in the calcaneus and less commonly the metaphyses of the long bones of the lower limb. Radiographically, it appears as a well-defined lytic lesion with a thin sclerotic margin often with a small central focus of dystrophic calcification (Fig. 90-44A).[20] The cardinal diagnostic feature is the identification of fat density on CT and fat signal intensity on MRI (see Fig. 90-44B). Many cases are an incidental finding on imaging performed for other purposes. Some cases, particularly those arising in the calcaneus, may present as a pathologic fracture owing to weakening of the bone. The differential diagnosis includes liposclerosing myxofibrous tumor and any benign bone tumor after curettage. In the latter, the ingrowth of host marrow around the margins of the lesion can simulate a fatty tumor. A focal form of lipomatosis, macrodystrophia lipomatosa, can cause focal gigantism in the hands and feet. Lipomas may also arise on the surface of bone (parosteal lipoma), presenting as a juxtacortical soft tissue mass of fat frequently stimulating some underlying coarse metaplastic periosteal new bone formation. Liposarcoma of bone is exceedingly rare and of questionable existence.

MISCELLANEOUS TUMORS

The miscellaneous category of primary bone tumors is reserved for adamantinoma, which remains of uncertain

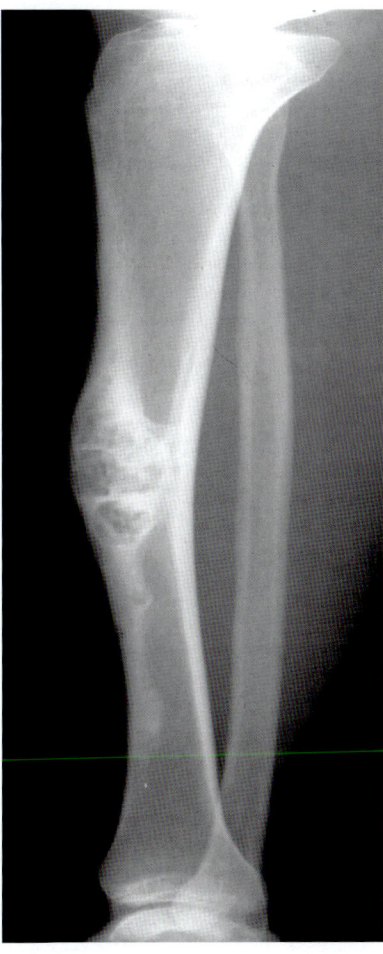

■ **FIGURE 90-45** Adamantinoma. Lateral radiograph shows a midtibial lesion. The anterior location and multilocular appearance are typical. The differential diagnosis would include fibrous dysplasia and osteofibrous dysplasia.

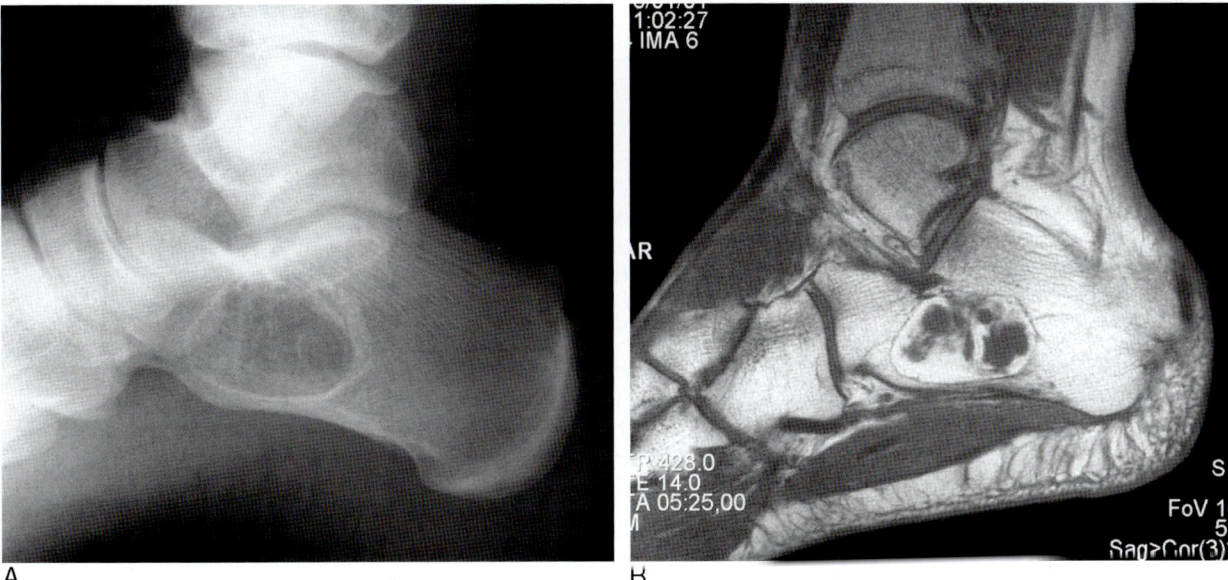

A   B

■ **FIGURE 90-44** Intraosseous lipoma. **A,** Lateral radiograph shows a well-defined lytic lesion in the calcaneus. **B,** Sagittal T1-weighted MR image reveals the lesion to be predominantly fatty with some cystic areas. Cystic change and dystrophic calcification are frequently found in this condition.

histogenesis. It is a rare, low-grade malignancy characterized by epithelial cells within a spindle cell stroma. It comprises less than 0.5% of all primary bone tumors; there is a large age range extending from the first to ninth decades. The mean age at presentation is around 25 years. Over 90% of cases arise anteriorly within the tibial diaphysis. Radiographically, it produces a multiloculated or "soap bubble" appearance with intervening areas of sclerosis (Fig. 90-45). There are frequently small satellite lesions that may be proximal or distal to the main tumor. The differential diagnosis includes fibrous dysplasia and osteofibrous dysplasia. Some investigators suggest that there is a spectrum of disease from benign osteofibrous-dysplasia to low-grade malignant adamantinoma, with an intervening category of osteofibrous dysplasia-like adamantinoma.

SUGGESTED READINGS

Choi JJ, Murphey MD. Angiomatous skeletal lesions. Semin Muscul Radiol 2000; 4:103–112.

Eggli KD, Quiogue T, Moser RP Jr. Ewing's sarcoma. Radiol Clin North Am 1993; 31:325–337.

Lopez C, Thomas DV, Davies AM. Neoplastic transformation in Paget's disease of bone: pictorial review. Eur Radiol 2003; 13:L151–163.

Murphey M, Choi J, Kransdorf MK, et al. From the archives of the AFIP: Imaging osteochondroma: variants and complications with radiologic-pathologic correlation. RadioGraphics 2000; 20:1407–1434.

Murphey MD, Nomikos GC, Flemming DJ, et al. From the archives of the AFIP: Imaging of giant cell tumor and giant cell reparative granuloma of bone: radiologic-pathologic correlation. RadioGraphics 2001; 21:1283–1309.

Murphey M, Walker EA, Wilson AJ, et al. From the archives of the AFIP: Imaging of primary chondrosarcoma: radiologic-pathologic correlation. RadioGraphics 2003; 23:1245–1278.

Seeger LL, Yao L, Eckardt JJ. State of the art: Surface lesions of bone. Radiology 1998; 206:17–33.

Smith SE, Kransdord MJ. Primary musculoskeletal tumors of fibrous origin. Semin Musculoskelet Radiol 2000; 4:73–88.

Williams HJ, Davies AM. The effect of x-rays on bone. Eur Radiol 2006; 16:619–633.

Woertler K. Benign bone tumors and tumor-like lesions: value of cross-sectional imaging. Eur Radiol 2003; 13:1820–1835.

REFERENCES

1. Davies M, Cassar-Pullicino VN, Davies AM, et al. The diagnostic accuracy of MR imaging in osteoid osteoma. Skeletal Radiol 2002; 31:559–569.
2. Liu PT, Chivers FP, Roberts CC, et al. Imaging of osteoid osteoma with dynamic gadolinium-enhanced MR imaging. Radiology 2003; 227:691–700.
3. Vanderschueren GM, Taminiau AHM, Obermann WR, Bloem JL. Osteoid osteoma: clinical results with thermocoagulation. Radiology 2002; 224:82–86.
4. Kroon HM, Schurmans J. Osteoblastoma: clinical and radiologic findings in 98 new cases. Radiology 1990; 175:783–790.
5. Rosenberg ZS, Lev S, Schmahmann S, et al. Osteosarcoma: subtle, rare, and misleading plain film features. AJR 1995; 165:1209–1214.
6. Bloem JL, Kroon HM. Osseous lesions. Radiol Clin North Am 1993; 31:261–278.
7. Andresen KJ, Sundaram M, Unni KK, Sim FH. Imaging features of low grade central osteosarcoma of the long bones and pelvis. Skeletal Radiol 2004; 33:373–379.
8. Ritts GD, Pritchard DJ, Unni KK, et al. Periosteal osteosarcoma. Clin Orthop 1987; 219:299–307.
9. Okada K, Unni KK, Swee RG, Sim FH. High grade surface osteosarcoma: a clinicopathologic study of 46 cases. Cancer 1999; 85:1044–1054.
10. Geirnaerdt MJA, Hermans J, Bloem JL, et al. Usefulness of radiography in differentiating enchondroma from central grade 1 chondrosarcoma. AJR Am J Roentgenol 1997; 169:1097–1104.
11. Yamamura S, Sato K, Sugiura H, Iwata H. Inflammatory reaction in chondroblastoma. Skeletal Radiol 1996; 25:371–376.
12. Geirnaerdt MJA, Hogendoorn PCW, Bloem JL, et al. Cartilaginous tumors: fast contrast-enhanced MR imaging. Radiology 2000; 214:539–546.
13. Mercuri M, Picci P, Campanacci M, Rulli E. Dedifferentiated chondrosarcoma. Skeletal Radiology 1995; 24:409–416.
14. Kumar R, David R, Cierney G III. Clear cell chondrosarcoma. Radiology 1985; 154:45–48.
15. Crim JR, Gold RH, Mirra JM, et al. Desmoplastic fibroma of bone: radiographic analysis. Radiology 1989; 172:827–832.
16. Murphey MD, Gross TM, Rosenthal HG. Musculoskeletal malignant fibrous histiocytoma: radiologic-pathologic correlation. RadioGraphics 1994; 14:807–826.
17. Bator SM, Bauer TW, Marks KE, Norris DG. Periosteal Ewing's sarcoma. Cancer 1986; 58:1781–1784.
18. Kirsch J, Ilaslan H, Bauer TW, Sundaram M. The incidence of imaging findings, and distribution of skeletal lymphoma in a consecutive patient population seen over 5 years. Skeletal Radiol 2006; 35:590–594.
19. Campanacci M, Baldini N, Boriani S, Sudanese A. Giant-cell tumor of bone. J Bone Joint Surg Am 1987; 69:106–114.
20. Campbell RSD, Grainger AJ, Mangham DC, et al. Intraosseous lipoma: a report of 35 new cases and a review of the literature. Skeletal Radiol 2003; 32:209–222.

CHAPTER 91

Myeloma

Andrea Baur-Melnyk

Myeloma typically is a multifocal, or diffuse, disease that is also called Kahler's disease, multiple myeloma, myelomatosis, and plasma cell myeloma. Solitary myeloma (plasmacytoma) is rare and must be differentiated from an early manifestation of what will eventually appear to be multiple myeloma and from benign plasma cell granuloma.

ETIOLOGY

Myeloma is a clonal B-lymphocyte neoplasm of terminally differentiated plasma cells. The cause of multiple myeloma remains unclear. Although not proven, infection, genetic predisposition, and various environmental factors such as radiation exposure, farm animals, various chemical dusts or gas, and electromagnetic waves/radar have been associated with myeloma.[1]

PREVALENCE AND EPIDEMIOLOGY

Multiple myeloma accounts for approximately 10% of all hematologic malignancies. The annual incidence in the United States is 3 to 4/100,000. The median age at diagnosis is 65 years. The disease has a higher incidence in men and blacks.

CLINICAL PRESENTATION

Clinical presentation is usually uncharacteristic. Patients may present with weakness, nausea, and weight loss. In most cases the disease is diagnosed by chance in a laboratory screening that shows an increased erythrocyte sedimentation rate and anemia. Further laboratory diagnostic workup includes immune electrophoresis and urine examination for Bence Jones protein content. The monoclonal strain of atypical plasma cells in the bone marrow secretes specific paraproteins, consisting of two heavy and two light chains. According to the heavy chains the type of myeloma is characterized as IgG (60%), IgA (25%), or, rarely, IgD and IgE. The myeloma cells also express light chains of λ or κ type. The paraproteins are detected in serum electrophoresis by a high peak in the α or γ region. In Bence Jones myeloma (20%), only light chains are secreted, which can be detected in urine electrophoresis. In nonsecretory myeloma (rare), no paraproteins are produced.

The myeloma cells displace normal hematopoiesis in bone marrow, resulting in anemia, leukopenia, and thrombocytopenia. Renal insufficiency and hypercalcemia are signs of progressive disease. Osteolyses and fractures can cause localized bone pain. Vertebral fractures with cord compression can cause neurologic impairment.

For the diagnosis of "multiple myeloma" three criteria have to be fulfilled: (1) greater than or equal to 10% atypical plasma cells in the bone marrow and/or the presence of biopsy-proven plasmacytoma, (2) monoclonal paraprotein present in the serum and/or urine, and (3) myeloma-related organ dysfunction (hypercalcemia, renal insufficiency, anemia, lytic bone lesions).[2]

Multiple staging systems have been created by various groups. The most widely accepted staging system is that of Durie and Salmon that was created in 1975 (Table 91-1).[3] In addition to the content of hemoglobin, the paraprotein component, the calcium value, the Bence Jones proteinuric excretion, and the findings of conventional radiographs are included. However, if available, the use of whole-body MRI is strongly recommended for a more precise evaluation of the bulk of disease.[2] In the Durie and Salmon PLUS staging system, the number of focal lesions and the extent of diffuse infiltration has to be determined using MRI and/or PET/CT (Table 91-2).

PATHOPHYSIOLOGY

Bone marrow biopsy or bone marrow aspirate is essential for the diagnosis of multiple myeloma. Multiple myeloma is a disease of terminally differentiated B lymphocytes. Different cell types, according to the stage of dedifferentiation, have been described (Fig. 91-1). At an initial stage it may be difficult to distinguish multiple myeloma from reactive plasmacytosis. The increase of the nucleus-plasma relationship and an atypical nucleus

KEY POINTS

- Multiple myeloma occurs in elderly patients with anemia and deteriorating general condition.
- Preliminary diagnosis is based on detection of paraproteins in serum and/or urine.
- Typical punched-out osteolytic lesions are seen on radiographs and CT.
- Focal and/or diffuse pattern of tumor infiltration is seen on MRI.
- Preferential location is red marrow (spine and pelvis).
- Osteopenia in patients with multiple myeloma may be secondary to osteoporosis and/or tumor- induced bone resorption.
- Assessment of extent of disease (staging) is important for prognosis and treatment.
- Durie and Salmon PLUS staging system including use of MR and/or FDG PET is superior to the old staging system (Durie and Salmon) using radiographs.
- Whole-body MRI is used to differentiate solitary plasmacytoma and MGUS from overt systemic multiple myeloma.

TABLE 91-2 Durie and Salmon PLUS Staging System

Classification	Whole-Body MRI and/or FDG PET
Monoclonal gammopathy of unknown significance (MGUS)	All negative
Stage IA (smoldering myeloma)	Normal skeletal survey or single lesion (limited disease)
Multiple myeloma	
Stage IB	< 5 focal lesions or mild diffuse disease*
Stage IIA/B	5–20 focal lesions or moderate diffuse disease†
Stage IIIA/B	> 20 focal lesions or severe diffuse disease‡

Subclassifications in stages II and III: (A) normal renal function, (B) abnormal renal function (serum creatinine > 2 mg/dL, extramedullary disease); stage was predictive of survival.

*Mild diffuse disease is a normal signal intensity or a slight homogeneous reduction of signal on T1-weighted spin-echo images and is often hard to detect.

†Moderate diffuse infiltration is a more apparent reduction in signal on T1-weighted spin-echo MR images.

‡Severe diffuse infiltration is a strong reduction in signal in which the signal intensity of bone marrow is almost equal to the intervertebral disc or the muscle on T1-weighted spin-echo images. Signal intensity on fat-suppressed images (e.g., STIR) is markedly increased.

Data from Durie BGM, Salmon SE. Myeloma management guidelines: a consensus report from the Scientific Advisors of the International Myeloma Foundation. Hematol J 2003; 4:379-398.

configuration are helpful signs for malignancy. Also the distribution of plasma cells in the marrow is important. In reactive plasmacytosis the plasma cells are distributed along vessels, whereas in multiple myeloma they are interstitially or focally distributed. In many institutions bone marrow biopsies are favored over bone marrow aspirates owing to methodologic problems of aspirates. In addition, in biopsies of bone marrow, quantification of plasmacytosis is more reliable. Hematopoiesis is reduced through direct replacement by myeloma cells and by release of hematopoiesis-inhibiting cytokines. In early stages, fat

can be increased, especially in the axial skeleton, and hematopoiesis (red marrow conversion) may increase in the peripheral skeleton as a reaction to decreased hematopoiesis in the axial skeleton. In more advanced disease, both yellow and red bone marrow are replaced by myeloma. Reduction of bone mass, seen on radiographs and CT as focal osteolysis, or general osteopenia is mainly caused by tumor-induced resorption of bone and not by mechanical destruction of bone by solid tumor. A crucial interaction between tumor and host, using complicated signaling pathways, develops, resulting in activation of osteoclasts and inhibition of osteoblasts. This interaction

TABLE 91-1 Durie and Salmon Staging System (1975)

Stage	Description

I	*All criteria need to be fulfilled:*
	Hemoglobin > 10 g/dL
	Serum calcium < 12 mg/dL
	Radiograph: normal bony structure < 2 osteolytic lesions
	M-gradient
	  IgG < 5 g/dL
	  IgA < 3 g/dL
	Bence Jones proteinuria: excretion < 4 g/24 hr

II	*Neither stage I nor stage III criteria are attributable.*

III	*One criteria need to be accomplished at minimum:*
	Hemoglobin < 8.5 g/dL
	Serum calcium > 12 mg/dL
	Radiograph: progressive osteolytic lesions
	M-gradient
	  IgG > 7 g/dL
	  IgA > 5 g/dL
	Bence Jones proteinuria: excretion > 12 g/24 hr

Subclassifications for I and III: (A) normal renal function (serum creatinine < 2.0 mg/dL, no extramedullary disease); (B) abnormal renal function (serum creatinine > 2 mg/dL, extramedullary disease).

Data from Durie BGM, Salmon SE. A clinical staging system for multiple myeloma: correlation of measured myeloma cell mass with presenting clinical features, response to treatment and survival. Cancer 1975; 36:842-854.

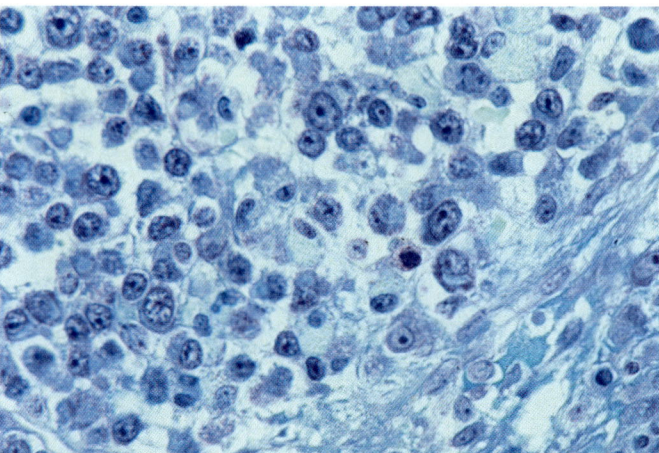

■ **FIGURE 91-1** Histology (Giemsa staining) of a patient with multiple myeloma of asynchronous type. The atypical plasma cells have a large, irregular, centrally located nucleus.

has a major impact on usefulness of imaging techniques. The impact of amyloid deposition in tumor on imaging is not well known. Amyloid deposition may also occur away from tumor, and this may be detected with MRI.

IMAGING TECHNIQUES

Techniques and Relevant Aspects

In patients with multiple myeloma the basic diagnostic workup in many institutions still consists of radiographs of the skull (two projections), the rib cage, the upper arms, the spine (two projections), the pelvis, and the upper legs. More and more cross-sectional imaging methods, such as multidetector CT (MDCT) and MRI, are used owing to the low sensitivity of radiography to demonstrate involvement by myeloma.[4,5]

Pros and Cons

Radiography versus Magnetic Resonance Imaging

Several studies demonstrated that radiographs often yield false-negative results, especially in the spine and pelvis secondary to superposition of complex osseous structures and soft tissues such as bowel. When radiographs are compared with MR images, high false-negative rates between 29% and 90% have been reported for radiographs in patients with multiple myeloma.[4,5] Even in asymptomatic patients (stage I according to the staging criteria of Durie and Salmon) with normal radiographs, MRI depicted diffuse or focal tumor infiltration in 29% to 50% of patients.[6,7] In approximately one third of patients the disease is understaged if MRI is not used.[8] However, disease stage would be underestimated in 10% of patients if conventional radiographs would have been replaced with limited MRI of the spine and pelvis because of lesions in the peripheral long bones, ribs, or skull.[9]

Current MR techniques allow a time-effective comprehensive skeletal survey using T1-weighted fast spin-echo and short tau inversion recovery (STIR) sequences in combination with dedicated receiver-coil elements, such as the total imaging matrix function in combination with parallel imaging (Siemens Medical Systems, Malvern, PA, USA) or the rolling table platform (AngioSURF Innovations, Essen, Germany). Thus, the entire bone marrow can be displayed, without patient repositioning, within approximately 35 minutes.

Computed Tomography versus Radiography

Computed tomography is more sensitive than radiography in detecting myeloma. Usually, radiographs show lesions and CT shows additional lesions but patients with combinations of negative radiographic surveys and positive CT scans have been reported.[10]

Multidetector Computed Tomography versus Magnetic Resonance Imaging

Magnetic resonance imaging (whole-body protocol at 1.5 T using T1-weighted and STIR sequences) is more sensitive than CT (16 or 64 detector rows using 0.75-mm collimation)

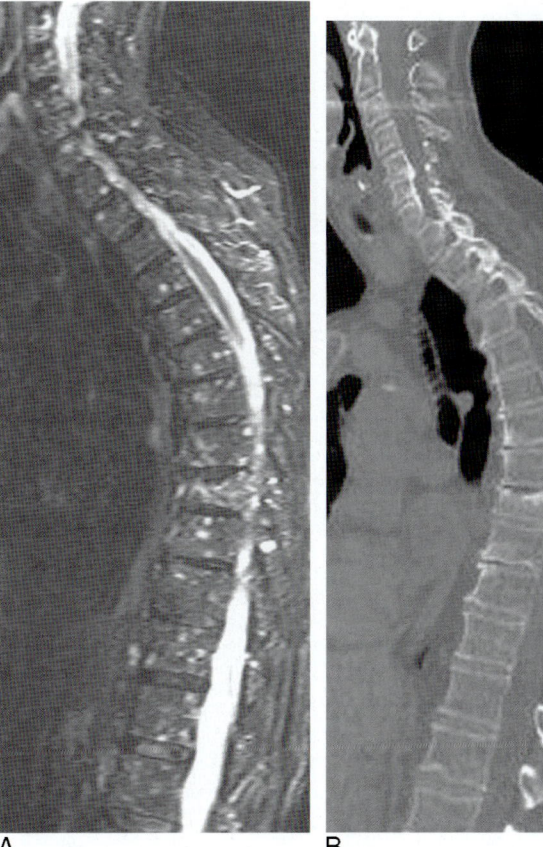

■ FIGURE 91-2 A, Sagittal STIR MR image of a female patient with multiple myeloma displaying many small foci and a fracture of the T9 vertebra. **B,** Sagittal reconstruction of the spine from a whole-body MDCT examination gave a false-negative finding.

in detecting myeloma infiltration (Fig. 91-2).[11] MRI displays tumor directly, whereas CT depends, like radiographs, on visualization of osseous destruction, resulting in a relatively high rate of false-negative results. Another consequence of this difference between MRI and CT is that after therapy, tumor load visualized on MR changes or even disappears while the secondary osseous changes seen on CT usually do not change. False-positive results in MDCT may be due to inhomogeneous osteoporosis. In a prospective study in 41 patients with multiple myeloma, MRT detected significantly more lesions than did MDCT. This resulted in significant understaging with MDCT alone.[11]

Controversies

A current issue is the choice of imaging modality in patients with multiple myeloma on a routine basis. Radiographs proved to be false negative in many studies; therefore, in many institutions whole-body MRI or whole-body MDCT is performed for primary diagnosis and for follow-up (Fig. 91-3). Up to now there is no consensus whether whole-body MRI or whole-body MDCT should be used. MDCT is more widely available, is a quick examination technique, and is especially useful for demonstration of osseous destructions and fractures. On the other hand, MRI is much more sensitive for evaluating early bone marrow involvement.

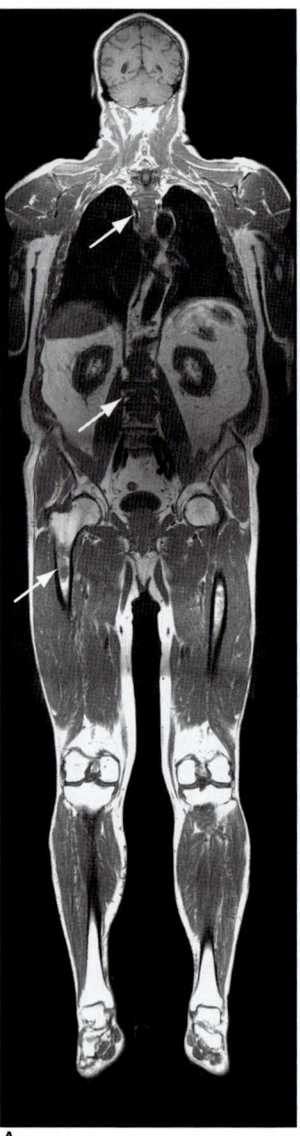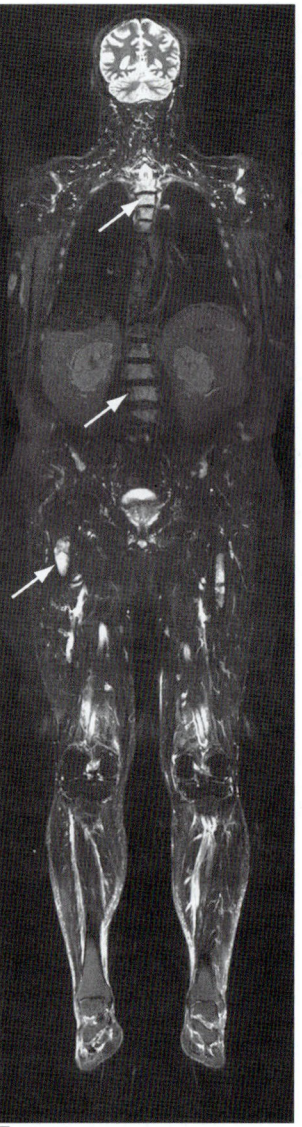

A   B

■ **FIGURE 91-3** Coronal composition of a whole-body MRI exam: T1-weighted spin-echo MR image (**A**) and STIR MR image (**B**). The patient has extensive infiltration of the spine, pelvis, and upper legs, demonstrated by low signal intensity on T1-weighted spin-echo and high signal intensity on STIR images (*arrows*).

MANIFESTATIONS OF THE DISEASE

Multiple myeloma is a primary disease of the bone marrow. Therefore, it affects first the bone marrow and second the bone itself in terms of osseous destruction. The bone is visualized with radiography and CT. With MRI, the tumor in the bone marrow is directly displayed. With PET/CT the utilization of glucose by tumor cells is determined. This is potentially important in monitoring treatment.

Rarely, atypical manifestations of multiple myeloma occur, such as peritoneal carcinomatosis, myeloma masses in the bowel wall, pleural carcinomatosis, pulmonary involvement due to myeloma or amyloidosis, hilar lymph nodes, liver lesions and myelomatous soft tissue masses in the sphenoidal sinus.[12]

Radiography

Predilection sites are the axial skeleton (spine and pelvis) but also the ribs, the shoulder region, the skull, and the proximal femur (Figs. 91-4 and 91-5). The appearance of multiple myeloma in radiographs is either focal circumscribed "punched out" osteolyses or diffuse inhomogeneous osteopenia, especially in the spine (Fig. 91-6). In the skull, multiple osteolytic lesions of similar size are found. In the long bones the osteolytic lesions are often, but not exclusively, centrally located (Figs. 91-7 and 91-8). With increasing size they lead to endosteal scalloping of the cortex. Large lesions may penetrate the cortex and demonstrate a soft tissue component. Enlargement may lead to apparent expansion of bone with a soap bubble appearance. Involvement of the ribs is usually seen as osteolyses or an inhomogeneous appearance of the spongiosa in combination with a circumscribed expansion of the bone. Differentiation of multiple myeloma from metastatic skeletal disease can be very challenging without the knowledge of laboratory parameters. The most important discriminating features of myeloma versus metastases are osteolytic rather than the combination of osteolytic and sclerotic lesions, diffuse osteopenia, lesions that are well defined and uniform in size, and cortical scalloping rather than cortical destruction.

Sclerotic lesions or osteolytic lesions with a sclerotic rim are rarely seen in myeloma.[13] Primary diffuse sclerosis of the skeleton is also rare (<3% of cases) and appears more often after therapy. Differential diagnoses in those cases include osteoblastic metastases, myelofibrosis, lymphoma, renal osteodystrophy, and mastocytosis.

Diffuse osteopenia due to myelomatous infiltration and tumor-induced osteoclast activity is difficult to distinguish from postmenopausal or senile osteoporosis. This is also true for vertebral fractures. Both osteoporotic fractures as well as neoplastic fractures are common in this patient group.

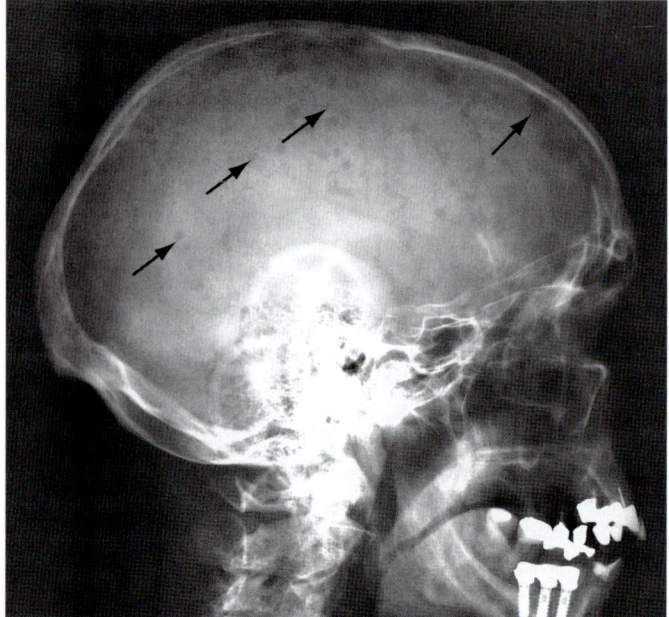

■ **FIGURE 91-4** Radiograph of the skull yields the typical multiple punched-out osteolytic lesions in a patient with multiple myeloma (*arrows*).

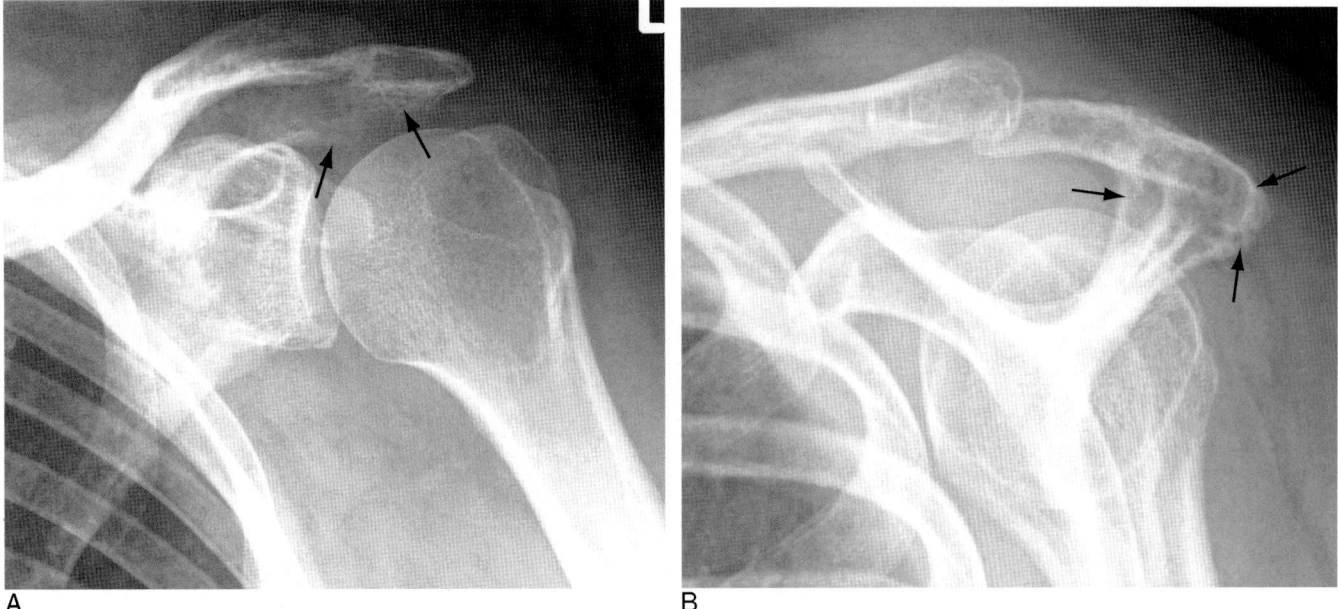

■ **FIGURE 91-5** Anteroposterior (**A**) and Y (**B**) radiographs show osteolytic destruction of the acromion in a patient with multiple myeloma (*arrows*).

■ **FIGURE 91-6** Anteroposterior (**A**) and lateral (**B**) radiographs of the thoracic spine in a patient with advanced multiple myeloma. Multiple vertebral fractures are indicative of multifocal and/or diffuse infiltration. However, radiographs are sometimes misleading, and differentiation from an osteoporotic spine with fractures may be challenging. MRI can exclude or demonstrate infiltration by myeloma.

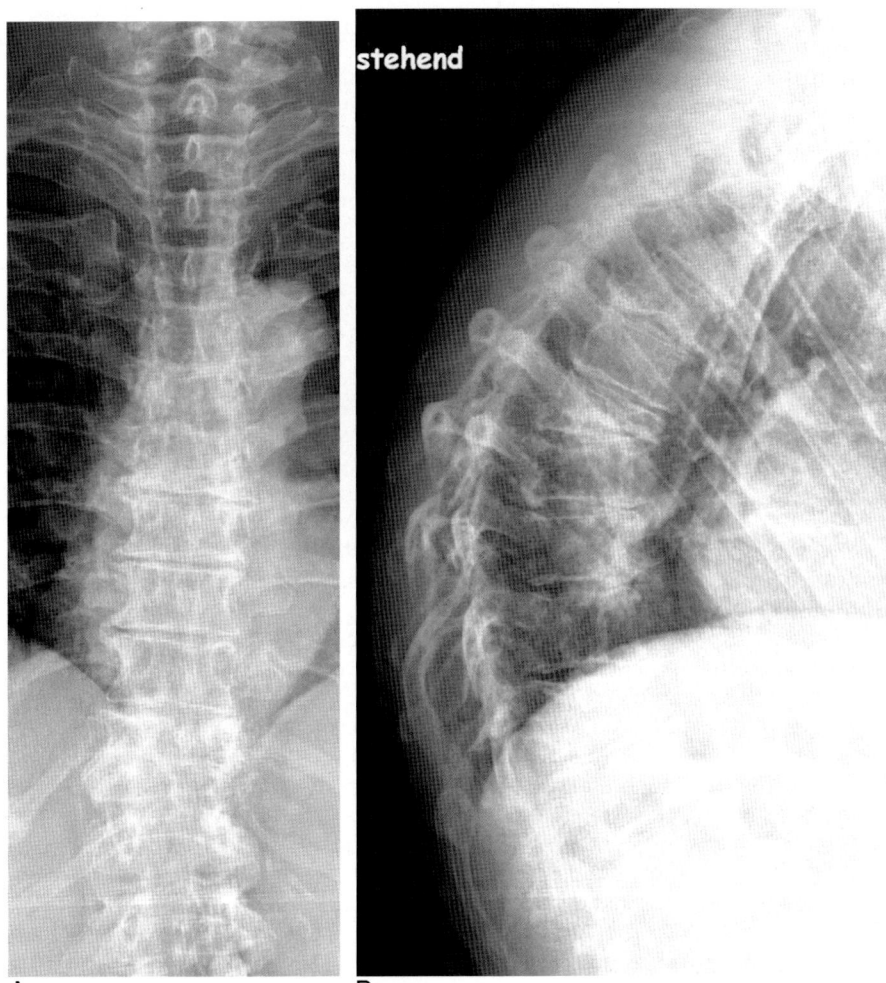

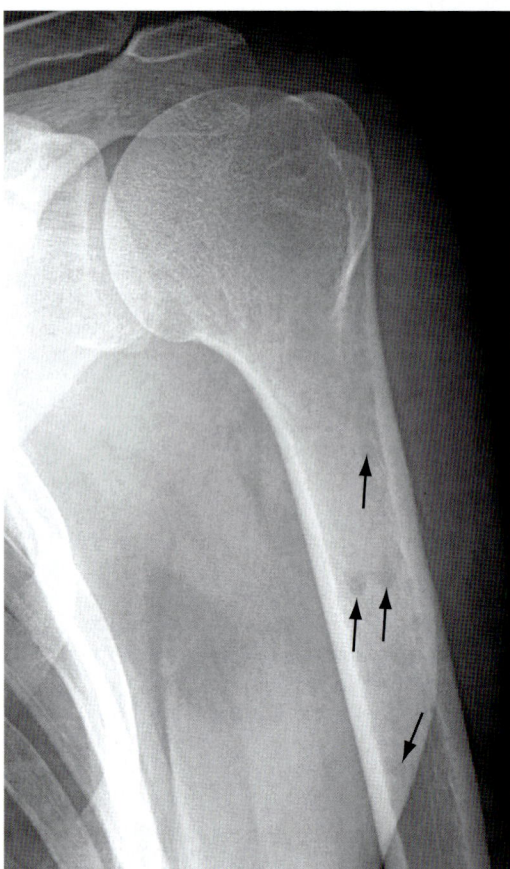

■ **FIGURE 91-7** Anteroposterior radiograph of an upper arm of a patient with multiple myeloma. Multiple punched-out osteolytic lesions can be seen (*arrows*).

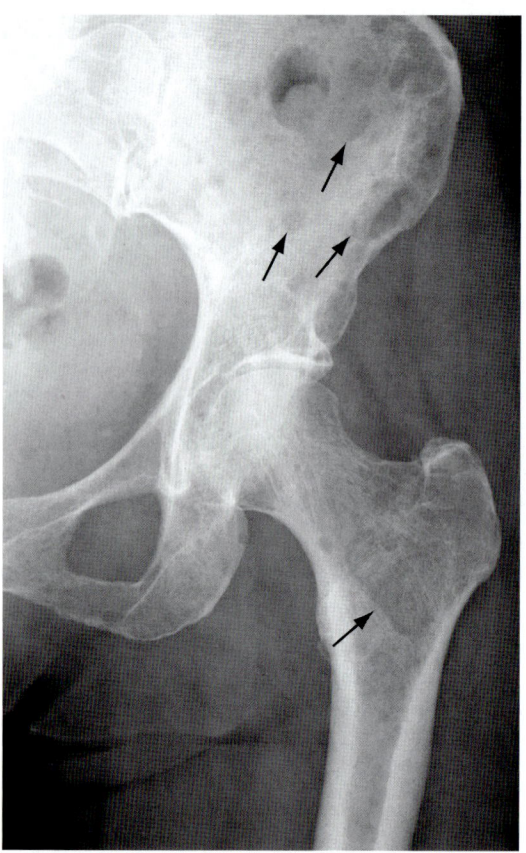

■ **FIGURE 91-8** Multiple osteolytic lesions of different size in the pelvis and the upper leg in a patient with multiple myeloma stage III (*arrows*).

In addition, the combination of the age of the patients and cortisone therapy favors bone loss. In these situations MRI can help in the differential diagnosis.

Magnetic Resonance Imaging

In patients with multiple myeloma, five patterns of infiltration patterns can be described by MRI.[4] First, in 28% of the patients a normal-looking bone marrow signal is found in all sequences with high signal intensity on T1-weighted images and an intermediate signal intensity on T2-weighted spin-echo images, as well as low signal intensity in fat-saturated sequences such as STIR. In histology, this corresponds to a slight interstitial plasma cell infiltration (<20 mg/dL in bone marrow biopsy). Normal bone marrow signal intensity in MRI does not exclude the diagnosis of multiple myeloma. However, these patients are eligible for a "watch and wait" strategy.

Second, focal myeloma can be found in approximately 30% of cases. Circumscribed areas of high signal intensity can be identified on gradient-echo, fat-suppressed T2-weighted and STIR MR sequences. These correspond to areas of low signal intensity on unenhanced T1-weighted spin-echo MR images (Figs. 91-9 to 91-11). In a few cases, isointense signal is found on T1-weighted spin-echo images. Contrast between the high signal intensity of normal yellow bone marrow on T2-weighted turbo or fast spin-echo sequences and high signal intensity of

focal myeloma is poor. Therefore, fat suppression should be used in combination with fast or turbo spin-echo sequences.[14] Frequency-selective fat saturation is effective in combination with T2 weighting when a small field of view is used in a magnet with a homogeneous magnetic field. However, when a large field of view (250 × 500 mm) is needed, as in skeletal surveys, STIR sequences offer more homogeneous fat suppression. Some authors employed chemical shift imaging by using opposed-phased gradient-echo sequences. By means of opposed phasing of fat- and, respectively, water-bound protons in normal bone marrow, multiple myeloma infiltrations are displayed as areas with high signal intensity.

Third, diffuse bone marrow infiltration is characterized by a homogeneous decrease of signal intensity on T1-weighted spin-echo MR images and of increased signal intensity on fat-suppressed MR images (Fig. 91-12). In cases of high-grade diffuse involvement (>50 volume % in bone marrow biopsy) the signal intensity on T1-weighted spin-echo MR images is nearly equal to that of the intervertebral disc or muscle (Figs. 91-13 and 91-14). In cases of intermediate grade of involvement (20 to 50 volume %) the signal reduction is only moderate and often hard to diagnose.[15] In those cases intravenous injection of gadolinium chelates is recommended to verify diffuse involvement. Enhancement of normal bone marrow varies between 3% and 40% (Fig. 91-15), with a mean of 17%, in patients older than 40 years of age. An increase of signal intensity after

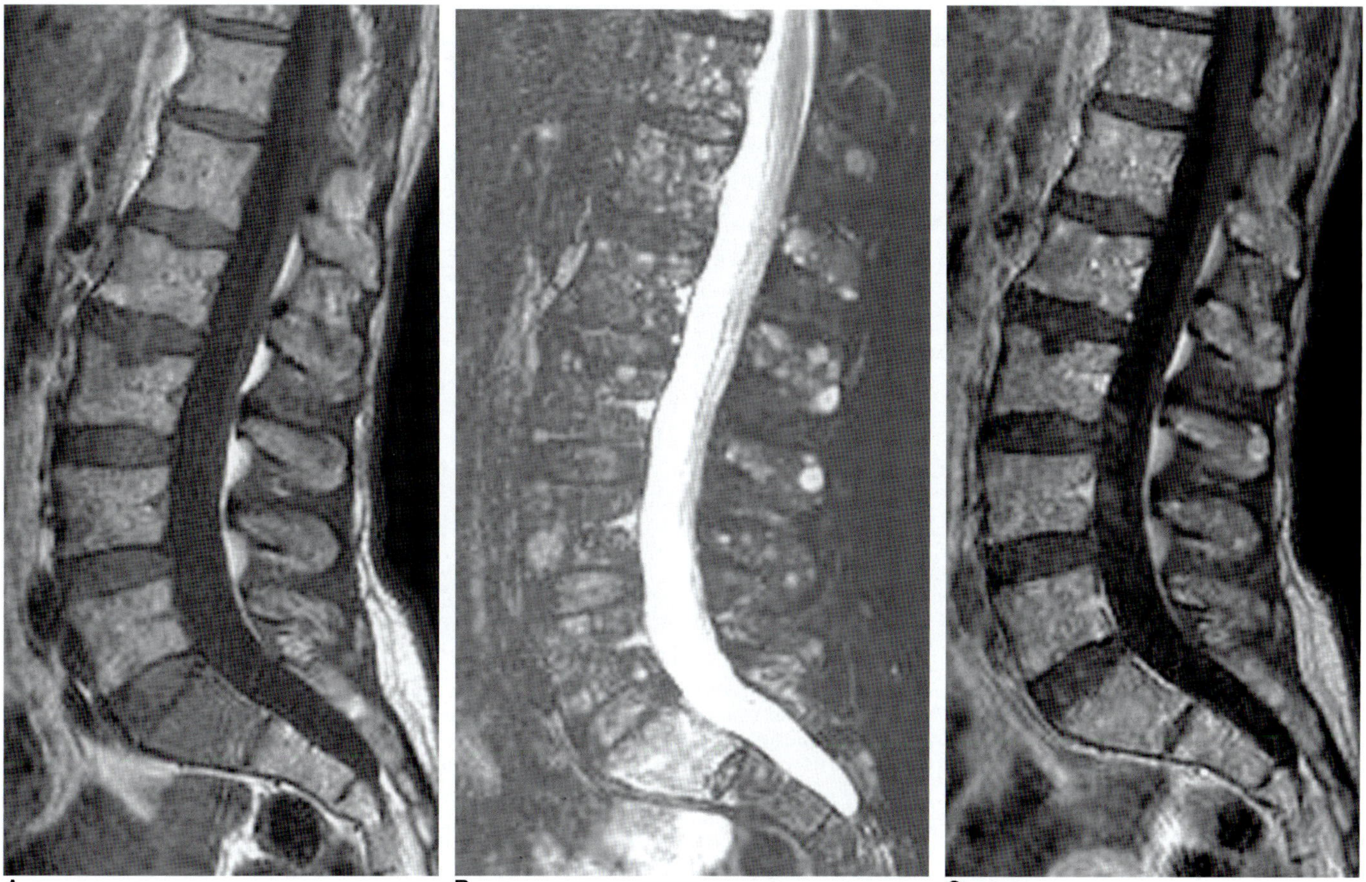

■ **FIGURE 91-9** Focal infiltration of the lumbar spine in a patient with advanced stage III disease. Focal areas of low signal intensity on a T1-weighted spin-echo MR image (**A**) correspond to areas of high signal intensity on a STIR MR image (**B**). Myeloma nodules enhance with Gd-DTPA (**C**).

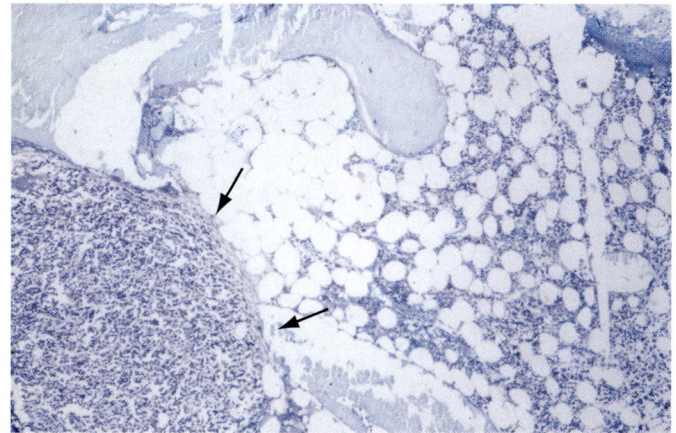

■ **FIGURE 91-10** Histology (Giemsa stain) of a patient with focal myeloma (*arrows*).

administration of gadolinium chelate exceeding the limit of 40% can be considered as pathologic.[16]

Fourth, a combined focal and diffuse infiltration pattern can be found in approximately 11% of patients. On T1-weighted spin-echo MR images the bone marrow signal intensity is diffusely decreased with additional foci interspersed (Fig. 91-16). Those foci are often better seen on STIR or gradient-echo MR images.

Fifth, in approximately 3% of cases a so-called salt-and-pepper pattern can be found.[4] On T1-weighted spin-echo images, but also on gradient-echo and T2-weighted spin-echo sequences, the bone marrow presents a very inhomogeneous patchy pattern. However, no hyperintense areas are demarcated in STIR sequences (Fig. 91-17). This corresponds to bone marrow with circumscribed fat islands beside normal bone marrow with a minor infiltration of plasma cells (<20 volume %, Fig. 91-18). In the early stage of multiple myeloma this special pattern is thought to be initiated by a hematopoiesis-inhibiting factor. Enhancement of bone marrow does not exceed 40%. These patients usually have stage I disease and do not require therapy.

Focal or diffuse signal alterations are not specific for myeloma. They may be found in a various other conditions, too. Differential diagnoses for focal lesions include metastases, lymphoma, atypical hemangiomas, and hematopoietic islands. Differential diagnoses for diffuse disease include metastases, lymphoma, leukemia, myelodysplastic syndrome, chronic myeloproliferative diseases, and stimulated bone marrow.

Prognosis

The time of survival in patients with multiple myeloma ranges between a few months to more than 10 years in so-called "smoldering myeloma." These large differences, which are

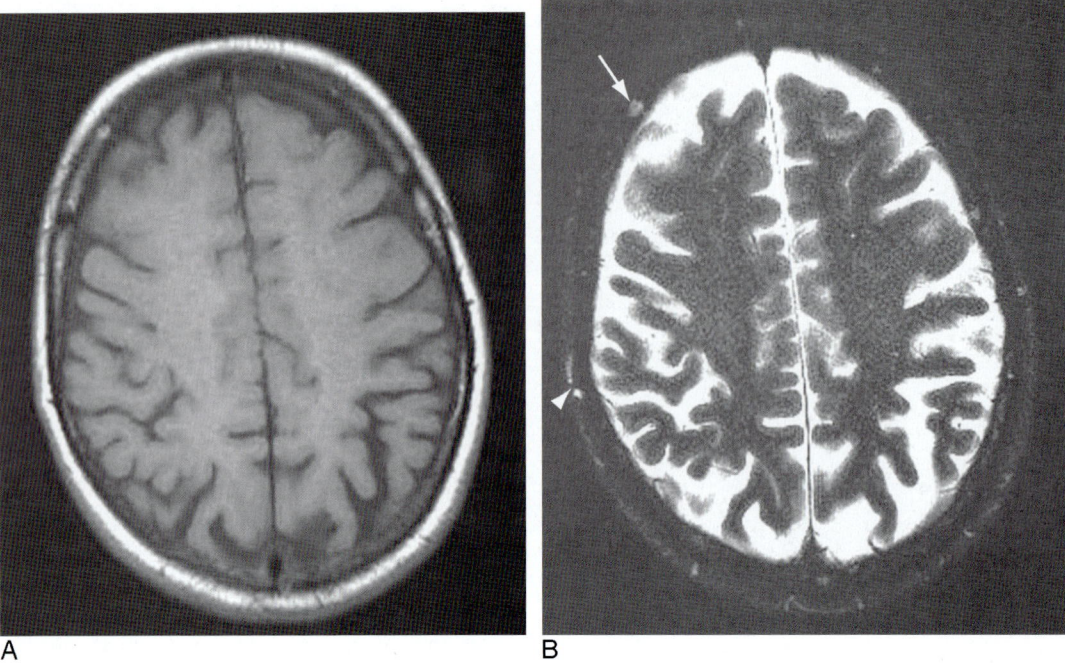

■ **FIGURE 91-11** Focal myeloma nodule in the right os frontale (*arrow*). T1-weighted spin-echo (**A**) and STIR (**B**) MR images. Myeloma nodules are situated in the diploë (marrow between tabula externa and interna). If small, the nodules have to be differentiated from pacchionian granulations (have a communication to the subarachnoid space, fluid-like signal) and vessel channels (can be followed as linear structures on several slices) (*arrowhead*).

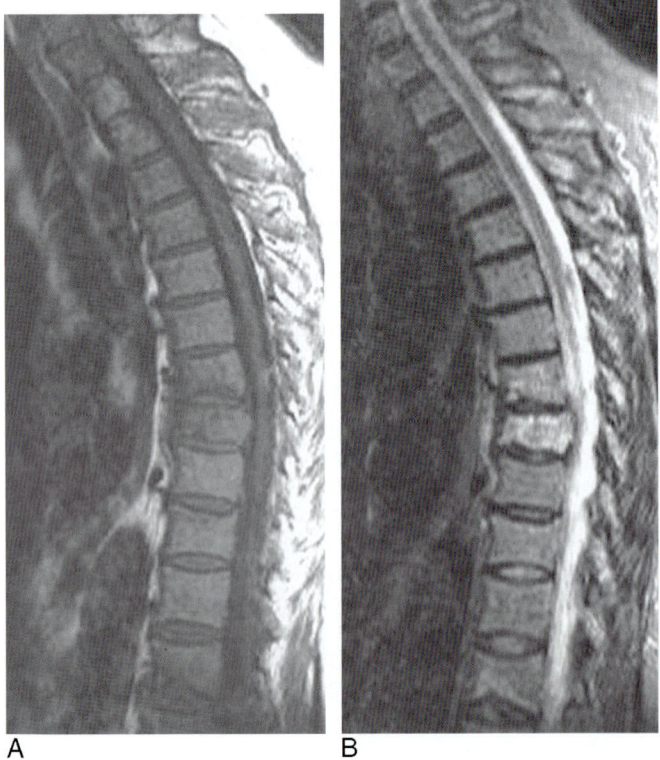

■ **FIGURE 91-12** Intermediate grade of diffuse infiltration of the spine is characterized by lowering of signal on T1-weighted spin-echo MR image (**A**) owing to reduction of fat cells and replacement by myeloma cells. However, there is still contrast in signal to the low signal of the intervertebral disc (high water content) on T1-weighted spin-echo images. In a STIR MR image (**B**) the signal is slightly elevated when compared with that of normal bone marrow. Note also the pathologic fracture of the T8 vertebral body.

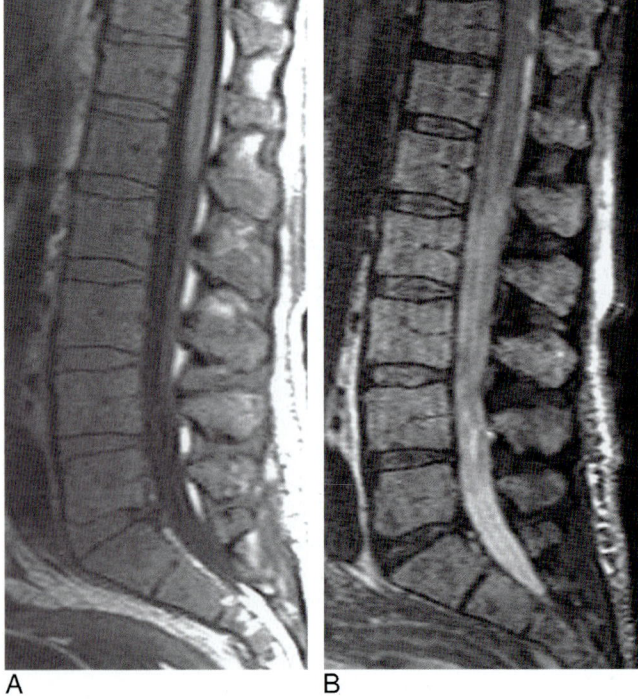

■ **FIGURE 91-13** High-grade diffuse infiltration of the lumbar spine. In patients with high-grade diffuse infiltration on a T1-weighted spin-echo MR image (**A**) the signal intensity of the bone marrow is almost the same as that of the intervertebral disc. On a STIR MR image (**B**) the signal intensity is markedly increased.

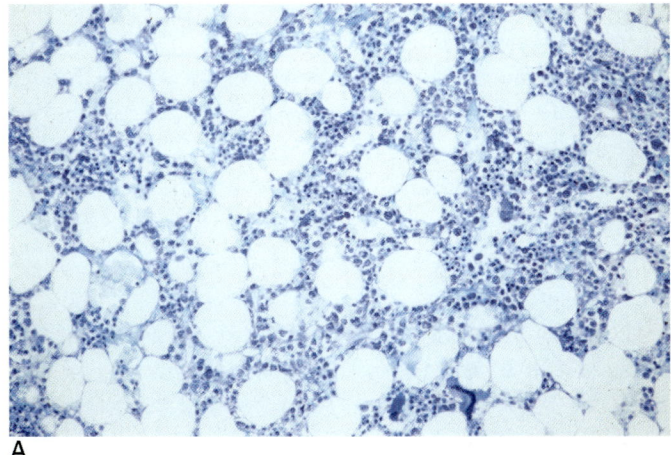
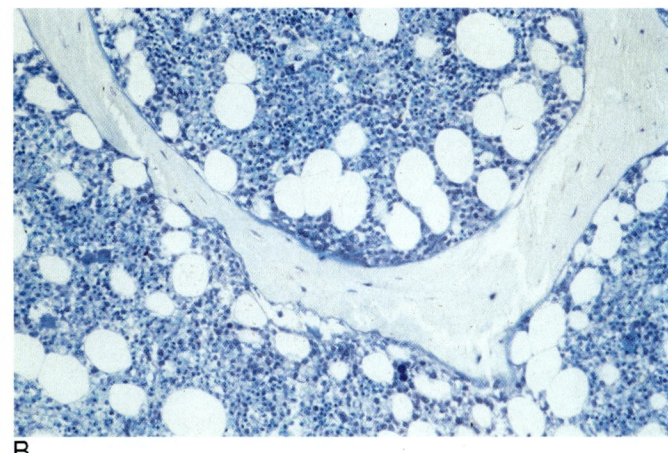
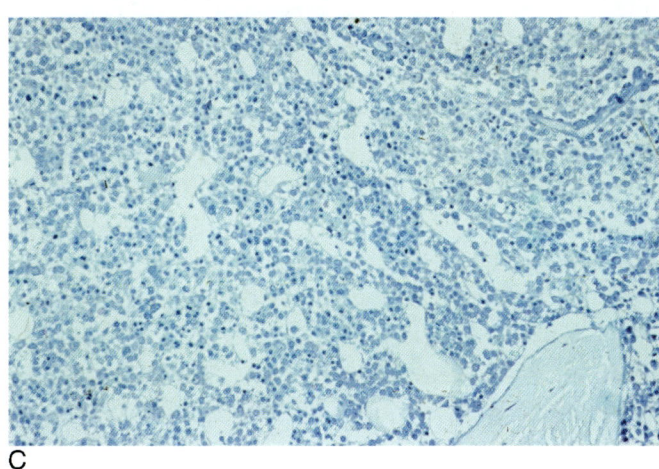

■ FIGURE 91-14 Low-grade (**A**), intermediate-grade (**B**), and high-grade (**C**) diffuse infiltration in histology (Giemsa stain). In low-grade diffuse infiltration there is 10 to 20 Volume % of interstitial infiltration with atypical plasma cells. Hematopoiesis is still normal; the fat cell content can be normal or increased. MRI is normal in those cases. In intermediate-grade (20 to 50 Volume % plasma cells) and high-grade (>50 Volume % plasma cells) diffuse infiltration the fat cell content and hematopoiesis are more and more reduced.

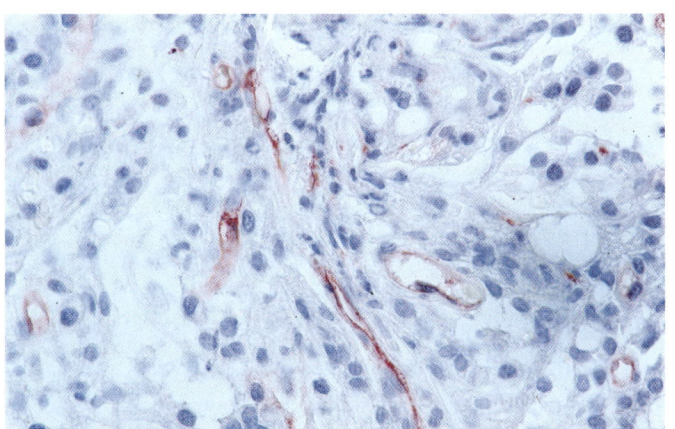

■ FIGURE 91-15 High-grade diffuse infiltration of the bone marrow. With increasing infiltration, increasing neovascularization of the bone marrow can be depicted (anti-CD 34+ immuno-stain).

associated with specific therapeutic options, indicate the need for prognostic parameters. Laboratory parameters, such as elevated levels of β_2-microglobulin, decreased levels of serum albumin, and deletion of chromosome 13, are predictors for time to progression and survival.[17] Paraprotein greater than 3g/dL, a type IgA plasmacytoma, and uric acid excretion of Bence Jones proteins more than 50mg/day have the greatest influence on prognosis as independent variables.[18]

MRI also has prognostic value.[6,7,8] The time to progression in patients with stage I disease and normal results of MRI has been reported to be significantly longer (44 months) than in patients with stage I disease and MR abnormalities in keeping with myeloma (11 months).[7] Also, in populations stratified according to laboratory risk factors, MR adds prognostic value, increasing time to progression from 21 months (abnormal MRI) to 57 months (normal MRI) in a population with intermediate laboratory risk factors.[18] The survival time in patients with a salt-and-pepper pattern of involvement is longer than in patients with diffuse or focal infiltrates.[8] In patients with diffuse or focal infiltrates, the extent of infiltration, and not the type of infiltration, is the prognostic factor.

Patients with abnormal MRI have lower 5-year survival rates (30%) than patients with normal MRI results (80%).[19] It seems that patients with pathologic MRI findings require earlier treatment.

Multidetector Computed Tomography

Multidetector CT is the method of choice for assessing fracture risk and loss of bone mass. Whole-body MDCT is now often used instead of radiographs, because sensitivity is higher and examination time is reduced to 1 to 2 minutes with 16- or 64-row CT scanners. Complex biochemical mechanisms and the secretion of osteoclast-activating factors lead to bony destruction. Osteolyses in multiple

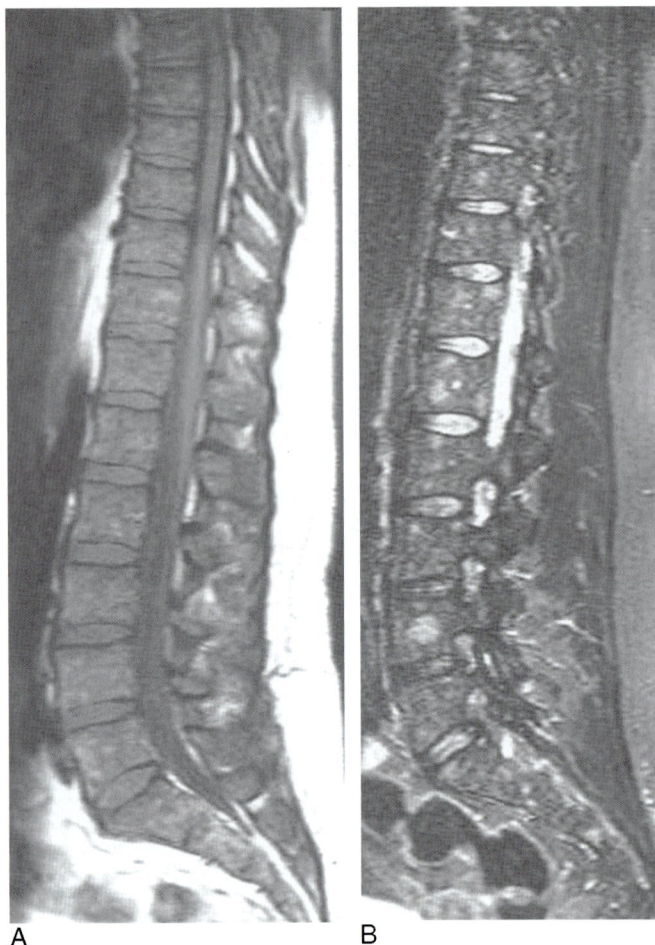

■ **FIGURE 91-16** Combined diffuse and focal infiltration of the spine in a patient with multiple myeloma. Diffuse lowering of signal on T1-weighted spin-echo MR image (**A**) combined with focal deposits, which are better depicted on the STIR MR image (**B**).

A   B

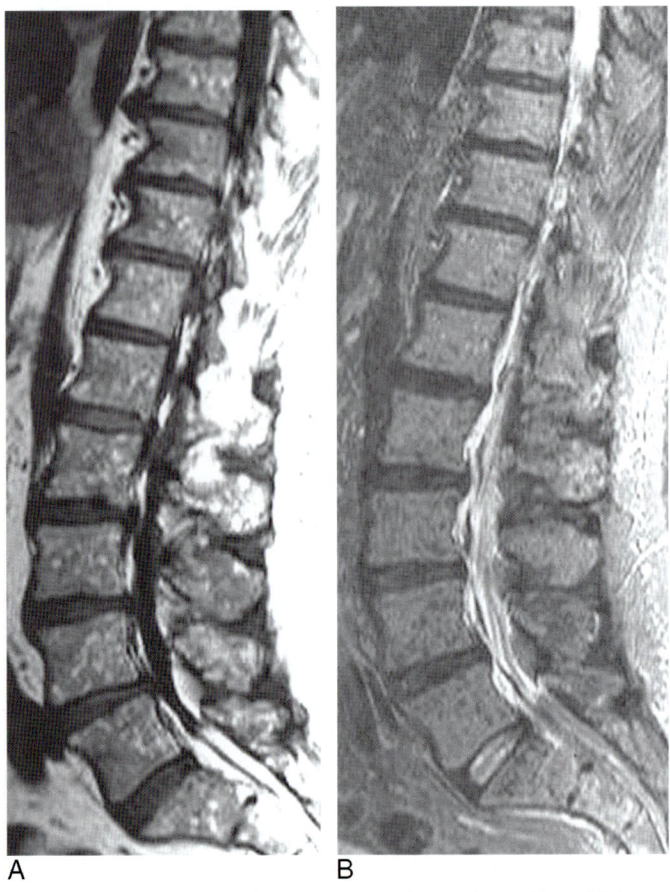

■ **FIGURE 91-17** Salt-and-pepper pattern in a patient with multiple myeloma. **A,** The signal intensity on a T1-weighted spin-echo MR image is patchy. The hyperintense areas represent fatty islands. **B,** However, on a STIR MR image no focal nodules can be seen.

A   B

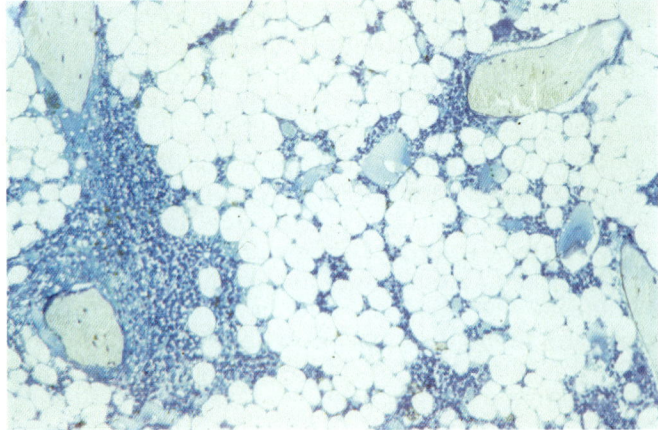

■ **FIGURE 91-18** Histology of a patient with salt-and-pepper pattern. Note normal bone marrow with only low-grade diffuse infiltration, beside focal fat islands. This can lead to the patchy appearance on MRI. These patients usually have stage I disease and do not require any therapy.

myeloma are usually well circumscribed and have a small zone of transition (Fig. 91-19). Osteolytic lesions usually have Hounsfield units of soft tissue density (~40–80 HU). Osteolytic lesions are initially situated within the trabecular bone. When tumor volume increases, cortical destruction and soft tissue extension may ensue (Figs. 91-20 and 91-21). In the skull, punched-out lesions within the tabula externa and interna are typically seen (Fig. 91-22). In the diaphyses of the long tubular bones, where only sparse trabecular bone is present, early osteolysis may be missed when only bony windows are used. Circumscribed soft tissue alterations within the normal fatty marrow are highly suggestive of myeloma. Comparison to the other side may be helpful in evaluating marrow involvement (Fig. 91-23). Cortical scalloping in the long bones may be visible on axial or reformatted coronal or sagittal planes. Small lesions in the ribs are easily overlooked. Focal enlargement of the rib with soft tissue density within the lesion represents myeloma. The cortex may be normal or thinned (Fig. 91-24). If the tumor continues to grow, a pathologic fracture will result. Careful examination of every rib is necessary to not overlook a rib lesion. The shoulder girdle with its complex structures (e.g., acromion, coracoid process) is another site of predilection (Fig. 91-25).

As in radiographs, inhomogeneous osteopenia may represent diffuse involvement. MRI is the method of choice in differentiating osteopenia secondary to diffuse myeloma from osteoporosis.

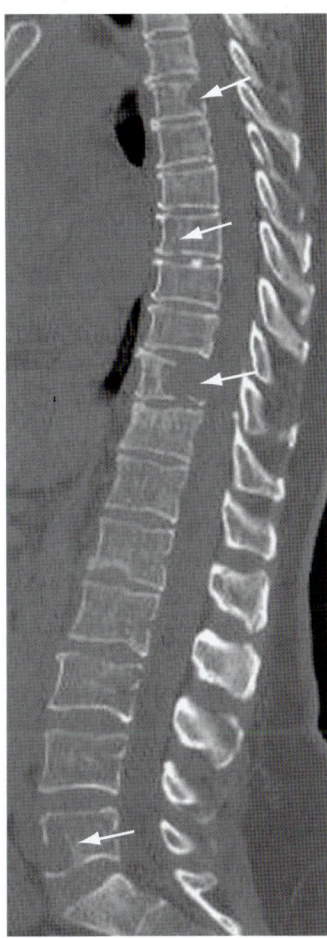

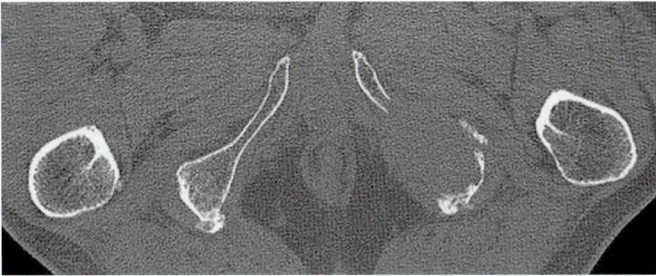

■ **FIGURE 91-21** Myeloma involvement of the left os ischii. Cortex is destroyed.

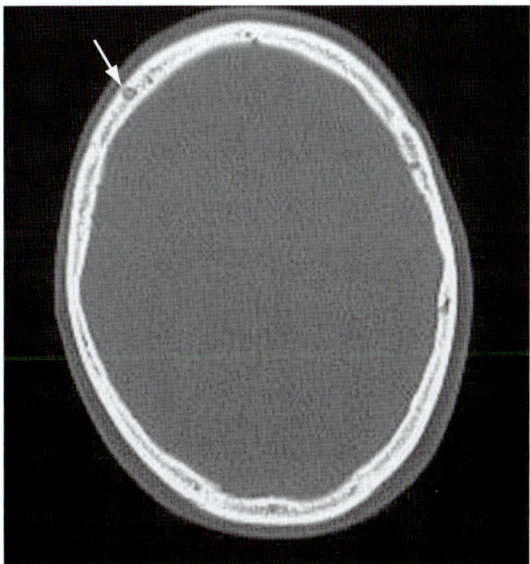

■ **FIGURE 91-19** Sagittal reconstructions of a 64-row MDCT examination of the spine. Multifocal osteolytic lesions are seen in a patient with multiple myeloma (*arrows*).

■ **FIGURE 91-22** Osteolyses of the right os frontale in a patient with multiple myeloma. Same patient as in Figure 91-12 (*arrow*).

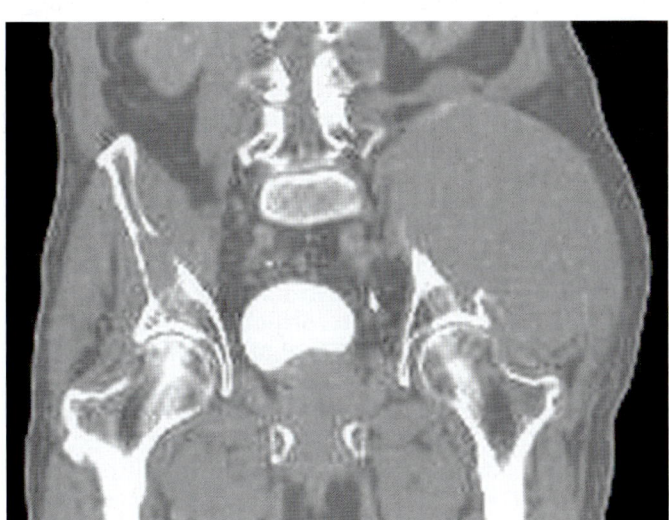

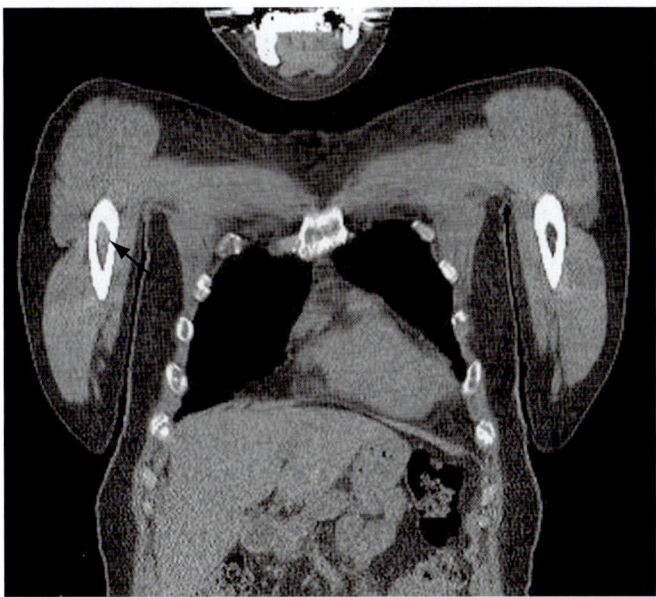

■ **FIGURE 91-20** Coronal reconstruction of the pelvis. Osteolytic lesions are evident in the left iliac bone. Sometimes myeloma can yield large soft tissue components as in this case.

■ **FIGURE 91-23** Coronal reconstruction of the thorax and arms shows marrow infiltration of the right upper arm (*arrow*). In contrast to the left upper arm, soft tissue is noted within the humerus. In the long bones, where no spongiose network is present, it is important to use soft tissue and bone windows.

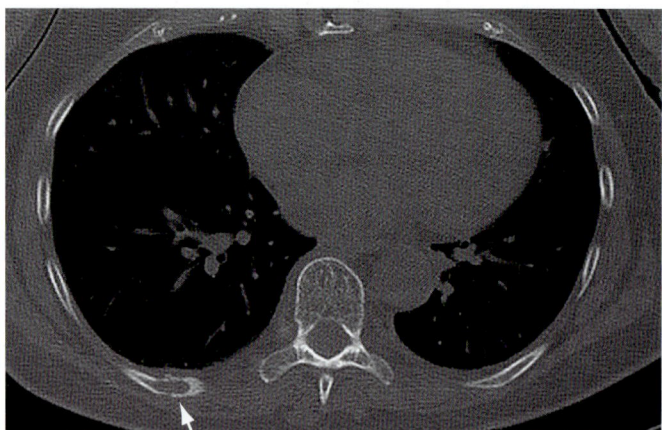

■ **FIGURE 91-24** Rib involvement in multiple myeloma (*arrow*). Note thinning of the cortex and enlargement of a circumscribed area of the rib. Soft tissue Hounsfield units are noted within the lesion. In contrast to osteoporotic or traumatic fractures of the rib no callus formation is seen. In a whole-body examination every single rib has to be screened by scrolling through it posteriorly to anteriorly.

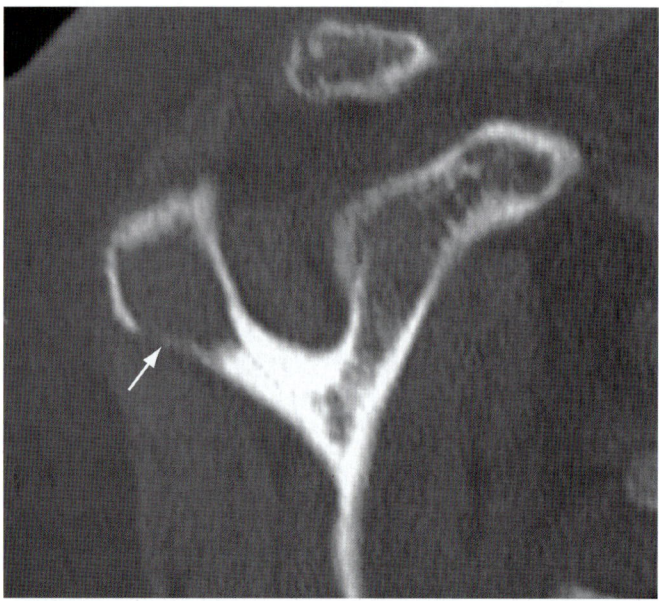

■ **FIGURE 91-25** Myeloma in the coracoid process shows endosteal thinning of the cortex. The shoulder girdle is a main site for myeloma infiltration (*arrow*).

Nuclear Medicine Studies

Multiple myeloma is primarily a neoplasm that produces osteolyses. Detection of bony involvement with technetium-99 m scintigraphy relies on an osteoblastic response of the skeletal system. This results in an underappreciation of the extent of disease and is not recommended for the diagnostic workup in patients with multiple myeloma.[20]

Positron Emission Tomography/ Computed Tomography

Recent efforts have been made toward direct imaging of tumor cells with fluorodeoxyglucose (FDG)-labeled PET.[21-23] Schirrmeister and colleagues examined 28 patients with multiple myeloma and 15 patients with solitary plasmacytoma of bone.[21] Focally increased tracer uptake was observed in 38 of 41 known osteolytic bone lesions. Another 71 bone lesions were detected that were negative on radiographs. As a result of FDG PET, clinical management was influenced in 5 patients. In a study of Durie and associates, 16 previously untreated patients with multiple myeloma had positive FDG PET scans, either focally or diffuse. Four of them had negative radiographs, and in another 4 patients extramedullary disease was detected.[22] In a study of Bredella and coworkers including 13 patients, sensitivity of FDG PET in detecting myeloma involvement was 85% and specificity was 92%.[23]

Classic Signs

- Punched-out osteolytic lesions are seen on radiographs and CT.
- Focal or diffuse tumor infiltration is evident on MRI.

DIFFERENTIAL DIAGNOSIS

Differential diagnosis includes metastases from other primary lesions, myeloproliferative disease, and leukemia. These differential diagnoses can be made by detecting a primary tumor and by biopsy. Imaging features as described in this chapter and in the chapters on metastatic disease and diffuse bone marrow disease are used to differentiate these disorders.

Monoclonal Gammopathy of Unknown Significance, Smoldering Myeloma

Primary differential diagnoses in case of elevated laboratory paraprotein are monoclonal gammopathy of unknown significance (MGUS) and smoldering myeloma. MGUS is a common cause of laboratory-discovered elevated paraprotein. It is usually an incidental finding. The incidence in patients older than 70 years of age is about 3%. Several laboratory parameters have to be fulfilled to diagnose MGUS. Follow-up examinations, which confirm stable disease, are necessary to diagnose MGUS rather than myeloma. No osteolyses should be present. Whole-body MRI is usually negative in MGUS and can be used as a tool to confirm the diagnosis (see Table 91-2). MGUS can evolve to manifest multiple myeloma, chronic lymphatic leukemia, lymphoma, Waldenström's macroglobulinemia, or amyloidosis. The majority of patients with a clinical diagnosis of MGUS but abnormal MRI will require treatment within 5 years.[24]

Smoldering, or stage Ia, myeloma is an intermediate category between MGUS and multiple myeloma (see Table 91-2). Such patients can have mild degrees of myeloma-related organ dysfunction (e.g., slight anemia). The bone marrow contains between 10 and 30 volume% plasma cells. The patients are eligible for supportive care measures such as administration of erythropoietin and bisphosphonates. Abnormalities on MRI or FDG PET indicate an increased risk of early disease progression.[2]

Solitary Plasmacytoma

Solitary bone plasmacytoma affects 2% to 3% of patients with plasma cell myeloma. Diagnostic criteria for solitary plasmacytoma of bone have varied over the years. Routine bone marrow biopsy usually is normal, and there should be no organ dysfunction. Radiographs typically show a singular lytic lesion with a narrow zone of transition. It may be also expansile with a soft tissue component. It may affect any bone but has a preference for the axial skeleton, in particular, the vertebrae (Fig. 91-26).[25] For therapy planning (surgery and or radiation) CT or MRI are required to display osseous destructions and the soft tissue component. In the spine, the soft tissue component may cause spinal cord or nerve root compression. A small, if any, M-protein component usually decreases after local radiation therapy. Several studies report that screening of patients with solitary plasmacytoma of bone with MRI revealed additional lesions. Some authors postulate that solitary plasmacytoma is multiple myeloma in which only one of multiple lesions is detected or is only a precursor for multiple myeloma. Thus, whole-body MRI is strongly recommended, because therapeutic regimens are different for solitary plasmacytoma and multiple myeloma.

Vertebral Fractures

Vertebral fracture is another important consideration in the differential diagnosis of myeloma. Vertebral fractures are common in the elderly population due to osteoporosis. They occur in 50% to 70% of patients within the clinical course of multiple myeloma and account for a large part of morbidity. In patients with multiple myeloma, vertebral fractures may be secondary to osteoporosis or to tumor. Osteoporotic fractures typically show a band-like pattern of bone marrow edema on MRI. In cases of extensive edema, small areas of normal fat-containing bone marrow, seen as areas of high signal intensity on T1-weighted images and of low signal intensity on STIR images, are still appreciated. In CT the presence of an intravertebral vacuum almost excludes a neoplastic origin of the fracture (Fig. 91-27). Neoplastic fractures often show an angling of end plates owing to asymmetric infraction and osteolytic destruction with soft tissue density on CT. A paravertebral soft tissue mass may or may not be present. Homogeneous decrease of signal intensity of the entire vertebral body on T1-weighted spin-echo images and increase in signal intensity on STIR images are the most reliable signs for neoplastic fractures on MRI.[26] Diffusion-weighted imaging may be an additional tool for the differentiation of acute benign from neoplastic vertebral fractures (Fig. 91-28).[27]

Although fractures occur earlier and more frequently in patients with diffuse disease, or with more than 10 focal lesions in the spine, MRI is not very useful in predicting collapse. Approximately two thirds of fractures occur in previously normal vertebral bodies, whereas in one third a preexisting lesion can be seen on MRI.

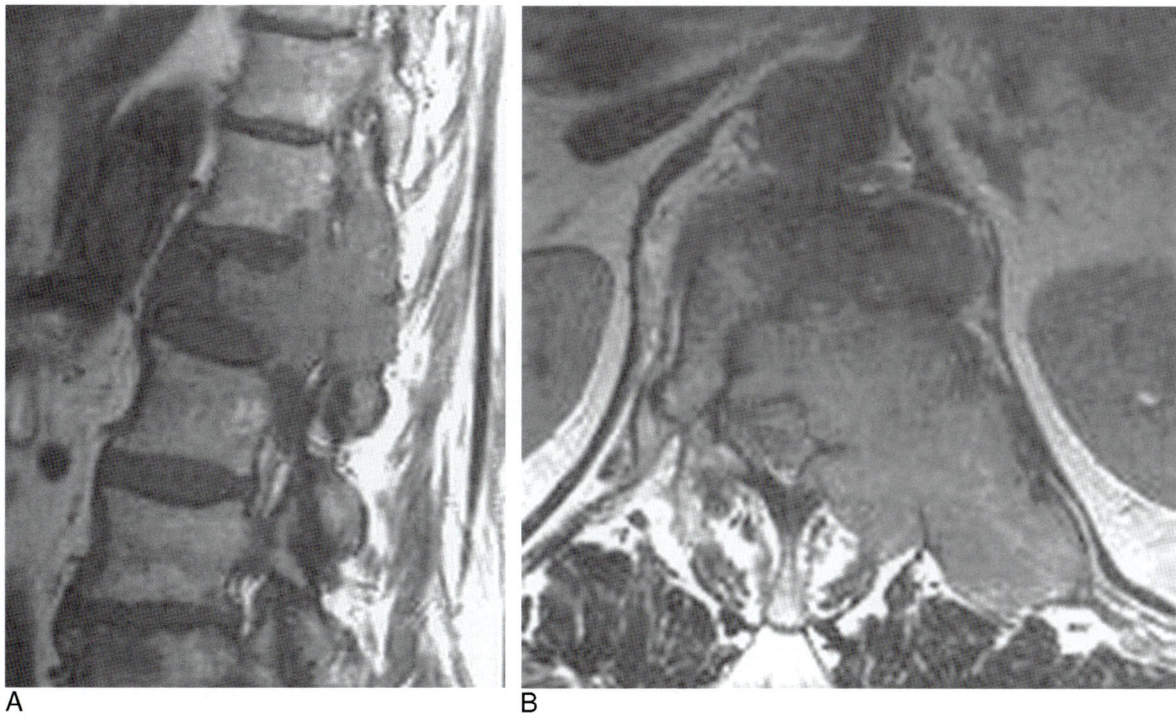

A   B

■ **FIGURE 91-26** Solitary plasmacytoma of bone with involvement of the first lumbar vertebral body. Sagittal T1-weighted spin-echo MR image (**A**) shows the hypointense tumor, which infiltrates the whole vertebral body and yields additionally a large soft tissue component. Axial T1-weighted turbo spin-echo MR image (**B**) shows the extent within the vertebral arch, paravertebral muscles, and the spinal canal. No other abnormal areas could be found on whole-body MRI.

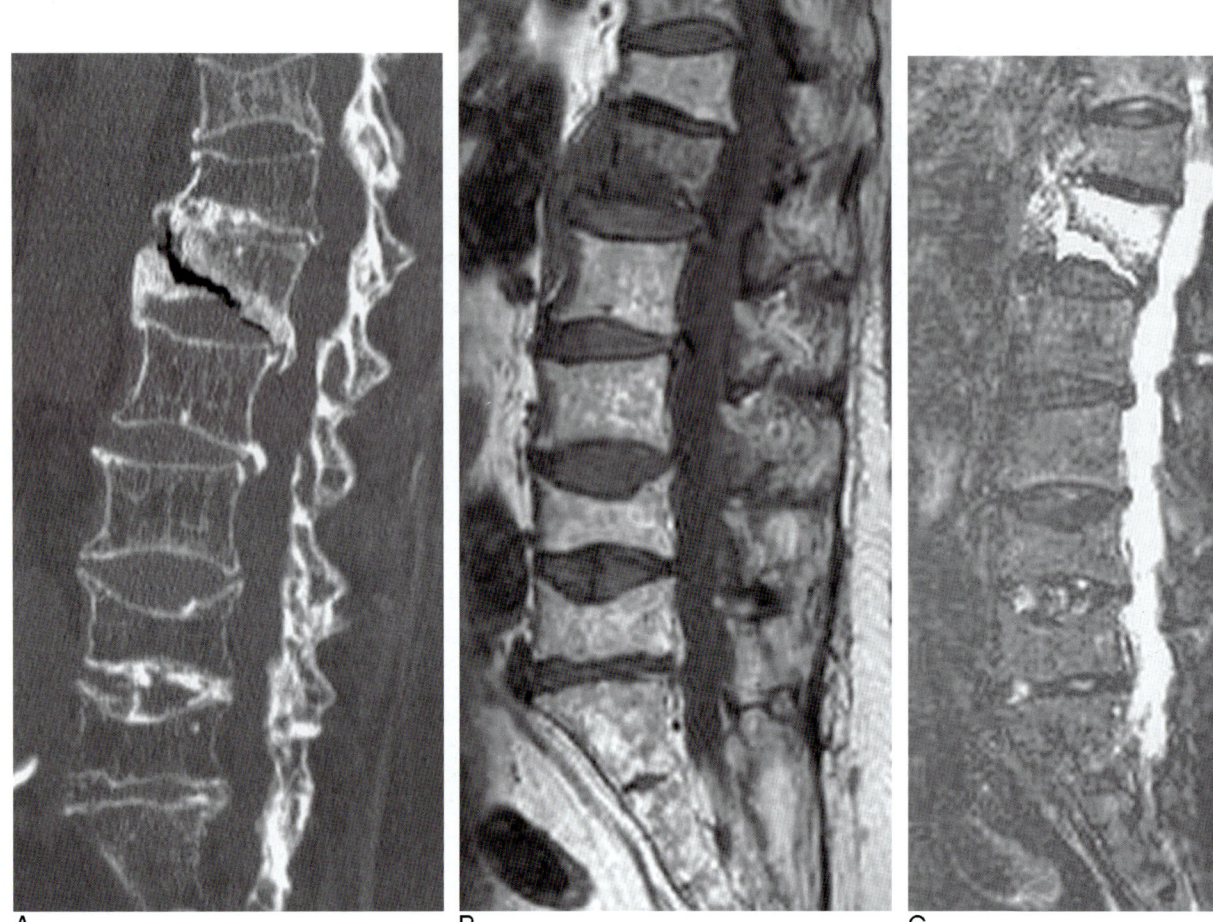

A   B   C

■ **FIGURE 91-27** A female patient presented with severe osteoporosis and multiple myeloma and pain at the upper lumbar spine. **A,** Sagittal reconstruction of the spine shows multiple end-plate fractures. The first lumbar vertebral body demonstrates an intravertebral vacuum phenomenon that extends into the disc space. This sign is indicative of a benign fracture. **B,** T1-weighted spin-echo MR image shows hypointense signal in the first lumbar vertebral body. **C,** STIR MR image shows strong hyperintense signal indicative of an acute fracture with edema. The fracture cleft is filled with fluid, which is also a sign of an osteoporotic fracture.

Vertebral fractures in patients with multiple myeloma may also be related to a combination of osteoporosis and tumor at the same time. Diffuse osteoporosis can be the result of the age of the patient, cortisone therapy, and/or the result of tumor-induced osteoclast activity. Interstitial tumor growth may be minimal and is hard to detect on MR images.

SYNOPSIS OF TREATMENT OPTIONS

Medical Treatment

Because of the complex situation and great variety in aggressiveness of the disease, management of patients with myeloma needs an interdisciplinary approach. At an initial stage without any detectable lesions patients can be followed according to a "watch and wait" consensus, because in this stage chemotherapy was found not to result in a prolonged time of survival. The treatment with bisphosphonates resulted in a reduced incidence of fractures and an increased quality of life.[28] The use of high-dose chemotherapy followed by autologous or a combined autologous and allogenic stem cell transplantation in patients with Durie and Salmon stage II and III disease has resulted in a significantly longer survival time compared with the classic Alexanian scheme with melphalan and prednisone.[29] In advanced stages, treatment of complications (e.g., renal insufficiency, anemia) and pain with medication and irradiation is important.

Surgical Treatment

Unstable pathologic fractures at the extremities and the spine are usually stabilized operatively with compound osteosynthesis or endoprosthesis. Those methods usually allow early mobilization.

Percutaneous vertebroplasty is one of the most promising new interventional procedures for relieving or reducing painful vertebra, with the injection of surgical polymethylmethacrylate or cement into vertebral bodies

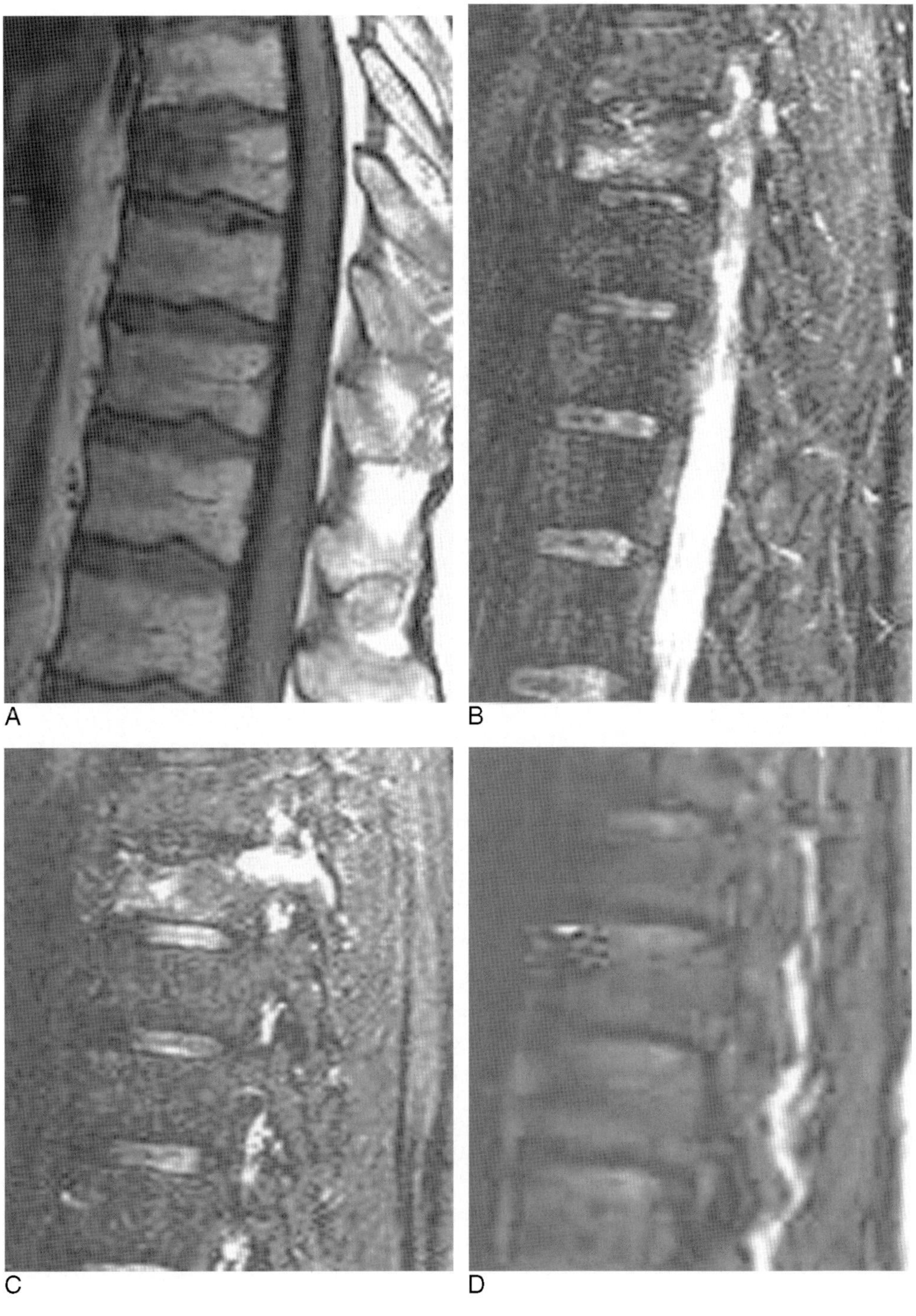

■ **FIGURE 91-28** Male patient with multiple myeloma who experienced an acute fracture in the T7 vertebral body while working in the garden. **A,** T1-weighted spin-echo MR image showed a focal zone of hypointensity in the anterior parts corresponding to hyperintensity in the STIR image in **B. C,** In the pedicles, on both sides, hyperintensity could be noted on a STIR MR image. The differential diagnosis is an acute osteoporotic fracture with edema extending in the pedicles or a pathologic fracture due to myeloma. **D,** Diffusion-weighted steady-state free precession (SSFP) imaging can help in those problematic cases showing isointense to hypointense signal in the affected areas consistent with edema. Tumor would show hyperintense signal.

in which bone is destructed or resorbed (Fig. 91-29). This imaged-guided technique, originally used to treat vertebral hemangioma, has more recently been used to treat metastases, osteoporotic compression fractures, and myeloma. The technique is especially useful in patients with multiple myeloma because fractures secondary to osteoporosis and myeloma-induced osteolysis are common and cause severe morbidity.

Percutaneous vertebroplasty is useful in patients with acute or subacute fractures who are not eligible for surgery and whose pain is not relieved by conservative treatment. Healed fractures without bone marrow edema at MRI are usually not an indication for percutaneous vertebroplasty, since pain in those patients mostly derives from other causes, such as muscle tension and osteochondrosis. About 30% of osteoporotic fractures show an intravertebral cleft filled with fluid or gas indicating motion between the opposing surfaces of the vertebral fracture cleft.[30] Placing cement into the cleft can reduce pain significantly, presumably from immobilizing those two fracture segments.[31] Patient selection is of utmost importance. Physical examination, including neurologic examination, should be performed in any patient to localize his or her pain. Any

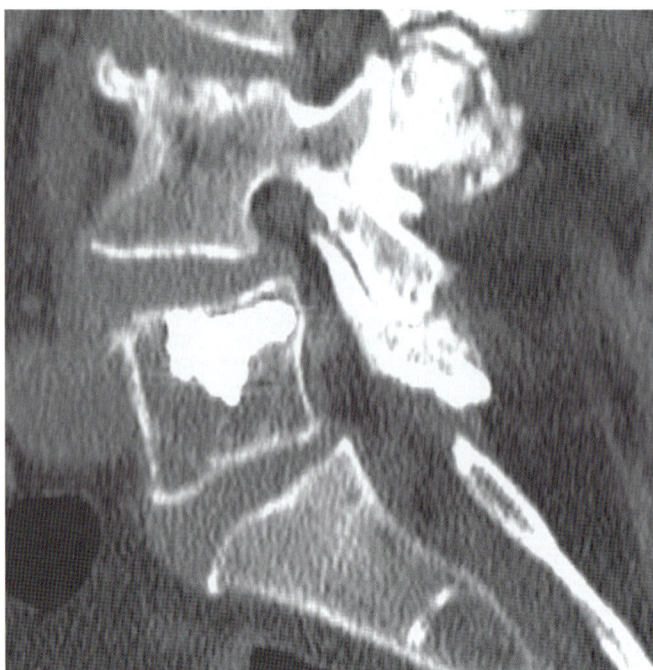

■ **FIGURE 91-29** Status post vertebroplasty at the L5 vertebral body in a patient with osteolyses due to multiple myeloma. CT-guided vertebroplasty is a quick and effective treatment of painful vertebral fractures and large osteolyses in patients with multiple myeloma.

discrepancy between the fracture site and the level of pain should be ruled out.

Another indication is extremely painful (requiring high doses of analgetic drugs) osteolysis or osteolysis at risk for fracture. The final treatment approach should be the result of a consensus between treating physician, spinal surgeon, and radiologist. Large tumor infiltrations can be pretreated by radiofrequency ablation before filling in the cement. Post-vertebroplasty radiotherapy can be added. Contraindications for vertebroplasty are presence of a marked defect in the posterior part of the vertebral body and soft tissue masses in the epidural space, owing to the risk of cement extrusion into the spinal canal resulting in spinal cord compression.

Evaluation of Relapse/Response to Therapy

According to the European bone marrow transplantation and International Bone marrow transplantation registry criteria, "Progressive disease, partial and complete response" is defined as follows[32]: *Progressive disease* requires the reappearance of serum and/or urine paraprotein, or an increase of 25% or more from the previous control, or more than 25% increased bone marrow plasma cell infiltration, or definite increase in size of osteolyses or soft tissue manifestations, or the development of new skeletal lesions. The development of new compression fractures is not a criterion for progressive disease. The definition of *partial response* to therapy requires all of the following: greater than or equal to 50% reduction

in serum paraprotein levels, 50% to 89% decrease of Bence Jones proteinuria, a 50% reduction in bone marrow plasma cell infiltration, greater than or equal to 50% reduction in the size of soft tissue plasmacytomas, and no increase in size or number of lytic bone lesions. *Complete response* requires all of the following: complete disappearance of serum and or urine monoclonal gammopathy with bone marrow plasma cell infiltration less than 5% for 2 months, no increase in size or number of lytic lesions, and disappearance of soft tissue plasmacytomas. Development of compression fractures does not exclude complete response.

Change of volume of plasmacytoma in soft tissues and change in size or number of lesions can be assessed most reliably by cross-sectional imaging, such as CT or MRI. Change in signal intensities on MR and enhancement patterns are only of limited value in assessing response to treatment.[33] Return of normal signal intensity of bone marrow signal or disappearance of peripheral or homogeneous enhancement of lesions has been described but is not seen in all patients with complete remission. Patients with partial response to therapy may show an overall decrease of abnormalities in bone marrow, with an increase in signal on T1-weighted spin-echo images due to an increase of fat cells. Carlson and colleagues calculated a tumor mass index in patients with focal disease at the time of initial diagnosis and after Alexanian I chemotherapy. The tumor mass index showed correlation with the extent of β_2-microglobulin. Patients with a low tumor mass at primary diagnosis had a longer survival time. The MRI tumor mass index correlated significantly with clinical response to therapy (no response, stable disease, progressive disease). In patients with diffuse infiltration, who responded to therapy, infiltrates were replaced by fatty marrow. This started in the extremities and progressed toward the axial skeleton. In patients not responding well to therapy, focal lesions changed into diffuse infiltrates mainly affecting the spine and the pelvis.[34]

Early results in small patient cohorts indicate that FDG PET might be a tool in monitoring relapse or response to therapy.[22,23] Negative PET scans reliably predicted stable MGUS. The development of new FDG-positive sites in the skeleton after therapy indicated relapse and poor prognosis.[22] Decreased tracer uptake has been reported in patients with good response.

SUGGESTED READINGS

Bartl R. Morphology of multiple myeloma. In Malpas JS, et al. Myeloma, Biology and Management, 2nd ed. Oxford, Oxford University Press, 1998, pp 89-121.

Durie B, et al. Myeloma management guidelines: a consensus report from the Scientific Advisors of the International Myeloma Foundation. Hematol J 2003; 4:379-398.

Baur A, Stäbler A, Nagel D, et al. MRI as a supplement for the clinical staging system of Durie and Salmon? Cancer 2002; 15:1334-1345.

REFERENCES

1. Durie BGM. The epidemiology of multiple myeloma. Semin Hematol 2001; 38:1-5.
2. Durie BGM, Salmon SE. Myeloma management guidelines: a consensus report from the Scientific Advisors of the International Myeloma Foundation. Hematol J 2003; 4:379-398.
3. Durie BGM, Salmon SE. A clinical staging system for multiple myeloma: correlation of measured myeloma cell mass with presenting clinical features, response to treatment and survival. Cancer 1975; 36:842-854.
4. Baur A, Stäbler A, Bartl R, et al. Infiltration pattern of plasmacytoma in MRI. Fortschr Röntgenstr 1996; 164:457-463.
5. Tertti R, Alanen A, Remes K. The value of MRI in screening myeloma lesions of the lumbar spine. Br J Haematol 1995; 9:658-660.
6. Van de Berg BC, Lecouvert F, Michaux L, et al. Stage I multiple myeloma: value of MRI of the bone marrow in the determination of the prognosis. Radiology 1996; 201:243-246.
7. Dimopoulos MA, Moulopoulos A, Smith TL, et al. Risk of disease progression in asymptomatic multiple myeloma. Am J Med 1993; 94:57-61.
8. Baur A, Stabler A, Nagel D, et al. Magnetic resonance imaging as a supplement for the clinical staging system of Durie and Salmon. Cancer 2002; 95:1334-1345.
9. Lecouvet F, Malghem J, Maldague B, et al. Skeletal survey in advanced multiple myeloma: radiographic versus MRI survey. Br J Haematol 1999; 106:35-39.
10. Mahnken AH, Wildberger JE, Gehbauer G. Multidetector CT of the spine in multiple myeloma: comparison with MR imaging and radiography. AJR Am J Roentgenol 2002; 178:1429-1436.
11. Baur-Melnyr A, Buhmann S, Becker C, et al. Whole-body-MRI versus whole-body-MDCT for the staging of patients with multiple myeloma. AJR 2007, accepted for publications.
12. Hess T, Egerer G, Kasper B, et al. Atypical manifestations of multiple myeloma: radiological appearance. Eur J Radiol 2006; 56:280-285.
13. Hall FM, Gore SM. Osteosclerotic myeloma variants. Skeletal Radiol 1988; 17:101-105.
14. Baur A, Stäbler A, Steinborn M, et al. MRI in plasmacytoma: value of different sequences in diffuse and focal infiltration patterns. Fortschr Röntgenstr 1998; 168:323-329.
15. Baur A, Stäbler A, Bartl R, et al. MRI gadolinium enhancement of bone marrow: age related changes in normals and in diffuse neoplastic infiltration. Skeletal Radiol 1997; 26:414-418.
16. Baur A, Bartl R, Pellengahr C, et al. Neovascularization of bone marrow in patients with diffuse multiple myeloma: a correlative study of MR-imaging and histopathologic findings. Cancer 2004; 101:2599-2604.
17. Bataille R, Durie BGM, Grenier J, Sany J: Prognostic factors and staging in multiple myeloma: a reappraisal. J Clin Oncol 1986; 4:80-87.
18. Weber DM, Dimopoulos MA, Moulopoulos LA, et al. Prognostic features of asymptomatic multiple myeloma. Br J Haematol 1997; 97:810-814.
19. Kusumoto S, Jinnai I, Itoh K, et al. MRI patterns in patients with multiple myeloma. Br J Haematol 1997; 99:649-655.
20. Woolfenden JM, Pitt MJ, Durie BGM, Moon TE. Comparison of bone scintigraphy and radiology in multiple myeloma. Radiology 1980; 134:723-728.
21. Schirrmeister H, Bommer M, Buck AK, et al. Initial results in the assessment of multiple myeloma using F18-FDG PET. Eur J Nucl Med Mol 2002; 29:361-366.
22. Durie BGM, Waxman AD, D'Agnolo A, Williams CM. Whole body F18-FDG PET identifies high risk myeloma. J Nucl Med 2002; 43:1457-1463.
23. Bredella MA, Steinbach L, Caputo G, et al. Value of FDG PET in the assessment of patients with multiple myeloma. AJR Am J Roentgenol 2005; 184:1199-1204.
24. Van de Berg BC, Lecouvet FE, Michaux L, et al. Nonmyelomatous monoclonal gammopathy: correlation of bone marrow MR images with laboratory findings and spontaneous clinical outcome. Radiology 1997; 202:247-251.
25. Dimopoulos MA, Moulopoulos LA, Maniatis A, Alexanian R. Solitary plasmacytoma of bone and asymptomatic multiple myeloma. Blood 2000; 96:2037-2044.
26. Cuenod CA, Laredo JD, Chevret S, et al. Acute vertebral collapse due to osteoporosis or malignancy: appearance on unenhanced and gadolinium enhanced MR images. Radiology 1996; 199:541-549.
27. Baur A, Stäbler A, Brüning R, et al. Diffusion-weighted MR Imaging of bone marrow: differentiation of benign versus pathologic vertebral compression fractures. Radiology 1998; 207:349-356.
28. Jantunen E. Bisphosphonates in multiple myeloma: current status, future perspectives. Br J Haematol 1996; 93:501-506.
29. Desikan R, Barlogie B, Sawyer J, et al. Results of high-dose therapy for 1000 patients with multiple myeloma: durable complete remission and superior survival in the absence of chromosome 13 abnormalities. Blood 2000; 95:4008-4010.
30. Baur A, Stäbler A, Arbogast S, et al. The fluid sign in acute osteoporotic and neoplastic vertebral compression fractures. Radiology 2002; 225:730-735.
31. Peh WCG, Gelbart MS, Gilula LA, Peck DD. Percutaneous vertebroplasty: treatment of painful vertebral compression fractures with intraosseous vacuum phenomena. AJR Am J Roentgenol 2003; 180:1411-1417.
32. Bladé J, Samson D, Reece D, et al. Criteria for evaluating disease response and progression in patients with multiple myeloma treated by high dose therapy and haematopoietic stem cell transplantation. Br J Haematol 1998; 102:1115-1123.
33. Rahmouni A, Divine M, Mathieu D, et al. MR appearance of multiple myeloma of the spine before and after treatment. AJR Am J Roentgenol 1993; 16:1053-1057.
34. Carlson K, Aström G, Nyman R, et al. MR imaging of multiple myeloma in tumour mass measurement at diagnosis and during treatment. Acta Radiol 1995; 36:9-14.

92

Tumor-like Lesions of Bone

A. Mark Davies

There is a large spectrum of bone conditions that can have similar imaging appearances to tumors. These can be broadly classified into two categories. First are the space-occupying lesions in bone that are macroscopic in appearance but non-neoplastic in nature. These include cystic lesions such as simple bone cyst (SBC) and aneurysmal bone cyst (ABC), fibrous lesions such as nonossifying fibroma and fibrous dysplasia, as well as Langerhans cell histiocytosis. The second category includes all those "nontumorous" disorders that may be mistaken for a bone tumor. What constitutes a tumor mimic depends very much on the expertise of the individual reviewing the imaging. The majority of these other cases can be classified as normal variants and metabolic, post-traumatic, and inflammatory conditions.

CYSTIC LESIONS

Simple Bone Cyst

The simple bone cyst (SBC), otherwise known as a solitary bone cyst or a unicameral bone cyst, is a common tumor-like osseous lesion that may present as an incidental finding or more frequently as a pathologic fracture. The annual prevalence of SBC has been reported to be approximately 0.30 per 100,000 population.[1] It is a true intraosseous cyst with a fluid-filled cavity lined by a thin layer of mesothelial-like cells. Most cases present in the first and second decades, with only 15% cases occurring later. There is a male preponderance, with 55% of cases arising in the proximal humeral metaphysis and 25% in the proximal femoral metaphysis (Fig. 92-1). Other sites, with exception of the anterior calcaneus, are uncommon (Fig. 92-2). Radiographically, SBC appears as a central, well-defined, mildly expansile, lytic lesion arising within a metaphysis usually bordering an open growth plate. A typical feature in the presence of a fracture is the "fallen fragment sign" in which a small segment of fractured cortex is seen to settle into the dependent part of the cyst seen in approximately 20% of cases (see Fig. 92-1). This sign is characteristic but, as with many signs in imaging, not pathognomonic because it may be seen in any bone

lesion with a fracture associated with a prominent cystic component. MRI will show the fluid nature of the lesions that are slightly hypointense on T1-weighted MR images and hyperintense on T2-weighted MR images (see Fig. 92-2). Debris and a solitary fluid-fluid level may be seen in the presence of a fracture due to internal hemorrhage. The cyst may heal after fracture alone. Other treatments advocated over the years include injecting corticosteroids and/or Ethibloc and curettage with or without bone grafting. In time the cyst will grow away from the physis and appear to migrate down the diaphysis as healthy new bone is laid down in the metaphysis. The precise appearance of the cyst on follow-up radiographs depends on the nature of the initial treatment. It is not unusual, particularly in active young boys, to see a cycle of fracture, partial consolidation, and re-fracture occurring over a period of several years as the SBC migrates down the shaft of the long bone that is frequently associated with a bowing deformity.

Aneurysmal Bone Cyst

Aneurysmal bone cyst (ABC) is a benign cystic lesion of bone composed of cystic blood-filled spaces divided by connective tissue septa containing giant cells, fibroblasts, and reactive woven bone. The cause of the lesion has long been debated. To date it has been generally considered a tumor-like lesion, possibly arising due to local hemodynamic problems or perhaps in response to trauma. Interestingly, theories are now going full circle, with increasing recent evidence that ABC is a true neoplasm and may therefore be classified in the future with the other true tumors of bone covered in Chapter 90. ABC constitutes approximately 4% of tumors and tumor-like lesions of bone, with 80% occurring in individuals younger than the age of 20 years. It has a similar annual prevalence to SBC of approximately 0.32 cases per 100,000 population.[2] Seventy percent arise de novo in bone, and 30% occur in association with other osseous tumors (secondary ABC), including giant cell tumor, chondroblastoma, osteoblastoma, and, less commonly, chondromyxoid fibroma and fibrous dysplasia (Fig. 92-3). ABC-like areas may be seen

KEY POINTS

- One third of ABCs arise in association with another bone lesion (e.g., giant cell tumor and chondroblastoma).
- Fluid-fluid levels are a typical MRI feature of ABCs but can be seen in many other osseous conditions (e.g., telangiectatic osteosarcoma, giant cell tumor, and brown tumor).
- Intraosseous ganglion may occur at any age but has a predilection for the fourth and fifth decades. It may be seen with or without degenerative joint disease.
- Fibrous cortical defect is a very common tumor-like lesion in children and young adults and is of little or no clinical significance.
- Thirty percent of cases of fibrous dysplasia are polyostotic with a tendency toward a monomelic or hemimelic distribution.
- Osteofibrous dysplasia is a benign lesion with a predilection preskeletal fusion of the anterior tibia. It may be a precursor of adamantinoma or the benign end of a spectrum of disease with adamantinoma at the malignant end.
- The localized form of Langerhans cell histiocytosis (eosinophilic granuloma) is a benign self-limiting disease that may mimic infection and Ewing's sarcoma.
- Brown tumor of hyperparathyroidism may be indistinguishable from a giant cell tumor on imaging and histologic examination.
- Fatigue-type stress fractures mimic osteomyelitis and Ewing's sarcoma but do not show cortical destruction or a soft tissue mass.

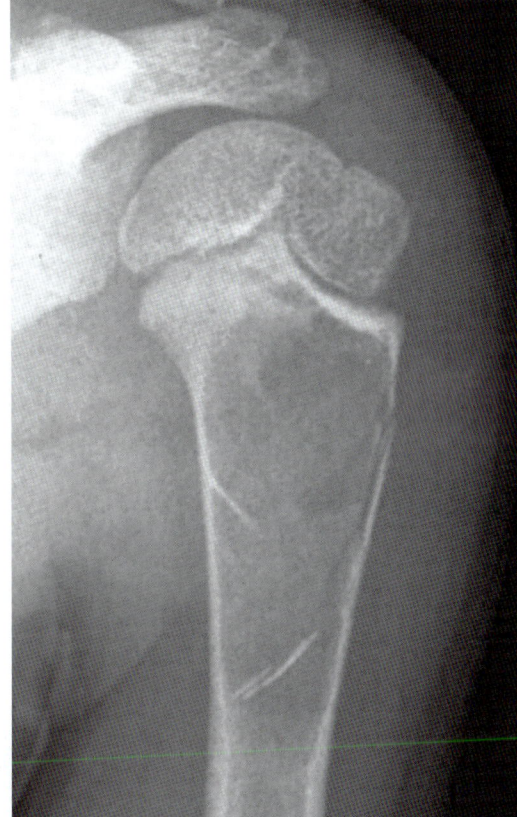

■ **FIGURE 92-1** Simple bone cyst. Anteroposterior radiograph shows a well-defined lytic lesion in the proximal humeral diaphysis with a "fallen fragment" sign.

in malignant bone tumors, notably telangiectatic osteosarcoma. It is therefore important to review all the imaging to see if there is any evidence of an antecedent bone lesion. Common sites of involvement include the long bones (50%) and posterior vertebral arch (20%). Eighty-five percent of cases arise within medullary bone, and 15% occur in a cortical or subperiosteal location.[2] The predominant radiographic features are those of a lytic, eccentric, multiseptated, markedly expansile lesion arising in the metaphysis of the long bone in a child or young adult (Fig. 92-4). There may be a thin-ridged or smooth peripheral shell of periosteal new bone formation around the margins of the lesion but, if the lesion is in a particularly active phase of growth, the peripheral shell may be absent, with marginal buttresses simulating Codman angles to give the lesion the overall appearance of a more aggressive, potentially malignant process (Fig. 92-5). Subperiosteal ABC can appear as a blowout surface lesion of bone and is more frequently diaphyseal in location (Fig. 92-6). The multicystic nature of ABC is confirmed with either CT or MRI. Fluid-fluid levels can frequently be visualized due to the layering out of blood products within the individual cysts (see Fig. 92-5B). The diagnostic value of identifying fluid-fluid levels has been debated in the literature. Studies have shown that the most common cause of a bone lesion in child showing multiple fluid-fluid levels is an ABC[3] and that lesions comprising a proportion greater than two thirds of fluid-fluid levels were

more likely to be a primary or secondary ABC rather than a malignancy.[4] However, a recent report correctly identifies the nonspecific nature of this sign when looking at a large series of both bone and soft tissue tumors.[5] Isolated cases of malignant transformation have been reported in ABC,[6] but the cynical observer might be tempted to suggest that these were ABC-like areas within an existing sarcoma (e.g., telangiectatic osteosarcoma) that took some time to manifest the true malignant nature of the underlying lesion. For the sake of completeness it should be noted that there are two further rare variants of ABC: the solid ABC and the soft tissue ABC, which are rarely diagnosed before biopsy.

Epidermal Inclusion Cyst

Epidermal inclusion cysts, otherwise known as implantation dermoid cysts, typically involve the distal phalanges of the hand and, to a lesser extent, the foot. They are seen in the skeletally mature and are attributed to penetrating injuries with intraosseous inoculation of skin epithelium. Histologically, the lesions are lined with squamous epithelium and contain keratin debris. The radiographic appearances are those of a well-defined, rounded lytic lesion with a sclerotic border arising within the terminal phalanx (Fig. 92-7). The lesion may or may not show expansion and is typically relatively asymptomatic unless presenting as a pathologic fracture. Similar appearances

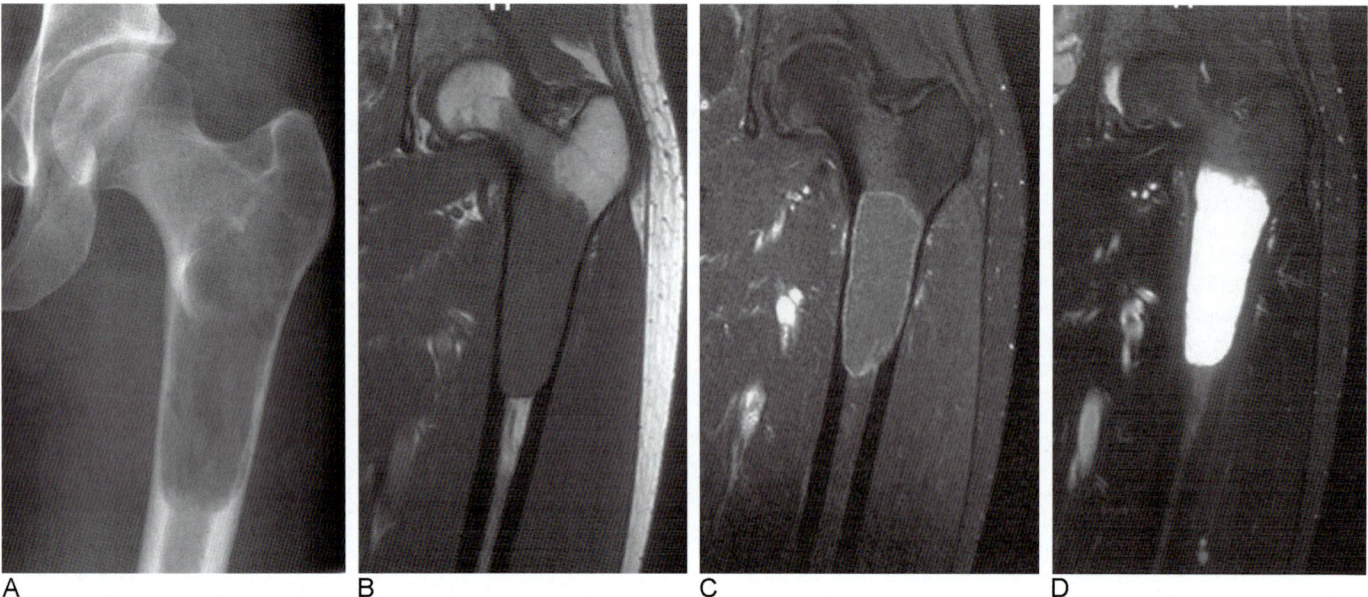

■ **FIGURE 92-2** Simple bone cyst in an adult. Anteroposterior radiograph (**A**) and coronal T1-weighted (**B**), coronal T1-weighted, fat-suppressed contrast-enhanced (**C**), and coronal STIR (**D**) MR images show a well-defined homogeneous lesion in the proximal femoral diaphysis with minor rim enhancement.

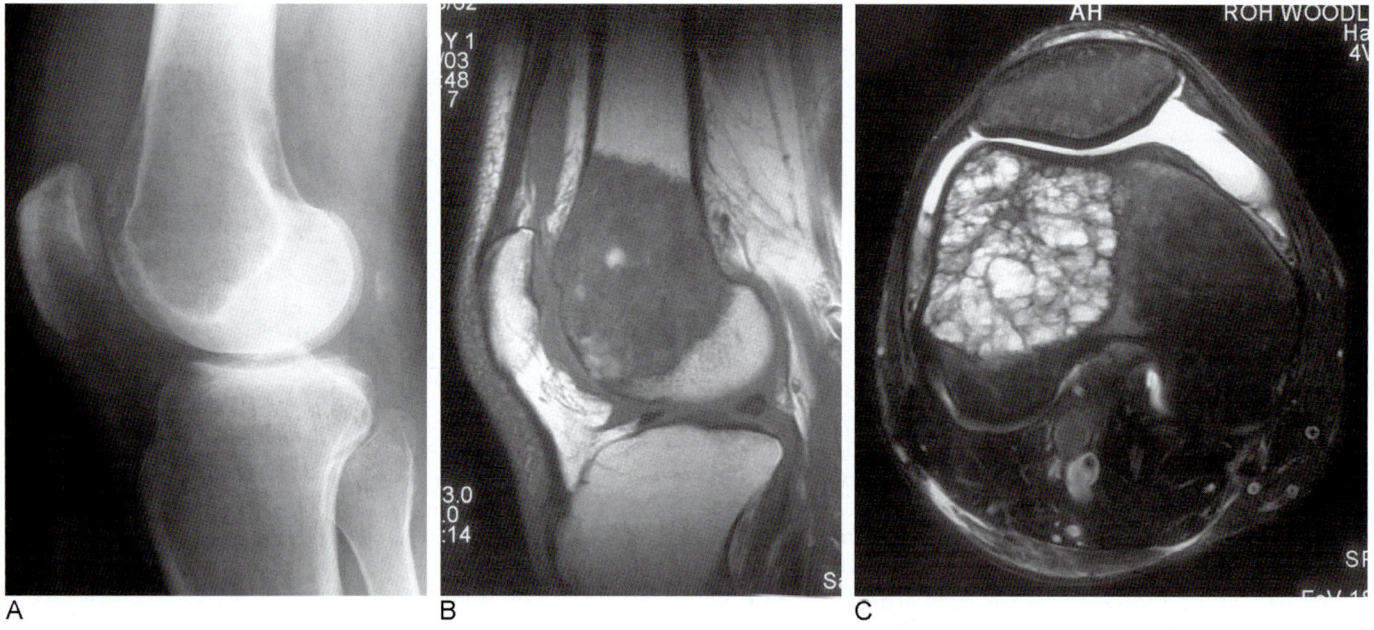

■ **FIGURE 92-3** Giant cell tumor with secondary aneurysmal bone cyst formation in a 42-year-old man. (**A**) Lateral radiograph shows typical features of a giant cell tumor. This would be an unusual age at which an aneurysmal bone cyst would present. Sagittal T1-weighted (**B**) and axial T2-weighted fat-suppressed (**C**) MR images show evidence of hemorrhage with multiple small cystic spaces containing fluid-fluid levels.

at this site may be seen with a glomus tumor, but this entity is usually painful and tender. Developmental epidermal cysts, as opposed to post-traumatic ones, typically arise in the skull vault of children.

Intraosseous Ganglion

Intraosseous ganglia are benign non-neoplastic bone lesions that are histologically similar to their soft tissue counterparts. They consist of a cavity or cavities of vary-ing size, without an epithelial or synovial lining, containing mucoid viscous material. Originally said to be rare they are increasingly recognized. Confusing nomenclature has undoubtedly contributed to the perception that they are uncommon. One article published more than 25 years ago identifies no fewer than 12 different names.[7] Today, the terms *intraosseous ganglion, subchondral cyst,* or *geode* are often applied interchangeably, although the latter two are more frequently used to describe juxta-articular lesions associated with degenerative or inflammatory joint

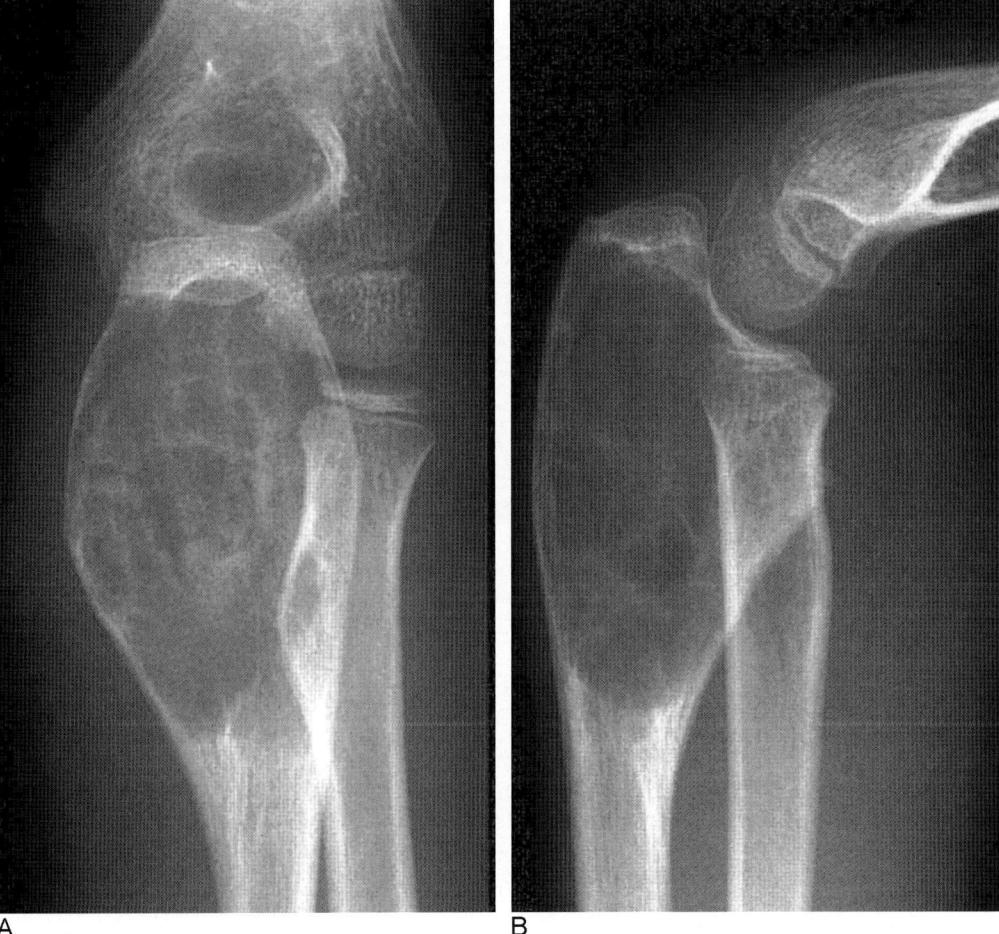

■ **FIGURE 92-4** Aneurysmal bone cyst. Anteroposterior (**A**) and lateral (**B**) radiographs show a central, mildly trabeculated, expansile lesion in the proximal ulna.

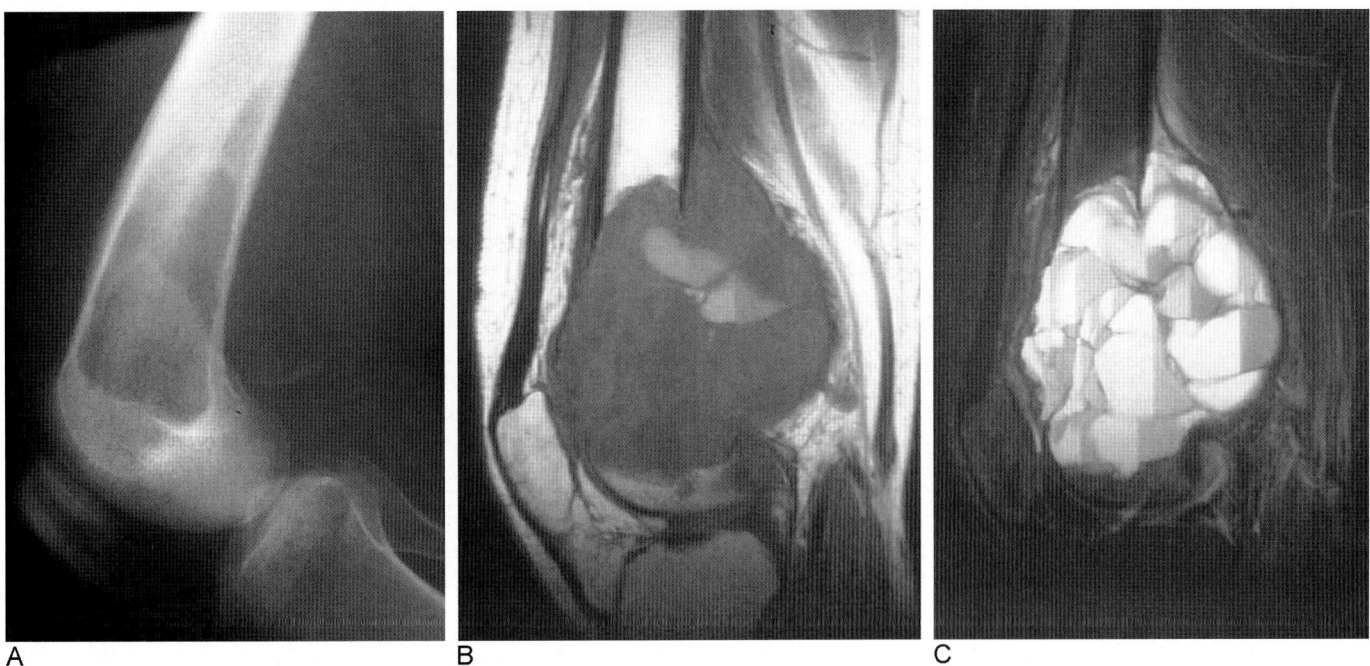

■ **FIGURE 92-5** Aneurysmal bone cyst. Lateral radiograph (**A**) and sagittal T1-weighted (**B**) and sagittal STIR (**C**) MR images show a lytic lesion in the distal femoral metadiaphysis extending posteriorly. Only the distal portion of a shell is visible, mimicking a Codman-Angle. The MR images show evidence of hemorrhage and multiple dependent fluid-fluid levels.

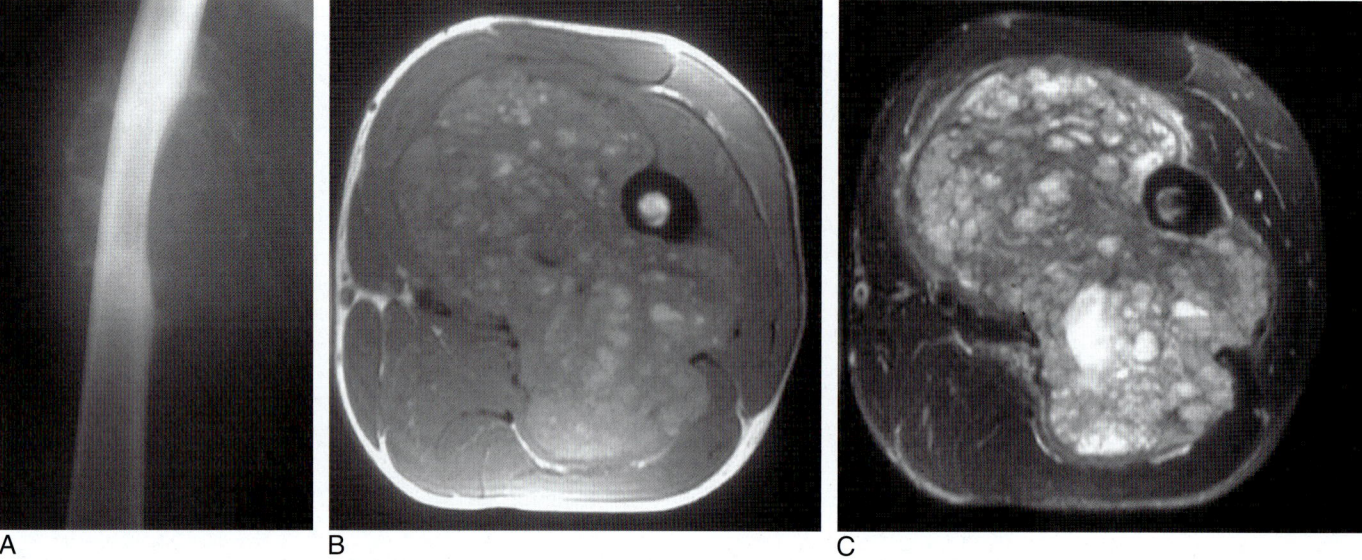

■ **FIGURE 92-6** Subperiosteal aneurysmal bone cyst. Lateral radiograph (**A**) and axial T1-weighted (**B**) and axial T2-weighted, fat-suppressed (**C**) MR images show a blowout surface lesion arising on the diaphysis of the femur containing multiple small cystic spaces. There is erosion of the underlying cortex with minor marrow edema.

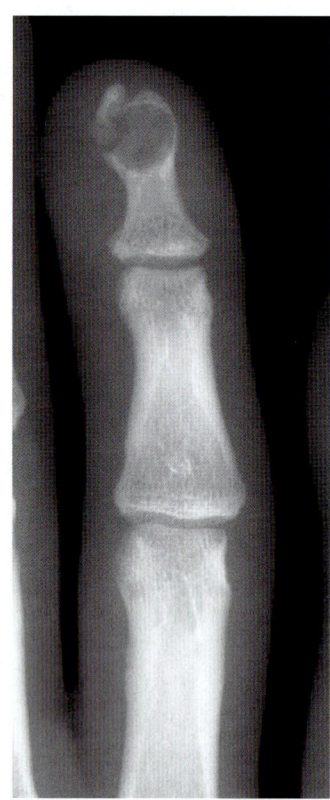

■ **FIGURE 92-7** Epidermal inclusion cyst. Posteroanterior radiograph shows a fracture through a well-defined, rounded, lytic lesion in the terminal phalanx of a finger.

disease. The etiology remains unknown. Several theories have been postulated to explain the pathogenesis. These include a primary or idiopathic form arising de novo in bone possibly due to intramedullary metaplasia followed by mucoid degeneration or secondary spread of a synovial cyst or intrusion of synovial fluid from an adjacent joint into the bone.

Intraosseous ganglia occur in the skeletally mature individual at all ages, with the peak incidence in the fourth and fifth decades. There is a predilection for the long bones of the lower limb, although the carpal bones are other well-recognized sites. The radiographic appearances are those of well-defined, lytic, oval or round, unilocular or multilocular lesions located in the epiphysis or metaphysis with or without cortical expansion and soft tissue extension (Fig. 92-8).[8] Periosteal new bone formation is not a feature. The majority of intraosseous ganglia are small, between 1 and 2 cm in diameter, with lesions over 5 cm uncommon. Large lesions may be mistaken as giant cell tumor, chondroma, and, in the older patient, chondrosarcoma, metastasis, and plasmacytoma. A diagnostic feature occasionally seen, more clearly identified on CT, is gas within the cyst that is sometimes referred to as an intraosseous pneumatocyst. Although these lesions tend to behave in an indolent manner, increased activity on bone scintigraphy is frequently seen due to osteoclastic and osteoblastic activity in the surrounding bone. The lesions appear hypointense or isointense to muscle on T1-weighted MR images and hyperintense on T2-weighted and STIR images, reflecting the mucoid/cystic nature of the contents (see Fig. 92-8B and C). There is marginal or, less commonly, heterogeneous enhancement with gadolinium (see Fig. 92-8D). Although there is no epithelial or synovial lining there is a fibrous membrane of varying thickness, which is presumably the structure showing peripheral enhancement. The heterogeneous enhancement may be due to connective tissue in earlier lesions undergoing myxoid transformation. Surrounding marrow edema may be seen in approximately 50% of cases, suggesting extension of the lesion into surrounding marrow or trabecular microfractures secondary to expansion of the lesion. Fluid-fluid levels have also been described in intraosseous ganglia.

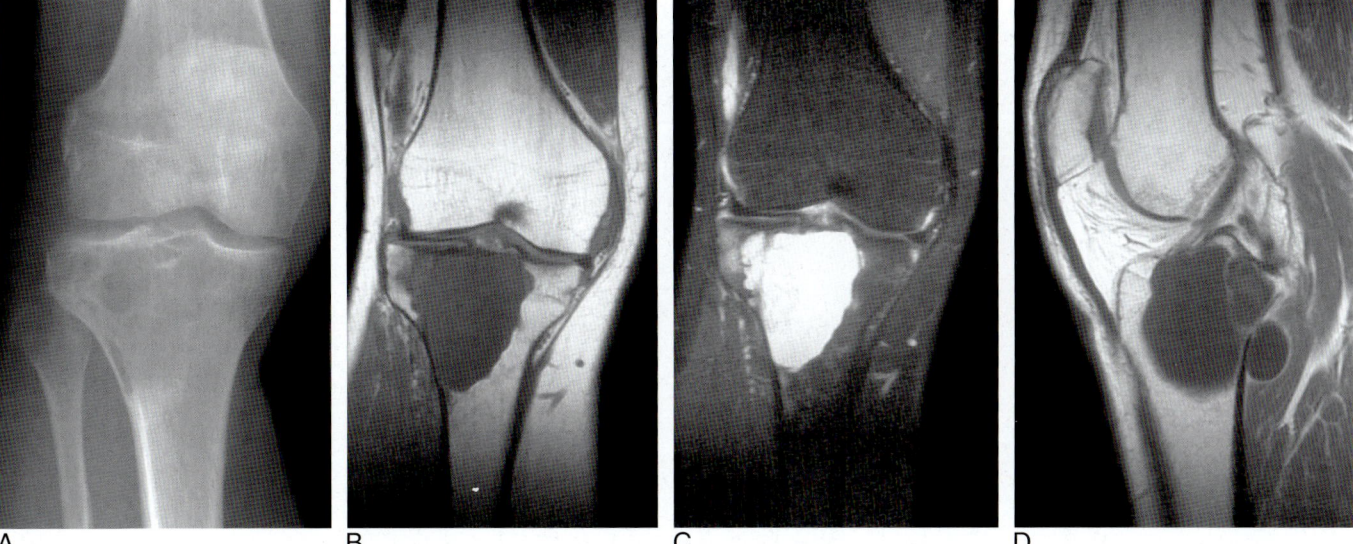

■ **FIGURE 92-8** Intraosseous ganglion. Anteroposterior radiograph (**A**) and coronal T1-weighted (**B**), coronal STIR (**C**), and sagittal T1-weighted, contrast-enhanced (**D**) MR images. The lytic lesion in the radiograph mimics a giant cell tumor or metastasis. The MR images show a relatively homogeneous lesion with minor rim enhancement. The soft tissue extension posteriorly evident on the sagittal image is not uncommon in this condition.

FIBROUS LESIONS

Benign tumor-like lesions of fibrous origin include fibrous cortical defect/nonossifying fibroma, fibrous dysplasia, osteofibrous dysplasia, and liposclerosing myxofibrous tumor. The first two conditions are relatively common and are frequently diagnosed as an incidental finding on radiographs obtained for other reasons.

Fibrous Cortical Defect/Nonossifying Fibroma

Fibrous cortical defect and nonossifying fibroma, also known in the older literature as fibroxanthoma, are histologically identical entities composed of storiform spindle cells with varying amounts of histiocytic cells and lipid-bearing xanthomatous cells. The only distinguishing features are their location and relative size. Small lesions (<15 mm in maximal length) confined to the cortex are generally called fibrous cortical defects, whereas larger lesions encroaching on the medulla are called nonossifying fibromas. These are lesions of childhood and adolescence, are more common in boys than girls, and tend to arise in the long bones of the lower limb, particularly around the knee. It is said that fibrous cortical defects may be seen in approximately one third of the normal population before skeletal fusion and can be multiple in less than 10% of cases. The radiographic appearances are usually diagnostic with a well-defined elliptical lytic lesion confined to the cortex of a long bone adjacent to a growth plate (Fig. 92-9). The long axis of the lesion is oriented with the long axis of the bone. Fibrous cortical defects are typically an incidental finding on radiographs and grow away from the growth plate with progressive skeletal maturation. Most will heal spontaneously to convert to normal bone or show healing with a sclerotic ghost of the original lytic defect (see Fig. 92-9B). Nonossifying

fibromas present as larger lesions, presumed to be due to persistent growth of a fibrous cortical defect. They also appear well-defined and eccentric, arising from a cortex but extend across the adjacent medullary cavity. The endosteal margin is typically sclerotic, and larger lesions may appear septated and/or trabeculated (Fig. 92-10). Matrix mineralization and periosteal new bone formation is not a feature, although they may be seen after pathologic fracture, which is a fairly common presenting feature of nonossifying fibroma. Lesions arising in small caliber bones may appear central. The lesions tend to appear as relatively low signal intensity on T1-weighted images and of variable signal intensity on T2-weighted images depending on the proportion of fibrous tissue (Fig. 92-11). Fibrous cortical defects do not require treatment. Nonossifying fibromas, if relatively small, may be followed up with serial radiographs to ensure no major growth. Larger lesions may require curettage with or without bone grafting and fracture fixation. Multiple nonossifying fibromas have been reported in association with neurofibromatosis.

Fibrous Dysplasia

Fibrous dysplasia is a benign fibro-osseous lesion of bone considered to be a developmental abnormality (i.e., a hamartomatous metaplasia). Histologically, there is replacement of the normal cancellous bone by abnormal fibrous tissue with varying amounts of immature woven bone. The lesions may be solitary (monostotic) or multifocal (polystotic), affecting one or more bones. The monostotic form accounts for approximately 70% of cases and typically affects the femur, notably the femoral neck, tibia, base of skull, and ribs (Fig. 92-12). The radiographic appearance reflects the relative amount of fibrous tissue to ossification. There is a spectrum from radiolucent, through the typical "ground glass," to heterogeneous with sclerotic areas (see Fig. 92-12). Skull base lesions tend to be at the sclerotic

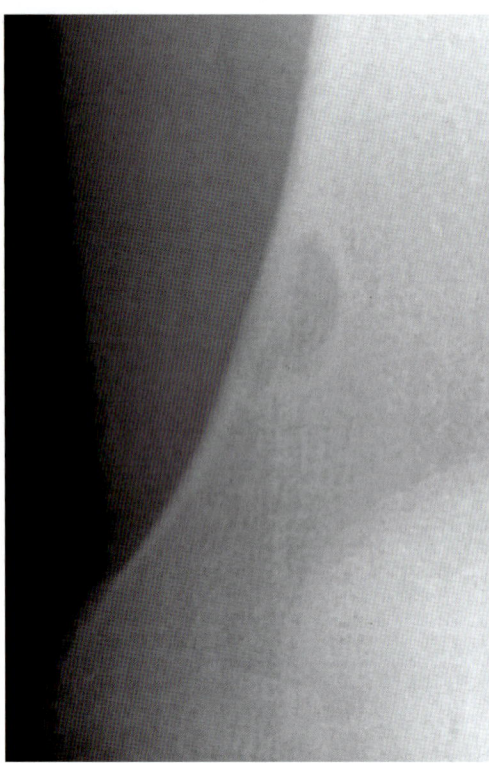
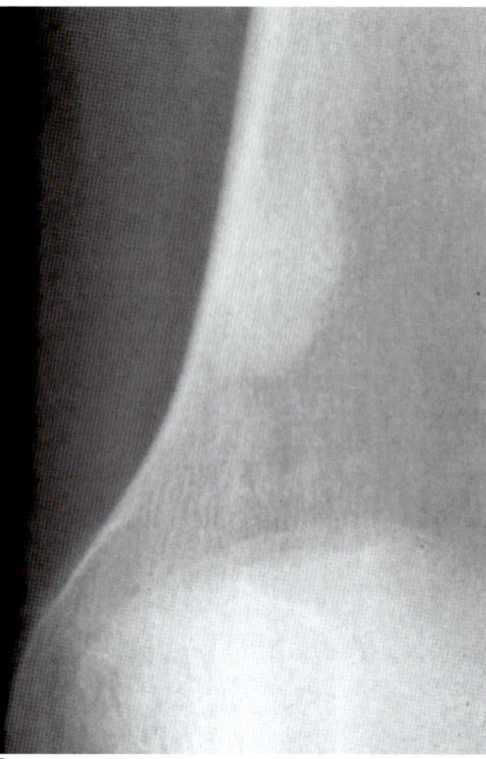

A   B

■ **FIGURE 92-9** Fibrous cortical defect. **A,** The initial anteroposterior radiograph shows a well-defined, oval lucency with a thin sclerotic border arising in the medial cortex of the distal femur. **B,** The follow-up radiograph obtained 7 years later shows the lesion to have healed with sclerosis.

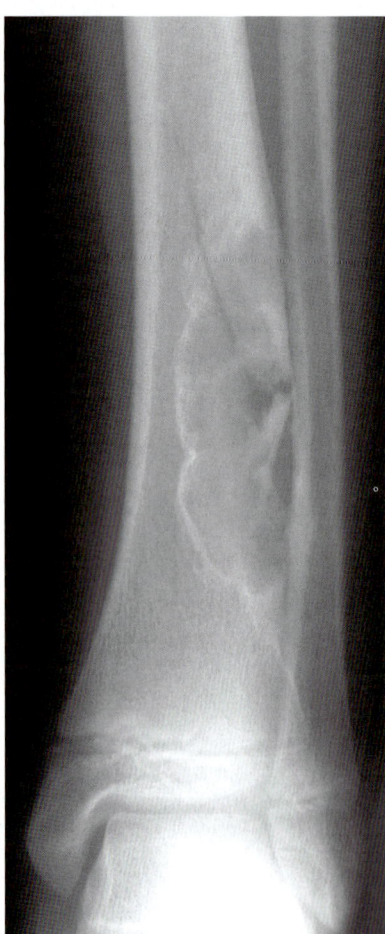

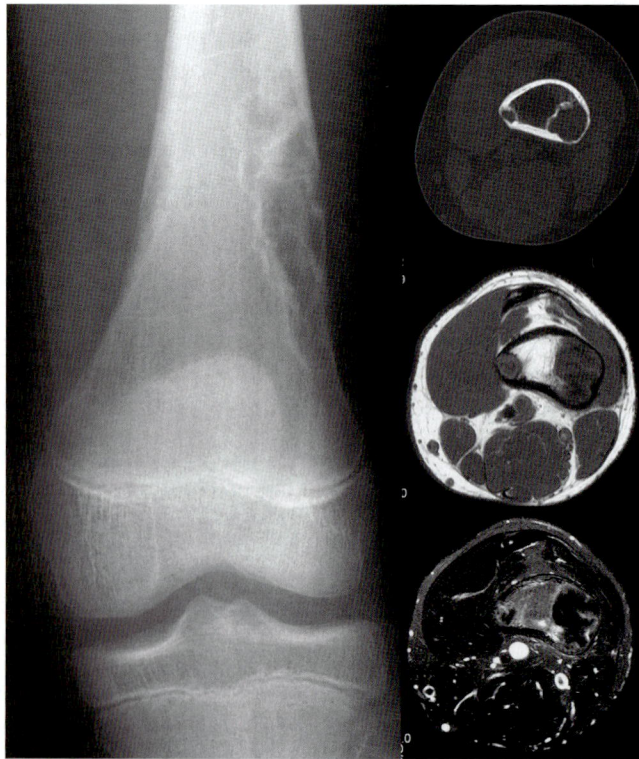

■ **FIGURE 92-10** Nonossifying fibroma. Anteroposterior radiograph shows a typical eccentric lesion arising in the distal tibia with a pathologic fracture.

■ **FIGURE 92-11** Nonossifying fibroma/fibrous cortical defect. Anteroposterior radiograph (**A**), axial CT scan (**B**), and axial T1-weighted (**C**) and T2-weighted, fat suppressed (**D**) MR images show a fibrous cortical defect arising medially and a nonossifying fibroma arising laterally in the distal femoral diaphysis. The CT scan confirms the cortical origin of both lesions, and the low signal intensity on the MR images indicates the predominantly fibrous nature of the matrix.

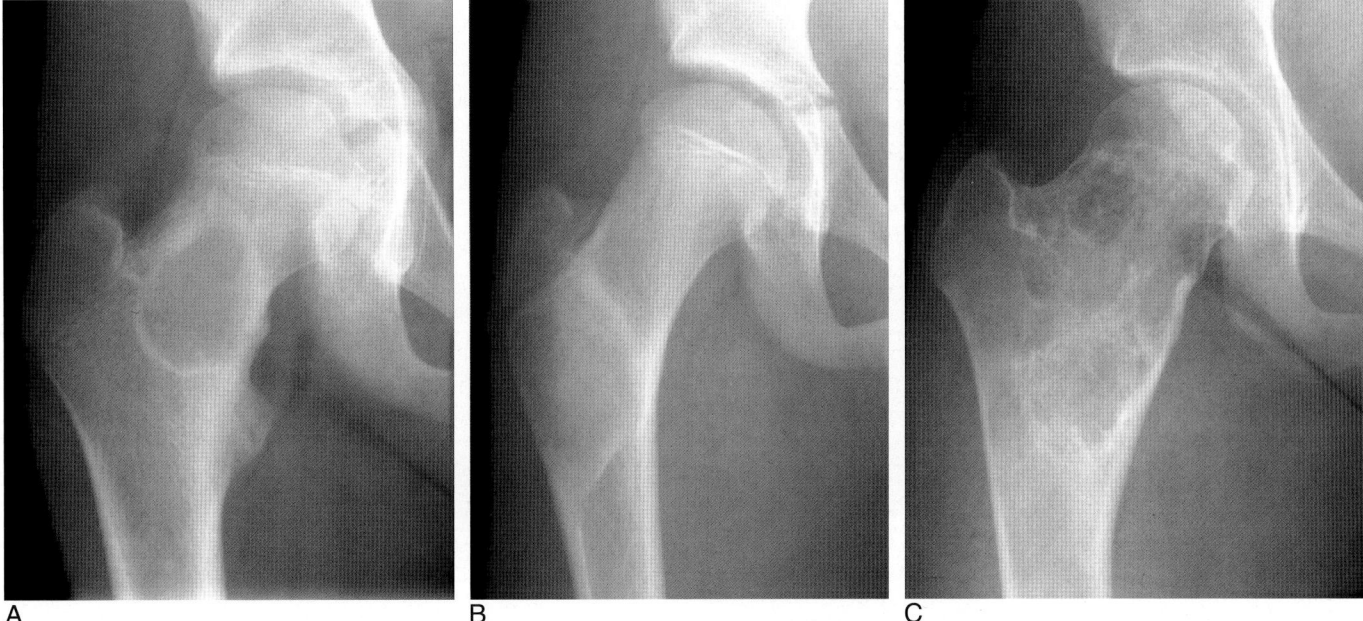

■ **FIGURE 92-12** Monostotic fibrous dysplasia: three different cases arising in the proximal femur. **A,** Predominantly lytic with a thin sclerotic border (rind sign) and a small medial cortical fracture. **B,** Intermediate density lesion showing classic ground-glass appearance. **C,** Mixed lesion with lysis and sclerosis and a long-standing modeling deformity.

end of the spectrum. Cortical thinning with bony expansion is seen in enlarging lesions affecting thin tubular bones such as the ribs. The endosteal margins tend to be well defined with a sclerotic border to give the so-called rind sign. Many cases are an incidental finding, with the remainder presenting as bone pain or pathologic fracture due to the structural weakness of the affected bone. Bone scintigraphy typically exhibits increased activity, and MRI shows decreased signal on T1-weighted images and heterogeneous signal intensity on T2-weighted images. Indeed, the lesion may appear relatively complex on T2-weighted images, with areas of low signal intensity fibrous tissue, mineralization, and rind as well as hyperintense cystic areas and foci of cartilaginous differentiation.

Thirty percent of cases of fibrous dysplasia are polyostotic, with the vast majority affecting the bones of one limb (monomelic) or one side of the body (hemimelic). This is altogether a different disease clinically in that most cases are symptomatic and present in the first decade of life with deformity, limb length inequality and pathologic fractures. Individual lesions radiographically resemble the monostotic form but tend to increase in size and number until skeletal fusion, with approximately 5% showing further growth in adult life. Structural weakness will cause softening of the affected bone, which may produce bowing deformity in the weight-bearing lower limb bones, such as the classic "shepherd's crook" deformity of the proximal femur (Fig. 92-13). Small incremental fractures, considered an insufficiency-type stress fracture, may develop in the convex cortex of expanded or bowed lesions (see Fig. 92-12A). These may heal in time or progress to complete pathologic fracture formation.

Endocrine abnormalities are well recognized in association with fibrous dysplasia. The classic example is the triad of McCune-Albright syndrome comprising polyostotic fibrous dysplasia (typically monomelic or hemimelic), cutaneous café-au-lait spots, and precocious puberty in girls. This syndrome may be seen in up to one third of females with polyostotic fibrous dysplasia, although all three elements of the triad are not usually present. Other forms of endocrine abnormalities may also occur in association with polyostotic fibrous dysplasia due to hypothalamic dysfunction. Mazabraud's syndrome is the rare association of polyostotic fibrous dysplasia and soft tissue myxomas. Malignant transformation of fibrous dysplasia to osteosarcoma or a spindle cell sarcoma is well documented but extremely rare (see Fig. 92-13C). Some of the cases reported historically were probably radiation-induced sarcomas because there was a vogue, long since discontinued, for treating fibrous dysplasia with radiotherapy in the mid-20th century.

Osteofibrous Dysplasia

Osteofibrous dysplasia, formerly known as ossifying fibroma and Kempson-Campanacci lesion, is a benign condition with a distinct predilection for the tibia. Histologically, this condition has many similarities with the much more common fibrous dysplasia in that there is a fibrous stroma with immature trabeculae. Distinction of the two entities requires identification of well-defined osteoblasts along the woven bone in osteofibrous dysplasia. Over 80% cases involve the anterior two thirds of the tibia, with a similar percentage showing mild tibial bowing. The majority of cases present in childhood or early adolescence. Radiographically the lesion is similar to that in fibrous dysplasia but eccentrically located, involving largely the anterior cortex (Fig. 92-14). There may be a predominantly lytic or mixed lytic-sclerotic appearance with or without satellite lesions extending down the

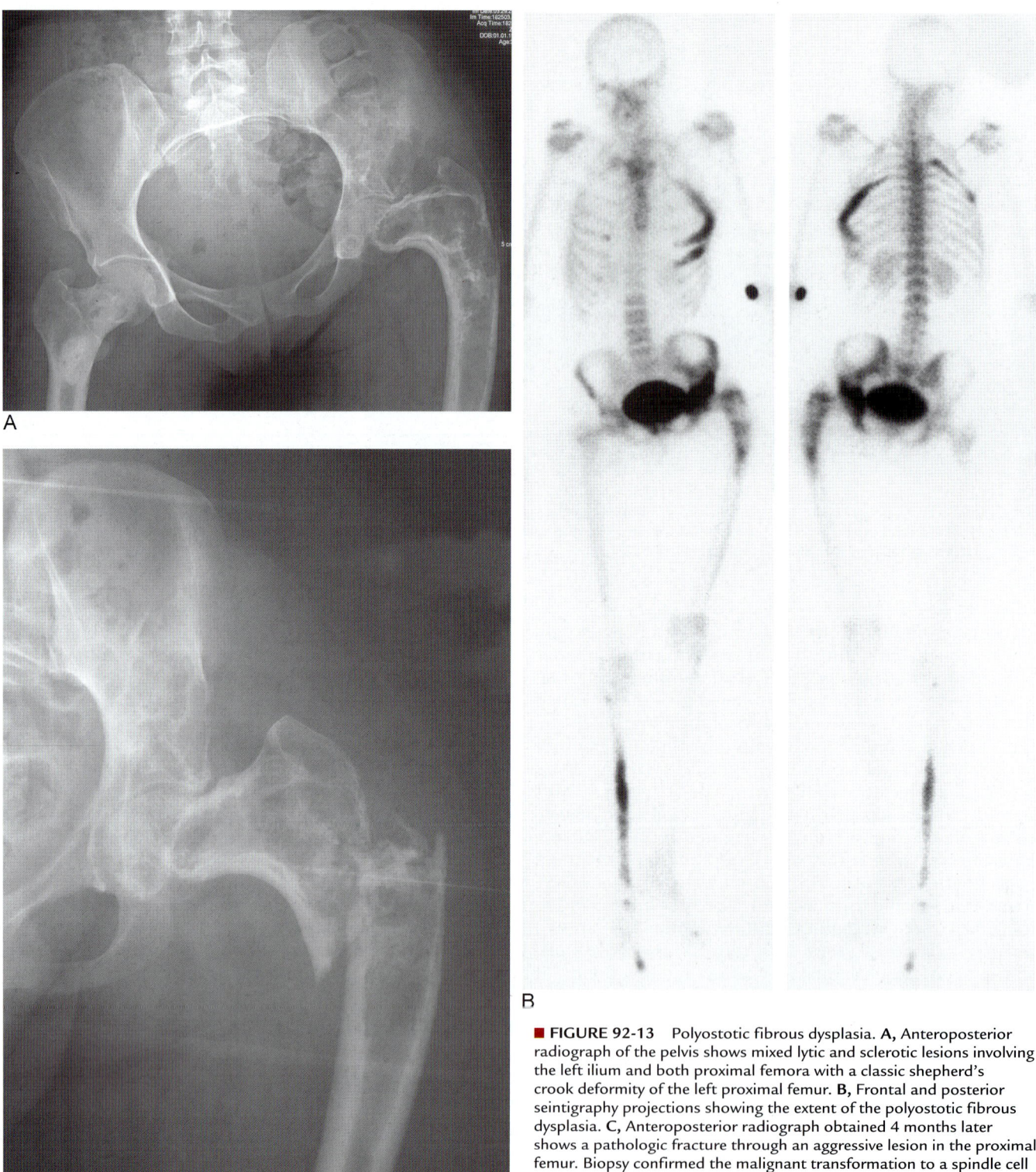

■ **FIGURE 92-13** Polyostotic fibrous dysplasia. **A,** Anteroposterior radiograph of the pelvis shows mixed lytic and sclerotic lesions involving the left ilium and both proximal femora with a classic shepherd's crook deformity of the left proximal femur. **B,** Frontal and posterior seintigraphy projections showing the extent of the polyostotic fibrous dysplasia. **C,** Anteroposterior radiograph obtained 4 months later shows a pathologic fracture through an aggressive lesion in the proximal femur. Biopsy confirmed the malignant transformation to a spindle cell sarcoma.

tibial diaphysis. The main imaging differential diagnosis is fibrous dysplasia, nonossifying fibroma, and adamantinoma. There are some histologic similarities between osteofibrous dysplasia and adamantinoma such that there is a school of thought that considers them the benign and malignant ends of the spectrum of the same disease. It is worth noting that osteofibrous dysplasia tends to present

in childhood and adamantinoma, mostly occur in a large age range after skeletal fusion.

Liposclerosing Myxofibrous Tumor

Liposclerosing myxofibrous tumor is a rare benign fibrous lesion containing varying amounts of fibrous,

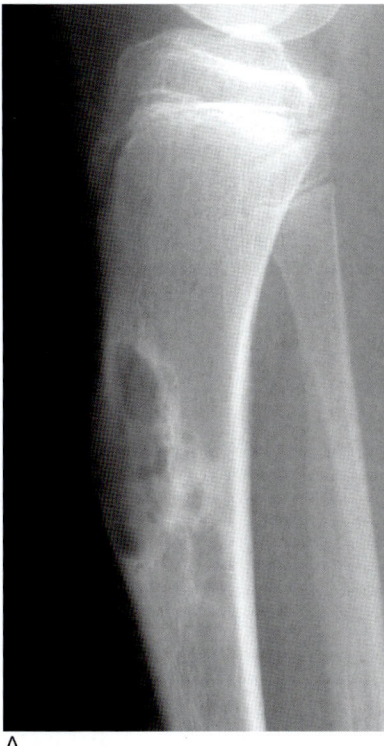

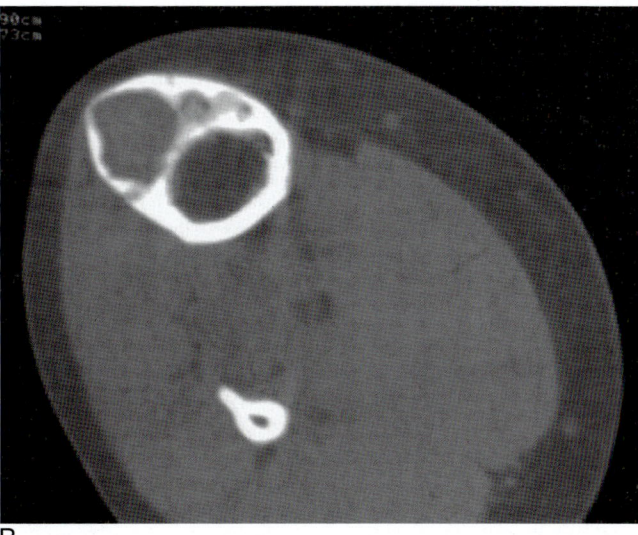

■ FIGURE 92-14   Osteofibrous dysplasia. Lateral radiograph (A) and CT scan (B) show the typical appearance of a mixed trabeculated lesion arising in the anterior cortex of the tibia with mild bowing in a patient with unfused growth plates.

myxoid, xanthomatous, and fatty elements. It is a lesion of the middle-aged and elderly, with 90% of cases arising in the intertrochanteric portion of the proximal femur.[9] Radiographically it appears as a well-defined lytic or ground-glass lesion with a sclerotic margin containing areas of calcified matrix mineralization. Because of the varying fatty and myxoid components the lesion can appear relatively heterogeneous on MRI. The imaging appearances can mimic those of fibrous dysplasia, intraosseous lipoma, and a cartilage tumor. Malignant transformation is reported in up to 10% of cases, but I cannot recall ever having seen such a case.[9]

LANGERHANS CELL HISTIOCYTOSIS

Langerhans cell histiocytosis (LCH) has replaced the term *histiocytosis X* to encompass all the clinical variants of this proliferation of histiocytes. There are three forms of the disease: LCH localized to one or several bones formerly known as eosinophilic granuloma, a chronic disseminated LCH (Hand-Schüller-Christian disease) with multiple bone lesions and extraskeletal involvement of the abdominal organs and lymph nodes, and a third acute or subacute LCH (Letterer-Siwe disease) with disseminated bone and organ involvement. The multifocal categories comprise less than 30% of cases of LCH, and the nonosseous manifestations usually predominate. The bony lesions tend to appear as multiple lytic lesions with little or no surrounding host bone response (Fig. 92-15). The differential diagnosis includes cystic angiomatosis and possibly marrow infiltration with leukemic deposits and neuroblastoma metastases, although involvement of

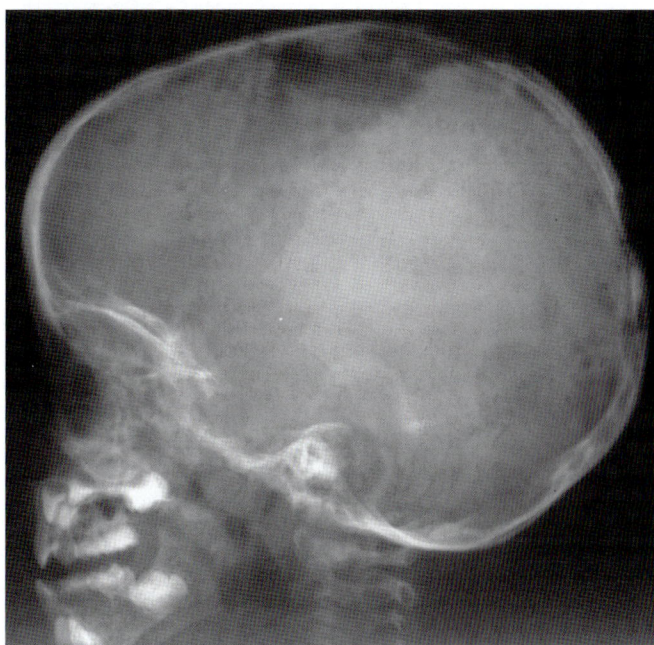

■ FIGURE 92-15   Subacute disseminated Langerhans cell histiocytosis (Letterer-Siwe disease). The lateral skull radiograph shows multiple lytic lesions throughout the skull vault with no surrounding sclerosis.

the medulla with the latter two disease processes is usually more permeative in appearance than geographic.

The localized form of LCH comprises approximately 70% of cases of this disease, with the majority presenting between 5 and 15 years of age. Unlike the disseminated forms of LCH the long-term prognosis is generally excellent. The flat bones of the skull, mandible, pelvis, and ribs are involved in about half the cases, with 30% of cases arising in the long bones and the final 10% in the spine. Typical sites of involvement of the long bones are the femur, humerus, and tibia, with approximately 60% of cases arising in the diaphysis (Fig. 92-16). The lesions in the long bones typically show a relatively well-defined lytic lesion, lacking a sclerotic margin, centrally located within the medulla, with an overlying intact lamellar periosteal reaction that, in time, will produce cortical thickening. Perilesional edema and inflammation can be a prominent feature on MRI, often pointing to the diagnosis (see Fig. 92-16B). The differential diagnosis of long-bone LCH includes osteomyelitis and, less likely, Ewing's sarcoma. The classic presentation in the spine is collapse with flattening of the vertebral body to produce the so-called vertebra plana appearance.

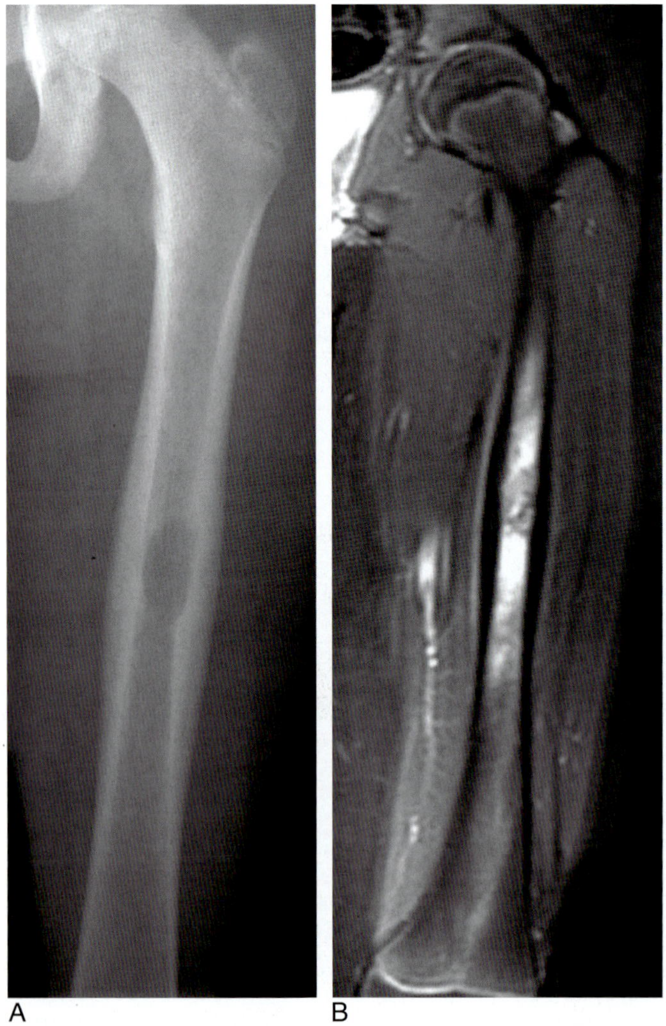

■ FIGURE 92-16 Solitary Langerhans cell histiocytosis (eosinophilic granuloma). **A,** Anteroposterior radiograph shows a well-defined lytic lesion in the midfemoral diaphysis with adjacent cortical hyperostosis. **B,** Coronal STIR MR image shows the lesion centrally with florid surrounding marrow edema and minor juxtacortical edema.

METABOLIC DISORDERS

The brown tumor of hyperparathyroidism is arguably the most "tumorous" of all tumor-like lesions of bone in that both imaging and histology may be indistinguishable from giant cell tumor, giant cell reparative granuloma of bone, and ABC. Brown tumors are associated with primary hyperparathyroidism in approximately 3% of cases and with secondary hyperparathyroidism in approximately 1.5% of cases. The name is attributed to the macroscopic color that results from the accumulation of hemosiderin released by interstitial hemorrhage. Raised parathormone levels stimulate osteoclast activity to produce irregular bone resorption, resulting in microfractures and hemorrhage. These cavities are filled with loose fibrous tissue containing osteoclast giant cells. The radiographic appearances of a brown tumor are of a lytic, usually expansile lesion with severe osteopenia (Fig. 92-17). The latter may readily be mistaken for disuse osteoporosis due to pain from a bone tumor if the metabolic nature of the underlying disease is not appreciated. Multiple brown tumors can mimic lytic metastases and myeloma. The MRI features of a brown tumor may resemble an ABC with fluid-fluid levels due to the hemorrhage.[10] It is important to actively exclude a brown tumor whenever faced with a benign giant cell–rich lesion of bone. On treatment of the underlying metabolic disorder brown tumors tend to heal with moderate sclerosis (see Fig. 92-17C).

NORMAL VARIANTS

The experienced radiologist will have a thorough knowledge of the diverse spectrum of normal skeletal variants and have on hand an atlas of bone disorders to consult if uncertain. Most problems arise when normal variants are confused with traumatic lesions. Less commonly, normal variants may simulate a tumor. These include the proximal metaphyseal notch of the humerus in children that may be normal but can also be seen in leukemia and Gaucher's disease. Also, ballooning of the ischiopubic synchondrosis in early adolescence may mimic a chondroma or cystic lesion. The lesion that repeatedly causes diagnostic problems is the periosteal or cortical desmoid. Also known as avulsive cortical irregularity and cortical irregularity syndrome it affects the posteromedial ridge of the distal femoral metaphysis in children and adolescents. On radiographs there is saucerization of the outer cortex with minor spiculated periosteal new bone formation (Fig. 92-18). It is thought to be due to mechanical stresses applied to the origin of the medial head of the gastrocnemius muscle or insertion of the adductor magnus. It could therefore be included in the post-traumatic disorders detailed later. However, bone scintigraphy typically demonstrates normal or only minimally increased activity that is somewhat against trauma. MRI may show some edema on the external surface of the cortex and occasionally in the underlying medulla that might tend to support a traumatic aetiology.[11] Pathologically there is evidence of reactive subperiosteal fibroblastic proliferation, thereby suggesting to some authors that the lesion should be included in the category of fibrous lesions. Either way, the typical radiographic appearance, bilateral in up to

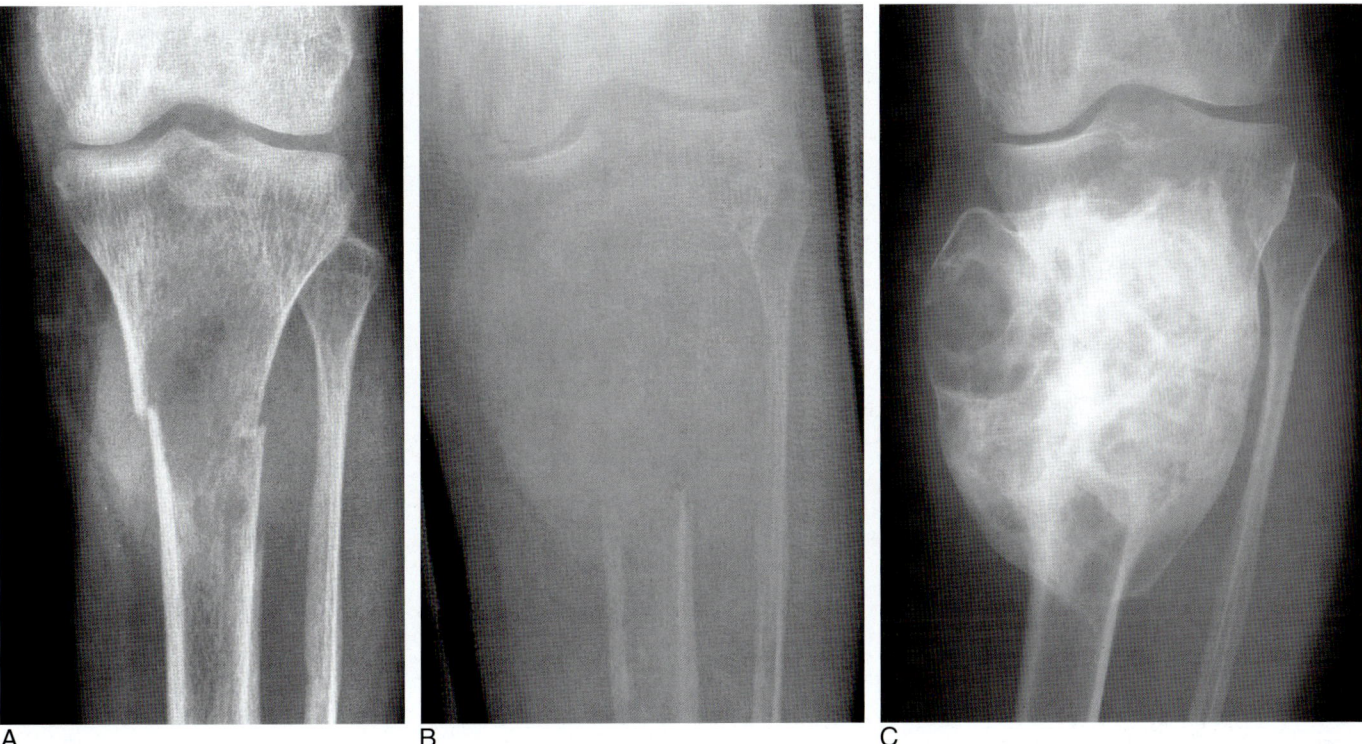

A   B   C

■ **FIGURE 92-17**   Brown tumor of secondary hyperparathyroidism. **A,** Anteroposterior radiograph at presentation with a pathologic fracture through a lytic lesion in the proximal tibial diaphysis. **B,** Anteroposterior radiograph taken 4 months later. The correct diagnosis had not been made, and the lytic lesion continued to grow with major demineralization. **C,** Anteroposterior radiograph 5 months later after commencement of medical treatment. The tumor has healed, and bone density has returned to normal.

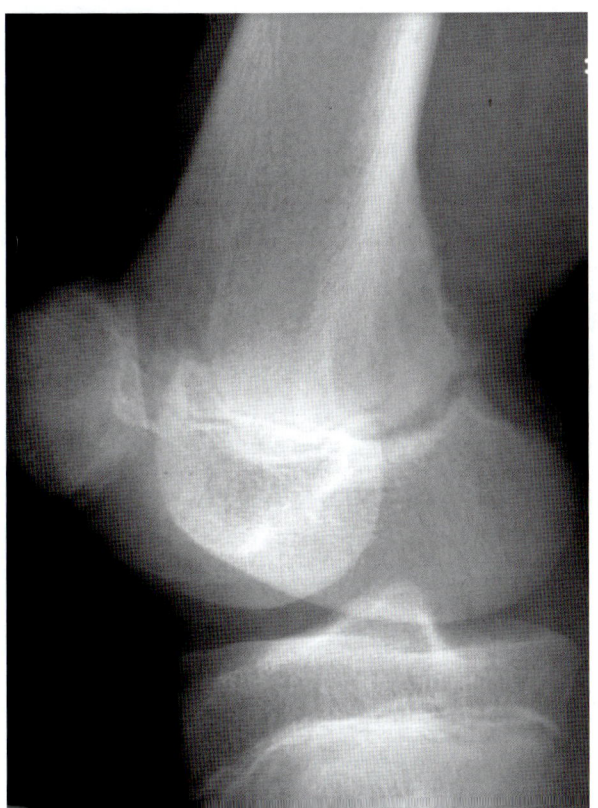

■ **FIGURE 92-18**   Periosteal/cortical desmoid (distal femoral cortical irregularity). Oblique radiograph of the knee in an adolescent showing irregularity of the posteromedial cortex of the distal femoral metaphysis.

40% of cases with virtually normal scintigraphic activity, allows for confident exclusion of other more significant pathologies. Because of the bilateralism and self-limiting nature of the condition I prefer to classify it as a normal variant.

POST-TRAUMATIC DISORDERS

Stress Fractures

Stress fractures are classified as either a fatigue fracture or insufficiency fracture (see Chapter 38). The fatigue-type arises due to abnormal loading on normal bone, whereas insufficiency type fractures occur due to normal physiologic stresses applied to weakened or abnormal bone. The fatigue type in the skeletally immature individual is frequently mistaken for a malignant lesion, particularly a primary sarcoma of bone. The proximal tibia is the most common site for fatigue fractures in the child and young adult and is also the most common site to be misinterpreted on imaging as a sarcoma of bone.[12,13] The periosteal new bone formation seen as ill-defined sclerosis en face and as a continuous lamella perpendicularly is all too frequently thought to be the early sign of Ewing's sarcoma, particularly if the typical history of increased physical activity is absent (Fig. 92-19). If the correct diagnosis is not considered on the radiographs, other imaging techniques, including MRI, may further confuse the unwary radiologist, with the adjacent medullary edema and hemorrhage mistaken for tumor infiltration. Close attention to image quality on

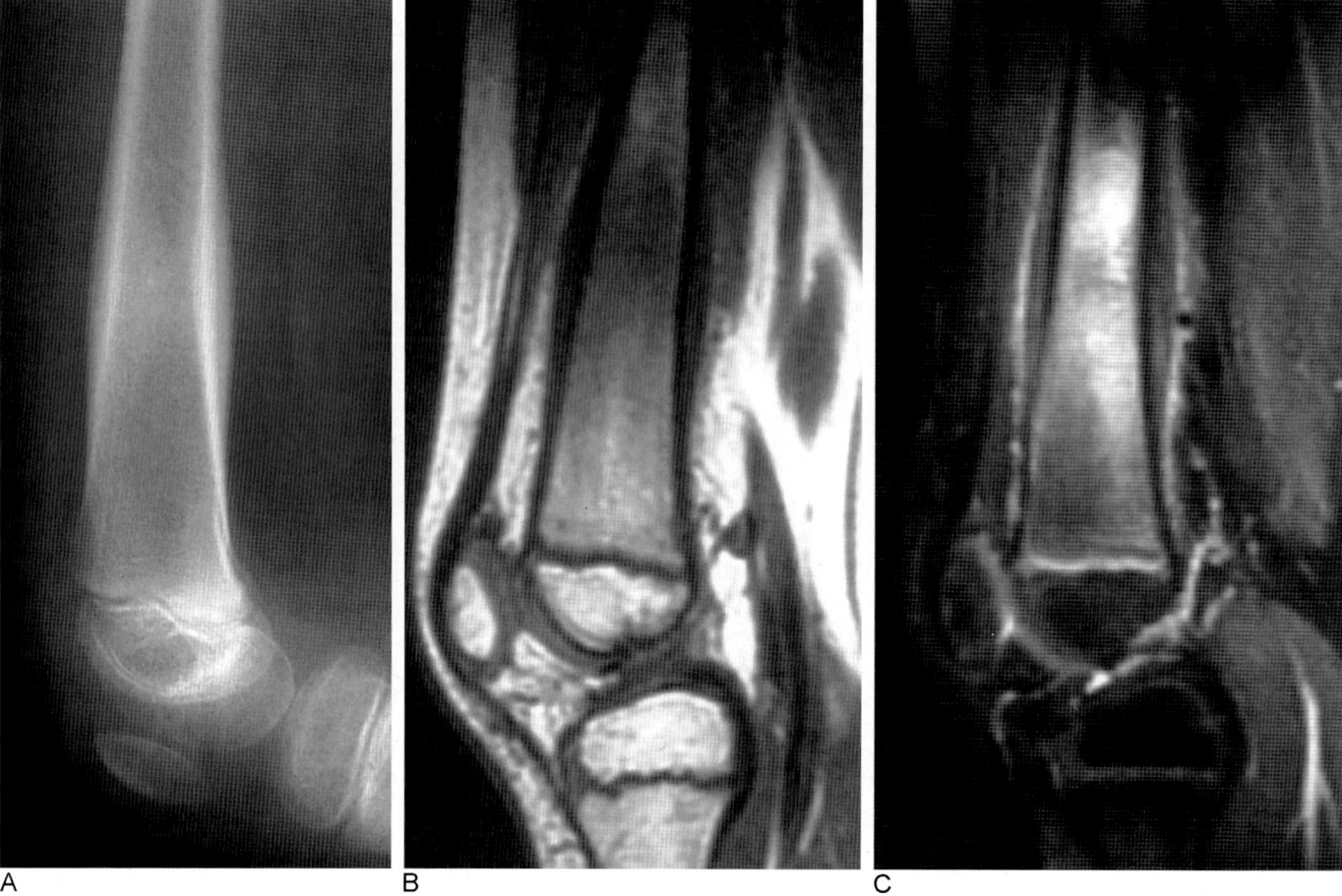

A   B   C

■ **FIGURE 92-19** Fatigue-type stress fracture of distal femoral diaphysis. Lateral radiograph (**A**) and sagittal T1-weighted (**B**) and sagittal STIR (**C**) MR images show a lamellar periosteal reaction and edema/hemorrhage in the underlying medullary bone that should not be misinterpreted as due to tumor infiltration.

CT and MRI will reveal the focal cortical radiolucency/low signal intensity line due to the fracture with the surrounding periosteal reaction. Features that are against a diagnosis of sarcoma are the absence of true cortical destruction and any evidence of a soft tissue mass. In my experience it is not unusual in fatigue fractures of the proximal tibia to see less marked marrow changes on MRI at the same site in the asymptomatic contralateral limb if it has been included in the scan field. Bilateral changes would be rare in malignancy unless there was multifocal disease that may be seen in malignant round cell tumors such as leukemia and Ewing sarcoma. However, there would usually be little difficulty in recognizing disseminated malignancy in this situation. Fatigue fractures are just one end of the spectrum of bone response to abnormal loading. MRI is sufficiently sensitive to subtle marrow abnormalities even when symptoms are absent or minimal. These nonspecific changes can be termed *stress reactions* or *stress phenomena*. They will typically resolve in several weeks, provided the source of the stress is removed. If the signs remain unaltered or show progression, then early sarcoma should be excluded.

Insufficiency-type stress fractures occur in association with a diverse group of conditions that weaken bone (see Chapter 38). The most frequently seen examples are in the postmenopausal osteoporotic female. Diagnostic problems are frequently experienced with fractures involving the pelvic ring where the reduced bone density, curvature of the bones, and overlying bowel gas/vascular calcifications may obscure the fractures on radiographs. It is not unusual in the elderly female patient for multiple insufficiency fractures of the pelvis to be misinterpreted on bone scintigraphy as indicative of metastatic disease, particularly if there is a history of prior malignancy elsewhere. There is a classic association between insufficiency fractures of the body of the pubis (parasymphyseal) and sacral ala. The H shape, also known as the Honda sign, of increased activity over the sacrum on bone scintigraphy is considered virtually pathognomonic of bilateral vertical sacral ala fractures joined by a horizontal fracture.

Avulsion Injuries

In the immature skeleton, particularly around the time of the adolescent growth spurt, the attachment of the apophyses to the underlying bone is relatively weak, rendering them susceptible to the effects of acute or chronic stress.[14] This is most frequently seen in the pelvis, with over 50% of cases involving the ischial apophysis (Fig. 92-20). Acute injuries are not usually a diagnostic problem. However, if

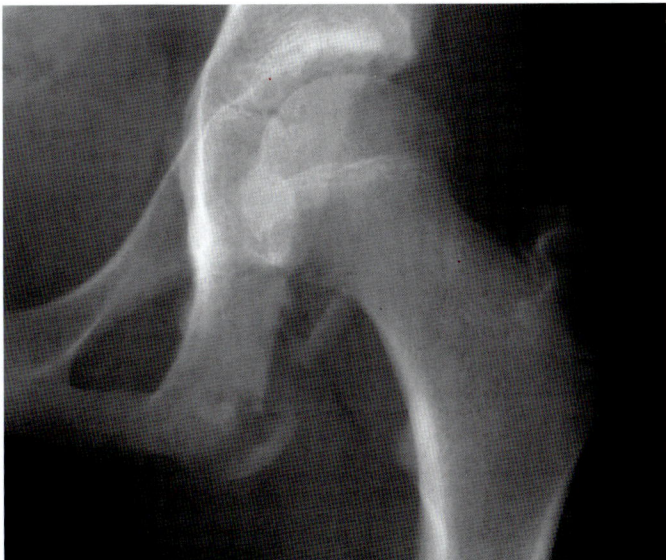

■ FIGURE 92-20   Acute-on-chronic ischial apophyseal avulsion. Anteroposterior radiograph of the hip in an adolescent showing the avulsed apophysis within the soft tissues and erosion of the underlying ischium mimicking a tumor arising from the surface of the bone.

there is a delay in diagnosis the immature amorphous callus may radiographically mimic an osteogenic surface lesion. The features are more pronounced in the presence of an acute-on-chronic injury in which MRI will show edema and hemorrhage in association with mineralization. If the ischial apophysis is acutely avulsed with its blood supply intact, it can continue to grow to present at a later stage with a large piece of mature bone in the soft tissues of the buttock.

Subperiosteal Hemorrhage and Hyperplastic Callus

Conditions resulting in loosely attached periosteum predispose to subperiosteal hemorrhage after minor trauma. In time the hematoma will ossify and, if particularly florid, may mimic a bone-forming tumor. Similar appearances occur with exuberant hyperplastic callus formation around fractures. Both may be seen with osteogenesis imperfecta, vitamin C deficiency (scurvy), and neuropathic disorders (Fig. 92-21).[15] A note of caution has to be expressed because osteosarcoma has been reported arising in patients with osteogenesis imperfecta, suggesting a possible relationship.[16] Cross-sectional imaging with MRI or CT may be helpful in extreme cases to distinguish benign callus from the aggressive appearances of a sarcoma with intramedullary invasion and soft tissue extension. Patients with a bleeding tendency such as hemophilia, if poorly controlled, may have repetitive spontaneous bleeding that can result in erosion of bone, producing the so-called hemophiliac pseudotumors.

Post-traumatic Bone Cysts

Penetrating injuries with foreign bodies may rarely be associated with the development of a chronic intraosseous cyst. Examples have been described after a stab wound with a bamboo cane and a bullet wound.[17] Approximately 20 cases

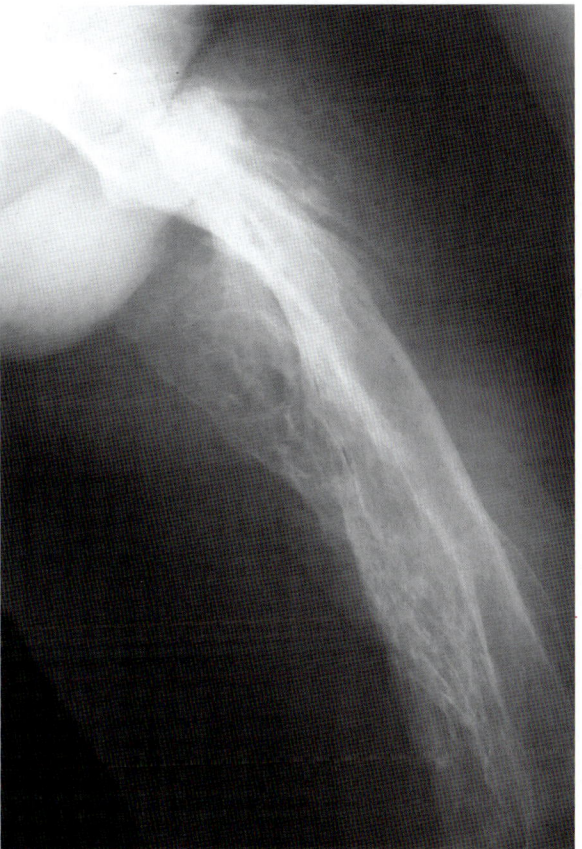

■ FIGURE 92-21   Osteogenesis imperfecta tarda. Lateral radiograph of the femur shows massive ossifying subperiosteal hematomas.

of radiolucent lesions appearing adjacent to fractures on follow-up radiographs have been described, although my experience of 3 such cases would suggest that it was not that uncommon.[18] The vast majority of cases are located in the distal radius after greenstick or torus fractures in children (Fig. 92-22).[19] It has been postulated that the lucency is due to the release of intramedullary fat beneath an intact periosteum. As the surrounding subperiosteal hematoma ossifies, the collection of fat appears as a relative eccentric lucency that seen en face may mimic a Brodie abscess or LCH. These cysts are of no clinical consequence and progressively disappear as the fracture consolidates.

INFECTION

The radiographic appearances of acute osteomyelitis are those of an aggressive bone lesion, including permeative bone destruction and complex periosteal new bone formation, thereby mimicking a malignant bone tumor such as Ewing's sarcoma. The two conditions cannot be reliably differentiated on clinic grounds because patients presenting with Ewing's sarcoma may show a systemic upset with raised inflammatory markers. One useful distinguishing feature is the rapidity of onset of radiographic changes. In acute osteomyelitis the radiographs frequently progress from relatively normal to grossly abnormal in only a couple of weeks (Fig. 92-23). Ewing's sarcoma is a locally aggressive tumor but will typically take several months to show a comparable degree of bone destruction. In any

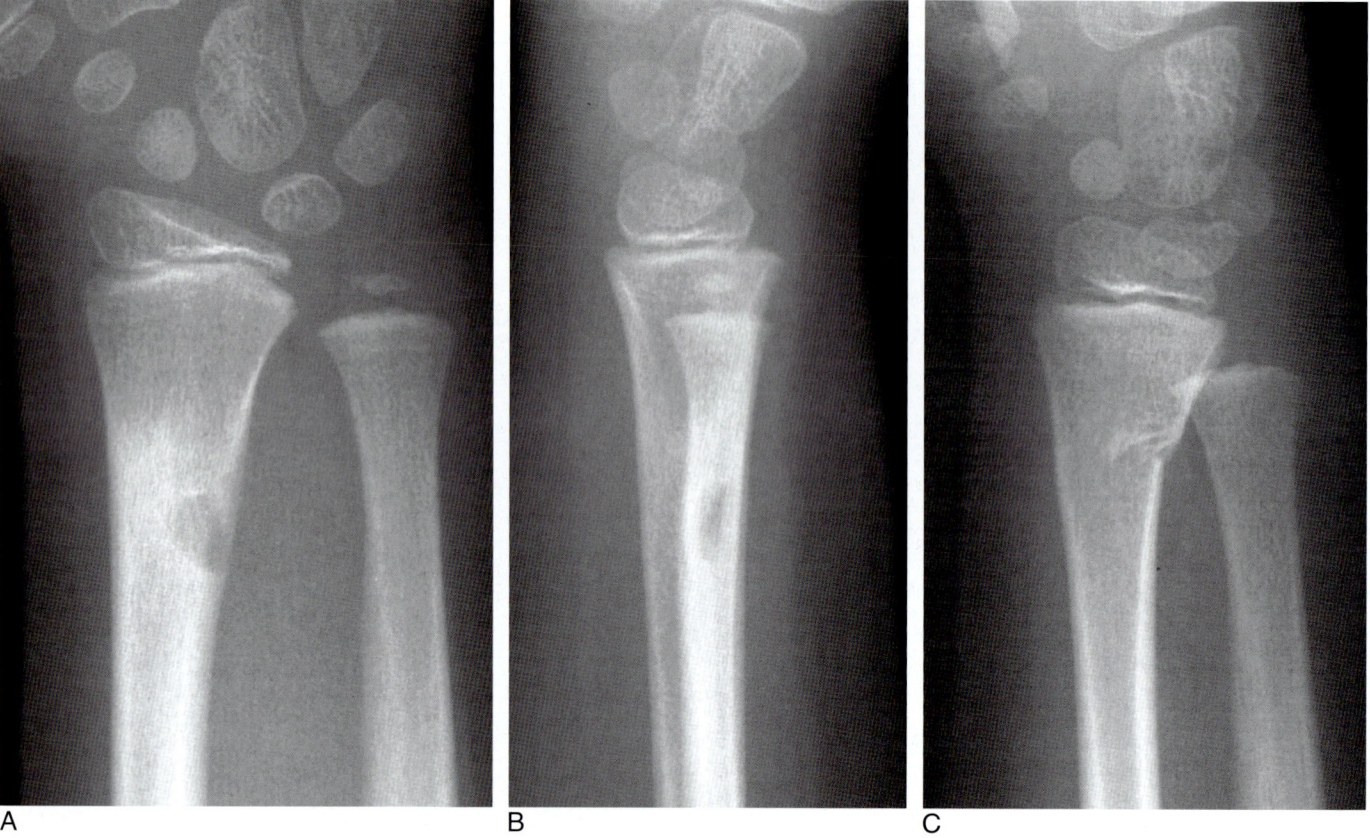

A   B   C

■ **FIGURE 92-22** Post-traumatic cyst of the distal radius. Posteroanterior (**A**) and lateral (**B**) radiographs of the wrist in a child show an eccentric lucency with mild surrounding sclerosis. **C,** Posteroanterior radiograph at presentation 7 months earlier shows a greenstick fracture of the distal radius.

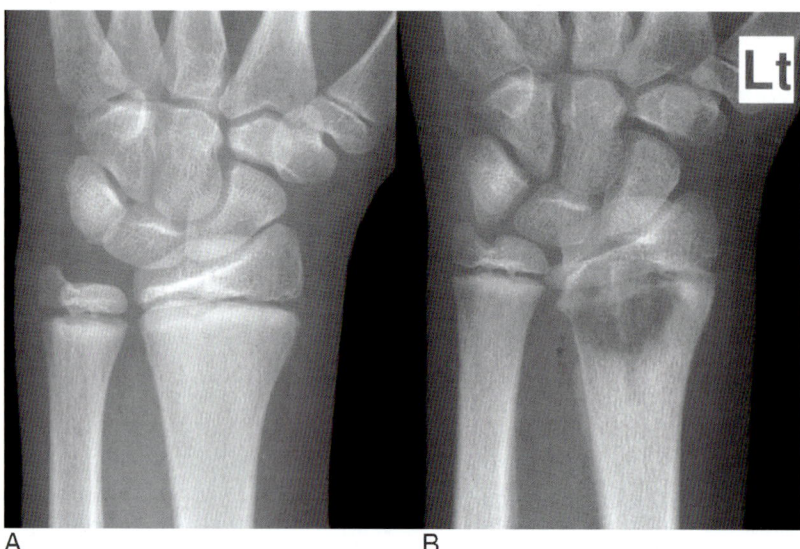

A   B

■ **FIGURE 92-23** Acute osteomyelitis. Posteroanterior radiograph at presentation (**A**) and 2 weeks later (**B**). The initial radiograph is normal. The follow-up radiograph shows a lytic lesion in the distal radial metaphysis with an interrupted lamellar periosteal reaction. The appearances are those of an aggressive lesion, but only infection is likely in view of the rapidity of onset of the changes.

case of suspected osteomyelitis, biopsy is usually required to identify the causative organism to ensure appropriate antibiotic therapy. If there is doubt as to the diagnosis the biopsy should be performed in such a manner as to not prejudice future limb salvage surgery if subsequently a primary sarcoma is identified.

Subacute osteomyelitis can be difficult to diagnose because the characteristic signs and symptoms of acute infection are absent (see Chapter 62). Frequently there is no systemic illness, no signs of infection locally, and normal laboratory values, with the exception of a mildly raised erythrocyte sedimentation rate. The radiographic appearances of subacute osteomyelitis are well documented, but all too often the condition can be mistaken for various benign and malignant bone tumors. It has been estimated that, in the pediatric age group, 50% of cases of subacute osteomyelitis are confused with tumor. The responsibility often falls on the radiologist to suggest the correct diagnosis, in which process MRI can be helpful. A "target" appearance has been described on MRI of a bone abscess in subacute osteomyelitis, the so-called

Brodie's abscess.[20] This comprises four layers (Fig. 92-24): (1) a central low-signal intensity on T1-weighted and high-signal intensity on T2-weighted and STIR images representing the abscess cavity; (2) an inner ring isointense to muscle representing the granulation layer; (3) an outer ring hypointense on all sequences due to reactive sclerosis; and (4) a peripheral halo of hypointense edema on T1-weighted images. In many of these patients the granulation layer appears particularly conspicuous on T1-weighted images owing to relative hyperintensity and has been called the penumbra sign. It is typically found in the metaphysis of a long bone, most commonly around the knee and may be unilocular or multilocular.

Breaching of the growth plate and secondary involvement of the epiphysis is common in osteomyelitis, whereas breaching of the growth plate is a relatively late feature of osteosarcoma and distinctly uncommon in Ewing's sarcoma. Primary epiphyseal osteomyelitis is unusual. The most common cause of a lytic epiphyseal lesion preskeletal fusion is a chondroblastoma.

Tuberculous infection of bone has always been recognized to be a great mimic of other pathologic processes, including bone tumors. It remains a diagnosis to be considered in these days of increased international travel, particularly in immigrants or visitors from endemic areas such as the Indian subcontinent as well as in the immunocompromised population. Multifocal disease can easily be mistaken for metastases or lymphoma (Fig. 92-25). Only 25% of cases of osseous tuberculosis show evidence of coexisting pulmonary disease.

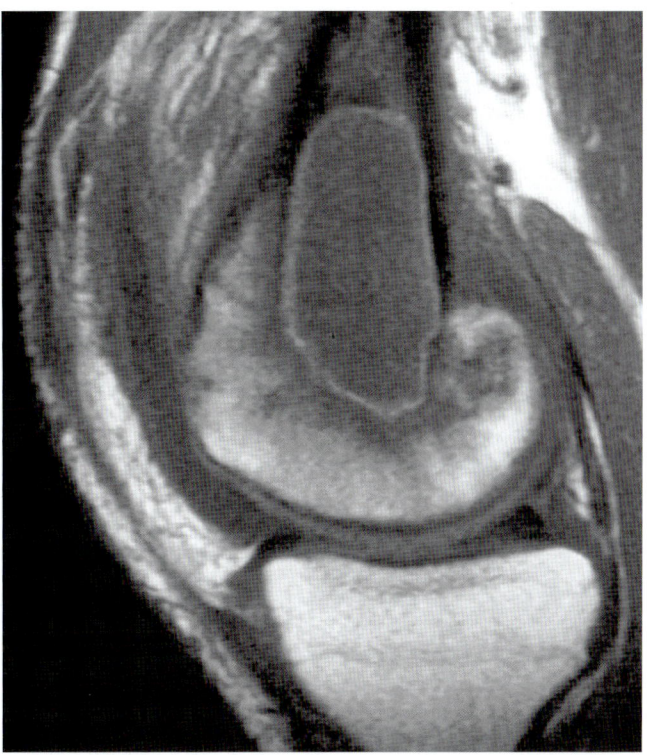

■ **FIGURE 92-24** Subacute osteomyelitis. The sagittal T1-weighted image shows the hypointense abscess cavity in the distal femoral metaphysis. There is a relatively hyperintense rim to the abscess (the penumbra sign) with surrounding hypointense sclerosis and marrow edema.

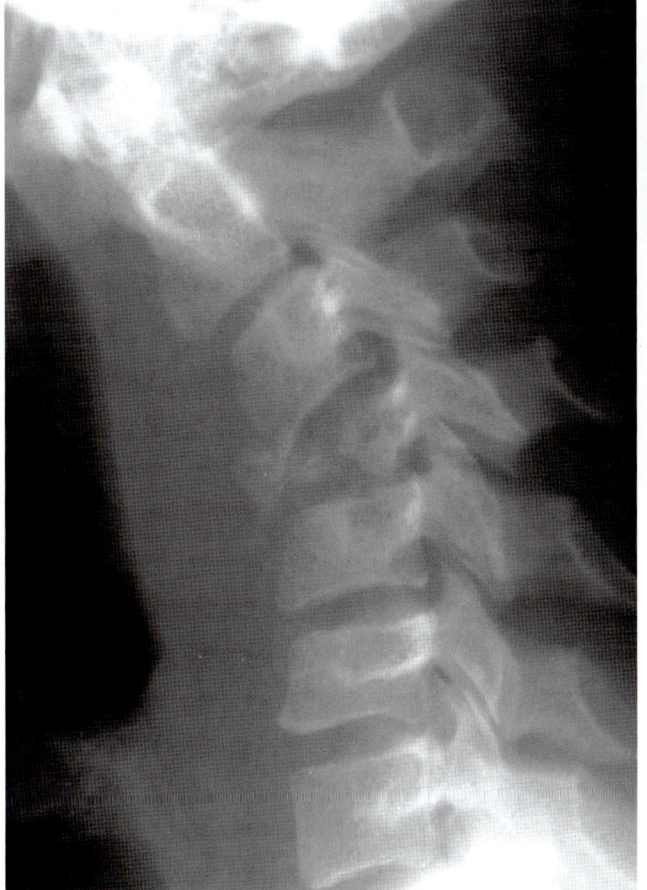

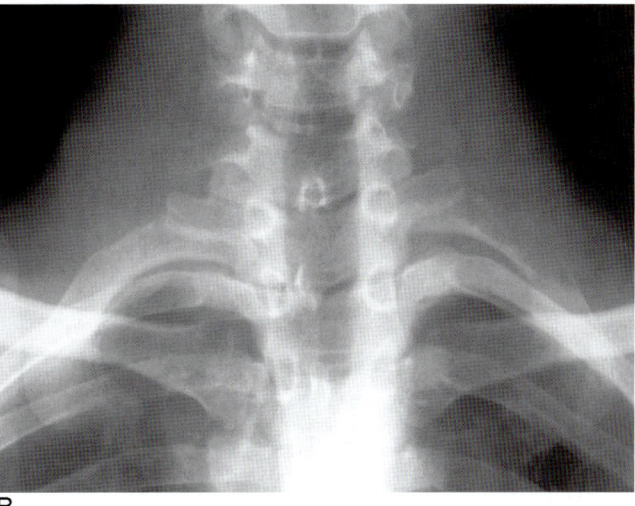

■ **FIGURE 92-25** Multifocal tuberculosis. **A,** Lateral radiograph of cervical spine shows destruction and collapse of the body of C4. **B,** Anteroposterior radiograph of lower cervical spine shows a destructive lesion in the left first rib. The differential diagnosis in an adult includes metastases and lymphoma.

A

B

Bone lesions occur in less than 3% of cases of echinococcosis (hydatid disease). The bone lesions tend to be lytic, expansile, and trabeculated, with a predilection for the spine, pelvis, and long bones. The radiographic manifestations are similar to those of plasmacytoma, fibrous dysplasia, giant cell tumor, and expansile metastases such as seen with renal or thyroid primary malignancies. CT and MRI will show cystic lesions in bone extending out into the soft tissues.

SUGGESTED READINGS

Conway WF, Hayes CW. Miscellaneous lesions of bone. Radiol Clin North Am 1993; 31:339–358.

David R, Oria RA, Kumar R, et al. Radiologic features of eosinophilic granuloma of bone. AJR Am J Roentgenol 1989; 153:1021–1026.

Hudson TM, Stiles RG, Monson DK. Fibrous lesions of bone. Radiol Clin North Am 1993; 31:279–293.

Kransdorf MJ, Smith SE. Lesions of unknown histiogenesis: Langerhans cell histiocytosis and Ewing sarcoma. Semin Musc Radiol 2000; 4:113–125.

Kumar R, Madewell JE, Lindell MM, Swischuk LB. Fibrous lesions of bone. RadioGraphics 1990; 10:237–256.

Meyer JS, Dormans JP. Differential diagnosis of pediatric musculoskeletal masses. MRI Clin North Am 1998; 6:561–577.

Nomikos GC, Murphey MD, Kransdorf MK, et al. Primary bone tumors of the lower extremities. Radiol Clin North Am 2002; 40:971–990.

Oudjhane K, Azouz EM. Imaging of osteomyelitis in children. Radiol Clin North Am 2001; 39:251–266.

Parman LM, Murphey MD. Alphabet soup: cystic lesions of bone. Semin Musc Radiol 2000; 4:89–101.

Smith SE, Kransdorf MJ. Primary musculoskeletal tumors of fibrous origin. Semin Musc Radiol 2000; 4:73–88.

REFERENCES

1. Zehetgruber H, Bittner B, Gruber D, et al. Prevalence of aneurysmal and solitary bone cysts in young patients. Clin Orthop 2005; 439:136–143.
2. Maiya S, Davies AM, Evans N, Grimer RJ. Surface aneurysmal bone cysts: a pictorial review. Eur Radiol 2002; 12:99–108.
3. Davies AM, Cassar-Pullicino VN, Grimer RJ. The incidence and significance of fluid-fluid levels on computed tomography of osseous lesions. Br J Radiol 1992; 65:193–198.
4. O'Donnell P, Saifuddin A. The prevalence and diagnostic significance of fluid-fluid levels in focal lesions of bone. Skeletal Radiol 2004; 33:330–336.
5. Van Dyck P, Vanhoenacker FM, Vogel J, et al. Prevalence, extension and characteristics of fluid-fluid levels in bone and soft tissue tumors. Eur Radiol 2006; 16:2644–2651.
6. Brindley GW, Greene JF, Frankel LS. Malignant transformation of aneurysmal bone cysts. Clin Orthop 2005; 438:282–287.
7. Schajowicz F, Clavel SM, Slullitel JA. Juxta-articular bone cysts (intraosseous ganglia): a clinicopathological study of 88 cases. J Bone Joint Surg Br 1979; 61:107–116.
8. Williams HJ, Davies AM, Allen G, et al. Imaging features of intraosseous ganglia: a report of 45 cases. Eur Radiol 2004; 14:1761–1769.
9. Kransdorf M, Murphey M, Sweet D. Liposclerosing myxofibrous tumor: a radiologic/pathologic distinct fibroosseous lesion of bone with a marked predilection for the intertrochanteric region of the femur. Radiology 212:693–698.
10. Davies AM, Evans N, Mangham DC, Grimer RJ. MR imaging of brown tumour with fluid-fluid levels: a report of three cases. Eur Radiol 2001; 11:1445–1449.
11. Posch TJ, Puckett ML. Marrow MR signal abnormality associated with bilateral avulsive cortical irregularities in a gymnast. Skeletal Radiol 1998; 27:511–514.
12. Davies AM, Evans N, Grimer RJ. Fatigue fractures of the proximal tibia simulating malignancy. Br J Radiol 1988; 61:903–908.
13. Davies AM, Carter SR, Grimer RJ, Sneath RS. Fatigue fractures of the femoral diaphysis in the skeletally immature simulating malignancy. Br J Radiol 1989; 62:893–896.
14. Donnelly LF, Bisset GS, Helms CA, Squire DL. Chronic avulsive injuries of childhood. Skeletal Radiol 1999; 28:138–144.
15. Dobrocky I, Seidl G, Grill F. MRI and CT features of hyperplastic callus in osteogenesis imperfecta tarda. Eur Radiol 1999; 9:665–668.
16. Gagliardi JA, Evans EM, Chandnani VP, et al. Osteogenesis imperfecta complicated by osteosarcoma. Skeletal Radiol 1995; 24:308–310.
17. Grainger AJ, Campbell RSD. Post-traumatic bone cyst: a case of the floating fragment. Skeletal Radiol 1998; 27:400–402.
18. Papadimitriou NG, Christophorides J, Beslikas TA, et al. Post-traumatic cystic lesion following fracture of the radius. Skeletal Radiol 2005; 34:411–414.
19. Dürr HR, Lienemann A, Stäbler A, et al. MRI of posttraumatic cyst-like lesions of bone after greenstick fracture. Eur Radiol 1997; 7:1218–1220.
20. Martí Bonmatí L, Aparisi F, Poyatos C, Vilar J. Brodie abscess: MR imaging appearance in 10 patients. J MRI 1993; 3:543–546.

93

Soft Tissue Tumors

Arthur de Schepper

In this chapter a pragmatic or analytical approach is presented for the detection, staging, grading, and tissue-specific diagnosis of soft tissue tumors (Fig. 93-1). Because of the large number of types of these tumors, classification in a few relevant categories is important. In the 2002 World Health Organization (WHO) classification of tumors it is recommended to divide soft tissue tumors into four categories, according to a lesion's biologic potential:

1. *Benign:* most benign soft tumor tissues do not recur locally and do not give rise to distant metastases.
2. *Intermediate* (locally aggressive): these tumors often recur locally and are associated with an infiltrative and locally destructive growth pattern without metastatic potential. The prototype in this category is desmoid or aggressive fibromatosis.
3. *Intermediate* (rarely metastasizing): soft tumor tissues in this category are often locally aggressive and show the ability to give rise to metastases to lymph nodes and lung in occasional cases.
4. *Malignant:* these tumors have the potential for locally destructive growth and recurrence and a significant risk of distant metastasis. Some low-grade sarcomas with a low metastatic risk may advance in grade in a local recurrence and thereby acquire a higher risk of distant spread.[1]

Substantial changes since the previous WHO classification include the following:

- *In the group of adipocytic tumors:* the recognition of atypical lipomatous tumor as a synonym for well-differentiated liposarcoma, the inclusion of chondroid lipoma, and the renaming of fibrolipomatous hamartoma as lipomatosis of nerve.
- *In the group of fibroblastic/myofibroblastic tumors:* the characterization of numerous previously undefined lesions, the clearer recognition of solitary fibrous tumor, the realization that most so-called hemangiopericytomas belong to this category and not to the group of tumors of vascular origin, as well as the reclassification of lesions formerly labeled myxoid malignant fibrous histiocytoma as myxofibrosarcoma.

- *In the group of fibrohistiocytic tumors:* the recognition of myxofibrosarcoma as a distinctive entity, the renaming of undifferentiated pleomorphic sarcoma as pleomorphic malignant fibrous histiocytoma as a diagnosis of exclusion accounting for less than 5% of sarcomas in adults, and the inclusion of localized and diffuse forms of giant cell tumor of tendon sheath.
- *In the group of vascular tumors:* the characterization of various newly recognized entities, especially in the group of hemangioendotheliomas, and the more frequent recognition of angiosarcomas by their epithelioid cytomorphology at deep soft tissue locations.
- *In the group of chondro-osseous tumors:* only soft tissue chondroma and extraskeletal osteosarcoma are retained under this heading. Myositis ossificans and fibrodysplasia ossificans progressiva move to the group of non-neoplastic processes or pseudotumors.
- *In the group of tumors of uncertain differentiation:* inclusion of synovial sarcoma in the malignant group, the addition of myoepithelioma, and the allocation of angiomatoid fibrous histiocytoma and extraskeletal myxoid chondrosarcoma to this category.

The relevance of these changes for the radiologist is of limited importance, but the list of soft tissue conditions that can be diagnosed on imaging, initially thought to be limited to a handful, will continue to grow in the near future.[2]

PREVALENCE AND EPIDEMIOLOGY

Although soft tissues constitute a large proportion of the human body (12%), soft tissue tumors account for less than 1% of all neoplasms. The annual clinical incidence of benign soft tissue tumors is 250 per 100,000 as compared with 3 per 100,000 for malignant ones. Moreover, according to Kransdorf, 70% of benign and 80% of malignant tumors can be classified in, respectively, six and seven "diagnostic categories" (Table 93-1).[3,4]

Age at presentation is a valuable diagnostic parameter. Seventy-nine percent of soft tissue tumors in children between birth and age 5 years are benign, as are 70%

KEY POINTS

- An analytical approach is preferred over an encyclopedic one for making a correct diagnosis or suitably ordered differential diagnosis in case of a soft tissue tumor.
- Although radiography, color Doppler ultrasonography, and CT may provide valuable information, MRI is the method of choice in analyzing soft tissue tumors (ACR appropriateness criteria).
- WHO recognizes four categories for STT: benign, intermediate (locally aggressive), intermediate (rarely metastasizing), and malignant. There is, however, no definite correlation between these four categories and findings on medical imaging.
- Differentiation between benign and malignant (grading) and making a tissue-specific diagnosis are based on combining parameters: prevalence, age at presentation, location, morphology, signal intensities on MRI, including fat suppression sequences, and administration of gadolinium chelates.
- Presence of intralesional calcifications/ossifications can indicate a correct tissue-specific diagnosis in a number of benign as well as malignant soft tissue tumors.
- Cytogenetics and molecular genetics play an increasing role in tissue-specific diagnosis. The radiologist is in a position to alert the treating physicians to the possibility that genetic studies may be indicated.
- A biopsy is necessary when the orthopedic surgeon and the radiologist believe they are dealing with a potentially malignant soft tissue tumors. Most biopsies are performed under imaging guidance, which requires close cooperation with the treating orthopedic surgeon, a thorough knowledge of compartmental anatomy, different biopsy techniques, and tissue sample fixation.

TABLE 93-1 Diagnostic Categories of Soft Tissue Tumors

80% of Malignant	70% of Benign
Myxofibrosarcoma	Lipoma(like)
Liposarcoma	Fibrous histiocytoma
Leiomyosarcoma	Nodular fasciitis
Malignant peripheral nerve sheath tumor	Hemangioma Fibromatosis
Synovial cell sarcoma	Neurofibroma-schwannoma
Fibrosarcoma	
Sarcoma NOS (not otherwise specified)	

Data from references 3 and 4.

TABLE 93-2 Most Common Tumors in Order of Prevalence

Children and Adolescents	Adults
Hemangioma	Lipoma
Fibrous hamartoma	Liposarcoma
Granuloma annulare	Myxofibrosarcoma
Lipoblastoma	
Fibrosarcoma	
Rhabdomyosarcoma	

TABLE 93-3 Preferential Sites of Soft Tissue Tumors

Tumor	Site
Giant cell tumor of tendon sheath	Hand (volar aspect)
Elastofibroma	Thoracic wall/subscapular region
Synovial hemangioma	Knee joint
Ganglion cyst	Periarticular wrist
Synovial cell sarcoma	Periarticular knee
Nodular fasciitis	Forearm
Fibrolipohamartoma	Median nerve
Abdominal desmoid	Rectus abdominis muscles
Xanthoma	Achilles tendon
Dermatofibrosarcoma protuberans	Subcutaneous compartment
Myxofibrosarcoma	Subcutaneous compartment
Glomus tumors	Subungual area of the finger tuft
Chondroma/osteochondroma	Infrapatellar fat pad
High-grade sarcomas	Thigh region
Alveolar soft part sarcoma	Anterior (extensor) compartment of the thigh

Data from De Schepper AM, Vanhoenacker F, Gielen J, Parizel P. Imaging of Soft Tissue Tumors, 3rd ed. Berlin, Springer Verlag, 2005.

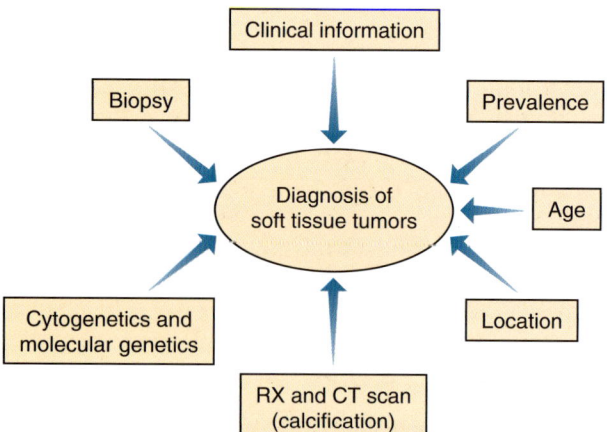

■ **FIGURE 93-1** Analytical approach to diagnosis of soft tissue tumors.

in those between 6 and 15 years of age. Fifty percent of the vascular tumors occur in patients younger than age 20 years. Embryonal rhabdomyosarcoma occurs almost exclusively in children, synovial sarcoma occurs mostly in young adults, whereas pleomorphic high-grade sarcoma, liposarcoma, and leiomyosarcoma dominate in the elderly.[1] Most common tumors are listed in Table 93-2.

A large number of soft tissue tumors have a preferential location in the human body (Fig. 93-2, Table 93-3; see reference 5 for a more complete list). The recognition of soft tissue tumors having a preferential location increases with the growing experience in the field, the organization of multi-institutional or national registries, and the publication of large series of specific tumor types.

CLINICAL PRESENTATION

Presence of clinical symptoms is related to the type of tumor (benign lesions are merely asymptomatic) and its location and extension. Small lesions are often asymptomatic and are discovered as incidental findings on CT or MRI.

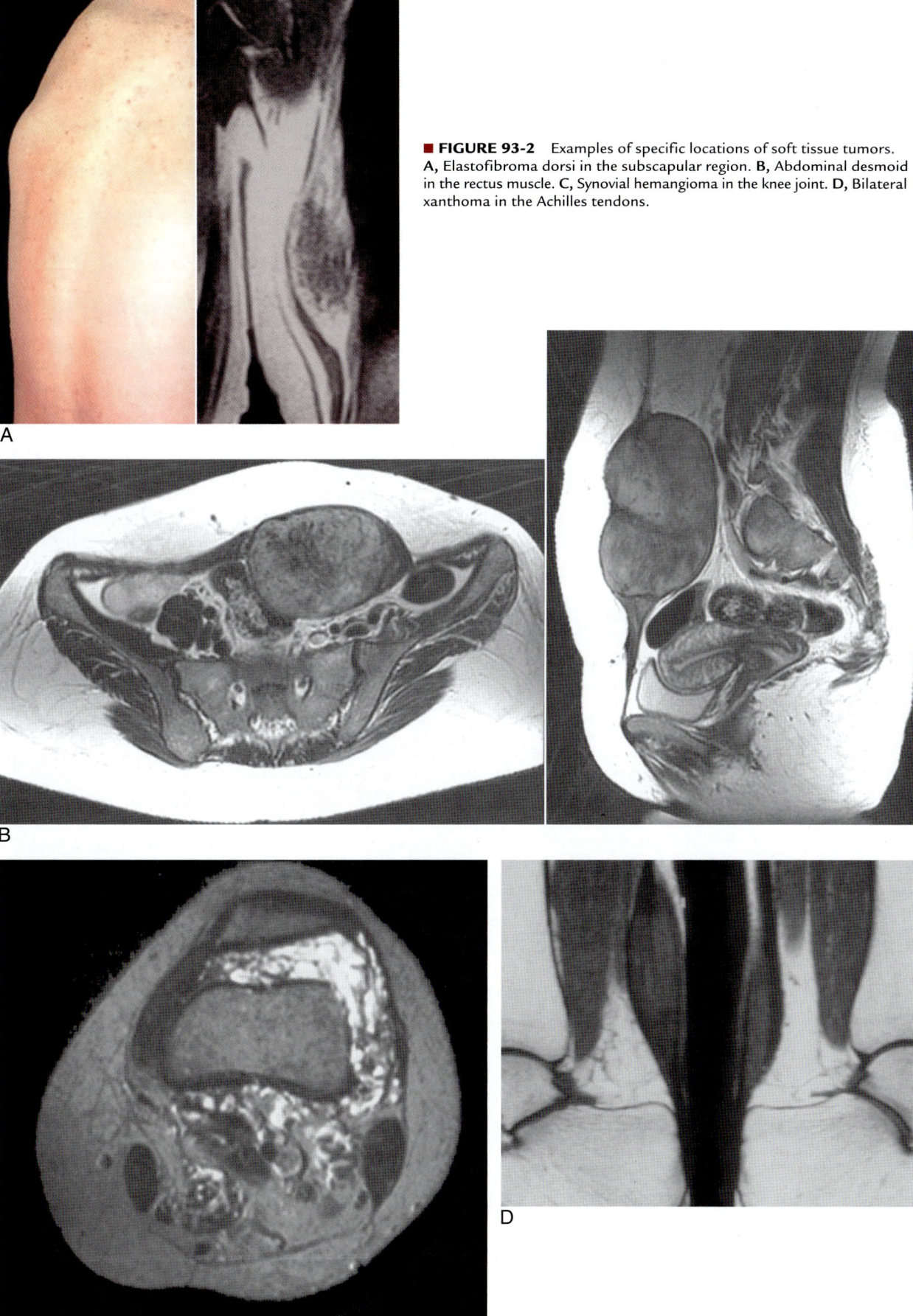

■ **FIGURE 93-2** Examples of specific locations of soft tissue tumors. **A,** Elastofibroma dorsi in the subscapular region. **B,** Abdominal desmoid in the rectus muscle. **C,** Synovial hemangioma in the knee joint. **D,** Bilateral xanthoma in the Achilles tendons.

Detection of a soft tissue nodule in a patient known to have a primary malignant tumor will raise the suspicion of a soft tissue metastasis.

Except for tumors of neurogenic origin, which may cause local or radiating pain and/or paresthesias, and except for metastases, multiple (angio)lipomas and angioleiomyomas,[1] which frequently present as locoregional pain, most soft tissue tumors, benign as well as malignant, tend to be painless. Clinical history may be relevant in Morton's neuroma (fibroma) and in systemic or concomitant diseases such as melanotic schwannoma in Carney's syndrome (cardiac myxoma, spotty pigmentation, and endocrine overactivity), cavernous hemangioma in Maffucci's syndrome (enchondromatosis), fibromatosis in Gardner's syndrome (intestinal polyposis, osteomata), xanthoma in familial hypercholesterolemia, myxoma in Mazabraud's syndrome (polyostotic fibrous dysplasia), amyloidoma in multiple myeloma, and neurofibromas and schwannomas in neurofibromatosis type II.

IMAGING TECHNIQUES

There is no controversy about the unequaled role of MRI along the whole diagnostic process of soft tissue tumors. Nevertheless, complementary information generated from other imaging modalities should not be neglected. In this regard, evaluation of a suspected soft tissue mass should always begin with conventional radiography. Valuable information may be derived from the presence of calcifications or ossifications, internal fatty components, and air and bone involvement. Although CT has been superseded by MRI for characterization of soft tissue tumors, it remains the best method for demonstrating subtle calcifications/ossifications (Figs. 93-3 and 93-4; Table 93-4). CT is also used for guiding biopsy and for the detection of (pulmonary) metastases.[5]

Ultrasonography is an important imaging technique in the initial assessment of a soft tissue swelling. In the majority of cases, it will establish the cystic/benign character of the swelling, obviating unnecessary further imaging workup. The drawback of ultrasonography is its nonspecificity in the setting of a hypoechoic, solid soft tissue mass. On the other hand, it is the most accessible and least time-consuming modality for imaged-guided biopsy (or aspiration) of superficially located lesions.[5] By depicting abnormal flow patterns, color Doppler ultrasonography may add specificity in the evaluation of soft tissue masses. Both high-systolic Doppler shifts with or without enhanced diastolic flow and low-impedance signals with little systolic-diastolic variation can be encountered in soft tissue sarcomas. Parameters based on changes in intratumoral blood flow and tumoral blood supply can be used

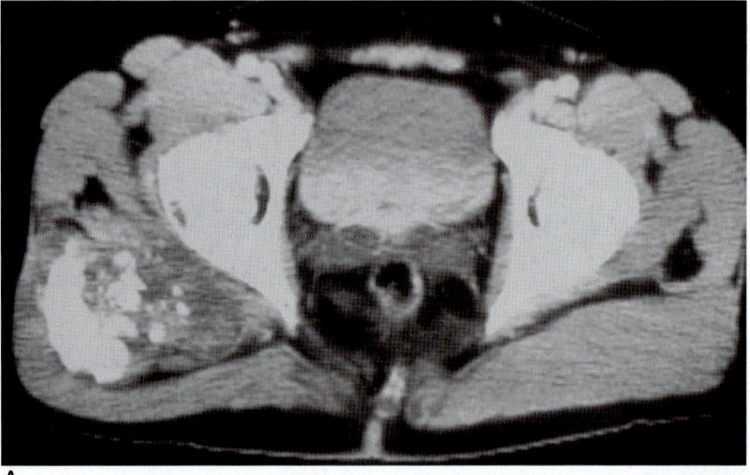

A

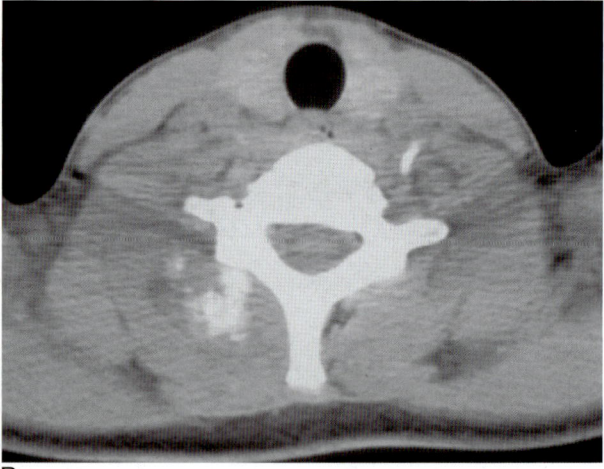

B

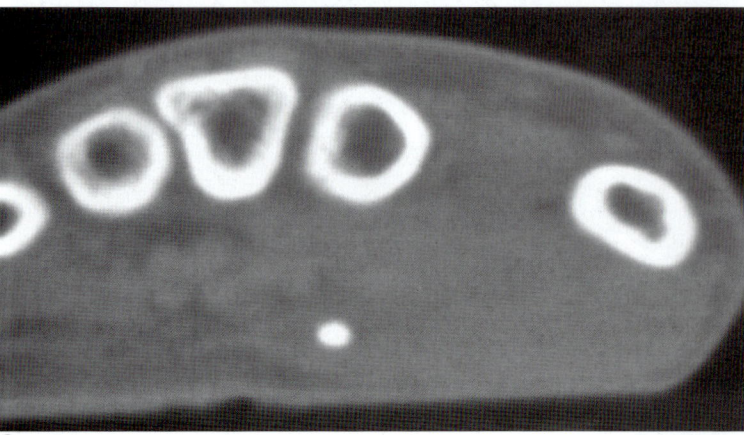

C

■ **FIGURE 93-3** **A,** Popcorn calcifications in a case of extraskeletal chondrosarcoma. **B,** Amorphous calcifications in a primitive neuroectodermal tumor involving the deep cervical muscles. **C,** Rounded phlebolith in a cavernous hemangioma.

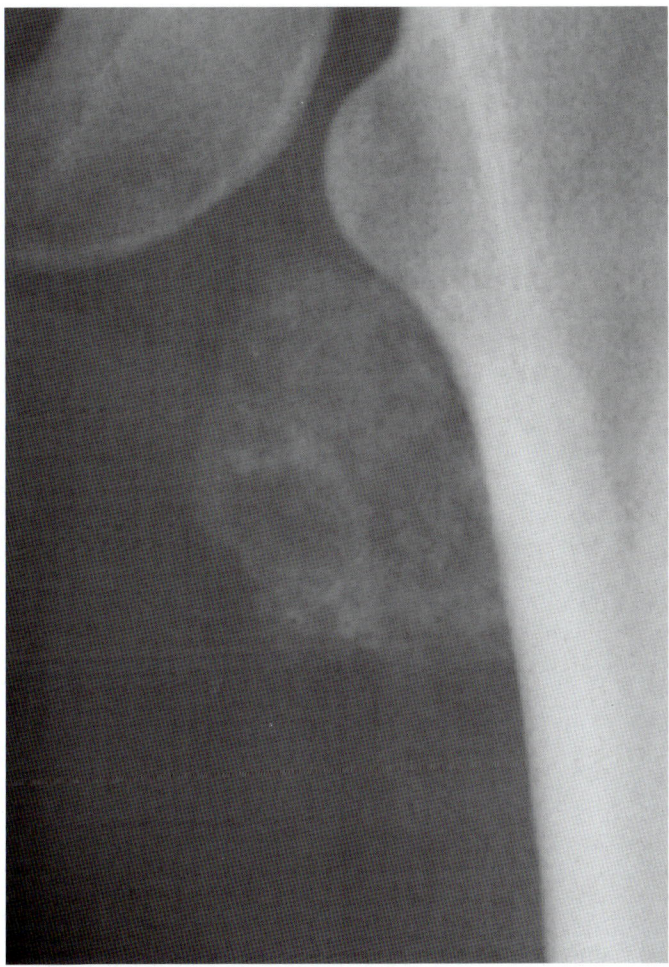

■ **FIGURE 93-4** Zonal calcification/ossification in a case of myositis ossificans.

to monitor the effect of preoperative systemic chemotherapy or isolated-limb perfusion in soft tissue sarcomas.[5] Angiography will only be used to preclude embolotherapy or in the case of isolated-limb perfusion chemotherapy.

The American College of Radiology (ACR) appropriateness criteria for diagnosis of a soft tissue mass vary according the clinical conditions. Radiography is the first appropriate imaging technique. If the radiograph is negative, MRI without (probably benign) or with (potentially malignant) contrast agent should be the next imaging technique used. If myositis ossificans is suspected on the radiograph, CT without contrast agents is appropriate if further analysis is needed. If the diagnosis of myositis ossificans cannot be confirmed, MRI including contrast enhancement has to be performed. When the mass is superficial or near a joint mass, MRI should also be performed. Ultrasonography could substitute for MRI, especially if a ganglion is suspected. In the case of an abdominal or chest wall soft tissue mass, radiography and contrast-enhanced CT are most appropriate. MRI may be less contributive owing to motion artifacts.

Although an MRI protocol for examining soft tissue tumors has to be flexible, use of a standard protocol is recommended (Table 93-5).

Differentiation between benign and malignant and definition of malignancy grade are also referred to as grading.[6] Histologic grading is considered the most powerful independent prognostic factor for local recurrence, metastasis, and overall survival in soft tissue tumors. Grading therefore also is important in treatment planning.

When a lesion is characterized by a high degree of cellularity, a small intercellular matrix, a high and atypical mitotic activity, extensive necrosis, vascular invasion, and high degree of pleomorphism, it is considered as a tumoral process with aggressive behavior (malignant). Using these histologic parameters, multiple grading systems have been conceived. Pathologic evaluation includes both macroscopic and microscopic inspection. Macroscopic examination, and MRI provide information on tumor size, relationship with adjacent anatomic structures, tumor heterogeneity, presence of necrosis, and hemorrhage. An integrated grading system, including MRI, however, does not exist. Still MR parameters that are indicative of malignancy have been identified and evaluated (Table 93-6).

The value of each individual parameter is too low, but sensitivity and specificity will increase by using a

TABLE 93-4	Calcifications/Ossifications in Soft Tissue Tumors and Pseudotumors	
Feature	**Benign Tumor**	**Malignant Tumor**
Popcorn, ring, and arc-like	Extraskeletal chondroma, synovial chondromatosis	Extraskeletal chondrosarcoma
Rounded or circular (phleboliths)	Hemangioma	
Peripheral	Myositis ossificans, panniculitis ossificans, fasciitis ossificans, extraskeletal aneurysmal bone cyst	
Ring-like	Calcific myonecrosis	
Cloud-like (mature trabecular bone)	Lipoma, low-grade liposarcoma, hemangioma	
Periosteal	Parosteal lipoma	
Amorphous	Chondroid lipoma and calcific tendinitis	Synovial sarcoma, extraskeletal osteosarcoma, primitive neuroectodermal tumor
Amorphous, cloud-like or stellar		Metastases of osteosarcoma
Multinodular	Tumoral calcinosis, juvenile hyaline fibromatosis, infantile myofibromatosis	
Linear and bridging	Fibroplasia ossificans progressiva	
Dense	Extraskeletal osteoma	
Stippled	Gout and pseudogout	

TABLE 93-5 Standard Protocol for Magnetic Resonance Imaging

Before Gadolinium Chelate Injection
Axial spin-echo T1 weighting
Axial spin-echo T1 weighting with fat suppression
Axial turbo spin-echo T2 weighting with fat suppression
After Gadolinium Chelate Injection
Dynamic Contrast Study
Axial spin-echo T1 weighting with fat suppression with subtraction
Sagittal or coronal spin-echo T1 weighting with fat suppression

TABLE 93-6 Magnetic Resonance Imaging Features in Favor of Malignancy

Large volume (>3 cm high sensitivity, >5 cm high specificity)
Located deep to fascia
Extracompartmental extension
Ill-defined margins
Broad contact with fascia
Inhomogeneity on all pulse sequences
High signal intensity on T2-weighted images
Invasion of bone and/or neurovascular bundle
Intralesional hemorrhage
Intralesional necrosis
Marked and merely peripheral enhancement (static contrast examination)
Fast enhancement, steep slope, long-standing plateau phase (dynamic contrast examination)

combination of multiple imaging parameters. In this regard, diagnostic accuracy, as reported in literature, is estimated between 30% and 80%. In a prospective study of 548 histologically verified soft tissue tumors, Gielen and colleagues obtained a sensitivity of 93%, a specificity of 82%, a negative predictive factor of 98%, and a positive predictive factor of 60% in differentiating between benign and malignant soft tissue tumors.[7] Even better results are obtained by van Rijswijk and associates, who used a multivariate logistic regression to identify the best combination of MRI parameters that might be predictive of malignancy and concluded that combined nonenhanced, static and dynamic contrast-enhanced MRI parameters were significantly superior to nonenhanced MRI parameters alone and to nonenhanced MRI parameters combined with static contrast-enhanced MRI parameters in prediction of malignancy. The most discriminating parameters were presence of liquefaction, start of dynamic enhancement (time interval between start of arterial and tumor enhancement), and the size of the lesion (diameter).[8]

In addition to differentiating benign from malignant soft tissue tumors, a specific diagnosis is also possible in specific circumstances. Kransdorf and colleagues stated in 1993 that "a correct histologic diagnosis reached on the basis of imaging studies is possible in only approximately one quarter of cases."[9] Gielen and coworkers, however, recently reported on a series of 548 histologically proven soft tissue tumors in which a correct tissue-specific diagnosis on MRI was made in 294 of 425 benign tumors (69%) and in 47 of 123 malignant tumors (38%).[7] It is important to realize that a specific diagnosis is more often possible in benign conditions than in malignant ones. Thus,

making a confident tissue-specific benign diagnosis may help in differentiating benign from malignant soft tissue tumors. The best results in tissue-specific diagnosis are obtained by using a combination of different parameters. The usefulness of prevalence, age at presentation, and zonal distribution (preferential location) has already been stressed. Morphology (i.e., the shape of the lesion) may be useful in making a specific diagnosis (Table 93-7).

Typically, soft tissue tumors have low signal intensity on T1-weighted images and high signal intensity on T2-weighted images. These common patterns are not helpful in making a specific diagnosis. Unusual signal intensities, that is, high signal intensity on T1 weighting and low signal intensity on T2 weighting, can frequently be used in making a specific diagnosis.

Intermediate to high signal intensity on T1 weighting, when compared with signal intensity of normal muscle, may indicate presence of fat (fatty components), methemoglobin in subacute hematomas, slow-flowing blood in cavernous hemangiomas and alveolar soft part sarcomas, high protein content in lymphangiomas, and melanin in metastases of malignant melanoma and clear cell sarcomas or deep-seated malignant melanomas.

A combination of low signal intensity on T1-weighted images and high signal intensity on T2-weighted images is seen in cystic lesions (ganglia) and all myxoid-containing tumors such as myxoma, fibromyxoid sarcoma, and the more frequent myxoid liposarcoma.[10]

Low signal intensity on T2-weighted images can be caused by fibrous tissue in desmoids and other fibromatoses, desoxyhemoglobin in acute hematomas, and hemosiderin in old hematomas, pigmented villonodular synovitis, and giant cell tumors of tendon sheath. Also, xanthomas and amyloidomas may present as low signal intensity on T2-weighted images. Low signal intensity can also be due to hypercellularity in high-grade malignancies and lymphomas. Calcifications (see also Table 94-4) or ossifications are seen in extraskeletal osteosarcomas, chondrosarcomas, and chondromatosis articularis and phleboliths occur in hemangiomas. Blooming effect on gradient-echo sequences is a consequence of susceptibility artifacts due to the presence of calcifications or ossifications or hemosiderin. Also, behavior after fat suppression can help in the identification of some tumors

TABLE 93-7 Morphology Related to Specific Diagnoses

Shape	Commonly Seen in
Fusiform, ovoid	Neurofibromas, lipomas
Multinodular, stellar, dumbbell	Desmoids
Moniliform	Neurofibromas, ganglion cysts
Rounded	Schwannomas, ganglion cysts
Serpiginous	Hemangiomas
Branching, finger-like	Plexiform neurofibromas
Broccoli-like, frond-like	Lipoma arborescens
Target sign*	Neurofibromas
Inverted target sign†	Nodular fasciitis, soft tissue metastases

*High signal intensity peripheral zone on T2-weighted images.
†Low signal intensity peripheral zone on T2-weighted images.

or tumor components. In this regard, myxoid-containing lesions show a relative decrease in signal intensity after fat suppression when compared with non–fat-suppressed T1-weighted imaging. Slow-flow hemangiomas, on the contrary, show a relative increase in signal intensity after fat suppression.[11]

Although a specific benign diagnosis can occasionally be made with high confidence, a biopsy is needed in the vast majority of patients. In general, a sample is taken using image guidance to allow a histologic diagnosis to be made. A biopsy is necessary when the orthopedic surgeon and the radiologist believe they are dealing with an unspecified, or even potentially malignant, soft tissue mass. Biopsy is not without risk because manipulation of the lesion may trigger different biologic behavior, such as dedifferentiation or progressive disease (e.g., in myositis ossificans) and complications related to all interventions (hemorrhage, infection). Moreover, biopsy of soft tissue tumors with large needles involves a risk of seeding malignant cells along the needle track. Because biopsy is considered part of the surgical therapy, en bloc resection of tumor and needle track is required. As a general rule, the shortest path between skin and the lesion should be chosen and the anticipated needle path should be discussed with the surgeon who will perform the definitive surgical treatment. The needle should not traverse uninvolved compartments.

Percutaneous musculoskeletal biopsy can be performed by fine-needle aspiration, core-needle biopsy, or open (incisional) biopsy. Excisional biopsy should be used only for small lesions (<3 cm) or when the radiologist is convinced that the lesion is benign.

Fine-needle aspiration biopsy essentially obtains cells without revealing their tissue architecture or matrix. Thus, one is able to study cytonuclear disturbances but no tumor differentiation or matrix components.[12] The pathologist is often only able to differentiate malignant from benign lesions. A core-needle biopsy, on the other hand, is able to provide tissue, including matrix, with preserved architecture. Open incisional biopsy also provides information about the reactive processes around the lesion.

The desired biopsy trajectory of a needle within the lesion itself depends on imaging features of the lesion. In homogeneous lesions, the trajectory is only dependent on compartmental anatomy. Therefore, knowledge of compartmental anatomy is mandatory for planning and executing percutaneous needle biopsies.[13] In nonhomogeneous lesions, a single long trajectory or two slightly angled trajectories that involve the same anatomic compartment are necessary. Biopsy samples have to be taken from contrast-enhancing areas, avoiding cystic, necrotic, or calcified components.

Fixation of the tissue sample is adapted to permit immunohistochemical characterization. A buffered 4% dilution of formalin (NF4) is recommended for tissue samples, and an alcoholic solution (Saccomano) is used for cell samples.

MANIFESTATIONS OF THE DISEASE

In this section, characteristics of the most important tumor types are presented in relation to imaging findings with emphasis on MRI.[5,14,15] Some non-neoplastic tumors

that are often included in the differential diagnosis of true soft tissue neoplasm are also discussed in this section. Most pseudotumors are discussed in Chapter 94.

Tumors of Connective Tissue

There is a large group of neoplastic and non-neoplastic mesenchymal tumors that share the presence of fibroblastic and/or myofibroblastic cells. The diversity of this group of tumors of connective tissue is important from a histologic perspective but less so from a radiologic perspective. The types are presented in Table 93-8, but only types that are relevant to radiology because of frequency or typical radiologic features are briefly discussed in this chapter.

Nodular Fasciitis

Nodular fasciitis is a benign non-neoplastic soft tissue lesion composed of fibroblastic-myofibroblastic cells that occurs mainly on the volar aspect of the upper arm in patients in their third to fourth decades of life.

The fascial type is the most common, the others being the subcutaneous and the intramuscular type. The MR signal intensity pattern reflects the cellular, myxoid, and fibrous components. More specific for nodular fasciitis is the "inverted target sign," which consists of a peripheral area of increased signal intensity on T1-weighted imaging,

TABLE 93-8 Tumors of Connective Tissue

Benign
Nodular fasciitis*
Proliferative fasciitis
Myositis ossificans
Fibro-osseous pseudotumor of digits
Ischemic fasciitis
Elastofibroma*
Inclusion body fibromatosis
Fibroma of tendon sheath
Desmoplastic fibroblastoma
Mammary type myofibroblastoma
Calcifying aponeurotic fibroma
Angiomyofibroblastoma
Cellular angiofibroma
Nuchal-type fibroma
Gardner fibroma
Calcifying fibrous tumor
Giant cell angiofibroma

Intermediate (locally aggressive)
Superficial fibromatosis*
Aggressive fibromatosis (desmoids)*
Lipofibromatosis

Intermediate (rarely metastasizing)
Solitary fibrous tumor*
Hemangiopericytoma
Inflammatory myofibroblastic tumor
Low-grade myofibroblastic sarcoma
Myxoinflammatory fibroblastic sarcoma
Infantile fibrosarcoma

Malignant
Adult fibrosarcoma*
Myxofibrosarcoma*
Low-grade fibromyxoid sarcoma
Sclerosing epitheloid fibrosarcoma

*Described in this chapter.

an inversion of signal intensity on T2-weighted imaging, and marked enhancement of the peripheral zone after administration of a contrast agent.[16]

Elastofibroma Dorsi

This benign pseudotumor consists of entrapped fat within a predominantly fibrous matrix. It occurs almost exclusively in the subscapular region, has an oval or lenticular shape, and can be bilateral in 10% to 60% of cases.

It is believed to be secondary to mechanical friction between the scapula and chest wall. MRI features consist of a nonhomogeneous but predominantly low signal intensity on all pulse sequences caused by intermingled fatty and fibrous components (see Fig. 93-2).[17]

Fibromatoses

Fibromatoses are non-neoplastic, fibroblastic proliferations that can be divided into superficial (mainly palmar and plantar fibromatosis) or deep fibromatosis (aggressive fibromatosis). The deep type, as opposed to the superficial types, displays a local aggressive growth pattern.

Palmar Fibromatosis

Palmar fibromatosis, also called Dupuytren contracture, affects adults, with a rapid increase in incidence with advancing age. It is bilateral in 40% to 60% of the cases. It consists of a nodule or cord in the palm of the hand that produces progressive flexion contracture of the fingers. Diagnosis is made by clinical history and examination. The cords have a uniformly low signal intensity on both T1- and T2-weighted MR images.

Plantar Fibromatosis

Plantar fibromatosis is located at the medial aspect of, and superficial to the plantar aponeurosis of the foot. It can be bilateral (20%) and multiple (32%). A male predominance is reported.

MR signal intensity pattern depends on the amount of fibrous versus cellular tissue and the age of the lesion. Most lesions are nonhomogeneous and of predominantly low signal intensity. Young lesions enhance moderately, older lesions to a lesser degree.[18]

Extra-abdominal Desmoid Tumors (Aggressive Fibromatosis)

This benign tumor with locally infiltrative growth is the most frequent tumor of connective tissue, with a peak incidence between 25 and 40 years of age. Its preferential locations are the deltoid muscle region, lower limb, and along the course of the sciatic nerve.

MRI presentation depends on age and composition of the lesion, but most of the lesions present as low signal intensity components, especially on T2-weighted imaging. These areas of low signal intensity, representing collagen, do not enhance after contrast agent administration. Areas of high signal intensity, representing more cellular components, show less or more prominent enhancement. A multicentric presentation with new lesions developing proximally in the limbs does occur. Because of the infiltrative growth pattern without a (pseudo)capsule, these lesions are microscopically connected. In that case, distal lesions are more collagenous (lower signal intensity on T2 weighting) whereas proximal lesions are more cellular and therefore biologically active (Figs. 93-5 to 93-9).[19]

Abdominal Fibromatosis

This rare fibroblastic lesion is commonly found within the musculoaponeurotic fascia of the anterior abdominal wall, especially of the rectus and oblique abdominal muscles. It mostly occurs in women. The lesion has a definite relationship with pregnancy, abdominal surgery, and

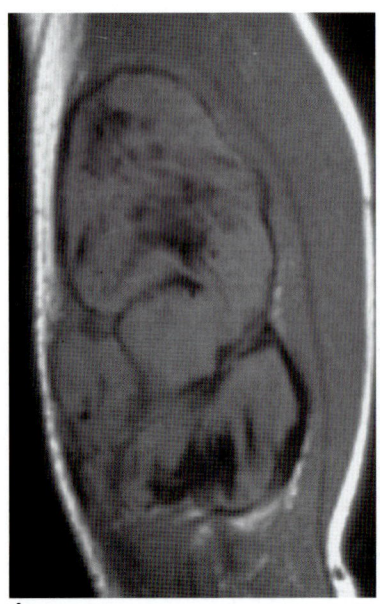 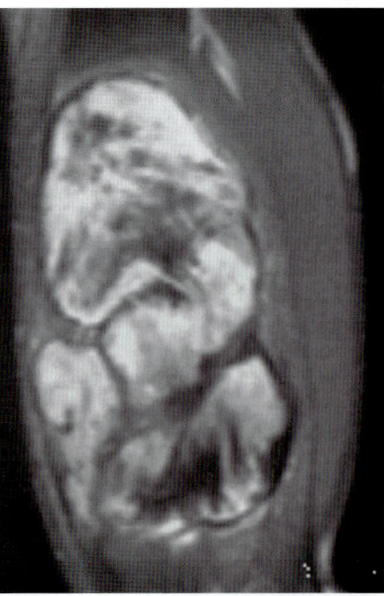

A   B

■ **FIGURE 93-5** Desmoid of the thigh. There are areas of low signal intensity on both T1- (**A**) and T2-weighted (**B**) sagittal MR images.

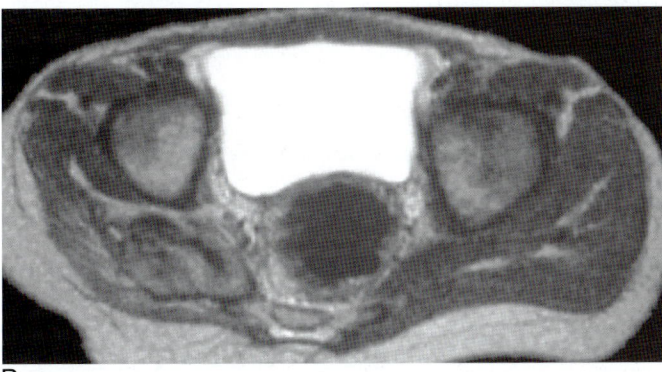

A

B

■ **FIGURE 93-6** Infantile fibromatosis in the right gluteal region in an 8-year-old boy. There are low signal intensity areas on both T1- (**A**) and T2-weighted (**B**) MR images. There is associated hypotrophy of the right gluteal muscles.

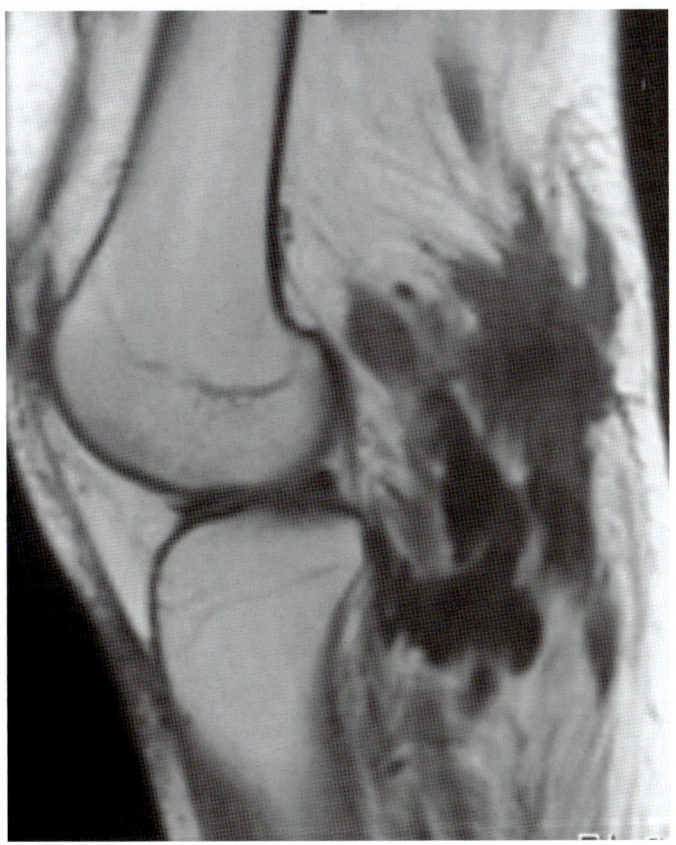

■ **FIGURE 93-7** Desmoid tumor of the popliteal fossa infiltrating toward the muscles, the subcutaneous compartment, and the paraperiosteal tissue. Although histologically benign, the lesion has an aggressive behavior (aggressive fibromatosis).

trauma. On MRI the lesion is of intermediate or low signal intensity on T2 weighting (see Fig. 93-2B).

Solitary Fibrous Tumor

This tumor belongs to the group of intermediate-grade fibromyoblastic tumors and consists of a mixture of hypocellular and hypercellular areas separated by thick bands of collagen and branching vessels. MRI features are nonspecific with intermediate signal intensity on both T1- and T2-weighted images.

Adult Fibrosarcoma

Fibrosarcomas are malignant soft tissue tumors composed of fibroblasts with variable collagen production. Preferential age for their occurrence is between 30 and 55 years, and they most often affect the thigh and knee region.

Differentiation between low- (well differentiated) and high-grade (poorly differentiated) fibrosarcoma is based on the degree of cellularity, cellular maturity, the amount of collagen produced by the tumor, and the presence of necrosis and/or intralesional hemorrhage.

MRI presentation consists of a low to intermediate signal intensity on T1 weighting and low signal intensity areas on a background of moderate to high signal intensity on T2 weighting. On postcontrast MR images there is frequently a peripheral and sometimes a "spokewheel" pattern of enhancement.

Myxofibrosarcoma

This tumor was formerly known as malignant fibrous histiocytoma and is one of the most frequent soft tissue tumors in adults. The mean age at presentation is 66 years. The subcutaneous compartment is the preferential location in more than 70% of the cases. Low-grade myxofibrosarcoma is defined by a large amount of myxoid tissue (>30%) and is more frequently superficially located. High-grade myxofibrosarcoma is defined by hypercellularity, high mitotic activity, pleomorphism, and intralesional necrosis and is usually located deep to the fascia.

MRI of low grade lesions reflects the high myxoid content and presents as low signal intensity on T1-weighted imaging and high signal intensity on T2-weighted imaging. High-grade lesions are indistinguishable from other pleomorphic soft tissue sarcomas (Figs. 93-10 and 93-11).[20]

Fibrohistiocytic Tumors

The neoplastic and non-neoplastic fibrohistiocytic tumors are subdivided into three categories (Table 93-9), but only types that are relevant to radiology because of frequency or typical radiologic features are briefly discussed in this chapter.

Giant cell tumor of tendon sheath and pigmented villonodular synovitis are the most frequent in the group of benign lesions, whereas dermatofibrosarcoma protuberans is the most frequently one seen in the group of intermediate malignancy.

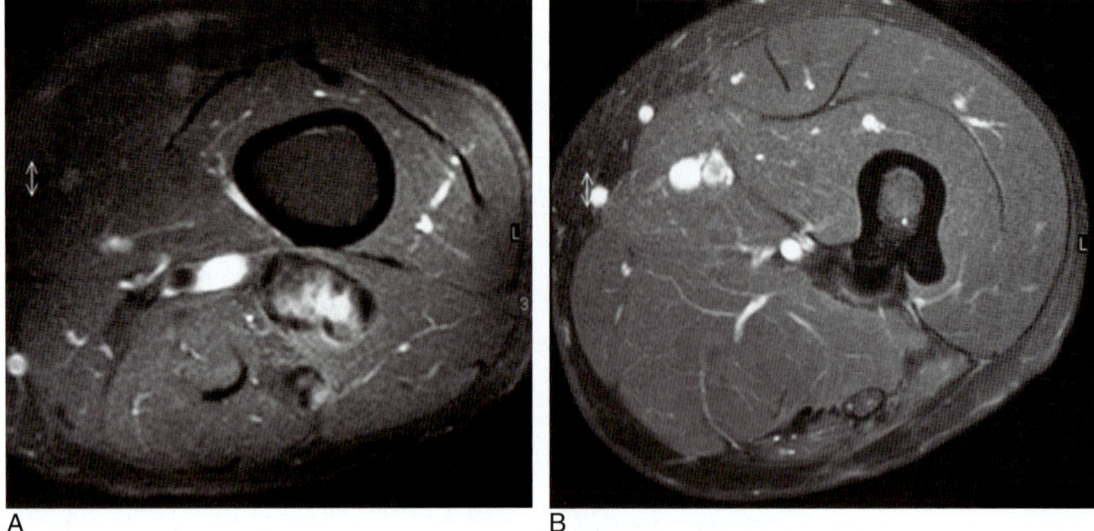

■ **FIGURE 93-8** **A,** Desmoid tumor of the flexor compartment of the thigh, with characteristic low signal intensity areas on a T2-weighted MR image. At a higher level there is a second desmoid tumor, superficially at the hamstrings. **B,** At the same level there is an exostosis at the posterior aspect of the femoral diaphysis. The association of multiple desmoids and an exostosis is seen in Gardner's syndrome.

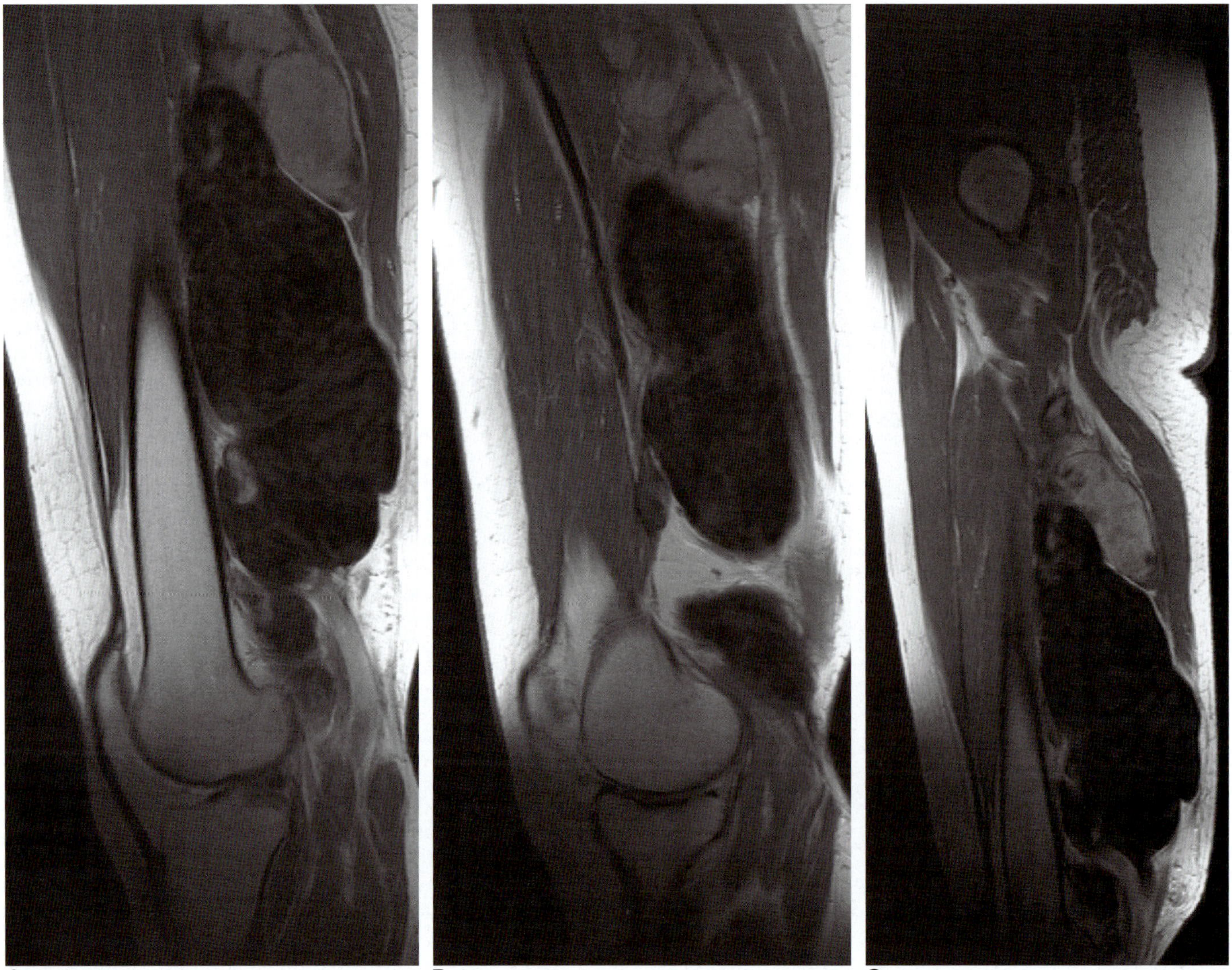

■ **FIGURE 93-9** A to C, Desmoid tumor at the flexor compartment of the thigh with a characteristic evolution from highly cellular to collagenous and also with a characteristic centripetal migration pattern. All three images are obtained after intravenous administration of contrast material. There is enhancement of the proximal, noncollagenous components and no enhancement of the distal, collagenous components.

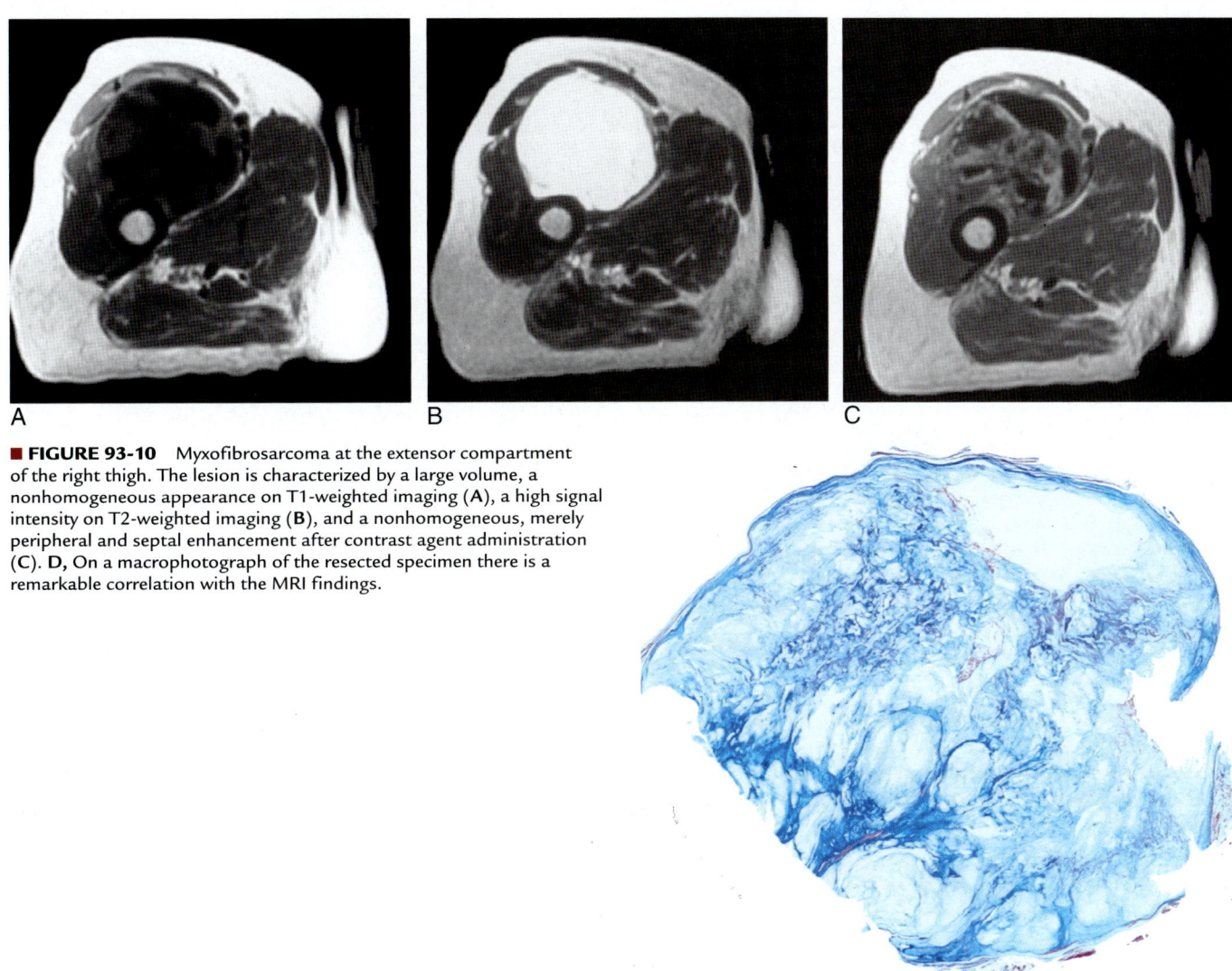

■ **FIGURE 93-10** Myxofibrosarcoma at the extensor compartment of the right thigh. The lesion is characterized by a large volume, a nonhomogeneous appearance on T1-weighted imaging (**A**), a high signal intensity on T2-weighted imaging (**B**), and a nonhomogeneous, merely peripheral and septal enhancement after contrast agent administration (**C**). **D,** On a macrophotograph of the resected specimen there is a remarkable correlation with the MRI findings.

Giant Cell Tumor of Tendon Sheath

This tumor consists of a circumscribed proliferation of synovial-like mononuclear cells, accompanied by a variable number of multinucleate osteoclast-like cells, foam cells, siderophages (hemosiderin deposition), and inflammatory cells, histologically similar to pigmented villonodular synovitis. The lesion is hypervascular with numerous proliferative capillaries in the collagenous stroma and is covered by a fibrous capsule. It is a small (0.5 to 4 cm), nodular, or polylobular, painless, slowly growing mass, mostly located at the flexor tendons of the fingers (67%-85%), adjacent or circumferential to the synovium of the tendon sheath. It mostly occurs in the third to fourth decade, with a 2:1 female predominance.

Findings on radiography and CT are soft tissue mass, pressure erosion/atrophy (15%) on adjacent osseous structures, true bone invasion, cortical defect, extension into the medullary cavity, cystic changes, periosteal reaction, and, rarely, intralesional calcification. Findings on MRI are a round, oval, or polylobular solid mass, eccentric to, or enveloping, the tendon sheath, with intermediate signal intensity on T1-weighted images, low signal intensity on T2-weighted images (reflecting the presence of collagen and hemosiderin), and marked enhancement on contrast enhanced T1-weighted images (Figs. 93-12 and 93-13).[21]

Pigmented Villonodular Synovitis

There is a diffuse, intra-articular form of pigmented villonodular synovitis that is monarticular and involves the knee in 80% of cases; a localized, more nodular and extra-articular form has a predilection for the infrapatellar fat

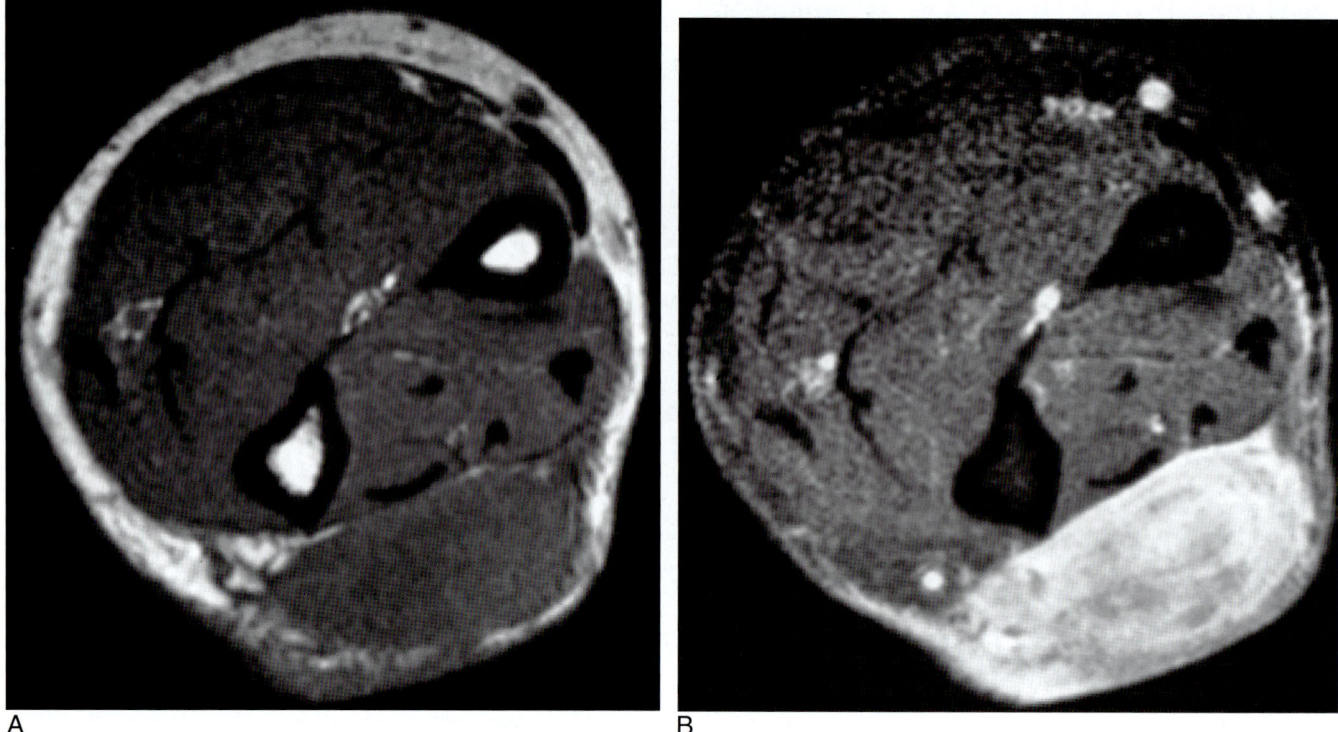

A   B

■ **FIGURE 93-11** Myxofibrosarcoma at the subcutaneous compartment of the forearm. The lesion is of low signal intensity on T1 weighting (**A**) and high signal intensity on T2 weighting (**B**) and is heterogeneous on both sequences.

TABLE 93-9	Fibrohistiocytic Tumors

Benign
Giant cell tumor of tendon sheath*
Pigmented villonodular synovitis*
Xanthoma*
Juvenile xanthogranuloma
Reticulohistiocytoma
Benign fibrous histiocytoma
Intermediate Malignancy
Dermatofibrosarcoma protuberans*
Bednar tumor
Plexiform fibrohistiocytic tumor
Giant cell fibroblastoma
Angiomatoid fibrous histiocytoma
Giant cell tumor of soft tissues
Malignant
Atypical fibroxanthoma
Malignant fibrous histiocytoma*

_____

*Described in this chapter.

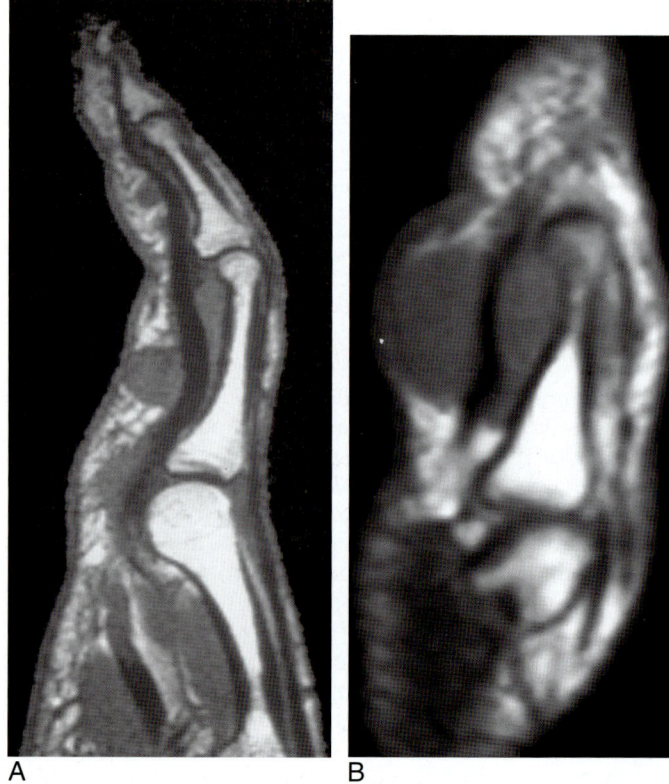

A   B

■ **FIGURE 93-12** **A** and **B,** Two examples of giant cell tumor of tendon sheath, adjacent to or wrapped around the flexor tendons of the fingers. All lesions are of low to intermediate signal intensity on T2 weighting.

pad. Pigmented villonodular synovitis, which is histologically similar to giant cell tumors of the tendon sheath, presents as finger-like hyperplasia of the synovium (diffuse form) or with a more nodular appearance (localized form). Both kinds of lesions contain intracellular and extracellular hemosiderin (yellow to yellow-brown).

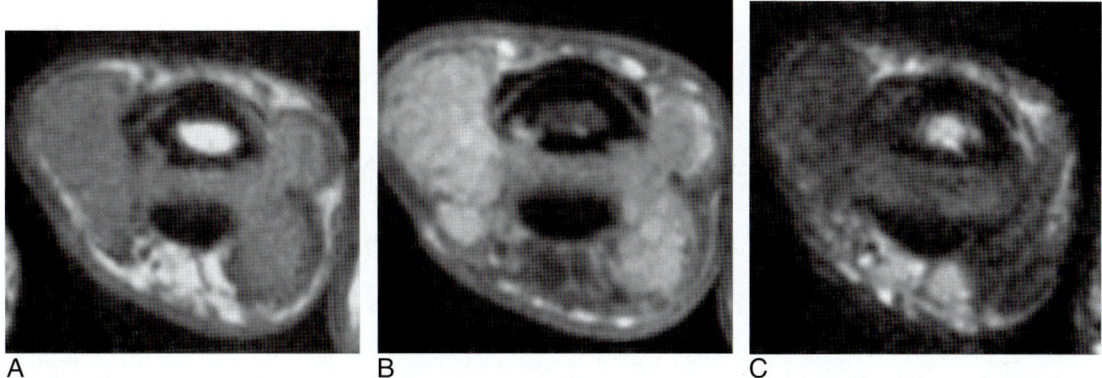

■ **FIGURE 93-13** Giant cell tumor of tendon sheath. Dumbbell-shaped lesion in between bone and flexor tendon of the finger. The lesion is of intermediate signal intensity on T1 weighting (**A**), enhances markedly after contrast agent administration (**B**), and has a low signal intensity on T2 weighting (**C**).

On radiography, concomitant bone erosions with sclerotic margins may be present and are more obvious in joints with a tight capsule, such as the hip (Fig. 93-14).

There are characteristic MRI features due to the abundance of hemosiderin, causing low signal intensity on all pulse sequences, especially on T2-weighted images, and a "blooming" effect on gradient-echo sequences. This is more pronounced at high field strengths and a consequence of signal loss due to local changes in susceptibility. After contrast agent administration lesions enhance to a moderate or marked degree (Fig 93-15; also see Fig 93-14).[22]

Xanthoma

Tendinous xanthomas especially of the Achilles tendons are the hallmark of familial hypercholesterolemia. On histology, the picture is dominated by collagenous fibers, separated by broad sheets of foamy histiocytes that contain cholesterol, cholesterol esters, triglycerides, and phospholipids.

Ultrasonography will depict the number and extent of focal intratendinous lesions. MRI findings consist of a mass of low signal intensity in which a reticulated or speckled network of high signal intensity can be appreciated on T2-weighted images. Normal tendon and cholesterol are of low signal intensity, whereas the high signal intensity lines are secondary to presence of triglycerides. On fat-suppressed, T1-weighted MRI the signal of xanthomas is only partly suppressed because 80% of the lesion is made up of liquid cholesterol and cholesterol esters.

Dermatofibrosarcoma Protuberans

Dermatofibrosarcoma protuberans accounts for 6% of all soft tissue sarcomas. Preferential locations are the trunk, head, and neck. The lesions are originally located in the dermis and subcutis. The "protuberant" character is seen at the end stage. Patients are mostly in the first to fifth decade, and there is a definite male preponderance. On histology, lesions present with myxoid components and hemorrhagic and cystic changes. The lesion has a tendency to recur in 50% of patients after surgery.

The MRI presentation is, apart from location and morphology of the exophytic components, nonspecific, showing low signal intensity on T1-weighted images and high signal intensity on T2-weighted images.

Malignant Fibrous Histiocytoma

As a result of recent cytogenetic studies, the term *malignant fibrous histiocytoma* has been partly abandoned in the new WHO classification of soft tissue neoplasms and the formerly named *malignant fibrous histiocytomas* are now renamed as undifferentiated pleomorphic sarcomas (formerly giant cell malignant fibrous histiocytoma) and myxofibrosarcoma (formerly myxoid malignant fibrous histiocytoma). The MRI appearance is not specific.

Lipomatous Tumors

Lipoma

Lipoma is the most common mesenchymal tumor. It is a painless, slow growing, well-circumscribed, encapsulated mass composed of mature fat. It affects patients in the fifth to seventh decades. It may be superficially or deeply located and intermuscular or intramuscular. Parosteal lipoma (Fig. 93-16), also called periosteal lipoma, is located adjacent to cortical bone with or without concomitant bony excrescence.

On ultrasonography the lesion is compressible and mostly hyperechogenic (75%). It has a low attenuation value (−100 HU) on CT. On MRI, the lesion is of homogeneous high signal intensity on T1 weighting and intermediate signal intensity on T2 weighting, and does not enhance after contrast agent administration. Thin septa between the fatty lobules may be seen on CT as well on MRI and may enhance slowly (>6 seconds after arterial enhancement) (Fig. 93-17).[23]

Chondroid Lipoma

Chondroid lipoma is a rare lipomatous tumor, containing fatty, myxoid, and cartilaginous components and, more

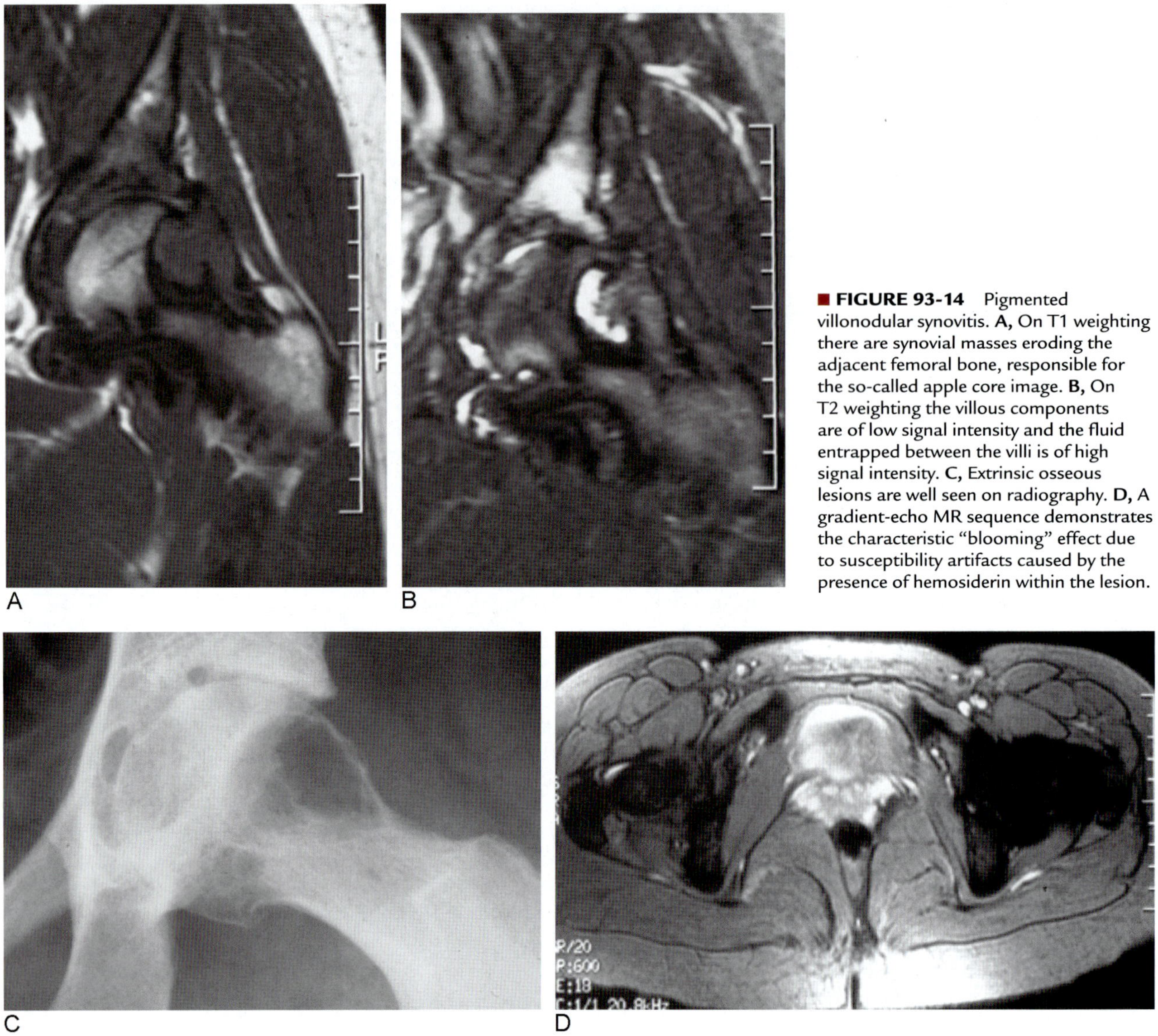

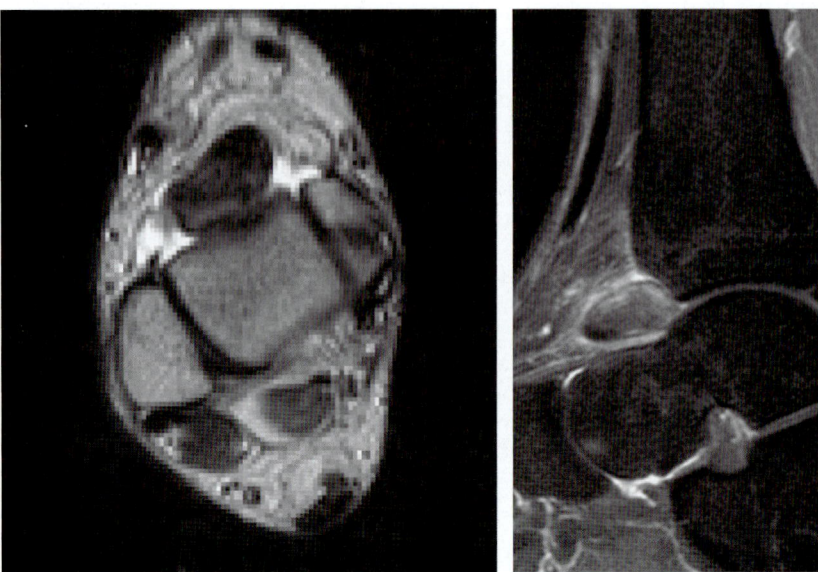

■ **FIGURE 93-14** Pigmented villonodular synovitis. **A,** On T1 weighting there are synovial masses eroding the adjacent femoral bone, responsible for the so-called apple core image. **B,** On T2 weighting the villous components are of low signal intensity and the fluid entrapped between the villi is of high signal intensity. **C,** Extrinsic osseous lesions are well seen on radiography. **D,** A gradient-echo MR sequence demonstrates the characteristic "blooming" effect due to susceptibility artifacts caused by the presence of hemosiderin within the lesion.

A

B

C

D

■ **FIGURE 93-15** Localized form of pigmented villonodular synovitis of the anterior recess of the ankle joint. The lesion is of low signal intensity on axial T2 weighting (**A**) and has low signal intensity areas on the sagittal, fat-suppressed, T2-weighted image (**B**).

A

B

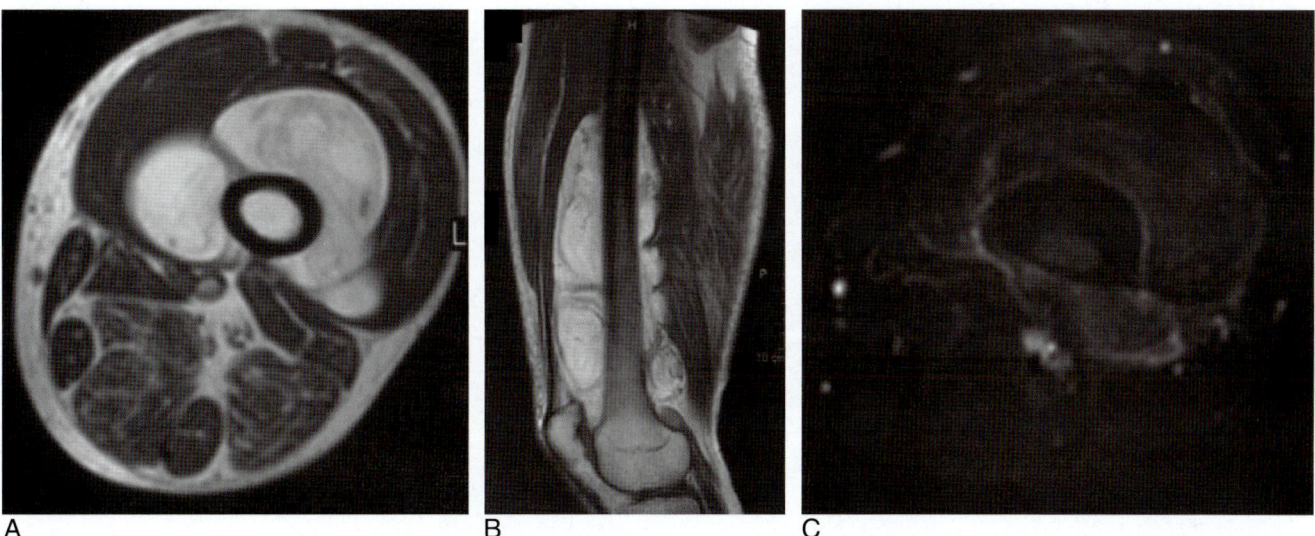

■ **FIGURE 93-16** Parosteal, low-grade liposarcoma. Axial (**A**) and sagittal spin-echo (**B**) T1-weighted MR images show polylobular mass lesion enveloping the femoral diaphysis without osseous or surrounding soft tissue involvement. Interlobular septa are of lower signal intensity. **C,** Axial, fat-suppressed, spin-echo T1-weighted MR image after administration of gadolinium shows area of high signal intensity components suppressed; intervening septa enhance moderately and remain of intermediate signal intensity.

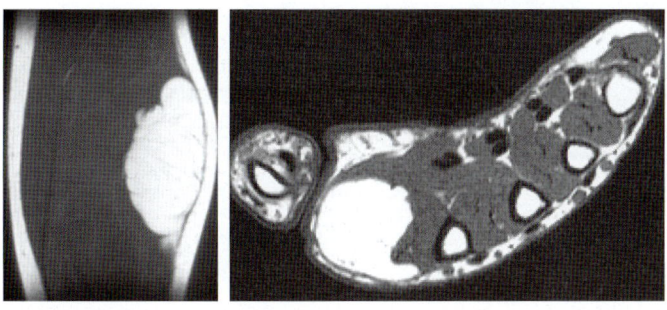

■ **FIGURE 93-17** Two cases of usual lipoma. Both lesions are superficially located, homogeneous, well delineated and of high signal intensity comparable with signal intensity of normal fat on T1-weighted MRI.

specifically, irregular and curvilinear calcifications. It may mimic myxoid liposarcoma.

It is mostly of low signal intensity with a few high signal intensity components (fat) on T1-weighted images. Signal intensity is inhomogeneous and high on T2-weighted images. Enhancement is nonhomogeneous and slow (>6 seconds after arterial enhancement) (Fig. 93-18).[24]

Lipoblastoma

Lipoblastoma is a well-encapsulated lesion, confined to the subcutis and containing lipoblasts in different stages of development. When it is more infiltrative it is called lipoblastomatosis. Eighty-eight percent occur in patients younger than 3 years of age, and boys are more affected than girls. It is a painless lesion, mostly seen in the extremities.

Presentation on MRI varies according to the amount of lipomatous versus nonlipomatous components. It is mostly hyperintense on both T1- and T2-weighted imaging. Myxoid components present with rather low signal intensity on T1-weighted imaging and high signal intensity on T2-weighted imaging. There is little and slow (>6 seconds after arterial enhancement) enhancement after contrast agent administration (Fig. 93-19).[25]

Lipoma of Tendon Sheath and Joint

The first form is a lipomatous mass spreading along the tendon sheaths; the second form is an intra-articular lipomatous lesion consisting of hypertrophic synovial villi distended by fat that replaces the subsynovial tissue. This lesion, called "lipoma arborescens," is more common than the tendon sheath variety. The first form is preferentially located at the wrist, the second form at the knee (Fig. 93-20). On MRI the first form presents as a peritendinous fatty mass, with signal intensity characteristics of a usual lipoma; the second form is a frond-like fatty mass arising from the synovium and associated with joint effusion.[26]

Lipomatosis of Nerve (Fibrolipomatous Hamartoma)

This lesion consists of a proliferation of fatty and fibrous components surrounding the thickened nerve bundles that infiltrate both the epineurium and the perineurium. It occurs mainly at the volar aspect of the hand and wrist and usually involves the median nerve. It may be associated with macrodactyly. On MRI, the contrast between the low signal intensity of the nerve fascicles and surrounding high-signal fat results in a so-called fascicular appearance on axial images and a spaghetti-like appearance on longitudinal planes (Fig. 93-21).[27]

Diffuse Lipomatosis

This is a group of rare diseases in which multiple symmetric lipomatosis or Madelung's disease is the most frequent. It is characterized by massive symmetric deposition of mature fat in the neck.

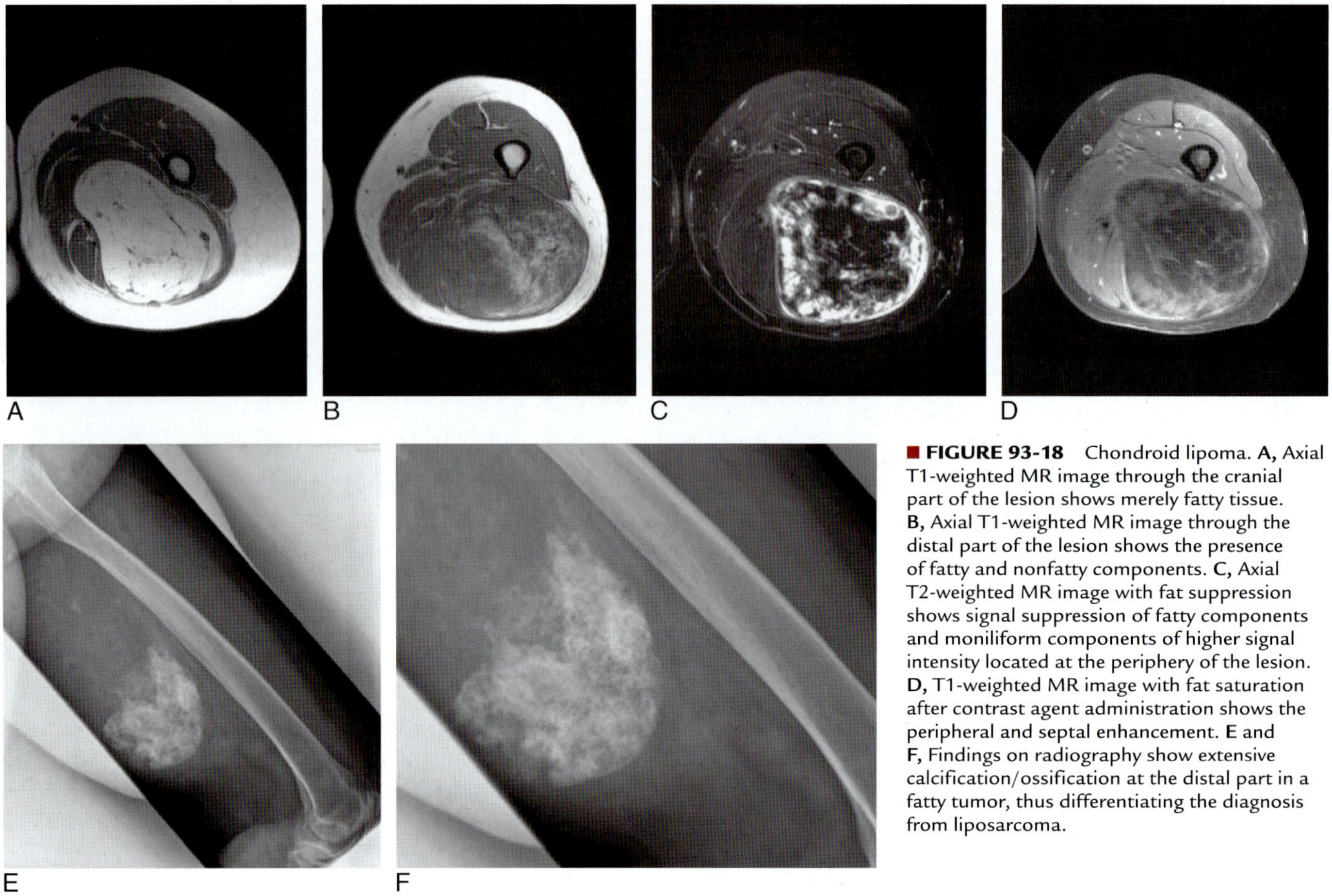

■ **FIGURE 93-18** Chondroid lipoma. **A,** Axial T1-weighted MR image through the cranial part of the lesion shows merely fatty tissue. **B,** Axial T1-weighted MR image through the distal part of the lesion shows the presence of fatty and nonfatty components. **C,** Axial T2-weighted MR image with fat suppression shows signal suppression of fatty components and moniliform components of higher signal intensity located at the periphery of the lesion. **D,** T1-weighted MR image with fat saturation after contrast agent administration shows the peripheral and septal enhancement. **E** and **F,** Findings on radiography show extensive calcification/ossification at the distal part in a fatty tumor, thus differentiating the diagnosis from liposarcoma.

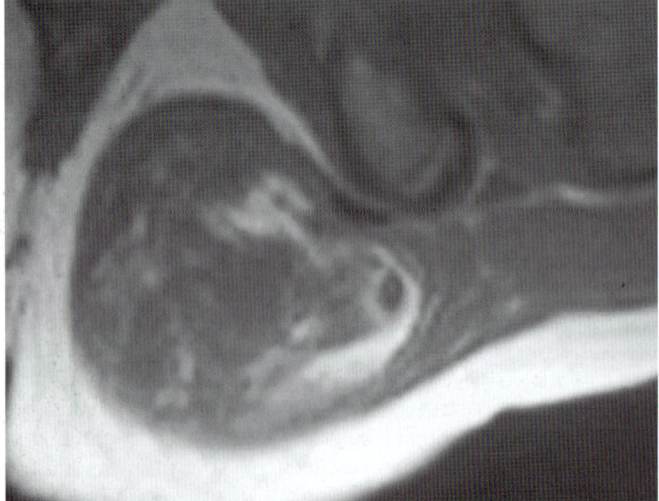

■ **FIGURE 93-19** Lipoblastoma at the gluteus muscle protruding into the ischiorectal fossa. On this T1-weighted MR image the lesion is nonhomogeneous with interspersed areas of high signal intensity that are similar to that of fat.

Hibernoma

This rare benign tumor contains brown fat, which on MRI presents as a heterogeneous or septated mass, with high signal intensity on T1-weighted images. The signal intensity, however, is lower than that of normal fat. The signal intensity is variable on T2-weighted images. Enhancement is nonhomogeneous and moderate. The clue to the diagnosis is that fat-suppression techniques fail to suppress the signal of fat because of the nature and the amount of lipids (Fig. 93-22).[28]

Malignant Lipomatous Tumors

Liposarcoma is the second most common soft tissue sarcoma. There are four subtypes, but in up to 10% of cases at least two histologic types are combined into the fifth subtype: mixed type liposarcoma. Liposarcomas are mostly located deep to the fascia and enhance fast (within 6 seconds after arterial enhancement on dynamic MRI), and the amount of fat that can be identified on MRI decreases from almost exclusively fatty tissue to no fat exhibited on MRI when moving from low- to high-grade liposarcoma. The well-differentiated subtypes are more common than the high-grade subtypes (atypical lipoma, 48%; myxoid liposarcoma, 21%).

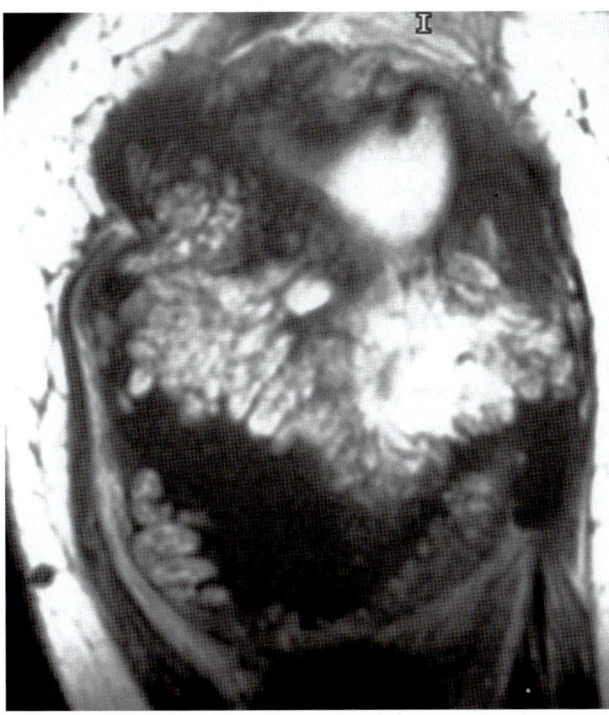

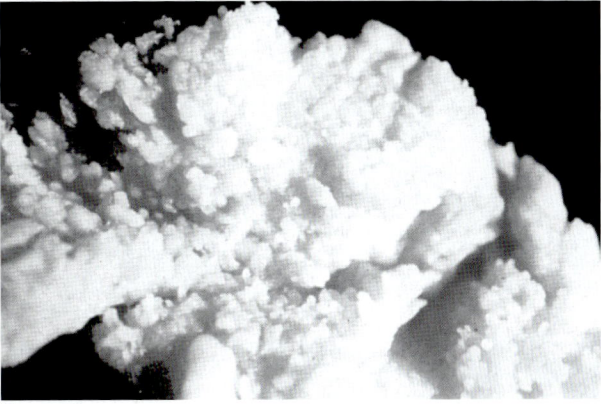

■ **FIGURE 93-20** Lipoma arborescens. **A,** On a coronal T1-weighted MR image there is a frond-like synovial mass that has the same signal intensity as subcutaneous fat. **B,** A macrophotograph shows the villous synovial proliferations.

■ **FIGURE 93-21** Lipomatosis of the median nerve (fibrolipohamartoma). Fibrous and fatty components are responsible for the mixed signal intensity of the lesion on T1- (**A**) and T2-weighted (**B**) MR images. Longitudinally coursing nerve bundles are responsible for the fascicular sign on axial images (**A**, **B**) and for the spaghetti-like appearance on the longitudinal image (**C**). **D,** Perioperative photograph shows the enlarged median nerve.

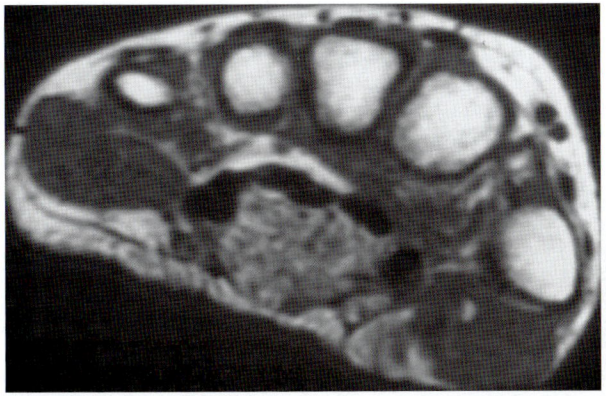

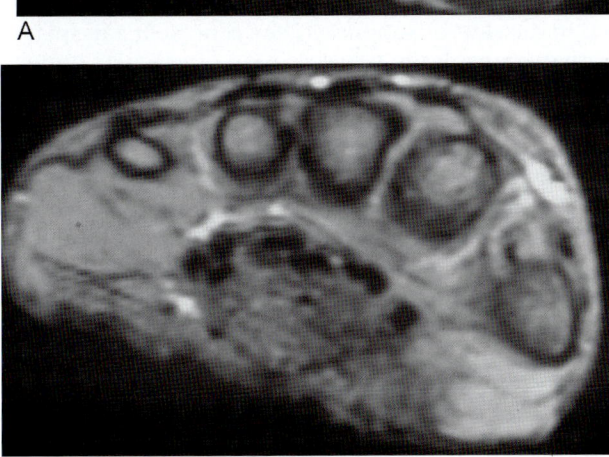

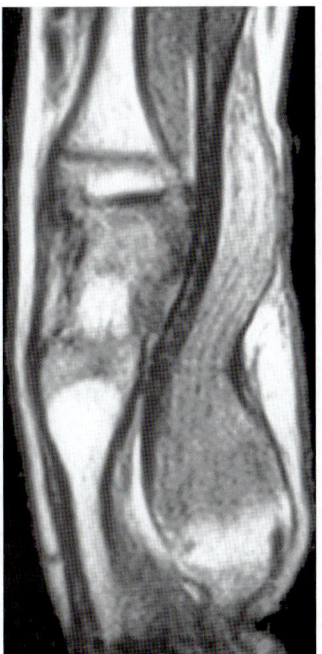

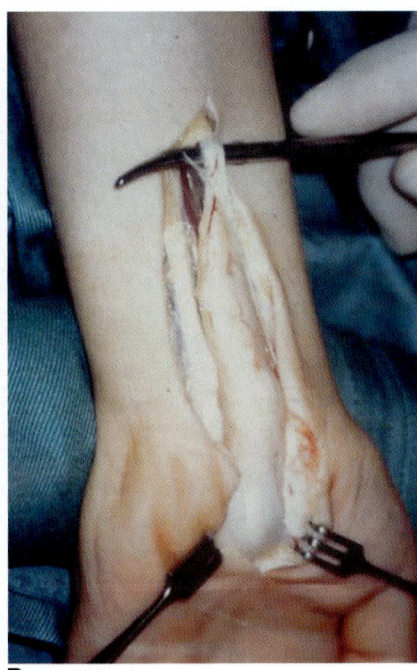

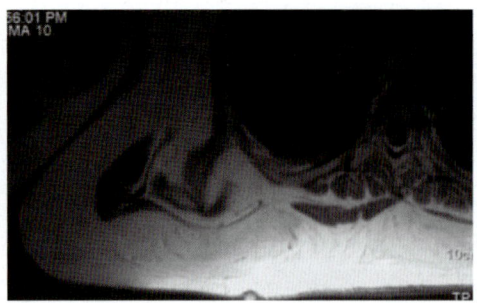

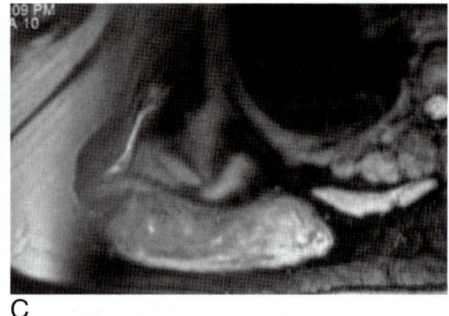

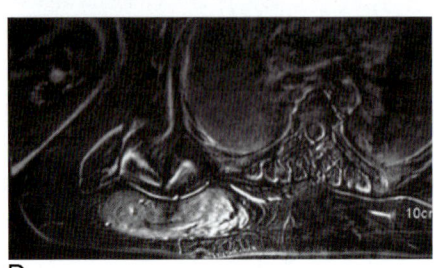

■ **FIGURE 93-22**   Hibernoma of the trunk. **A,** On T1 weighting the lesion is slightly hypointense when compared with signal intensity of normal subcutaneous fat. **B,** Degree and pattern of enhancement are difficult to judge on contrast-enhanced T1 weighting without fat saturation. **C,** Enhancement is well appreciated on T1 weighting with fat suppression. **D,** Enhancement is confirmed on a subtraction image. Signal intensities and behavior after contrast agent administration allow the differentiation of the lesion from a usual lipoma.

Atypical Lipomatous Tumor, Well-Differentiated Liposarcoma, or Lipoma-like Liposarcoma

This tumor grossly resembles lipoma, but besides variably sized fat cells (>75%) it consists of scattered lipoblasts, broad fibrous septa, and thick-walled blood vessels. On MRI the bulk of the tumor has signal intensities comparable with signal intensities of normal fat. Thick, or even nodular fibrous septa of low signal intensity on T1-weighted imaging and of high signal intensity on T2-weighted imaging are appreciated. These thick septations enhance fast (within 6 seconds after arterial enhancement) after contrast agent administration.

Myxoid Liposarcoma

This tumor is characterized by a basophilic myxoid matrix or ground substance that accounts for more than 90% of the tumoral mass. The thigh and buttocks are preferential locations. Frequently, there is no radiologic evidence of fat because of the small amount of mature fat in this subtype. This makes a tissue-specific diagnosis difficult. On MRI, minute fatty components present as signal intensities of normal fat; myxoid components are of low signal intensity on T1-weighted images and very high signal intensity on T2-weighted images. After contrast agent injection, there is a variable degree of enhancement allowing differentiation with cystic (non-enhancing) lesions (Fig. 93-23).

Pleomorphic and Round Cell Liposarcoma

These high-grade subtypes contain variable amounts of fatty, myxoid, and cellular tissue. Round cell liposarcoma is currently classified as a subgroup of myxoid liposarcoma (high-grade myxoid liposarcoma with round cell component). MR signal intensities reflect their mixed composition. They are heterogeneous on all pulse sequences and show a marked, also nonhomogeneous enhancement (Fig. 93-24).

Dedifferentiated Liposarcoma

Dedifferentiation occurs as a late complication of a preexisting, well-differentiated liposarcoma, most commonly of the retroperitoneum, mediastinum, or groin. Dedifferentiation mostly occurs into myxofibrosarcoma and should be suspected when areas within a preexisting tumor exhibit signal intensities other than those commonly seen in fatty tissue.[29]

Tumors of Vascular Origin

The majority of vascular tumors are benign and are located in the skin or subcutis. They represent a dysplasia rather than a neoplasm. Classification of vascular tumors is compromised by confusion secondary to the various classification systems that are being used. The oldest classification system is that of Mulliken, which was updated in 1992 by the International Society for the Study of Vascular Anomalies (ISSVA). It is based on endothelial growth characteristics and correlates well with clinical and imaging findings. It distinguishes between hemangioma (cellular proliferation, small or absent at birth, rapid growth during infancy, spontaneous involution during childhood) and vascular malformations (dysplastic vessels, present at birth, grows with the child, no spontaneous regression). Vascular malformations can be subdivided into subtypes depending on composition: capillary, venous, arterial,

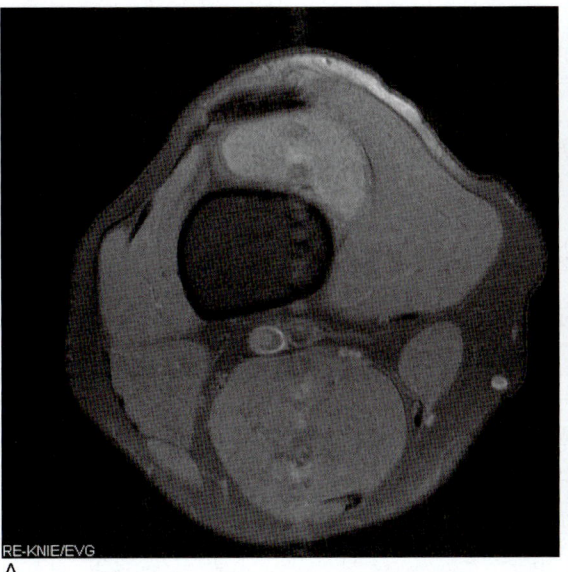 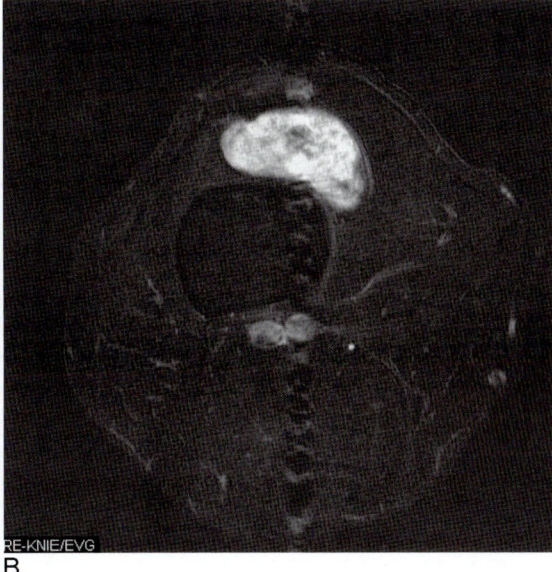

■ **FIGURE 93-23** Myxoid liposarcoma. **A,** There are no obvious fatty components within the lesion and as a consequence, no tissue signal suppression on T1 weighting with fat suppression. **B,** The lesion is of high signal intensity on T2 weighting owing to the abundance of myxoid substance.

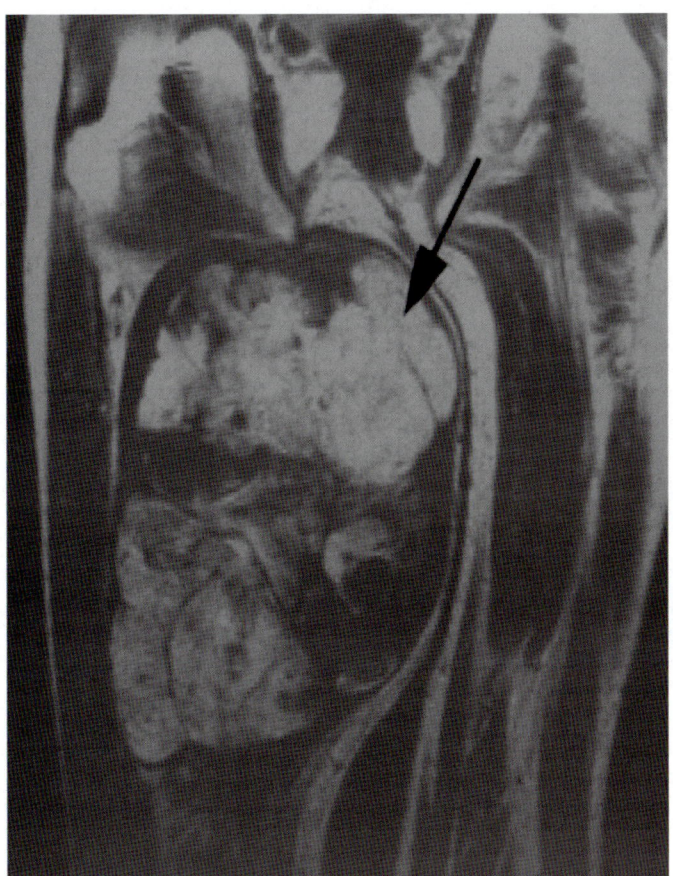

■ **FIGURE 93-24** Pleomorphic liposarcoma of the thigh region with components of high (*arrow*), intermediate, and low signal intensity on T1 weighting.

and lymphatic. Usually, combinations occur. Vascular malformations can also be subdivided into high- or low-flow lesions.

In the second classification system, the clinical perspective is replaced by a histologic perspective. All lesions, including the vascular malformations of Mulliken, are called hemangiomas. Hemangioma is defined as a benign, but nonreactive process in which there is an increase in the number of normal- or abnormal-appearing vessels. The two classification systems using this approach are those of Enzinger and the WHO. Both are very similar and distinguish between benign, intermediate, and malignant subgroups. The WHO classification is used in this chapter.[30]

Benign Vascular Tumors

Hemangiomas of the subcutis/deep soft tissue and capillary, cavernous, arteriovenous, venous, intramuscular, and synovial types of hemangioma (Figs. 93-25 to 93-28), as well as angiomatosis and lymphangioma (vascular and lymphatic endothelium are indistinguishable), belong to this group.

Hemangiomas may present as intralesional phleboliths on radiographs and CT and osseous changes such as periosteal reaction or erosion. Color Doppler ultrasonography may differentiate between low flow (no Doppler signal) and high flow (low resistance flow pattern) vascular malformations.

On MRI, hemangiomas are characterized by their high signal intensity on T2-weighted images and intermediate (between that of muscle and fat) signal intensity on T1-weighted images. They are frequently multilobular, resembling a "bunch of grapes." Fluid-fluid levels are merely seen in cavernous hemangiomas. Areas of high signal

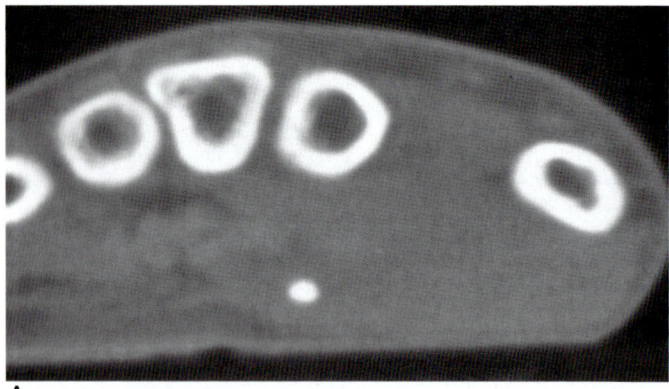

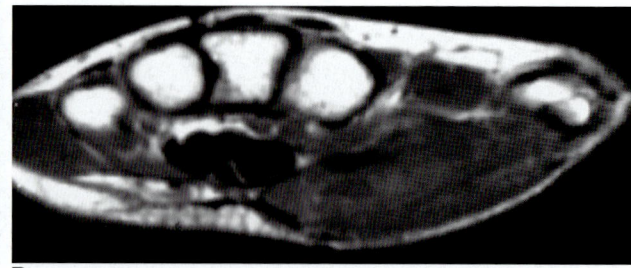

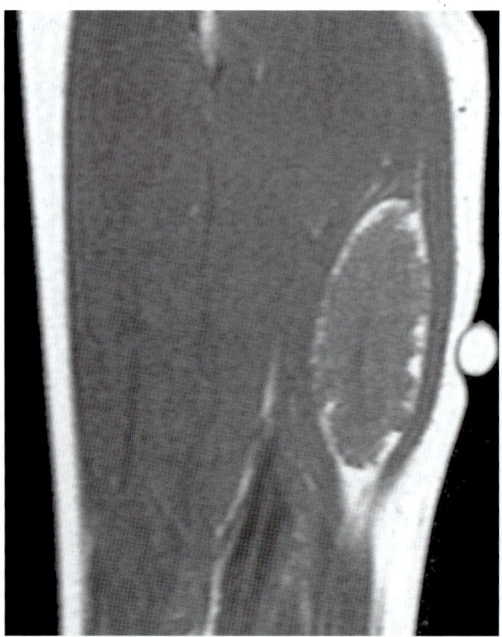

■ **FIGURE 93-25** Cavernous hemangioma of the thenar eminence. **A,** There is a phlebolith on the CT scan. The lesion is nonhomogeneous on T1 weighting (**B**) and shows multiple small fluid-fluid levels with high signal intensity of the supernatans on T2 weighting (**C**).

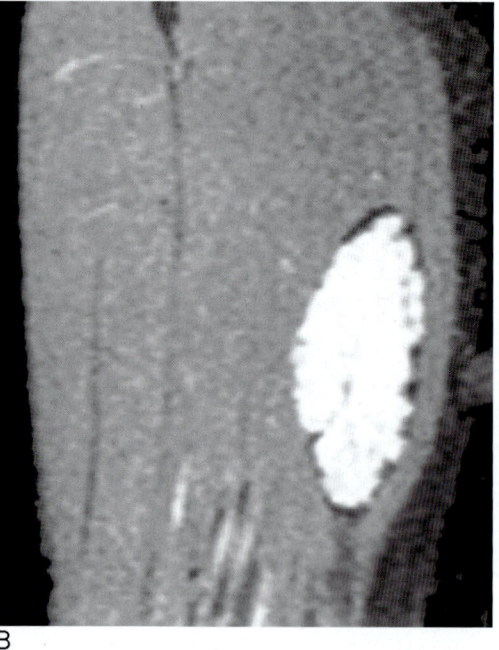

■ **FIGURE 93-26** Hemangioma showing intermediate signal intensity on T1 weighting (**A**) and high signal intensity on T2 weighting with fat suppression (**B**) with perilesional fat induction.

intensity corresponding to fat are seen at the periphery of the lesions ("fat induction" phenomenon). High-flow lesions may show signal voids on all pulse sequences. After contrast agent administration they exhibit a serpiginous, marked enhancement, seen within 6 seconds after enhancement of feeding arteries. The identification of low-flow venous hemangiomas, characterized by the presence of large venous convolutes in combination with late enhancement, is especially important, because these patients can be treated with percutaneous techniques without using diagnostic arterial angiography.[31]

Synovial hemangioma presents as the same MRI features and also as pressure erosions at adjacent osseous structures.

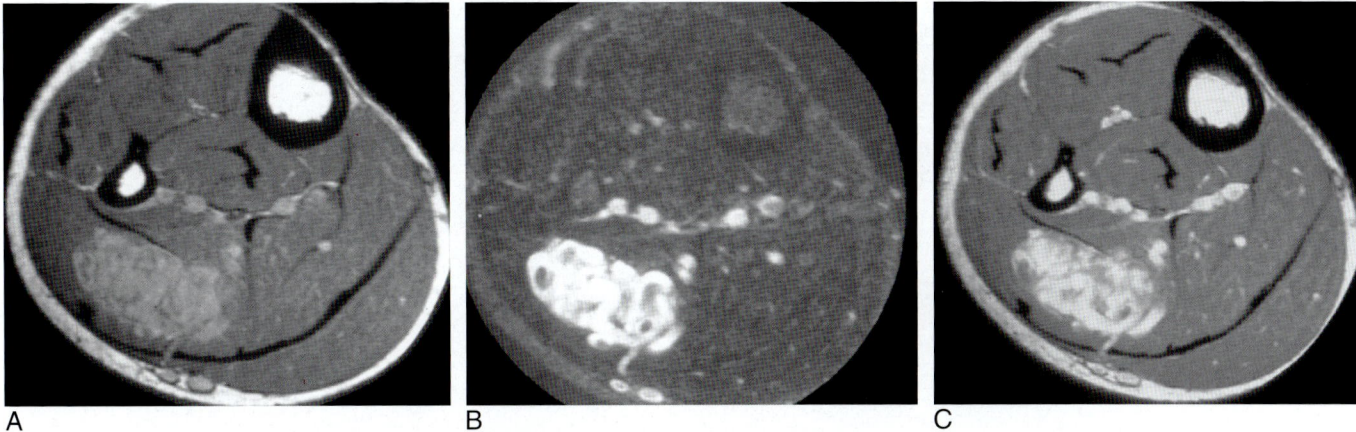

A   B   C

■ **FIGURE 93-27** Arteriovenous malformation (hemangioma) within the soleus muscle, showing a serpiginous morphology on all pulse sequences and draining veins toward the superficial vena saphena parva. The lesion is of high signal intensity when compared with the signal intensity of normal muscle on T1 weighting (**A**), is of very high signal intensity on T2 weighting with fat suppression (**B**), and enhances markedly after contrast agent administration (**C**).

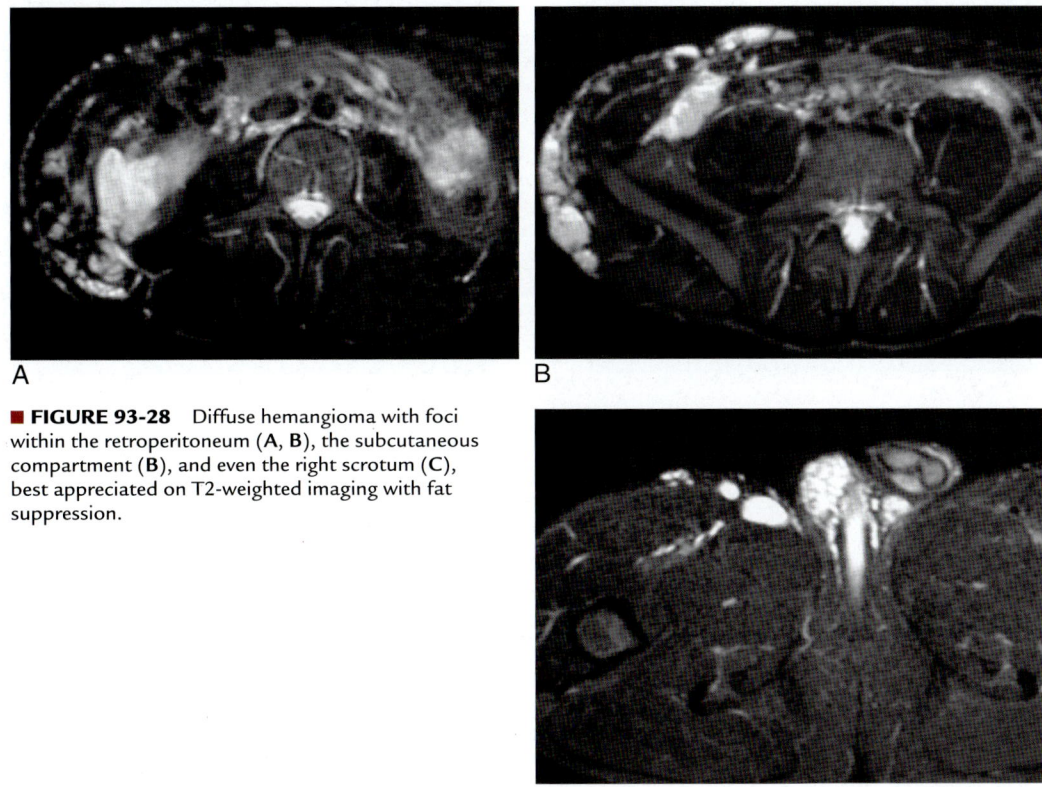

A   B

■ **FIGURE 93-28** Diffuse hemangioma with foci within the retroperitoneum (**A, B**), the subcutaneous compartment (**B**), and even the right scrotum (**C**), best appreciated on T2-weighted imaging with fat suppression.

C

Angiomatosis only differs from this solitary component by its multiplicity.

Glomus tumors are lesions consisting of cells resembling cells of the normal glomus body. They are subungually located and cause radiating pain, elicited by changes in temperature. An associated bone erosion with sclerotic borders is frequently noted. On MRI, glomus tumors are seen as homogeneous lesions with high signal intensity on T2-weighted images (Fig. 93-29).

Vascular Tumors of Intermediate Malignancy Grade

Hemangioendothelioma and angiosarcomas are very rare and have no specific imaging characteristics. Angiosarcoma is most common in the lower extremity and pelvis region and may be multifocal, surrounding the hip.

Tumors of Lymphatic Origin

Tumors of lymphatic origin are rare and are usually detected early in childhood. They have been reported in every type of tissue except in neural tissue. MRI is the imaging method of choice to demonstrate the full extent of the lesion, especially on fat-suppressed images.

Signal intensities of lymphangioma are nonspecific and are similar to those of hemangioma. On T1-weighted images with fat suppression, lymphangioma is of low signal intensity

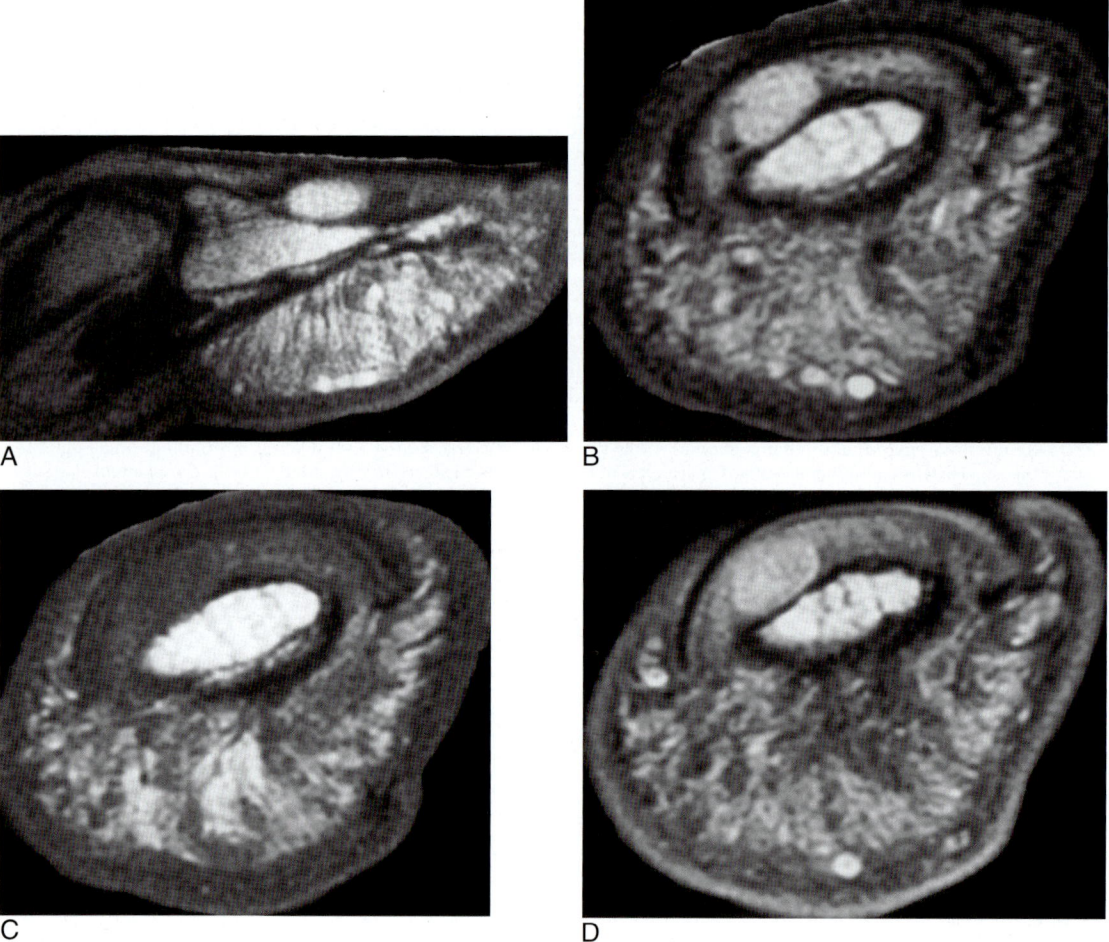

■ **FIGURE 93-29** Glomus tumor at the subungual region. Oval lesion of high signal intensity on T2-weighted imaging (**A, B**), intermediate signal intensity on T1-weighted imaging (**C**), and marked enhancement after contrast agent administration (**D**).

whereas hemangioma is of high signal intensity. On T2-weighted images, both lesions are of high signal intensity. Differentiation can be facilitated by the presence of phleboliths, by flow voids arising from feeding arteries or draining veins in hemangioma, and by a less pronounced and less homogeneous enhancement in lymphangioma. A special entity and by far the most frequent is the cystic lymphangioma or cystic hygroma. It consists of a lobulated, fluctuating mass in the supraclavicular fossa, the posterior triangle, or the axillary region that is not attached to the skin but fixed to the deep tissues of the neck. About 60% of these lesions are found at birth, and as many as 90% are noticed within the first 2 years of life. Intralesional hemorrhage may be responsible for the presence of fluid-fluid levels.[32]

Tumors of Muscular Origin

Smooth muscle tumors have no specific imaging features except for vascular leiomyosarcoma, which mostly occurs within the inferior vena cava. Leiomyosarcoma mostly presents as large, spindle-shaped masses with variable signal intensities, central necrosis, and marked peripheral and septal enhancement. Benign striated muscle tumors

are extremely rare. Rhabdomyosarcoma is the most common soft tissue tumor in children, the embryonal subtype being by far the most frequent (Fig. 93-30).

Synovial Tumors

Cystic soft tissue lesions can be divided into four groups based on the combination of their anatomic location and histologic composition: synovial cyst, ganglion cyst, bursa de novo, and permanent bursa. The diagnosis of a cystic lesion is usually straightforward on ultrasonography and/or MRI. If there is any doubt, however, of the true cystic nature of the lesion, contrast-enhanced MRI should be performed to exclude a pseudocystic benign or malignant tumor (Table 93-10).

Baker's cyst is the prototype of the synovial cyst. Ganglion cysts may occur anywhere but are frequently seen in fatty tissue. Meniscal and labral cyst also belong to the group of ganglion cysts. The most common example of a bursitis de novo is the bursa developing at the medial side of the first metatarsal head secondary to mechanical friction. A bursa is a normal structure that is only seen when it enlarges secondary to friction, inflammation, or

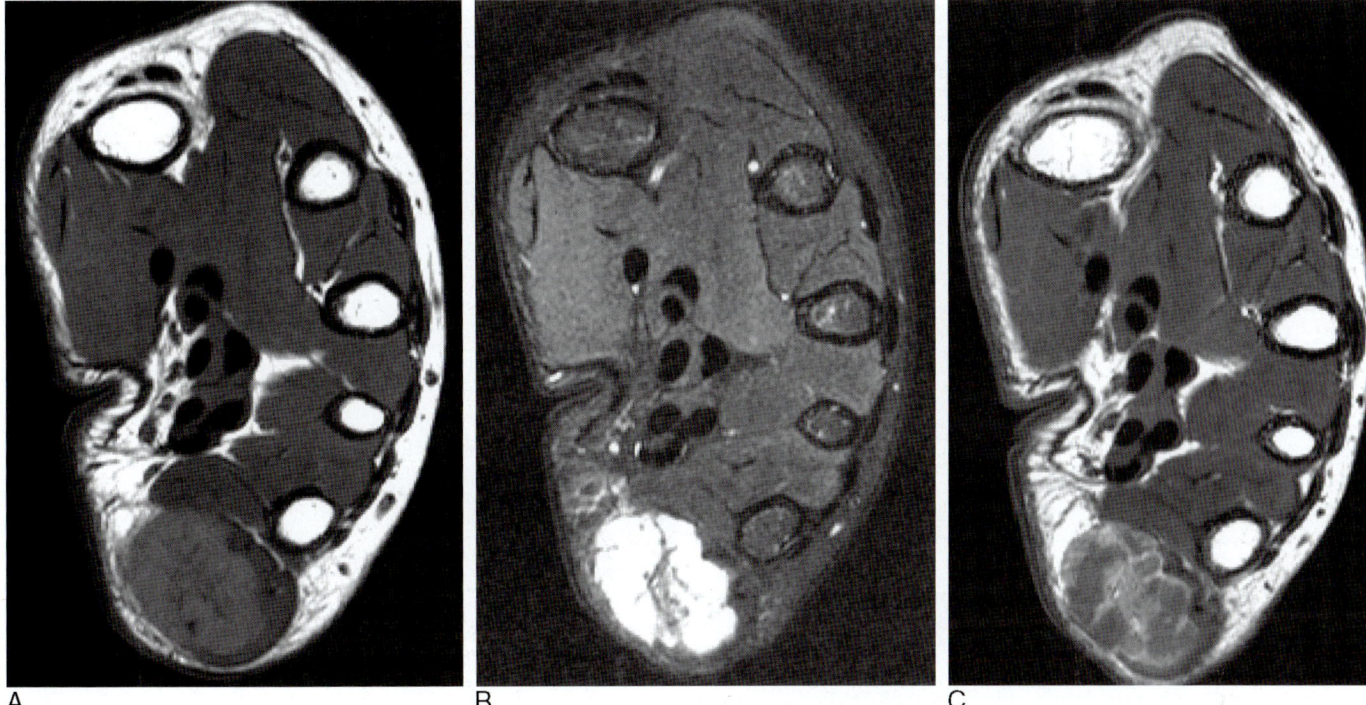

A   B   C

■ **FIGURE 93-30** Alveolar rhabdomyosarcoma of the hypothenar eminence. On T1-weighted imaging there is a large mass within the hypothenar muscles (abductor digiti minimi) that is inhomogeneous and slightly hyperintense to adjacent normal muscle. **A,** Infiltration is seen toward the muscle belly. **B,** On T2-weighted imaging with fat suppression the lesion is ill defined and of very high signal intensity, with a scar-like central component of lower signal intensity. **C,** On T1-weighted imaging after contrast agent administration there is a septal and peripheral enhancement. Although features are in favor of a malignant soft tissue tumor, MRI does not allow a more tissue-specific oriented diagnosis in this case.

TABLE 93-10 Classification of Para-articular Cystic Lesions

Lesion	Communication with Joint	Wall Composition	Cell Lining	Content
Synovial cyst	Yes	Continuous mesothelial lining	True cells	Mucinous fluid
Ganglion cyst	May be present	Discontinuous mesothelial lining	Flattened pseudo-synovial cells	Mucinous fluid
Bursitis de novo	Absent	Fibrous wall lining	No mesothelial lining	Fibrinoid necrosis
Permanent bursa	Absent	Continuous mesothelial lining	True synovial cells	Mucoid fluid

new communication with a joint (subdeltoid bursa filling secondary to rotator cuff tear).

According to the most recent WHO classification, giant cell tumors of tendon sheath and pigmented villonodular synovitis are categorized in the group of fibrohistiocytic tumors. Lipoma arborescens belongs to the group of lipomatous tumors, whereas synovial cell sarcoma is included in the group of tumoral lesions of uncertain differentiation.[5,33]

Tumors of Peripheral Nerves

This group comprises schwannomas, neurofibromas, and malignant peripheral nerve sheath tumors. Benign neurogenic tumors (schwannomas, neurofibromas) are well demarcated, round or fusiform lesions located on the course of a peripheral nerve. Other imaging features suggestive of a neurogenic tumor are findings of an entering/exiting nerve, the so-called target sign (high signal intensity peripheral area and low signal intensity center on T2-weighted images), the fascicular sign (transverse image of enlarged longitudinally coursing nerve bundles), the split fat sign, and associated muscle atrophy (Figs. 93-31 and 93-32).

Although neurofibromas occur centrally in the nerve and schwannomas have a more peripheral (nerve sheath) location, differential diagnosis between a schwannoma and a neurofibroma cannot be reliably made on imaging studies. This is relevant because schwannomas allow, because of their peripheral location relative to the nerve, resection without damaging the nerve. MRI features suggestive of a schwannoma include a fascicular appearance on T2-weighted images, a thin, hyperintense rim on T2-weighted images, and diffuse enhancement after contrast agent administration. Imaging findings suggestive of neurofibroma include a target sign on T2-weighted imaging, central enhancement, or a combination of both findings (Figs. 93-33 to 93-35). Criteria that can help in establishing the diagnosis of malignant peripheral nerve sheath tumors include a large mass (>5 cm) with mass

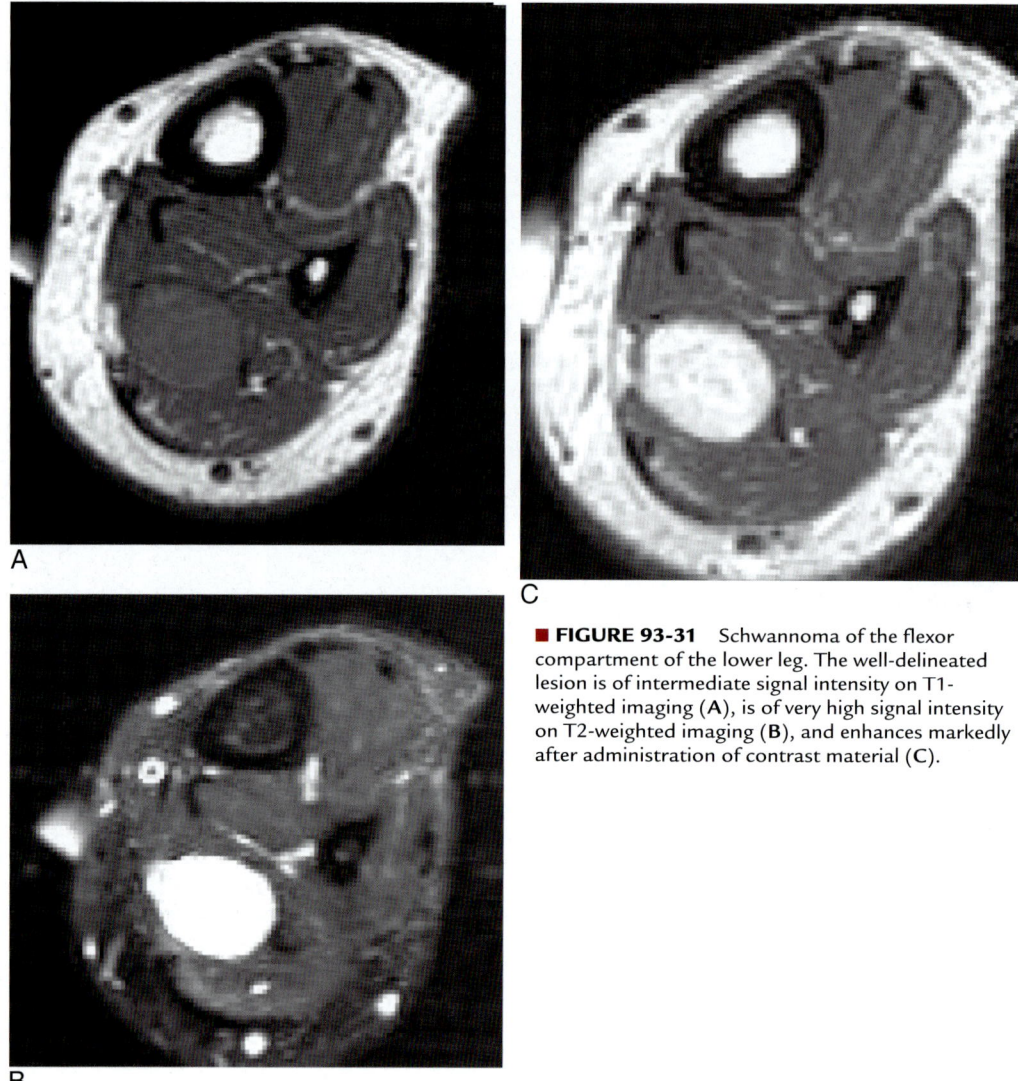

■ **FIGURE 93-31** Schwannoma of the flexor compartment of the lower leg. The well-delineated lesion is of intermediate signal intensity on T1-weighted imaging (**A**), is of very high signal intensity on T2-weighted imaging (**B**), and enhances markedly after administration of contrast material (**C**).

effect, inhomogeneous tumor architecture (due to areas of necrosis and hemorrhagic foci), ill-defined margins, perilesional edema, fast (within 6 seconds after arterial enhancement) heterogeneous enhancement, destruction of adjacent bony structures, and involvement of regional lymph nodes (Figs. 93-36 and 93-37). Schwannomas, neurofibromas, and malignant peripheral nerve sheath tumors can all occur in patients with neurofibromatosis (Fig. 93-38).

Schwannomatosis is a rare tumor syndrome characterized by the presence of multiple schwannomas arising on cranial, spinal, and peripheral nerves, without clinical or radiologic evidence of neurofibromatosis. These patients do not develop vestibular tumors. The hallmark of this condition is chronic pain.[5,34]

Extraskeletal Cartilaginous and Osseous Tumors

Extraskeletal chondroma consists of mostly small, well-defined nodules composed of focal areas of cartilage, without any connection to bone, periosteum, or articular synovium. Some of them may have undergone focal fibrosis or ossification. Hands and feet are preferential locations. They present as a specific intermediate signal intensity on T1-weighted images and high signal intensity on T2-weighted images. "Ring and arc" enhancement may be seen on contrast-enhanced MRI.

Para-articular chondroma is a very rare tumor, composed of hyaline cartilage with variable endochondral ossification in the central area and preferentially located at Hoffa's fat pad of the knee.

Synovial Osteochondromatosis

The primary form is characterized by the formation of numerous, metaplastic cartilaginous or osteocartilaginous nodules of small size, originating in the outer lining of the synovial membrane of joint or tendon sheath. Knees and hips are most affected. When the entire synovial membrane becomes involved, communication with the joint cavity is established and nodules will detach and form loose bodies in the joint space.

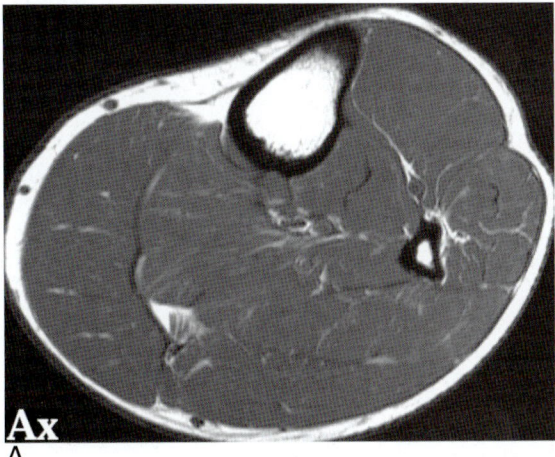

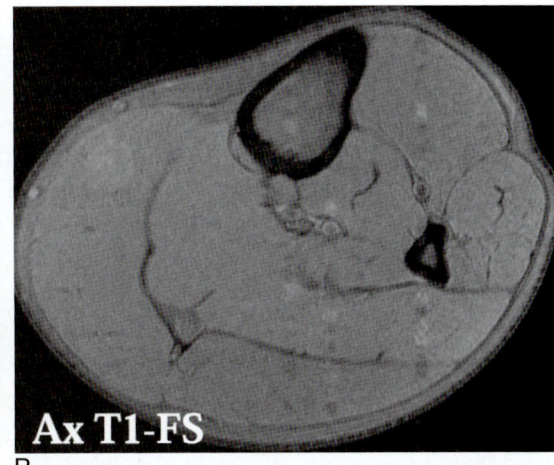

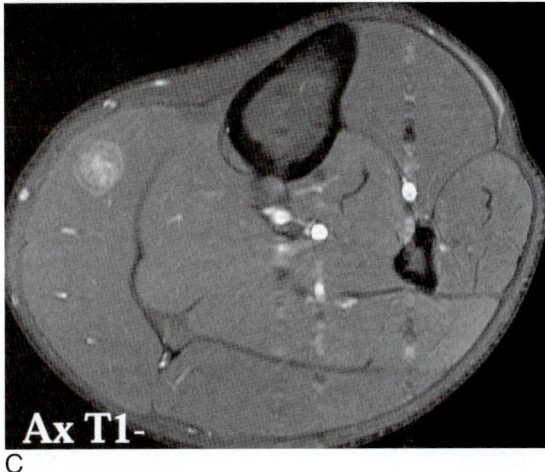

■ **FIGURE 93-32** Schwannoma at the left medial gastrocnemius muscle. **A,** The lesion is isointense with muscle and as a consequence hardly visible on T1-weighted imaging. It becomes better visible after fat suppression (**B**) and enhances moderately after contrast agent administration, merely at the center of the lesion (**C**).

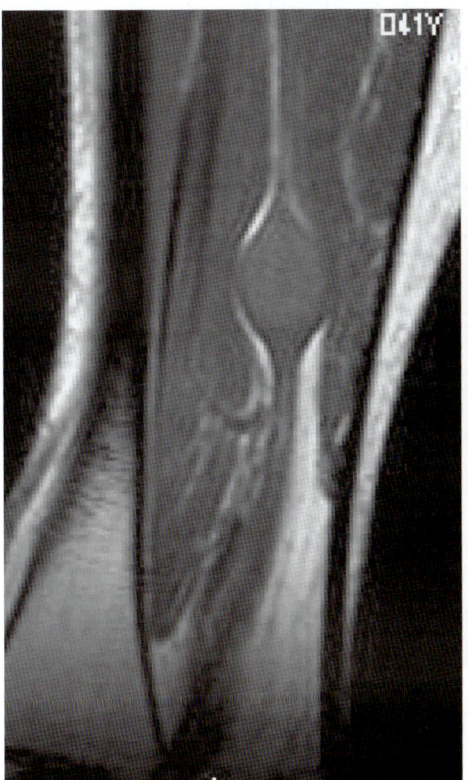

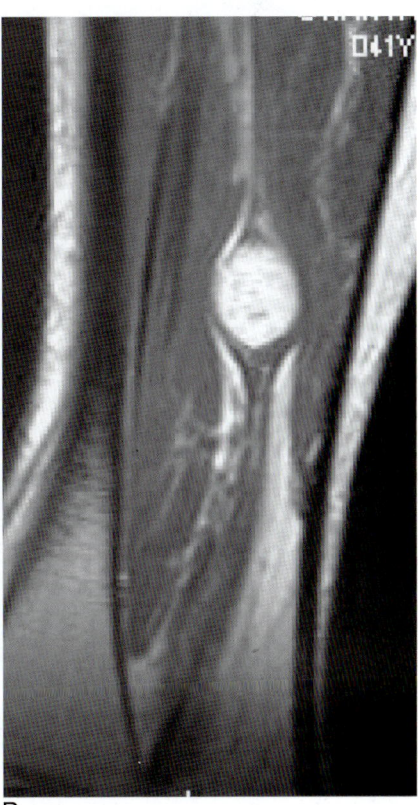

■ **FIGURE 93-33** Neurofibroma of the sciatic nerve. The lesion is located on the course of a major nerve and has a central position within the nerve. **A,** On T1-weighted imaging the lesion is isointense to muscle. **B,** It enhances markedly after contrast agent administration.

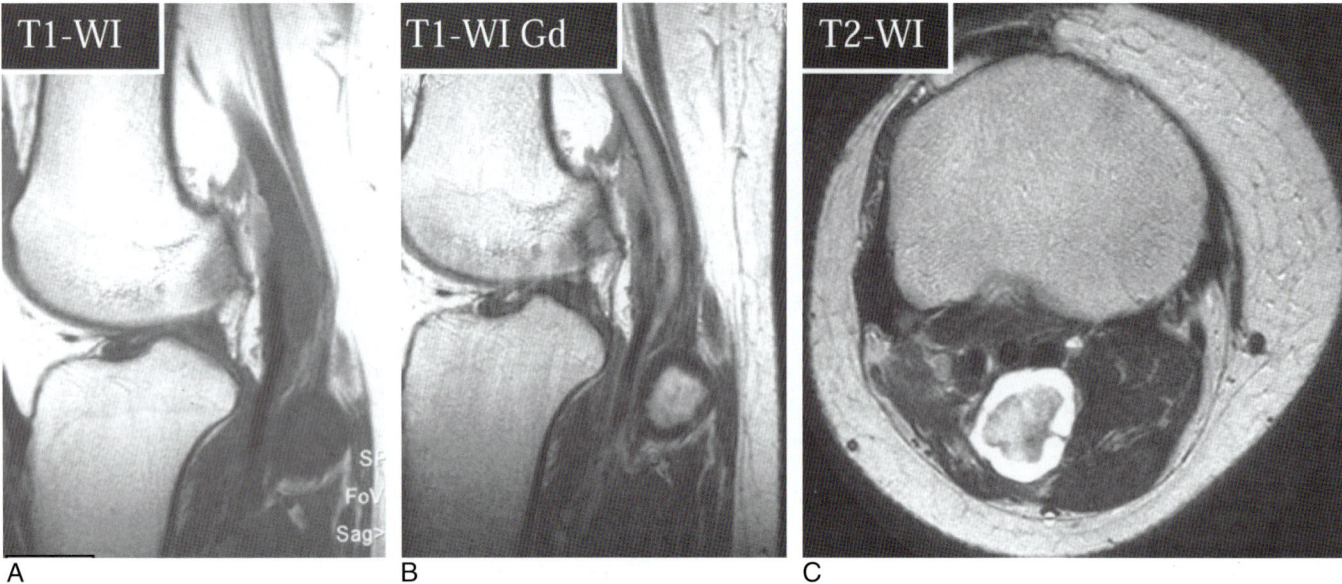

■ **FIGURE 93-34**   Neurofibroma of the tibial nerve. The lesion presents as a characteristic "target" sign consisting of a low signal intensity peripheral rim on T1 weighting before (**A**) and after (**B**) contrast agent administration. **C,** On T2 weighting the peripheral rim is of high signal intensity.

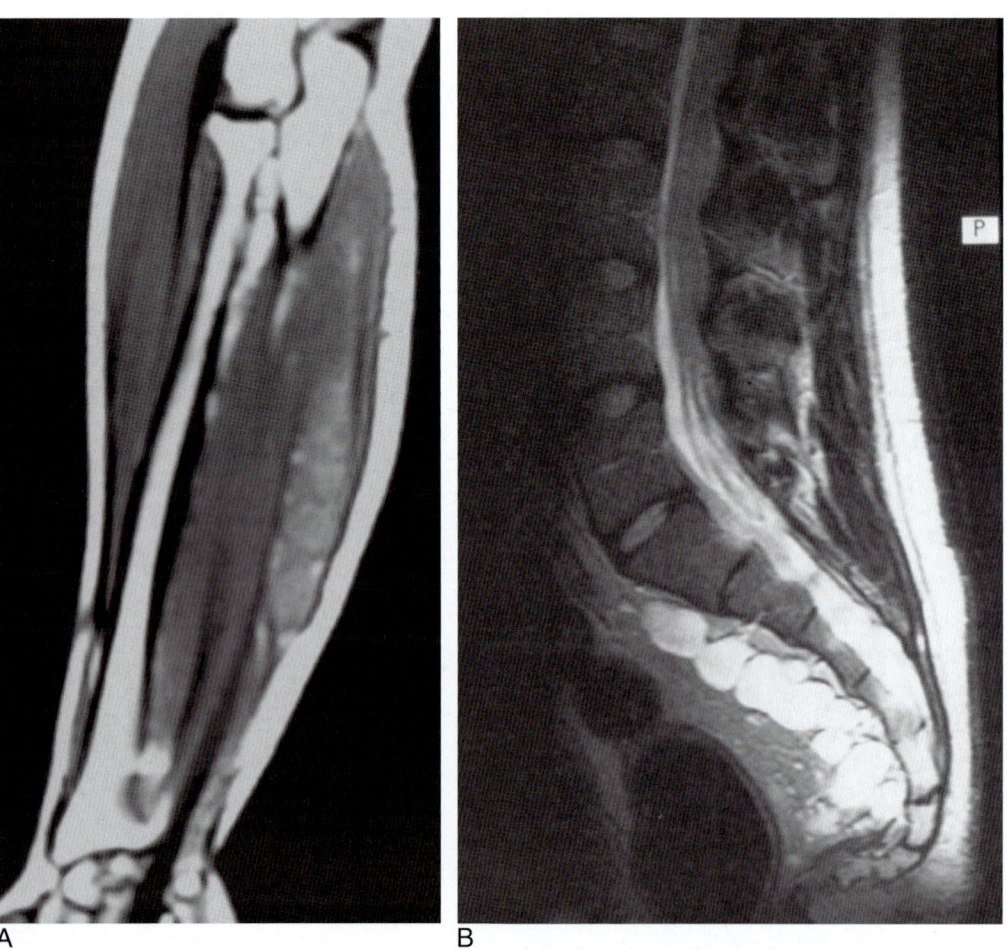

■ **FIGURE 93-35**   Plexiform neurofibroma of the ulnar nerve (**A**) and presacral plexus (**B**). Both lesions present with the characteristic moniliform aspect.

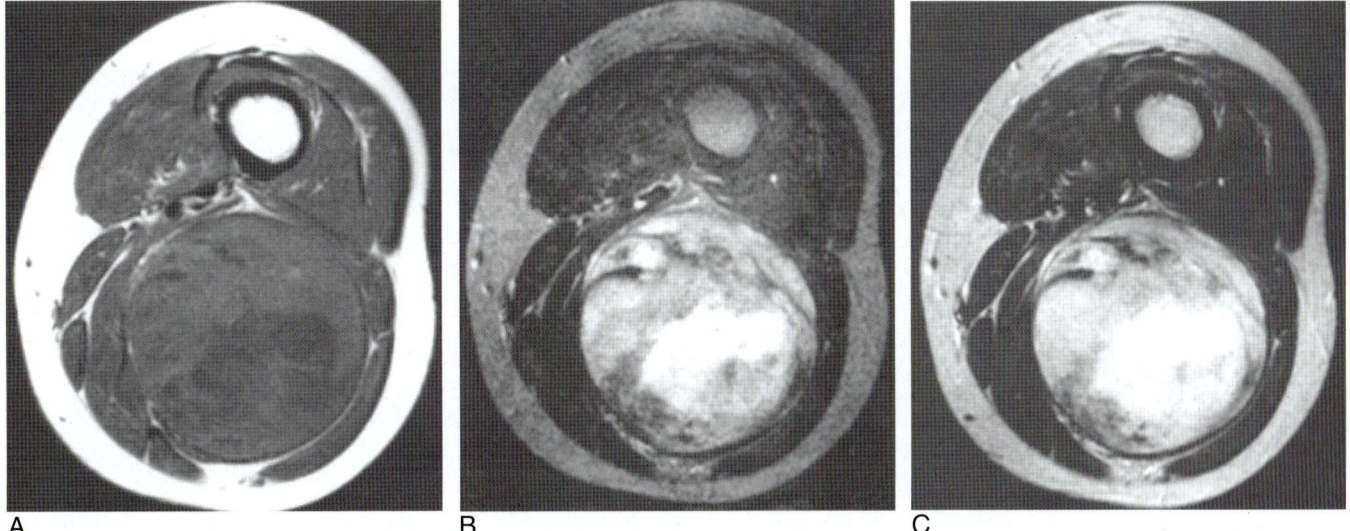

■ FIGURE 93-36 Malignant peripheral nerve sheath tumor on the course of the sciatic nerve. Axial MR images of the thigh. The lesion is highly inhomogeneous on T1-weighted sequence (**A**), T2-weighted sequence with fat saturation (**B**), and T1-weighted sequence after gadolinium contrast administration (**C**).

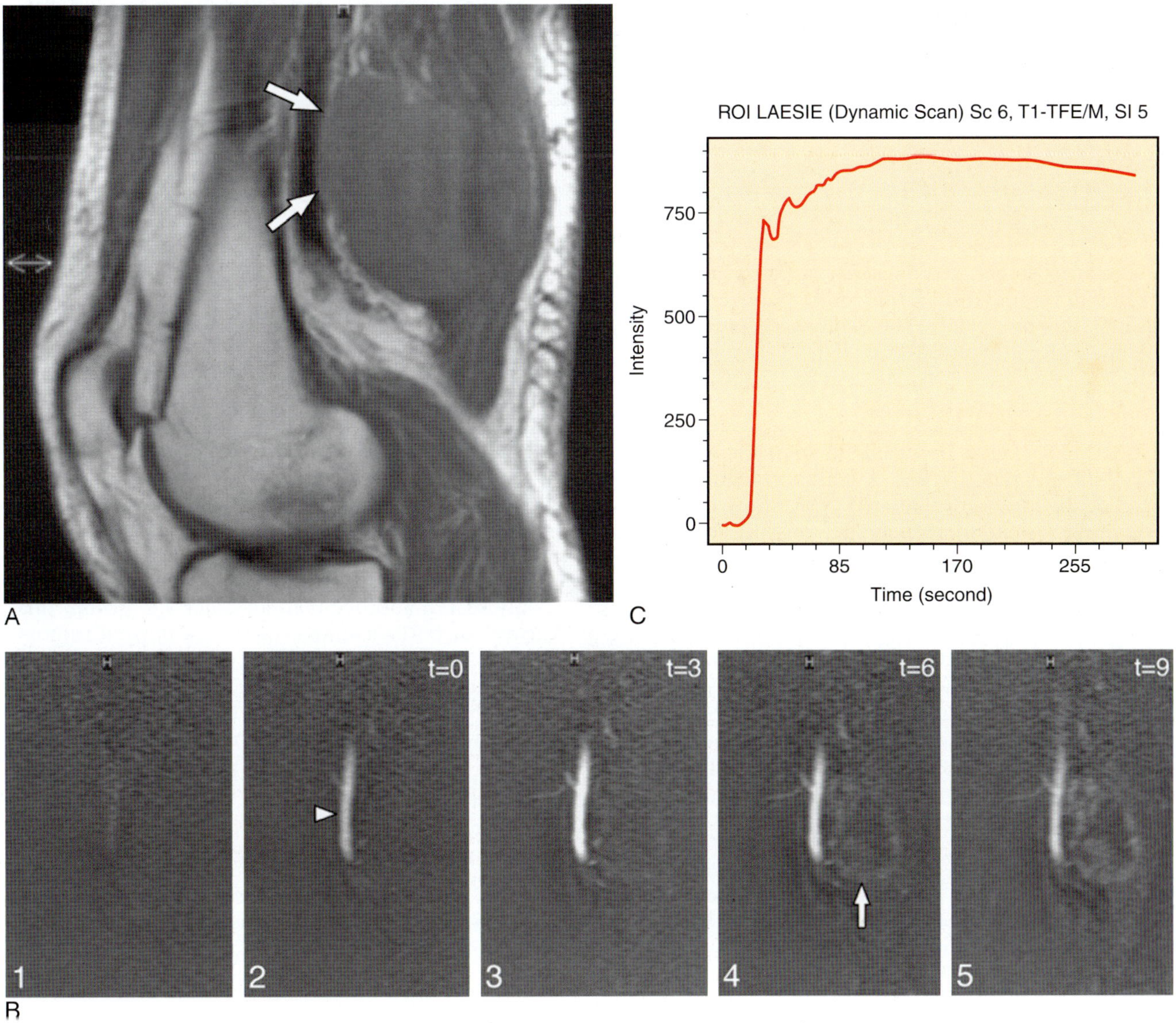

■ FIGURE 93-37 **A,** Dynamic sagittal, contrast-enhanced, T1-weighted MR image of a malignant peripheral nerve sheath tumor (*arrows*) in the lower extremity. **B,** Subtracted images of the dynamic series. Every 3 seconds one section is imaged. Arrival of contrast agent in the artery (2, *arrowhead*). Six seconds later distinct tumor enhancement (4, *arrow*) is seen. **C,** The graph depicts the early enhancement of the lesion and the rapid progression of enhancement in time.

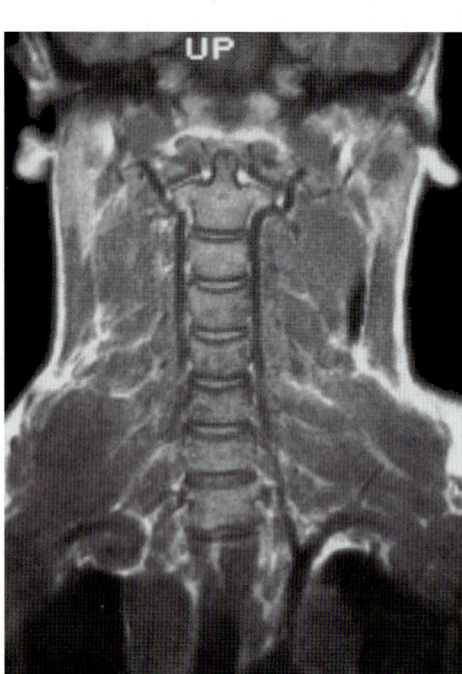
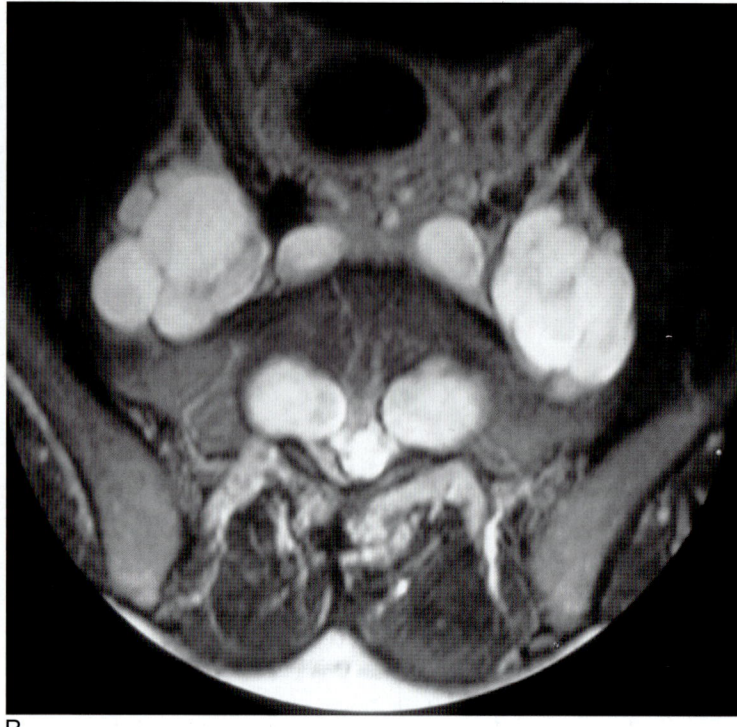

■ **FIGURE 93-38**   Neurofibromatosis with plexiform neurofibromas of the cervical spinal nerves (**A**) and of the presacral nerve plexus (**B**).

Secondary osteochondromatosis is much more common and develops inside the joint when cartilage is released in the joint cavity. The diagnosis is preferentially made on radiography or CT.

Extraskeletal Chondrosarcoma

A distinction is made between myxoid, mesenchymal, and well-differentiated types. A common feature is that all, except the well-differentiated type, show only minimal cartilage formation. Appearance on MRI depends on the type of and any related tumoral components, such as high signal intensity of myxoid types on T2-weighted images (Fig. 93-39).[35]

Benign extraskeletal osseous tumors comprise myositis ossificans (see Chapter 94); fibrodysplasia ossificans progressiva, which is a rare inheritable disorder characterized by progressive ossification of connective tissue and muscles and by osseous anomalies (abnormalities best seen on radiography and CT); and extraskeletal osteoma, which may be the end stage of myositis ossificans.

Extraskeletal Osteosarcoma

This is a mesenchymal neoplasm that forms osteoid or bone. It is located in soft tissues and is not attached to underlying bone or periosteum. This tumor is mostly located in the lower extremities and retroperitoneum. Calcifications within the tumor are observed on plain radiography and CT in about half of all cases. Signal intensity is low and nonhomogeneous on T1-weighted images and high and also nonhomogeneous on T2-weighted images.[36]

Primitive Neuroectodermal Tumors

These tumors form part of the heterogeneous group of small, round (blue) cell tumors of childhood and adolescence, which also includes conventional neuroblastoma, rhabdomyosarcoma, lymphoma, and Ewing's sarcoma. They occur preferentially in the thoracopulmonary region, abdomen, pelvis, and lower extremities. A special entity of primitive neuroectodermal tumors is the Askin tumor, which is mostly located at the chest wall. Both are highly aggressive soft tissue tumors. Extraskeletal Ewing's sarcoma is histologically indistinguishable from the osseous form. In contrast to the osseous form, these tumors are deeply seated and occur in an older age group. Imaging features of both primitive neuroectodermal tumors and Ewing's sarcoma are similar to those of other malignant soft tissue tumors. They frequently exhibit areas of cystic degeneration, necrosis, and hemorrhage. They mostly present with intermediate, nonhomogeneous signal intensity on spin-echo sequences and with heterogeneous, fast enhancement after contrast agent administration.[37]

Tumors of Uncertain Differentiation

Myxoma and synovial cell sarcoma are by far the most frequent representatives of this group.

Myxoma is benign and histologically characterized by the presence of abundant, avascular myxoid stroma in which a small number of cells are embedded. It is a tumor of adults. Areas most frequently involved are the large muscles of the thigh, shoulder, buttocks, and upper arm (Fig. 93-40). There is an association with polyostotic

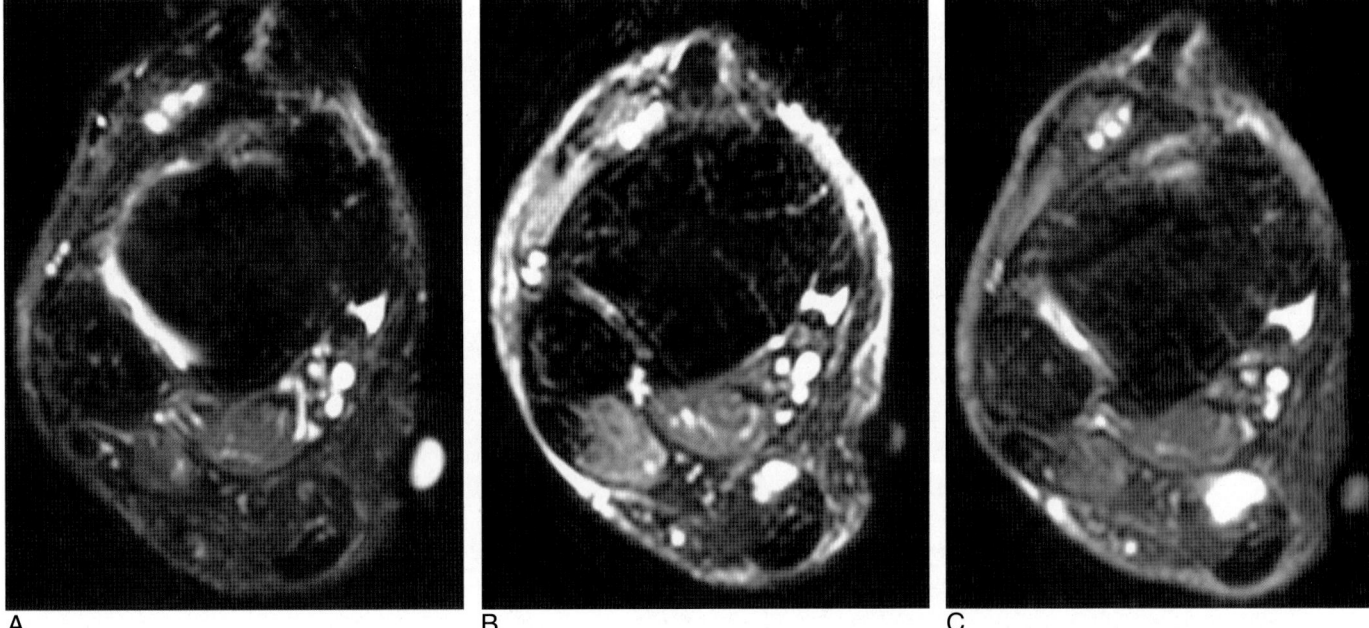

A   **B**   **C**

■ **FIGURE 93-39**   Recurrence of a soft tissue chondrosarcoma. **A,** No recurrent tumor on a control MRI, 6 months after surgery for a soft tissue chondrosarcoma. **B,** Small recurrent lesion anterior to the Achilles tendon on a control examination after 1 year. **C,** Second control examination 6 months later. Recurrent tumors are best detected on T2-weighted imaging with fat suppression.

fibrous dysplasia (bones involved are usually in the vicinity of the myxoma) in so-called Mazabraud's syndrome. On MRI, myxomas present as very low signal intensity on T1-weighted images (lower than signal intensity of normal muscle) and as high signal intensity on T2-weighted images (higher than signal intensity of fat). There may be moderate, central enhancement after contrast agent administration, having a "smoke"-like appearance.[38]

In the group of malignant lesions of uncertain differentiation, synovial cell sarcoma is by far the most frequent. Synovial cell sarcoma occurs primarily in the para-articular region, usually in close relationship with tendon sheaths, bursae, and joint capsules, with the knee region being most often affected. It is most prevalent in adolescents and young adults between 15 and 40 years of age. The term *synovial cell sarcoma* is a misnomer because it is not related to normal synovial structures. Intra-articular synovial sarcoma does occur but is extremely rare. The name is derived from the microscopic resemblance to normal synovium, the real origin being undifferentiated mesenchymal tissue. Chromosomal rearrangements have been reported in association with synovial cell sarcoma. On radiography, focal calcifications/ossifications are seen in 20% to 30%, and osseous invasion in 5% to 30%. On MRI lesions are isointense to muscle on T1-weighted images but areas of increased signal intensity are frequently seen and due to intralesional hemorrhage. On T2-weighted images large lesions are nonhomogeneous and have a so-called "triple signal" sign, consisting of a mixture of low, intermediate, and high signal intensity. Here also fluid-fluid levels are seen and are a consequence of intratumoral bleeding. After contrast agent administration there is an early, marked enhancement that is homogeneous in small lesions and nonhomogeneous in large lesions.

Because of location and cyst-like signal intensities on nonenhanced MRI, synovial cell sarcomas are frequently mistaken for para-articular cysts.[39,40]

Alveolar soft part sarcoma constitutes less than 1% of all soft tissue sarcomas. Its histology mimics the alveolar pattern of the respiratory alveoli. It is a highly vascular lesion surrounded by tortuous blood vessels and minute amounts of fat. It occurs between 11 and 40 years of age and has a female predominance. The lesion is highly aggressive with a metastatic potential of more than 50% at the moment of detection. Preferential location is the anterior portion of the thigh. On MRI the lesion is nodular with internal septations and high signal intensity on both T1- and T2-weighted images, due to abundant slow flowing blood. The lesion is nonhomogeneous on all pulse sequences and also on postcontrast images (Fig. 93-41).[41]

Epithelioid sarcoma, which is the most common malignant neoplasm of the hand, presents as noncharacteristic malignant features on MRI.

Clear cell sarcoma or malignant melanoma of soft parts is a slow-growing malignant tumor, the cells of which are capable of producing melanin. It arises deeply in the soft tissues of the limbs in the vicinity of tendons, aponeuroses, and fasciae. Young adults between the ages of 20 and 40 years are most frequently affected. All lesions present on T1-weighted MR images with hyperintensity relative to normal muscle; this results from the shortening of the T1-relaxation time, which is due to the paramagnetic effect of intralesional melanin. Although melanin also shortens T2-relaxation time, most lesions are of high signal intensity on T2-weighted images, which is due to the high water and myxoid content of the lesions. Marked enhancement after contrast agent administration is the rule (Fig. 93-42).[42]

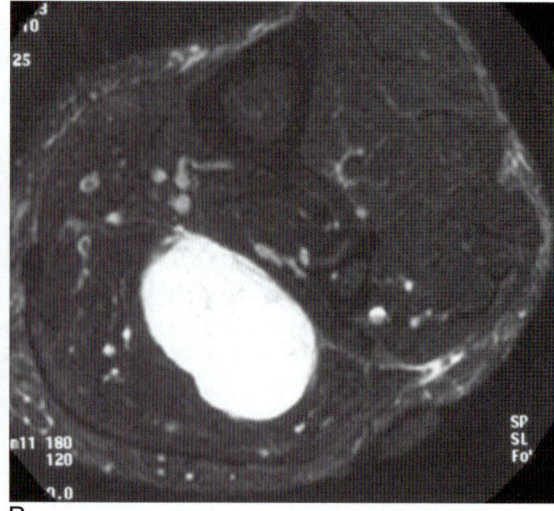

■ FIGURE 93-40 Myxoma of the lower leg (soleus muscle). Signal intensity on T1-weighted imaging (**A**) is lower than the signal intensity of normal muscle. **B,** Note very high signal intensity on T2-weighted imaging. **C,** Subtle, smoke-like, central enhancement after contrast agent administration.

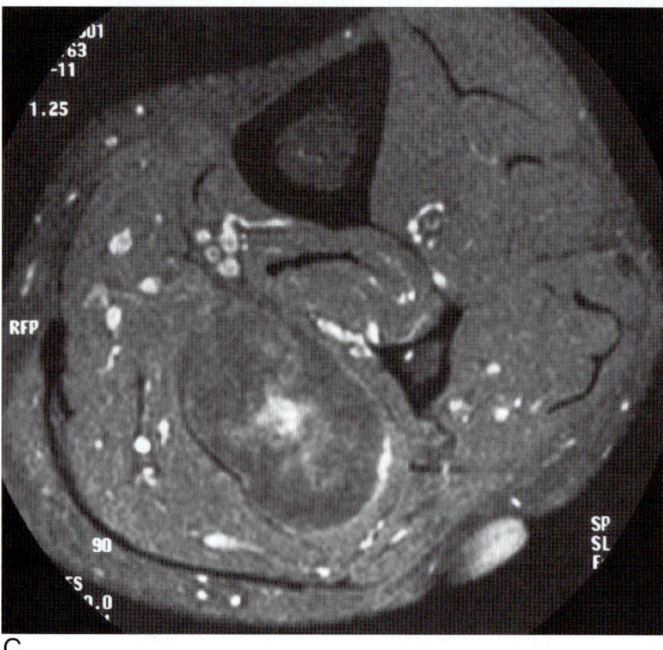

Soft Tissue Metastases

Although skeletal muscle metastases are relatively rare, they are not uncommon, especially in end-stage cancer. Primary tumors responsible for soft tissue metastases are adenocarcinomas and squamous cell carcinomas, mostly originating from lung, kidney, and gastrointestinal tract.

Soft tissue metastases are frequently painful lesions, in contradistinction to primary soft tissue tumors, which are mostly painless.

Most metastases have nonspecific features on imaging, except for metastases of osteosarcoma (intralesional ossification), and melanosarcoma (increased signal intensity on T1-weighted MR images). MR findings of low to intermediate signal intensity on T2-weighted images, owing to hypercellularity and increased nuclear-cytoplasmic index, and especially the "inverted target sign" (high central signal on T2-weighted images with low signal intensity of the peripheral rim, and inversion of signal intensities after contrast administration, i.e., peripheral enhancement and lack of central enhancement, due to central necrosis) are more specific features seen in soft tissue metastases (Fig. 93-43).[43,44]

Pediatric Soft Tissue Tumors

Soft tissue tumors are rare in childhood and adolescence. They are mostly benign. Hemangiomas are the most common benign tumors of childhood, and rhabdomyosarcomas are the most common malignant soft tissue tumors.

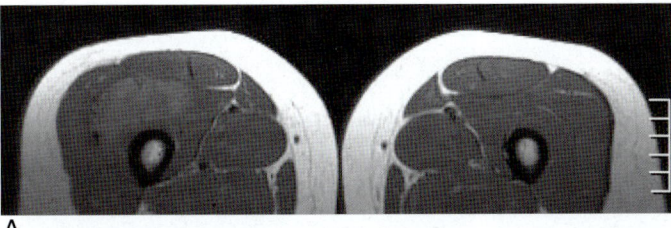

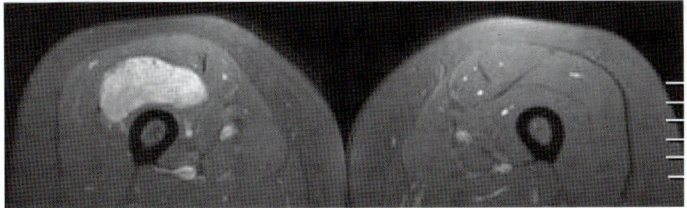

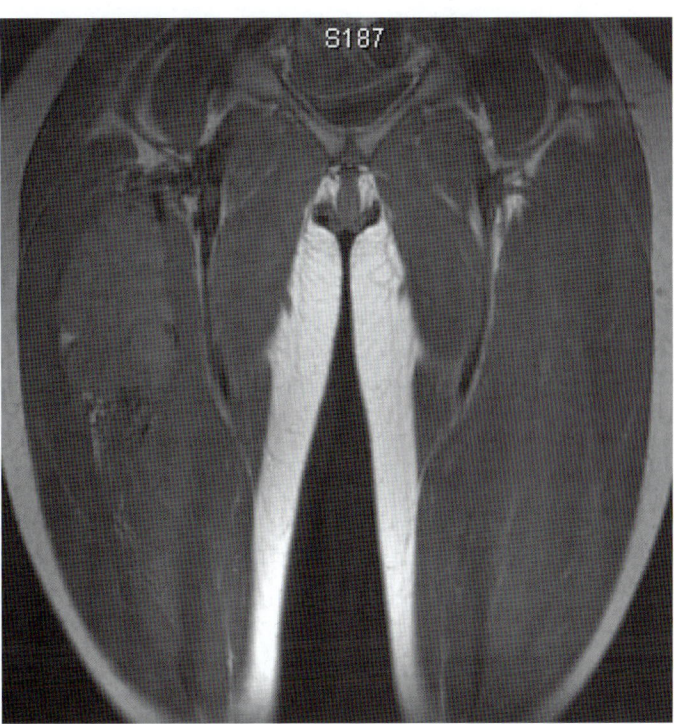

■ **FIGURE 93-41** Alveolar soft part sarcoma. Characteristic MRI features of this rare tumor are its preferential location in the extensor compartment of the thigh, its high signal intensity on T1-weighted imaging, due to abundant slow flowing blood within the lesion (**A**), and the presence of prominent vessels at both poles of the lesion (**B**). **C,** There is marked enhancement as seen on T1-weighted imaging after contrast agent administration and with fat suppression.

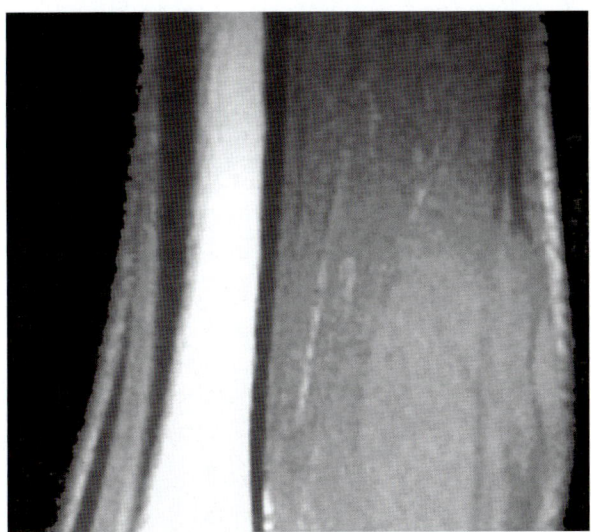

■ **FIGURE 93-42** Clear cell sarcoma or deeply seated melanoma characterized by an intermediate to high signal intensity on this T1-weighted MR image.

Because long-term survival of children with malignant soft tissue tumors is strongly related to disease stage at the time of diagnosis, early detection is mandatory.

Notwithstanding the limitations of ultrasonography, it remains the first diagnostic modality to use in children suspected of having a soft tissue tumors. Plain radiography and CT are best suited for demonstration of calcified lesions or intralesional calcifications. MRI is also used in children as the main modality for grading, staging, and characterizing soft tissue tumors.

In rhabdomyosarcomas a specific staging system is used in which the TNM classification, anatomic site, and clinical status at presentation are major parameters.

Tissue-specific diagnosis by imaging is possible in many benign tumors but difficult in the malignant group.

Children with a soft tissue tumor should be treated in specialized centers during diagnosis and for treatment and follow-up.[45]

DIFFERENTIAL DIAGNOSIS

Cytogenetics and Molecular Genetics of Soft Tissue Tumors

Human tumors are primarily caused by anomalies affecting two types of genes: (1) dominantly acting oncogenes, whose protein products serve to accelerate cell growth and whose functions are altered by increased gene dosage (amplification) or by activating mutations or participation in fusion genes, resulting from chromosomal translocations, inversions, or insertions; and (2) tumor suppressor genes, whose products normally serve as brakes on cell growth and runaway cell proliferation and whose inactivation leads to uncontrolled cell proliferation and downregulation of apoptosis (programmed cell death). Specific translocations are diagnostic of the tumors in which they are found; they have not been observed in other tumor types and can be of crucial value in establishing the correct diagnosis in confusing cases. Tumors for which the cytogenetic and/or molecular changes are diagnostic are listed in Table 93-11.

The radiologist is in an unique position for determining which soft tissue tumor may require cytogenetic

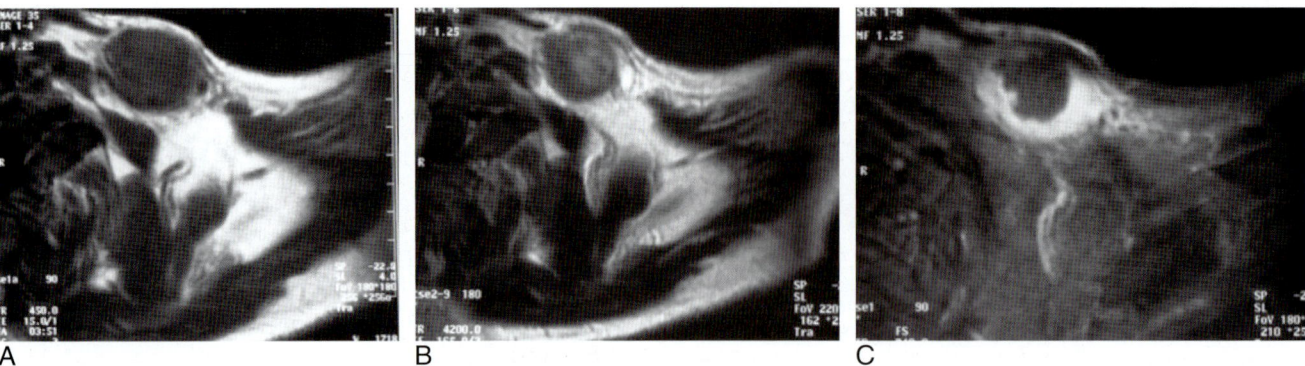

■ **FIGURE 93-43** Metastasis of a squamous cell carcinoma showing the "inverted target sign." Note the hyperintense, peripheral rim on a T1-weighted MR image (**A**), the hypointense peripheral rim and hyperintense center on a T2-weighted MR image (**B**), and peripheral enhancement after contrast agent administration on a T1-weighted MR image (**C**).

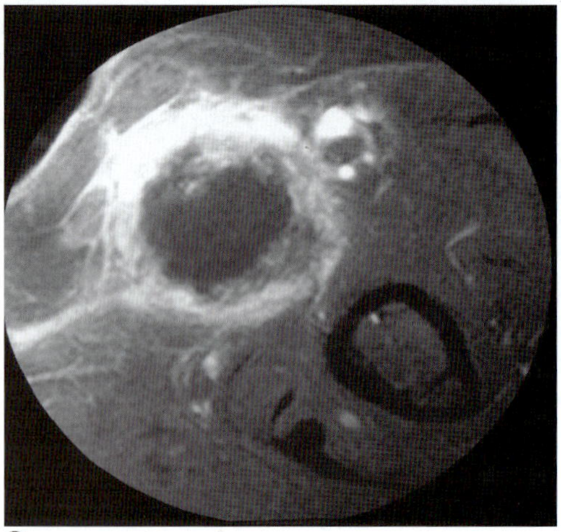

■ **FIGURE 93-44** Metastasis of a papillary renal carcinoma showing the "inverted target sign." Note the hyperintense peripheral rim on a T1-weighted MR image (**A**), hypointense peripheral rim and hyperintense center on a T2-weighted MR image (**B**), and peripheral enhancement after contrast agent administration on a T1-weighted MR image (**C**).

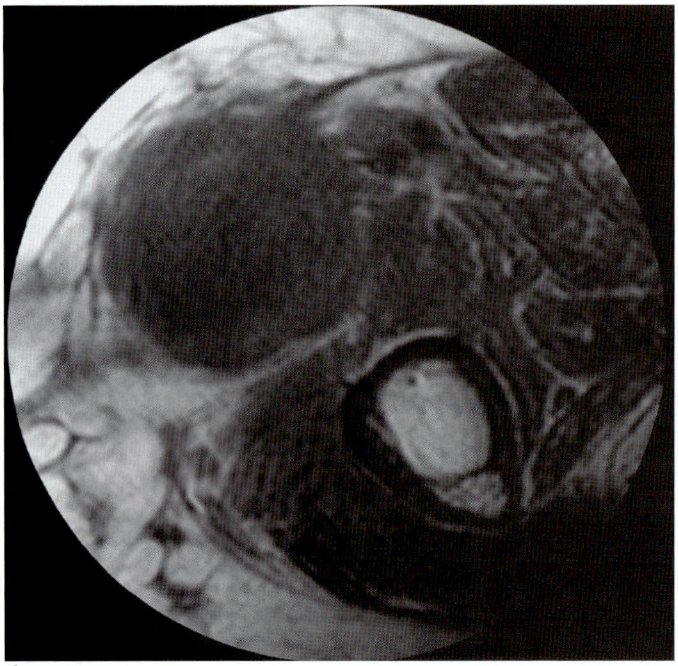

and/or molecular diagnostic studies. When the radiologic findings are confusing and raise uncertainty regarding the exact diagnosis, the radiologist is in a position to alert the responsible surgeons and physicians before surgical or therapeutic procedures are initiated to the possibility that genetic studies may be indicated. This is particularly true if cytogenetic analysis is contemplated, because fresh (not fixed) tissue is required for such an analysis and may be obtained at the time of surgery or biopsy. Emphasis must be placed on the combined use of cytogenetic and

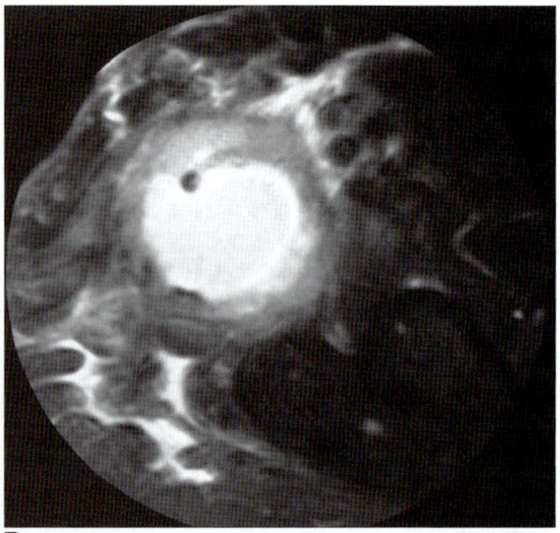

TABLE 93-11 Tumors with Specific Cytogenetic and/or Molecular Changes

Synovial sarcoma
Liposarcoma
Extraskeletal Ewing's sarcoma
Rhabdomyosarcoma
Clear cell sarcoma (malignant melanoma of soft parts)
Desmoplastic round-cell tumor
Dermatofibrosarcoma protuberans
Congenital (infantile) fibrosarcoma
Inflammatory myofibroblastic tumor
Extraskeletal chondrosarcoma
Alveolar soft part sarcoma
Malignant peripheral nerve sheath tumor
Desmoid tumor
Leiomyosarcoma
Chondroma

molecular techniques in obtaining an optimal and full picture of diagnostic value of the genetic changes in tumors, because tumors may have molecular changes exceeding in number that of the cytogenetic anomalies and at the same time present cytogenetic changes not reflected in the molecular abnormalities. Particularly useful in that regard are fluorescence in-situ hybridization (cytogenetic changes) and reverse transcriptase polymerase chain reaction (molecular changes).[12]

SYNOPSIS OF TREATMENT OPTIONS

Treatment strategies are discussed in Chapter 88. The importance of multidisciplinary approach and treatment planning is addressed in Chapter 89. The role of MRI in local staging is discussed in Chapter 98.

What the Referring Physicians Needs to Know

- Is there a soft tissue tumor or pseudotumor?
- Is the lesion benign or (potentially) malignant?
- Is there a tissue-specific diagnosis?
- Is additional imaging needed?
- Is biopsy needed?
- In which compartments does the lesion extend? (see Chapter 98)

REFERENCES

1. Fletcher CD, Unni KK, Mertens F. World Health Organization Classification of Tumours. Pathology and Genetics. Tumours of Soft Tissue and Bone. Lyon, IARC Press, 2002.
2. Enzinger F, Weiss S, Goldblum J. Enzinger and Weiss's Soft Tissue Tumors, 4th ed. St. Louis, CV Mosby, 2001.
3. Kransdorf M. Malignant soft tissue tumors in a large referral population: distribution of specific diagnoses by age, sex and location. AJR Am J Roentgenol 1995; 164:129-134.
4. Kransdorf M. Benign soft tissue tumors in a large referral population: distribution of specific diagnoses by age, sex and location. AJR Am J Roentgenol 1995; 164:395-402.
5. De Schepper AM, Vanhoenacker F, Gielen J, Parizel P (eds). Imaging of Soft Tissue Tumors, 3rd ed. Berlin, Springer Verlag, 2005.
6. Oliveira AM, Nascimento AG. Grading in soft tissue tumors: principles and problems. Skeletal Radiol 2001; 30:543-559.
7. Gielen JL, De Schepper AM, Vanhoenacker F, et al. Accuracy of MRI in characterization of soft tissue tumors and tumor-like lesions: a prospective study in 548 patients. Eur Radiol 2004; 14:2320-2330.
8. van Rijswijk CS, Geirnaerdt MJ, Hogendoorn PCW, et al. Soft tissue tumors: value of static and dynamic gadopentate dimeglumine-enhanced MR imaging in prediction of malignancy. Radiology 2004; 233:493-502.
9. Kransdorf M, Jelinek J, Moser R. Imaging of soft tissue tumors. Radiol Clin North Am 1993; 31:359-372.
10. Sundaram M. MR imaging of soft tissue tumors: an overview. Semin Musculoskelet Radiol 1999; 3:15-20.
11. Gielen J, De Schepper AM, Parizel PM, et al. Additional value of magnetic resonance with spin echo T1-weighted imaging with fat suppression in characterization of soft tissue tumors. J Comput Assist Tomogr 2003; 27:434-441.
12. Sandberg AA. Cytogenetics and molecular genetics in soft tissue tumors. In De Schepper AM, Vanhoenacker F, Gielen J, Parizel P (eds). Imaging of Soft Tissue Tumors, 3rd ed. Berlin, Springer Verlag, 2005.
13. Anderson MW, Temple HT, Dussault RG, Kaplan PA. Compartmental anatomy: relevance to staging and biopsy of musculoskeletal tumors. AJR Am J Roentgenol 1999; 173:1663-1671.
14. Kransdorf MJ, Murphey MD, Smith SE. Imaging of soft tissue neoplasms in the adult: benign tumors. Semin Musculoskeletal Radiol 1999; 3:21-37.
15. Kransdorf MJ, Murphey MD, Smith SE. Imaging of soft tissue neoplasms in the adult: malignant tumors. Semin Musculoskeletal Radiol 1999; 3:39-58.
16. Wang XL, De Schepper AM, Vanhoenacker F, et al. Nodular fasciitis: correlation of MRI findings and histopathology. Skeletal Radiol 2002; 31:155-161.
17. Lang P, Suh KJ, Grampp S, et al. CT and MRI in elastofibroma: a rare benign soft tissue tumor. Radiologe 1995; 35:611-615.
18. Morrison W, Schweitzer M, Wapner K, Lackman R. Plantar fibromatosis: a benign aggressive neoplasm with a characteristic appearance on MR images. Radiology 1994; 193:841-845.
19. Vandevenne J, De Schepper AM, De Beuckeleer L, et al. New concepts in understanding evolution of desmoid tumors: MR imaging of 30 lesions. Eur Radiol 1997; 7:1013-1019.
20. Rosenberg AE. Malignant fibrous histiocytoma: past, present, and future. Skeletal Radiol 2003; 32:613-618.
21. De Beuckeleer L, De Schepper A, De Belder F. Magnetic resonance imaging of localized giant cell tumor of tendon sheath. Eur Radiol 1997; 7:198-201.
22. Llauger J, Palmer J, Roson N, et al. Pigmented villonodular synovitis and giant cell tumors of the tendon sheath: radiological and pathological features. AJR Am J Roentgenol 1999; 172:1087-1091.
23. Kransdorf MJ, Bancroft LW, Peterson JJ, et al. Imaging of fatty tumors: distinction of lipoma and well-differentiated liposarcoma. Radiology 2002; 224:99-104.
24. Green RA, Cannon SR, Flanagan AM. Chondroid lipoma: correlation of imaging findings and histopathology of an unusual benign lesion. Skeletal Radiol 2004; 33:67-73.

25. Reiseter T, Nordshus T, Borthne A, et al. Lipoblastoma: MRI appearances of a rare paediatric soft tissue tumor. Pediatr Radiol 1999; 29:542-545.

26. Soler T, Rodriguez E, Bargiela A, Da Riba M. Lipoma arborescens of the knee: MR characteristics in 13 joints. J Comput Assist Tomogr 1998; 22:605-609.

27. Maron EM, Helms CA. Fibrolipomatous hamartoma: pathognomonic on MR imaging. Skeletal Radiol 1999; 22:260-264.

28. Seynaeve P, Mortelmans L, Kockx M, et al. Hibernoma of the left thigh. Skeletal Radiol 1994; 23:137-138.

29. Peterson JJ, Kransdorf MJ, Bancroft LW, O'Connor MI. Malignant fatty tumors: classification, clinical course, imaging appearance and treatment. Skeletal Radiol 2003; 32:493-503.

30. Teo EHJ, Strause PJ, Hernandez RJ. MR imaging differentiation of soft tissue hemangiomas from malignant soft tissue masses. AJR Am J Roentgenol 2000; 174:1623-1628.

31. van Rijswijk CS, van der Linden E, van der Woude HJ, et al. Value of dynamic contrast-enhanced MR imaging in diagnosing and classifying peripheral vascular malformations. AJR Am J Roentgenol 2002; 178:1181-1187.

32. Schuster T, Grantzow R, Nicolai T. Lymphangioma colli: a new classification contributing to prognosis. Eur J Pediatr Surg 2003; 13:97-102.

33. Vanhoenacker FM, Van de Perre S, De Vuyst D, De Schepper AM. Cystic lesions around the knee. JBR-BTR 2003; 86:302-304.

34. Simoens WA, Wuyts FL, De Beuckeleer LH, et al. MR features of peripheral nerve sheath tumors: can a calculated index compete with radiologist's experience? Eur Radiol 2001; 11:250-257.

35. Okamoto S, Hara K, Sumita S, et al. Extraskeletal myxoid chondrosarcoma arising in the finger. Skeletal Radiol 2002; 31:296-300.

36. Vanhoenacker FM, Van de Perre S, Van Marck E, et al. Extraskeletal osteosarcoma: a report of a case with unusual features and histopathological correlation. Eur J Radiol Extra 2004; 49:97-102.

37. Ibarburen C, Haberman JJ, Zerhouni EA. Peripheral neuroectodermal tumors: CT and MRI evaluation. Eur J Radiol 1996; 21:225-232.

38. Peterson KK, Renfrew DL, Feddersen RM, et al. Magnetic resonance imaging of myxoid containing tumors. Skeletal Radiol 1991; 20:245-250.

39. Jones BC, Sundaram M, Kransdorf MJ. Synovial sarcoma: MR imaging findings in 34 patients. AJR Am J Roentgenol 1993; 161:827-830.

40. van Rijswijk CS, Hoogendoorn PC, Taminiau AH, Bloem JL. Synovial sarcoma: dynamic contrast-enhanced MR imaging features. Skeletal Radiol 2001; 30:25-30.

41. Lorigan JG, O'Keefe FN, Evans HL, Wallace S. The radiologic manifestations of alveolar soft part sarcoma. AJR Am J Roentgenol 1989; 153:335-339.

42. De Beuckeleer LH, De Schepper AM, Vandevenne JE, et al. MR imaging of clear cell sarcoma (malignant melanoma of the soft parts): a multicenter correlative MRI-pathology study of 21 cases and literature review. Skeletal Radiol 2000; 29:187-195.

43. Glockner JF, White LM, Sundaram M, McDonald DJ. Unsuspected metastases presenting as solitary soft tissue lesions: a fourteen-year review. Skeletal Radiol 2000; 29:270-274.

44. Damron TA, Heiner J. Distant soft tissue metastases: a series of 30 new patients and 91 cases from the literature. Ann Surg Oncol 2000; 7:526-534.

45. Harms D. Soft tissue malignancies in childhood and adolescence: pathological and clinical relevance based on data from the Kiel pediatric tumor registry. Handchir Mikrochir Plast Chir 2004; 36:268-274.

94

Tumor-like Soft Tissue Lesions

Rodrigo Salgado and Arthur de Schepper

Every radiologist occasionally will be confronted with a mass of undetermined imaging characteristics. Eventually, many of these lesions turn out to be non-neoplastic. These non-neoplastic masses belong to a large and heterogeneous group usually named "pseudotumors." Soft tissue pseudotumors are a frequent clinical problem and can present at any age, occur in any location, and affect both men and woman. Many of these lesions share a common feature, being essentially reactive in nature and therefore mostly self-limiting without the need for further investigation and significant intervention. Nevertheless, other lesions (e.g., necrotizing fasciitis) are acute life-threatening conditions in which prompt recognition and subsequent intervention are essential for the survival of the patient.

It is the aim of this chapter to provide an overview of the most commonly encountered soft tissue pseudotumors, ranging from pure anatomic variants to posttraumatic lesions to metabolic conditions and other origins. Knowledge of the existence and common presentation of these entities, in combination with relevant clinical findings, can direct the radiologist and physician to the correct diagnosis, thereby limiting the need for invasive procedures in these often reactive benign lesions.

NORMAL ANATOMIC VARIATIONS AND MUSCULAR ANOMALIES

Normal anatomic variants presenting as soft tissue tumors are occasionally seen in clinical practice. Many of these occur in specific locations, facilitating their diagnosis (Table 94-1; Fig. 94-1). In this chapter, normal variants that may mimic soft tissue tumors are briefly discussed.

In the lower extremities, anatomic variants occur almost exclusively in the soleus muscle. Although present from birth, an accessory soleus muscle (or low lying muscle belly of the normal soleus muscle) usually becomes clinically apparent in the late adolescent age secondary to increased physical activity. This occurs especially in athletes and other professions requiring increased physical activity. It presents as a soft tissue mass, arising either from the anterior surface of the soleus muscle or from the

soleal line of the tibia and fibula, clinically appearing as an asymptomatic soft tissue mass medial to the calcaneus (Fig. 94-2). Symptoms, when present, have been attributed to closed compartment ischemia and are accentuated by exercise.

The accessory breast or nipple presents along the primitive milk line above or below the normal breast location (Fig. 94-3). Because the primitive milk line extends from the axilla to the groin, these masses may occasionally also be found in the axilla, scapula, thigh, and labia majora. It is the most frequently encountered congenital anomaly of the breast. These accessory breasts are subject to the same physiologic and pathologic changes as proper breast tissue. Although they are often dismissed as cosmetic curiosities, they have nevertheless potential for pathologic degeneration and may be associated with significant congenital abnormalities.

INFLAMMATORY AND INFECTIOUS LESIONS

In general, differentiation between infection and sarcoma may be easy in typical cases, but it may be impossible to differentiate the two in atypical cases. Epidemiologic data

KEY POINTS

- Soft tissue pseudotumors encompass a vast range of pathologic processes, varying from normal anatomic variants, inflammatory and infectious lesions, posttraumatic masses, and other lesions.
- Knowledge of the common presentation of these entities in combination with relevant clinical findings can direct the clinician to the correct diagnosis, thereby limiting the need for invasive procedures in these often reactive benign lesions.
- The radiologic approach of soft tissue pseudotumors is no different than for their "true" tumoral counterparts. When there is doubt, a biopsy should be performed.
- Finally, always consider an infectious or reactive origin for a mass with undetermined imaging characteristics.

TABLE 94-1 Common Anatomic Variants Presenting as Soft Tissue Masses

Structure	Location
Accessory palmaris longus muscle	Upper extremity
Duplication of hypothenar muscle	Upper extremity
Anomalous extensor indicis	Upper extremity
Langer's axillary arch*	Upper extremity
Soleus muscle; low position muscle belly	Lower extremity
Accessory breast, nipple	Primitive milk line

*Langer's arch is a musculotendinous structure that usually extends from the latissimus dorsi to the pectoralis major muscle.

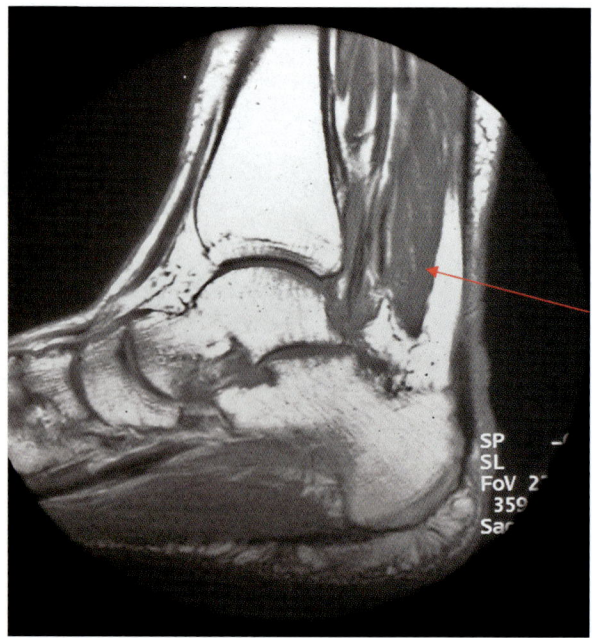

■ **FIGURE 94-2** Accessory soleus muscle in an adult man. On this sagittal, spin-echo, T1-weighted MR image there is a muscle belly (*arrow*) within Kagher's fat triangle, anterior to the Achilles tendon. Signal intensity and location of this abnormality are in favor of an accessory soleus muscle. *(Courtesy of Dr. Filip Vanhoenacker.)*

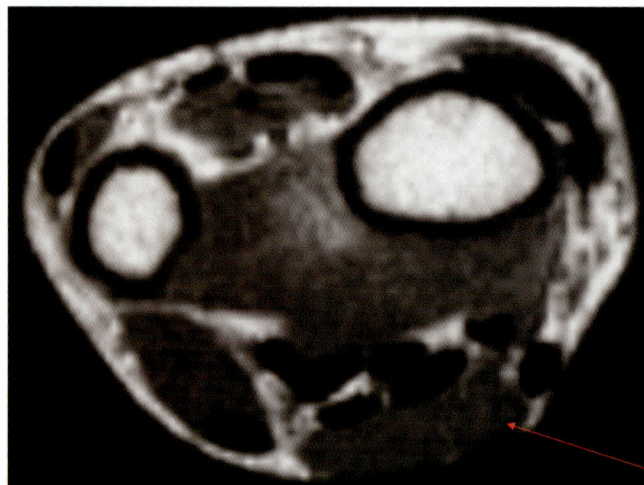

■ **FIGURE 94-1** Accessory palmaris longus muscle in a 15-year-old boy. Axial T1-weighted MR image after intravenous contrast medium administration. The additional mass located superficially to the flexor digitorum tendons (*arrow*) can be identified as accessory muscle because of its signal intensity and texture that are identical to that of skeletal muscle. *(From Salgado R, Alexiou J, Engelholm JL. Pseudotumoral lesions. In De Schepper AM [ed]. Imaging of Soft Tissue Tumors, 3rd ed. Berlin, Springer-Verlag, 2006, pp 415–446.)*

such as location, morphology, and sometimes MRI characteristics may be helpful in differentiating infection from sarcoma. Dynamic contrast-enhanced MRI is not very helpful in differentiating infection from sarcoma because both will display rapid, aggressive enhancement.

Necrotizing Fasciitis

Necrotizing fasciitis is a rare, rapidly evolving and life-threatening soft tissue infection that, unlike cellulitis, typically extends into deep fascial planes. The causative

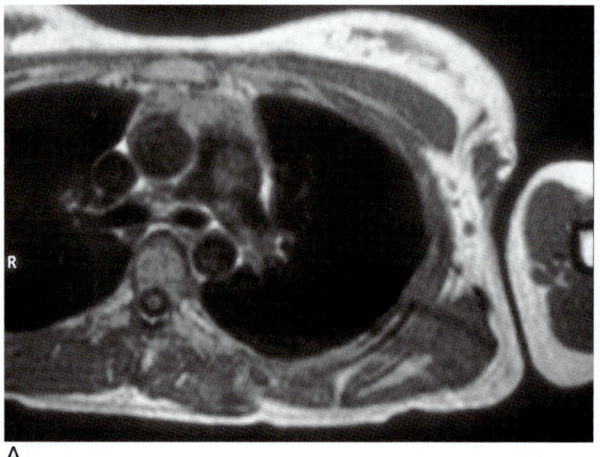

A

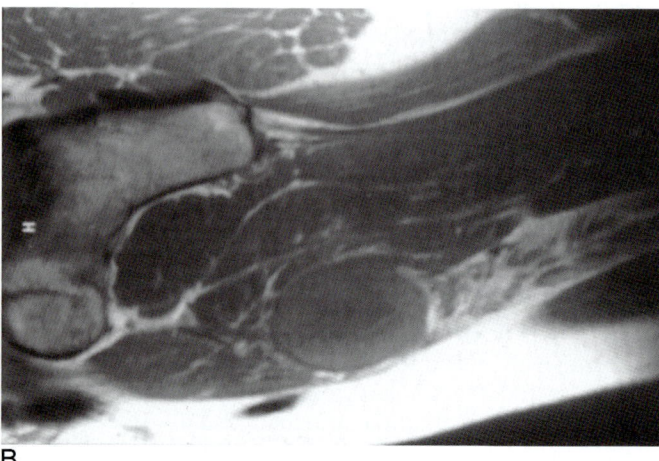

B

■ **FIGURE 94-3** Accessory breast in a 17-year-old girl. Axial, spin-echo, T1-weighted (**A**) and axial, turbo spin-echo, T2-weighted (**B**) MR images demonstrate a small soft tissue mass lateral to the left pectoralis muscle with signal intensities similar to the signal intensity of normal adjacent breast. *(From Salgado R, Alexiou J, Engelholm JL. Pseudotumoral lesions. In De Schepper AM [ed]. Imaging of Soft Tissue Tumors, 3rd ed. Berlin, Springer-Verlag, 2006, pp 415–446.)*

organisms are mostly group A hemolytic streptococci and *Staphylococcus aureus*, on occasion acting in synergy. Other both aerobic and anaerobic pathogens may also be involved. Known predisposing factors include older patients, especially in combination with malignancy, poor nutrition, and alcohol or drug abuse. It can also be found after trauma or around foreign bodies in surgical wounds. However, it can also appear in otherwise healthy subjects with no known risk factors (Fig. 94-4). The clinical course can be fulminant, with reported mortality rates as high as 73%. Early recognition is mandatory, because survival depends on prompt surgical intervention.

On MRI, this condition shows as hyperintense signal intensity on T2-weighted images extending into the deep fasciae with fluid collections. After intravenous administration of a contrast agent, peripheral enhancement is clearly seen. However, this presentation can be seen in other non-necrotizing conditions. When no deep fascial involvement is revealed, necrotizing fasciitis can be excluded.

Abscess

A soft tissue abscess is a well-delineated fluid collection surrounded by a well-vascularized fibrous pseudocapsule. Although in many cases there will be a suggestive preceding event (e.g., puncture) or underlying illness, it can also occur without a suggestive history or symptoms. Therefore, when confronted with a mass with undetermined imaging characteristics one must always consider a possible infectious origin. Abscesses can be multiple and can distort normal muscle anatomy and fascial planes due to their inflammatory nature. Their margins can be well defined or infiltrating, depending on the organism involved.

Conventional radiography has no or little value in the imaging workup. It may occasionally show gas within the lesion. Ultrasonography reveals an elongated or lobulated fluid collection and can assist in guiding an aspiration biopsy or percutaneous catheter drainage. On MRI, an abscess is hypointense to isointense compared with muscle tissue on T1-weighted images. On T2-weighted images, the central portion of the abscess is usually hyperintense but the capsule may display an isointense or hypointense signal intensity relative to subcutaneous fat. On T1-weighted images the pseudocapsule can have a variable signal intensity compared with skeletal muscle. After intravenous contrast medium injection, a peripheral rim of enhancement is seen, corresponding to the inflammatory and cellular component of the abscess (Fig. 94-5). When occurring near bone, an association with osteomyelitis or a periosteal reaction can be seen.

Inflammatory edematous changes in the surrounding tissues (muscle, subcutaneous tissue) are seen as a hyperintense signal intensity on T2-weighted images. Inhomogeneity on T2-weighted sequences may be a consequence of intralesional gas bubbles and/or necrotic material.

However, imaging characteristics may be different in an immunocompromised host. The peripheral edema usually seen on T2-weighted images is sometimes absent. Similarly, T1-weighted images will not always show the pseudocapsule. The infected fluid in the center of the abscess can have an inhomogeneous signal intensity. If the content is sufficiently viscous, it can even show mild increased signal intensity on T1-weighted images. Enhancement after intravenous contrast medium injection can also be absent.

Pyomyositis

Pyomyositis, also known as bacterial myositis, is a rare cause of single or multiple abscesses of skeletal muscle of unknown etiology. In general, normal skeletal muscle has a

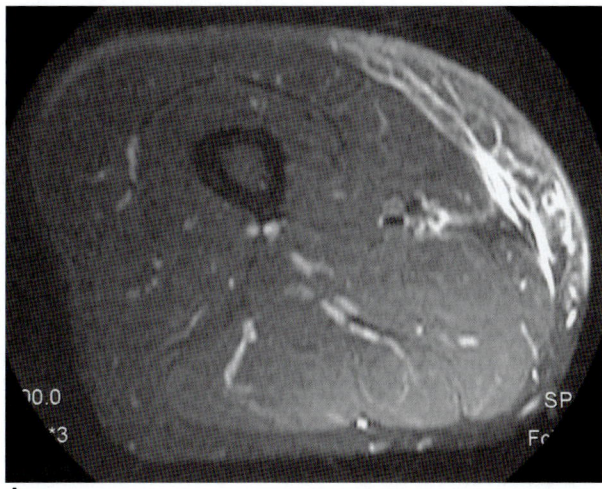
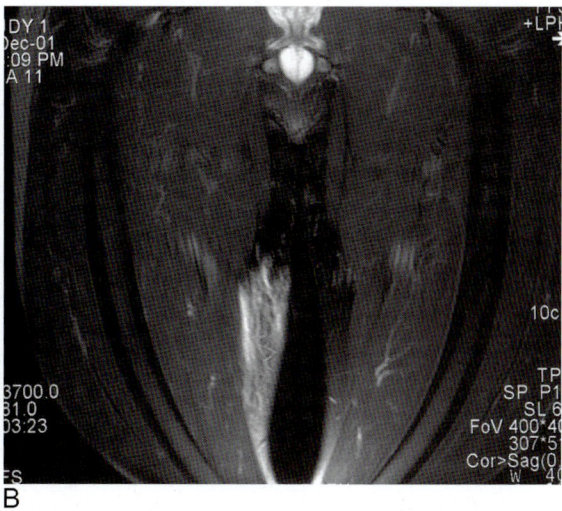

A

B

■ **FIGURE 94-4** A 36-year-old previously healthy man presented with a rapidly spreading skin infection and swelling of the right upper leg. Axial, turbo spin-echo, T2-weighted MR image with fat suppression (**A**) and coronal, turbo spin-echo, T2-weighted MR image with fat suppression (**B**) are shown. In contrast to cellulitis, this case shows extensive subcutaneous thickening and reticular infiltration, extending to the superficial adductor fascia. No signal changes in the muscles are seen, which is an important finding in the preoperative planning. The combination of both clinical and imaging findings were consistent with this surgically proven necrotizing fasciitis. *(From Salgado R, Alexiou J, Engelholm JL. Pseudotumoral lesions. In De Schepper AM [ed]. Imaging of Soft Tissue Tumors, 3rd ed. Berlin, Spinger-Verlag, 2006, pp 415–446.)*

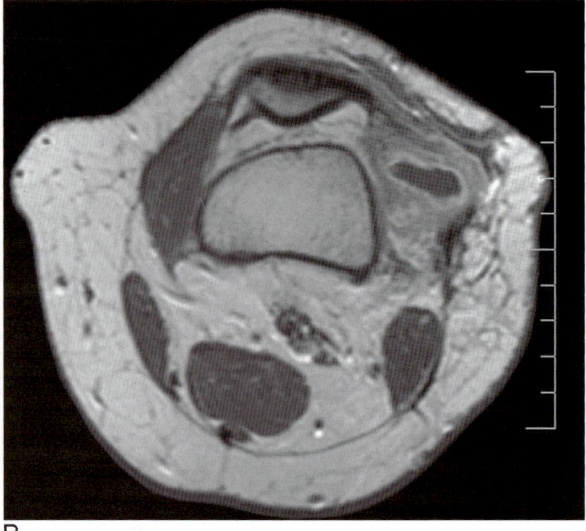

■ **FIGURE 94-5** A 40-year-old woman presented with a swelling at the left knee. **A,** Axial, spin-echo, T1-weighted MR image shows an ill-defined mass at the vastus lateris muscle of the left knee. **B,** On axial, spin-echo, T1-weighted MR image after gadolinium contrast medium administration a clear peripheral enhancement of an irregular mass is seen, with concomitant diffuse perilesional enhancement. The center of the lesion remains unchanged. The imaging characteristics are consistent with those of an intramuscular abscess.

high intrinsic resistance to bacterial infection and abscess formation. Therefore, some authors suggest that underlying muscle damage may facilitate the onset of pyomyositis.

Whereas pyomyositis was initially mainly found in tropical regions (e.g., after minor trauma or insect bite), in recent years there has been an increased incidence of this disease in industrialized regions with a more temperate climate. This is due to the presence of predisposing immune-compromising conditions including diabetes, human immunodeficiency virus infection, and malignancy. Pyomyositis is considered one of the most common musculoskeletal complications of the acquired immunodeficiency syndrome (AIDS). The causative organism is mostly *S. aureus*, although a number of other pathogens such as *Streptococcus pyogenes* and *Mycobacterium tuberculosis* have also been reported.

The clinical course can be divided into three stages. Initially, there is localized pain in one muscle group with induration of the overlying skin. This is accompanied by signs of systemic inflammation such as low-grade fever and mild elevation of the white blood cell count. Subsequently, in the second stage there is development of pus in the lesion, with increasing pain, fever, and edema of the affected muscle. Finally, a clear abscess develops with necrosis of the affected muscle. Blood cultures are positive in only 5% of cases, and in 1.8% the outcome is fatal due to sepsis and shock. Nevertheless, many of these symptoms may be absent when the lesion is deep seated. The muscles of the thigh and gluteus region are most often affected (Fig. 94-6), although the infection can appear in many other locations. In AIDS patients, pyomyositis may present as multiple lesions. However, multiplicity in this setting is not very specific for pyomyositis, because it may be found in other pathologic conditions, such as polymyositis, Kaposi sarcoma, and lymphoma.

On T1-weighted images the abscess collection has a low signal intensity compared with surrounding muscle tissue. On occasion, a high intensity peripheral rim is noted, probably representing blood breakdown products or granulation tissue. This has been described as very specific for infection.[1,2]

Pus in the abscess can have an intermediate to high signal on T1-weighed images depending on the protein content. T2-weighed images reveal a hyperintense collection in the affected muscle, with increased signal in the surrounding muscle tissue representing edema, organized phlegmonous collections, or hyperemia. Intravenous administration of contrast material can further discriminate between viable and necrotic muscle tissue, with the latter lacking enhancement.

On occasion, the imaging presentation of pyomyositis can be confused with a sarcomatous lesion, especially when further clinical and biochemical information is inconclusive. Key elements in the differential diagnosis favoring an infectious origin are the extent of the perilesional inflammatory reaction and the possible association of cellulitis (in the absence of previous surgery or local radiotherapy). Gallium scintigraphy is very sensitive for detection, on occasion also revealing additional distant abscesses. Because no anatomic detail is obtained, it must be reserved for those cases in which in spite of very suggestive clinical findings CT or MRI gives no additional relevant information.

Hydatid Cystic Disease

Hydatid cystic disease is a parasitic disease usually caused by the tapeworm parasite *Echinococcus granulosus*. Infection by *E. multilocularis* is more rare but has a more invasive nature sometimes mimicking a malignant

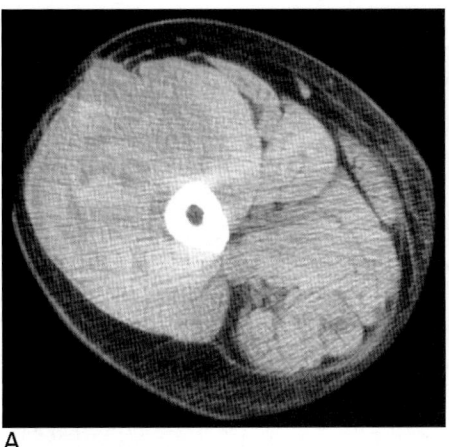
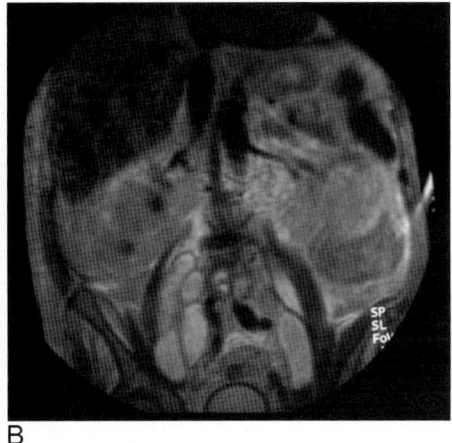
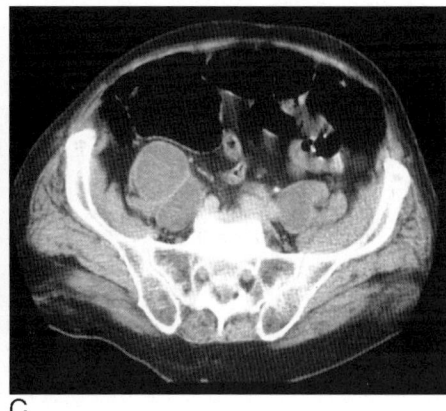

A   B   C

■ **FIGURE 94-6** Pyomyositis in a 48-year-old man (**A**) and a 72-year-old man (**B, C**), both after minor trauma during travel in tropical regions. **A,** CT scan in the first patient shows a distinctive increase in size of the vastus medialis, intermedius, and lateralis muscles of the right leg, with multiple ill-defined low-density areas. **B,** Similar findings can be seen in the second patient, with an ill-defined collection located between the L4-L5 intervertebral disc and the right psoas muscle. **C,** This is better illustrated on the coronal T2-weighted MR image, which shows bilateral, descending, soft tissue abscesses between the spine and the psoas muscles. These two cases demonstrate the typical history, location, and imaging characteristics of pyomyositis. *(From Salgado R, Alexiou J, Engelholm JL. Pseudotumoral lesions. In De Schepper AM [ed]. Imaging of Soft Tissue Tumors, 3rd ed. Berlin, Spinger-Verlag, 2006, pp 415–446.)*

lesion.[3] Hydatid cystic disease is a rare finding in Western countries. It is more common in parts of South America, the Middle East, Africa, Australia, and Mediterranean areas with sheep rearing, where the parasite is endemic. Although it may affect any organ, soft tissue involvement is unusual (1.75%-2.42%) because intramuscular growth of a cyst is countered by muscle contractility and lactic acid. Soft tissue hydatid cysts are nevertheless usually intramuscular and most frequently found in the head, neck, trunk, and the root of the extremities. A subcutaneous localization is also possible.

The imaging characteristics of soft tissue involvement resemble those of hydatid cysts found in the liver, showing a multiseptated or multicystic mass surrounded by a rim. Typically, the lesion consists of a mother cyst, containing multiple daughter cysts. On T1-weighted images these daughter cysts are seen as hypointense cysts within the intermediate signal of the mother cyst. The signal intensity of the daughter cysts on T2-weighted images can be high or low, with some authors suggesting a relation with the presence and absence, respectively, of viable scolices.[4] Still, the value of MRI in determining the viability of the cysts remains controversial.

A rim of low and/or high signal intensity on T2-weighted images surrounds the lesion. This rim is composed of three layers: an endocyst, ectocyst, and pericyst. The pericyst develops as a reaction after compression and inflammation of surrounding tissue. It is well vascularized, enhancing after intravenous contrast injection, and has thus an appearance like a pseudocapsule of sarcoma.[4]

MRI has proven superior over ultrasonography in detecting this multivesicular structure. More solid appearances are also possible, making it sometimes difficult to differentiate it from other soft tissue tumors.[5] Even in these cases, MRI can often reveal the vesicular nature of the lesion.

Focal Myositis

Focal myositis is a relative rare, usually self-limiting soft tissue pseudotumor. Although it can occur in many locations, it is usually found in the lower extremities, with 50% of the cases being located in the thigh and 25% in the lower leg. There is no sex or age preference. Approximately one third of the patients with focal myositis evolve to polymyositis or a polymyositis-like syndrome,[6] suggesting that focal myositis may be a localized form of polymyositis.

Focal myositis usually presents as a sometimes painful local intramuscular soft tissue mass, which can rapidly grow in a few weeks (Fig. 94-7). While the process is normally limited to a single muscle, involvement of multiple muscles has been reported. MRI reveals a heterogeneous signal pattern, with increased signal intensity on T2-weighted images, in one or more affected muscle groups. It can also clearly depict the extensive surrounding edema. A focal mass, when visualized, may enhance less than the surrounding edema.

Diabetic Muscle Infarction

Diabetic muscle infarction is a rare complication of diabetes mellitus. Patients with poorly controlled type 1 insulin-dependent diabetes mellitus and severe end-organ damage are most frequently affected, although it may occur in a well-controlled patient without known diabetic complications. Although the pathogenesis is still to be completely clarified, the most likely hypothesis is that muscle infarction is secondary to vascular disease such as arteriosclerosis and diabetic microangiopathy.

MRI can detect subclinical muscle infarction months before the onset of clinical symptoms. Whether MRI in conjunction with additional clinical and biochemical

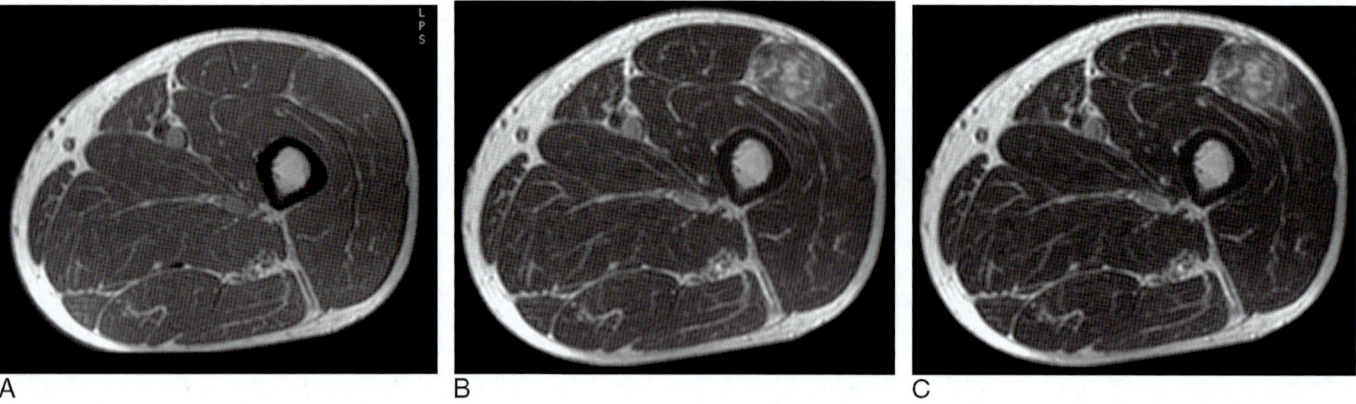

■ FIGURE 94-7 A 45-year-old man presented with a recently detected, nonpainful lesion at the anterior aspect of the left thigh. There was no history of trauma. Axial, spin-echo, T1-weighted (**A**), axial, turbo spin-echo, T2-weighted (**B**), and axial spin-echo, T1-weighted, contrast enhanced (**C**) MR images are shown. The T1-weighted MR images reveal a hardly visible lesion at the rectus femoris muscle. The lesion is clearer on the T2-weighted image, which shows the inhomogeneous and ill-defined aspect of this lesion. After intravenous contrast administration there is marked inhomogeneous and mainly peripheral enhancement with a nonenhancing central core. This case illustrates a biopsy-proven case of focal myositis.

information can reliably establish the diagnosis remains nevertheless unclear. As a consequence, the place of a biopsy in the diagnosis remains controversial.

MR images display enlargement of the involved muscles, with uniform increased signal intensity on T2-weighted and short tau inversion recovery (STIR) images, demonstrating the edematous and inflammatory changes (Fig. 94-8). T1-weighted images show normal or decreased signal intensity in the involved muscles, with the swelling being sometimes less appreciated on this sequence. The role of intravenous contrast medium injection in the differentiation with other entities such as pyomyositis, muscle abscess, or a necrotic tumor is not yet clearly established.

Bursitis

Bursae are defined as spaces near joints containing small amounts of fluid, thereby reducing friction between different structures. Whereas more than 140 different bursae have been described, the most frequently affected ones are the trochanteric, subdeltoideal, ischiogluteal, pes anserina, iliopsoas, and retrocalcaneal and olecranon bursae.

The amount of fluid may increase due to inflammation, which can have a infectious or noninfectious origin (overuse, direct trauma). In *noninfectious* bursitis repeated movements cause microtrauma in the tendon, tendon sheaths, and/or bursae. It may also be a first presentation of rheumatoid arthritis.

Infectious bursitis is a rarer pathologic process, usually associated with *S. aureus* infection or, on rare occasions, with β-hemolytic streptococci. It frequently affects the olecranon and prepatellar and infrapatellar bursa, probably because of their superficial location, which makes them susceptible to trauma and subsequent infection. Nevertheless, a clear history of trauma is not always found.

On MRI the increased fluid is hypointense on T1-weighted images and hyperintense on T2-weighted images. After intravenous administration of contrast medium, enhancement of hypertrophied synovium and surrounding soft tissue edema can be seen in both infectious and noninfectious bursitis.

Although no single imaging feature is able to reliably distinguish infectious from noninfectious bursitis, the combination of bone erosions with marrow edema is more suggestive for septic bursitis. Other features favoring an infectious origin are marked synovial thickening, synovial edema, soft tissue edema, and a complex appearance of the lesion. On occasion, the differentiation with a soft tissue sarcoma may be difficult, especially when the lesion has a complex appearance. However, the anatomic location of bursitis is often characteristic (e.g., iliopsoas bursitis) (Fig. 94-9), further adding to the correct diagnosis.

Sarcoidosis

Muscle involvement in sarcoidosis is rare, reported in only 1.4% to 6% of patients with known sarcoidosis.[7] Three main clinical presentations of muscular sarcoidosis can be distinguished: an acute myositic form, a diffuse atrophic form, and a nodular form. However, a diagnosis of sarcoid is typically not yet made and specific symptoms are often absent when a patient presents with a mass secondary to sarcoid infection. The acute myositis type occurs exclusively in the early stage of sarcoidosis, presenting as myalgia secondary to inflammation. MRI is usually negative, presumably because of the sparse distribution and small size of epithelioid cell granulomas.

In the diffuse atrophic myopathic form, patients can present with myalgia, muscle weakness, and atrophy. The muscles of the proximal portions of the extremities are frequently involved. MRI findings are nonspecific, revealing proximal muscle atrophy with fatty replacement. Differentiation from a corticoid myopathy is mainly based on clinical and laboratory findings.

The least common form is the nodular presentation, presenting as single or multiple, often bilateral, sarcoid nodules (Fig. 94-10). They may, or may not be, clinically

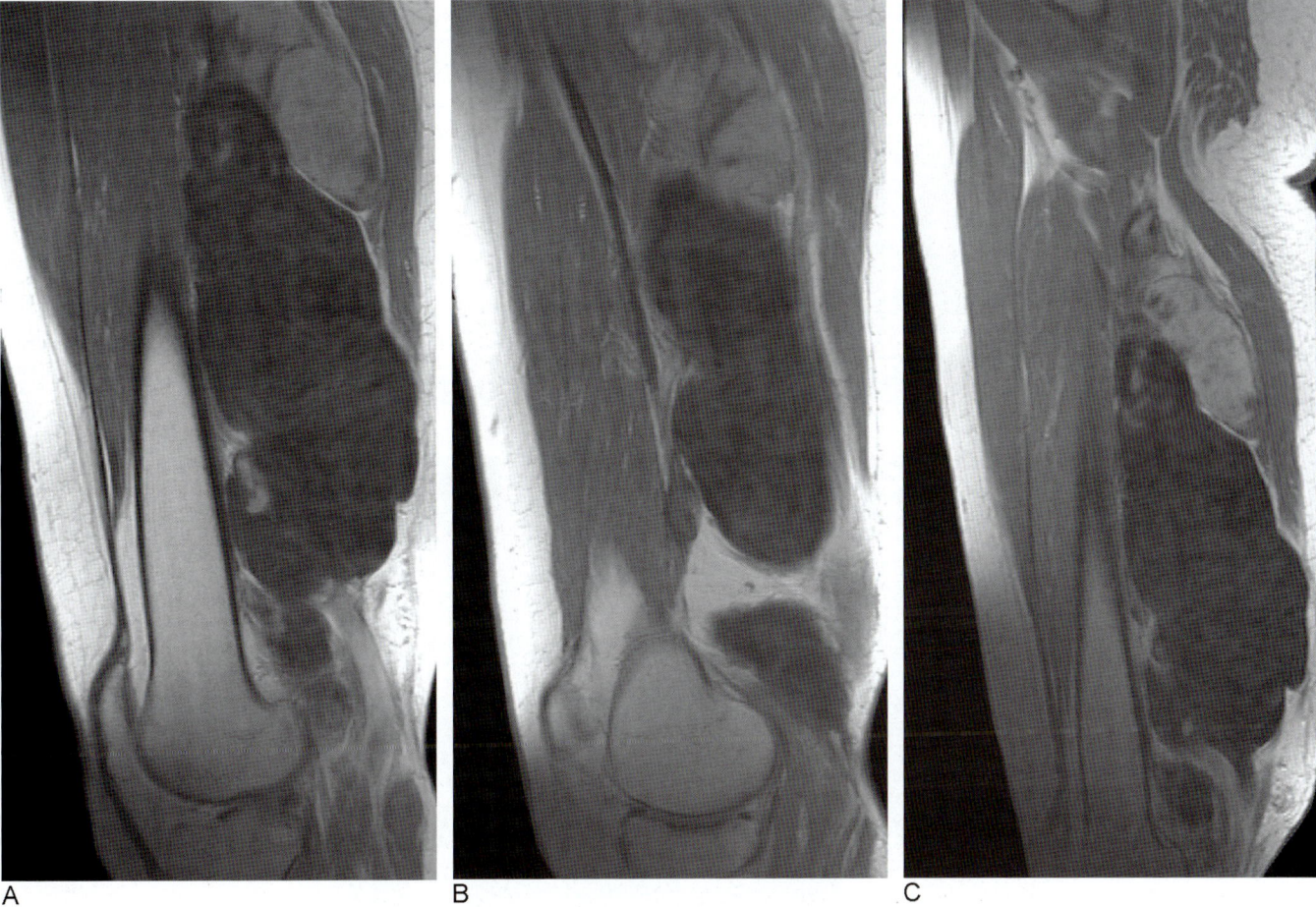

A   B   C

■ **FIGURE 94-8** Desmoid tumor at the flexor compartment of the thigh with a characteristic evolution from highly cellular to collagenous and also with a characteristic centripetal migration pattern. **A** to **C**, All three images are performed after intravenous administration of contrast material. There is enhancement of the proximal, noncollagenous components and no enhancement of the distal, collagenous components.

palpable. These nodules appear elongated and extend along muscle fibers. On ultrasound examination, sarcoid nodules present as a hyperechoic center and a hypoechoic peripheral zone. They may also present with well-defined borders and an overall hypoechogenic aspect.

On MRI, the nodules may have a star-shaped hypointense center on all axial pulse sequences ("dark star" sign) that is believed to correspond with fibrous tissue, which does not enhance after intravenous administration of a contrast agent.[8,9] However, this central structure is not present in the acute stage of the disease. It can also be absent in small nodules (<10 mm), presumably because of the short time of granulomatous inflammation in these small structures.

The peripheral area of the nodules is slightly hyperintense compared with muscle on T1-weighted images and has homogeneous high signal intensity on T2-weighted images. There is homogeneous enhancement after intravenous administration of a contrast medium, secondary to the high cellularity of granulomas and edema.

Coronal and sagittal images may show the "three stripes" sign, consisting of a hypointense inner stripe and hyperintense outer stripes. After corticosteroid therapy the sarcoid nodules may disappear, or only the inner stripe may be visualized.

Cat-Scratch Disease

Cat-scratch disease is a benign, self-limiting cause of regional lymphadenitis affecting mostly children and young adults. In more than 90% of the cases there is a history of recent contact with cats, a cat scratch, or both. In contrast, the site of inoculation is not always found. A gram-negative bacillus, *Bartonella henselae*, is the microorganism most often incriminated. In an otherwise healthy host, the adenitis resolves spontaneously within 3 weeks to several months, even without antibiotic therapy.

Cat-scratch disease has a wide spectrum of clinical manifestations, ranging from regional lymphadenitis to disseminated infection. Common locations include the neck, groin, and epitrochlear region. A typical case includes skin lesions and an associated enlarged painful reactive adenopathy commonly presenting along a single lymph node chain. Involved glands can have diameters up to 5 cm. Single-node involvement is most common, but multiple-node involvement at a single site is also possible. Disseminated infection is rare (5%-10%) but when present is most frequently seen in immunocompromised patients. Neurologic involvement is uncommon. Histologically, the soft tissue masses resemble granulomatous disease.

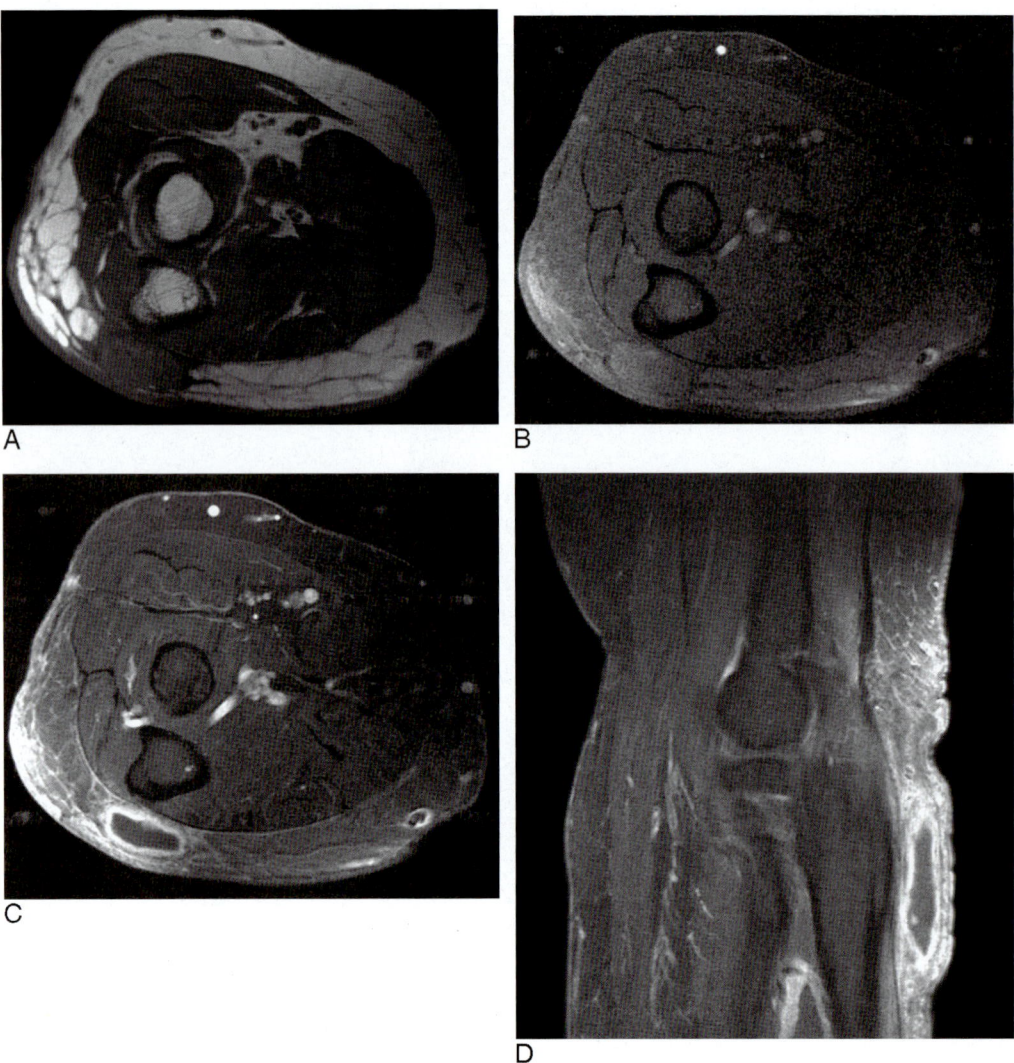

■ **FIGURE 94-9** A 60-year-old man with swelling at the right elbow for 2 months presented with redness of the overlying skin. Axial, spin-echo, T1-weighted (**A**), axial, spin-echo, fat-suppressed T1-weighted (**B**), axial, spin-echo, fat-suppressed contrast-enhanced T1-weighted image (**C**), and sagittal, spin-echo, fat-suppressed, contrast-enhanced T1-weighted (**D**) MR images. All of the images show an oval lesion at the posteromedial aspect of the right elbow, with perilesional stranding. After intravenous contrast administration there is clear peripheral and perilesional enhancement. These findings are concurrent with infected or inflammatory olecranon bursitis.

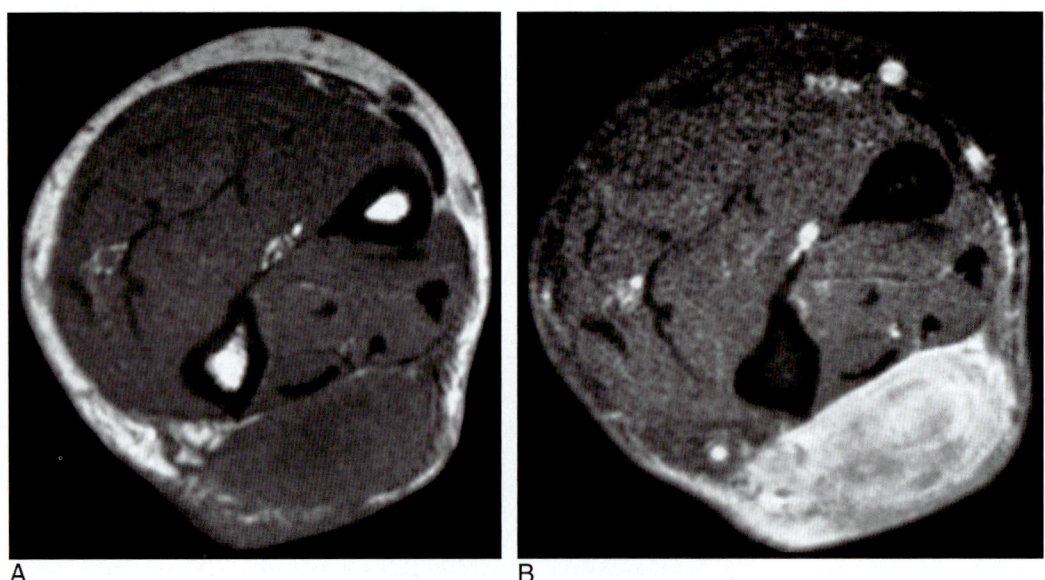

■ **FIGURE 94-10** Myxofibrosarcoma at the subcutaneous compartment of the forearm. The lesion is of low signal intensity on T1-weighted (**A**) imaging and high signal intensity on T2-weighted (**B**) imaging and nonhomogeneous with spin-echo sequences (not shown).

CT shows the enlarged, involved lymph nodes. Central necrosis can be seen as a low attenuation. MR images reveal the regional lymphadenopathy as homogeneous or heterogenic masses surrounded by edema. T1-weighted images show a homogeneous isointense signal intensity compared with muscle (Fig. 94-11). On T2-weighted images the area of the mass and surrounding edema becomes hyperintense. After intravenous contrast injection there may be homogeneous or slight peripheral enhancement of the involved lymph nodes and adjacent soft tissue edema.

Bone involvement is rare, usually presenting as lytic lesions. A periosteal reaction and associated sclerosis can be found. A single osteolytic lesion can simulate Langerhans cell histiocytosis.[10]

Actinomycosis

Actinomycosis is a chronic, suppurative, and granulomatous bacterial infection, usually caused by *Actinomycosis israelii*. Clinically, a cervicofacial, abdominopelvic, or pulmonary form can be distinguished. Soft tissue

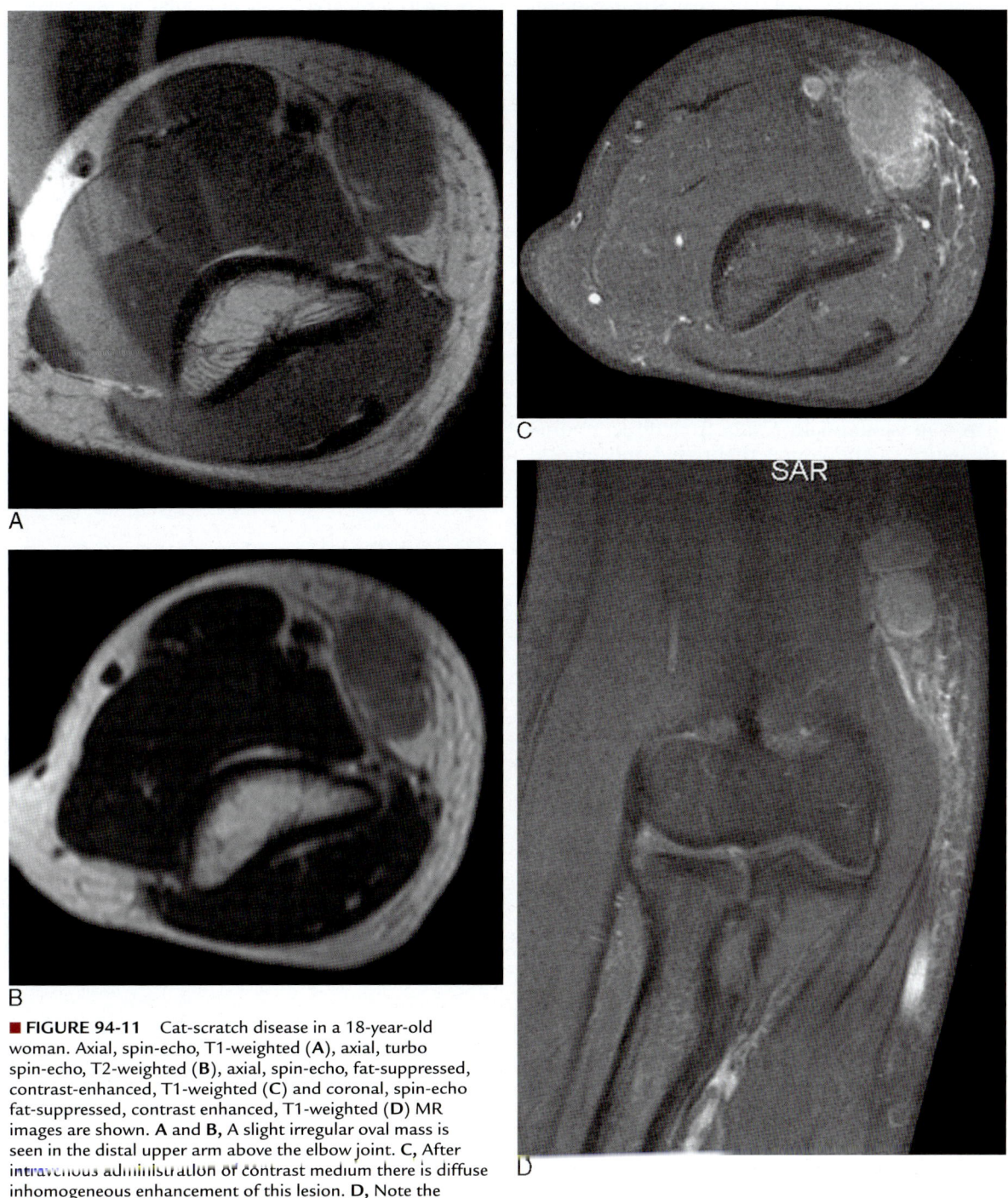

■ **FIGURE 94-11** Cat-scratch disease in a 18-year-old woman. Axial, spin-echo, T1-weighted (**A**), axial, turbo spin-echo, T2-weighted (**B**), axial, spin-echo, fat-suppressed, contrast-enhanced, T1-weighted (**C**) and coronal, spin-echo fat-suppressed, contrast enhanced, T1-weighted (**D**) MR images are shown. **A** and **B,** A slight irregular oval mass is seen in the distal upper arm above the elbow joint. **C,** After intravenous administration of contrast medium there is diffuse inhomogeneous enhancement of this lesion. **D,** Note the perilesional extensive surrounding lymphedema, a feature not commonly seen with soft tissue sarcoma.

manifestation often presents as a subacute cellulitis. On clinical examination a wooden, hard, palpable mass is often found. It commonly evolves to abscess formation. More unusual presentations can mimic tuberculosis, aspergillosis, or a malignant tumor (e.g., Ewing's sarcoma in the thoracic wall).

It can affect the head and neck, thorax, spine, abdomen, and skin. Histologically, the presence of "sulfur granules" containing colonies of *Actinomyces* is considered pathognomonic, although their absence does not rule out the infection.

Ultrasonography is useful in identifying the abscess formation and guides aspiration for culture of the organism. MRI characteristics are not specific, resembling abscess formation or a centrally necrotizing tumor (Fig. 94-12). MRI further illustrates the infiltrative nature, often showing a lesion that invades and crosses tissue planes.

TRAUMATIC LESIONS

Hematoma and Contusion

In every radiology department, trauma is a very common indication for further diagnostic imaging. Therefore, it is important for the radiologist to be familiar with the different presentations of post-traumatic soft tissue lesions.

Muscle contusion is generally caused by rupture of the small capillaries causing bleeding between the tissue muscle fibers. Muscle fibers are pushed apart rather than being torn. A contusion usually results from direct trauma with crush injury of the connective tissue and muscle fibers. This evokes subsequent edema and an inflammatory reaction with sometimes volume increase of the affected muscle. Contusions are not always painful, may be located deep in the muscle belly, and often produce late skin discoloration. MR images reveal a diffuse interstitial infiltration due to edema that is hyperintense on T2-weighted images but without associated architectural muscle distortion. These two features are uncommon in sarcoma.

In the workup of soft tissue hematomas ultrasonography is often the first imaging modality performed. An acute hematoma is usually hyperechoic, but echogenicity tends to decrease as the hematoma becomes older (Fig. 94-13). The margin may be well defined or irregular. The MRI appearance of muscular hematomas has many similarities with that of intracranial hemorrhage, sharing a similar pathophysiology of forming hemoglobin breakdown products (Table 94-2). The magnetic properties of these degradation products are mostly related to the oxidation and binding state of iron in the heme unit, closely correlated with the age of the hematoma. Nevertheless, other factors such as anatomic location, local partial pressure of oxygen, pH, presence of an underlying lesion, and field strength of the MR unit also influence the resulting image. Furthermore, there is no definite proof that blood within muscle tissue behaves exactly as an intracranial hematoma. Finally, more often than not, the age is not known, and signal characteristics are confusing at best (Fig. 94-14).

In intact erythrocytes, hemoglobin alternates freely between oxyhemoglobin and deoxyhemoglobin. In both forms the iron in the heme ring is in its reduced or ferrous form (+2 oxygenation state), a prerequisite for oxygen exchange. The relatively hypoxic environment of an acute hematoma (hours to days) promotes the release

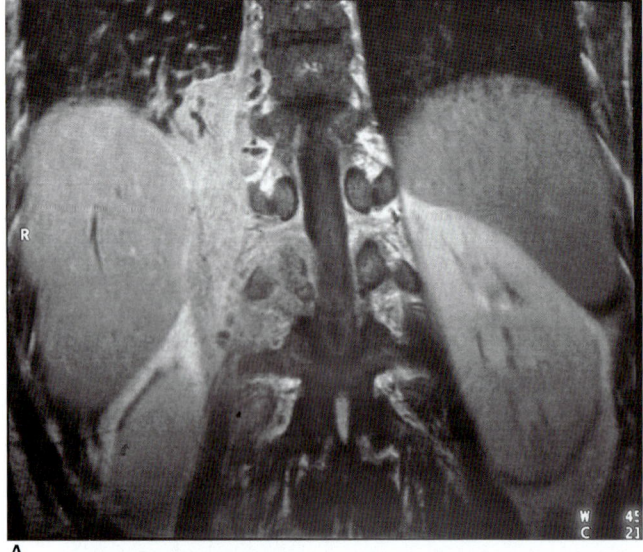
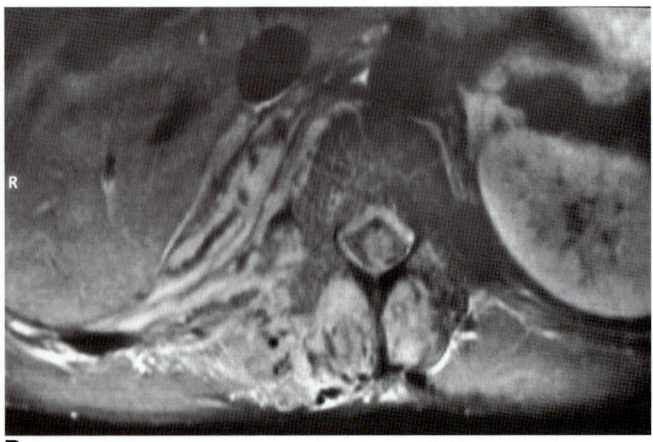

■ **FIGURE 94-12** Actinomycotic abscess in a 23-year-old man. Coronal, spin-echo, T1-weighted (**A**) and axial, turbo spin-echo, fat-suppressed, T2-weighted (**B**) MR images are shown. Note ill-defined structure of homogeneous intermediate signal intensity on the T1-weighted image at the level of the paraspinal muscles on a low thoracic level. The lesion extends both cranially and caudally, invading the right psoas muscles and the spine. *(From Salgado R, Alexiou J, Engelholm JL. Pseudotumoral lesions. In De Schepper AM [ed]. Imaging of Soft Tissue Tumors, 3rd ed. Berlin, Springer-Verlag, 2006, pp 415–446.)*

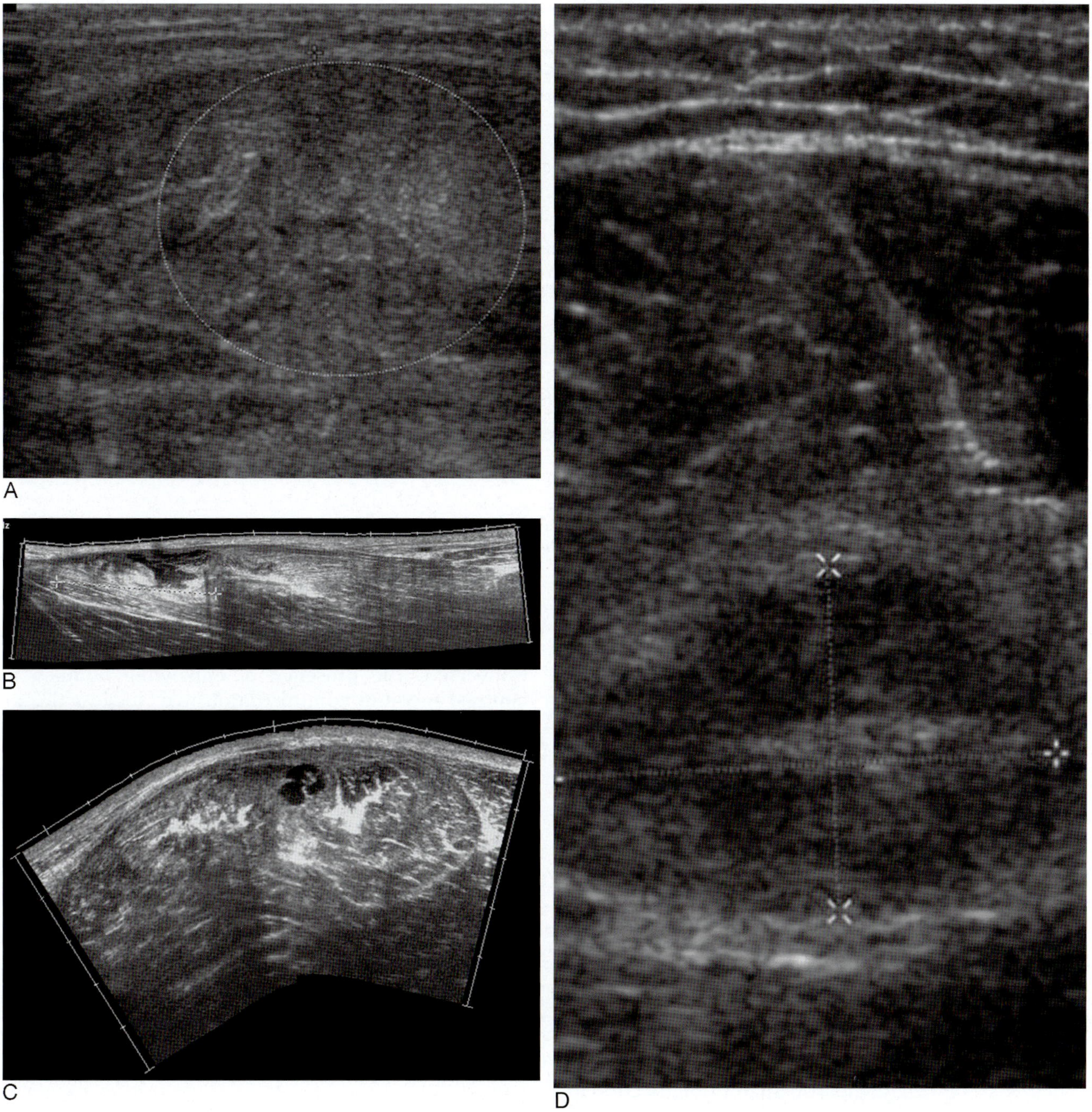

■ **FIGURE 94-13** Various stages of hematoma shown on ultrasound evaluation. **A,** Hyperacute hematoma in a 22-year-old man. The transverse image of the right biceps brachii muscle shows a hyperacute grade I injury, with several small areas of low and high reflectivity adjacent to one of the intramuscular septa in the long axis of the muscle belly (*dotted circle*). **B** and **C,** Post-traumatic hematoma in a 36-year-old man. Panoramic images of a grade II adductor longus muscle injury are seen in longitudinal and axial planes. There is a subacute partial tear at the muscle at the proximal myotendinous junction with an organizing hematoma. The torn end is evident by the presence of retracted muscle fibers ("clapper bell" sign). Perimysium tear with extramuscular fluid is evident. **D,** Follow-up of a subacute hematoma in a 25-year-old man. The ultrasound appearance reflects an aging hematoma (*cursors*), with an hypoechoic center and a slight hyper-reflective periphery. *(Images courtesy of Dr. Jan Gielen.)*

of oxygen, thereby disturbing this balance and quickly transforming oxyhemoglobin into deoxyhemoglobin.

In an early subacute hematoma (a few days), the shortage of oxygen as an energy source causes mitochondrial respiration to cease, thereby inactivating antioxidant metabolic pathways. This causes oxidation of deoxyhemoglobin into methemoglobin, which is in the ferric form (+3 oxygenation state).

So far, these processes have taken place in intact red blood cells. However, in a late subacute hematoma (7 days to 1 month) integrity of the cell membrane is lost, allowing methemoglobin to migrate extracellularly. This extracellular methemoglobin is further transformed into compounds named hemichromes. The final iron-containing degradation product is hemosiderin, which is formed by lysosomal degradation in macrophages.

TABLE 94-2   Evolution of MR-signal characteristics of hematomas according to their age

	Hyperacute hemorrhage	Acute hemorrhage	Early subacute hemorrhage	Late subacute hemorrhage	Chronic hemorrhage
Elapsed time after event	A few hours	Hours—days	<1 week	+/− 7 days— one month	Weeks—years
Hemoglobine degradation state	Intracellular oxyHb	Intracellular deoxy-Hb	Intracellular met-Hb (first at periphery of collection)	Extracellular met-Hb	Hemosiderin (accelerated at periphery of collection)
Magnetic properties	Diamagnetic	Paramagnetic	Paramagnetic	Paramagnetic	FeOOH is superparamagnetic
SI on T1-weighted images	Intermediate to low	Intermediate or low	High	High	Intermediate to low
SI on T2-weighted images	High	Low	Low	High	Low

A *hyperacute* hematoma (a few hours old) is seldom investigated with MRI. Because the transition from oxyhemoglobin into deoxyhemoglobin happens very fast, imaging of oxyhemoglobin as the main compound only occurs in rare instances, (e.g., in an aneurysm). This translates in a high signal on T2-weighted images, reflecting high water content of the collection.

In an *acute* hematoma the signal characteristics are dominated by intracellular deoxyhemoglobin. Because there is no proton-electron dipole-dipole (PEDD) interaction, the hematoma is isointense or slightly hypointense on T1-weighted images compared with muscle. Susceptibility effects also lead to low signal on T2-weighted images and are only well seen on high field strength systems.

A hematoma in the *early subacute* stage is characterized by the presence of intracellular methemoglobin, which has PEDD interaction. This produces a high signal intensity on T1-weighted images, often visualized as a high-intensity peripheral rim (Fig. 94-15A). This high-intensity rim is a useful sign because it may be the only clue that the mass is a hematoma. Susceptibility effects persist on T2-weighted images.

When loss of cell compartmentalization occurs in *late subacute* hematomas, extracellular methemoglobin is present. PEDD interaction is still at hand, giving T1 shortening. However, T2-weighted images now reveal a high signal intensity (see Fig. 94-15B). Diffuse edema is also present within the muscle in acute and subacute hematomas. Therefore, on T2-weighted images, the hematoma may be outlined by an area of high signal intensity.

Finally, hemosiderin in a *chronic* hematoma has no PEDD effect and also produces susceptibility effects on T2-weighted images. This results in low signal intensity on T1-weighted images and particularly on T2-weighted images. Furthermore, this phenomenon is accelerated at the periphery of the collection, resulting in a peripheral hypointense rim whereas the central portion of the hematoma may remain hyperintense (Fig. 94-16).

On occasion, a hematoma can be confused with a hemorrhagic tumor, because hemorrhage may obscure an underlying tumor. T1-weighted images with fat suppression can thereby aid in the differentiation, discriminating methemoglobin from fatty tissue. Overall, the best features in favor of a hematoma are the progressive decrease in size of the lesion, the presence of fluid-fluid levels, and the time-dependent signal intensity changes. Conversely, the presence of enhancing nodules after contrast medium administration may suggest the presence of tumor.[11] Nevertheless, organized hematomas can show some enhancement (see Fig. 94-14). In contrast to fast enhancement in soft tissue sarcoma, enhancement of hematoma is slow (>6 seconds after arterial enhancement).

A chronic expanding hematoma is an entity characterized by its persistence and increasing size for more than 1 month after the initial hemorrhage.[12] Its pathogenesis is poorly understood, the increase in size possibly due to the irritant effects of blood and its breakdown products, causing repeated episodes of bleeding from capillaries in the granulation tissue. MRI reveals a heterogeneous signal intensity on both T1- and T2-weighted images, with a peripheral rim of low signal intensity.

Foreign Body Reactions

Foreign bodies such as plastic, wood, glass, and silica may penetrate the soft tissues and induce an inflammatory granulomatous reaction. Clinically, this initially appears as a painful soft tissue swelling. After a quiescent period of weeks or months the symptoms may reappear. If not removed immediately, the foreign body can become encapsulated with fibrous tissue and a granuloma is subsequently formed. Histologically, histiocytes and giant cells with a surrounding inflammatory reaction are seen.

Different imaging methods each have their advantages and limitations in the evaluation of foreign bodies. Radiopaque bodies of sufficient size can be demonstrated on conventional radiographs (Fig. 94-17A). When the lesion is in or near bone, radiographs may show an

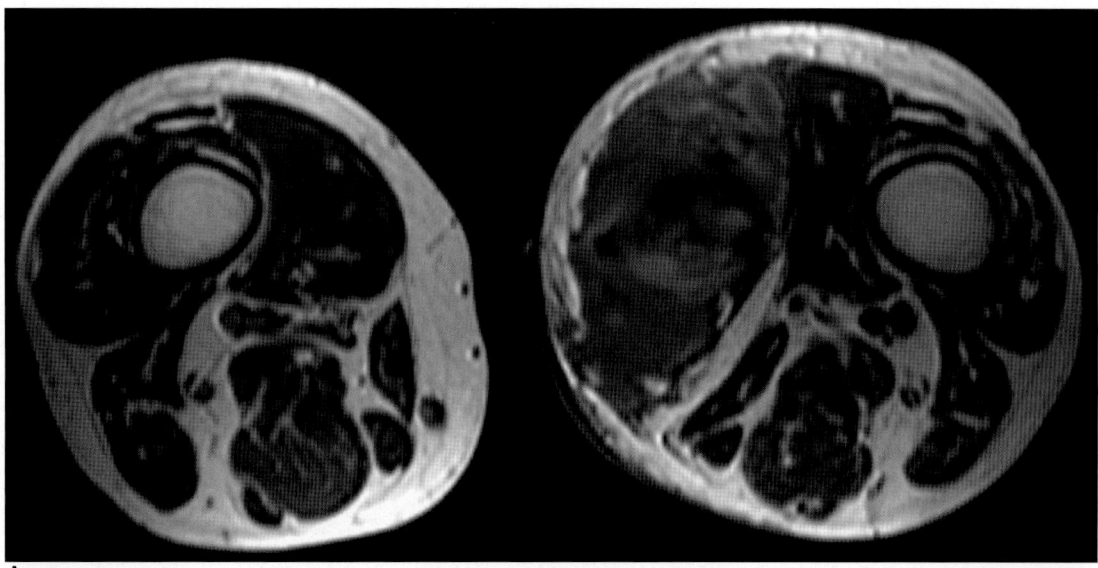

A

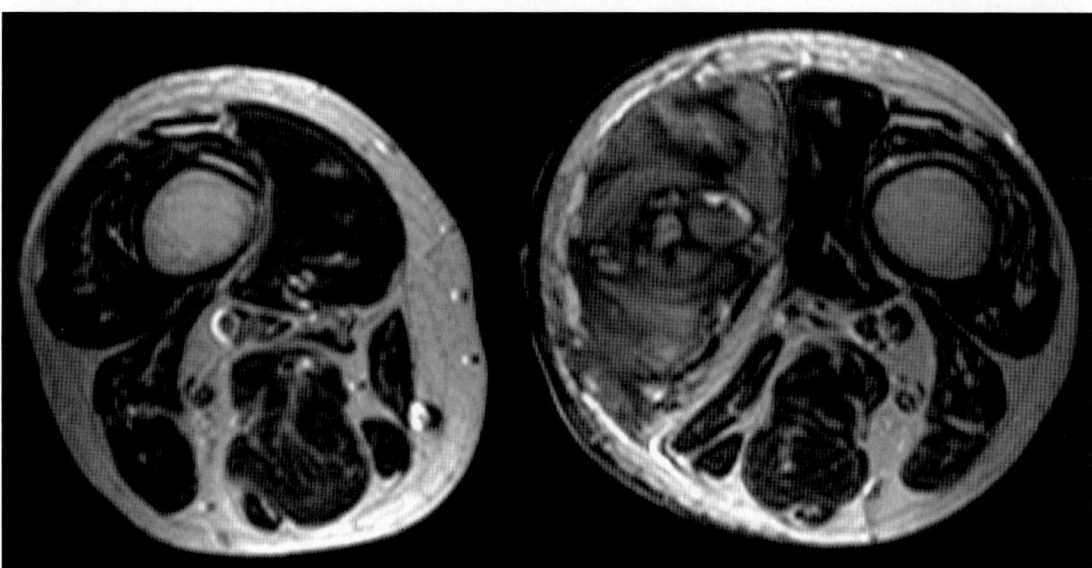

B

■ **FIGURE 94-14** A 60-year-old man presented with a complex mass on the medial aspect of the left thigh. Both axial, spin-echo, T1-weighted (**A**) and axial, turbo spin-echo, T2-weighted (**B**) MR images show a mix of high, intermediate, and low signal intensities with ill-defined margins. **C,** On the coronal spin-echo, fat-suppressed, contrast-enhanced T1-weighted image there is persistent inhomogeneous aspect of the lesion with subtle peripheral enhancement. Surgery confirmed a complex hematoma with blood products in different stages of degradation.

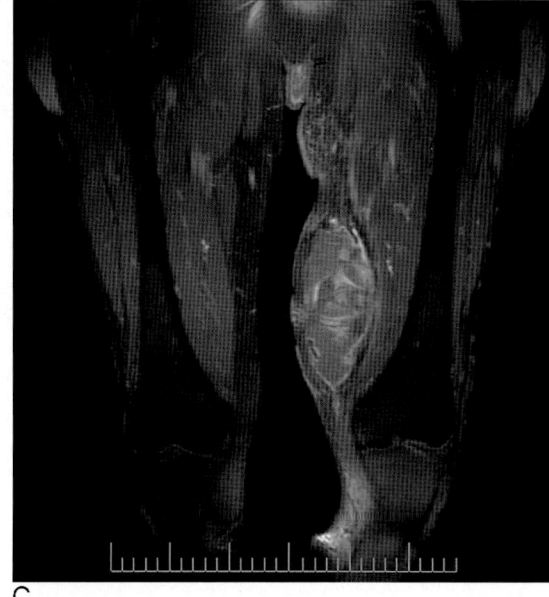

C

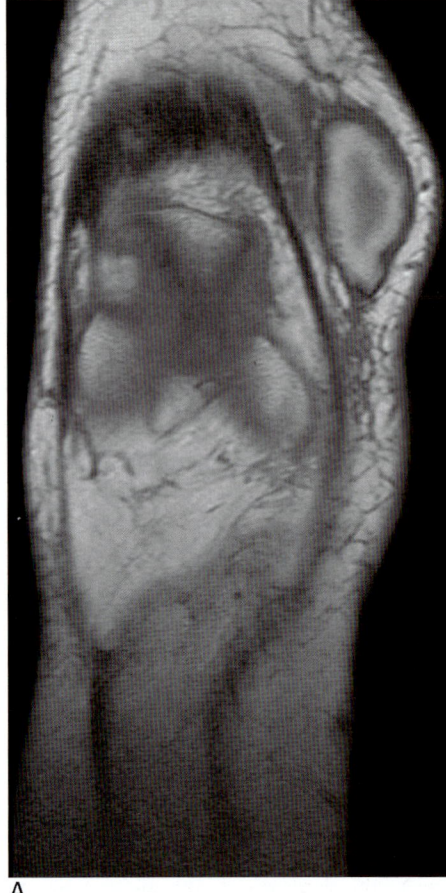

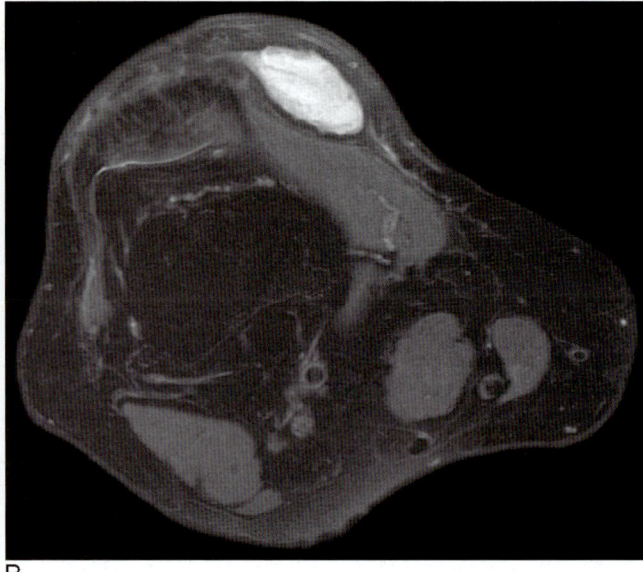

■ **FIGURE 94-15** Subacute hematoma above the knee in a 45-year-old woman with persistent pain. **A,** There is an oval mass within the subcutaneous tissue above the knee. Intermediate signal intensity of the center, high signal intensity of the periphery (representing methemoglobin), and low signal intensity of a small peripheral rim (representing hemosiderin) on this coronal, spin-echo, T1-weighted MR image result from different stages of hemoglobin breakdown products. **B,** On the axial, turbo spin-echo, T2-weighted MR image with fat suppression, overall signal intensity is very high, with exception made for a low signal intensity peripheral rim caused by hemosiderin. Signal intensities are characteristic of a subacute hematoma.

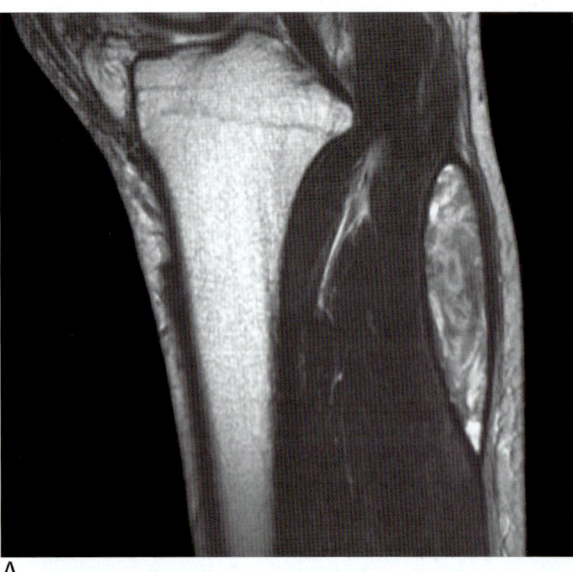

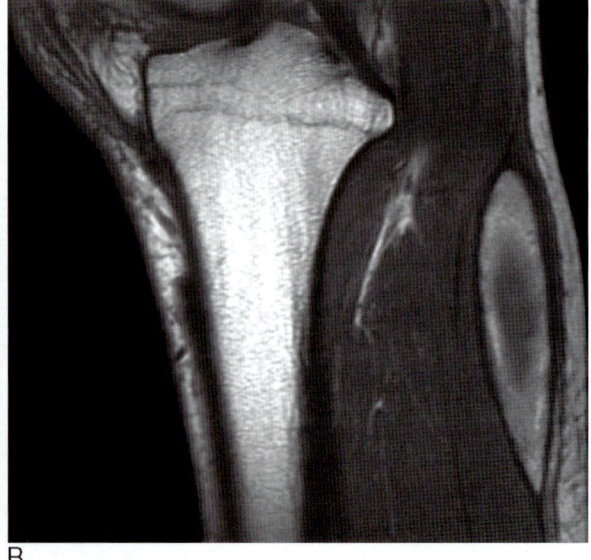

■ **FIGURE 94-16** Long-standing swelling posterior in the lower leg in a 30-year-old man. **A,** On a sagittal, spin-echo, T1-weighted MR image different strands of high signal intensity are seen, corresponding to extracellular methemoglobin. **B,** The central lower signal intensity on the sagittal, turbo spin-echo, T2-weighted MR image is caused by susceptibility effects. A clear low signal intensity hemosiderin ring is clearly demonstrated on both images. These signal characteristics correspond to a chronic hematoma. *(From Salgado R, Alexiou J, Engelholm JL. Pseudotumoral lesions. In De Schepper AM [ed]. Imaging of Soft Tissue Tumors, 3rd ed. Berlin, Spinger-Verlag, 2006, pp 415–446.)*

osteolytic and/or osteoblastic bone lesion.[13] A positive history of penetrating trauma is not always obvious, and some lesions can be radiolucent, making a clear diagnosis difficult.

Ultrasonography is a primary imaging tool when conventional radiographs fail in detecting the foreign object. Its use in the detection and guided retrieval of a suspected foreign body has been well established. Ultrasonography shows large differences in acoustic impedance between hyperechoic foreign bodies and hypoechoic surrounding inflammatory tissue (see Fig. 94-17B).

On MRI studies the foreign body itself is usually low, owing to the presence of few mobile protons in the commonly found foreign materials (e.g., glass, wood, metal). However, dispersed oil droplets can induce a granulomatous reaction and present as subcutaneous soft tissue masses with high signal on T1-weighted images.

The foreign body reaction appears isointense to muscle on T1-weighted images and hyperintense compared with subcutaneous fat on T2-weighted images. It is usually seen as an elongated mass without well-defined margins and surrounded by edema, which is best seen on T2-weighted images. The foreign body itself is hypointense both on T1-weighted images and T2-weighted images (Fig. 94-18).

Calcific Myonecrosis

Calcific myonecrosis is an uncommon and late sequela of trauma. The reported delay after the initial traumatic event ranges from 10 to 64 years, with an average age at the time of diagnosis of 56 years. Over time, a fusiform soft tissue mass develops in the traumatized compartment and may mimic a neoplastic process.[14] It is almost

exclusively found in the lower extremities, especially in the anterior and lateral compartments of the leg. Other reported more unusual locations include the foot and upper extremities.

The exact pathogenesis is still unknown. The initial event seems mostly to be local trauma, with subsequent development of compartment syndrome possibly leading to decreased regional circulation with necrosis and fibrosis. However, it has also been reported after neurovascular injury without compartment syndrome. Eventually, cystic degeneration occurs in the involved muscle, with plate-like calcification of a rind of fibrous tissue around the central liquefaction zone or hematoma. The expansive character of the lesion is believed to be secondary to intralesional hemorrhage. Some investigators believe that pathologic processes such as post-traumatic cysts of soft tissue, chronic expanding hematoma, and calcific myonecrosis share a common pathophysiologic mechanism. Therefore, Mentzel proposes the unifying term of *ancient hematoma* to describe these entities.[15]

Plain radiographs show a fusiform mass with plate- or plaque-like peripheral calcifications, which may precipitate in the cystic area of the lesion (Fig. 94-19A). In the presence of nearby bone, smooth bone erosions may occur, usually with no or minimal periosteal reaction. On occasion, these erosions can be extensive, thereby mimicking a soft tissue sarcoma. A liquid center can be seen on CT.

MRI signal characteristics range from a homogeneous to heterogeneous soft tissue mass on T1- and T2-weighted images (see Fig. 94-19B to E), with blood breakdown products contributing to the heterogeneity of the lesion. T1-weighted images reveal a fusiform mass with usually intermediate signal intensity in the central fluid region. The mass appears rather heterogeneous on T2-weighted

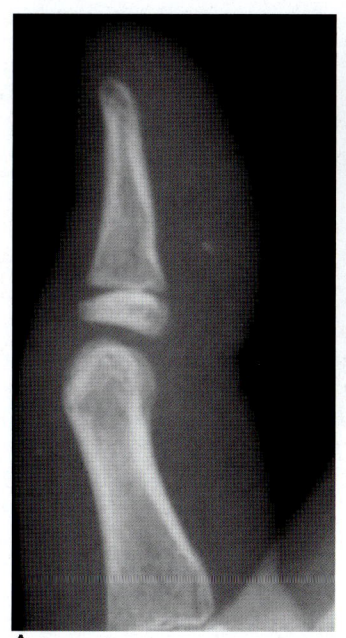

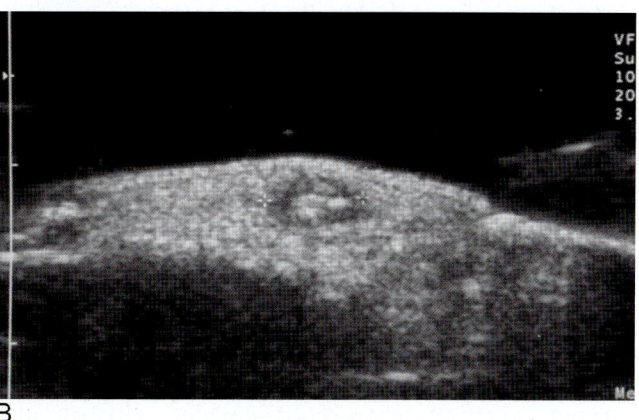

■ **FIGURE 94-17** A 14-year-old girl presented with a foreign body (wood) in her thumb. **A,** Radiograph reveals a small radiopaque foreign body in the thumb's soft tissue. **B,** The subsequently performed ultrasound examination shows a central hyperechoic wood fragment surrounded by a hypoechoic inflammatory reaction.

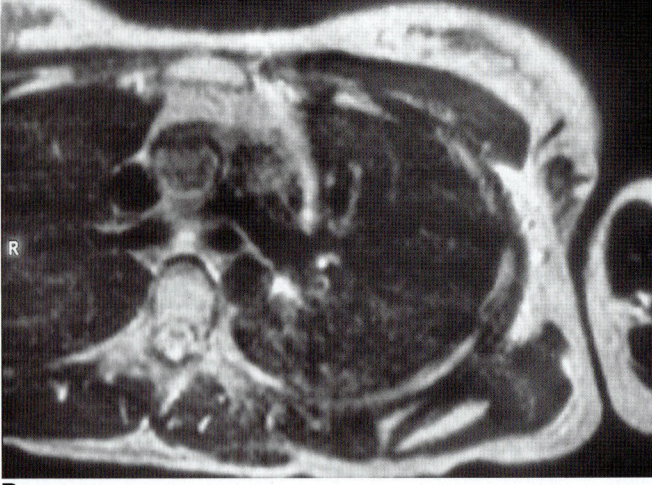

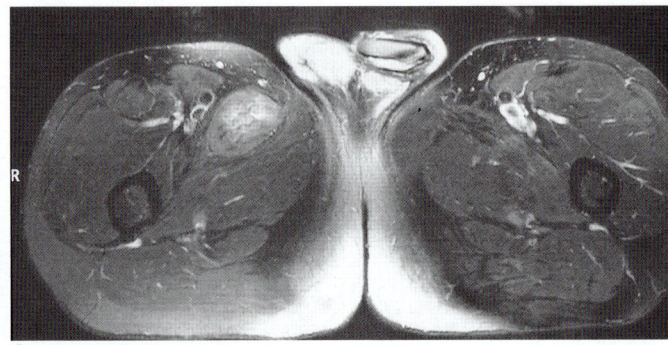

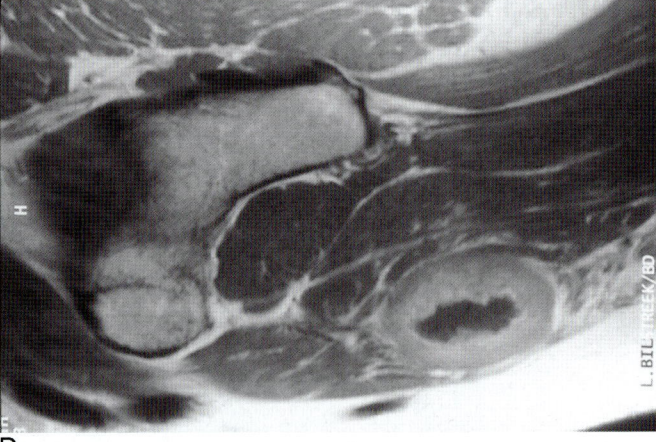

■ **FIGURE 94-18**   Foreign body in a 31-year-old man with a textiloma (gossypiboma) 3 years after orthopedic surgery. **A,** Radiograph of the right proximal thigh shows a foreign body, corresponding to a retained surgical sponge. **B,** On a sagittal, spin-echo, T1-weighted MR image a well-circumscribed nodular lesion is seen at the anteromedial aspect of the right thigh, with a slight hypointense center. **C,** On a T2-weighted MR image the lesion is inhomogeneous and has a predominantly intermediate signal intensity. No sign of necrosis is observed. **D,** A sagittal spin-echo, T1-weighted MR image after gadolinium contrast administration demonstrates strong enhancement of the periphery of the lesion. *(From Salgado R, Alexiou J, Engelholm JL. Pseudotumoral lesions. In De Schepper AM [ed]. Imaging of Soft Tissue Tumors, 3rd ed. Berlin, Springer-Verlag, 2006, pp 415–446.)*

images, with focal bright areas of high signal consistent with fluid while the rest of the lesion demonstrates an intermediate signal intensity. The calcified outer layer is reflected by a signal void. Usually there is no enhancement after intravenous administration of a contrast agent.

Infection of the mass without recent surgical intervention is rare.

Hypothenar Hammer Syndrome

The hypothenar hammer syndrome is a rare clinical entity, initially described by Guttani (1772) and Von Rosen (1934), while the term was more recently coined by Conn (1970). Typically there is unilateral digital ischemia due to embolic digital artery occlusion from a thrombosed palmar ulnar artery. It is commonly found in men around the age of 40 who usually in an occupational context repeatedly strike an object with the heel of the palm of the dominant hand. This causes damage to the superficial division of the distal ulnar artery as it passes over the hamate bone in the hypothenar region (Fig. 94-20).

Although most cases are unilateral, Ferris and associates found in a large series a striking incidence of similar changes in the asymptomatic and less traumatized hand.[16] Therefore, they hypothesized that there may be a preexisting fibrodysplasia of the palmar ulnar artery, making

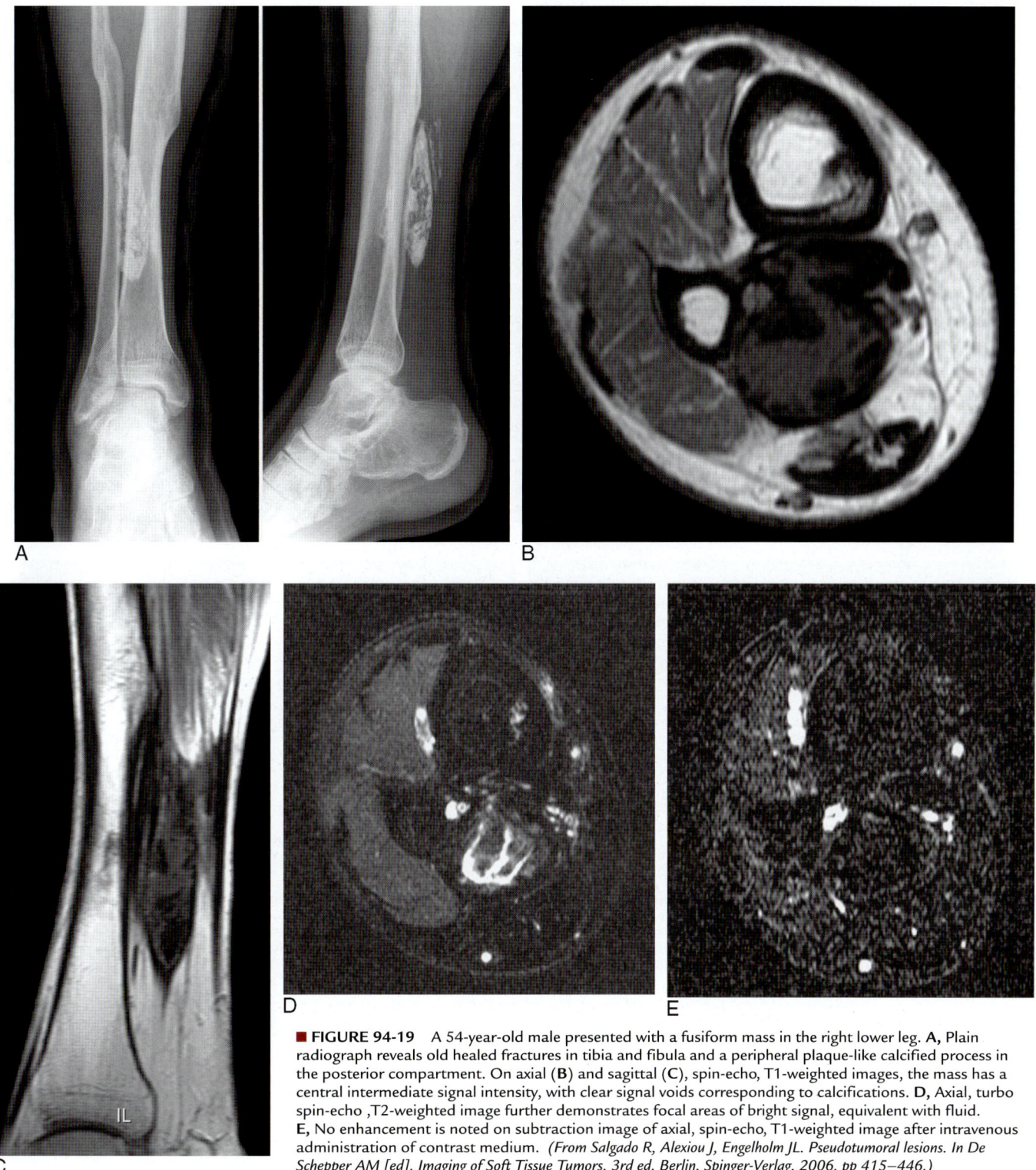

■ **FIGURE 94-19** A 54-year-old male presented with a fusiform mass in the right lower leg. **A**, Plain radiograph reveals old healed fractures in tibia and fibula and a peripheral plaque-like calcified process in the posterior compartment. On axial (**B**) and sagittal (**C**), spin-echo, T1-weighted images, the mass has a central intermediate signal intensity, with clear signal voids corresponding to calcifications. **D**, Axial, turbo spin-echo ,T2-weighted image further demonstrates focal areas of bright signal, equivalent with fluid. **E**, No enhancement is noted on subtraction image of axial, spin-echo, T1-weighted image after intravenous administration of contrast medium. *(From Salgado R, Alexiou J, Engelholm JL. Pseudotumoral lesions. In De Schepper AM [ed]. Imaging of Soft Tissue Tumors, 3rd ed. Berlin, Spinger-Verlag, 2006, pp 415–446.)*

this vessel more susceptible to arterial damage when subjected to repetitive local trauma.

The diagnosis is mainly based on clinical history and physical findings of unilateral digital ischemia. Angiography shows either segmental ulnar artery occlusion in the affected palm or "corkscrew" elongation with alternating stenoses and ectasia. Multiple digital artery occlusions are further demonstrated.

Treatment is mostly conservative, with surgery only used in rare instances.

Muscle Herniations

Muscle herniations may present as indeterminant soft tissue masses. They often appear in young persons who are subject to strenuous exercise (e.g., athletes, soldiers)

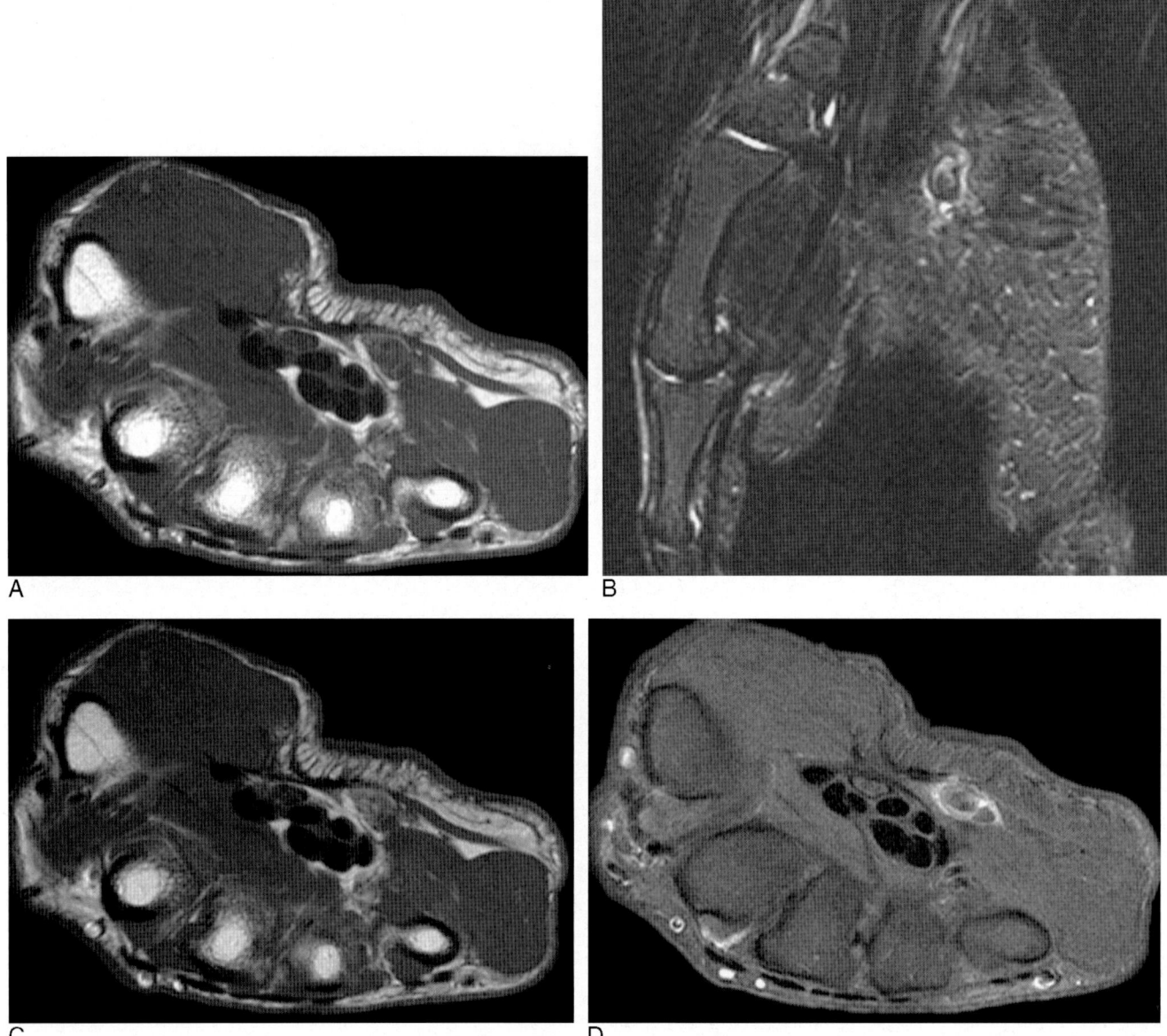

■ FIGURE 94-20 A 52-year-old man presented with painful soft tissue swelling on the right hand. Axial, spin-echo, T1-weighted (**A**) and coronal (**B**) STIR MR images show a nodular inhomogeneous lesion in Guyon's canal at the course of the ulnar artery, on the radial side of the ulnar nerve. **C,** On axial spin-echo T1-weighted imaging after intravenous contrast administration there is a marked enhancement of the peripheral part and of the perilesional area. **D,** This is better seen on a fat-suppressed image. The central part remains of low sign intensity with a low peripheral rim. Because sarcoma could not be excluded, surgery was performed, revealing damage to the ulnar artery consistent with hypothenar hammer syndrome.

and can be multiple and bilateral. The diagnosis is mainly based on knowledge of the most common locations and can be confirmed by ultrasonography and MRI. Here the soft tissue mass has the same echographic and MRI signal characteristics as normal muscular tissue. Dynamic examination is possible on both imaging modalities, revealing the changes in shape and size of the lesion. MRI can further depict adjacent edema or contusion and can, on occasion, reveal the fascial defect (Fig. 94-21).

Myositis Ossificans

Myositis ossificans is a well-known benign, self-limiting entity, typically presenting as a solitary soft tissue mass.

The mass may, however, be connected to bone. It is the most common bone-forming lesion of soft tissue and is most frequently found in young males. Although the exact pathogenesis in not really known, in around 50% of cases there is a history of trauma. The limbs are most commonly affected, presumably because they are most prone to trauma. Other precipitating factors include paraplegia or quadriplegia, burns, and other neuromuscular disorders.

In the acute stage the most frequent complaint is pain, tenderness, and soft tissue swelling in the affected region. Over 2 to 3 weeks, the lesion becomes gradually more circumscribed and indurated to eventually evolve into a firm hard mass that can vary in size between 3 and 6 cm. These stages are reflected in a varying imaging appearance.

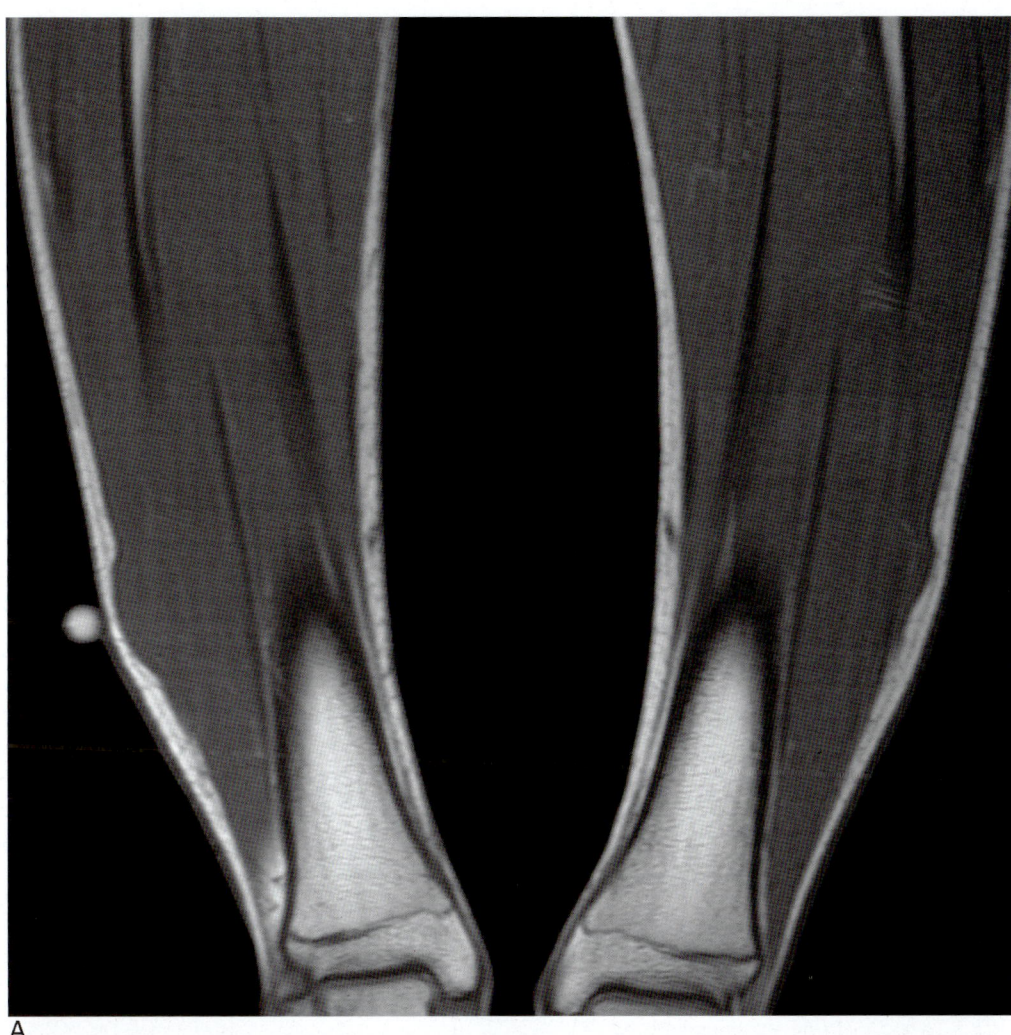

A

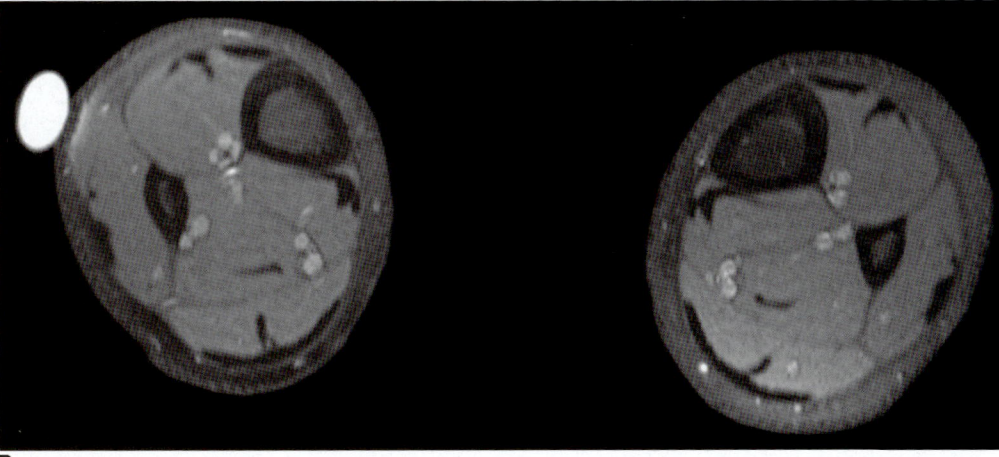

B

■ **FIGURE 94-21** Long-standing bilateral muscle herniation in a 15-year-old boy. Coronal, spin-echo, T1-weighted (**A**) and axial, turbo spin-echo, fat-suppressed, T2-weighted (**B**) MR images show a focal bulging of the peroneus muscle compartment that is more pronounced on the right side. As expected, this protruding mass has the same signal characteristics of normal muscle tissue. *(From Salgado R, Alexiou J, Engelholm JL. Pseudotumoral lesions. In De Schepper AM [ed]. Imaging of Soft Tissue Tumors, 3rd ed. Berlin, Spinger-Verlag, 2006, pp 415–446.)*

The initial acute phase is mainly characterized by an increased vascularization of the region, with increased density of soft tissues. No ossification is present. On MRI a focal mass can be seen that is isointense to slightly hyperintense on T1-weighted images compared with muscle and hyperintense on T2-weighted images. Marked surrounding inflammation and edema can also be appreciated. After intravenous administration of a contrast agent, an enhancing peripheral rim, surrounded by the reactive zone can be seen (Fig. 94-22). However, other enhancement patterns in active lesions can also been seen mimicking other inflammatory masses or a malignant lesion (Fig. 94-23).

In the more intermediate/subacute phase, there is only a slight hyperintense signal on T2-weighted images whereas the lesion remains isointense on T1-weighted images. This reflects the central fibrous transformation. After 4 to 6 weeks a thin peripheral rim of floccular and

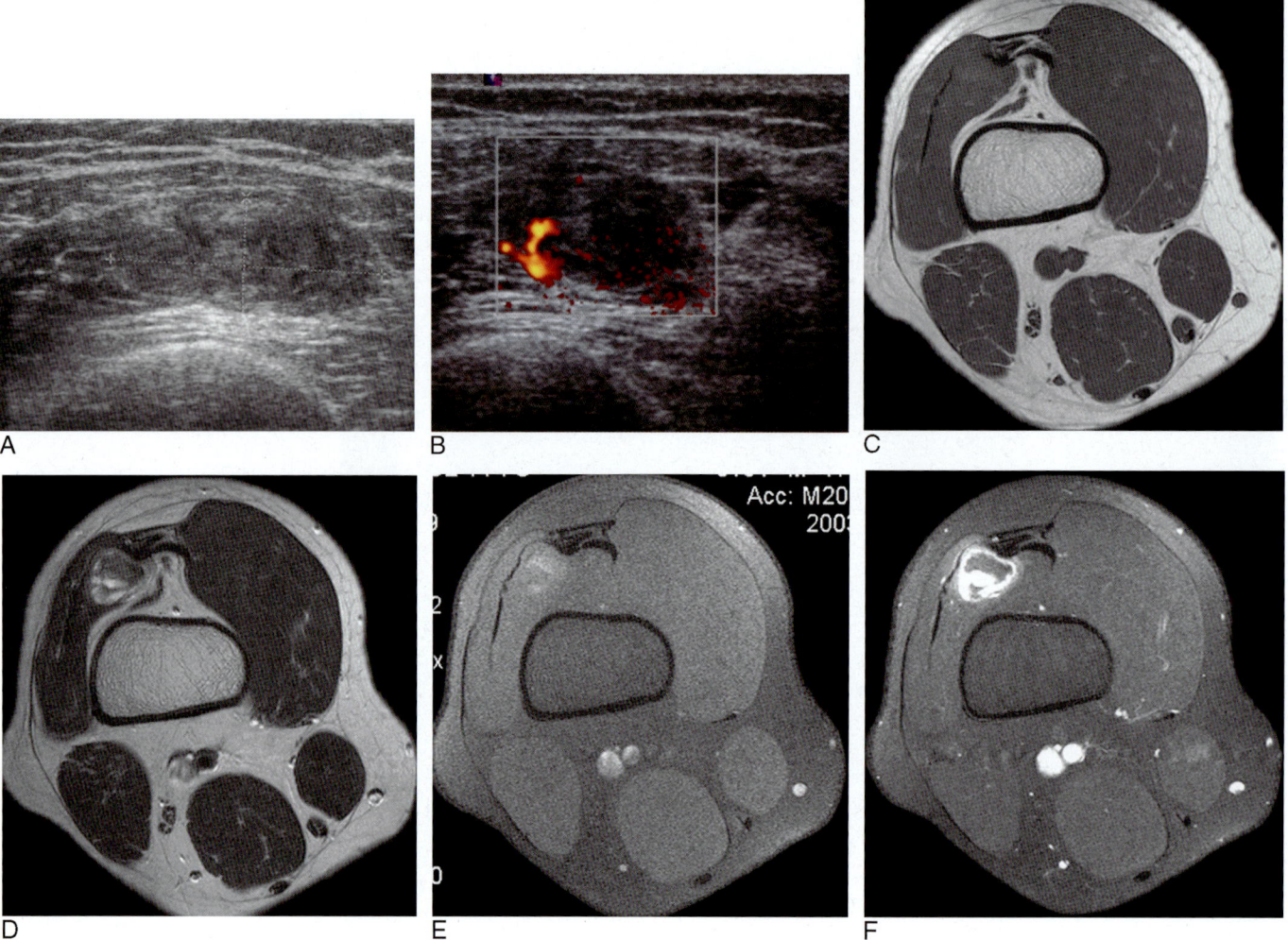

■ FIGURE 94-22 A 17-year-old young man presented with a suddenly noticed, firm mass at the right upper leg. A fusiform inhomogeneous but overall hypoechoic mass is clearly seen on ultrasound (**A**, *cursors*), with some peripheral vascular signal on power Doppler examination (**B**). **C** to **F**, The MR images further show a small, nonhomogeneous lesion at the distal musculotendinous junction of the vastus intermedius muscle. It is almost invisible on the conventional axial spin-echo T1-weighted image (**C**) but better appreciated on a fat-suppressed image (**E**), where it has a hyperintense center with an isointense periphery. **D**, The axial turbo, spin-echo, T2-weighted image reveals a hypointense center and intermediate to high signal at the periphery. **F**, A marked peripheral enhancement is noted after intravenous administration of contrast medium. This case shows typical imaging findings, with little reactive changes, of myositis ossificans in a more mature stage.

irregular-shaped calcifications may begin to form, giving small signal voids on all pulse sequences. Signs of hemorrhage can also be seen.

In the chronic or mature phase, the calcification-ossification has further developed, giving significant signal void on all pulse sequences (Fig. 94-24). This bone-forming process follows a centrifugal pattern or "zoning" phenomenon, with lamellar bone forming at the periphery (highest cell maturation) and proceeding toward the immature center. When a biopsy is taken from this immature center only, an erroneous histologic diagnosis of sarcoma can be made. This calcification-ossification progression can be seen with ultrasonography but is better depicted with CT or conventional radiography (Fig. 94-25) and can give the lesion an onionskin appearance. The MRI appearance of the various stages usually allows a confident diagnosis of myositis ossificans to be made. Biopsy can be replaced by follow-up in these cases. This is important because biopsy may trigger progression of disease. Especially in osteogenesis imperfecta, callus

formation and myositis ossificans may mimic osteosarcoma both on imaging and histology.

Although malignant transformation to an extraskeletal osteosarcoma has been suggested, this has not been proven. Consequently, myositis ossificans has an excellent prognosis.

Injection Granulomas

Injection granulomas are most often encountered in the upper outer quadrant of the buttocks and in the deltoid muscle. The typical location and the absence of muscle distortion are the clues to the diagnosis. On CT, they appear as small well-defined nodules, often containing calcifications. These lesions are hypointense on T1-weighted MR images and hyperintense or hypointense on T2-weighted images, depending on whether the major pattern of the lesion is inflammatory or fibrous. This pattern depends on the time elapsed after injection.

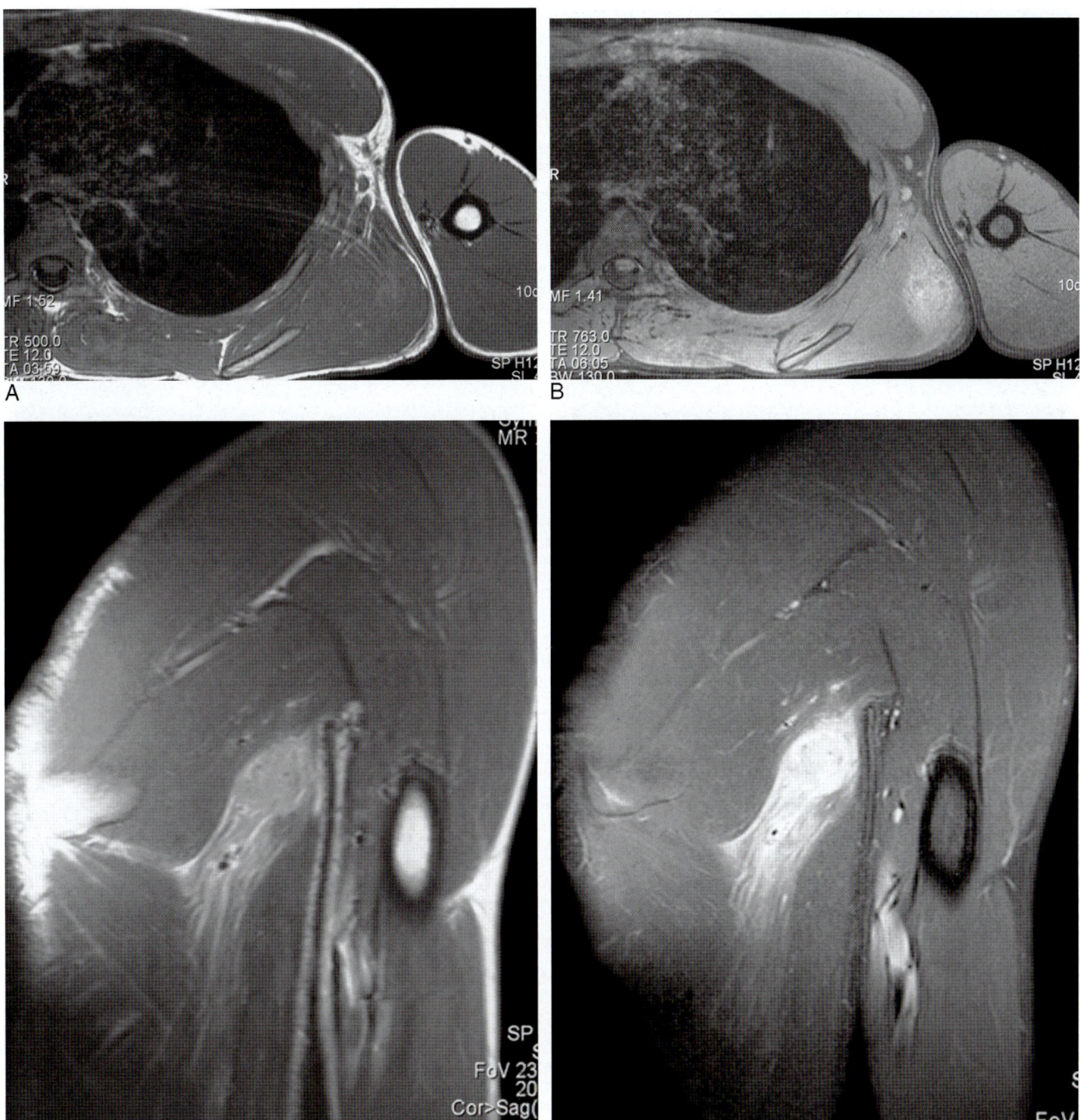

■ **FIGURE 94-23** Shoulder mass since 3 weeks in a 18-year-old swimmer with no history of trauma. The different images show an oval, slight ill-defined lesion within the latissimus dorsi region. It is hardly visible on the standard axial spin-echo T1-weighted image (**A**) but is overall slightly hyperintense on the fat-suppressed T1-weighted image (**B**). **C,** The center of the lesion is nonhomogeneous on the coronal, turbo spin-echo, T2-weighted image, with a slightly higher signal at the periphery and perilesional edema and inflammation. **D,** After intravenous administration of a contrast medium there is strong enhancement of the nodule and the surrounding reactive changes on this coronal, spin-echo, T1-weighted image. This case illustrates a histologically proven case of myositis ossificans in the acute stage, with diffuse increased vascularity but without detectable ossification.

SKIN LESIONS

Pilomatricoma

A pilomatricoma is a benign, slow-growing superficial tumor of the hair follicle most commonly seen in children and young adults. Various terms have been previously used to indicate this pathology, including calcifying epithelioma of Malherbe and pilomatrixoma, the latter better indicating its histologic origin from hair matrix cells. Clinically it presents as a solitary subcutaneous calcified mass, most often found (in decreasing order of prevalence) in the head, neck, upper extremities, trunk, and lower extremities. Calcification is not mandatory. Most lesions are less than 3 cm, but larger masses have

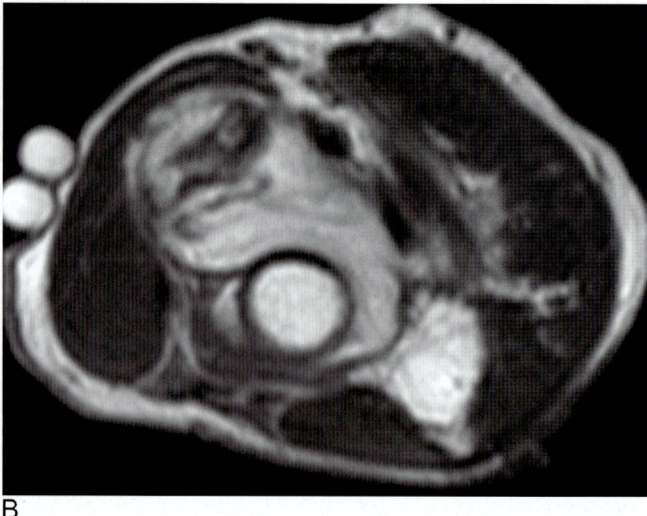

A   B

■ **FIGURE 94-24** A 75-year-old woman had a long-standing mass in the upper arm. A comma-shaped, sharply delineated mass is seen anterior to the head of the radial bone and adjacent to the biceps tendon. **A,** Signal characteristics on the axial, spin-echo, T1-weighted image are equal that of normal fat except for a central hypointense component. **B,** On the axial, turbo spin-echo, T2-weighted image the central component is more hyperintense with a low signal periphery. There was no enhancement after intravenous administration of contrast medium (not shown). The imaging findings are consistent with long-standing mature myositis ossificans with calcification-ossification and no obvious vascularity.

been reported. A rare association of multiple pilomatrico-mas with myotonic dystrophy, Steinert's disease, Turner's syndrome, sarcoidosis, and Gardner's syndrome has been described.

MR images reveal a well-defined subcutaneous tumor with intermediate signal intensity on T1-weighted images and low-to-intermediate signal intensity on gradient-echo and T2-weighted images (Fig. 94-26). T2-weighted fat-suppressed images may show bands of hyperintense signal radiating away from a lower signal intensity center toward the periphery. Enhancement is possible but not necessary. Amorphous calcification of the tumor may give the lesion an inhomogeneous aspect.

A pilomatrix carcinoma is an uncommon aggressive form, representing up to 9% of benign pilomatricomas at any age. Local invasion is possible, but distant metastasis is rare.

Granuloma Annulare

Granuloma annulare is a benign inflammatory idiopathic disorder of the dermis characterized by formation of dermal papules mostly in young children. Its pathogenesis is still unknown. It typically presents as a rapidly growing, solitary, painless, subcutaneous nodule without calcification. According to Kransdorf, in children it is the most sampled benign soft tissue mass of the lower extremity.[17]

It has various clinical presentations, in which four forms can be distinguished: three cutaneous forms (erythematous, perforating and generalized) and the subcutaneous form, the latter presenting as a soft tissue mass. Radiographs have little value, revealing only an increased density in the subcutaneous compartment

without evidence of bone involvement or mineralization. Ultrasonography shows an ill-defined solid mass that is hypoechoic to surrounding fat. It excludes a vascular or cystic lesion.

The MRI characteristics of subcutaneous granuloma annulare have been described by several authors.[18] T1-weighted images show an ill-defined subcutaneous mass, isointense to muscle, with a slightly hypointense signal intensity compared with fat on T2-weighted images (Fig. 94-27). T2-weighted images may show a heterogeneous hyperintense lesion. After intravenous contrast injection a diffuse enhancement can be seen.

Epidermal Inclusion Cyst (Infundibular Cyst)

Epidermal inclusion cysts are common benign subcutaneous cysts formed by the cystic enclosure of epithelium within the dermis. They contain a mixture of keratin and lipid-rich debris. Commonly, they are iatrogenic, resulting from mechanical obstruction, scarring, or inflammation. Many locations have been described, but this cyst commonly is found in the head, neck, and trunk. Less than 10% occur in the extremities. Although most lesions are small, some can grow into large masses.

The MRI findings resemble that of a simple cyst, with signal characteristics varying with the protein content of the cyst (Fig. 94-28). High protein content can appear hyperintense to muscle on T1-weighted images. Cysts may rupture, provoking a foreign body reaction, granulomatous reaction, or abscess formation. On occasion, they may be multiloculated.

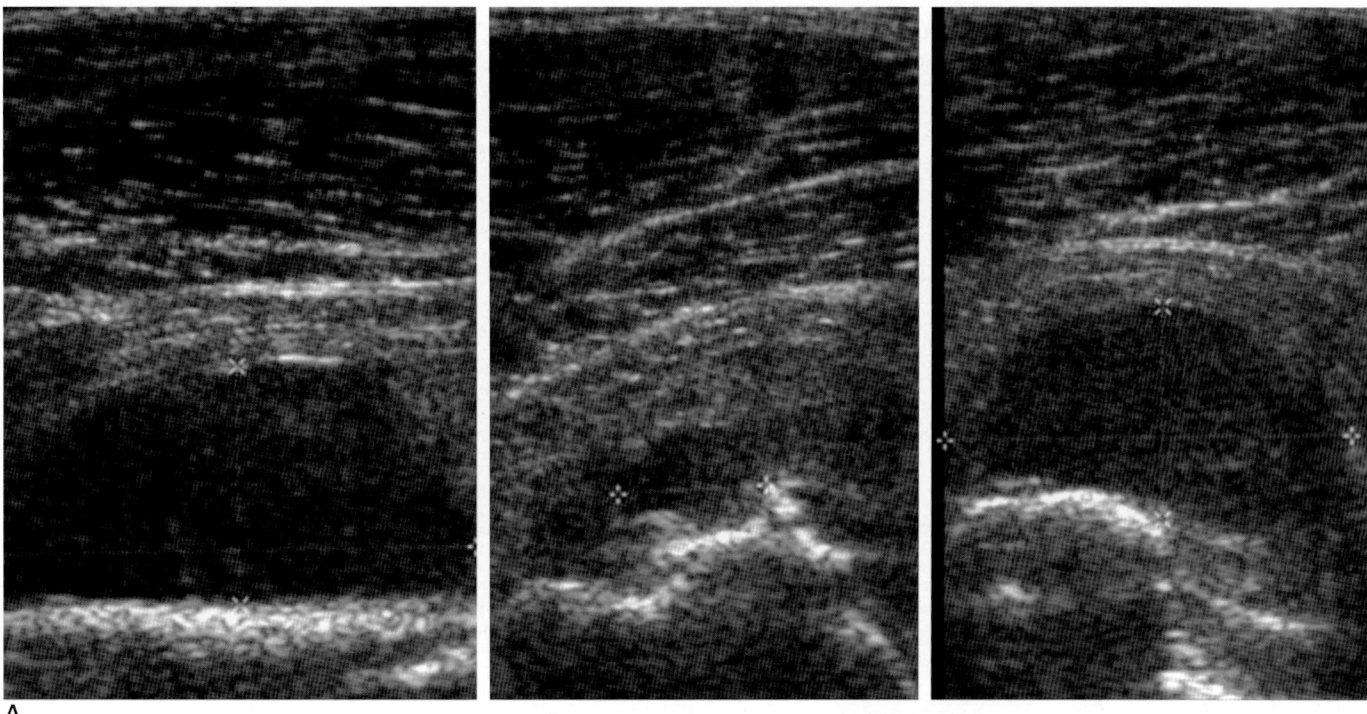

A

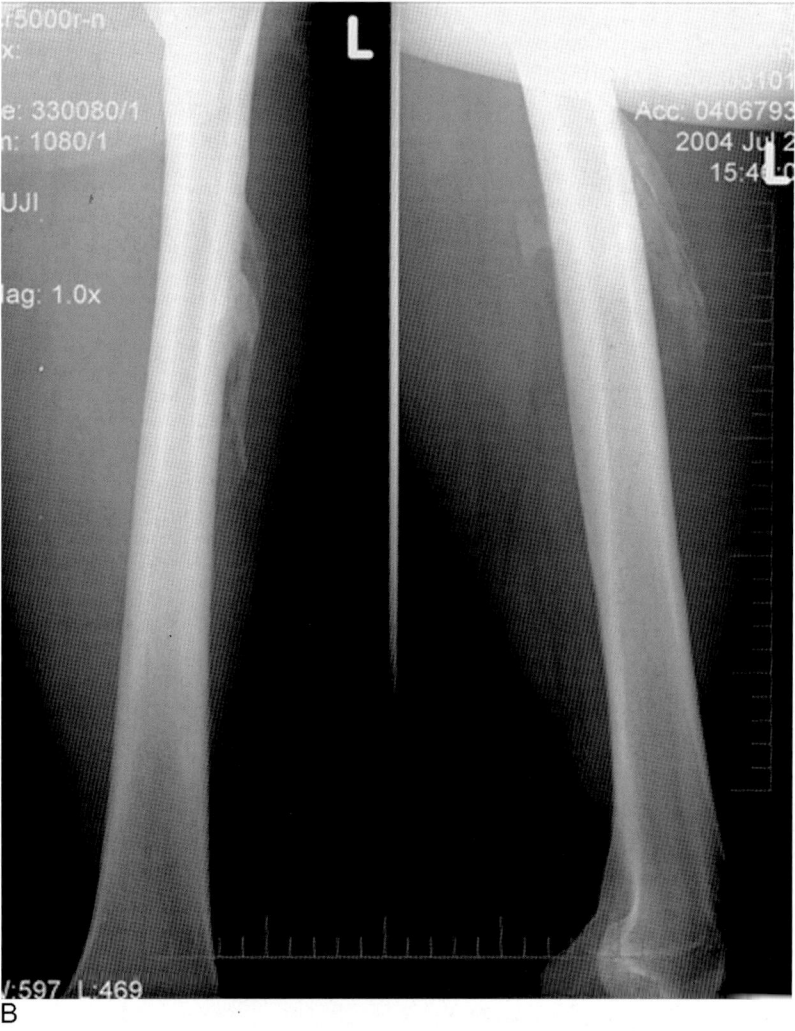

B

■ **FIGURE 94-25** Palpable mass in the thigh of a 35-year-old man, 4 months after injury. **A,** Longitudinal (*left*) and axial (*middle* and *right*) ultrasound images of the thigh reveal a focus of calcification and posterior acoustic shadowing that corresponded to a palpable soft tissue mass at the vastus intermedius muscle. **B,** Radiograph obtained on the same day demonstrates a huge focus of mature ossification. These appearances are compatible with late myositis ossificans.

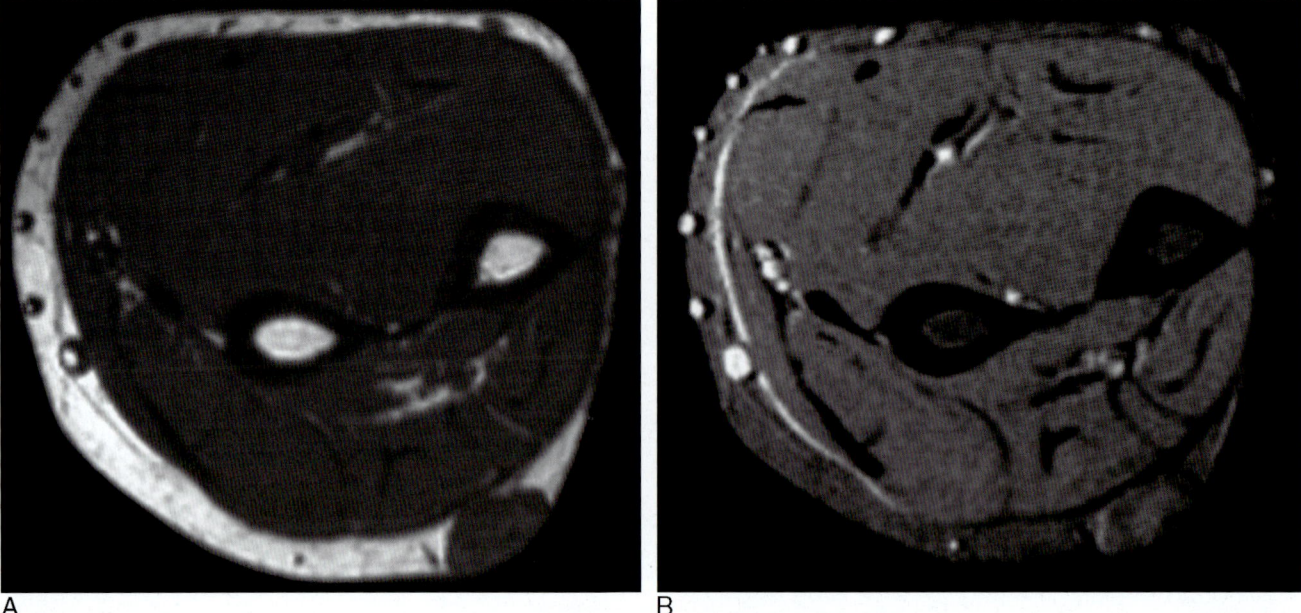

A
B

■ **FIGURE 94-26** A 60-year-old man presented with a subcutaneous lesion in the left lower arm. Axial, spin-echo, T1-weighted (**A**) and axial, gradient-echo (**B**) T2-weighted MR images reveal a well-defined nodular mass in the subcutaneous fat, with no specific signal characteristics. A biopsy confirmed the diagnosis of a pilomatricoma. *(From Salgado R, Alexiou J, Engelholm JL. Pseudotumoral lesions. In De Schepper AM [ed]. Imaging of Soft Tissue Tumors, 3rd ed. Berlin, Spinger-Verlag, 2006, pp 415–446.)*

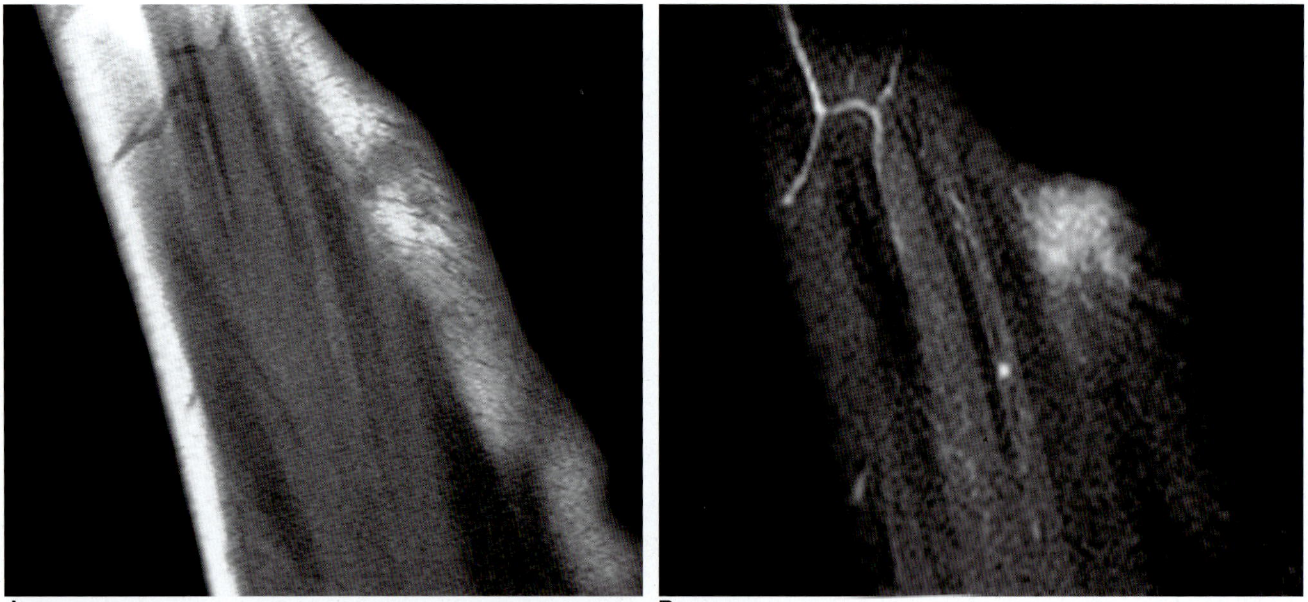

A
B
C 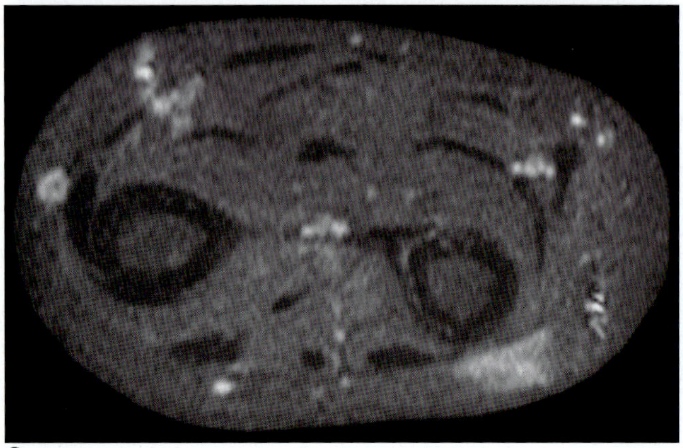

■ **FIGURE 94-27** A 12-year-old boy had noncontinuous pain at the left forearm for about 1 year. Coronal, spin-echo, T1-weighted (**A**), coronal, turbo spin-echo, fat-suppressed T2-weighted (**B**), and axial, spin-echo, fat-suppressed, contrast-enhanced T1-weighted (**C**) MR images show an ill-defined lesion in the subcutaneous compartment posterior to the middle third of the radius, with a broad contact with the superficial fascia. The lesion is hyperintense on the T2-weighted image, with moderate enhancement after intravenous contrast administration. Age, location, and MR presentation are in favor of a granuloma annulare, which was eventually proven on biopsy.

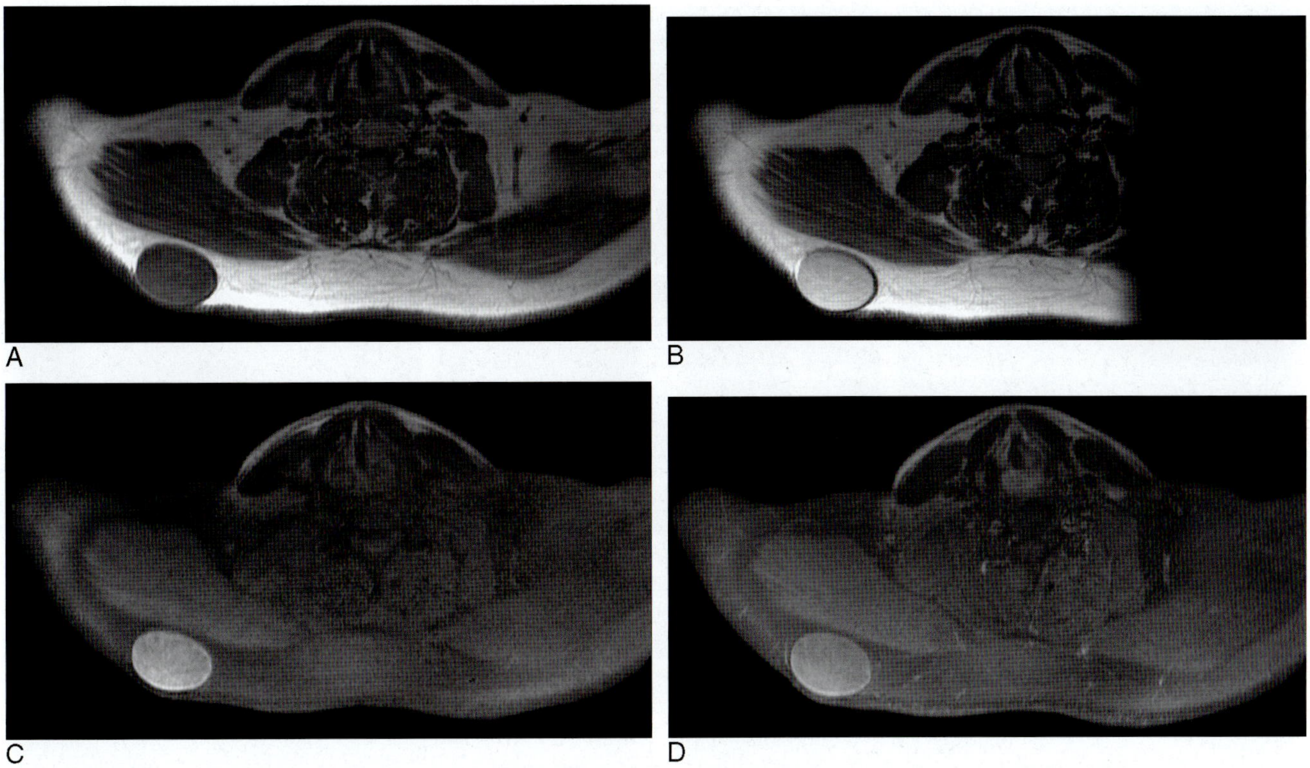

■ FIGURE 94-28 A 40-year-old man had a painless soft tissue mass at the dorsal aspect of the right shoulder. The images reveal a homogeneous mass lesion superficially within the subcutaneous tissue posterocranially at the right shoulder. **A,** On the axial, spin-echo, T1-weighted image there is an intermediate signal intensity comparable with normal muscle. **B,** On the axial, turbo spin-echo T2-weighted image the lesion has an uniform intermediate signal intensity. **C,** The signal appears hyperintense on the axial, turbo spin-echo, fat-suppressed T1-weighted image. **D,** No enhancement is seen on the axial, spin-echo fat-suppressed, contrast-enhanced T1-weighted image. This case shows the imaging characteristics of a large epidermoid inclusion cyst.

CRYSTAL DEPOSITIONS

Gout and Pseudogout

Gout is a metabolic disorder characterized by hyperuricemia and deposits of monosodium urate monohydrate crystals in periarticular soft tissues. In pseudogout, depositions consist of calcium pyrophosphate dihydrate (CPPD). The disorders most frequently affect the first metatarsophalangeal joint, followed by the ankle, knee, wrist, fingers, and elbow. Clinical and radiographic findings are usually diagnostic (Fig. 94-29). On occasion, these conditions may present as a soft tissue mass. Calcification of the mass is possible and more frequently seen in pseudogout.

The MRI features of gouty arthritis include synovial thickening and joint effusion. Both conditions display a low to intermediate signal intensity on T1-weighted images. T2-weighted images characteristics vary from a heterogeneously hypointense to hyperintense mass on T2-weighted images, depending on the degree of inflammation. Diffuse enhancement after intravenous injection of a contrast agent may be seen.

Calcific Tendinosis

Calcific tendinosis, also known as calcific tendonitis or calcium hydroxyapatite disease, is a self-limiting inflammatory disorder characterized by the deposition of hydroxyapatite crystals in tendons and periarticular soft tissue. It mostly occurs in the shoulder, but the hip, hand, and wrist may also be affected.

In an initial phase, calcium deposits are contained within the tendons, producing no significant clinical symptoms. As the deposits increase in size, the resulting increased tension in the tendon leads to pain. Acute onset (periarticular inflammation secondary to shading of crystals in joint or bursa) causes severe pain. An adhesive periarthritis can subsequently develop.

Radiography has an important role, revealing amorphous calcification or a radiopaque dense mass at the suspected site. Bone erosion of the adjacent cortical bone is not common but has been reported,[19] presumably secondary to inflammation at the tendon insertion or mass effect. This can lead to the wrong diagnosis of an aggressive neoplasm, especially when previous imaging studies are not available. Although periarticular calcifications are typically encountered at the tendon attachment sites, they can occur in and around ligamentous structures with concomitant inflammation.

Both T1- and T2-weighted images demonstrate a signal void in the area of calcification. A high signal intensity in surrounding muscles related to edema can be seen on T2-weighted images (Fig. 94-30). Bone marrow edema can also incidentally be found, on occasion mimicking an osseous metastasis.

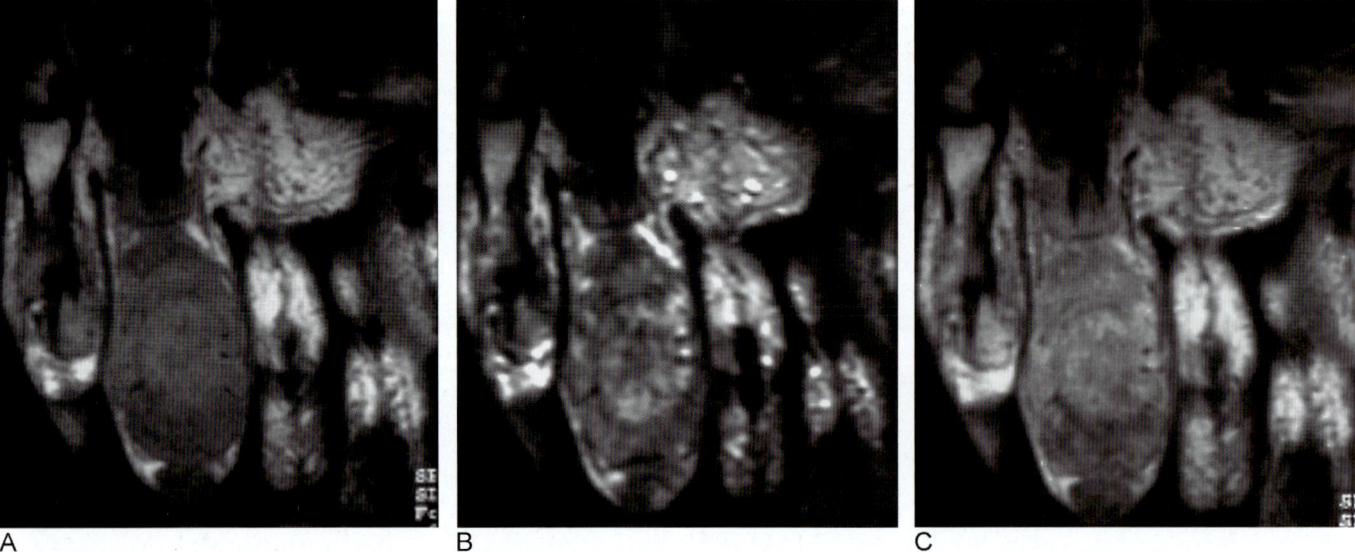

■ FIGURE 94-29   Gout of both hands in a 65-year-old man. The tophi have an intermediate signal intensity on both coronal T1-weighted (**A**) and T2-weighted (**B**) MR images. **C**, Enhancement is evident on gadolinium contrast administration. Imaging is characteristic of gouty tophi in a patient with clinical and biochemical evidence of gout. *(From Salgado R, Alexiou J, Engelholm JL. Pseudotumoral lesions. In De Schepper AM [ed]. Imaging of Soft Tissue Tumors, 3rd ed. Berlin, Spinger-Verlag, 2006, pp 415–446.)*

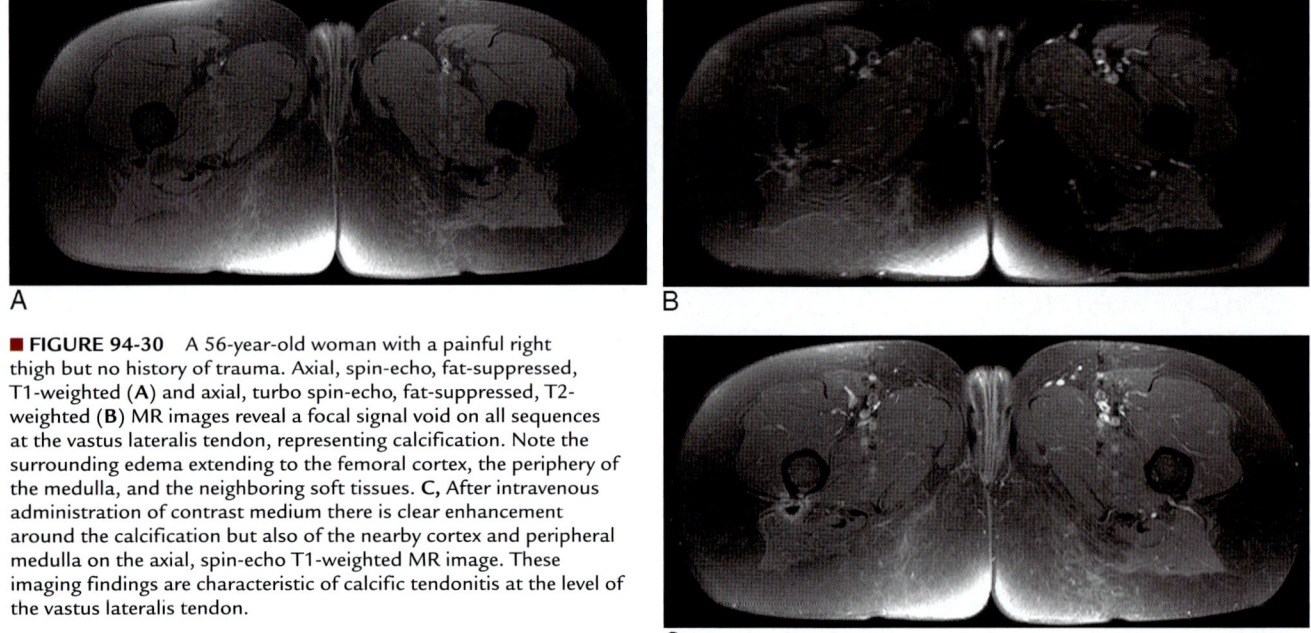

■ FIGURE 94-30   A 56-year-old woman with a painful right thigh but no history of trauma. Axial, spin-echo, fat-suppressed, T1-weighted (**A**) and axial, turbo spin-echo, fat-suppressed, T2-weighted (**B**) MR images reveal a focal signal void on all sequences at the vastus lateralis tendon, representing calcification. Note the surrounding edema extending to the femoral cortex, the periphery of the medulla, and the neighboring soft tissues. **C**, After intravenous administration of contrast medium there is clear enhancement around the calcification but also of the nearby cortex and peripheral medulla on the axial, spin-echo T1-weighted MR image. These imaging findings are characteristic of calcific tendonitis at the level of the vastus lateralis tendon.

OTHER VASCULAR LESIONS

Adventitial cystic disease of the popliteal artery is an unusual condition of uncertain etiology in which a mucin-containing cyst forms within the adventitia of the popliteal artery, narrowing the arterial lumen and causing symptoms of intermittent lower extremity claudication. Early recognition and treatment is mandatory to prevent progression to popliteal thrombosis and ischemia of the lower leg. However, diagnosis of the condition is difficult, with sometimes misleading clinical features, such as the presence of normal peripheral pulses and normal ankle pressures.

Arteriography shows a focal, smoothly tapered stenosis of the popliteal artery at the level of the femoral condyles.

CT may show a nonenhancing cyst-like mass causing extrinsic compression of an enhancing arterial lumen, with rim enhancement after intravenous contrast administration. Today, both CT and MR angiography are valuable noninvasive imaging modalities in the evaluation of these lesions (Fig. 94-31). MRI may reveal cyst-like structures closely invested in a compressed artery, without specific signal intensity (Fig. 94-32). Aneurysms secondary to impingement of osteochondroma on arteries may be found.

On occasion, a vascular aneurysm may present as a soft tissue mass. The presence of a pulsatile mass with bruit in close proximity to an artery in a patient with a history of trauma suggests the correct diagnosis. Likewise, when a soft tissue tumor entirely surrounds and obliterates a major artery, an aneurysm or a pseudoaneurysm should be considered. Pseudoaneurysm formation is also the most frequent vascular complication of osteochondroma. The most common location is the popliteal artery, although it has also been described in the superficial femoral, brachial, and posterior tibial arteries. It typically appears around the time of skeletal maturity as the soft cartilage cap becomes hardened by calcification or ossification. Chronic abrasion and eventually laceration of the adjacent arterial surface during normal movement or repetitive trauma can lead to a pseudoaneurysm in the adjacent vessel. Other less common complications are vessel displacement, stenosis, and occlusion. Peripheral arterial aneurysms are most commonly found in the popliteal artery, often in association with widespread atherosclerotic disease.

An aneurysm or pseudoaneurysm is recognized on MRI by signal void in regions of flowing blood, hyperintensity on T1-weighted images and T2-weighted images due to subacute hemorrhage, and hypointense areas caused by hemosiderin deposits. Moreover, MRI demonstrates a characteristic flow-related artifact in the direction of the phase-encoding gradient. A major vein engulfed by or adjacent to a mass should evoke a lesion of venous origin.

Congenital arteriovenous malformations are characterized by dilated, tortuous blood vessels that infiltrate muscles. Post-traumatic acquired arteriovenous malformations have also been reported. On MRI, the appearance of an arteriovenous malformation is similar on T1-weighted images and T2-weighted images and is characterized by hypointense, serpiginous blood vessels of low signal intensity due to flow-void effects.

MISCELLANEOUS

Tumoral Calcinosis

The term *tumoral calcinosis* has been a source of confusion and misinterpretation in the medical literature and is still often liberally misused by both radiologists and clinicians.[20] On conventional radiography the calcifications have an amorphous to cystic morphology with a periarticular distribution often more concentrated on the extensor side of the affected joint. Fluid-fluid levels

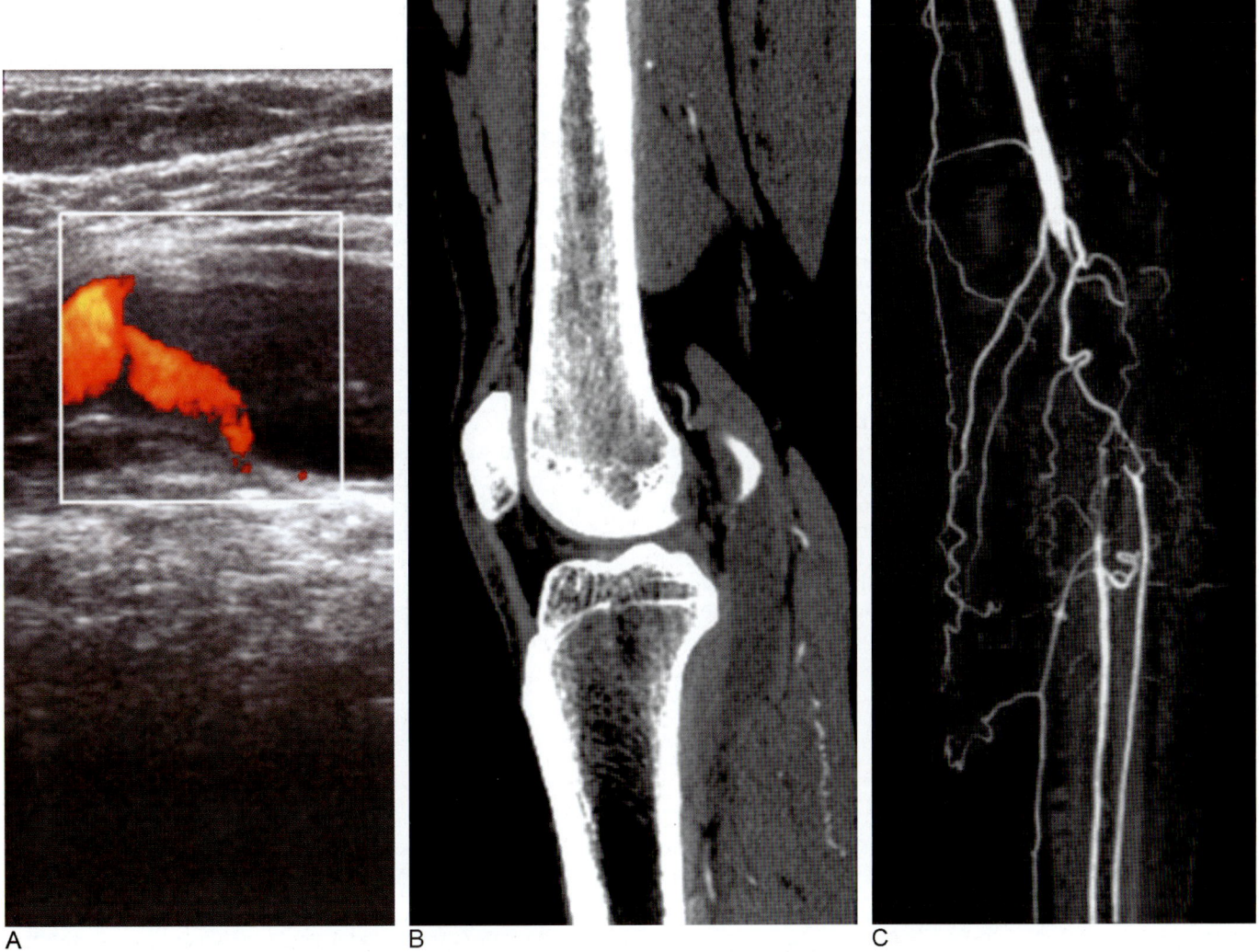

A   B   C

■ **FIGURE 94-31** A 35-year-old man had rapidly progressing pain in the left calf. **A,** The initial ultrasound examination revealed a cyst-like structure in the left knee pit, compressing the popliteal artery. **B,** A subsequent multislice sagittal CT examination further showed a long cyst, abutting and occluding the popliteal artery. **C,** This was documented with an angiographic maximal intensity projection CT image. There are typical findings of an adventitial cyst arising from the popliteal artery with arterial occlusion and rapidly evolving claudication.

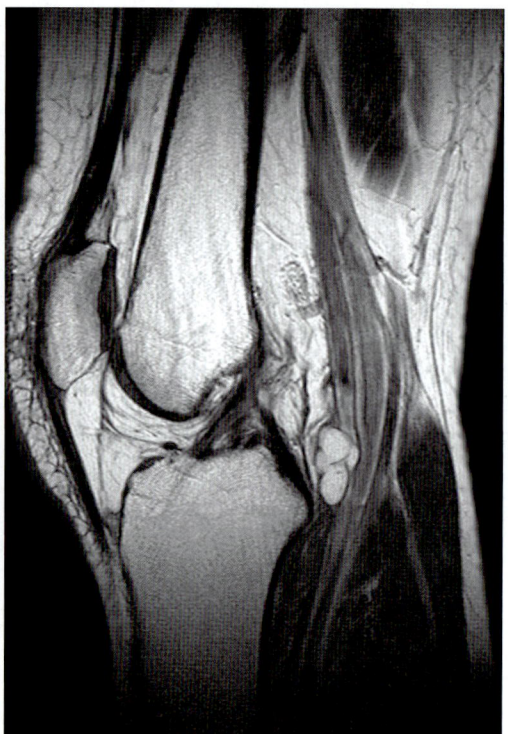

A   B

■ **FIGURE 94-32** A 52-year-old man presented with intermittent claudication. Sagittal, spin-echo, T1-weighted (**A**) and sagittal, turbo, spin-echo T2-weighted (**B**) MR images reveal a well-defined multicystic process around the popliteal artery. It is isointense on T1-weighted imaging and hyperintense on T2-weighted imaging. When these findings are encountered an adventitial cyst around the popliteal artery should always be considered.

can be seen, a finding referred to as the "sedimentation sign." The cortex of the adjacent bone remains unaffected. Nevertheless, an association with calcific myelitis has been described, showing patchy areas of calcification in long bones and the calvaria.

On MRI these lesions have an inhomogeneous low signal intensity on T1-weighted images but a remarkable high signal on T2-weighted images despite their calcified component.

Many other diseases can mimic the radiologic presentation of tumoral calcinosis. These diseases include connective tissue diseases, degenerative and metabolic diseases such as CPPD deposition and chronic renal failure, as well as neoplastic processes such as synovial sarcoma and chondrosarcoma. It is often impossible to make an accurate distinction between these entities and tumoral calcinosis based solely on imaging findings. In such cases a firmer diagnosis can be established combining the radiologic presentation with the patient's history and serum chemistry levels (including markers of phosphate metabolism).

Amyloid Tumor of Soft Tissue

The majority of soft tissue amyloid tumors are manifestations of secondary amyloidosis, associated with underlying conditions such as multiple myeloma, chronic infections, and a variety of inflammatory diseases, such as tuberculosis and rheumatoid arthritis.

On the other hand, primary soft tissue amyloidosis is extremely rare, usually presenting late in life with a predilection for the male gender. Macromorphologically they have a lobulated appearance, with a white or yellow-like waxy surface. The most affected areas include the groin, abdominal wall, breast, neck, and orbit.

Unfortunately, imaging characteristics of these rare lesions are nonspecific, thereby indicating the need for a biopsy to establish the diagnosis. On MRI, these lesions show a low to intermediate signal intensity on both T1- and T2-weighted images, varying between that of fibrocartilage and muscle. There is no enhancement after intravenous administration of a contrast agent.

SUGGESTED READINGS

Beltran J. MR imaging of soft tissue infection. Magn Reson Imaging Clin North Am 1995; 3:743–751.

Jelinek J, Kransdorf MJ. MR imaging of soft tissue masses: mass-like lesions that simulate neoplasms. Magn Reson Imaging Clin North Am 1995; 3:727–741.

Kransdorf MJ. Imaging of soft tissue tumors: masses that may mimic soft tissue tumors. In: Kransdorf MJ (ed). Imaging of Soft Tissue Tumors. Philadelphia, WB Saunders, 1997, pp 373–420.

Lebon C, Malghem J, Lecouvet F, et al. Pseudotumeurs des Parties Molles. Paris, Editions Scientifiques et Médicales Elsevier SAS, 2003.

Salgado R, Alexiou J, Engelholm JL. Pseudotumoral lesions. In De Schepper AM (ed). Imaging of Soft Tissue Tumors, 3rd ed. Berlin, Spinger-Verlag, 2006, pp 415–446.

REFERENCES

1. Major NM, Tehranzadeh J. Musculoskeletal manifestations of AIDS. Radiol Clin North Am 1997; 35:1167-1189.
2. Beltran J. MR imaging of soft tissue infection. Magn Reson Imaging Clin North Am 1995; 3:743-751.
3. Polat P, Kantarci M, Alper F, et al. Hydatid disease from head to toe. RadioGraphics 2003; 23:475-494; quiz 536-477.
4. Garcia-Diez AI, Ros Mendoza LH, Villacampa VM, et al. MRI evaluation of soft tissue hydatid disease. Eur Radiol 2000; 10:462-466.
5. Tacal T, Altinok D, Yildiz YT, Altinok G. Coexistence of intramuscular hydatid cyst and tapeworm. AJR Am J Roentgenol 2000; 174:575-576.
6. Flaisler F, Blin D, Asencio G, et al. Focal myositis: a localized form of polymyositis? J Rheumatol 1993; 20:1414-1416.
7. Heckmann JG, Stefan H, Heuss D, et al. Isolated muscular sarcoidosis. Eur J Neurol 2001; 8:365-366.
8. Otake S, Imagumbai N, Suzuki M, Ohba S. MR imaging of muscular sarcoidosis after steroid therapy. Eur Radiol 1998; 8:1651-1653.
9. Vanhoenacker P, Brijs S, Geusens E, et al. MR imaging of primary muscular sarcoidosis. Case report. Rofo 1994; 161:570-571.
10. Berg LC, Norelle A, Morgan WA, Washa DM. Cat-scratch disease simulating histiocytosis X. Hum Pathol 1998; 29:649-651.
11. Jelinek J, Kransdorf MJ. MR imaging of soft tissue masses: mass-like lesions that simulate neoplasms. Magn Reson Imaging Clin North Am 1995; 3:727-741.
12. Liu PT, Leslie KO, Beauchamp CP, Cherian SF. Chronic expanding hematoma of the thigh simulating neoplasm on gadolinium-enhanced MRI. Skeletal Radiol 2006; 35:254-257.
13. Sakayama K, Fujibuchi T, Sugawara Y, et al. A 40-year-old gossypiboma (foreign body granuloma) mimicking a malignant femoral surface tumor. Skeletal Radiol 2005; 34:221-224.
14. Zohman GL, Pierce J, Chapman MW, et al. Calcific myonecrosis mimicking an invasive soft tissue neoplasm: a case report and review of the literature. J Bone Joint Surg Am 1998; 80:1193-1197.
15. Mentzel T, Goodlad JR, Smith MA, Fletcher CD. Ancient hematoma: a unifying concept for a post-traumatic lesion mimicking an aggressive soft tissue neoplasm. Mod Pathol 1997; 10:334-340.
16. Ferris BL, Taylor LM Jr, Oyama K, et al. Hypothenar hammer syndrome: proposed etiology. J Vasc Surg 2000; 31:104-113.
17. Kransdorf MJ. Benign soft tissue tumors in a large referral population: distribution of specific diagnoses by age, sex, and location. AJR Am J Roentgenol 1995; 164:395-402.
18. Shehan JM, El-Azhary RA. Magnetic resonance imaging features of subcutaneous granuloma annulare. Pediatr Dermatol 2005; 22:377-378.
19. Chung CB, Gentili A, Chew FS. Calcific tendinosis and periarthritis: classic magnetic resonance imaging appearance and associated findings. J Comput Assist Tomogr 2004; 28:390-396.
20. Olsen KM, Chew FS. Tumoral calcinosis: pearls, polemics, and alternative possibilities. RadioGraphics 2006; 26:871-885.

95

Tumoral Calcinosis

Bryan T. Jennings, Michael S. Gibson, and Mark D. Murphey

Tumoral calcinosis is a distinct disease characterized by calcium deposition in the para-articular soft tissues.[1,2] In 1899, Duret described a disorder in a 17-year-old girl and her younger brother with multiple calcifications around the elbow and hip joints.[3] Inclan coined the term *tumoral calcinosis* to describe this condition in 1943.[4]

ETIOLOGY

Variable expression of an autosomal dominant inheritance pattern is suggested.[5] Although the exact underlying biochemical defect is not known, it is thought to be related to formation of 1,25-dihydroxyvitamin D. Mild hyperphosphatemia and elevated 1,25-dihydroxyvitamin D levels are commonly found in patients with tumoral calcinosis.[5,6]

PREVALENCE AND EPIDEMIOLOGY

Tumoral calcinosis predominately involves otherwise healthy patients during childhood or adolescence, typically in the first or the second decade of life. There is no sex predilection. An increased incidence is noted in patients of African American descent,[3,5-7] and 50% of children with tumoral calcinosis have an affected sibling. Tumoral calcinosis cases are familial in 30% of cases.[5] Multiple areas are usually affected, with three sites of involvement found on average in each patient.[5]

CLINICAL PRESENTATION

Tumoral calcinosis presents as para-articular masses about the large joints. Joints commonly involved include the hips, buttocks, scapula, shoulders, and elbows.[5,6] There is less frequent involvement of the hands, feet, and knees. The extensor surface is frequently affected, particularly with a lesion about the elbow. The site of origin is considered to be bursal about joints. However, the pathologic proof of bursal origin is lacking. Destruction of bursal synovial tissue is thought to be secondary to the underlying calcific process.[5] Lesions generally present as slowly growing firm, painless masses. Although

these lesions may be cosmetically deforming, limitations in range of joint motion do not typically occur because of the extra-articular location of the lesions. Lesions of sufficient size may ulcerate the overlying skin and drain a chalky, milky fluid.[5] Clinical abnormalities can also include skin and vascular calcifications as well as retinal involvement in association with pseudoxanthoma elasticum.[5] Dental abnormalities with intrapulp calcification and root enlargement have also been described.[5]

PATHOPHYSIOLOGY

Gross pathologic specimens demonstrate firm, rubbery masses that extend to involve adjacent tendons and muscles.[3] Lesions typically measure 5 to 15 cm in diameter and are composed of numerous small deposits of hydroxyapatite calcium salts.[3] Margins are variable; some lesions have a well-defined pseudocapsule, whereas some infiltrate the surrounding tissues.[6] Microscopy in the active phase demonstrates a foreign body response with a rim of chronic inflammatory cells, giant cells, and macrophages surrounding the calcific deposits.[3] Dense fibrous material is present surrounding the central calcified material in the inactive phase.[3]

MANIFESTATIONS OF THE DISEASE

Radiography

Radiographs demonstrate well-defined calcified para-articular masses that may be multiloculated or lobular (Fig. 95-1). Intersecting lucent lines may course through the otherwise densely opacified mass in what has been called a "cobblestone" or "chicken wire" pattern.[8] These lucent areas reflect fibrous septa.[3] Calcium fluid levels may be present within the lesions on upright, horizontal-beam radiographs. Some authors contend that the presence of calcium fluid levels indicates an active lesion that is more likely to respond to phosphate depletion therapy.[3,8] Involvement of the adjacent bone with erosions may rarely be present.[9] Periosteal reaction or calcifications within the adjacent bone have also rarely been described.[5]

KEY POINTS

- Typically otherwise healthy young patients (in the first or second decades) present with juxta-articular masses without range-of-motion abnormalities.
- Involvement of three or more sites at presentation is common.
- The disorder is familial in 30% of cases, and up to 50% of a patients have an affected sibling. Transmission is autosomal dominant with variable expression.
- A "cobblestone" or "chicken wire" pattern has been described on radiographs or CT in which lucent lines course through an otherwise calcified mass.
- On MRI, lesions are predominately of low signal intensity on both T1- and T2-weighted images, although higher signal intensity in septations and the peripheral rim are common.
- MRI may demonstrate peripheral and septal enhancement.
- The diagnosis remains one of exclusion in older patients. Collagen vascular disease, hyperparathyroidism, milk-alkali syndrome, and renal failure can also have juxta-articular calcifications.

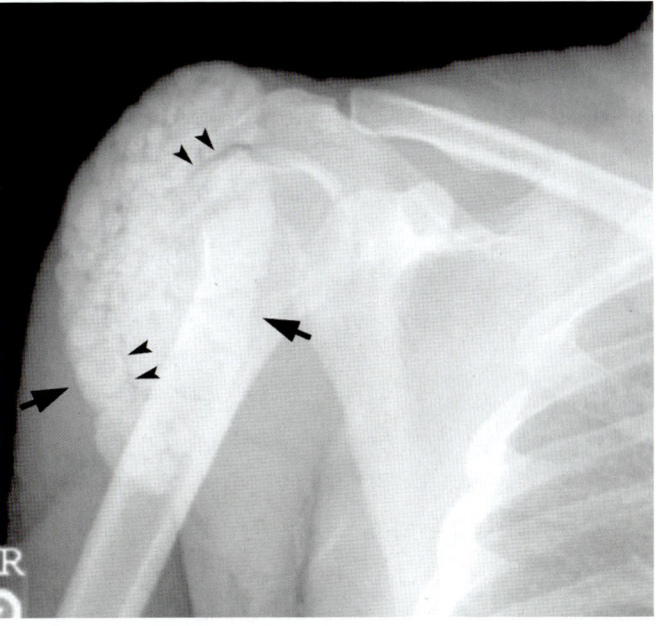

■ **FIGURE 95-1** A radiograph of the shoulder demonstrating a large multiloculated calcified mass (*arrows*) with radiolucent septations (*arrowheads*) causing a "cobblestone" pattern.

Magnetic Resonance Imaging

Magnetic resonance imaging of tumoral calcinosis can have variable appearances based on the metabolic activity of the lesion. Metabolically active lesions may demonstrate heterogeneously increased signal intensity on T2-weighted images owing to the granulomatous foreign body reaction at the lesion site. Inactive lesions tend to demonstrate signal intensity that is more typical of the underlying calcifications, with predominately low signal intensity on both T1- and T2-weighted images, although higher signal intensity in septations and the peripheral rim is common (Figs. 95-2 and 95-3). In our experience the latter pattern is most frequent. A fatty rim may surround the lesion with increased signal intensity on both T1- and T2-weighted images.[5-7] Vascularized tissue sur-

rounding the calcium salt deposits may produce a peripheral and septal enhancement pattern after the intravenous administration of gadolinium (see Fig. 95-2).[9] Periosteal reaction may be seen on MRI as a high signal rind about the cortex on T2-weighted images.[5] On MRI, marrow involvement shows decreased T1-weighted signal and increased T2-weighted signal interspersed with multiple punctate areas of decreased T2-weighted signal (corresponding to small calcifications).[5]

Multidetector Computed Tomography

Computed tomography demonstrates calcified para-articular lesions within the fatty planes deep to muscles. Lesions may present either as a solid mass with interspersed septa of low attenuation (the "chicken wire" appearance) or as a

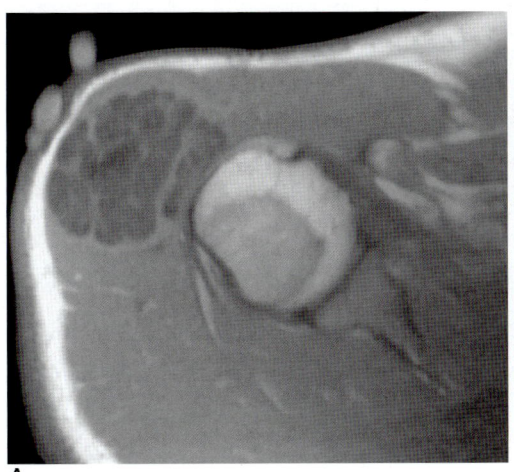
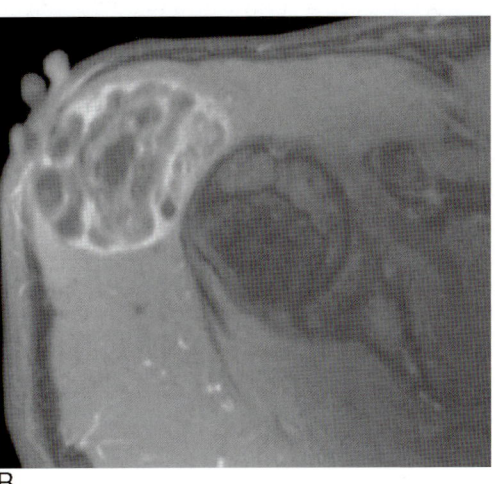

A   B

■ **FIGURE 95-2** Axial T1-weighted MR images both before (**A**) and after intravenous administration of gadolinium with fat saturation (**B**) demonstrate a shoulder mass with low signal intensity with a peripheral and septal enhancement pattern.

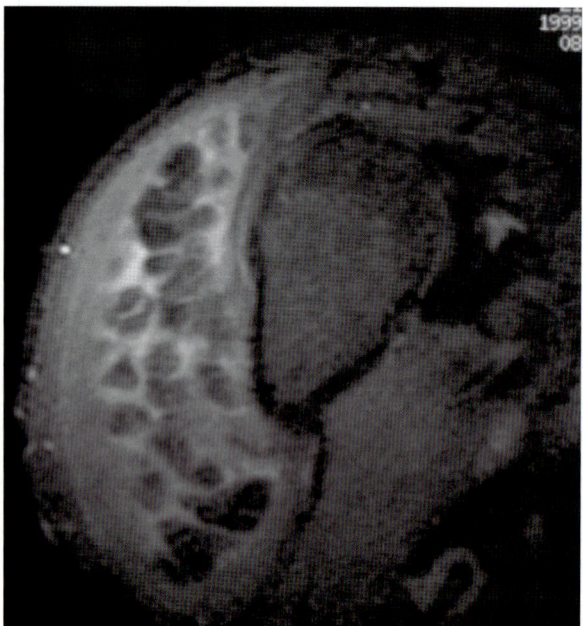

■ **FIGURE 95-3** A coronal T2-weighted image of the shoulder demonstrates a mass with predominately low signal intensity, with higher signal intensity in the periphery and septa representing a "chicken wire" pattern of the fibrovascular reactive tissue about the calcific deposits.

cystic lesion with calcified walls.[5] The degree of calcification varies from lesion to lesion. Calcium fluid levels may also be present, but they are not specific for tumoral calcinosis and may be present in milk-alkali syndrome or renal failure.

Nuclear Medicine

Bone scintigraphy is a simple, reliable method for detecting and localizing the extent of tumoral calcinosis within the body, often demonstrating multiple sites of involvement with marked increased radionuclide uptake.[5] However, it should be noted that very small lesions may not be demonstrated on scintigraphy.[5]

DIFFERENTIAL DIAGNOSIS

The differential diagnosis of para-articular calcifications includes hyperparathyroidism, collagen vascular disease, milk-alkali syndrome, and renal failure. Calcification in these entities may be considered secondary tumoral calcinosis. Only once these entities have been ruled out should the diagnosis of primary tumoral calcinosis be entertained.[9] Metastatic disease rarely calcifies (mucinous gastrointestinal tumor or thyroid primary tumor), and a para-articular location is unusual.

SYNOPSIS OF TREATMENT OPTIONS

Treatment focuses on reduction of serum phosphate through restriction of dietary intake and oral phosphate binders.[10] Medical management alone often results in clinical improvement and reduction in size of the masses. Surgery in combination with medical therapy may be performed for large lesions.[10]

What the Referring Physician Needs to Know

- Is the confidence level of the diagnosis of primary or secondary tumoral calcinosis high enough to refrain from taking a biopsy?
- What is the differential diagnosis for causes of secondary tumoral calcinosis?

ACKNOWLEDGMENT

The views expressed in this chapter are those of the authors and do not necessarily reflect the official policy or position of the Department of the Navy, Department of Defense, or the U.S. Government.

SUGGESTED READING

Martinez S, Vogler JB 3rd, Harrelson JM, Lykes KW. Imaging of tumoral calcinosis: new obervations. Radiology 1990; 174:215–222.

REFERENCES

1. Miettinen M. Cartilage- and bone-forming tumor and tumor-like lesions. In: Diagnostic Soft Tissue Pathology. New York, Churchill Livingstone, 2003, pp 403–425.
2. Enzinger F, Weiss SW. Soft tissue tumors: benign soft tissue tumors and pseudotumors of miscellaneous type. In Enzinger F, Weiss S, Goldblum J (eds). Enzinger and Weiss's Soft Tissue Tumors, 4th ed. St. Louis, CV Mosby, 2001, pp 1419–1483.
3. Enzinger F, Weiss S, Goldblum J. Enzinger and Weiss's Soft Tissue Tumors, 4th ed. St. Louis, CV Mosby, 2001.
4. Inclan A, Leon P, Camejo M. Tumoral calcinosis. JAMA 1942; 121:490–495.
5. Martinez S, Vogler JB 3rd, Harrelson JM, Lyles KW. Imaging of tumoral calcinosis: new observations. Radiology 1990; 174:215–222.
6. Slavin RE, Wen J, Kumar D, Evans EB. Familial tumoral calcinosis: a clinical, histopathologic, and ultrastructural study with an analysis of its calcifying process and pathogenesis. Am J Surg Pathol 1993; 17:788–802.
7. Chew FS, Crenshaw WB. Idiopathic tumoral calcinosis. AJR Am J Roentgenol 1992; 158:330.
8. Steinbach LS, Johnston JO, Tepper EF, et al. Tumoral calcinosis: radiologic-pathologic correlation. Skeletal Radiol 1995; 24:573–578.
9. Geirnaerdt MJ, Kroon HM, van der Heul RO, Herfkens HF. Tumoral calcinosis. Skeletal Radiol 1995; 24:148–151.
10. Giardina F, Sudanese A, Bertoni F, et al. Tumoral calcinosis of the popliteal space. Orthopedics 2004; 27:1104–1107.

96

Metastatic Disease

Michael Mulligan, Donald Flemming, and Mark D. Murphey

ETIOLOGY

The formation of osseous metastases follows a complicated series of events that is dependent on the intrinsic properties of the cancerous cells that comprise the primary malignancy. First, the neoplastic cells must not be too cohesive so that they may break free from the primary site of disease and enter a vascular or lymphatic structure. The cell must survive transport through the vascular tree and attacks from the host immune system and then be able to cross the vascular barrier at the end organ. The cell must then survive in the local environment of the host tissue, replicate, and establish its own blood supply. Regarding these steps, one important agent is osteopontin. Osteopontin is a glyco-phosphoprotein secreted by cancer cells that has effects on cell adhesion, chemotaxis, host immune suppression, and angiogenesis.[1] The vascular barrier in bone is not as impregnable as in other sites because there are large gaps in the walls of the marrow vessels. These gaps exist to allow the large hematopoietic precursor cells to enter circulation from their marrow development sites. Local environmental factors such as oxygen tension, pH, food substrate, and hormones, as well as properties of the metastatic cell including tumor adhesion, are important to the establishment of a metastasis and may explain why metastatic disease to muscle, spleen, and the muscular layers of hollow viscera is rare. Fewer than 0.1% of cells survive the transport process to form distant metastases. The bone marrow microenvironment possesses unique features that enable circulating cancer cells to deposit, survive, and develop. The skeleton holds stores of many different growth factors, as well as massive quantities of calcium and phosphorus, which all seem to play important roles in the establishment of a metastasis.

PREVALENCE AND EPIDEMIOLOGY

It is imperative for radiologists to have a thorough understanding of both the typical and atypical presentations of metastatic disease to bone because it is the most common malignant process in the skeleton, presenting 25 to 35 times more commonly than primary osseous neoplasms and resulting in approximately 140,000 new cases in the United States annually. It has been estimated that 350,000 patients die each year in the United States with skeletal metastases.[2] Five primary carcinomas account for 80% of these cases in adults, including cancers of the prostate, thyroid, breast, lung, and kidney. Neuroblastoma and leukemia represent the most common primary malignancies to metastasize to bone in children. The true incidence of metastatic disease to bone is difficult to ascertain owing to the inherent difficulty of performing pathologic examination of the entire skeleton at autopsy. Bone metastases may have a significant impact on quality of life, with complications including pain, fracture, spinal cord and nerve root compression, hypercalcemia, and marrow suppression. Bone follows only lung and liver in frequency as a site of metastatic disease and may be the only location of metastatic disease. When the skeleton is the only location of metastatic involvement, breast cancer

---

KEY POINTS

- Any new lesion in an adult older than age 40 is a metastasis until proven otherwise.
- Metastases can appear in any form.
- Advanced imaging studies (MR, CT, PET) help with diagnosis and staging.
- Pathologic fractures sometimes can be predicted and prevented.
- The missing pedicle is a specific, but late, sign of metastasis.
- Although common in Paget's disease, an ivory vertebra may reflect metastasis.
- Thick, solid, smooth or undulating periosteal new bone formation and parallel track pattern on bone scan are signs of hypertrophic osteoarthropathy.
- "Cookie cutter" and "cookie bite" signs are seen with cortical metastases.
- Transverse fracture lines are suggestive of pathologic fracture.

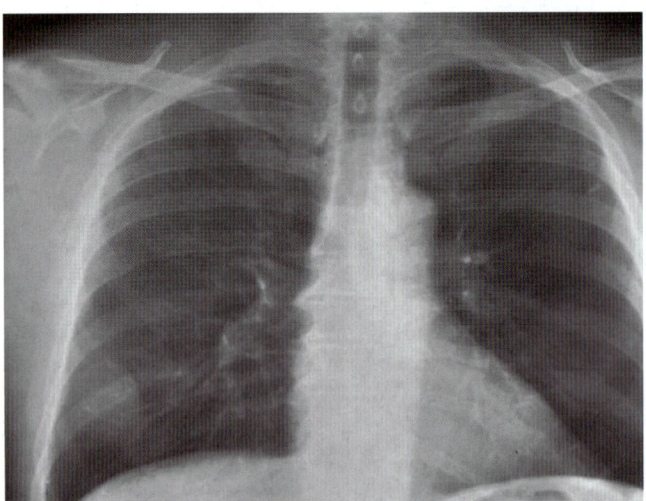

■ FIGURE 96-1 A 65-year old man, with no known primary cancer, presented with chest wall pain. Chest radiograph shows abnormal ventral right sixth rib, with expansion and lytic destruction. This was resected for diagnosis and proven a metastasis from a subsequently discovered primary esophageal carcinoma.

patients have a better prognosis than those with additional visceral metastases.[3] Although most patients have a known primary tumor at the time of discovery of osseous metastases, bone may be the first site of presentation of malignancy in up to 15% of cancer patients (Fig. 96-1) and in up to 60% of patients a primary lesion may never be found.[4]

CLINICAL PRESENTATION

Pain is one of the most common presenting symptoms and one of the most significant clinical consequences associated with skeletal metastases, but the relationship between pain and osseous metastatic disease is not well understood. In a study examining the relationship between pain and scintigraphic abnormalities in patients with breast or prostate carcinoma Palmer and associates found that 20% of patients with osseous metastases reported no pain and 36% of patients with breast cancer reported pain without scintigraphic abnormality.[5] In this same study there was poor correlation between site of scintigraphic abnormality and complaint of pain but lumbar spine lesions were most likely to be reported as painful (45%). Therefore, lack of pain does not exclude the diagnosis of osseous metastatic disease and pain in and of itself is a poor predictor of metastatic disease.

Hypercalcemia of malignancy is a paraneoplastic syndrome seen in 10% of patients with cancer. It is most commonly associated with osseous metastatic disease but may be seen without lesions in bone. The symptoms may be protean, and this condition carries a very poor prognosis, with median survival of only 3 months after recognition of hypercalcemia.[6] Hypercalcemia of malignancy is seen without elevated parathyroid hormone, although the disease has many features of a hyperparathyroid state. A parathyroid hormone–related peptide (PTHrP) considered to be responsible for hypercalcemia of malignancy has been discovered that shares many of the biologic effects of native parathormone. It is detectable in 80% to 90% of patients with hypercalcemia of malignancy. Numerous other potential osteolytic cytokines may be produced by tumor cells, including transforming growth factor, tumor necrosis factor, pro-cathepsin D, interleukin-1 and interleukin-6, colony-stimulating factor, and prostaglandins of the E series.[7] These substances may all contribute to a hypercalcemic state.

PATHOPHYSIOLOGY

Anatomy

Distant metastatic disease occurs as a result of transport of cells through a vascular or lymphatic structure. Osseous metastases most commonly result from invasion into and transport through the venous system. Lymphatic and arterial spread are of lesser importance. Direct invasion of the arterial system with spread of tumor distal to site of penetration is very rare except for bronchogenic carcinoma. Access to the arterial system usually occurs when tumor gains entry to a pulmonary vein, as in the case of bronchogenic carcinoma or in the rare case of intracardiac or extracardiac right-to-left shunt. Predictably, lung is the most common tumor to produce the rare case of metastatic disease in the distal limbs (below the elbow or knee) reflective of arterial spread of tumor (Fig. 96-2).

The lung and liver are efficient filters of particles such as tumor cells, which explains in part why these organs are the most likely to manifest metastatic disease. The relatively low incidence of gastrointestinal tumors metastasizing to bone is partially due to tumor trapping by the liver.

Bone involvement also may occur from local contiguous spread of disease. Two examples are spread of a Pancoast tumor to the adjacent ribs or vertebrae (Fig. 96-3) and direct spread from malignant paravertebral lymph nodes to the adjacent vertebrae.

Osseous metastatic disease can occur without disease in the liver or lung, although transpulmonary migration of tumor cells through the vasculature of the lung is thought to be rare. These observations led to the idea that a vascular system existed that bypasses the venae cavae and the lungs. Such a pathway was described by Batson in 1940 in a landmark article[8] that delineated a complex valveless plexiform network of paraspinal veins, now known as Batson's plexus. After injecting the dorsal vein of the penis in male cadavers with colored dyes, Batson's careful dissections showed direct communication of the pelvic veins to the paraspinal veins. Subsequent experiments with injection of female breast veins showed communication with the same venous plexus. The plexus likely exists so that blood may return to the chest cavity during Valsalva maneuvers, as demonstrated by Batson in experiments on live monkeys. Batson's plexus extends from the proximal femur and caudal base of the spine to the dural sinuses in the skull (Fig. 96-4) and consists of a richly interconnecting series of veins in and around the spine and spinal canal that communicates with veins in the azygous system, intercostal veins, posterior bronchial veins, and parietal pleural veins.

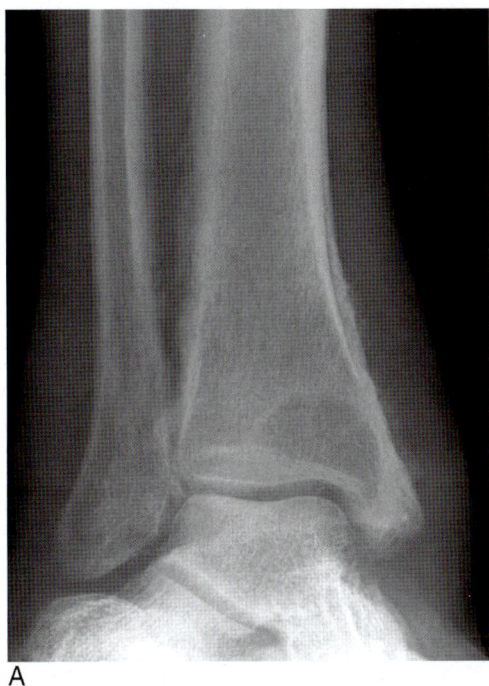
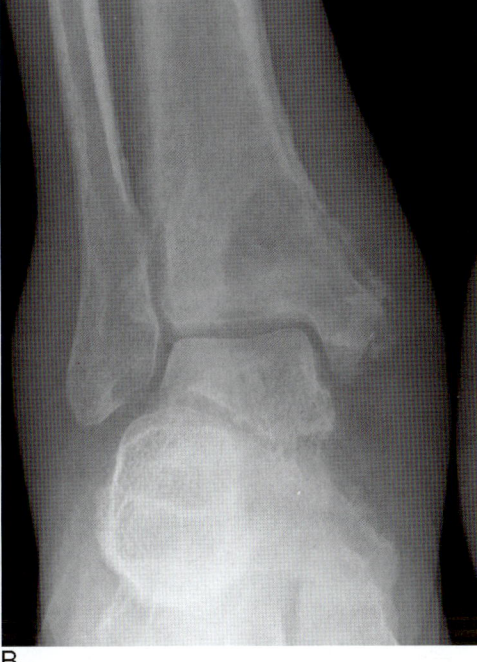

A   B

■ **FIGURE 96-2** **A,** A 38-year old man presented with right lower limb pain 3 years after initial diagnosis of lung cancer. Ankle radiographs show focal lytic lesion in the distal tibia and hypertrophic periosteal reaction of tibia and fibula. **B,** Appearance 14 months after first radiograph. This was the only site of metastatic involvement.

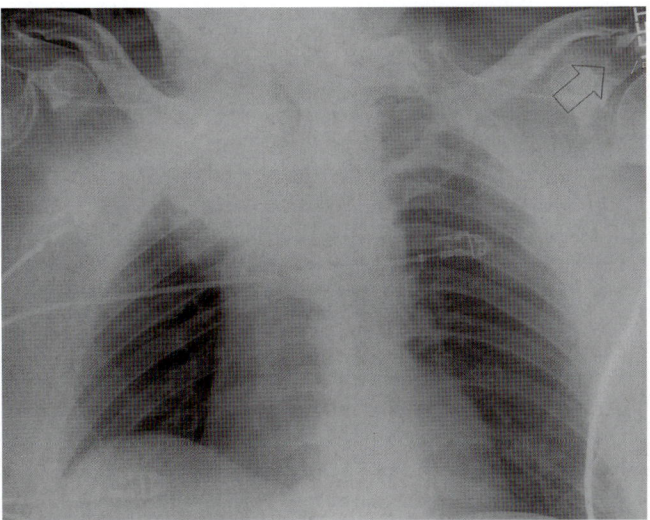
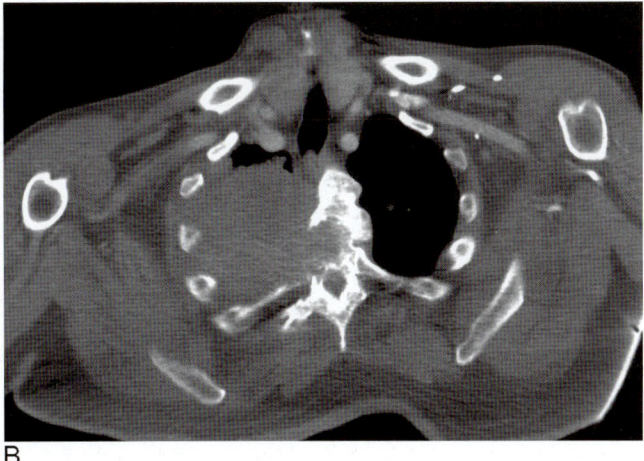

A   B

■ **FIGURE 96-3** **A,** A 69-year old man presented after a motor vehicle accident. A right apical lung mass was noted incidentally on an initial chest radiograph. **B,** Axial CT shows large Pancoast tumor with contiguous spread into the thoracic vertebrae. Also note the cortical destruction in adjacent ribs.

Valveless veins of the limbs also have been shown to communicate with this plexus as well as occasional interconnections with renal veins and the pelvic viscera. Batson's plexus may explain in some measure why metastatic disease in bone predominates in the axial skeleton. Although Batson was not a radiologist, his work was so important to radiologists that he was invited to give the Caldwell lecture at the 1956 annual meeting of the American Roentgen Ray Society.

Pathology

Why are most metastases lytic whereas others have blastic changes? The answer depends largely on factors that balance bone homeostasis between bone destruction or bone production. One of the first steps that occurs in the destructive phase of normal bone remodeling is activation of osteoclasts and the synthesis of collagenase by osteoclasts. Osteoclast-activating factor is a cytokine produced by normal white blood cells that helps initiate the process of osteoclastic resorption of bone. Similar cytokines, called osteoclast-stimulating factors, have been isolated from primary bone tumors (myeloma and lymphoma) and in cases of metastases.[9] These cytokines aid in the normal development, differentiation, and activation of osteoclasts. In metastasizing tumors, PTHrP is one of the most important cytokines. It is considered to be the major factor responsible for hypercalcemia in

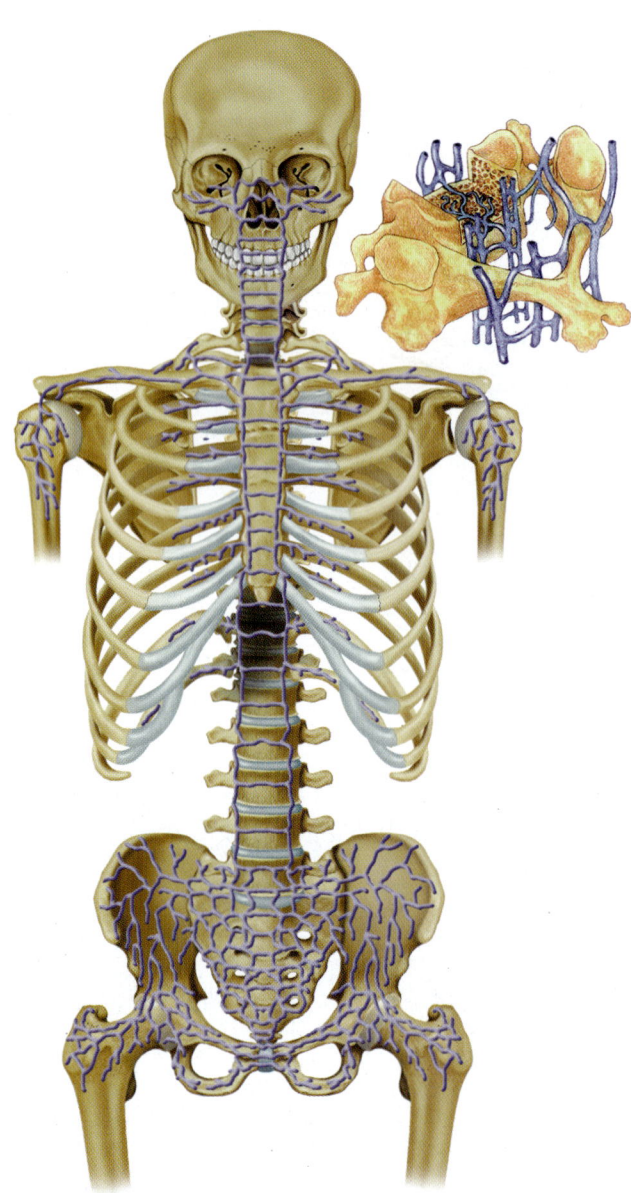

■ **FIGURE 96-4** Diagram of full extent of Batson's plexus.

patients with metastatic disease, as described earlier. Overproduction of these cytokines or an inability to regulate them leads to osteoclastic destruction out of proportion to new bone formation, resulting in lytic lesions on radiographs. Tumor-driven osteolysis is exacerbated by bone resorption associated with prolonged immobility in these severely ill patients. These cytokines are dependent on many factors, including prostaglandin E; therefore, prostaglandin inhibitors and other cytokine antagonists (interferon) have been investigated as a way to reduce or obliterate lytic bone destruction in these patients. Another treatment approach involves the use of bisphosphonates to interfere with osteoclast function.

Blastic lesions result when the homeostatic balance is tipped toward new bone production. Indeed, a humoral factor that stimulates osteoblasts has been found in patients with prostate carcinoma. Another osteoblastic

response mediator is endothelin-1. Endothelin-1, produced by tumor cells, mediates an osteoblastic response by stimulating osteoblastic cellular proliferation and hence new bone formation.[10] This osteoblastic stimulation results in new woven bone formation. The addition of this woven bone to the existing trabeculae causes increased radiographic density (Fig. 96-5). Another component of the increased radiographic density is normal reactive bone formation that is seen as a response to any pathologic process.

The lytic-blowout pattern also has a pathophysiologic explanation. Many of these lesions show extreme hypervascularity (Fig. 96-6). Active hyperemia (hypervascularity) is one factor that tips the homeostatic balance to osteoclastic resorption. The prominent hypervascularity of these lesions likely accounts for their extreme degree of lytic destruction.

The involvement of normal osteoclasts in the destruction of the host bone of a cancer patient is a unique feature of skeletal metastatic disease.[21]

IMAGING TECHNIQUES

Technical Aspects

An adult patient older than the age of 40 who presents with a new bone lesion is considered to have metastatic disease until proven otherwise. The final determination requires a good history, physical examination, and appropriate laboratory tests. Imaging studies should be based on pertinent findings gleaned from the history and physical and laboratory results. For example, if the patient is a heavy smoker with a chronic cough, then chest radiographs and perhaps chest CT would be appropriate. If a woman has a breast lump detected on physical examination, then mammography is certainly indicated. If an elderly man's prostate-specific antigen value is elevated, further imaging studies of the prostate and prostate biopsy would be useful. One could cite many other examples. The point is that directed imaging studies must be done. The "shotgun" search with CT or MRI from head to toe does a disservice to the patient. It is not cost effective and in today's managed care environment is not tolerated. Head-to-toe CT or MRI will not reveal all of the primary lesions. Indeed, in some series, 60% of the primary tumors could not be found despite an extensive workup, including exploratory laparotomy.[4] Imaging studies should be done with the intent of establishing a diagnosis of primary tumor or metastasis and to determine the extent of disease.

Radiography

Metastases can look like anything is the typical generalized statement most radiology residents hear when they are taught about the appearances of metastatic disease in the skeleton. The generalization is quite true. Skeletal metastases range in appearance from purely lytic to purely blastic with mixed lytic/blastic types and lytic blowout patterns in between.[11] Lytic metastases are most common and again span the range of appearances from geographic to permeative types of destruction (Fig. 96-7).

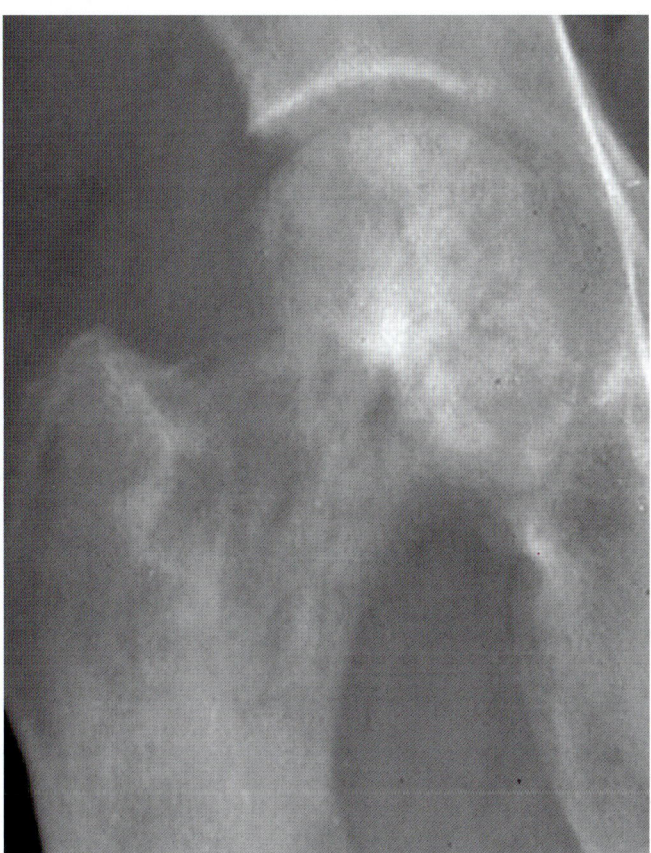

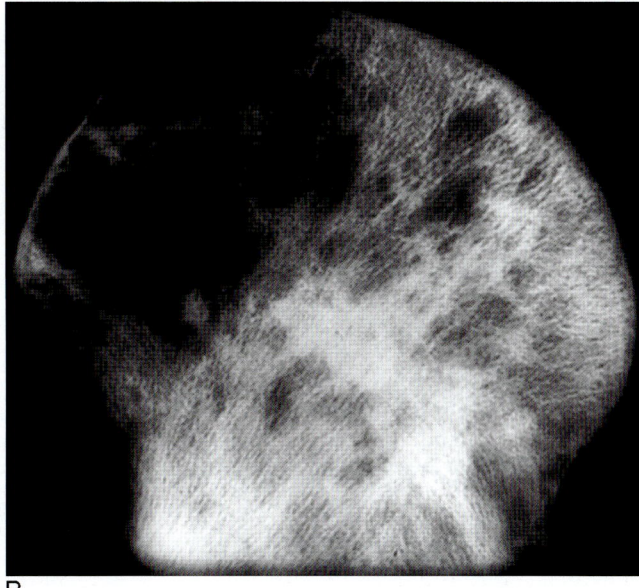

■ **FIGURE 96-5** A 65-year old man presented with metastatic prostate cancer. Right hip radiograph (**A**) and specimen radiograph (**B**) after resection show patchy increased density in femoral head due to deposition of new bone on top of existing trabeculae. In the radiograph in **B** note the patchy increased density in the femoral head due to deposition of new bone on top of existing trabeculae.

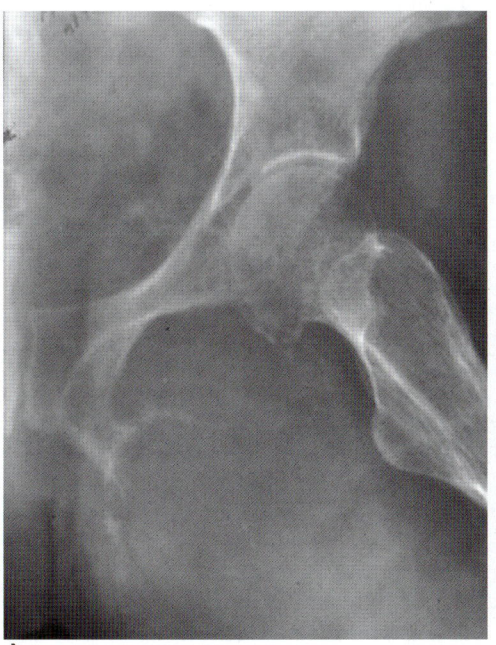

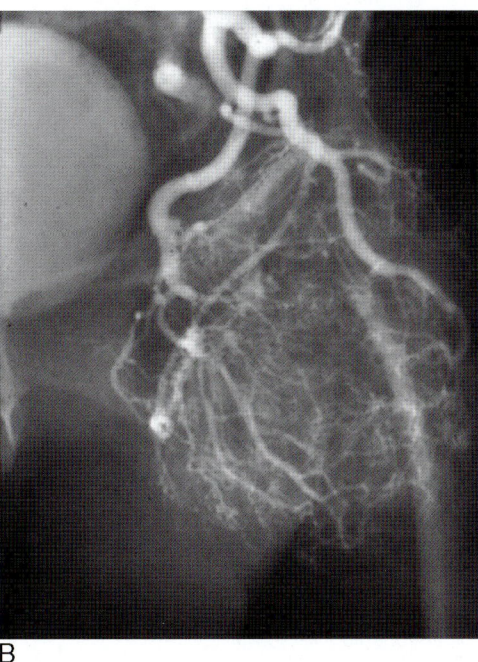

■ **FIGURE 96-6** A 67-year old woman presented with metastatic thyroid cancer. **A,** Left hip radiograph shows lytic blowout lesion of the ischium. **B,** Angiogram shows lytic blowout lesion of the ischium and extensive hyperemia with neovascularity.

Lytic metastases are not specific as to the site of origin of the primary tumor. The two most common primary sites of malignancy are the breast or lung. Lytic lesions with a blowout pattern are somewhat more specific for the site of the primary tumor. Renal cell and thyroid carcinomas account for most of these lesions, although the pattern also may be seen with breast and lung carcinomas. A mixed lytic/blastic pattern (Fig. 96-8) is sometimes seen particularly with breast, lung, and gastrointestinal tract primary tumors.

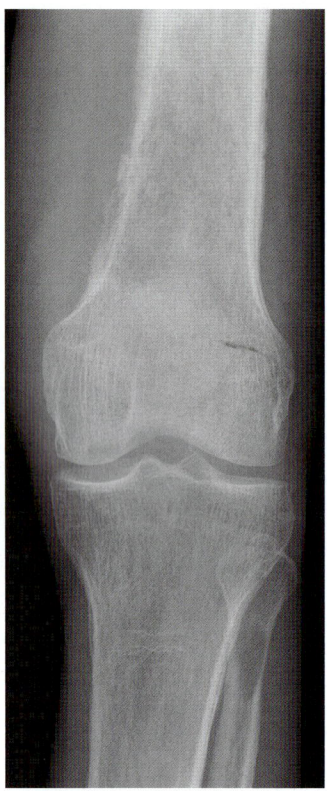

■ **FIGURE 96-7** Radiograph of a 57-year old man with metastatic lung cancer shows a variety of appearances of metastases from geographic in the fibula to permeative in the distal femur.

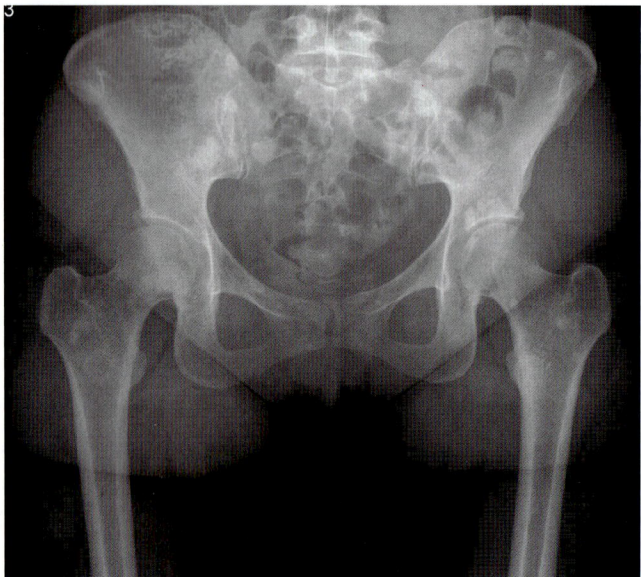

■ **FIGURE 96-8** Mixed lytic/blastic pattern in a 49-year old woman with metastatic breast cancer. Pelvic radiograph shows multiple foci of blastic metastases as well as some lytic and mixed foci, most notable in the proximal right femur.

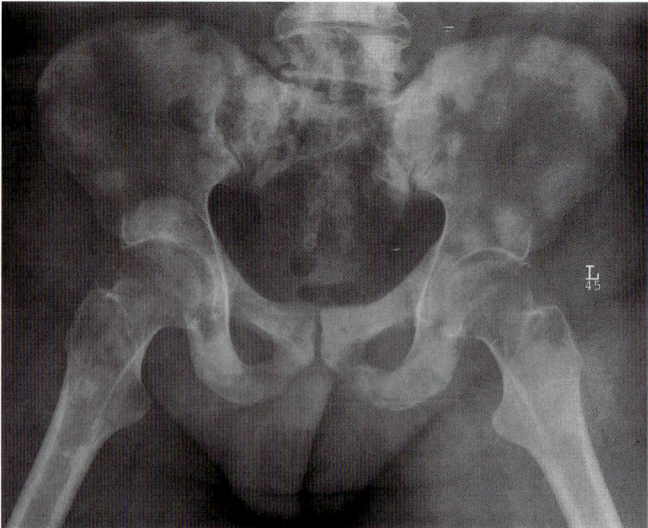

■ **FIGURE 96-9** Purely blastic metastases in a 55-year old man with metastatic carcinoid lung tumor. Pelvic radiograph shows multiple foci of blastic metastatic involvement.

TABLE 96-1	Metastatic Patterns of Primary Carcinomas		
Lytic	**Lytic Blowout**	**Mixed**	**Blastic**
Breast	Renal	Breast	Prostate
Lung	Thyroid	Lung	Breast
Head/neck	Breast	Prostate	Carcinoid
Neuroblastoma	Lung	Gastrointestinal tract	Small cell lung
Gastrointestinal tract		Neuroblastoma	Medullo- blastoma
Genitourinary tract		Carcinoid	
Reproductive organs			
Skin			

Purely blastic metastases (Fig. 96-9) are most often seen with prostate carcinomas, although carcinoid tumors, medulloblastomas, and breast and small cell lung carcinomas also may have blastic metastases (Table 96-1).

The amount of lytic destruction needed before a lesion becomes evident on radiographs depends on the specific location of the lesion within bone. Cortical or intracortical lesions are readily evident even when the lesions are very small (Fig. 96-10).

On the other hand, intramedullary lesions without cortical involvement (Fig. 96-11) can be quite large before they are readily detectable on radiographs.

It has been experimentally shown that vertebral body lesions may not be detectable, on lateral radiographs, until 50% to 75% of the vertebral body has been destroyed.[12] Even more bone destruction is needed for vertebral lesions to be evident on anteroposterior radiographs. Pedicle involvement is readily detectable and should always be looked for on anteroposterior films of the spine (Fig. 96-12). However, pedicle involvement is a late finding.

Magnetic Resonance Imaging

The basic sequences usually done to evaluate a patient with known or suspected metastatic disease include combined T1-weighted and fat saturated T2-weighted or inversion recovery in standard axial, coronal, and sagittal planes. Chemical fat saturation is dependent on many factors specific to certain magnets and manufacturers.

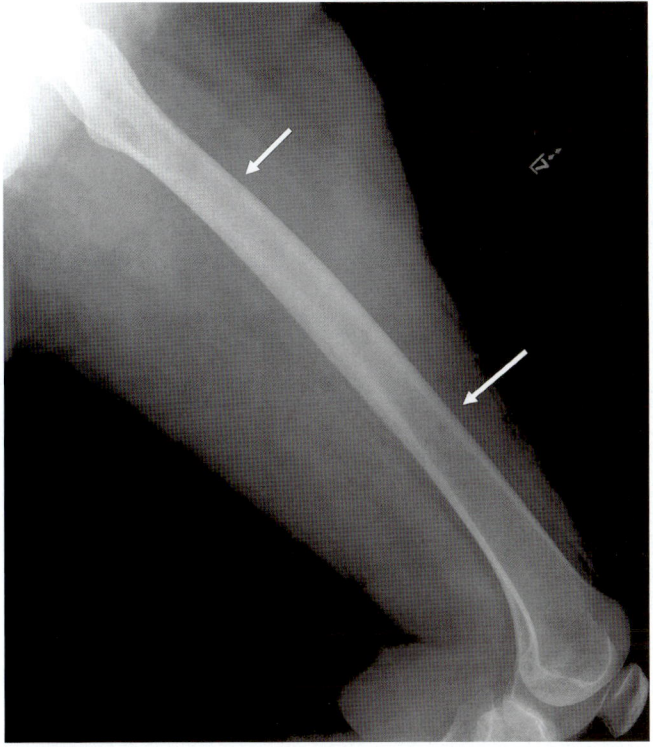

■ FIGURE 96-10 Cortical metastases in a 57-year old woman with metastatic breast cancer. Radiographs of left femur readily show small areas of metastatic involvement (*arrows*) because they involve the cortical bone.

Inversion recovery sequences are often more satisfactory especially for large fields of view, in the presence of metallic artifacts and other instances of field inhomogeneity. Other imaging sequences that may be used include diffusion weighted imaging and in- and out-of-phase imaging.

Multidetector Computed Tomography

Computed tomographic technology continues to evolve rapidly. Scanners in clinical use today include those with 4-, 16-, and 64-slice capabilities. Dual scanners and those with up to 256-slice capabilities are just becoming available. The increased speed of image acquisition offered by these machines is not as critical for detecting metastatic disease within the skeleton as it is for detecting disease within the coronary arteries. For skeletal metastatic disease the basic technique involves acquisition of images with isotropic voxels so coronal and sagittal reformatted images can be obtained without degradation of image quality. Coronal and sagittal reformatted images are obtained routinely to better demonstrate the extent of disease, especially in the pelvis and appendicular skeleton.

Ultrasonography

Routine ultrasonography does not have a direct role in the evaluation of skeletal metastatic disease. Indirectly, quantitative ultrasound studies might be done in some patients to monitor bone mineral density during treatment with

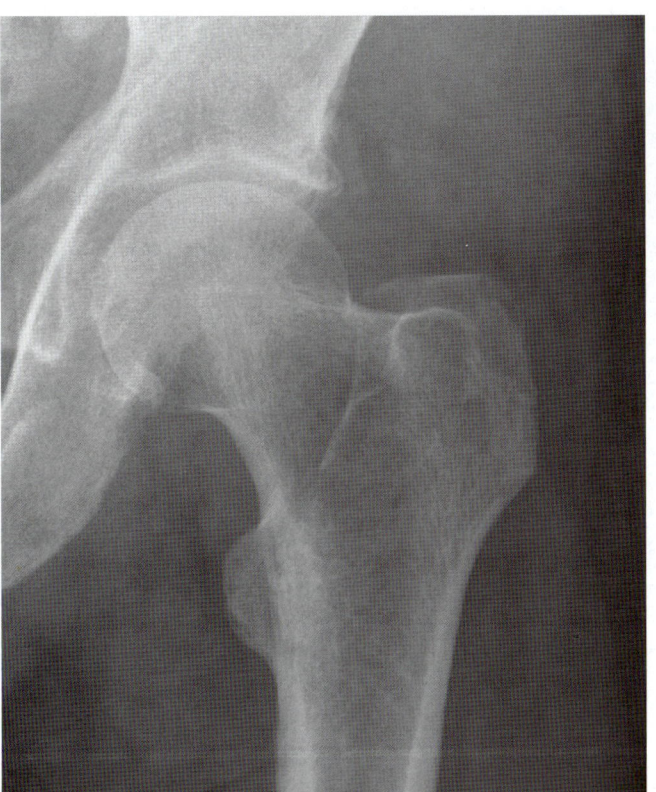

A

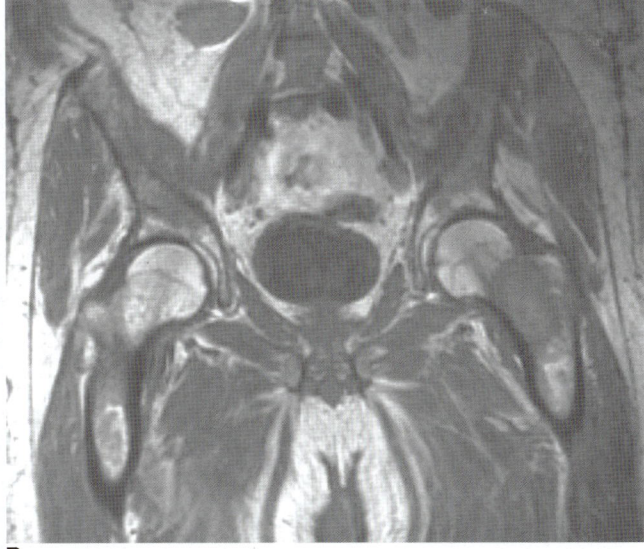

B

■ FIGURE 96-11 A 63-year old man with known metastatic renal cell cancer presented with a complaint of left hip pain. Hip radiograph (**A**) fails to reveal large metastasis shown on coronal T1-weighted MR image (**B**) obtained 6 days later because it involves only medullary bone.

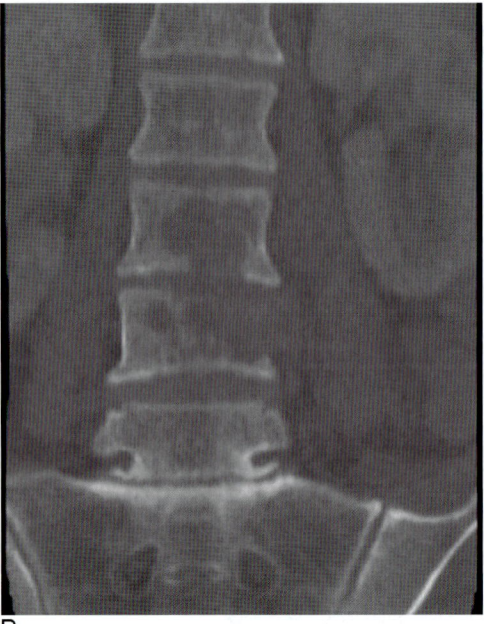

■ FIGURE 96-12 A 56-year old man with metastatic squamous cell carcinoma of the tongue complained of new back pain. **A,** Lumbar spine radiograph shows absent pedicle on the left at L4. **B,** Coronal CT reformatted image shows destructive lesions in L3 and L4. The L3 lesion is not evident, even in retrospect, on the frontal radiograph.

A   B

bisphosphonates. Ultrasonography may be the first imaging study done to evaluate a soft tissue mass. Metastatic disease must be remembered as an uncommon cause of soft tissue masses in adult patients.

Nuclear Medicine

Bone scintiscans with technetium-99m (^{99m}Tc) are performed in many patients to establish the total number of lesions. If multiple lesions are found (Fig. 96-13), the likelihood of metastatic disease increases.

Other conditions with involvement of multiple bones include Langerhans cell histiocytosis, fibrous dysplasia, multiple myeloma, Paget's disease, brown tumors, primary lymphoma of bone, and multifocal osteomyelitis. Even if the initial lesion is shown to be solitary, one must still consider metastatic disease, because 10% to 17% of solitary rib lesions shown on bone scintigraphy represent metastases and up to 80% of solitary lesions (Fig. 96-14) at other sites (particularly the spine) will be due to metastatic disease.[13,14]

Positron Emission Tomography/ Computed Tomography

Positron emission tomography/computed tomography is currently the imaging study of choice for the staging and follow-up of patients with cancers of the head/neck region (including the thyroid and esophagus), lung, breast, and ovary as well as for those patients with lymphoma and melanoma. PET/CT can play a role in the detection of unknown primary tumors as well. Besides initial staging, PET and PET/CT are very useful for monitoring treatment response. With regard to skeletal metastases per se there are conflicting reports in the literature regarding the accuracy

of FDG PET/CT versus traditional ^{99m}Tc bone scintigraphy.[15] However, the differences are tumor specific and PET/CT will certainly improve in the future with newer agents such as ^{18}F-fluoride and advances in the scanner hardware and the associated software programs. One recent report has shown ^{18}F-fluoride-PET/CT to be more sensitive and specific than standard ^{99m}Tc-methylene diphosphonate planar scintigraphy, SPECT, and FDG-PET for the detection of prostate cancer metastases.[16] Lytic lesions have higher FDG uptake than sclerotic lesions, so one should be careful not to rely simply on the standardized uptake value when assessing individual lesions (Fig. 96-15).

Pros and Cons

One imaging study is not necessarily better than another. The choice of an imaging study depends on the individual patient, the specific primary cancer, and the site of known or suspected metastatic involvement.

Controversies

Which Whole-Body Imaging Technique is Best for Initial Staging and Subsequent Monitoring?

For an individual patient, the answer to this question will depend on what imaging techniques are available where care is received and what the primary cancer diagnosis is. The treating physician and local radiologist will also influence which whole-body examination is preferred. Current choices of whole-body techniques include PET, PET/CT, MRI, CT, and various nuclear scintigraphic agents, including monoclonal antibodies. The ideal imaging technique rapidly and accurately identifies all sites of active disease. None of our current techniques satisfies all of these criteria in all circumstances.

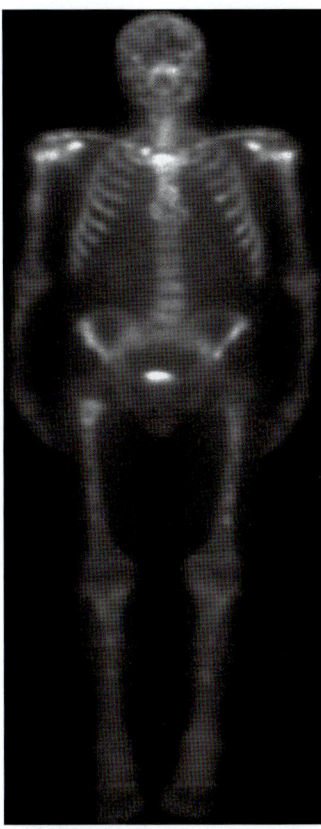

■ FIGURE 96-13 A 58-year-old man presented with prostate cancer. Whole-body ^{99m}Tc bone scan shows multiple foci of increased uptake typical of widespread metastatic disease.

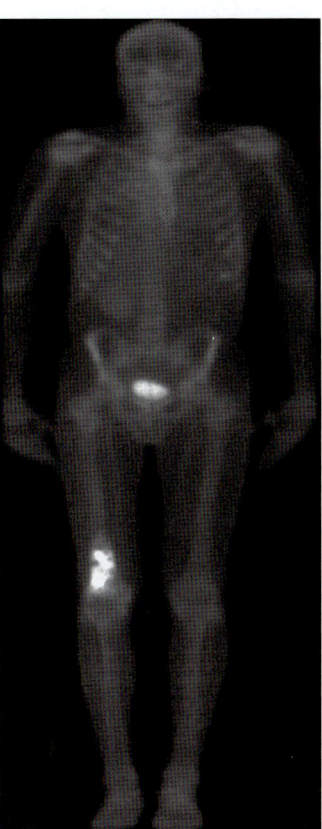

■ FIGURE 96-14 Whole-body ^{99m}Tc bone scan of a 44-year-old man who presented with solitary metastasis from renal cell carcinoma.

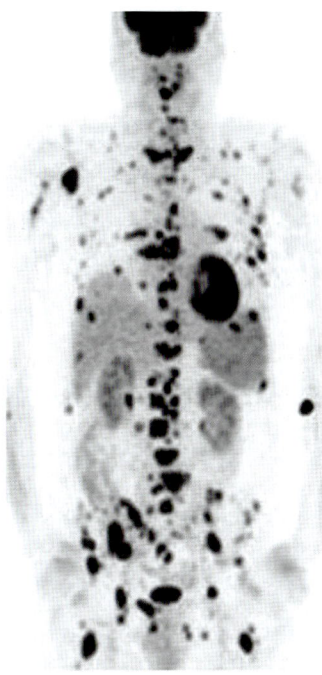

■ FIGURE 96-15 Whole-body FDG PET in a 56-year-old man with head/neck cancer shows multiple foci of avid FDG activity typical of widespread metastatic disease.

Does Magnetic Field Strength Matter?

For most patients with known or suspected skeletal metastatic disease the magnetic field strength is not the most important consideration. Radiologists have become quite skilled at acquiring excellent images with MR scanners at all field strengths from low (0.35 T) to high (3.0 T). Whole-body imaging is usually only available on newer machines operating at 1.5 to 3.0 T, but whole-body imaging is not needed in all instances.

Are Intravenous Contrast Agents Needed?

Intravenous contrast agents are not routinely needed for CT or MR examinations when the question is the presence or absence of metastatic involvement of specific skeletal sites. If the evaluation of the skeleton is combined with evaluation of visceral organs, then intravenous contrast will be used in most cases.

MANIFESTATIONS OF THE DISEASE

Spinal Involvement

Red bone marrow, and the spine in particular, is the most common site of skeletal metastatic disease on pathologic examination. Clinical presentations range from asymptomatic patients to those with back and/or radicular pain, weakness, sensory deficit, bowel/bladder dysfunction, pathologic fracture, cord compression, and paralysis. Cord compression occurs in approximately 5% of patients with metastatic disease due to intradural and/or extradural disease. Imaging of a patient with known malignancy and suspected spinal cord compression should be performed emergently because the disease may progress rapidly. Radiographs should be performed initially. The thoracic and lumbar vertebrae are the most commonly involved spine segments, and the vertebral body is more frequently affected than the posterior elements. The classic radiographic finding of an absent pedicle is a late feature representing extension from posterior vertebral body disease into the pedicle. Disc involvement, including direct invasion of the disc by tumor, disc degeneration, and Schmorl's node formation, can be seen as a manifestation of metastatic disease to the spine. Visualization of associated soft tissue mass and compression of the thecal sac requires myelography, CT, or MRI.

Radiography

Vertebral collapse is a common manifestation of metastatic disease that can be a source of clinical and radiographic confusion because up to 30% of patients with metastatic disease have a nonmalignant cause for the compression fracture.[17] Although it may be impossible to radiographically differentiate benign from malignant collapse there are some important diagnostic clues that may be helpful. The presence of intravertebral gas in a collapsed vertebral body almost invariably indicates avascular necrosis and virtually excludes the diagnosis of neoplasm. Benign compression fracture in the cervical and upper thoracic spine (above T6 particularly without multiple compressions of the lower thoracic spine) is rare. Fractures in these regions should raise concern for neoplasm. Angular end-plate deformity and osseous destruction (Fig. 96-16) are not typically associated with benign osteoporotic compression fractures. These latter findings should suggest the presence of a pathologic process such as metastatic disease.

Magnetic Resonance Imaging

Magnetic resonance imaging is the single best method to detect metastatic disease in the spine because it allows accurate, multiplanar assessment of bone marrow, epidural and intradural spaces, and the spinal cord (Table 96-2). Marrow involvement typically presents as areas of replacement of fat with tumor demonstrating intermediate signal on T1-weighted images and high signal on T2-weighted images (Fig. 96-17).

Sclerotic metastases may demonstrate low signal on both T1- and T2-weighted images. The entire vertebral body may be involved, or focal rounded areas of marrow replacement may be seen. Involvement of red marrow particularly in children is better appreciated on T2-weighted images or post-gadolinium T1-weighted images with fat saturation. MRI may help distinguish benign from malignant compression fracture. A benign osteoporotic fracture is suggested when a retropulsed bone fragment is seen, when fat signal is preserved on T1-weighted images throughout the body and there is no high signal on T2 weighted images (Fig. 96-18), and when horizontal band-like areas representing the fracture plane are seen after administration of gadolinium.

A malignant etiology of collapse is suggested when the posterior cortex is convex toward the spinal canal,

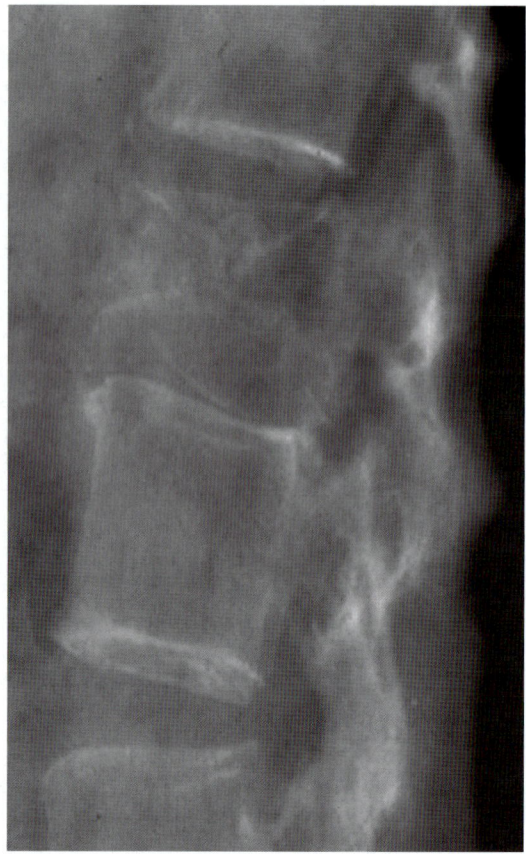

■ **FIGURE 96-16** A 61-year-old woman presented with breast cancer and back pain. Lateral radiograph shows angular deformity of superior end plate of L2 with some collapse of this vertebral body as well. (*Reproduced with permission of American Registry of Pathology.*)

an epidural mass is seen, when the entire vertebral body or pedicles are replaced by low signal on T1-weighted images, and high or heterogeneous signal is seen (Fig. 96-19) within the body after gadolinium injection or on T2-weighted images.[18]

MRI with dynamic gadolinium enhancement and evaluation of time-intensity curves has been shown to be

TABLE 96-2	Magnetic Resonance Imaging Features of Benign vs. Malignant Spine Lesions	
MRI Feature	**Benign Process Favored When:**	**Malignant Process Favored If:**
Bone marrow pattern	Not focal	Focal or geographic
T1-weighted spin echo	Low to intermediate signal	Low to intermediate signal
T2-weighted spin echo	High (bright) signal	High (bright) signal
Inversion recovery	High (bright) signal	High (bright) signal
Dynamic intravenous contrast	No or slow enhancement or rapid wash in with equilibrium	Rapid wash-in and early wash-out or rapid wash-in with second slow peak
Morphology	Horizontal band-like	Rounded, diffuse, or irregular
	Abnormal signal intensity	Abnormal signal intensity
	Posterior cortex of vertebral body has acute angle	Posterior cortex of vertebral body is smooth, convex toward canal
	Retropulsed bone fragment	Soft tissue and/or epidural mass
Diffusion-weighted	Low (slow)	High (fast)
Dual-phase chemical shift (In and out of phase)	In phase: low signal Out of phase: low signal	In phase: low signal Out of phase: high signal

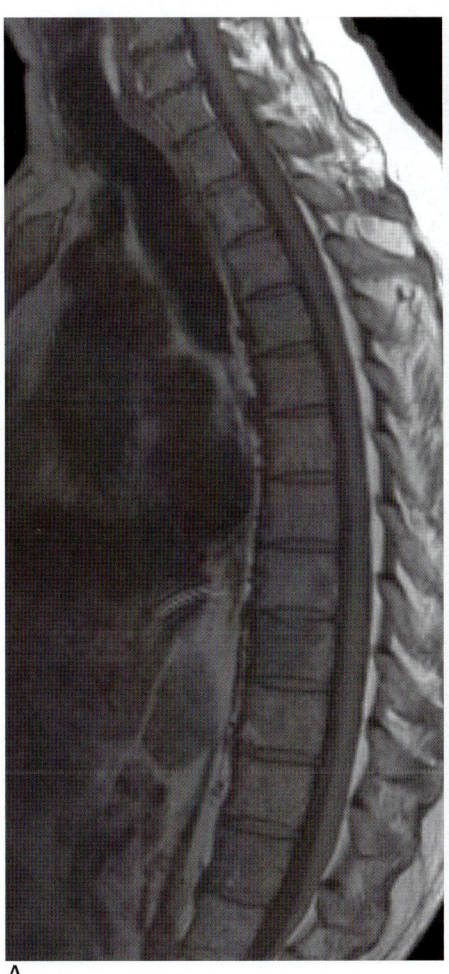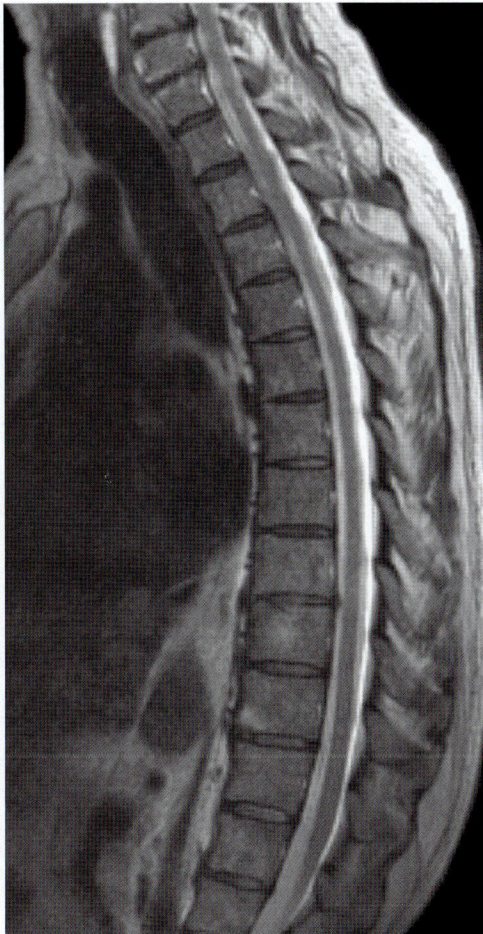

A   B

■ **FIGURE 96-17** Sagittal T1-weighted (**A**) and T2-weighted (**B**) MR images show multifocal metastases at T8, T9, and T12 in a 64-year-old man with prostate cancer.

valuable.[17] Chen and coworkers showed that rapid contrast wash-in with early wash-out had a 100% positive predictive value for metastatic involvement. Chemical-shift imaging may allow accurate differentiation of edema due to fracture from tumor replacement of marrow by nulling the signal from water in a local fatty environment. Diffusion-weighted imaging techniques also have been reported to be able to reliably distinguish benign compression fractures from those due to malignant processes. Another helpful distinguishing feature for focal lesions is the halo sign. This sign of malignancy is said to be present when a rim of high T2 signal intensity is seen surrounding a lesion. Whole-body MRI techniques are now available. Their clinical usefulness and cost effectiveness are being studied. One report indicates a better sensitivity for whole-body MRI (Fig. 96-20) compared with PET/CT for the detection of skeletal metastases.[19]

Multidetector Computed Tomography

Computed tomography is a useful tool to help differentiate benign from malignant compression fractures, and it is important to understand the utility of CT because some patients may not be able to safely undergo MRI examination, which is frequently the imaging modality of choice. In one study,[20] CT findings suggesting benign

fracture included retropulsed posterior fragment, cortical fragments without destruction, identifiable fracture lines within cancellous bone (Fig. 96-21), intravertebral vacuum phenomenon, and a thin diffuse paraspinal soft tissue mass. Malignant indicators included destruction of cortical or cancellous bone in a pedicle or body, focal paraspinal soft tissue mass, and epidural mass (Fig. 96-22).

Nuclear Medicine

Typical bone scintigraphic findings are scattered foci of increased uptake (see Fig. 96-13) that are not linear and not along the vertebral end plates or in the area of the facet joints.

Ivory Vertebra

Homogeneously dense vertebral bodies are referred to as ivory vertebrae (Fig. 96-23). The term was coined by Souques, Lafourcade, and Terris.[21] Their initial case report was published in 1925. They observed an ivory vertebra in a woman with breast carcinoma. Because this case was reported 15 years before Batson published his work on the vertebral plexus as discussed earlier, the authors had a difficult time explaining the pathway of spread in this

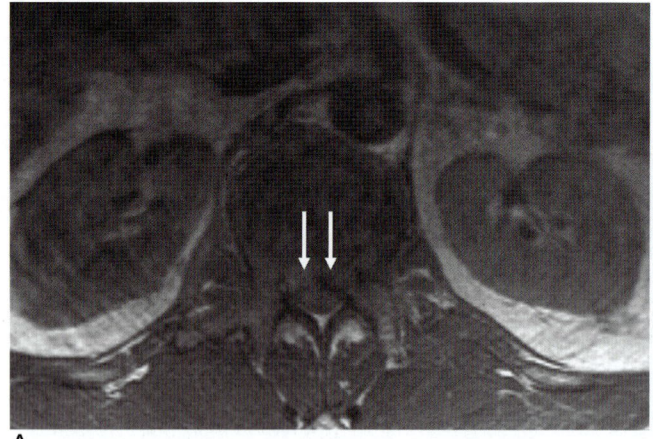

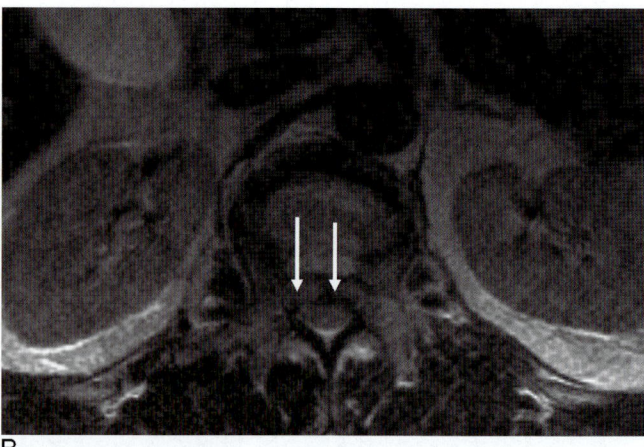

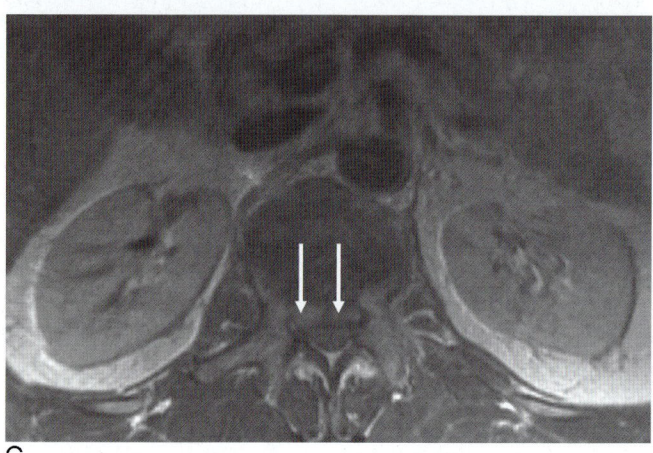

■ **FIGURE 96-18** Axial T1-weighted (**A**), T2-weighted (**B**), and T1-weighted post-gadolinium (**C**) MR images show retropulsed fracture fragment in the spinal canal but no other soft tissue mass in this 26-year-old male patient with traumatic L1 burst fracture.

woman who had no other evidence of metastatic disease. An ivory vertebra is not specific for metastatic disease. Pagetic involvement is said to account for approximately 50% of cases of ivory vertebrae.[22] Nearly 30% of cases are due to metastatic Hodgkin's lymphoma, with other blastic metastases accounting for most of the remaining cases. Rarely, chordomas and unusual cases of vertebral osteomyelitis may give an ivory vertebra appearance.

Hypertrophic Osteoarthropathy

Hypertrophic osteoarthropathy, also called Marie-Bamberger disease, may be primary (idiopathic) or secondary. Secondary hypertrophic osteoarthropathy is a condition affecting bone that is, most commonly, a manifestation of pulmonary disease, including malignancy. It is seen in 3% to 10% of all patients with bronchogenic carcinoma.[23] Tumors of the pleura (mesothelioma) have a higher overall association with hypertrophic osteoarthropathy (35% of cases) but are much less common than primary lung cancers. Originally described in patients with chronic lung disease, this entity has now been described in numerous conditions, including congenital heart disease, inflammatory bowel disease, and abdominal neoplasms. The etiology of this condition is unclear, but theories include humoral factors and neurogenic-mediated increased blood flow via the vagus nerve. Reports have documented, by immunohistochemical analysis, the production of growth hormone–releasing hormone by lung cancer cells.[24] Interestingly, surgical or chemical vagotomy may produce relief of symptoms and thoracotomy or thoracoscopy alone can relieve symptoms when chest disease is the cause of hypertrophic osteoarthropathy. Clinically, the patients may present with clubbing and/or articular pain and swelling.

Radiography

Radiographically, periostitis is most pronounced (Fig. 96-24) along the paired long bones of the distal upper and lower limbs, that is, the radius, ulna, tibia, and fibula. The femur, humerus, and the small bones of the hands and feet less commonly show radiographic changes. The periostitis is typically thick, solid, smooth, or undulating and extends for a variable distance along the length of the diaphysis and metaphysis. It does not usually involve the epiphyseal area.

Nuclear Medicine

Bone scintigraphy is more sensitive than radiography. Findings consist of increased uptake in a parallel track pattern (Fig. 96-25) along all long bones, reflecting increased blood flow and periosteal reaction. The scintigraphic

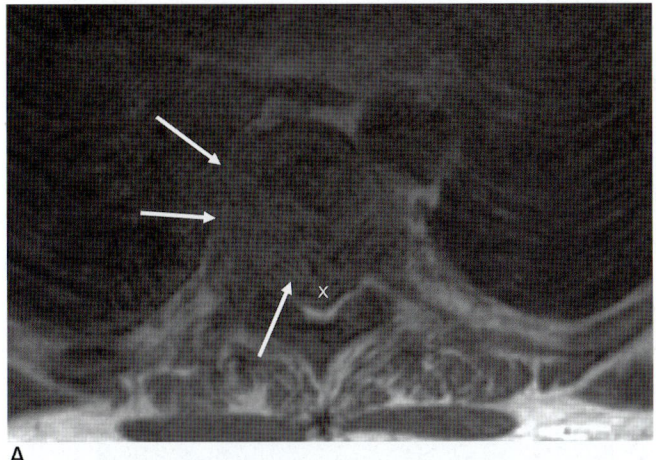

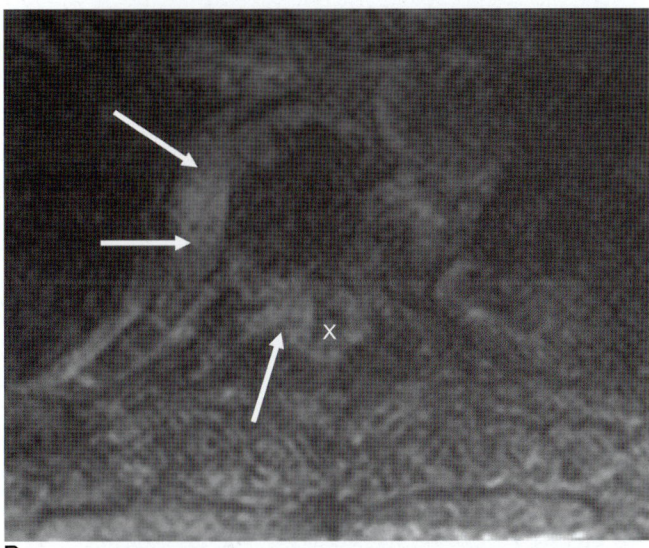

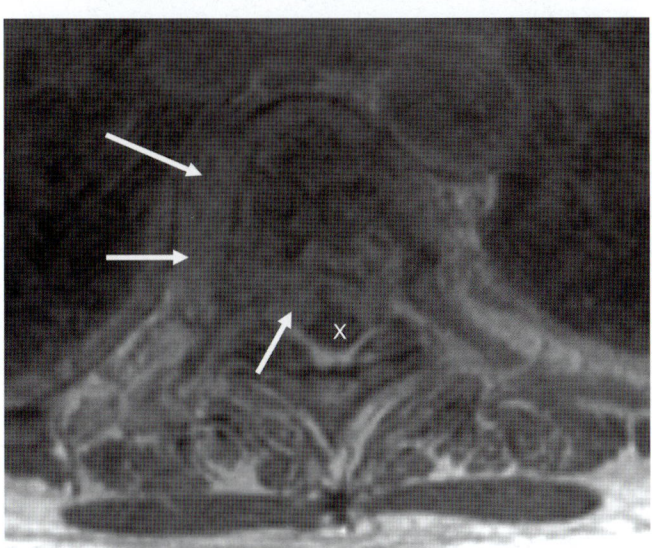

■ **FIGURE 96-19** Axial T1-weighted (**A**), T2-weighted (**B**), and T1-weighted post-gadolinium (**C**) MR images show soft tissue mass along right side of vertebral body and encroaching on the spinal cord in a 49-year old woman with unknown primary cancer.

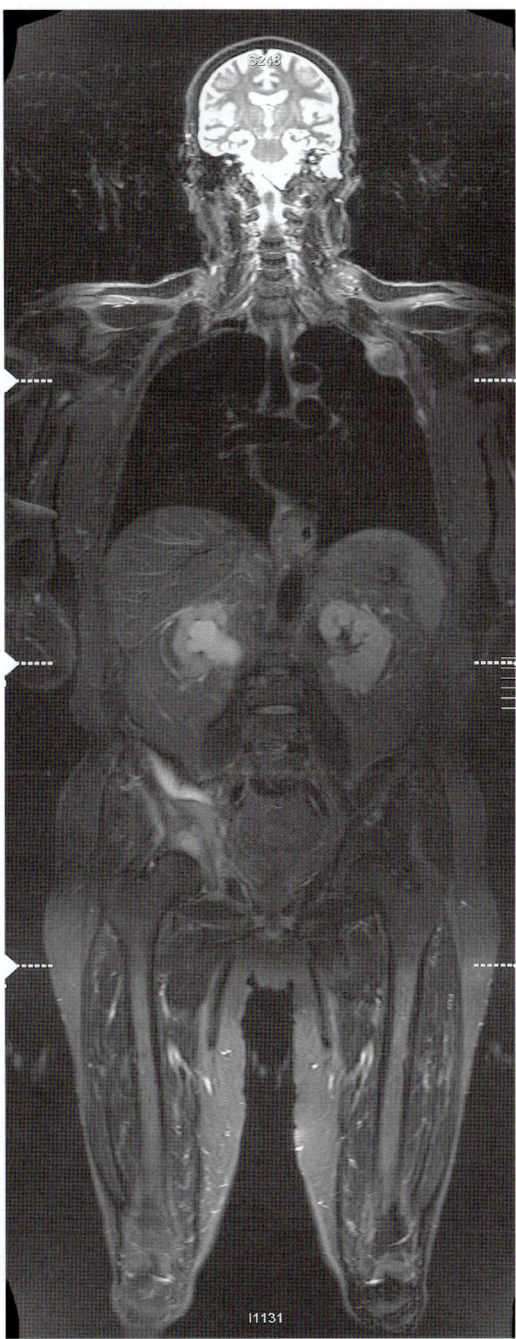

■ **FIGURE 96-20** Coronal whole-body MR image in a 64-year-old man with prostate cancer shows foci of bright signal intensity on this fast inversion recovery image typical of metastatic disease. Lesions are most readily seen involving the left upper ribs and right acetabulum.

findings may be more extensive and more pronounced than can be appreciated with radiographs.

Focal Periosteal Reaction

A focal proliferative periosteal reaction is an uncommon manifestation of metastatic disease. With an underlying dense lesion, however, it may be florid enough to simulate

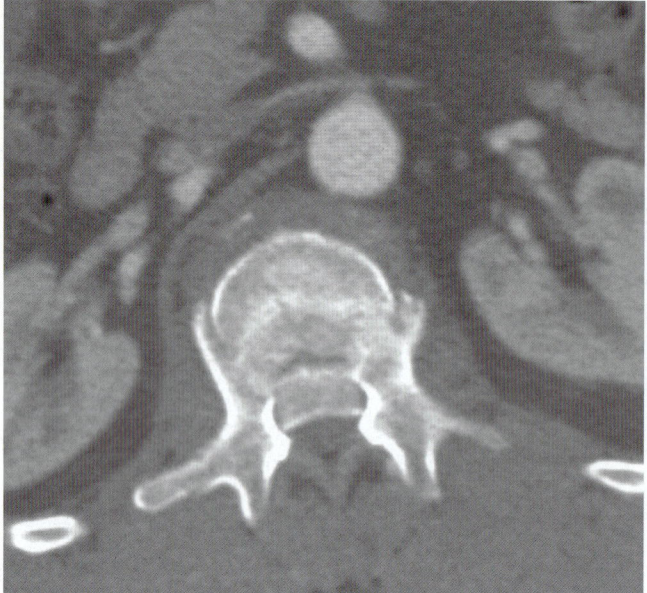

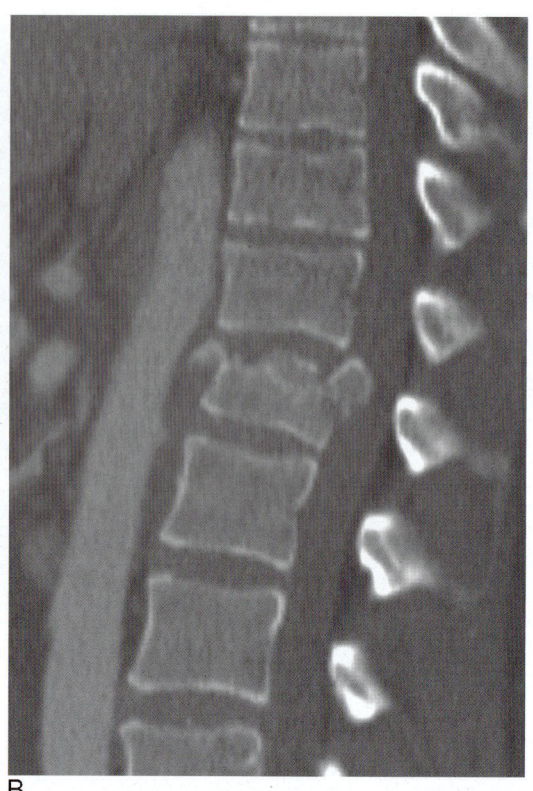

■ **FIGURE 96-21** Axial (**A**) and sagittal reformatted (**B**) CT images in the same patient as in Figure 96-18 show typical acute traumatic burst fracture at L1. There is no destruction of vertebral walls, only fracture fragmentation.

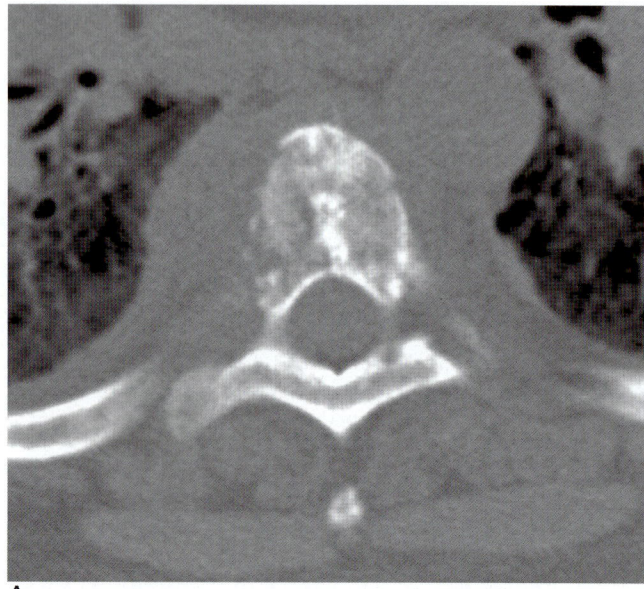

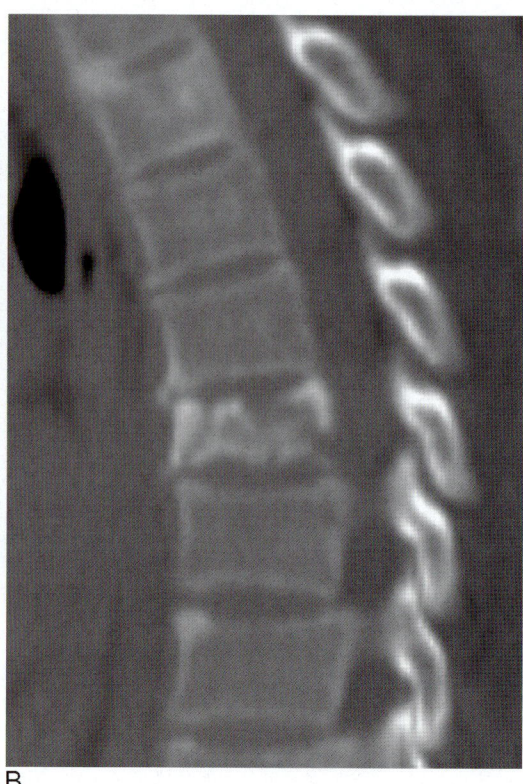

■ **FIGURE 96-22** Axial (**A**) and sagittal reformatted (**B**) CT images in the same patient as in Figure 96-19 show destruction of right and left vertebral body walls as well as portions of superior and inferior end plates in this pathologic fracture.

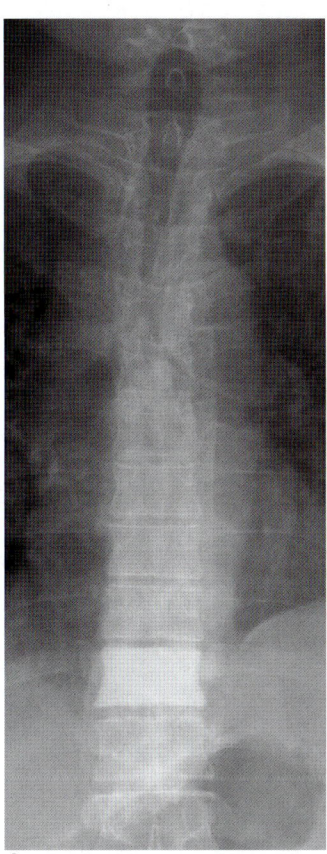

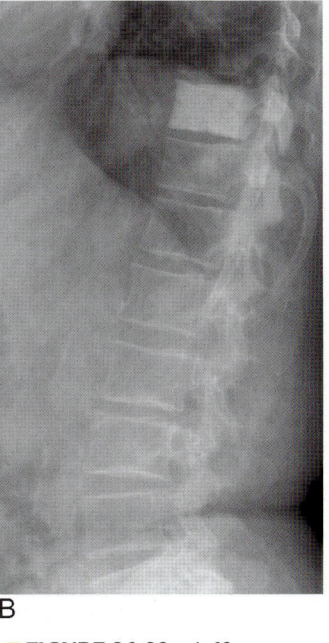

■ FIGURE 96-23 A 69-year-old man presented with prostate cancer and a rising prostate-specific antigen value. **A** and **B,** Spine radiographs show ivory vertebra at T10 level.

a primary osteosarcoma and is most commonly associated with metastatic prostate carcinoma (Fig. 96-26).

Other primary tumors that may have metastases with significant local periosteal reaction (Fig. 96-27) include neuroblastoma, bronchogenic carcinoma, and gastrointestinal tract malignancies.

Cortical Metastases

Bronchogenic carcinoma is the most common source of cortical or intracortical metastases (Fig. 96-28). Large cortical lesions often have a "cookie cutter" or "cookie bite" appearance.[25] If there is more than 50% cortical destruction the risk of impending pathologic fracture is said to be about 66%.

Multiple small cortical lesions also are seen most commonly in patients with lung cancer. When multiple, cortical metastases can mimic primary bone malignancies such as angiosarcomas.

Soft Tissue Mass

Small subcutaneous lesions are not uncommon in patients with widespread metastatic disease (Fig. 96-29). In contradistinction, large, solitary, deep soft tissue masses are an uncommon manifestation of metastatic disease, although carcinomas can present in this way, particularly bronchogenic carcinomas. However, one should consider

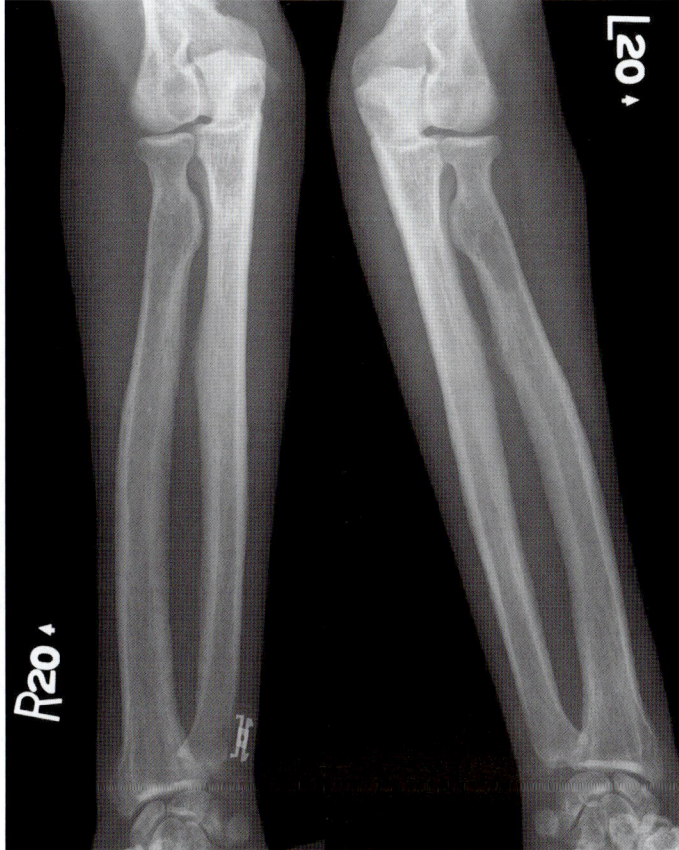

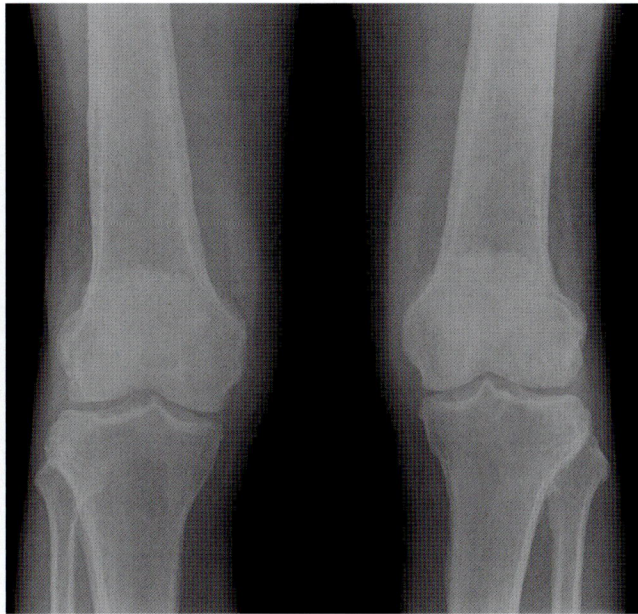

■ FIGURE 96-24 **A,** Forearm radiographs in a 39-year old man with lung cancer, done as part of bone survey, show typical periosteal changes of hypertrophic osteoarthropathy, especially along both ulnas. **B,** Knee radiographs in same patient show typical periosteal changes of hypertrophic osteoarthropathy.

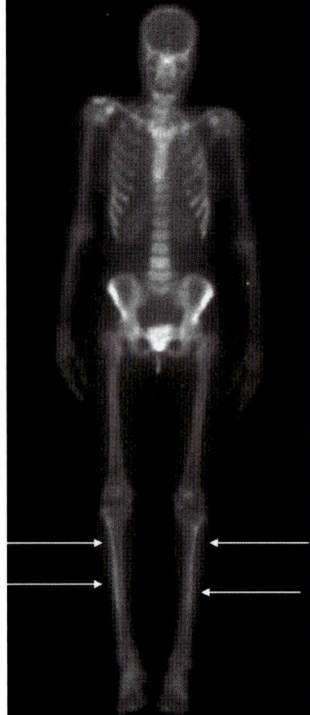

■ **FIGURE 96-25** ⁹⁹ᵐTc scintiscan of a 48-year-old woman with non–small cell lung cancer shows typical linear uptake along shafts of both tibias indicative of hypertrophic osteoarthropathy.

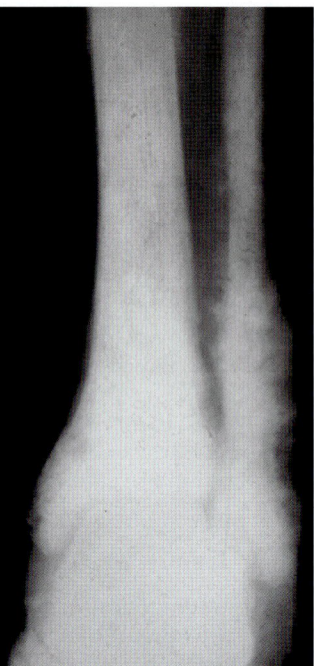

■ **FIGURE 96-26** Radiograph of left ankle shows very florid periosteal reaction around the distal fibula due to adjacent metastatic focus within the bone in a 76-year old man with prostate cancer. (*Reproduced with permission of American Registry of Pathology.*)

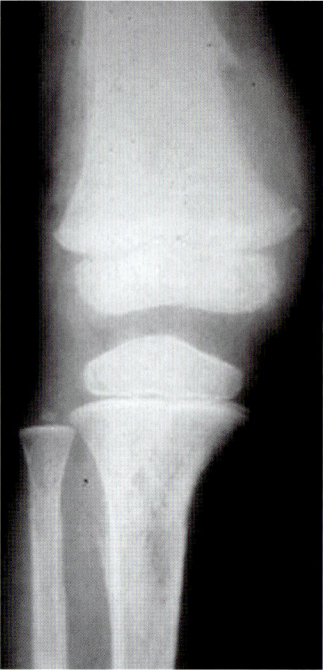

■ **FIGURE 96-27** Knee radiograph of a 3-year-old boy with neuroblastoma shows aggressive periosteal reaction around distal femur and proximal tibia due to metastatic involvement in the same areas of the medullary portion of the femur and tibia.

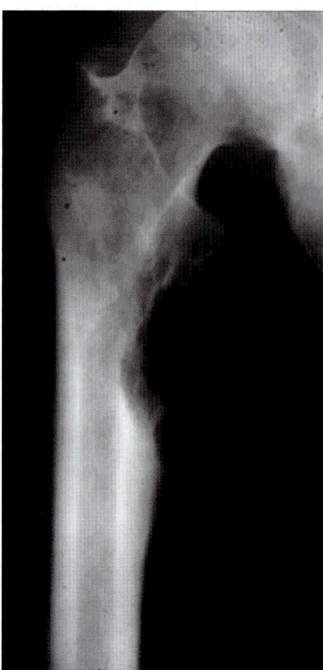

■ **FIGURE 96-28** Femur radiograph in a 55-year old man with lung cancer shows large medial cortical "cookie bite" metastasis. (*Reproduced with permission of American Registry of Pathology.*)

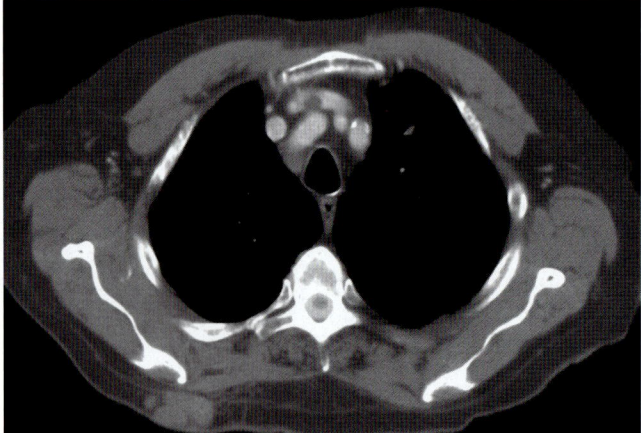

■ **FIGURE 96-29** Axial CT scan through the upper chest of a 74-year old man with known head/neck cancer shows lobular soft tissue metastasis in right posterior subcutaneous tissues.

a primary soft tissue tumor as a more likely explanation than metastatic disease in this clinical setting.

Magnetic Resonance Imaging

The findings on MRI are nonspecific. Generally there is low signal intensity on T1-weighted sequences with increased signal intensity on T2-weighted sequences.

Multidetector Computed Tomography

Findings are nonspecific.

Ultrasonography

Findings are nonspecific and may be hypovascular or hypervascular on Doppler examination.

Synovial Involvement

Metastatic involvement of the synovium is rare. It may occur by direct extension from disease in the adjacent bones or by hematogenous routes. Breast and lung primary lesions account for most of the cases that have been reported. The knee is the most commonly affected joint. Very rarely arthropathy due to synovial metastatic disease is the initial manifestation of malignancy. Imaging findings are nonspecific. Joint effusion and thickening of the synovium (Fig. 96-30) have been described. Rarely, synovial calcifications are seen, particularly with mucinous adenocarcinomas. If a destructive process is evident in the adjacent osseous structures, then the joint abnormalities are more suspicious. The joint abnormalities also may be due to a reactive synovitis without malignant infiltration. Aspiration of serosanguineous joint fluid is suspicious for metastatic involvement in this clinical setting. Synovial biopsy is usually definitive. Metastatic involvement of the synovium reportedly has a poor prognosis.[26]

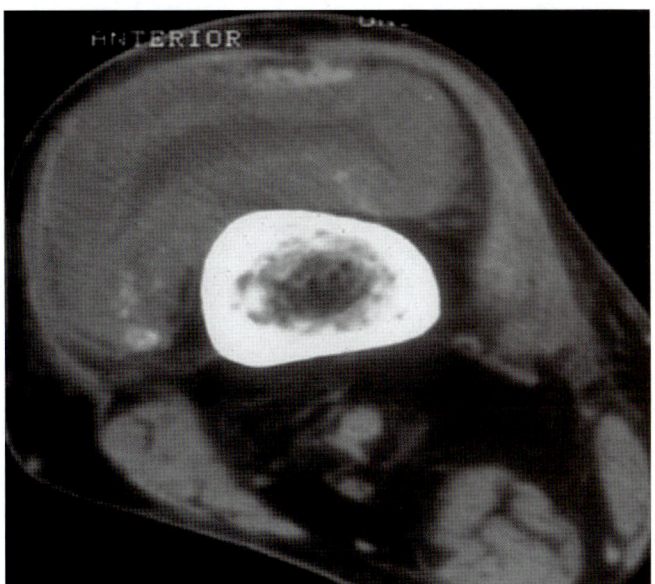

■ **FIGURE 96-30** Axial CT scan in a 61-year old man who first complained of pain in his knee shows marked thickening of the synovium subsequently proven to represent metastatic involvement from a primary colon cancer. *(Case courtesy of Dr. Steve Hatem, Cleveland Clinic, Cleveland, OH.)*

Pathologic Fracture

Pathologic fracture may have a significant impact on the quality of life of a cancer patient (Fig. 96-31) as improvements in oncologic care have led to the prolonged survival of patients with metastatic disease.

The incidence of pathologic fracture is between 7% and 27% of patients with metastatic disease[27] to bone when rib and spine lesions are considered in addition to long bone lesions. Pathologic fracture is more likely to occur with breast metastases (53%-59%) than other primary tumors. Melanoma rarely produces pathologic fracture.[28] Pathologic fracture is more common in the lower than upper extremity and should always be considered when a transverse fracture is seen (Fig. 96-32), with nontraumatic avulsion of the lesser trochanter,[29] and when little or no trauma results in a fracture.

Pathologic fractures must be differentiated from stress fractures, and particularly from insufficiency fractures, to avoid unnecessary biopsy because resorptive and reparative changes may mimic malignancy histologically. Resorptive and reparative changes can be particularly prominent in areas of previously irradiated bone. The linear or band-like morphology of insufficiency fractures, particularly in the public rami and sacrum where the H-shaped ("Honda") sign[30] is seen (Fig. 96-33), can be helpful in distinguishing insufficiency fractures from pathologic fractures due to metastases. This sign also can be appreciated on coronal CT and MR images.

Healing of pathologic fractures occurs in less than 35% of all cases[31] but is more likely in the setting of breast and prostate cancer, with life expectancy greater than 6 months, with internal fixation, and with local radiation dose of less than 30 Gy. Identifying an impending pathologic fracture is important not only to avoid pain and decreased mobility but also because pathologic fractures

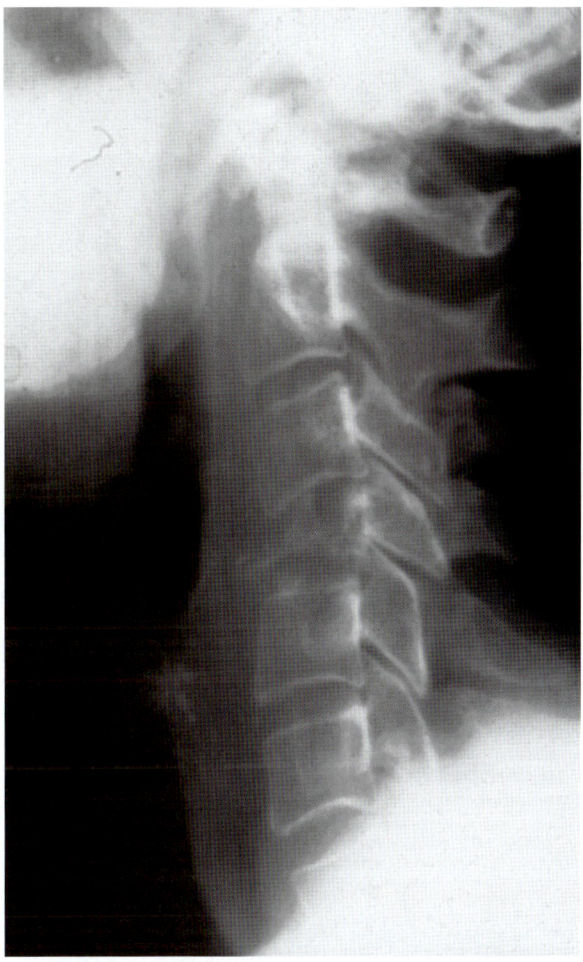

■ **FIGURE 96-31** A 35-year-old cancer patient with pathologic compression fracture of the C4 vertebral body.

may be associated with increased risk of later development of pulmonary metastases that may be minimized by prophylactic fixation after irradiation.[32] Two criteria for prophylactic fixation of an impending long bone fracture include (1) a well-defined lucent defect greater than 2.5 cm in dimension that involves the cortex or is painful and (2) 50% total cortical destruction combined on anteroposterior and lateral radiographs.[33] Both criteria are based on routine radiographic examinations and may be poor predictors of fracture. The lesion dimension of 2.5 cm applies only to the femur, requires a well-defined lytic lesion, and does not account for baseline mineralization of the affected patient. The criterion of 50% cortical destruction suffers from difficulty of assessing extent of cortical involvement accurately on radiographs and difficulty of determining extent of poorly defined lesions. Neither criterion addresses blastic lesions. Because of these limitations, other scoring systems have been developed to help the orthopedic surgeon decide when surgery might be needed for a long bone lesion. One such scoring system was developed by Mirels[34] and includes lesion location (upper vs. lower extremity), size, appearance (blastic vs. lytic), and presence or absence of pain. A weighted scoring is done (Table 96-3). Lesions with a score of 7 or lower are managed nonoperatively, whereas those with a score of 8 or higher are typically treated with surgery.

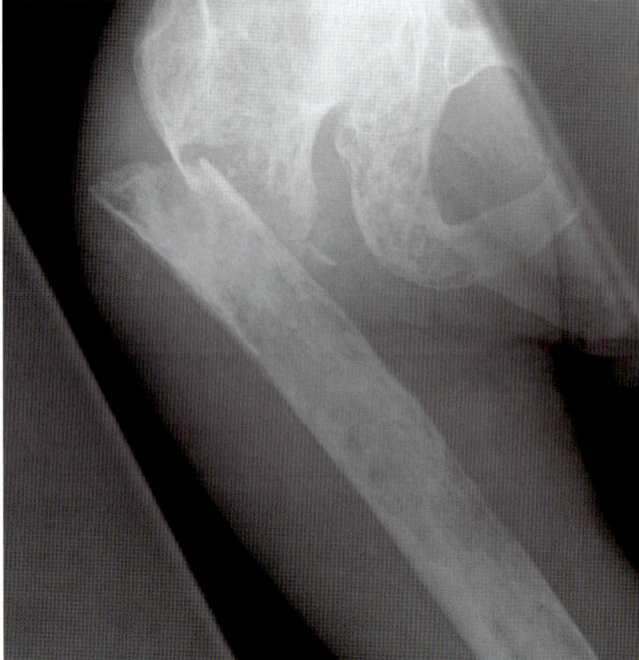

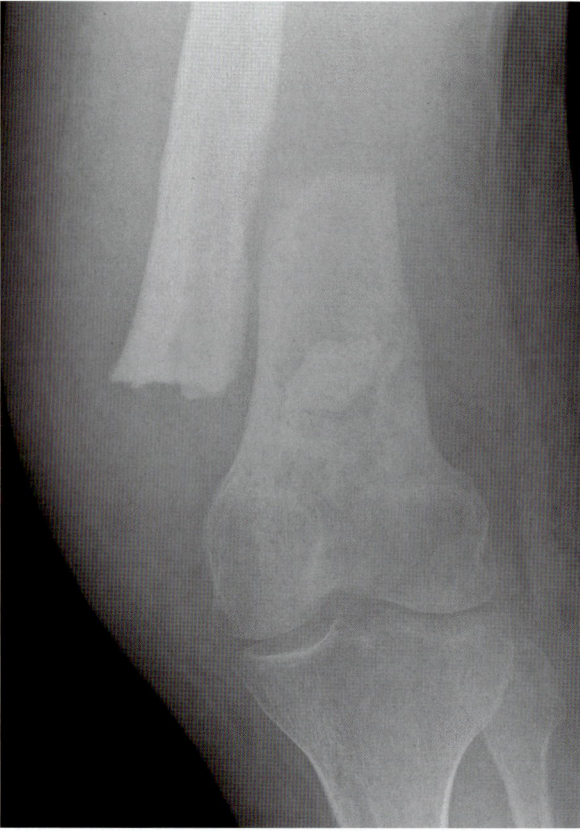

■ **FIGURE 96-32** Two patients with pathologic fractures, one (**A**) in the proximal femoral subtrochanteric region and the other (**B**) in the distal femoral shaft. Note that both fractures are transversely oriented.

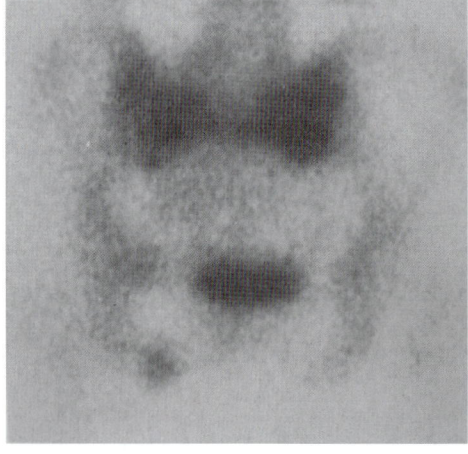

■ **FIGURE 96-33** ^{99m}Tc bone scan spot view of the pelvis show typical H-shape ("Honda" sign) of increased uptake vertically in both sacral alae and transversely across the body of the sacrum.

For the flat bones, treatment criteria are not as well defined, except for acetabular lesions. Harrington categorizes acetabular defects as follows: class I defects are small, with intact acetabular walls and cortices, class II defects are larger (Fig. 96-34) with involvement of the medial wall, and class III defects are massive (Fig. 96-35) with additional involvement of the lateral cortex and dome.[35] Radiologists should pay particular attention to these areas when evaluating imaging studies of the pelvis.

Radiography

Simple transverse fracture through an underlying area of lytic, blastic, or mixed disease should suggest the diagnosis of pathologic fracture.

Magnetic Resonance Imaging

The CT and MRI features that should suggest a pathologic fracture include well-defined areas of marrow replacement, endosteal scalloping, and surrounding soft tissue mass.[36] CT and MRI findings are usually definitive.

DIFFERENTIAL DIAGNOSIS

The differential diagnosis includes the following:
● Multiple myeloma/plasmacytoma
● Primary bone tumor
● chronic recurrent multifocal osteomyelitis
● Polyostotic fibrous dysplasia
● Polyostotic Paget's disease
● Multiple brown tumors
● Langerhans cell histiocytosis
● Insufficiency fracture

SYNOPSIS OF TREATMENT OPTIONS

Medical Treatment

Currently, options range from simple pain control to utilization of various chemotherapy regimens. Bisphosphonates are

TABLE 96-3 Mirels' Scoring System

Point Value	1	2	3
Location	Upper limb	Lower limb	Peritrochanteric
Appearance	Blastic	Mixed	Lytic
Pain	Mild	Moderate	Severe

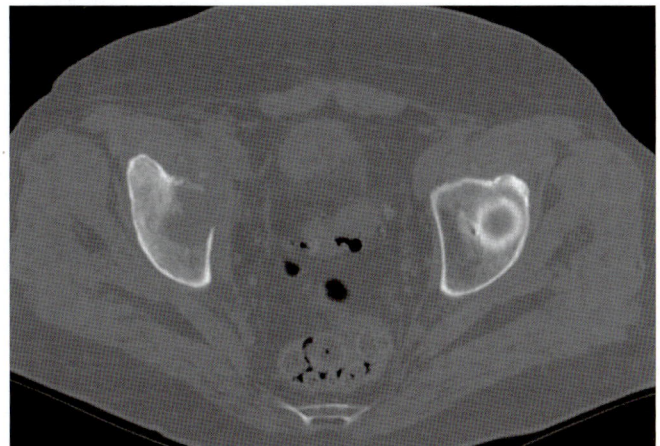

■ **FIGURE 96-34** Harrington class 2 lesion in a 64-year old man with prostate cancer. Acetabular metastasis shows destruction of medial cortex on axial CT.

the current treatment of choice for reduction of osteoclastic activity and for prevention of additional lytic bone destruction. Strontium-89, phosphorus-32, hormonal therapies, and/or various chemotherapies have been used to combat painful diffuse skeletal disease, depending on the origin of the primary lesion. Pain control for focal lesions is usually attempted initially with an outpatient course of external-beam radiation. In the future we will see the development of monoclonal antibodies directed against specific tumor factors such as PTH-rP.

Outpatient external-beam radiation therapy is an important tool for the management of small, solitary, painful metastases. Outpatient treatment is preferred to help to maintain the patient's quality of life. There is debate about the optimal treatment regimen, including total dose to be given and the fractionation schedule. For the patient with multiple lesions, there also is debate about use of half-body radiation versus single-lesion therapy.

Surgical Treatment

Despite the medical therapies described previously, some patients still require further intervention. This can range from percutaneous interventional procedures, performed by radiologists, to full operative procedures, performed by orthopedic surgeons. In one reported series, 20% of breast cancer patients with metastases to the skeleton required surgery for problems related to pathologic fractures or neurologic deficits.[37] Embolization of vascular metastases (particularly renal) is a percutaneous procedure that has been performed, by radiologists, for more than 20 years. Vertebroplasty and kyphoplasty now are well-established useful procedures for treatment of painful spinal metastases. Newer interventional techniques include percutaneous radiofrequency ablation for appendicular metastases or ablation combined with vertebroplasty for some spine lesions.[38] Surgical options include a vast array of rods, nails, plates, and prosthetic implants.

What the Referring Physician Needs to Know

● Is it a metastasis or a primary bone tumor?
● How many lesions are present?
● Is there a risk of pathologic fracture?
● What is the best imaging study for staging and monitoring response to treatment?

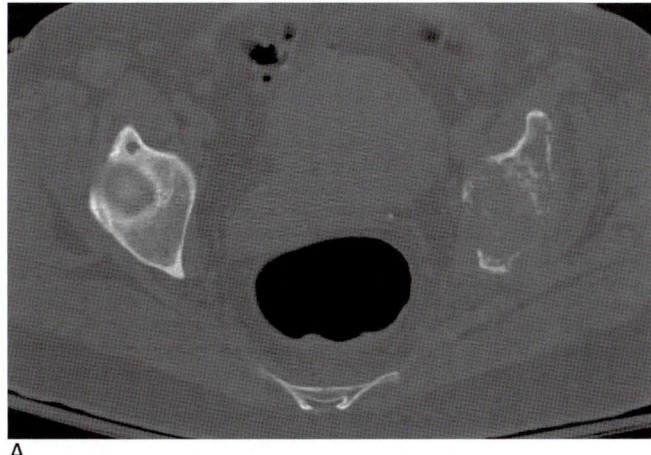
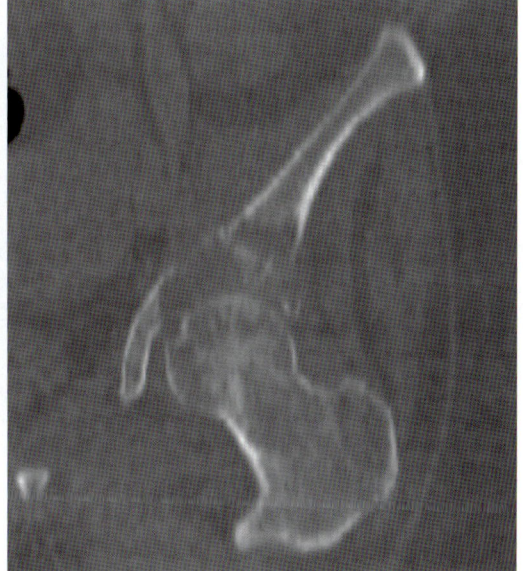

■ **FIGURE 96-35** Harrington class 3 lesion in a 61 year old woman with breast cancer. Axial (**A**) and coronal reformatted (**B**) CT scans show acetabular metastases with extensive destruction of roof, as well as medial and lateral cortices.

SUGGESTED READINGS

Avril N, Weber W. Monitoring response to treatment in patients utilizing PET. Radiol Clin North Am 2005; 43:189–204.

Fogelman I, Cook G, Israel O, Van der Wall H. Positron emission tomography and bone metastases. Semin Nucl Med 2005; 35:135–142.

Ghanem N, Uhl M, Brink I, et al. Diagnostic value of MRI in comparison to scintigraphy, PET, MS-CT and PET/CT for the detection of metastases of bone. Eur J Radiol 2005; 55:41–55.

Glockner J, White L, Sundaram M, McDonald D. Unsuspected metastases presenting as solitary soft tissue lesions: a fourteen-year review. Skeletal Radiol 2000; 29:270–274.

Koutsilieris M. Skeletal metastases in advanced prostate cancer; cell biology and therapy. Crit Rev Oncol Hematol 1995; 18:51–64.

Posteraro A, Dupuy D, Mayo-Smith W. Radiofrequency ablation of bony metastatic disease. Clin Radiol 2004; 59:803–811.

Roodman G. Mechanisms of bone metastasis. N Engl J Med 2004; 350:1655–1664.

Walls J, Bundred N, Howell A. Hypercalcemia and bone resorption in malignancy. Clin Orthop Relat Res 1995; 312:51–63.

Weber K, Lewis V, Randall R, et al. An approach to the management of the patient with metastatic bone disease. Instr Course Lect 2004; 53:663–676.

Yoneda T, Hiraga T. Crosstalk between cancer cells and bone microenvironment in bone metastasis. Biochem Biophys Res Commun 2005; 328:679–687.

REFERENCES

1. Wai P, Kuo P. The role of osteopontin in tumor metastasis. J Surg Res 2004; 121:228–241.
2. Mundy G. Metastasis to bone: causes, consequences and therapeutic opportunities. Nat Rev Cancer 2002; 2:584–593.
3. Sherry M, Greco F, Johnson D, Hainsworth J. Metastatic breast cancer confined to the skeletal system: an indolent disease. Am J Med 1986; 81:381–386.
4. Simon M, Bartucci E. The search for the primary tumor in patients with skeletal metastases of unknown origin. Cancer 1986;58:1088–1095.
5. Palmer E. Henrikson B, McKusick K, et al. Pain as an indicator of bone metastasis. Acta Radiol 1988; 29:445–449.
6. Walls J, Ratcliffe W, Howell A, Bundred J. Response to intravenous biophosphonate therapy in hypercalcemic patients with and without bone metastases: the role of parathyroid hormone-related protein. Br J Cancer 1994; 70:169–172.
7. Walls J, Bundred N, Howell A. Hypercalcemia and bone resorption in malignancy. Clin Orthop Relat Res 1995; 312:51–63.
8. Batson O. The function of the vertebral veins and their role in the spread of metastases. Ann Surg 1940; 112:138–149.
9. Kitazawa S, Maeda S. Development of skeletal metastases. Clin Orthop Relat Res 1995; 312:45–50.
10. Mohammad K, Guise T. Mechanisms of osteoblastic metastases: role of endothelin-1. Clin Orthop Relat Res 2003; 415(Suppl): S67-S74.
11. Mulligan M. Skeletal metastases, myeloma, lymphoma. In Koeller K, et al (eds). Radiologic Pathology, 3rd ed. Washington, DC, American Registry of Pathology, 2004, pp 868–874.
12. Edelstyn G, Gillespie P, Grebbell F. The radiological demonstration of osseous metastases. Clin Radiol 1967; 18:158–162.
13. Tumeh S, Beadle G, Kaplan W. Clinical significance of solitary rib lesions in patients with extraskeletal malignancy. J Nucl Med 1985; 26:1140–1143.
14. Corcoran R, Thrall J, Kyle R, et al. Solitary abnormalities in bone scans of patients with extraosseous malignancies. Radiology 1976; 121:663–667.
15. Peterson J, Kransdorf M, OConnor M. Diagnosis of occult bone metastases: positron emission tomography. Clin Orthop Relat Res 2003; 415(Suppl):S120–S128.
16. Even-Sapir E, Metser U, Mishani E, et al. The detection of bone metastases in patients with high-risk prostate cancer: 99 m Tc-MDP planar bone scintigraphy, single- and multi-field-of-view SPECT, ^{18}F-fluoride PET, and ^{18}F-fluoride PET/CT. J Nucl Med 2006; 47:287–297.
17. Chen W, Shih T, Chen R, et al. Blood perfusion of vertebral lesions evaluated with gadolinium-enhanced dynamic MRI: in comparison with compression fracture and metastasis. J Magn Reson Imaging 2002; 15:308–314.
18. Cuenod C, Laredo J, Chevret S, et al. Acute vertebral collapse due to osteoporosis or malignancy: appearance on unenhanced and gadolinium-enhanced images. Radiology 1996; 199: 541–549.
19. Ghanem N, Uhl M, Brink I, et al. Diagnostic value of MRI in comparison to scintigraphy, PET, MS-CT and PET/CT for the detection of metastases of bone. Eur J Radiol 2005; 55:41–55.
20. Laredo JD, Lakhdari K, Bellaiche L, et al. Acute vertebral collapse: CT findings in benign and malignant non-traumatic cases. Radiology 1995; 194:41–48.
21. Souques A, Lafourcade J, Terris E. Vertebre divoire dans un cas de cancer metastatique de la colonne vertebrale. Rev Neurol 1925; 32:3–10.
22. Dennis J. The solitary dense vertebral body. Radiology 1961; 77:618–621.
23. Coury C. Hippocratic fingers and hypertrophic osteoarthropathy: a study of 350 cases. Br J Dis Chest 1960; 54:202–209.
24. Mito K, Maruyama R, Uenishi Y, et al. Hypertrophic pulmonary osteoarthropathy associated with non-small cell lung cancer: demonstrated growth hormone-releasing hormone by immunohistochemical analysis. Intern Med 2001; 40:532–535.
25. Deutsch A, Resnick D, Niwayama G. Case report 145. Skeletal Radiol 1981; 6:144–148.
26. Benhamou C, Tourliere D, Brigant S, et al. Synovial metastasis of an adenocarcinoma presenting as a shoulder monoarthritis. J Rheum 1988; 15:1031–1033.
27. Tubiana-Hulin M. Incidence, prevalence, and distribution of bone metastases. Bone 1991;12(Suppl 1):S9–S10.
28. Paul G, Craig C, Banks H. Pathologic fracture from metastatic malignant melanoma. Clin Orthop Relat Res 1973; 90:255–261.
29. Phillips C, Pope T, Jones J, et al. Nontraumatic avulsion of the lesser trochanter a pathognomonic sign of metastatic disease? Skeletal Radiol 1988; 17:106–110.
30. Ries T. Detection of osteoporotic sacral fractures with radionuclides. Radiology 1983; 146:783–785.
31. Gainor B, Buchert P. Fracture healing in metastatic bone disease. Clin Orthop Relat Res 1983; 178:297–302.
32. Bouma W, Mulder J, Hop W. The influence of intramedullary nailing upon the development of metastases in the treatment of an impending pathological fracture: an experimental study. Clin Exp Metastasis 1983; 1:205–212.
33. Bealis R, Lawton G, Snell W. Prophylactic internal fixation of the femur in metastatic breast cancer. Cancer 1971; 28:1350–1354.

34. Mirels H. Metastatic disease in long bones: a proposed scoring system for diagnosing impending pathologic fractures. Clin Orthop Relat Res 1989; 249:256-264.
35. Harrington K. The management of acetabular insufficiency secondary to metastatic malignant disease. J Bone Joint Surg Am 1981; 63:653-664.
36. Fayad L, Kamel I, Kawamoto S, et al. Distinguishing stress fractures from pathologic fractures: a multimodality approach. Skeletal Radiol 2005; 34:245-259.
37. Wedin R, Bauer H, Rutqvist L. Surgical treatment for skeletal breast cancer metastases. Cancer 2001; 92:257-262.
38. Posteraro A, Dupuy D, Mayo-Smith W. Radiofrequency ablation of bony metastatic disease. Clin Radiol 2004; 59:803-811.

97

Treatment Strategies for Musculoskeletal Tumors and Tumor-like Lesions

Davide Donati

Surgical treatment of a patient with a musculoskeletal tumor is aimed against the disease but often also affects functional ability of the patient for the rest of his or her life. Disability related to treatment can be minimal in small, benign tumors located in the extremities, or it can be devastating after surgical treatment of axial malignant tumors. The outcome is in many ways uncertain. The result of treatment can be unexpected owing to tumor aggressiveness and/or surgical or medical complications. A correct approach to treatment depends on two main aspects: knowledge of the patient's functional expectations and the exact diagnosis.

FUNCTIONALITY

After tumor resection, the choice of the best musculoskeletal reconstruction depends on the patient's current life style and future expectations. Gender, age, condition, functional needs of work, and recreational activity are the most important issues to consider when making the final decision. Patients with knee fusion are known to dislike this functional limitation during daily life activity, such as driving a car or sitting in narrow spaces. However, the same reconstruction can allow the patient's recreational activity, such as playing tennis or volleyball, without the risk of damaging the reconstruction. On the other hand, a perfect working knee, achieved with a modular prosthesis, cannot be used for various recreational activities, whereas it is very much appreciated for activities of daily living. Young patients usually have more demanding functional needs. In younger patients the type of reconstruction also needs to last for a longer life time.

DIAGNOSIS

The diagnostic process starts from the first contact between patient and doctor in the outpatient clinic. Key elements are determined by medical history, physical examination, laboratory tests, and imaging. However, it is the biopsy that gives the final confirmation of the suspected diagnosis.

It is important to note that the hypothesis starts from the first suggestion by the patient while describing the symptoms and then additional elements can support or change the initial assumption. The final diagnosis depends on the correlation of all the elements. None of these elements should be underestimated; otherwise, a diagnostic error may be the result.

Patient History

The interview is the first step. It is important to differentiate symptoms and events that are related to the tumor from those that are not. Similar occurrences in parents and relatives, previous events, initial pain and its course, changes in daily life activity, and tenderness and numbness can be important for the diagnosis.

Physical Examination

Presence of a mass is one of the most important signs. Pain, mobility of the mass, and superficial versus deep location are the three most important parameters. The range of motion of the joints close to the tumor and the vascular and neurologic integrity of the extremity are to be carefully evaluated. Pain and large volume of an extraosseous mass are not always indicative of malignancy (Fig. 97-1).

KEY POINTS

- Because symptoms are often not specific, and concomitant trauma also tends to hide the real cause of pain, a high level of suspicion is needed.
- Biopsy, in combination with imaging and other signs and symptoms, is frequently the only way to make the diagnosis.
- Biopsy is a simple surgical procedure, but it is better performed by the treating surgeon or radiologist, who are part of the multidisciplinary team.
- In benign and low-grade sarcoma, surgery is the only cure, whereas in high-grade sarcoma (neo)-adjuvant therapies are used in combination with surgical treatment.
- For the cure of bone and soft tissue sarcoma it is better to refer the patient to a center with the availability of specialized pathology, radiology, oncology, and orthopedic surgery services.
- In the presence of limb pain, which continues for 5 to 6 days despite anti-inflammatory drugs, additional analysis with radiographs and, if negative, ultrasonography is needed.
- In areas of bone remodeling or soft tissue swelling a needle biopsy should be considered; this can be performed by the orthopedic oncologist or radiologist skilled in invasive techniques.
- Staging is part of an integrated multidisciplinary process that should be done in the center that is going to treat the patient.
- Biopsy samples should be analyzed by pathologists with experience in musculoskeletal oncology.
- Do not underestimate symptoms or attribute them to minor trauma, especially in young patients: musculoskeletal tumors are rare but can be fatal. A radiograph or ultrasound study can obviate most surprises.
- Do not perform an incisional biopsy when the patient is not going to be treated in this hospital.
- Do not remove the "nodule" from the soft tissues under local anesthetic when unsure whether the lesion is benign.
- Do not drain the hematoma in an elderly adult patient without making sure a consistent trauma has occurred.
- Do not make all diagnoses based on radiologic results only but only with specific exceptions that can be identified by specialized radiologists; diagnosis is based on multidisciplinary cooperation and biopsy is part of this process.

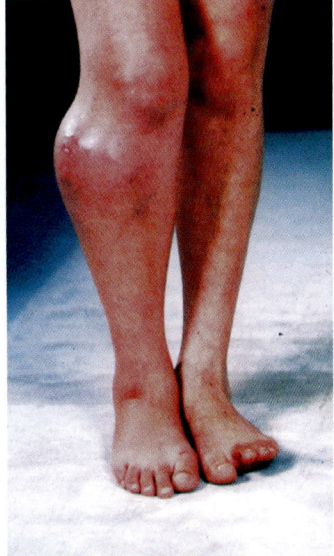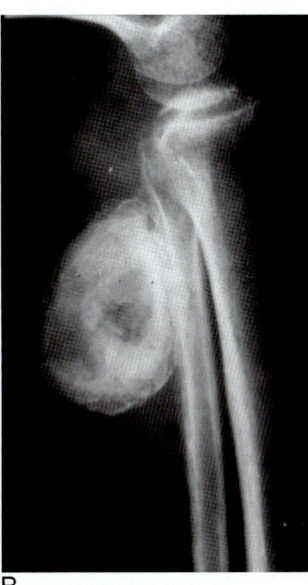

A   B

■ FIGURE 97-1 **A,** Painful enlarging mass in the lateral gastrocnemius muscle in a 23-year-old woman. Marked swelling, tenderness, and thinning of the skin were found. **B,** Lateral radiograph shows the ossified mass diagnosed as myositis ossificans. An open biopsy confirmed the diagnosis.

Laboratory Tests

Sometimes laboratory tests are performed at the first examination. Although increased alkaline phosphatase may be seen in association with osteolysis, the absence of specific markers limits the contribution of laboratory tests.

Imaging

Imaging contributes to the diagnosis and is important in staging and thus planning the surgical approach.

Radiographs are usually the first test and are important in making a diagnosis. When of poor quality,[1] or if poorly centered, or if not recent enough, mistakes are easily made.[2,3]

Bone scintigraphy is still needed in primary and secondary malignant bone tumors to identify multifocality. Its use in patients with soft tissue tumors is questionable because they very rarely present with bone metastases. Nowadays, single photon emission CT (SPECT) can be considered as an additional improvement in some cases whereas positron emission tomography (PET) is still not reliable in intermediate malignant bone tumors. PET has been demonstrated to be reliable in the detection of recurrence of aggressive malignant bone and soft tissue tumors.

CT is still valuable in demonstrating osseous morphology in 2D and 3D reconstructions. CT may also reveal highly vascularized soft tissue lesions. Angio-CT is able to show vascular structures in great detail.

MRI has largely replaced CT in tumor imaging. Its specificity and, most of all, sensitivity make this examination the first to be applied in defining the local extent of a neoplastic lesion. Technical improvements have enabled the surgeon to recognize the exact extension of musculoskeletal tumors. MRI is the primary tool in visualizing osseous and soft tissue tumors, including satellite nodules, in relation to surrounding structures such as adjacent neurovascular bundles, and joints. Sequential MRI examinations can be performed to evaluate the effect of (neo)-adjuvant therapy, such as arterial embolization, radiotherapy, and chemotherapy. Finally, MRI is now routinely used for the detection of local recurrence during follow-up.

The role of ultrasonography in orthopedic oncology is limited, mainly because of the use of MRI. There remains, however, a place for ultrasound imaging (see later).

Biopsy

In the majority of cases, a biopsy is essential in making a correct diagnosis. Biopsy is a critical procedure due to potential local, or distant, spread of tumor cells. It can be done with a needle or by open surgery. In both cases strict rules have to be honored. When biopsy is planned, surgical treatment options should also be considered. This is important because when the tumor is resected the surgical incision and approach need to allow resection not only of the tumor but also of all contaminated tissue.[4,5] The biopsy tract and wound, including hemorrhage, are considered to be contaminated. Usually, a vertically oriented wound scar is easier to resect than a horizontal one.

Chances of hematoma developing should be minimized, because hematoma will be the most likely carrier of tumor cells to the surrounding tissues. If bleeding is difficult to control during surgery, leaving a wound drain is suggested to avoid cell diffusion.

Concerning the deeper part of the biopsy approach, particular care has to be taken not to invade the joint or fat surrounding a neurovascular bundle. Passage through muscle is preferred because this route does not involve the major nerves and vessels. Muscle can be excised when the tumor is resected (Fig. 97-2). If violated, structures such as nerves and vessels will have to be resected together with the tumor, resulting in severe morbidity and loss of function (Fig. 97-3).

When a tumor is located close to a joint, the risk of cell dispersion can be minimized by selecting a route through the bone, similar to the procedures in the vertebral pedicle or neck of the femur.

Finally, it is very important to obtain a diagnostic specimen. Because of the small wound and sometimes profuse bleeding of tumor, there is the risk of not harvesting enough tissue or of harvesting tissue that is not representative of the tumor. We have to differentiate viable tumor from surrounding reactive soft tissue as well as necrotic tissue (Fig. 97-4).

PRINCIPLES OF TREATMENT

Treatment consists mainly of surgery with or without additional therapy. Benign tumors are nearly always treated with surgery only, whereas malignant and metastatic tumors are often treated in combination with adjuvant (after surgery) or neoadjuvant (before surgery) therapy. Image-guided focal ablation of lesions is discussed elsewhere in this book. Neoadjuvant and adjuvant therapy can be applied to reduce or destroy the primary tumor and/or metastases or in the case of neoadjuvant therapy to provide an easier approach for surgery. The choice of therapy is mainly based on the type and grade of tumor. In a great number of patients with metastatic disease, the treatment is not intended to be curative but palliative. In this section we address the concept of compartments and staging in relation to the principles of achieving systemic and local control.

Staging and Compartments

In the early 1980s Enneking revised the TNM staging classification by giving clearer criteria for a surgical staging system in musculoskeletal tumors (Table 97-1).[6] There are two types of criteria in the system: tumor grading and local staging. Tumor grading is based on histologic analysis. Local staging, meaning determination of local extension, is based on radiology.

Because tumors of mesenchymal origin have the tendency to invade rather than infiltrate, as carcinomas do, the concept of compartments and their margins is important. A compartment is an anatomically defined space. A tumor growing inside the medullary canal without penetrating the cortex is, by definition, intracompartmental (Fig. 97-5). The cortex acts as a barrier.

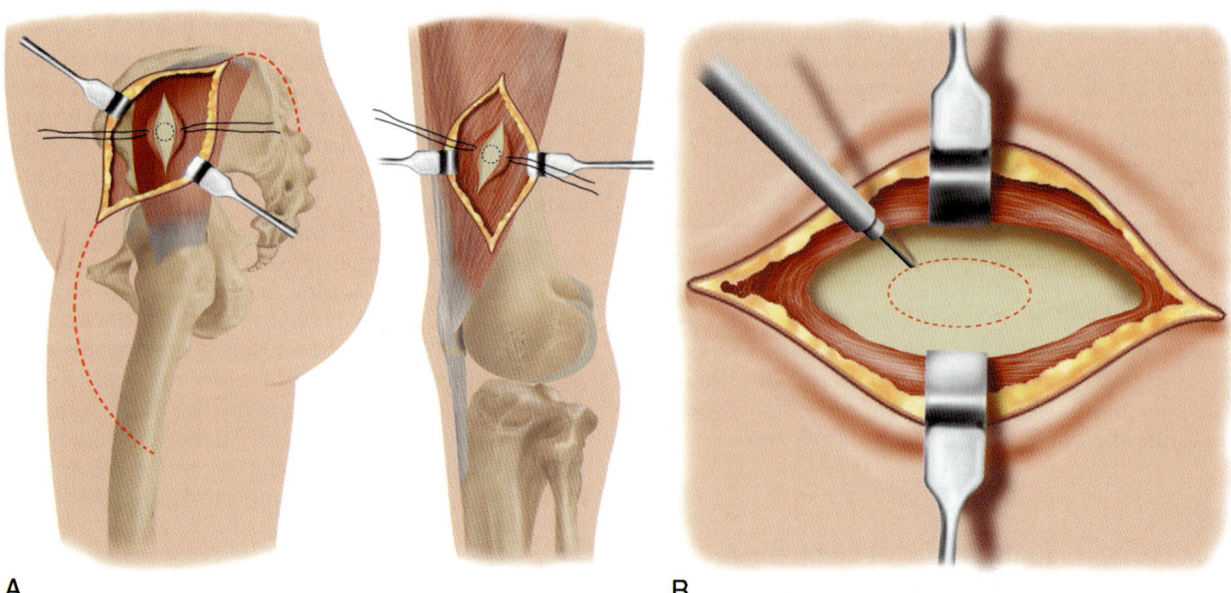

A   B

■ **FIGURE 97-2** Drawings illustrating two examples of the correct approach of an open biopsy. **A,** The skin incision has to follow the definitive surgical approach of final surgery, because the biopsy scar needs to be excised with all contaminated soft tissue. **B,** The deep tract will be through a muscle to avoid major vessel contamination and to achieve easier control of the hematoma.

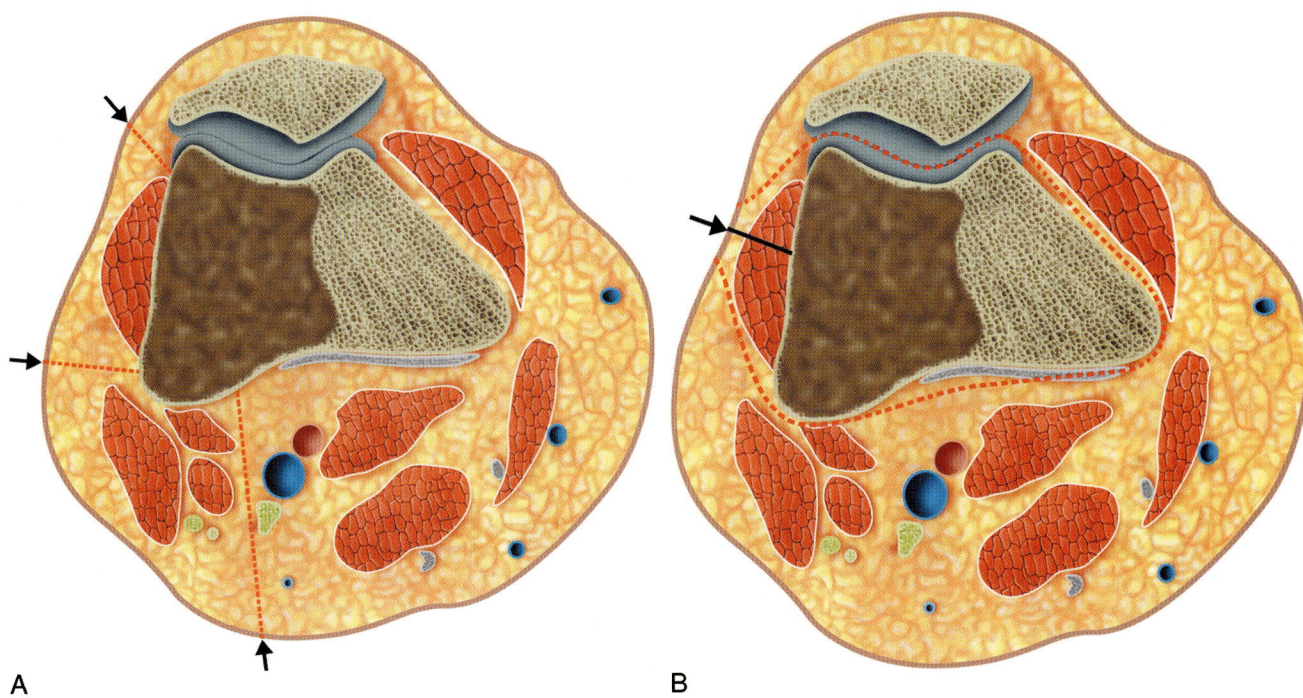

A

B

■ **FIGURE 97-3** **A,** Wrong biopsy approach. These three projected routes (*arrows*) contaminate critical structures. **B,** The correct biopsy tract (*arrow*) should pass through a muscle, avoiding contaminating the joint and soft tissue around the neurovascular bundle.

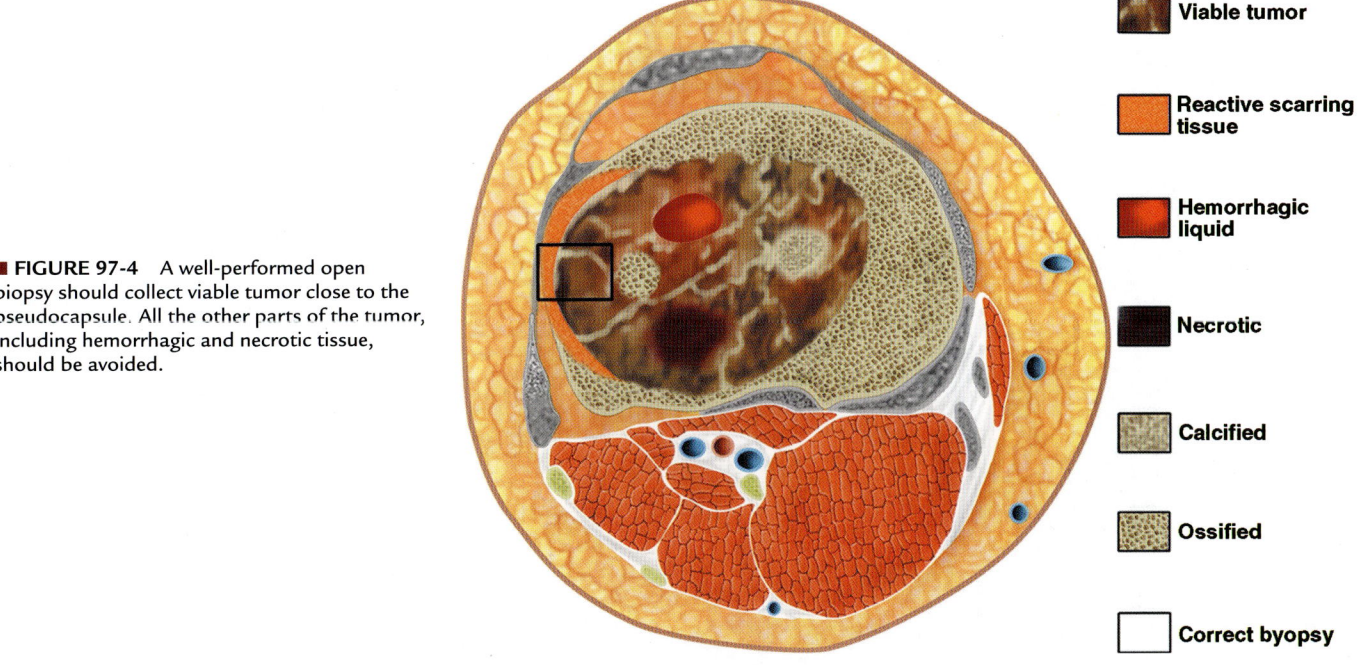

■ **FIGURE 97-4** A well-performed open biopsy should collect viable tumor close to the pseudocapsule. All the other parts of the tumor, including hemorrhagic and necrotic tissue, should be avoided.

Viable tumor

Reactive scarring tissue

Hemorrhagic liquid

Necrotic

Calcified

Ossified

Correct byopsy

It is important to realize what kinds of tissues can be strong enough to contain tumor. Both benign aggressive and malignant tumors develop over time the capability to destroy the natural compartmental barriers and break out into the next compartment. Tumors can be confined inside the pseudocapsule, as in benign bone tumors; however, the more malignant in grade, the easier the tumor can invade adjacent space, thus overcoming the usual anatomic barrier. At the same time, high-grade malignant tumors have the ability to produce tumor satellites and skip metastasis. Some structures are certainly more resistant than others. Fascia, septa, and capsule, among soft tissues, can contain the tumor for a long time.[7] When the tumor reaches these anatomic barriers it tends to proceed by growing in less-resistant directions.

TABLE 97-1 Surgical Staging System for Musculoskeletal Malignant Tumors

Stage	Grade*	Tumor Extension†	Metastasis‡
IA	1	1	0
IB	1	2	0
IIA	2	1	0
IIB	2	2	0
III	Any	Any	1

*Histologic grade: 1, low grade; 2, high grade.
†Tumor extension: 1, intracompartmental; 2, extracompartmental.
‡Presence of metastasis: 0, no; 1, yes.

We can define compartmental anatomy with general and specific distribution in upper and lower limbs as well as the pelvis.[8] In general, if a tumor is confined inside a bone, a muscle, or joint we can consider it as intracompartmental. On the other hand, throughout the body there are spaces with indefinite anatomic margins, such as the head and neck, paraspinal and paraclavicular tissue, axilla, antecubital and popliteal fossae, as well as the groin, ankle, and dorsa of foot and hand. Specific compartments in the upper limb can be considered: periscapular tissue, anterior or posterior upper arm, dorsal or volar forearm, and palmar hand.[8] In the lower limb compartments include the anterior, posterior and medial thigh; anterior, posterior, deep posterior and lateral lower leg; and plantar tissue of the foot.[8] Recognizing these anatomic compartments is very important in planning and executing biopsy and resection of tumor with all the potentially contaminated tissues. However, this general outline of the major compartments in the body is usually insufficient in the individual patient. In each individual patient the treatment options are based on all available clinical, histologic, and radiologic information. Finally, the experience of the surgeon also plays an important role in choosing the optimal therapy.

Ideally, resection of the entire compartment is preferred to be sure to eradicate the tumor. However, the vast majority of high-grade malignant tumors are extracompartmental as they cross from one compartment to another. In this case the safest surgical procedure will be the excision of both compartments. This type of surgery is defined as radical and often necessitates amputation. Because the use of (neo)-adjuvant therapy can help control cell diffusion, a less aggressive surgical procedure is acceptable; this is called a wide resection. In this case the surgeon removes the tumor as well as the pseudocapsule with a consistent layer of surrounding healthy tissue in order to include tumor satellites in the resected tissues. All other types of surgery (marginal, intralesional) are not suitable for malignant bone and soft tissue tumors (Fig. 97-6).

We also have to recognize areas without consistent barriers where the tumor can easily extend. These are the biopsy tract, bone marrow, fat surrounding the neurovascular bundles, and small veins around the tumor (tumor thrombi). In addition, it is difficult to detect tumor extending into these areas at an early stage. When tumor is suspected to extend to these sites more aggressive surgery in combination with local (neo)-adjuvant therapy is suggested.

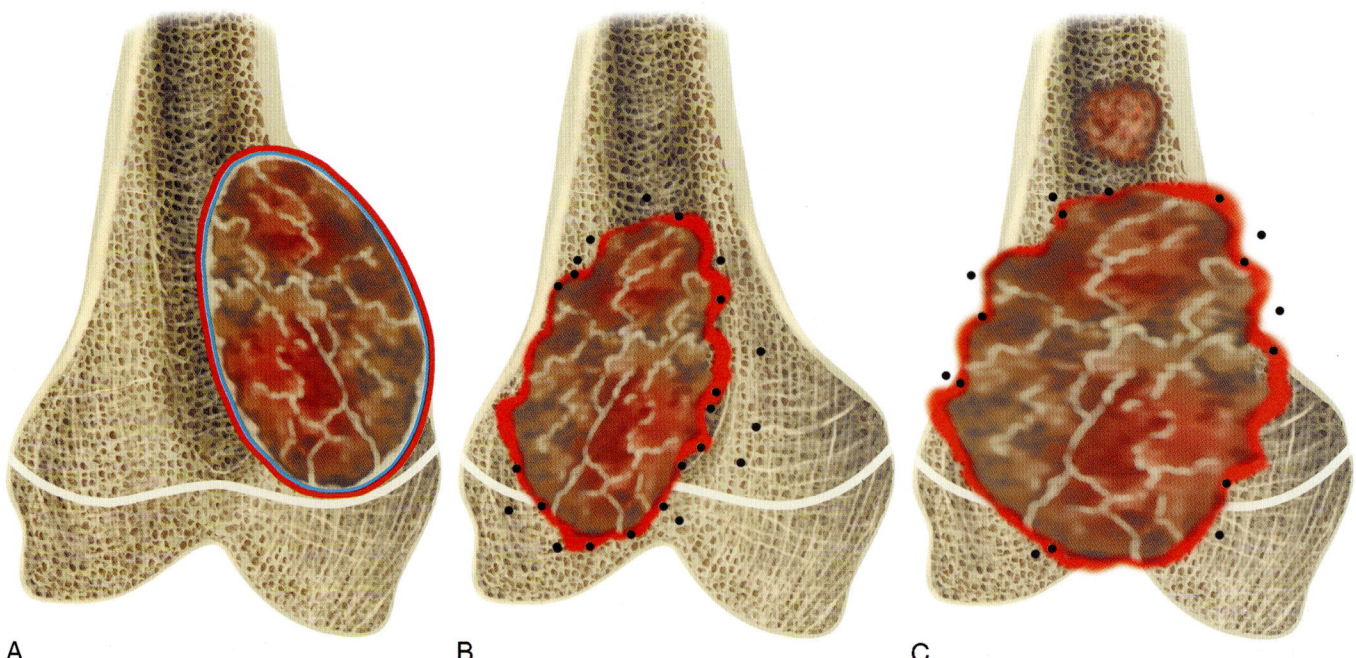

A   B   C

■ **FIGURE 97-5** Schematic drawing of different bone tumor manifestations. **A,** Benign bone tumor is classified as active; the tumor expands to the metaphyseal cortex without passing through it. The reactive bone (*internal blue line*) and pseudocapsule (*external red line*) are regular and intact and are successful in containing the tumor. **B,** Malignant bone tumor is confined to the osseous compartment (intracompartmental). Its malignant behavior is represented by the production of satellites (*black dots*) located outside the pseudocapsule that is irregular and uneven. **C,** Extracompartmental malignant bone tumors are still able to produce local satellites but also skip metastases, as represented in the proximal part of the medullary canal.

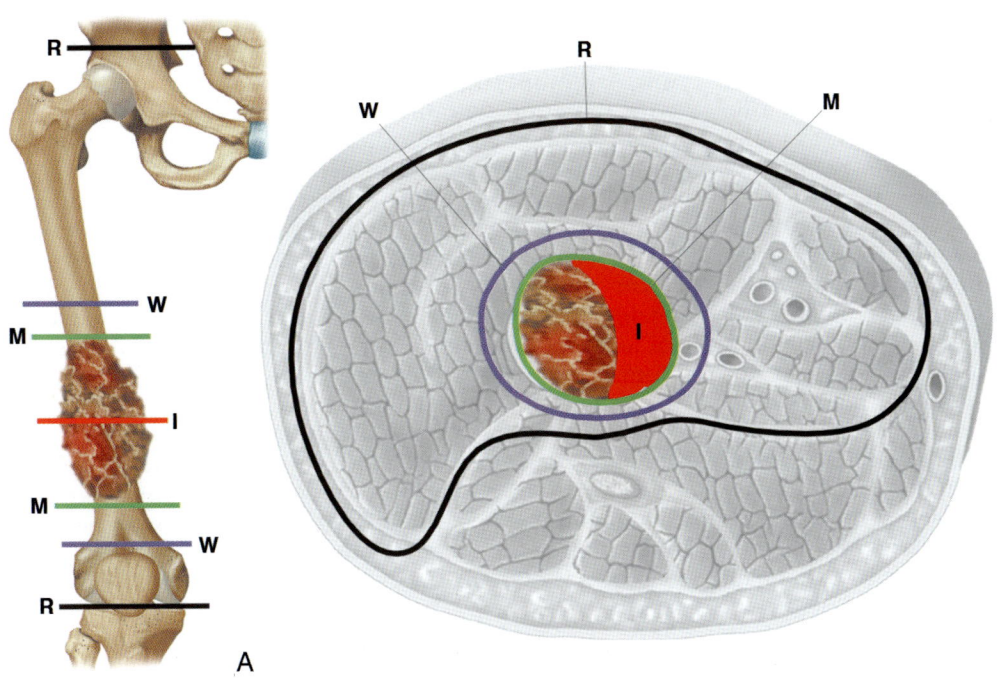

A

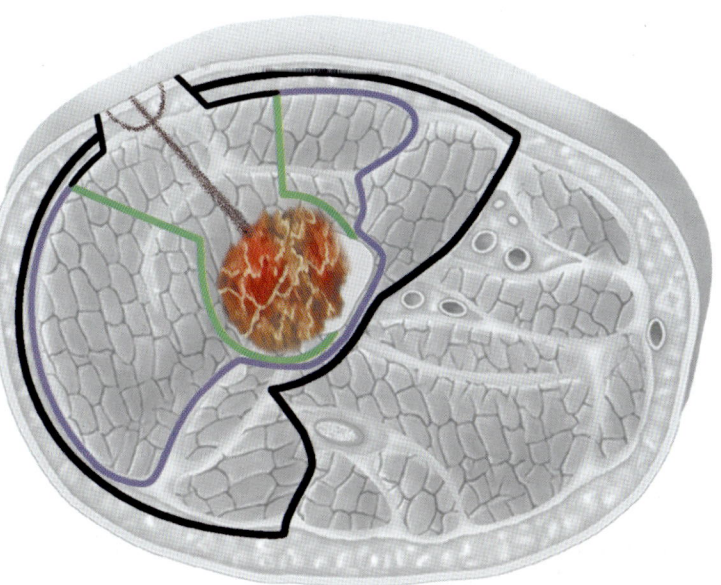

B

■ **FIGURE 97-6** Drawing of the type of margins used in bone and soft tissue tumor surgery. **A,** When the excision passes through the tumor the margin is called intralesional (I); if the cutting edge is close to the tumor it is called marginal (M). Both types of margins are considered inadequate in resection of malignant bone tumors. Adequate margins are achieved when a part of healthy tissue is excised all around the tumor. The margin may be wide (W) or radical (R). In a radical procedure the entire compartment containing the tumor is resected. **D,** In malignant tumors, as a rule, biopsy-contaminated tissues have to be excised to reduce the risk of local recurrence.

Systemic Control

Systemic control of sarcoma is mainly dependent on the efficacy of (neo)-adjuvant therapy. Local control, depending mainly on surgical treatment, also is important in achieving systemic control, because local recurrence is often associated with the onset of systemic illness. Major orthopedic referral institutes report a 5% local recurrence rate in high-grade malignant tumors.[9] Due to the natural local aggressiveness of malignant bone and soft tissue tumors, it seems to be impossible to reduce this rate.[10]

The occurrence of pulmonary metastasis is a treatable event. In recent studies we demonstrated no difference in survival chances between patients with an event-free course and patients who develop one to two nodules in the same lung 3 years after the initial diagnosis.[11] The role

of pulmonary surgery has become more important in the treatment of these patients. It provides, in combination with aggressive chemotherapy, significantly higher chances of survival. Prognosis is less favorable when osseous metastases are detected. Osseous metastases occur typically together with pulmonary metastases in patients with local recurrence. Still, when one or two osseous metastases are detected without metastases at other sites we resect the osseous lesions.

Local Control

Surgery

In our institution more than 90% of patients with high-grade malignant tumor in the extremities are surgically treated with limb salvage. Diagnostic imaging, systemic tumor control, orthopedic internal devices, and biologic means of reconstruction (graft and transplant) enable the surgeon to perform extensive reconstructions after major bone and soft tissue resection. However, as malignant tumors increase in size they are able to produce local invasion that eludes the imaging techniques. Local extension into small veins and lymphatic vessels not visible on MRI is more likely to occur when the mass is bigger. This is especially true when the tumor originates or extends in ill-defined anatomic regions such as the axial skeleton, the pelvis, the groin, and the popliteal fossa. In these cases various structures often need to be excised and sometimes functional reconstruction is not possible. We can substitute a number of structures, such as bone, joint, and vessels, but muscle and major nerves are still irreplaceable. On the other hand if the tumor clearly invades the pelvic area as well as the spine there is very little chance, even after mutilating procedures such as hindquarter amputation, of an oncologically adequate procedure aimed at cure.

Based on the just-described information obtained from clinical analysis, imaging, histology, biologic behavior, and treatment options, the surgeon is still faced with a difficult decision. What is a good balance between safety and functional and cosmetic outcome? How much tissue has to be excised to be wide enough? In malignant bone tumors a wide resection has to include Codman's triangle along with at least 2 cm of bone from beyond the intramedullary tumor margin. Rules for soft tissue extension are more difficult to define. A tumor may, for instance, touch the neurovascular bundle without enwrapping it (Fig.

97-7). How much healthy tissue remains between tumor and vessels? How much is enough? Once again the use of (neo)adjuvant therapy is critical to allow an oncologically safe resection without sacrificing an excessive number of structures. On the other hand, safety is our primary concern. We first need to determine the most adequate oncologic solution; limb salvage is a secondary concern. Only amputation can give the ultimate assurance against local recurrence. Should we go back to the past and perform amputation in all the patients with a high-grade malignant tumor? As stated earlier the usual percentage of local recurrence is 5% to 10% in high-grade bone sarcomas, whereas it is 5% to 20% in soft tissue sarcomas.[12] Patients are informed about these figures as well as the possibility to have a potentially safer procedure with an amputation. However, in recent studies the percentage of long-term survival between amputees and limb-salvaged patients was not statistically different. Even without local recurrence the general prognosis in musculoskeletal sarcoma is 60% to 70% disease-free survival at 5 years.

(Neo)-adjuvant Therapies

The local effect of (neo)-adjuvant therapies is usually a shrinkage of the tumor extension detectable with CT or MRI. It is important to stress that any application of local (neo)-adjuvant therapy always produces definite damage to the surrounding bone and soft tissues. The use of combination therapies such as chemotherapy and radiotherapy produces more extensive damage. It is important to take this into account in the evaluation of the patient's ability to recover from surgery.

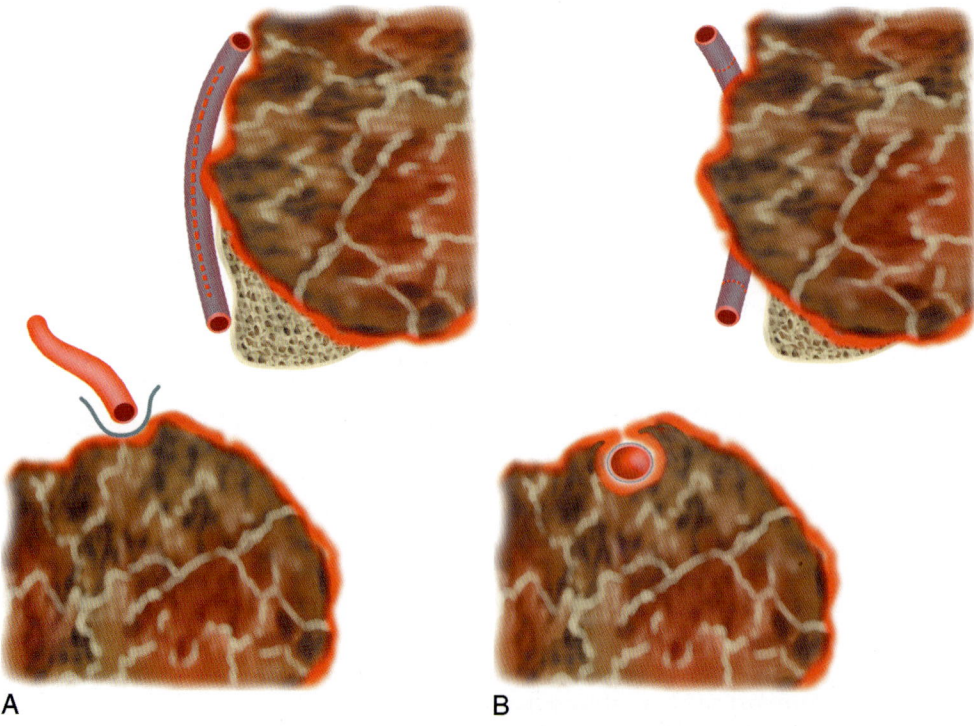

A   B

■ **FIGURE 97-7**   Drawing of involvement of vessels by the tumor. **A,** The tumor is in contact with the vessels; in this case the external sheath of the artery is considered to be an adequate barrier to the tumor invasion. **B,** If the malignant tumor enwraps the artery, this is an indication to excise and replace it.

Antiblastic Chemotherapy

The local effect of antiblastic chemotherapy is related to the aggressiveness of the tumor. The faster the tumor grows, the more effective the antiblastic effect is in terms of tumor necrosis. Round cell tumors such as Ewing's sarcoma are known to have a marked response to the antiblastic chemotherapy; spindle cell sarcomas, on the other hand, are less responsive. The use of preoperative antiblastic chemotherapy has been the rule for the past 20 years, although oncologists are now discussing this principle. There is concern about delaying the resection. Typically, neoadjuvant chemotherapy takes more than 3 months. This is considered too long when chemotherapy is not effective enough. The risk of having systemic diffusion of cells in nonresponsive patients during this time can be unacceptable. However, even if the tumor is not responding, usually the surgeon has an operating field that has less edema (Fig. 97-8) as well as a better healing of the biopsy region. When resection is performed soon after biopsy, the biopsy-produced hematoma is very difficult to excise.

Isolating Limb Perfusion

This is a technique using local antiblastic chemotherapy through the cannulation of the main artery and vein of the limb. An extracorporeal circulation is created to enhance the dose of chemotherapy only in the desired anatomic district. This is usually applied in very large tumors with the hope of achieving a marked reduction in tumor volume, thus giving the opportunity to change the indication from an amputation to a limb salvage resection. There are two major problems: the first is that there is no systemic delivery and therefore no systemic treatment; and the second is marked soft tissue damage in the perfused limb. The second disadvantage is usually related to a high number of local complications mostly related to failure of wound closure.

Radiation Therapy

Radiation therapy has now gained importance in the treatment of musculoskeletal malignant tumors. The relative ease of application in combination with its effectiveness makes radiotherapy an important tool for local tumor control. It seems to be more effective in residual tumors (postoperative application) and in superficially located tumors away from the nervous system, such as in the gastrointestinal tract, urinary bladder, and lungs. It is routinely applied in high-grade soft tissue sarcoma as preoperative treatment with the same aims described for chemotherapy in malignant bone tumors. There are several techniques of application: external-beam therapy combined, or not, with interstitial therapy or intraoperative radiation treatment (IORT). The intraoperative radiation treatment applied to the surgical field before closing the wound has the advantage of hitting directly the contaminated tissues without compromising the adjacent healthy tissues, but this application needs an expensive facility rarely present in clinical settings.

Proton beam therapy allows better targeting of the tumor without compromising adjacent healthy soft tissues and bone.

Arterial Embolization

This technique is used mainly in well-vascularized lesions and in difficult operative regions, such as the pelvis and spine. It has two advantages: increase of tumor cell necrosis and reduction of bleeding during surgery. This treatment is often applied the day before surgery, because a larger

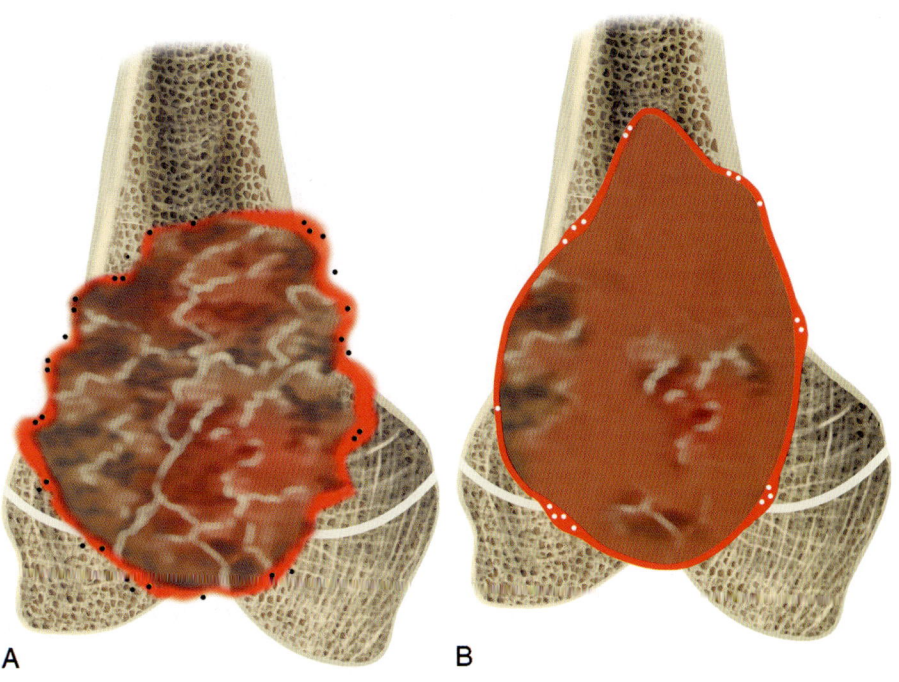

■ **FIGURE 97-8** **A,** Drawing of the margin of a high-grade malignant tumor located in the distal femur before antiblastic chemotherapy showing an irregular margin in red with microscopic tumor foci (*black dots*) within and beyond the pseudocapsule. **B,** The same tumor after preoperative chemotherapy exhibits a well-defined tumor pseudocapsule of adjacent reactive soft tissues including the tumor satellites.

A   B

time interval will allow revascularization of tumor. In metastatic tumors arterial embolization is often combined with radiation therapy. These two methods of local tumor control are the main tools for curing these lesions. Local ablation of tumors is discussed elsewhere in this book.

Surgical Treatment

The orthopedic surgeon has to face two major issues—how to eradicate the tumor while maintaining as much function as possible.

Benign Bone and Soft Tissue Tumors

Benign bone tumors are frequently present in young patients and can present in a variety of ways from a small lytic lesion located in the epiphysis of a long bone to a large metaphyseal tumor presenting as a pathologic fracture and bleeding, thereby contaminating adjacent soft tissues. In any event the majority of benign bone tumors occur very close to a joint. Therefore, two issues are important: what is the best surgical approach and how to preserve the joint (Fig. 97-9).

The standard surgical treatment for benign bone tumors is intralesional curettage. This type of surgery has the major advantage of greatly limiting intraoperative and secondary reconstructive complications. Bone mechanical stability is widely preserved; therefore, reconstruction consists of filling the defect instead of providing mechanical support (Fig. 97-10).

Usually only one surgical procedure is needed to heal the lesion and the final functional outcome is close to normal. Local recurrence can occur in the first 3 follow-up years in 8% to 30% of cases. When local recurrence occurs near the cement in bone, it is not necessary to resect the joint; a new curettage can heal the new lesion (Fig. 97-11).

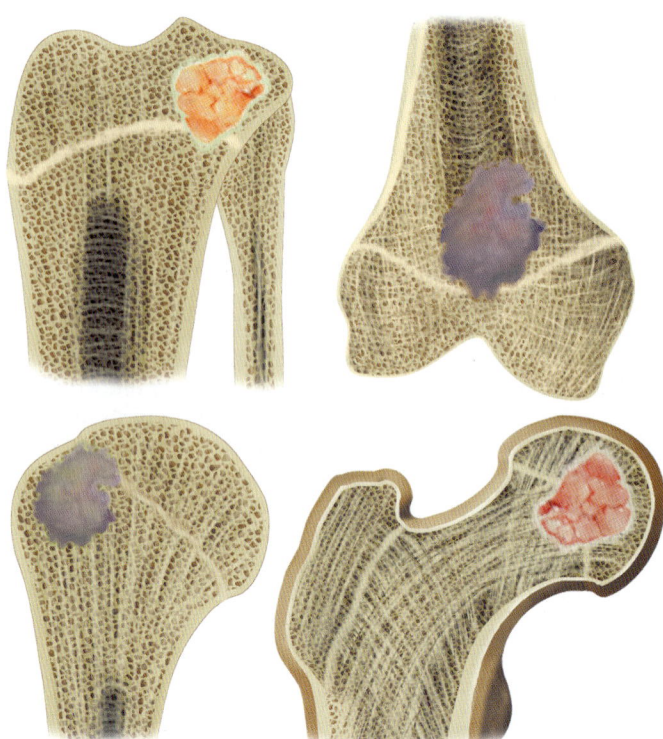

■ **FIGURE 97-9** The usual locations of a chondroblastoma in the intra-articular part of the epiphysis. The surgical approach needs to take into consideration the possibility of easy curettage as well as avoiding damage to the epiphysis vascular supply.

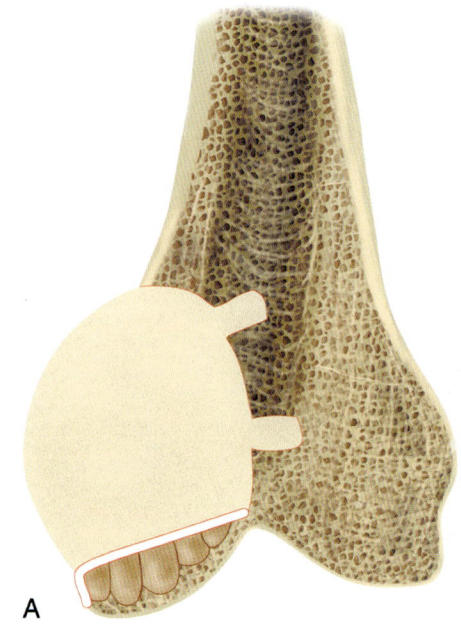

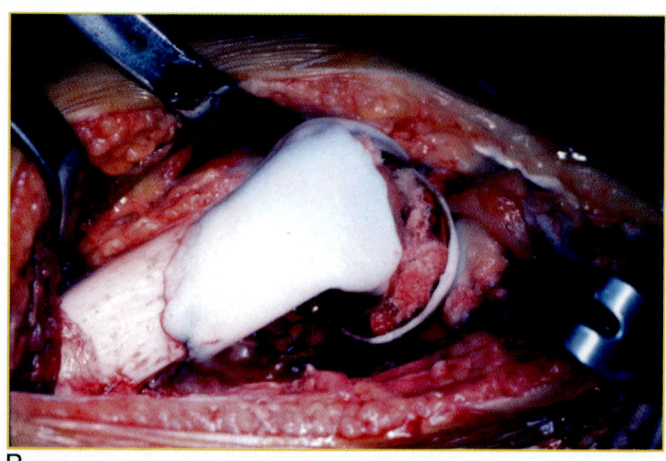

■ **FIGURE 97-10** Drawing (**A**) and operative photograph (**B**) of bone filling after an extensive curettage of the medial condyle of the distal femur for a giant cell tumor. The subchondral bone has been supplemented by autograft cancellous bone, whereas the majority of the cavity has been filled with bone cement.

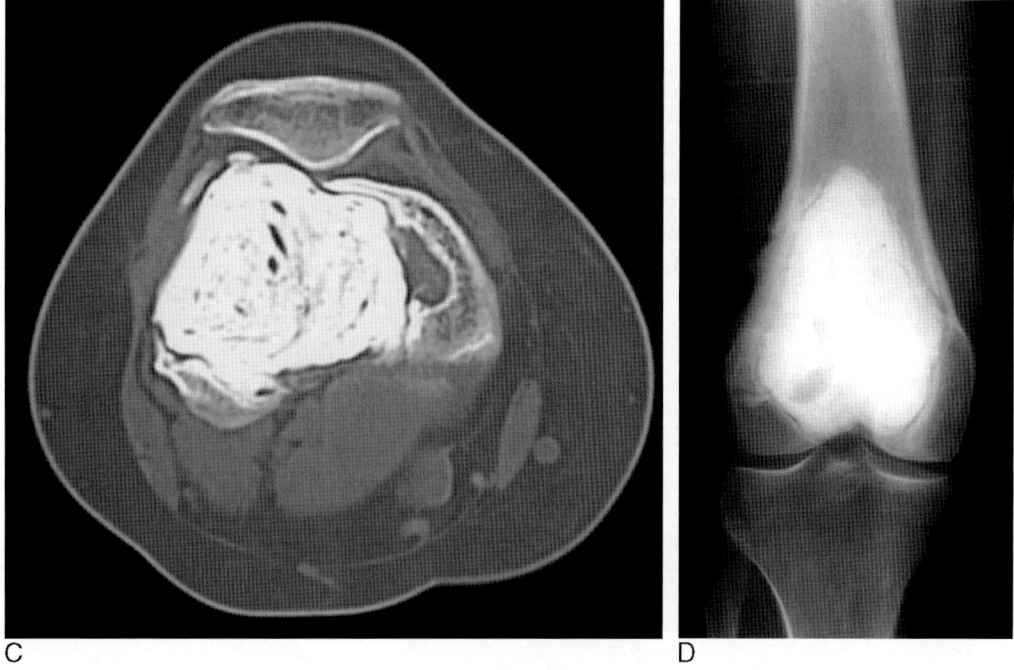

■ **FIGURE 97-11** **A,** Anteroposterior radiograph of extensive intralesional curettage of a giant cell tumor of the distal femur filled with cement only. Eighteen months later a local recurrence on the medial site, seen as a lucency, is easily detected on radiography (**B**) and CT (**C**). **D,** Radiograph shows results of the same case after new curettage of the local recurrence and again cement filling.

However, in the presence of an articular fracture, intra-articular recurrence or marked bone loss, a resection, and articular reconstruction is strongly advised.[13]

Despite creating a large osseous window, and the use of a high speed bur, intralesional surgery by definition can leave remnants of tumor cells in the surgical area, causing a local recurrence. The use of local adjuvants, such as phenol, liquid nitrogen, and methylmethacrylate thermal reaction, can cause necrosis on the surrounding cells, thus reducing the occurrence of a local recurrence. Radiation therapy is, because of the risk of second-ary radioinduced malignancy, not suggested in benign tumors. However, in axial tumors, where the compart-ment barriers are less clear and a recurrence could be very difficult to eradicate, adjuvant radiotherapy is sometimes applied.

Benign tumors in the soft tissues are often easy to eradi-cate, they do not need adjuvant therapy, damage to sur-rounding tissue does not occur, and no reconstruction is needed. Unfortunately, a low-grade malignant tumor is easily misdiagnosed as a benign one. Hence, a tentative wide exci-sion is usually suggested. Lipoma is an exception because it is a frequently encountered superficial tumor that is easily resected. Local recurrence is very rare (Fig. 97-12).

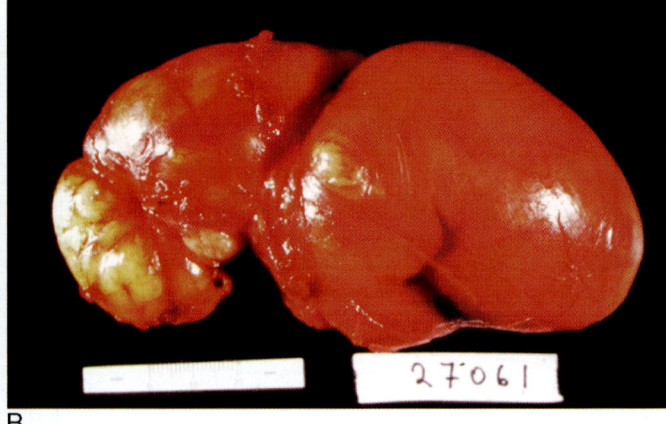

■ **FIGURE 97-12** Large lipoma of the posterior compartment of the thigh. **A,** The usual aspect on CT scan characterized by density equal to the subcutaneous fat and interdigitation among the surrounding muscles. **B,** Gross appearance of the tumor after excision: a thin layer of fibrous tissue usually covers the bulky structure of the multilobulated mass.

Malignant Bone and Soft Tissue Tumor

Musculoskeletal sarcomas are, in contrast to, for instance, multiple myeloma, focal lesions. In low-grade sarcoma antiblastic therapy is usually not effective and is therefore not added to the surgical procedure. The surgical resection should, in contrast to the treatment of benign lesions, at least be wide. In this type of tumor a local recurrence can threaten the patient's life because distant metastases are more likely to occur in recurrent cases. Normally, the reconstruction technique is the same as it is for a high-grade malignant tumor. The only difference is that reconstructions are in general easier because the resections are less extensive than in high-grade sarcomas. High-grade malignant tumors are, because of their potential to metastasize, also treated with chemotherapy and/or radiation therapy. In soft tissue sarcoma, preoperative radiation therapy is still widely used to control the local extension of the tumor satellites better. The reasonable combination of the two adjuvant therapies allows the surgeon to excise the tumor much closer to the pseudo-capsule, thus avoiding the sacrifice of important adjacent structures, such as bone, nerve, and vessels (Fig. 97-13).

Bone Metastases

Bone metastases occur in at least 35% of carcinomas. Sometimes they are evident at the first presentation; others occur later during follow-up. Bone metastases are quite often referred to the orthopedic surgeon with the aim of achieving local control of the lesion. The aims are to prevent a pathologic fracture and to reduce pain and disability. Orthopedic treatment planning is based on the general oncologic situation with respect to prognosis, clinical condition, systemic treatment, histology, and local circumstances such as location and aggressiveness of the lesion. Various tools are available including bisphosphonates, arterial embolization, radiation therapy, and surgical

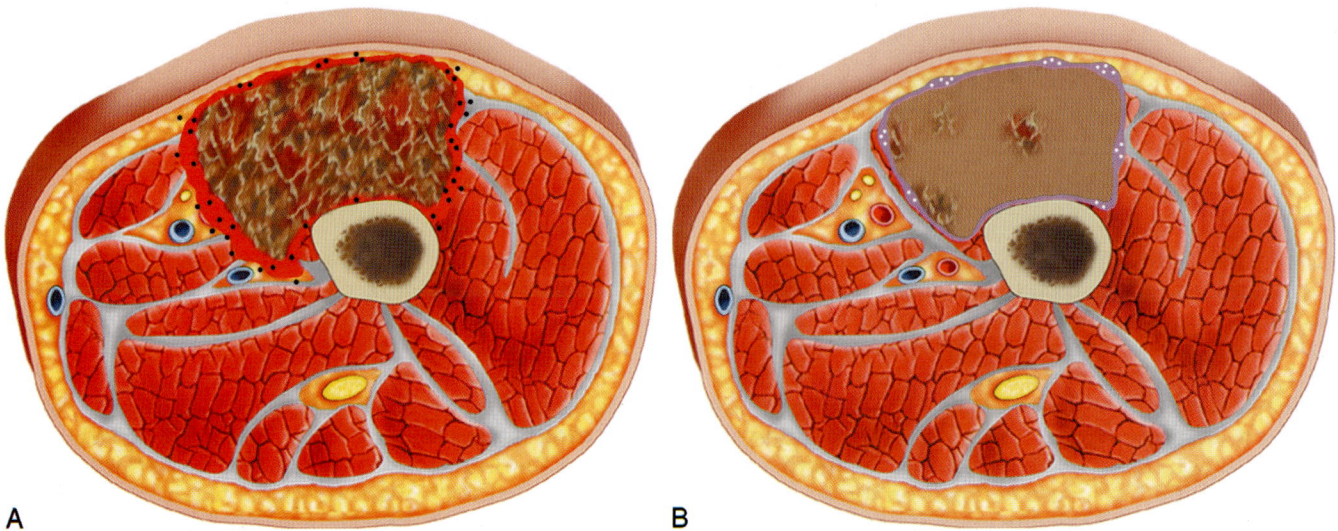

■ **FIGURE 97-13** **A,** Schematic view of a soft tissue tumor of the medial thigh. **B,** Reduction in size and induction of necrosis occur after neoadjuvant therapy. Resection will be easier, allowing salvage of the medial compartment along with the femoral neurovascular bundle.

therapy. The goal is to improve the patient's quality of life and when possible to locally eradicate the tumor, while maintaining mechanical stability. The presence of visceral metastases in liver, lung, and especially the brain is usually the reason to limit surgical intervention. In this case use of braces for pain relief is the rule.[14]

Surgical Techniques

As a general rule we have to bear in mind that a bad and painful reconstruction is more demanding for the patient than amputation.[15] A reconstruction should only be considered when the chance of success is reasonably high. The excision of a number of structures, such as bone, joint, skin, and vessels, in patients older than 60 years of age is frequently followed by a high number of complications. One of the worst is usually infection. When large orthopedic devices are involved by infection, it can be a very difficult experience for the patient and a challenging event for the surgeon.

Amputation

Although amputation is a less demanding procedure for surgeon and patient, it is nowadays not accepted by the patients, even when strongly recommended by the physician. The older the patient, the more difficult the acceptance of this operation is. In addition, younger patients have the ability to perform better functionally with artificial limbs. In the lower limb, improvements have been made in prosthetic limb manufacturing. Technical development, such as electronically assisted joints, new exter-

nal and internal materials, and lighter structural alloys make the use of an artificial limb easier than it was in the past. We can appreciate how good the functional results are when we observe sport competitions in disabled athletes. The same results cannot be achieved with internal reconstruction.[16,17]

Limb Salvage

In the majority of patients limb salvage is the rule; therefore, the main task is skeletal reconstruction. However, sometimes also skin, fascia, and muscle may need to be replaced, as well as vessels and nerves. The type of skeletal reconstruction needed depends on the amount of bone resected and on involvement of other structures such as joint capsules, ligaments, tendons, and muscles.

Prosthetic Device

In orthopedic oncology, prosthetic devices are called modular prostheses. Because we no longer make reconstruction devices tailored to the patients, orthopedic companies have produced modular components to be assembled in different lengths and sizes in the surgical field. Usually they are able to substitute part of a diaphyseal bone and the connected joint. Modular prostheses have a stem that is inserted in the host diaphyseal bone and connected to the body of a prosthesis, which in turn is connected to an articular device. The articular device is connected to the stem inserted in the opposite site of a joint (Fig. 97-14).

The current systems can be used around several joints, such as knee, hip, shoulder, and elbow. There are plans

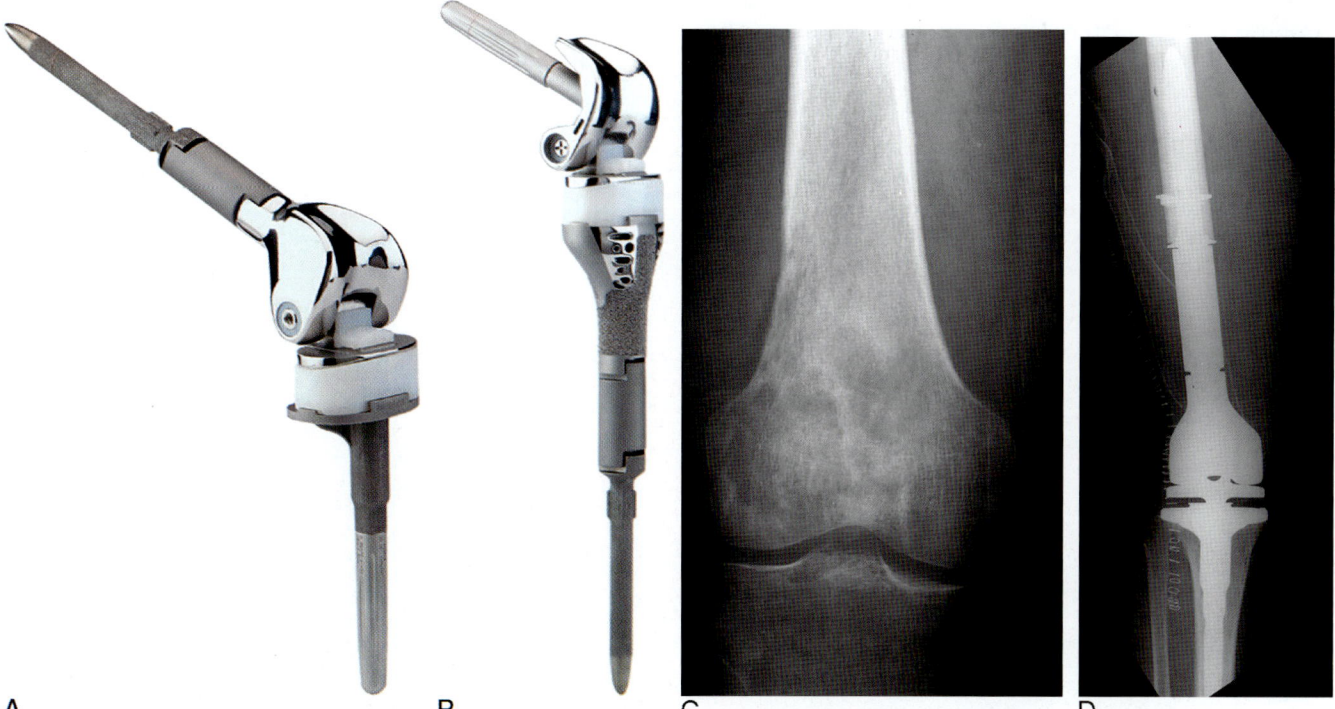

A   B   C   D

■ **FIGURE 97-14** A and B, Current modular prosthetic device for distal femur and proximal tibia reconstruction. The prosthesis is composed of intramedullary stems, bodies, and articular components. In this prosthesis the articular component rotates, thus allowing axial movement between femur and tibia components; the bearing articular surface is constructed of high-density polyethylene. C, Distal femur fibrosarcoma resected and replaced with the modular prosthesis (D).

to replace even a whole bone, such as femur or humerus. There are special customized prostheses with an expendable system that can be used in young skeletally immature patients with the aim of limb elongation. One of the advantages is the ease of application, thus reducing surgical time and related blood loss and risk of infection. Another favorable element is the possibility to combine modular prostheses with radiotherapy. Reconstructions using modular prostheses also have benefits in older patients or in any circumstances in which the capability of host bone to integrate is decreased.

The reliability of the device depends on the method of fixing the stem in the host bones and the efficiency of the joint mechanism. Over time, the polyethylene part of the joint in particular can wear and fail. However, survival of modular prostheses is mainly affected by infection.

Wide excision of metaphyseal bone along with joint and surrounding muscles can lead to complications in wound healing, even a deep infection. Part of the incidence of wound slough and failure is due to the use of postoperative chemotherapy. The reduced biologic activity in the surroundings of the implant increases the risk of infection. Moreover, the use of an indwelling catheter can improve the risk of transient bacteremia that, coupled with a decrease in defensive blood cells, can be another jeopardizing factor related to drug administration in the postoperative period. Thus, all precautions that can reduce the general and local risk of contamination have to be used. Nonetheless, an early deep infection is present in 3% to 8% of our prosthetic reconstructions. The proximal tibia is by far the most common site of infection. In this region muscular and skin flaps are recommended to improve the local biologic conditions.[18]

Mechanical failure should be more and more reduced by the use of new materials and prosthetic design. The use of rotating joints that allow a more physiologic movement and better stem design results in less mechanical failure.

There are still some weak points in modular prosthetic reconstruction: the use of cement in the fixation of the stems, the wearing of the articular joint, and the lack of reliable attachment devices for the major tendons. In some locations, insertion of tendons on prosthetic material is difficult. This is the case in proximal femur reconstructions, where sectioned glutei tendons cannot be efficiently reinserted on the prosthesis. Similarly, insertion of the patellar tendon on the prosthesis in proximal tibia resections is difficult.

Bone Allograft

Autograft bone is no longer used after oncologic resection. Allograft bone, from sterile human donation and stored in a deep freeze at −80 °C, has been increasingly used in reconstructive surgery. The use of biologic material provides a stable and long-lasting reconstruction, and the bone and other implanted tissues are completely integrated in the body. Allografts are also used for small or partial reconstructions, as in partial diaphyseal resection, where the structural integrity of the bone is still present, or in condyle replacement (Figs. 97-15 and 97-16).

Allografts are also preferred in joints in which modular prostheses are not effective, such as in forearm, distal tibia, hand, and foot replacement. Osteoarticular allografts allow a better reattachment of soft tissue and tendons, making the postoperative functional activity largely better than that achieved with modular prostheses. That is the reason why we prefer allograft replacement in the upper extremity and in children; however, in the lower limb, osteochondral allograft replacement has been almost entirely abandoned because of the relative fragility of the subchondral bone. The main indication for allograft replacement is a diaphyseal reconstruction without resection of joint (surfaces). Long-term results are good, and these patients regain almost complete functionality. The role of host immunogenetic reactions is not yet clear, but it seems to play a small part in the remodeling of the graft. In general, allografts are only partially integrated over time, and even after 10 or more years, in massive replacements, only a small percentage of the bone is renewed, whereas 50% to 80% is still the old implanted necrotic bone. Therefore, allografts should be mechanically protected for the life of the patient; still, they can deteriorate and fracture even after long-term follow-up (Fig. 97-17).

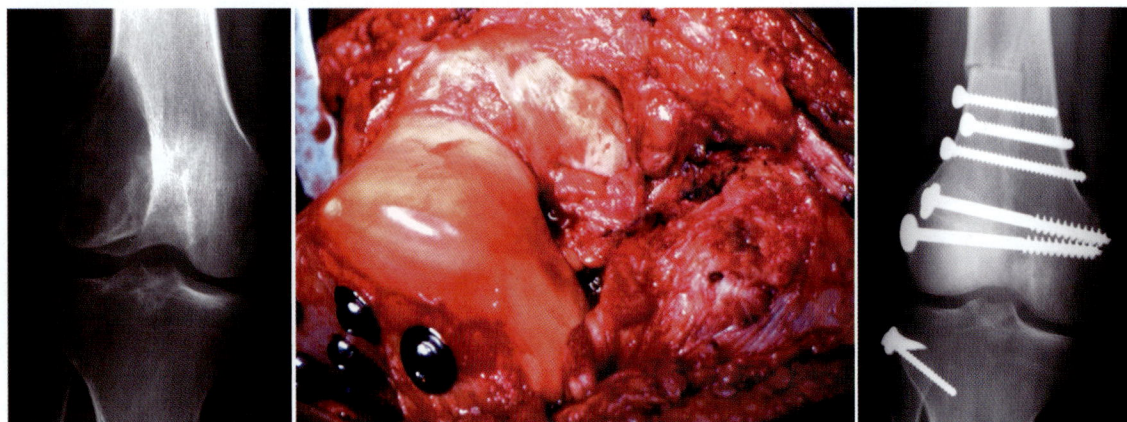

■ **FIGURE 97-15**   Giant cell tumor of the distal femur. The lateral condyle was resected and replaced with an osteochondral allograft. Correct matching of the new and old condyles is critical in constructing a congruent joint.

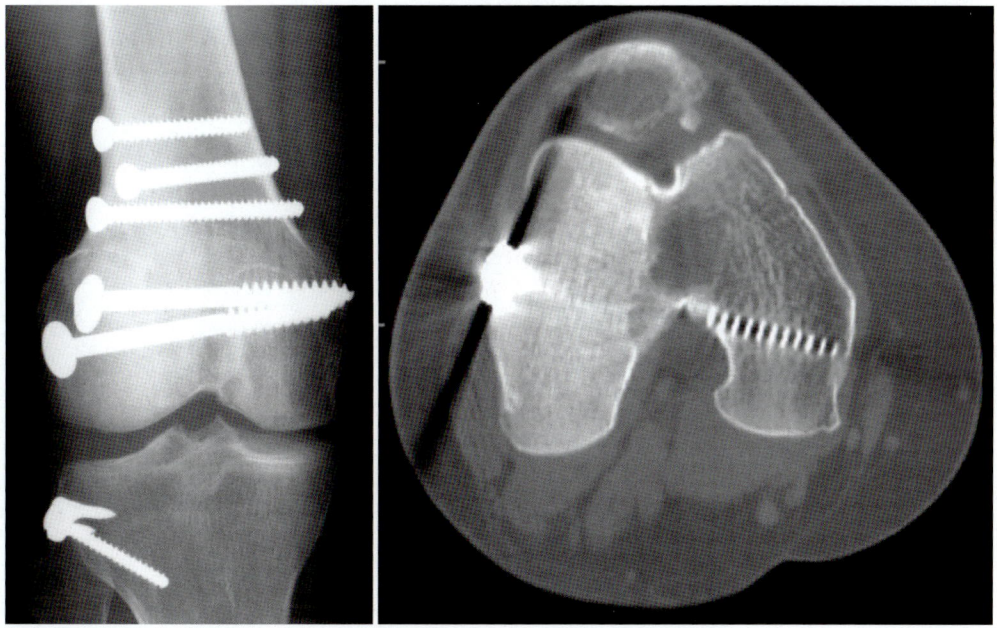

■ **FIGURE 97-16** Appearance 8 years later of same case as in Figure 97-15. Note the good morphologic result both on radiography and CT.

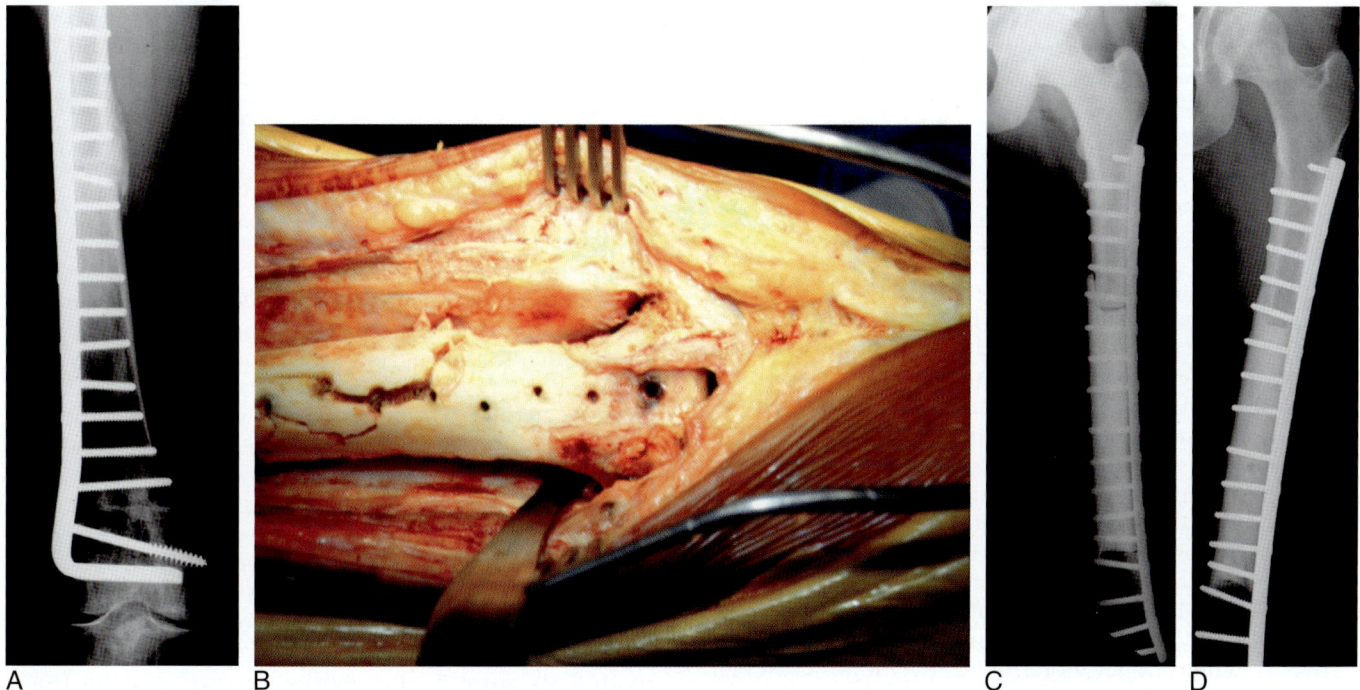

A   B   C   D

■ **FIGURE 97-17** **A** and **B,** Massive intercalary femoral reconstruction with allograft. The graft is weakened by the many screw holes in the cortex. After 22 months a fracture was evident. **C** and **D,** Postoperative and late follow-up anteroposterior view of a massive intercalary allograft reconstruction in the mid-diaphysis of the femur. Acrylic cement has been introduced in the medullary canal to avoid fracture of the allograft.

Allograft Prosthetic Composite

To prevent joint deterioration and failure a standard prosthesis can be inserted in the allograft. With this procedure we can have the benefit of a better soft tissue reattachment onto the allograft while at the same time providing more structural stability to the joint and allograft diaphysis. This type of reconstruction is called an allograft prosthetic composite, and it is particularly indicated in the proximal femur[19] and tibia, where the need for tendon reinsertion is more demanding. In both sites we use a standard revision prosthesis with a long stem cemented in the allograft and press-fit in the host bone (Fig. 97-18).

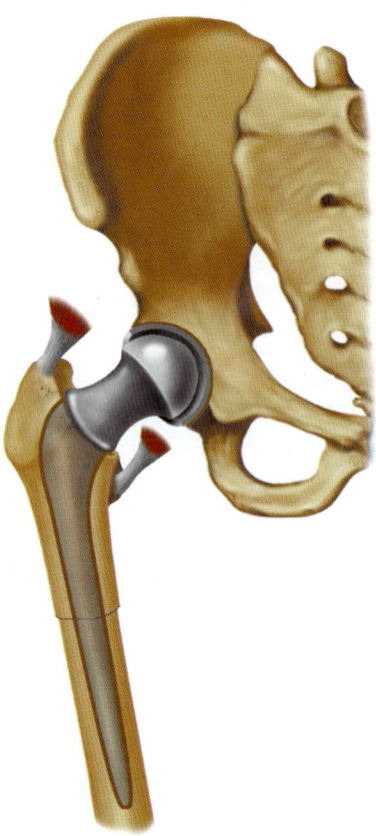

A

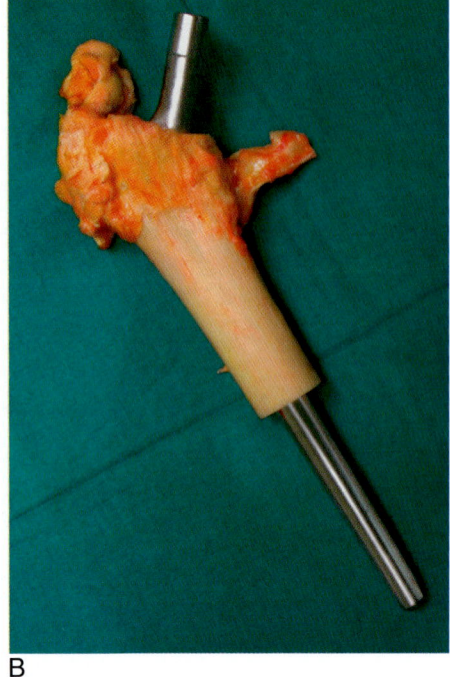

B

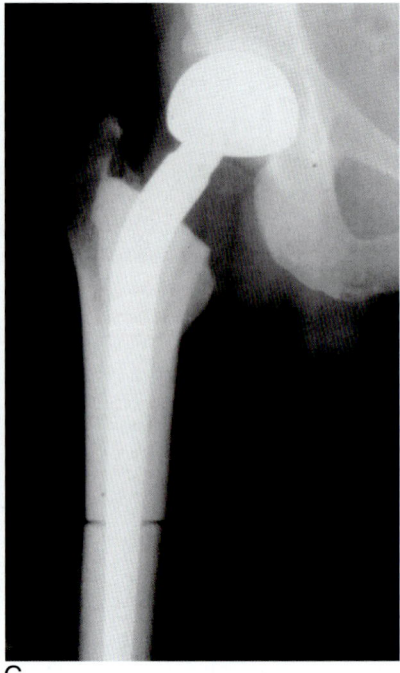

C

■ **FIGURE 97-18** **A,** Schematic drawing of the noncemented revision of a hip prosthesis inserted in the allograft and host bone. **B,** The allograft is complete with medial gluteus and iliopsoas tendon reattachment. **C,** Postoperative anteroposterior radiograph shows cement between the allograft and prosthesis, while this composite is press-fit into the host bone. The cup is a bipolar reconstruction.

Bone Transplant

Allogenic transplantation is still experimental, and there is little chance of it being used in the future, whereas auto transplants are a well-recognized type of reconstruction. The bone widely used is the fibula due to its ability to supply the structural need of an intercalary resection. The advantage in using a bone transplant is the possibility of having new self-regenerating bone. On the other hand, the need of microvascular anastomosis, requiring long surgical procedures, tends to limit this type of application. For this reason, its indication is mainly restricted to difficult situations in which a standard method would be unsuccessful, for example, when we have an irradiated field in the tibial diaphysis, or failure of a previous allograft. However, when applied alone in the lower limb, a vascularized fibula graft needs a very long time to become strong enough to allow a free function of the limb without support. Thus, in the majority of cases the use of a vascularized fibula graft is combined with the use of an allograft.[20] This combination has the advantage of achieving integration due to the contribution of the transplanted fibula, coupled with the good mechanical support provided by the allograft (Fig. 97-19).

Choosing a Type of Reconstruction

An orthopedic oncology referral center needs to be able to offer all the possible types of reconstruction available. Orthopedic surgeons need to be familiar with standard and special orthopedic devices, and they have to be able to perform the best reconstruction tailored to the patient's characteristics and needs. Both adult prosthetic reconstruction as well as traumatology need to be in the bag of tools of the orthopedic oncology surgeon. Nonetheless, over time we have established preferences as a general guideline for preferred types of reconstruction in various circumstances. These preferences are based on the site and type of resection (amount of bone loss and soft tissue involvement) and on tumor staging, age of the patient, and (neo)-adjuvant therapies (Tables 97-2 and 97-3). As a general rule, more biologic reconstructions are preferred in young patients whereas adult patients with strong working needs are treated by joint fusion with allograft and/or fibula transplant. In older patients, cemented stem modular prostheses are often indicated. Any type of partial resection of a joint is usually treated by an osteochondral reconstruction.

The Patient's Choice

Finally, it is important to stress that the final choice is up to the patient. The task of the treating physician is to make the patients aware of the illness by discussing with them their future life from a positive, realistic perspective. Usually, the physician cannot propose many alternatives to the patient but the goal is to make the

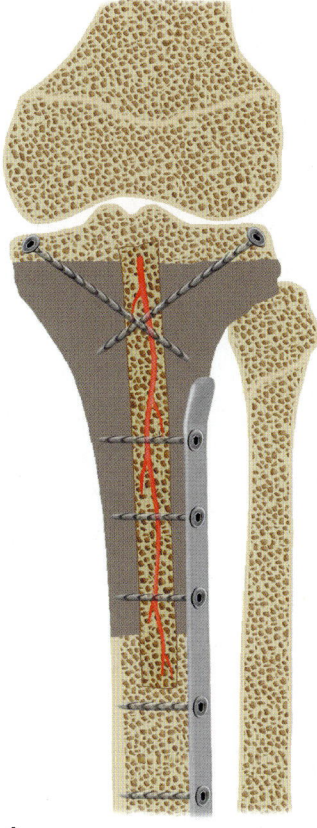 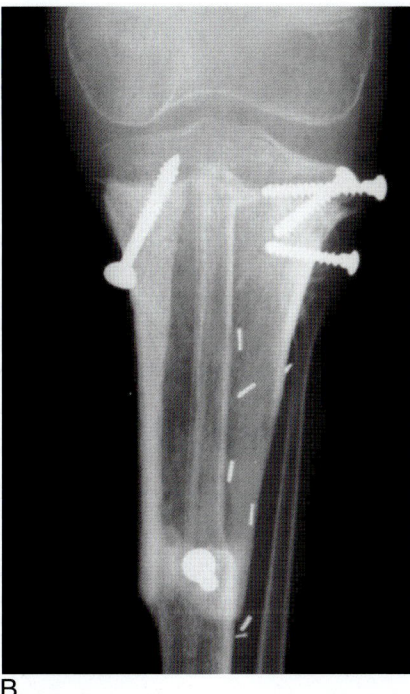 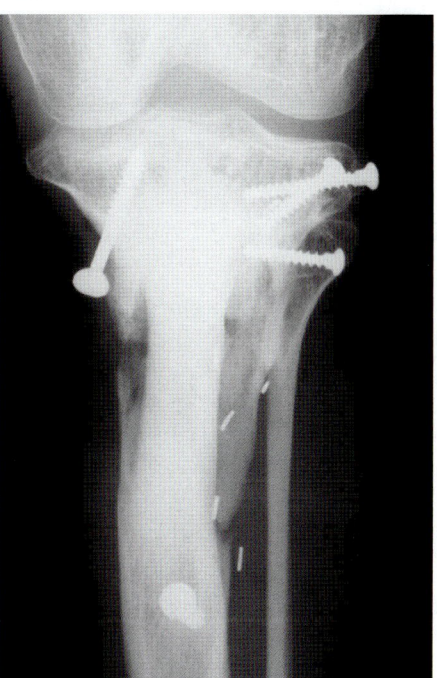

■ **FIGURE 97-19** **A,** Schematic drawing of an intercalary reconstruction of the proximal part of the tibia. In this case only a small part of the tibial plateau could be saved after tumor resection. **B,** Anteroposterior radiograph of the reconstruction shows biologic (fibula transplant) and mechanical (allograft) contribution. **C,** As the living transplant will get bigger and stronger over time the contribution of the allograft to mechanical integrity will decrease.

A   B   C

TABLE 97-2	Surgical Reconstructions in Upper Extremity Orthopedic Oncologic Surgery					
Site	**Age**	**Stage**	**Soft Tissue Involvement**	**Radiation Therapy**	**Reconstruction**
Proximal humerus		IA IIA	Axillary bundle not involved	No	Osteochondral allograft filled with cement
		III*	Axillary bundle involved*	Yes*	Modular prosthesis
		IA IIA	Major soft tissues preserved including axillary bundle	No	Osteochondral allograft filled with cement
		III	Major soft tissue excised*	Yes*	Modular prosthesis*
Humerus intercalary	Adult		Standard bone involvement		Intercalary allograft
	Young		Adult with extended bone involvement		Fibula transplant
Distal humerus					Modular prosthesis
Intercalary ulna/radius					Allograft
Distal radius			Standard soft tissues involvement	No	Osteochondral allograft
			Extended soft tissues involvement*	Yes*	Arthrodesis with allograft

*Only one of the variables is enough to achieve the index indication.

patient comfortable with his or her choice. Patients, and their relatives, usually make the choice based on how much they trust the physician's experience. For this reason it is very important to make the patients confident with their future hopes by letting them know that any problems can be solved together. We therefore work with the patients on awareness of the situation, and our dedicated staff works with them in the postoperative period and the intensive physical rehabilitation programs.

TABLE 97-3 Surgical Reconstruction in Lower Extremity Orthopedic Oncologic Surgery

Site	Age	Stage	Soft Tissue Involvement	Radiation Therapy	Reconstruction
Proximal femur	Young	IA IIA	Glutei and iliopsoas tendon preserved	No	Allograft prosthetic composite
	Adult	III*	Short tendon remnants to be reattached*	Yes*	Modular prosthesis
Total femur					Modular prosthesis
Femur intercalary	Adult		Standard bone involvement		Intercalary allograft filled with cement
	Young		Adult with extended bone involvement		Fibula transplant associated to allograft
Distal femur	Adult				Modular prosthesis
	Young				Growing prosthesis
Proximal tibia	Adult				Modular prosthesis
	Young			No	Allograft prosthetic composite
Tibia intercalary			Short resection		Intercalary allograft filled with cement
	Young	IA IIA	Long resection		Fibula transplant associated to allograft
Distal tibia					Arthrodesis with allograft

*Only one of the variables is enough to achieve the index indication.

ACKNOWLEDGMENT

I would like to remember my teacher Professor Mario Campanacci with whom I began to study and cure bone tumors. A special thank you to Giliola Gamberini and Cristina Ghinelli for their assistance with the medical drawings.

SUGGESTED READINGS

Bacci G, Lari S. Current treatment of high grade osteosarcoma of the extremity: review. J Chemother 2001; 13:235-243.

Falkmer U, Jarhult J, Wersall P, Cavallin-Stahl E. A systematic overview of radiation therapy effects in skeletal metastases. Acta Oncol 2003; 42:620-633.

Ghanem N, Uhl M, Brink I, et al. Diagnostic value of MRI in comparison to scintigraphy, PET, MS-CT and PET/CT for the detection of metastases of bone. Eur J Radiol 2005; 55:41-55.

Heare TC, Enneking WF, Heare MM. Staging techniques and biopsy of bone tumors. Orthop Clin North Am 1989; 20:273-285.

Jadvar H, Gamie S, Ramanna L, Conti PS. Musculoskeletal system. Semin Nucl Med 2004; 34:254-261.

Mendenhall WM, Zlotecki RA, Scarborough MT, et al. Giant cell tumor of bone. Am J Clin Oncol 2006; 29:96-99.

Pommersheim WJ, Chew FS. Imaging, diagnosis, and staging of bone tumors: a primer. Semin Roentgenol 2004; 39:361-372.

Saifuddin A. The accuracy of imaging in the local staging of appendicular osteosarcoma. Skeletal Radiol 2002; 31:191-201 [Epub Feb 9, 2002].

Veth R, van Hoesel R, Pruszczynski M, et al. Limb salvage in musculoskeletal oncology. Lancet Oncol 2003; 4:343-350.

Wafa H, Grimer RJ. Surgical options and outcomes in bone sarcoma. Exp Rev Anticancer Ther 2006; 6:239-248.

REFERENCES

1. Finnbogason T, Ringertz HG. The changed preliminary report: a repeatedly missed paediatric tibial tumour. Eur Radiol 2000; 10:867-869.
2. Campanacci M, Mercuri M, Gasbarrini A, Campanacci L. The value of imaging in the diagnosis and treatment of bone tumors. Eur J Radiol 1998; 27(Suppl 1):S116-S122.
3. Fabiny R. Bone tumour simulators: problems and pitfalls in radiology. Acta Orthop Scand Suppl 1997; 273:14-20.
4. Campanacci M, Mercuri M, Gamberini G. Biopsy. Chir Organi Mov 1995; 80:113-123.
5. Campanacci M. The wrong approach to tumors of the musculo skeletal system: what should not be done. Chir Organi Mov 1999; 84:1-17.
6. Enneking WF, Spanier SS, Goodman MA. A system for the surgical staging of musculoskeletal sarcoma. Clin Orthop Relat Res 2003; (415):4-18.
7. Toomayan GA, Robertson F, Major NM. Lower extremity compartmental anatomy: clinical relevance to radiologists. Skeletal Radiol 2005; 34:307-313 [Epub 2005; Apr 16].
8. Anderson MW, Temple HT, Dussault R, Kaplan PA. Compartmental anatomy: relevance to staging and biopsy of musculoskeletal tumors. AJR Am J Roentgenol 1999; 173:1663-1671.
9. Bacci G, Longhi A, Versari M, et al. Prognostic factors for osteosarcoma of the extremity treated with neoadjuvant chemotherapy: 15-year experience in 789 patients treated at a single institution. Cancer 2006; 106:1154-1161.
10. Picci P, Sangiorgi L, Rougraff BT, et al. Relationship of chemotherapy induced necrosis and surgical margins to local recurrence in osteosarcoma. J Clin Oncol 1994; 12:2699-2705.
11. Ferrari S, Briccoli A, Mercuri M, et al. Postrelapse survival in osteosarcoma of the extremities: prognostic factors for long-term survival. J Clin Oncol 2003; 21:710-715.

12. Eilber FC, Rosen G, Nelson SD, et al. High-grade extremity soft tissue sarcomas: factors predictive of local recurrence and its effect on morbidity and mortality. Ann Surg 2003; 237:218–226.
13. Lackman RD, Hosalkar HS, Ogilvie CM, et al. Intralesional curettage for grades II and III giant cell tumors of bone. Clin Orthop Relat Res 2005; 438:123–127.
14. Nathan SS, Healey JH, Mellano D, et al. Survival in patients operated on for pathologic fracture: implications for end-of-life orthopedic care. J Clin Oncol 2005; 23:6072–6082.
15. Bacci G, Ferrari S, Lari S, et al. Osteosarcoma of the limb: amputation or limb salvage in patients treated by neoadjuvant chemotherapy. J Bone Joint Surg Br 2002; 84:88–92.
16. Rougraff BT, Simon MA, Kneisl JS, et al. Limb salvage compared with amputation for osteosarcoma of the distal end of the femur: a long-term oncological, functional, and quality-of-life study. J Bone Joint Surg Am 1994; 76:649–656.
17. Zahlten-Hinguranage A, Bernd L, Ewerbeck V, Sabo D. Equal quality of life after limb-sparing or ablative surgery for lower extremity sarcomas. Br J Cancer 2004; 91:1012–1014.
18. Hardes J, Gebert C, Schwappach A, et al. Characteristics and outcome of infections associated with tumor endoprostheses. Arch Orthop Trauma Surg 2006; [Epub ahead of print].
19. Donati D, Giacomini S, Gozzi E, Mercuri M. Proximal femur reconstruction by an allograft prosthesis composite. Clin Orthop Relat Res 2002; (394):192–200.
20. Donati D, Di Liddo M, Zavatta M, et al. Massive bone allograft reconstruction in high-grade osteosarcoma. Clin Orthop Relat Res 2000; (377):186–194.

98

Staging Bone and Soft Tissue Tumors

Hans L. Bloem and Herman M. Kroon

Staging encompasses determination of local tumor extent and identification or exclusion of distant spread. Information on local extent and distant spread is a requisite for treatment planning, as discussed in Chapter 98. MRI is the preferred technique for local staging and should be performed before the lesion is sampled because postbiopsy changes such as hemorrhage can exaggerate the extent of the tumor. The second advantage of doing MRI before biopsy is that the results can be used to plan the biopsy and target the most representable part of the lesion. Surgery is the cornerstone of the treatment strategy. The biologic aggressiveness of the sarcoma, indicated by histologic grading, is the key factor in the selection of the surgical margin required to achieve local control.[1,2] Four different surgical procedures, implying four different margins, are recognized: intralesional, marginal, wide, and radical (see Chapter 98 for details and other factors used to determine treatment strategy). Local staging gives the answer to the question how a required tumor-free margin can be obtained. Both these factors (grade and local extent) are used in the staging system of the Musculoskeletal Tumor Society (see Chapter 98).

Surgery is often used in combination with other forms of treatment such as chemotherapy. The role of imaging in monitoring the effect of neoadjuvant (prior to surgery) chemotherapy is addressed in Chapter 100. Information obtained from these imaging studies is also used in local staging before surgery.[3-5] Thus, local staging is typically based on multiple imaging studies taken at different points in time. The surgeon and radiologist should confer, when planning the customized surgical procedure, to make sure that all relevant imaging information is used.

Musculoskeletal sarcoma metastasizes first to the lungs. Therefore, chest radiographs and multidetector row CT (MDCT) are used to identify or exclude pulmonary metastases. Locoregional lymph node metastases do occur, especially around the foot, and should be looked for when the primary tumor is imaged. Bone marrow biopsies are used in detecting diffuse spread of Ewing's sarcoma.

IMAGING TECHNIQUES

Magnetic Resonance Imaging

Magnetic resonance imaging has gained a prominent position in the diagnosis and management of patients with musculoskeletal sarcoma. It directly exhibits the lesion in relationship to surrounding normal structures with exquisite anatomic detail (Fig. 98-1).[6] The MR protocol for bone and soft tissue sarcoma can be identical. We routinely use fast, or turbo, spin echo for all sequences. A longitudinal T1-weighted sequence is used to exclude or determine intraosseous extent because high contrast between low signal intensity of tumor and relatively high signal intensity of normal fatty or hematopoietic marrow is combined with excellent spatial resolution. It is important to include an anatomic point of reference in the field of view, usually the nearest joint. The coronal plane is preferred around the shoulder, wrist, pelvis, and hip because it best displays tumor and tumor-containing osseous

---

KEY POINTS

- Osseous sarcoma usually extends beyond its original compartment and invades soft tissues.
- Synovial sarcoma is the only soft tissue sarcoma that commonly invades bone.
- The neurovascular bundle is not commonly invaded.
- MRI has a tendency to overstage tumors (providing false-positive findings).

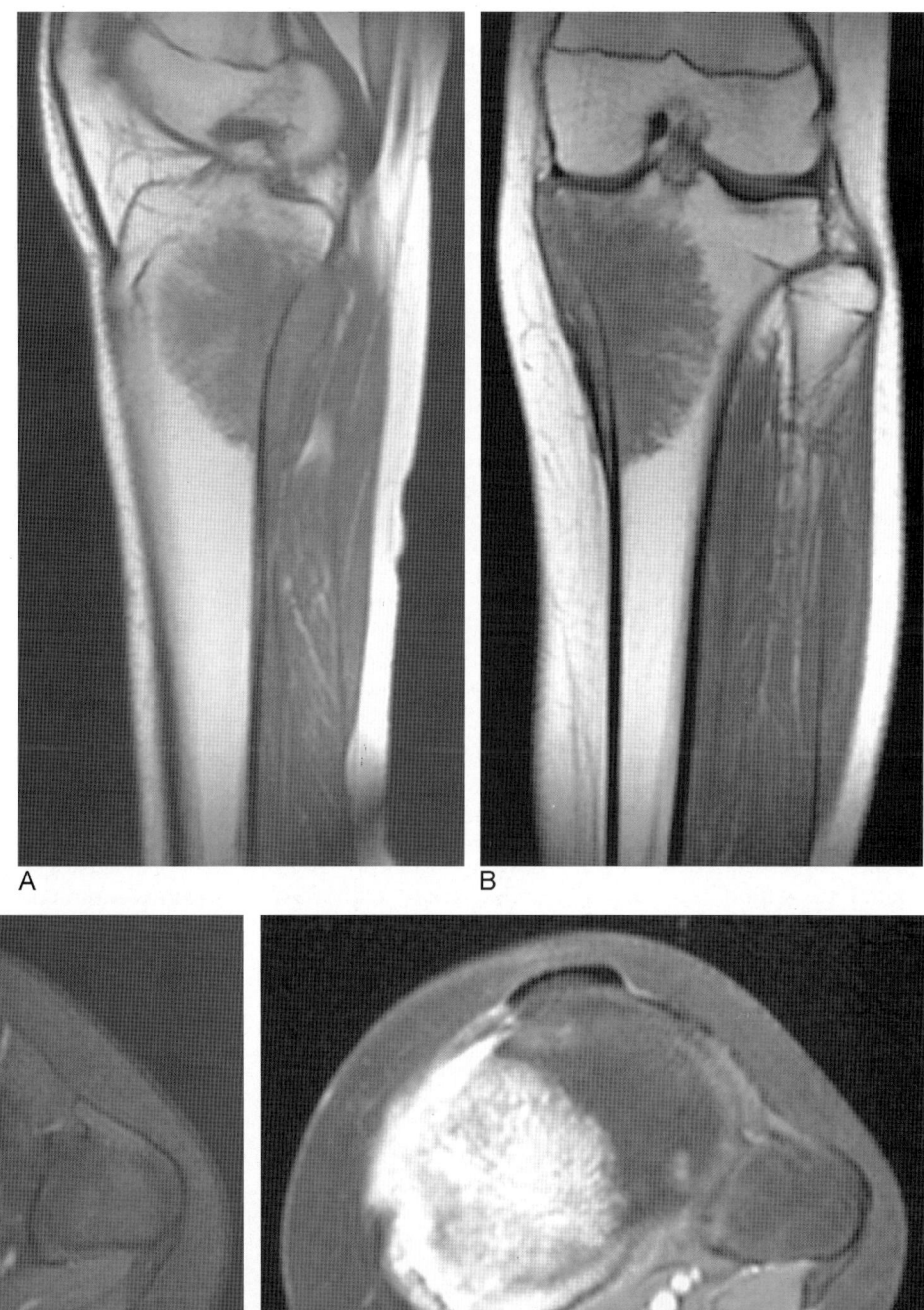

■ **FIGURE 98-1** Staging of osteosarcoma in the proximal tibia of a 21-year-old man. **A,** Sagittal T1-weighted image shows high contrast between low signal intensity of tumor and high signal intensity of normal marrow. **B,** T1-weighted image coronal image shows extent in the other direction; this is an alternative to an axial T1-weighted image. Axial fat-suppressed T2-weighted (**C**) and fat-suppressed Gd-DTPA enhanced (**D**) MR images show high signal intensity tumor extending into the soft tissues medially (medial collateral band, tendons of sartorius and gracilis muscles) and posteriorly (popliteus muscle). Note that the femoral artery and vein are free of tumor.

structures relative to the joints. For the same reason the sagittal plane is the preferred longitudinal plane around the knee. The plane that best displays the tumor in relation to bone is chosen around the elbow and ankle. In the spine the sagittal plane often is preferred over the coronal plane because it usually shows the relationship between a lesion and the spinal canal to the best advantage.

A fat-suppressed, T2-weighted sequence is used for imaging in the axial plane. The axial plane displays the relationship between tumor (cortical), bone, and soft tissues such as muscle compartments and neurovascular bundles. The axial and longitudinal planes are both used to evaluate the relationship between tumor and the curved joint surfaces. When fat-suppressed, T2-weighted sequences cannot be obtained, for instance because of field inhomogeneity, a short tau inversion recovery (STIR) sequence can be used.

For comparison with the contrast-enhanced images a T1-weighted sequence is also obtained in the axial plane. This also has the advantage of having a second plane to evaluate intraosseous extent. Depending on location, a coronal plane may be used instead of the axial plane (see Fig. 98-1).

A gadolinium chelate (e.g., gadopentetate dimeglumine [Gd-DTPA])–enhanced T1-weighted image displays additional information because the generated contrast between the various tissue types depends on vascularity, permeability of tumor vessels, volume of interstitial space, and interstitial pressure.[7] Gadolinium is paramagnetic and thus reduces both T1 and T2 relaxation times. The dominant effect is concentration dependent. In normal tissue and in tumor the T1 effect is dominant, and an increase of signal intensity is observed in enhancing tissue. Signal drop, because of T2 shortening, can be observed only when concentration is high, such as in the artery when the first bolus passes or when the Gd-chelate accumulates in the bladder.

The additional information of Gd-chelate–enhanced MR images is therefore best displayed on fat-suppressed T1-weighted sequences, which have an intrinsic high spatial resolution (see Fig. 98-1). Gd-chelate–enhanced images are therefore taken in both a longitudinal and axial plane 3 to 5 minutes after bolus injection of 0.2 mL of Gd-chelate per kilogram of body weight, administered intravenously with a flow of 2 mL/s. Because of the small volume (a patient of 60 kg will receive only 12 mL) a saline flush is administered directly after the administration of the contrast agent. Cellular areas such as in viable tumor will enhance more than normal tissue or liquefied necrotic tumor. This, combined with the high spatial resolution, contributes to identifying small nests of viable tumor in critical areas. In addition to confluent necrotic and liquefied areas, viable tumor with a high interstitial pressure, usually located centrally, will enhance not at all, or very late (Table 98-1).

A similar observation can be made in cartilaginous tumors, where we can appreciate very late enhancement because of diffusion of contrast agent into the tumor matrix. In general, sarcoma with low cellularity and/or large tumor matrix, such as osteoid in osteosarcoma, and well-differentiated cartilage with mucoid in well-differentiated chondrosarcoma will enhance poorly and/or late. On the other hand, angiogenesis in the margin of necrotic areas and the reactive tissue zone will enhance. These differences in enhancement patterns are a function of time, and it is for this reason that dynamic Gd-chelate–enhanced imaging is used to increase the accuracy in identifying viable tumor. As a rule of thumb, tissue that enhances within 6 seconds after arterial enhancement observed close to the tumor represents viable tumor and tissue that enhances later represents a reactive tissue zone. These differences

TABLE 98-1 Enhancement of Tissue Relative to Arterial Enhancement on Dynamic Gd-Chelate–Enhanced MRI

	Enhancement < 6 Seconds after Artery	Enhancement > 6 Seconds after Artery
Cellular tumor High interstitial	X	
Pressure within tumor		X
Tumor liquefaction		No enhancement
Necrosis		X, margin may enhance fast
Osteoid		X, or no enhancement
Well-differentiated cartilage		X, diffusion takes minutes
Septations in chondrosarcoma	Enhancement < 10 seconds	
Reactive tissue zone		X
Physeal vessels	X	
Woven bone	X	

in the start of enhancement are best appreciated on subtraction images. The subtraction images can also be used to place regions of interest for more quantitative analysis of enhancement curves (see Chapter 99). Because of this time frame it is important to have a temporal resolution of at least 3 seconds. Spatial resolution and number of sections sampled in this time frame should be as high as possible but should not be increased at the cost of the temporal resolution. The temporal resolution and the cutoff value of 6 seconds are based on empirical evidence as well as on theoretical pharmacokinetic modeling.[8] Gd-chelate–enhanced MR angiography may be used as an additional sequence to evaluate involvement of the neurovascular bundle.

Computed Tomography

Multidetector row CT is the optimal modality in identifying, or excluding, pulmonary metastases. The 3D dataset is obtained with small collimation (e.g., 1 mm), and axial reconstructions of 3 to 5 mm are analyzed in cine mode and multiplanar reconstructions on a viewing station (Figs. 98-2 and 98-3). The thicker reconstructions facilitate differentiation between vessels and nodules. Multiplanar reconstructions may increase accuracy because they allow a second look and because the periphery of the lung, the area where metastases preferentially occur, can be analyzed in planes that are orthogonal on bordering structures such as the diaphragm. Unless conventional chest radiographs show metastatic disease, CT should be obtained before treatment to diagnose, or exclude, metastatic disease. Because of the high sensitivity of CT, many small benign nodules are also detected; therefore, histologic proof of pulmonary metastases is needed when a few small nodules are found.[9] The use and timing of CT relative to radiographs in follow-up is discussed in Chapter 99.

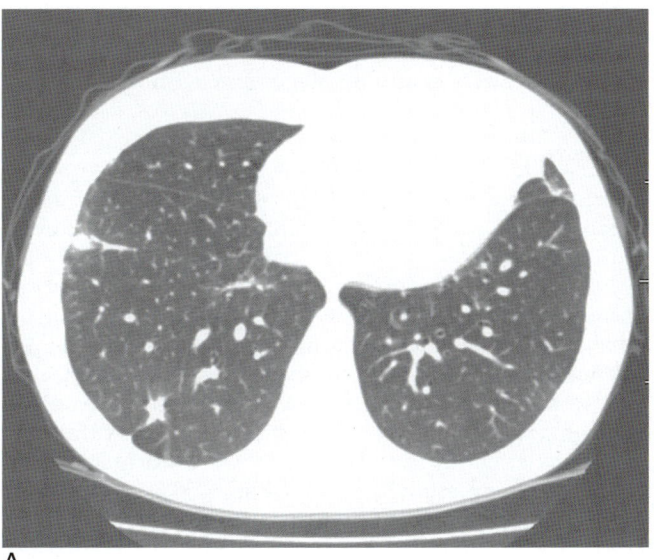

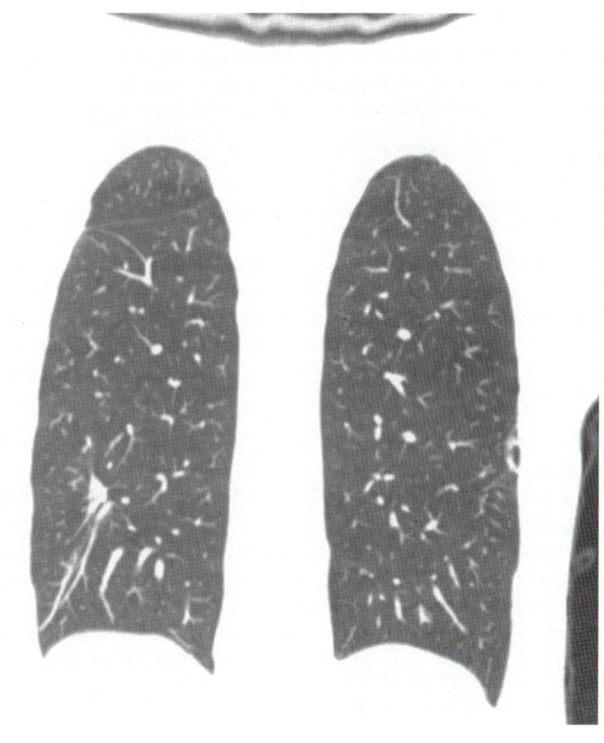

■ **FIGURE 98-2** Axial (**A**) and coronal (**B**) images show, respectively, two metastases and one metastasis in a patient with osteosarcoma.

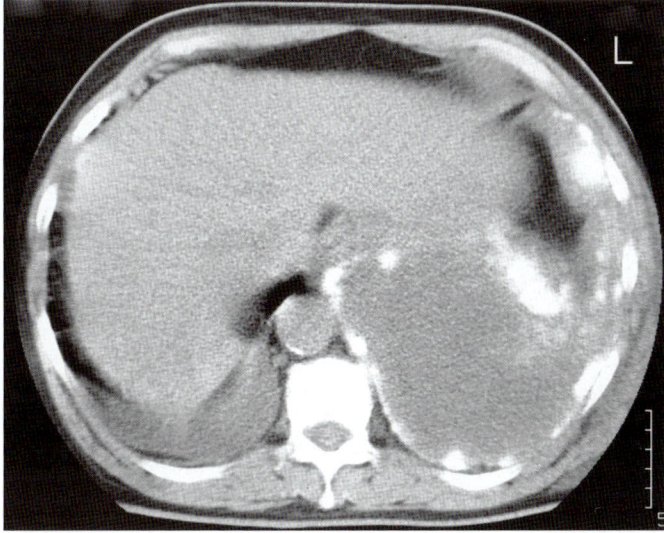

■ **FIGURE 98-3** Axial image of patient with pleuritis carcinomatosis. Note the pleural effusion and the multiple ossified nodules in the pleura.

The role of CT in local staging is limited to a small number of specific situations. The anatomic detail that CT offers is useful when anatomic information is needed preoperatively in osseous benign tumors and tumor-like conditions. CT is routinely used in planning and executing percutaneous therapy and biopsy procedures.

Bone Scintigraphy

Technetium-99m methylene diphosphonate (^{99m}Tc-MDP) has been the method of choice for screening for osseous metastases because of its capability to image the entire skeleton. However, whole-body MRI using T1-weighted and STIR sequences and a floating table has become available and has the advantage of superior sensitivity and specificity compared with planar bone scintigraphy (see Chapter 97).[8]

Positron Emission Tomography/ Computed Tomography

Because of limited spatial resolution, PET with or without CT has no role in local staging of musculoskeletal tumors. Its role in detecting sarcoma metastases is not yet determined (see also Chapter 97).

Controversies

The use of the extracellular, interstitial contrast agent Gd-chelate in imaging musculoskeletal tumors is somewhat controversial. There is ample evidence that it adds clinically relevant information in specific situations, such as in monitoring therapy (see Chapter 99), in differentiation between benign and malignant soft tissue tumors (see Chapter 93), in diagnosing some bone tumors, such as low-grade chondrosarcoma and giant cell tumor, and in specific problems related to local staging. Usually, staging can be accurately done without the use of contrast agents. In some situations, for instance, tumor extending toward structures that are critical for surgical planning, the high-resolution Gd-chelate–enhanced images provide essential information. For this reason we routinely use Gd-chelates in the workup of musculoskeletal tumors. It can be argued that contrast agents should only be administered when problems arise on the native MR studies. This approach has two disadvantages. First, some patients need to be rescheduled, or the needed second-look examination is not obtained because of practical reasons. Second, there is no dynamic Gd-chelate–enhanced dataset allowing follow-up of chemotherapy (see Chapter 99).

MANIFESTATIONS OF THE DISEASE

Magnetic resonance imaging has had a dramatic impact on the accuracy of local staging and has contributed to replacement of ablative by limb-salvage surgery. Only after meticulous preoperative staging is it possible to execute limb-saving surgery, resulting in control of the primary tumor and satisfactory residual function. Anatomic compartments are used in analyzing local tumor extent on MRI. As discussed in Chapter 97, the surgeon uses surgical compartments that often encompass multiple anatomic compartments such as individual muscles.[10] Knowledge of these surgical compartments and communication between surgeon and radiologist is important in focusing on clinically relevant problem areas when planning surgical intervention.[11-13]

Although risks cannot be taken, it is important to realize that MRI is so sensitive in visualizing tumor extent that equivocal findings are more often than not negative for tumor invasion. Also because most sarcomas grow in an expansile fashion, contact of an anatomic structure with the tumor does not necessarily mean that the structure is invaded. Invasion is more likely in high-grade malignancies, and knowledge of biologic behavior of tumors, as described later, will be useful in differentiating between invasion and displacement without invasion.

Bone Marrow Involvement

Magnetic resonance imaging is superior to other imaging techniques in displaying bone marrow involvement.[14,15] MRI has an almost perfect correlation with pathologic/morphologic examination of the resected specimen (Fig. 98-4). The osseous tumor margin may be obscured by the presence of accompanying intraosseous edema (Fig. 98-5). Often, a double margin can be visualized. The margin nearest to the center of the tumor represents the true tumor margin, whereas the outer margin represents the margin of the edematous reactive zone toward normal bone marrow.[4] Differentiation between tumor and reactive zone can be facilitated by using intravenous Gd-DTPA or similar Gd-chelates. Tumor and edematous reactive zone display different enhancement patterns: a well-vascularized tumor will enhance more rapidly than the reactive zone on dynamic sequences.[4,5] The intraosseous reactive zone is usually not a clinical problem, because it disappears after one or two cycles of chemotherapy. The true tumor margin is then easily identified. The extent of bone marrow involvement should thus be evaluated on the post-chemotherapy MR images obtained before surgery. Because cartilage is a relatively difficult barrier to cross for most tumors, an open growth plate is not easily crossed. The main exception

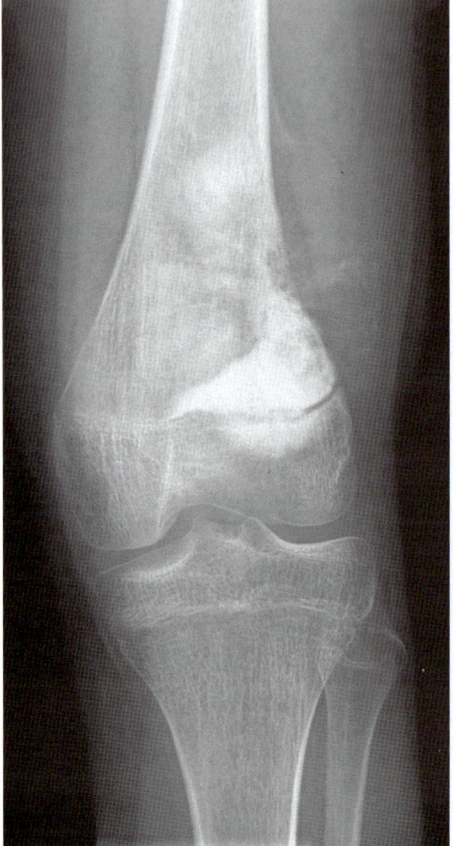
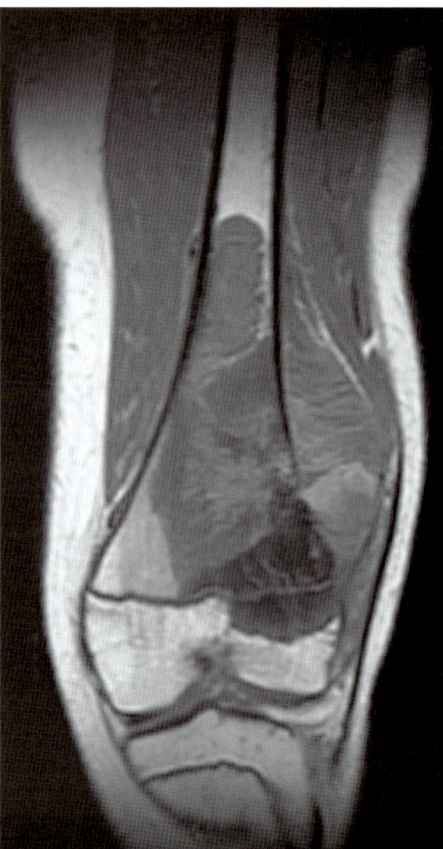

■ **FIGURE 98-4** Osteosarcoma in a 14-year-old girl. **A,** Anteroposterior radiograph shows classic signs of osteosarcoma: osteoid formation in tumor, irregular cortical destruction, and interrupted periosteal reaction including Codman's triangle. Note that tumor ossification extends into the epiphysis. **B,** T1-weighted coronal MR image shows precise tumor margin in bone. These proximal and distal tumor margins are used to plan osteotomy planes close to the tumor. *(Courtesy of Netherlands Committee of Bone Tumors.)*

A   B

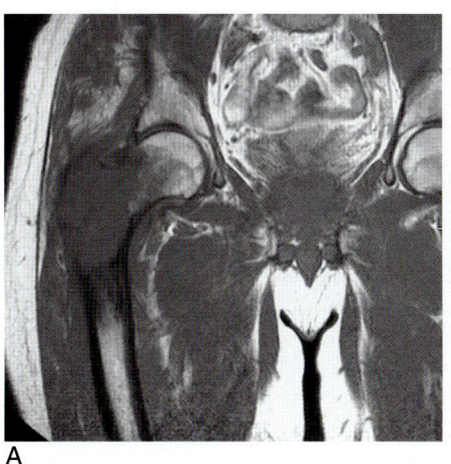
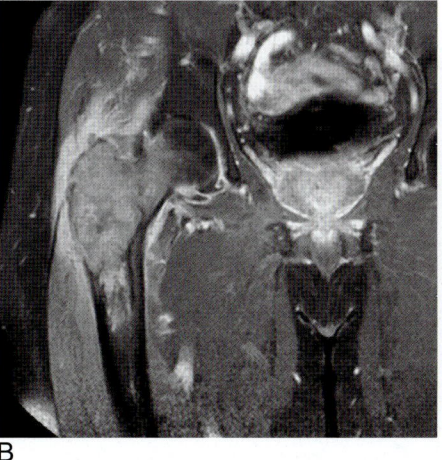
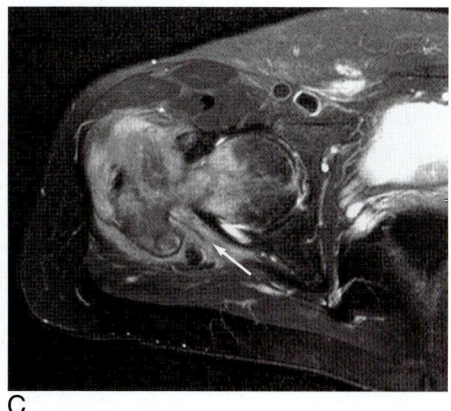

A   B   C

■ **FIGURE 98-5**   Osteosarcoma in the proximal femur. **A,** Coronal T1-weighted image shows marrow extension and cortical breakthrough on the lateral site. Note ill-defined reactive changes in the bone marrow distally and proximally. **B** and **C,** Soft tissue extension (lateral in fascia lata and anterior in gluteus minimus, medius, vastus lateralis) and ill-defined reactive changes in gluteal muscle compartment, short rotator muscles (*arrow*) (gemelli superior, inferior, and quadratus femoris muscle) are well demonstrated on the fat-suppressed, Gd-DTPA–enhanced coronal (**B**) and axial fat-suppressed, T2-weighted (**C**) MR images.

is osteosarcoma. When a tumor located in the metaphysis crosses the physis and extends into the epiphysis, an osteosarcoma is very likely. Ewing's sarcoma, on the other hand, usually bypasses the physis by extending into the soft tissues, invading the epiphysis via the soft tissues.

Caution is needed in the diagnosis of skip metastases in osteosarcoma and Ewing's sarcoma because they should also be resected together with the primary tumor (Fig. 98-6). Presence of skip metastases adversely affects prognosis. The prevalence of skip metastases in osteosarcoma has been reported to be up to 10% in osteosarcoma and 6% in Ewing's sarcoma.[16,17] Because Ewing's sarcoma is considered to be a systemic disease, bone marrow biopsies are taken from the iliac crest. Skip metastases can be detected with bone scintigraphy unless the size is below the detection threshold. Skip lesions of less than 5 mm may thus pose a diagnostic problem and are usually detected by MRI proximal to the tumor. Imaging the entire bone on T1-weighted images using a large field of view may be of help.

Cortex

Destruction of cortical bone can be evaluated with plain radiographs, CT scans, or MR images. Invasion of cortex by tumor is best shown on fat-suppressed T2-weighted or fat-suppressed Gd-chelate–enhanced T1-weighted images as a disruption of the cortical line and replacement of cortex by high signal intensity of tumor (see Figs. 98-1 and 98-5). Ewing's sarcoma and lymphoma may permeate cortical bone without displaying gross destruction (Fig. 98-7). MRI is usually as accurate as CT in displaying involvement of cortical bone. It only has an advantage over CT in densely ossified osteosarcoma or when permeation of cortex by lymphoma or Ewing's sarcoma is subtle.[2] Invasion by sarcoma is the rule when sarcoma originates in bone. Soft tissue sarcoma rarely invades bone, with the exception of synovial sarcoma. Also rare is osseous sarcoma extending into soft tissue and invading a second bone. This occurs occasionally when joints are immobile, such as in sacroiliac or tibiofibular joints (Fig. 98-8)

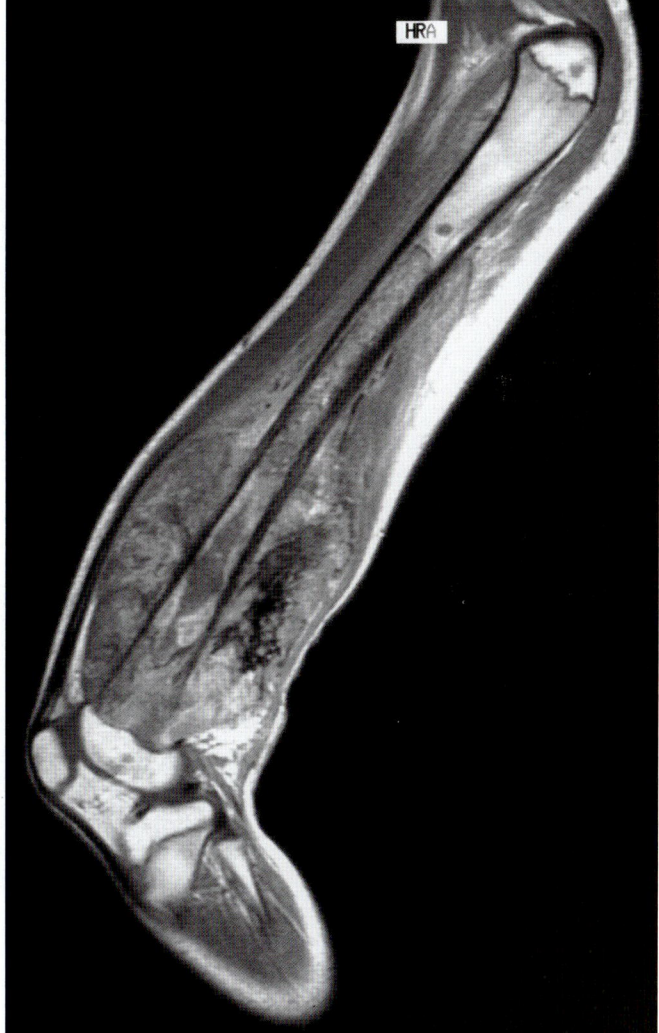

■ **FIGURE 98-6**   Sagittal T1-weighted image of osteosarcoma in the femur. The distal physis is the distal margin; the proximal margin is well demarcated and seen in the proximal diaphysis. Note the three rounded low-signal-intensity skip lesions: in the distal epiphysis, proximal to the proximal margin, and in the trochanter apophysis.

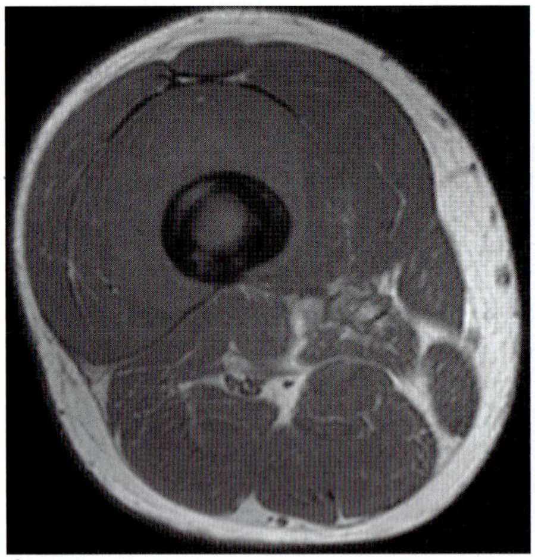

A

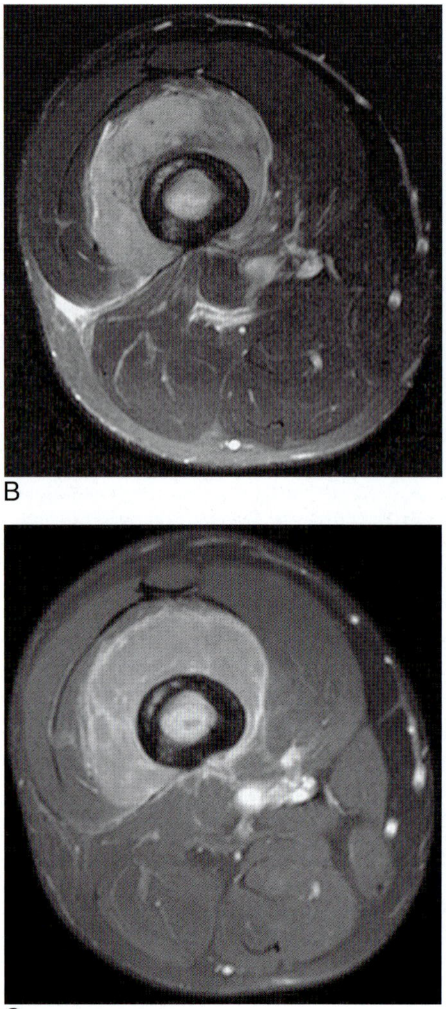

B

■ **FIGURE 98-7** Permeative, rather than gross, cortical destruction is demonstrated in this patient with osseous lymphoma showing the osseous component, areas of abnormal signal intensity within cortex that is mainly preserved, and the large soft tissue component in the vastus intermedius muscle on T1-weighted (**A**), T2-weighted (**B**), and Gd-chelate–enhanced (**C**) axial images. Note the continuity between the vastus intermedius (containing tumor), vastus lateralis, and vastus medialis, due to absence of fascia between these three muscles. In contrast, the rectus femoris muscle is separated from the vastus muscles by its own fascia. **D,** The corresponding lateral radiograph depicts thickened abnormal cortex with lucent areas but no massive destruction.

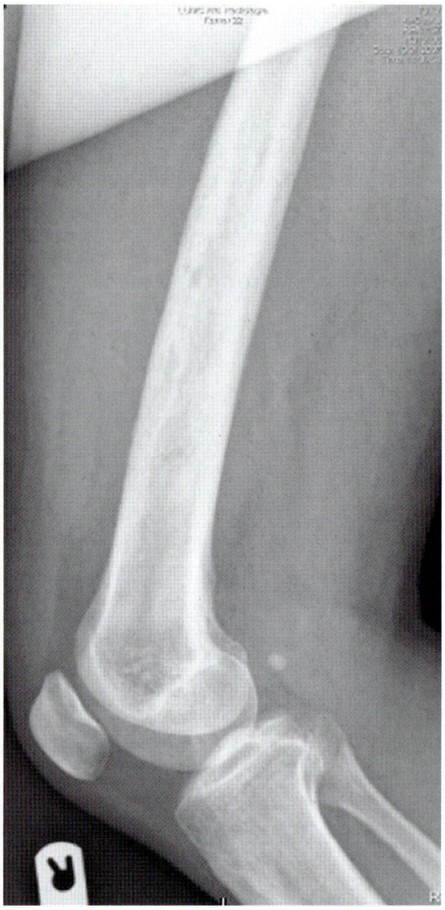

C

D

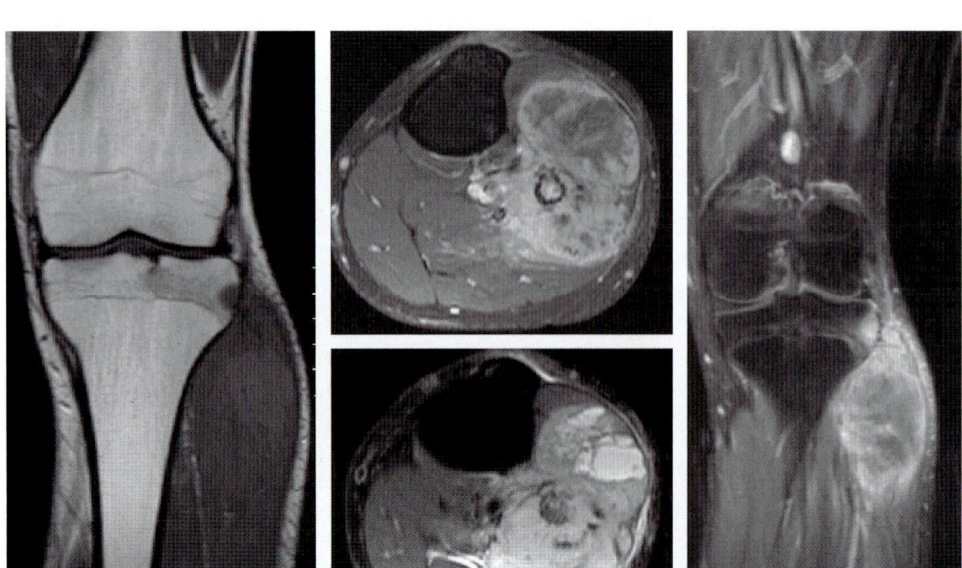

■ **FIGURE 98-8** Osteosarcoma originating in the fibula of a 22-year-old man before chemotherapy. Axial fat-suppressed, T2-weighted (*middle bottom*) and fat-suppressed, Gd-DTPA–enhanced (*middle top*) images show circumferential soft tissue extension (extensor digitorum longus, peroneus longus, posterior tibial, and soleus muscles) of osteosarcoma of the fibula. The tumor extends toward the neurovascular bundle but does not encase it. Superior extension is seen invading the tibia on coronal T1-weighted (*left*) and fat-suppressed Gd-DTPA–enhanced (*right*) images.

and in severe osteoarthritis. Osseous tumor types most frequently exhibiting this behavior are osteosarcoma, giant cell tumor, chondrosarcoma, and chordoma (leaving one vertebral body and invading another one at a different level).

Periosteum

When an osseous tumor breaches the periosteum, it extends beyond its original compartment and becomes thus an extracompartmental tumor. Ossified periosteum, especially when periosteal reaction is present as a result of tumor activity within the medullary canal and/or cortex, is well seen on radiographs, and especially

on CT. When not yet mineralized, the cellular layer or cambium of the periosteum is very well seen on MRI, especially when it is lifted off the bone by the tumor (Fig. 98-9).

Muscular Compartments

Magnetic resonance imaging is highly accurate and significantly superior to other imaging techniques in identifying muscle compartments containing tumor (see Figs. 98-1, 98-5, 98-7, 98-8, 98-10, and 98-11).[2] For tumors, muscular fascia is a relatively difficult border to cross. Macroscopically, tumors tend to grow in an expansile, rather than an invasive, fashion. Therefore, muscle is initially

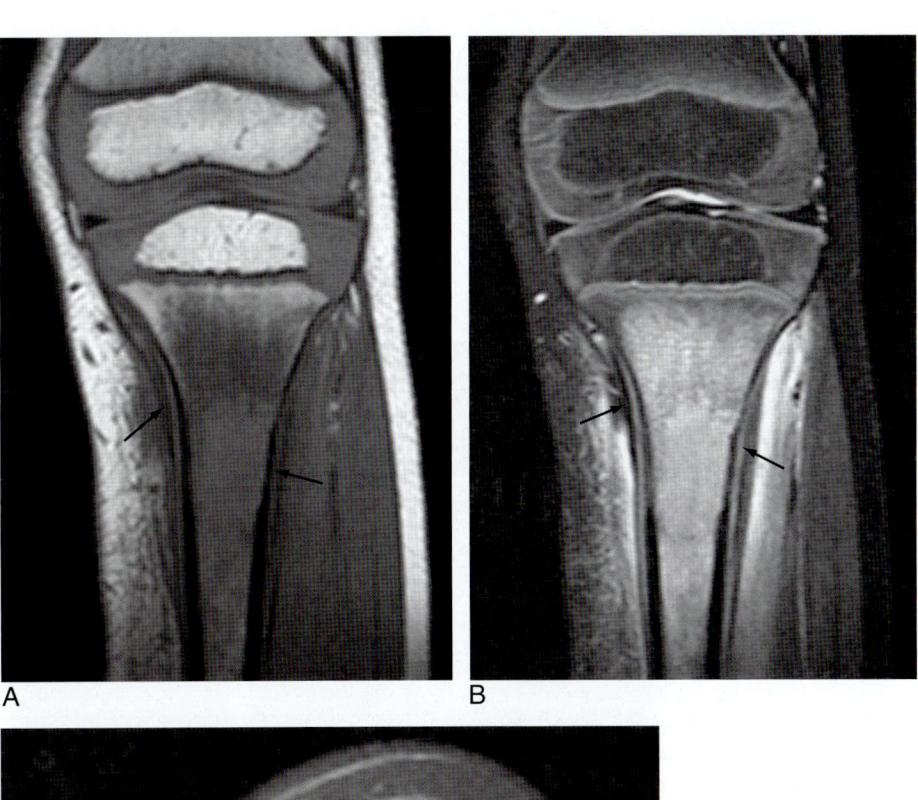

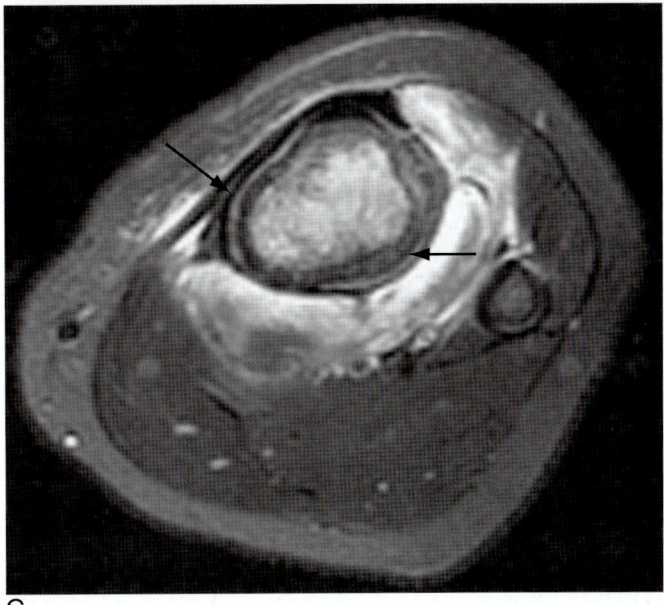

■ **FIGURE 98-9** T-cell lymphoma in a 4-year-old boy. The intraosseous tumor and soft tissue extension are easily appreciated. Cortical bone and ossified periosteum is black (signal void). Note the continuous cellular periosteal reaction (*arrows*), which has an intermediate signal on T1-weighted (**A**) and high signal intensity on STIR (**B**) and fat-suppressed T2-weighted (**C**) MR images. *(Courtesy of Netherlands Committee of Bone Tumors.)*

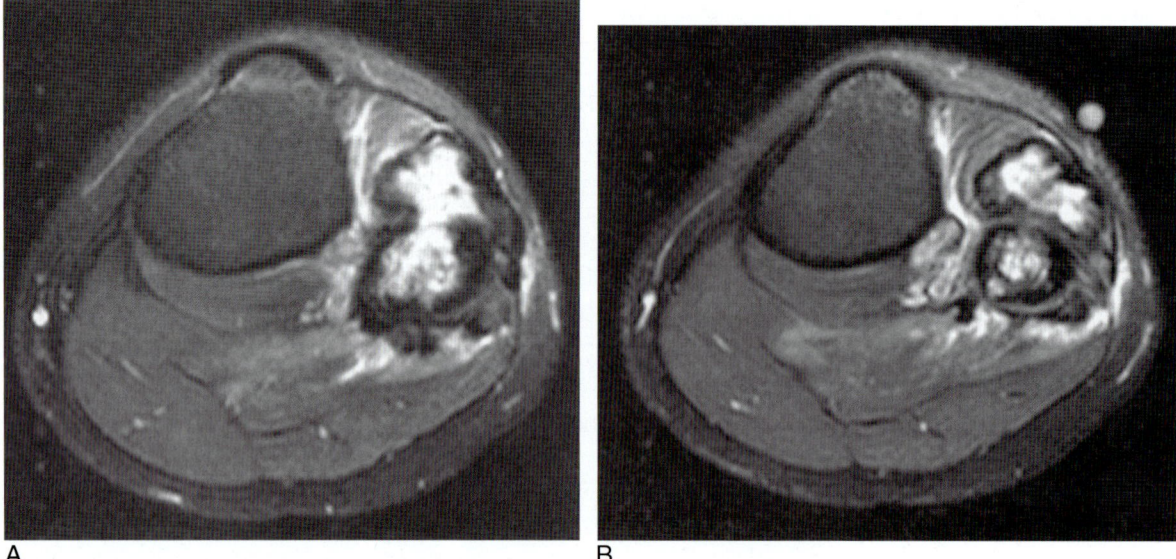

■ **FIGURE 98-10**　Same patient as in Figure 98-8 with images obtained after chemotherapy. **A** and **B,** Axial fat-suppressed T2-weighted images at two levels. Tumor is well defined and is seen to extend in the peroneus longus and extensor digitorum longus muscles. Reactive changes are seen in the anterior and posterior tibialis muscles and in the soleus muscle. Neurovascular bundle is free of tumor.

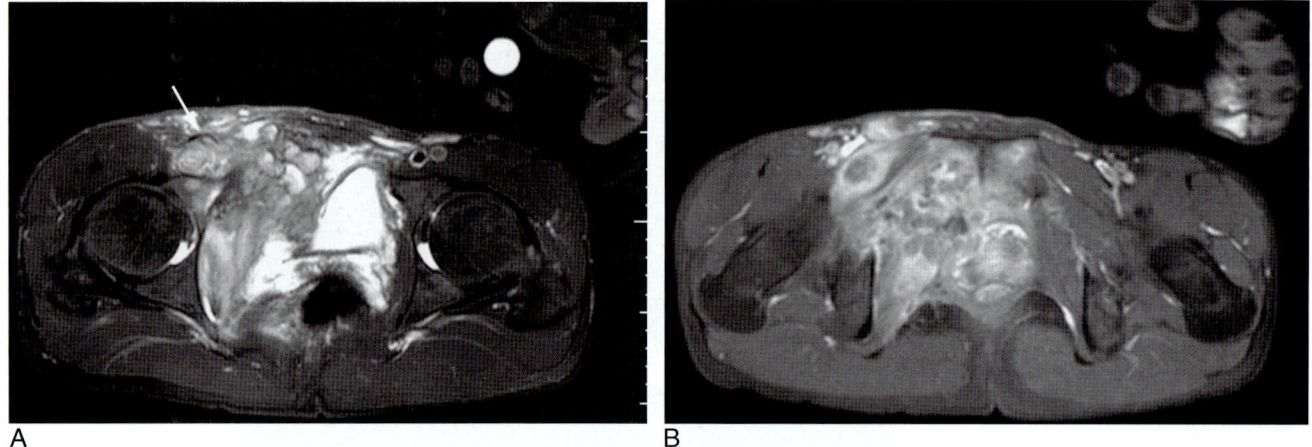

■ **FIGURE 98-11**　Large Ewing's sarcoma in the pelvis. Axial fat-suppressed, T2-weighted (**A**) and fat-suppressed, Gd-chelate–enhanced (**B**) MR images at the different levels. The tumor originates from the acetabulum and extends into the pelvis (internal obturator muscle), displaces and compresses the urinary bladder, extends into the pectineus and iliopsoas muscles anteriorly, and compresses the femoral vein, which is flattened (*arrow*). The femoral artery (lateral to the vein) is not compressed, but tumor is seen anterior to the artery and vein (on **A**).

displaced and invasion is a late event. The presence or absence of fascia is the reason that tumor located in one of the vastus muscles extends easily in the other vastus muscles but does not easily invade the rectus femoris muscle. The reason for this is that no fascia is present between the three vastus muscles, whereas the rectus femoris muscle has its own fascia (see Fig. 98-7). The expansile mode of growth results in the presence of a well-defined pseudocapsule, which is often surrounded by a reactive zone that may contain microscopic tumor, especially in high-grade sarcoma.[18] When the lesion has an infiltrative growth pattern (e.g., in aggressive fibromatosis) rather than the usual expansile pattern, strings of tumor, not visible on MRI, extend beyond the macroscopically detectable tumor margins. The reactive zone, when present, is well seen on MRI outside the well-defined pseudocapsule of the tumor. It is as a rule easily identified because of slightly different signal intensity as compared with that of the tumor and because of the fading outward margins (see Fig. 99-5). When needed, using multiple echos can highlight differences between tumor and reactive zone or Gd-chelate–enhanced MRI. Especially dynamic Gd-chelate–enhanced imaging may provide additional information. The soft tissue component of osseous or soft tissue sarcoma typically enhances within 6 seconds of arterial enhancement in the area of the tumor, whereas the reactive zone enhances later.

Neurovascular Bundle

The neurovascular bundle is invaded by tumor in approximately 10% of patients. It is reported to be higher in soft tissue sarcoma than in bone sarcoma.[19] Neurovascular bundles are more often displaced than encased by tumor. When a fat plane is seen between tumor and neurovascular bundle, the neurovascular bundle is free of tumor. Evaluation is challenging when the fat plane has disappeared and the tumor is in contact with the neurovascular bundle but does not yet encase the bundle (see Figs. 98-8 and 98-10). When contact between tumor and vessels or nerves is less than 180 degrees of the circumference, invasion usually is not present and the nerve, or even vessels, are not fixed to the tumor. In these cases MR angiography may be of help. When no stenosis is seen, invasion of the neurovascular bundle is unusual. The neurovascular bundle may be lifted from the pseudocapsule during surgery, but, especially in high-grade sarcoma, the resection is usually not radical (see Chapter 97).

Encasement of vessels or nerves is rare; but when it occurs, no surgical cleavage plane between these structures and tumor is present (see Figs. 98-11 and 98-12).

The neurovascular bundle is seen to be surrounded by tumor, and on MR angiography a stenosis is typically seen.

The major vessels are easily identified on MRI. The nerves are not always well depicted. It is important to realize that around the knee, where most tumors occur, the sciatic nerve and its branches are located posterior to the popliteal artery and vein. This means that a soft tissue tumor that is located posterior to the popliteal vessels and that is in contact with, or even displaces, these vessels may very well encase the sciatic nerve and its branches. When, however, the tumor lies anterior to the popliteal vessels, the tumor typically does not invade the nerve, because the vessels are between tumor and nerve. Also, the perineurium is a border that is difficult to breach. Invasion of small veins surrounding the tumor are not consistently well visualized with MRI. This is not a clinical problem because these do not extend beyond the reactive zone.

Joints

Joints are invaded in approximately 30% of patients. CT and especially MRI are able to demonstrate joint involvement with high accuracy (Fig. 98-13).[2] False-positive findings can be avoided if pitfalls related to biologic behavior of the tumor are recognized. Anterior to the distal femur,

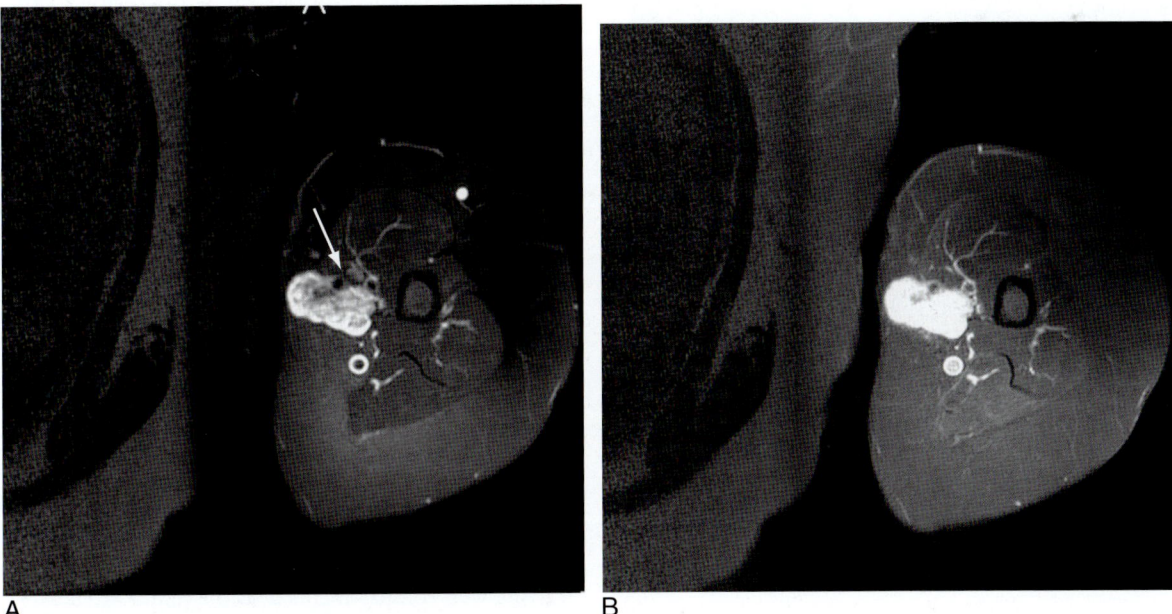

A   B

■ **FIGURE 98-12** The wall of the brachial artery (**A**, *arrow*) is part of this vascular soft tissue tumor (myopericytoma). The tumor surrounds the artery for more than 50%, and there is no cleavage plane visible on T2-weighted, fat-suppressed (**A**) or T1-weighted, fat-suppressed, Gd-chelate–enhanced (**B**) MR images.

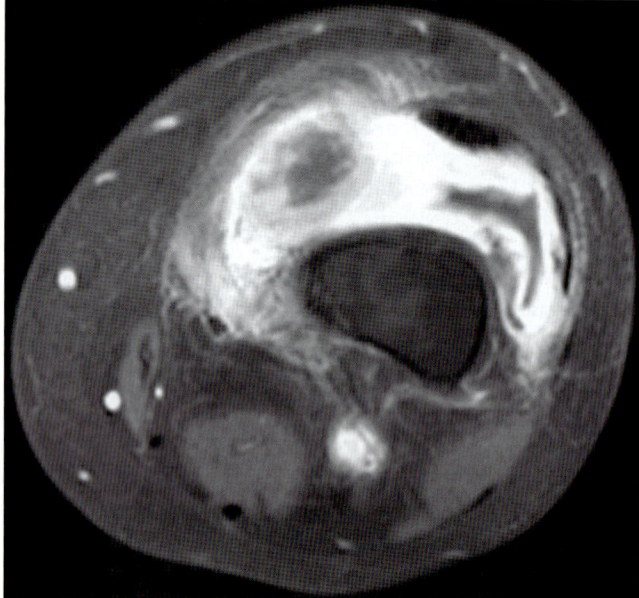

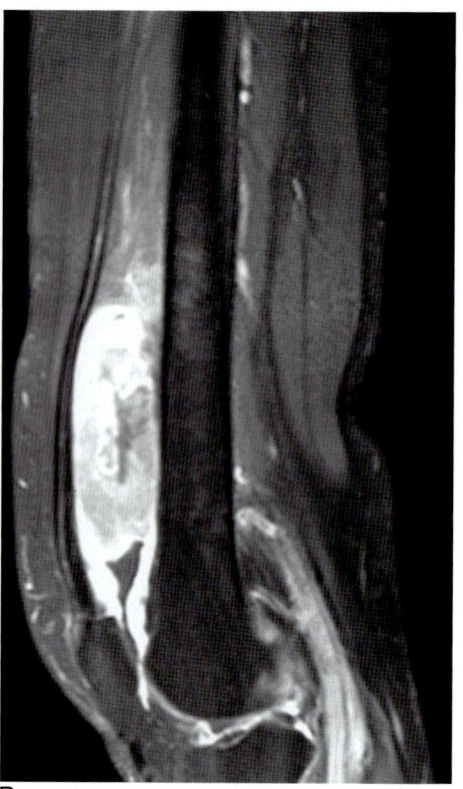

■ **FIGURE 98-13** Leiomyosarcoma in a 69-year-old woman. The enhancing soft tissue tumor invades the enhancing synovium as demonstrated on these axial (**A**) and sagittal (**B**) fat-suppressed, Gd-DTPA–enhanced images. Note the low signal intensity of the synovial fluid. This intra-articular space is distorted.

B

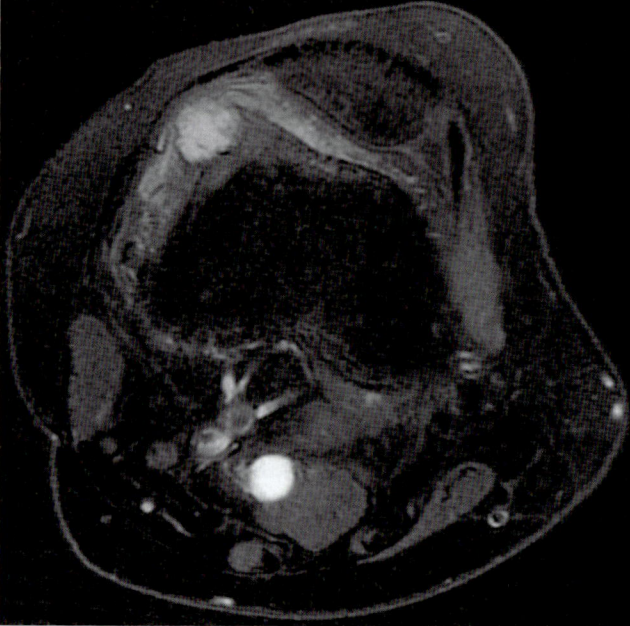

■ **FIGURE 98-14** Juxtacortical chondroma of the distal femur in 53-year-old woman extends into prefemoral fat but does not reach into the articular space, as demonstrated on this axial fat-suppressed, T2-weighted MR image. *(Courtesy of Netherlands Committee on Bone Tumors, Leiden.)*

sarcoma easily extends into the prefemoral fat. This is an extra-articular compartment posterior to the patellar recess. Extension of tumor in the prefemoral fat is frequently mistaken for intra-articular involvement (Fig. 98-14). Insertion of tendons and ligaments are vulnerable areas, because these structures function as scaffolds for soft tissue extension. Cartilage is an effective barrier that is not easily crossed by most tumors. However, osteosarcoma and giant cell tumor have, in contrast to Ewing's sarcoma, the capability to cross cartilage. When joints are immobile, because of either anatomy (sacroiliac joints) or pathology (severe osteoarthritis), tumor crossing such a joint and invading the opposite bone may occur (see Fig. 98-8). Joint effusion with or without hemorrhage can be reactive and is not always a secondary sign of a contaminated joint.

What the Referring Physician Needs to Know

- In what compartments does the tumor extend?
- What is the level of confidence?
- Are there pulmonary metastases?

SUGGESTED READINGS

Berquist TH, Dalinka MK, Alazraki N, et al. Bone tumors. American College of Radiology. ACR Appropriateness Criteria. Radiology 2000; 215(Suppl):261–264.

Bloem JL, van der Woude HJ, Geirnaerdt M, et al. Does magnetic resonance imaging make a difference for patients with musculoskeletal sarcoma? Br J Radiol 1997; 70:327–337.

REFERENCES

1. Enneking WF, Spanier SS, Goodman MA. The surgical staging of musculoskeletal sarcoma. J Bone and Joint Surg Am 1980; 62:1027–1030.
2. Enneking WF, Spanier SS, Goodman MA. A system for the surgical staging of musculoskeletal sarcoma. Clin Orthop Relat Res 2003; 415:4–18.
3. Holscher HC, Bloem JL, Vanel D, et al. Osteosarcoma: chemotherapy-induced changes at MR imaging. Radiology 1992; 182: 839–844.
4. MacVicar AD, Olliff JFC, Pringle J, et al. Ewing's sarcoma: MR imaging of chemotherapy-induced changes with histologic correlation. Radiology 1992; 184:859–864.
5. Van der Woude HJ, Bloem JL, Verstraete KL, et al. Osteosarcoma and Ewing's sarcoma after neoadjuvant chemotherapy: value of dynamic MR imaging in detecting viable tumour before surgery. AJR Am J Roentgenol 1995; 165:593–598.
6. Bloem JL, Taminiau AHM, Eulderink F, et al. Radiologic staging of primary bone sarcoma: MR imaging, scintigraphy, angiography, and CT correlated with pathologic examination. Radiology 1988; 169:805–810.
7. Verstraete KL, van der Woude HJ, Hogendoorn PCW, et al. Dynamic contrast-enhanced MR imaging of musculoskeletal tumours: basic principles and clinical applications. JMRI 1996; 6:311–321.
8. Tofts PS, Brix G, Buckley DL, et al. Estimating kinetic parameters from dynamic contrast-enhanced T1-weighted MRI of a diffusable tracer: standardized quantities and symbols. JMRI 1999; 10:223–232.
9. Grampp S, Bankier AA, Zoubek A, et al. Spiral CT in the lung in children with malignant extra-thoracic tumors: distribution of benign vs malignant pulmonary nodules. Eur Radiol 2000; 10:1318–1322.
10. Anderson MW, Temple HT, Dussault RG, Kaplan PA. Compartmental anatomy relevance to staging and biopsy of musculoskeletal tumors. AJR Am J Roentgenol 1999; 173:1663–1671.
11. van Trommel MF, Kroon HM, Bloem JL, Taminiau AH. MR imaging based strategies in limb salvage surgery for osteosarcoma in the distal femur. Skeletal Radiol 1997; 26(11): 636–641
12. Toomayan GA, Robertson F, Major NM. Lower extremity compartmental anatomy: clinical relevance to radiologists. Skeletal Radiol 2005; 34:307–313.
13. Toomayan GA, Robertson F, Major NM, Brigman BE. Upper extremity compartmental anatomy: clinical relevance to radiologists. Skeletal Radiol 2006; 35:195–201.
14. Onikul E, Fletcher BD, Parham DM, Chen G. Accuracy of MR imaging for estimating intraosseous extent of osteosarcoma. AJR Am J Roentgenol 1996; 167:1211–1215.
15. Gillespy T, Manfrini M, Rugierri P, et al. Staging of intraosseous extent of osteosarcoma: Correlation of preoperative CT and MR imaging with pathologic macroslides. Radiology 1988; 167:765–767.
16. Sajadi KR, Heck RK, Neel MD, et al. The incidence and prognosis of osteosarcoma skip metastases. Clin Orthop Relat Res 2004; 426:92–96.
17. Jiya TU, Wuisman PL. Long-term follow-up of 15 patients with non-metastatic Ewing's sarcoma and a skip lesion. Acta Orthop 2005; 76:899–903.
18. Beltran J, Simon DC, Katz W, Weis LD: Increased MR signal intensity in skeletal muscle adjacent to malignant tumours: pathologic correlation and clinical relevance. Radiology 1987; 162:251–255.
19. Panicek DM, Go SD, Healey JH, et al. Soft tissue sarcoma involving bone or neurovascular structures: MR imaging prognostic factors. Radiology 1997; 205:871–875.

99

Monitoring Therapy in Bone and Soft Tissue Tumors

Catharina S. P. van Rijswijk and Hans L. Bloem

The objectives of treatment of bone and soft tissue sarcomas are described in Chapter 97. Information on effectiveness of treatment plays an important role in the quest for these objectives. Monitoring the response to local or systemic chemotherapy comprises accurate identification and quantification of the proportion of therapy-induced necrosis and residual viable tumor. This may have an impact on prognosis, modification of neoadjuvant (presurgical) treatment protocols, timing and planning of surgery, planning of radiation therapy, and selection of postoperative radiation therapy and/or chemotherapy regimens. Secondly, imaging modalities strongly influence the therapeutic strategies by revealing absence or presence and location of recurrent local, regional, or distant tumor after initial treatment. In this chapter we address histopathologic changes occurring after chemotherapy and radiotherapy as they pertain to imaging response to treatment and identification of recurrent tumor, as well as the corresponding imaging findings and required imaging strategies.

PATHOPHYSIOLOGY

The histologic response to neoadjuvant chemotherapy is one of the most important prognostic factors for patients with bone or soft tissue sarcoma who are scheduled for surgical treatment. Patients whose tumors show little necrosis relative to the fraction of viable tumor after neoadjuvant chemotherapy have poorer survival than patients with tumors that have more chemotherapy-induced necrosis. The amount of spontaneous, or non–chemotherapy-induced necrosis as a result of the tumor outgrowing its blood supply can be quite substantial. Therefore, both histologic and radiologic techniques focus on determination of the fraction of the entire tumor that is still viable

instead of the fraction that is necrotic. Historically, only one or two macrosections of the resected tumor have been used in the pathologic laboratory to determine the fraction of viable tumor. To avoid sample errors that are secondary to this limited analysis, MRI can presently be used by the pathologist to target components of the tumor that are viable, thereby avoiding these errors.

Although the principle of classifying response of musculoskeletal sarcoma to therapy, based on fraction of viable tumor, is the same for all sarcomas, some differences do exist. The basis for the classification system has initially been described for osteosarcoma (Table 99-1).[1] Residual viable tumor in osteosarcoma preferentially persists within the soft tissues, cortical bone and endosteal surface, zones adjacent to cartilage, ligaments, and areas around zones of liquefaction.

KEY POINTS

- DCE MRI allows differentiation between good and poor response.
- Clinical evaluation is key in detecting recurrent tumor.
- MRI is superior to clinical evaluation when physical examination is difficult (retroperitoneum, head and neck) and in aggressive fibromatosis.
- DCE MRI and ultrasonography are pivotal tools in diagnosing recurrent sarcoma.
- Always sample a suspicious mass that was found with MRI.
- Chest CT for lung metastases is required when local recurrence of a sarcoma is proven.
- Timing of follow-up imaging should depend on the patient's risk factors at presentation.

TABLE 99-1 Histologic Classification of Response to Chemotherapy in Osteosarcoma

Grade	Necrosis (%)	Histologic Appearance
I	0–49	Little or no necrosis
II	50–89	Areas of acellular tumor osteoid and/or fibrotic material attributable to the effect of chemotherapy, with other areas of viable tumor
III	90–99	Predominant areas of acellular tumor osteoid and/or fibrotic material attributable to the effect of chemotherapy, with only scattered foci of viable tumor cells
IV	100	No pathologic evidence of viable tumor within the specimen

Data from Huvos AG, Rosen G, Marcove RC. Primary osteogenic sarcoma: pathologic aspects in 20 patients after treatment with chemotherapy en bloc resection, and prosthetic bone replacement. Arch Pathol Lab Med 1977; 101:14–18.

TABLE 99-2 Histologic Classification of Response to Chemotherapy in Ewing's Sarcoma of Bone

Poor Response

Class I	Minimal or no effect of chemotherapy: ≥90% of viable tumor, <10% tumor necrosis
Class II	Moderate effect: solid areas of viable tumor remnants, 10%–90% tumor necrosis or loose hypocellular fibrous tissue

Good Response

Class IIIa	Minimal residual disease: less than 10% viable tumor, localized in small clusters subperiosteally between trabeculae of reactive periosteal bone formation and/or in the soft tissues
Class IIIb	Minimal residual disease: less than 10% viable tumor, localized in small clusters in the intramedullary tumor compartment only
Class IV	No viable tumor cells, only necrosis and/or vascularized fibrous tissue

Data from van der Woude HJ, Bloem JL, van Oostayen JA, et al. Treatment of high-grade bone sarcomas with neoadjuvant chemotherapy: the utility of sequential color Doppler sonography in predicting histopathologic response. AJR Am J Roentgenol 1995; 165:125–133.

The grading system is slightly modified for Ewing's sarcoma (Table 99-2).[2] Sites of predilection for persistence of minimal residual viable tumor in Ewing's sarcoma comprise the subperiosteal area, the intramedullary compartment, the soft tissues, and the zones adjacent to hemorrhagic areas.

Although analysis of resected soft tissue tumors is hampered by the absence of osseous support and structure of the specimen, a similar grading system has been used for soft tissue sarcoma.[3]

Recurrence of tumor is typically diagnosed when residual tumor is detected by imaging techniques or when it becomes symptomatic secondary to growth. Recurrences of both osseous and soft tissue sarcoma typically occur in the soft tissues of the surgical bed. Recurrences of benign osseous tumors are frequently also found in bone because resection margins are smaller than in sarcoma surgery.

IMAGING TECHNIQUES

Dynamic Contrast-Enhanced Magnetic Resonance Imaging

Dynamic contrast-enhanced (DCE) MRI has evolved into an adjunct imaging technique that can be integrated into a standard morphologic imaging protocol. The small molecular contrast agent gadolinium diethylenetriamine-pentaacetic acid (Gd-DTPA) passes from the intravascular space into the interstitium at a rate determined by the permeability of the capillaries, total vascular cross-sectional area, interstitial pressure, volume of extracellular space, contrast agent injection rate, and cardiac output. In DCE MRI, rapid imaging techniques are used to acquire serial images before, during, and after a small, intravenous bolus injection of Gd-chelates such as Gd-DTPA to evaluate the initial distribution of the contrast agent in the capillaries and interstitial space (Fig. 99-1). Gd-chelates decrease, depending on concentration, T1 and T2 relaxation times. At high concentrations T2 shortening is dominant, whereas at lower concentrations T1 shortening is dominant. Because the concentration of Gd-chelate is initially high, first-pass T2-weighted imaging is sensitive to blood flow and blood volume. T1-weighted imaging is sensitive to the low concentrations of Gd-chelates that permeate through the capillary walls and is thus used to measure parameters that reflect permeability. Directly after MR data acquisition is started, a bolus injection of Gd-chelate with a concentration of 0.2 mL/kg at an injection rate of 4 mL/s is intravenously administered. An imaging frequency (temporal resolution) of at least one image per 3 seconds is initially needed to produce at least two data points in the first part of the enhancement curve, with its potentially rapid rise of concentration of the contrast agent in the tumor. The entire first phase lasts 7 to 15 minutes. In addition to obtaining information on the initial enhancement, information on distribution of the contrast agent is obtained by sampling for approximately 5 minutes with a temporal resolution that can be lower than the initial one. Adequate tumor sampling with multiple slices, high spatial resolution, and high temporal resolution are competing parameters. Higher temporal resolution appears to improve the specificity of examinations because of better delineation of differences of signal intensity on the time-intensity curves. High spatial resolution imaging with sufficient high temporal resolution and adequate tumor coverage may improve the detection of small foci of residual viable tumor. Fast or ultrafast MR sequences such as turbo field echo (Philips, Best, the Netherlands), turbo fast low-angle shot (FLASH) (Siemens, Erlangen, Germany), and inversion recovery prepared fast gradient-recalled acquisition in the steady state (GRASS) (General Electric, Milwaukee, WI, USA) allow fast imaging with a sufficiently high temporal and spatial temporal resolution.

Enhancement on T1-weighted DCE MRI can be assessed in two ways: by the analysis of signal intensity changes

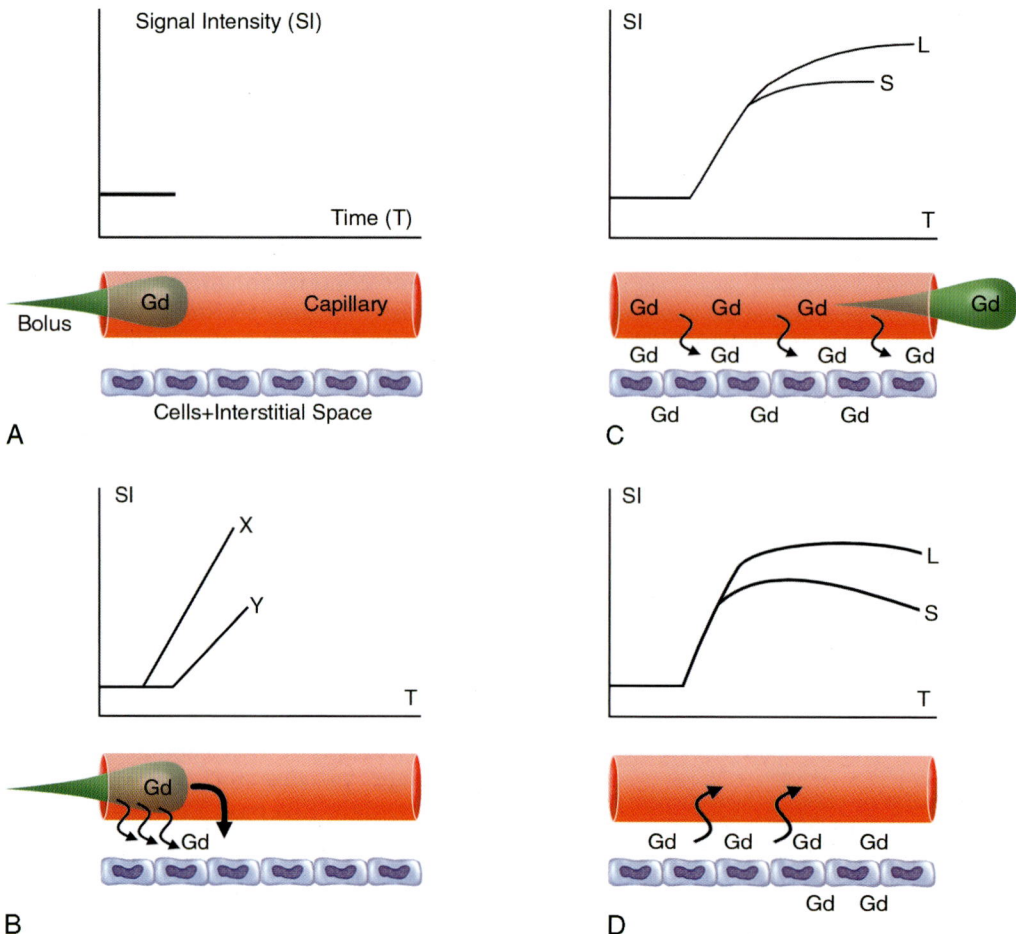

■ **FIGURE 99-1   Factors determining early tissue enhancement.** The lower parts of **A** to **D** show what occurs at the level of the capillary and the interstitial space after intravenous bolus injection; the upper parts graphically display the changes in signal intensity (SI) interval between the intravenous bolus injection and arrival of the bolus in the capillary, which is determined by the injection rate, the heart rate, the localization of the lesion, and the local capillary resistance (tissue perfusion). **C,** The enhancement rate during the first pass of the contrast agent is determined by number of vessels (tissue vascularization), local capillary resistance (tissue perfusion), and capillary permeability. Tissues with high vascularization, perfusion, and capillary permeability (X) will enhance earlier and faster than tissues with less vessels, higher capillary resistance, and lower capillary permeability (Y). **C,** After the first pass of the bolus, the signal intensity increases further until the concentration of the gadolinium contrast medium in the blood and the interstitial space of the tissue are equal. In tissues with a small (S) interstitial space, this equilibrium is reached earlier than in tissues with a larger (L) interstitial space. **D,** As the arterial concentration of the contrast medium decreases, the SI drops while the gadolinium is progressively washed out from the interstitial space. This process occurs faster in tissues with a small (S) interstitial space than in tissues with a large (L) interstitial space. *(Reproduced with permission from Vanhoenacker F, DeSchepper AM, Parizel PM, Gielen J (eds). Imaging Soft Tissue Tumors, 3rd ed. New York, Springer, 2006.)*

(semiquantitative) and/or by quantifying contrast agent concentration change using pharmacokinetic modeling techniques. Signal enhancement can be visually evaluated with the use of subtraction techniques and by using the region of interest (ROI) method. Subtraction images are created by subtraction of precontrast MR images from the gadolinium-chelate enhanced MR images. On these subtraction images, areas within the tumor that enhance fast relative to enhancement of nearby arteries can be identified. By selection of ROIs encircling the whole lesion and the earliest enhancing tumor areas, the signal intensity within this ROI is plotted against time in time-intensity curves (Fig. 99-2). Semiquantitative parameters can be derived from these time-intensity curves. These

parameters include curve shape, onset time (time from arrival of contrast agent in an artery relative to arrival of contrast agent in the tissue of interest), slope of enhancement curves, time to maximum enhancement, maximum enhancement, and wash-out (Fig. 99-3). However, these simplified methods of analyzing enhancement curves in DCE MRI are limited because they may not accurately reflect concentration of contrast agent and are influenced by scanner settings and cardiac output and because comparison between patients and between systems is difficult. Another limitation of the region of interest analysis is the operator-dependent positioning of the ROI that yields only averaged enhancement of the pixels within the area of interest.

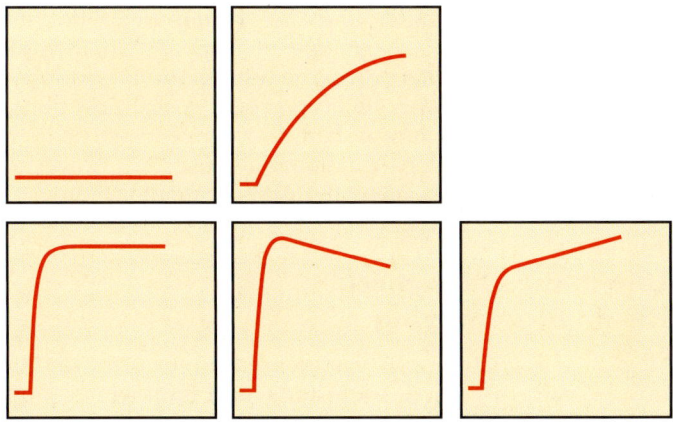

■ **FIGURE 99-2** Classification for subjective assessment of time-intensity curves: type I, no enhancement; type II, gradual increase of enhancement; type III, rapid initial enhancement followed by a plateau phase; type IV, rapid initial enhancement followed by a washout phase; and type V, rapid initial enhancement followed by sustained late enhancement.

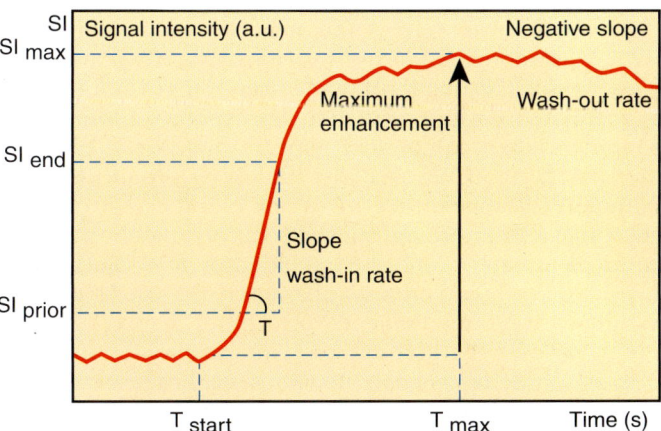

■ **FIGURE 99-3** Time-intensity curve (TIC). In a TIC, the temporal change of the signal intensity in a region of interest (ROI; or pixel) is plotted against time. At T_{start} when the bolus enters the ROI, the signal intensity rises above the baseline signal intensity (SI_{base}). The steepest slope represents the highest enhancement rate during the first pass (wash-in rate) and is mainly determined by tissue vascularization, perfusion, and capillary permeability. At T_{max}, the time of maximum enhancement, capillary and interstitial concentrations reach equilibrium. The time period between the end of the first pass and the maximum enhancement is mainly determined by the volume of the interstitial space. The washout rate can be calculated from the negative slope of the curve. a.u., arbitrary units; T, time interval between SI_{end} and SI_{prior}. *(Reproduced with permission from Vanhoenacker F, DeSchepper AM, Parizel PM, Gielen J [eds]. Imaging Soft Tissue Tumors, 3rd ed. New York, Springer, 2006.)*

Quantitative techniques using pharmacokinetic modeling are preferred. Signal intensity values observed during dynamic acquisition can be used to estimate contrast agent concentration at each time point. Mathematically fitting these data to pharmacokinetic models yields quantitative kinetic parameters. Pharmacokinetic modeling of data in each voxel has been used to quantify the hemodynamic parameters. In first-pass or slope images, all pixels are displayed with intensity equal to the highest enhancement rate (i.e., during the first pass).

A two-compartment model relating the change of tissue tracer concentration to the difference between arterial plasma and interstitial fluid concentrations is most often used. A detailed discussion on pharmacokinetic modeling techniques is beyond the scope of this chapter and can be found elsewhere.[4] A transfer constant K^{trans} (s^{-1}) describes the transendothelial transport of the small molecular contrast agent from the vascular to the interstitial space. Three major factors determine the behavior of the contrast agent in tissues during the first few minutes after injection: blood perfusion, transport of contrast agent across vessel walls, and diffusion of contrast medium in the interstitial space. Changes in the semiquantitative parameters can be used to assess changes in microcirculation during chemotherapy.

Diffusion-Weighted Magnetic Resonance Imaging

In addition to information based on intrinsic MR contrast mechanisms and contrast-enhanced MRI, diffusion-weighted MRI is able to provide an estimate of molecular diffusion in tissues. Diffusion-weighted MRI uses a pulse sequence that is sensitive to motion of protons, also called brownian motion. The extracellular, intracellular, and transcellular random motion of water molecules as well as microcirculation (perfusion) contribute to the MR signal in diffusion MRI. The extracellular component and perfusion contribute most to the signal on diffusion-weighted MRI.[5,6] However, diffusion-weighted sequences not only are sensitive to molecular motion but also are sensitive to bulk motion (moving patient), pulsation of vessels, and intrinsic contrast mechanisms such as T2 contrast (the so-called T2 shine-through). These contrast mechanisms and artifacts can be reduced by special measures in pulse sequence design such as electrocardiographic triggering to reduce pulsation artifacts, fast scanning to reduce bulk motion artifacts, and short echo time (TE) to reduce T2 shine-though, but they have also to be taken into account when analyzing diffusion-weighted images. Different diffusion-weighted sequences have been described: spin-echo, echo-planar imaging, and steady-state free precession (SSFP) sequences.[5]

Recent work with animal models has demonstrated accurate differentiation between viable and necrotic tumor in soft tissue sarcoma and osteogenic sarcoma by the use of diffusion-weighted MRI.[7] There is more diffusion in necrotic tissue than in viable tumor, because there are more cell boundaries and there is a smaller extracellular space in viable tumor relative to necrotic tissue. More diffusion means more destructive dephasing of spins, resulting in lower signal intensity. Increased diffusion in necrotic tissue can be displayed as signal loss on diffusion images relative to images without the gradient settings that introduce sensitivity to diffusion. Alternatively, an increase in diffusion can be displayed as an increase in signal on apparent diffusion coefficient images. This technique has been used in experimental settings and may become an additional tool to allow monitoring of response to treatment.

Ultrasonography

Color Doppler ultrasonography can provide clinically relevant information related to tumor vasculature but is currently not widely used for monitoring response to chemotherapy in musculoskeletal tumors. Ultrasonography is a low-cost, noninvasive, and readily available modality, but considerable operator expertise is required and the technique is prone to interobserver and intraobserver variation. Doppler ultrasonography can only depict blood flow in relatively large vessels and is not sensitive to blood vessels smaller than 100 μm in diameter.[8] Absence of detectable intratumoral blood flow can thus not only reflect absence of flow but also may be secondary to flow that is below the minimal threshold of detection.

In malignant tumors, two different Doppler signals have been identified that may coexist in the same tumor. The first is a high-systolic Doppler shift corresponding to high peak-systolic velocities with or without enhanced diastolic flow arising from arteriovenous shunting. The second Doppler signal is a low impedance signal with little or no variation between systole and diastole and spectral broadening, which is associated with low-resistance flow secondary to the presence of thin-walled sinusoidal spaces. Angiogenesis results in the formation of tumor vessels that lack a muscular wall and that are therefore incapable of building up hemodynamic resistance. Both Doppler signals thus relate to the histologic structure and hemodynamic properties of tumor circulation. Abnormal newly formed tumor vessels are most prevalent at the tumor periphery but can also be encountered in the center of the tumor.

Recent technical improvements of instrumentation with higher signal-to-noise ratio as well as the advent of micron-sized gas-filled microbubble based contrast agents that are true intravascular contrast agents will improve the threshold to lower blood volume and slower flow and give direct and indirect information on tumor neovascularity and response to therapy. The results of estimating blood volume by ultrasound imaging using microbubble contrast agents have been shown to correlate with estimates derived from MR data.[9] Visualization of the vasculature may further be enhanced with the use of harmonic imaging, which utilizes the ability of microbubbles to oscillate nonlinearly. In addition, microbubbles labeled with agents that bind to angiogenic markers, such as $\alpha_v\beta_3$ integrin, are useful for molecular imaging of angiogenic vasculature. Animal studies and phase 1 clinical trials have demonstrated differences in flow and vascular volume in tumors at different stages during antiangiogenic therapy. Prospective clinical studies are needed to determine whether this will result in real diagnostic improvement.

MONITORING THERAPY

Conventional Radiography

Conventional radiographs are not uniformly considered to be useful in monitoring chemotherapy. Although gross increase in volume, associated with progressive destruction of normal bone, usually is indicative of poor response, other changes such as changes in host reaction (periosteal reaction, calcification) or changes within the tumor itself (calcification, ossification, fracture, hemorrhage) do not correlate with histologic grading of response. In Ewing's sarcoma, a marked reduction of the soft tissue tumor component in association with solidification of periosteal new bone, reconstitution of the cortical shaft, and reappearance of intramedullary trabeculations is commonly observed. However, this also does not correlate with histologic grading.[10,11]

Unenhanced Magnetic Resonance Imaging

Magnetic resonance criteria such as tumor size, definition of margins, signal intensities, and homogeneity on T1- and T2-weighted MR images have been used in assessing response to chemotherapy. However, it is currently not proven that we can accurately predict response prior to, or shortly after, the start of chemotherapy using unenhanced MRI. Only an increase in tumor volume not caused by massive hemorrhage within the tumor correlates with a poor histologic response. An unchanged or decreasing tumor volume is not predictive for a good response. Even the earlier described, marked reduction of the soft tissue component observed in the majority of patients with Ewing's sarcoma is not indicative of good response. The presence of a residual soft tissue mass after chemotherapy is correlated with poor histologic response. Also, microscopic residual tumor foci may be multi-drug resistant and are therefore associated with a poor prognosis. Only complete disappearance of tumor is indicative of good response and improved survival. Unfortunately, minimal residual disease cannot be excluded by MRI. Because of overlapping signal intensity characteristics on T1- and T2-weighted MRI, unenhanced MRI cannot be used to accurately predict the amount of tumor necrosis. Although necrosis, based on signal intensities, cannot be accurately differentiated from other tissue types, an increase of signal intensity on T2-weighted MR images after chemotherapy in Ewing's sarcoma may represent tumor necrosis, cystic hemorrhage, or replacement of tumor by a hypocellular mucomyxoid matrix. Mucoid may be the cause of high signal intensity on T1-weighted images and is more frequently seen on post- than on pre-chemotherapy images. The increase of signal intensity on T2-weighted images, basically reflecting liquefaction, may indicate a favorable histologic response. Increase of peritumoral (outside the low signal intensity pseudocapsule) edema has been correlated with poor histologic response. Decrease of peritumoral edema is a common finding that is not correlated with a favorable histologic response.[12,13]

Contrast-Enhanced Magnetic Resonance Imaging

Comparison of unenhanced and contrast-enhanced MR images after intravenous administration of Gd-chelates improves distinction of different components within the tumor. These contrast-enhanced MR images generally assist in identifying solid enhancing tumor parts and nonenhancing cystic, liquefied, hemorrhagic, or necrotic components. However, these contrast-enhanced MR images are not sufficiently specific because remnant viable tumor tissue cannot be differentiated from early immature granulation tissue, neovascularity in necrotic areas, and reactive hyperemia. Moreover, the small molecular agent Gd-DTPA passes from the intravascular space to the interstitium of tissues, resulting in an overestimation of the amount of residual viable tumor and, thus, inaccurate discrimination between good and poor histologic response.[14]

Fast DCE MRI has been reported to be a valuable technique for the identification and localization of residual viable tumor after chemotherapy and improves differentiation between good and poor response in bone and soft tissue sarcomas. Under therapy, changes in capillary permeability (time intensity curve shape and slope) and vascular density (maximum enhancement) are often observed before changes in tumor volume. Direct visual inspection of the (subtraction) images before and after chemotherapy allows easy detection of highly vascular and/or highly perfused viable tumor tissue. When more than 10% of the total tumor volume enhances early (defined as enhancement within 6 seconds after arterial enhancement), a poor response with more than 10% of tumor tissue remaining viable should be suspected. This subjective assessment should be verified by producing time-intensity curves by the ROI method. Areas of early and rapidly progressive enhancement (steep slopes) confirmed by type III, IV, or V time-intensity curves (see Fig. 99-2) correspond with more rapid uptake of the contrast agent, owing to increased vascularization and perfusion associated with presence of viable tumor. Areas within the tumor demonstrating late and gradual or absence of enhancement confirmed by type I or II time-intensity curves reflect the presence of nonviable tumor tissue (Figs. 99-4 and 99-5; Table 99-3).

There are several pitfalls to take into account. In the early phase of chemotherapy young granulation tissue replacing tumor necrosis may enhance early. Small, early, and rapidly progressive enhancing lines may represent (subperiostally) arterioles or small physeal vessels. Scattered tumor cells without formation of tumor nests cannot be depicted because of limitations of spatial resolution. This is more important for Ewing's sarcoma than for osteosarcoma, because of the earlier described histopathologic response. In first-pass or slope images, all pixels are displayed with intensity equal to the highest enhancement rate (i.e., during the first pass). Using this method, an estimate of the relative volume of residual viable tumor in osteosarcoma and Ewing's sarcoma after neoadjuvant chemotherapy can be made.[15,16] Moreover, according to recent literature, alterations of the transfer constant K^{trans} seems to be the most important parameter of therapy response, indicating the importance of pharmacokinetic modeling.

Ultrasonography

The value of color Doppler ultrasonography with spectral analysis has been demonstrated in patients with osteogenic or Ewing's sarcomas with an associated soft tissue mass. Blood flow parameters that can be measured by spectral analysis include peak velocity, mean velocity, volume flow rate, pulsatility index, and resistive index

([peak systolic velocity/end-diastolic velocity]/peak systolic velocity). Response to neoadjuvant chemotherapy can be reliably predicted after two cycles but not sooner (Fig. 99-6). In a good respondent a vascular tumor with low vascular resistive index in feeding arteries changes into a system with an increase, or even normalization, of resistive index and a decrease of flow and shunting in the tumor. In good respondents, the resistive indices calculated in the tumor-feeding artery are almost equal to the resistive indices in the contralateral reference artery. Apparently, increase of peripheral resistance corresponds to the reduction or disappearance of intratumoral high-velocity Doppler shifts, which indicates the reduced need for attracting blood from the host's circulation in chemotherapy-sensitive tumors (Table 99-4).[17]

Early studies demonstrate the potential of Doppler ultrasonography with microbubble-based contrast agents in evaluating tumor response to chemotherapy. A decrease of contrast uptake the day after isolated limb perfusion with high-dose chemotherapy and tumor necrosis factor has been reported to correlate with a favorable histologic response. No ultrasound parameters have been reported that can predict the response to therapy before the start of treatment.

Positron Emission Tomography

Because of the increased glucose metabolism in sarcoma, ^{18}F-deoxyglucose positron emission tomography (FDG-PET) has been advocated as a method to assess response to chemotherapy. Changes in tumor accumulation of FDG during and after neoadjuvant therapy have been reported to reflect tissue viability (Fig. 99-7). However, a recent meta-analysis of the results of FDG-PET concluded that routine use in the standard treatment of sarcomas is currently unjustified. The exact value is still unclear and needs to be further explored. False-positive FDG uptake has been observed in complete respondents as a result of uptake within benign therapy-induced fibrous tissue. Moreover, significant FDG uptake has also been observed at sites of uncontaminated incisional biopsy. Other disadvantages of FDG-PET in routine clinical monitoring of response to chemotherapy are its limited availability and high cost. The limited spatial resolution requires complementary CT or MRI (image fusion or CT-PET, respectively MR-PET) to localize an area of increased accumulation.

IMAGING POST-THERAPEUTIC CHANGES AND RECURRENCES

Benign Bone Tumors

Imaging of the postoperative recurrence of benign bone lesions basically follows the same principles as imaging of the primary lesions. Special considerations have to be made in the diagnosis of recurrent giant cell tumor, osteoid osteoma, and benign cartilaginous tumors. The accepted therapy for the majority of benign bone tumors is curettage and filling of the surgical defect with bone graft or cement. In the locally aggressive tumors, such as giant cell tumors, the use of adjuvant agents as phenol or liquid nitrogen has been recommended after curettage. The incidence of local recurrence of giant cell tumor

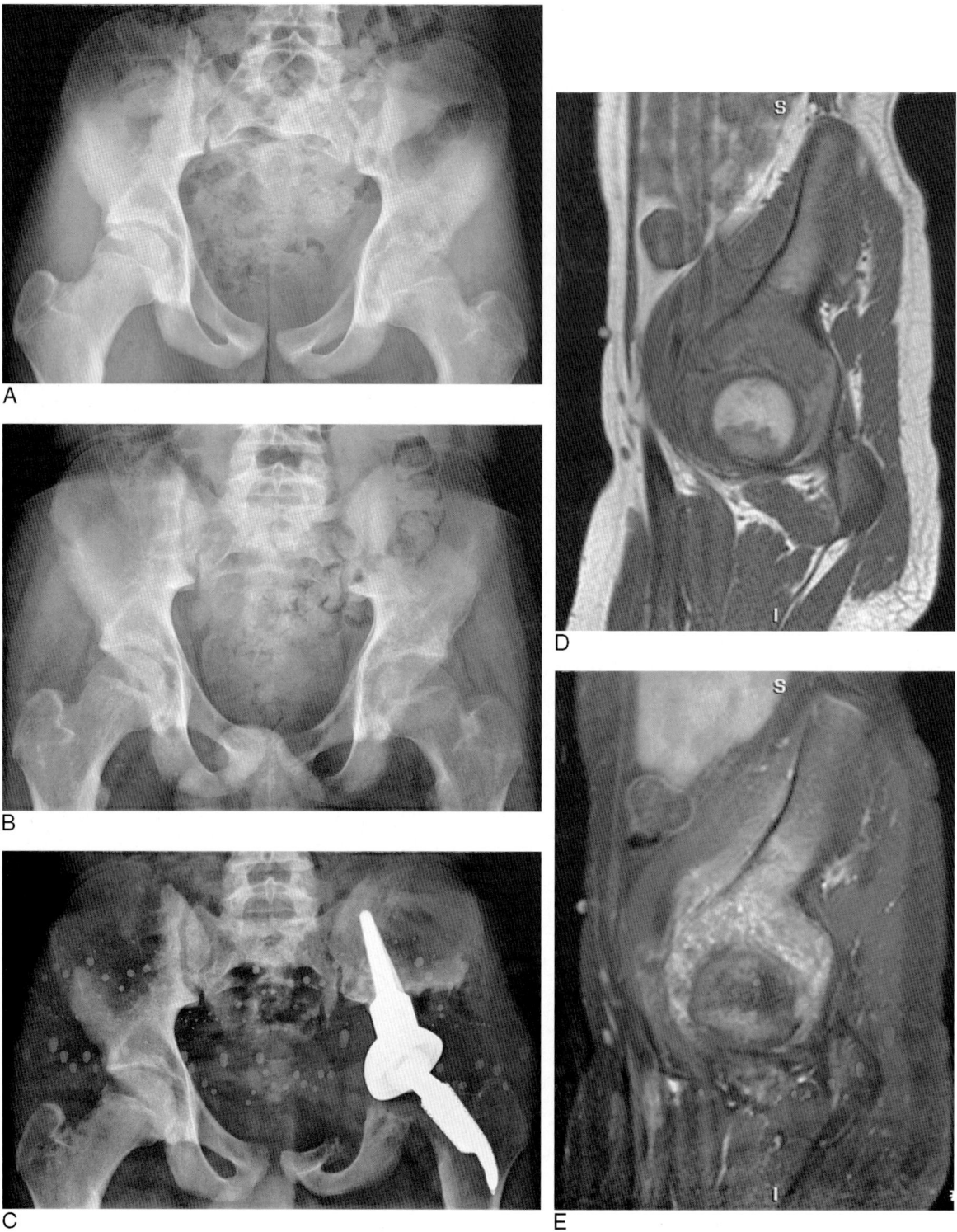

■ **FIGURE 99-4** A 14-year-old boy presented with Ewing's sarcoma in the left acetabulum that responded well to chemotherapy. Conventional radiographs of the pelvis before treatment (**A**), after six cycles of neoadjuvant chemotherapy (**B**), and after radical excision and reconstruction with Pedestal cup prosthesis (**C**). Sagittal T1-weighted MR images before (**D**) and after (**E**) contrast medium injection at initial presentation. Note minor tumor extension in the surrounding soft tissues.

(Continued)

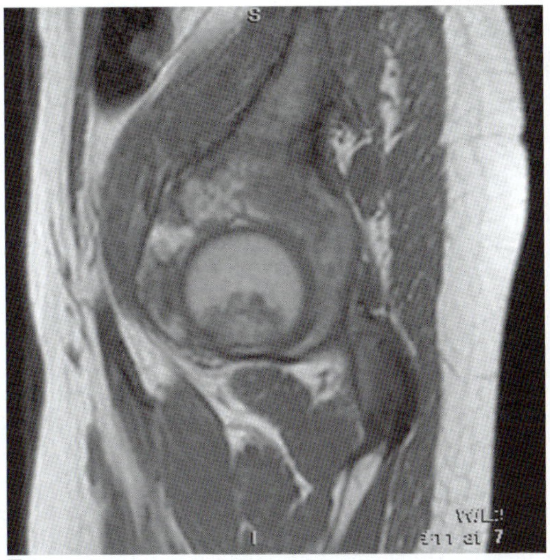

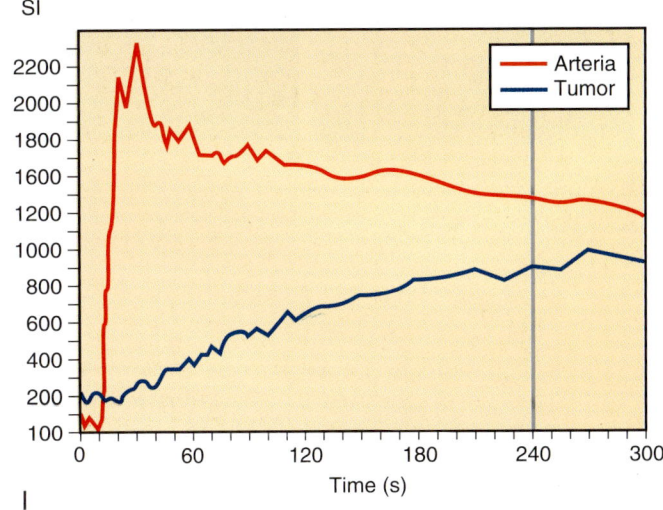

■ **FIGURE 99-4—Cont'd** Sagittal T1-weighted MR images before (**F**) and after (**G**) contrast medium injection after six cycles of neoadjuvant chemotherapy. **H,** Consecutive sagittal dynamic contrast-enhanced subtraction MR images taken every 3 seconds demonstrate no early tumor enhancement suggestive of nonviable tumor tissue. Only enhancement of the artery is seen on the early images. **I,** The time-intensity curve of a region within the tumor demonstrates gradual enhancement. Only tumor necrosis and fibrofatty vascular tissue without viable tumor were found at histopathologic examination of the resected tumor.

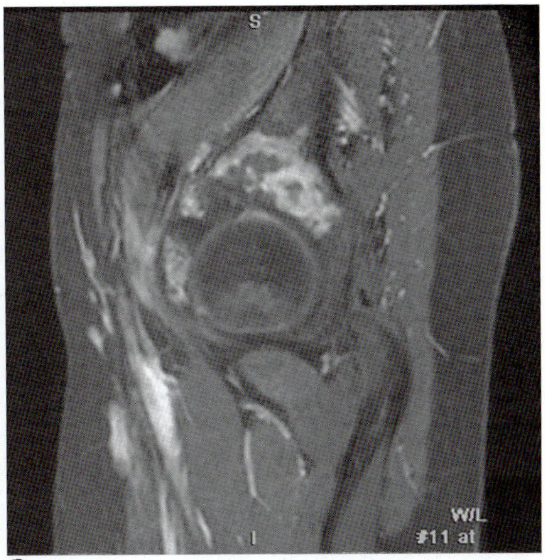

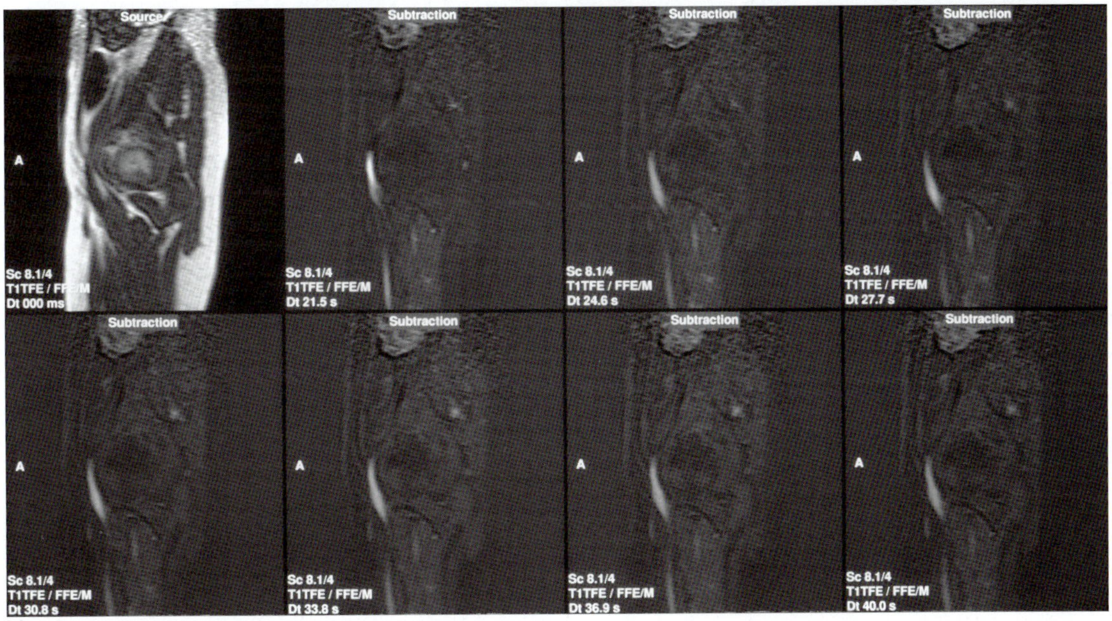

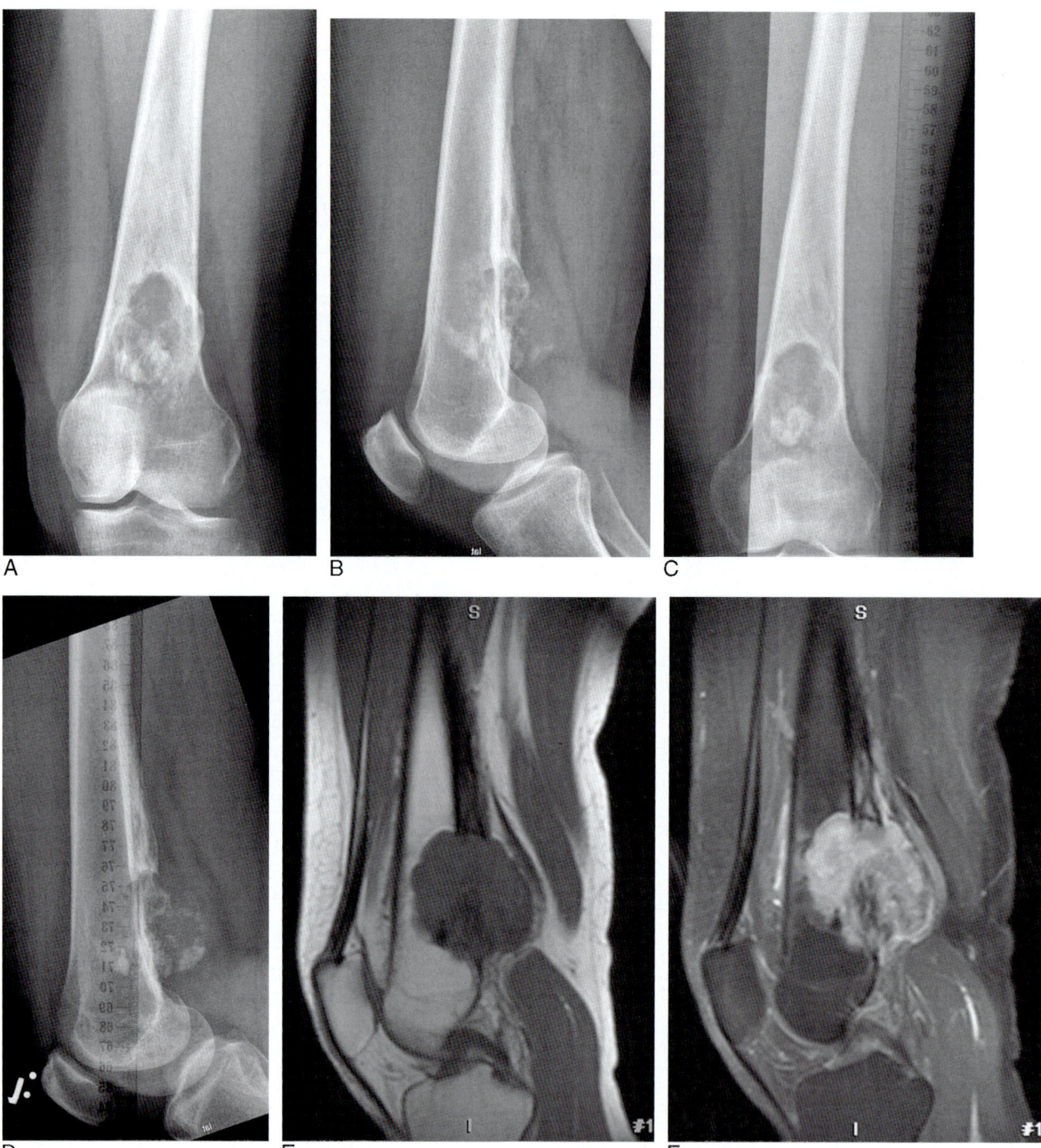

■ **FIGURE 99-5** A 45-year-old woman presented with an osteosarcoma in the left distal femur that did not respond well to chemotherapy. Conventional radiographs of the distal femur before treatment (**A** and **B**) and after 3 cycles of neoadjuvant chemotherapy (**C** and **D**). Sagittal T1-weighted MR images before (**E**) and after (**F**) contrast medium injection obtained at initial presentation.

(Continued)

after curettage has been reported to be 20% to 50%. Most of them occur in the first 2 years after treatment, but late recurrences after 5 years do occur. Local recurrence can be diagnosed when progressive or new focal bone destruction at the previous resection margin and/ or bone-cement interface is detected. Progressive resorption of the bone graft material seen on sequential conventional radiographs is also a sign of recurrence. This must be distinguished from the normal smooth and symmetric radiolucent zone (usually < 2 mm) surrounding the cement. This lucent zone is secondary to retraction and the cytotoxic effect of hot cement at the bone-cement interface. Normally, the radiolucent area demonstrates a surrounding rim of sclerosis and does not progress after 6 to 8 months postoperatively.[18] Moreover, bone grafts may normally demonstrate resorption or incomplete

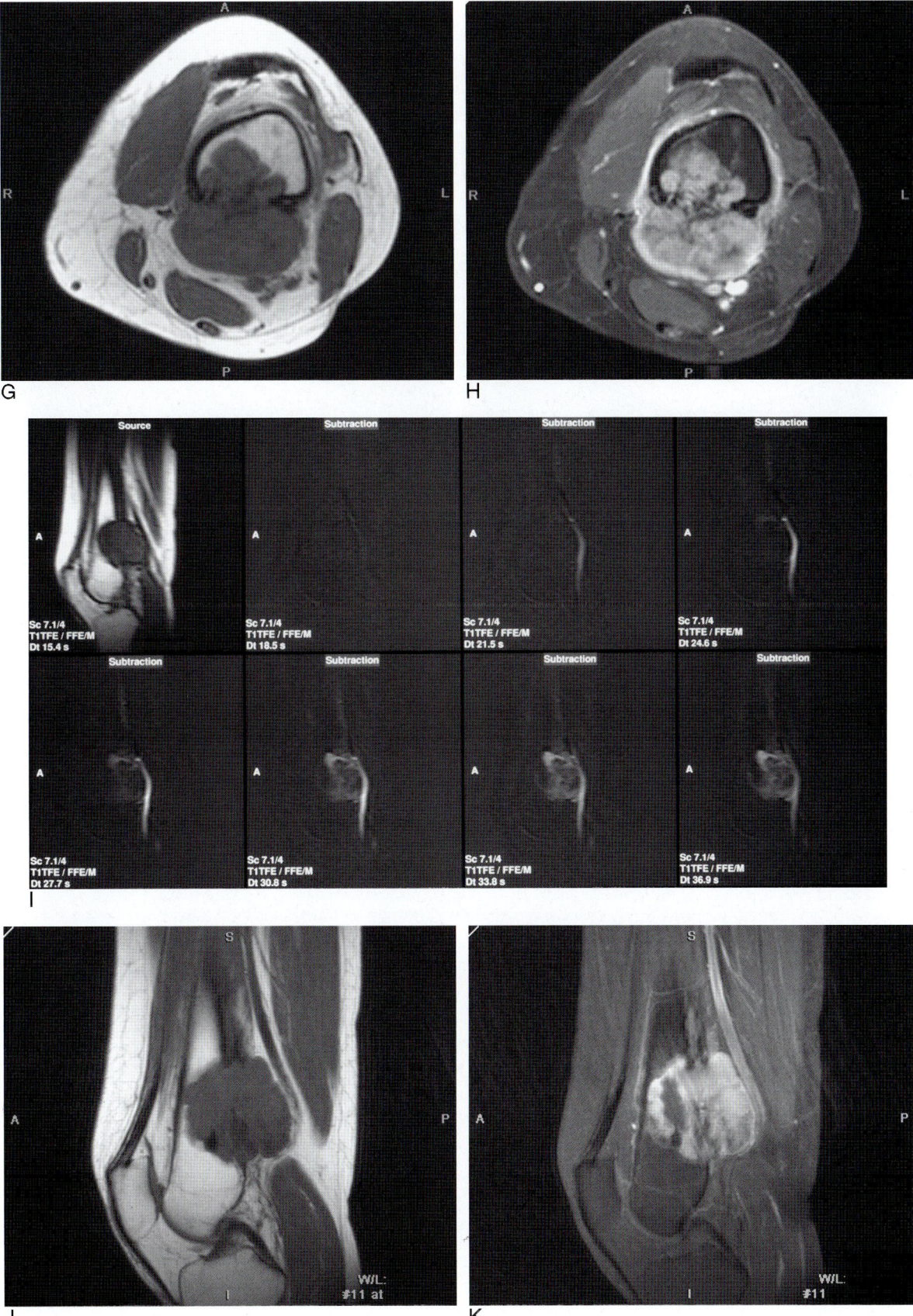

■ **FIGURE 99-5—Cont'd** Transverse T1-weighted MR images before (**G**) and after (**H**) contrast medium injection obtained at initial presentation. **I,** Consecutive sagittal dynamic contrast-enhanced subtraction MR images demonstrate extensive areas with early tumor enhancement. Sagittal T1-weighted MR images before (**J**) and after (**K**) contrast medium injection obtained after three cycles of neoadjuvant chemotherapy.

(Continued)

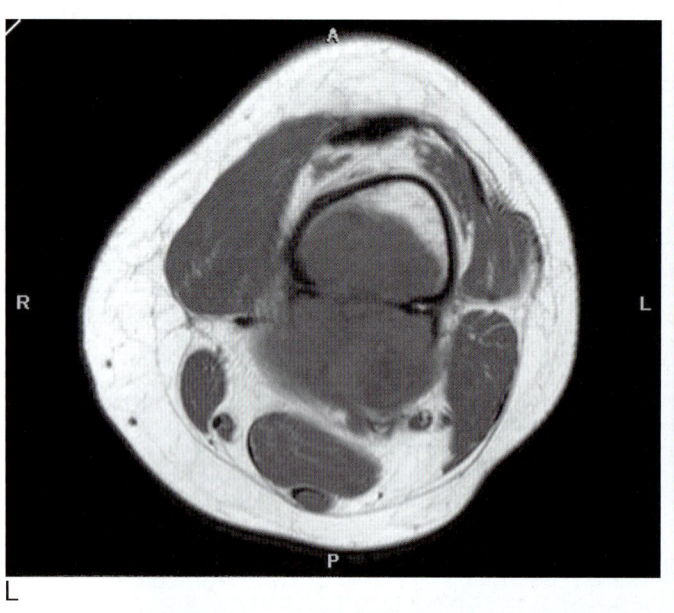

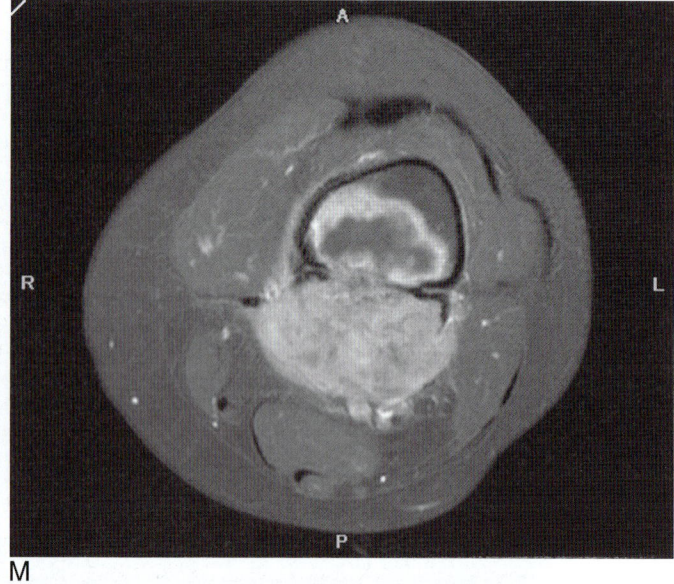

L M

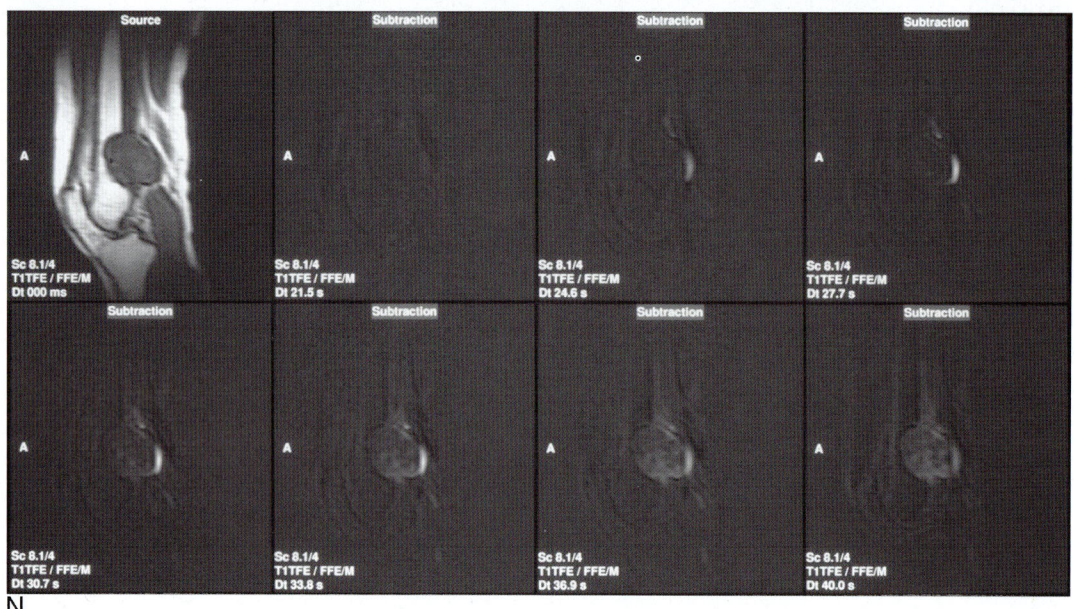

N

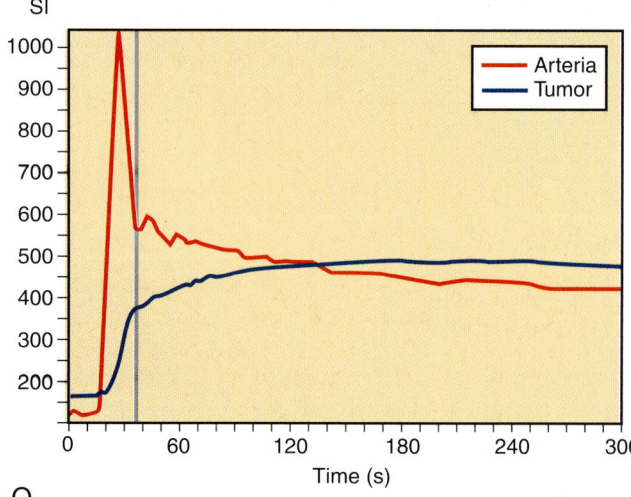

O

■ **FIGURE 99-5—Cont'd** Transverse T1-weighted MR images before (**L**) and after (**M**) contrast medium injection obtained after three cycles of neoadjuvant chemotherapy. **N,** Consecutive sagittal dynamic contrast-enhanced subtraction MR images demonstrate extensive areas with early tumor enhancement indicating viable tumor. **O,** The time-intensity curve of a region within early enhancing tumor demonstrates rapidly progressive enhancement followed by a plateau phase. Histopathologic examination of the resected specimen demonstrated poor response.

TABLE 99-3 Correlation of MR Parameters with Response to Neoadjuvant Chemotherapy in Ewing's and Osteogenic Sarcomas

MR Parameters	Response to Neoadjuvant Chemotherapy	
	Good	Poor
Ewing's Sarcoma		
Tumor volume	No tumor detectable	Residual or increase of soft tissue mass
Signal intensity	Increase of intramedullary homogeneous signal intensity on T2-weighted MRI	No correlation
Early enhancement on DCE MRI indicating viable tumor	Complete disappearance of viable tumor or minimal residual tumor	More than 10% viable tumor
Osteosarcoma		
Tumor volume	No correlation	Increase
Peritumoral edema	No correlation	Increase
Early enhancement on DCE MRI indicating viable tumor	Less than 10% viable tumor	More than 10% viable tumor

Good response is defined as less than 10% viable tumor (Classification III and IV).

incorporation with radiolucent areas at radiography. Both CT and MRI are helpful in identifying the progressive bone destruction that is expected in recurrent giant cell tumors. However, MRI is more specific in differentiating early recurrence of giant cell tumors from postoperative changes such as fibrous scarring and granulation tissue at the bone-cement interface or heterogeneous marrow changes seen in incomplete bone graft incorporation. Recurrent giant cell tumor is diagnosed, using DCE MRI, when solid nodules displaying rapid (within 6 seconds after arterial enhancement) contrast enhancement in combination with immediate wash-out on time intensity curves are seen. The enhancement characteristics are identical to those of untreated giant cell tumor. Incomplete bone graft incorporation will demonstrate more heterogeneous diffuse marrow changes.[19]

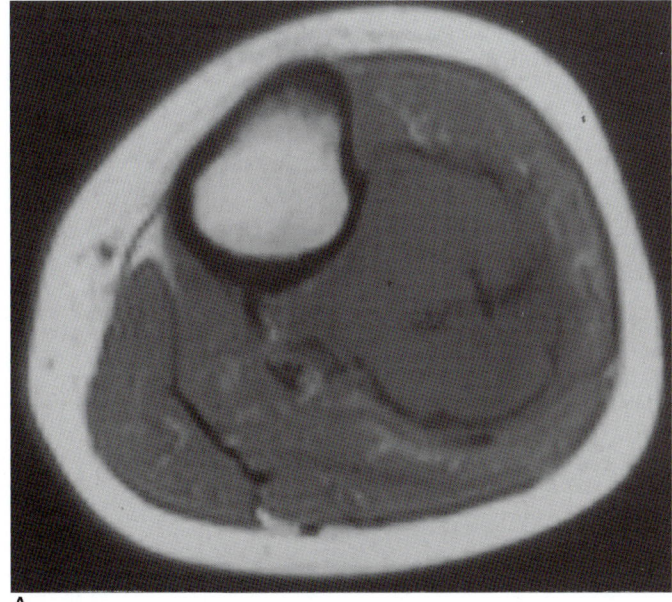

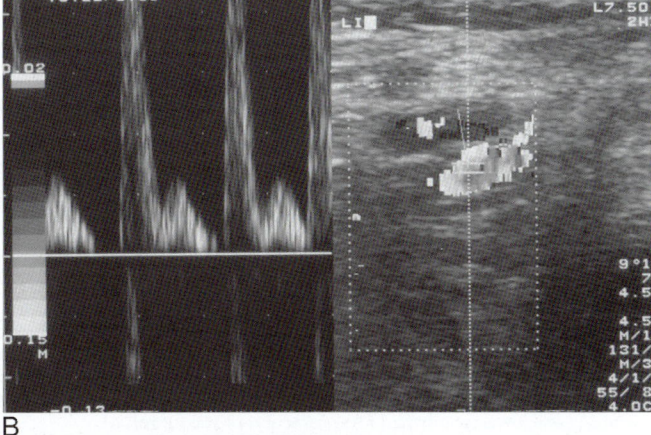

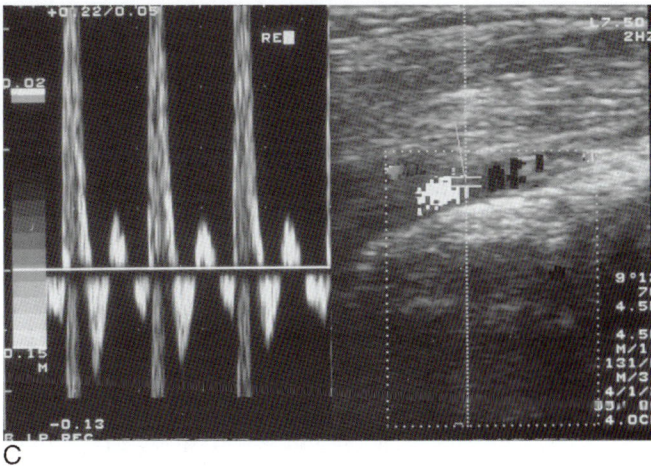

■ **FIGURE 99-6** A 17-year-old young woman presented with osteosarcoma of proximal fibula that did not respond well to chemotherapy. **A,** T1-weighted turbo spin-echo MR image demonstrates the tumor with intermediate signal intensity compared with muscle with a large accompanying soft tissue mass. **B,** Doppler spectrum obtained in the popliteal artery feeding the tumor-bearing lower leg. There is a biphasic flow pattern with positive diastole, consistent with presence of significant low-resistance tumor. **C,** Flow spectrum in contralateral popliteal artery shows normal triphasic pattern, with flow in the opposite direction during diastole.

(Continued)

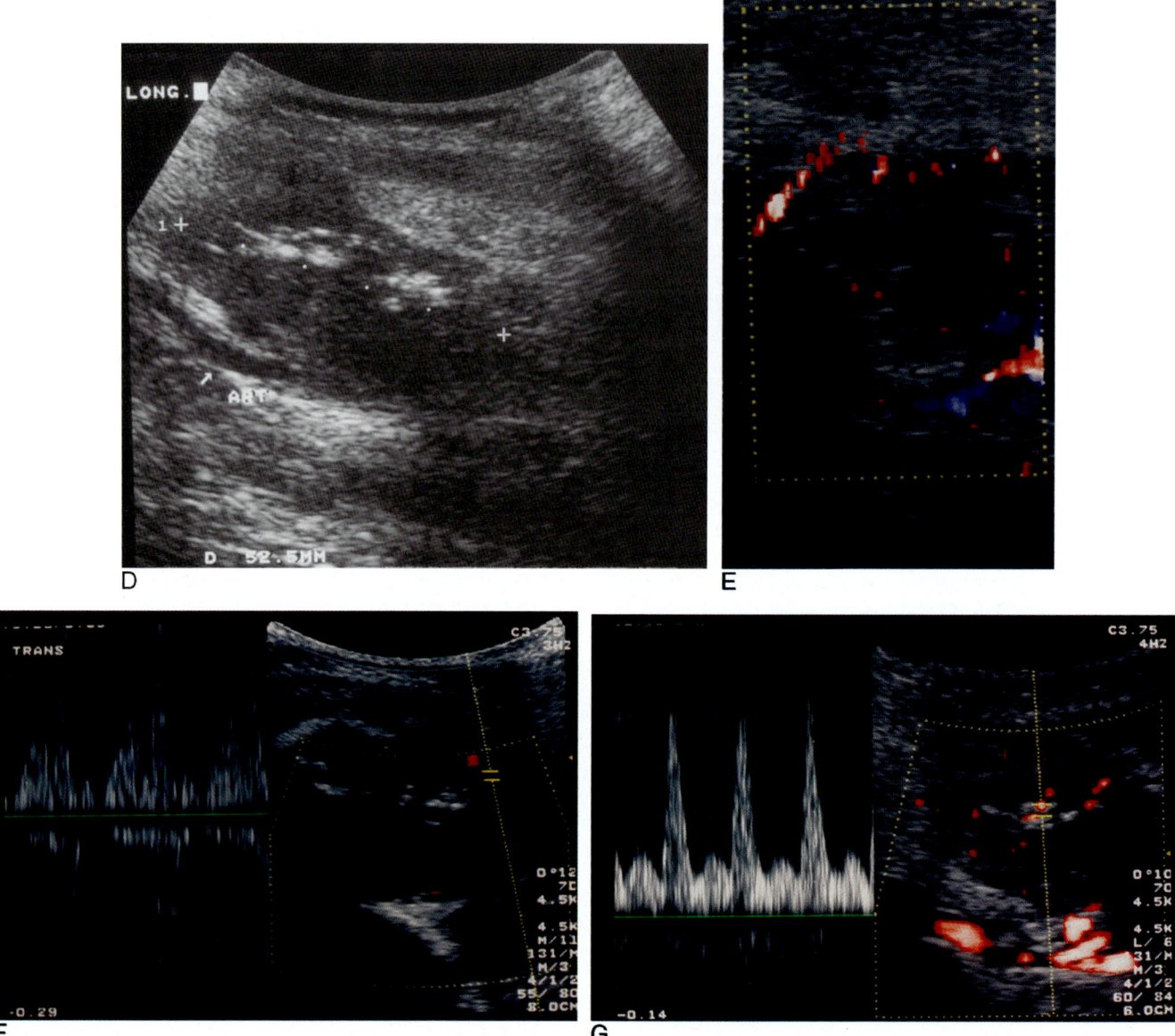

■ **FIGURE 99-6—Cont'd   D,** Heterogeneous sonographic appearance of the soft tissue mass before chemotherapy. **E,** Color Doppler flow image of the soft tissue mass before chemotherapy shows peripheral (capsular) vessels with high-velocity signals (*white color*). **F,** Abnormal Doppler shifts within the soft tissue mass with high velocities in both systole and diastole (aliasing due to high velocities) before chemotherapy. **G,** After three cycles of chemotherapy there are persistent abnormal signals within remaining large soft tissue mass, consistent with incomplete (poor) histologic response, which was confirmed after resection of the tumor.

TABLE 99-4   Doppler Ultrasound Parameters in Ewing's or Osteogenic Sarcomas with an Associated Soft Tissue Mass Related to Response to Neoadjuvant Chemotherapy

Ultrasound Parameters	Response to Neoadjuvant Chemotherapy	
	Good	Poor
Intratumoral flow	Decrease	Increase or unchanged
Arteriovenous shunting	Decrease of high systolic Doppler shifts	Persistence of high systolic Doppler shifts
Flow pattern in feeding artery	Normalization to triphasic	Biphasic with positive end-diastolic velocity
Resistive index in feeding artery	Increase or normalization	Decrease or no change

Good response is defined as less than 10% viable tumor (Classification III and IV).

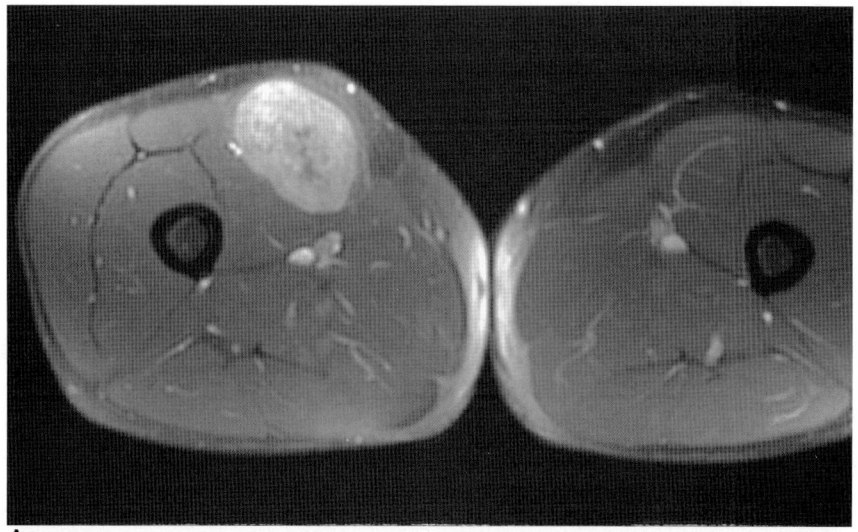

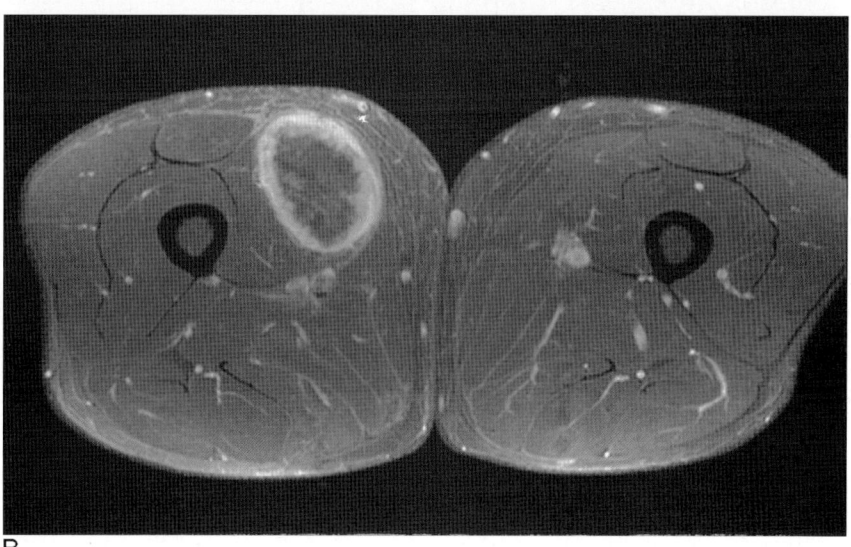

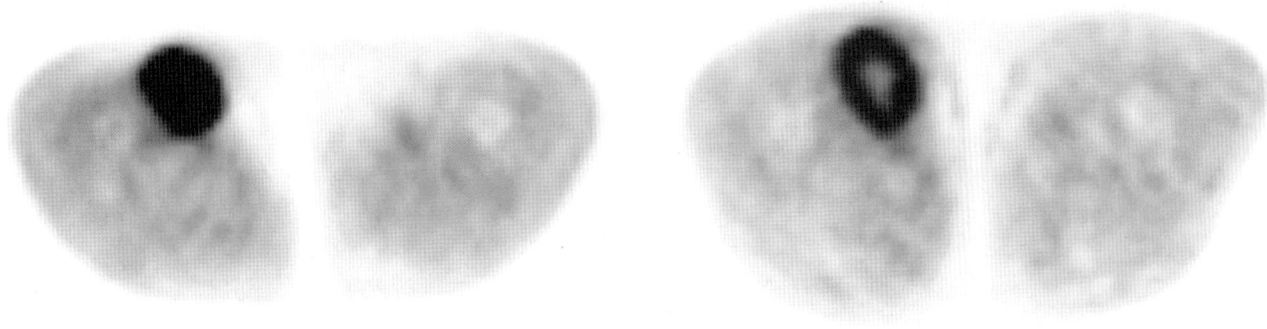

■ FIGURE 99-7 A 48-year-old man presented with an extraskeletal mesenchymal chondrosarcoma in the upper leg. Transverse T1-weighted MR images with fat suppression after injection of Gd-DTPA before (**A**) and after (**B**) 50 Gy of radiation therapy. A large soft tissue mass is displayed with marked enhancement before radiation therapy. After radiation therapy there is no significant reduction of tumor volume but the central part of the tumor no longer enhances. **C,** Transverse FDG PET image reveals homogeneous increased accumulation before radiation therapy. **D,** Absence of central accumulation in the mass reflects necrosis after radiation therapy (activity decrease of 30%), confirmed on histologic examination after local resection. *(Case courtesy of Dr. M. Kartachova, Antoni van Leeuwenhoek Hospital, Amsterdam.)*

Recurrence of osteoid osteoma after surgical resection or percutaneous ablation with radiofrequency is characterized by persistence and/or reappearance of pain or impaired function, identical to or resembling the presenting complaints. Morphologic criteria such as remodeling are not very useful because these changes toward normal structure occur at a pace that is much slower than persistence or recurrence of symptoms. Only rapid enhancement within 3 to 6 seconds after arterial enhancement seen on DCE MRI allows a confident radiologic diagnosis of recurrence to be made. Thin-section CT is used to identify the treated, but symptomatic nidus, allowing targeting for repeated thermal ablation (Fig. 99-8).

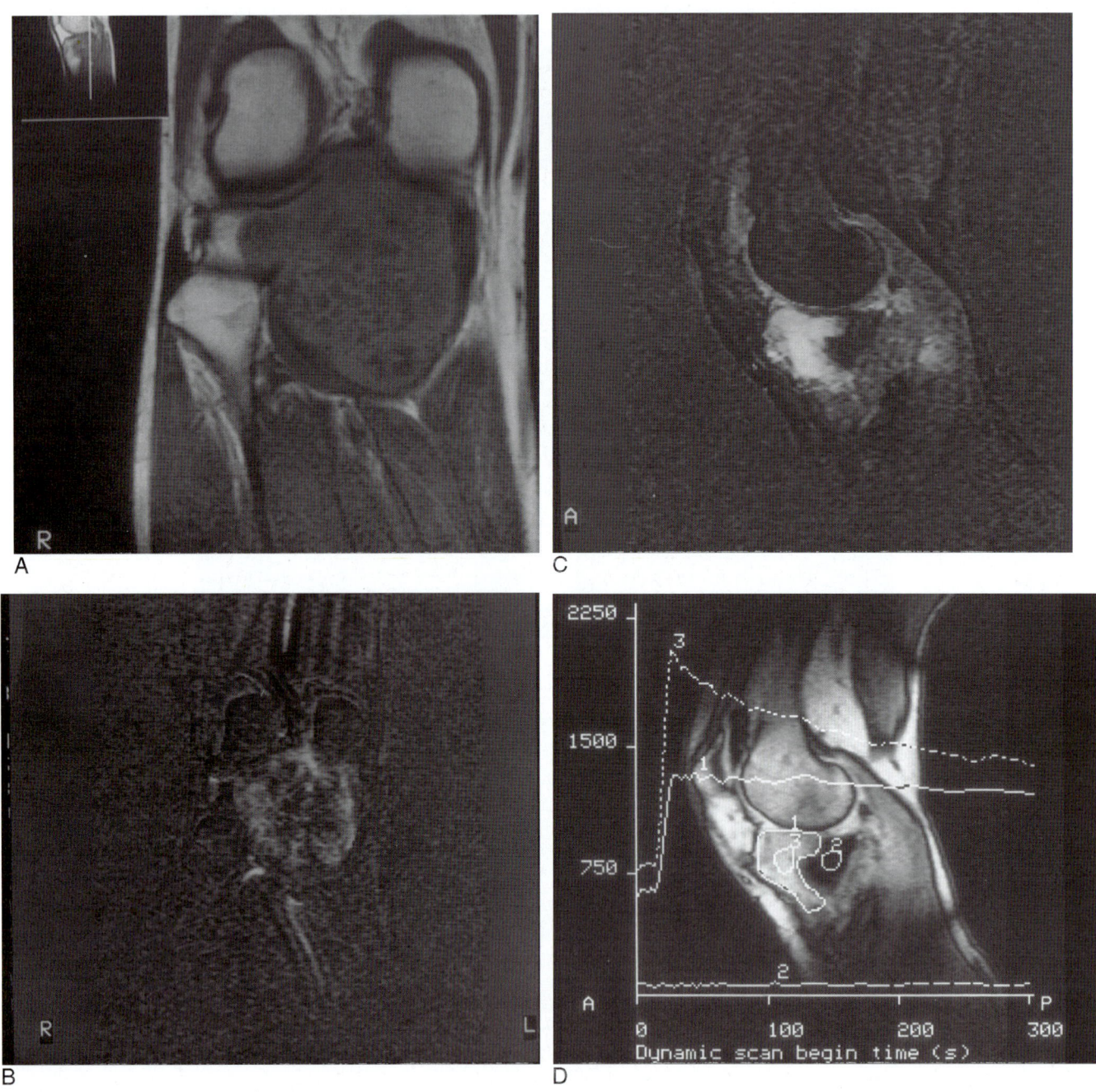

■ **FIGURE 99-8** A 28-year-old man presented with recurrent giant cell tumor of the proximal tibia. **A,** Coronal T1-weighted turbo spin-echo MR image showed a tumor in the epi-metaphysis with destruction of articular subchondral bone. **B,** Coronal subtraction dynamic contrast-enhanced T1-weighted gradient-echo MR image shows rapidly progressive enhancement, synchronously with arterial enhancement (image acquired 17 seconds after injection of gadolinium). **C,** Same patient, 6 months after curettage of giant cell tumor and phenol application. The bone defect has been filled with cement. Sagittal subtraction dynamic contrast-enhanced T1-weighted gradient-echo MR image reveals enhancing tissue both anteriorly and posteriorly to the cement (image acquired 20 seconds after injection Tumof gadolinium). **D,** The time-intensity curve obtained from the enhancing tissue anteriorly shows rapidly progressive enhancement with early wash-out consistent with recurrent or residual giant cell tumor (2, nonenhancing cement).

Enchondromas and osteochondromas rarely recur after surgical treatment by curettage or complete resection, respectively. The overall recurrence rate after resection of osteochondromas has been estimated at 2%. Recurrences of osteochondromas occur especially in the soft tissues, where they arise from perichondrium left behind. MRI is most valuable to detect recurrence and has the potential to demonstrate typical morphologic features of a cartilage-forming lesion (Fig. 99-9).

Sarcomas

The risk of local recurrence of bone and soft tissue sarcoma depends on the histologic type, biologic grade of the primary tumor, surgical margins, and presence of satellite or skip lesions. Locally recurrent bone sarcoma will usually occur within the soft tissues at the site of initial surgery. Radiography, ultrasonography, CT, and especially MRI can be used to detect local recurrence of

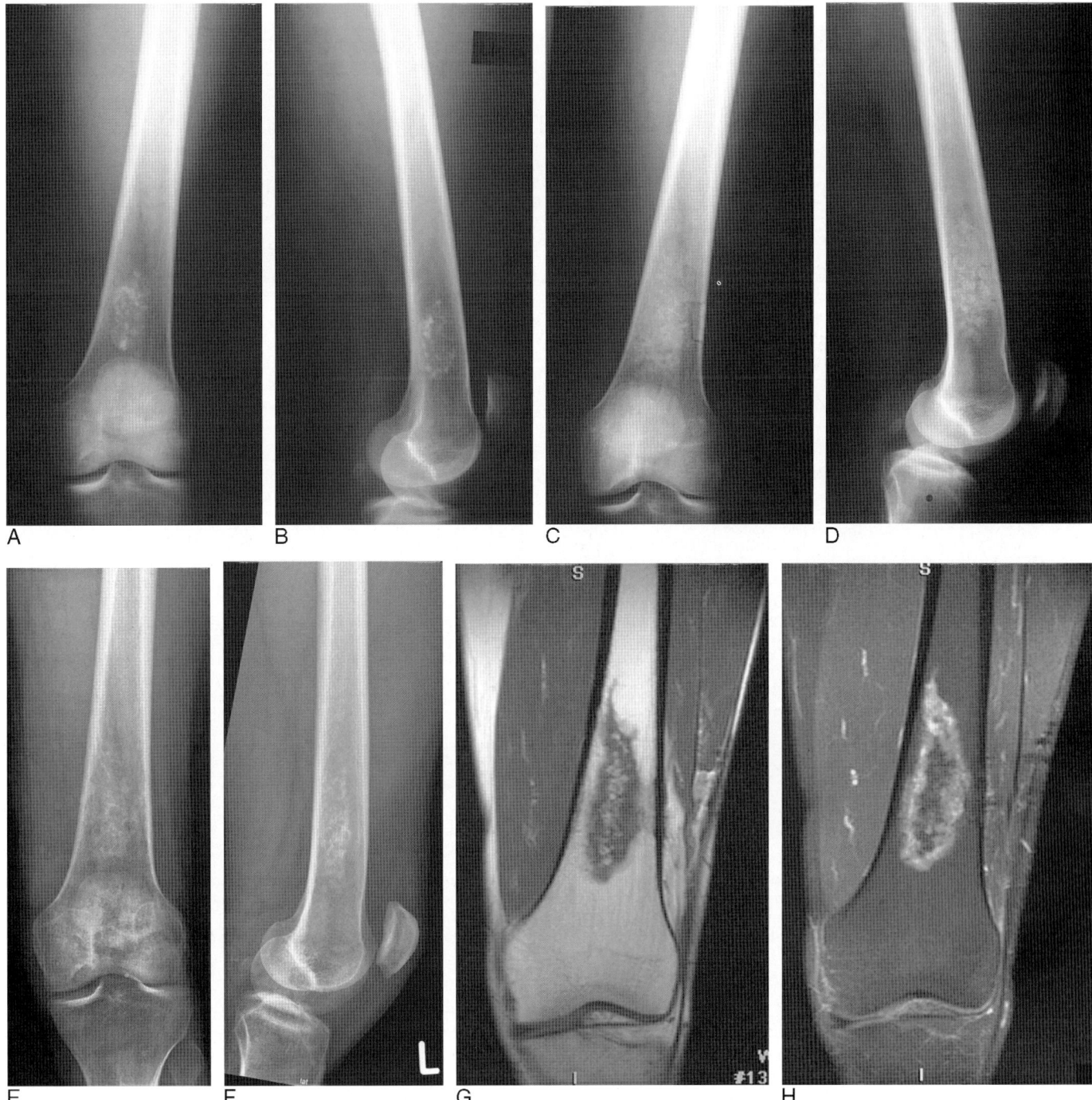

■ **FIGURE 99-9** **A** and **B,** Low-grade chondrosarcoma in the distal femur diaphysis. **C** and **D,** First postoperative conventional radiographs after curettage with adjunct chemical ablation and bone grafting of the defect. **E** and **F,** Conventional radiographs performed 18 months after treatment show normal appearance of the bone graft with no focal osteolysis. **G,** Coronal T1-weighted MR image performed 1 year after treatment. **H,** coronal T1-weighted MR image with fat suppression after intravenous injection of gadolinium chelate.

(Continued)

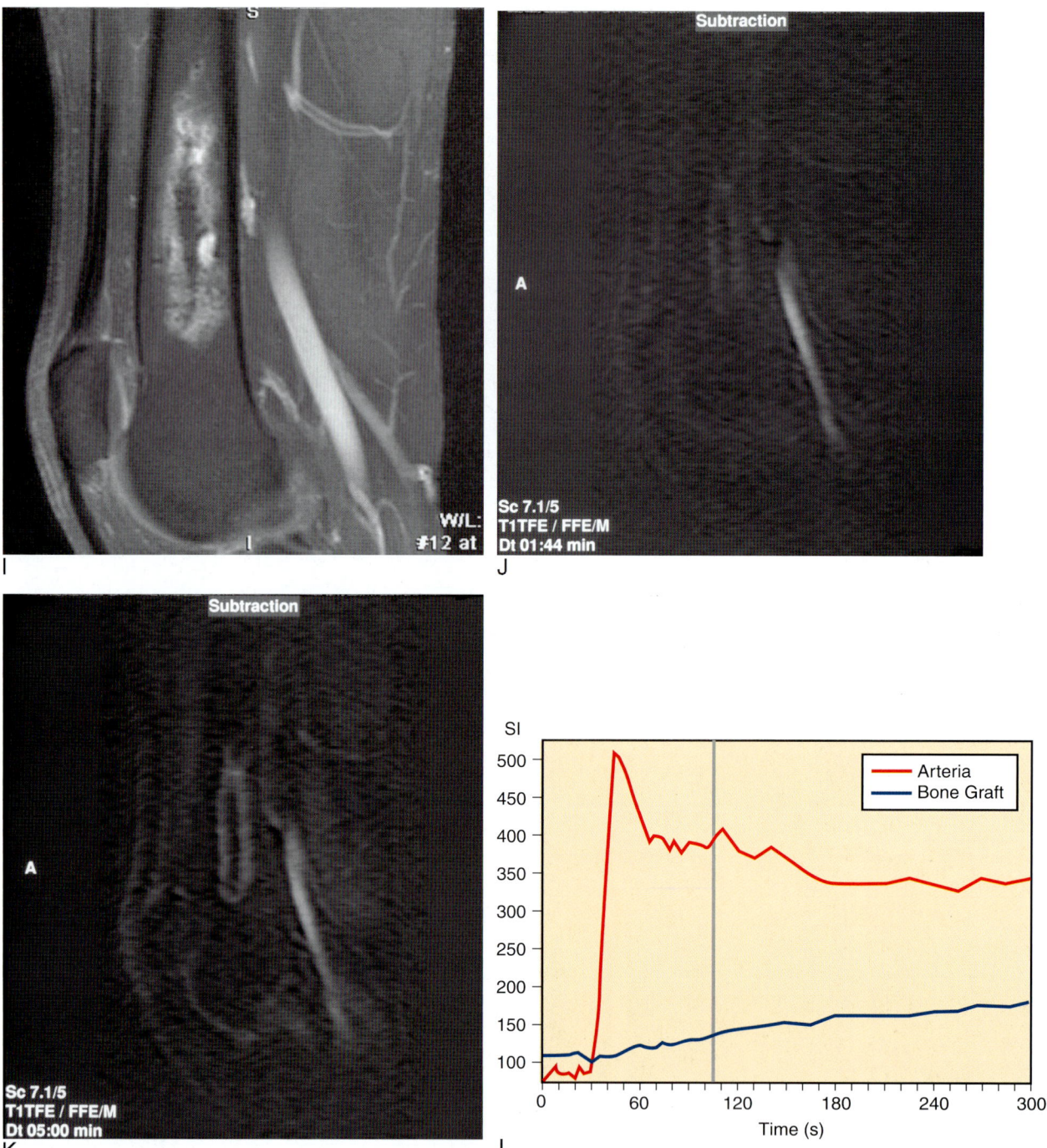

■ **FIGURE 99-9—Cont'd** **I,** Sagittal T1-weighted MR image with fat suppression after intravenous injection of gadolinium chelate. MRI of curetted bone lesions can give a confusing appearance due to variable amounts of fibrous scarring, granulation tissue, and sometimes cystic areas occupying the bony defect. **J** and **K,** Sagittal dynamic subtraction MR images obtained 90 seconds and almost 5 minutes after arterial enhancement, respectively, demonstrate normal incorporation of the bone graft with surrounding granulation tissue. No recurrent focal early enhancing lesions were identified. **L,** The time-intensity curve obtained from the endomedullary enhancing tissue shows gradual enhancement consistent with granulation tissue.

bone and soft tissue sarcoma. Recurrence may be detected on radiographs as a soft tissue mass with or without bone destruction. Mineralization of matrix facilitates detection on radiographs.

An MRI algorithm for the management of a suspected recurrent sarcoma has been proposed by Vanel and colleagues.[20] Post-therapeutic MR evaluation should at least include T1- and fat-suppressed T2-weighted or short tau inversion recovery (STIR) MR sequences. If MRI is negative for recurrence (Table 99-5), tumor appears to be present in only 1% of cases (false-negative MRI). High signal intensity without mass effect generally represents post-therapy changes or inflammation, whereas high signal intensity mass-like lesions on T2-weighted or

TABLE 99-5   **MRI Evaluation of Post-therapeutic Changes**

MRI Feature	Inflammation	Granulation Tissue	Hygroma/ Seroma	Recurrence
High SI on T2-weighted MRI	Yes	Yes	Yes	Yes
Low SI on T1-weighted MRI	Yes	Yes	Yes	Yes
Mass effect	No	Yes	Yes	Yes
Enhancement on contrast-enhanced MRI	Diffuse	Diffuse	No or minor rim	Diffuse or inhomogeneous
Enhancement on DCE MRI	Late and gradual	Late and gradual	No	Early and rapidly progressive
Signal loss on diffusion-weighted MRI	NE	NE	High	Low

SI, signal intensity; NE, not evaluated.

STIR images are suspect and require further examination with an intravenous gadolinium chelate. The most common cause of high signal intensity mass on T2-weighted or STIR images after surgery for a sarcoma is a localized fluid collection such as a seroma or hygroma.

Although recurrent tumor usually is characterized by high signal intensity on T2-weighted images and marked enhancement, knowledge of the imaging characteristics of the tumor before therapy can prevent pitfalls. Densely mineralized tumors (e.g., osteosarcomas) or hypocellular tumors (e.g., fibromatosis) will demonstrate mass effect, but the predominant signal intensity on T2-weighted MR images may be lower than usually encountered. Hypovascular tumors will demonstrate high signal intensity lesions on T2-weighted MR images but may show only peripheral enhancement after injection of Gd-chelate, simulating a seroma.[19]

Evaluation of bone marrow after treatment for a bone tumor can be challenging. Granulocyte colony-stimulating factors are increasingly used as an adjunct to chemotherapy in patients with bone tumors, resulting in red bone marrow conversion primarily in the pelvis and proximal long bones. Distinguishing recurrent or metastatic disease from reconversion (rebound) hematopoietic marrow may be difficult, because both tend to have intermediate signal intensity on T1-weighted images and high signal intensity on T2-weighted MR images. Recurrent tumor, however, is typically more nodular and focal, whereas hematopoietic marrow is more serpiginous and widespread. Opposed-phase gradient-echo images and DCE MRI may further assist in differentiating tumor from hematopoietic marrow. Sarcoma will have a higher signal intensity on opposed-phase gradient-echo images than hematopoietic marrow. Hematopoietic marrow enhances slowly on DCE MRI (more than 6 seconds after arterial enhancement), whereas sarcoma often, but not always, enhances faster.

After radiotherapy, the initial response of bone marrow is congestion and edema, resulting in high signal intensity on T2-weighted and STIR images. Subsequently, hematopoietic tissue disappears and partial conversion to fatty marrow as early as 8 days post treatment and complete fatty replacement by 8 weeks with high signal intensity are observed on T1-weighted spin-echo MR images, with intermediate signal intensity on T2-weighted, spin-echo MR images, signal characteristics that are typical of adipose tissue.

Fixation devices used in reconstructive surgical procedures causing susceptibility artifacts on MRI may hamper the diagnosis of recurrences. The type of material, object orientation, and imaging parameters affect these metallic artifacts. For example, titanium is more suitable for MRI than stainless steel; and gradient-echo and echo sequences should be avoided. Fast spin-echo pulse sequences with long echo trains show less metal artifact than conventional spin-echo sequences. Moreover, aligning the long axis of the metallic object with the main magnetic field and the frequency encoding direction can reduce artifacts. Further improvements can be obtained by increasing the read-out bandwidth. Because metal distorts the local magnetic field, typical frequency-selective fat saturation techniques (SPIR) give only limited fat suppression. Instead, STIR sequences can be used to obtain fat suppression without frequency-selective fat saturation. However, STIR sequences cannot be used for post-contrast MRI because these sequences perform a nonselective suppression of fat as well as other tissues with short T1 values. STIR sequences will tend to obscure gadolinium enhancement, because Gd-containing tissues may have T1 values shortened into the fat range.

When an equivocal lesion is detected on MRI, follow-up imaging, biopsy, or other imaging studies such as ultrasonography may be helpful. Ultrasonography may be used to detect local soft tissue recurrences, particularly when interpretation of MR images is hampered by artifacts of metallic fixation devices. Presence of a hypoechoic soft tissue mass highly suggests recurrent sarcoma, but differentiation from seroma, hematoma, abscess, and/or granulation tissue may be difficult, particularly in the early postoperative phase. A baseline MRI examination obtained 3 months after surgery can be very helpful in interpreting subsequent scans. In each case of a suspected recurrence on MRI, pathologic confirmation should be obtained. Ultrasonography can be used to guide fine-needle aspiration or Tru-Cut biopsy. Because of the heterogeneity of sarcomas for accurate histopathologic examination, it is important to avoid necrotic or hemorrhagic areas. When ultrasonography is used, a high yield of solid, representative tissue can be achieved. Routine restaging of the tumor of a patient with the use of chest CT is required when local recurrence of a sarcoma is proven.

Positron Emission Tomography in Detection of Recurrence

Only a few studies have addressed the potential of FDG-PET in the evaluation of tumor recurrence. The diagnostic accuracy of FDG PET in the evaluation of post-therapeutic changes is still questionable because the range of standardized uptake values from the accumulation of FDG in inflammatory tissue overlaps that of residual or recurrent tumor. However, FDG-PET in conjunction with MRI seems particularly useful in patients with extensive histories of surgery, often with metallic artifacts from limb salvage prostheses and radiation therapy.

IMAGING AS SURVEILLANCE STRATEGY

Prognosis of bone and soft tissue sarcoma is dominated by presence or absence of local recurrence and distant metastasis. The overall survival mainly depends on the development of metastatic disease. Subsequently, early detection of pulmonary metastases is an important component of surveillance. The benefit of early detection of local recurrence depends on the availability of therapeutic options that can prolong survival. Radical compartmental resection with or without adjuvant radiotherapy and/or chemotherapy may provide long-term salvage in patients with a local recurrence.

Several guidelines have been recommended for the follow-up of bone and soft tissue sarcoma, including a combination of clinical history, physical examination, blood tests, chest radiographs, CT, and MRI. Most institutions rely on consensus-based guidelines, owing to the absence of evidence-based guidelines. Surveillance strategies that, through early detection and treatment, improve survival and quality of life while minimizing costs have yet to be identified in randomized clinical trials. Only few studies have reported on the efficacy of surveillance strategies for the follow-up of bone soft tissue sarcoma. Clinical assessment and physical examination have been reported as the most useful tools for evaluating locoregional recurrence, whereas routine MRI of the primary tumor site and laboratory blood tests appear ineffective strategies. However, MRI has been shown to be useful in patients in whom physical examination is hampered by location (e.g., retroperitoneal sarcomas or radiotherapy changes).

A rational and practical surveillance algorithm should include routine office visits (with clinical assessment and chest radiograph) every 4 months for 2 years, followed by two visits with an interval of 6 months in the third year. An annual visit is often recommended thereafter. In addition, the patient should be instructed to contact the treating physician when symptoms such as pain or swelling develop. Additional MRI should be performed based on the reliability of physical examination and suspicion for recurrence within the perspective of patients' risk factors. Consequently, patients with retroperitoneal, or head or neck sarcomas may require MRI for routine follow-up. Moreover, close follow-up is also mandatory in patients with large high-grade primary tumors and patients with intralesional or marginal initial surgical resections.

Local recurrence rates of aggressive fibromatosis (desmoid-type fibromatosis) are similar to those of soft tissue sarcoma and have been reported to range from 25% to 77% depending on location and tumor size. The prognostic significance of positive surgical margins is still controversial. After resection, routinely close follow-up with MRI should be considered for early detection of local recurrence of aggressive fibromatosis because of the infiltrative growth pattern and high incidence of postsurgical recurrence. Moreover, these recurrences are often clinically silent.

What the Referring Physician Needs to Know

- How much of the tumor is viable after chemotherapy and where is it located?
- Is local recurrence excluded or proven?
- Are pulmonary metastases present or absent?

SUGGESTED READINGS

Blomley MJK, Eckersley RJ. Functional ultrasound methods in oncological imaging. Eur J Cancer 2002; 38:2108–2115.

Delorme S, Knopp MV. Non-invasive vascular imaging: assessing tumour vascularity. Eur Radiol 1998; 8:517–527.

Forsberg F, Ro RJ, Potoczek M, et al. Assessment of angiogenesis: implications for ultrasound imaging. Ultrasonics 2004; 42:325–330.

Griebel J, Mayr NA, de Vries A, et al. Assessment of tumor microcirculation: a new role of dynamic contrast MR imaging. J Magn Reson Imaging 1997; 7:111–119.

Knopp MV, Giesel FL, Marcos H, et al. Dynamic contrast-enhanced magnetic resonance imaging in oncology. Top Magn Reson Imaging 2001; 12:301–308.

Padhani AR, Husband JE. Dynamic contrast-enhanced MRI studies in oncology with an emphasis on quantification, validation and human studies. Clin Radiol 2001; 56:607–620.

Tofts PS, Brix G, Buckley DL, et al. Estimating kinetic parameters from dynamic contrast-enhanced T(1)-weighted MRI of a diffusable tracer: standardized quantities and symbols. J Magn Reson Imaging 1999; 10:223–232.

REFERENCES

1. Huvos AG, Rosen G, Marcove RC. Primary osteogenic sarcoma: pathologic aspects in 20 patients after treatment with chemotherapy en bloc resection, and prosthetic bone replacement. Arch Pathol Lab Med 1977; 101:14–18.

2. van der Woude, Bloem JL, Schipper J, et al. Changes in tumor perfusion induced by chemotherapy in bone sarcomas: color Doppler flow imaging compared with contrast-enhanced MR imaging and three-phase bone scintigraphy. Radiology 1994; 191:421–431.

3. Eilber FC, Rosen G, Eckardt J, et al. Treatment-induced pathologic necrosis: a predictor of local recurrence and survival in patients receiving neoadjuvant therapy for high-grade extremity soft tissue sarcomas. J Clin Oncol 2001; 19:3203-3209.

4. Tofts PS, Brix G, Buckley DL, et al. Estimating kinetic parameters from dynamic contrast-enhanced T(1)-weighted MRI of a diffusable tracer: standardized quantities and symbols. J Magn Reson Imaging 1999; 10:223-232.

5. Baur A, Reiser MF. Diffusion-weighted imaging of the musculoskeletal system in humans. Skeletal Radiol 2000; 29:555-562.

6. van Rijswijk CSP, Kunz P, Hogendoorn PCW, et al. Diffusion-weighted MRI in the characterization of soft-tissue tumors. J Magn Reson Imaging 2002; 15:302-307.

7. Lang P, Wendland MF, Saeed M, et al. Osteogenic sarcoma: noninvasive in vivo assessment of tumor necrosis with diffusion-weighted MR imaging. Radiology 1998; 206:227-235.

8. Taylor GA, Perlman EJ, Scherer LR, et al. Vascularity of tumors in children: evaluation with color Doppler imaging. AJR Am J Roentgenol 1991; 157:1267-1271.

9. Kiessling F, Krix M, Heilmann M, et al. Comparing dynamic parameters of tumor vascularization in nude mice revealed by magnetic resonance imaging and contrast-enhanced intermittent power Doppler sonography. Invest Radiol 2003; 38:516-524.

10. Taber DS, Libshitz HI, Cohen MA. Treated Ewing sarcoma: radiographic appearance in response, recurrence, and new primaries. AJR Am J Roentgenol 1983; 140:753-758.

11. Holscher HC, Hermans J, Nooy MA, et al. Can conventional radiographs be used to monitor the effect of neoadjuvant chemotherapy in patients with osteogenic sarcoma? Skeletal Radiol 1996; 25:19-24.

12. Erlemann R, Sciuk J, Bosse A, et al. Response of osteosarcoma and Ewing sarcoma to preoperative chemotherapy: assessment with dynamic and static MR imaging and skeletal scintigraphy. Radiology 1990; 175:791-796.

13. Holscher HC, Bloem JL, Vanel D, et al. Osteosarcoma: chemotherapy-induced changes at MR imaging. Radiology 1992; 182:839-844.

14. van der Woude HJ, Bloem JL, Verstraete KL, et al. Osteosarcoma and Ewing's sarcoma after neoadjuvant chemotherapy: value of dynamic MR imaging in detecting viable tumor before surgery. AJR Am J Roentgenol 1995; 165:596-598.

15. Verstraete KL, De Deene Y, Roels H, et al. Benign and malignant musculoskeletal lesions: dynamic contrast-enhanced MR imaging—parametric "first-pass" images depict tissue vascularization and perfusion. Radiology 1994; 192:835-843.

16. Egmont-Petersen M, Hogendoorn PC, van der Geest RJ, et al. Detection of areas with viable remnant tumor in postchemotherapy patients with Ewing's sarcoma by dynamic contrast-enhanced MRI using pharmacokinetic modeling. Magn Reson Imaging 2000; 18:525-535.

17. van der Woude HJ, Bloem JL, van Oostayen JA, et al. Treatment of high-grade bone sarcomas with neoadjuvant chemotherapy: the utility of sequential color Doppler sonography in predicting histopathologic response. AJR Am J Roentgenol 1995; 165:125-133.

18. Murphey MD, Nomikos GC, Flemming DJ, et al. From the archives of AFIP. Imaging of giant cell tumor and giant cell reparative granuloma of bone: radiologic-pathologic correlation. RadioGraphics 2001; 21:1283-1309.

19. Davies AM, Vanel D. Follow-up of musculoskeletal tumors: I. Local recurrence. Eur Radiol 1998; 8:791-799.

20. Vanel D, Shapeero LG, De Baere T, et al. MR imaging in the follow-up of malignant and aggressive soft-tissue tumors: results of 511 examinations. Radiology; 190:263-268.

Clinically Relevant Developmental Dysplasias

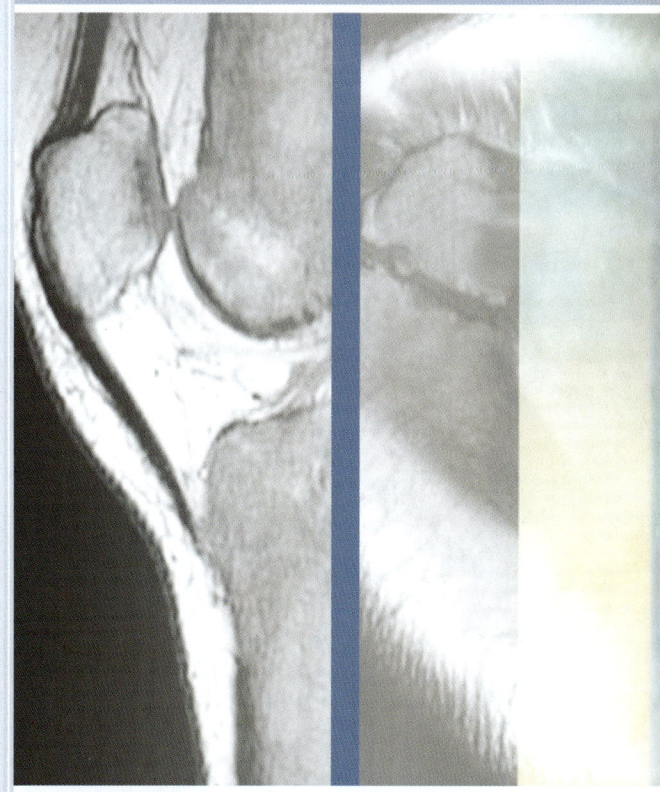

100

Focal Growth Disturbances

F. M. Vanhoenacker, W. Courtens, and A. Snoeckx

ETIOLOGY

Teratologic factors due to drugs taken during pregnancy are the best known cause of focal growth disturbances (e.g., thalidomide-associated phocomelia), but sporadic cases of unknown cause are now more frequent. This is due principally to the greater precautions taken in prescribing medications during pregnancy.[2]

Some malformations involving limb reductions are genetically determined, and these usually have an autosomal dominant pattern of inheritance.

Prevalence and Epidemiology

Fortunately, focal limb disturbances are very rare as individual occurrences. The prevalence varies from disease to disease.

Clinical Presentation

Focal malformations of the limbs include absence of bone, hypoplastic bones, fusion with segmentation anomalies, and abnormal bowing.

They may be associated with abnormalities of other organ systems, such as the skin, heart, abdominal viscera, or central nervous system.[1,2]

Pathophysiology

The embryologic limb buds appear bilaterally at about the 26th day of gestation at Wolff's crest (Fig. 100-1). By the 30th day the upper limb has started differentiating into three segments (upper arm, forearm, and hand), and in the lower limb the same process occurs shortly afterward. By the end of the sixth gestational week the embryo has acquired a recognizable human form.[3] Therefore, most congenital anomalies occur in the third through the seventh weeks, when the tissues are rapidly developing.[4] After the seventh week, certain types of insult may still result in limb anomalies, because the upper limb is only fully formed by 12 weeks' gestation and the lower limb by 14 weeks' gestation.[3]

IMAGING TECHNIQUES

Techniques and Relevant Aspects

Defects in limb formation are most often recognized by ultrasound during pregnancy.[5-7] After birth, conventional radiography remains the "gold standard" for assessment of focal growth anomalies. Ultrasonography and MRI may be useful in delineating unossified cartilage or associated soft tissue abnormalities.

MANIFESTATIONS OF THE DISEASE

Various classification systems of limb deficiencies have been proposed, but none is completely satisfactory.[3] Some of them are very complex and are therefore difficult to use in routine daily practice. For the sake of simplicity, congenital focal growth anomalies are classified here based on the number of bones (absence vs. extra bones), morphology (hypoplasia, bowing), segmentation, and location (upper vs. lower limb). Only the most common and clinically important entities are discussed in this chapter. Unusual and atypical cases may be analyzed with the more detailed texts described in Suggested Readings.

KEY POINTS

- Focal malformations of the limbs include absence of bone, hypoplastic bones, fusion with segmentation anomalies, and abnormal bowing.
- Look always for associated abnormalities of other organ systems, such as the skin, heart, abdominal viscera, or central nervous system.
- During pregnancy, defects in limb formation are most often recognized by ultrasound.
- After birth, plain radiography is the gold standard for assessment of focal growth anomalies.
- Ultrasonography and MRI may be useful in showing unossified cartilage or associated soft tissue abnormalities.

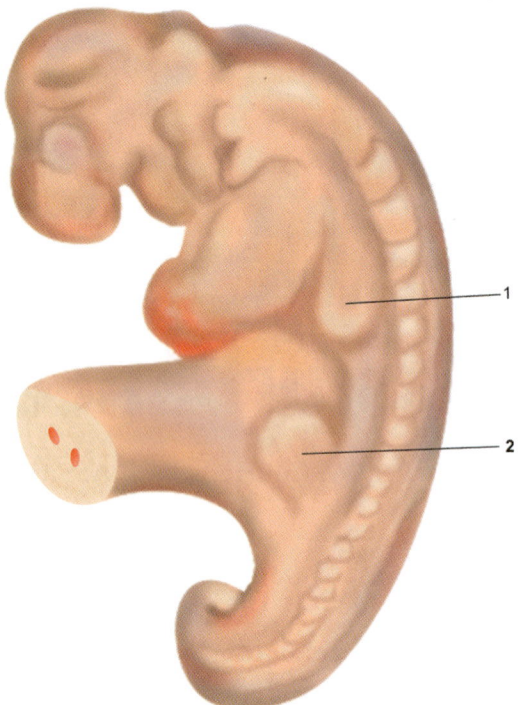

■ **FIGURE 100-1** Schematic drawing of the embryologic limb buds at Wolff's crest. 1, upper limb bud; 2, lower limb bud.

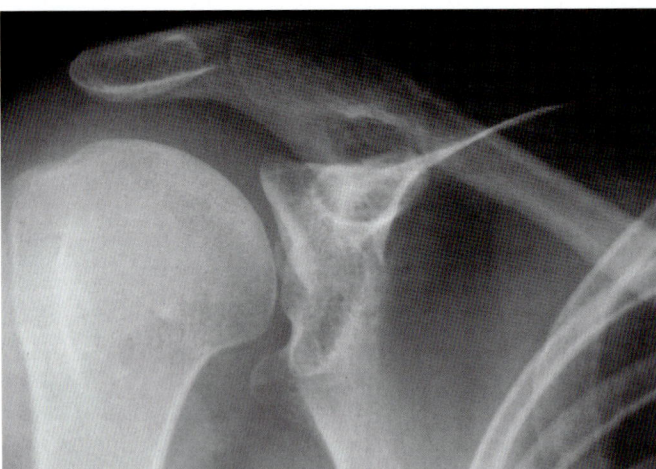

■ **FIGURE 100-2** Glenoid hypoplasia. The standard radiograph of the right shoulder shows a dentate articular surface of the glenoid and a decreased ossification of the scapular neck. The glenohumeral joint appears widened inferiorly, and there is slight hypoplasia of the humeral head.

Absent or Hypoplastic Bones (Deficiency)

Complete absence of a limb is called *amelia*, almost complete absence (with only a stub remaining) is called *phocomelia*, and partial absence is *ectromelia*. Defects may be transverse or axial.

Glenoid Hypoplasia

Glenoid hypoplasia or dysplasia of the scapular neck is a congenital anomaly characterized by an ossification failure of the lower two thirds of the glenoid and adjacent scapula.[8]

Radiographic Findings

The usual radiographic findings consist of hypoplasia of the scapular neck with a typical dentate or notched appearance of the articular surface of the glenoid. The inferior glenohumeral joint is usually widened. Additional findings may include hypoplasia of the humeral neck and head, varus deformity of the proximal portion of the humerus, and sometimes enlargement and bowing of the acromion and clavicle (Fig. 100-2).

MRI Arthrography

MR arthrography confirms a deformed and angulated bony glenoid fossa, with thick articular cartilage and a large posterior and anteroinferior portion of the labrum.

Radial or Ulnar Ray Deficiency

Absence or hypoplasia of the radius may occur as an isolated entity (Fig. 100-3) or may be associated with

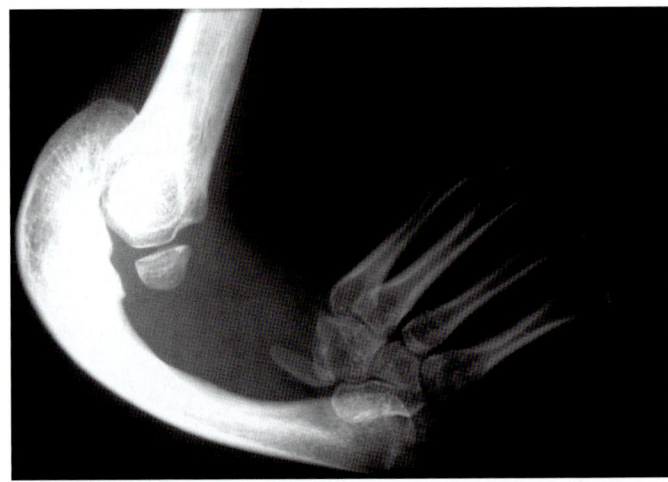

■ **FIGURE 100-3** Radial deficiency. Plain radiograph of the left forearm showing absence of the diaphysis of the radius, with small residual remnant at the radial head and distal radius. Note associated carpal fusion and absence of the thumb ("radial ray syndrome").

visceral anomalies (e.g., cardiovascular anomalies in Holt-Oram syndrome) or certain blood dyscrasias (e.g., thrombocytopenia–absent radius syndrome [TAR syndrome]). The elbow is often abnormal, and the thumb may be missing.

Hypoplasia of the distal end of the ulna is much less frequent and is usually part of a more extensive syndrome (e.g., hereditary multiple exostosis syndrome, Fig. 100-4).

Amputations of Limbs

Transverse congenital amputations of limbs may be due to amniotic (Streeter) bands (Fig. 100-5) and can also be seen in thalidomide embryopathy syndromes and in other syndromes (e.g., Möbius, Cornelia de Lange, and aglossia-adactyly).

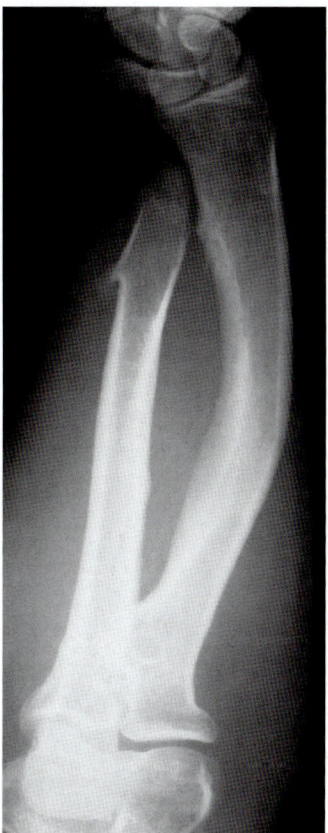

■ **FIGURE 100-4** Ulnar deficiency in a patient with hereditary multiple exostosis syndrome. Plain radiograph of the right forearm. There is shortening of the ulna with secondary bowing of the radius.

Proximal Femoral Focal Deficiency

Proximal femoral focal deficiency (PFFD) is a developmental defect of the proximal femur and acetabulum (Fig. 100-6). PFFD includes a spectrum of findings ranging from mild femoral shortening with varus deformity to complete absence of both acetabulum and proximal femur with only a small distal fragment.[9]

The most common associated abnormalities of the ipsilateral limb include fibular deficiency (see Fig. 100-6) (50%), tibial shortening, equinovalgus deformity of the ankle, and deficiencies of the lateral rays of the foot. All the hip muscles are smaller than normal with exception of the sartorius muscle, which is hypertrophied.

Radiographic Findings

Although the clinical diagnosis of PFFD is usually straightforward, correct classification may be difficult if one relies solely on clinical findings. Most attempts to classify the severity of the abnormality are based on the radiographic findings. Conventional radiography is somewhat limited because it only examines the bony structures.

Ultrasonography and MRI

Ultrasonography and MRI[9,10] have been proposed as additional tools in assessment of PFFD. In particular, the absence or presence of unossified cartilage and associated soft tissue findings can be determined. This will have an impact on surgical corrections.

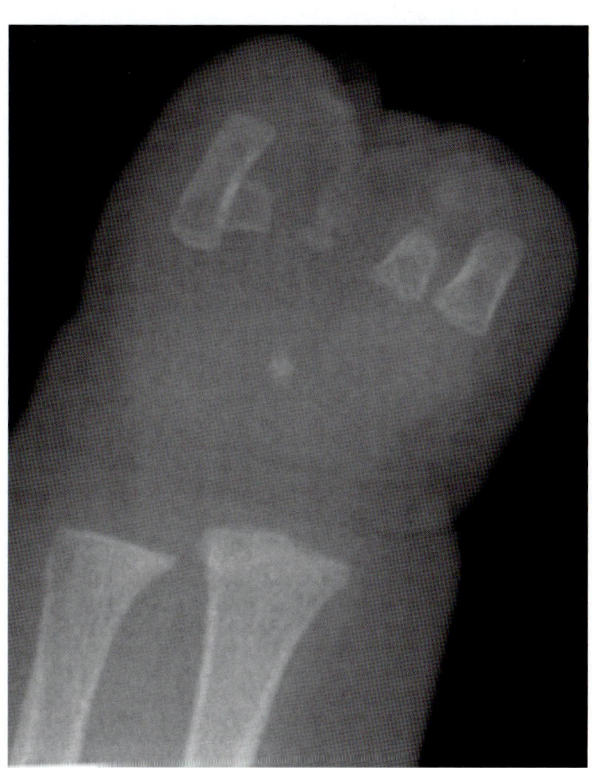

■ **FIGURE 100-5** Amniotic bands syndrome. Radiograph of the left hand. Note transverse amputation of the digits at the metacarpal level due to Streeter's bands.

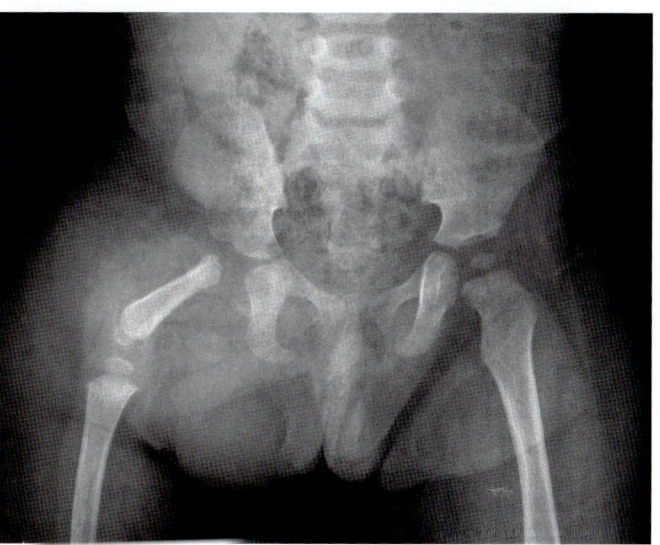

■ **FIGURE 100-6** Proximal femoral focal deficiency. Standard radiograph of the pelvis showing a short right femur with absence of the proximal segment. There is lack of ossification of the proximal femoral epiphysis. Note also associated absence of the right fibula.

Tibial and Fibular Deficiency

Congenital absence of the tibia is extremely rare and is usually associated with other anomalies of the limbs.

Hypoplasia of the fibula causes only slight shortening or deformity of the lower limb (Fig. 100-7), whereas complete absence of the fibula leads to considerable shortening and deformity with bowing of the tibia and valgus deformity of the unsupported ankle. There may be concomitant absence of the fourth and fifth rays of the foot.

Nail-Patella Syndrome

Nail-patella syndrome or hereditary onycho-osteodysplasia is an autosomal dominant disorder, affecting the nails, kidneys, pelvis, knees, and elbows. Iliac horns are seen at the posterior aspect of the iliac wings of the pelvis. When they occur as an isolated finding, the disorder is described as Fong's disease (Fig. 100-8). The iliac wings may be small and squared. The patellae may be absent or hypoplastic as well and laterally subluxed. The lateral femoral condyles are usually small and flattened. Elbow abnormalities include hypoplasia and posterior dislocation or subluxation of the radial heads.

Radiographic Findings

Iliac horns are seen at the posterior aspect of the iliac wings of the pelvis. When they occur as an isolated finding, the disorder is described as Fong's disease (Fig. 100-8). The iliac wings may be small and squared. The patellae may be absent or hypoplastic and laterally subluxed. The lateral

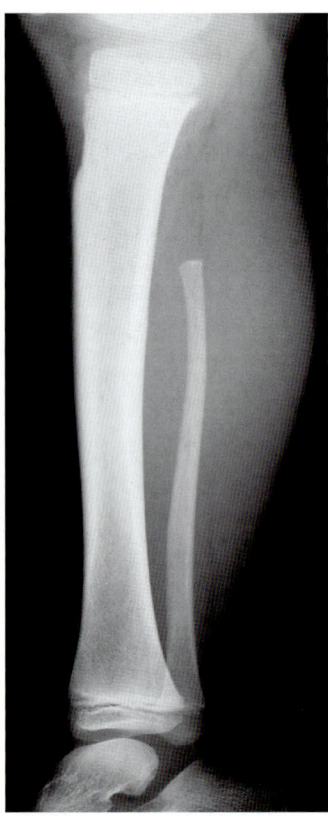

■ **FIGURE 100-7** Fibular deficiency. Lateral plain radiograph of the right lower leg demonstrating focal hypoplasia of the proximal segment of the fibula.

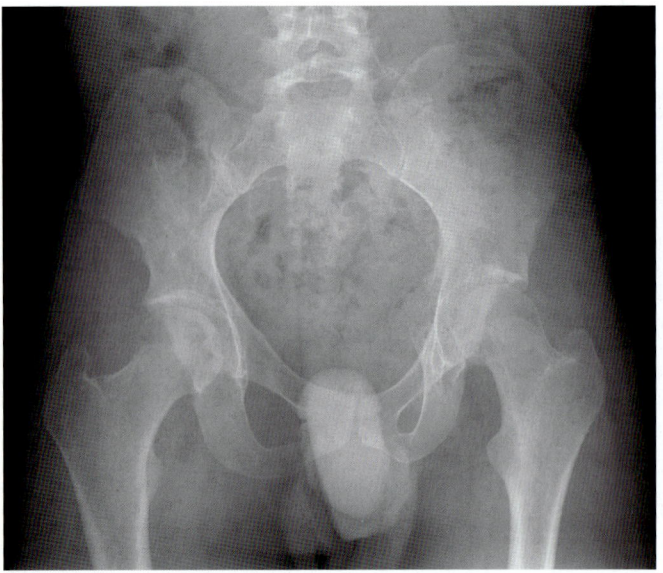
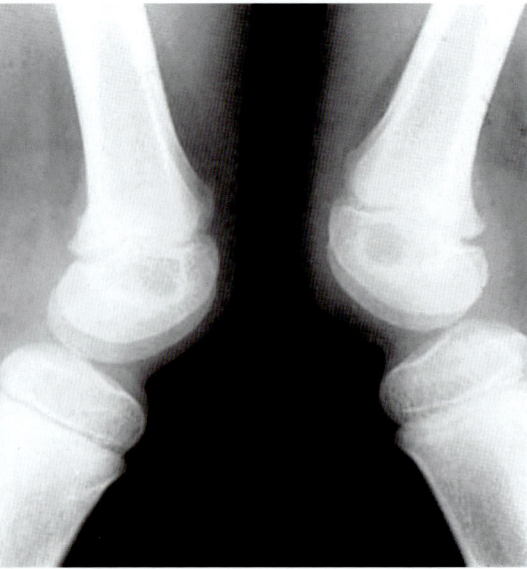

A   B

■ **FIGURE 100-8** Nail-patella syndrome. **A,** Radiograph of the pelvis showing hypoplastic pelvic wings (more pronounced on the right side) and a small iliac horn on the right ilium. **B,** Lateral knee radiographs. Note absence of the patellar bones. *(From Vanhoenacker FM. Congenital skeletal abnormalities: an introduction to the radiological semiology. Eur J Radiol 2001; 40:168–183).*

femoral condyles are usually small and flattened. Elbow abnormalities include hypoplasia and posterior dislocation or subluxation of the radial heads.

Hands and Feet Anomalies

Oligodactyly (lack of digits) may be on one or the other side of the hand and may be part of either radial or ulnar deficiency syndromes. Absence of middle digits may result in split-hand deformity or ectrodactyly.

Shortening of various phalanges, thumbs, and metacarpals (brachydactyly) is seen in a number of congenital genetic diseases. Shortening of the metacarpals of the ring and small fingers, resulting in a positive metacarpal sign, is the hallmark of many systemic congenital disorders.[1]

Acro-osteolysis is the term used for distal phalangeal resorption, which may be the result of congenital, genetic, or acquired disorders (e.g., vinyl chloride acro-osteolysis, frostbite, burns, rheumatologic cause, Raynaud's phenomenon) (Fig. 100-9).

Extra Bones

A condition characterized by too many fingers is designated as polydactyly, which can be either preaxial (on the radial side) or postaxial (on the ulnar side) and occurs in various genetic syndromes such as acrocallosal syndrome and Bardet-Biedl syndrome. Polydactyly in association with short ribs occurs in a number of polydactyly–short rib syndromes (Fig. 100-10). A triphalangeal thumb can be associated with congenital anemia and cardiovascular abnormalities (e.g., Fanconi's pancytopenia) and can be seen in some genetic disorders.

Fusion Anomalies and Segmentation Deformities

Congenital Pseudarthrosis

Congenital pseudarthrosis of the limb most commonly involves the tibia, although various combinations of bones including fibula, radius, ulna, clavicle, and humerus have all

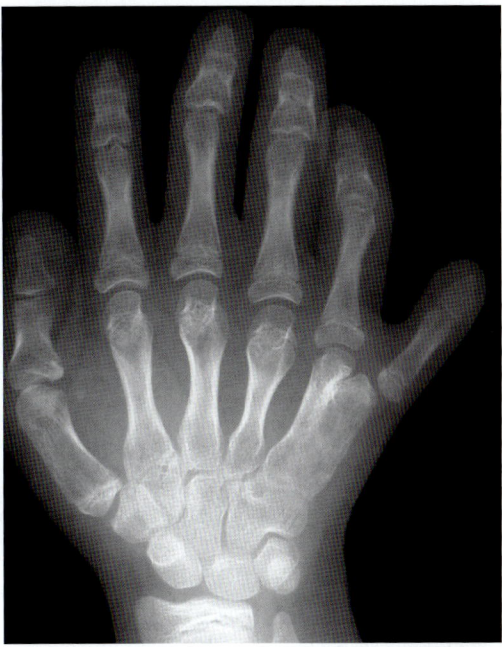

FIGURE 100-10 Postaxial polydactyly in a patient with chondroectodermal dysplasia (Ellis-van Creveld syndrome). The plain radiographs show an extra digit on the ulnar side of the right hand. Note also bony fusion of the fifth metacarpal digit and the metacarpal of the extra digit (bony syndactyly).

been described.[11] Congenital pseudarthrosis of the tibia or fibula has been classically associated with neurofibromatosis type 1[12] but has also been described in osteofibrous dysplasia.[13]

Congenital pseudarthrosis of the clavicle is a rare condition of unknown cause, usually presenting as a painless mass in the clavicular region.[14] According to some authors, it may be due to pressure by the subclavian artery on the developing bone.[3,14]

Synostosis

Abnormal fusion may occur between various bones (radioulnar, tibiofibular, carpal, or tarsal) They are discussed more in detail in Chapter 102: Coalitions.

Syndactyly and Symphalangism

Fusion occurring between two (adjacent) fingers is called syndactyly (see Fig. 100-10), whereas symphalangism (Fig. 100-11) refers to fusion between two phalanges within the same ray. Syndactyly can be membranous, bony, or combined. Symphalangism can be "proximal" (at the proximal interphalangeal joint) or "distal" (at the distal interphalangeal joint) or "variable" (distally and proximally located within the same patient).[1]

Bowing Deformities

Congenital bowing of the tibia is most frequent. Posteromedial tibial bowing has a benign course with spontaneous resolution being the rule.

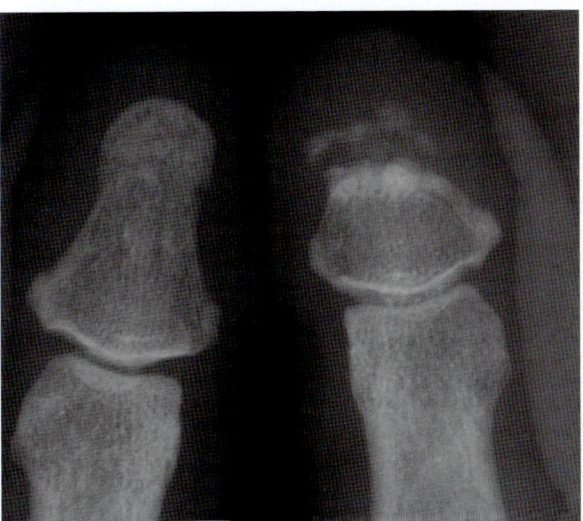

FIGURE 100-9 Congenital acro-osteolysis in a patient with Hajdu-Cheney syndrome. Plain radiographs of the thumb show resorption of the tuft of the distal phalanx on the right side.

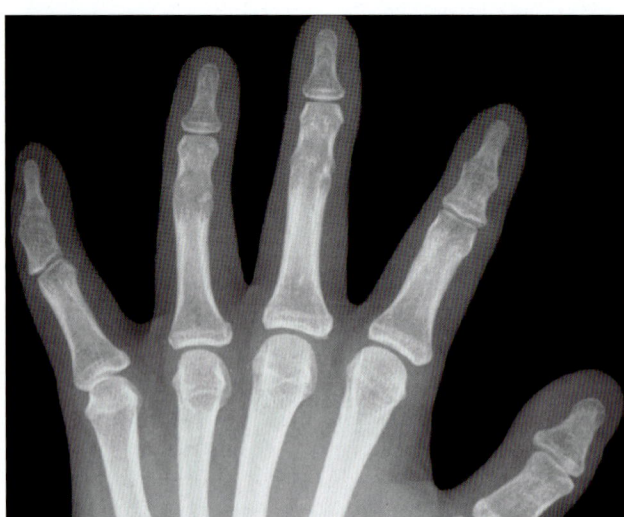

■ **FIGURE 100-11** "Variable" symphalangism in a patient with Pfeiffer's disease. Plain radiograph of the left hand shows fusion of the proximal interphalangeal joints of the third and the fourth finger and of the distal interphalangeal joint of the second digit.

Anteromedial bowing is almost always associated with fibular deficiency and congenital defects of the foot or some types of femoral dysplasia. Anterolateral tibial bowing is prone to fracture with persistent pseudarthrosis of the tibia.[3]

Generalized bowing may be associated with osteogenesis imperfecta.

SYNOPSIS OF TREATMENT OPTIONS

Medical Treatment

Curative medical treatment is currently not available in most disorders. Conservative orthopedic treatment with an orthosis and braces aims to maintain limb function and stability.

Surgical Treatment

Operative reconstructive surgery depends on the complexity of the disorder and requires a multidisciplinary approach.

What the Referring Physician Needs to Know

- Genetic counseling for inherited disorders is always mandatory.
- Correct diagnosis and management is usually the result of intensive teamwork and cooperation among the referring physician, the radiologist, the orthopedic surgeon, and the expert in medical genetics.

SUGGESTED READINGS

Hall CM and the International Nomenclature Group on Constitutional Disorders of Bone. International nosology and classification of constitutional disorders of bone (2001). Am J Med Genet 2002; 113:65–77.

Kozlowski K, Beighton P, (eds): Gamut index of skeletal dysplasias: an aid to radiodiagnosis. 3rd ed. London, Springer-Verlag, 2001.

Offiah AC, Hall CM. Radiological diagnosis of the constitutional disorders of bone; as easy as A, B, C? Pediatr Radiol 2003; 33:153–161.

Vanhoenacker FM, Van Hul W, Gielen J, De Schepper AM. Congenital skeletal abnormalities: an introduction to the radiological semiology. Eur J Radiol 2001; 40:168–183.

REFERENCES

1. Vanhoenacker FM, Van Hul W, Gielen J, De Schepper AM. Congenital skeletal abnormalities: an introduction to the radiological semiology. Eur J Radiol 2001; 40:168–183.
2. Wilson D, Cheung R. Congenital and developmental disorders. In Wilson D (ed). Paediatric Musculoskeletal Disease. Berlin, Springer, 2005, pp 1–17.
3. Solomon L, Warwick DJ, Nayagam S. Genetic disorders, skeletal dysplasias and malformations. In Solomon L, Warwick DJ, Nayagam S (eds). Apley's System of Orthopaedics and Fractures, 8th ed. London, Arnold, 2001, pp 133–165.
4. Beatty E. Upper limb tissue differentiation in the human embryo. Hand Clin 1985; 1:391–403.
5. Ryu JK, Cho JY, Choi JS. Prenatal sonographic diagnosis of focal musculoskeletal anomalies. Korean J Radiol 2003; 4:423–251.
6. Camera G, Dodero D, Parosi M, et al. Antenatal ultrasonographic diagnosis of a proximal focal deficiency. J Clin Ultrasound 1993; 21:475–479.
7. Seow KM, Huang LW, Lin YH, et al. Prenatal three-dimensional ultrasound diagnosis of a camptomelic dysplasia. Arch Gynecol Obstet 2004; 269:142–144.
8. Vanhoenacker FM, Van de Perre S, De Schepper AM. Glenoid hypoplasia. JBR-BTR 2003; 86:27.
9. Anton CG, Applegate KE, Kuivila TE, Wilkes DC. Proximal femoral focal deficiency (PFFD): More than an abnormal hip. Semin Musculoskelet Radiol 1999; 3:215–226.
10. Bernaerts A, De Ridder K, Pouillon M, Vanhoenacker FM. Value of magnetic resonance imaging in early assessment of proximal femoral focal deficiency (PFFD). JBR-BTR 2006; 89:325–327.
11. Yang KY, Lee EH. Isolated congenital pseudarthrosis of the fibula. J Pediatr Orthop B 2002; 11:298–301.
12. Mariaud-Schmidt RP, Rosales-Quintana S, Bitar E, et al. Hamartoma involving the pseudarthrosis site in patients with neurofibromatosis type 1. Pediatr Dev Pathol 2005; 8:190–196.
13. Hisaoka M, Hashimoto H, Ohguri T, et al. Congenital (infantile) pseudarthrosis of the fibula associated with osteofibrous dysplasia. Skeletal Radiol 2004; 33:545–549.
14. Dzupa V, Bartonicek J, Zidka M. Fracture of the clavicle after surgical treatment for congenital pseudarthrosis. Med Sci Moni 2004; 10: CS1-CS4.

Developmental Dysplasia of the Hip

David Wilson

ETIOLOGY AND PREVALENCE

Congenital dislocation of the hip is a condition that presents in infancy in approximately 1 in 9000 live births. Although childhood presentation of the condition is uncommon, the occult form of developmental dysplasia occurs frequently. This consists of a shallow acetabulum that is potentially unstable, thereby leading to a premature degeneration and osteoarthritis seen in early adult life (Fig. 101-1). There are no precise statistics to indicate its incidence, but it can be stated that the vast majority of patients who undergo total-hip replacement when younger than the age of 55 suffer from developmental dysplasia that predisposed to premature arthropathy.

The condition is highly disabling if it presents in infancy with a true dislocation of the hip. Mild subluxation of the hip leading to instability produces little in the way of symptoms that can be identified in infancy and it is only in later life that these lead to degeneration.

There is a window of opportunity in the first 6 to 12 weeks of life in which treatment with splint therapy has been shown to be effective in increasing the depth of the acetabulum and thereby diminishing the risk of dislocation and subluxation and possibly reducing the incidence of early osteoarthritis in the long term. In the early stages of the disease the aim of the clinician and imaging team will be to identify those children who would benefit from early splint therapy. Infants with the much rarer and more severe cases in which there is true dislocation will need operative reduction and probably surgery to confine the hip within the acetabulum and allow the child to walk normally at approximately 1 year of age.

MANIFESTATIONS OF THE DISEASE

Radiography

Before an infant is 3 months old the majority of the hip and acetabulum are unossified and as a result radiographs are of little or no value in the assessment of children for developmental dysplasia or congenital dislocation. If there is a true and substantial dislocation, malalignment of the femur may be visible, but in cases of this severity the problem is usually clinically apparent and the radiograph adds little to the diagnosis. It does exclude other lesions such as proximal femoral deficiency and sacral agenesis.[1]

Computed Tomography

A CT examination would show the cartilage and structures modestly well. However, this would involve a significant radiation dose and would be very difficult to achieve without anesthesia to keep the child still. It is, therefore, of no value in the screening procedures and of some limited value in the patient with a more complex problem.

Magnetic Resonance Imaging

Magnetic resonance imaging has similar constraints to CT. General anesthesia or heavy sedation would be required, even more so than with a CT examination. The absence of ionizing radiation is a distinct advantage in infants, but, again, MRI is not a practical screening procedure. MRI may be indicated in a few children in which a complex problem has been identified. It is probably the best method of demonstrating major deficiencies and deformity of the pelvis and proximal lower limb.

Both MR and CT have a role in the assessment of children undergoing treatment after surgery and this is discussed later in this chapter.

Ultrasonography

Ultrasonography has proven to be the most effective imaging technique in both screening and primary assessment of children with potential dislocation, subluxation, and

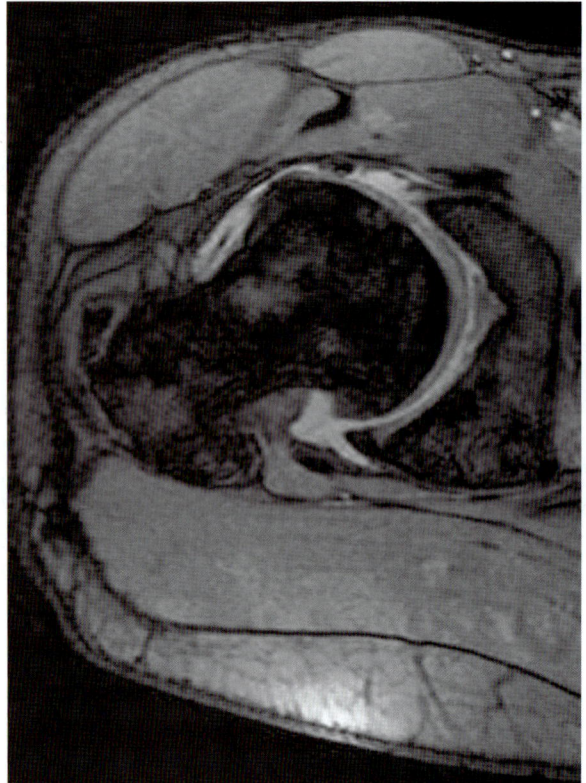

■ **FIGURE 101-1** MR arthrography of the hip of a 24-year-old patient with acetabular dysplasia. This is the late presentation of developmental dysplasia of the hip.

TABLE 101-1	Clinical Signs of Hip Dysplasia
Sign	**Predictive Value**
Reduced mobility	93%
Asymmetry	19%
Click	16%
Breech presentation	21%
Family history	16%

hip dysplasia.[2] Its principal advantages are that it allows the direct imaging of the cartilage, which appears as a relatively echo-free structure. Small canaliculi and blood vessels within the cartilage will show as reflective dots on a generally dark background. Bone reflects all sounds and is therefore seen as a sharp line at the advancing edge of ossification; the femoral shaft and the pelvis are clearly identified. Ultrasonography is a dynamic examination that allows the child to move while still achieving reasonably good image quality. It does not use any ionizing radiation, and it is accepted by parents, patients, and clinical staff. Ultrasound machines are also significantly less expensive than CT and MRI equipment. The ability to examine the hip dynamically is important in some of the techniques that I describe later. Subluxation may be a transient event that only occurs in certain positions or motions, and the real-time dynamic nature of an ultrasound examination is ideal for investigation of these abnormalities.

SYNOPSIS OF TREATMENT OPTIONS

Clinical Examination

The most common method applied is for a well-trained clinical observer to examine all infants shortly after birth. In the United Kingdom this is normally undertaken by a Senior House Officer in Paediatrics who will examine all infants before they are discharged from hospital. This will be supplemented by examination by visiting nurses at routine visits and sometimes review by the general practitioner.

The signs that the examiner looks for are listed in Table 101-1 and are derived from the work of Zieger and Schultz.[3] Note that the symptom most commonly associated with congenital dislocation or dysplasia of the hip—the clicking hip—is one of the least sensitive signs. Reduction in mobility of the joint is of far greater importance. Unfortunately, the detection of this stiffness or reduced mobility is one that requires considerable training on the part of the observer. There is, therefore, a significant observer error, particularly when whole populations are surveyed. In the hands of an experienced clinical examiner the majority of children with subluxatable or dislocated hips will be detected. Indeed, it is very rare for a child with a total-hip dislocation to be missed on clinical examination. However, there is a significant error rate even in the hands of a pediatric orthopedic surgeon, and children who have identifiable subluxation of the hip seen on imaging will be normal in a small percentage of cases.[4]

The arguments in favor of providing a routine imaging investigation are that a small percentage of treatable cases are overlooked by an experienced clinical examiner and that imaging provides support to the less able practitioner.

Ultrasound Techniques

There are three broad techniques applied when using ultrasound to examine children with potential hip dysplasia.[5] These may be summarized as (1) anatomic (morphology) measurement, (2) dynamic stability testing, and (3) combined clinical maneuver and ultrasound examination (a variant of dynamic assessment).

The strategy that is most commonly used is that developed by the Austrian orthopedic surgeon Reinhardt Graf. His method is a shape or morphology assessment. The infant is placed in a lateral decubitus position with the hips flexed. Rolled towels are placed in front and behind the infant, or, alternatively, the child lies in a trough made of soft padded material. These stabilizing devices have the advantage of keeping the infant still and also tend to reassure the crying child. The ultrasound probe, which should be a linear array producing a rectangular image, is placed in a true coronal plane along the lateral aspect of the hip. Because the child is in a decubitus position, this means that the probe is held vertically (Fig. 101-2). Young infants tend to have a very straight lumbar spine, and the probe can be orientated to be parallel to the spine, placing the fingers of the examiner's hand along the spine while using the thumb and first finger to grip the probe.

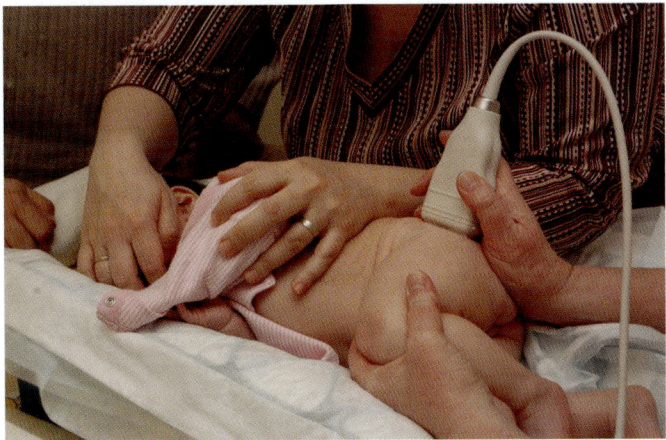

■ FIGURE 101-2 Ultrasound examination of an infant's hip.

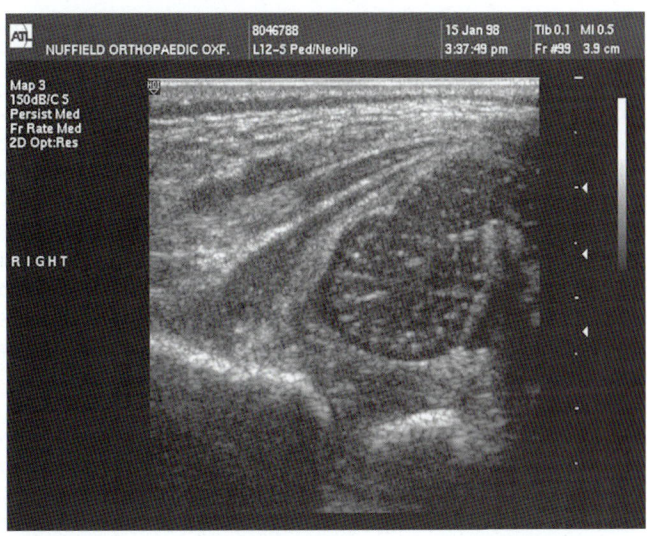

■ FIGURE 101-4 Coronal ultrasound of a dislocated hip. The femoral head no longer sits in the acetabular cup.

For this assessment it is important to produce a coronal image (Figs. 101-3 and 101-4). If the probe is rotated or tilted, then anomalous results will follow.

Anatomic (Morphology) Measurement

Once a true coronal image is obtained, then measurements may be made to assess the size and depth of the acetabulum. There are two common techniques. The first is that developed by Graf and his coworkers.[6,7] The first line (baseline) is drawn along with the lateral aspect of the bony ileum. In most infants this is seen as a relatively straight echogenic line, although there may be a slight curvature in a concave direction. If this is the case, the lower part of the ileum is used to construct the baseline. The second (roof) line is drawn from the supralateral corner of the acetabulum along the osseous margin where the advancing ossification of the ileum creates an echogenic white line. This is not a true representation of the position of the roof of the acetabulum because the line sits deep to the unossified cartilage within the acetabulum. The angle that this line makes to the baseline is termed the *α angle*. A second line is then constructed from the most inferior corner of the acetabulum at a tangent to the femoral head to intersect the tip of the hyaline cartilage of the labrum. This is referred to as the labral line. The angle described by this line to the baseline is the *β angle* (Fig. 101-5).

The hip is described by a classification that depends on the comparison of these two angles and on the age of the patient. In children whose hips fall into the category 2b or above there is perceived risk, and they are usually reviewed at 2 to 3 weeks. If the hip is not maturing to a category 1 (normal), then treatment is instituted.

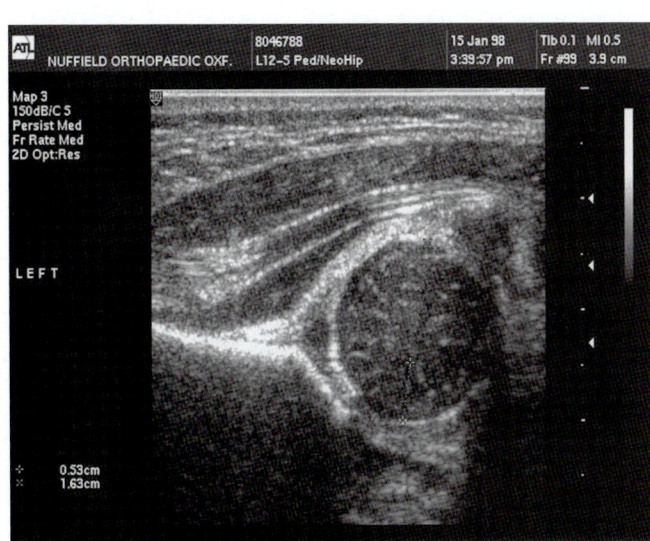

■ FIGURE 101-3 Coronal ultrasound image of a hip with a shallow acetabulum. Less than half of the femoral head is covered by the bony acetabulum.

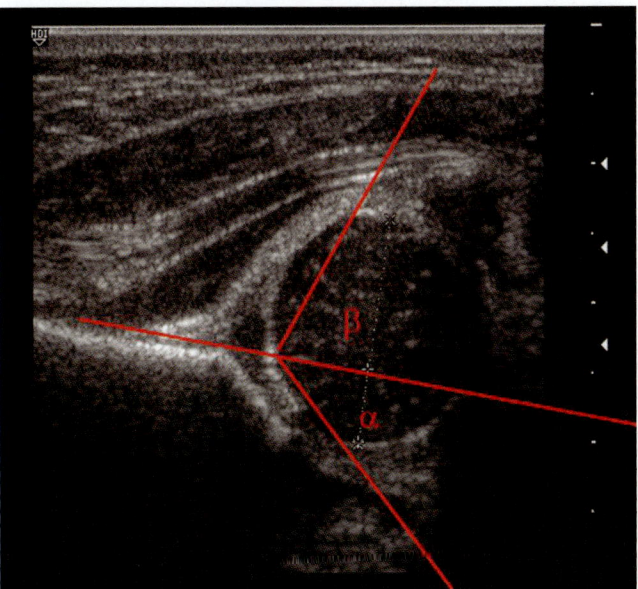

■ FIGURE 101-5 An ultrasound image with Graf measurement lines applied. The α and β angles are indicated.

A potential criticism of this technique is the difficulty in reproducing the points and position for the description of these angles. There is a particular problem in describing cartilaginous labral line. However, the roof line is relatively easy to reproduce, and in practice this is an effective technique. A further potential criticism of the method is that treatment is affected by minor variations in measurement. If the upper angle is greater than 43 degrees, this is considered abnormal; if it is less than 43 degrees, then it is normal. Therefore, a variation of 1 or 2 degrees can affect the management group. In practice, most workers will take this as guidance and if it is a borderline case they will clinically review the patient with further clinical and ultrasound follow-up.

An alternative ultrasound measurement technique is to produce the same image in a coronal plane and then to measure the percentage cover of the femoral head by the acetabulum. The same baseline is drawn, and then a circle is described around the unossified cartilage of the femoral head. The percentage of the circle that lies inside, or deep to, the baseline is calculated by measurements of the amount of the head inside and outside of the line (Fig. 101-6). Infants with 50% or more of the femoral head covered are considered to be entirely normal; those with 45% to 50% coverage are borderline, and those with less than 45% coverage are considered shallow. There are similar criticisms of this technique based on the positioning of lines, although it does prove relatively easy to place the circle when in comparison to the roof and labral lines of the Graf technique.

Dynamic Stability Testing

Subluxation of the hip may be a transient phenomenon. It has been noted that a hip that is looser or slacker than normal may be predisposed to subluxation. Therefore, some workers have suggested a dynamic assessment

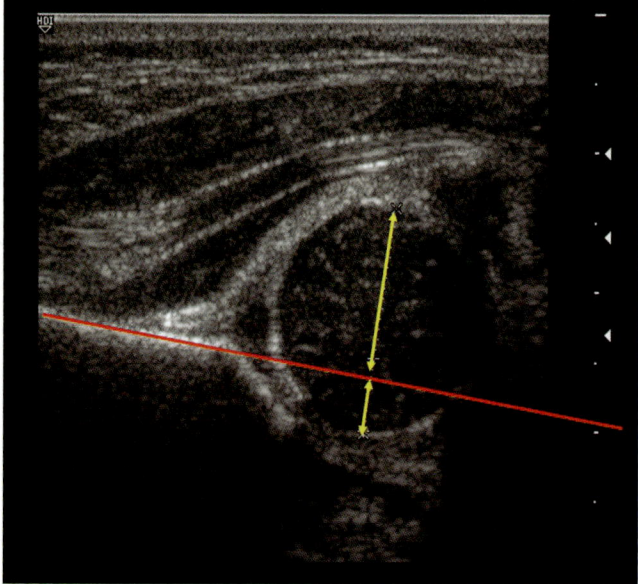

■ **FIGURE 101-6** Morin measurements applied to the ultrasound image. The ratio of the amount of the femoral head outside the line to that inside gives an index of femoral head coverage.

using gentle pressure to attempt to lift the femoral head out of the acetabulum as a means of assessing this potential for subluxation. A common technique that is used is to place the patient in the same decubitus position with the ultrasound probe aligned to achieve a coronal image. The probe must be placed with light pressure only. The examiner's hand is then placed under the child's thigh, and gentle pressure is exerted in the lateral direction in an attempt to slightly elevate the femoral head within the acetabulum. Observation of movement on the ultrasound image is recorded. Greater than 1 mm of movement of the femoral head away from the acetabulum is regarded as abnormal. This technique depends on the child being relaxed and comfortable. The crying infant will tense the muscles and tend to hold the femoral head in situ whatever the integrity of the acetabulum. As infants mature from birth to 3 months the capsule of the joint becomes tighter and this form of transient subluxation is less frequent. Persisting subluxation at follow-up appointments is regarded as a significant abnormality.

Most workers who recommend dynamic assessment will also use some form of morphologic assessment, and indeed many of those who originally had relied totally on morphologic assessment are now using a dynamic element to discriminate between the cases where there is difficulty in deciding on the next management step. Dynamic assessment is therefore particularly useful in those hips that are borderline in depth.

Combined Clinical and Ultrasound Examination

The clinical examinational techniques of Ortolani and Barlow are designed to allow the examiner to exert pressure on the femur and hip to attempt to subluxate the hip. The fingers of the examining hand detect this motion, and they may also detect the relocation of the hip as it moves back into place. Some workers use ultrasound as an adjunct to this examination. The child lies supine; the Ortolani and Barlow maneuvers are undertaken in the normal way while placing the ultrasound probe along the hip. A transverse (axial) plane of imaging is used. The combination of clinical and ultrasound observation is used to assess the stability of the hips.[8] This technique has the advantage that it combines a well-tried clinical method with a probably more sensitive means of assessing movement. However, it is difficult to quantify and measure and therefore difficult to audit its effectiveness.

Late Presentation

Children who present beyond the age of 3 months with symptoms or signs that are suggestive of hip dysplasia are probably best examined by plain radiographs. In the 3- to 6-month-old child ultrasound examination may assist the plain film assessment, although the degree of ossification in the femoral head varies and the more ossified the femoral head and the metaphysis are the harder it is to use ultrasound. However, because it is a noninvasive test it is also reasonable to use this in the first instance in the younger infant because if ultrasound examination is possible it will give more information than the plain radiograph.

The signs that are suggestive of development dysplasia in this age group are failure to walk at the normal milestones and abnormal skin folds or creases on clinical examination.

Assessment of acetabular depth on a plain radiograph is achieved by drawing a line between the obturator foramen (see Fig. 101-5) and then projecting a tangent along the bony acetabular roof. This describes the acetabular angle. An acetabular angle in excess of 25 degrees is considered to be abnormal. Simple measuring devices incorporating spirit levels have been used to make this easy from plain radiographs, but now with the advent of computer-based images it is a measurement easily performed at a workstation.

Postoperative imaging of osteotomies is also best achieved with plain radiographs. Occasionally the addition of a CT examination may be of value. MRI may be misleading because the metalwork involved often produces considerable metal artifacts. CT with metal suppression will allow reasonable assessment of the three-dimensional shape of the acetabulum and proximal femur. Care should be taken not to use CT excessively because of the radiation dose in young infants in a highly radiation sensitive part of the body.

The final assessment is of the young adult who presents with a premature osteoarthritis. Most clinicians will judge degrees of acetabular dysplasia by simply judging the overall appearance of the acetabulum, declaring it to be shallow or normal. Measurements may be taken of depth, but they are usually of little predictive value. Most important is the detection of narrowing of the joint space in a weight-bearing area, subchondral sclerosis, and subchondral cyst formation. These are the same signs looked for when examining for conventional degenerative arthropathy.

Patients who have shallow hips but otherwise normal joints may present with pain. An MR examination may be very useful in detecting subchondral edema, which will occur much earlier than radiographic bony changes. Articular surface fissuring and cracks may be detected best on MR arthrography in those in borderline cases. In cases of doubt a trial of local anesthetic placed in the joint may be diagnostic.

Screening Strategies

There is considerable debate as to how to screen populations for developmental dysplasia of the hip. It is generally agreed that clinical examination should be performed on all newborn infants, and there is considerable literature and evidence that this is effective in detecting the majority of cases of hip dislocation and a significant proportion of those with unstable hips. However, there is also evidence that a significant minority will be overlooked by plain clinical examination alone. In some centers a high-risk screening policy using ultrasound has been instituted. Factors that place an infant at higher risk of developmental dysplasia are listed in Table 101-2.

This screening policy will include well over 98% of those children who have hip anomalies, but there are still occasional patients who present with late dislocation because they did not fall into these high-risk categories.

TABLE 101-2	Risk Factors for Developmental Dysplasia of the Hip
Family history
Breech delivery
Prematurity
Other congenital anomalies
Any abnormality detected by health care workers

Ultrasonography has a modest positive predictive value (62%) but a high negative predictive value (99%).[9] Therefore a negative study should be reassuring.

In some countries (Germany, Austria, Switzerland) ultrasound examination of the newborn infant is compulsory if the parents are to receive child benefit.[10] This policy has been instituted for several years, and it will be very interesting to see in the long term whether these countries have a lower instance of premature osteoarthritis in the young or early middle-aged adult. It is notable that the incidence of splint therapy is very high in these practices. To date there have been no reports to suggest that the incidence of osteonecrosis or complications of splint therapy have increased; however, it is unclear whether this problem has been sought actively. Critics of the system say that children developing with other hip disorders such as Legg-Calvé-Perthes disease may have occult cases of osteonecrosis or femoral head damage caused by splint therapy. Proponents of the policy point out that the incidence of major surgery of the correction of developmental dysplasia of the hip and congenital dislocation has been massively reduced in the countries with a population screening policy. They also point out that the use of ultrasound screening reduces the rate of potentially damaging splint therapy.[11] In a recent review of the literature it was found that there was no hard evidence in favor of screening policies and these authors in common with others in European countries use ultrasound only to examine infants at risk.[12,13]

Follow-Up

In some institutions, infants who have borderline shallow hips or minor degrees of subluxation will be treated by early splinting. However, there are small, but significant, risks of splint therapy. Excessive confinement of the hip may lead to osteonecrosis and long-term permanent damage. This fortunately rare event is more likely to happen when the splint therapy is not controlled by a physiotherapist and when it is used for excessive periods. Less striking in terms of damage to the infant is the effect on the family dynamics of telling the parents that the child has an abnormality that needs treatment. This will alter the parents' approach to the infant and may have some psychological impact. It is generally believed that the minimal and least amount of treatment necessary is the best course. If minor degrees of dysplasia (shallow hip) and subtle degrees of dynamic subluxation are used to institute splint therapy, then a substantial proportion of normal newborns would be treated by splints. In some series this has reached 25% of newborns. Most workers will now use a follow-up examination to reduce the need for splint therapy. As the child matures, the hip will become stiffer and a properly confined femoral head will encourage the acetabulum to develop. This occurs quite rapidly, and even a short interval of a week may be sufficient to show change toward normal. Follow-up examination by clinical examination and ultrasound study is very useful in predicting this return to normalcy. It is often possible, in the borderline hip with minor subluxation, to avoid splint therapy by careful monitoring. Splint therapy should start by the age of 6 weeks for it to have a reasonable chance of success; therefore, there is a short opportunity in the relatively young infant for follow-up studies. Once the child is older than 6 weeks, then most workers would use a shallow hip or modest degrees of subluxation as indication for splint therapy.

True Dislocation

True dislocation, whether detected by clinical means and then confirmed by ultrasound or detected on ultrasound examination alone, is an indication for urgent referral to a pediatric orthopedic surgeon. The timing of surgical reduction and corrective osteotomies will depend on the individual and local surgical practice. Ultrasonography may be used to assess the depth of the acetabulum to which the hip will be reduced and in the detection of thickening of the ligamentum teres, which may prevent easy reduction. However, because the management of these cases is usually surgical, ultrasonography does not have a major role beyond initial diagnosis.

Postoperative Imaging

Most surgeons will perform operative reduction with the infant under general anesthesia in the operating suite using an arthrogram (contrast medium injected into the hip) to assess the location, size, and effectiveness of reduction. Once the hip is reduced, whether it be with the assistance of a pelvic osteotomy or not, then its correct location is at first determined by a combination of palpation and clinical judgment. It is then necessary to confirm the position of the hip by imaging. Plain radiographs are potentially misleading because the child will be in a hip plaster spica and the quality of the image will be poor. In addition, posterior dislocation, which may follow surgery, will be difficult to interpret on a single projection radiograph. Indeed, the alignment of the femur compared with the pelvis may look entirely normal when the femoral head, which is as yet unossified, is markedly dislocated.

Both CT and MRI have a role in these circumstances. The child is usually recovering from anesthesia and therefore relatively sedated. In addition, he or she is in a hard plaster spica, which immobilizes the child. It is therefore easy to perform either a CT examination, which will show up the residual contrast in the joint, or an MR study, which achieves the same effect without radiation (Figs. 101-7 to 101-10). Axial images will best demonstrate the location of the femoral head with respect to the shallow acetabulum.[14]

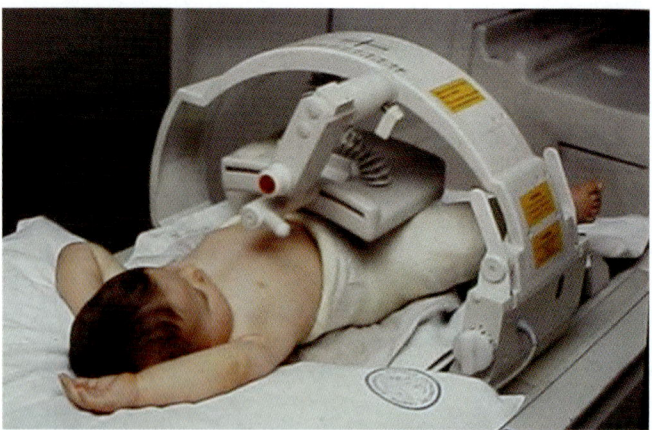

■ **FIGURE 101-7** After operative reduction of a dislocated hip the child is placed in a hip spica and MR examination is straightforward.

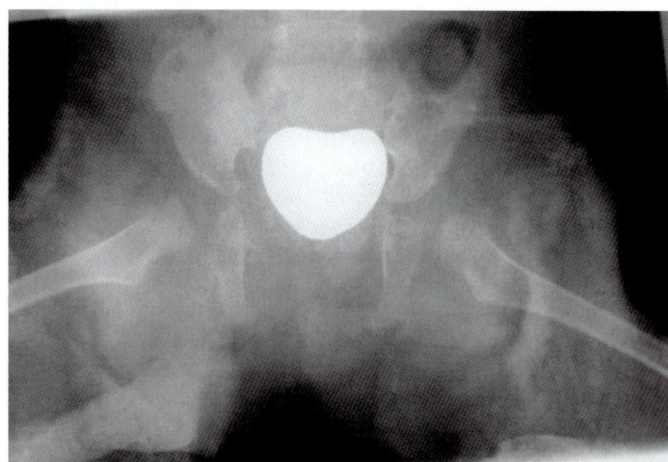

■ **FIGURE 101-8** Plain radiographs taken postoperatively are misleading because most cases of subluxation are in a posterior direction. This is the same case as Figure 101-10.

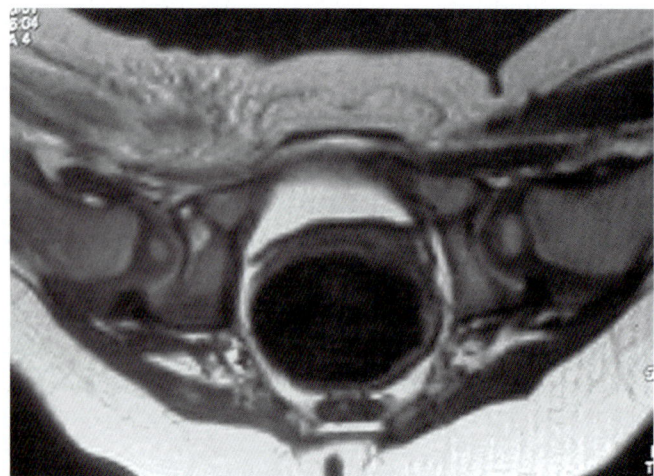

■ **FIGURE 101-9** On the postreduction MR axial image the femoral heads should align with the acetabulum as in this case.

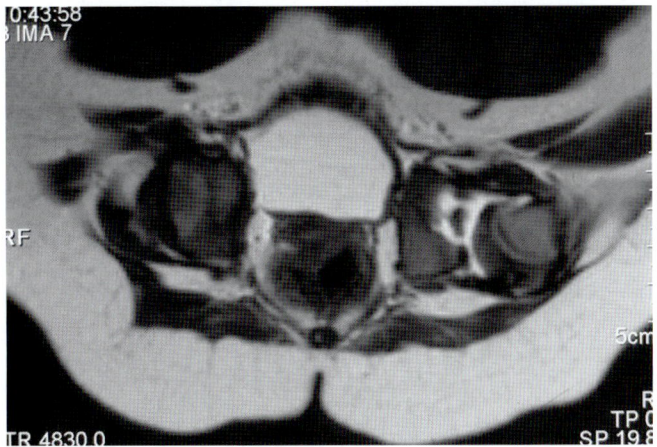

■ **FIGURE 101-10** This postoperative MR image is from the same case as in Figure 101-8. The plain radiograph failed to show that the hip was subluxated posteriorly, and further surgery was indicated.

SUMMARY

Ultrasound examination is the principal imaging method for detecting hip dysplasia when there is clinical doubt. There are advocates for its use in screening all infants. Splint therapy should begin before the age of 6 weeks. In the older child and young adult suspected of premature degeneration due to hip dysplasia, plain radiographs may be supplemented by CT, MRI, MR arthrography, and local anesthetic injection.

REFERENCES

1. Donaldson JS, Feinstein KA. Imaging of developmental dysplasia of the hip. Pediatr Clin North Am 1997; 44:591–614.
2. Gerscovich EO. A radiologist's guide to the imaging in the diagnosis and treatment of developmental dysplasia of the hip: II. Ultrasonography: anatomy, technique, acetabular angle measurements, acetabular coverage of femoral head, acetabular cartilage thickness, three-dimensional technique, screening of newborns, study of older children. Skeletal Radiol 1997; 26:447–456.
3. Zieger M, Schulz RD. Ultrasonography of the infant hip: III. Clinical application. Pediatr Radiol 1987; 17:226–232.
4. Rosenberg N, Bialik V. The effectiveness of combined clinical-sonographic screening in the treatment of neonatal hip instability. Eur J Ultrasound 2002; 15:55–60.
5. Allen G, et al. [Paediatric musculoskeletal ultrasound]. J Radiol 2005; 86:1924–1930.
6. Graf R. [Profile of radiologic-orthopedic requirements in pediatric hip dysplasia, coxitis and epiphyseolysis capitis femoris]. Radiologe 2002; 42:467–473.
7. Ozcelik A, et al. Assessment of the use of hip ultrasonography by Graf's method between 1 and 6 years of age. J Pediatr Orthop B 2005; 14:97–100.
8. Harcke HT. Imaging methods used for children with hip dysplasia. Clin Orthop Relat Res 2005; (434):71–77.
9. Woolacott NF, et al. Ultrasonography in screening for developmental dysplasia of the hip in newborns: systematic review. BMJ 2005; 330:1413.
10. Dorn U, Neumann D. Ultrasound for screening developmental dysplasia of the hip: a European perspective. Curr Opin Pediatr 2005; 17:30–33.
11. Gardner F, et al. The hip trial: psychosocial consequences for mothers of using ultrasound to manage infants with developmental hip dysplasia. Arch Dis Child Fetal Neonatal Ed 2005; 90: F17–F24.
12. U.S. Preventive Services Task Force. Screening for developmental dysplasia of the hip: recommendation statement. Am Fam Physician 2006; 73:1992–1996.
13. Paton RW, Hinduja K, Thomas CD. The significance of at-risk factors in ultrasound surveillance of developmental dysplasia of the hip: a ten-year prospective study. J Bone Joint Surg Br 2005; 87:1264–1266.
14. Westhoff B, et al. Magnetic resonance imaging after reduction for congenital dislocation of the hip. Arch Orthop Trauma Surg 2003; 123:289–292.
15. Godward S, Dezateux C. Surgery for congenital dislocation of the hip in the UK as a measure of outcome of screening. MRC Working Party on Congenital Dislocation of the Hip. Medical Research Council. Lancet 1998; 351:1149–1152.

CHAPTER 102

Coalitions

Michele Calleja and Simon Ostlere

Coalition represents abnormal fusion between two or more bones; it occurs more commonly in the bony tarsus but is also seen in the carpal bones. The condition may be congenital or acquired. Coalitions may be complete or incomplete and are bony (synostosis), cartilaginous (synchondrosis), or fibrous (syndesmosis).

Carpal coalition is often an incidental finding, although fused bones are known to be more prone to fracturing. On the other hand, patients with tarsal coalition usually present in the second and third decades of life with foot pain.

ETIOLOGY

Both tarsal and carpal coalitions may be *acquired* secondary to trauma; this may be secondary to injury or may be surgically induced (arthrodesis). It may also result from infection (including osteomyelitis and tuberculosis) or articular disorders such as juvenile chronic arthritis and osteoarthritis.[1]

Early research by Pfitzner, Sloman, Badgley, Harris, and others favored a theory of incorporation of accessory ossicles into adjacent tarsal bones as an explanation for *congenital* coalition. This theory was later disproved by the discovery that coalition was present in fetuses. After Leboucq's initial proposition in 1890 and its subsequent confirmation by Harris' anatomic studies on fetal cadavers in 1955, it is now universally accepted that congenital or developmental coalition represents a disorder of organization of primitive mesenchyme in the fifth week of life.[2-4]

A tarsal-carpal coalition syndrome exists. This is transmitted as an autosomal dominant condition and is characterized by fusion of carpals, tarsals, and phalanges and short first metacarpals, causing brachydactyly and humeroradial fusion.

Both carpal and tarsal coalition occur in various syndromes: Ellis-van Creveld syndrome, symphalangism, arthrogryposis multiplex congenita, hand-foot-uterus syndrome, Apert's syndrome, gonadal dysgenesis (Turner's syndrome), Nievergelt's syndrome, fetal alcohol syndrome, Holt-Oram syndrome, as well as diastrophic dwarfism.

In some cases of tarsal coalition, a family history of identical abnormalities is obtained. Leonard reported that 39% of 98 first-degree relatives of 31 patients with peroneal spastic flat foot and partial coalition had some type of fusion themselves, although the pattern varied among the patients and their relatives. He proposed that the disorder was of autosomal dominant inheritance with genetic variability of expression.[5]

PREVALENCE AND EPIDEMIOLOGY

Coalitions have been part of the human gene pool for centuries. In 1965, Harris discovered a coalition in a Mayan archeological specimen found in Guatemala. In 1969, Heiple and Lovejoy demonstrated the presence of bilateral talocalcaneal coalitions in a pre-Columbian Indian specimen.[3]

The earliest mention of coalition in the literature was made in 1829, when Cruveilhier produced the first known anatomic description of calcaneonavicular coalition.[4] It was Holl, in 1880, who first theorized the relationship between tarsal coalition and peroneal spastic flatfoot.

The true prevalence of tarsal coalitions is not known; estimates range from far less than 1% of the population to 1% to 2%, although they may well be higher because patients

---

KEY POINTS

- Tarsal coalition is not an uncommon condition, with a quoted prevalence of 1% to 2%, although higher estimates are quoted.
- Although often asymptomatic in the earlier years, tarsal coalition may present as midfoot pain during the period in which ossification of cartilaginous precursors occurs.
- Calcaneonavicular and talocalcaneal coalitions are most commonly encountered.
- Carpal coalition is often asymptomatic and discovered incidentally.
- A combination of imaging modalities, including plain radiography, CT, and MRI, is often necessary for accurate diagnosis and surgical planning.

are commonly asymptomatic. A recent dissection and CT study of cadaveric feet found that the incidence of nonosseous tarsal coalition is around 12.7%, much higher than previously thought.[5] There is a slight male preponderance. The condition is bilateral in around 50% of cases.

The prevalence of isolated carpal coalition is quoted at 0.08% to 0.13%. It tends to occur more commonly in the black population, and there is a strong female predilection. Carpal fusions are frequently bilateral.

CLINICAL PRESENTATION

Tarsal Coalition

Although some patients may be asymptomatic, patients typically present in the second or third decade of life with vague pain in the foot, which is often aggravated by minor trauma or unusual athletic activity. An earlier age at onset is rare, perhaps because, at this time, the fusion is fibrous or cartilaginous. Symptoms usually become more pronounced with progressive ossification of the coalition.

Physical examination can reveal pes planus, limited subtalar motion (worse with talocalcaneal coalition), and shortening with persistent or intermittent spasm of the peroneal muscles. The rigid foot may be held in valgus, although a varus deformity can be seen with anterior tibial spasm. A cavus foot may also be seen at presentation.

Carpal Coalition

This is mostly an asymptomatic condition. It may produce symptoms by virtue of alteration of the normal biomechanics of the wrist. This can then predispose the affected joints and surrounding soft tissues to abnormal stress, leading to discomfort or pain during repetitive strain, such as while playing musical instruments or racquet sports. Partial coalitions and cystic changes are associated with an increased incidence of pain. Fused carpal bones also incur an increased risk of fracture. Patients with congenital lunatotriquetral coalition may poorly tolerate stress loading or trauma, resulting in symptoms similar to degenerative arthritis or pseudarthrosis. Kienböck's disease may also present in conjunction with carpal coalition.

Activities posing a high stress demand on the wrist movement, especially in sportsmen, result in progressive loading and thus early degenerative arthritis or pseudarthrosis, leading to earlier presentation.

MANIFESTATIONS OF THE DISEASE

Tarsal Coalition

Isolated coalitions can be classified according to the bones that are affected—*calcaneonavicular, talocalcaneal, talonavicular,* and *calcaneocuboid* in decreasing order of frequency—although improved detection using CT and MRI has shown that talocalcaneal coalition is at least as common as is the calcaneonavicular type.

Tarsal fusions occurring as part of a syndrome may have atypical patterns or may even involve the whole tarsus.

Calcaneonavicular Coalition

This is one of the most frequent types of coalitions and may be bilateral. The anatomy of calcaneonavicular coalition was described by Cruveilhier in 1829,[4] nearly a century before its clinical relationship to peroneal spastic flatfoot was radiographically shown by Sloman in 1921. It may present as part of the rigid flatfoot or may be asymptomatic. Calcaneonavicular coalition is defined as abnormal coalescence of the calcaneus with the tarsal navicular bone. As with the other coalitions, it may be described as osseous (synostosis) or nonosseous (synchondrosis or syndesmosis), but it is probably best to consider these categories as points in a histopathologic continuum.[6] The normal morphologic relationship between the calcaneus and the navicular can be described as a slender gap between the two articulated bone structures, and this occurs in a statistically normal distribution in the general population. At either end of the spectrum is found a broader gap between the two and completely continuous osseous ossification.

Radiography

Osseous calcaneonavicular coalition is clearly visualized as a continuous bony bar bridging the calcaneus and the navicular. It is best diagnosed by using three standard radiographic views of the foot; these should ideally include a 45-degree medial or lateral oblique view, which is considered to be the best view for detection of the coalition (Fig. 102-1). The diagnosis can be overlooked on the standard anteroposterior and lateral projections, although a study by Crim and Kjeldsberg[7] has shown that in a substantial number of coalition cases this osseous bar can be seen if the lateral margin of the navicular bone is examined carefully on a standard anteroposterior film. The theory behind this is that the shape of the navicular bone is altered by an underlying coalition. The anteroposterior radiograph will thus often show that the proximal border of the navicular is wider than the talonavicular joint. Occasionally, a fracture may occur across the coalition.

Cartilaginous or fibrous coalitions are harder to diagnose; there are various radiographic pointers that should raise the level of suspicion:

1. Close proximity of the calcaneus to the navicular
2. Flattening and widening of the calcaneus as it approaches the navicular
3. Eburnation or sclerosis of the two cortical surfaces
4. Elongation of the anterosuperior portion of the calcaneus—the "anteater nose" sign.
5. Hypoplasia of the talar head (secondary sign)
6. A proximal portion of the navicular that is wider than the talonavicular joint
7. A tapered elongated appearance to the navicular bone

CT and MRI are not usually necessary for the diagnosis of calcaneonavicular coalition. When all the radiographic pointers just described are used, radiographic sensitivity for diagnosis of calcaneonavicular coalition was 100% with 97% specificity in one study.[7] Cross-sectional imaging may occasionally be used for further characterization and for presurgical planning. The transverse and coronal planes provide the best delineation of this form of coalition.

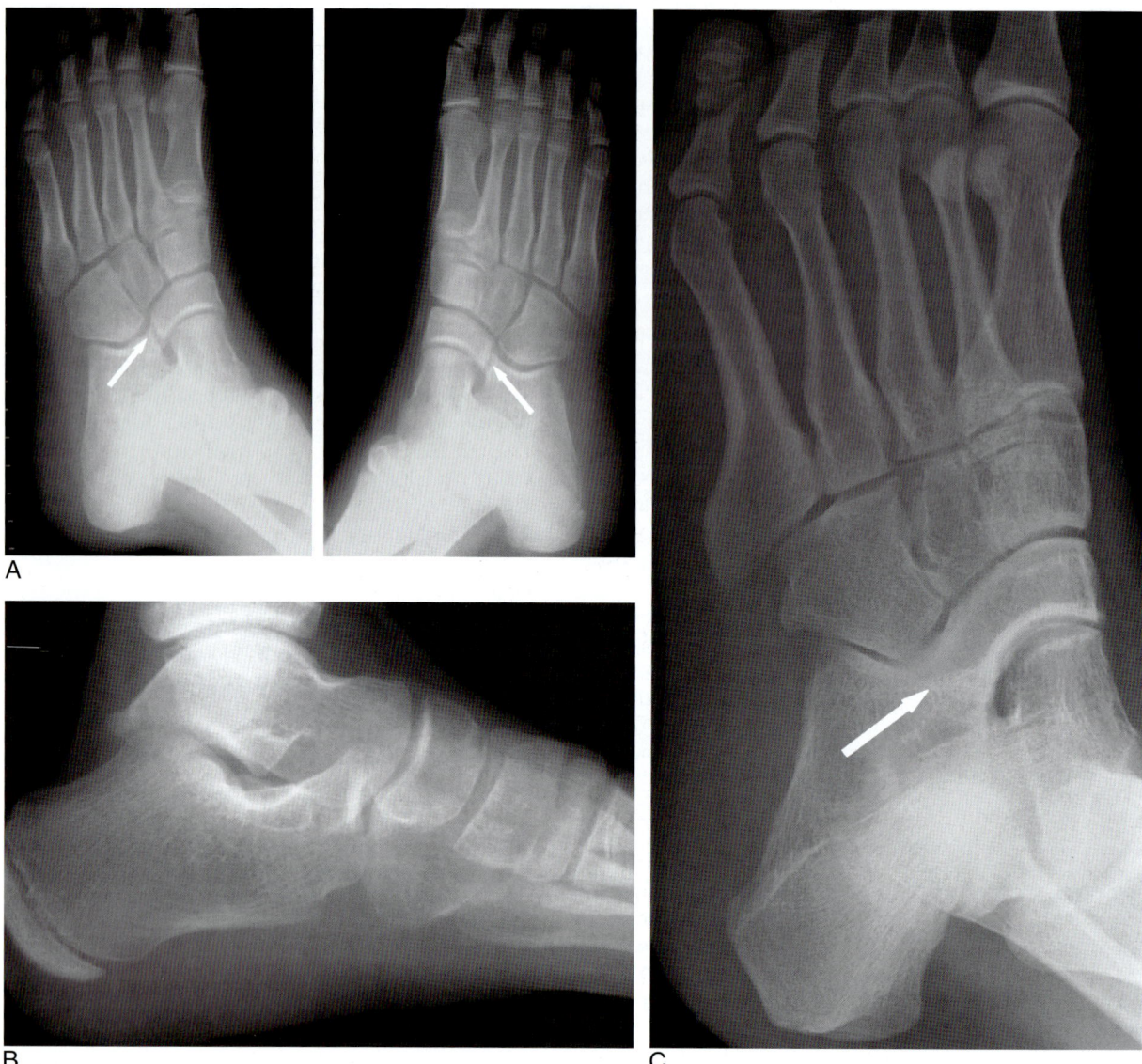

■ **FIGURE 102-1** **A,** Medial oblique radiograph of both feet shows a calcaneonavicular coalition. There are defects in the bony bar indicating that these represent the fibrous or cartilaginous type of coalition. **B,** Lateral radiograph of the same patient shows the "anteater nose" sign—elongation of the anterior process of the calcaneus. **C,** Oblique radiograph shows a complete osseous bar (*arrow*) across the calcaneonavicular joint.

Axial CT sections in a plane parallel to the ankle joint and long axis of the foot show broadening of the medial aspect of the anterior and dorsal calcaneus as it lies close to the navicular. There may be narrowing and reactive sclerosis of the apposing bony surfaces.

Talocalcaneal Coalition

This is the other common type of talar coalition. Understanding the complex articular anatomy of the subtalar joint is crucial to understanding this type of coalition. Although the talus and calcaneus articulate by means of three facets (anterior, middle, and posterior), the anatomic (posterior) subtalar joint consists only of the articulation between the posterior calcaneal facet of the

talus and the posterior talar facet of the calcaneus. These posterior facets are separated from the middle and anterior facets by the sinus tarsi.

The anterior and middle facets of the calcaneus articulate with the corresponding talar facet in a separate synovial articulation. This anteromedial subtalar joint is continuous with the talocalcaneonavicular joint. Rarely, the posterolateral subtalar joint and the anteromedial talocalcaneonavicular joints may become confluent.

Talocalcaneal fusion most commonly involves the middle facet, between the talus and the sustentaculum tali.[8]

Coalitions centered just posterior to the sustentaculum are rare but have been reported both in children and in adults.[9] In these cases, the abnormal articulation lies posterior to the sustentaculum, and it comprises a pseudarthrosis between a bony overgrowth of the middle tubercle of the talus and a bony exostosis lying between the posterior and middle subtalar facets.

Anterior facet ankylosis may also occur but are far less frequent.

Talocalcaneal coalition is more common in boys and is bilateral in 20% to 25% of patients.

Radiography

Because of the complex nature of the subtalar joint, this coalition type may be difficult to diagnose on the three standard views of the foot. Early reports of imaging for tarsal coalition emphasized the axial (Harris-Beath) projection of the hindfoot. However, this is not normally part of a routine foot series. Thus, a number of secondary radiographic signs have been described. Some of these develop due to altered hindfoot biomechanics secondary to the coalition and include:

1. *A talar beak:* this refers to a flaring of the superior margin of the talar head seen on lateral radiographs. It is caused by rigidity at the subtalar joint leading to dorsal subluxation of the navicular and subsequent elevation of the periosteum beneath the talonavicular ligament. A similar excrescence occurs on the adjacent navicular. Fracture of the beak may occur after trauma. It is important to stress that a talar beak is not always present with talocalcaneal coalition. Conversely, a hypertrophied talar ridge may occur in the absence of coalition, for example, in patients with diffuse idiopathic skeletal hyperostosis, acromegaly, or rheumatoid arthritis and in certain athletes.
2. *Narrowing of the posterior subtalar joint:* this often represents degenerative arthropathy and is seen in 50% to 60% of cases.
3. *Broadening of the lateral talar process:* this is present in 40% to 60% of patients.
4. *Classic or continuous C sign of Lateur:* originally described by Lateur and associates,[10] this is seen on the lateral view and is a C-shaped line formed by the medial outline of the talar dome and a bony bridge between the talar dome and the sustentaculum tali (Fig. 102-2). The C sign may be observed in both osseous and nonosseous coalitions and is reported by some authors to be a sensitive and specific sign of talocalcaneal coalition,[10] although both false-positive (in pes planovalgus) and false-negative (in sustentacular aplasia) findings occur. Several studies have, in fact, reported a 20% incidence of the C sign in patients who had a flatfoot deformity but no tarsal coalition.[7,11] In normal persons, the C line is noncontinuous because it is broken by the posterior margin of the sustentaculum. Various authors have reported different sensitivities (88%-98%) for this sign.
5. *Absent middle facet sign:* this refers to the finding of an osseous density bridging the subtalar middle facets that can be seen on standing lateral radiographs. Liu and associates[12] found that this sign has a higher sensitivity and a specificity nearly equal to the C sign and talar beak sign for the diagnosis of subtalar coalition.
6. *Ball-and-socket tibiotalar joint:* this is seen in severe cases of juvenile coalition and occurs as a consequence of adaptation of the ankle joint to provide the inversion and eversion function that is restricted at the subtalar joint by the coalition.[12] A ball-and-socket ankle joint is usually fully developed by 5 years of age. Incidentally, this anomaly may also occur in conjunction with other congenital and acquired disorders of the midfoot.
7. *Dysmorphic sustentaculum tali:* this occurs when the sustentaculum tali is enlarged and has an ovoid configuration on lateral radiographs. This sign was described by Crim and Kjeldsberg[7] and was found to have a sensitivity of 82% but a specificity of only 70%; it tended to vary depending on the angle of the radiographic beam.[7]

In posteromedial subtalar coalition, the radiographic features are more subtle and there is absence of the features usually associated with middle facet coalition. On the lateral radiograph, the middle facet remains visible, although abnormal ossification between the middle and posterior facets may be seen.[9]

Computed Tomography

Computed tomography is extremely valuable in the diagnosis of this type of coalition because of its ability to display the complex bony anatomy of the hindfoot. It may also be used for surgical planning, when it assists in determining whether resection of the coalition is feasible or whether an arthrodesis is required. However, some studies have found that spiral CT has a low sensitivity in the detection of nonosseous coalitions, and fibrous unions may be completely missed; thus its routine use is questionable when tarsal coalition is suspected.[13,14]

Conventional multiplanar CT is used in some institutions. Alternatively, spiral CT may be performed with reconstructions in both coronal and axial planes. The coronal plane is perpendicular to the ankle joint and long axis of the foot, although Wechsler and associates[15] described a slightly different orientation that is perpendicular to the plane of the subtalar joint. The axial plane is parallel to the ankle joint and long axis of the foot. It is crucial to image both feet simultaneously because of the potential bilaterality of the condition and also for accurate comparison.

Magnetic Resonance Imaging

Magnetic resonance images of the foot and ankle should be acquired in three planes: axial or oblique axial, coronal, and sagittal. T1-, T2- and proton density–weighted fast spin-echo sequences are generally adequate. For adequate assessment of bone marrow edema, at least one fat-suppressed sequence is used (e.g., short tau inversion recovery [STIR] or frequency-selective fat-suppressed proton density– or T2-weighted imaging), usually in the coronal or sagittal plane. These sequences will also help assess soft tissue edema and inflammatory changes. The sagittal plane nicely shows the secondary osseous changes such as talar beaking.

With MRI, talocalcaneal coalitions can be seen directly, whether they are osseous, cartilaginous, or fibrous (see Fig. 102-2). The fat-suppressed sequences are very sensitive at detecting marrow edema at the sites of coalition. The T1-weighted sequences may show bone marrow continuity across a bony coalition, and marginal reactive changes may also be noted.

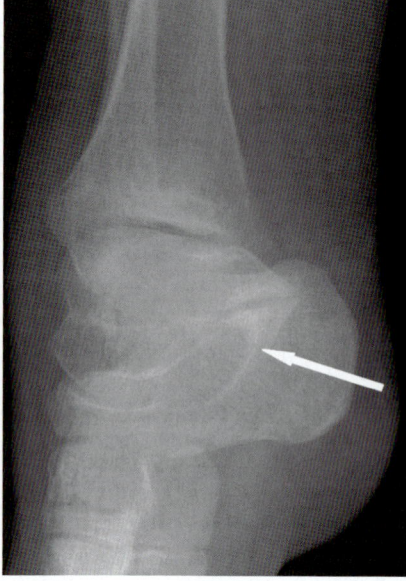

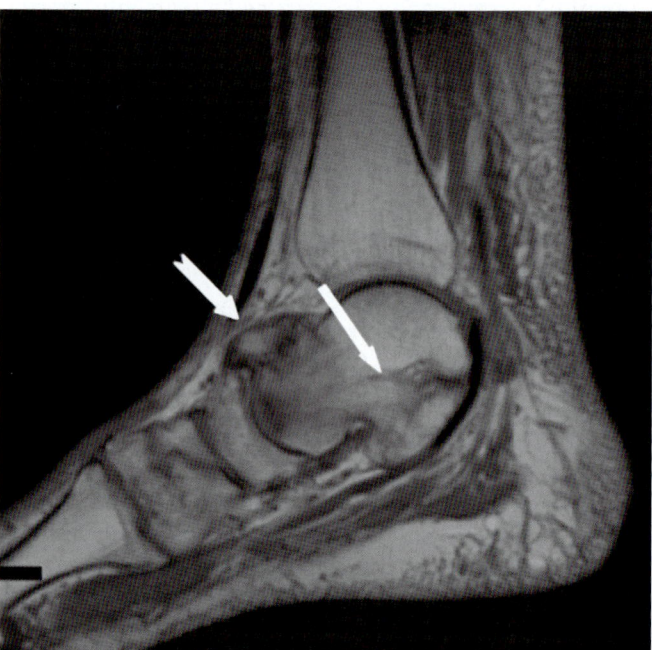

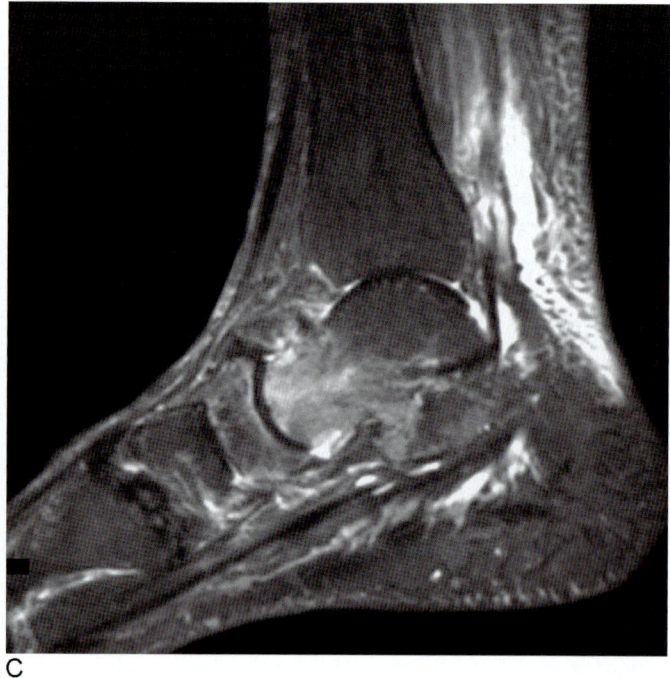

■ **FIGURE 102-2** The "continuous C-sign of Lateur" is demonstrated on a lateral radiograph (**A**, *arrows*). It is formed by the medial outline of the talar dome, the edge of bony coalition, and the enlarged sustentaculum tali. Sagittal T1-weighted (**B**) and STIR (**C**) MR images of the ankle of a 30-year-old man with chronic midfoot pain. The T1-weighted image shows bone marrow continuity across the bony coalition of the middle facet, between the talus and the sustentaculum (*straight arrow*). There is secondary talar beaking (*notched arrow*). On the STIR image there is bone edema mainly related to secondary degenerative changes at the talonavicular joint.

(Continued)

Moreover, MRI allows assessment of accompanying abnormalities (e.g., peroneal tendon disease).

Both cross-sectional imaging methods can be used to observe patients after surgical resection of the osseous, cartilaginous, or fibrous bar.

Talonavicular Coalition

Talonavicular coalition is uncommon and may be inherited as an autosomal dominant or recessive trait. It may also be associated with anomalies of the little finger. Patients are often asymptomatic,[15] although they may present early (around age 5 years) with some pain or peroneal spasm.

Isolated talonavicular synostosis in the developing foot may result in marked impairment of subtalar range of motion and may even lead to the development of a ball-and-socket ankle joint. Bony protuberance at the level of the navicular bone may also be observed.

Acquired talonavicular coalition has been reported after avascular necrosis of the navicular bone.

Radiography

Plain radiography usually clearly shows the osseous bridge. Both CT and MRI may be useful when the diagnosis is in doubt (Fig. 102-3).

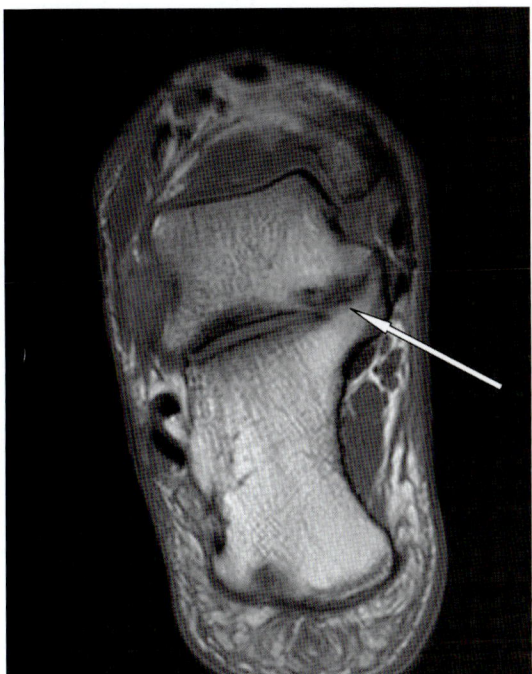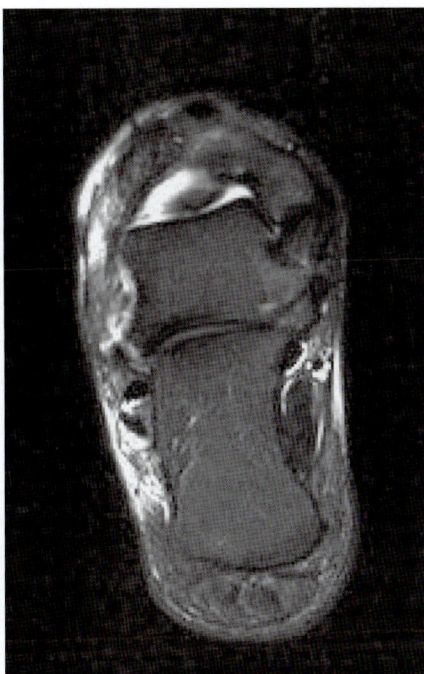

D

■ FIGURE 102-2—Cont'd D, These coronal T1-weighted (*left*) and proton density–weighted, fat-saturated (*right*) images show nonosseous coalition across the middle facet (*arrow*). There is surrounding bone marrow stress change that is well seen on the fat-saturated image.

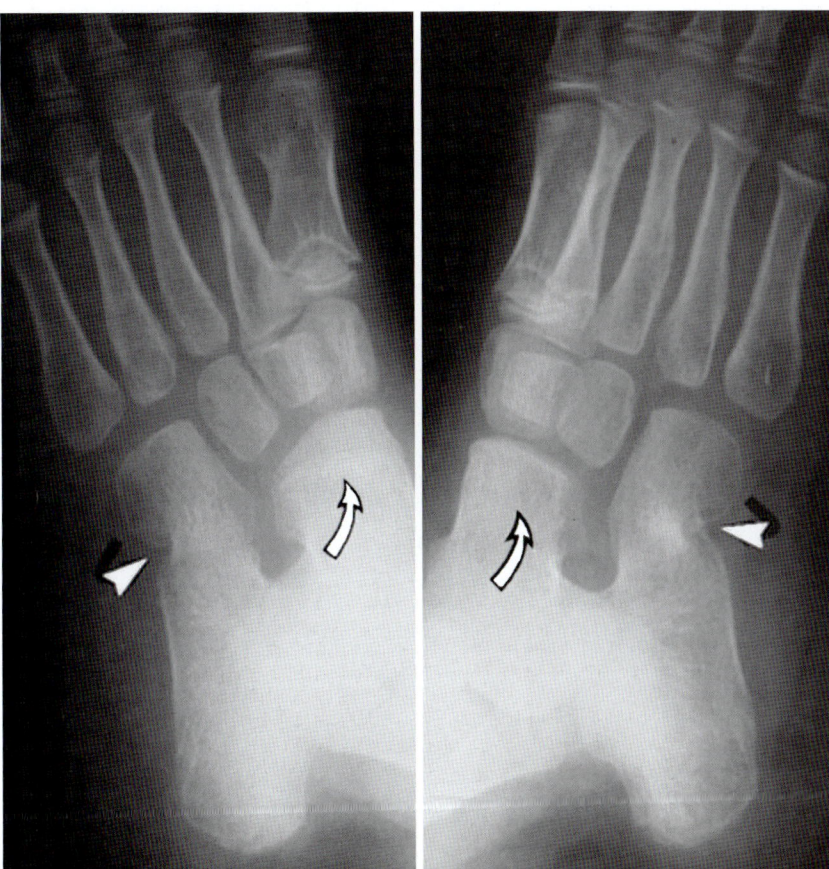

■ FIGURE 102-3 Oblique radiographs of both feet in a 10-year-old child show bilateral osseous talonavicular (*curved arrows*) and calcaneocuboid (*arrowheads*) coalitions. These were part of a syndromic manifestation.

Other Coalitions

Calcaneocuboid and cubonavicular coalitions are very rare. Navicular/first cuneiform coalitions have also been reported, and some authors have suggested that the actual incidence may be higher than previously thought. Around 25% of patients diagnosed with the condition were symptomatic, with mild midfoot pain. Some had been erroneously diagnosed as having osteoarthritis. CT is useful in diagnosing the condition.

CARPAL COALITIONS

Synostosis of carpal bones is usually an incidental finding on carpal radiographs taken for totally unrelated reasons. It may be congenital, in which there is a common association with syndromic disorders, or secondary to inflammatory arthropathy.

Congenital carpal fusions are thought to develop from failure of segmentation and cavitation at the site of a future joint space with subsequent chondrification and ossification rather than union of separate carpal bones.[16] The ossification process is not affected by the cartilaginous segmentation; hence, the fused bones still retain their shape.

Isolated fusion has a prevalence of around 0.1% in the white population and 1.6% in the black population, with an incidence of up to 8% reported in native Nigerians.[17] There is a strong female predilection, and the lesion is frequently bilateral, usually involving adjacent bones in the same carpal row (Fig. 102-4).

Conversely, *syndrome-related fusion* affects bones in different rows.[18] Massive carpal fusions and fusions between the carpal bones and radius and ulna are generally associated with additional malformations. These include tarsal coalitions or one of the congenital syndromes such as acrocephalosyndactyly, arthrogryposis, diastrophic dwarfism, Ellis-van Creveld syndrome, Holt-Oram syndrome, Turner's syndrome, or symphalangism.

Drug-induced fusion has been reported with thalidomide-induced embryopathy in which congenital multiple carpal fusion is a recurring feature. In fetal alcohol syndrome, capitate-trapezoid and radioulnar synostoses have been described.[1]

Acquired carpal fusion may be seen after injury. Traumatic conditions cause ligamentous ruptures or may lead to chronic periostitis, both of which may eventually result in bony union in the affected joints. Surgically induced carpal fusion (arthrodesis) may be performed to improve hand function and provide pain relief in conditions such as degenerative disease, subluxation, dislocation, fracture, nonunion, avascular necrosis, and so on. Acquired fusions are also common in arthritis, particularly in rheumatoid arthritis and juvenile chronic arthritis, where they are easily distinguished from congenital fusion. There is a distinct pattern of intra-articular osseous fusion occurring mostly bilaterally and commonly involving midcarpal joints.

Most cases of isolated carpal fusion are asymptomatic, although pain has been observed in some cases. Partial coalitions and cystic changes produce a higher incidence of pain. Fused carpal bones also carry a definite increased risk of fracture.

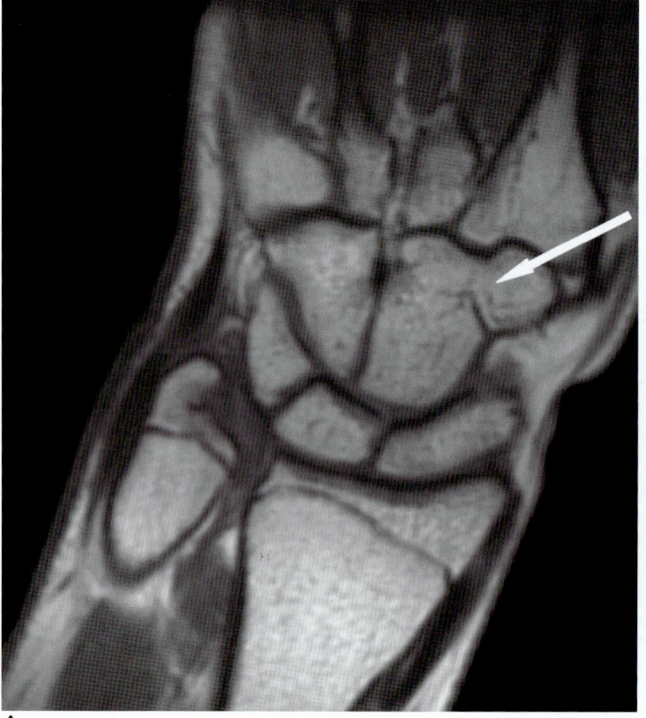
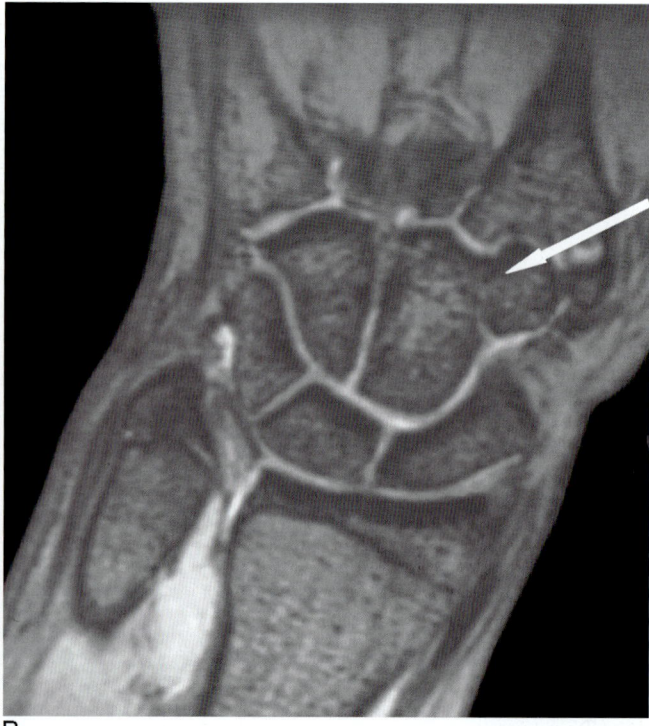

A   B

■ **FIGURE 102-4**   Coronal T1-weighted (**A**) and proton density–weighted, fat-saturated (**B**) MR images in a 16-year-old girl with a year's history of wrist pain show an incomplete osseous fusion between the distal portion of the capitate and the trapezoid bones (*arrows*). A small proximal cleft persists. This was an incidental finding. She was also found to have abnormality of the triangular fibrocartilage complex.

Lunotriquetral Coalition

This is the most common isolated carpal coalition. It was first described in an anatomy text in the late 18th century by Sandifort,[19] although the earliest clinical case was reported approximately 120 years later by Corson.[20] The condition is most commonly bilateral, but if unilateral it tends to be left sided. The highest incidence is in people of West African descent, with a 10% to 20% higher incidence in blacks than whites.

Lunate-triquetral coalition may show incomplete fusion (type I), proximal osseous bridge with a distal notch (type II), complete fusion (type III), or fusion with associated carpal abnormalities (type IV) (Fig. 102-5).

Patients with congenital lunotriquetral coalition, especially type I fusions, may poorly tolerate trauma or stress loading; and this may result in a symptomatic state similar to degenerative arthritis or pseudarthrosis. This is an uncommon cause for ulnar-sided wrist pain. In these cases, MRI will demonstrate evidence of bone edema and there is gadolinium-enhancing fibrovascular tissue in the synovium and subarticular cysts. Traumatic disruption of a fibrocartilage lunate-triquetral coalition has been described in the literature.

In around 46% of patients with congenital lunate-triquetral coalition there is an abnormally widened scapholunate joint space with, however, an intact scapholunate ligament. This finding is thought to be a normal variant and not disease.[21]

Capitate-Hamate Fusion

This is the second most common pattern of carpal fusion and was first reported by Dwight in 1907.[22] It is most frequently bilateral, and the lowest incidence reported is in East Africans, with the highest incidence (0.4%-0.8%) reported in West Africans. There is a syndromic association, although it may also occur secondary to any of the causes listed earlier. Although generally asymptomatic, isolated capitate-hamate fusion may present as sequelae of neuropathy, arthritis, or fracture.

Iatrogenic (surgically induced) capitate-hamate fusion is commonly used as treatment for Kienböck's disease of the lunate. The rationale behind this is that once the capitate and hamate are fused there is an increase in the radioscaphoid mean pressure, with a subsequent decrease in the radiolunate mean pressure. There is overall little effect on the radiocarpal mean pressure, and patients with Kienböck's disease benefit by means of an increase in grip strength.[23]

Radiography

Because this type of coalition may be incomplete, multiple radiographic projections may be necessary for assessment of the synostosis. Sometimes intraosseous cysts are seen adjacent to the area of coalition. Cross-sectional imaging is only used when the diagnosis is in doubt and the radiographic findings are subtle.

Pisiform-Hamate Fusion

This is a rare anomaly and only a few cases have been reported in the literature. It is thought to be due to metaplastic conversion of ligament into bone and not due to failure of formation of articular interzones.

SYNOPSIS OF TREATMENT OPTIONS
Medical Treatment

Symptomatic calcaneonavicular coalition is initially managed with a trial of reduced activity or cast immobilization. This may render patients asymptomatic. Intermittent casting for short periods may also be useful. Molded firm arch supports may be used especially during activities.

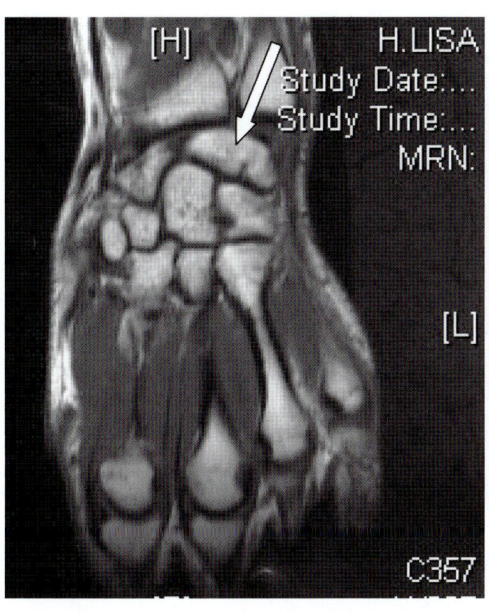
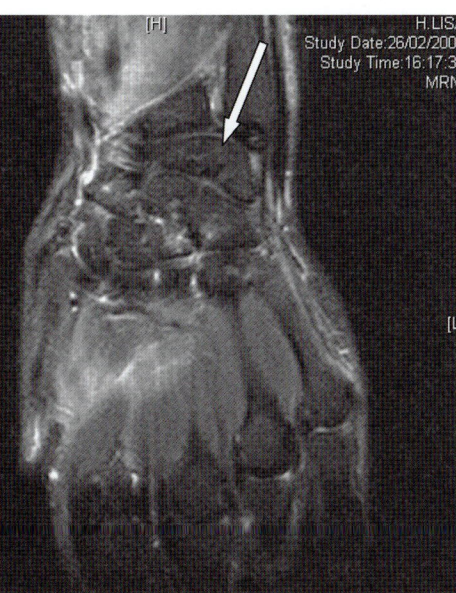

■ **FIGURE 102-5** These coronal T1-weighted (*left*) and STIR (*right*) MR images through the hand of a young adult with persistent wrist pain show almost complete bony lunotriquetral fusion (*arrows*), with persistence of a tiny distal cortical cleft.

An initial trial of conservative treatment is also recommended for talocalcaneal coalitions. This includes reduced activity, 4 to 6 weeks in a short-leg walking cast, followed by a period wearing arch supports. Corticosteroid injection into the sinus tarsi may be useful.

Surgical Treatment

The most commonly accepted surgical treatments for calcaneonavicular coalition are resection of the calcaneonavicular bar with interposition of fat at the site of resection, subtalar arthrodesis, or triple arthrodesis.

For talocalcaneal coalition, resection of the fibrous or bony talocalcaneal bar is recommended as an initial treatment of middle facet subtalar coalition. Better results are obtained in the younger population, although excellent results have been achieved in patients in their 20s and 30s. In older patients, especially those in whom degenerative changes are pronounced, triple arthrodesis is indicated.[24]

REFERENCES

1. McCredie J. Congenital fusion of bones: radiology, embryology and pathogenesis. Clin Radiol 1975; 26:47-51.
2. Resnick D: Additional Congenital or Heritable Anomalies and Syndromes. In Resnick D (ed): Diagnosis of Bone and Joint Disorders, 4th ed. Philadelphia, WB Saunders, 2002, pp 4592-4599.
3. Heiple KG, Lovejoy CO. The antiquity of tarsal coalition: bilateral deformity in a pre-Columbian Indian skeleton. J Bone Joint Surg Am 1969; 51:979-983.
4. Cruveilhier J. Anatomie Pathologique du Corps Humain. Paris, Bailliere, 1829, vol 1.
5. Solomon LB, Ruhli FJ, Taylor J, et al. A dissection and computer tomography study of tarsal coalitions in 100 cadaver feet. J Orthop Res 2006; 21:352-358.
6. Lysack JT, Fenton PV. Variations in calcaneonavicular morphology demonstrated with radiography. Radiology 2004; 230:493-497.
7. Crim JR, Kjeldsberg KM. Radiographic diagnosis of tarsal coalition. AJR Am J Radiol 2004; 182:323-328.
8. Sartoris DJ, Resnick DL. Tarsal coalition. Arthritis Rheum 1985; 28:331-338.
9. McNally EG. Posteromedial subtalar coalition: imaging appearance in three cases. Skeletal Radiol 1999; 28:691-695.
10. Lateur LM, Van Hoe LR, Van Ghillewe KV, et al. Subtalar coalition: diagnosis with the C sign on lateral radiographs of the ankle. Radiology 1994; 193:847-851.
11. Brown RR, Rosenberg ZS, Thornhill BA. The C sign: more specific for flatfoot deformity than subtalar coalitions. Skeletal Radiol 2001; 30:84-87.
12. Liu PT, Roberts CC, Spencer Chivers F, et al. Absent middle facet: a sign on unenhanced radiography of subtalar coalition. AJR Am J Roentgenol 2003; 181:1565-1572.
13. Lamb D. The ball and socket ankle joint: a congenital abnormality. J Bone Joint Surg Br 1958; 40:240-243.
14. Solomon LB, Ruhli FJ, Taylor J, et al. A dissection and computer tomography study of tarsal coalitions in 100 cadaver feet. J Orthop Res 2006; 21:352-358.
15. Wechsler RJ, Schweitzer ME, Deely DM, et al. Tarsal coalition: depiction and characterization with CT and MR imaging. Radiology 1994; 193:447-452.
16. Kumai T, Tanaka Y, Takakura Y, Tamai S. Isolated first naviculocuneiform joint coalition. Foot Ankle Int 1996; 17:635-640.
17. Hughes PCR, Tanner JM. The development of carpal bone fusion as seen in serial radiographs. AJR Am J Roentgenol 1966; 39:943-949.
18. Garn SM, Burdi AR, Babler WJ. Prenatal origins of carpal fusions. Am J Phy Anthropol 1976; 45:203-208.
19. Cope JR. Carpal coalition. Clin Radiol 1974; 25:261-266.
20. Sandifort E. Observationum anatomico pathologicarum. Batavia 1779; 3:136.
21. van Schoonhoven J, Prommersberger KJ, Schmitt R. Traumatic disruption of a fibrocartilage lunate-triquetral coalition: a case report and review of literature. Hand Surg 2001; 6:103-108.
22. Dwight T. Variations of Bones of Hands and Feet: A Clinical Atlas. Philadelphia, JB Lippincott, 1907.
23. Viola RW, Kiser PK, Bach AW, et al. Biomechanical analysis of capitate shortening with capitate hamate fusion for the treatment of Kienböck's disease. J Hand Surg (Am) 1998; 23:395-401.
24. Murphy G. Pes Planus. In Canale TS (ed): Campbell's Operative Orthopaedics, 10th ed. vol 4, Philadelphia, Mosby, 2002, pp 4029-4039.

103

Dysplasias

Amaka Offiah

ACHONDROPLASIA

Achondroplasia belongs to group 1 (the achondroplasia group) of the osteochondrodysplasias, as listed in the International Classification of Constitutional Disorders of Bone.[1] It is one of the more common skeletal dysplasias, with a prevalence ranging from 1:15,000 to 1:40,000 live births.[2,3] Achondroplasia is usually inherited as a sporadic autosomal-dominant condition. The incidence increases with increasing paternal age.[2] The homozygous condition is lethal.

Achondroplasia arises from a point mutation in the fibroblast growth factor receptor-3 (*FGFR3*) gene, as do hypochondroplasia, thanatophoric dysplasia (types 1 and 2), San Diego platyspondylic dysplasia, severe achondroplasia with developmental delay and acanthosis nigricans (SADDAN), Muenke's coronal craniosynostosis, and Crouzon's syndrome with acanthosis nigricans.[2,4]

Antenatal diagnosis (by ultrasonography) is possible by detecting shortening of the long bones. Short limbs (specifically short femora) are not apparent until toward either the end of the first trimester (homozygous disease) or the end of the second trimester (heterozygous disease).[5]

Complications include restrictive and obstructive lung disease, otitis media, hearing loss, speech problems, tibial bowing, apnea, cervicomedullary compression, and neurologic signs attributable to spinal stenosis.[6] To this list should be added complications of orthopedic procedures such as limb lengthening.

Radiologic findings from the skeletal survey include:

1. *Skull*: Large vault; small foramen magnum (Fig. 103-1)
2. *Spine*: Bullet-shaped vertebral bodies; short pedicles with interpedicular distances narrowing from L1 to L5; posterior vertebral scalloping; horizontal sacrum with exaggerated lumbar lordosis (Figs. 103-2 and 103-3)
3. *Chest*: Small thorax with short ribs
4. *Pelvis*: Medial and lateral acetabular spurs (trident acetabula); horizontal acetabular roof; squared iliac wings; small sacrosciatic notch (Fig. 103-4)
5. *Long bones*: Predominantly rhizomelic shortening (Fig. 103-5); long distal fibula relative to tibia (causing progressive varus deformity); chevron deformity of growth plates (V-shaped notches); characteristic sloping metaphyses (especially of the proximal femora) seen only in infancy (Fig. 103-6)
6. *Hands*: Trident; bullet-shaped phalanges (Fig. 103-7)

Classic Signs

- Autosomal-dominant inheritance
- Antenatal diagnosis of heterozygous achondroplasia (based on femoral length) possible from approximately the 24th gestational week.
- Lethal if homozygous
- Narrowing of interpedicular distances from L1 to L5 (not seen in infants)
- Posterior vertebral scalloping
- Trident acetabulum
- Characteristic sloping metaphyses with oval radiolucency of proximal femora (in infants)

HYPOCHONDROPLASIA

Hypochondroplasia belongs to the achondroplasia group of osteochondrodysplasias.[2,4] It is allelic to achondroplasia and, like achondroplasia, is inherited as an autosomal-dominant trait. The degree of short stature is variable, and the phenotype may range from nearly normal to almost as severe as achondroplasia. Although there are reports of antenatal diagnosis,[7] it is more common for the (radiologic) diagnosis to be made in early or even middle childhood when mild short stature or failure of the pubertal growth spurt is noted. Genotype phenotype correlation studies have revealed different *FGFR3* mutations in those with milder radiologic changes than in those whose radiologic findings are more severe.[8] Clinical features include short limbs with or without bowing of the lower limbs, a muscular build, lumbar hyperlordosis, and macrocephaly with frontal bossing.

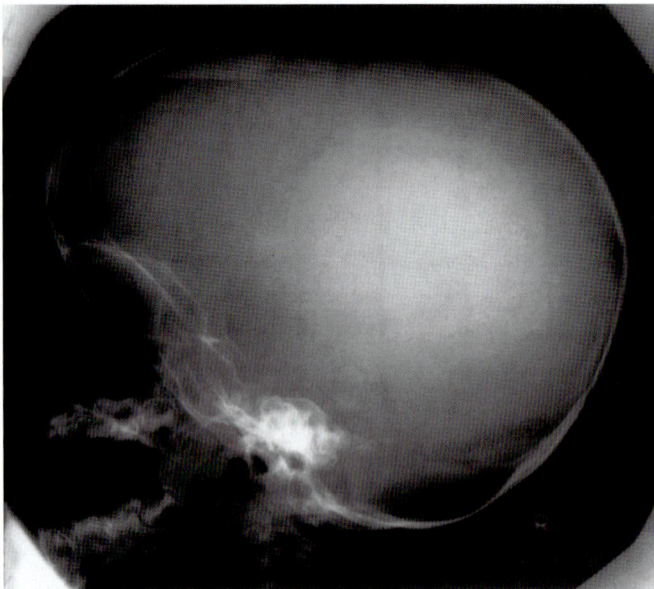

■ **FIGURE 103-1** Achondroplasia. Lateral radiograph of skull shows large skull vault and small foramen magnum.

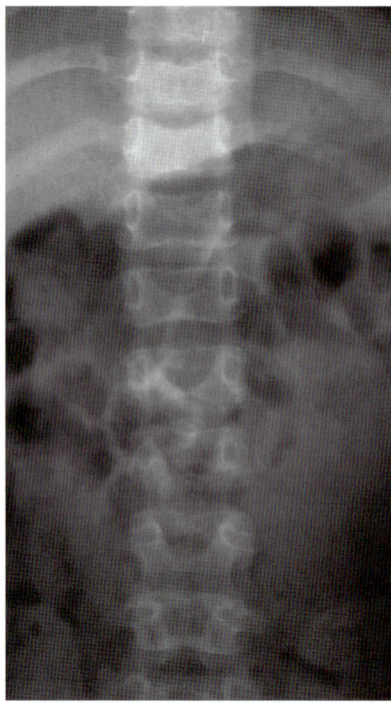

■ **FIGURE 103-3** Achondroplasia. Anteroposterior radiograph of the spine. There is abnormal narrowing of the interpedicular distances from L1 to L5 (should get progressively wider). This narrowing is not seen in infants.

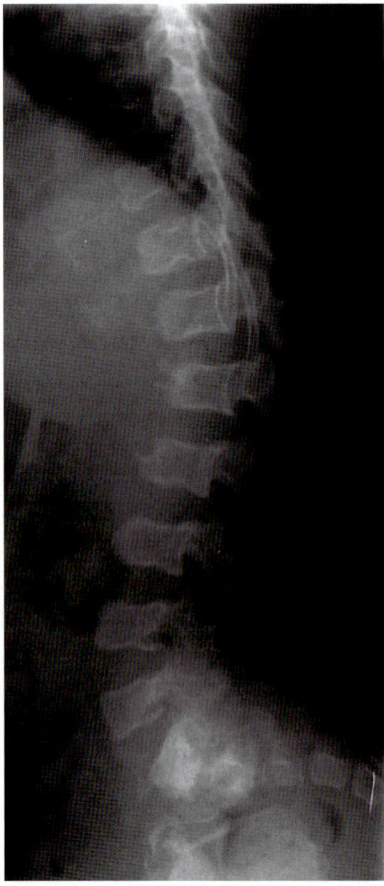

■ **FIGURE 103-2** Achondroplasia. Lateral radiograph of spine. Note posterior scalloping, bullet-shaped vertebral bodies, short pedicles, and horizontal orientation of the sacrum.

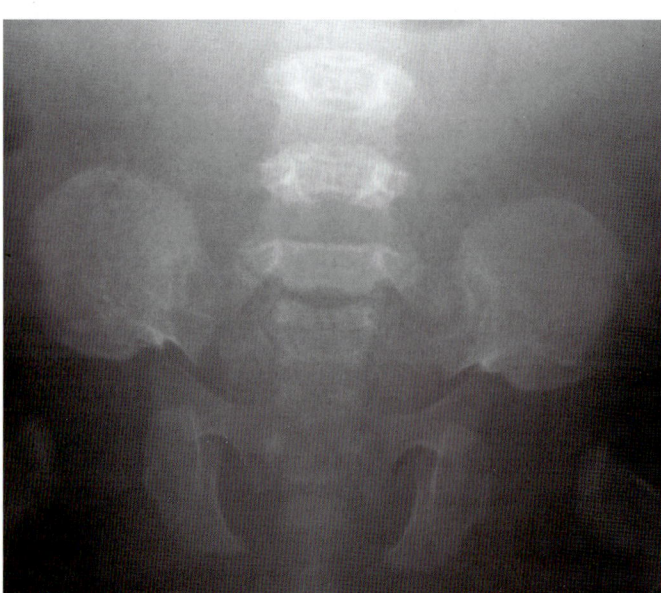

■ **FIGURE 103-4** Achondroplasia. Anteroposterior radiograph of the pelvis. Typical changes include horizontal acetabular roofs, trident acetabula, and square iliac wings.

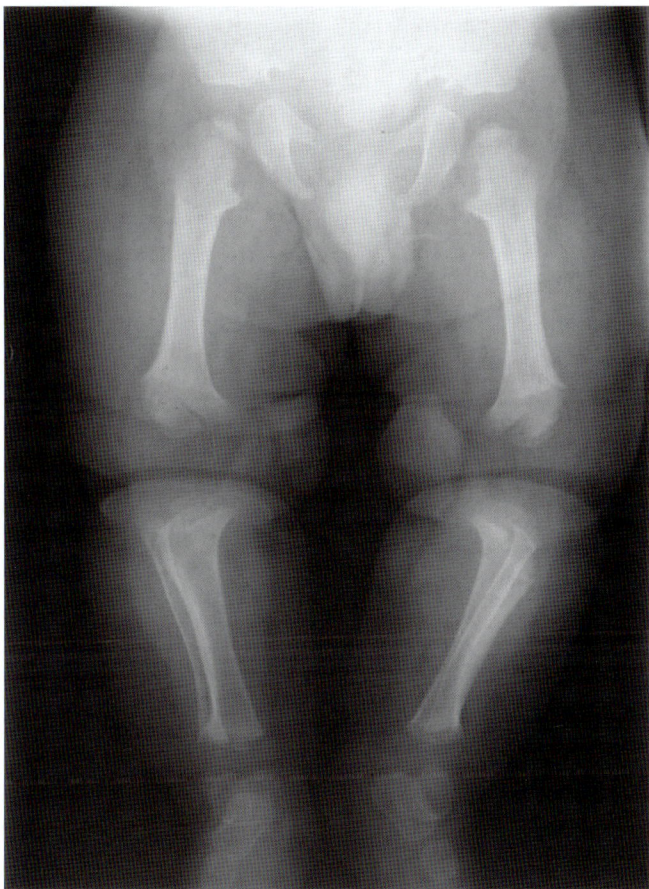

■ **FIGURE 103-5** Achondroplasia. Anteroposterior radiograph of lower limbs shows rhizomelic shortening.

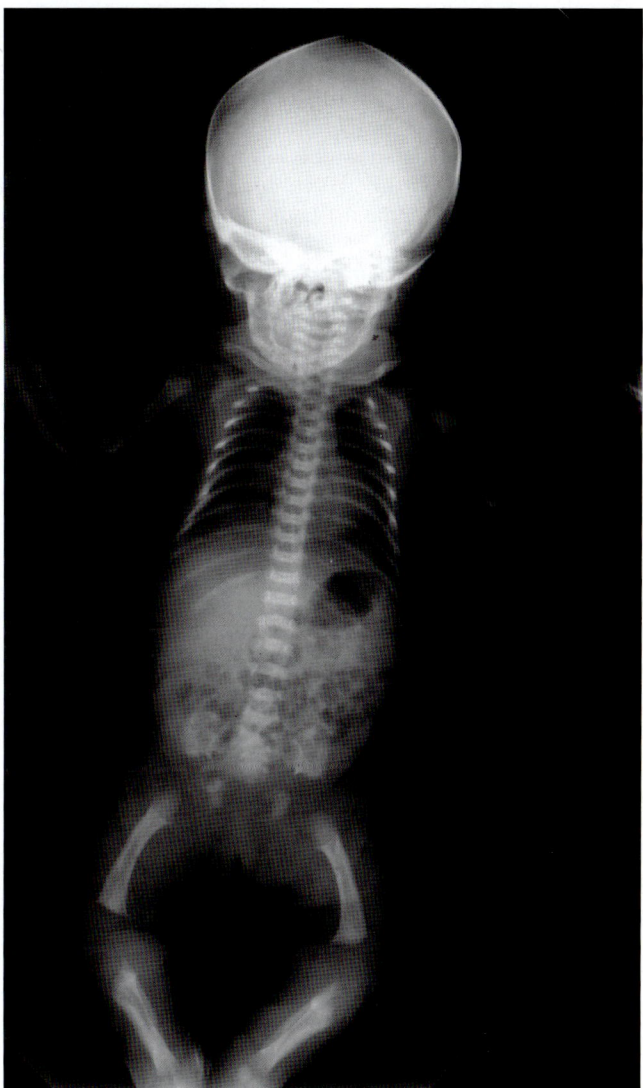

■ **FIGURE 103-6** Achondroplasia. Anteroposterior "babygram." Note the characteristic oval radiolucency of the proximal femora, which is a result of the sloping metaphyses.

Radiologic findings from the skeletal survey are similar to, but milder than, those seen in achondroplasia. They include:

1. *Spine*: Loss of the normal widening of the interpedicular distance from L1 to L5
2. *Pelvis*: Short, square iliac wings
3. *Long bones*: Short and relatively broad with prominence of sites of muscular insertion; relatively long distal fibula; long ulna styloid process
4. *Hands*: Brachydactyly (not inevitable)

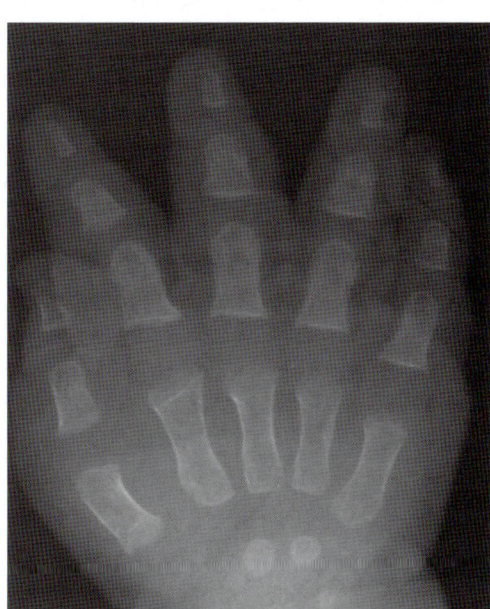

■ **FIGURE 103-7** Achondroplasia. Anteroposterior radiograph shows a trident hand and bullet-shaped phalanges.

Classic Signs

- Autosomal-dominant inheritance
- Usually less severe than achondroplasia
- No change or decrease in interpedicular distance from L1 to L5
- Short, relatively broad long bones
- Long distal fibula

THANATOPHORIC DYSPLASIA

"Thanatophoric" comes from the Greek for "death bearing." This is the most common lethal osteochondrodysplasia and belongs to the achondroplasia group (group 1) of the International Classification of Constitutional Disorders of Bone.[1] It results from a sporadic autosomal-dominant *FGFR3* mutation. Antenatal diagnosis is based on identification of short, bowed femora in association with a small thorax. The role of 3D compared with 2D ultrasonography in the antenatal diagnosis of skeletal dysplasias including thanatophoric dysplasia continues to be evaluated.[9]

Radiologic findings from the skeletal survey include:

1. *Skull*: Relative macrocephaly; in type I (Fig. 103-8) the skull is of normal shape; in type II (Fig. 103-9) there is premature fusion of the temporoparietal sutures and frontal bossing, giving rise to the "cloverleaf" skull or *Kleeblattschadel*.
2. *Spine*: Severe platyspondyly with "wafer thin" or H-shaped vertebral bodies on lateral (Fig. 103-10) and anteroposterior (Fig. 103-11) spine radiographs, respectively
3. *Chest*: Small thorax; short horizontal ribs with cupped costochondral junctions (Fig. 103-12)
4. *Pelvis*: Small, square iliac wings; small sacrosciatic notch; trident acetabula

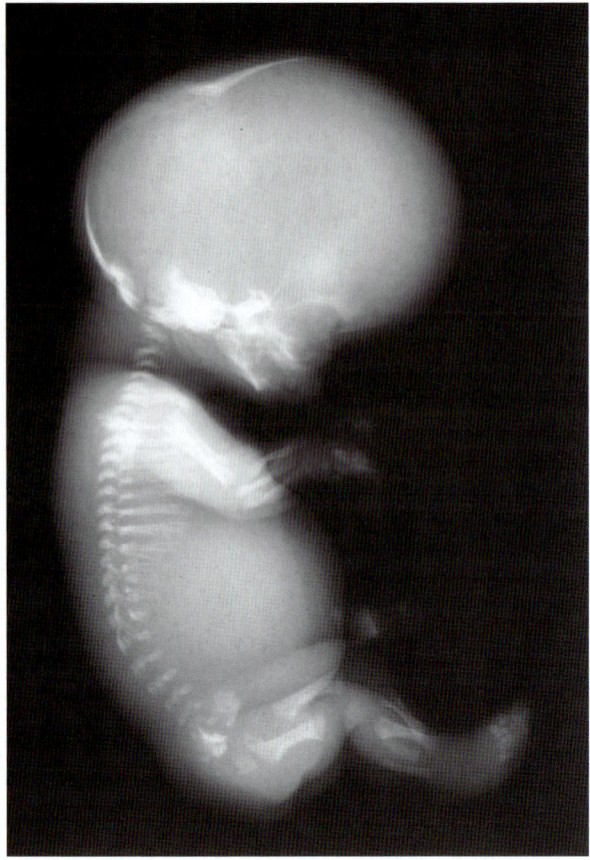

■ **FIGURE 103-9** Lateral "babygram": Thanatophoric dysplasia type II. Cloverleaf skull as seen on lateral radiograph. Note frontal bossing.

5. *Long bones*: Significant micromelia; irregular, flared metaphyses; bowed "telephone receiver" femora, but not in all cases (Fig. 103-13; also see Fig. 103-12)
6. *Hands*: Short, broad tubular bones

Classic Signs

■ Most common lethal osteochondrodysplasia
■ Type I has normal skull shape
■ Type II has "cloverleaf" skull
■ Classic bowed ("telephone receiver") femora not seen in all cases

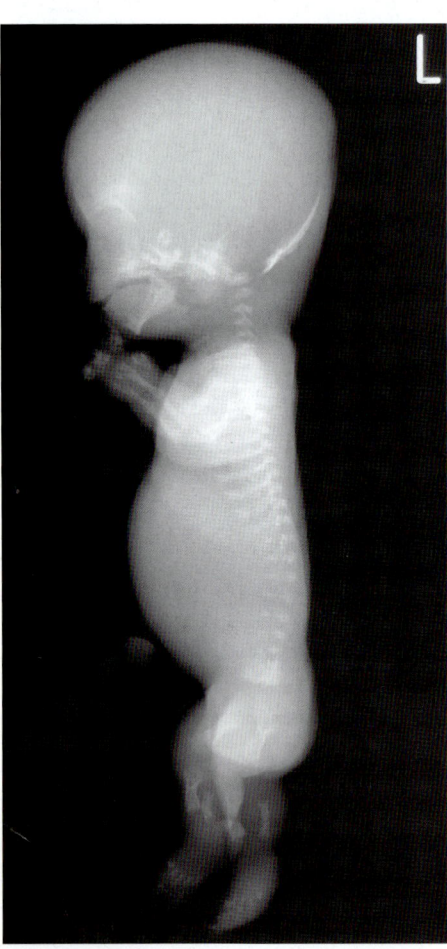

■ **FIGURE 103-8** Thanatophoric dysplasia. Lateral "babygram." The normal skull classifies this as type I.

ASPHYXIATING THORACIC DYSTROPHY

This autosomal-recessive disorder belongs to group 4 of the osteochondrodysplasias—the short rib conditions with or without polydactyly. Asphyxiating thoracic dystrophy and chondroectodermal dysplasia are nonlethal, compared with short rib dysplasia types I/III, IV, and II, which are perinatally lethal.

Asphyxiating thoracic dystrophy may be diagnosed antenatally[10] with identification of a small thorax and postaxial polydactyly (in 10% of cases).

Death is usually a result of respiratory distress associated with the small thorax and hypoplastic lungs. Midsternal

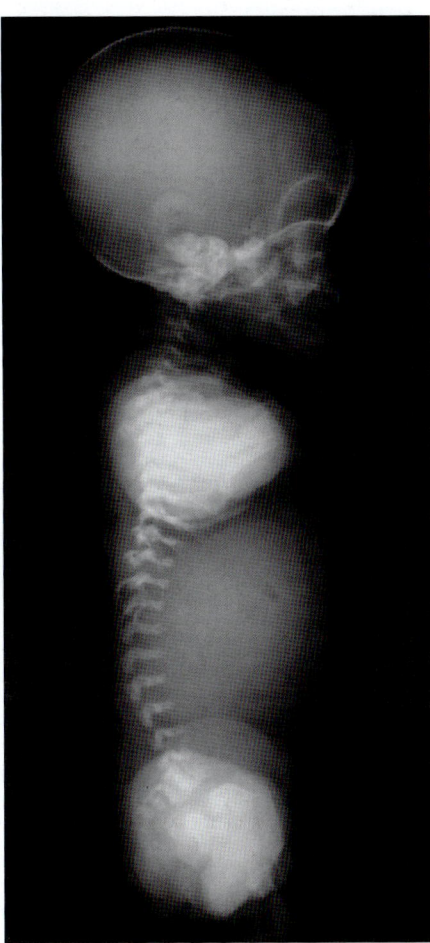

■ FIGURE 103-10   Thanatophoric dysplasia. Lateral "babygram." Note severe platyspondyly with "wafer-thin" vertebral bodies.

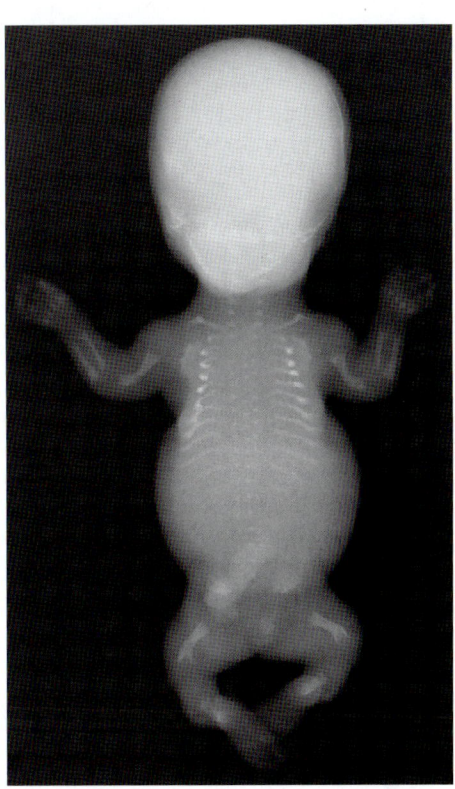

■ FIGURE 103-12   Thanatophoric dysplasia. Anteroposterior "babygram" shows small chest and short horizontal ribs with anterior cupping. Note straight femora in this fetus.

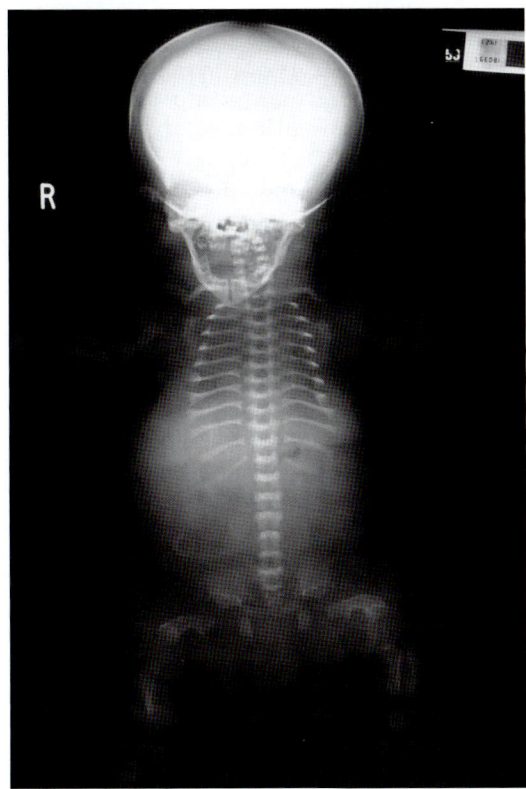

■ FIGURE 103-11   Thanatophoric dysplasia. Anteroposterior "babygram." There is severe platyspondyly with H-shaped vertebral bodies.

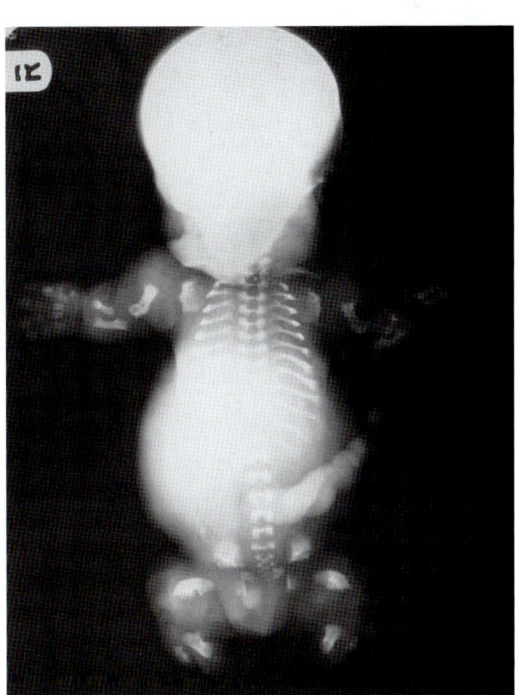

■ FIGURE 103-13   Thanatophoric dysplasia. Anteroposterior "babygram." Micromelia with bowed long bones and "telephone receiver" femora can be seen.

expansion[11] and lateral thoracic[12] thoracoplasty are surgical techniques devised to increase chest size and, therefore, the survival rate in patients with asphyxiating thoracic dystrophy.

Pancreatic cysts, retinal abnormalities, and hepatic complications have also been described.[13]

Long-term survivors develop renal cystic disease and will not survive without renal transplantation.[14]

Radiologic findings from the skeletal survey include:

1. *Chest*: Small thorax; short horizontal ribs (Fig. 103-14)
2. *Pelvis*: Short iliac bones; trident acetabula with medial and lateral spurs
3. *Long bones*: Mild micromelia; bowed; metaphyseal spurs; premature ossification of proximal femoral epiphyses
4. *Hands*: Cone-shaped epiphyses of phalanges (Fig. 103-15); postaxial polydactyly (10%)

It is worth noting that in survivors these features resolve, with the only radiographic abnormalities that

---

Classic Signs

- Nonlethal, autosomal-recessive, short rib syndrome; perinatal death from lung hypoplasia may occur
- Those who survive infancy develop renal cystic disease and may die of renal failure
- Trident acetabula
- Postaxial polydactyly in 10% of patients
- Metaphyseal spurs
- Cone-shaped epiphyses of hands

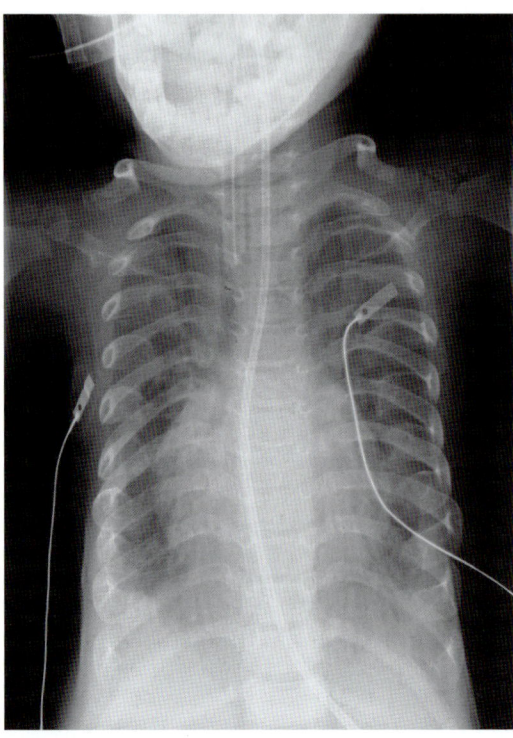

■ **FIGURE 103-14** Asphyxiating thoracic dystrophy. Anteroposterior radiograph of the chest shows a small thorax with short horizontal ribs. Note the endotracheal tube.

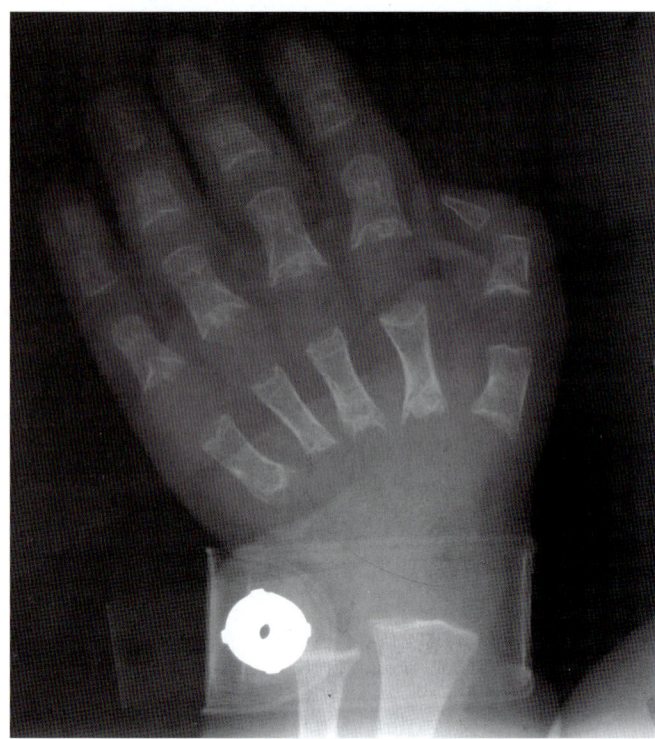

■ **FIGURE 103-15** Asphyxiating thoracic dystrophy. Radiograph shows cone-shaped epiphyses. No polydactyly is evident (only seen in 10%).

persist into childhood being short middle and distal phalanges associated with cone-shaped epiphyses.

ELLIS-VAN CREVELD SYNDROME

This is an autosomal-recessive nonlethal short rib syndrome with polysyndactyly occurring in 90% of patients. It belongs to the same group (group 4) of osteochondrodysplasias as asphyxiating thoracic dystrophy. The small thorax and polydactyly in addition to mesomelic shortening and an atrial (occasionally ventricular) septal defect allow antenatal diagnosis.[15]

Clinical findings include natal teeth, abnormally shaped microdontic teeth, dystrophic nails, fusion of the upper lip to the gingival margin, and oral frenula.

As with asphyxiating thoracic dystrophy, perinatal death may result from pulmonary hypoplasia.

Radiologic features from the skeletal survey include:

1. *Chest*: Small thorax; short horizontal ribs
2. *Pelvis*: Short iliac bones; trident acetabula with medial and lateral spurs; narrow sacrosciatic notch
3. *Long bones*: Mesomelic shortening; smooth rounded metaphyses (Fig. 103-16); deficient ossification of the lateral aspect of the proximal tibial metaphysis leading to gradual genu valgum
4. *Hands*: Cone-shaped epiphyses of middle and distal phalanges; short middle and distal phalanges; postaxial polysyndactyly in up to 90% of patients (Fig. 103-17)

The chest and pelvic changes improve with age (similar to asphyxiating thoracic dystrophy), leaving the older child with residual mesomelic shortening (most pronounced in the lower limbs) and short middle and distal phalanges with cone-shaped epiphyses.

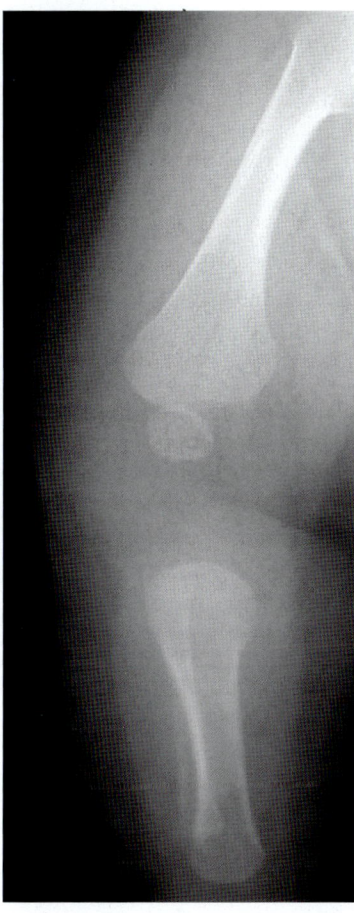

■ **FIGURE 103-16** Ellis-van Creveld syndrome. Anteroposterior radiograph of lower limb shows smooth rounded epiphyses, which are characteristic.

KNIEST'S DYSPLASIA

Kniest's dysplasia belongs to group 8 of the osteochondrodysplasias—the type II collagenopathies. Other type II collagenopathies include achondrogenesis type II, hypochondrogenesis, spondyloepiphyseal dysplasia congenita (SEDC), and Stickler's syndrome type I.

Kniest's dysplasia is inherited as an autosomal-dominant trait.

Clinical features include short stature, enlarged joints, cleft palate, severe myopia, retinal detachment, hearing loss from recurrent ear infections, and tracheomalacia.

Histopathologic examination of unossified cartilage reveals a characteristic "Swiss cheese" appearance that has also been documented on MRI.[16]

Radiographic findings from the skeletal survey include:

1. *Spine*: Mild platyspondyly; irregular end plates; coronal clefts; kyphoscoliosis in older children and adults
2. *Chest*: Short, broad thorax
3. *Pelvis*: Sloping acetabular roofs
4. *Long bones*: Short; wide metaphyses giving a "dumbbell" appearance; delayed ossification of epiphyses; stippled epiphyses
5. *Hands*: Pseudoepiphyses of proximal and middle phalanges

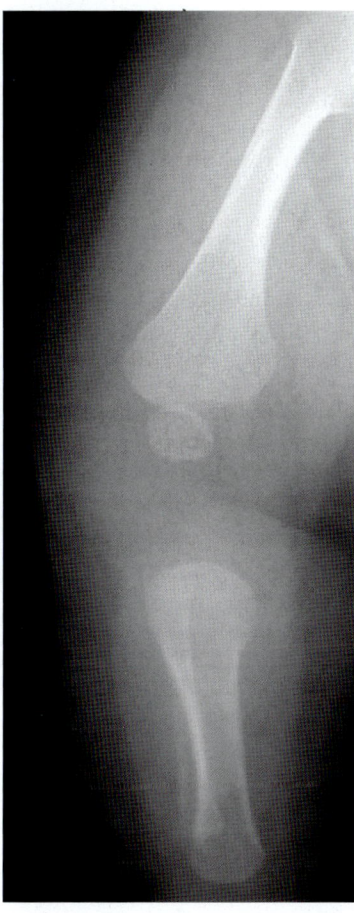

■ **FIGURE 103-17** Ellis-van Creveld syndrome. Radiograph of the hand shows postaxial polysyndactyly.

SPONDYLOEPIPHYSEAL DYSPLASIA CONGENITA

Like Kniest's dysplasia, SEDC is an autosomal-dominant type II collagenopathy. Affected patients are short at birth with a flat face and may have a cleft palate. There is severe myopia, and retinal detachment may develop.[17] Respiratory complications requiring tracheostomy have been described.[18]

Radiologic findings from the skeletal survey include:

1. *Spine*:
   a. Infancy: Platyspondyly; anisospondyly with L1 being larger than L5 (Fig. 103-18); oval vertebral bodies;

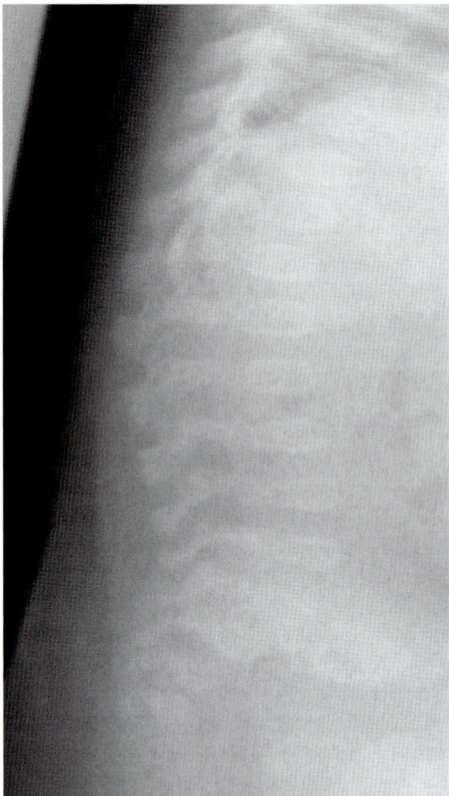

■ **FIGURE 103-18** Spondyloepiphyseal dysplasia congenita. Lateral lumbar spine shows anisospondyly with L1 being significantly larger than L5.

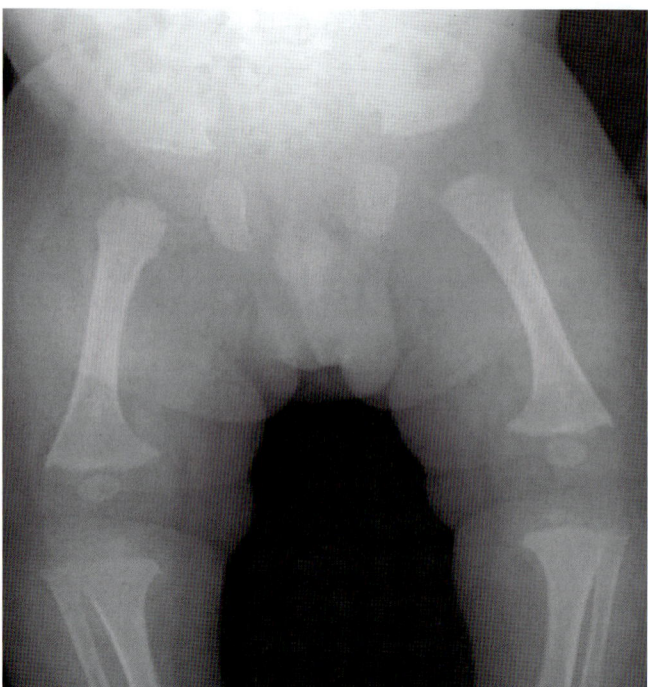

■ **FIGURE 103-19** Spondyloepiphyseal dysplasia congenita in a 6-month-old child. Anteroposterior radiograph of pelvis and lower limbs shows delayed ossification of femoral heads, micromelia, and metaphyseal spurs.

hypoplastic peg and/or cervical vertebral body (usually C3)
  b. Childhood: Pear-shaped vertebral bodies; cervical kyphosis and instability as a result of a hypoplastic peg/vertebral body; progressive kyphoscoliosis may develop
2. *Chest*: Small thorax with short ribs
3. *Pelvis*: At birth there is absent ossification of the pubic rami; horizontal acetabular roofs
4. *Long bones*: Absent ossification of epiphyses of the knees at birth; micromelia; short or absent femoral necks; delayed ossification of proximal femoral epiphyses (Fig. 103-19); significant coxa vara deformity with waddling gait and high-riding greater trochanters; posterior dislocation of the hips
5. *Hands*: Delayed maturation of carpal bones on the radial side of the hand

Classic Signs

■ Autosomal-dominant type II collagenopathy
■ Cleft palate, myopia, and respiratory complications
■ Delayed appearance of epiphyseal centers
■ Severe coxa vara
■ Odontoid hypoplasia with cervical instability
■ Anisospondyly (in infancy)

STICKLER'S SYNDROME

Stickler's syndrome is an autosomal-dominant disorder with characteristic eye and facial features, deafness, and arthritis.

There are three types, with Stickler's dysplasia type I belonging to group 8—type II collagenopathies and Stickler's dysplasia types II and III belonging to group 9—type XI collagenopathies. Types II and III are differentiated by the absence of ocular involvement in the former.

Clinical features include midface hypoplasia with a depressed nasal bridge and micrognathia. Midline abnormalities may be absent or range from a cleft soft palate to the Pierre Robin sequence. Patients have a congenital non-progressive high myopia, and the associated abnormality of the vitreous gel is said to be pathognomonic. Retinal detachment is a recognized complication. Sensorineural deafness is another finding. There is joint hypermobility that improves with age, but early osteoarthritis may develop.

Patients are usually of normal stature and normal intelligence.

Infants with the Zweymuller-Weissenbacher (ZW) syndrome (Pierre Robin sequence, mild platyspondyly, and flared metaphyses) are later diagnosed (around the age of 3 years) either with Stickler's syndrome or with oto-spondylomegaepiphyseal dysplasia (OSMED), but not all patients with Stickler's syndrome will have had the ZW phenotype.

Radiologic findings in Stickler's syndrome (all types) may be subtle and include:

1. *Spine*: Mild platyspondyly (localized or generalized); irregular end plates; kyphoscoliosis
2. *Pelvis*: Tilted acetabular roofs (Fig. 103-20)
3. *Long bones*: Flared, wide metaphyses in infancy (ZW syndrome); wide femoral necks; early osteoarthritis
4. *Hands*: Accelerated bone age (Fig. 103-21)

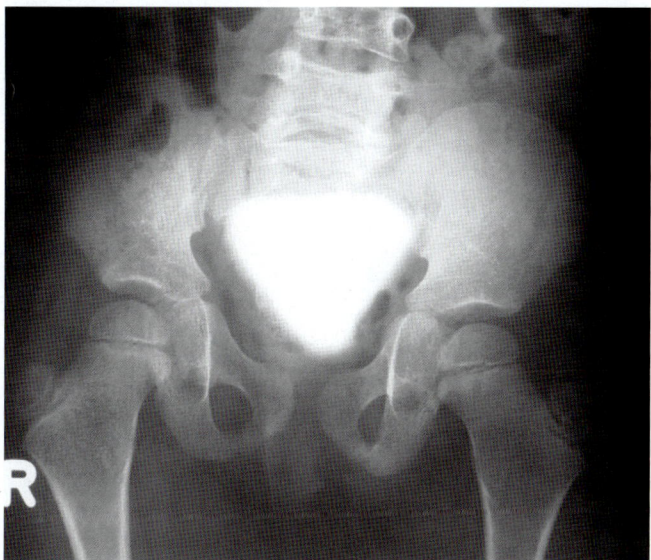

■ FIGURE 103-20 Stickler's syndrome. Anteroposterior radiograph of pelvis. Tilted acetabular roofs render easy visualization of posterior wall.

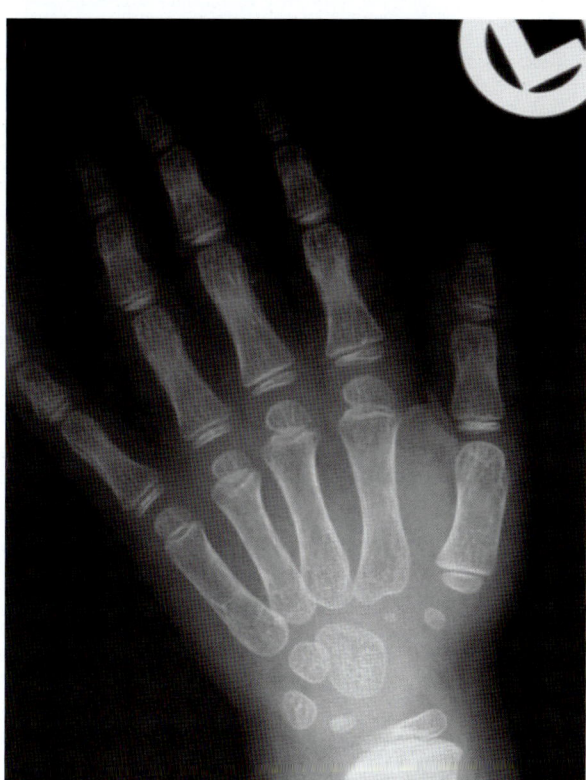

■ FIGURE 103-21 Stickler's syndrome in a 3-year-old child. Radiograph of left hand. Note accelerated bone age.

Classic Signs

- Autosomal-dominant type II or type XI collagenopathy
- Myopia with pathognomonic abnormality of the vitreous
- Cleft palate with or without the Pierre Robin sequence
- Sensorineural deafness
- Broad femoral necks with tilted acetabular roofs
- Mild platyspondyly
- Normal stature with accelerated bone age

X-LINKED SPONDYLOEPIPHYSEAL DYSPLASIA TARDA

X-linked spondyloepiphyseal dysplasia tarda belongs to group 10 of the classification system—other spondyloepi-(meta)-physeal dysplasias.

Clinically, affected males (early childhood) are of short stature with arm span exceeding height (i.e., short trunks). They have a barrel-shaped chest and complain of back stiffness and pain as well as hip pain due to premature osteoarthritis.

The characteristic radiographic finding is in the spine.

1. *Spine*: Characteristic vertebral body humps consisting of dense mounds of bone affecting the posterior two thirds of the superior and inferior end plates (Fig. 103-22).
2. *Long bones*: Mild flattening of proximal femoral epiphyses with premature osteoarthritis.

Classic Signs

- Spondyloepiphyseal dysplasia tarda comprises a heterogeneous group of conditions.
- X-linked SEDT presents in early childhood.
- Affected males have arm span greater than height (short trunk).
- The main symptoms are back and hip pain and stiffness.
- The characteristic radiographic finding is humps in the posterior two thirds of the vertebral bodies (best seen between ages 4 and 12 years).

MULTIPLE EPIPHYSEAL DYSPLASIA

There are various types of multiple epiphyseal dysplasia (MED) each caused by a specific mutation. Autosomal-recessive MED belongs to group 6 of the classification system (the diastrophic dysplasia group); other autosomal-dominant forms of MED belong to group 11 of the classification system (multiple epiphyseal dysplasias and pseudoachondroplasia) and are due to mutations in *COMP* (as is pseudoachondroplasia), type IX collagen, and matrilin-3.

Clinically, patients are of normal intelligence. They may be of normal height or have mild short stature. They present with prominent, stiff painful joints with contractures and premature osteoarthritis.

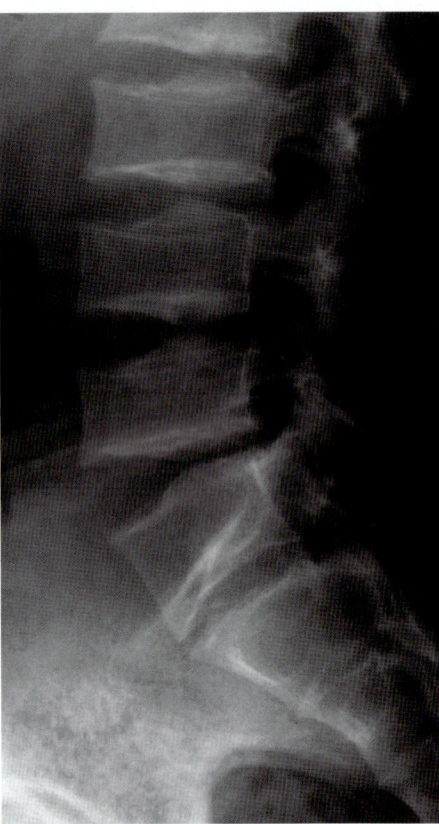

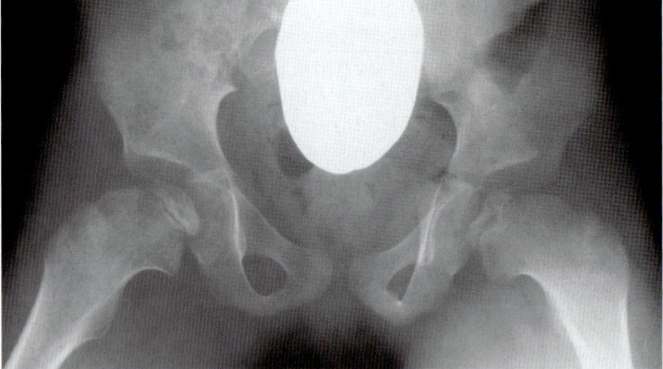

■ **FIGURE 103-23** Multiple epiphyseal dysplasia. Anteroposterior radiograph of the pelvis shows small irregular femoral epiphyses.

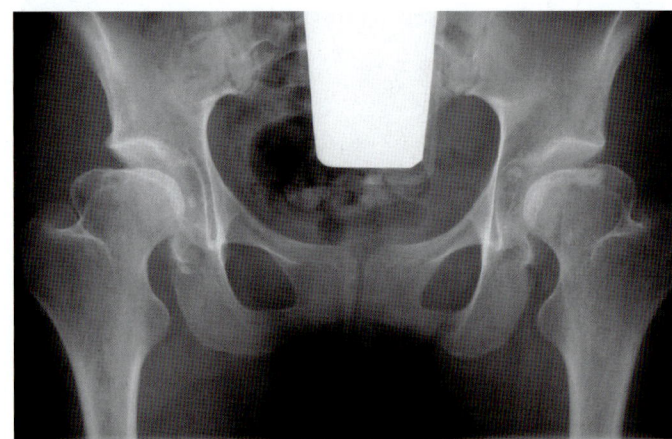

■ **FIGURE 103-22** X-linked spondyloepiphyseal dysplasia tarda. Lateral radiograph of lumbosacral spine shows characteristic vertebral humps, which become less apparent with increasing age and are best seen between the ages of 4 and 12 years.

■ **FIGURE 103-24** Multiple epiphyseal dysplasia. Flattened sclerotic femoral heads are seen on this anteroposterior radiograph.

Genotype/phenotype studies have revealed significant patterns[19]; however, in all cases radiologic findings mainly involve hips, knees, and hands.
1. *Hips*: Small, flattened, fragmented, irregular and sclerotic proximal femoral epiphyses (Figs. 103-23 and 103-24). The differential diagnosis is bilateral Legg-Calvé-Perthes disease (however this disorder is rarely synchronous).
2. *Knees*: Small, flattened epiphyses; multilayered patellae (Fig. 103-25) in autosomal-recessive MED; these patients may also have brachydactyly and talipes.

3. *Hands*:
   a. Children (Fig. 103-26): Delayed appearance of epiphyses; small irregular/angulated epiphyses
   b. Adults (Fig. 103-27): Small broad tubular bones; flattened joint surfaces; premature osteoarthritis; contractures
4. *Spine*: Normal; mild changes including end plate irregularity; platyspondyly; dorsal wedging

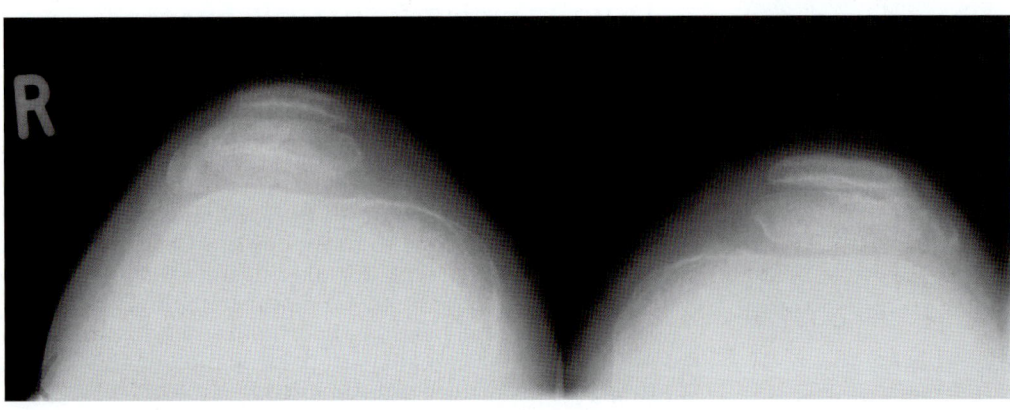

■ **FIGURE 103-25** Multiple epiphyseal dysplasia. "Skyline knees." Multilayered patellae are characteristic of the autosomal-recessive type of this disease.

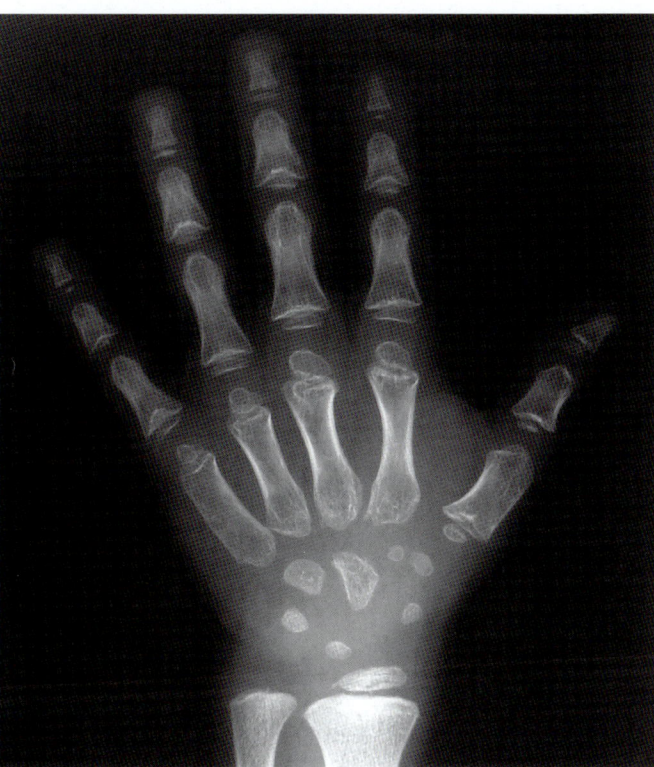

■ FIGURE 103-26 Multiple epiphyseal dysplasia. Radiograph shows small irregular/angulated epiphyses in a child.

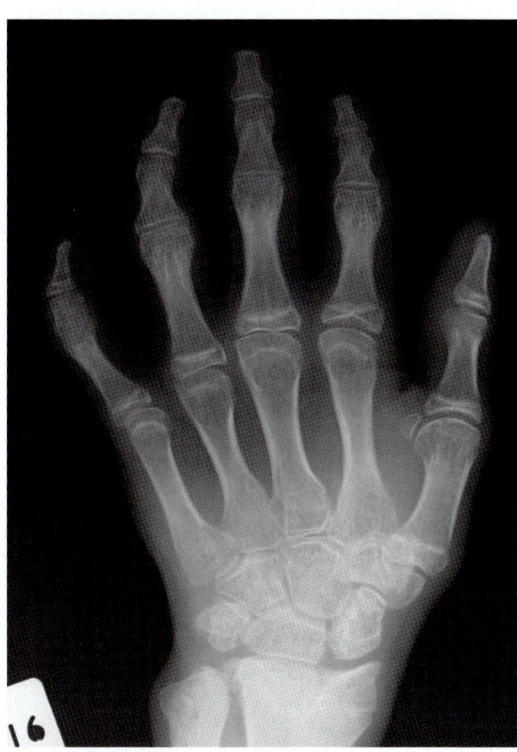

■ FIGURE 103-27 Multiple epiphyseal dysplasia. Radiograph shows broad tubular bones and flattened joint surfaces in an adult. Early osteoarthritis is present.

Classic Signs

■ There are autosomal-recessive and autosomal-dominant forms of MED
■ Patients present with joint stiffness, pain, and premature osteoarthritis
■ There is delayed appearance of small fragmented epiphyses of hips, knees, and hands
■ A multilayered patella is characteristic of autosomal-recessive MED
■ The differential diagnosis is bilateral Legg-Calvé-Perthes disease (however this disorder is rarely synchronous)

PSEUDOACHONDROPLASIA

Pseudoachondroplasia belongs to group 11 of the osteochondrodysplasias (multiple epiphyseal dysplasias and pseudoachondroplasia). It is inherited as an autosomal-dominant trait and, like some cases of MED, is due to a mutation in the *COMP* gene.[20] The phenotype is more severe than MED.

Patients present around the age of 2 years with short-limbed short stature, ligamentous laxity, and a waddling gait. Like patients with MED, they develop premature osteoarthritis.

Radiographic findings from the skeletal survey include:

1. *Long bones*: Small, flattened, irregular epiphyses; flared irregular metaphyses
2. *Spine*: In children there is mild platyspondyly; biconvex end plates; anterior tongues of the vertebral bodies
3. *Pelvis*: Wide triradiate cartilage
4. *Chest*: Cupping of the posterior rib ends

Classic Signs

■ Autosomal-dominant condition similar to but more severe than MED
■ Patients present around the age of 2 years
■ Short stature, waddling gait, joint stiffness and pain, premature osteoarthritis
■ Small irregular epiphyses
■ Wide triradiate cartilage

CHONDRODYSPLASIA PUNCTATA

X-linked dominant (Conradi-Hünermann syndrome), X linked recessive (brachytelephalangic), autosomal-dominant (tibia metacarpal), and autosomal-recessive (rhizomelic) types of chondrodysplasia punctata (CDP) are recognized. They belong to group 12 (stippled epiphyses group) of the osteochondrodysplasias.

Prenatal diagnosis in Conradi-Hünermann type CDP is made by identifying stippled calcification and asymmetric limb shortening.

Affected patients are usually female (more severe/lethal disease in males). They have a depressed nasal bridge and may have ichthyosis and cataracts. Patients with severe perinatally lethal disease may show features overlapping with hydrops ectopic calcification motheaten (HEM) dysplasia,[21] which also belongs to the stippled epiphyses group.

Radiologically there is stippled calcification of cartilage.

1. *Spine*: Stippling of any part of the vertebral body; other features include coronal and sagittal clefts (Fig. 103-28); calcification of the anterior and posterior longitudinal ligaments; kyphoscoliosis; cervical instability
2. *Chest*: Stippling of the cartilaginous anterior portions of the ribs; stippling of the laryngeal cartilages
3. *Pelvis*: Stippling of the triradiate cartilage
4. *Long bones*: Asymmetric epiphyseal stippling; asymmetric shortening of the long bones (Fig. 103-29)

Classic Signs

- X-linked dominant condition (Conradi-Hünermann)
- Antenatal diagnosis is possible
- Characterized radiologically by stippled calcification of cartilage
- Stippling of the long bones is asymmetric, leading to asymmetric long-bone shortening

---

SCHMID METAPHYSEAL CHONDRODYSPLASIA

This autosomal-dominant condition belongs to group 13 of the osteochondrodysplasias—the metaphyseal chondrodysplasias. It is due to a mutation in the *COL10A1* gene and is the mildest and most common condition in this group (others include cartilage hair hypoplasia, Jansen-type metaphyseal chondrodysplasia, and Schwachmann-Diamond chondrodysplasia).

Clinically, patients present with short stature, bowed legs, and a waddling gait.

Radiographic changes are most severe in the lower limbs.

1. *Lower limbs*: Coxa vara, flared irregular metaphyses, normal bone density (Fig. 103-30)
2. *Spine*: Mild platyspondyly with irregular end plates in 10%[22]
3. *Hands*: Subtle hand changes, including mild shortening and metaphyseal cupping[23] (Fig. 103-31)
4. *Chest*: Splaying of the anterior rib ends

Classic Signs

- This is the mildest and most common metaphyseal chondrodysplasia
- Major differential diagnosis is rickets, but bone density is normal
- Lower limbs are most severely affected

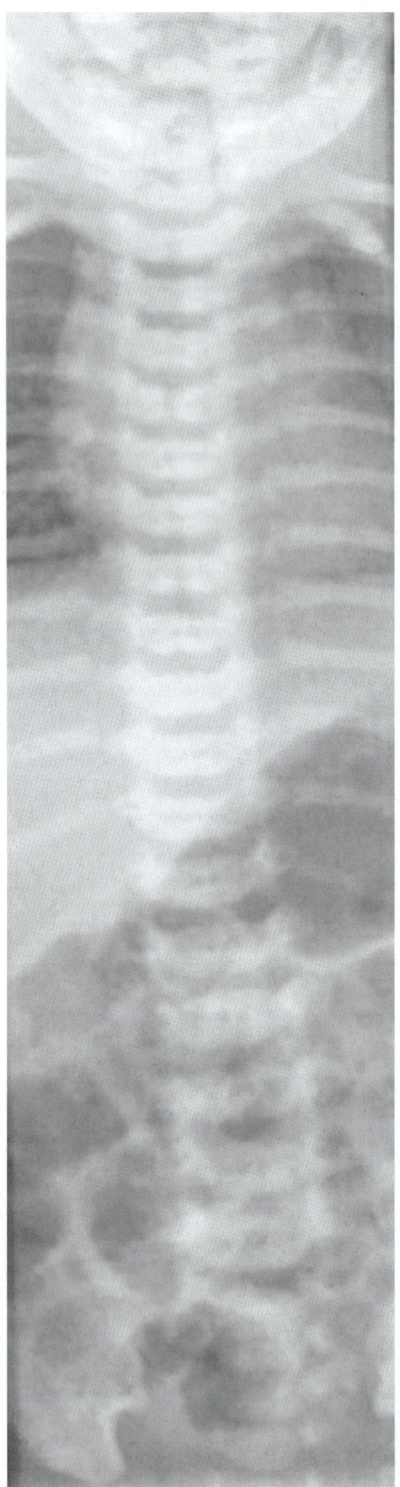

■ **FIGURE 103-28** Chondrodysplasia punctata. Anteroposterior radiograph of the spine shows sagittal cleft vertebral bodies with stippled calcification at some levels.

DYSCHONDROSTEOSIS

Dyschondrosteosis is a mesomelic dysplasia, belonging to group 16 of the classification system. It is the mildest and most common mesomelic dysplasia. It is inherited as an autosomal-dominant trait (although females are more

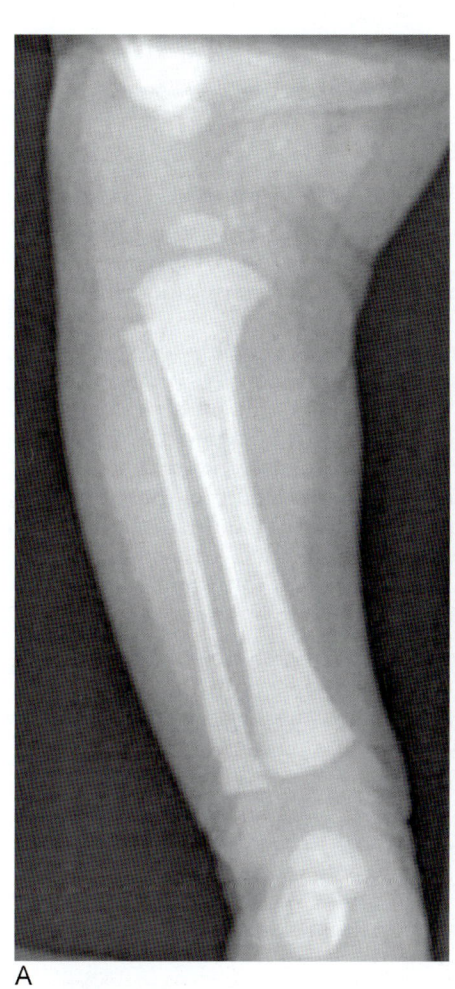
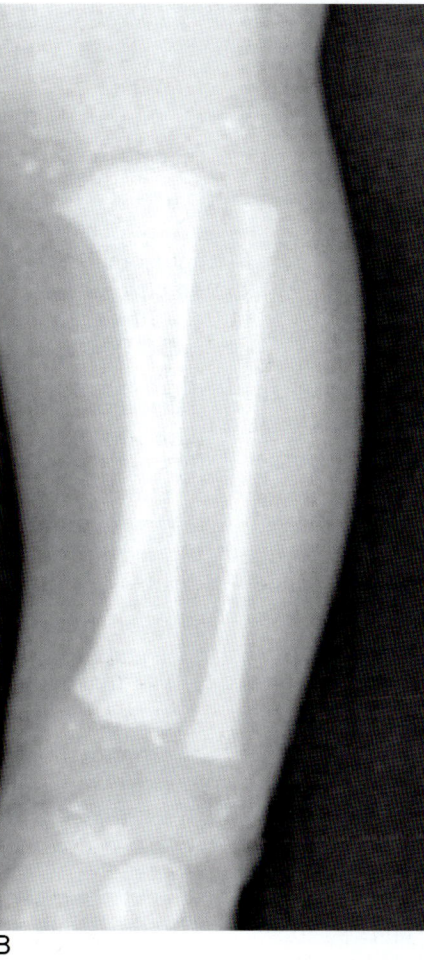

A

B

■ FIGURE 103-29 Conradi-Hünermann syndrome. Anteroposterior radiographs of right (**A**) and left (**B**) lower limbs Note asymmetrical stippling with the left more severely affected than the right. The distal left tibia is shortened.

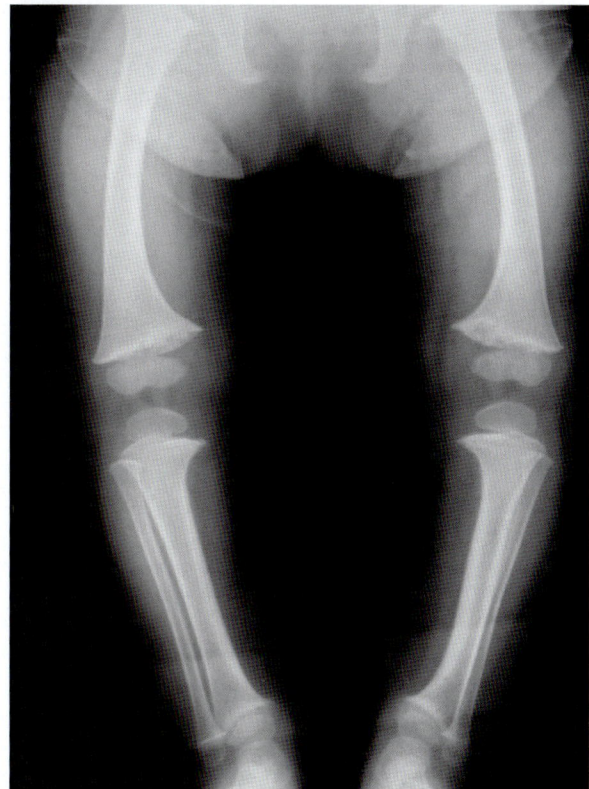

■ FIGURE 103-30 Schmid metaphyseal chondrodysplasia. Anteroposterior radiograph of lower limbs shows flared irregular metaphyses with widened growth plates. This patient has coxa vara and normal bone density.

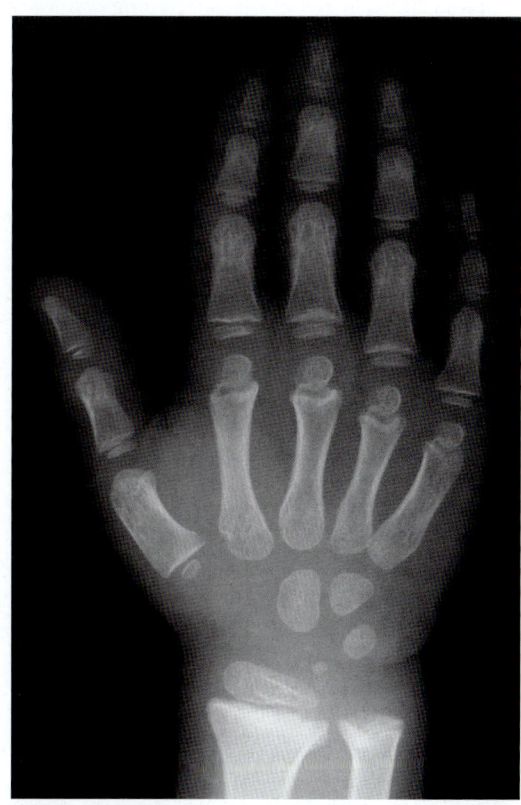

■ FIGURE 103-31 Schmid metaphyseal chondrodysplasia. Radiograph shows subtle metaphyseal cupping of short tubular bones (particularly proximal phalanges). Note absence of osteopenia.

severely affected) and is due to a mutation in the *SHOX* gene. Homozygous inheritance of the abnormal gene causes Langer-type mesomelic dysplasia.

Dyschondrosteosis is characterized by mesomelic short stature and Madelung deformity usually presenting around the age of 7 years.

1. *Long bones*: Mesomelic shortening
2. *Wrists*: Madelung deformity (Fig. 103-32). This is due to premature fusion of the medial half of the distal radial physis. The result is a reduction in the carpal angle and a relatively long distal ulna that subsequently dislocates. The morphology has been studied using conventional radiographs, CT, and MRI.[24]

Madelung deformity may occur in isolation (i.e., without the mesomelic shortening that occurs in Leri-Weill syndrome). Madelung deformity should not be confused with conditions in which the distal ulna is shortened (e.g., Ollier's disease, hereditary multiple exostoses, trauma, infection). The abnormality in these circumstances is described as a reverse-Madelung deformity (see Fig. 103-61).

CAMPTODACTYLY-ARTHROPATHY-COXA VARA-PERICARDITIS (CACP) SYNDROME

CACP syndrome belongs to group 17 of the osteochondrodysplasias—the group of acromelic dysplasias. It is an autosomal-recessive condition due to an abnormal gene on chromosome 1.

Clinically, patients present in early childhood with camptodactyly (finger contractures) and features of a noninflammatory arthropathy with cold joints and no laboratory signs of inflammation. Confusion with systemic-onset juvenile idiopathic arthropathy (JIA) is possible, but radiologic findings in this condition are quite distinct from those of JIA.[25]

The radiologic findings are those of a nonerosive arthropathy with minimal synovial thickening. Loss of joint space is a relatively late finding. Fusion across joints (e.g., in the carpus) does not occur and the cervical spine is spared.

1. *Pelvis*: Coxa vara, short femoral necks, interosseous acetabular cysts (which connect with the joint spaces; Fig. 103-33). Similar cysts may also be seen at the knees.
2. *Hands*: Camptodactyly, squaring of the metacarpals and phalanges

Differentiation from JIA is essential to prevent relatively toxic or aggressive treatment to which patients with CACP will not respond.

Classic Signs

- Inheritance is autosomal-dominant with variable expression, and it is more severe in females
- The homozygous condition is Langer's mesomelic dysplasia
- It is characterized by mesomelic shortening and Madelung deformity
- Madelung deformity may occur as an isolated condition
- Do not confuse Madelung with reverse-Madelung deformity

Classic Signs

- Autosomal-recessive disorder with abnormal gene on chromosome 1
- Noninflammatory, nonerosive arthropathy
- Large acetabular cysts that in the correct clinical setting are pathognomonic

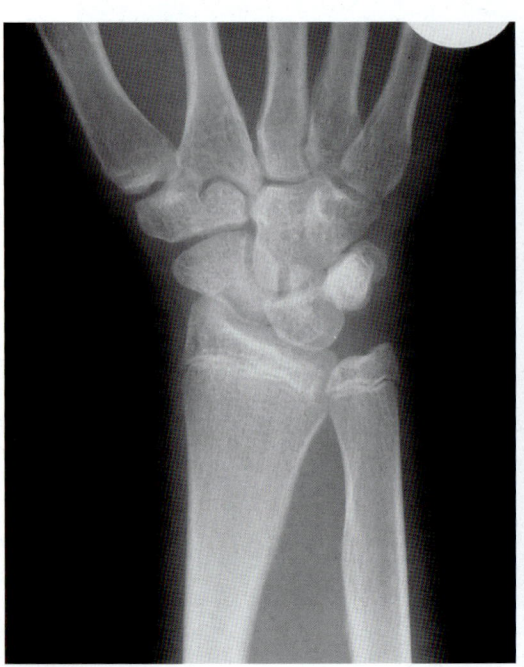
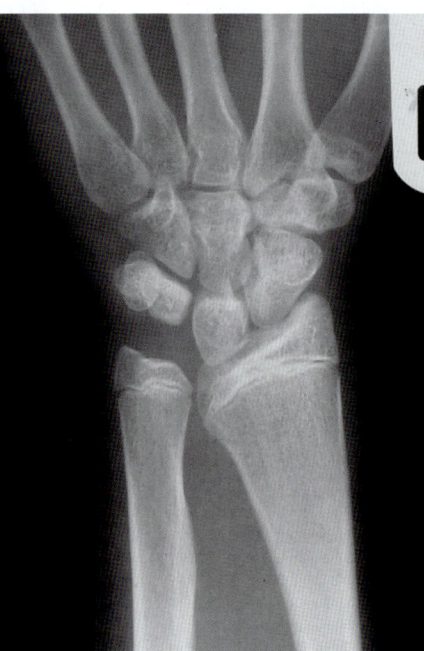

■ **FIGURE 103-32** Dyschondrosteosis. Anterior radiographs of wrist show bilateral Madelung deformity.

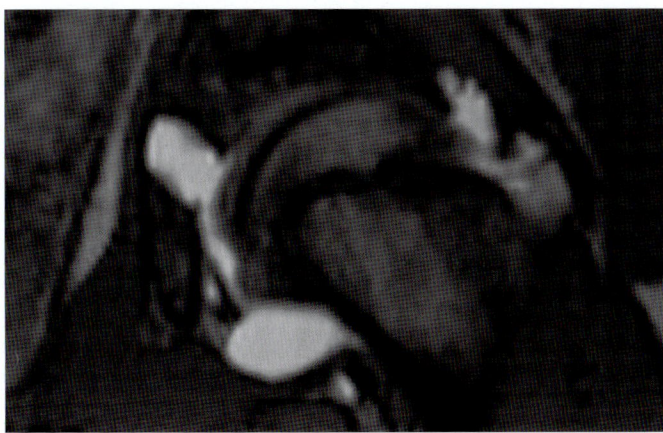

■ **FIGURE 103-33** CACP T2-weighted MR image of left hip. Joint fluid is continuous with an acetabular cyst.

CLEIDOCRANIAL DYSPLASIA

This is an autosomal-dominant condition with the abnormal gene located on chromosome 6.[26] It belongs to group 19 of the classification system—dysplasias with predominant membranous bone involvement.

Clinically, patients have short stature; the diagnosis is made based on the following radiographic findings:

1. *Skull*:Wide sutures; delayed closure of wide fontanelles; multiple wormian bones (Fig. 103-34); supernumerary teeth
2. *Chest*: Hypoplastic or absent clavicles (Fig. 103-35); pseudarthrosis of middle third of clavicle
3. *Pelvis*: Narrow iliac bones; short pubic rami; wide symphysis pubis; short femoral necks; coxa valga; "chef's hat" configuration of proximal femoral epiphyses (Fig. 103-36)
4. *Hands*: Short middle phalanges with cone-shaped epiphyses (Fig.103-37); pseudoepiphyses of metacarpals; acro-osteolysis
5. *Long bones*: Pseudarthoses (rare)

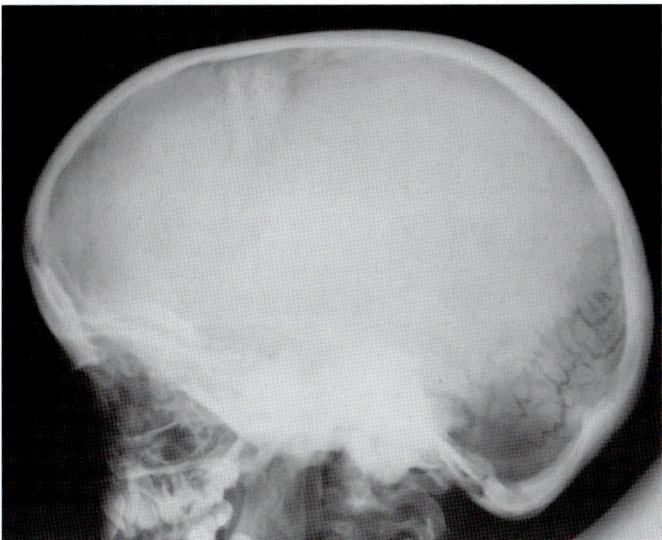

■ **FIGURE 103-34** Cleidocranial dysplasia. Lateral radiograph of the skull. Note multiple wormian bones (more than 10 wormian bones is considered pathologic).

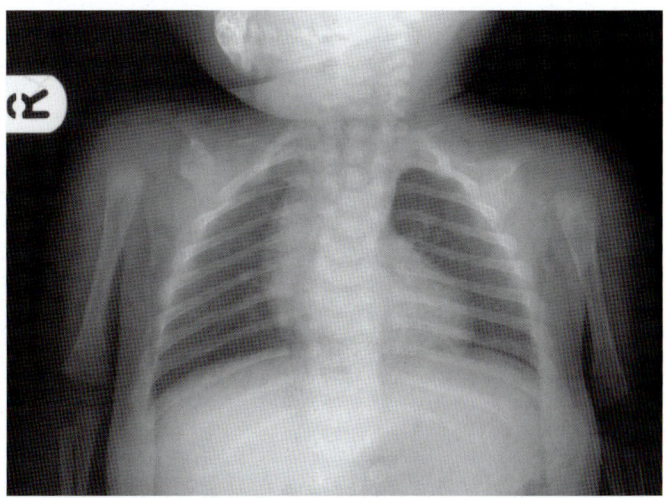

■ **FIGURE 103-35** Cleidocranial dysplasia. Anteroposterior chest radiograph. The right clavicle is absent, and the left clavicle is hypoplastic.

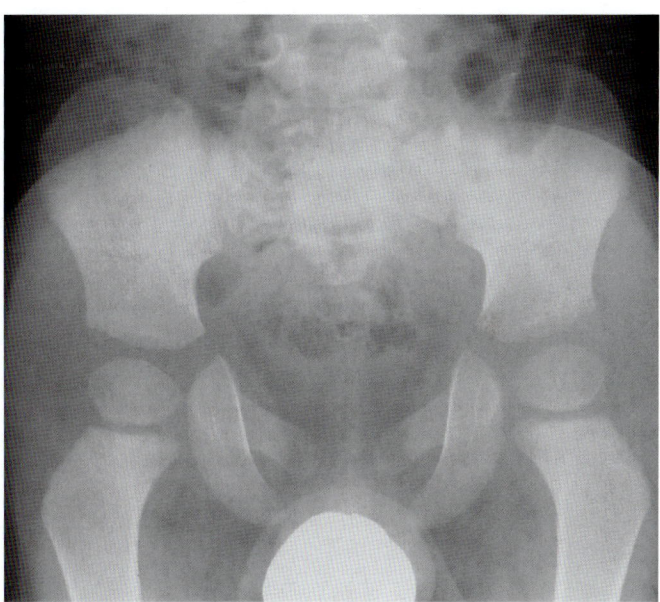

■ **FIGURE 103-36** Cleidocranial dysplasia. Anteroposterior radiograph of the pelvis shows the "chef's hat" configuration of proximal femoral epiphyses with wide symphysis pubis.

Classic Signs

- Autosomal-dominant disorder
- Predominant involvement of membranous bone
- Wide-open sutures with multiple wormian bones
- Absent or hypoplastic clavicles
- Wide symphysis pubis

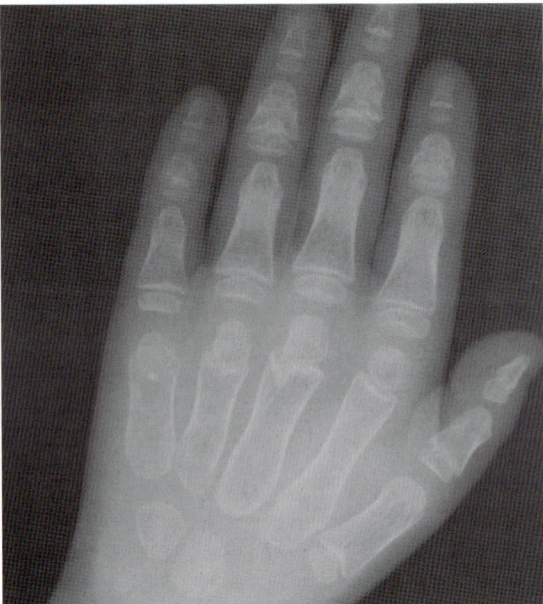

■ **FIGURE 103-37**   Cleidocranial dysplasia. On this radiograph, note the short middle phalanges with cone-shaped epiphyses.

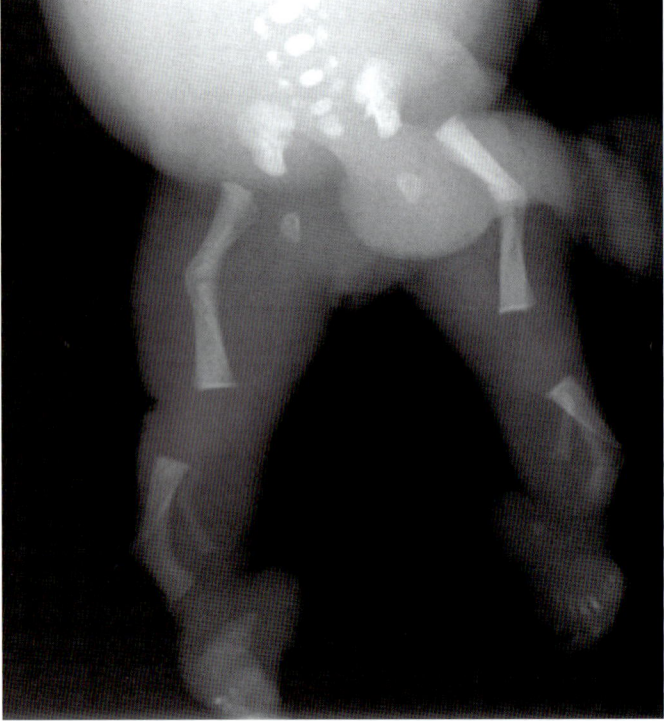

■ **FIGURE 103-38**   Campomelic dysplasia. Anteroposterior "babygram." Characteristic angulation of femora and tibiae, with narrow iliac wings.

CAMPOMELIC DYSPLASIA

This autosomal-dominant condition belongs to group 20 of the osteochondrodysplasias—the bent-bone dysplasia group. It is usually perinatally lethal due to severe respiratory insufficiency.

Some patients diagnosed as having the ischiopubic-patella syndrome have been shown to have mild or mosaic mutations of the *SOX9* gene and are actually survivors of campomelic dysplasia. The majority of survivors with a male karyotype have partial or complete sex reversal.[27,28]

Radiologic findings from the skeletal survey include:

Neonate

1. *Long bones*: Characteristic angulation (Fig. 103-38) of the femora (junction of upper and middle thirds) and tibiae (junction of middle and lower thirds); short fibulae
2. *Pelvis*: Dislocated hips; narrow iliac wings (see Fig. 103-38)
3. *Chest*: 11 pairs of ribs; absent wings of scapulae (Fig. 103-39)
4. *Spine*: Cervical kyphosis; hypoplastic pedicles of the dorsal spine (see Fig. 103-39)
5. *Skull*: Prominent occiput; small mandible

Survivors

1. *Long bones*: Bowing of tibia and fibula; short fibula; hypoplastic patella
2. *Chest*: 11 pairs of ribs; hypoplastic wings of scapula
3. *Pelvis*: Absent ossification of the inferior pubic rami
4. *Spine*: Severe kyphoscoliosis, spinal dysraphism
5. *Hands*: Short middle phalanges with cone-shaped epiphyses

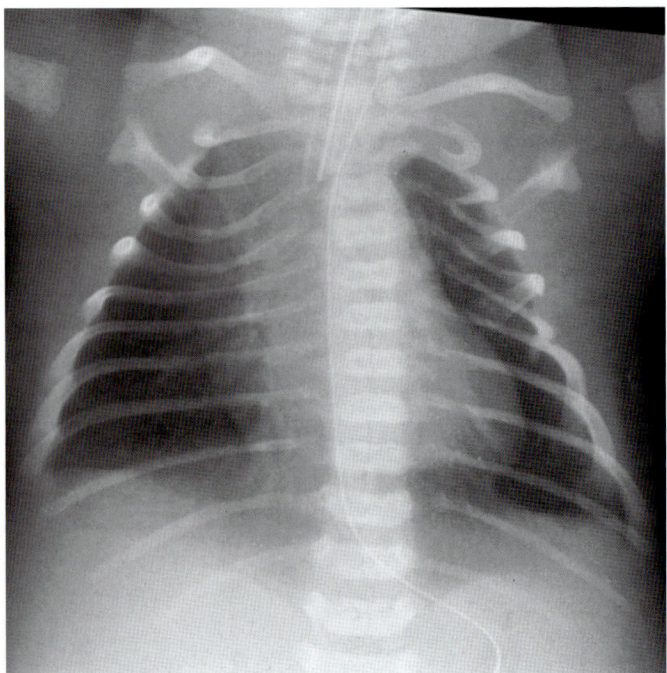

■ **FIGURE 103-39**   Campomelic dysplasia. Anteroposterior radiograph of the chest shows 11 pairs of ribs. The wings of the scapulae are absent as are the pedicles of the upper dorsal spine.

Classic Signs

- Autosomal-dominant disorder caused by mutation in *SOX9* gene
- Often perinatally lethal due to respiratory insufficiency
- Survival may occur in those with mild or mosaic mutations
- Angulated long bones (with no shortening) and absent wings of scapulae in neonates
- Hypoplastic patellae, absent ossification of inferior pubic rami, hypoplastic scapular wings, and kyphoscoliosis in survivors

1. *Skull*: Macrocephaly; ground-glass opacity of the skull vault; elongated/J-shaped sella turcica (Fig. 103-40)
2. *Face*: Flattening of mandibular condyles
3. *Chest*: Broad ribs with posterior constriction—"oar/paddle-shaped" ribs (Fig. 103-41); broad clavicles
4. *Spine*: Hypoplasia at thoracolumbar junction; kyphosis; oval vertebral bodies with central tongues or inferior beaking (Fig. 103-42); posterior scalloping; platyspondyly severe in type IV (Fig. 103-43); hypoplastic odontoid peg in type IV (Fig. 103-44)

MUCOPOLYSACCHARIDOSES

Group 22 of the International Classification includes the storage disorders of which the mucopolysaccharidoses are one. Others are fucosidosis, mannosidosis (α and β), aspartylglucosaminuria, mucolipidosis (types II and III), sialic acid storage disease, multiple sulfatase deficiency, and the several different forms of GM_1 gangliosidosis, sialidosis, and galactosialidosis.

All the storage disorders in group 22 are autosomal recessive except for mucopolysaccharidosis type II (Hunter's disease), which is X-linked recessive.

Various therapies exist or are being researched for the lysosomal and storage disorders, including enzyme replacement, bone marrow transplantation, substrate reduction therapy, and gene therapy.[29]

The mucopolysaccharidoses as a group are the most common of the storage disorders (Table 103-1).

The constellation of radiographic findings is known collectively as "dysostosis multiplex." These findings include:

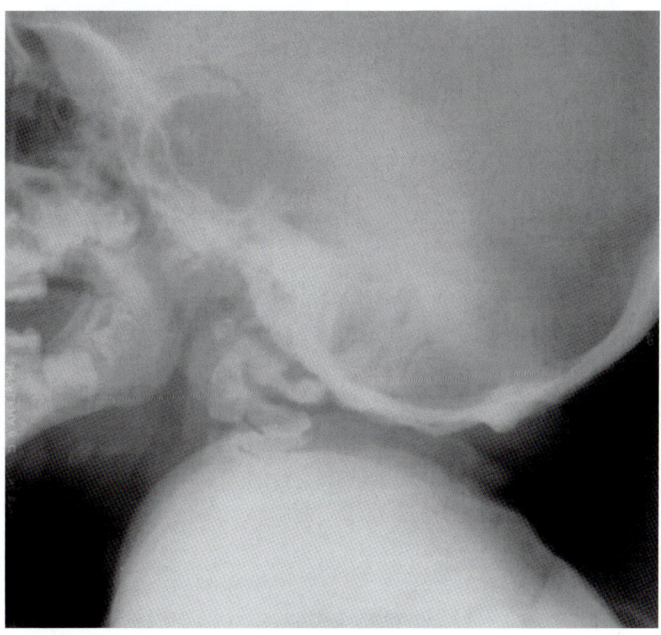

■ **FIGURE 103-40** Mucopolysaccharidosis. Radiograph of lateral skull shows elongated/J-shaped sella turcica.

TABLE 103-1   Clinical Features of the Mucopolysaccharidoses

Disorder	Inheritance	Enzyme Deficiency	Severity	Age at Presentation	Comment
Type I-H (Hurler)	AR	α-L-iduronidase	Severe	1-2 years	Mental retardation, corneal clouding
Type I-S (Scheie)	AR	α-L-iduronidase	Mild	Childhood	Normal intelligence, corneal clouding, stiff joints, previously type V
Type II (Hunter)	XLR	Iduronate-2-sulfatase	Moderate	2-4 years	Mental retardation
Type III (San Filippo)	AR	IIIA: heparan sulfate sulfatase IIIB: *N*-Ac-α-D-glucosaminide IIIC: Ac-CoA: α-glucosaminidase-*N*-acetyltransferase IIID: *N*-Ac-glucosamine-6-sulfatase	Mild/moderate	Early childhood	No coarse features, severe neurologic degeneration, behavioral disturbance
Type IV (Morquio)	AR	IVA: galactose-6-sulfatase IVB: β-galactosidase	Variable (mild to severe)	1-3 years	Normal intelligence, normal skull, severe platyspondyly, odontoid hypoplasia
Type VI (Maroteaux-Lamy)	AR	Arylsulfatase B	Moderate	2-4 years	Normal intelligence, corneal clouding
Type VII (Sly)	AR	β-glucuronidase	Variable (mild to severe)	Infancy/childhood	May present in utero as hydrops fetalis

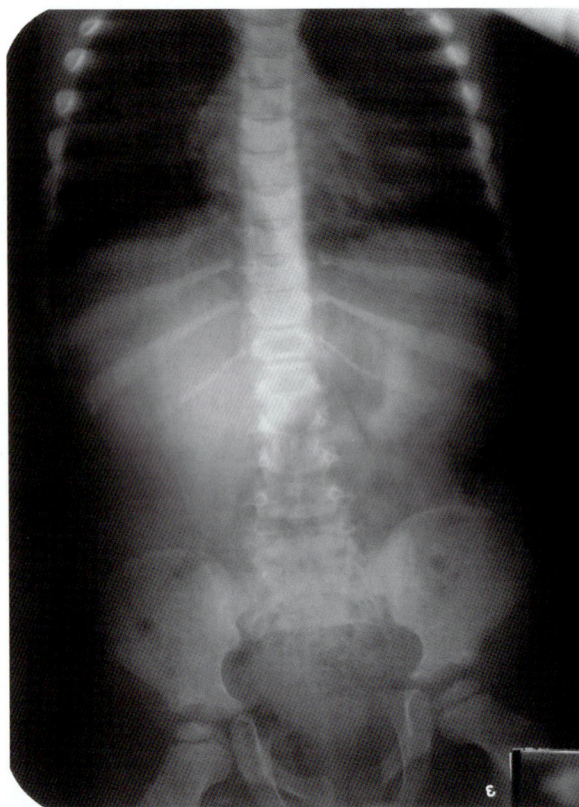

■ **FIGURE 103-41** Mucopolysaccharidosis. Anteroposterior radiograph of abdomen. Note posterior constriction of lower ribs, giving rise to so-called paddle-shaped ribs.

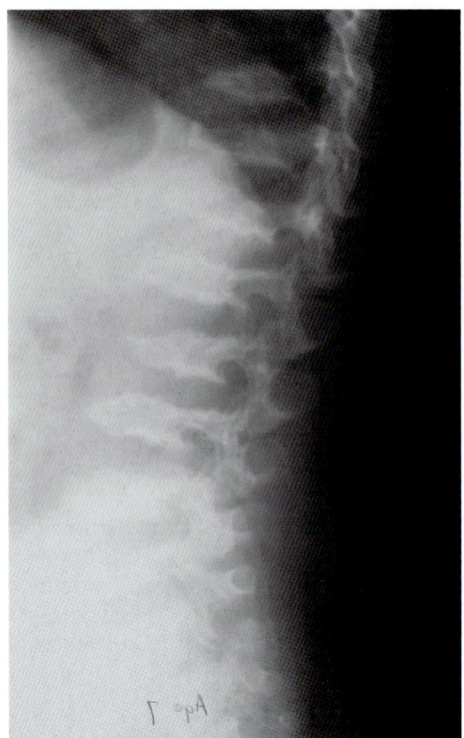

■ **FIGURE 103-43** Mucopolysaccharidosis type IV. Lateral radiograph of lumbar spine. Severe platyspondyly is a feature of Morquio's syndrome.

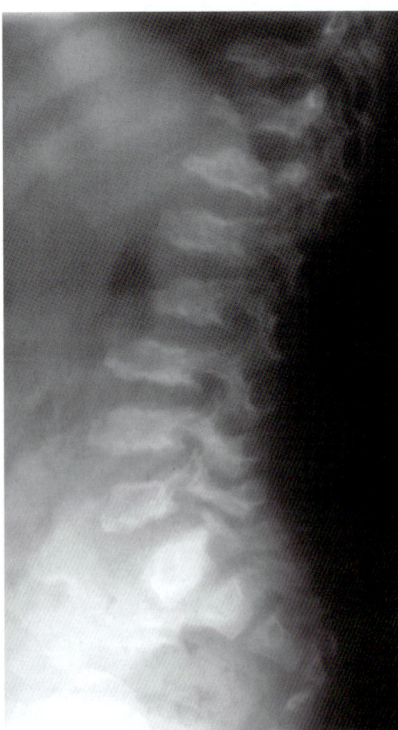

■ **FIGURE 103-42** Mucopolysaccharidosis. Lateral radiograph of lumbar spine shows hypoplastic vertebral body at thoracolumbar junction, central tongues and inferior beaking, posterior scalloping, and broad ribs.

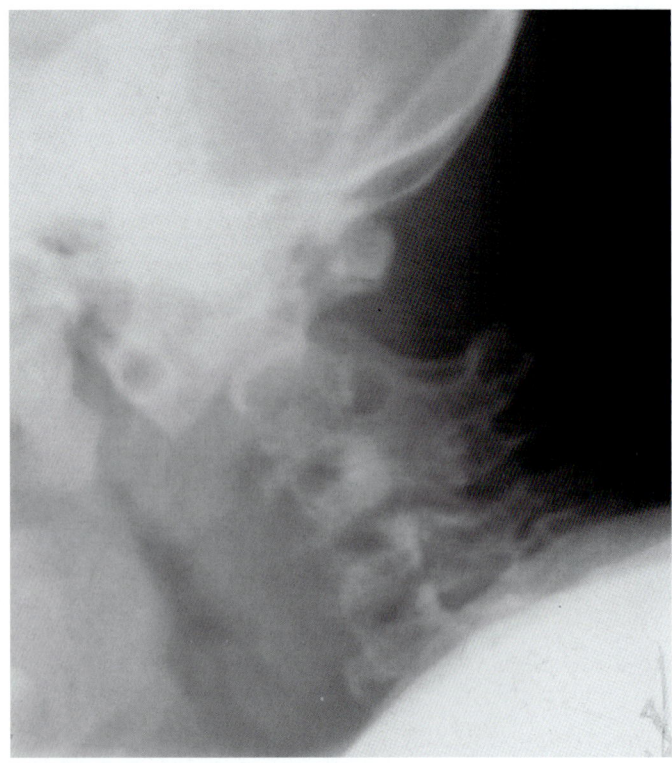

■ **FIGURE 103-44** Lateral radiograph of the craniocervical junction. Odontoid hypoplasia with cervical instability is a feature of Morquio's syndrome.

5. *Pelvis*: Narrow; flared iliac wings; dysplastic acetabula (Fig. 103-45)
6. *Long bones*: Generalized epiphyseal dysplasia; fragmented proximal femoral epiphyses (see Fig. 103-45); coxa valga; elongated femoral necks (Fig. 103-46); genu valgum in type IV (Fig. 103-47)
7. *Hands*: Reduced carpal angle; short broad ("sugarloaf") metacarpals; short broad phalanges; pointed base of second to fifth metacarpals (Fig. 103-48)

OSTEOGENESIS IMPERFECTA

Group 24 of the classification system consists of those dysplasias associated with decreased bone density and includes the various forms of osteogenesis imperfecta (OI), Bruck's dysplasia (OI plus joint contractures), and idiopathic juvenile osteoporosis among others. Osteogenesis imperfecta is heritable; idiopathic juvenile osteoporosis is not. In OI there is reduced bone density with normal calcium and phosphate metabolism.

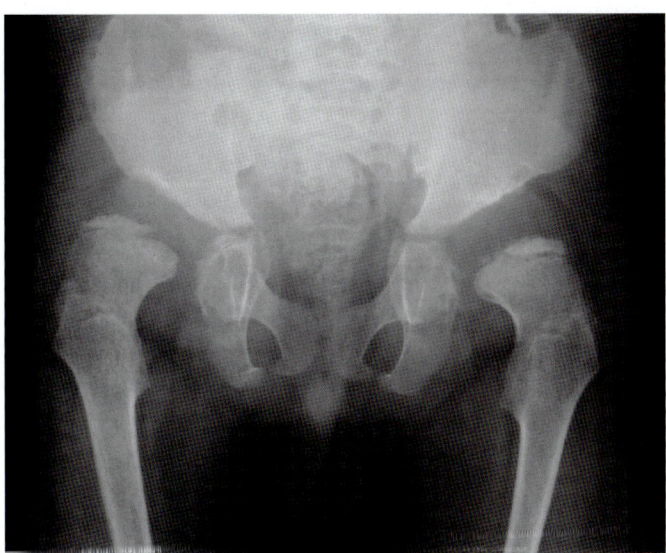

■ **FIGURE 103-45** Mucopolysaccharidosis. Anteroposterior radiograph of pelvis shows dysplastic acetabula, flared iliac wings, and fragmented proximal femoral epiphyses.

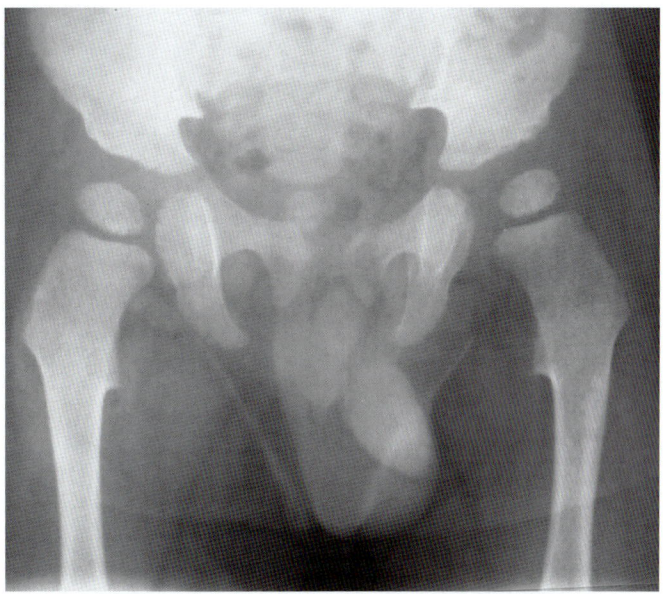

■ **FIGURE 103-46** Mucopolysaccharidosis. Anteroposterior radiograph demonstrates coxa valga and elongated femoral necks.

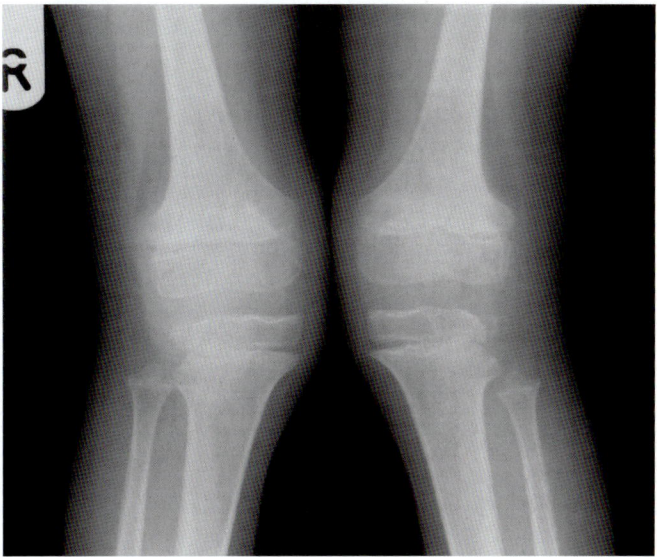

■ **FIGURE 103-47** Mucopolysaccharidosis type IV. Anteroposterior radiograph of the knees shows genu valgum.

There are currently seven subtypes of OI,[30] some but not all of which are associated with a disorder of type I collagen. Table 103-2 summarizes the salient clinical points of each type.

The characteristic radiologic features of OI are reduced bone density, multiple fractures, slender ribs and long bones, and multiple wormian bones.

The increased tendency to fracture in type I OI becomes less apparent after puberty.

The three subgroups of OI type II are summarized in Table 103-3.

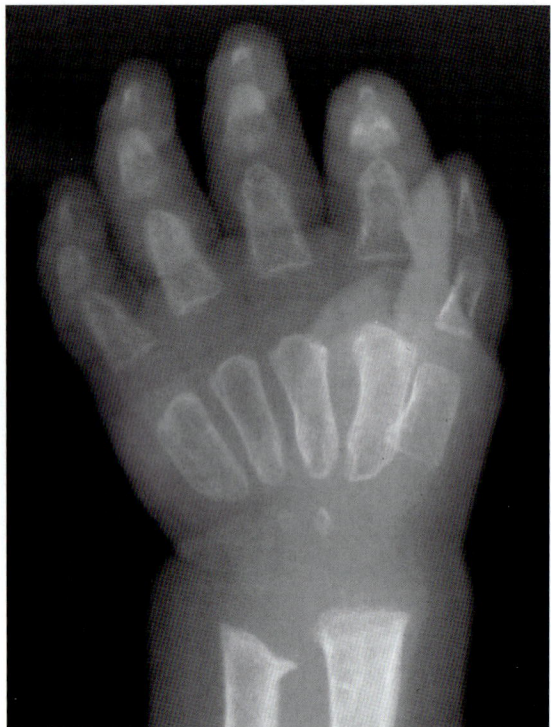

■ **FIGURE 103-48** Mucopolysaccharidosis. Radiograph of the hand shows reduced carpal angle; short, broad phalanges; and pointed base of metacarpals.

Radiologic findings of type III (severe deforming) OI include:

1. *Skull*: Deficient mineralization; wide sutures; multiple wormian bones; tam-o'-shanter skull with platybasia, basilar invagination, and cord compression (Fig. 103-51)
2. *Long bones*: Extremely slender; multiple fractures on minimum handling; limb deformities
3. *Spine*: Codfish vertebrae (Fig. 103-52); kyphoscoliosis
4. *Pelvis*: Protrusio acetabuli

Bisphosphonate therapy is increasingly being used in children with OI, and radiologists should recognize the

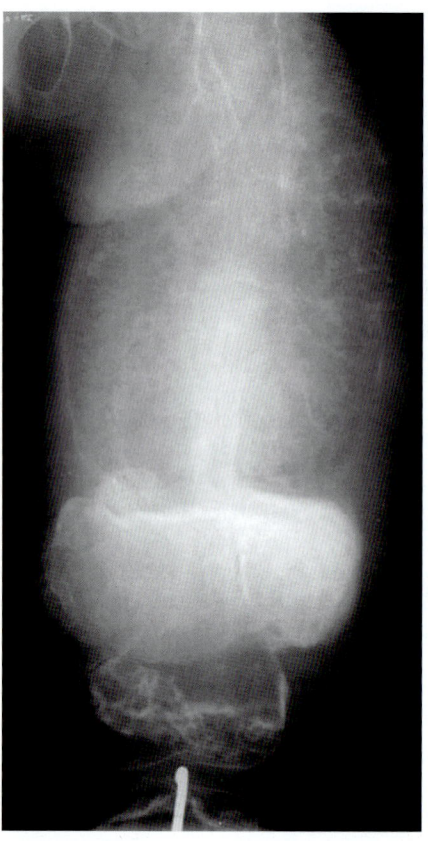

■ **FIGURE 103-49** Osteogenesis imperfecta type V. Anteroposterior radiograph of the femur shows hyperplastic callus at fracture sites in which callus has been replaced with fatty marrow.

dense metaphyseal bands that arise from individual pulses of bisphosphonate (Figs. 103-53 and 103-54).

Nonaccidental injury (NAI) is an important differential diagnosis in infants with type IV OI and multiple fractures. The key point to note is that bone density is normal in NAI and, by the time fractures have begun to occur, bone density is sufficiently reduced in type IV OI to be detected on radiographs.

TABLE 103-2	Types of Osteogenesis Imperfecta					
Type	**Inheritance**	***COL1* Mutation**	**Sclerae**	**Teeth**	**Skull**	**Comment**
I	AD	Common	Blue	IA: normal IB: dentinogenesis imperfecta	Multiple wormian bones	Mildest; most common; deafness may develop
II	AD	Common	—	—	—	Perinatally lethal
III	AD and AR forms	Common	Blue/gray	Normal	Multiple wormian bones	Most severe type that is compatible with life; early deafness; bisphosphonate therapy is beneficial
IV	AD	Common	Normal	IVA: normal IVB: dentinogenesis imperfecta	Normal	Varies in severity from mild (overlap with type I) to severe (overlap with type III)
V	AD	Absent	Normal	Normal	Normal	Hypertrophic callus (Fig. 103-49); calcification of forearm interosseous membrane; dense metaphyseal bands
VI	AD	Absent	Normal	Normal	Normal	Characteristic histologic appearance of bone lamellae with excess osteoid
VII	AR	Absent	Normal	Normal	Normal	Rhizomelic shortening of long bones

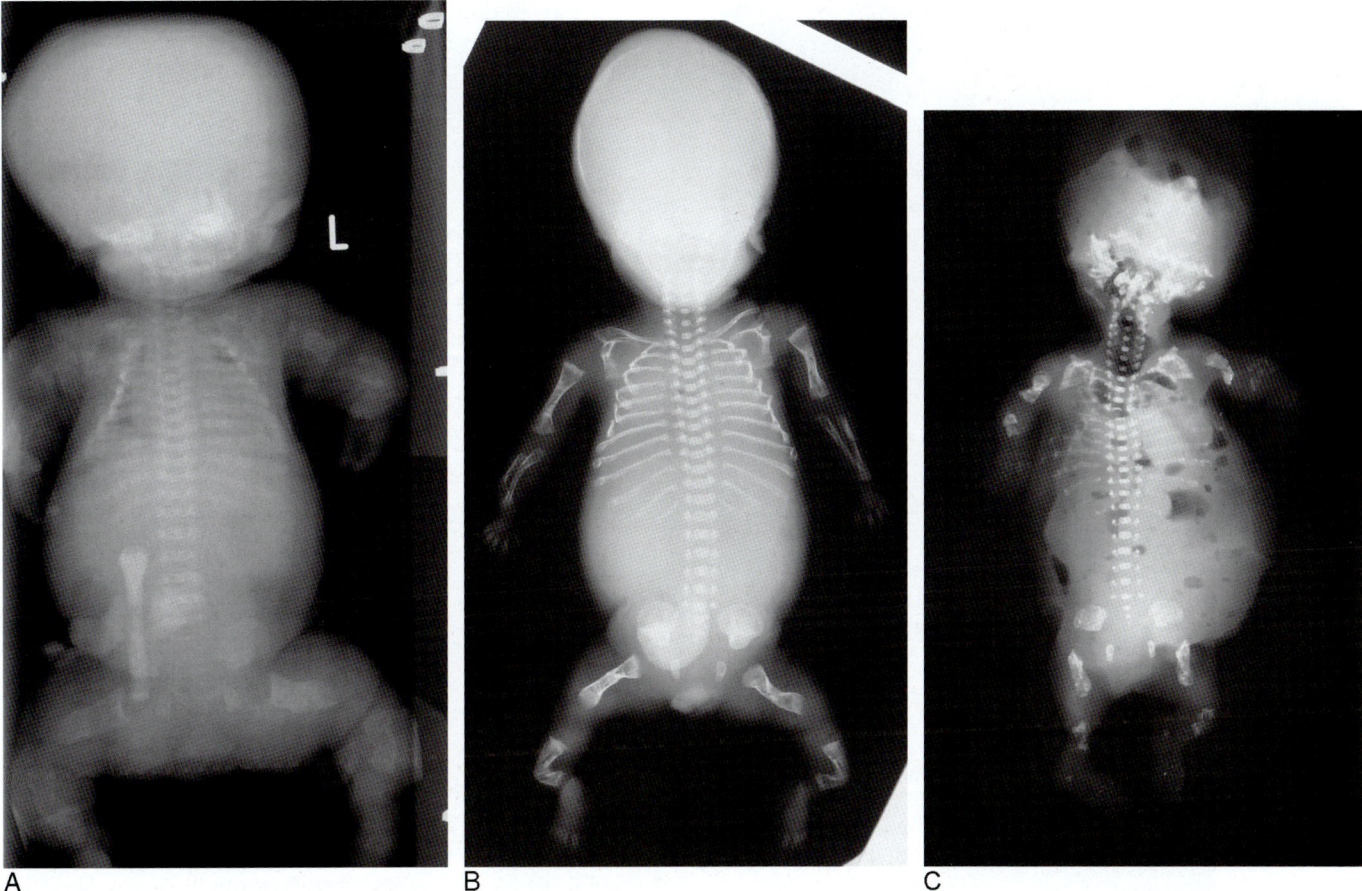

■ **FIGURE 103-50** Anteroposterior "babygrams." **A,** Osteogenesis imperfecta type IIA. Note concertina femora with no distinction between metaphyses and diaphyses. **B,** Osteogenesis imperfecta type IIB. Note ossified skull vault, discrete rib fractures, and angulated tibiae. Type IIB overlaps with severe type III. **C,** Osteogenesis imperfecta type IIC. There is unusual dense stippling of the skeleton.

TABLE 103-3	Subgroups of Osteogenesis Imperfecta Type II (Fig. 103-50)				
Subgroup	**Skull**	**Ribs**	**Femora**	**Vertebral Fractures**	**Comment**
A	Absent ossification	Broad (multiple fractures)	Short crumpled; no distinction between metaphyses and diaphyses (see Fig. 103-50)	Common	Most severe subgroup
B	Ossified	Beaded (discrete healing fractures)	Short crumpled; recognizable metaphyses and diaphyses	Rare	Confused with type III OI in the perinatal period
C	Absent ossification	Fractures (no beading)	Unusual dense stippling throughout the skeleton	Rare	

Classic Signs

- All seven subtypes of OI are autosomal dominant except type III (AD and AR forms) and type VII (AR)
- Blue sclerae occur in type I (mild)
- Type II is perinatally lethal
- Type III is the severe deforming type
- White sclerae occur in type IV (ranges from mild to severe)
- The presence of normal teeth or dentinogenesis imperfecta divides types I and IV into subtypes A and B, respectively

- If fractures are occurring in infants with type IV OI, then reduced bone density should be apparent on radiographs (normal bone density in NAI)
- Type V is associated with hypertrophic callus formation
- Type VI has characteristic histology
- Type VII is associated with rhizomelic shortening
- Bisphosphonate therapy leads to characteristic dense metaphyseal bands

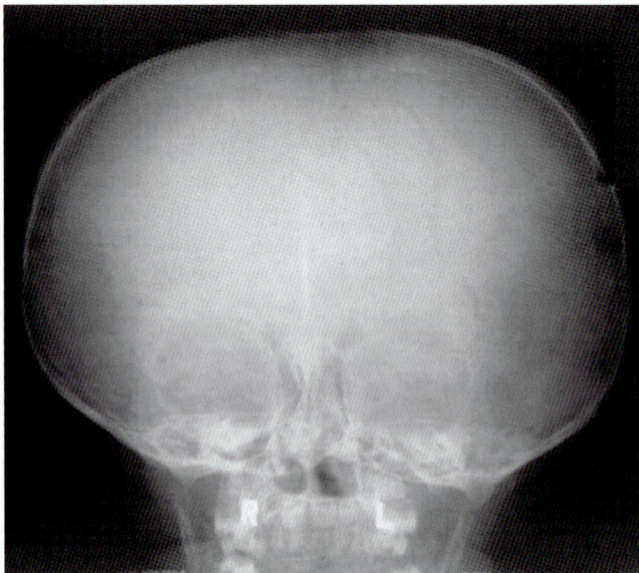

■ **FIGURE 103-51** Osteogenesis imperfecta type III/severe IV. Radiograph shows tam-o'-shanter skull (brachycephaly, increased biparietal diameter, platybasia, and basilar invagination).

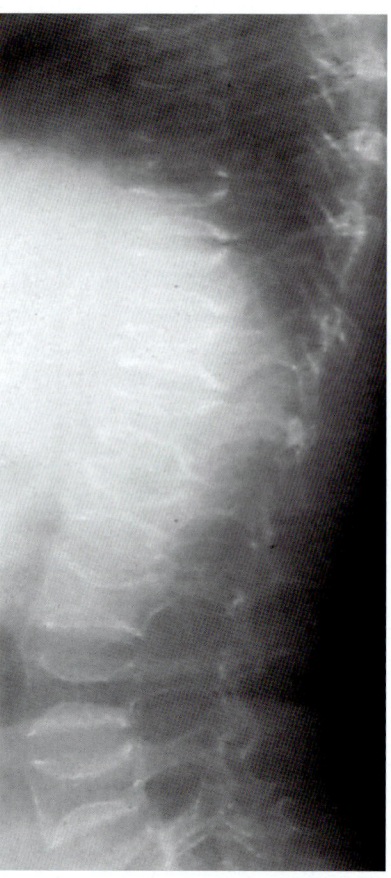

■ **FIGURE 103-52** Osteogenesis imperfecta type III. Lateral radiograph of the spine shows osteopenia with biconcave end plates giving rise to "codfish" vertebrae.

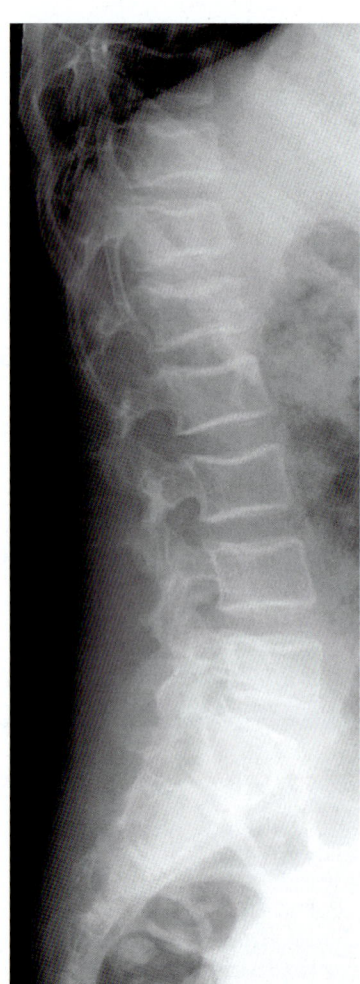

■ **FIGURE 103-53** Osteogenesis imperfecta. Dense vertebral end plates are evident in a patient on pamidronate therapy. Note loss of vertebral body height in keeping with crush fractures secondary to reduced bone mass.

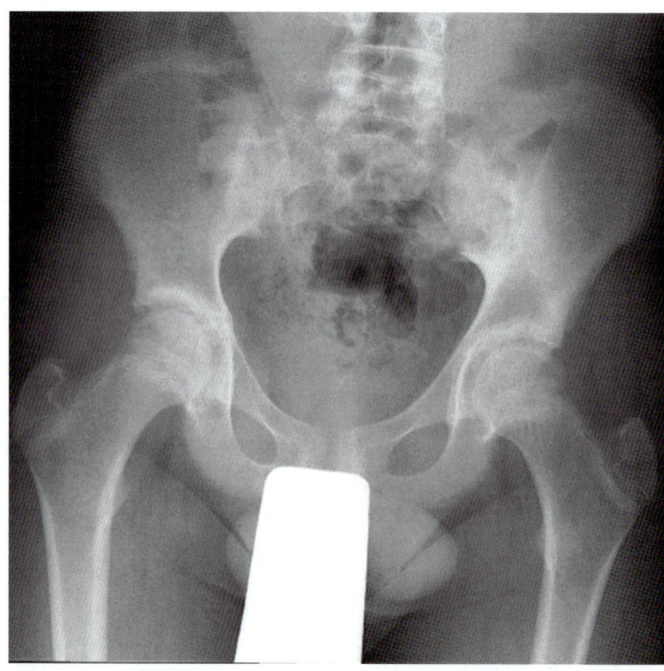

■ **FIGURE 103-54** Osteogenesis imperfecta. Bisphosphonate lines. Dense metaphyseal lines of proximal femoral metaphyses, and apophyses of the greater trochanters and iliac wings due to pamidronate therapy. The relatively radiolucent gaps between the lines represent interval growth between pulses of pamidronate.

OSTEOPETROSIS

Group 26 of the classification (increased bone density without modification of bone shape) includes osteopetrosis (various forms), dysosteosclerosis, pyknodysostosis, melorheostosis, osteopathia striata, osteopoikilosis, osteosclerosis (Stanescu type), osteomesopyknosis, cranial osteosclerosis with bamboo hair, and mixed sclerosing bone dysplasia.

There are three main subtypes of osteopetrosis: severe infantile (autosomal-recessive), intermediate juvenile (autosomal-recessive), and mild adult (autosomal-dominant) types.

Severe autosomal-recessive osteopetrosis presents at birth with generalized osteosclerosis (there may be relative osteopenia of the metaphyses; Fig. 103-55); progressive bone marrow failure with anemia and hepatosplenomegaly; early, progressive blindness (optic nerve compression and retinal degeneration) and early death. Timely bone marrow transplantation (by providing precursors for normally functioning osteoclasts) is curative.

The intermediate (juvenile) type of osteopetrosis is characterized radiographically by a "bone-in-bone" appearance (Fig. 103-56) of all bones. There is an increased tendency to fracture. A small proportion of these patients have an abnormality in the carbonic anhydrase II (*CAII*) gene, and osteopetrosis in these patients is associated with intracranial calcification.[31]

Autosomal-dominant (adult) osteopetrosis may present as an increased tendency to fracture or may be diagnosed as an incidental finding. Type I has generalized osteosclerosis most pronounced in the cranial vault; it is not associated with an increased tendency to fracture. Sclerosis in type II typically affects the spine ("rugger jersey" spine; Fig. 103-57), pelvis, and skull base; there is an increased tendency to fracture and to mandibular osteomyelitis and dental abscesses.

Classic Signs

- Increased bone density with fragile bones due to abnormal osteoclast function
- Timely bone marrow transplantation in the severe infantile autosomal-recessive type is curative
- Intermediate type is characterized by "bone-in-bone" appearance of entire skeleton
- Adult type may be an incidental finding; those with type I autosomal-dominant osteopetrosis do not have an increased tendency to fracture

PYKNODYSOSTOSIS

Like osteopetrosis, this condition belongs to group 26—conditions with increased bone density without modification of bone shape. It is autosomal recessive with the abnormal gene located on chromosome 1.

Patients are of short stature and have a generalized increase in bone density with an increased tendency to fracture.

The artist Henri de Toulouse Lautrec is said to have had this condition.

Radiographic features from the skeletal survey include:

1. *Skull*: Prominent vault; multiple wormian bones; wide open sutures and fontanelles; obtuse or absent mandibular angle
2. *Chest*: Resorption of lateral ends of clavicles; slender clavicles
3. *Pelvis*: Narrow iliac bones with normal ossification of pubic bones (compare with cleidocranial dysplasia)

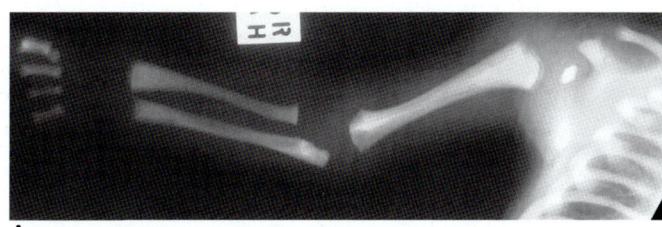
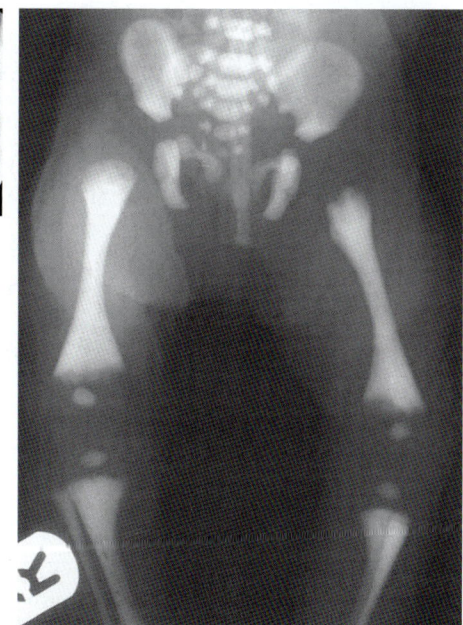

■ **FIGURE 103-55** Infantile osteopetrosis. Anteroposterior radiographs of upper (**A**) and lower (**B**) limbs. Note dense bones with relative radiolucency of metaphyses

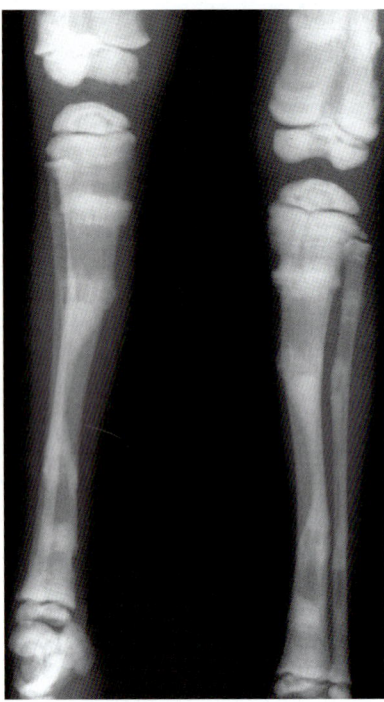

■ **FIGURE 103-56** Juvenile osteopetrosis. Anteroposterior radiograph of the legs shows significant "bone-in-bone" appearance.

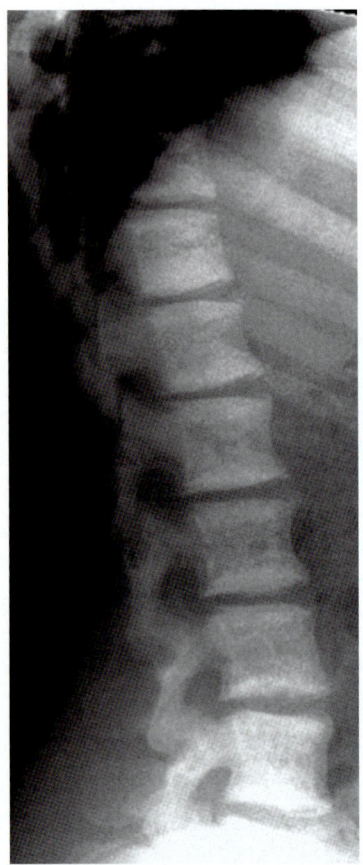

■ **FIGURE 103-57** Adult osteopetrosis. Lateral radiograph of the spine. Dense vertebral end plates give rise to the "rugger-jersey" appearance in type II adult osteopetrosis.

4. *Spine*: Dense vertebral bodies, with or without spondylolisthesis
5. *Hand*: Resorption of the terminal phalanges

Classic Signs

- Autosomal-recessive disorder
- Generalized increase in bone density with an increased tendency to fracture
- Multiple wormian bones
- Resorption of terminal phalanges and lateral ends of clavicles
- Normal ossification of pubic bones

DIAPHYSEAL DYSPLASIA

Group 27 of the International Classification system consists of those osteochondrodysplasias with increased bone density with diaphyseal involvement, of which diaphyseal dysplasia (Camurati-Engelmann disease) is one.

It is an autosomal-dominant condition due to mutation of a gene on chromosome 19. The condition demonstrates "anticipation," which is earlier onset of symptoms and increased severity with successive generations.

Clinical symptoms usually begin in childhood, the most common being pain in the affected limbs. Others include muscle weakness with increased fatigability and a waddling gait. Anemia and hepatosplenomegaly may coexist.

Radiographs reveal cortical thickening and sclerosis of the diaphyses with sparing of metaphyses and epiphyses (Fig. 103-58). The axial skeleton is also involved, but the skull base only occasionally. As the patients get older, differentiation from fibrous dysplasia becomes difficult.

Bone scintigraphy is said to demonstrate hot spots before bone sclerosis is detectable on radiographs[32] and therefore may be an important screening tool in apparently normal individuals with affected family members.

Classic Signs

- Autosomal-dominant disorder
- Shows "anticipation"
- Painful cortical thickening usually in childhood and adolescence
- Epiphyses and metaphyses are spared
- Skull base is only occasionally involved
- In older patients differentiation from fibrous dysplasia may be difficult
- Bone scintigraphy shows hot spots before radiologic evidence of sclerosis

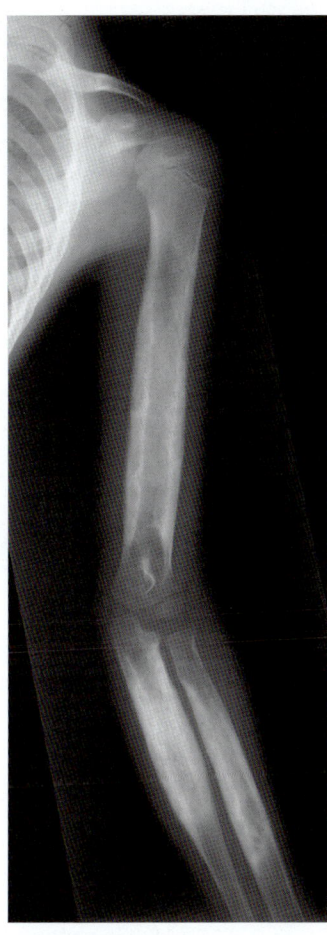

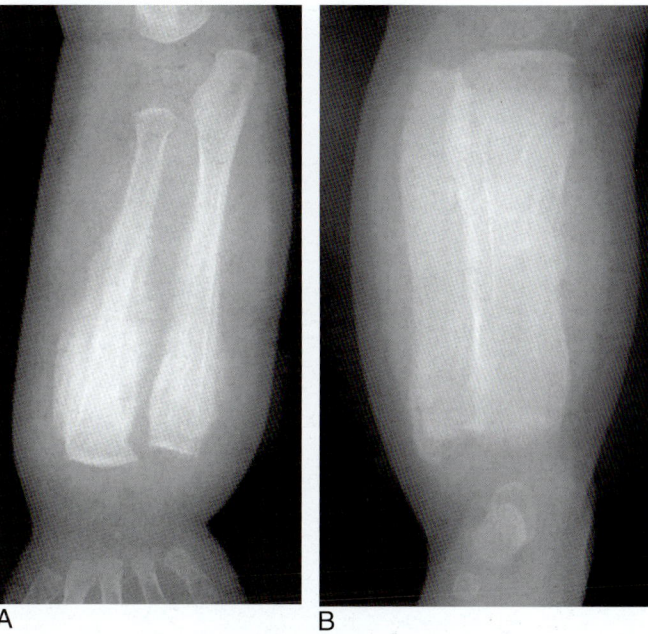

■ **FIGURE 103-59** Infantile cortical hyperostosis. Anteroposterior radiographs of forearm (**A**) and leg (**B**). Marked periosteal reaction and diaphyseal widening particularly of the lower limb can be seen. Note the associated soft tissue swelling.

■ **FIGURE 103-58** Diaphyseal dysplasia. Anteroposterior radiograph of left arm. Cortical thickening and sclerosis of diaphyses are seen. The metaphyses and epiphyses are relatively spared.

Classic Signs

- Prenatal autosomal-recessive form is severe and lethal
- Prenatal autosomal-dominant type is milder
- Postnatal autosomal-dominant type has median onset at 9 weeks of age
- There is painful swelling of affected sites with associated systemic symptoms
- Jaw, ribs, and long bones are commonly affected
- Radiographs reveal florid periosteal reactions

INFANTILE CORTICAL HYPEROSTOSIS

Like progressive diaphyseal dysplasia, infantile cortical hyperostosis (Kenny-Caffey dysplasia) belongs to group 27 of the International Classification system—increased bone density with diaphyseal involvement.

Prenatal and postnatal onset forms of the disease are recognized.

There are two forms of prenatal disease: mild (autosomal-dominant) and severe (autosomal-recessive).[33] The severe antenatal form is diagnosed before 35 weeks' gestation and is associated with polyhydramnios, angulated bones, lung disease, and prematurity. This severe form is lethal.

The postnatal onset form of disease commonly presents around 9 weeks of age (certainly before 5 to 7 months[34]) with irritability and general malaise, fever, and poor feeding. This is followed by firm soft tissue swelling, which is painful. Characteristically, the disease is self-limiting but may wax and wane. Bridging across paired long bones is a recognized complication. Commonly affected sites include the jaw, scapulae, ribs, and upper and lower limbs. Disease may be symmetric.

Radiographs reveal multifocal layered periosteal reactions of the affected sites (Fig. 103-59) with associated soft tissue swelling.

HEREDITARY MULTIPLE EXOSTOSES

Also termed *diaphyseal aclasis*, this condition belongs to group 31 of the International Classification system—the group with disorganized development of cartilaginous and fibrous components of the skeleton.

The syndrome of hereditary multiple exostoses is inherited as an autosomal-dominant condition with sporadic mutation in 33% and incomplete penetrance in females. Disease severity, number of exostoses, and risk of malignant transformation varies between, and even within, affected families. Several chromosomes have been identified: 8, 11, and 19 with the gene loci being termed *EXT1*, *EXT2*, and *EXT3*, respectively.

Clinically, patients present with nontender lumps and bumps, angular deformities of joints, and local pain (compression of nerves, other structures).

The cartilage-capped exostoses are seen on radiographs to arise from the metaphysis and point away from the adjacent joint (Fig. 103-60). With continued growth

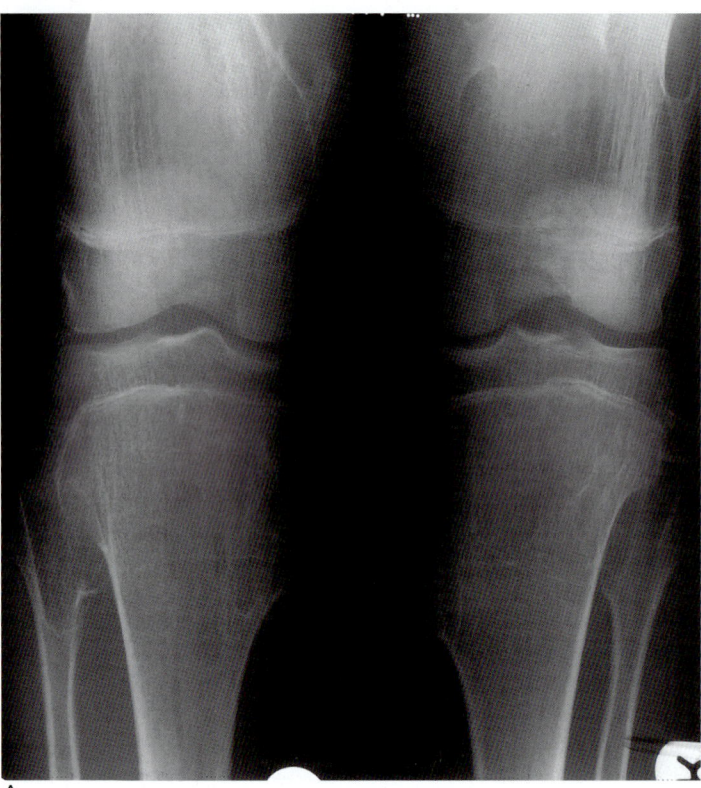

A

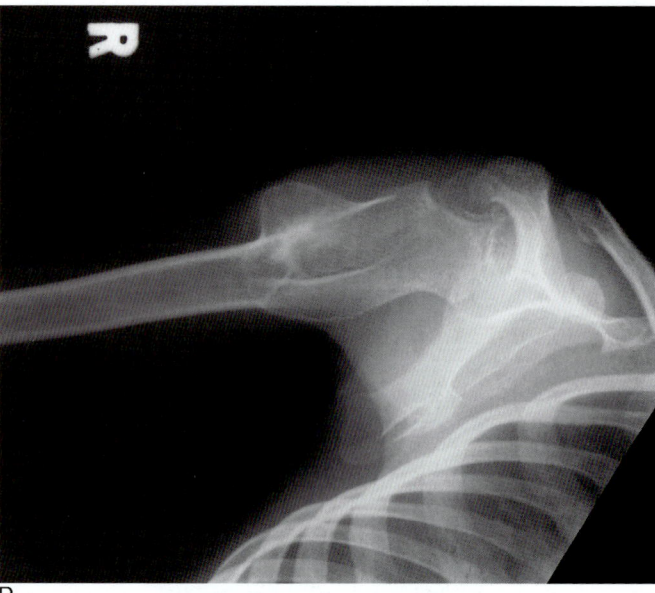

B

■ **FIGURE 103-60** Hereditary multiple exostoses. Anteroposterior radiographs of the knees **(A)** and shoulder **(B)**. Exostoses arise from the metaphyses and point away from the adjacent joint.

there may be compression of adjacent structures and joint subluxation/dislocation. When affecting the distal ulna, a reverse-Madelung deformity may result (Fig. 103-61). Males are said to have more severe and more frequent complications.[35]

The condition has an age-related penetrance (number of exostoses increases with age), with children younger than 10 years of age having significantly fewer exostoses than older children and adults.[36] In affected families, a member who does not present by the age of 12 years will not manifest the disease.[37] Growth of exostoses ceases after skeletal maturity.

Malignant degeneration is usually to a chondrosarcoma in the cartilage cap, although very rarely osteosarcoma may occur at the base of the stalk of the exostosis. Malignancy in childhood is rare. The reported rate of malignant degeneration is variable (0.6% to 5%); and although it has been reported as high as 8.3% in one family,[38] there is as yet no reliable screening method, which is particularly important for lesions in the axial skeleton that cannot be observed clinically. The risk of malignant degeneration does not appear to be associated with disease severity; however, families with the *EXT1* mutation have a risk of malignancy equal to the risk of breast cancer in the elderly screened population. Families with the *EXT2* mutation have a smaller risk,[36] and those with the *EXT3* mutation do not appear to be at any increased risk.

Malignant degeneration is most likely in central lesions (particularly pelvis, hips, and shoulders). Clinical indicators of malignant transformation include rapid growth,

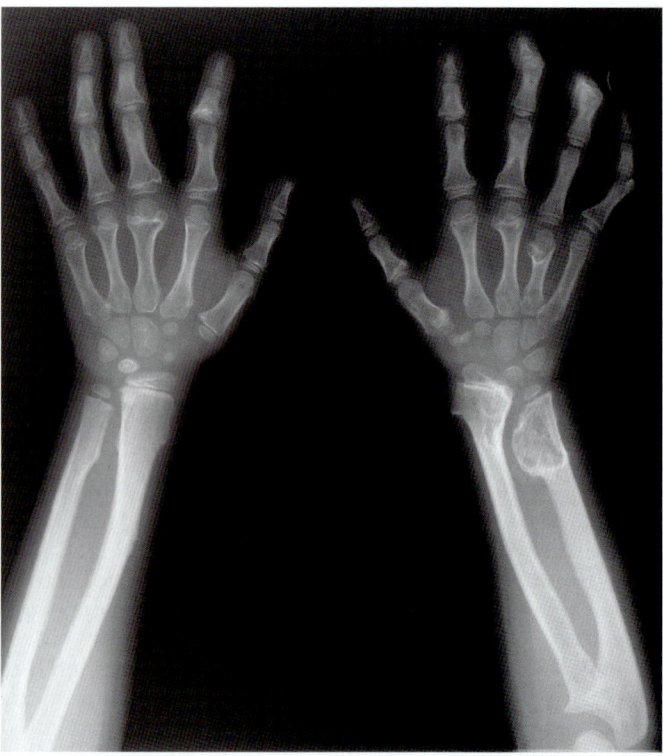

■ **FIGURE 103-61** Hereditary multiple exostoses. Radiograph of hands/forearms. Multiple exostoses arise from the short tubular bones of hands. There is an exostosis of the right distal ulna with reverse-Madelung deformity. Note the growth disturbance and shortening of right fourth metacarpal.

growth after skeletal maturity, and unusual pain (particularly after skeletal maturation).

Radiographic findings that suggest malignancy[39] include:

1. Growth of a previously static osteochondroma after skeletal maturation
2. Surface of the exostosis that is irregular or indistinct
3. Focal regions of radiolucency within the lesion
4. Erosion or destruction of adjacent bone
5. A significant soft tissue mass (especially if associated with scattered/irregular calcification)
6. A cartilage cap more than 1.5 cm thick (as shown by ultrasonography, CT or MRI)

Classic Signs

- Autosomal-dominant disorder
- Exostoses arise from the metaphyses and point away from the adjacent joint
- Growth ceases with skeletal maturity
- Reverse-Madelung deformity
- Malignant transformation to chondrosarcoma occurs in up to 8%

MULTIPLE ENCHONDROMATOSIS

Also known as Ollier's disease, multiple enchondromatosis belongs to the group of disorganized development of cartilaginous and fibrous components of bone (group 31 of the classification). It occurs as a sporadic mutation on chromosome 19 and is not a familial disorder.

Clinically, patients present with asymmetric limb lengths and unsightly lumps and bumps.

Radiographs reveal unilateral or asymmetric bilateral abnormality with multiple irregular elongated or oval radiolucent lesions of the short tubular bones (Fig. 103-62) and/or striated metaphyses of the long bones. The ribs and pelvic bones (Fig. 103-63) may also be affected. Complications include shortening of the affected bone (limb-length discrepancy may require orthopedic intervention) and pathologic fractures. Ollier's disease is a cause of the reverse-Madelung deformity.

Maffucci's syndrome is the association of multiple enchondromas with venous malformations. Radiographs may reveal calcification of rounded phleboliths within the hemangioma. Absence of calcification does not mean absence of venous malformations.

The risk of malignant transformation is significant in Ollier's disease (particularly chondrosarcoma of the skull base and ovarian granulosa cell tumors); however, in Maffucci's syndrome the risk approaches 100% (including intracranial chondrosarcoma and spindle cell hemangioendothelioma.[40]

Classic Signs

- Ollier's disease and Maffucci's syndrome are nonhereditary sporadic conditions
- Maffucci's syndrome is the association of multiple enchondromas with venous malformations
- The incidence of malignancy is increased in both conditions, reaching 100% in older patients with Maffucci's syndrome
- The most common malignancies include chondrosarcoma of the skull base, ovarian granulosa cell tumor, and spindle cell hemangioendothelioma

---

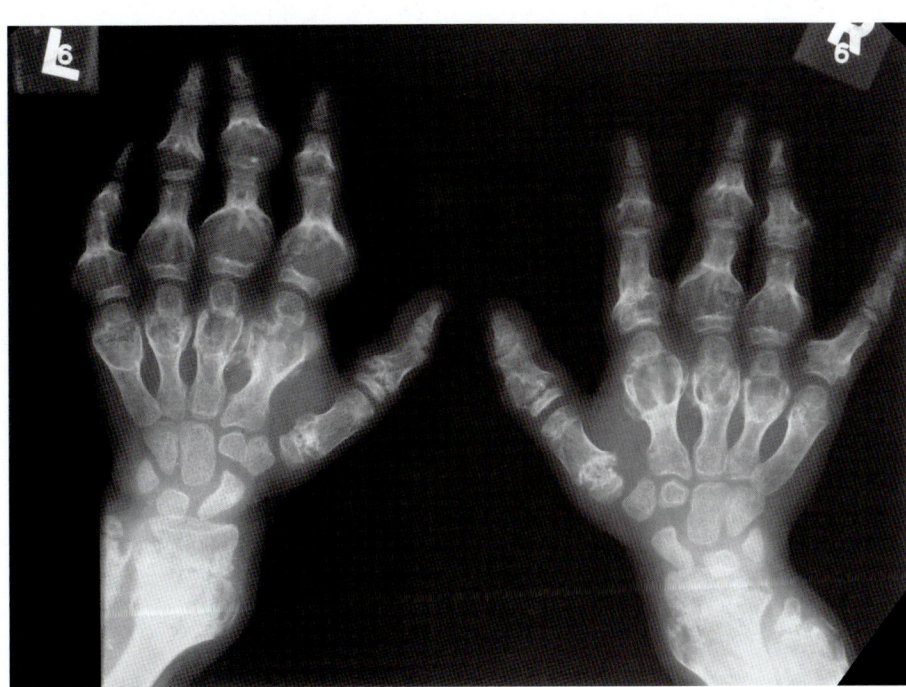

■ **FIGURE 103-62** Multiple enchondromatosis. Multiple rounded/oval nonaggressive lucent lesions of short tubular bones. Note striated appearance of distal radial and ulnar metaphyses.

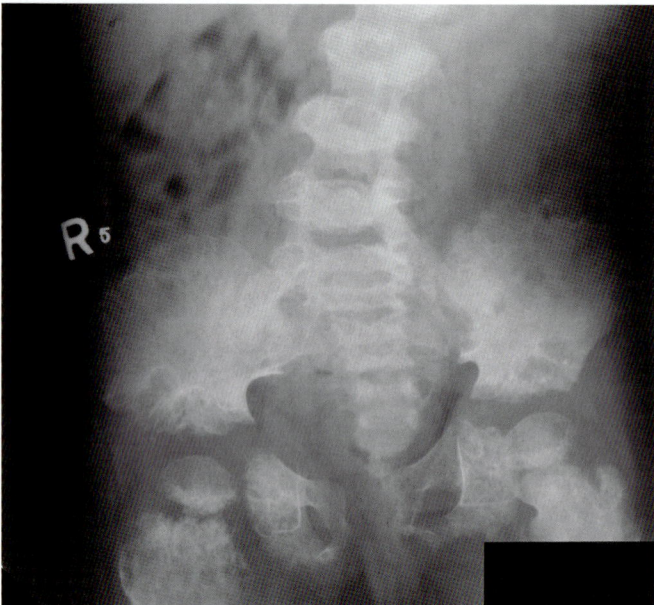

■ **FIGURE 103-63** Multiple enchondromatosis. Anteroposterior radiograph. Note striations of proximal femoral metaphyses and involvement of pelvic bones.

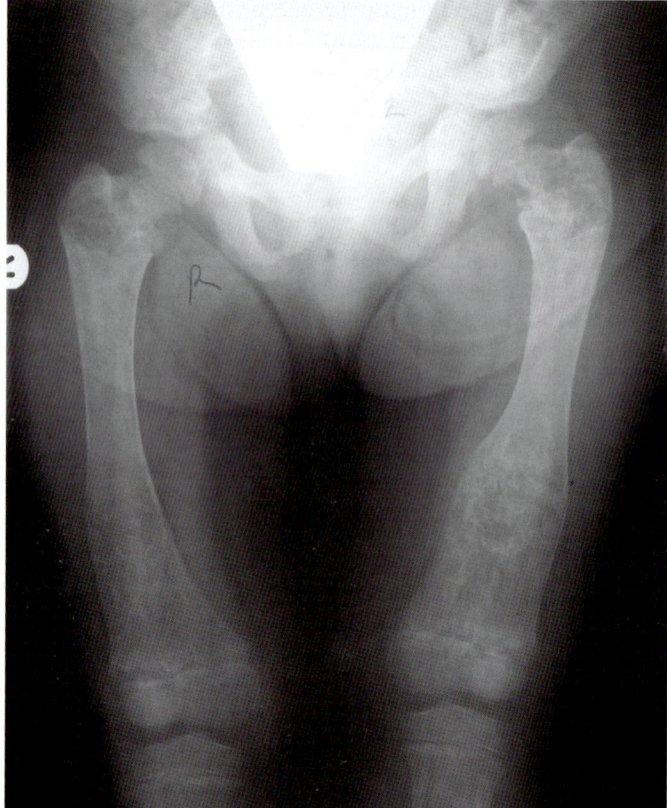

■ **FIGURE 103-64** Polyostotic fibrous dysplasia. Anteroposterior radiograph of femora. Note bilateral coxa vara (shepherd's crook deformity).

FIBROUS DYSPLASIA

Fibrous dysplasia (including McCune-Albright and other types) occurs as a result of sporadic (mosaic) mutation on chromosome 20. It belongs to the group of disorganized development of cartilaginous and fibrous components of bone (group 31) of the International Classification.[1] In patients with fibrous dysplasia, normal bone marrow is replaced by fibro-osseous material.

Clinical presentation is variable; there may be multiple café-au-lait macules, precocious puberty in up to 50% of affected females with polyostotic fibrous dysplasia, and other endocrine disturbances, including hyperthyroidism and Cushing's syndrome.

Radiologic findings are those of patchy bone destruction and sclerosis. The lytic lesions are expanded with a narrow zone of transition and central ground-glass opacification. Endosteal scalloping is a feature (Fig. 103-64). Overgrowth of affected bones may occur.

An exophytic form of fibrous dysplasia (fibrous dysplasia protuberans) has also been described.[41]

Specific descriptive terms include:

1. *Leontiasis ossea*: overgrowth of skull and facial bones
2. *Shepherd's crook deformity*: progressive bilateral coxa vara deformity as a result of bone softening

Other complications include protrusio acetabuli, pathologic fractures, and tumor rickets.

MRI reveals lesions to be of low or intermediate signal on T1-weighted images and of high signal intensity on T2-weighted images with peripheral enhancement.[42]

Classic Signs

- Sporadic condition
- May be associated with multiple café-au-lait macules
- May be associated with endocrine disturbances, including precocious puberty in females, hyperthyroidism, and Cushing's syndrome
- Nonaggressive expansile lesions with well-defined sclerotic margins and central ground-glass opacification
- Overgrowth of bones is a feature leading to leontiasis ossea when skull and facial bones are affected
- Bone softening leads to bilateral progressive coxa vara (shepherd's crook deformity)

APERT'S SYNDROME

The International Classification of Osteochondrodysplasias[1] divides the localized skeletal malformations (dysostosis) into three groups:

Group A: predominant facial and cranial involvement
Group B: predominant axial involvement
Group C: predominant involvement of the extremities

Apert's syndrome, along with the other acrocephalo-syndactyly syndromes, belongs to group A. It is inherited as an autosomal-dominant trait and is due to a mutation in the *FGFR2* gene on chromosome 10.

Patients with Apert's syndrome present at birth with a high arched or cleft palate and brachyturricephaly with proptosis as a result of premature fusion of the coronal suture.

Radiographic features predominantly affect the hands, feet,[43] and skull, although the cervical spine may also be involved.

1. *Skull*: Brachyturricephaly—premature fusion of coronal suture (Fig. 103-65)
2. *Hands and feet*: Complex or simple[44] progressive bony and soft tissue syndactyly that may involve the tips of the distal phalanges—so-called "sock" and "mitten" appearance (Fig. 103-66); progressive carpal/tarsal fusions; broad thumbs (attempted preaxial polydactyly); progressive symphalangism
3. *Long bones*: Progressive fusions of large joints; hypoplastic glenoid fossa; dislocated radial head
4. *Spine*: Progressive fusion of cervical spine particularly at C5-C6 (Fig. 103-67)

Classic Signs

- Autosomal-dominant acrocephalosyndactyly
- Complex "sock" and "mitten" polysyndactyly of feet and hands
- Premature fusion of coronal suture causing brachyturricephaly
- Progressive fusion of joints including cervical spine

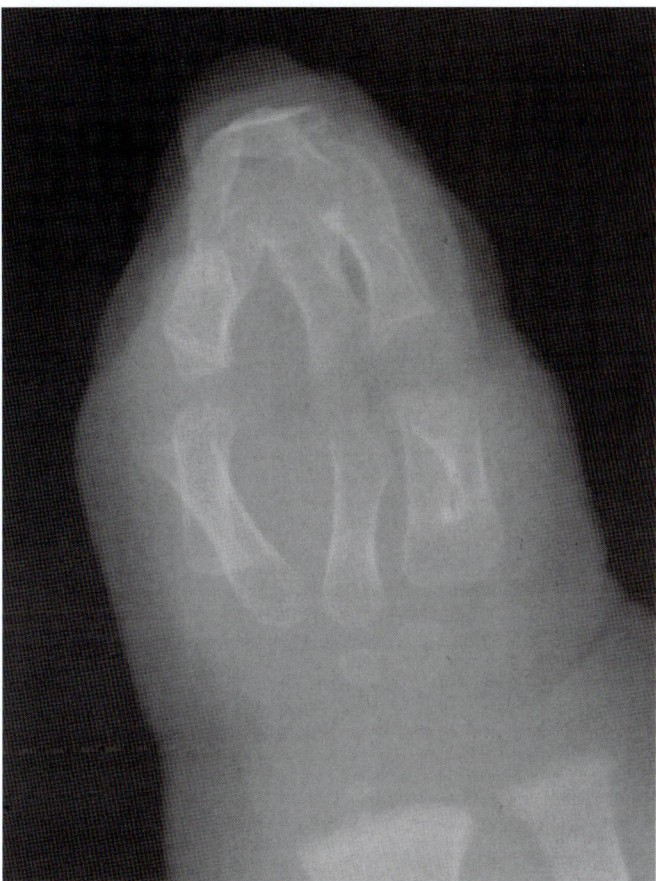

■ **FIGURE 103-66** Apert's syndrome. Radiograph of the hand. "Mitten" polysyndactyly of soft tissues and bones.

TREACHER COLLINS SYNDROME

Treacher Collins syndrome belongs to group A of the dysostoses—those with predominant facial and cranial involvement. It is inherited as an autosomal dominant trait and is due to a mutation on chromosome 5.

The condition involves structures derived from the first and second branchial arches. It is characterized by symmetric abnormalities of the external ear, malar hypoplasia, antimongoloid slanting palpebral fissures, lateral coloboma of the lower eyelids, and cleft palate. Choanal atresia is a less common finding.[45]

Radiologic findings include narrowing/atresia of the external auditory meatus and hypoplasia of the jaw bones.

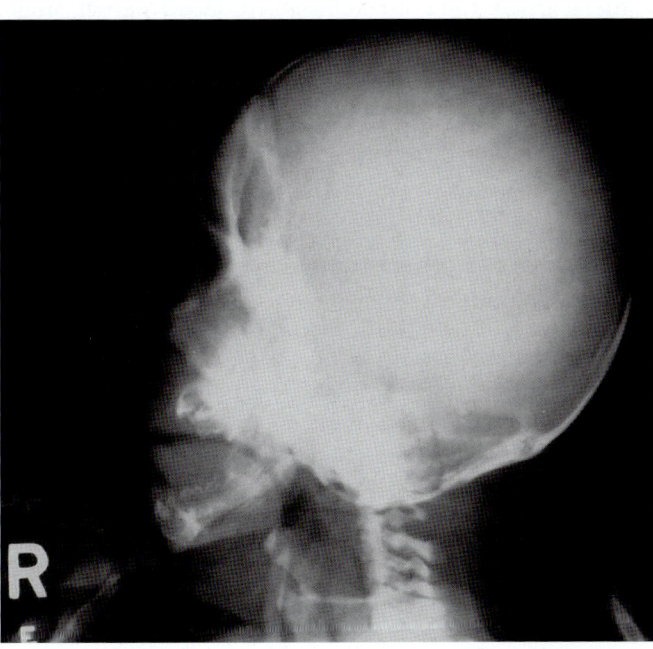

■ **FIGURE 103-65** Apert's syndrome. Lateral radiograph of the skull shows brachyturricephaly secondary to premature fusion of coronal sutures.

Classic Signs

- Autosomal dominant disorder
- Involves structures that derive from the first and second branchial arches
- Radiology demonstrates narrowing of the auditory canals and hypoplastic jaw bones

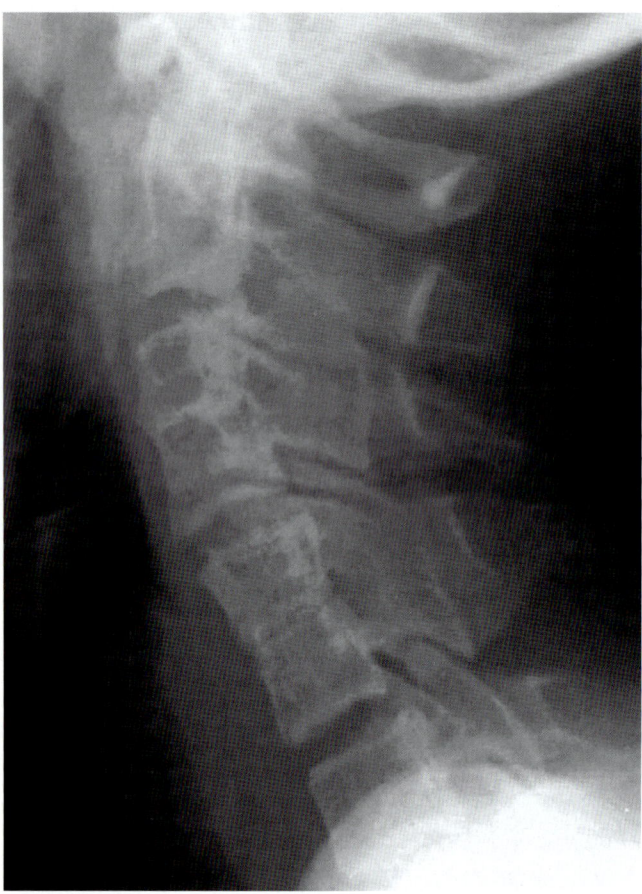

■ **FIGURE 103-67** Apert's syndrome. Lateral radiograph of the cervical spine. Progressive fusion of the cervical spine is a recognized feature of this condition.

TRISOMY 21 (DOWN SYNDROME)

This is the most common chromosomal disorder. Antenatal diagnosis with ultrasonography is possible by assessing nuchal translucency thickness and the length of the nasal bone.[46]

Postnatally, patients present with short stature, a characteristic facies, and varying degrees of mental retardation. Older patients have reduced bone mass.

Radiographic findings from the skeletal survey include:

1. *Skull*: Microcephaly
2. *Spine*: Hypoplastic C1 arch; widened atlantoaxial distance; atlantoaxial instability (despite these findings, neurologic complications are uncommon[47]); ossification of the posterior longitudinal ligament
3. *Chest*: 11 pairs of ribs; double ossification center for the manubrium sterni
4. *Pelvis*: "Elephant ear" iliac wings—flared, decreased acetabular index, increased iliac index
5. *Hands*: Clinodactyly; brachydactyly; negative metacarpal sign

6. *Cardiac*: Congenital heart disease (usually atrioventricular septal defect)
7. *Gastrointestinal tract*: Duodenal atresia; annular pancreas; Hirschsprung's disease

Classic Signs

- Most common chromosomal disorder
- Antenatal diagnosis possible (nuchal thickness, length of nasal bone)
- Neurologic complications uncommon despite abnormalities of cervical spine
- "Elephant ear" iliac wings
- 11 pairs of ribs, two ossification centers for manubrium
- Associated congenital heart disease, duodenal atresia, Hirschsprung's disease, and annular pancreas

TURNER'S SYNDROME

In this condition (also known as gonadal dysgenesis) there is monosomy of chromosome X. Although most females will present at birth or in early childhood, it is said that nearly one fourth present to adult services with primary or secondary amenorrhea.[48]

Clinically, patients are of short stature with a webbed neck and cubitus valgus. Lymphedema is a recognized association.

In addition to generalized osteopenia, radiographs reveal:

1. *Spine*: Irregular vertebral end plates; kyphosis; atlantoaxial abnormalities
2. *Chest*: Shield chest
3. *Hands*: Positive metacarpal sign (i.e., short fourth/fifth metacarpals (and metatarsals); reduced carpal angle; prominent phalangeal tufts
4. *Knees*: Exostoses of medial tibial plateaus; large medial femoral condyles
5. *Cardiovascular system*: Coarctation of the aorta
6. *Genitourinary system*: Horseshoe kidneys; ovarian dysgenesis

Classic Signs

- Monosomy of chromosome X
- Up to 25% of females may present as adults with primary or secondary amenorrhea
- Associated with short stature, webbed neck, and cubitus valgus
- Short fourth/fifth metacarpals and metatarsals
- Coarctation of the aorta, lymphedema, and horseshoe kidneys are recognized findings

REFERENCES

1. Superti-Furga A, Unger S: Nosology and classification of genetic disorders: 2006 revisions. Am J Med Genet A 2007; 143: 1–18.
2. Vajo Z, Francomano CA, Wilkin DJ. The molecular and genetic basis of fibroblast growth factor receptor 3 disorders: the achondroplasia family of skeletal dysplasias, Muenke craniosynostosis and Crouzon syndrome with acanthosis nigricans. Endocr Rev 2000; 21:23–39.
3. Aviezer D, Golembo M, Yayon A. Fibroblast growth factor receptor-3 as a therapeutic target for achondroplasia—genetic short limbed dwarfism. Curr Drug Targets 2003; 4:353–365.
4. Cohen MM Jr. Some chondrodysplasias with short limbs: molecular perspectives. Am J Med Genet 2002; 112:304–313.
5. Patel MD, Filly RA. Homozygous achondroplasia: ultrasound distinction between homozygous, heterozygous and unaffected fetuses in the second trimester. Radiology 1995; 196:541–545.
6. Hunter AG, Bankier A, Rogers JG, et al. Medical complications of achondroplasia: a multicentre patient review. J Med Genet 1998; 35:705–712.
7. Bonnefoy O, Delbosc JM, Maugey-Laulom G, et al. Prenatal diagnosis of hypochondroplasia: three-dimensional multislice computed tomography findings and molecular analysis. Fetal Diagn Ther 2006; 21:18–21.
8. Ramaswami U, Rumsby G, Hindmarsh PC, Brook CG. Genotype and phenotype in hypochondroplasia. J Paediatr 1998;133:5–6.
9. Garjian KV, Pretorius DH, Budorick NE, et al. Fetal skeletal dysplasia: three-dimensional ultrasound—initial experience. Radiology 2000; 214:717–723.
10. Tongsong T, Chanprapaph P, Thongpadungroj T. Prenatal sonographic findings associated with asphyxiating thoracic dystrophy (Jeune syndrome). J Ultrasound Med 1999;18:573–576.
11. Aronson DC, Van Nierop JC, Taminiau A, Vos A. Homologous bone graft for expansion thoracoplasty in Jeune's asphyxiating thoracic dystrophy. J Pediatr Surg 1999; 34:500–503.
12. Davis JT, Long FR, Adler BH, et al. Lateral thoracic expansion for Jeune syndrome: evidence of rib healing and new bone formation. Ann Thorac Surg 2004; 77:445–458.
13. Yerian LM, Brady L, Hart J. Hepatic manifestations of Jeune syndrome (asphyxiating thoracic dystrophy). Semin Liver Dis 2003; 23:195–200.
14. Amirou M, Bourdat-Michel G, Pinel N, et al. Successful renal transplantation in Jeune syndrome type 2. Pediatr Nephrol 1998; 12:293–294.
15. Sergi C, Voigtlander T, Zoubaa S, et al. Ellis-van Creveld syndrome: a generalised dysplasia of enchondral ossification. Paediatr Radiol 2001; 31:289–293.
16. Dwek JR. Kniest dysplasia: MR correlation of histologic and radiographic peculiarities Paediatr Radiol 2005; 35:191–193.
17. Ikegawa S, Iwaya T, Taniguchi K, Kimizuka M. Retinal detachment in spondyloepiphyseal dysplasia congenita. J Pediatr Orthop 1993; 13:791–792.
18. Harding CO, Green CG, Perloff WH, Pauli RM. Respiratory complications in children with spondyloepiphyseal dysplasia congenita. Paediatr Pulmonol 1990; 9:49–54.
19. Unger SL, Briggs MD, Holden P, et al. Multiple epiphyseal dysplasia: radiographic abnormalities correlated with genotype. Paediatr Radiol 2001; 31:10–18.
20. Kennedy J, Jackson G, Ramsden S, et al. COMP mutation screening as an aid for the clinical diagnosis and counselling of patients with a suspected diagnosis of pseudoachondroplasia or multiple epiphyseal dysplasia. Eur J Hum Genet 2005; 13:547–555.
21. Offiah AC, Mansour S, Jeffrey I, et al. Greenberg dysplasia (HEM) and X-linked dominant Conradi-Hünermann chondrodysplasia punctata (CDPX2): Presentation of two cases with overlapping phenotype. J Med Genet 2003; 40:e129.
22. Savarirayan R, Cormier-Daire V, Lachman RS, Rimoin DL. Schmid type metaphyseal chondrodysplasia: a spondylometaphyseal dysplasia identical to the "Japanese" type. Paediatr Radiol 2000; 30:460–463.
23. Elliott AM, Field FM, Rimoin DL, Lachman RS. Hand involvement in Schmid metaphyseal chondrodysplasia. Am J Med Genet A 2005; 132:191–193.
24. Cook P, Yu JS, Wiand W, et al. Madelung deformity in skeletally immature patients: morphologic assessment using radiography, CT, and MRI. J Comput Assist Tomogr 1996; 20:505–511.
25. Offiah AC, Woo P, Prieur AM, et al. Camptodactyly–arthropathy–coxa vara–pericarditis syndrome versus juvenile idiopathic arthropathy. AJR Am J Roentgenol 2005; 185:522–529.
26. Mundlos S. Cleidocranial dysplasia: clinical and molecular genetics J Med Genet 1999; 36:177–182.
27. Mansour S, Offiah AC, McDonald J, et al. The phenotype of survivors of campomelic dysplasia. J Med Genet 2002; 39:597–602.
28. Offiah AC, Mansour S, McDonald J, et al. Surviving campomelic dysplasia has the radiological features of the previously reported ischio-pubic-patella syndrome. J Med Genet 2002; 39:e50.
29. Ellinwood NM, Vite CH, Haskins ME. Gene therapy for lysosomal storage diseases: the lessons and promise of animal models. J Gene Med 2004; 6:481–506.
30. Roughley PJ, Rauch F, Glorieux FH. Osteogenesis imperfecta: clinical and molecular diversity. Eur Cell Mater 2003; 5:41–47.
31. Tolar J, Teitelbaum SL, Orchard PJ. Osteopetrosis. N Engl J Med 2004; 351:2839–2849.
32. Jansenns K, Vanhoenacker F, Bonduelle M, et al. Camurati Engelmann disease: review of the clinical, radiological and molecular data of 24 families and implications for diagnosis and treatment. J Med Genet 2006; 43:1–11.
33. Schweiger S, Chaoui R, Tennstedt C, et al. Antenatal onset of cortical hyperostosis (Caffey disease): case report and review. Am J Med Genet A 2003; 120:547–552.
34. Glorieux FH. Caffey disease: an unlikely collagenopathy. J Clin Invest 2005; 115:1142–1144.
35. Wicklund CL, Pauli RM, Johnston D, Hecht JT. Natural history study of hereditary multiple exostoses. Am J Med Genet 1995; 55:43–46.
36. Porter DE, Lonie L, Fraser M, et al. Severity of disease and risk of malignant change in hereditary multiple exostoses: a genotype-phenotype study. J Bone Joint Surg Br 2004; 86:1041–1046.
37. Legeai-Mallet L, Munnich A, Maroteaux P, Le Merrer M. Incomplete penetrance and expressivity skewing in hereditary multiple exostoses. Clin Genet 1997; 52:12–16.
38. Kivioja A, Ervasti H, Kinnunen J, et al. Chondrosarcoma in a family with multiple hereditary exostoses. J Bone Joint Surg Br 2000; 82:261–266.
39. Murphey MD, Choi JJ, Kransdorf MJ, et al. Imaging of osteochondroma: variants and complications with radiologic-pathologic correlation. Radiographics 2000; 20:1407–1434.
40. McDermott AL, Dutt SN, Chavda SV, Morgan DW. Maffucci's syndrome: clinical and radiological features of a rare condition. J Laryngol Otol 2001; 115:845–847.
41. Dorfman HD, Ishida T, Tsuneyoshi M. Exophytic variant of fibrous dysplasia (fibrous dysplasia protuberans). Hum Pathol 1994;25:1234–1237.
42. Shah ZK, Peh WC, Koh WL, Shek TW. Magnetic resonance imaging appearances of fibrous dysplasia. Br J Radiol 2005;78:1104–1115.
43. Anderson PJ, Hall CM, Evans RD, et al. The feet in Apert's syndrome. J Pediatr Orthop 1999; 19:504–507.
44. al-Qattan MM, al-Husain MA. Classification of hand anomalies in Apert's syndrome. J Hand Surg Br 1996; 21:266–268.
45. Andrade EC, Junior VS, Didoni AL, et al. Treacher Collins syndrome with choanal atresia: a case report and review of disease features. Rev Bras Otorrhinolaryngol [Engl Ed] 2005; 71:107–110.
46. Cicero S, Bindra R, Rembouskos G, et al. Integrated ultrasound and biochemical screening for trisomy 21 using fetal nuchal translucency, absent fetal nasal bone, free beta-hCG and PAAP-A at 11 to 14 weeks. Prenat Diagn 2003; 23:306–310.
47. Frost M, Huffer WE, Sze CI, et al. Cervical spine abnormalities in Down syndrome. Clin Neuropathol 1999; 18:250–259.
48. Conway GS. Considerations for transition from paediatric to adult endocrinology: women with Turner's syndrome. Growth Horm IGF Res 2004; 14(Suppl A):S77–S84.

Spinal Deformity

James J. Rankine

CLASSIFICATION AND DEFINITIONS

Many different classification systems have been described for spinal deformities. Over the years some of these classifications have fallen out of favor while new descriptive terms have been applied. To accurately diagnose a spinal deformity it is important to understand the definitions of the terms used.

Spinal deformities are described in relation to the position of the deformity within the spine, the characteristics of the curve pattern, the size of the curve, the etiology of the deformity, and the age at onset. Deformity of the spine is described in relation to the three anatomic planes of the body, which are the coronal (frontal) plane, the sagittal (lateral) plane, and the horizontal (transverse or axial) plane. The spine is usually straight in the frontal plane; and if it is not, then coronal asymmetry exists, which is termed *scoliosis*. This rather simplistic view of scoliosis is a result of the plain radiograph being a two-dimensional projection of a three-dimensional structure. CT and MRI have demonstrated that far from being a simple coronal plane deformity scoliosis results in deformity in all three planes.[1,2] Nevertheless, if the spine is not straight on a frontal radiograph then scoliosis exists.

In the sagittal plane there are normal physiologic curves: a lordosis in the cervical and lumbar regions and a thoracic and sacral kyphosis.

The terms *structural* and *nonstructural curves* are used to differentiate a potentially progressive curve from a less important nonprogressive one. The term *structural* is applied to those curves in which there is a fundamental problem of growth and is most commonly seen in the idiopathic type of scoliosis. The key feature of this is deformity in all three planes, and this is recognized on the frontal radiograph by rotation of the spinous processes toward the concavity of the curve, indicating transverse plane deformity (Fig. 104-1). It is apparent that if the spinous processes are lying in the concavity of the curve they must take a shorter route than the vertebral bodies, leading to a relative lordosis (Fig. 104-2). Indeed, the growth disturbance in idiopathic scoliosis is a relative overgrowth of the anterior spine, which results in a buckling and deformity in all three planes. One of the basic principles of anterior corrective surgery is to prevent continued anterior growth by removing the intervertebral discs and end plates and fusing the spine between the vertebral bodies. The term *kyphoscoliosis* is therefore inaccurate because this is actually a *lordoscoliosis*. The apparent clinical kyphosis is a result of the rib hump that occurs due to the transverse rotation. Axial CT is helpful to determine to what

---

KEY POINTS

SCOLIOSIS

- Scoliosis is deformity of the spine in the coronal plane.
- Nonstructural scoliosis is a secondary response of the spine to a separate pathology. The deformity occurs only in the coronal plane.
- Idiopathic scoliosis is a growth abnormality of the spine that results in deformity in all three planes.
- Rotation of the spinous processes toward the concavity of the curve is evidence of the transverse plane deformity.
- Idiopathic scoliosis is a nonpainful condition. The presence of pain with a scoliosis requires urgent investigation for underlying neoplasia.
- Arnold-Chiari type 1 malformation and spinal cord syringomyelia are commonly associated with idiopathic scoliosis.

CONGENITAL SPINAL DEFORMITY

- Vertebral anomalies result from failure of formation, failure of segmentation, or a combination of the two.
- The anomaly may result in a scoliosis, kyphosis, or kyphoscoliosis.
- The risk of progression of the deformity is related to the presence of intact end plates.
- Whole-spine MRI is required to investigate underlying spinal dysraphism.
- CT with multiplanar reformats may be required to define the anatomy before surgical correction.

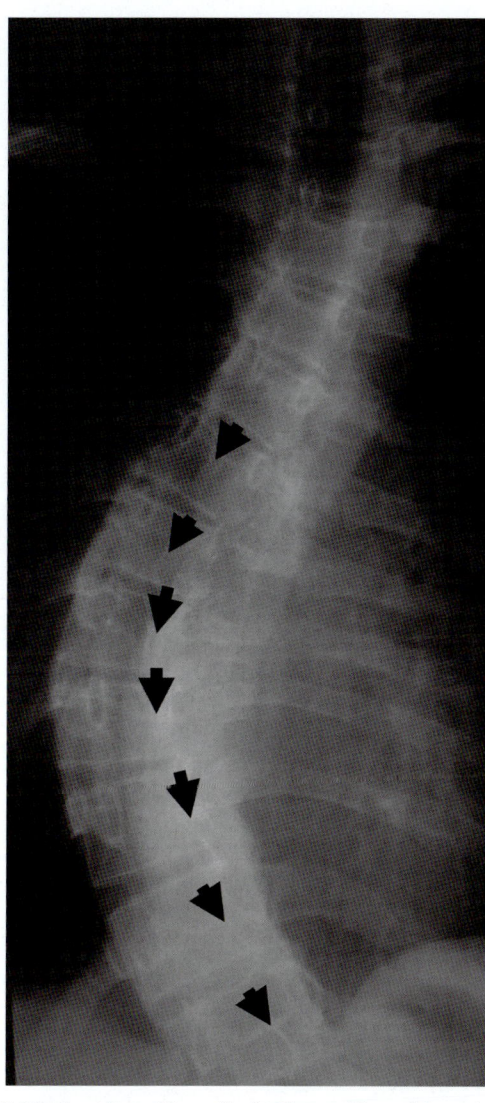

■ **FIGURE 104-1** Idiopathic scoliosis. The position of the spinous processes is indicated by the *arrows*. The spinous processes turn into the concavity of the curve, indicating a deformity in the transverse plane.

extent the ribs contribute to the deformity and select which patients would benefit from *costoplasty*, which is a surgical removal of the ribs at the site of the rib hump (Fig. 104-3).

The term *nonstructural scoliosis* is applied to non-progressive curves in which the scoliosis is a second-ary feature and not the consequence of an intrinsic growth problem. The most common cause of this is pelvic-tilt scoliosis secondary to leg-length inequality (Fig. 104-4). The key features are a lumbar scoliosis with the sacrum at the bottom of the curve and the spinous processes not rotated into the curve, indicating the lack of a transverse deformity. The next most common cause of a nonstructural scoliosis is an irritating focus within the spine. A painful scoliosis is a strong clinical indica-tor of an irritating focus because idiopathic scoliosis is not a painful condition. Therefore, the presence of pain with scoliosis always warrants further investigation. MR sequences that are sensitive to edema may localize the problem, although MRI can easily miss a small osteoid

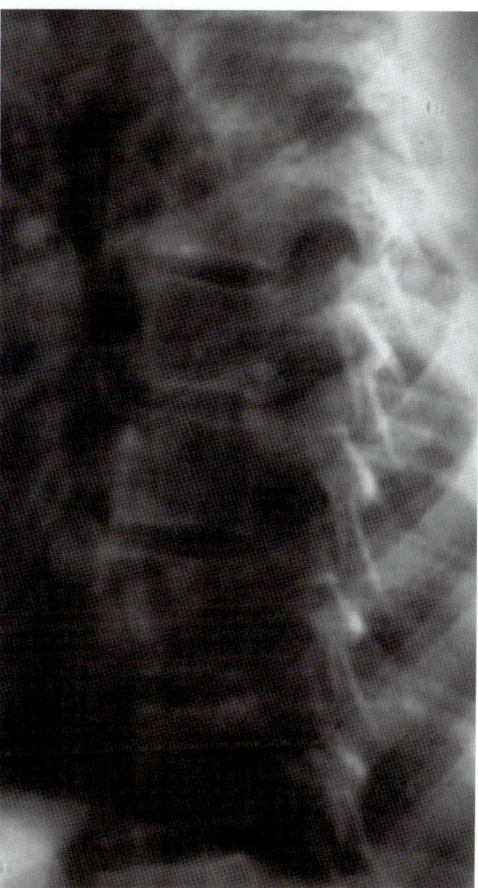

■ **FIGURE 104-2** Lateral thoracic radiograph in a patient with idiopathic scoliosis. There is a relative lordosis, resulting in a straightening of the spine in the sagittal plane. The rib hump deformity is therefore not the result of a kyphosis but due to the transverse plane deformity.

osteoma because sections performed in the standard ana-tomic sagittal and axial planes will cut obliquely through a spine with a scoliotic deformity (Fig. 104-5). In many cases, bone scintigraphy is the most sensitive method of isolating the lesion and allowing cross-sectional imaging to target the area of abnormality. Even if the radiologic features suggest an idiopathic scoliosis the presence of pain warrants further investigation. Idiopathic scoliosis is a relatively common condition in adolescent girls, and another cause for the pain should be sought because the scoliosis may be an incidental finding (Fig. 104-6).

Curve Characteristics

By convention, a curve is described as right or left sided according to the side of convexity of the curve. The end vertebrae are those vertebrae at the top and bottom of the curve that are maximally tilted into the curve. The stan-dard method of measurement of the curve is the Cobb angle. A line is drawn along the upper end plate of the upper end vertebrae and along the lower end plate of the lower end vertebrae (Fig. 104-7). The angle where these lines intersect is the Cobb angle. Protractors with a freely hanging needle are available that allow measurement of the angle without actually marking the film. Although the Cobb angle is a crude measurement of curve severity that

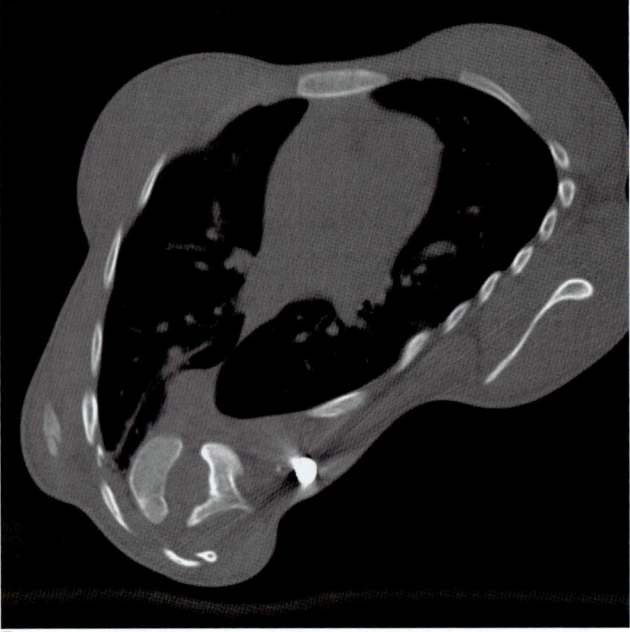

A   B

■ **FIGURE 104-3** **A,** Axial CT in a patient with residual deformity after previous spinal correction surgery. The rib hump is the result of the axial rotation of the spine. The posterior aspect of the right ribs lies at the deformity. The patient underwent a costoplasty with removal of the posterior aspect of a number of the right ribs, resulting in a partial correction of the deformity. **B,** Axial CT in a patient with a previous surgical correction for idiopathic scoliosis and residual deformity. The metal hardware is a "growing rod." There is marked axial rotation resulting in the spine lying within the rib hump deformity. Costoplasty cannot be performed because removal of the ribs would have little effect on the deformity.

records only the coronal plane deformity, it is an easy and reproducible method of recording curve progression.

The vertebra in the middle of the curve is termed the *apical vertebra*. This is the vertebra whose spinous process will be maximally rotated into the curve. The position of this apical vertebra determines the curve type. If the apex lies between T2 and T11, it is defined as a thoracic curve. A thoracic curve is the most common pattern and usually has an apex at T8 or T9. If the apex is at T12 or L1, it is defined as a thoracolumbar curve. A curve apical below L1 is termed a lumbar curve, and at C7 or T1 it is a cervicothoracic curve. The major curve is the one with the largest Cobb angle. A single major curve will have compensatory curves above and below it correcting the vertical alignment of the spine. In this case the spine is said to be in balance. Occasionally, the whole spine will list toward the convexity of the major curve, if the compensatory curves progress beyond that which makes the spine vertical. This is an important observation to make if surgery is being considered because correction of the major curve may throw the patient further out of balance, resulting in tilting of the shoulders. A common curve pattern is a thoracic curve with a thoracolumbar or lumbar curve below.

ETIOLOGY, CLINICAL PRESENTATION, AND IMAGING TECHNIQUES

Spinal deformity can further be defined in terms of the etiology. The most common group are the idiopathic deformities, which comprise idiopathic scoliosis and

idiopathic kyphosis, which is more commonly known as Scheuermann's disease.

Idiopathic Scoliosis

The etiology of scoliosis is unknown, and although it is the most common cause of spinal deformity it is essentially a diagnosis of exclusion. Clinically, there should be no evidence of a neuromuscular disorder, including neurofibromatosis, and radiologically there should be no evidence of a congenital spinal anomaly. Traditionally, idiopathic scoliosis has been further subdivided into infantile, juvenile, and adolescent, depending on the age at onset.[3] More recently, it has been argued that the distinction between infantile and juvenile is arbitrary and of no clinical significance.[4] A more clinically relevant classification is early and late onset with the threshold at 5 years. Early-onset scoliosis usually begins in infancy and can be associated with severe cardiorespiratory symptoms because a severe thoracic deformity can prevent normal development of the lung, resulting in pulmonary hypoplasia. After the age of 5 the lung has fully developed and a late-onset scoliosis does not result in cardiopulmonary dysfunction.[5] Although there may be associated psychosocial distress, surgical correction of a late-onset scoliosis really amounts to a cosmetic operation.

Early-Onset Idiopathic Scoliosis

The incidence of early-onset scoliosis has markedly declined over the past 50 years, and the precise reasons for this are

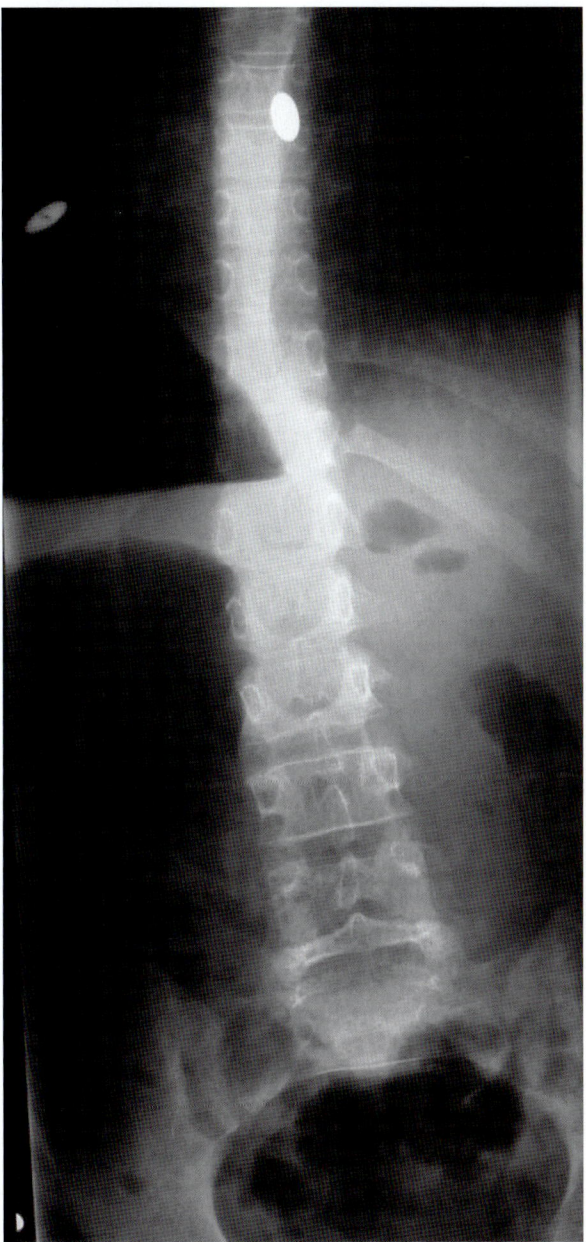

■ **FIGURE 104-4** Anteroposterior standing erect radiograph of the thoracic and lumbar spine. The air-fluid level in the stomach is acting as an in-built spirit level and demonstrates that the pelvis is tilted, which is the result of leg-length inequality. The scoliosis occurs secondarily to the pelvic tilt, the degree of deformity directly related to the degree of pelvic tilt. Note that the spinous processes are not rotated toward the concavity of the curve; this is a nonstructural scoliosis and there is no transverse plane deformity.

unknown. It now accounts for less than 1% of all cases of scoliosis. It is more common in males, with a left thoracic curve pattern being the most common. This is in distinction to adolescent scoliosis, which is far more common in females with a predominant right thoracic curve pattern.

Radiographs of the full thoracic and lumbar spine should be performed using anteroposterior and lateral projections. This can usually be accommodated on a standard 35 × 43-cm cassette when conventional radiography is used. Digital radiography with the ability to manipulate the window levels lends itself very well to imaging the

spine, particularly as the overlying soft tissue densities vary between the thoracic and lumbar spine.

Interpretation of the radiograph is principally directed at excluding a congenital vertebral body abnormality. Some minor lateral wedging of the vertebrae may be evident on the anteroposterior projection at the apex of the curve. This reflects the growth abnormality, but there should not be any evidence of a hemivertebra.

If there are no clinical features to suggest a neuromuscular disorder, with a child who is progressing normally through the developmental milestones and no evidence of a congenital anomaly on the radiograph, no further investigation is required. Any suggestion of pain, abnormal neurology, or a rapidly progressive curve warrants further investigation with MRI of the whole spine because of the possibility of an associated neuromuscular or congenital abnormality.

Late-Onset Idiopathic Scoliosis—Adolescent Scoliosis

This is the most common spinal deformity in children. The etiology is unknown, but there is an increased incidence with a positive family history and there is a female predominance. That this is a growth abnormality is evident by the development of the abnormality during the pubertal growth spurt.

As with early-onset idiopathic scoliosis this is essentially a diagnosis of exclusion. The deformity should be painless, and there should be no neurologic abnormality.

The standard radiographs are standing anteroposterior and lateral views of the entire thoracic and lumbar spine. Radiographs performed in the supine position can underestimate the degree of deformity because it is well recognized that the scoliotic deformity worsens in the erect position. In conventional radiography, long 60-cm cassettes are used. Many modern digital systems use "stitching software," which allows the whole spine to be demonstrated on a single image. Additional radiographs may be used to plan surgical correction. These include lateral bending and traction films to assess curve flexibility.

As with the interpretation of the radiograph in early-onset scoliosis, it is important to assess the spine for the presence of congenital abnormalities. Lateral wedging may occur as part of the growth disturbance, but there should be no congenital abnormalities for this to be an idiopathic curve. These are much less likely to be encountered than in early-onset scoliosis. An associated neuromuscular condition should be considered, and features to suggest neurofibromatosis (see later) should be sought.

Provided there are no clinical features to suggest a neuromuscular condition, and a typical idiopathic curve pattern, no further investigation is required. If a surgical correction is planned, then an MRI is performed. An associated neurologic abnormality, most commonly a spinal cord syrinx, can occur without clinical neurologic abnormality. Because the spinal cord may be put under traction during spinal correction surgery, a spinal cord abnormality increases the risks of spinal cord injury.

The spinal deformity of scoliosis presents particular problems when imaging with MRI using standard spinal sequences. Sequences performed in the sagittal plane cut

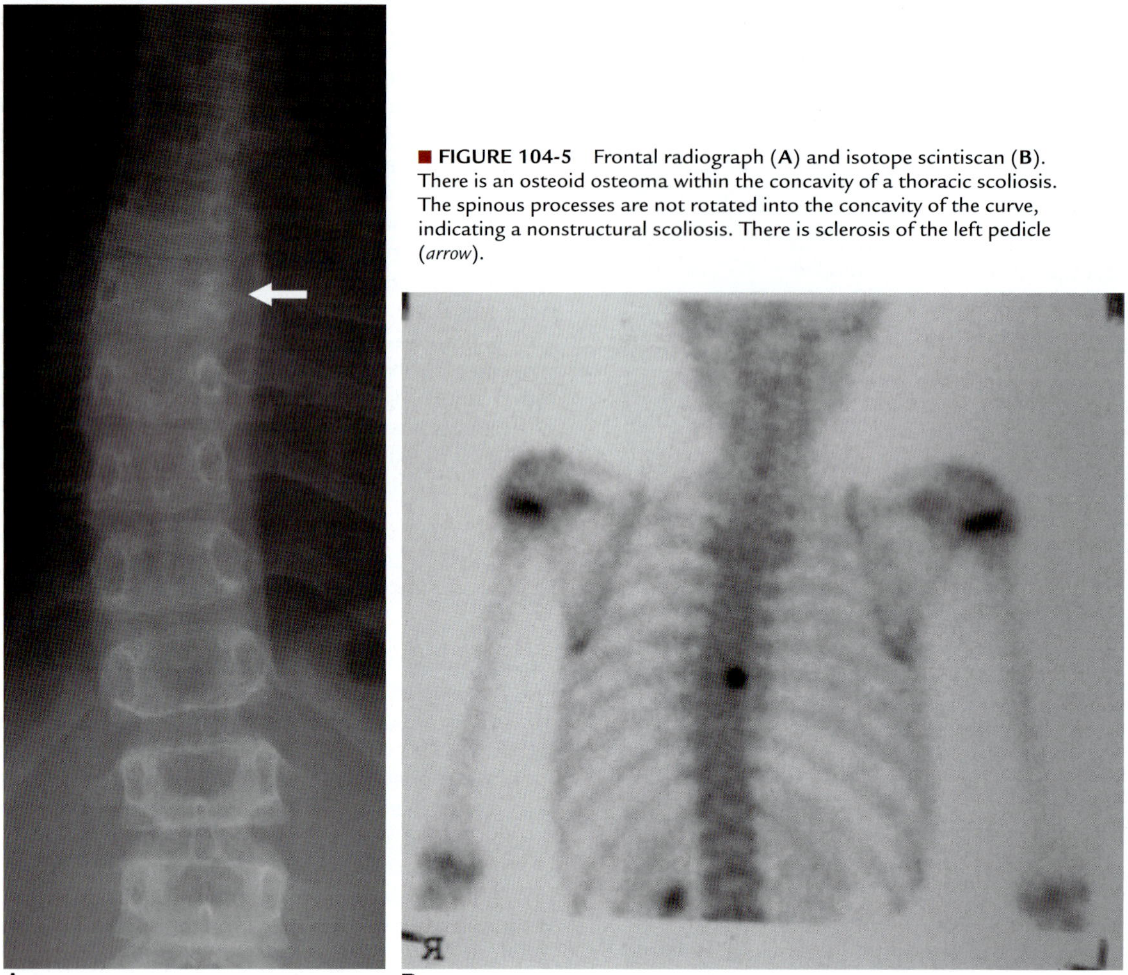

■ **FIGURE 104-5** Frontal radiograph (**A**) and isotope scintiscan (**B**). There is an osteoid osteoma within the concavity of a thoracic scoliosis. The spinous processes are not rotated into the concavity of the curve, indicating a nonstructural scoliosis. There is sclerosis of the left pedicle (*arrow*).

obliquely through the spine due to the degree of lateral plane deformity. There is little deformity in the coronal plane; indeed, there is straightening of the thoracic kyphosis due to a relative lordosis, and it makes more sense to image the spine in the long axis with coronal sequences. The whole of the spine from the craniocervical junction to the sacrum should be covered. The cervical spine can be imaged with sagittal sequences because there is little in the way of lateral plane deformity at this level. The most common abnormality encountered at the craniocervical junction is an Arnold-Chiari type 1 malformation, which is found in 14% of patients with idiopathic scoliosis.[6] The diagnosis of an Arnold-Chiari malformation is made when the cerebellar tonsils herniate more than 5 mm through the foramen magnum (Fig. 104-8). The hindbrain structures otherwise appear normal, distinguishing this from an Arnold-Chiari type 2 malformation. The type 2 malformation usually presents in the newborn with an associated myelomeningocele and is characterized by caudal displacement of the fourth ventricle and a caudally displaced brain stem in addition to the tonsillar herniation seen in the type 1 malformation.

The demonstration of an Arnold-Chiari malformation may require a posterior fossa decompression before scoliosis correction surgery to prevent neurologic injury.

In approximately 10% of cases of idiopathic scoliosis there is a syringomyelia (Fig. 104-9). This will often be detected on the coronal sequences, but axial sections should be performed to demonstrate the size and extent of the syrinx. This can vary from a small localized slit in the cord to extensive dilatation of the central canal extending along the full length of the cord.

A tethered spinal cord is diagnosed when the conus lies below the level of L2-3. There may be associated thickening of the filum terminale, and a diameter exceeding 2 mm is considered abnormal. In this situation the filum terminale frequently contains fat. A tethered cord occurs occasionally as a feature of idiopathic scoliosis but is more commonly a feature of spinal dysraphism.

Congenital Spinal Deformities

Congenital scoliosis is caused by anomalies in vertebral development. There are essentially two types of anomalous development: failure of formation and failure of segmentation. When a vertebra fails to form on one side this forms a triangular hemivertebra. Identifying the number of pedicles present is a useful way of detecting a hemivertebra on a frontal radiograph. The hemivertebra may be fully segmented, that is, have a disc space above and below

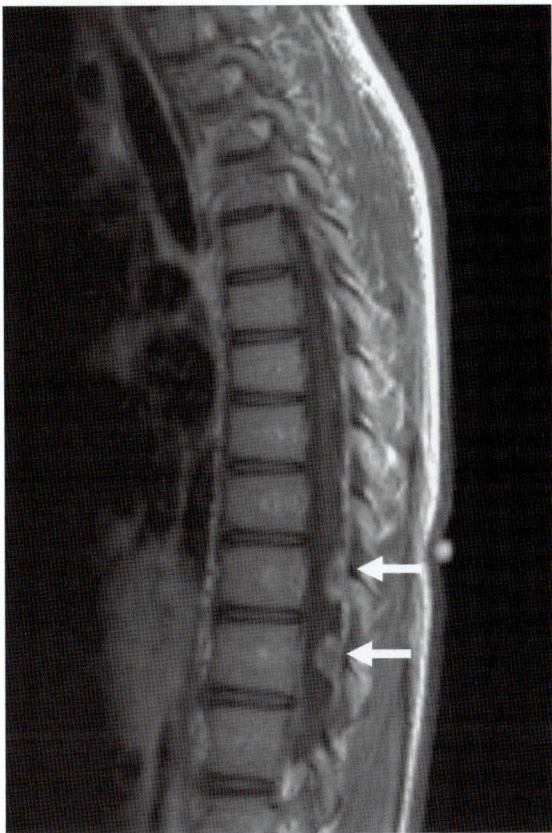

■ FIGURE 104-6   T1-weighted post-gadolinium sagittal MR image in a 14-year-old girl evaluated for painful scoliosis. There are leptomeningeal metastases at the site of the pain (*arrows*). MRI of the brain revealed a suprasellar glioma. She had a typical idiopathic curve pattern that was thought to predate the development of the glioma metastases. The idiopathic scoliosis occurred coincidentally with the tumor. Idiopathic scoliosis should never be painful, and another cause for pain should always be sought.

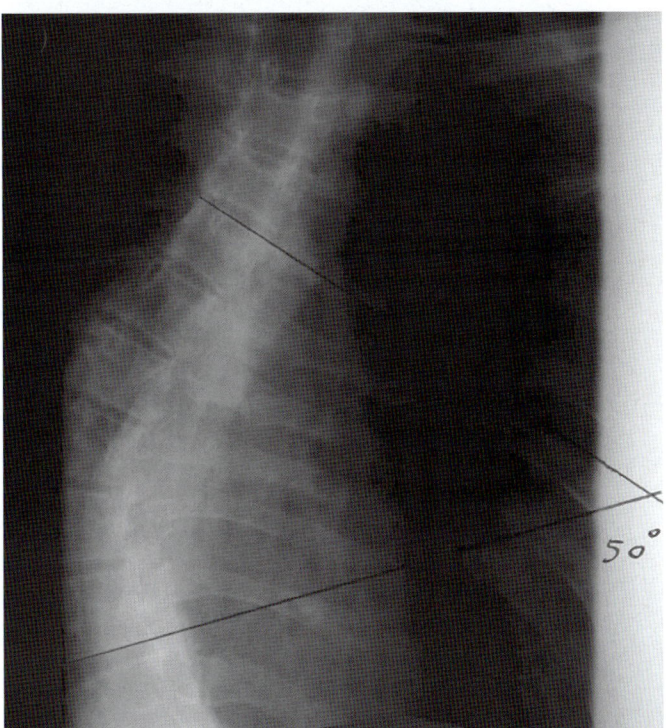

■ FIGURE 104-7   Measurement of the Cobb angle. The upper and lower end vertebrae are identified as the last vertebrae at the ends of the curve that tilt in toward the curve. The Cobb angle is measured between the upper end plate of the upper vertebra and the lower end plate of the lower vertebra.

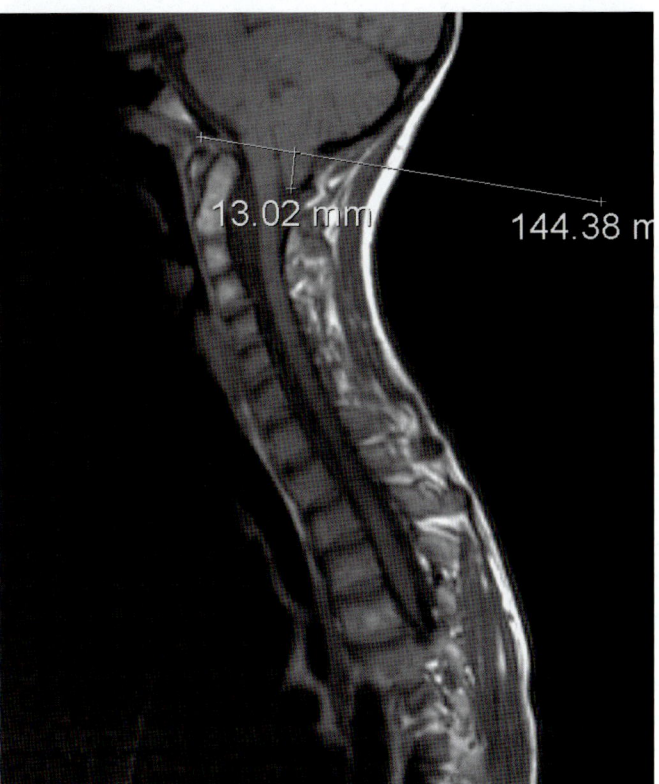

■ FIGURE 104-8   Sagittal T1-weighted MR image. Type 1 Arnold-Chiari malformation. A line drawn along the base of the foramen magnum allows the degree of herniation of the cerebellar tonsils to be measured. Herniation of greater than 5 mm is abnormal.

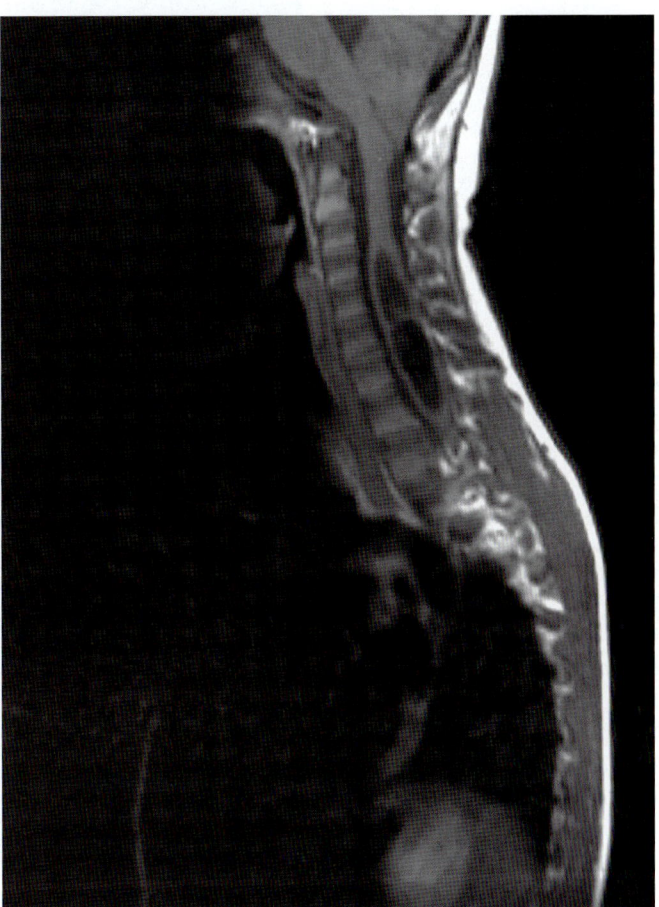

■ FIGURE 104-9   Sagittal T1-weighted MR image. Large-volume spinal cord syrinx that is expanding the cord. There is also an Arnold-Chiari type 1 malformation.

it, be partially segmented where one side is fused to the adjacent vertebra, or be nonsegmented where it is fused to the vertebra above and below it. Because the growth potential depends on an intact end plate and intervertebral disc, a fully segmented hemivertebra has the greater potential for progression. When predicting the potential for progression of the deformity it is therefore important to identify the number of disc spaces present. Because it is not always possible to determine this on the radiograph, MRI can be useful (Fig. 104-10). The principal reason, however, for performing MRI is to investigate associated spinal cord abnormalities and spinal dysraphism.

Congenital spinal anomalies may be associated with more widespread congenital anomalies in other body systems. The VATER association[7] describes the association of vertebral anomalies with anal atresia, tracheoesophageal fistula, and renal and radial anomalies. More recently, this acronym has been expanded to the VACTERL association to include cardiac and limb anomalies.

Spinal Dysraphism

Spinal dysraphism represents an embryologic failure of midline fusion of the spine, which can involve the bony structures and the neural elements. There is a strong association between congenital scoliosis and the presence of spinal dysraphism. Many patients, however, with congenital scoliosis do not have features of spinal dysraphism, and, conversely, many patients with spinal dysraphism have normal vertebral body development and therefore do not present with a spinal deformity. The presence of a congenital scoliosis does warrant the investigation of the patient by MRI for the presence of spinal dysraphism. The timing of this investigation can be delayed in a child who does not require a surgical correction and is otherwise neurologically normal. It is not justified to subject a young child to an MRI, which may require a general anesthetic, when the demonstration of spinal dysraphism does not make any immediate change to their management. In such children the MRI can be delayed until an age when the child is able to tolerate the examination without sedation or anesthesia, usually at about 6 years of age. Any suggestion clinically of neurologic abnormality, however, warrants immediate investigation, because surgical intervention may limit the neurologic deterioration.

Spinal dysraphism presents a wide spectrum, from the open defect of myelomeningocele evident at birth and increasingly diagnosed antenatally with ultrasound to the closed spina bifida occulta. Spina bifida occulta refers to the unfused posterior elements of the lower lumbar spine,

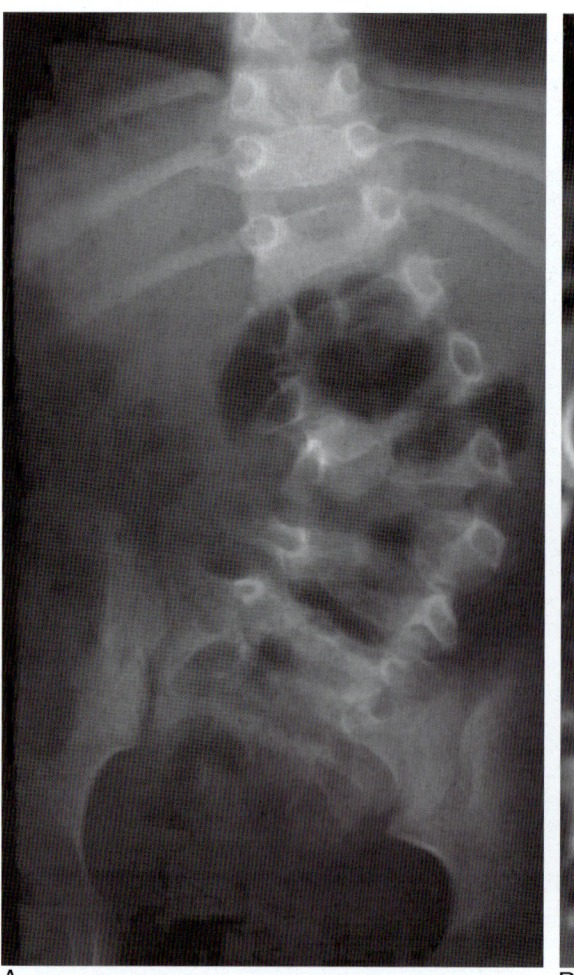
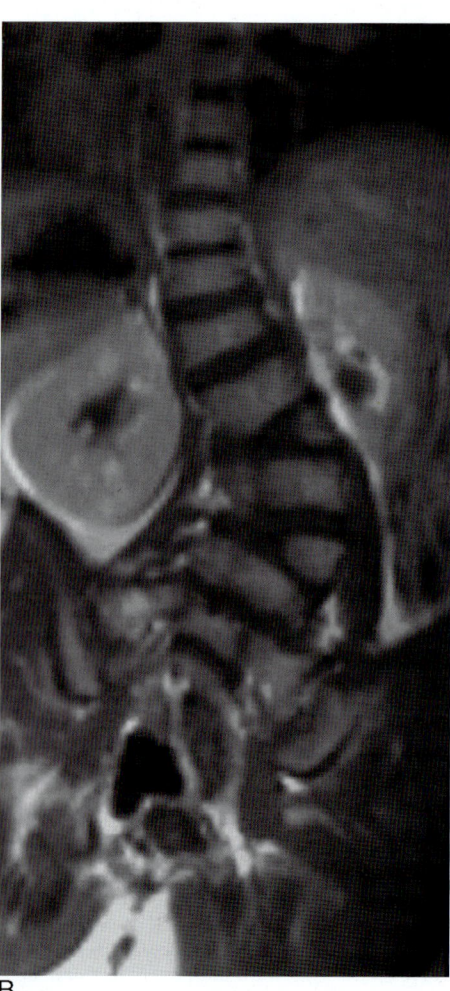

■ **FIGURE 104-10** Antero-posterior radiograph (**A**) and coronal T1-weighted MR image (**B**) in a patient with congenital scoliosis. Failure of formation on the right side has resulted in two left-sided hemivertebrae. The hemivertebrae have disc spaces above and below them and are therefore fully segmented. This increases the risk of progression of the deformity.

A

B

usually the L5 or S1 levels. There is no clinical neurologic abnormality, and this is such a common finding that it can be considered a normal variant.

Occult spinal dysraphism commonly has features of one or more of the following: diastematomyelia, low-lying conus, and intraspinal tumors, usually lipomas and dermoid tumors. A common feature of spinal dysraphism is a widened spinal canal. In many cases this is not due to the presence of an occult spinal bifida because the canal can be very widened in the presence of intact posterior elements. Diastematomyelia is a longitudinal split in the spinal cord that separates into two cords. The two cords may be contained within a single dural sac, or the dura may split into two separate sacs. The split usually occurs in the lower thoracic spinal cord. An osseous bony spur may be present between the two parts of the cord. Occasionally, this bony spur is visible on a plain radiograph, but MRI is required to make the diagnosis (Fig. 104-11).

Neuromuscular Scoliosis

There is a wide spectrum of neuromuscular conditions in which a scoliotic deformity can be a prominent feature. Most common among these conditions are cerebral palsy, muscular dystrophy, and spinal cord trauma. Although the curve pattern may be indistinguishable from an idiopathic curve, the characteristic appearance is of a long thoracolumbar or S-shaped double curve that extends down to an oblique pelvis. In general, the more neurologically dysfunctional the child is, the more severe the spinal deformity.

Scoliosis Associated with Neurofibromatosis

Skeletal deformity is common in neurofibromatosis type 1, occurring in up to 40% of cases. The scoliosis is classically described as a short angular thoracic curve (Fig. 104-12). In fact, many patients with neurofibromatosis will have a curve pattern indistinguishable from a typical idiopathic curve. There may be associated vertebral and rib dysplasias. Diagnostic features include posterior vertebral wall scalloping, enlarged foramina, and ribbon rib deformities. On MRI, dural ectasia and neurofibromas may be observed (Fig. 104-13).

Kyphosis

Because the normal thoracic spine has a kyphotic curve, a kyphotic deformity refers to a hyperkyphosis of this curve. This results clinically in a round-back deformity.

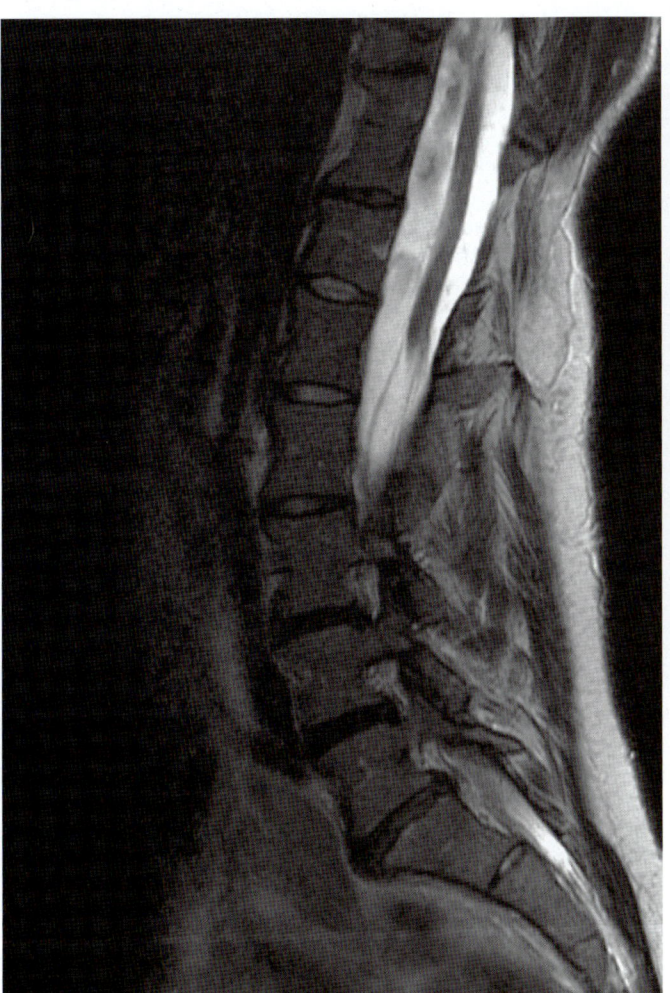

A

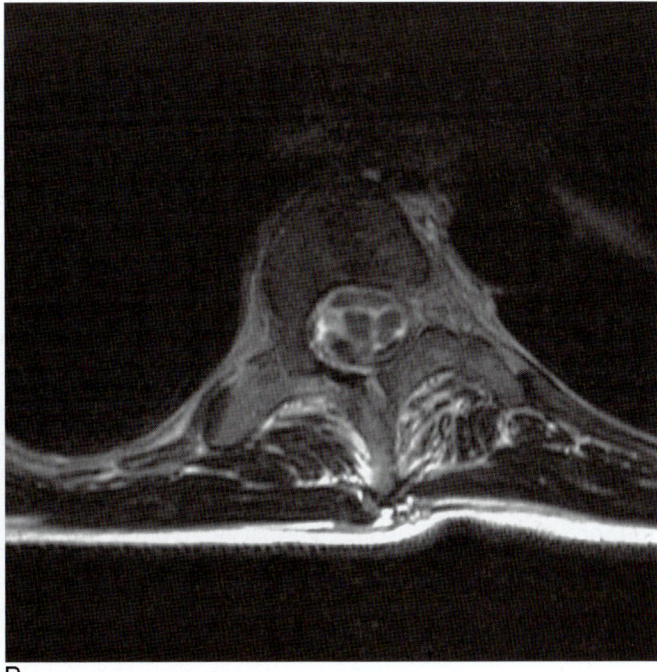

B

■ **FIGURE 104-11** Sagittal T1-weighted (**A**) and axial T2-weighted (**B**) MR images. The wide spinal canal seen on the sagittal sequence gives a clue to the presence of spinal dysraphism. The axial T2-weighted sequence shows the presence of diastematomyelia in the lower thoracic cord, with the cord splitting into two, contained within a single dural sac. Marked flow void artifact is seen within the cerebrospinal fluid. This is a particularly prominent feature when the spinal canal is widened, and there is an increased amount of cerebrospinal fluid.

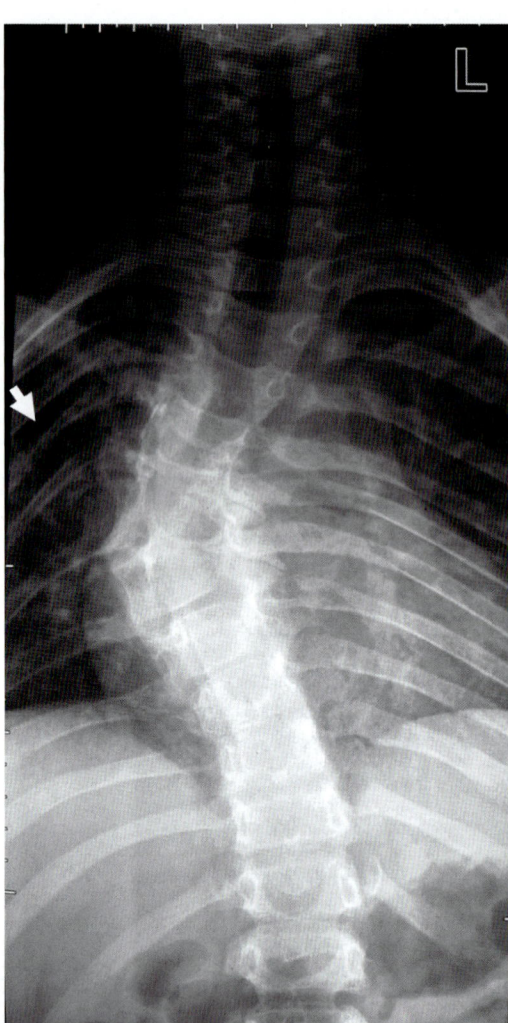

■ FIGURE 104-12 Scoliosis in a patient with type 1 neurofibromatosis. Characteristic appearance of a high thoracic, short angular curve. Note a thin dysplastic right rib (*arrow*).

Because the center of gravity of the body lies in front of the fourth lumbar vertebral body any vertebral body collapse will result in a kyphotic deformity. Any process that destroys a vertebral body, be it trauma, tumor, or infection, can therefore result in a kyphotic deformity. The other common types of kyphosis are idiopathic hyperkyphosis, which is termed *Scheuermann's disease*, and congenital kyphosis due to a vertebral anomaly.

Scheuermann's Disease

Scheuermann's disease is defined as a minimum of three adjacent thoracic vertebrae that are kyphotically wedged by 5 degrees or more. Hereditary factors are thought to be important in the development of the disease, which occurs most often in adolescent boys. In many ways Scheuermann's disease is analogous to idiopathic scoliosis, being a growth disturbance of the spine. Idiopathic

scoliosis results from anterior overgrowth of the spine resulting in buckling and deformity in all three planes. Scheuermann's disease, on the other hand, is an underdevelopment of the anterior spine. Thoracic hyperkyphosis is rotationally stable, being behind the axis of spinal column rotation, so the kyphotic deformity occurs without the lateral or transverse plane deformity encountered in idiopathic scoliosis.[8] The classic form, as described by Scheuermann, occurs at the same site as idiopathic scoliosis, namely T7 to T10, and has been termed type I Scheuermann's disease (Fig. 104-14). Type II Scheuermann's disease, also termed *atypical Scheuermann's disease*, occurs at the thoracolumbar junction. There is evidence that type II disease occurs more often in adolescent athletes, suggesting that mechanical factors are important. It is of no surprise that mechanical factors should have their greatest effect on the spine at the thoracolumbar junction, because this is the site of greatest mobility in the thoracic and lumbar spine.

Features of Scheuermann's disease are anterior wedging, end-plate irregularities, and Schmorl's nodes. These features are seen on plain radiographs, but MRI can show edema associated with the acute formation of a Schmorl node, which correlates with episodes of back pain (Fig. 104-15). Acute Schmorl's nodes are not visible on a radiograph because it may take several months for the sclerotic edge to develop that renders them visible. Once the changes develop in adolescence they are present throughout adult life. End-plate irregularities and Schmorl's nodes are such a common finding on MRI examinations in the general population that it is important not to label someone as having Scheuermann's disease in the absence of the kyphotic deformity. Such Scheuermann-type end-plate irregularities in the absence of kyphosis are of no clinical relevance.

In contradistinction to idiopathic scoliosis, which is a painless condition, patients with Scheuermann's disease frequently have back pain, particularly those with type II disease. Extension bracing and surgical correction can be used in treating the condition, but adolescent boys with Scheuermann's disease are much less likely to submit to surgical correction for cosmetic deformity than adolescent girls with idiopathic scoliosis.

Congenital Kyphosis

Congenital kyphosis is most frequently the result of anterior failure of formation, resulting in a dorsal hemivertebra. Less commonly, it may result from anterior failure of segmentation (Figs. 104-16 and 104-17). It results in a short angular kyphotic deformity, which can lead to neurologic injury from spinal cord compression. Frequently, there are complex vertebral anomalies that include lateral hemivertebrae, which give a scoliotic deformity, and dorsal hemivertebrae, which result in a kyphotic deformity. This is the only true form of kyphoscoliosis. CT can be helpful in defining the anatomy before surgical correction (Fig. 104-18). Whole-spine MRI should be performed to detect an associated spinal dysraphism.

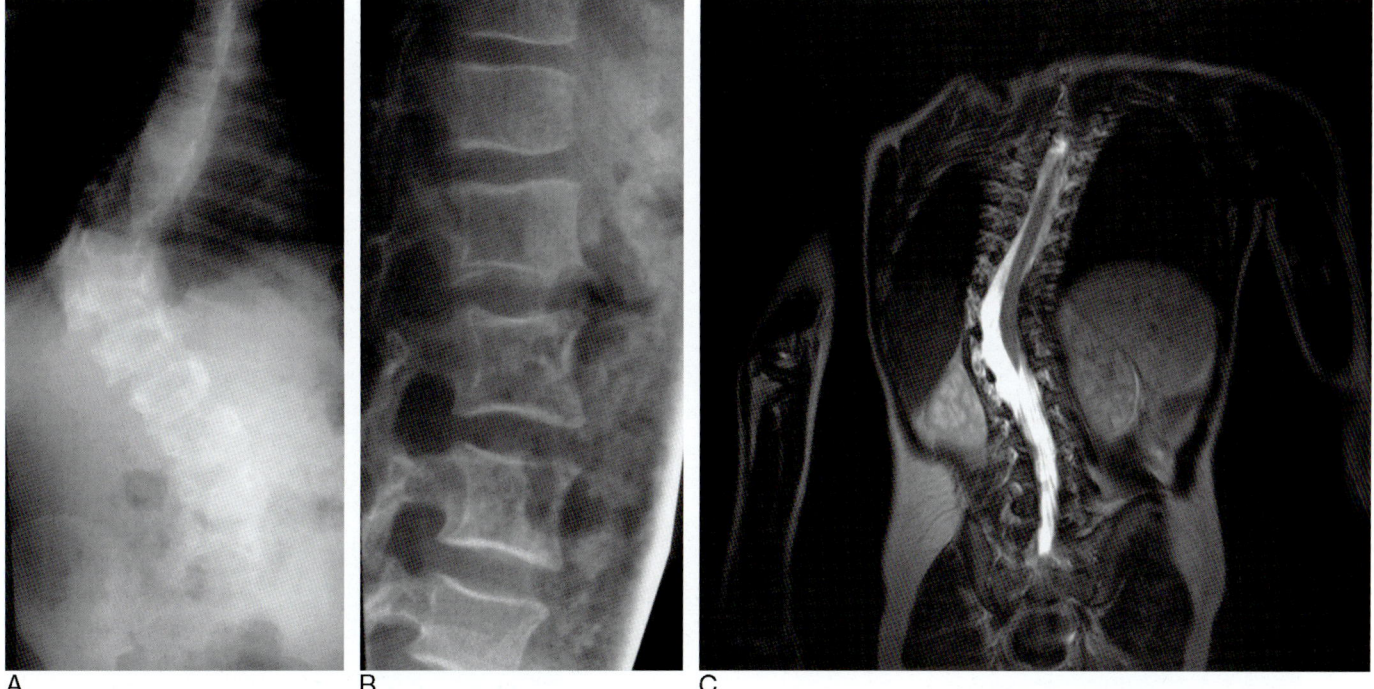

■ **FIGURE 104-13** Type 1 neurofibromatosis with a short angular thoracolumbar curve as seen on an anteroposterior radiograph (**A**), lateral radiograph (**B**), and coronal T2-weighted MR image (**C**). There is scalloping of the posterior vertebral body wall and enlargement of the exit foramen. The MR image demonstrates dural ectasia with a widened spinal canal.

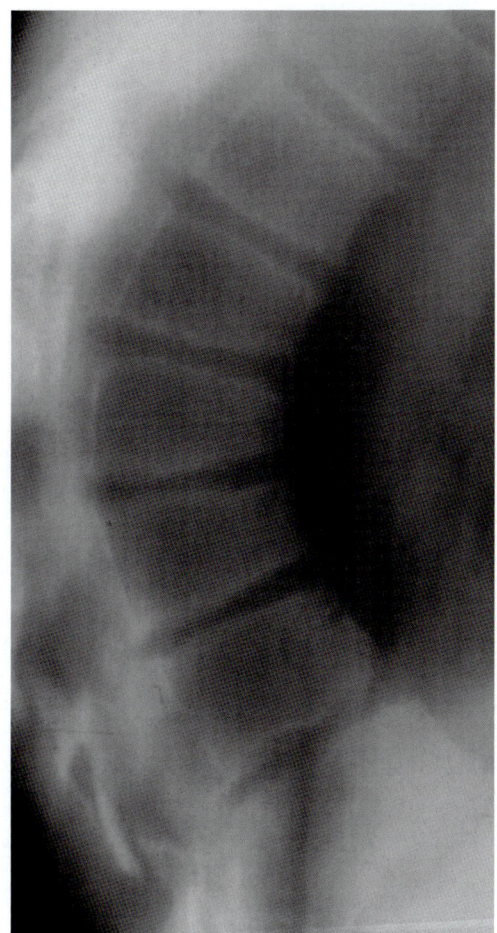

■ **FIGURE 104-14** Lateral thoracic radiograph showing typical appearances of type I Scheuermann's disease with end-plate abnormalities and anterior wedging resulting in a kyphotic deformity.

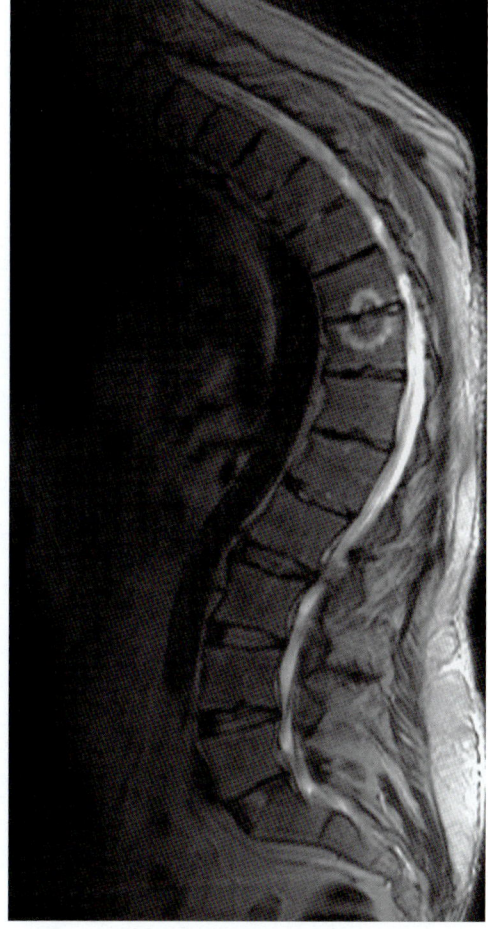

■ **FIGURE 104-15** Sagittal T2-weighted MR image in Scheuermann's disease. Multiple Schmorl's nodes and anterior wedging with thoracic deformity. Semicircular edema adjacent to the D10 and D11 end plates is the result of acute Schmorl's node formation.

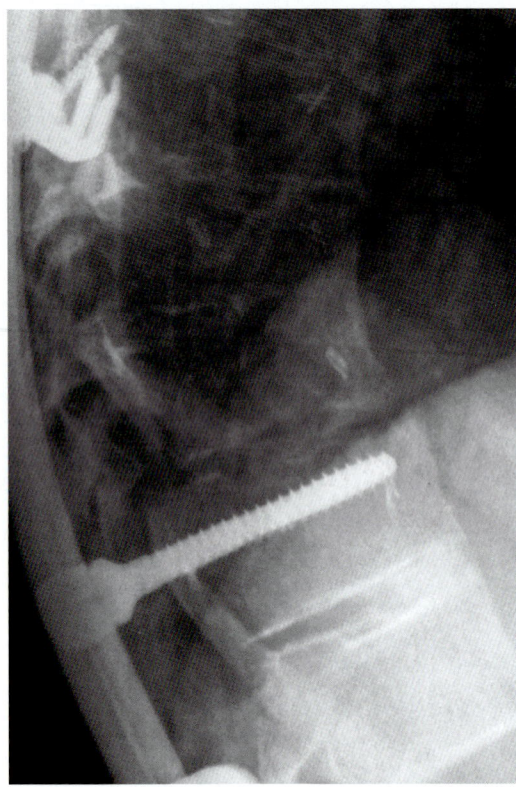

■ **FIGURE 104-16** Partial failure of segmentation with fusion of the anterior aspect of two thoracic vertebrae. Continued growth posteriorly has resulted in a kyphotic deformity. A concave anterior surface to the spine is typical of a congenital fusion and distinguishes this from an acquired fusion.

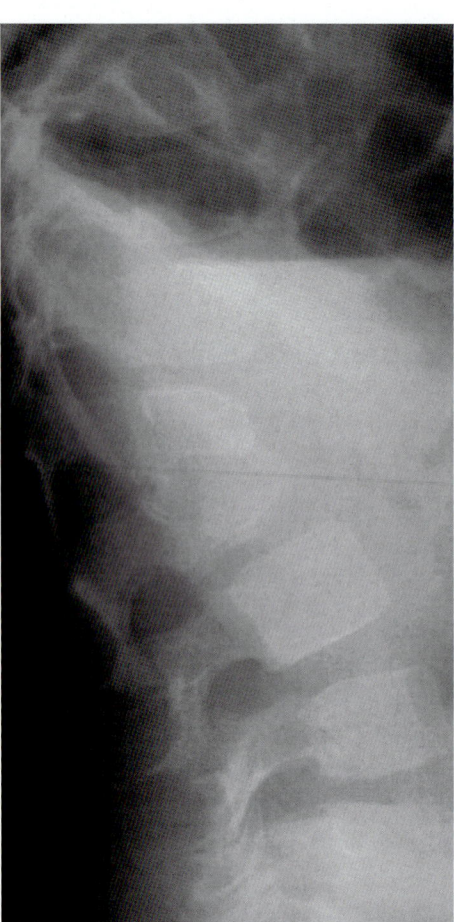

■ **FIGURE 104-17** Complete failure of segmentation resulting in a kyphotic deformity at the thoracolumbar junction. MR image showed an associated spinal cord syrinx.

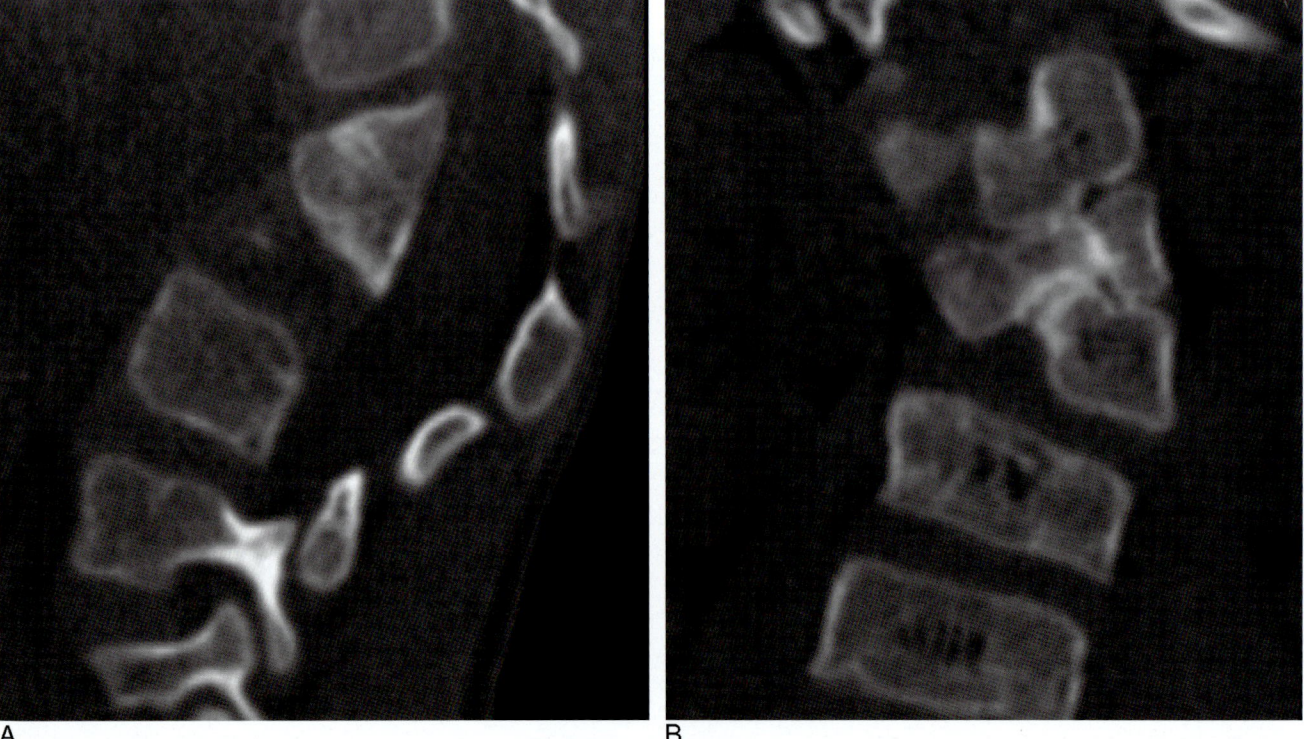

A   B

■ **FIGURE 104-18** Multiplanar reformatted CT in kyphoscoliosis. Sagittal (**A**) and coronal (**B**) reformatted images are shown. Failure of anterior formation results in a dorsal hemivertebra and a kyphotic deformity. Left-sided hemivertebrae give a scoliotic deformity. The hemivertebrae are not fully segmented, which limits the potential for progression of the deformity.

REFERENCES

1. Deacon P, Flood BM, Dickson RA. Idiopathic scoliosis in three dimensions: a radiographic and morphometric analysis. J Bone Joint Surg Br 1984; 66:509-512.
2. Birchall D, Hughes DG, Hindle J, et al. Measurement of vertebral rotation in adolescent idiopathic scoliosis using three-dimensional magnetic resonance imaging. Spine 1997; 22:2403-2407.
3. James JIP. Idiopathic scoliosis: the prognosis, diagnosis and operative indications related to curve patterns and the age at onset. J Bone Joint Surg Br 1954; 38:36-49.
4. Dickson RA. Conservative treatment of idiopathic scoliosis. J Bone Joint Surg Br 1984; 67:176-181.
5. Branthwaite MA. Cardiorespiratory consequences of unfused idiopathic scoliosis. Br J Dis Chest 1986; 80:360-369.
6. Inoue M, Minami S, Nakata Y, et al. Preoperative MRI analysis of patients with idiopathic scoliosis: a prospective study. Spine 2005; 30:108-114.
7. Quan L, Smith DW. The VATER association. Vertebral defects, Anal atresia, T-E fistula with esophageal atresia, Radial and Renal dysplasia: a spectrum of associated defects. J Pediatr 1973; 82:104-107.
8. Dickson RA. The aetiology of spinal deformities. Lancet 1988; 1:1151.

Postsurgical Imaging and Complications

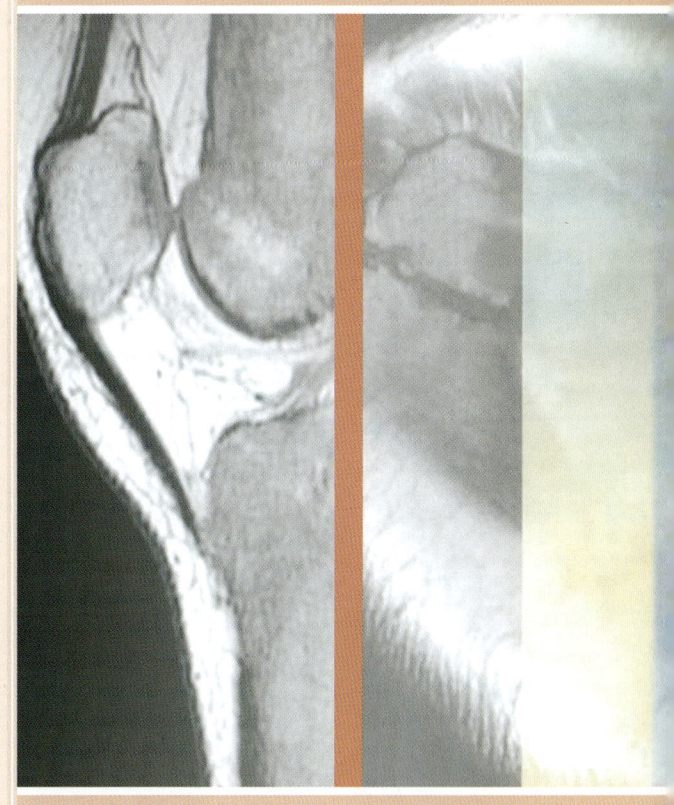

105

General Principles of Fixation, Fusion, and Joint Replacement

Kirkland W. Davis

Evaluating the postoperative patient is integral to the practice of musculoskeletal radiology. Most of the subsets of musculoskeletal pathology, including trauma, neoplasia, arthritis, sports medicine, and congenital and developmental maladies, encompass many diagnoses and entities that lead to surgical intervention. The radiologist must combine knowledge of normal and abnormal reparative processes with understanding of the pathology, surgical procedures, and various implants and devices to render adequate service to referring surgeons. The subsequent chapters in this section review musculoskeletal surgical procedures, their effects on tissues, and the associated hardware and complications by anatomic divisions. This chapter provides a general overview of basic principles of fixation and reconstruction with comments on hardware, complications, and imaging in specific postoperative situations. A special focus will be the continuing evolution of fixation techniques and newer implants. All available implants will not be reviewed, but the devices discussed here are a representative sample of the devices used by musculoskeletal surgeons.

PLATES AND SCREWS

Plates and screws are central in the armamentarium of any surgeon who operates on bones. They are used not only in open and percutaneous fixation of fractures but also to aid osteosynthesis in cases of osteotomies, fusions, and tumor resection. Basic principles of plates and screws apply across all these uses but are probably easiest to understand in the setting of fracture fixation. Certainly, many types of fractures are best treated with closed techniques, but plate osteosynthesis is central to the treatment of many other fractures.

Cortical Plates

Plate and screw technology, although seemingly simple at first glance, is an apt example of the evolution of principles of orthopedic surgery. As our knowledge of physiology, pathology, and material science has progressed, plates and screws have become more sophisticated and individualized for specific tasks. The first plates were simple cortical plates, often referred to as flat plates. Although plates have variable functions of compression, stabilization, tension, neutralization, buttressing, and bridging, they all provide at least some stability and serve to hold bones in apposition to allow healing to occur. Cortical plates create their stability by being tightly screwed to the surface of the bone, with friction at the bone surface performing the work. The screws achieve this tight application of the plate to the bone. To accomplish this, the screws for most cortical plates are bicortical, crossing both the near and far cortex.

The simple cortical plate has undergone a remarkable evolution, incorporating designs for specific anatomic sites

---

KEY POINTS

- Cortical plates achieve stability by friction between the plate and the cortex.
- Contouring, buttressing, low contact profile, and dynamic compression are all specialized features of plates that take advantage of physical and physiologic principles to improve healing and decrease complication rates.
- Locking plates utilize locking screws, which become fixed into the plates and provide rigid fixation. Locking screws are recognized by their shallow threads and narrow pitch.

and designs to satisfy different physical and physiologic principles, to the point that today it is difficult to find a simple flat rectangular plate with round holes. For instance, many plates have been manufactured to fit certain anatomic sites. The one-third tubular plate (Fig. 105-1) is primarily used to fix distal fibular fractures and osteotomies. Its short axis is an arc, although curiously not one third of a tube or 120 degrees. It is also a relatively thin plate. These features make the one-third tubular plate an ideal design for the distal fibula, a bone that is so small that its cortex is noticeably curved, not flat, and that is nearly subcutaneous in all but the largest persons, requiring a thin plate. In this same family of plates are the smaller one-quarter tubular plate, occasionally used in metacarpals and metatarsals, especially in children, and the larger semitubular plate, which is rarely used today.

Other cortical plates are also contoured for specific sites. This feature is especially common in buttress plates. The term *buttress plate* is generally applicable to any plate near a joint that flares out or widens as it nears the articular surface. They perform a buttress function, in that they provide a broad surface to support and bolster a comminuted fracture where the cortex is thin. This situation is especially common in fractures involving the distal radius, femur, and tibia and the tibial plateau. Each of these sites has several buttress plates specific to it. Buttress plates are often named by their shape and appearance (Fig. 105-2).

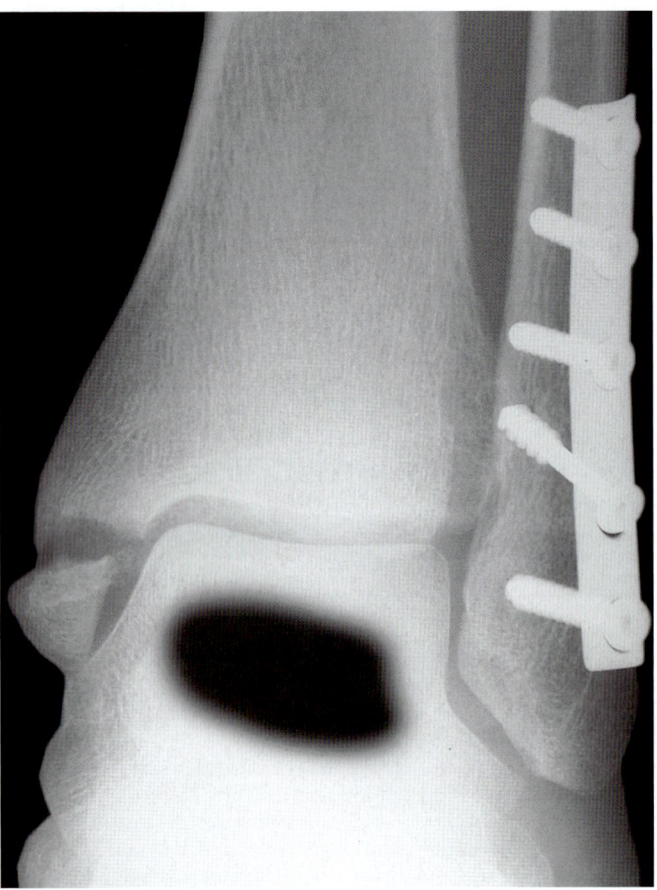

■ FIGURE 105-1 One-third tubular plate fixing a prior distal fibular fracture. The plate is slightly curved to match the surface of the fibula and is very thin.

Another specialized plate is the reconstruction plate. Sometimes called malleable plates, these plates are manufactured with notches along the sides, in between each screw hole. When viewed en face, these plates have wavy margins (Fig. 105-3). This notching weakens the plate enough to allow it to be contoured to fit the exact shape of the bone at the time of implantation. Because these plates require tools to be shaped, they are better termed *contoured plates* instead of malleable plates, which might imply flimsiness in situ. *Reconstruction plate* is the preferred term, because these plates are employed to provide significant structural support to fracture sites, most commonly in the pelvis.

Another modification of some plates is to use them to apply compression across a fracture. Appropriate compression of fracture margins augments healing. Whether this effect is due to the function of keeping the two ends in constant, close apposition, even in the presence of resorption of the fracture margins or due to actual acceleration of the healing response, remains uncertain. Either way, compression techniques allow more rapid healing when used appropriately. Several fracture characteristics obviate the use of compression: these include fractures with more than minimal comminution; fractures involving the metaphysis, osteoporotic bone, or otherwise weak cortex; pathologic fractures; and fractures involving an articular surface. Hence, the ideal fracture in which to use compression is a diaphyseal traumatic fracture in a younger adult patient. Fracture compression can be achieved in several ways. First, human anatomy and physiology provide several sites where stabilization of a fracture naturally creates tension on one side of a bone but resultant compression on the other side. The classic example of this is the femur, about which the lateral musculature is stronger than the medial musculature, and placement of a plate on the lateral side converts the tension there to compression on the medial side. This is truly a dynamic compression whenever the muscles are in use. Another way to provide compression is to use axial loading from weight bearing and gravity to compress a fracture that is not fully fixed in the axial plane, such as femoral neck fractures secured by a dynamic compression screw, spine fusions with plates that allow some craniocaudal translation, and long bone fractures stabilized by nails or rods without locking screws (all discussed later in the chapter). Compression also may be applied with special devices at the time of open reduction. A plate then secures the fragments in static compression.

A final method of fracture compression involves a specific design feature of some plates. These plates contain oval screw holes. The holes have sloped margins. If the surgeon places the screw eccentrically in the hole, farthest from the fracture, the rounded head of the screw will contact the slope of the hole, forcing the screw (and the bone it is entering) toward the fracture. When this eccentric screw placement technique is carried out on either side of the fracture, the fracture margins are brought into compression (Fig. 105-4). Despite the fact that this compression is static, these plates are called dynamic compression (DC) plates.

The latest advances in plate designs have been based more on biologic principles. These plates are occasionally grouped under the term *biologic plates*. The first signifi-

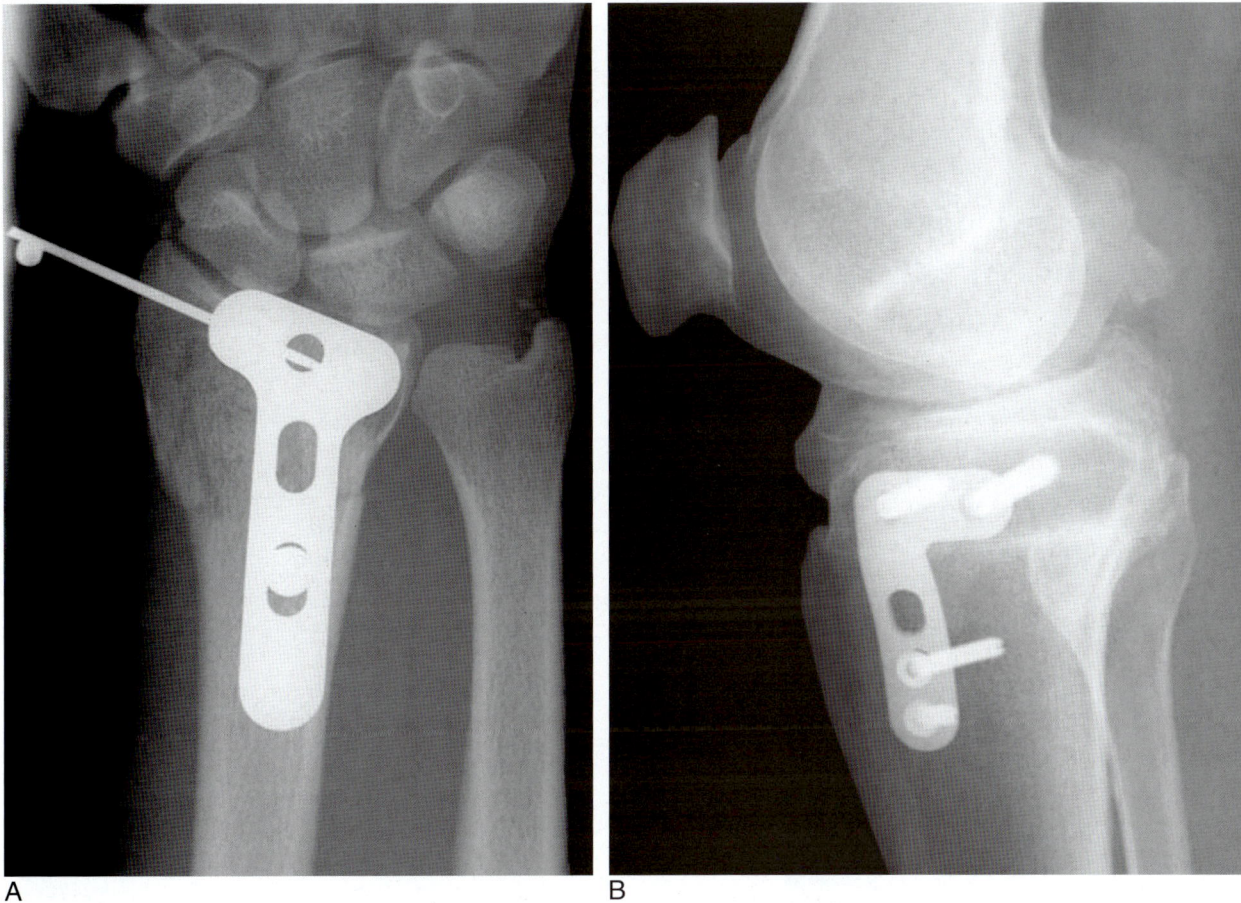

A   B

■ **FIGURE 105-2** Buttress plates. Posteroanterior view of the wrist (**A**) demonstrates a distal radial T plate. Lateral view of the knee (**B**) shows an L plate securing a tibial osteotomy.

cant improvement based on biology was to limit the surface contact of the plate. Cortical plates pressed onto the surface of bones create a zone of devitalization, primarily involving the periosteum. Optimal fracture (or osteotomy) healing requires maximum vascularity, but cortical plates reduce vascularity. The concept that improving vascularity would improve bone healing and reduce infection rates led to the design of cortical plates that only contact bone where they must, adjacent to the screw holes. Unlike reconstruction plates, these plates are notched or cut out along the deep surface, not the sides. This creates an undulating profile to these plates when one views them from the side (Fig. 105-5). This plate design is termed *limited contact* or *low contact*. This feature is often present in DC plates, creating the low-contact dynamic compression (LCDC) plate.

Locked Plates

The most recent advances in plate technology that take biologic principles into account are the locked plates. The primary differing feature of locked plates is that some or all of their screws are locking screws. A locking screw has a threaded head that locks the screw into place in the plate, which has threaded holes (Fig. 105-6). This design feature is helpful in that it makes locking screws into rigid, fixed-angle devices, which will not toggle or back

out of the plate. As such, locking plates should markedly reduce the incidence of loss of fixation and plate-screw failure. On radiographs, one can recognize locking screws because their threads are very shallow, meaning they take a small "bite" into the bone; and the thread pitch, or spacing between each thread, is quite narrow. Standard cortical and cancellous screws have a wider pitch and deeper threads (Fig. 105-7). Plates that use locking screw technology include less invasive stabilization system (LISS) plates, combination plates, and locked condylar plates.

There are a couple other important features of these plates. First, because locking screws are fixed into the plate, they cannot compress the plate down on the periosteum and cortex. Their main principle of fixation and stabilization, then, is not friction of the plate on the cortex, as with cortical plates, but is along the shanks of the screws. These locking screws act like pins from external fixators, and this whole class of plates is often referred to as internal fixators. The fixation they provide is quite rigid. Second, many of these plates are inserted in a minimally invasive fashion; the surgeon makes a short incision and then attaches a guide to assist in sliding the plate in to its final, submuscular position. The guide is also a template for inserting the screws percutaneously. When the surgeon can choose a minimally invasive insertion, tissue damage is minimized and the local healing environment at the fracture is improved. LISS plates are best able

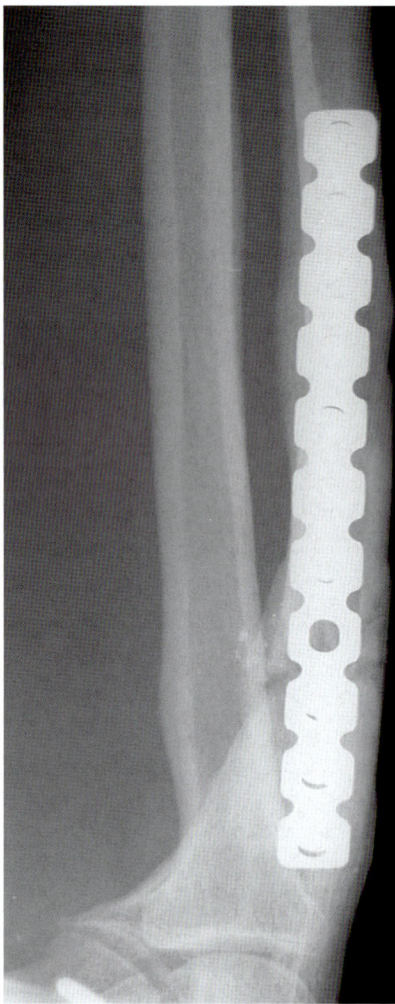

■ **FIGURE 105-3** Reconstruction plate fixing a proximal ulnar fracture in the forearm. Notching allows the plate to be contoured in the operating room.

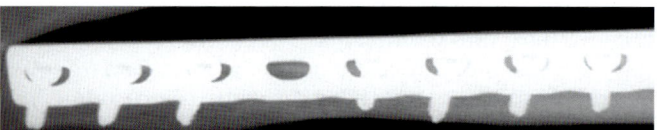

■ **FIGURE 105-4** Anteroposterior view of a dynamic compression plate in place, demonstrating eccentric placement of screws away from the original fracture site, creating the compression force.

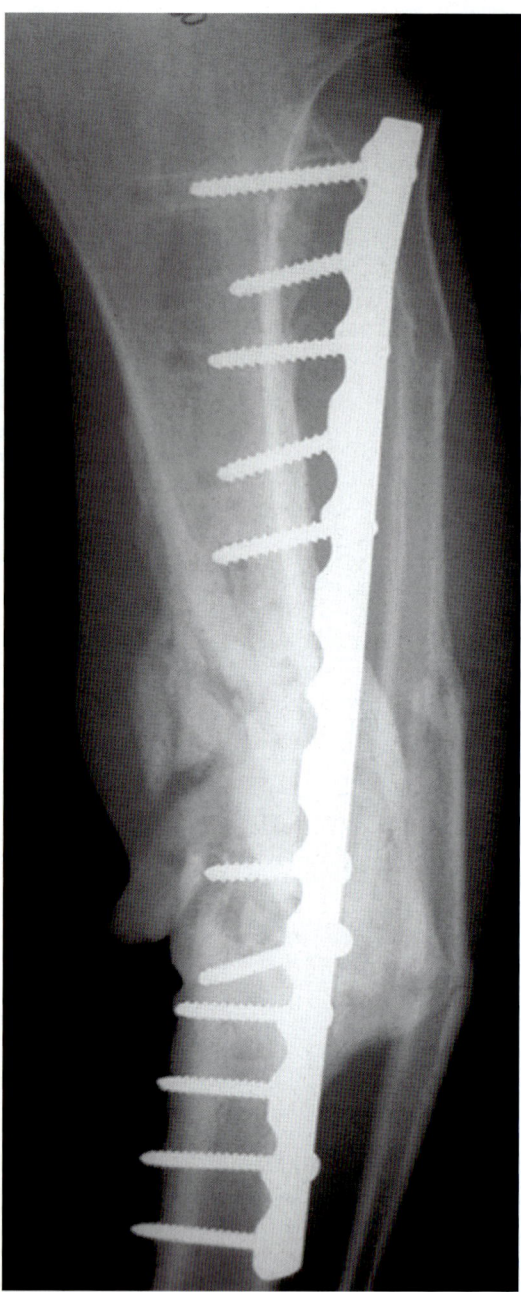

■ **FIGURE 105-5** Anteroposterior view of a tibial low-contact plate showing the undulating deep surface, limiting the amount of the plate that contacts the surface. Note obvious pullout of the screws and plate liftoff, termed *catastrophic failure*.

to take advantage of minimally invasive techniques, but almost all locking plates have smooth, tapered, rounded ends to allow minimally invasive insertion, rather than open fixation, when appropriate.

The LISS plates are specialized locking plates available only for the distal femur and proximal tibia. They are contoured to fit the shape of the lateral margins of these bones, and they come in three lengths and right and left versions. LISS plates are designed for intra-articular fractures about the knee with significant comminution, especially when there is associated diaphyseal involvement. The rigid fixation and fixed-angle locked screws resist the tendency of these fractures to fall into varus malalignment. These plates are especially beneficial in patients

with osteoporosis, in whom fracture fixation about the knee is otherwise fraught with hardware pullout and failure of fixation. One can recognize these plates by three features (Fig. 105-8): they are used only in the distal tibia and proximal femur; the screws are locking screws; and the holes in the plate are all single, circular, locking holes (unlike the combination holes described later). Also, because these plates are inserted in a submuscular fashion and act as internal fixators, there is a gap between most of the plate and the underlying cortex.

Combination (combi) plates have hybrid screw holes. These holes are usually shaped like the number 8. The

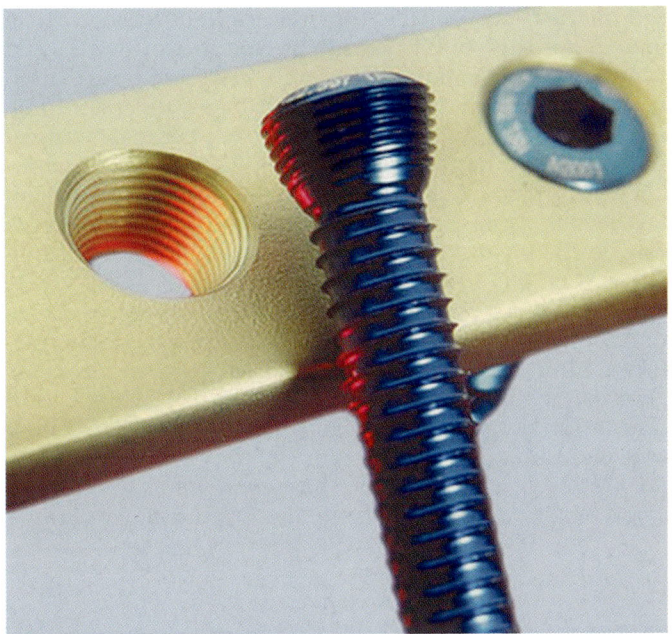

■ **FIGURE 105-6** Locking screws have threads on their heads, which lock them into the plate's threaded holes. *(Reproduced by permission of Synthes, copyright © Synthes, West Chester, PA.)*

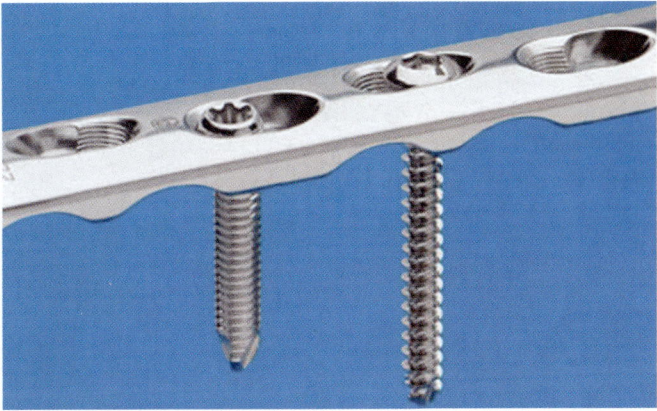

■ **FIGURE 105-7** Combi plate with cortical (*right*) and locking screws in place, demonstrating the difference in their threads. *(Reproduced by permission of Synthes, copyright © Synthes, West Chester, PA.)*

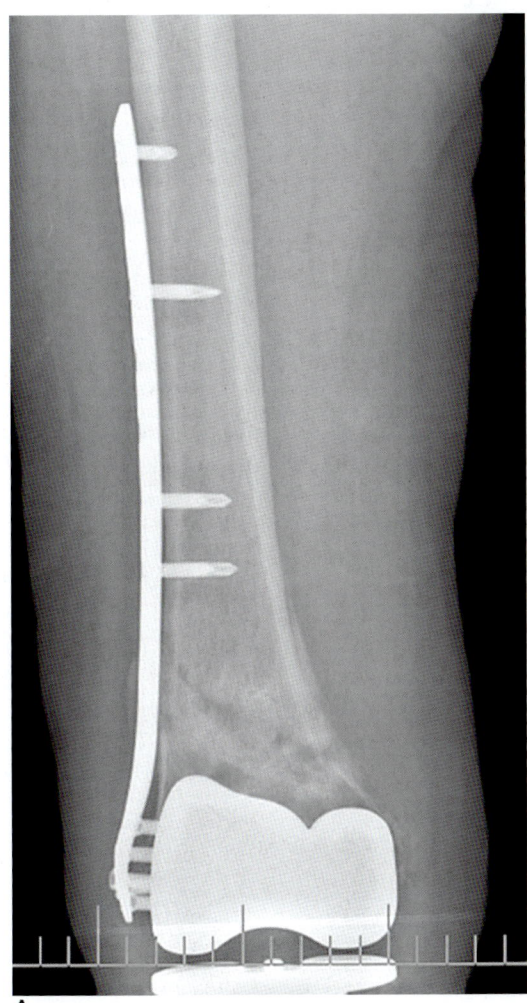

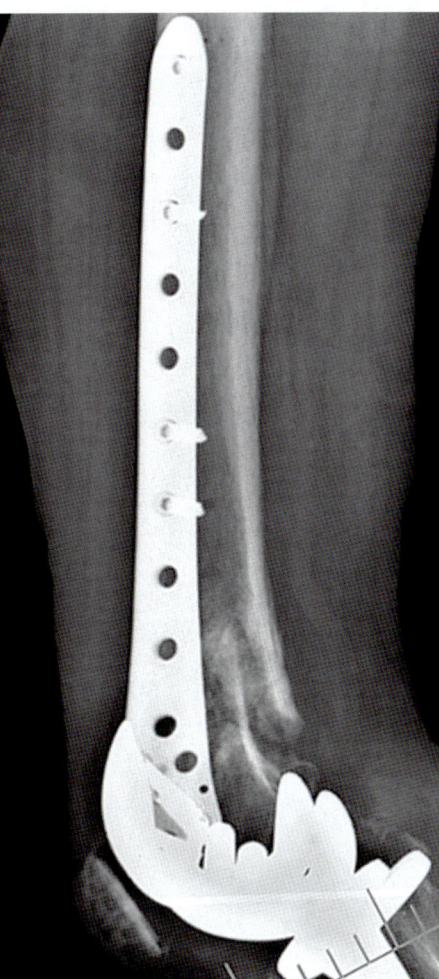

■ **FIGURE 105-8** Anteroposterior (**A**) and lateral (**B**) views of an LISS plate demonstrate its characteristic features: only locking screws are used; the holes are all circular; the location is the distal femur; and there is a gap between much of the plate and the underlying bone.

A   B

smaller half of the hole is a locking hole. The larger half is a hole for a regular (cortical or cancellous) screw. These holes allow the surgeon flexibility regarding when to place locking screws. If locking screws are in place, the surgeon cannot use the screw and plate to manipulate and further reduce a fracture, because the locking mechanism rigidly fixes the bone and plate in place. Similarly, locking screws will not allow the application of "dynamic" compression. Using a combi plate, surgeons may use regular screws to achieve a DC configuration and further reduce the fracture and then place the final locking screws to fix everything in place rigidly. These plates are used in diaphyseal fractures and are recognized by the "8"-shaped combi holes (Fig. 105-9; also see Fig 105-7).

Locked condylar plates, also called locked periarticular plates, are for fixation of intra-articular and juxta-articular fractures. These plates flare out as they near the articular surface. In this, they resemble buttress cortical plates, but they often provide no significant buttressing function because of their locking screws and limited contact. The periarticular, wider portion of the plate only uses locked screws, with circular holes. In the diaphyseal portion, there are combi holes, allowing the surgeon to choose to place locking or regular screws. These design features allow easy recognition of these plates, which are now available in designs for the ends of most of the long bones (Fig. 105-10).

Locking screw technology has revolutionized the techniques of internal fixation of numerous types of fractures. While they have not supplanted cortical plates for all uses, the improved healing and reduced complication rates afforded by locking plates has brought them quick and widespread acceptance in the surgical community. Locking screw technology has even been applied to some old standbys, such as the one-third tubular plate.

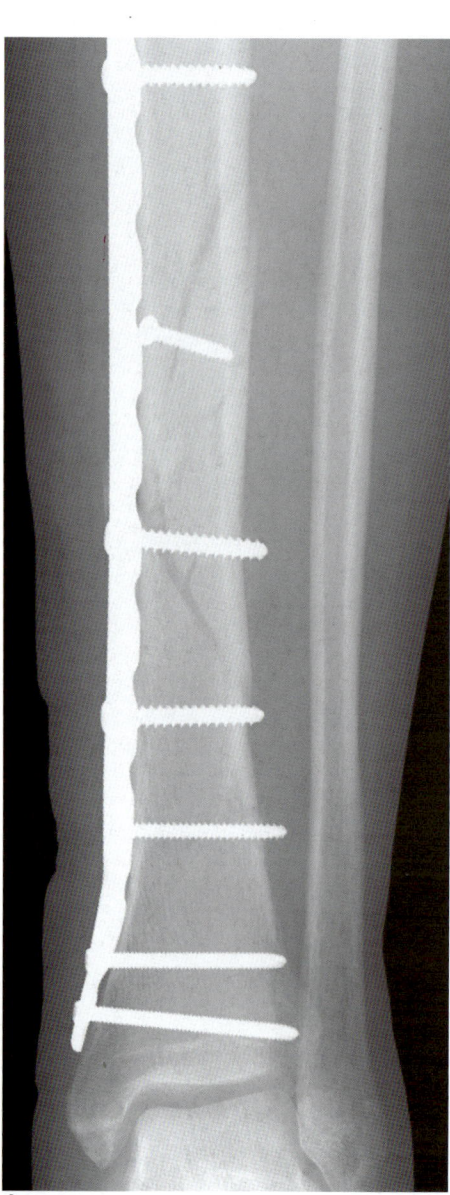
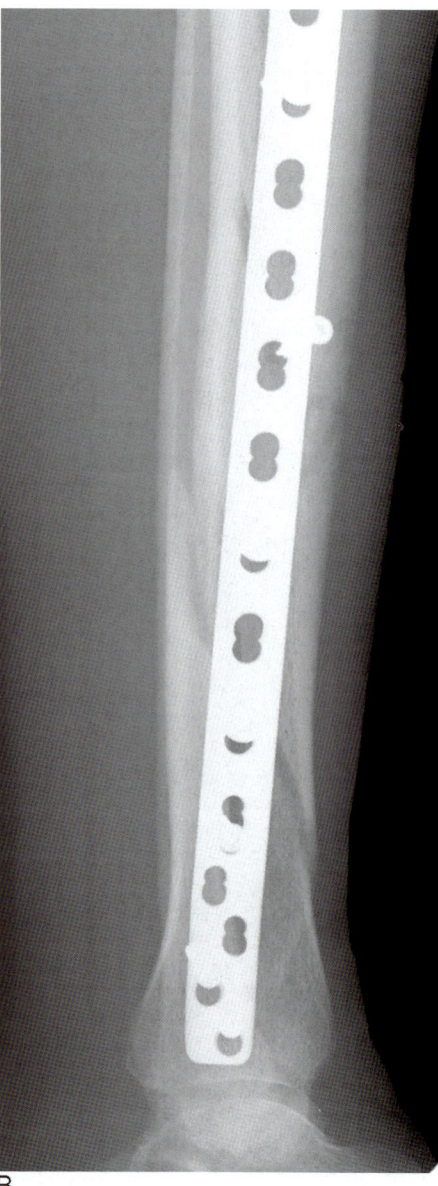

■ **FIGURE 105-9** Anteroposterior (**A**) and lateral (**B**) views of the left ankle demonstrating a combi plate. The lowest two screws demonstrate the characteristic profile of locking screws, whereas the remainder are bicortical screws. The combi holes are "8" shaped.

A

B

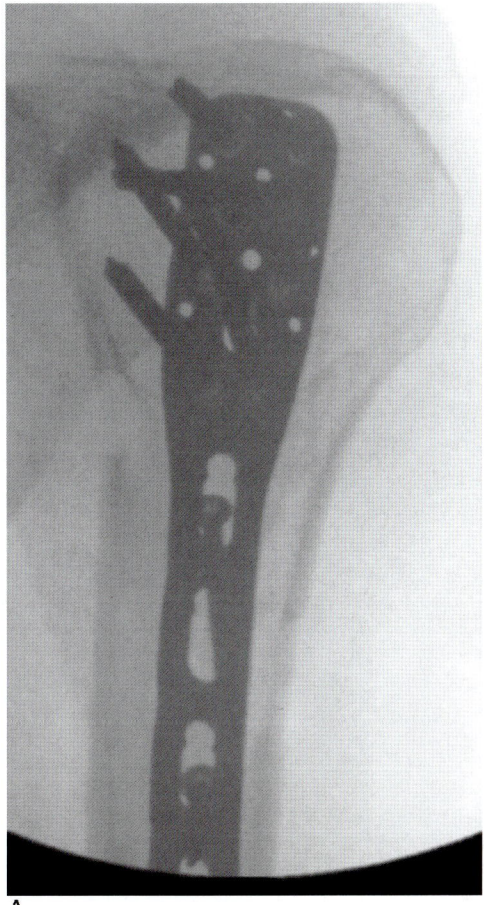

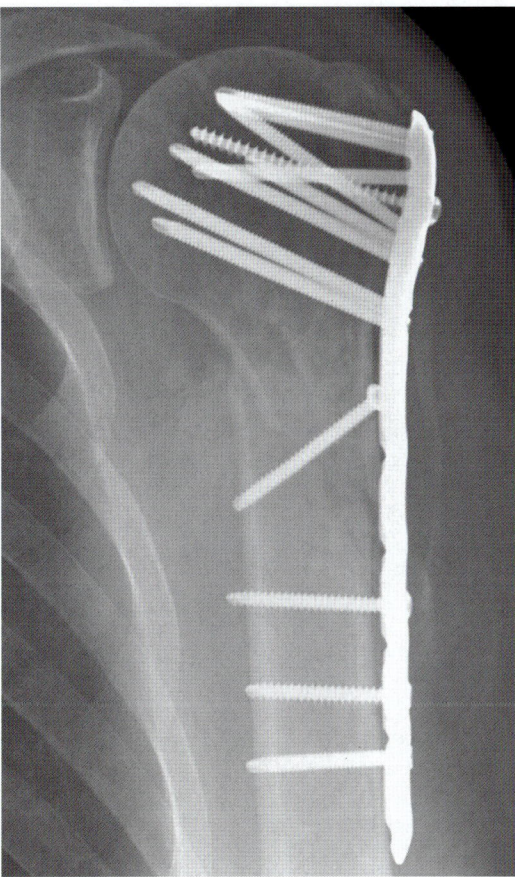

A

B

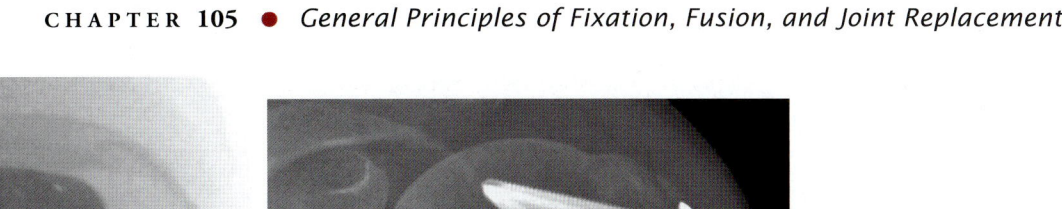

■ **FIGURE 105-10**
Anteroposterior fluoroscopic image (A) and lateral radiograph (B) demonstrating a locked proximal humeral plate. All of the proximal screws are locking, but some of the distal ones, passing through "8"-shaped holes, are cortical screws.

SCREWS

A working knowledge of fixation hardware includes familiarity with screw types. Locking screws are described in the previous section. The other basic screws in use are cortical and cancellous screws. Cortical screws have shallower threads and a narrower thread pitch relative to cancellous screws (Fig. 105-11), although both are wider and deeper than a locking screw. The thread design of cortical screws takes advantage of the dense bone of the cortex for fixation, whereas the thread design of cancellous screws allows them to achieve fixation in the relatively porous center of a bone. Cortical screws are usually placed across the near and far cortex of a bone and are termed *bicortical*.

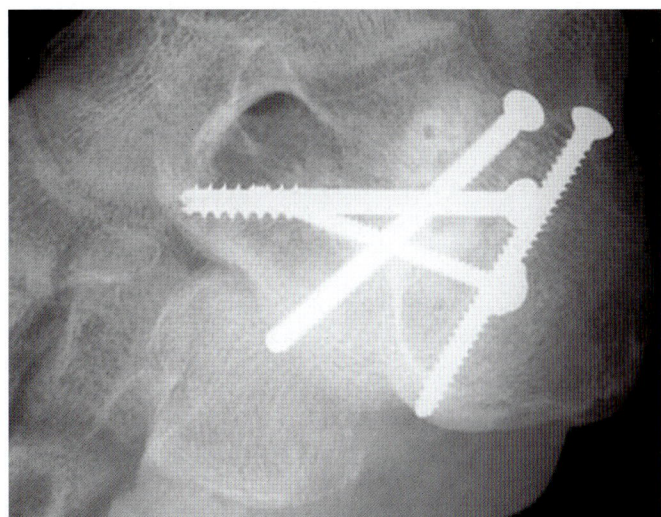

■ **FIGURE 105-11** Oblique view of the calcaneus demonstrates the narrower pitch of the threads of a cortical screw (*right*) and the wider pitch of a partially threaded cancellous screw (*left*).

KEY POINTS

■ Cortical screws usually are placed across the near and far cortex (bicortical) and their threads are relatively shallow and have a narrow pitch.
■ Cancellous screws have deeper threads and a wider pitch.
■ The term lag screw refers to the function of compressing the distant fragment of bone into the near one, not any particular screw design.

The term *lag screw*, derived from carpentry, refers to the function of a screw, not one specific design. A screw performs a lagging function when it is placed across two fragments of bone and the threads in the distal piece pull it and compress it against the proximal piece. There are

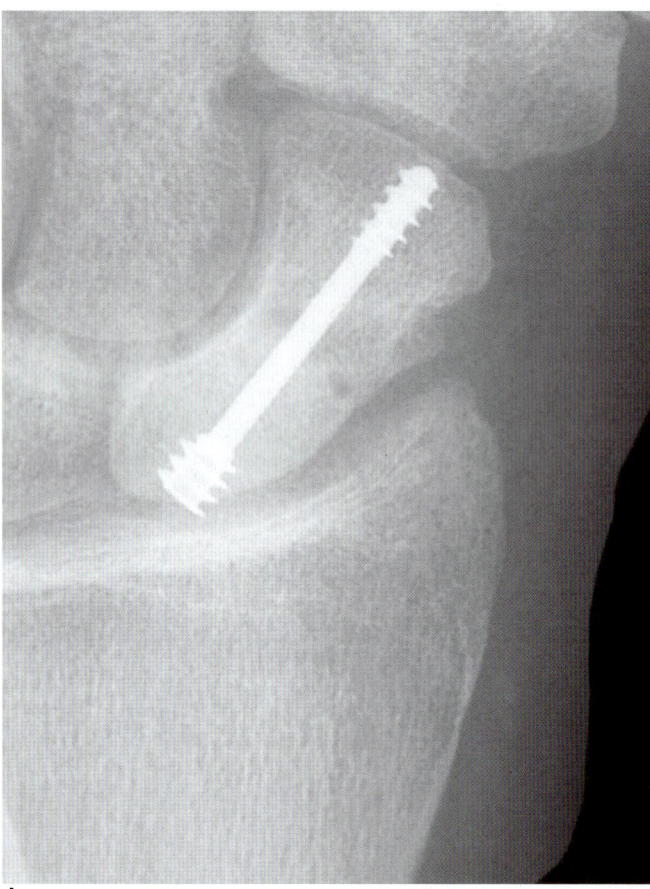

A

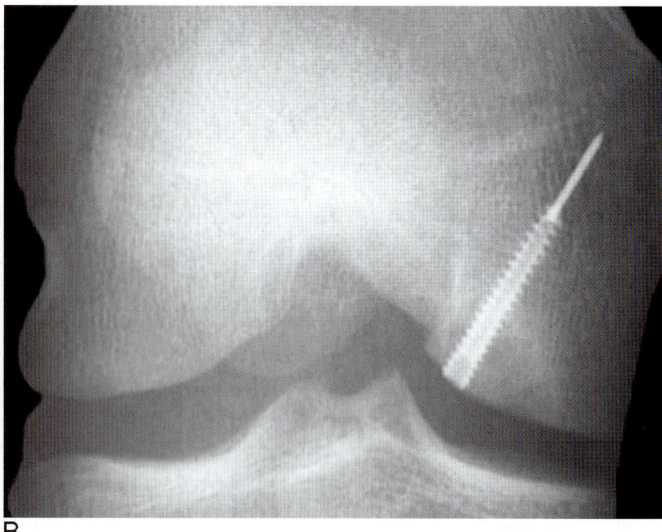

B

■ **FIGURE 105-12** Headless variable compression screws: Herbert screw fixing a scaphoid waist fracture (**A**) and Acutrak screw fixing a femoral osteochondral fragment (**B**) demonstrate the variable thread pitch that provides the unique function of these screws.

several ways to achieve this function. One is to use a partially threaded screw, with no threads on the proximal shank. As one inserts the screw and the screw head contacts the near piece of bone, progressive turning of the screwdriver advances the threads into the distal piece, drawing it toward the proximal piece and creating compression. The same effect can be achieved with a fully threaded screw, if one overdrills the screw hole in the proximal fragment such that the screw threads do not engage it. Again, the distal threads pull the distal piece toward the proximal one.

Another way to achieve a lag function is with headless variable compression screws. The most familiar of these is the Herbert screw, but the Acutrak screw has supplanted the Herbert screw for many purposes. These screws do not have heads, but they are slotted for screwdrivers. The threads on the distal portion of these screws have a wider pitch than the proximal threads. As the screw is driven, the wider pitch of the distal threads draws the distal fragment toward the proximal one. These screws are most common in fixation of scaphoid waist fractures and fractures and osteochondral lesions of the femoral condyles (Fig. 105-12).

One implant that has features of plates, screws, and intramedullary devices is the dynamic compression screw (DCS). These are most commonly seen in the proximal femur for fixation of some femoral neck and peritrochanteric fractures (dynamic hip screw [DHS]), but there also is a version for the distal femur intercondylar fractures (dynamic condylar screw). In the DHS, a wide-bore, partially threaded cancellous screw is driven up into the femoral head via the neck. This screw slides into a sleeve that is connected to a side plate; the plate is placed along the lateral cortex of the proximal femur (Fig. 105-13). As the patient begins to bear weight on the extremity, the femur fracture compresses along the shaft of the screw. Invariably, there is progressive impaction of the fracture as healing progresses and the screw telescopes into the sleeve.

INTRAMEDULLARY DEVICES

Nails, rods, pins, and wires fit into this category. There is some overlap in these terms, leading to some confusion when reporting on these devices. Nails are used for diaphyseal fractures of long bones and fill the medullary cavity at its narrowest point. They are typically tapped into place from the proximal (antegrade) or distal (retrograde) end of the bone. Large-bore nails are usually implanted with proximal and distal interlocking screws (Fig. 105-14). This adds rotational and axial stability to the construct but eliminates the possibility of fracture compression. When nails are implanted without interlocking screws or if the screws are removed, known as dynamizing the nail, the fracture margins will compress against each other, similar to the mode of the DCS. Most nails seen in daily practice are the large-bore nails that are used in the adult femur and tibia. The treatment for children 5 to 15 years old with long-bone diaphyseal fractures is often

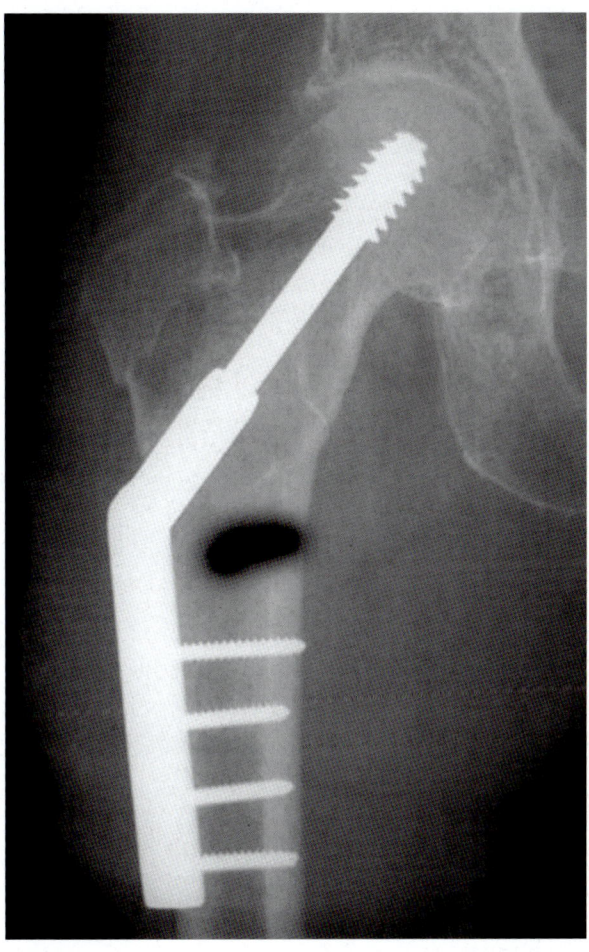

■ **FIGURE 105-13** Dynamic hip screw (DHS): as the femoral fracture heals, it may subside. The screw will telescope into the sleeve.

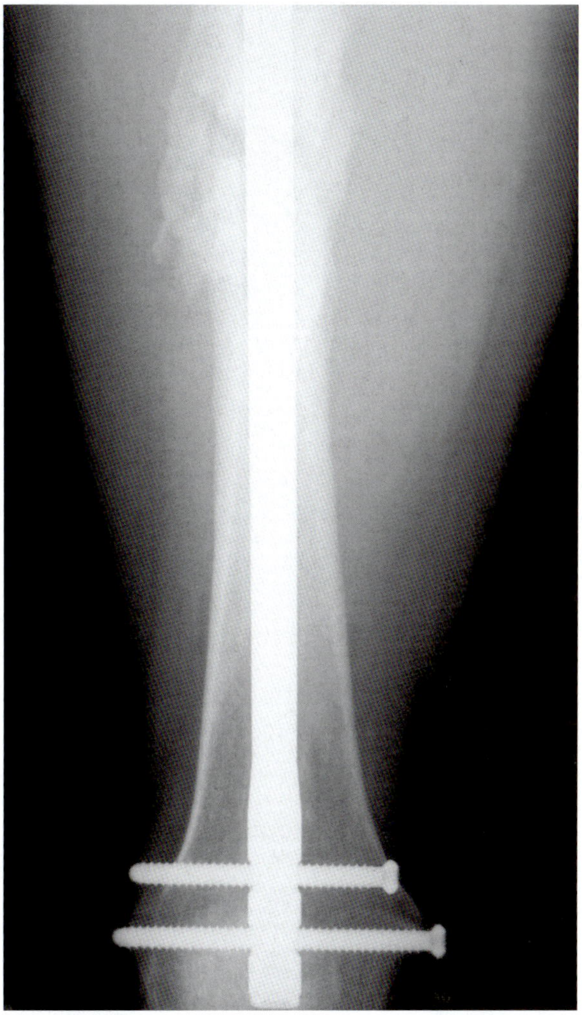

■ **FIGURE 105-14** Anteroposterior view of the distal aspect of a retrograde interlocking intramedullary nail.

KEY POINTS

- Intramedullary devices are used to stabilize some long-bone fractures and include nails, rods, pins, and wires.
- Nails usually fill the medullary canal at its narrowest point and are tapped into place.
- Whereas Kirschner wires usually are inserted percutaneously and end within the marrow, malleable wire is used in cerclage settings, as a tension band, and to anchor posterior spine fusion hardware and external fixators.

the elastic intramedullary nail, which is moderately flexible but is curved in its native state (Fig. 105-15). The prototype of this nail was the Ender nail, and that name usually is still applied to these nails. Although one of these nails rarely fills the medullary cavity in the long bone of even a young (normal) child, the application of two or three of these nails in concert will fill the marrow space and provide extra stability. The proximal and distal ends are anchored through the cortex of the bone, adding rotational stability.

One of the recent advances in this arena is the development of cephalomedullary nails for specific proximal femur and humerus fractures. These are modifications of standard femoral nails, with the addition of a blade plate, screw, or pins passing up the femoral neck into the head. The common example of this is the trochanteric fixation nail (TFN), which is inserted through the greater trochanter and has a large-bore screw (akin to a DCS screw) or blade plate passing up into the femoral head (Fig. 105-16). These devices are designed to be implanted for proximal femur fractures involving the intertrochanteric region but with complicating features, such as extensive comminution, reverse obliquity, or extension into the diaphysis. Piriformis-starting nails are nearly identical devices except the insertion site is different, slightly medial to the trochanter on an anteroposterior radiograph. There are other examples of the cephalomedullary technology, and it has even been applied to the proximal humerus in the form of a proximal humeral spiral blade nail.

Rods are also used to stabilize long-bone fractures, but they are narrower devices. Because a single Ender nail is a narrow device, it is sometimes referred to as an Ender rod. The classic rod in use for the last few decades is the

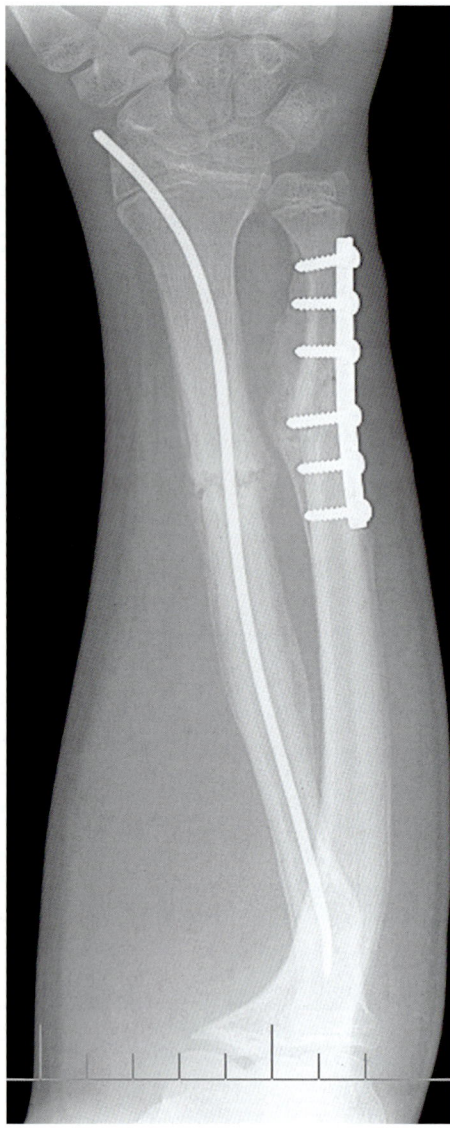

■ **FIGURE 105-15** Anteroposterior view of the forearm demonstrating the flexible Ender nail crossing the radial shaft fracture. Also note the one-third tubular plate on the distal radius.

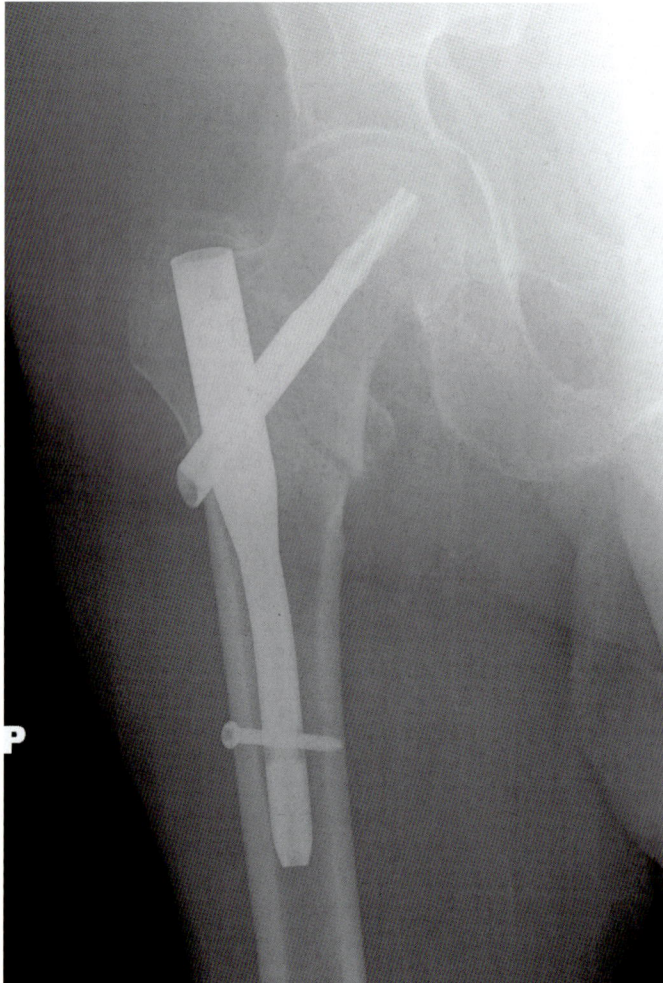

■ **FIGURE 105-16** Anteroposterior view of the hip shows a short trochanteric fixation nail. This model uses a spiral blade to achieve stabilization across the femoral neck.

Rush rod. This implant is straight except for a tight curve on the end, resembling a crochet needle (Fig. 105-17). The curved portion may serve as an anchor and allows for easy retrieval. These rods are often the best device to stabilize fractures of narrower long bones such as the fibula or the pediatric radius, and they play an important part in stabilizing long bones of patients with osteogenesis imperfecta.

Pins are narrow, shorter devices that have their pointed, often threaded end buried in bone across a fracture site. The back end of the pin protrudes out of bone, sometimes just through the cortex and sometimes outside the whole body. It is common to speak of pinning fractures, in which the surgeon inserts or screws the device across the fracture percutaneously. Some pins are threaded and are essentially screws, whereas others are pointed on the end but not threaded (Fig. 105-18). When threads are present on pins, the width of the threads often does not exceed that of the unthreaded shank.

There are two types of wires in common usage. Kirschner wires (K wires) are relatively rigid, straight devices that are typically employed in the mode of a pin (Fig. 105-19). They are rigid enough to provide stability in fracture fixation but are often bent and truncated in the operating room with tools. The other type of wire is malleable wire provided on a spool. This type of wire is commonly seen as cerclage wires around hip prostheses, tension band wires at the olecranon, and in association with posterior spine instrumentation, especially Luque instrumentation. Cable, in which smaller strands of wire are prebraided together, also serves these purposes.

PEDIATRIC FIXATION

Fractures

Because of the ability of younger bones to remodel significant displacements and modest angular deformities and because of the rapid healing of children's bones, most pediatric fractures are reduced in a closed fashion and treated with casts, splints, or slings. There are several exceptions to this concept in routine pediatric fracture treatment. First, the weight-bearing long bones will often be treated

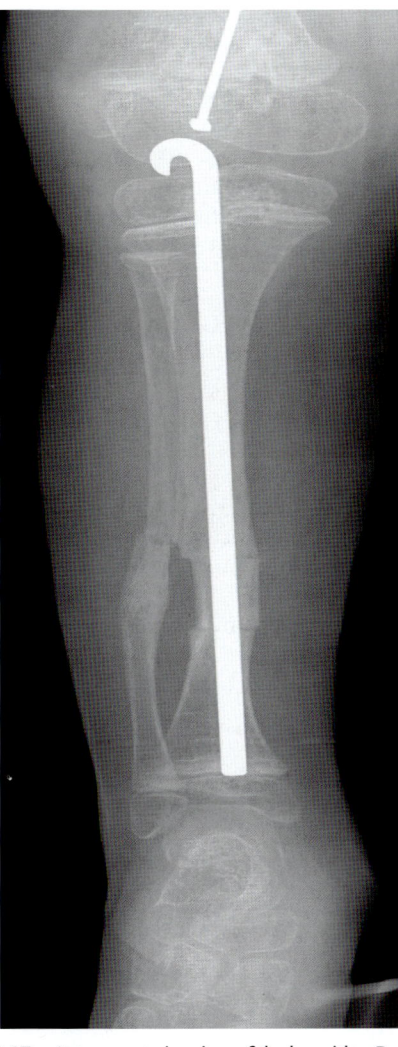

■ FIGURE 105-17   Anteroposterior view of the leg with a Rush rod securing tibial osteotomies. The patient suffers from osteogenesis imperfecta.

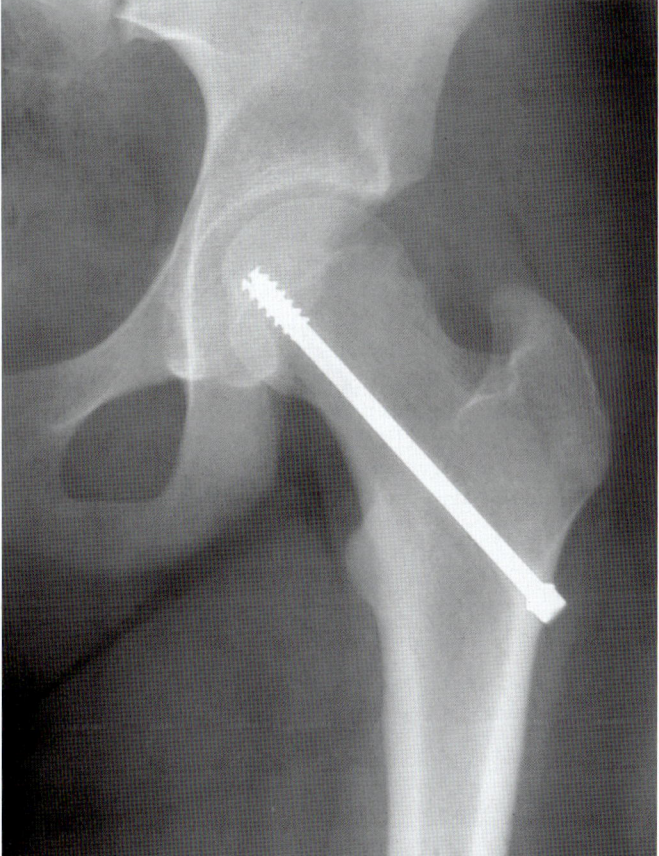

■ FIGURE 105-18   Anteroposterior view of the hip demonstrates prior pinning of the femoral head in a child with slipped capital femoral epiphysis. This pin is a cannulated, partially threaded cancellous screw.

KEY POINTS

- Pediatric fractures often require only closed reduction and fixation techniques to achieve a favorable result.
- External fixators are available in unilateral, planar, and ring types.
- Osteotomies may be employed to rectify malunions and nonunions and to correct angular deformities.

---

with one or more elastic intramedullary nails if the child is 5 to 15 years old and the fracture is transverse, oblique, or a simple spiral fracture. Second, plate and screw fixation is reserved for older teenagers and overweight children. Third, although displacement is of lesser concern in diaphyseal fractures, anatomic reduction is critical in epiphyseal and transphyseal fractures, to ensure a functional articular surface and to ward off growth disturbances resulting from growth plate disruption. These fractures are often fixed with Kirschner wires; the classic example is the Salter-Harris IV lateral condyle fracture of the distal humerus. Fourth, markedly unstable lower extremity fractures are often best served by external fixation.

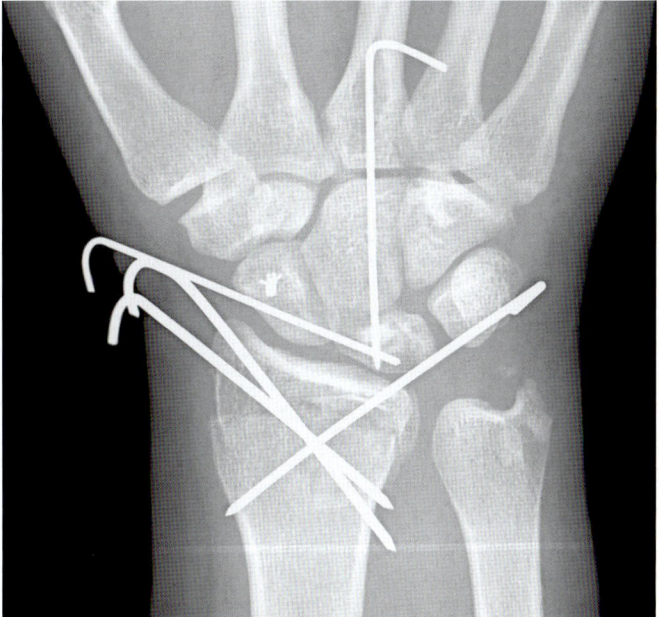

■ FIGURE 105-19   Posteroanterior view of the wrist shows multiple Kirschner wires pinning a complex fracture-dislocation. The external ends of the wires have been curved to limit unnecessary contact.

External Fixators

External fixators are used in both pediatric and adult patients for fracture treatment and stabilization of rotational osteotomies, lengthening, and bone transfer. This type of fixation is the most rigid available. Unilateral external fixators consist of half-pins (penetrating one side of the extremity but not exiting the other) connected by graphite or metal rods on one side of the extremity (Fig. 105-20). Planar external fixators use the same building blocks but occupy more than a 90-degree arc around the extremity. Ring fixators, first developed by Ilizarov, consist of a series of rings that surround the extremity and are connected to each other by rods. The whole construct is anchored into the bone by wires or fully threaded pins (Fig. 105-21). External fixators that cross a joint are termed *spanning fixators* (vs. nonspanning), and they often will be constructed with angular capability across the joint. Similar angulation, which can be changed over time, is used when external fixators are employed to gradually rotate an osteotomy to overcome a preexisting angular deformity.

Several decades ago, Ilizarov pioneered the first effective and reliable system for lengthening long bones. These techniques continued to be refined, but the principles are largely those that he developed. Lengthening is often employed in patients with limb-length discrepancy due to childhood trauma, infection, or congenital/developmental deformity. Another use is limb lengthening for dwarfs. The basic steps of the technique include creating a corticotomy, which is a careful osteotomy in which the periosteum is left largely intact, with placement of a ring external fixator; an initial 5- to 10-day latency period to start the healing process; gradual distraction of the corticotomy in tiny increments totaling no more than 1 mm/day; and a consolidation phase at least as long as the distraction phase, to allow new bone to fill the defect while the extremity is protected by the fixator. Radiographs usually are obtained every 7 to 14 days (Fig. 105-22). The radiologist should scrutinize the images to describe the amount of interval lengthening, document the presence and increasing consolidation of new bone in the gap after lengthening, and alert the

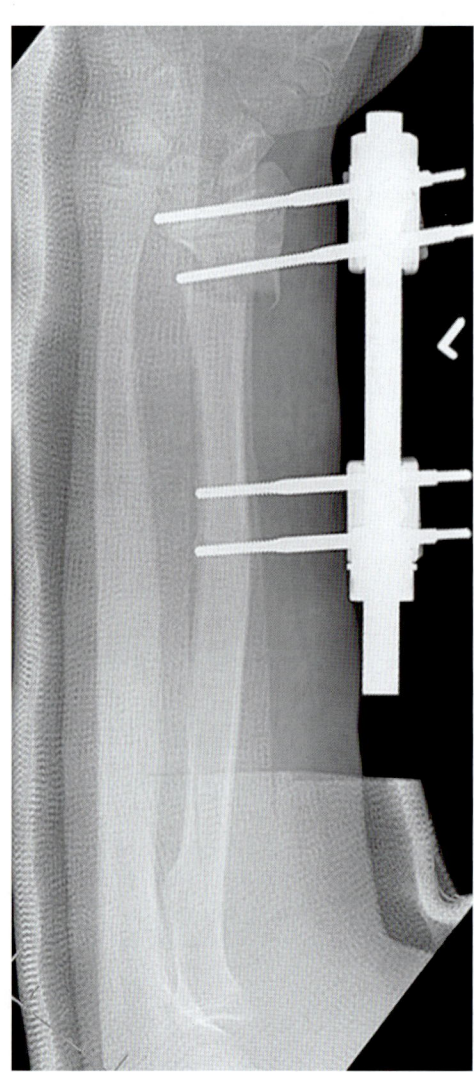

■ **FIGURE 105-20** Anteroposterior view of the forearm reveals an external fixator across the distal radial osteotomy. The child had a prior fracture that had resulted in premature arrest of growth of the radius.

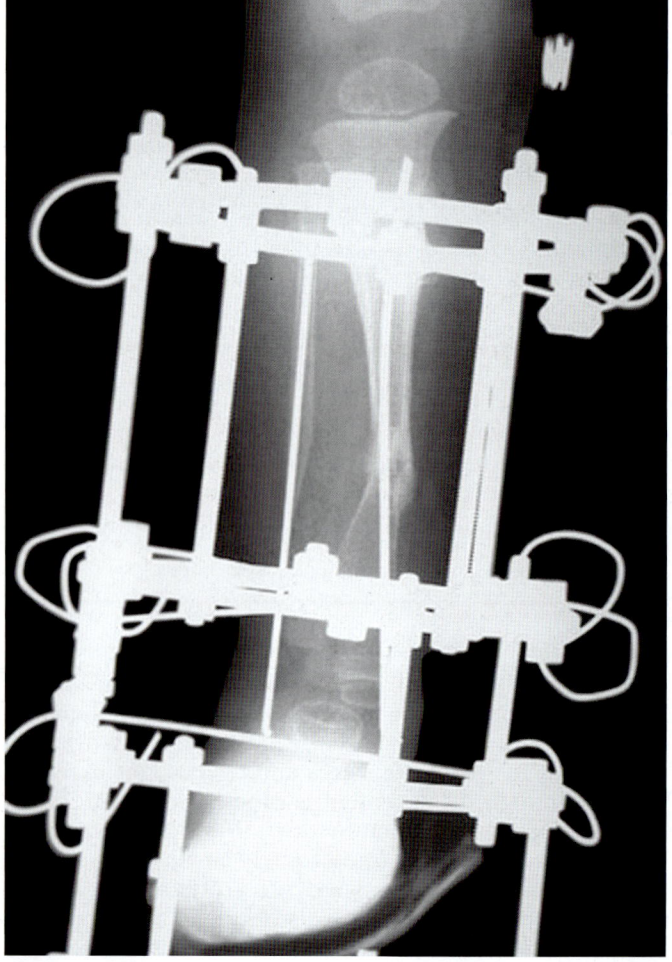

■ **FIGURE 105-21** Ring external fixator securing a congenital pseudarthrosis of the tibia. Bone transfer will occur shortly.

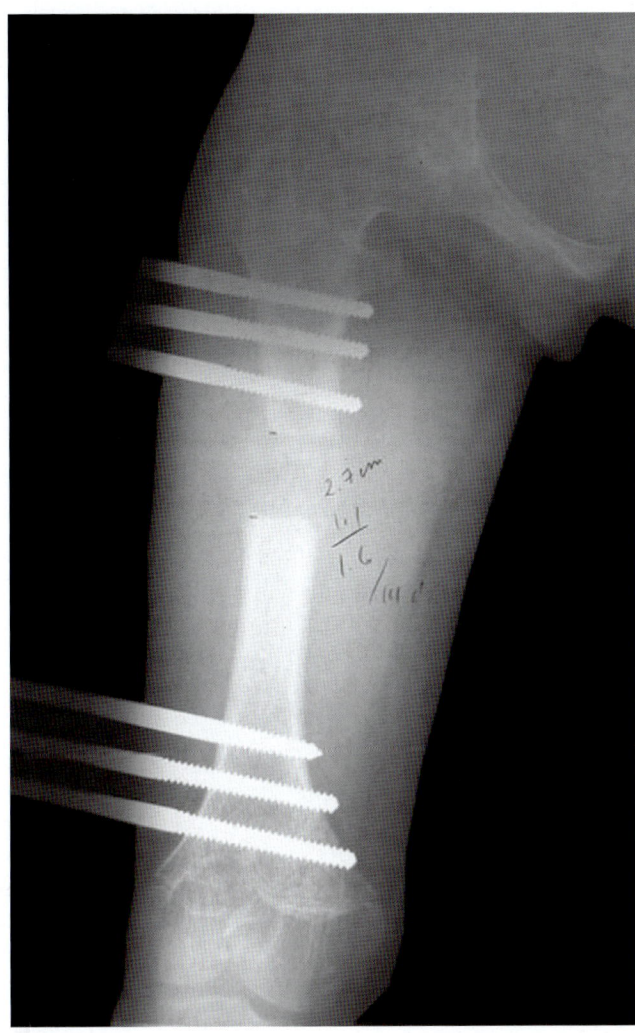

■ **FIGURE 105-22** Proximal femoral lengthening site demonstrates moderate new bone developing in the gap, secured by a unilateral external fixator.

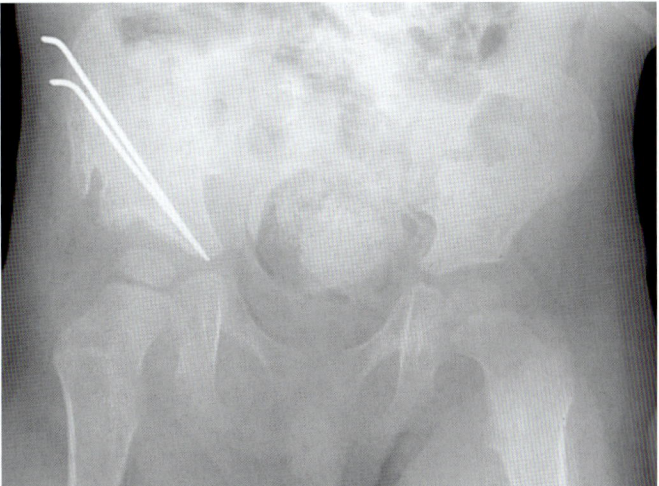

■ **FIGURE 105-23** Two Kirschner wires pin the site of the previous supra-acetabular osteotomy, performed to correct developmental dysplasia of the hip.

surgeon to complications, such as fracture through the new bone, progressive angular deformity or buckling, or infection along the pin tracks. Similar processes now are employed to correct some angular long bone deformities and to achieve bone transfer to fill a bone gap left behind after fracture, infection, or congenital pseudarthrosis.

Osteotomies and Epiphysiodesis

Osteotomies are used in both children and adults to correct angular deformities and to allow surgeons to re-set malunited fractures (see Fig. 105-17). The osteotomy is secured by internal hardware or an external fixator. The most common use of osteotomies in children is in the setting of developmental dysplasia of the hip. In these children, the femoral head is laterally subluxated or dislocated and the acetabulum develops abnormally as a result. To provide improved coverage of the femoral head, the child may undergo one of a number of periacetabular osteotomies, usually fixed with several pins (Fig. 105-23), or a varus derotational osteotomy of the proximal femur, secured by an angled blade plate.

The previous paragraphs allude to a number of situations in which adults undergo osteotomy. One of the classic adult osteotomies is the opening wedge osteotomy of the proximal tibia. This is performed in young or middle-aged adults with isolated medial compartment arthrosis of the knee. These patients and their surgeons wish to avoid total-knee arthroplasty as long as possible. By realigning the proximal tibia, the surgeon re-creates the normal mild valgus at the knee and unloads the degenerated medial compartment by shifting the mechanical axis laterally. This may buy some time before the patient's first total-knee replacement, but the procedure is falling out of favor as techniques evolve. Many of these patients now undergo a medial unicompartmental arthroplasty instead (Fig. 105-24). This procedure had been largely abandoned for awhile but is gaining popularity again with improved devices and techniques. These implants are proving nearly as durable as total knee prostheses, yet the operation and recovery are much less rigorous and it does not preclude the patient from undergoing standard total-knee arthroplasty in the future.

Another reconstructive procedure for children is epiphysiodesis. This procedure is for children with open growth plates and either limb-length discrepancy or developing angular deformity across a growth plate, often due to injury of the epiphysis. The surgeon disrupts the growth plate cartilage and secures it with either a staple, plates and screws, or a bone dowel (Fig. 105-25).

ARTHROPLASTY AND ARTHRODESIS

These topics are covered in more detail in the specific anatomic chapters that follow. Arthroplasty is the replacement of a native joint. One usually thinks of replacing the joint with hardware, especially in the hip and knee. However, other types of arthroplasty include interposition arthroplasty, in which a tendon or man-made spacer takes the place of a joint, and resection arthroplasty, in which some or all of the articular surfaces are removed but not replaced. An example of interposition arthroplasty is the resection of the

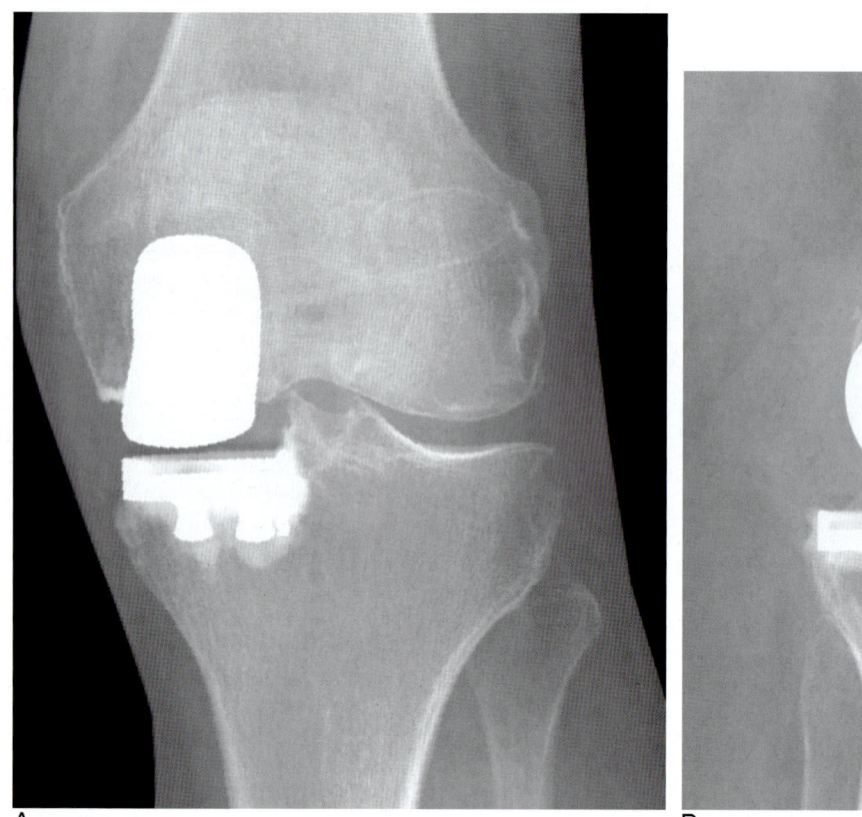
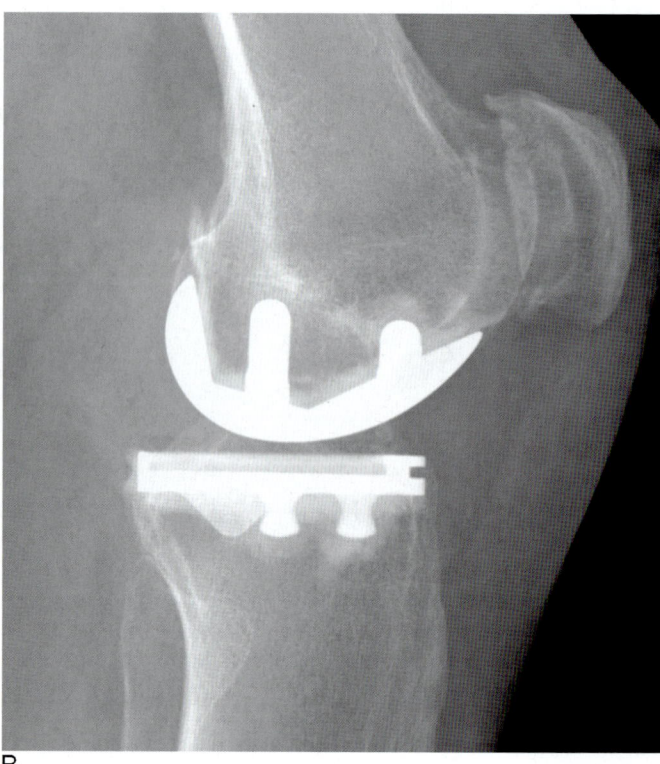

A
B

■ **FIGURE 105-24** Anteroposterior (**A**) and lateral (**B**) views of the knee show a medial unicondylar prosthesis.

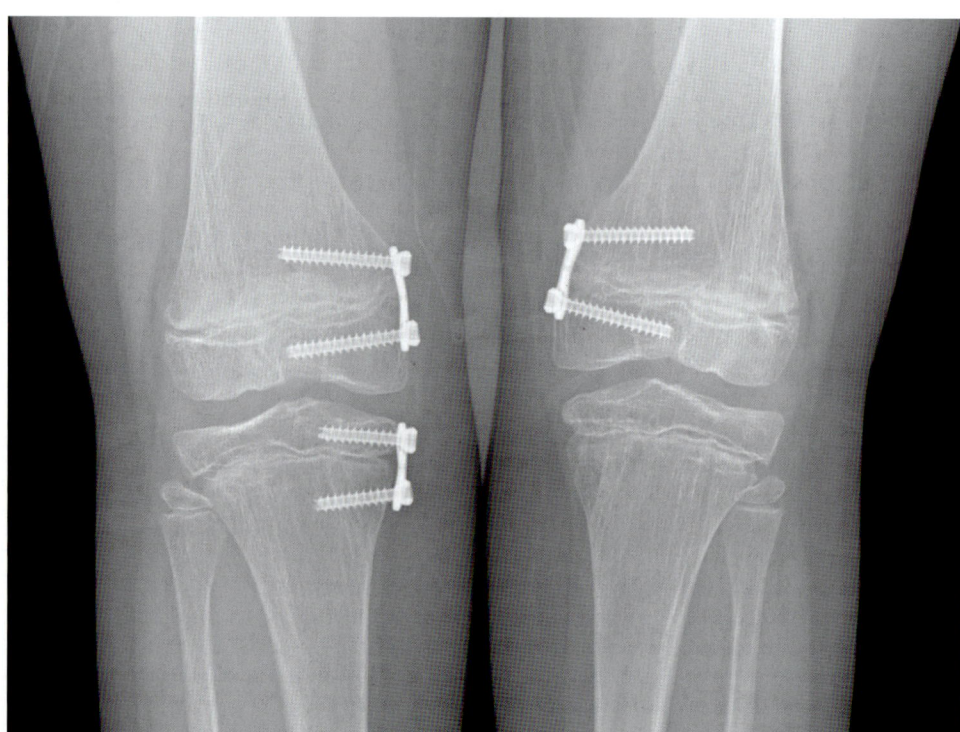

■ **FIGURE 105-25** Anteroposterior view of both knees demonstrates plate and screw devices in place in a child who has undergone epiphysiodesis.

trapezium in cases of severe first carpometacarpal joint arthrosis with interposition of a tendon to maintain appropriate length in the first ray (Fig. 105-26). Alignment is initially maintained by a Kirschner wire. The classic example of resection arthroplasty is the Girdlestone procedure, in which the femoral head and neck are resected but not replaced. Initially developed to treat tuberculous septic arthritis, occasional patients still undergo this procedure for multiply failed hip prostheses and in some cases of fracture in which the patient is too unstable for a full joint replacement procedure.

A total joint replacement requires replacement of all the surfaces that are within the synovial cavity of the joint. A hemiarthroplasty is a procedure in which only half the joint is replaced; the most common examples are the proximal femur and the proximal humerus (Fig. 105-27). Limited joint resurfacing is also occasionally a choice. This is another arena for evolution of hardware and techniques. Femoral head resurfacing had been abandoned some time ago due to high com-

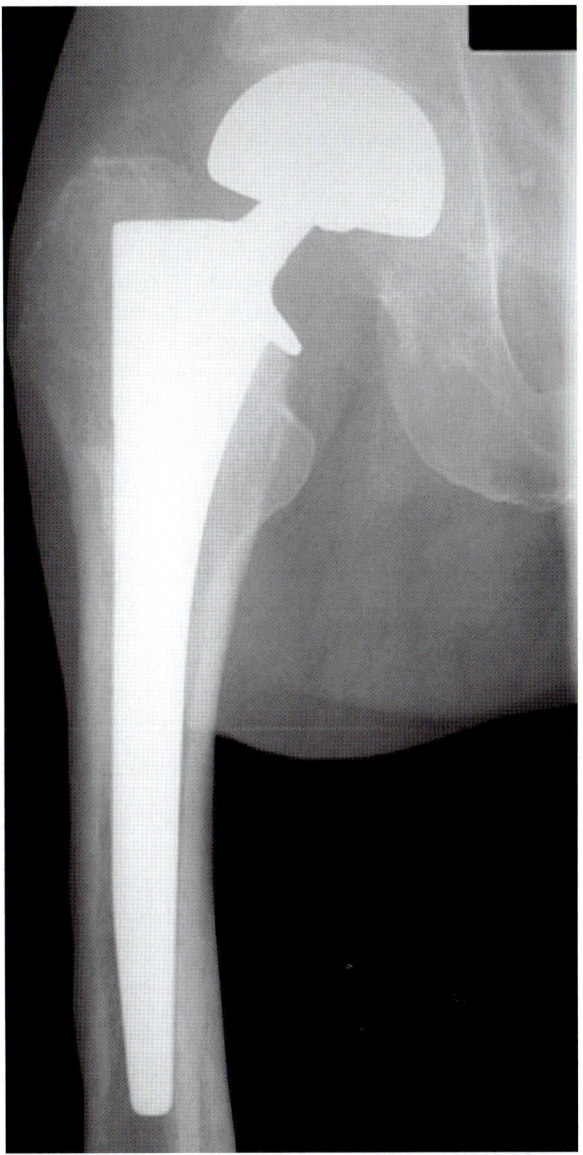

■ FIGURE 105-27 Anteroposterior view of a bipolar hemiprosthesis, with a femoral stem and head covered by a cup but with acetabular cortex intact.

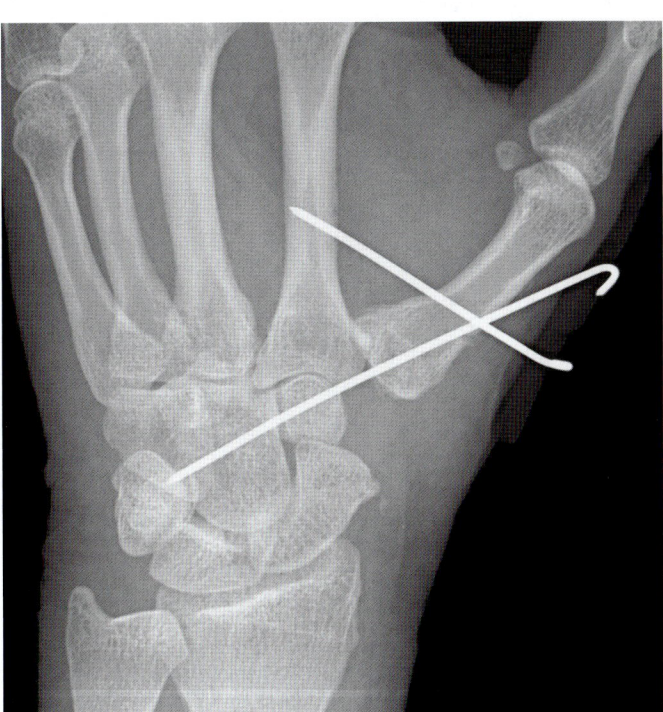

■ FIGURE 105-26 Oblique wrist image in a patient who has undergone resection of the trapezium for arthritis. There has been tendon interposition and two Kirschner wires temporarily stabilize alignment and position.

plication rates and low patient satisfaction. However, improved devices and techniques, including adding a medullary peg to stabilize the femoral head resurfacing, and additional resurfacing of the acetabulum, have revived this procedure. Because of the lack of long-term follow-up studies and the lingering skepticism regarding this procedure, it should be several years before it gains widespread use.

Evolution of arthroplasty continues for other joints. Improved devices and techniques have brought both total elbow and total ankle arthroplasty back into use and made them viable options for patients suffering pain and/or stiffness due to degenerative or post-traumatic arthrosis or inflammatory arthritis. Both of these joints exhibited dismal results in the early days of arthroplasty. The physiology and function of each joint were poorly understood. Hinged elbow prostheses had a high rate of pullout, and 1970s-era ankle replacements often experienced loosening of the tibial component or subsidence of the talar component. Just recently, improved understanding of the normal motion and function of these joints, in combination with improved materials and techniques, has allowed some patients to have these joints replaced rather than fused or ignored (Fig. 105-28).

There has been continual evolution regarding how best to treat the severely symptomatic wrist and the joints of the hand and foot. Replacements for the smaller joints are typically made of silicone or Silastic, sometimes with metal grommets or backing. Swanson has contributed a large number of designs, and some of these remain popular. However, relatively high rates of failure continue to encourage new designs (Fig. 105-29). Wrist prostheses have progressed from Swanson's initial silicone single-piece implant to metal and polymer joint replacements. Still, fusion of the wrist (arthrodesis) remains a common choice, as does resection arthroplasty, in which the proximal carpal row is removed. Arthrodesis remains the mainstay of treatment of recalcitrant painful degenerative joint disease of the hindfoot and midfoot, as there are no suitable prostheses for these sites. In fact, ankle arthrodesis (Fig. 105-30), typically a very effective salvage procedure to palliate pain, is still more common than the resurgent arthroplasty techniques.

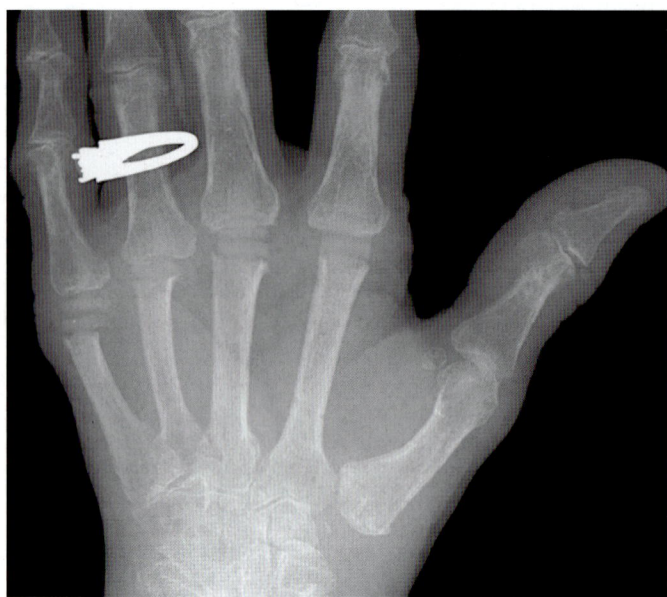

■ **FIGURE 105-29** Two-part silicone metacarpophalangeal joint prostheses are in place.

SPINE HARDWARE

Neck and back pain are ubiquitous in humans, and there are numerous nonoperative and operative treatments for maladies of the spine. Although complication and failure rates of spine surgery are relatively high, many patients find themselves resorting to this option, often multiple times. As with extremity operations, the imperfect outcomes of spine surgery continue to drive innovation in hardware and techniques. These devices and procedures are more completely covered in a subsequent chapter, with an overview of the advancements presented here.

The first effective posterior instrumentation to augment correction and fusion in scoliosis consisted of the Harrington distraction rods, soon to be coupled with Harrington compression rods (Fig. 105-31). Luque instrumentation, with rods secured to the vertebrae by sublaminar wires, and Cottrell-Dubousset rods, anchored by laminar hooks, have been joined by the Texas Scottish Rite Hospital (TSRH) and Isola systems, and current instrumentation often is a hybrid of these

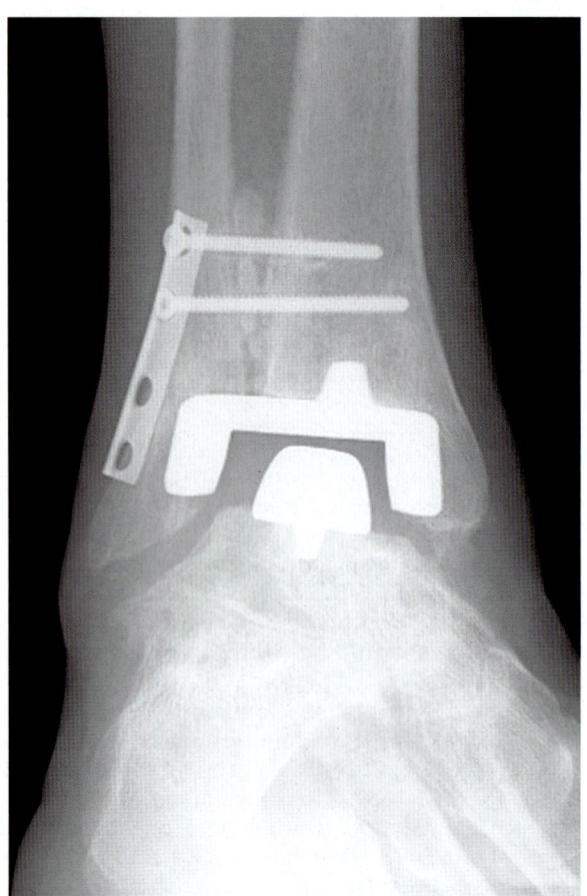

■ **FIGURE 105-28** Total ankle arthroplasty has been performed in this patient. Polyethylene tibial insert is radiolucent.

KEY POINTS

- Recent developments in lumbar spine are trending toward restoring anatomy and function, rather than just discectomy and fusion.
- Some of the newer devices include disc prostheses, interbody cages, and interspinous spacers.
- Standard plate and screw devices are no longer in use in the cervical spine. Modern cervical plates include methods to capture the screws and often allow some settling of the spine to accommodate physiologic healing.

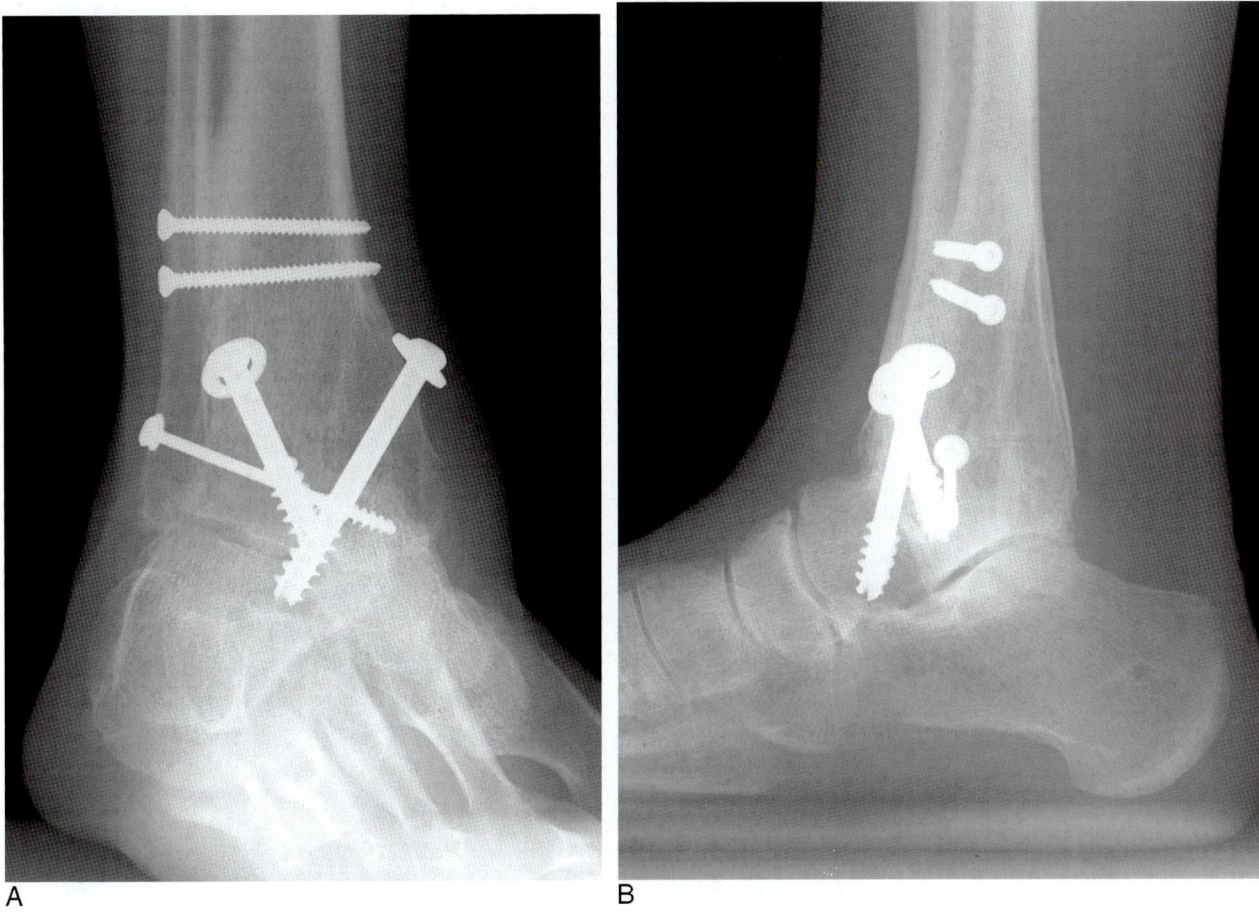

■ FIGURE 105-30   Oblique (**A**) and lateral (**B**) views of the ankle demonstrate solid arthrodesis of the ankle joint. Three cancellous screws were used for stabilization while the fusion healed.

designs. Long-segment anterior fusion systems, such as Dwyer instrumentation and Zielke instrumentation, are no longer widely used.

Lessons learned from long-segment thoracic and lumbar fusions have been adapted to shorter segments, and there is a strong trend toward posterior instrumentation to augment fusion to accompany spinal canal decompressions (Fig. 105-32). As understanding of normal spine mechanics and physiology improves, some innovations attempt to preserve or restore motion or anatomy. For instance, it is thought that many people suffering from painful degenerative disc disease have multiple causes for pain. Although the degenerated disc may be painful, abnormal motion there worsens pain. Moreover, the loss of height across the disc space and posterior elements contributes to radiculopathy. A relatively recent approach to this combination of problems has been to perform a discectomy but then restore disc height with two threaded interbody cages. If the cages are tapered, with the narrower aspect placed posteriorly, this will also restore natural lordosis at the site (Fig. 105-33). The X-stop interspinous spacer (Fig. 105-34) is a new device that restores height, especially posteriorly, and decompresses the neural foramina. Its ease of implantation and good short-term results suggest it may be a helpful first option for patients with positional neurogenic

claudication. To restore natural motion and one hopes lessen the risk of adjacent segment degeneration, effective intervertebral disc prostheses have been developed. A number of these devices for the lumbar and cervical spine are in various stages of the approval process by the U.S. Food and Drug Administration, and early and intermediate results are promising (Fig. 105-35).

Cervical spine procedures also have undergone recent evolution. Cervical disc arthroplasty mirrors the development of lumbar disc prostheses. Plate and screw technology for anterior fusion have made vast improvements since the early 1990s. There are several plates available now that have captured screw technology. In these plates, the screws will not back out or extrude. Flat plates without captured screw technology, such as the Caspar plate, are an anachronism. Additionally, some of these plates allow variable angling or translation of their screws, permitting some natural subsidence of the spine as there is resorption of the ends of interbody bone grafts, a common part of the normal healing process. Another advance has been the development of laminoplasty for patients with long-segment cervical canal stenosis. In this procedure, the canal is decompressed by hinging the posterior elements and opening up the canal without removing the posterior elements. Osteotomies are secured with small plates or suture in this procedure.

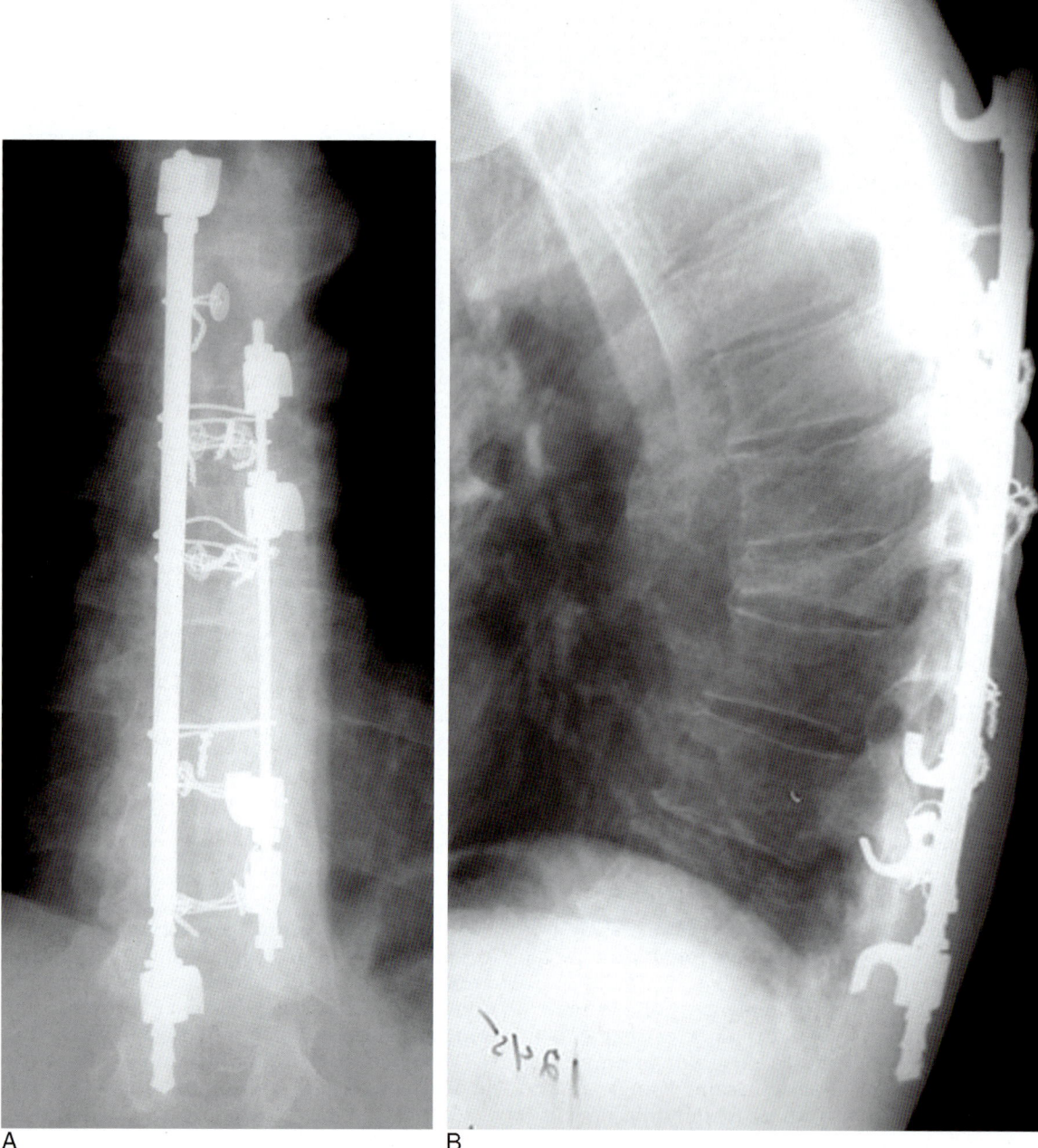

A   B

■ **FIGURE 105-31**   Anteroposterior (**A**) and lateral (**B**) views of the lumbar spine in a patient instrumented with Harrington distraction (*right*) and compression rods. On the lateral view, note the pullout of the superior laminar hook.

BIOLOGIC IMPLANTS

There is a growing trend toward using devices and substances that are biodegradable and/or augment bone healing and fusion.

Bone Graft Substitutes

Bone graft is extremely useful in filling voids, providing structural support, and augmenting osseous fusion. However, allograft (from another person) is in limited supply and engenders risks of using allogeneic material while

KEY POINTS

- Calcium phosphate and calcium sulfate are bone graft substitutes, resembling bone cement, but they are eventually reabsorbed by the body, with bone taking their place.
- Bone morphogenetic protein is another bone graft substitute, which encourages the speed of osseous fusion.
- Bioabsorbable implants are being used more frequently. They are radiolucent on radiographs but are of uniformly low signal intensity on MRI.

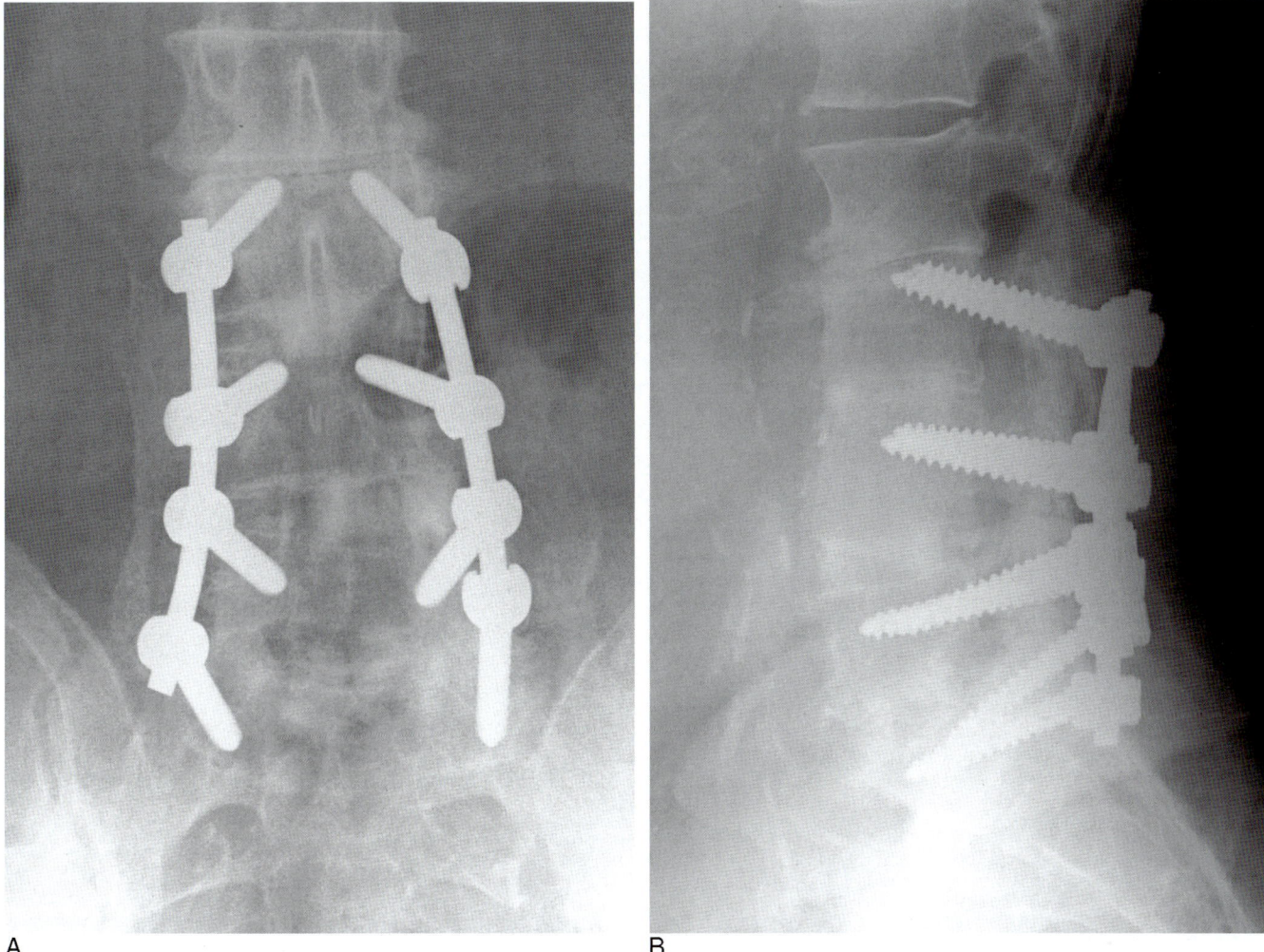

A   B

■ **FIGURE 105-32**   Anteroposterior (**A**) and lateral (**B**) views of the lumbar spine in a patient who has undergone posterior decompression supplemented by posterior fusion from L3 through the sacrum. Note the adjacent segment degeneration at the L2-L3 disc, which was new in the last year.

harvesting autograft from the patient often leaves donor site morbidity. The search for substitutes has resulted in a number of options. Three of the most popular are bone morphogenetic protein (BMP-2 and -7 are in use), which primarily serves to hasten osseous fusion, and calcium phosphate and calcium sulfate putty. The latter two are used to fill osseous voids, commonly in depressed calcaneal and tibial plateau fractures (Fig. 105-36). Both resemble polymethyl methacrylate (PMMA) bone cement but are eventually absorbed by the body and replaced by bone marrow, with calcium sulfate remaining in place for just a few months, as opposed to a few years for calcium phosphate. Calcium sulfate also may be formed into bioabsorbable antibiotic-impregnated beads and joint spacers for the treatment of chronic osteomyelitis or septic arthritis.

Bioabsorbable Hardware

There have been great advances in the development of bioabsorbable devices. These are implants that are used to stabilize bone or soft tissue defects until the body heals the injury. With time, the body breaks down and absorbs these devices. As such, these implants need to be stable

long enough to ensure healing of the defect and strong enough to withstand the considerable forces that daily activities put on many body parts. Yet their chief advantage is in their eventual disappearance and the lack of a need to be retrieved. Additionally, because of their dissolution, they will not generate stress shielding in the bone. Another touted advantage is their marked reduction in artifact generation on postoperative CT and MRI. Their imaging characteristics are a mixed blessing for radiologists, however, because they may be unaware that one of these radiolucent devices is even present!

The longest standing and most widely used devices in this category are absorbable sutures, such as PDS. Just in the past few years, bioabsorbable implants have been developed and approved for a wide range of applications, including darts and tacks to repair tears of the knee menisci and glenoid labral tears; suture anchors, most widely used in rotator cuff reattachments; numerous small and even a few large plate and screw devices, mostly used in craniofacial surgery; lumbar intervertebral cage devices; and a variety of small nails and tacks for securing small fracture fragments and osteochondral lesions. Current polymers in use in this field are mostly

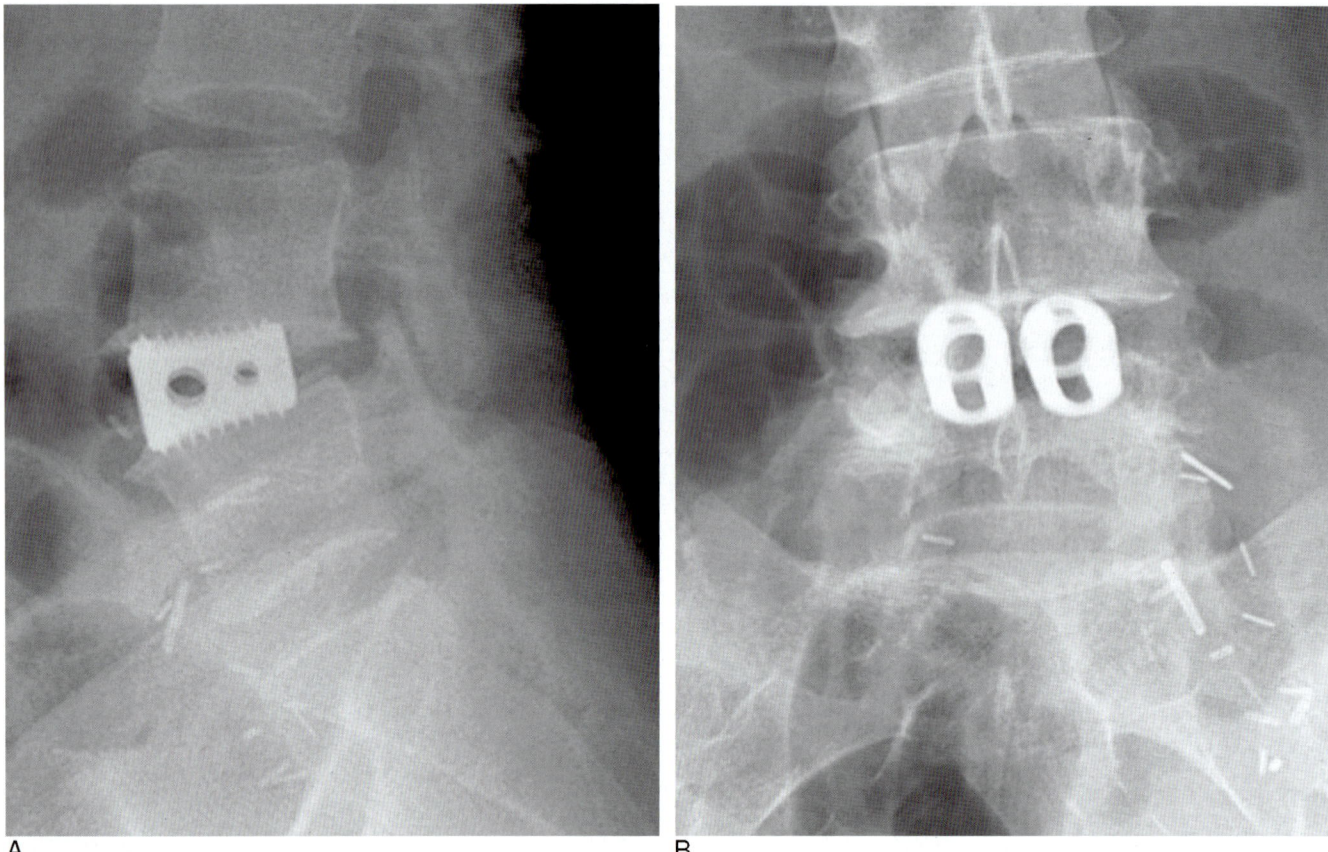

■ **FIGURE 105-33** Anteroposterior (**A**) and lateral (**B**) views of a pair of tapered, threaded LT interbody cages at the L4-5 level. Note the restoration of disc space height and lordosis at this level.

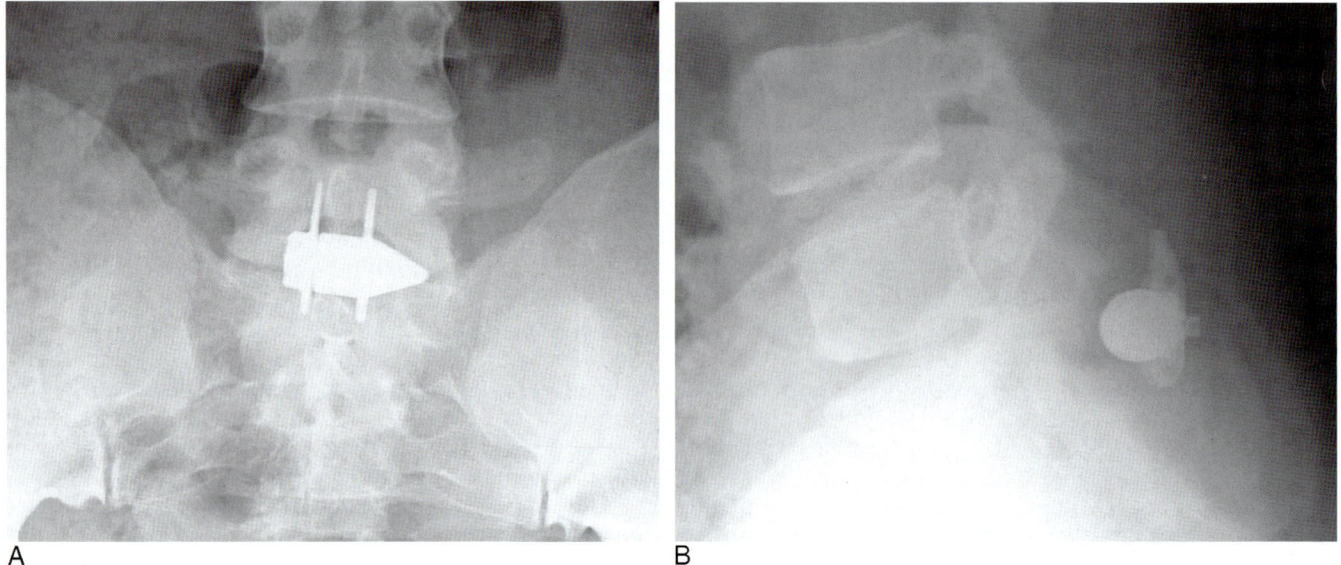

■ **FIGURE 105-34** Anteroposterior (**A**) and lateral (**B**) views of the lower lumbar spine reveal an X-stop interspinous spacer placed between the spinous processes of L5 and S1. The S1 vertebra is anomalous and has a larger spinous process than is typical.

polymers of polylactic acid (PLA) and polyglycolic acid (PGA). These are lucent on radiographs. On CT, they usually have attenuation in the range of soft tissue. At MR, these devices are uniformly low signal on all sequences and do not exhibit susceptibility artifact (blooming) on gradient-recalled-echo sequences unless there is adjacent micrometallic debris. The main imaging findings of concern with these devices are failure of fixation, which should be obvious; dislodgement, such as with rotator cuff anchors and Smart Nails securing knee osteochondral lesions; and aggressive synovitis, more commonly seen with the more rapidly resorbing PGA than with PLA.

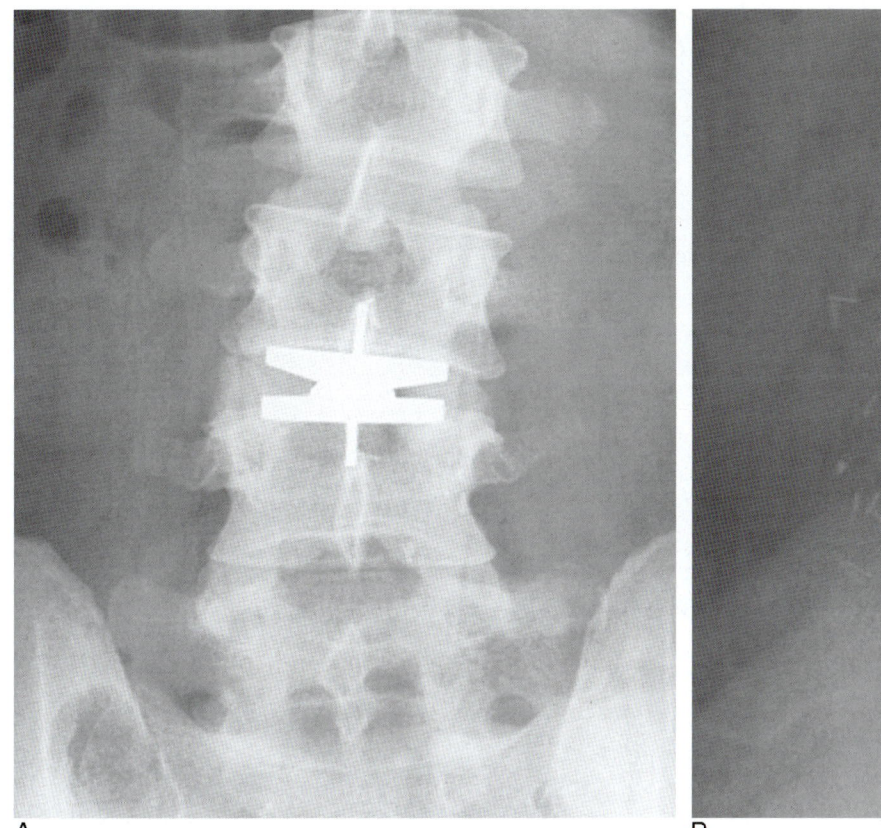
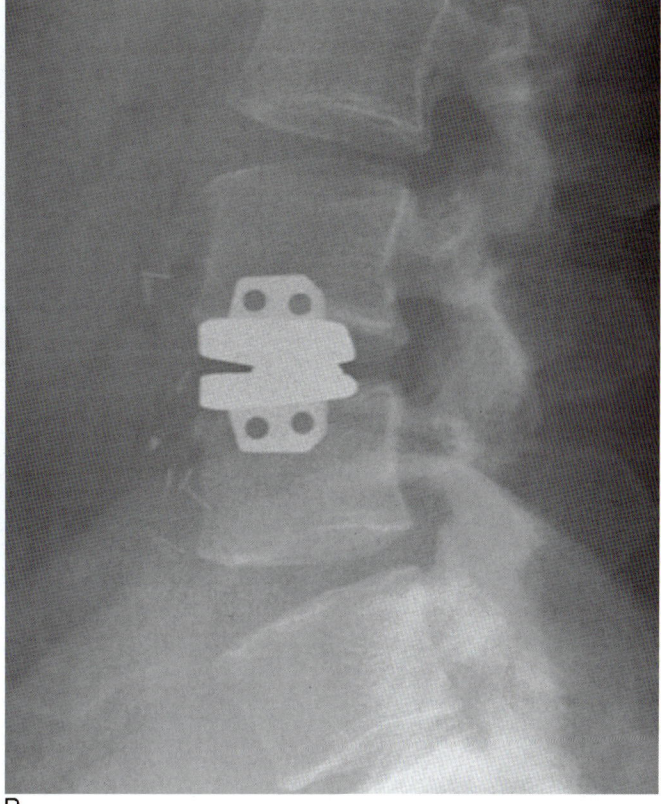

A   B

■ **FIGURE 105-35** Anteroposterior (**A**) and lateral (**B**) views of a Maverick lumbar disc prosthesis at L3-L4. The sagittal keels on the device anchor the pieces into the end plates and provide immediate stability. This is a metal-on-metal prosthesis.

POSTOPERATIVE IMAGING AND COMPLICATIONS

Postoperative Imaging

In most settings, radiographs will be the first and only imaging study needed to evaluate a patient's postoperative status. Even when there are specific complaints raising questions of complications, radiographs are usually indicated first and may provide all the necessary information. Ultrasonography is a powerful tool in certain situations, but this technique is not widely used for this purpose by radiologists, especially in the United States. Various scintigraphic techniques are sometimes quite helpful.

For many years, the literature has been replete with statements that CT and MRI are poor choices to evaluate patients with significant metallic implants, due primarily to beam hardening (CT) and susceptibility (MR) artifacts. That has been the mantra of radiologists and our referring colleagues until recently. However, with recent advances in CT technology and MR sequences and knowledge, many metallic implants can be imaged without significant loss of relevant information. One excellent review of this topic is the article by White and Buckwalter listed in the suggested readings section of this chapter. Most of the suggestions are summarized here.

With the development and evolution of modern multidetector CT scanners and improved multiplanar reformat

capability, current CT scanners produce much less beam-hardening artifact than prior generations of scanners. For CT, geometry of the implant matters. The less metal in any one axial image, the less artifact there will be. Therefore, positioning an implant with its long axis perpendicular to the axial plane will reduce artifact. Unfortunately, most

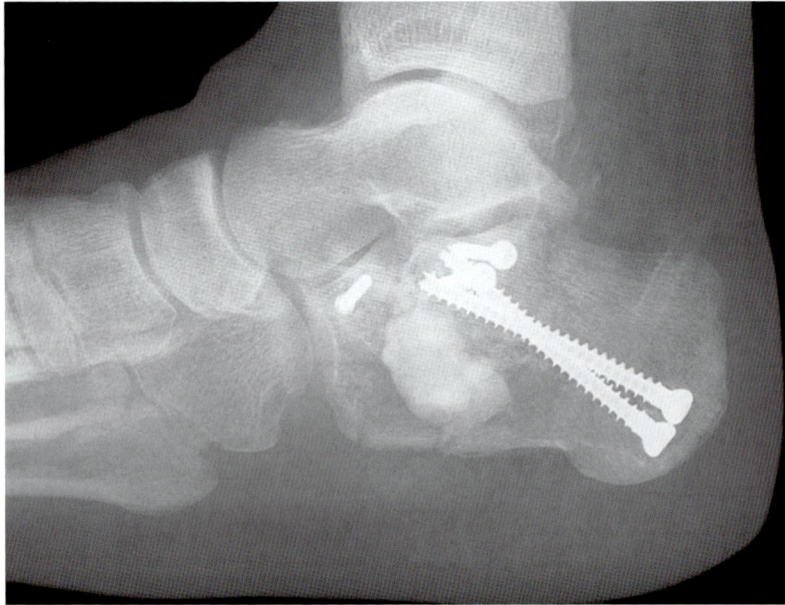

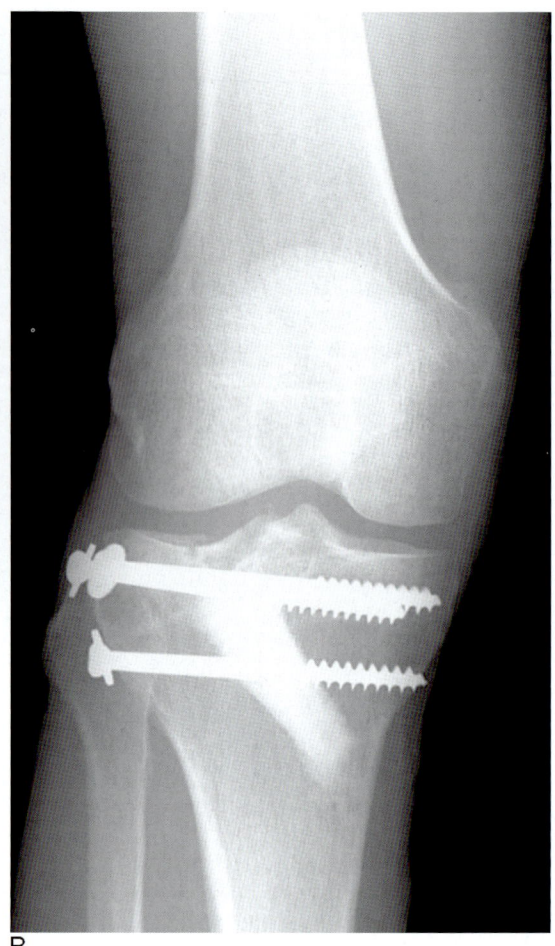

■ **FIGURE 105-36** Bone graft substitute: lateral view of the calcaneus (**A**) and anteroposterior view of the knee (**B**) show dense calcium phosphate filling osseous defects after reduction of fractures.

implanted hardware allows little leeway regarding patient positioning. An additional consideration to reduce scatter artifact at CT is to increase the exposure factors. This is achieved better with significantly increasing the mAs than the kVp. It is also known that using a soft tissue/ standard reconstruction algorithm, and then viewing in bone windows, will diminish beam-hardening artifact. In fact, widening the windows will aid further in inspecting the regions nearest the metal implant. Finally, reviewing the multiplanar reformatted images that are routine with modern multidetector scanners helps to evaluate even the tissues closest to an implant.

For MRI of metallic implants, positioning again affects the scan. The longitudinal axis of the device should be aligned with the direction of B_o, the main magnetic field. Gradient-recalled-echo sequences markedly enhance susceptibility artifact and should be avoided when hardware is in the field. Fast or turbo spin-echo sequences are superior to spin-echo, and T2-weighted sequences suffer more than T1-weighted sequences. Frequency-selective fat suppression worsens susceptibility artifact, so one should use inversion recovery to serve as a fluid-sensitive sequence with fat suppression. Misregistration artifact propagates in the direction of the frequency-encoding axis but not the phase-encoding axis, so switching these axes may allow inspection of tissues near an implant. Increasing the

receiver bandwidth is another parameter adjustment that may be helpful. These hints for limiting artifacts on MRI and CT are certainly useful, but some portions of bone and soft tissues adjacent to metallic implants may be impervious to advanced imaging and may require the implant to be removed before adequate images are possible.

Infection

Osteomyelitis next to an implant often looks like osteomyelitis in an unoperated bone, except for associated artifact on CT or MRI. However, infection can behave differently when it is associated with hardware. When an implant or other foreign body is colonized by microbes, they change their phenotype and create a biofilm. This biofilm offers a protective effect against natural host defenses and creates additional barriers to penetration by antimicrobial medications. These features render eradication of the organism difficult. This is compounded by the typical reduced vascular supply in close proximity to implants. These effects are the reason that most implants must be removed to eliminate an established infection.

Infection around an implant occasionally is fulminant and will give obvious systemic clues to the process. More often, these infections are relatively indolent and cause modest alterations in laboratory values and low fevers at most. Likewise, local bone destruction around orthopedic implants is often relatively mild and the appearance seemingly innocuous. Diagnosis of these infections remains difficult at times. Certainly, sampling the local environment with microbiologic analysis is usually preferred. However, joint aspirations and bone and tissue biopsies are complicated by false-negative results, an occasional false-positive finding from a skin contaminant, reduced sensitivity in the setting of recent antibiotics, and occasional difficulty accessing the site. Of note, any time a joint aspiration is performed, some of the fluid should be submitted for cell count and differential. In an undiluted specimen, more than 2500 white cells, especially with a majority of granulocytes, indicates infection and will require removal of the prosthesis or implant regardless of the microbiologic results.

Radiographs are the first line of radiologic investigation. They are frequently negative for any signs of infection. When positive evidence is present, it usually is fairly unimpressive, consisting of mild degrees of lucency around the implant at its interface with bone (Fig. 105-37). Although extensive areas of osteolysis and aggressive periosteal reaction, or any periosteal reaction, for that matter, are strong indicators of infection, they rarely are present. When local tissue sampling is not an option due to difficult access, patient instability, or ongoing antimicrobial treatment, and the radiographs are not illuminating, scintigraphy can be very helpful. Currently, the best tool in nuclear medicine remains an indium-111–labeled white blood cell scan, although investigations into the use of positron emission tomography to evaluate for infection are showing promise.

Loosening

Loosening of an implant carries different implications based on the nature of the device. Loosening of plates, screws, and other fixation devices will often portend a lack of effective osteosynthesis at the site. A cardinal rule of hardware is that all hardware that bears a load or stress will eventually fail unless the body fuses or heals at the site. Fixation hardware is rarely intended to be a permanent solution. Instead, it provides stability and apposition of structures until they can heal. As such, when loosening of devices is discovered, one should assume that the fracture, osteotomy, or other defect is ununited or malunited.

On radiographs, loose implants are recognizable by a lucency surrounding them. This is especially true when the lucency exceeds 2 mm or increases in size after the first year (Fig. 105-38). Loose screws will often gradually retract and may eventually become expelled from the bone entirely. One of the most dramatic examples of this is cutout of a dynamic hip screw, in which the screw within the femoral head migrates through the head and into the hip joint (Fig. 105-39). Certainly, any motion of hardware between images, other than intended effects such as settling of a DHS, indicates loosening.

Catastrophic Failure

When an implant grossly breaks or the device becomes largely dissociated from the underlying bone, it is termed

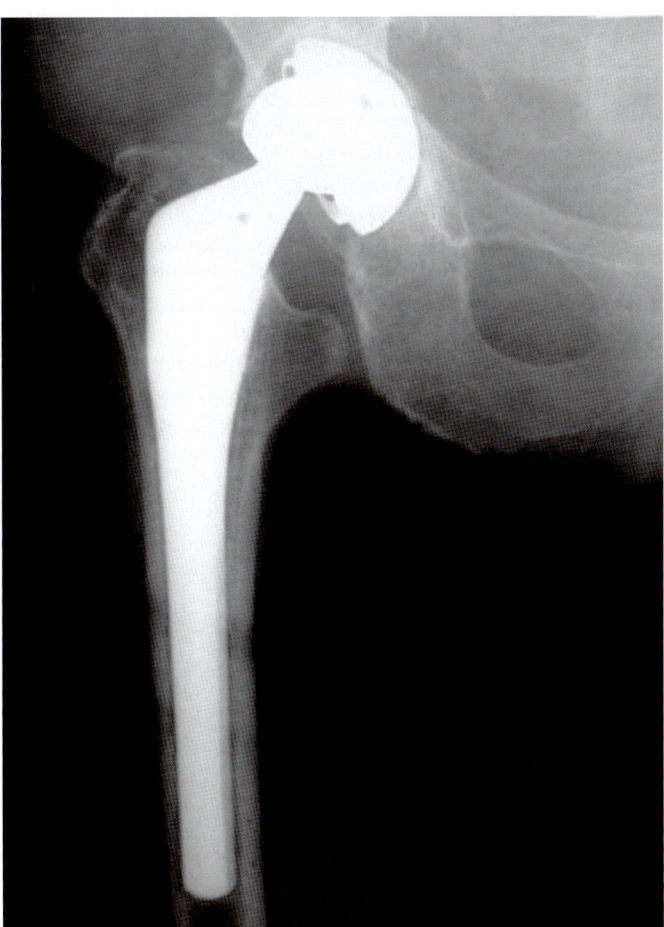

■ **FIGURE 105-37** Infection: the acetabular component is clearly too vertical and is obviously loose, but the picture is not an aggressive one and could be due to bland loosening or particle disease. Cultures at the time of revision were positive.

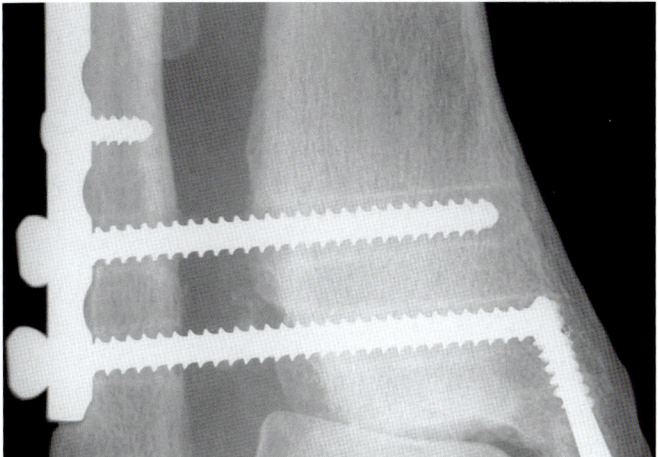

■ **FIGURE 105-38** Coned-down anteroposterior view of the ankle demonstrates failure of fixation, with lucency surrounding the syndesmotic screws, which are pulling out, and widening of the syndesmosis.

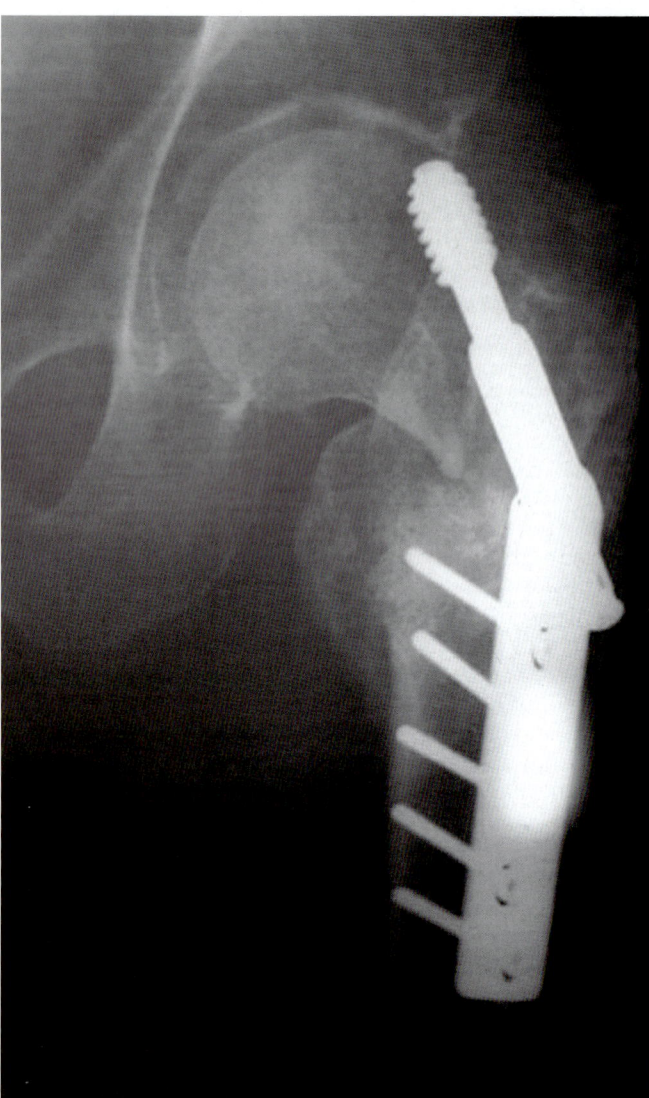

■ **FIGURE 105-39** Anteroposterior view of the hip shows nonunion of the intertrochanteric fracture with failure of fixation. The DHS screw has cut out of the femoral head.

catastrophic failure (see Fig. 105-5). The findings in these cases are obvious and merit little discussion. However, there are two significant points in this situation. First, liftoff of a plate, gross breakage of an implant, dissociation of spine fusion rods from the spine, and other such catastrophic hardware failures should raise strong suspicion for lack of fusion or fracture nonunion. The surgeon should assume such is the case and take appropriate corrective action. Second, one should at least suspect infection when there is a remarkable hardware failure.

Complications of Joint Replacements

Complications related to prostheses will be discussed in their respective anatomic chapters that follow, but because prostheses are so ubiquitous, they deserve some general comments here.

Periprosthetic fractures are most common at the distal femur, just above a knee prosthesis (Fig. 105-40). Nevertheless, because of implant-related stress shielding and the advanced age of many patients who have joint replacements (implying higher rate of osteoporosis), fractures occasionally occur around almost all types of joint replacements. They are more common at certain sites because of the inherent stresses involved and at times the surgical technique. For instance, many distal femoral periprosthetic fractures occur because the anterior femur is inappropriately notched at the time of surgical implantation, creating a stress riser that later fractures.

Loosening of joint prostheses typically causes lucency, just as is seen around other types of implants. However, loosening can also be manifest as breakage of PMMA cement, which is never normal; gross subsidence of the implant; change in alignment of the implant, or shedding of tiny metallic beads that are part of an uncemented device's porous coating (Fig. 105-41).

Infection of arthroplasty hardware most often looks normal on radiographs or resembles bland loosening. Thus, if one observes abnormal lucencies around a device on a radiograph, infection should remain in the differential diagnosis along with loosening.

Particle disease and *osteolysis* are two terms applied to a foreign body granulomatous reaction that occurs around prostheses. A whole prosthesis does not incite these chronic inflammatory responses. Instead, the culprit is microscopic debris, including PMMA particles, particles of polyethylene, and small particles of metal. Again, this reaction may manifest only with radiographic signs of loosening. However, this process often leads to more focal, large granulomas, which appear as multifocal, bubbly lucencies around a device. Eventually, particle disease leads to failure of the prosthesis, requiring surgical revision. Because the osteolysis creates large defects that complicate revision arthroplasty, and because the size of the lucencies is underestimated by radiographs, surgeons often resort to cross-sectional imaging to find and characterize known or suspected osteolysis (Fig. 105-42). With modern equipment and techniques, both CT and MR have been shown to be accurate at this task, with CT slightly better at accurate measurement of the defects and MR slightly better at demonstrating smaller lesions.

Implant-Related Sarcoma

Numerous metals have been shown to be carcinogenic when implanted into humans. Still, the occurrence of implant-related sarcoma is a true rarity. When these neoplasms occur, they are most commonly malignant fibrous histiocytomas and osteosarcomas. These sarcomas are usually quite aggressive locally and often metastasize. They must be differentiated from other aggressive but benign processes, such as infection and extensive particle disease.

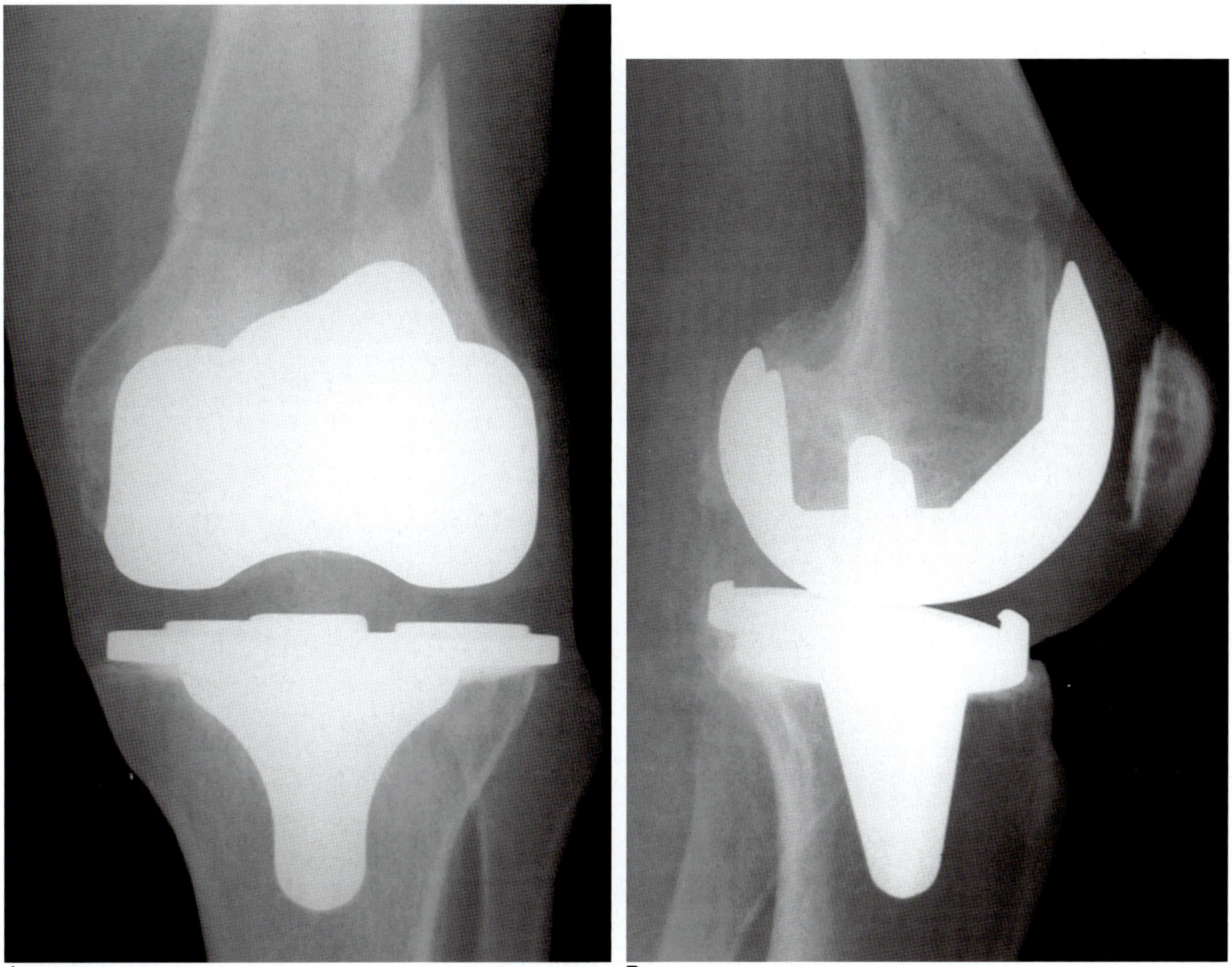

■ **FIGURE 105-40**   Anteroposterior (**A**) and lateral (**B**) views of the knee demonstrate a fracture just above the knee prosthesis. This is the most common site of all periprosthetic fractures.

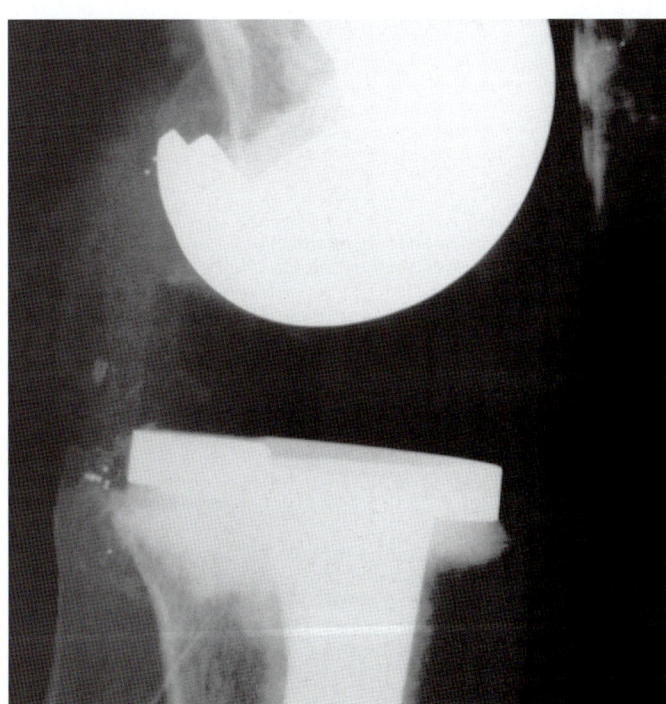

■ **FIGURE 105-41**   Lateral view of a revision knee prosthesis demonstrates tiny metallic beads that have been shed from the porous coating of the original device and now lie posterior to the tibial tray. These beads portend loosening.

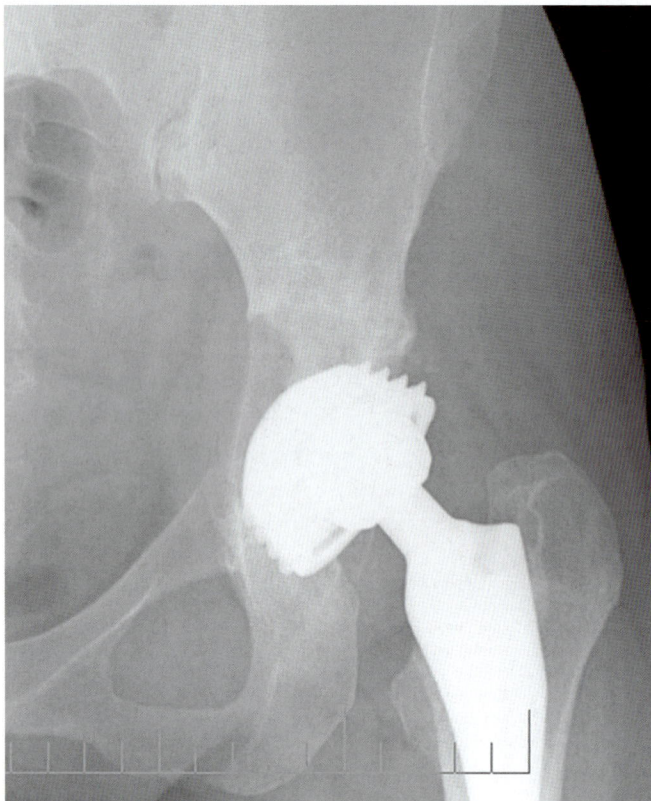

A

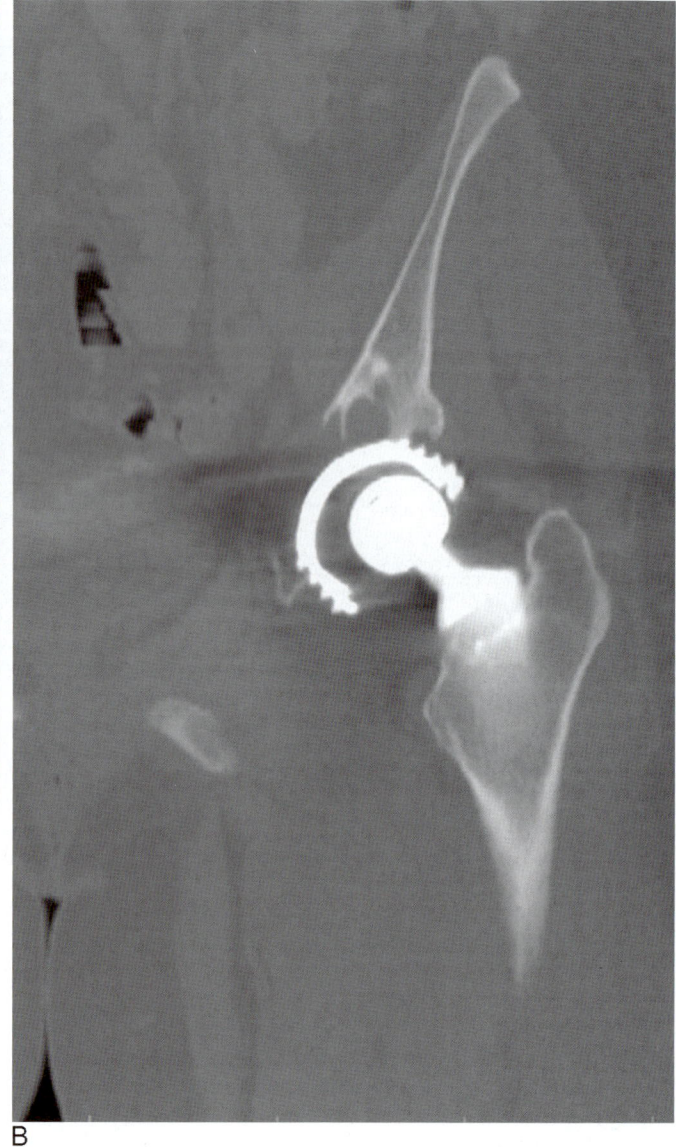

B

■ **FIGURE 105-42** Anteroposterior radiograph (**A**) and coronal reformatted CT scan (**B**) of the left hip: there is extensive osteolysis in the acetabulum deep to the prosthesis. Despite the hardware, the CT images are exquisite.

SUGGESTED READINGS

Allen AM, Ward WG, Pope TL Jr. Imaging of the total knee arthroplasty. Radiol Clin North Am 1995; 33:289–303.

Anderson DG, Albert TJ. Bone grafting, implants, and plating options for anterior cervical fusions. Orthop Clin North Am 2002; 33:317–328.

Andrews CL. Evaluation of the postoperative spine: spinal instrumentation and fusion. Semin Musculoskelet Radiol 2000; 4:259–279.

Boden SD, Balderston RA, Heller JG, et al. Disc replacements: this time will we really cure low-back and neck pain? J Bone Joint Surg Am 2004; 86:411–422.

Brems JJ. Complications of shoulder arthroplasty: infections, instability, and loosening. Instruct Course Lect 2002; 51:29–39.

Chiang PP, Burke DW, Freiberg AA, Rubash HE. Osteolysis of the pelvis: evaluation and treatment. Clin Orthop Relat Res 2003; (417):164–174.

Ciccone WJ 2nd, Motz C, Bentley C, Tasto JP. Bioabsorbable implants in orthopaedics: new developments and clinical applications. J Am Acad Orthop Surg 2001; 9:280–288.

Conway JD, Mont MA, Bezwada HP. Arthrodesis of the knee. J Bone Joint Surg Am 2004; 86:835–848.

Eustace S, Shah B, Mason M. Imaging orthopedic hardware with an emphasis on hip prostheses. Orthop Clin North Am 1998; 29:67–84.

Herbert AJ, Herzenberg JE, Paley D. A review for pediatricians on limb lengthening and the Ilizarov method. Curr Opin Pediatr 1995; 7:98–105.

Keel SB, Jaffe KA, Petur Nielsen G, Rosenberg AE. Orthopaedic implant-related sarcoma: a study of twelve cases. Mod Pathol 2001; 14:969–977.

King GJ. New frontiers in elbow reconstruction: total elbow arthroplasty. Instruct Course Lect 2002; 51:43–51.

Kostuik JP, Connolly PJ, Esses SI, Suh P. Anterior cervical plate fixation with the titanium hollow screw plate system. Spine 1993; 18:1273–1278.

Krego PJ, Stannard JA, Zlowodzki M, Cole PA. Treatment of distal femur fractures using the less invasive stabilization system. J Orthop Trauma 2004; 18:509–520.

Manaster BJ. From the RSNA refresher courses. Total hip arthroplasty: radiographic evaluation. RadioGraphics 1996; 16:645–660.

Marks RM. Arthrodesis of the first metatarsophalangeal joint. Instruct Course Lectures 2005; 54:263–268.

Miller TT. Imaging of knee arthroplasty. Eur J Radiol 2005; 54:164-177.

Mohaideen A, Nagarkatti D, Banta JV, Foley CL. Not all rods are Harrington—an overview of spinal instrumentation in scoliosis treatment. Pediatr Radiol 2000; 30:110-118.

Palestro CJ, Love C, Tronco GG, Tomas MB. Role of radionuclide imaging in the diagnosis of postoperative infection. RadioGraphics 2000; 20:1649-1660; discussion 1660-1643.

Sanders WP, Truumees E. Imaging of the postoperative spine. Semin Ultrasound CT MR 2004; 25:523-535.

Slongo TF. The choice of treatment according to the type and location of the fracture and the age of the child. Injury 2005; 36:S-A12-S-A19.

Stover MD, Beaule PE, Matta JM, Mast JW. Hip arthrodesis: a procedure for the new millennium? Clin Orthop Relat Res 2004; (418):126-133.

Syed AA, Agarwal M, Giannoudis PV, et al. Distal femoral fractures: long-term outcome following stabilization with the LISS. Injury 2004; 35:599-607.

Taljanovic MS, Jones MD, Hunter TB, et al. Joint arthroplasties and prostheses. RadioGraphics 2003; 23:1295-1314.

Temmerman OP, Raijmakers PG, Berkhof J, et al. Accuracy of diagnostic imaging techniques in the diagnosis of aseptic loosening of the femoral component of a hip prosthesis: a meta-analysis. J Bone Joint Surg Br 2005; 87:781-785.

Vinh DC, Embil JM. Device-related infections: a review. J Long Term Eff Med Implants 2005; 15:467-488.

Walde TA, Weiland DE, Leung SB, et al. Comparison of CT, MRI, and radiographs in assessing pelvic osteolysis: a cadaveric study. Clin Orthop Relat Res 2005; (437):138-144.

White LW, Buckwalter KA. Technical considerations: CT and MR imaging in the postoperative orthopedic patient. Semin Musculoskelet Radiol 2002; 6:5-17.

Yu GV, Vincent AL, Khoury WE, Schinke TL. Techniques of digital arthrodesis: revisiting the old and discovering the new. Clin Podiatr Med Surg 2004; 21:17-50.

Zdeblick TA, Phillips FM. Interbody cage devices. Spine 2003; 28: S2-S7.

106

Postoperative Imaging of the Shoulder

Babu Paruchuri and Michael Zlatkin

Recurrent or persistent pain is a common complaint after shoulder surgery. MRI is often performed in the postoperative setting as a noninvasive means of determining the etiology of postoperative pain. Numerous surgical and arthroscopic techniques are available to the surgeon, and many of these procedures result in a change to the normal anatomy of the shoulder. An accurate interpretation of a postoperative shoulder MR image requires a thorough understanding of the surgical techniques and their effect on the local anatomy. In this chapter we describe the commonly performed surgical procedures used to treat impingement, rotator cuff disease, and shoulder instability. The normal expected postoperative MR appearance is then described, followed by a discussion of the MR appearance of recurrent pathologic processes and surgical complications.

Shoulder surgery is usually performed as either an open or an arthroscopic procedure or occasionally as a combination procedure referred to as a mini-open procedure. An arthroscopic procedure utilizes several small incisions as portals for the arthroscopic instruments, whereas an open procedure is much more invasive, typically requiring detachment of the deltoid from the acromion to gain access to the shoulder. The advantages of open surgery over arthroscopy include better long-term results, improved visualization of both the rotator cuff and the subacromial space, and ease of performance for those more familiar with this approach. The disadvantages include increased perioperative morbidity and the need for detachment of the deltoid muscle. Arthroscopic procedures offer the advantage of fewer complications, better intra-articular visualization, and less postoperative pain and morbidity.[1] Mini-open procedures combine elements of both arthroscopy, and the open surgical approach and may be used by a surgeon less experienced with the arthroscope in complicated shoulder surgeries that they believe cannot be easily completed with arthroscopy alone (Tables 106-1 and 106-2).

IMAGING TECHNIQUES

With use of a dedicated shoulder coil, images are typically acquired in the axial, oblique, coronal, and oblique sagittal planes. Postoperative MRI and MR arthrography protocols from our institutions for a 1.5-Tesla magnet are included (Tables 106-4 to 106-6). MR arthrography is performed after the injection of approximately 12 mL of a 1/200 mL gadolinium solution. If infection is suspected, intravenous gadolinium may be utilized. In situations in which use of intra-articular gadolinium injection is not feasible, intravenous MRI arthrography may be used as an alternative.

Susceptibility artifact from screws, suture anchors, and staples can create significant artifact. For this reason, gradient-echo sequences tend to have significant blooming artifact (Fig. 106-1). Instead, turbo and fast spin-echo imaging are useful because multiple 180-degree pulses help to minimize the degree of magnetic susceptibility artifact. Fat saturation will also tend to be less reliable owing to the presence of magnetic susceptibility effects from adjacent metal and thus reduced magnetic field homogeneity. Fast spin-echo inversion recovery may provide a better solution in these circumstances. These artifacts will typically be more prominent in the frequency encoding direction, and adjustments should be made according to the area of interest in a particular study.

Subacromial Decompression

Description

Via an open[3] or arthroscopic approach,[4] a combination of shavers and burs are used to remove the anteroinferior aspect of the acromion from the level of the acromioclavicular (AC) joint to the level of the deltoid insertion (see Fig. 106-1). The subacromial bursa, if inflamed, is often resected at the time of the subacromial decompression. The coracoacromial ligament, if thickened, may be

KEY POINTS

- In the postoperative shoulder, gradient-echo sequences and fat-saturation sequences tend to have significant magnetic susceptibility. Turbo and fast spin-echo imaging as well as STIR sequences have less magnetic susceptibility artifact.
- MR arthrography is an excellent means of assessing capsulolabral structures and tendon integrity after repair.
- Subacromial decompression usually involves acromioplasty, subacromial bursa removal, coracoacromial ligament partial resection, osteophyte removal and, at times, AC joint removal. This procedure is often performed in conjunction with cuff repair and débridement.
- Changes in the acromion configuration to a flatter undersurface, scar tissue, metallic artifact, acromion fibrosis, absence of the subacromial bursa, or persistent subacromial fluid are all normal postoperative MRI findings after subacromial decompression.
- Potential complications of subacromial decompression include inadequate acromioplasty, progression of underlying rotator cuff disease, failure to recognize an os acromiale, or secondary impingement due to anterior instability.
- Rotator cuff repair technique depends on the degree of tendon tear, symptomatology, and age of the patient and may range from simple débridement to tendon-to-bone or tendon-to-tendon repair.
- Normal postoperative findings after cuff repair include tendon medialization, creation of a surgical trough, granulation tissue formation, and metallic/suture artifact.
- Potential complications of cuff repair include recurrent cuff tear, iatrogenic tears, inadequate acromioplasty, and failure to recognize AC joint arthrosis or chondral defects that may mimic cuff pathology.
- Instability repair may be accomplished via direct or indirect repair. Direct repair includes reattachment of capsulolabral structures (e.g., Bankart repair) or capsulorrhaphy. Indirect repair involves indirect tightening of the joint capsule without actual repair of the detached labrum/capsule and is less frequently performed, owing to a high rate of complications and patient dissatisfaction.
- Anterior instability is typically treated with surgical repair via Bankart repair. Multidirectional and posterior instability are usually treated surgically only after conservative measures, including physical therapy and activity modification, have failed.
- MR arthrography and ABER positioning may be particularly useful in assessing the integrity of the capsulolabral complex.
- Complications for instability repair include recurrent labral tear, overtight repair, or detached staples or tacks.
- Complications common to subacromial decompression, rotator cuff repair, and glenohumeral instability include deltoid detachment, adhesive capsulitis, synovitis, abscess formation, osteomyelitis, chondrolysis, and hematoma formation.

TABLE 106-1 Open versus Arthroscopic Procedures

	Advantages	Disadvantages
Open Procedures	Better long term results	Increased perioperative morbidity
	Improved visualization of cuff and subacromial space	Detachment of deltoid
	Ease of performance	
Arthroscopic Procedures	Fewer perioperative complications	Lack of experience on the part of the surgeon
	Improved intra-articular visualization	Poorer long-term results
	Less perioperative morbidity	

TABLE 106-2 Indications for Subacromial Decompression

- Symptoms and physical signs consistent with impingement
- Failure of conservative management through rehabilitation
- Presence of severe coexisting cuff disease requiring subacromial decompression in combination with cuff repair
- Young active patients may require earlier intervention.
- Preoperative MRI findings consistent with impingement including severe acromioclavicular joint degenerative disease, type 3 acromion, and thick coracoacromial ligament

along with the distal 2.5 cm of the clavicle, referred to as a Mumford procedure (Fig. 106-2). Prominent osteophytes may also be resected.

Indications, Contraindications, Purpose, and Underlying Mechanics

The basic goal of subacromial decompression is to treat extrinsic impingement of the rotator cuff by resecting those areas of the osseous outlet and acromion that result in narrowing of the supraspinatus outlet. Pain over the anterolateral and superior aspect of the shoulder may be elicited or exacerbated by passive forward elevation of the arm (Neer sign) or by internal rotation that brings the greater tuberosity beneath the anterior aspect of the acromion (Hawkins sign). The impingement test involves injection of lidocaine into the subacromial space. Significant relief of symptoms after injection is considered specific in ascribing pain to rotator cuff pathology that may benefit from subacromial decompression.[5]

Nonoperative management of overuse syndromes includes rehabilitation such as capsular stretching, rotator cuff and scapulothoracic strengthening, and patient education with regard to alterations in athletic participation and training or job modification. Modification of activity is geared to reducing repetitive overhead use of the arm. Oral anti-inflammatory agents or corticosteroid injections may help reduce inflammation associated with impingement. Chronic rotator cuff problems often lead to limitations of movement and may require capsular stretching exercises as a prelude to eventual rotator cuff strengthening. Nonoperative management is typically less successful for

resected at the level of its attachment to the acromion. Many orthopedic surgeons, however, will choose to débride rather than resect the ligament, especially in younger patients, in an attempt to prevent superior migration of the humeral head. In the setting of advanced AC joint degenerative change, the AC joint may be resected

TABLE 106-3 Routine Postoperative Shoulder Sequences

Plane	Sequence	TR	TE	FOV	Slice Thickness	Slice Spacing	Matrix	Nex
Axial	MPGR	600	22	14	3	0	256×160	2
Axial	FSE FS dual echo*	2500	17/50	14	4	0.5	320×224	2
Sagittal	FSE	3000	50	14	4	0.5	320×224	2
Coronal	FSE FS dual echo*	3000	20/50	14	4	1.0	320×224	1

TR, repetition time, TE, echo time; FOV, field of view; FS, fat suppression, FSE, fast spin-echo, MPGR, multiplanar gradient-recalled-echo sequence.
*Short tau inversion recovery (STIR) imaging may be utilized if fat suppression fails.

TABLE 106-4 MR Arthrogram Protocol for Labrum Assessment

Plane	Sequence	TR	TE	FOV	Slice Thickness	Slice Spacing	Matrix	Nex
Axial	FSE FS	500	17	12	3	0.0	256×256	2
Coronal	FSE FS	4000	35–45	12	3	0.5	384×224	2
Sagittal	FSE	3000	55	14	3	0.0	320×224	2
Axial	FSE	600	15	12	2	0.0	512×256	2

TR, repetition time, TE, echo time; FOV, field of view; FS, fat suppression, FSE, fast spin-echo.
Note: Abduction and external rotation (ABER) imaging may also be performed with TR/TE 600/15, matrix 256×192, slice thickness 3 mm, Nex 2, and FOV 14.

TABLE 106-5 MR Arthrogram Protocol for Rotator Cuff Assessment

Plane	Sequence	TR	TE	FOV	Slice Thickness	Slice Spacing	Matrix	Nex
Axial	FSE FS	500	17	12	3	0.0	256×256	2
Axial	FSE FS	4000	35	12	3	0.5	384×224	2
Sagittal	FSE	3000	55	14	4	1.0	320×224	2
Coronal	FSE	600	15	12	2	0.0	512×256	2

TR, repetition time, TE, echo time; FOV, field of view; FS, fat suppression, FSE, fast spin-echo.

TABLE 106-6 Relative Contraindications to Subacromial Decompression

- Advanced age of the patient
- Minimal activity level
- Poor surgical candidate
- Unrealistic patient expectations of surgery
- Occult instability as etiology of symptoms

those younger patients with a rotator cuff tear. Small chronic rotator cuff tears in older, less active patients with normal range of motion may respond more favorably to nonoperative management. Failure to respond to nonoperative management is an indication for subacromial decompression.[5]

Preoperative MR findings of the coracoacromial arch associated with the clinical syndrome of impingement include extensive capsular hypertrophy or a large inferiorly directed osteophyte at the level of the AC joint, resulting in mass effect on the underlying cuff. Anatomic abnormalities of the anterior aspect of the acromion that can be associated with impingement include a subacromial spur or

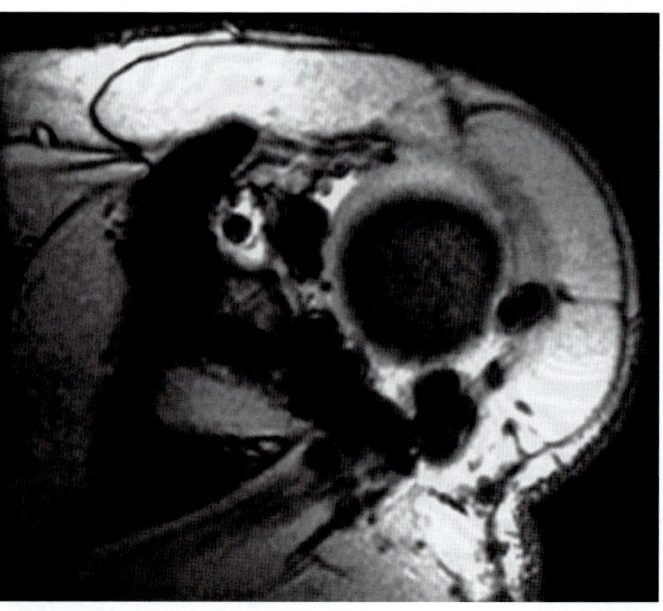

■ **FIGURE 106-1** Axial gradient-echo image reveals extensive blooming artifact after rotator cuff repair.

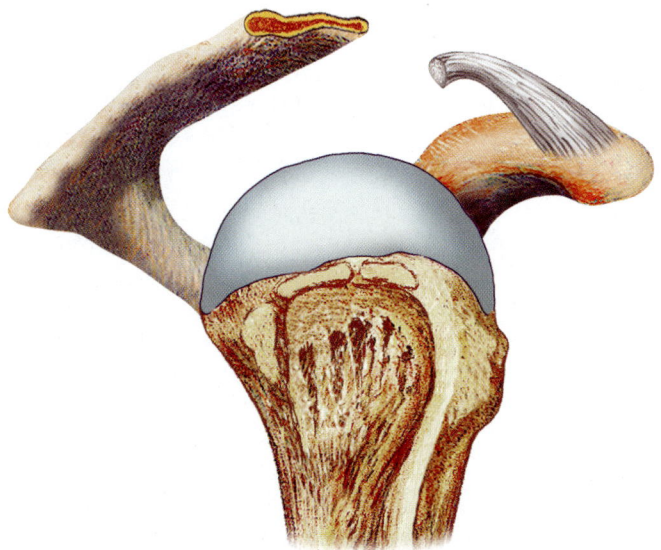

■ **FIGURE 106-2** Anterior acromioplasty. A portion of the anterior acromion has been removed along with the attachment of the coracoacromial ligament. *(From Zlatkin MB. MRI of the Shoulder, 2nd ed. Philadelphia, Lippincott Williams & Wilkins, 2003. Diagram by Salvador Beltran, MD.)*

a type 3 acromial configuration. Finally, thickening of the coracoacromial ligament (>3mm) may also predispose to impingement of the anterior rotator cuff.

Although there are no absolute contraindications to subacromial decompression, some factors such as age, activity level, general medical condition, patient expectations, and the severity of disease will determine the likelihood of proceeding to surgery. The partial-thickness tear in a young throwing athlete must be approached cautiously and examined for occult instability leading to

eccentric loading of the rotator cuff or internal glenoid impingement.[6] Acromioplasty is not indicated in this patient with occult instability unless bursal pathology is also present (see Tables 106-2 and 106-6).

Expected Appearance on Relevant Modalities

Comparison with preoperative imaging studies is of particular importance in accurately assessing the postsurgical changes as they relate to impingement. Understanding of the patient's presurgical anatomy enables the radiologist to give a more accurate description of the changes to the osseous outlet. After acromioplasty, MRI may demonstrate a change from a curved or hooked acromial configuration to a flat undersurface (see Fig. 106-3).[7] Low signal artifact from small metal fragments is often present as a result of burring of the acromion, and typically the anterior third of the acromion is not visualized due to resection (Fig. 106-4). Residual microscopic metal shavings resulting from burring of the acromion often result in extensive susceptibility artifact on MRI. If AC joint pathology was considered the source of impingement, postoperative changes may include absence of the distal 1.5 to 2.0cm of the clavicle (Mumford procedure) or widening of the AC joint (Fig. 106-5). Fibrosis often develops at the site of acromioplasty, resulting in low T1- and T2-weighted signal within the remaining acromion (Fig. 106-6).

If inflamed, the subacromial/subdeltoid bursa is often resected at the time of acromioplasty, resulting in scar tissue and residual fluid in the region of the bursa. As a result, fluid in the location of the bursa is not a useful secondary sign of cuff injury or bursal inflammation after acromioplasty (Fig. 106-7).[8] The coracoacromial ligament may also be lysed or débrided at the time of the surgery, typically near its attachment to the acromion (Fig. 106-8).

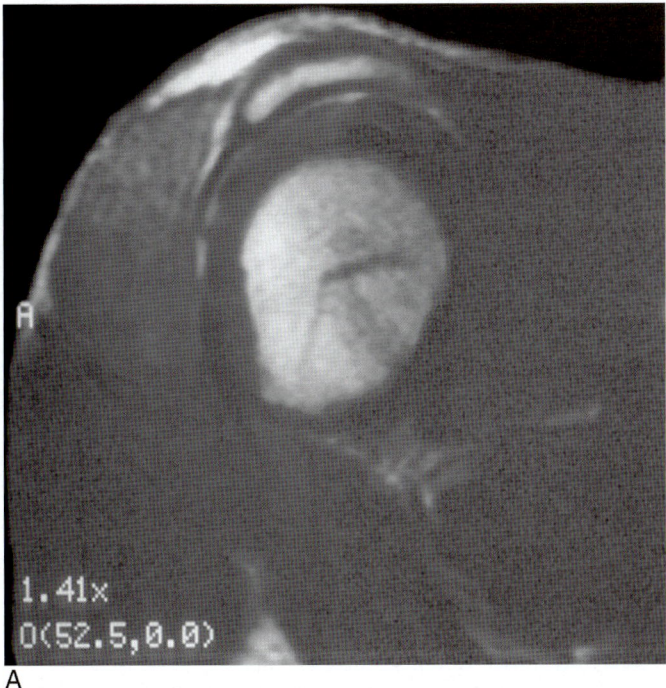

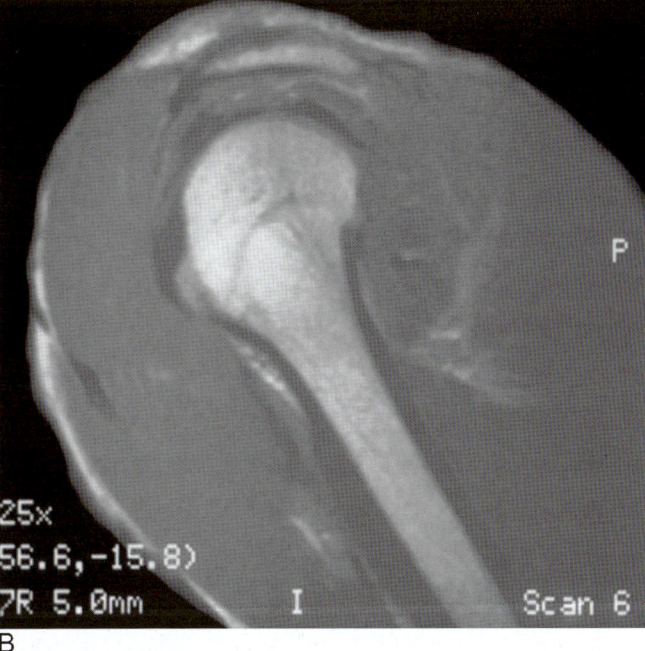

■ **FIGURE 106-3** **A,** Preoperative sagittal oblique T1-weighted MR image demonstrates a type 3 acromial configuration. **B,** After acromioplasty, an oblique sagittal T1-weighted MR image demonstrates conversion to a type 1 acromial configuration (flat undersurface).

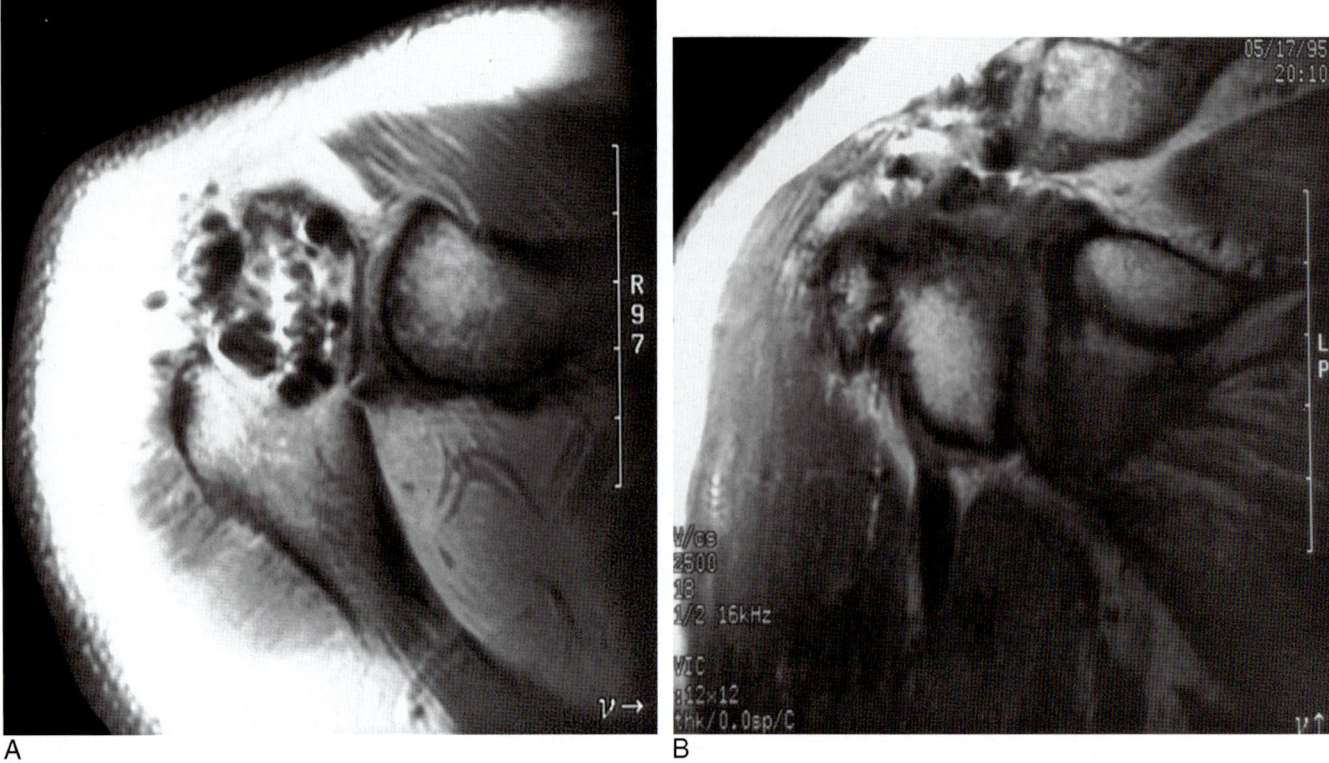

A   B

■ **FIGURE 106-4** **A,** After acromioplasty, an axial proton density–weighted image shows postsurgical artifact along the anterior aspect of the acromion. **B,** After acromioplasty, a coronal oblique proton density–weighted image shows absence of the anterior portion of the acromion.

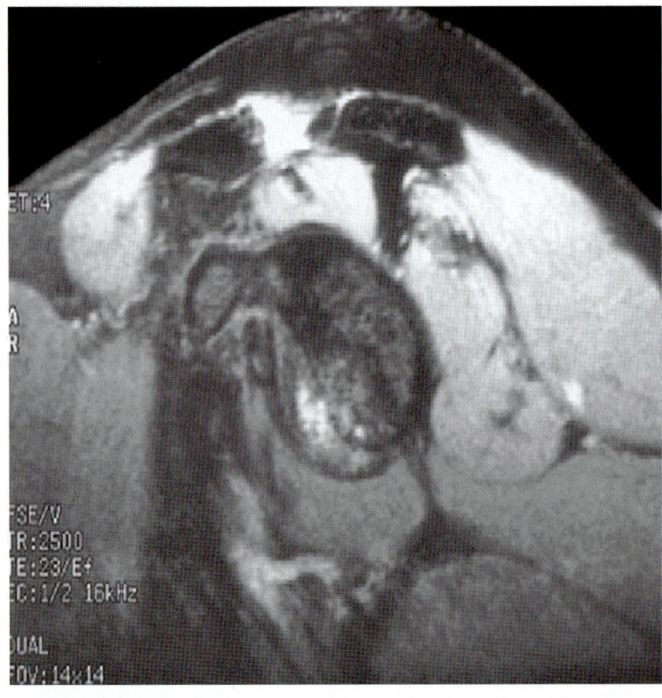

■ **FIGURE 106-5** Oblique sagittal proton density–weighted image reveals widening of the acromioclavicular joint after joint excision.

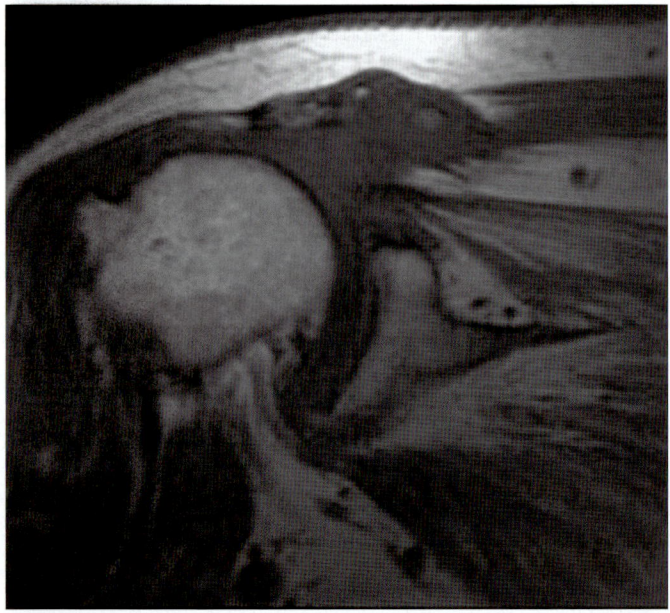

■ **FIGURE 106-6** Acromion fibrosis. Coronal T1-weighted MR image reveals decreased signal in the acromion as a result of fibrosis after acromioplasty. The patient also has a full-thickness tear of the supraspinatus with tendon retraction and fatty atrophy.

After subacromial decompression without rotator cuff repair there may be slight improvement in the altered MR signal intensity seen within the rotator cuff tendon and peritendinous tissues; however, most changes of tendinosis and additional alterations in the tendon such as bursal or articular surface fraying or partial tear usually persist.[9]

Potential Complications and Radiologic Appearance

There are many potential sources of continued or recurrent pain after subacromial decompression. One source of pain is inadequate acromioplasty. Sagittal and coronal MR images are typically most helpful in assessing for the presence of persistent anatomic changes of the osseous outlet that may be associated with continued impingement, such as residual spur formation along the undersurface of the acromion that indents the supraspinatus muscle or tendon (Fig. 106-9). After acromioplasty, the patient may continue to have pain because of osteoarthritis of the AC joint that was not addressed at the time of surgery or progression of disease in the region of the AC joint (Fig. 106-10).[10] An additional cause for persistent impingement would be the formation of extensive postoperative scarring interposed between the cuff tendon and the remaining acromion.

The persistence or progression of rotator cuff disease is also a common source of pain after acromioplasty (Fig. 106-11).[8] This may occur because of inadequate decompression or the natural progression of cuff disease not treated at the time of acromioplasty. Because many of these patients have coexisting disease of the rotator cuff disease to some degree, MRI is indicated in the setting

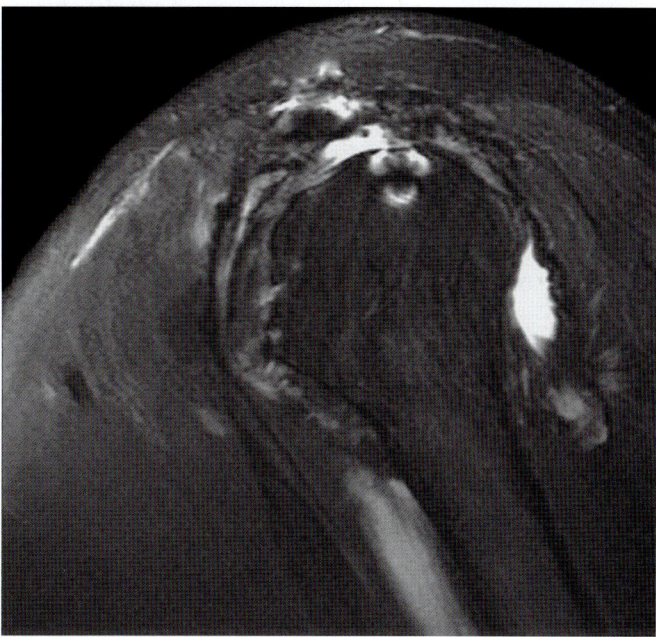

■ **FIGURE 106-8** Postoperative appearance of the coracoacromial ligament. Oblique sagittal fat-saturated proton density–weighted MR image shows resection of the coracoacromial ligament at its distal attachment to the acromion after acromioplasty.

of persistent postoperative symptoms. Clinical findings such as night pain, loss of motion, and weakness are not considered to be specific. Rotator cuff tendinosis may progress to a tear, or unrecognized partial or small complete tears may extend (see Fig. 106-11).

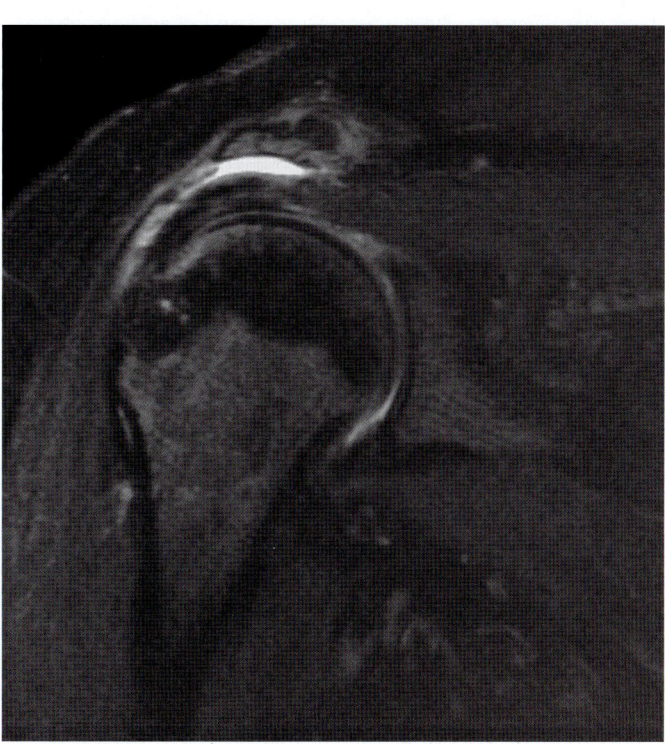

■ **FIGURE 106-7** Subacromial fluid is noted after acromioplasty on this oblique coronal fat-saturated T2-weighted MR image. This does not suggest a cuff tear or bursitis.

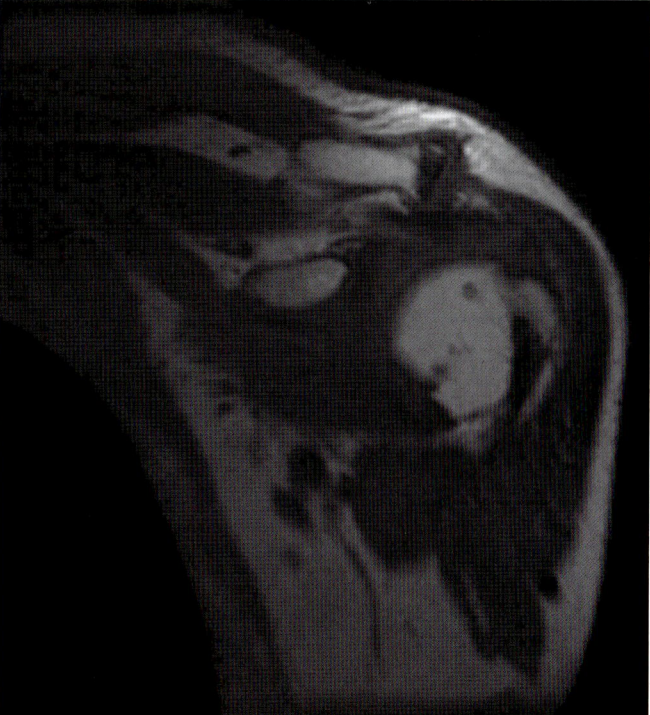

■ **FIGURE 106-9** Post-acromioplasty pain. Oblique coronal T1-weighted image shows persistent mass effect on the supraspinatus muscle from an osteophyte arising along the undersurface of the clavicle after acromioplasty.

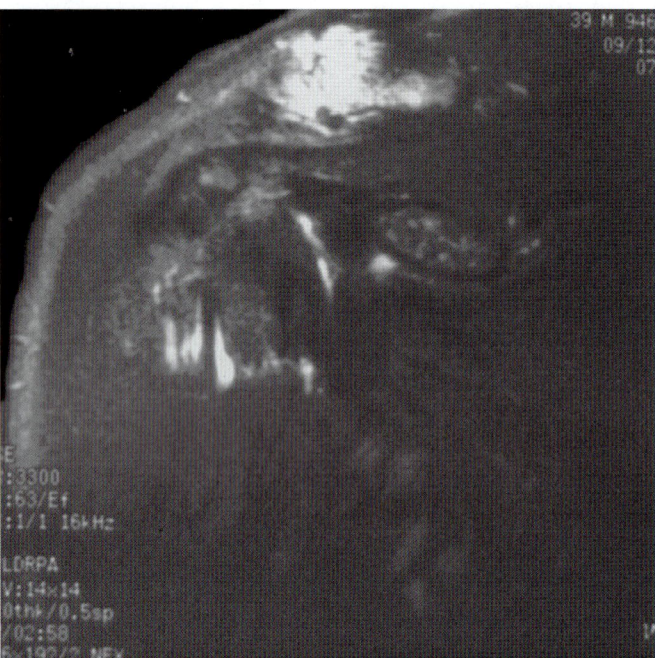

■ **FIGURE 106-10** Post-acromioplasty pain. Oblique coronal T2-weighted fast spin-echo MR sequence with fat saturation after acromioplasty shows persistent acromioclavicular joint arthritis with marginal edema and joint space fluid. There has also been interval development of a small partial-thickness undersurface tear.

The assessment of cuff integrity after surgery is complicated by the fact that there may be persistent signal in the cuff tendons after acromioplasty. However, MRI remains sensitive but not as specific in this setting for the assessment of cuff tear. It is fairly sensitive (84%) and specific (87%) for residual impingement according to a study by Magee and associates.[11] The typical criteria for a cuff tear in which there is tendon discontinuity and a fluid signal defect on long repetition time/echo time (TR/TE) sequences still applies. MR arthography may also be helpful in further evaluating for more subtle cuff tears because contrast agent extravasation though a cuff defect may be more readily apparent.[12]

Another potential cause of unsuccessful acromioplasty is failure to recognize and treat an unstable os acromiale. A persistent unstable os acromiale can lead to continued impingement on the rotator cuff during deltoid contraction and continued symptoms of impingement (Fig. 106-12). Finally, in some patients, symptoms of impingement result from unrecognized glenohumeral instability rather than from extrinsic impingement, and acromioplasty can, in fact, worsen the situation in these patients.[6]

Open surgical procedures for subacromial decompression and rotator cuff repair carry the risk of deltoid detachment or atrophy because this procedure involves a deltoid takedown in an open approach or a deltoid-splitting procedure in a mini-open approach (Fig. 106-13). The mini-open procedure may carry a lower risk of this complication (Table 106-7).

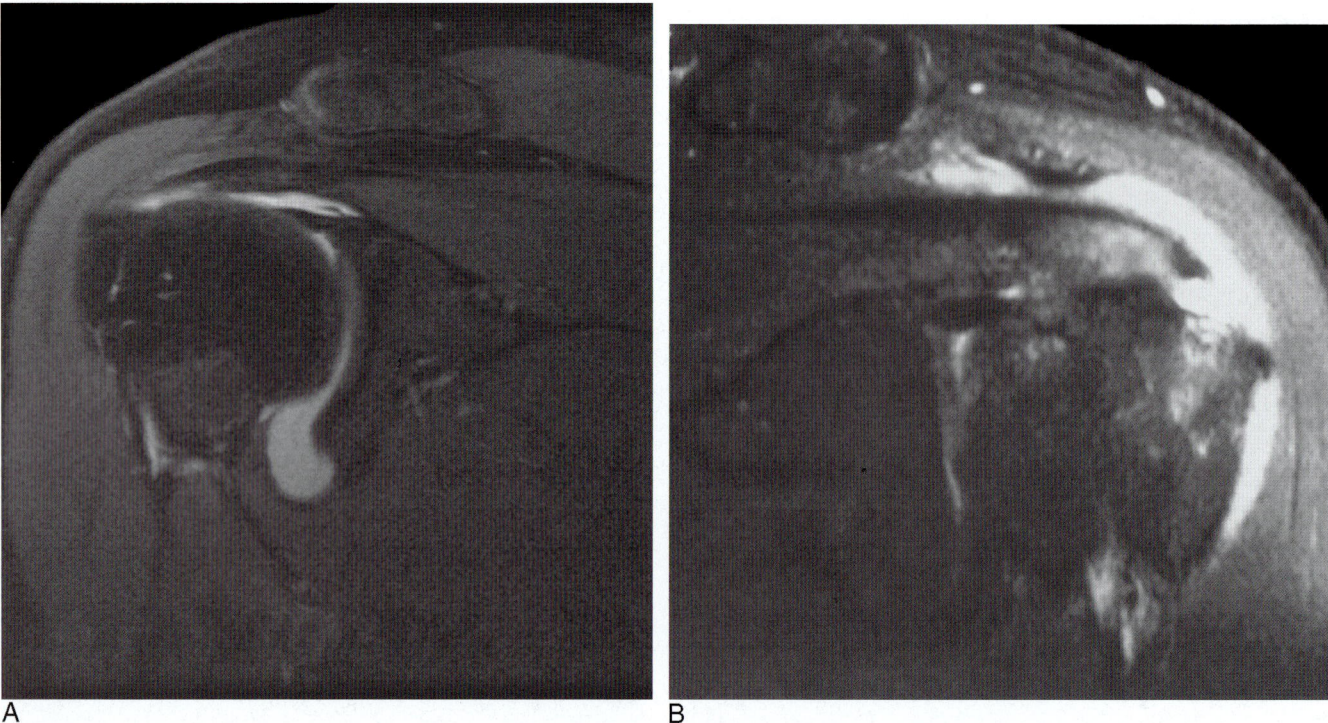

A

B

■ **FIGURE 106-11** **A,** Progression of rotator cuff disease after acromioplasty. Oblique coronal T2-weighted fast spin-echo image with fat saturation shows the interval development of a articular surface partial tear after acromioplasty. **B,** Progression of rotator cuff disease. Coronal oblique, turbo inversion recovery sequence in another patient. Status post acromioplasty there had been interval development of a full-thickness tear of the supraspinatus tendon anterodistally.

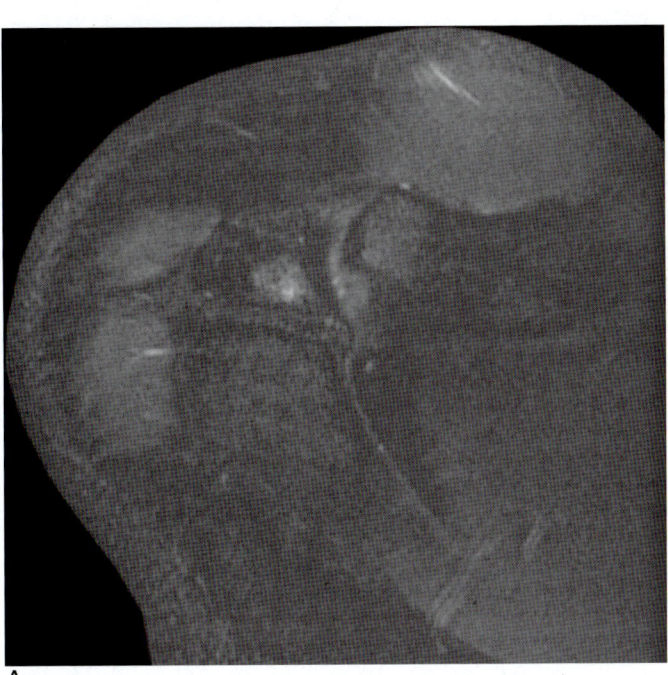
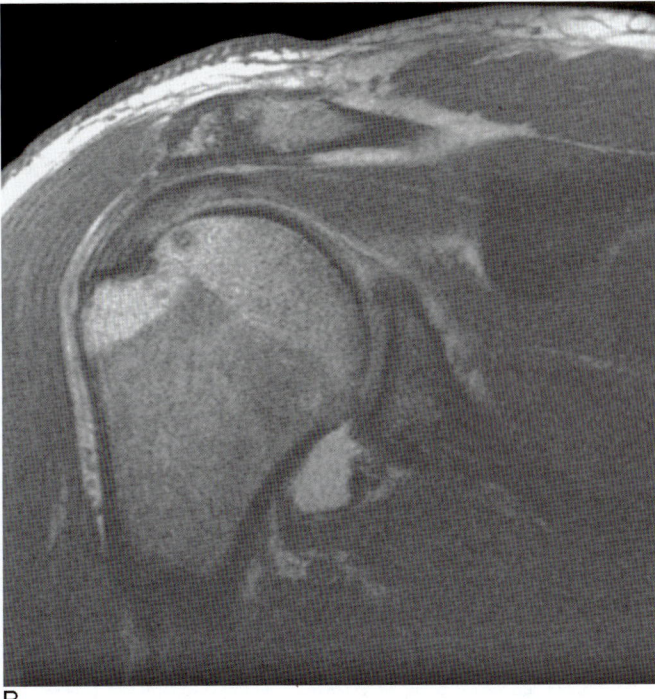

A   B

■ **FIGURE 106-12** **A,** Persistent os acromiale after acromioplasty. Axial proton density–weighted MR sequence with fat saturation reveals the presence of marginal edema within a previously unrecognized os acromiale after acromioplasty. **B,** Persistent os acromiale after acromioplasty. Oblique coronal proton density–weighted MR image shows a flat undersurface of the acromion after acromioplasty, but a persistent os acromiale is noted that may contribute to continued impingement.

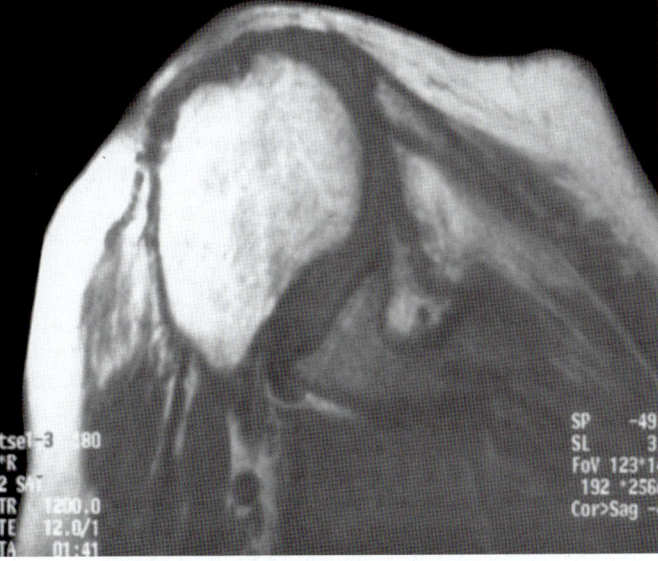

■ **FIGURE 106-13** Detachment and atrophy of the deltoid muscle after acromioplasty. Oblique coronal proton density–weighted image reveals retraction and fatty atrophy of the deltoid muscle. Deltoid detachment in combination with a large rotator cuff tear and acromioplasty has led to superior migration of the humeral head.

Rotator Cuff Repair or Débridement

Description

Several surgical techniques are available for repair of the rotator cuff, and a general knowledge of the most commonly used methods can be helpful when attempting to understand the postoperative anatomy of the shoulder.

TABLE 106-7	Complications of Subacromial Decompression

- Inadequate acromioplasty
- Failure to recognize acromioclavicular joint degenerative change
- Postoperative scarring interposed between the cuff and acromion
- Failure to address an os acromiale
- Unrecognized instability as the cause of symptoms
- Deltoid detachment
- General postoperative complications: adhesive capsulitis, synovitis, abscess formation, osteomyelitis, chondrolysis, and hematoma formation

The general principle of rotator cuff repair is subacromial decompression, rotator cuff mobilization, and repair of the tendon if possible back to the tuberosity (Fig. 106-14). Most open repairs are performed via an anterosuperior approach through a takedown of the proximal deltoid whereas mini-open repairs involve a split of the deltoid without a takedown. Arthroscopic procedures involve the use of three bursal portals: anterior, lateral, and posterior. Small full-thickness tears are typically repaired using a side-to-side suturing technique. Distal small tears may be repaired with a tendon-to-bone repair. Larger tears with retraction also require the reattachment of tendon to bone. In the past, a trough was created in the greater tuberosity for tendon-to-bone reattachment; however, most surgeons now typically freshen the articular-tuberosity junction for tendon to bone reattachment.[13] Cuff repairs can be performed with suture material or suture anchors that can be made of ferromagnetic metal,

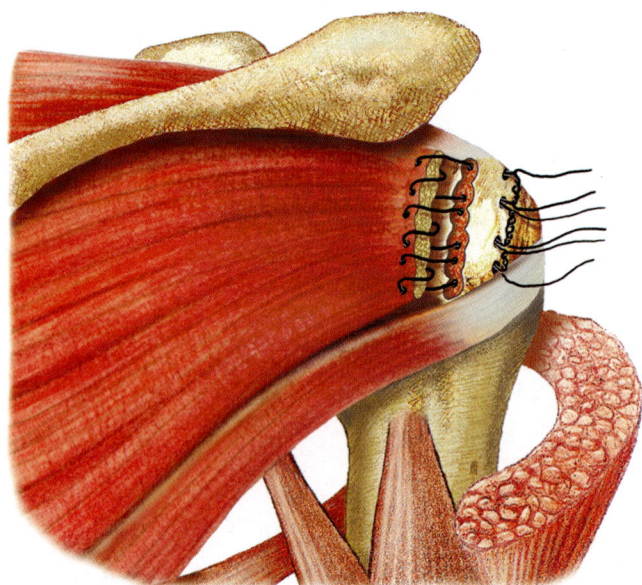

■ **FIGURE 106-14** Tendon-to-bone rotator cuff repair using a trough. The edge of the torn tendon is sutured into the trough using a combination of drill holes and nonabsorbable sutures. *(From Zlatkin MB. MRI of the Shoulder, 2nd ed. Philadelphia, Lippincott Williams & Wilkins, 2003. Diagram by Salvador Beltran, MD.)*

nonferromagnetic material such as titanium, plastic, or bioabsorbable polymers.

Massive tears may require mobilization of the remainder of the rotator cuff or incorporation of the long head of the biceps and subscapularis tendons to achieve an effective repair, and for these reasons open surgery is usually indicated. Recently, some surgeons have even advocated an all arthroscopic approach for repair of these lesions.[14] In massive tears where coverage of the humeral head cannot be achieved even with these techniques, synthetic meshes have been placed by some. Subacromial decompression is often performed in conjunction with rotator cuff repair and may be performed using either an open or arthroscopic approach.[15] Finally, a bursal release may also be performed at the time of rotator cuff repair to relieve the cuff of adhesions from chronic inflammation.

Indications, Contraindications, Purpose, and Underlying Mechanics

The decision to treat a rotator cuff tear depends on the size and character of the tendon tear in combination with the severity of impingement. The surgeon will typically evaluate whether the patient's pain is secondary to rotator cuff pathology related to impingement, by assessing for impingement signs and a positive impingement test (described earlier). Shoulder pain worsened by overhead activity, crepitus, weakness, and decreased range of motion can all be seen as a result of rotator cuff pathology. Atrophy in the supraspinatus and infraspinatus fossa may further suggest a large chronic tear.[5]

Simple débridement may be utilized for younger patients without significant bony changes about the coracoacromial arch or with cuff injuries related to instability or internal impingement. Débridement tends to be less effective in older patients or in those with high-grade

tears. Partial tears either along the bursal or articular surface are typically treated based on the grade of the tear. High-grade tears may be completed with excision of the damaged tissue and then treated as a full-thickness tear. This more aggressive repair is often used for more active patients younger than 40 years of age. Intermediate-grade tears can be débrided, and the bridge formed by the débridement may be sutured with treatment of the underlying cause of the partial tear. Low-grade tears may simply be débrided and the underlying cause treated. Subacromial decompression may also be undertaken if there is a bursal surface tear or if there are changes in the coracoacromial arch (e.g., osteophytes, type 3 acromion) that predispose to impingement.[1,4,14]

The basic principle of cuff repair is complete closure of the defect without tension at the repair site. Often, smaller tears may be managed with arthroscopic decompression and cuff repair while larger tears may be managed by open decompression and cuff repair. Large chronic tears may be managed by tendon transfer (e.g., a latissimus dorsi transfer), although at times an aggressive subacromial decompression alone may also result in an improvement in symptoms.[16]

The patient with a full-thickness tear who has good strength and a normal range of motion will typically first have nonoperative treatment. If the pain does not resolve after conservative treatment for 3 to 6 months, surgery may then be suggested. Pain is the primary indication for treatment of a full-thickness tear in an older patient. As was mentioned earlier, younger functional patients will have early repair of a full-thickness tear.[5] Although there are no absolute contraindications to rotator cuff repair, patients with movement disorders, poor surgical candidates, and those with severe underlying osteoarthritis or underlying muscle atrophy limiting motion may be considered as having relative contraindications (Tables 106-8 and 106-9).

Expected Appearance on Relevant Modalities

Comparison with preoperative examinations and correlation with surgical notes (if available) is suggested to render a reliable evaluation of postoperative findings. After repair of a high-grade partial- or full-thickness tear, the tendon may be medialized. A surgical trough may be seen on the greater tuberosity in many older repairs (Fig. 106-15). In the event of an end-to-end repair, there may only be some distortion of the tendon and peritendinous structures due to suture placement (Fig. 106-16). Artifacts due to soft tissue metal and suture artifacts can occur due to nonabsorbable sutures and anchors.[7] Large balloon artifact may occur, particularly if ferromagnetic sutures are employed. These suture anchor artifacts will often be in close proximity to the site of reattachment created in the greater tuberosity and can impair evaluation of the tendon integrity (Fig. 106-17).[17]

Extensive granulation tissue often surrounds the sutures and may result in intermediate-to- high T2-weighted signal intensity in the peritendinous tissues. Within the cuff tendon, granulation tissue may mimic a tear, especially in the early postoperative period. Granulation tissue will demonstrate intermediate signal intensity on both T1- and proton density-weighted images and may enhance

TABLE 106-8   Indications for Cuff Repair

- Positive physical signs and symptoms of cuff disease or impingement
- Degree of tear and patient activity level typically dictate surgical approach with high-grade tears usually excised and treated as full-thickness tears, intermediate-grade tears débrided with suturing of the defect created by débridement, and low-grade tears treated with simple débridement.
- Full-thickness tears are usually managed aggressively unless the patient has normal strength and/or range of motion as well as minimal cuff-related symptoms.
- Subacromial decompression is often added especially in the presence of bursal tears.

TABLE 106-9   Relative Contraindications for Cuff Repair

- Severe cuff muscle atrophy or severe tendon retraction
- Poor surgical candidates
- Minimal activity level
- Patients with movement disorders or advanced age

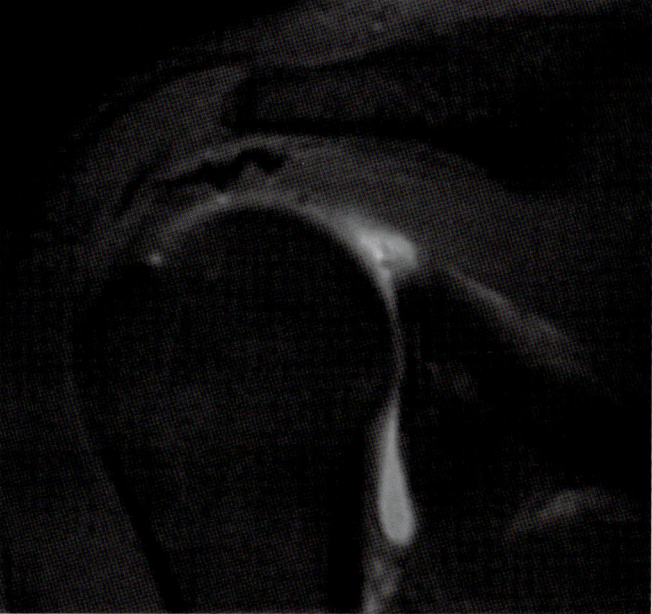

■ **FIGURE 106-16**   Tendon distortion after an end-to-end tendon repair. Coronal oblique T1-weighted MR image with fat suppression and intra-articular administration of gadolinium shows suture artifact at the level of tendon repair. The repair is watertight and contrast agent remains within the joint.

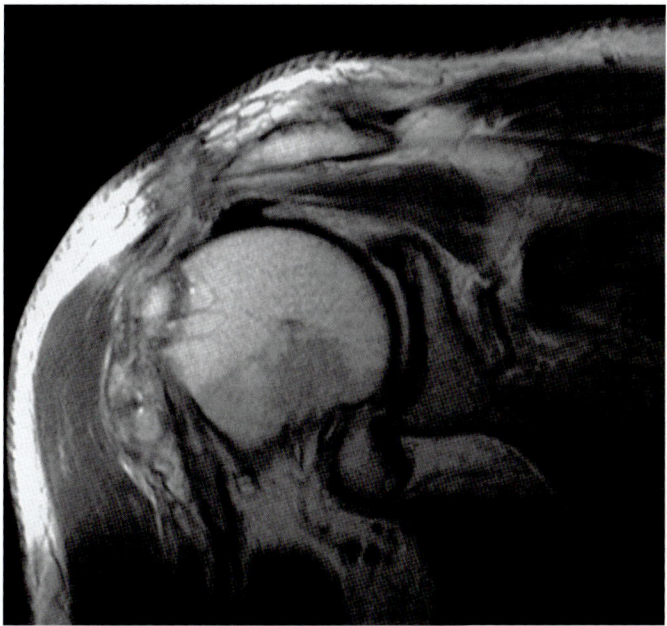

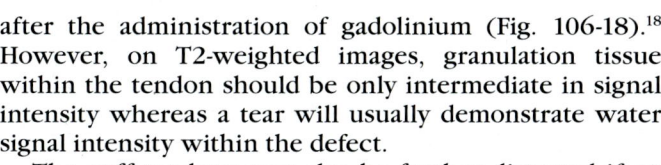

■ **FIGURE 106-15**   Medialization of the repaired tendon end. Coronal oblique proton density–weighted MR image shows a tendon-to-bone rotator cuff repair with medialization of the supraspinatus tendon. A surgical trough is also seen laterally.

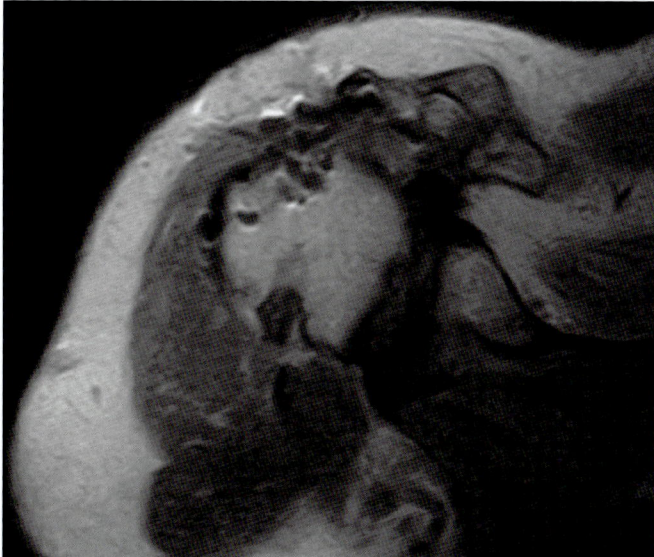

■ **FIGURE 106-17**   Metallic artifact resulting from suture material within a surgical trough. Coronal oblique proton density–weighted sequence reveals extensive metallic artifact at the site of the surgical trough and cuff repair.

after the administration of gadolinium (Fig. 106-18).[18] However, on T2-weighted images, granulation tissue within the tendon should be only intermediate in signal intensity whereas a tear will usually demonstrate water signal intensity within the defect.

The cuff tendons may also be further distorted if an allograft is utilized or if there is transfer of other tendons. Superior migration of the humeral head (often thought of as a secondary sign of cuff tear) may also occur in the

postoperative setting as a result of scarring, bursectomy, cuff atrophy, or capsular tightening.[12] Decreased acromiohumeral distance may not predict a tear of the rotator cuff but may increase the stress on the cuff by humerus. After bursectomy, there may be nonvisualization of subdeltoid fat or fluid (Fig. 106-19). As with subacromial decompression, the presence of fluid in the subacromial space does not imply a cuff tear or bursitis but may simply be the sequela of recent bursal resection or leakage of fluid from

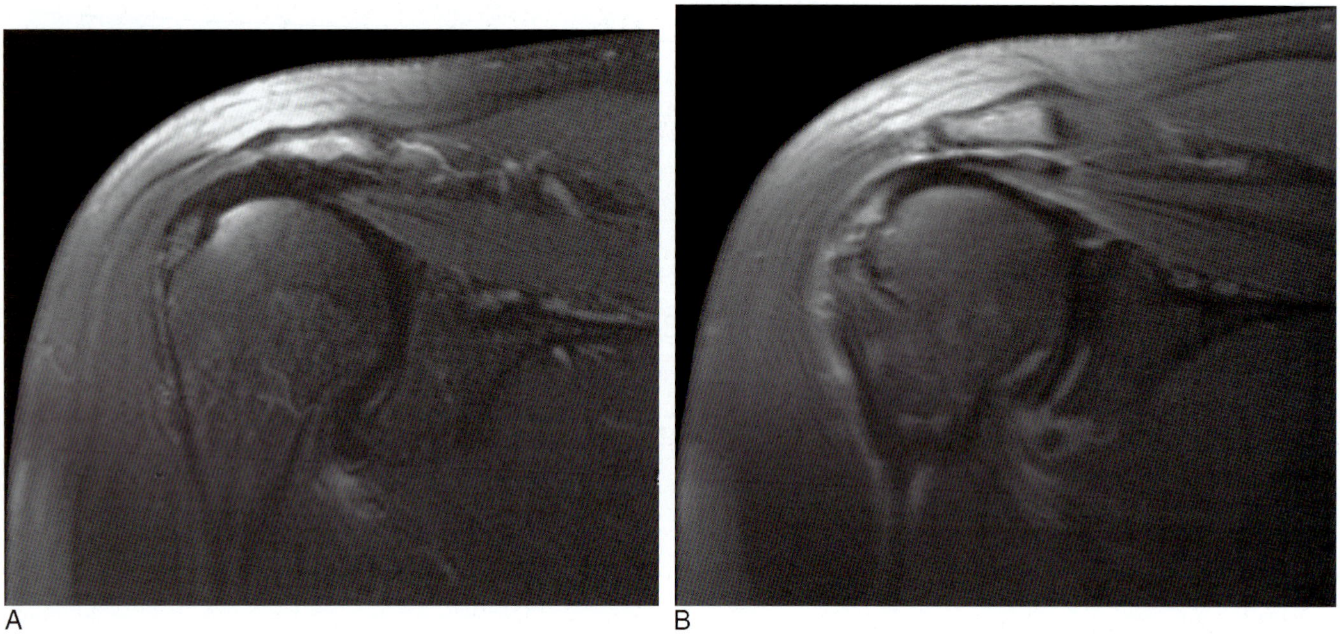

■ **FIGURE 106-18** **A,** Granulation tissue. Coronal oblique fat-saturated T2-weighted MR image shows intermediate T2-weighted signal intensity (not fluid signal) within the distal supraspinatus tendon representing granulation tissue at the site of repair. **B,** Granulation tissue. Oblique coronal T1-weighted image with fat saturation shows enhancement of granulation tissue after the intravenous administration of gadolinium.

the joint in a cuff repair that is not watertight (see Fig. 106-7).[19] Bone marrow edema in the humeral head is also another common finding that may persist for years after surgery.

Potential Complications and Radiologic Appearance

Recurrent rotator cuff tear is a common complication after rotator cuff repair and can occur as a result of untreated impingement, premature resumption of activity, poor tendon tissue quality, suture fixation failure, or excessive tension at the anastomotic site.[8] The presence of fluid signal on T2-weighted images within a tendon defect is the most reliable indicator of tendon tears in the postoperative setting (Fig. 106-20).[7] The most specific finding is absence or retraction of the tendon. Magee and associates found the sensitivity and specificity for rotator cuff tears (partial and complete) after repair were 100% and 87%,

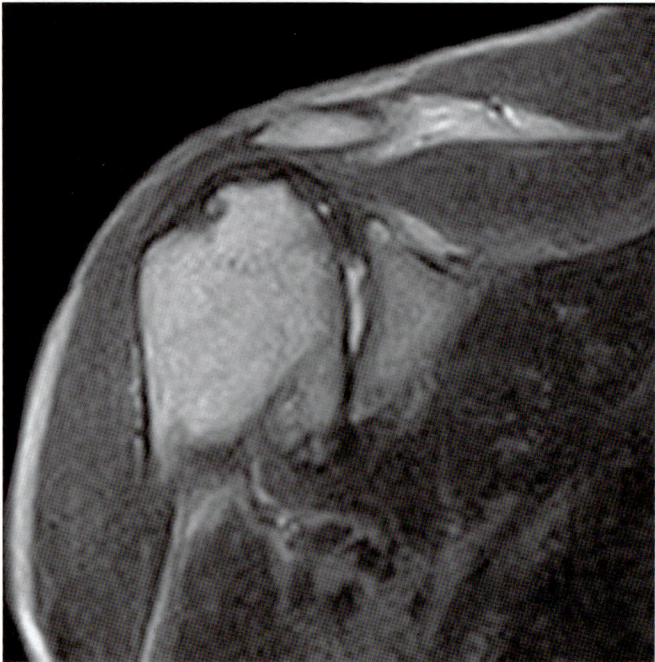

■ **FIGURE 106-19** Nonvisualization of the subdeltoid bursa or fat after bursectomy. Coronal T2-weighted MR image in a patient status post bursectomy shows nonvisualization of the subacromial bursa and fat with some mild superior migration of the humeral head.

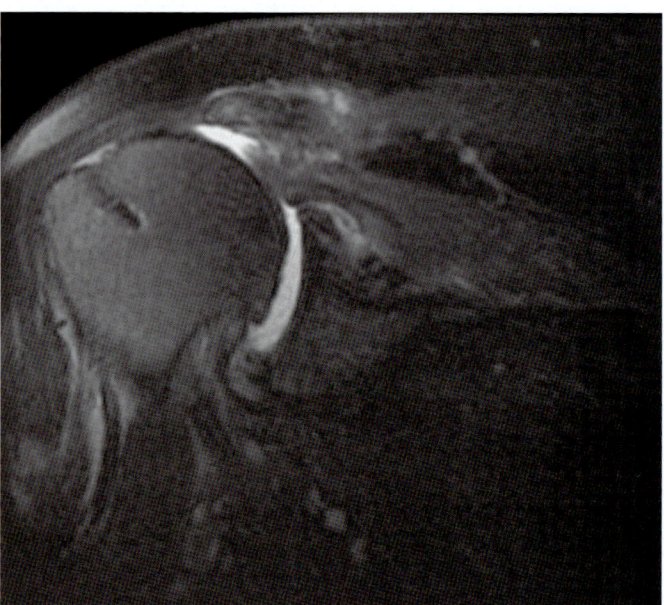

■ **FIGURE 106-20** Full-thickness tear after cuff repair. Coronal oblique T2-weighted MR image with fat suppression demonstrates a full-thickness tear of the supraspinatus tendon with retraction to the level of the glenohumeral joint and extensive fraying of the tendon edges.

respectively. For partial-thickness tears alone, the sensitivity and specificity dropped to 83% and 83%.[11] In some cases the incidence of low signal tear may increase owing to the presence of chronic granulation tissue. In this setting, secondary signs such as muscle atrophy and tendon retraction (see Fig. 106-6) along with comparison with a baseline postoperative study may be of benefit.

Given the alterations in the tendon appearance after surgery, direct MR arthrography may be of particular value in demonstrating leakage of contrast agent through either a partial- or full-thickness tendon defect. It may better characterize the extent of a tendon tear that can be obscured by postoperative artifact (Fig. 106-21). Characterization of the rotator cuff recurrent tear in terms of muscle atrophy, tendon retraction, and fragmentation is necessary to determine the feasibility of revision of the postoperative cuff. It should be noted that the location of the musculotendinous junction may not be a reliable secondary finding of rotator cuff tear because its position can change if the cuff has been mobilized during repair.

Additional potential causes of failure of rotator cuff repair include deltoid detachment (see Fig. 106-13), axillary or suprascapular nerve injury, inadequate acromioplasty, and unidentified symptomatic AC joint arthritis (see Fig. 106-10). Interestingly, defects of the articular cartilage along the humeral head or glenoid are also a common mimicker of subacromial impingement syndrome and cuff pathologic processes that may also be missed (Fig. 106-22). Occasionally, cuff tears may be produced iatrogenically, especially during arthroscopy, in some cases due to aggressive débridement (Table 106-10).[20]

Repairs for Glenohumeral Instability

Description

Glenohumeral instability may be unidirectional, bidirectional, or multidirectional and can occur in the anterior, posterior, inferior, or, rarely, superior directions. Unidirectional instability is usually traumatic and can result from a single traumatic event or after repetitive microtrauma, as occurs in activities such as throwing or weight lifting. Approximately 95% of all cases of glenohumeral instability are anterior in direction, with most occurring after a dislocation. Associated injuries include avulsion or tear of the anterior labrum, capsule, or glenohumeral ligaments (anteroinferior labroligamentous complex), and these lesions are referred to as the Bankart lesion and its variants.[21]

Surgical repair techniques are classified as either direct or indirect. A direct repair is one in which the labral or capsular injury is directly repaired in an attempt to prevent recurrent instability, whereas an indirect repair alters the anatomy in ways such as capsular tightening to prevent recurrent instability without specifically addressing the underlying lesion of the labroligamentous complex. Because of frequent patient dissatisfaction and a high rate of recurrence, indirect repairs are rarely performed today.

Direct repairs can be accomplished via either an open or arthroscopic[22] approach, with the latter resulting in less damage to the surrounding tissues and less scarring. Regardless of the approach, repair is typically performed by placing suture anchors at the 3-, 4-, and 5-o'clock positions with subsequent reattachment of the labrum (Fig. 106-23). The suture anchors can be ferromagnetic or instead made of plastic or bioabsorbable materials. A second type of direct

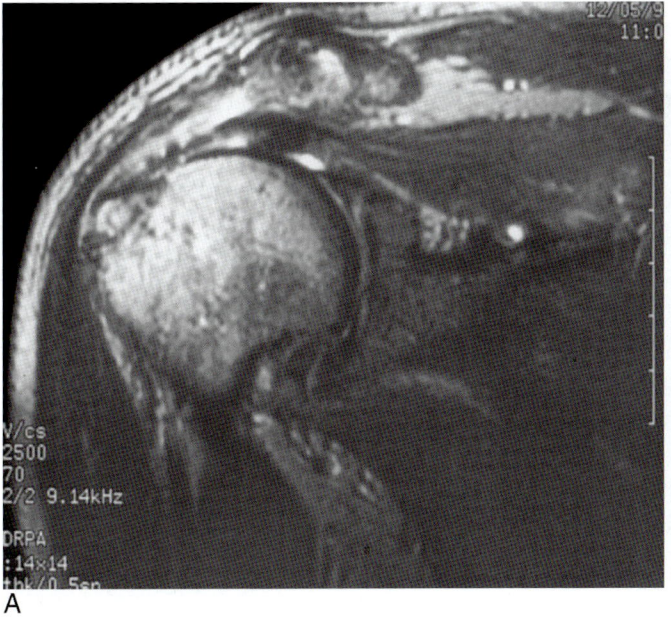
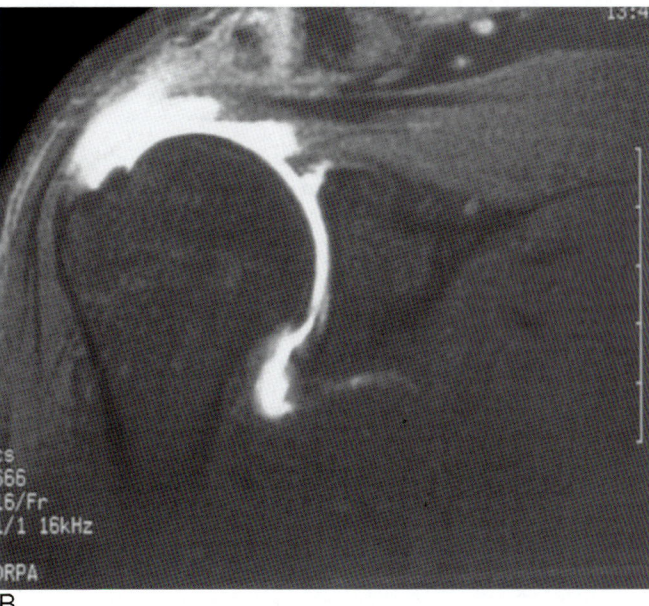

A   **B**

■ **FIGURE 106-21**   **A,** Recurrent rotator cuff tear. Coronal oblique T2-weighted MR image reveals a probable recurrent tear of supraspinatus tendon that is obscured due to artifact from prior repair. **B,** Recurrent rotator cuff tear. MR arthrography on the same patient better shows the extent of this full-thickness tear as well contrast agent imbibition into the degenerated tendon edges.

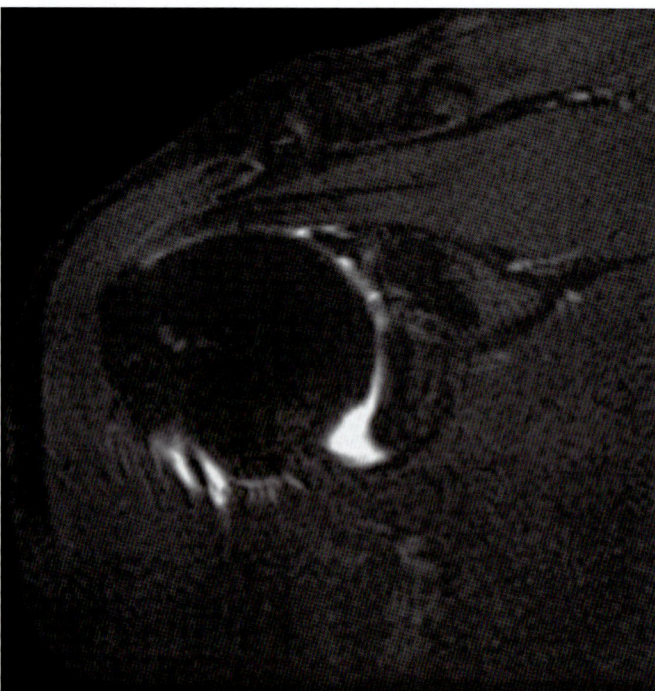

■ **FIGURE 106-22**   Focal chondral defects of the glenoid. Coronal oblique T2-weighted sequence with fat suppression reveals multiple chondral defects along the superior aspect of the glenoid.

TABLE 106-10   Complications of Rotator Cuff Repair

- Recurrent rotator cuff tear
- Axillary or suprascapular nerve injury
- Inadequate acromioplasty or failure to recognize acromioclavicular joint arthritis
- Chondral defects of the glenoid mimicking impingement and cuff disease
- Iatrogenic tears of the cuff during aggressive débridement
- Deltoid detachment
- General postoperative complications: adhesive capsulitis, synovitis, abscess formation, osteomyelitis, chondrolysis, and hematoma formation

repair is the capsulorrhaphy, which can also be performed as an open or arthroscopic procedure. Capsulorrhaphy may be performed in conjunction with labral repair; or if no labral lesion is identified, capsulorrhaphy may be performed as an isolated procedure. Sutures are used to tighten or plicate the capsule. In the past, staple or thermal capsulorrhaphy has been performed, but these techniques have largely fallen out of favor because of either a high rate of failure or as a result of other associated complications.

Techniques for indirect repair include the Putti-Platt procedure, in which the subscapularis tendon is divided 2.5 cm proximal to its insertion. The lateral stump is then attached to the glenoid while the medial stump is imbricated over the lateral stump, in effect shortening the subscapularis and capsule (Fig. 106-24). The Magnuson-Stack procedure involves transfer of the subscapularis from the lesser tuberosity to the greater tuberosity. Finally, the Bristow procedure involves transfer of the coracoid process with the conjoined tendon to the anteroinferior

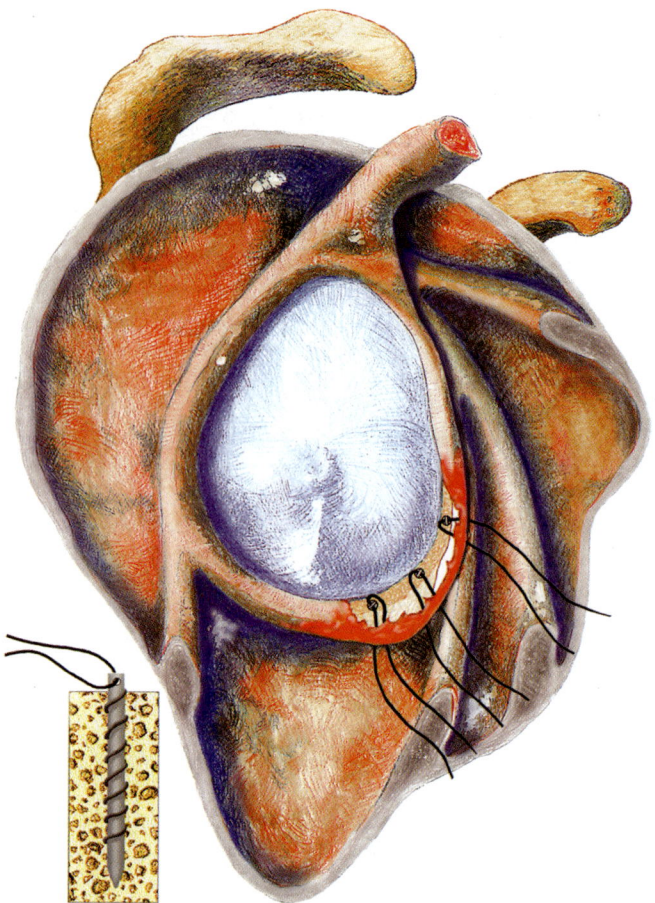

■ **FIGURE 106-23**   Bankart repair. Suture anchors are placed at the 3, 4, and 5-o'clock positions. *(From Zlatkin MB. MRI of the Shoulder, 2nd ed. Philadelphia, Lippincott Williams & Wilkins, 2003. Diagram by Salvador Beltran, MD.)*

glenoid to create a bony block, thus preventing anterior instability (Fig. 106-25).

Posterior instability is treated similar to anterior instability with direct repair of the labral lesion and posterior capsular plication or shift. Bone deficiency of either the anterior or posterior glenoid is treated with a bone graft (Laterjet procedure) or an opening wedge osteotomy.

Multidirectional instability often results from ligamentous laxity, and it is frequently bilateral. These patients are first treated with rehabilitation to strengthen the dynamic stabilizers (rotator cuff) of the glenohumeral joint. Surgical repair with an inferior capsular shift is reserved for individuals not responsive to conservative therapy. A T-shaped incision of the anterior capsule is performed via the deltopectoral interval, and the inferior capsule is advanced in a superior direction with resultant capsular tightening (Fig. 106-26).[23]

Isolated labral tears such as SLAP lesions may be independent of instability and can be treated with débridement of loose tissue and staple/suture repair of the labrum back down to the bony glenoid. Labral fraying may also occur posterosuperiorly in patients with internal impingement. Paralabral cyst formation may be an additional complication of a labral tear and can extend into the spinoglenoid or suprascapular notch. These cysts may be removed arthroscopically, but if they become too large, they may

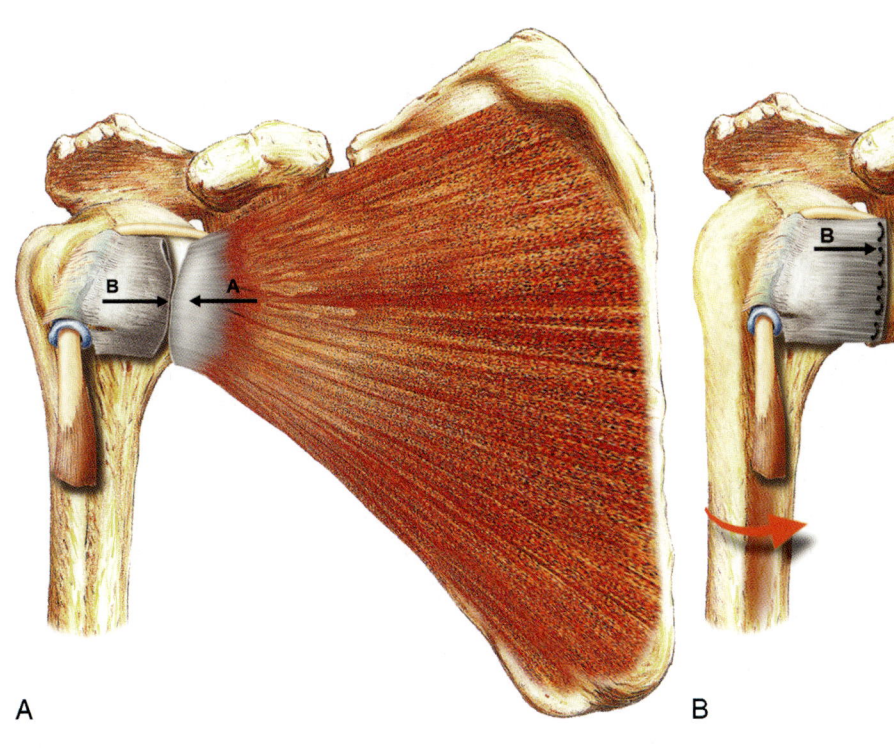

A

B

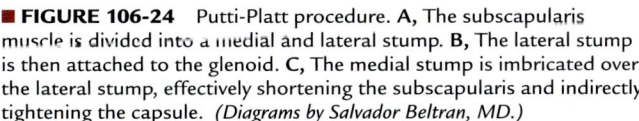

■ **FIGURE 106-24** Putti-Platt procedure. **A,** The subscapularis muscle is divided into a medial and lateral stump. **B,** The lateral stump is then attached to the glenoid. **C,** The medial stump is imbricated over the lateral stump, effectively shortening the subscapularis and indirectly tightening the capsule. *(Diagrams by Salvador Beltran, MD.)*

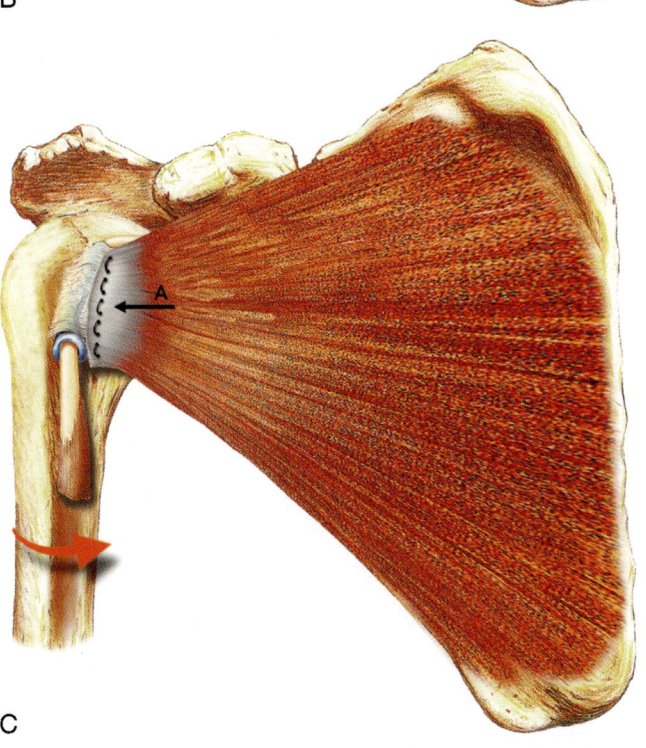

C

be unroofed and decompressed. Large cysts may also be excised in an open procedure.

Indications, Contraindications, Purpose, and Underlying Mechanics

Nonoperative management depends on the type and direction of instability as well as the age and level of activity of the patient. Initially, the patient may be treated with 2 to 3 weeks of immobilization after closed reduction with a specific rehabilitation program to strengthen the dynamic stabilizers of the cuff and scapula. However, young active patients who have sustained a Bankart lesion have a high rate of recurrence even with conservative treatment and will often require surgical intervention either direct or indirect. The goal of surgical repair is anatomic repair of the capsular ligaments to the glenoid rim in Bankart repair. Early Bankart repair may also be performed in those young patients aiming to return to their previous level of activity. Open procedures may be performed for those in contact sports, whereas in first-time dislocators arthroscopic repair may be best.[5] The presence of a

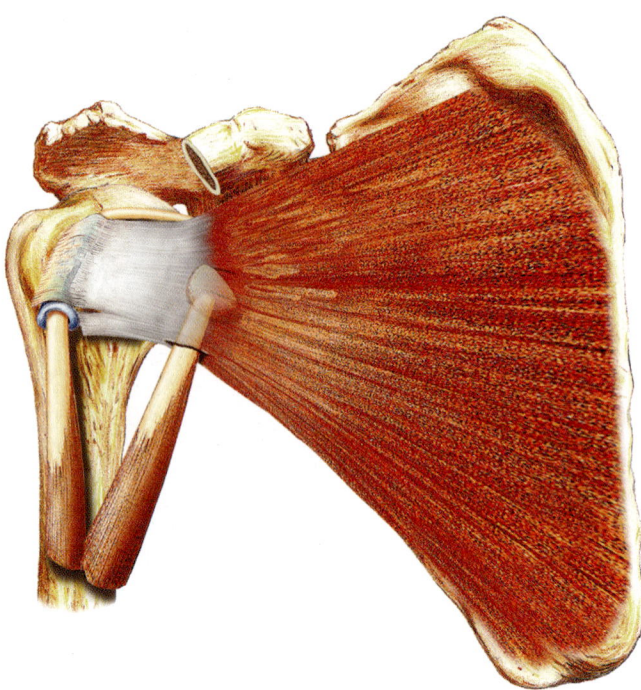

■ FIGURE 106-25 Bristow procedure. The coracoid process with the conjoined tendon is transferred to the anterior inferior glenoid through a split in the subscapularis. *(Diagram by Salvador Beltran, MD.)*

bony glenoid deficiency involving more than 25% of the articular surface (inverted pear–shaped glenoid) with associated instability is considered an indication for open surgery, with reduction of a bone fragment if present or bone grafting to fill the defect. If there is redundancy of the anterior capsule and inferior capsular recess, a capsular shift will also be performed.

In contrast to anterior instability, nonoperative treatment is favored as the initial treatment for posterior, multidirectional, and atraumatic unidirectional instability. Strengthening of the cuff, deltoid, and scapular stabilizing muscles along with activity modification are successful in 80% to 90% of cases. These measures are typically exhausted before surgery is considered. Surgery for traumatic posterior instability typically focuses on repair of the posterior labrum. Posterior capsulorrhaphy may also be performed. If there is coexisting anterior and posterior instability, both may be addressed at the time of surgery. Multidirectional instability in those who have failed conservative treatment is usually approached from the side of greatest instability. The inferior capsular shift procedure aims to decrease the capsular volume, thicken the capsule on the side of the approach, and, as a result, provide tension to the capsule on the opposite side. Volitional dislocators are considered a contraindication to surgical repair (Tables 106-11 and 106-12).[5]

Expected Appearance on Relevant Modalities

At the time of Bankart repair, suture anchors are placed along the anteroinferior margin of the glenoid rim and these anchors result in varying degrees of artifact, depending on their composition (Fig. 106-27).[8] Scar or granulation tissue is often present in the region of incision and may result in the loss of fat planes and decreased tissue contrast. After direct repair, the labrum and capsule should demonstrate a normal anatomic position but subtle changes are often noted in their morphology. The labrum may appear thickened or blunted but should remain firmly attached to the glenoid with no evidence of detachment. MR arthrography is particularly useful in demonstrating the altered capsular and labral anatomy and in identifying subtle areas of recurrent detachment. Abduction and external rotation (ABER) imaging is useful

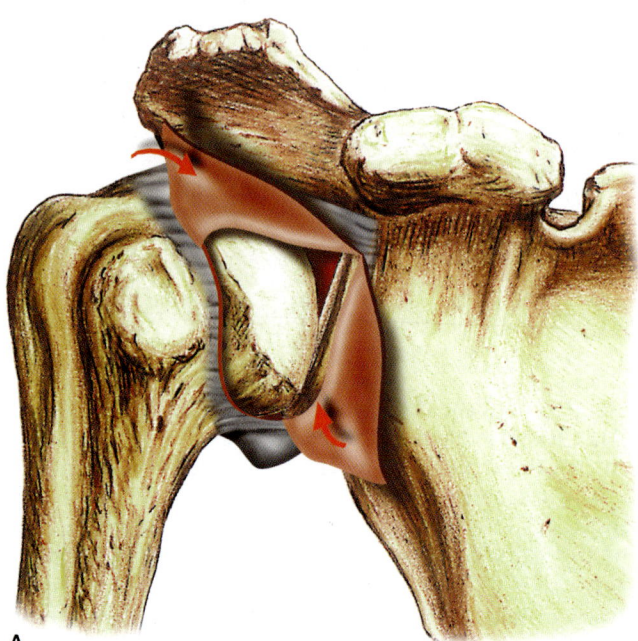

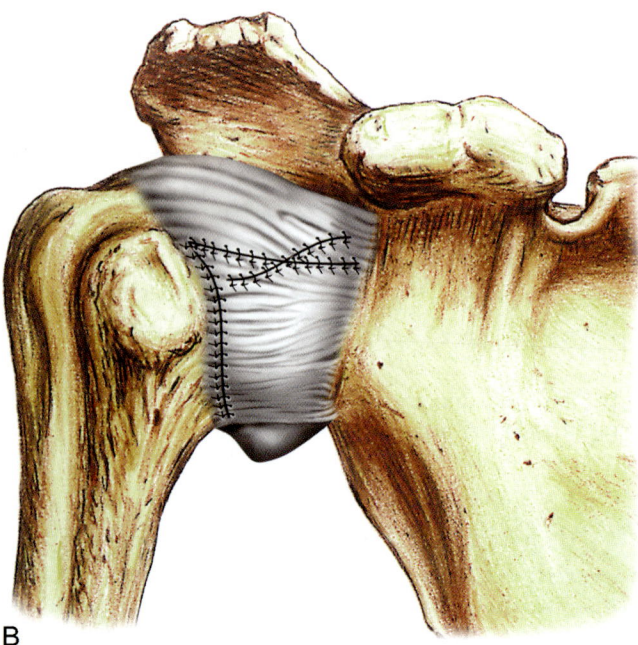

A   B

■ FIGURE 106-26 **A,** Inferior capsular shift. A horizontal T-shaped incision is made and the capsule is opened. **B,** Inferior capsular shift. The inferior capsule is advanced in a superior direction and oversewn, with resultant tightening of the anterior capsule.

TABLE 106-11 Indications for Repair of Glenohumeral Instability

- Anterior instability generally requires surgical intervention in a young active patient due to a high rate of recurrence.
- Capsular redundancy may require concomitant capsular shift at the time of surgery.
- Bony defect of the glenoid involving more than 25% of the articular surface is an indication for open surgery.
- Repair of posterior and multidirectional instability is performed only after failure of an exhaustive rehabilitation program.

TABLE 106-12 Contraindications to Glenohumeral Instability Repair

- Volitional dislocators
- Posterior, multidirectional and atraumatic instability repair not indicated unless conservative therapy has failed
- Advanced age and minimal activity level of the patient
- Poor surgical candidates

in better visualizing the anterior band of the inferior glenohumeral ligament and its glenoid attachment.[24]

Although rarely performed today, indirect repairs will show alteration in shoulder anatomy depending on the specific procedure performed, but the labral pathology will remain clearly evident because it is not addressed or repaired in these procedures. Following the Putti-Platt procedure, the subscapularis tendon or anterior capsule will appear thickened (Fig. 106-28).[25] A transfer of the subscapularis tendon from the lesser to the greater tuberosity will be seen after a Magnuson-Stack procedure (Fig. 106-29).

Repairs of multidirectional instability typically demonstrate thickening of the anteroinferior capsule on MRI. Coronal images will demonstrate a decrease in the size of the axillary pouch (Fig. 106-30), and suture material is often seen as low signal foci located in the region of the anterior capsule and subscapularis tendon. Distention of the joint using MR arthrography is ideal for evaluation of residual capsular redundancy after capsular plication. Some have postulated that an anterior-to-posterior capsular width ratio of less than 1 after arthrography predicts a good outcome, particularly after capsulorhaphy.[8]

Potential Complications and Radiologic Appearance

The recurrence rate for instability procedures performed as an open procedure varies between 1% and 10%. Arthroscopic procedures have recurrence rates on the order of 15% to 20%. Because of potential artifact, scarring, and the possibility of residual untreated lesions, MR arthrography (either direct or indirect) provides better visualization of recurrent lesions (Fig. 106-31). Signs indicative of a recurrent labral tear include detachment or displacement of the labrum seen on MRI as fluid signal intensity or contrast agent extension into or beneath the labrum. Wagner and colleagues studied 24 patients who had MRI after instability repair and retrospectively

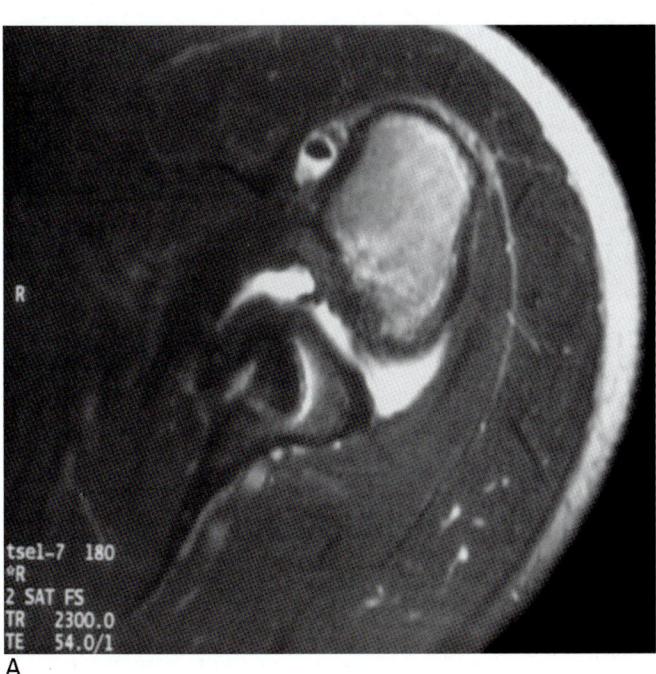
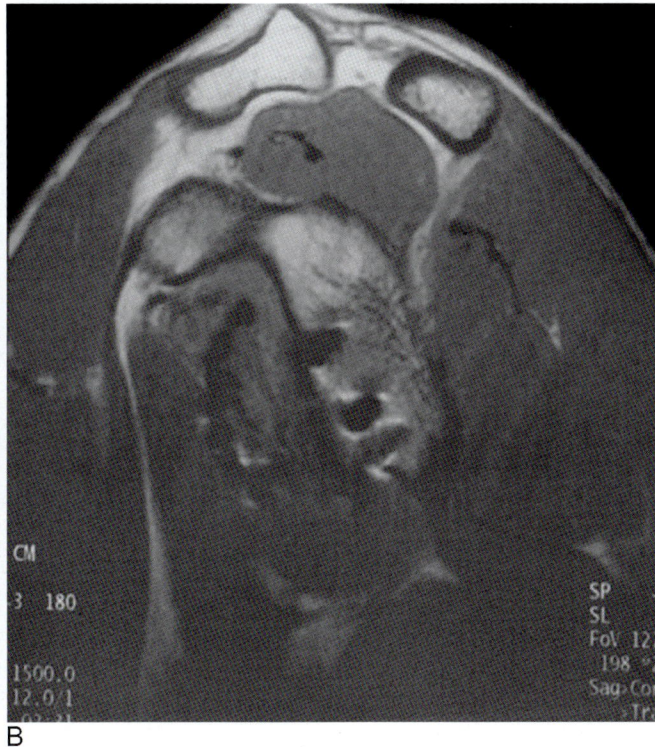

A   B

■ **FIGURE 106-27** **A,** Post Bankart repair. Axial turbo spin-echo MR image. Artifact is seen from the suture anchor in the anterior inferior glenoid. Note the scar tissue at the site of capsular reattachment to the glenoid. **B,** Suture anchor artifact. Sagittal oblique proton density–weighted MR image shows artifact along the site of fixation of the labrum to the anterior glenoid rim, from the 3 to 5 o'clock positions.

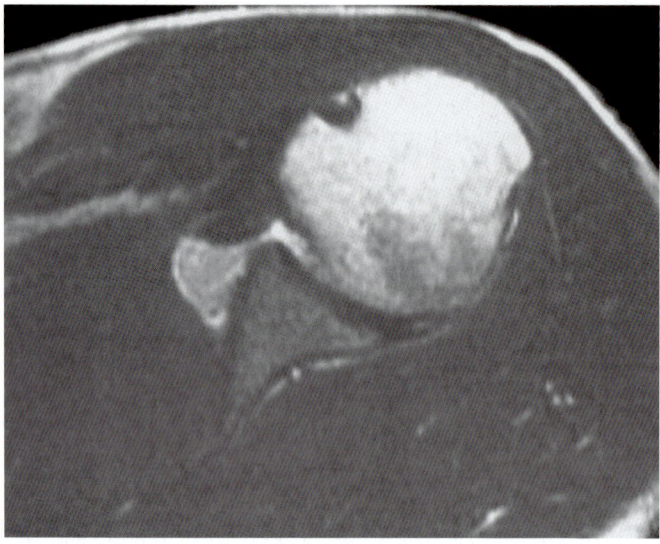

■ **FIGURE 106-28** Post Putti-Platt repair. Axial T2-weighted MR image demonstrates thickening and deformity of the subscapularis tendon. The anterior labrum is absent in this nonanatomic indirect repair.

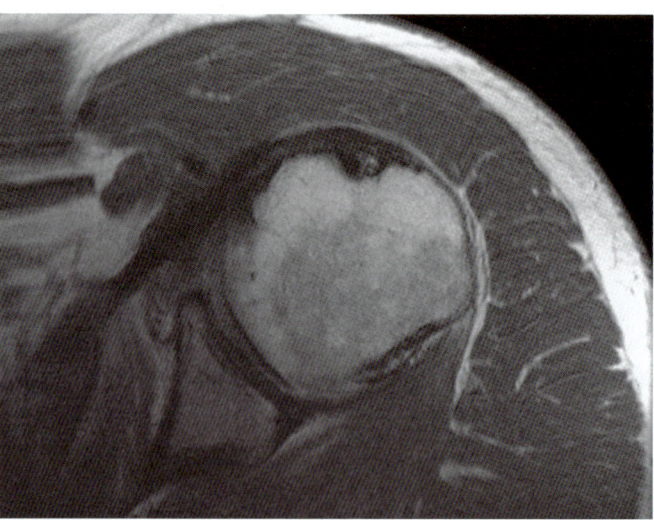

■ **FIGURE 106-29** Magnuson-Stack procedure. Axial proton density–weighted MR sequence. The subscapularis tendon has been transferred from the lesser to the greater tuberosity as part of an indirect repair.

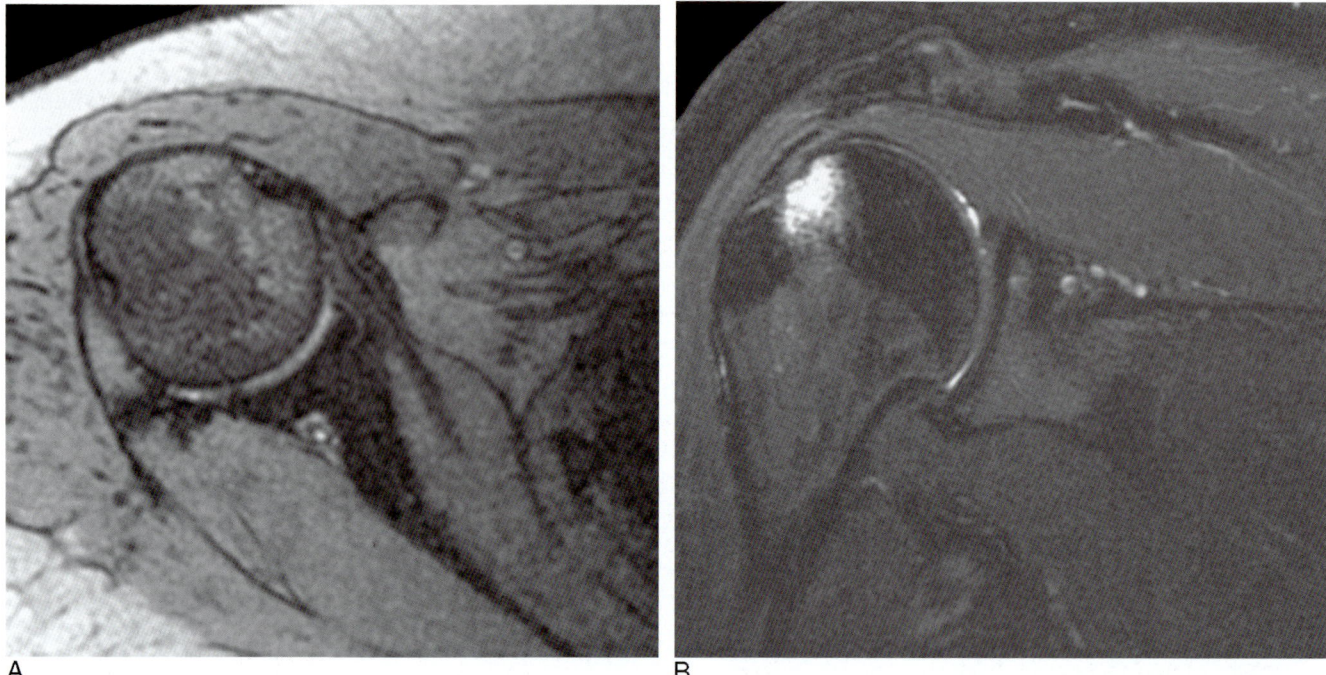

A   B

■ **FIGURE 106-30** **A,** Capsular plication. Axial gradient-echo MR sequence reveals thickening of the capsule and a decrease in the volume of the glenohumeral joint anteriorly and posteriorly after capsular plication in a patient with multidirectional instability. **B,** Capsular plication. Coronal oblique proton density–weighted MR sequence reveals a decrease in the size of the axillary pouch in a patient who is status post inferior capsular shift.

reviewed these studies for the presence of recurrent labral tear. The accuracy was on the order of 79% in demonstrating recurrent labral tear.[26] It should be noted that after repair the capsule may become stretched out and redundant. A capsular detachment may be suggested if the capsular attachment is more medial than would be expected for a type 3 capsular attachment.

Paralabral cyst may arise as a result of a recurrent labral tear or may be a cause of persistent symptoms if not ade-

quately excised (Fig. 106-32).[27] Damage to the suprascapular nerve or artery is another potential complication of paralabral cyst excision and may manifest as atrophy of the supraspinatus and infraspinatus muscle bellies, depending on the site of injury. MRI or MR arthrography may also visualize recurrent SLAP lesions after débridement or repair. MR arthrography may best accomplish this by revealing contrast agent extending between the labrum and the subjacent site of repair to the bony glenoid (Fig. 106-33).

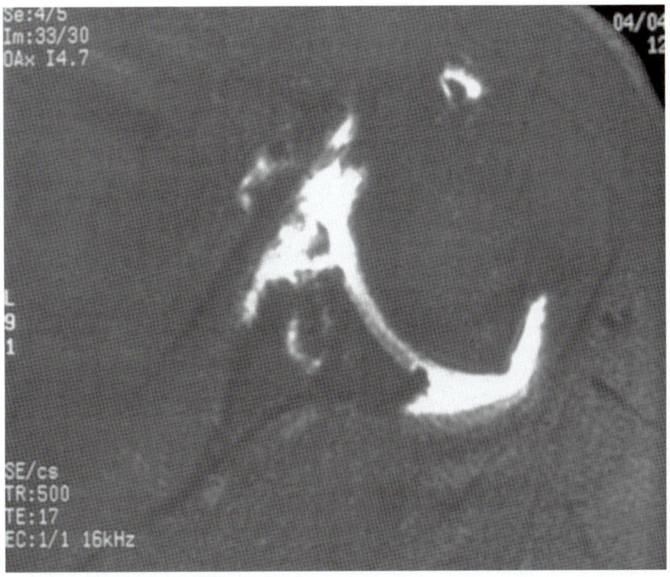

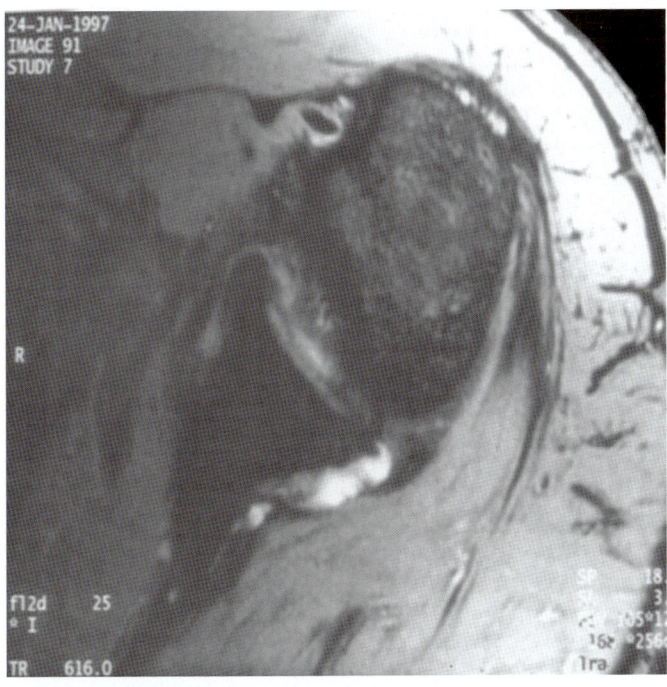

■ **FIGURE 106-31** Post Bankart repair, recurrent labral tear and degenerative change. MR arthrogram, axial T1-weighted image with fat saturation shows the anterior inferior labrum to be detached and blunted. There is also early articular cartilage loss of the glenohumeral joint with minimal osteophyte formation along the posterior margin of the humeral head. A Hill-Sachs lesion is noted posteriorly.

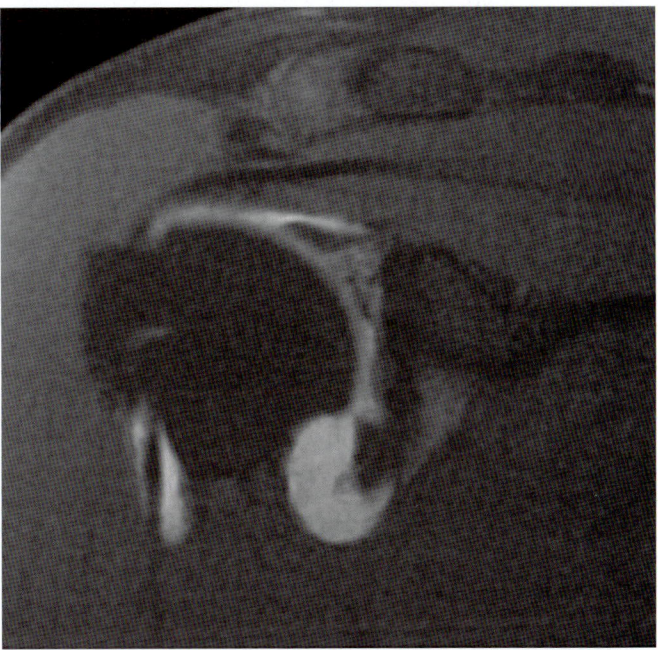

■ **FIGURE 106-33** Recurrent SLAP tear. MR arthrogram reveals the presence of a recurrent SLAP tear in the superior and posterior labrum after repair.

■ **FIGURE 106-32** Paralabral cyst. Axial T2-weighted image. There is paralabral cyst formation arising from the posterior labrum with some extension to the spinoglenoid notch.

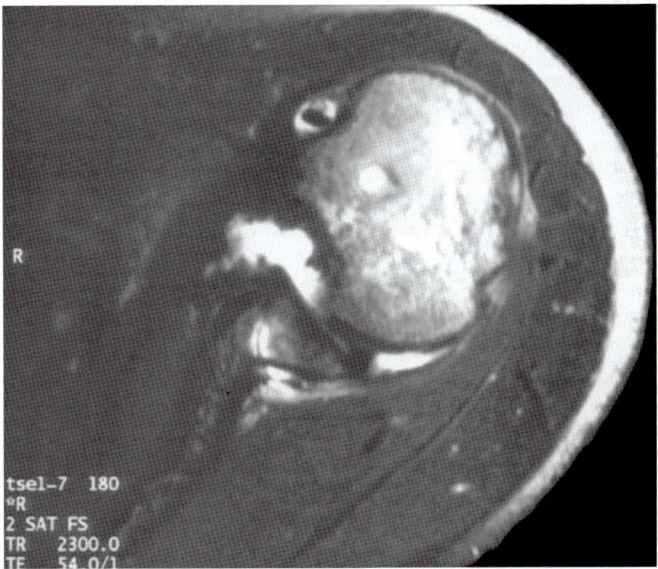

■ **FIGURE 106-34** Overtight repair of the anterior capsule. Axial T2-weighted image demonstrates mild posterior subluxation and degenerative change of the glenohumeral joint.

In addition to a recurrent tear of the labrum, an additional cause of recurrent/persistent instability may include an inadequate or incorrect surgical procedure to address the specific type of instability. It is also possible that anterior and posterior instability may coexist, with one masking the other. Treatment addressing only one form of instability may unmask the other, resulting in instability in the opposite direction.

Overtightening of the capsule can lead to degenerative change of the glenohumeral joint or to instability in the opposite direction (Fig. 106-34). This complication is more common after indirect repairs. Inferior capsular shift may also be overtightened, resulting in either loss of the axillary pouch or posterior subluxation of the humeral head. At times, misplaced or detached staples, tacks, or suture anchors can result in recurrent pain and (if left untreated) can eventually lead to degenerative change (Fig. 106-35). Adhesive capsulitis is an uncommon complication after instability repair. The normal

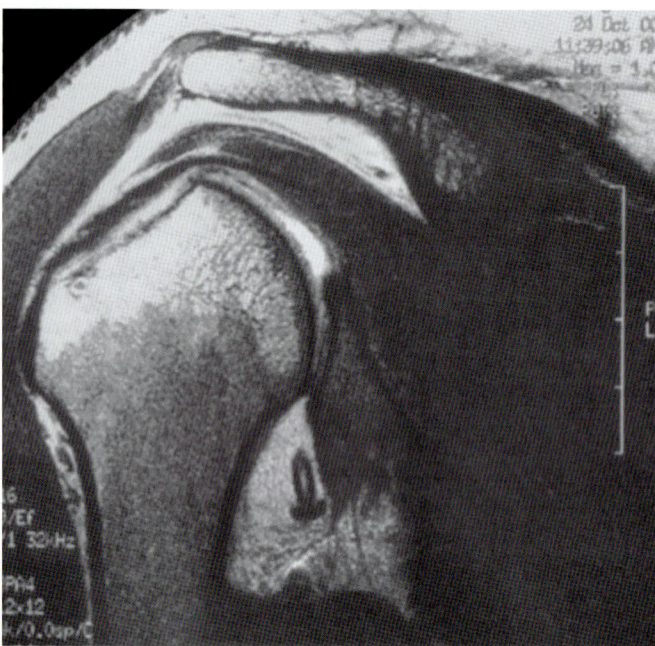

■ **FIGURE 106-35** Displaced tack. Coronal oblique image, fast spin-echo T1-weighted MR arthrogram without fat suppression shows a displaced tack in the axillary recess after a Bankart repair. A Hill-Sachs lesion is present.

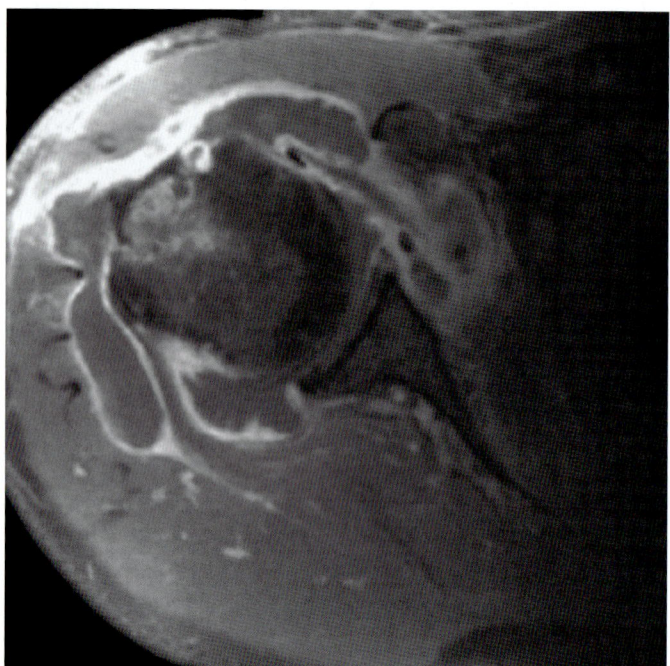

■ **FIGURE 106-36** Postoperative synovitis. Axial T1-weighted MR image with fat suppression demonstrates extensive enhancement and nodular thickening of the synovium as well as a large joint effusion.

postoperative capsule is usually 2 to 4 mm in thickness. A measurement of the capsule in the region of the axillary exceeding 4 mm in thickness suggests adhesive capsulitis when seen in the appropriate clinical setting.[28]

Reactive synovitis and postoperative infection can occur as a complication of any of the procedures described earlier. They have some overlap in terms of their imaging appearance. Synovitis is associated with joint effusions and nodular thickening of the joint capsule (Fig. 106-36). Intravenous gadolinium injection will often better demonstrate the thickening of the synovium. If synovitis is the result of infection, joint destruction may become evident with resultant cartilage loss, cysts, and erosions. The patient with synovitis may be difficult to differentiate from the inflammation that may be seen in the immediate postoperative period. In this case, often an interval follow-up may be necessary. Osteomyelitis may be suggested by the presence of marrow edema or abscess formation on short tau inversion recovery (STIR) and fat-saturated T2-weighted sequences as well as a loss of normal marrow signal intensity on the T1-weighted sequences (Fig. 106-37).

Additional complications that may occur with any of these procedures include hematoma formation, abscess formation, or avascular necrosis. The appearance of a hematoma will typically depend on its stage but in the early stages will typically be bright on T1- and T2-weighted sequences with fluid-fluid levels occasionally seen. Abscess formation will appear as a localized cavity similar in signal intensity to fluid but with a rim of tissue that demonstrates avid enhancement and may be bright on the T2-weighted or STIR images.

Rapid-onset chondrolysis of the glenohumeral joint is a devastating complication that has recently been reported with increasing frequency in young patients after shoulder reconstruction for glenohumeral instability.[29] The exact etiology is not certain, but one theory suggests that an immune response to some unknown inciting factor leads to the onset rapid of cellular death of all of the chondrocytes on both sides of the glenohumeral joint. Some have proposed that the use of thermal energy in the performance of capsulorrhaphy is a potential etiology; however, not all

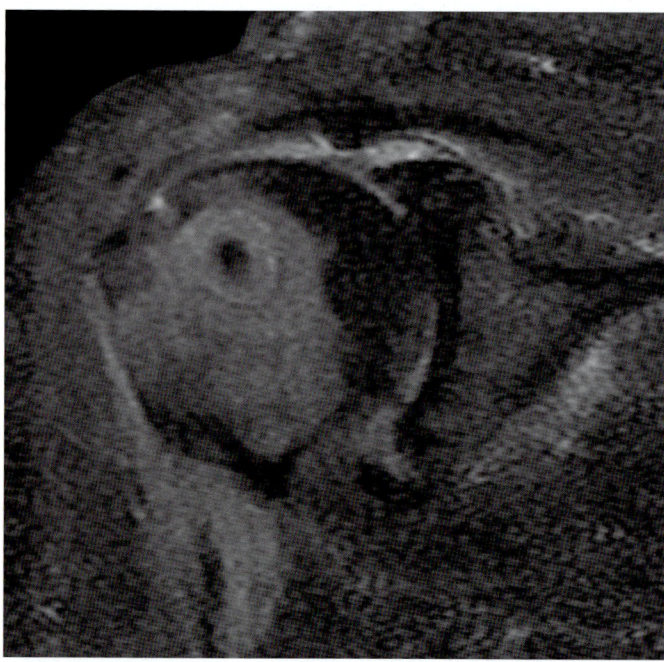

■ **FIGURE 106-37** Postoperative osteomyelitis. Coronal oblique T2-weighted image with fat saturation shows osteomyelitis and abscess formation surrounding a suture anchor in the humeral head.

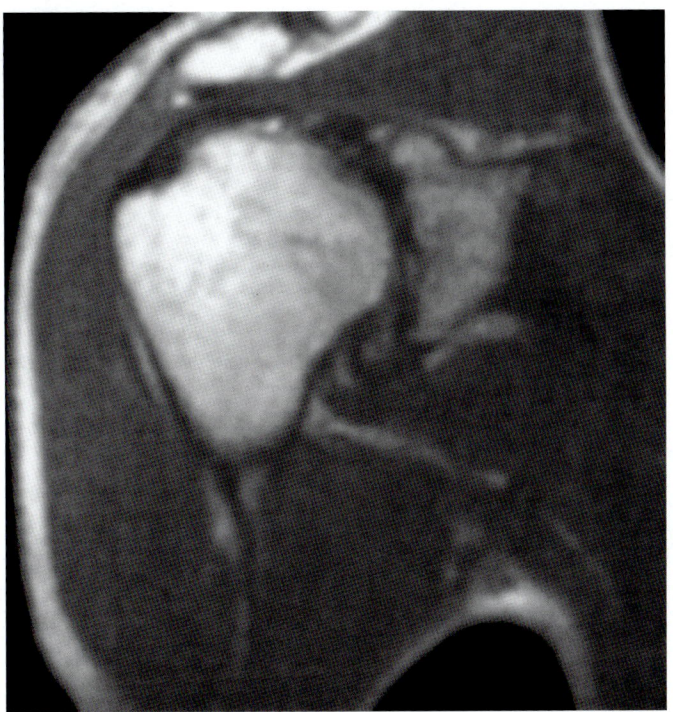

■ **FIGURE 106-38** Acute onset of chondrolysis after Bankart repair. Coronal T2-weighted image shows complete loss of the articular cartilage on both sides of the glenohumeral joint with subtle subchondral marrow edema involving the glenoid and humeral head. Note the lack of joint effusion and the lack of synovial thickening.

TABLE 106-13 Complications of Repair for Glenohumeral Instability

- Recurrent labral tear
- Inadequate paralabral cyst resection
- Suprascapular nerve injury during paralabral cyst resection
- Failure to address occult instability in another direction
- Overtight repair resulting in subluxation or degenerative change
- Detached staples, tacks, sutures
- General postoperative complications: adhesive capsulitis, synovitis, abscess formation, osteomyelitis, chondrolysis, and hematoma formation

patients have been exposed to thermal energy. Additional research is going to be required to determine the exact etiology. Patients developing rapid-onset chondrolysis typical develop shoulder pain and loss of normal range of motion at some time during the first 3 to 12 months after shoulder reconstruction. MRI demonstrates complete loss of the articular cartilage on both sides of the joint with subchondral sclerosis and marrow edema (Fig. 106-38). There is a conspicuous absence of osteophyte formation and usually a paucity of joint fluid and no synovial thickening, which helps in differentiating this entity from synovitis or acute infection (Table 106-13).

SUGGESTED READINGS

Feller JF, Howey TD, Plaga BR. MR imaging of the postoperative shoulder. In Steinbach LS, Tirman PFJ, Petrfy CG, Feller JF (eds). Philadelphia, Lippincott-Raven, 1998, pp 187–221.

Haygood TM, Oxner KG, Kneeland JB, Dalinka MK. Magnetic resonance imaging of the postoperative shoulder. MRI Clin North Am 1993; 1:143–155.

Longobardi RSF, Rafii M, Minkoff JM. MR imaging of the postoperative shoulder. MRI Clin North Am 1997; 5:841–859.

Mohana-Borges A, Chung C, Resnick D. MR imaging and MR arthrography of the postoperative shoulder: spectrum of normal and abnormal findings. RadioGraphics 2004; 24:69–85.

Owen RS, Iannotti JP, Kneeland JB, et al. Shoulder after surgery: MR imaging with surgical validation. Radiology 1993; 186:443–447.

Rand T, Trattnig S, Breitensher M, et al. The postoperative shoulder. Topics Magn Reson Imaging 1999; 10:203–213.

Zlatkin MB. MRI of the postoperative shoulder. Skelet Radiol 2002; 31:63–80.

REFERENCES

1. Matsen FA, Arntz CT, Lippitt SB. Rotator cuff. In Rockwood CE, Matsen FA (eds). The Shoulder. Philadelphia, WB Saunders, 1998, pp 755–795.
2. Yamaguchi K. Mini-open rotator cuff repair: an updated perspective. Instr Course Lect 2001; 50:53–61.
3. Rockwood CA, Lyons FR. Shoulder Impingement syndrome: diagnosis, radiographic evaluation, and treatment with a modified Neer acromioplasty. J Bone Joint Surg Am 1993; 75:409–424.
4. Beach WR, Caspari RB: Arthroscopic management of rotator cuff disease. Orthopedics 1993; 16:1007–1015.
5. Cameron BD, Iannotti JP. Clinical evaluation of the painful shoulder. In Zhatkin MB (ed). MRI of the Shoulder. Philadelphia, Lippincott Williams & Wilkins, 2003, pp 47–84.
6. Kvitne RS, Jobe FW. The diagnosis and treatment of anterior instability in the throwing athlete. Clin Orthop Relat Res 1993; (291):107–123.
7. Owen RS, Ianotti JP, Kneeland JB, et al. Shoulder after surgery: MR imaging with surgical validation. Radiology 1993; 186:443–447.
8. Longobardi RSF, Rafii M, Minkoff JM. MR imaging of the postoperative shoulder. MRI Clin North Am 1997; 5:841–859.
9. Gusmer PB, Potter HG, Donovan WD, O'Brien SJ: MR imaging of the shoulder after rotator cuff repair. AJR Am J Roentgenol 1997; 168:559–563.
10. Ogilvie-Harris D, Wiley A, Sattarian J: Failed acromioplasty for impingement syndrome. J Bone Joint Surg Br 1990; 72:1070–1072.
11. Magee TH, Gaenslen ES, Seitz R, et al. MR imaging of the shoulder after surgery. Am J Roentgenol AJR 1997; 168:925–928.
12. Rand T, Trattnig S, Breitensher M, et al. The postoperative shoulder. Topics Magn Reson Imaging 1999; 10:203–213.
13. Arroyo JS, Flatow EL. Management of rotator cuff disease: intact and repairable cuff. In Iannotti JP, Williams GR Jr (eds). Disorders of the Shoulder: Diagnosis and Management. Philadelphia, Lippincott Williams & Wilkins, 1999, pp 31–56.
14. Burkhart SS. Shoulder arthroscopy: new concepts. Clin Sports Med 1996; 15:635.

15. Budoff JE, Nirschl RP, Guidi EJ. Débridement of partial thickness tears of the rotator cuff without acromioplasty. J Bone Joint Surg Am 1988; 80:733-748.
16. Melilo AS, Savoie FH, Field LD. Massive rotator cuff tears: débridement versus repair. Orthop Clin North Am 1997; 28:117-124.
17. Haygood TM, Oxner KG, Kneeland JB, Dalinka MK: Magnetic resonance imaging of the postoperative shoulder. MRI Clin North Am 1993; 1:143-155.
18. Gaenslen ES, Stterlee CC, Hinson GA, Wetzel LH. Magnetic resonance imaging for evaluation of failed repairs of the rotator cuff: relationship to operative findings. J Bone Joint Surg Am 1996; 78:1391-1396.
19. Zanetti MD, Jost B, Hodler J. MR findings in asymptomatic patients after supraspinatus reconstruction. Radiology 1999; 213:157.
20. Norwood L, Fowler FH: Rotator cuff tears: a shoulder arthroscopy complication. Am J Sports Med 1989; 17:837-841.
21. Feller JF, Howey TD, Plaga BR. MR imaging of the postoperative shoulder. In Steinbach LS, Tirman PFJ, Peterfy CG, Feller JF (eds). Shoulder Magnetic Resonance Imaging. Philadelphia, Lippincott-Raven, 1998, pp 187-192.
22. Matthews LS, Pavlovich LJ Jr. Anterior and anteroinferior instability: diagnosis and management. In Iannotti JP, Williams GR Jr (eds). Disorders of the Shoulder: Diagnosis and Management. Philadelphia, Lippincott Williams & Wilkins, 1999, pp 251-294.
23. Neer CS, Foster CR. Inferior capsular shift for involuntary inferior and multidirectional instability of the shoulder: a preliminary report. J Bone Joint Surg Am 1980; 62:897-908.
24. Sugimoto H, Suzuki K, Mihara K, et al. MR arthrography of shoulders after suture-anchor Bankart repair. Radiology 2002; 224:105-111.
25. Hashiuchi T, Ozaki J, Sakurai G, Imada K. The changes occurring after the Putti-Platt procedure using magnetic resonance imaging. Arch Orthop Trauma Surg 2000; 120:286-289.
26. Wagner SC, Schweitzer ME, Morrison WB, et al. Shoulder instability: accuracy of MR imaging performed after surgery in depicting recurrent injury. Radiology 2002; 222:196-203.
27. Tirman PF, Feller JF, Janzen DL, et al. Association of glenoid labral cysts and tears and glenohumeral instability: radiological findings and clinical significance. Radiology 1994; 190:653-658.
28. Emig W, Scweitzer ME, Karasick D, Lubowtiz J. Adhesive capsulitis of the shoulder: MR diagnosis. Am J Roentgenol AJR 1994; 164:1457-1459.
29. Levine WN, Clark AM Jr, D'Alessandro DF, Yamaguchi K. Chondrolysis following arthroscopic thermal capsulorrhaphy to treat shoulder instability. J Bone Joint Surg Am 2005; 87:616-621.

107

The Postoperative Elbow, Wrist, and Hand

Lynne S. Steinbach and Christine B. Chung

Elbow, wrist, and hand surgery are frequently done to repair bone and soft tissues such as fractures and disruptions of ligaments and tendons. Nerves also traverse the area and are released from various tunnels. In this chapter we discuss common indications for surgery on various bone and soft tissue structures in and around these joints and describe some of the procedures with their postoperative imaging appearances.

Ulnar Collateral Ligament of the Elbow Reconstruction

DESCRIPTION, INDICATIONS, CONTRAINDICATIONS, PURPOSE, UNDERLYING MECHANICS

The ulnar collateral ligament (UCL) complex is composed of an anterior, a posterior, and a transverse bundle. Although the entire complex is charged with providing valgus stability to the elbow, it is the anterior bundle that has been shown to be the most important stabilizer against valgus stress at the joint from 30 to 120 degrees of flexion. Interestingly, a single acute traumatic episode to this ligament rarely leads to symptomatic instability in the majority of those injured.[1,2] Rather it is chronic repetitive microtrauma with recurrent valgus stress at the medial elbow, such as that encountered in the overhead throwing athlete, that has been implicated in symptomatic valgus instability.[3–9] It is the near-failure tensile stress encountered in the overhead throwing motion that results in the injury to the UCL and the need to expose an injured ligament to this stress that forms the basis for two of the indications for

surgical management. These include (1) throwing athletes with a complete UCL tear; (2) partial tears that have failed rehabilitation; and (3) symptomatic nonthrowing athletes after a minimum of 3 months of rehabilitation.[3,6,10]

There are six phases of throwing: wind up, early cocking, late cocking, acceleration, deceleration, and follow through. It is the combination of large valgus loads initiated in the late cocking phase with the rapid elbow extension generated in acceleration that produces compression overload laterally, sheer stress in the posterior compartment, and tensile overload medially. This phenomenon, termed *valgus extension overload syndrome* forms the basic pathophysiologic model behind most common elbow injuries in the overhead throwing athlete, including UCL injury.[11] This concept, although incompletely developed, was introduced in the literature in the late 1960s and was termed *medial elbow-stress syndrome*.[12] This marked the advent of a heightened awareness and new understanding of the pathophysiology of a major cause of elbow pain in the

---

KEY POINTS

- The anterior band of the ulnar collateral ligament is usually reconstructed rather than repaired.
- There are a variety of techniques used to reconstruct the ulnar collateral ligament, and it is important to understand which one was used.
- The ulnar nerve may be transposed during surgery and is occasionally injured.
- The reconstructed ligament should be evaluated for full-thickness and partial-thickness tears that may occur at any location.
- Metal hardware may dislodge after surgery.
- Metal suppression techniques and MR arthrography are useful for evaluating postoperative complications.

overhead throwing athlete, one that would clearly require operative treatment for a successful outcome.

In 1974, the first UCL reconstruction was performed by Dr. Frank Jobe, who gave his patient, Tommy John (a Los Angeles Dodgers pitcher), a 1% chance of avoiding retirement with the intervention. Tommy John returned to baseball 2 years later, and the successful procedure revolutioned the treatment of UCL reconstruction. Although early studies advocated primary repair of UCL injuries, the applicability of these studies to current patient populations is limited because they did not include high performance athletes or document the type or level of sports involvement.[13,14] Numerous recent studies have concluded that UCL reconstruction is more effective than primary repair in correcting medial elbow instability and returning overhead throwing athletes to a preinjury level of play in less than 1 year, the measure of a successful procedure.[5,15,16]

Figure-of-Eight Repair

The original UCL reconstruction was performed by Jobe and associates.[6] The ligament was exposed by detaching and elevating the flexor-pronator muscle mass from the medial epicondyle of the humerus. A submuscular ulnar nerve transposition was performed. The anterior bundle of the UCL was reconstructed with a harvested autograft (palmaris longus) in a figure-of-eight fashion through two drill holes in the ulna and three in the medial epicondyle (Fig. 107-1). The posterior cortex of the humerus was penetrated, and the graft was sutured to itself.

At 2-year follow-up, 63% of elite throwing athletes returned to a preinjury level of throwing for at least 1 year.[5,6] Despite the ground-breaking success of this procedure, the rate of complication was 31%. Postoperative dysfunction of the ulnar nerve was the most commonly cited complication, often requiring decompression. Similar results were seen in a subsequent larger study group with 68% of elite throwing athletes returning to a preinjury level

of throwing for at least 1 year.[1] In this group, postoperative ulnar nerve dysfunction occurred in 21% of patients, several of whom required revision decompression of the ulnar nerve. These results prompted the development of surgical modifications to simplify the technique, evade dissection and detachment of the flexor-pronator mass, and limit handling of the ulnar nerve.

Muscle-Splitting Modification

In 1996, Smith and associates described the "safe zone" of the medial elbow.[17] This zone refers to an internervous plane of exposure to the medial ulnohumeral articulation that extends from the medial epicondyle to 1 cm distal to the insertion of the UCL on the sublime tubercle of the ulna. It is between the median and ulnar nerve sites of innervation of surrounding muscles. Rather than completely detach the flexor-pronator mass from the medial epicondyle, the muscle group was split along its "safe zone," through the posterior third of the common flexor bundle (the most anterior fibers of the flexor carpi ulnaris), to access the joint and perform the ligament reconstruction using Jobe's original technique. This modified technique also obviated the need to transpose the ulnar nerve.

At 2-year follow-up, 82% of elite overhead throwing athletes returned to play.[18] In athletes without prior surgery, this number increased to 93%. In the immediate postoperative period, only 5% of the patients had transient ulnar nerve problems. All resolved without surgery.

American Sports Medicine Institute (ASMI) Modification

Andrews and colleagues modified Jobe's original technique by retracting the flexor carpi ulnaris anteriorly and by performing a subcutaneous rather than submuscular nerve transposition.[15,16] In a large retrospective review comparing primary ligament repair with this modified technique, 79% of patients undergoing reconstruction returned to a preinjury level of play an average of 9.8 months after surgery.[16] In comparison, only 63% of patients treated with direct repair returned to the same level of sport. Only one of the patients with ligament reconstruction developed transient postoperative ulnar nerve changes. Moreover, 9 of 10 patients who had preoperative ulnar neuritis experienced resolution of symptoms.

Suture Anchor Method

In the mid 1990s, suture anchors were introduced into the UCL reconstruction techniques in an attempt at further simplifying the procedure. A cadaveric study by Hechtman and associates compared the suture anchor and bone tunnel techniques in 31 cadaveric specimens (15 underwent reconstruction with bone tunnels, 16 with suture anchors).[19] The strength of each reconstruction was compared with the original strength of the ligament. Results of this study showed that there was no significant difference in reconstruction strength between the suture anchor (76.3%) and the bone tunnel (63.9%) techniques. Both methods produced reconstructions that were significantly

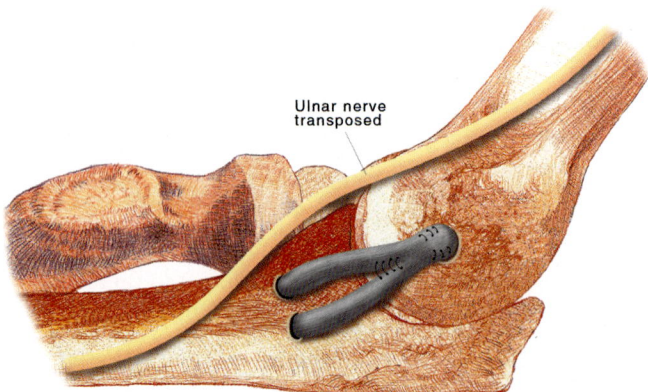

Ulnar nerve transposed

■ **FIGURE 107-1** Figure-of-eight repair, known as the Tommy John procedure, was the first ulnar collateral ligament reconstruction method. The ligament was exposed by detaching and elevating the flexor-pronator muscle mass from the medial epicondyle of the humerus. A submuscular ulnar nerve transposition was performed. The anterior bundle of the ligament was reconstructed with a harvested autograft (palmaris longus) in a figure-of-eight fashion through two drill holes in the ulna and three in the medial epicondyle.

weaker than a native UCL. It was apparent, however, that the suture anchor technique reproduced normal UCL anatomy and mechanical function more closely than bone tunnels. Despite the apparent success of this cadaveric work, the technique fell out of use when clinical applications yielded a failure rate of 30%.[9]

Docking Technique

In 1996, Altchek and coworkers implemented a muscle-splitting approach to modify the UCL reconstruction in a technique called the "docking procedure."[20] Unlike Jobe's technique, in which the graft is placed in a figure-of-eight position, in this technique the graft is placed in a triangular configuration through a single humeral tunnel and the limbs are brought out through separate bone tunnels and tied over a bone bridge. It has been suggested that the docking technique allows for better tensioning of the ligament graft. In an uncontrolled retrospective review by Rohrbough and associates, 92% of patients returned to a preinjury level of play for at least 1 year. No complications were reported.

Interference Technique

Ahmad and coworkers described an interference technique for fixation of the UCL graft. The goal was to reconstruct the central isometric fibers of the native UCL, which lie between the anterior one third and the posterior two thirds of the anterior bundle of the UCL.[21] Through a muscle-splitting approach, grafts are fixed with interference screws placed in single bony tunnels in the humerus and ulna. Unlike Jobe's original technique, only two bone tunnels are needed. The ulnar nerve is less at risk. Likewise, without an intervening bony bridge on the ulna, the risk of tunnel fractures between the two tunnels, is theoretically eliminated.

The biomechanical results of this technique have been mixed. In a cadaveric study comparing intact with reconstructed elbows using the interference technique, the normal elbow kinematics were restored with the interference fixation. The failure strength of the UCL reconstruction with interference fixation was reported to be similar to that of the native intact UCL.[22] In this study, the ligament was loaded once to failure. However, in a study in which a cyclic loading protocol is used to better replicate the clinical mechanism of injury, this technique as well as other reconstruction techniques showed reconstruction failure at significantly lower loads than the normal intact ligament.[23]

EXPECTED APPEARANCE ON IMAGING

Little has been written on imaging evaluation of ulnar collateral ligament reconstruction. Stress radiographs are limited for examination of the ulnar collateral ligament. Sometimes they are normal in the presence of a rupture. CT arthrography is also limited. In our experience, the reconstructed ligament is continuous and water tight, as demonstrated on MR arthrography (Fig. 107-2). The integrity of the ligament can be assessed with MRI, MR arthrography, or ultrasound. On MRI performed in the early stages, the ligament may demonstrate high signal intensity within its

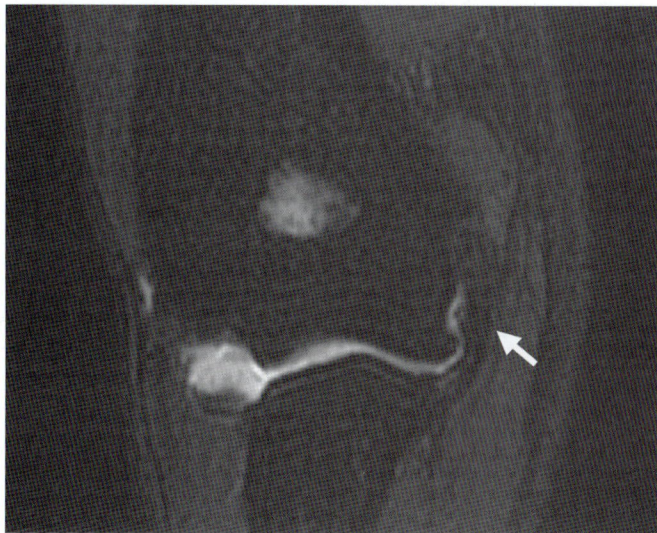

■ **FIGURE 107-2** This coronal T1-weighted MR arthrographic image of a pitcher's elbow demonstrates an intact ulnar collateral ligament 5 years after surgical reconstruction (*arrow*). (*Courtesy of William Morrison, MD, Philadelphia, PA.*)

substance related to suture material and granulation tissue. With time (approximately 6 months) the normal ligament decreases in signal intensity on all imaging sequences. It may be thickened (Fig. 107-3). There are often tunneling defects in the distal humerus and proximal ulna. Metal anchors and screws may be present. These metallic devices could interfere with assessment of the ligament on MRI (Fig. 107-4). Metal reduction techniques such as increasing bandwidth, avoiding fat-suppression and gradient-echo

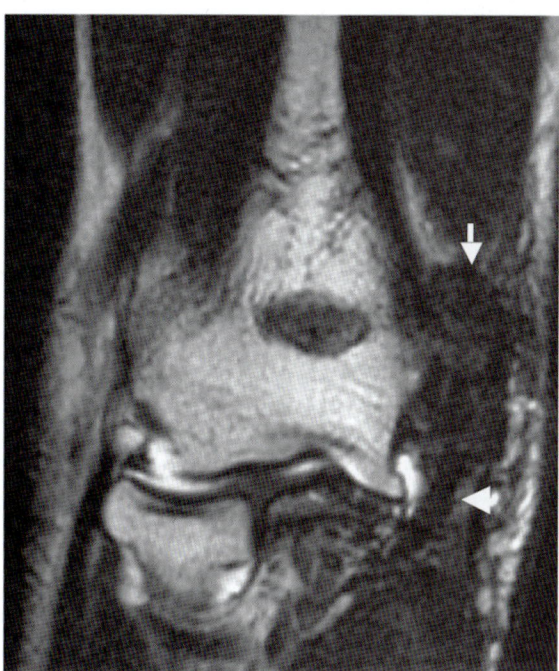

■ **FIGURE 107-3** Intact ulnar collateral ligament repair on a coronal T2-weighted MR image. Notice the normally thickened tendon graft (*arrowhead*) as well as the scarring above the graft (*arrow*). (*Courtesy of William Morrison, MD, Philadelphia, PA.*)

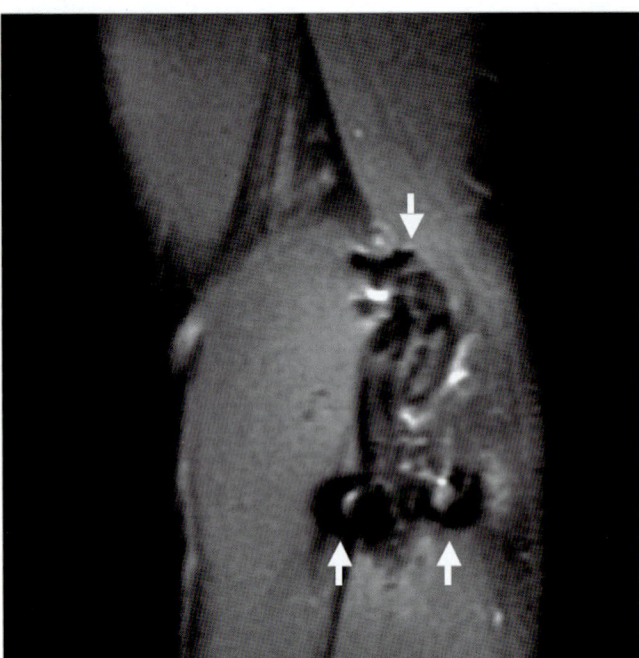

■ **FIGURE 107-4** Sagittal T2-weighted MR image of the elbow demonstrates artifact from screws at both ends of an ulnar collateral ligament reconstruction. The ligament was intact. *(Courtesy of William Morrison, MD, Philadelphia, PA.)*

techniques, and using lower magnetic field strength aid in evaluation of the ligament reconstruction. MR arthrography is useful for evaluation of the intact ligament. The ulnar nerve may have been transposed from the cubital tunnel and placed in a submuscular or subcutaneous location. One should assess the nerve signal and size related to itself in other locations or to other nerves around the elbow to determine if it is abnormal.

POTENTIAL COMPLICATIONS AND RADIOLOGIC APPEARANCE

The success rates of reconstruction vary between 63% and 97%, depending on the technique. Reported complication rates are less than 10%. Despite the variability in techniques, the unifying features are that decreased dissection of the flexor-pronator mass and decreased handling of the ulnar nerve leads to improved outcomes.[7]

As noted previously, four UCL reconstruction techniques have been compared biomechanically (docking, interference screw fixation, figure-of-eight, single-stranded UCL reconstruction using an EndoButton [Smith & Nephew, London, England] for ulnar fixation).[23] Cadaveric specimens were subjected to pneumatic cyclic valgus loading. All techniques showed significantly lower peak load to failure than the intact native ligament. No difference in strength was found between the docking and single-stranded UCL reconstruction using EndoButton fixation. Both of these techniques were stronger than the interference screw or figure-of-eight techniques.

For the 20 intact specimens in the study, complete disruption of the ligament occurred at the humeral attachment in 9 specimens, the ulnar attachment in 4, and the midsubstance of the anterior bundle of the medial collateral ligament in 2.[23] In the remaining five specimens the joint gapped 5 mm without complete visual disruption of the ligament. In the reconstruction, no complete disruption occurred for any technique. For the docking, EndoButton, and figure-of-eight procedures, the mode of failure was the suture pulling out of the suture/ligament interface. For the interference screw reconstruction, the tendon pulled out at the tendon/screw interface.

Regarding visualization of complications on imaging, one should evaluate the elbow for abnormal valgus angulation and dislodgement of hardware on radiographs, ultrasonography, and MRI. The tendon or graft should be assessed for discontinuity, laxity, thinning, and irregularity. MR arthrography is helpful for evaluating continuity of the ligament and for outlining the undersurface of the ligament for irregularity or laxity related to partial tears. Median, radial, and ulnar nerve injury is a complication of elbow surgery due to laceration or compression. One should look for other postoperative changes such as excessive scar tissue, infection, synovial fistula formation, and instruments or other hardware left in the joint.

SUGGESTED READINGS

Cain EL, Dugas JR, Wolf RS, Andrews JR. Elbow injuries in throwing athletes: a current concepts review. Am J Sports Med 2003; 31:621–635.

Jobe FW, Start H, Lombardo SF. Reconstruction of the ulnar collateral ligament in athletes. J Bone Joint Surg Am 1986; 68:1158.

Kaplan LJ, Potter HG. MR imaging of ligament injuries to the elbow. Magn Reson Imaging Clin North Am 2004; 12:221–232.

O'Holleran JD, Altchek DW. The throwers elbow: arthroscopic treatment of valgus extension overload syndrome. HSS J 2006; 2:83–93.

REFERENCES

1. Morrey BF, An KN. Articular and ligamentous contributions to the stability of the elbow joint. Am J Sports Med 1983; 11:315–319.
2. Schwab GH, Bennett JB, Woods GW, Tullos HS. Biomechanics of elbow instability: the role of the medial collateral ligament. Clin Orthop Relat Res 1980; (146):42–52.
3. Chen FS, Rokito AS, Jobe FW. Medial elbow problems in the overhead-throwing athlete. J Am Acad Orthop Surg 2001; 9:99–113.
4. Ciccotti MG, Jobe FW. Medial collateral ligament instability and ulnar neuritis in the athlete's elbow. Instr Course Lect 1999; 48:383–391.
5. Conway JE, Jobe FW, Glousman RE, Pink M. Medial instability of the elbow in throwing athletes: treatment by repair or reconstruction of the ulnar collateral ligament. J Bone Joint Surg Am 1992; 74:67–83.
6. Jobe FW, Stark H, Lombardo SJ. Reconstruction of the ulnar collateral ligament in athletes. J Bone Joint Surg Am 1986; 68:1158–1163.
7. Langer P, Fadale P, Hulstyn M. Evolution of the treatment options of ulnar collateral ligament injuries of the elbow. Br J Sports Med 2006; 40:499–506.
8. Pappas AM, Zawacki RM, Sullivan TJ. Biomechanics of baseball pitching: a preliminary report. Am J Sports Med 1985; 13:216–222.
9. Williams RJ 3rd, Urquhart ER, Altchek DW. Medial collateral ligament tears in the throwing athlete. Instr Course Lect 2004; 53:579–586.
10. David TS. Medial elbow pain in the throwing athlete. Orthopedics 2003; 26:94–103; quiz 104–105.
11. Wilson FD, Andrews JR, Blackburn TA, McCluskey G. Valgus extension overload in the pitching elbow. Am J Sports Med 1983; 11:83–88.

12. King J, Brelsford HJ, Tullos HS. Analysis of the pitching arm of the professional baseball pitcher. Clin Orthop Relat Res 1969; 67:116-123.
13. Kuroda S, Sakamaki K. Ulnar collateral ligament tears of the elbow joint. Clin Orthop Relat Res 1986; (208):266-271.
14. Norwood LA, Shook JA, Andrews JR. Acute medial elbow ruptures. Am J Sports Med 1981; 9:16-19.
15. Andrews JR, Timmerman LA. Outcome of elbow surgery in professional baseball players. Am J Sports Med 1995; 23:407-413.
16. Azar FM, Andrews JR, Wilk KE, Groh D. Operative treatment of ulnar collateral ligament injuries of the elbow in athletes. Am J Sports Med 2000; 28:16-23.
17. Smith GR, Altchek DW, Pagnani MJ, Keeley JR. A muscle-splitting approach to the ulnar collateral ligament of the elbow: neuroanatomy and operative technique. Am J Sports Med 1996; 24:575-580.
18. Thompson WH, Jobe FW, Yocum LA, Pink MM. Ulnar collateral ligament reconstruction in athletes: muscle-splitting approach without transposition of the ulnar nerve. J Shoulder Elbow Surg 2001; 10:152-157.
19. Hechtman KS, Tjin A, Zvijac JE, et al. Biomechanics of a less invasive procedure for reconstruction of the ulnar collateral ligament of the elbow. Am J Sports Med 1998; 26:620-624.
20. Rohrbough JT, Altchek DW, Hyman J, et al. Medial collateral ligament reconstruction of the elbow using the docking technique. Am J Sports Med 2002; 30:541-548.
21. Ochi N, Ogura T, Hashizume H, et al. Anatomic relation between the medial collateral ligament of the elbow and the humero-ulnar joint axis. J Shoulder Elbow Surg 1999; 8:6-10.
22. Ahmad CS, Lee TQ, El Attrache NS. Biomechanical evaluation of a new ulnar collateral ligament reconstruction technique with interference screw fixation. Am J Sports Med 2003; 31:332-337.
23. Armstrong AD, Dunning CE, Ferreira LM, et al. A biomechanical comparison of four reconstruction techniques for the medial collateral ligament-deficient elbow. J Shoulder Elbow Surg 2005; 14:207-215.

Lateral Collateral Ligament of the Elbow Reconstruction

DESCRIPTION, INDICATIONS, CONTRAINDICATIONS, PURPOSE, UNDERLYING MECHANICS

The lateral collateral ligament (LCL) complex consists of four components: the annular ligament, the radial collateral ligament, the lateral ulnar collateral ligament, and the accessory annular ligament.[1] The ligament complex originates from the undersurface of the lateral epicondyle at a point through which the center of rotation passes. Therefore, it is isometric throughout the normal range of flexion and extension. The radial collateral ligament has a distal point of attachment on the annular ligament, stabilizing the proximal radioulnar joint. The lateral ulnar collateral ligament also attaches to the annular ligament but has a point of attachment distally at the supinator crest of the ulna.[2] Because this ligament crosses the articulation and has both a proximal and distal osseous attachment, it is considered to be a major stabilizer of the lateral elbow. In 1991, O'Driscoll and associates first described posterolateral rotatory instability of the

elbow.[3] The cause for this condition was thought to be a laxity of the lateral ulnar collateral ligament allowing a transient rotatory subluxation of the ulnohumeral joint and a secondary dislocation of the radiocapitellar joint. Ordinarily, the LCL complex maintains these joints in a reduced position. A mechanism for elbow subluxation and dislocation was then described in which there was increasing ligamentous and capsular damage progressing from lateral to medial across the joint.[4] Dislocation was the final of three sequential stages of elbow instability resulting from posterolateral rotation.

Presentation and Indications for Operative Treatment

Most patients with lateral elbow instability present with symptoms after an elbow dislocation. Less commonly, there is a history of surgery to the lateral side of the elbow. Although most studies indicate that both medial and lateral collateral ligament complexes are disrupted after dislocation, residual instability more commonly involves the lateral side.[5] The clinical presentation is quite variable, although patients often present with a history of recurrent painful clicking, catching, or snapping of the elbow. Symptoms typically occur in the extension portion of the motion arc with the forearm in supination. The classic activity that reproduces a patient's symptoms is pushing down on the armrest when rising from a chair. The physical examination may be unremarkable. The classic physical examination finding is that of a positive pivot shift maneuver. The elbow is supinated by applying torque at the wrist, and a valgus moment is applied to the elbow during flexion. This action results in a typical apprehension response with reproduction of the patient's symptoms and a sense that the elbow is about to dislocate.[3] Reproducing the actual subluxation and the clunk that occurs with reduction can usually be accomplished only with the patient under general anesthesia.[6]

Indications for surgical treatment of the LCL complex include patients with symptomatic instability. Reconstruction of the LCL complex has been recommended to restore stability of the elbow in patients with posterolateral rotatory instability.[3,7-9] Although there are no absolute contraindications to surgical treatment

---

KEY POINTS

■ The lateral collateral ligament complex can be repaired or reconstructed.
■ There are a variety of techniques used to reconstruct the lateral collateral ligament, and it is important to understand which one was used.
■ The reconstructed ligament should be evaluated for full-thickness and partial-thickness tears that may occur at any location.
■ Metal hardware may dislodge after surgery.
■ Metal suppression techniques and MR arthrography are useful for evaluating postoperative complications.

there are relative ones. Children with open epiphyseal plates should not have their ligaments reconstructed with tendon grafts across the physis.[9] Instead, the existing lateral collateral ligament tissues are imbricated and reattached to bone iosmetrically. The absence of a radial head adversely affects the prognosis of surgical therapy but is not a contraindication.

Primary Ligament Repair

As on the medial side, the LCL complex can be treated with a primary repair or reconstruction. Sanchez-Sotelo and coworkers reported that reconstruction using a tendon graft seemed to provide better results than ligament repair for the treatment of posterolateral rotatory instability of the elbow.[10] Osborne and Cotterill first described repair of the lateral capsuloligamentous structures of the elbow for recurrent dislocation.[9] Currently, acute ligament repair is recommended only for gross instability after reduction of the elbow or in conjunction with open reduction of fracture-dislocations. This is particularly indicated when there has been internal fixation of the radial head and or coronoid process.[11] In such cases, the ligamentous and muscular origins have usually been avulsed from the lateral epicondyle and can be repaired directly back down to bone, thereby reestablishing lateral elbow stability. Most authors believe that acute ligament repairs should be augmented with a heavy suture along the course of the lateral ulnar collateral ligament.[12] This serves to stress-shield the repair during the early postoperative period. The LCL complex can also be augmented using three fan-shaped arcades of suture secured through holes drilled in the lateral epicondyle.[13] The first arcade follows the path of the lateral ulnar collateral ligament, the second follows the path of the lateral collateral ligament and engages the annular ligament, and the third engages the posterior capsule and anconeus muscle.

Lateral Collateral Ligament Complex Reconstruction

While there is little in the way of long-term results of this treatment, the procedure appears successful. O'Driscoll and associates briefly mention results in five patients in their initial description of the posterolateral rotatory instability of the elbow.[3] In 1992, Nestor and colleagues reported results of LCL complex reconstruction in 11 patients with an average of 42 months' follow-up.[14] Stability was obtained in 10 patients, 7 of whom had an excellent functional result. The 4 patients with less than excellent results had had previous surgery. If the radial head has been excised or there is degenerative change in the joint, the satisfactory result decreases, although stability is usually achieved.[11] More recently, Sanchez-Sotelo and associates described the intermediate results of lateral ligamentous reconstruction for posterolateral rotatory instability of the elbow. Surgery restored stability in all except 5 patients. In 2 of the 5, the elbow became stable after a second procedure. Better results were obtained in patients with a post-traumatic etiology, subjective symptoms of instability at presentation,

and those who had an augmented reconstruction using a tendon graft.[10]

Most LCL complex reconstructions use the technique introduced by O'Driscoll, or some modification of it.[3] This technique begins with a 10-cm incision between the epicondyle and olecranon. The deep fascia is incised along the supracondylar ridge and distally between the anconeus and extensor carpi ulnaris muscles. The triceps and anconeus are reflected in continuity off the posterior humerus and capsule, exposing the lateral side of the ulna. The common extensor origin is partially reflected to expose the capsule. Capsuloligamentous attenuation is assessed and laxity confirmed. The capsule is opened along the capitellum in an arc to permit inspection of the joint and later imbrication of the capsule. The insertion site for the tendon graft is then prepared by creating two drill holes in the ulna, one near the tubercle on the supinator crest and the other 1.25 cm proximally at the base of the annular ligament. The underlying bone is channeled. Suture is passed through the holes, and the isometric ligament insertion is determined by flexing and extending the elbow to see if the suture moves. No movement occurs when suture and hemostat are on the isometric point. A hole for the graft entry site on the humerus is then created. If the hole is placed distal or posterior, the graft will be lax in extension and tight in flexion. An exit for the graft is created just posterior to the supracondylar ridge about 1.5 cm proximally with a tunnel extending between the entry and exit sites. A third and final hole is placed in the distal humerus and is referred to as the reentry site. It is located just posterior to the initial entry site hole, and a tunnel will extend between it and the entry site. The graft will pass through this tunnel and will be sutured to itself at the entry site.[3,10,14]

EXPECTED APPEARANCE ON IMAGING

On MRI, the ligament should be continuous after primary repair or graft reconstruction. It will be heterogenous in signal intensity at first but should decrease in signal intensity with time. It may be helpful to see this ligament using the 20-degree posterior oblique axis with regard to the elbow joint from a sagittal scout image.[16]

POTENTIAL COMPLICATIONS AND RADIOLOGIC APPEARANCE

Delayed laxity, recurrent dislocation, and reinjury have been observed after lateral collateral ligament complex reconstruction (Fig. 107-5). Complications associated with graft harvesting are possible. Iatrogenic fracture of the osseous tunnels can occur but are generally not problematic with careful surgical technique. Mild flexion contracture can be accepted as the most vulnerable position of instability in full extension. As always, infection is also a possible complication of surgery (Fig. 107-6).

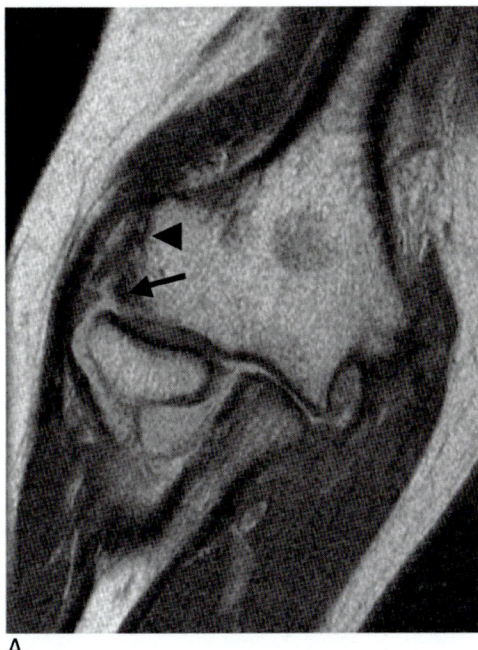

A

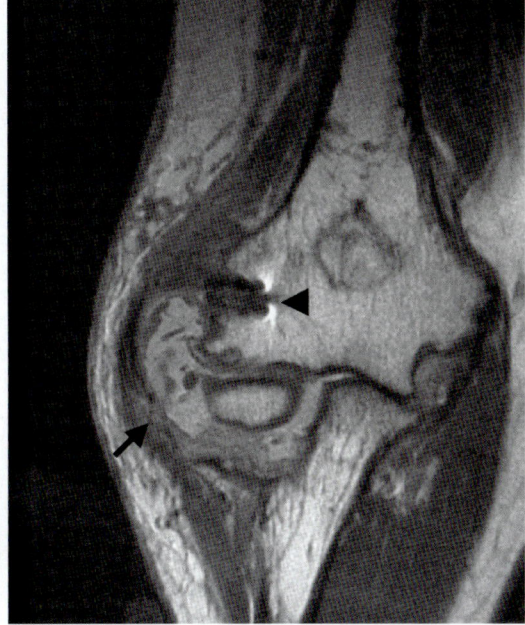

B

■ **FIGURE 107-5** Lateral ulnar collateral ligament tear with repair. **A,** There is a high-grade partial tear of the origin of the lateral ulnar collateral ligament at the lateral epicondyle (*arrow*) on this coronal proton density–weighted MR image of the elbow. Also note the torn common extensor tendon (*arrowhead*). **B,** The lateral ulnar collateral ligament tore again after repair, this time in the mid- distal aspect (*arrow*). Notice the metallic hardware (*arrowhead*) and the joint debris. (*Courtesy of the Department of Radiology and Imaging, Hospital for Special Surgery, New York, NY.*)

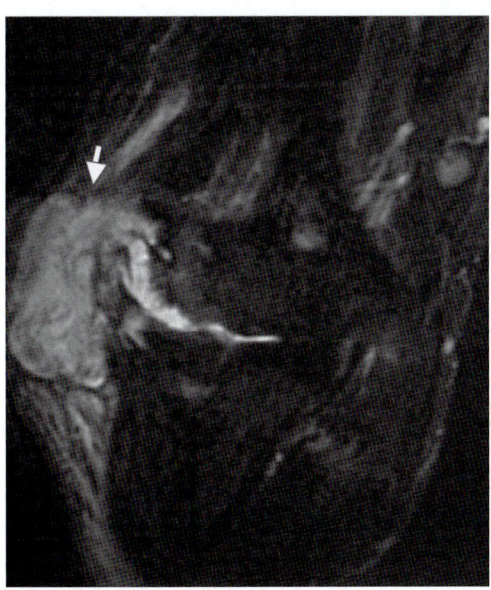

A

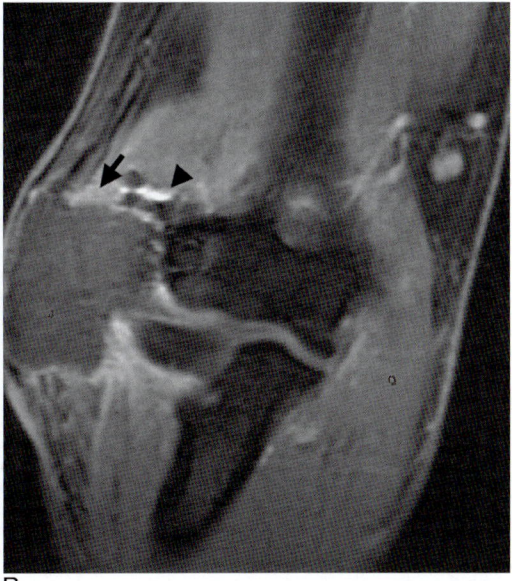

B

■ **FIGURE 107-6** **A,** Coronal, fat-suppressed, T2-weighted MR image of the elbow demonstrates a high signal intensity abscess (*arrow*) communicating with the elbow joint after surgery on the lateral ulnar collateral ligament. **B,** The abscess rim enhances on the fat-suppressed, coronal, T1-weighted MR image after intravenous administration of gadolinium (*arrow*). Notice the postoperative metallic artifact (*arrowhead*). (*Courtesy of William Morrison, MD, Philadelphia, PA.*)

SUGGESTED READINGS

Kaplan LJ, Potter HG. MR imaging of ligament injuries to the elbow. Magn Reson Imaging Clin North Am 2004; 12:221–232.

O'Driscoll S, Morrey BF. Surgical reconstruction of the lateral collateral ligament. In Morrey BF (ed). The Elbow, 2nd ed. Philadelphia, Lippincott Williams & Wilkins, 2002, pp 249–263.

REFERENCES

1. Morrey BF, An KN. Functional anatomy of the ligaments of the elbow. Clin Orthop Relat Res 1985; (201):84–90.
2. O'Driscoll SW, Morrey BF, Carmichael SW. Anatomy of the ulnar part of the lateral collateral ligament of the elbow. Clin Anat 1992; (5):296–303.
3. O'Driscoll SW, Bell DF, Morrey BF. Posterolateral rotatory instability of the elbow. J Bone Joint Surg Am 1991; 73:440–446.
4. O'Driscoll SW, Morrey BF, Korinek S, An KN. Elbow subluxation and dislocation: a spectrum of instability. Clin Orthop Relat Res 1992; (280):186–197.
5. Josefsson PO, Johnell O, Wendeberg B. Ligamentous injuries in dislocations of the elbow joint. Clin Orthop Relat Res 1987; (221):221–225.
6. Ball CM, Galatz LM, Yamaguchi K. Elbow instability: treatment strategies and emerging concepts. Instr Course Lect 2002; 51:53–61.
7. Olsen BS, Sojbjerg JO. The treatment of recurrent posterolateral instability of the elbow. J Bone Joint Surg Br 2003; 85:342–346.
8. Olsen BS, Sojbjerg JO, Nielsen KK, et al. Posterolateral elbow joint instability: the basic kinematics. J Shoulder Elbow Surg 1998; 7:19–29.
9. Osborne G, Cotterill P. Recurrent dislocation of the elbow. J Bone Joint Surg Br 1966; 48:340–346.

10. Sanchez-Sotelo J, Morrey BF, O'Driscoll SW. Ligamentous repair and reconstruction for posterolateral rotatory instability of the elbow. J Bone Joint Surg Br 2005; 87:54–61.
11. O'Driscoll SW, Jupiter JB, King GW, et al. The unstable elbow. Instr Course Lect 2001; 50:89–102.
12. O'Driscoll SW. Elbow instability. Hand Clin 1994; 10:405–415.
13. King JC, et al. Lateral ligamentous instability: techniques of repair and reconstruction. Tech Orthop 2000; (15):93–104.
14. Nestor BJ, O'Driscoll SW, Morrey BF. Ligamentous reconstruction for posterolateral rotatory instability of the elbow. J Bone Joint Surg Am 1992; 74:1235–1241.
15. Rijke AM, Goitz HT, McCue FC, et al. Stress radiography of the medial elbow ligaments. Radiology 1994; 191:213–216.
16. Cotton A, Jacobson J, Brossmann J, et al. Collateral ligaments of the elbow: conventional MR imaging and arthrography with coronal oblique plane and elbow flexion. Radiology 1997; 204:806–812.

Ulnar Nerve Decompression

DESCRIPTION, INDICATIONS, CONTRAINDICATIONS, PURPOSE, UNDERLYING MECHANICS

Ulnar nerve entrapment at the elbow is the second most common peripheral nerve compression neuropathy. At the level of the elbow, the ulnar nerve is housed in the cubital tunnel. The cubital tunnel is a fibro-osseous conduit along the posterior aspect of the medial epicondyle. This fibro-osseous space is formed by the medial epicondyle anteriorly and the medial margin of the trochlea and olecranon laterally. The posterior bundle of the ulnar collateral ligament forms the floor of the cubital tunnel and the arcuate ligament the roof. The arcuate ligament may be absent in up to 23% of subjects.[1] Fatty tissue usually surrounds the ulnar nerve and posterior recurrent ulnar artery as they pass through the cubital tunnel.

The ulnar nerve innervates the skin and muscles of the ulnar side of the forearm and hand. This includes the flexor carpi ulnaris and half of the flexor digitorum profundus muscles. Several provocative tests can be used to identify the presence of ulnar nerve compression. Percussion over the ulnar nerve can elicit paresthesias or numbness, resulting in a positive "Tinel" sign. The elbow flexion test is analogous to the Phalen test in diagnosing carpal tunnel syndrome. With the elbow maximally flexed, forearm in supination, and wrist in full extension, patients with cubital tunnel syndrome can experience paresthesias and numbness along the distribution of the nerve.[2] Unfortunately, false-positive results can occur in approximately 10% of normal individuals.[3] Numbness along the small and ulnar half of the ring finger commonly can be due to ulnar nerve compression at the level of the elbow or as the nerve passes Guyon's canal. Sensory deficits over the dorsal ulnar aspect of the hand and the dorsum of the small finger can help in determining the level of compression. This area is innervated by the dorsal sensory branch of the ulnar nerve arising proximal to Guyon's canal, implying compression at the elbow.

Indications for Operative Ulnar Nerve Treatment

The clinical evaluation of ulnar nerve entrapment is crucial to guiding treatment, predicting success rates for treatment, as well as assessing post-therapy success. Although it appears that there is no uniformly accepted grading system to evaluate ulnar nerve entrapment, most assessments are based on subjective symptoms, muscle strength, and sensory disturbance. Some very detailed classification systems, such as the Yokohama City University scoring system, also consider the presence of finger deformity.[4] In general, surgical indications include patients with fixed sensory loss, pain, weakness, or significant denervation on electromyography.[5] Patients presenting with transient paresthesias and normal clinical findings are generally managed conservatively with behavioral modification that includes minimizing elbow flexion and prolonged pressure on the elbow.[6] Not only does the initial clinical assessment of ulnar nerve dysfunction serve as the basis for conservative versus operative treatment, it may indicate prognosis. Reports have suggested that prognosis may be more closely related to the level of preoperative damage of nerves and the period between the occurrence and surgery than to surgical methods.[4,7]

Surgical Therapy for Ulnar Nerve Decompression

Operative procedures for ulnar nerve entrapment at the elbow can be divided into two groups: decompression with transposition of the ulnar nerve and decompression without transposition of the ulnar nerve. The latter is also referred to as decompression in situ or a simple decompression.

Simple Decompression of the Ulnar Nerve

The operative procedure for simple decompression was described by Osborne.[6] An 8-cm long curved skin incision is made posterior to the medial epicondyle of the humerus.

KEY POINTS

- Ulnar neuropathy at the elbow can be treated with simple decompression of the arcuate ligament, medial epicondylectomy, or decompression with transposition.
- With transposition, the ulnar nerve is repositioned in an anterior subcutaneous, submuscular, or intramuscular location.
- The ulnar nerve should be evaluated for abnormal enlargement with MRI and ultrasonography.
- Abnormal high signal intensity in the nerve on MRI or hypoechogenicity on ultrasonography are postoperative signs of ulnar neuropathy.
- Scar tissue may cause complications for ulnar nerve surgery.
- Muscles should be evaluated for denervation.

The subcutaneous tissues are dissected, and the nerve is identified. The cubital tunnel retinaculum or arcuate ligament of Osborne is released. This is followed by widening of the entrance to the cubital tunnel between the two heads of the flexor carpi ulnaris muscle. Those who argue for simple decompression point out the potential for ischemia when the nerve is separated from its primary blood supply. The vascular stripping incurred during transposition may cause a significant decrease in regional blood flow.[8] Animal studies have shown that a devascularized nerve is more susceptible to pressure than a normal nerve.[9] One major aim of the simple decompression is to preserve the vascularity of the nerve.[10] Several studies have compared the simple decompression to both anterior submuscular transposition as well as anterior subcutaneous transposition.[6,11-14] In general, no statistically significant differences existed between outcomes of the simple decompression versus either transposition method. Because the simple decompression carries less risk of complication, many authors favor it.

Another method to decompress the ulnar nerve includes medial epicondylectomy. This procedure, the modified King's method, consists of a medial epicondylectomy of the humerus with resection of the fibrous band bridging the two heads of the flexor carpi ulnaris (arcuate ligament). Some advocate the use of a subtotal medial epicondylectomy with resection of 50% of the epicondyle.[2] The advantages of this procedure include removing or releasing all the compressing structures, creating minimal additional trauma to the nerve with preservation of the native blood supply, and allowing the nerve to follow a course of least resistance. The disadvantages can include bone tenderness at the site of osteotomy, nerve subluxation, flexor-pronator weakness, flexion contracture, and valgus instability. Numerous studies reporting the effectiveness of medial epicondylectomy for cubital tunnel syndrome have been published.[2,15,16] Geutjens and coworkers conducted the only randomized prospective study of 52 patients comparing medial epicondylectomy and anterior transposition. In this study, better results were found with medial epicondylectomy. This study found no evidence of ligamentous instability after removal of the medial epicondyle.

Ulnar Nerve Transposition

The issue of nerve transposition is a controversial one. It has two main advantages. The first, depending on the cause of the nerve entrapment, is that the nerve may be removed from an unfavorable environment.[17,18] This may occur when the etiology is scar tissue, fibrosis, or other lesions within the epicondylar groove.[19,20] The second advantage is that by transposing the nerve into a new pathway volar to the axis of elbow flexion, the nerve is effectively lengthened, thereby decreasing tension on it. Most authors intuitively agree that the presence of a structural abnormality of the elbow, as noted earlier, or hypermobility of the nerve constitute good indications for a transposition.[13]

There are three types of anterior transposition: subcutaneous, submuscular, and intramuscular. All are widely used. Subcutaneous transposition is the most commonly used method of ulnar nerve transposition because of its technical ease, high success rate, and low complication rate.[17] With this procedure, the anterior subcutaneous soft tissues are dissected to form a "bed" for the nerve. The nerve is transposed and retained in the bed with a fascial sling raised from the underlying muscle fascia that is sutured to the dermis.[6] This is an effective procedure, particularly in the elderly and patients who have a thick layer of adipose tissue. The disadvantages are risk of failure to decompress the nerve at the most distal site of the cubital tunnel.[21] In addition, the nerve is most vulnerable to direct trauma after subcutaneous transposition. In one series, unsatisfactory results were reported in up to 15% of cases after this procedure.[22]

Submuscular anterior transposition has become established in the management of chronic ulnar neuropathy, but its success rate in published series has varied considerably.[23,24] This procedure is generally achieved through a modified Learmonth technique (similar to that described by Kline and colleagues).[25] A curved incision extends from the distal arm to the volar aspect of the medial elbow and into the forearm. The ulnar nerve is identified and a 360-degree neurolysis is performed at the level of the elbow and distal to the cubital tunnel. A plane of dissection is created on the lateral edge of the pronator teres, taking care to avoid injury to the median nerve. A submuscular plane is created with the median nerve serving as the lateral boundary. The ulnar nerve is transposed into the submuscular bed, and the muscle is subsequently repaired. The advantages of this procedure are that potential sites for nerve compression are definitely explored and released and the nerve lies in an unscarred anatomic plane not subject to traction forces.[5,21,26,27] This procedure can cause more scarring than others and is usually contraindicated if there is scarring of the joint capsule or distortion of the joint due to arthritis or a malunited fracture.[5] One study comparing submuscular transposition with subcutaneous transposition found that submuscular transposition achieved better results.[6]

Intramuscular transposition is the most controversial of the three methods of ulnar transposition.[28-30] One study evaluating intramuscular transpositions reported 15% of patients with no improvement.[31]

EXPECTED APPEARANCE ON IMAGING

With simple decompression, the ulnar nerve should be located in the cubital tunnel. If there has been transposition, the ulnar nerve will be repositioned anteriorly between muscles (Fig. 107-7) or in the subcutaneous tissues (Fig. 107-8). In all cases, the size of the ulnar nerve should be normal on MRI and ultrasonography and should not deviate from that above or below the region of surgery. The signal intensity should be intermediate on MRI. With medial epicondylectomy, there will be absence of a portion of the medial epicondyle.

POTENTIAL COMPLICATIONS AND RADIOLOGIC APPEARANCE

The ulnar nerve may sublux or dislocate out of the cubital tunnel in cases of simple decompression (Fig. 107-9) or medial epicondylectomy. Adjacent vascular structures

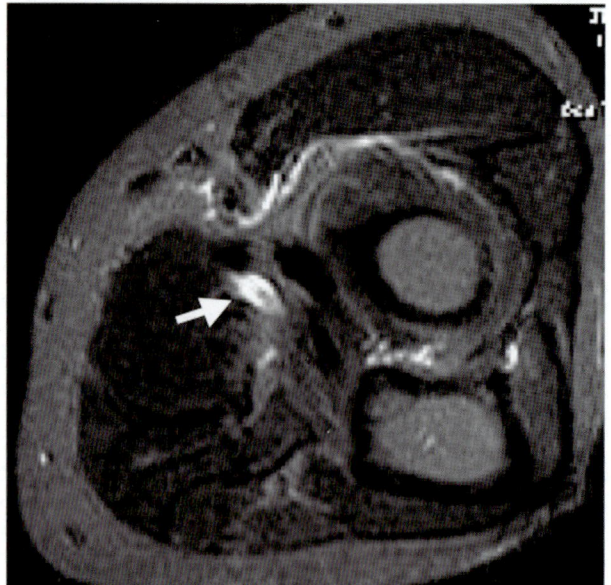

■ **FIGURE 107-7** Axial, fat-suppressed, T2-weighted MR image shows the ulnar nerve transposed anteriorly underneath the pronator muscle (*arrow*). (*Courtesy of Javier Beltran, MD, Brooklyn, NY.*)

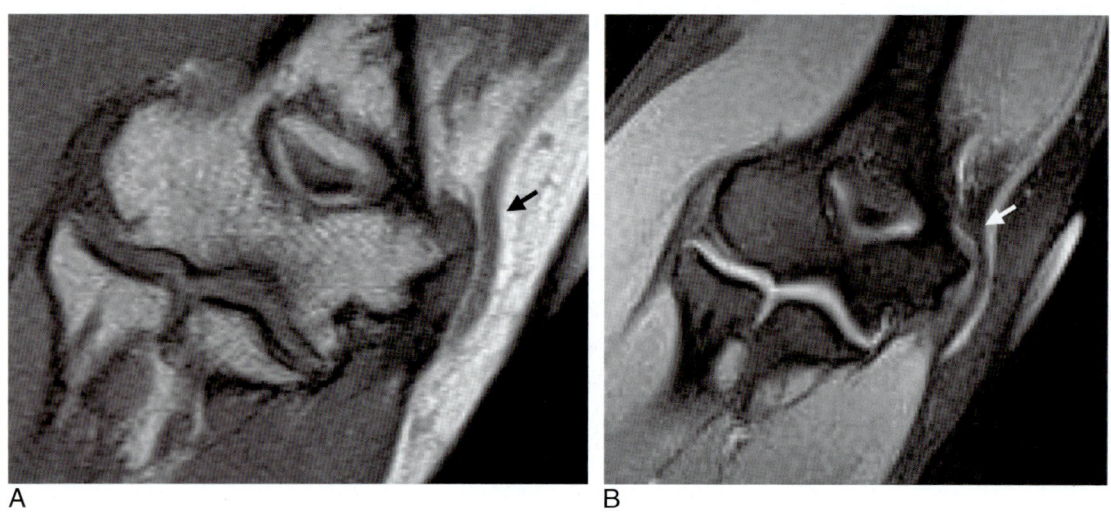

A   B

■ **FIGURE 107-8** Coronal, T1-weighted (**A**) and gradient-echo (**B**) MR images of the elbow after ulnar nerve transposition. The nerve lies superficial in the subcutaneous fat (*arrows*). (*Courtesy of Javier Beltran, MD, Brooklyn, NY.*)

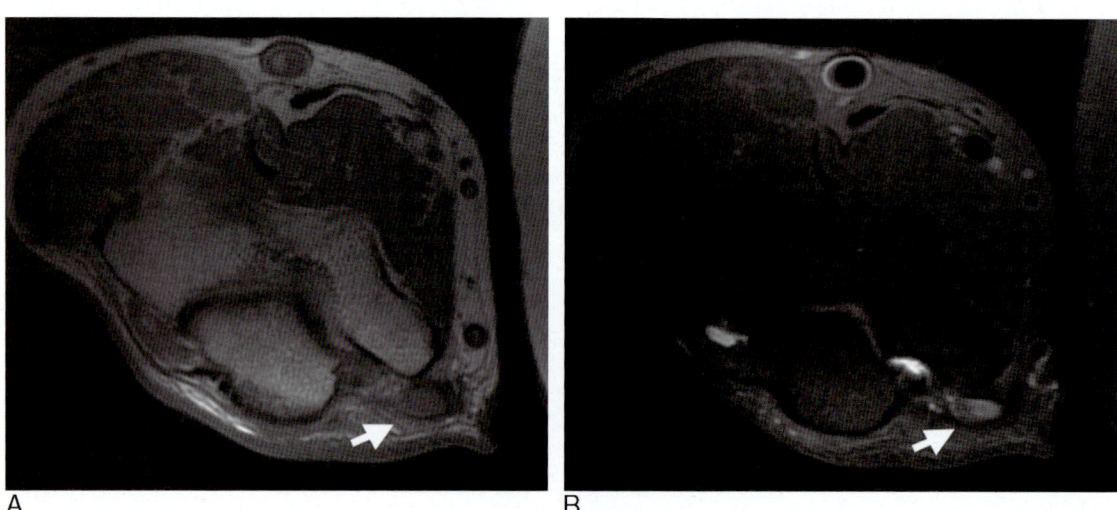

A   B

■ **FIGURE 107-9** Ulnar nerve decompression with retinacular release. Axial T1-weighted (**A**) and fat-suppressed, T2-weighted (**B**) MR images of the elbow show the enlarged ulnar nerve subluxed out of the cubital tunnel (*arrow*) that has undergone a retinacular release. The nerve is abnormally high in signal intensity on the T2-weighted image.

should also be assessed for patency and absence of damage. Excessive scar tissue can interfere with nerve function. The muscles innervated by the ulnar nerve should be evaluated for denervation changes. Infection or inflammatory changes may present with increased signal intensity on MRI in the area of surgery. Abscesses or seromas will be identified as rim-enhancing collections of fluid in the region on post-contrast MRI and as hypoechoic areas of fluid on ultrasonography.

SUGGESTED READINGS

Bordalo-Rodrigues M, Rosenberg ZS. MR imaging of entrapment neuropathies at the elbow. Magn Reson Imaging Clin North Am 2004; 12:247-263.

Izzi J, Dennison D, Noerdlinger M, et al. Nerve injuries of the elbow, wrist, and hand in athletes. Clin Sports Med 2001; 20:203-217.

Keefe DT, Lintner DM. Nerve injuries in the throwing elbow. Clin Sports Med 2004; 23:723-742.

REFERENCES

1. Dellon AL. Musculotendinous variations about the medial humeral epicondyle. J Hand Surg [Br] 1986; 11:175-181.
2. Dinh PT, Gupta R. Subtotal medial epicondylectomy as a surgical option for treatment of cubital tunnel syndrome. Tech Hand Up Extrem Surg 2005; 9:52-59.
3. Rayan GM, Jensen C, Duke J. Elbow flexion test in the normal population. J Hand Surg [Am] 1992; 17:86-89.
4. Yamamoto K, Shishido T, Masaoka T, et al. Postoperative clinical results in cubital tunnel syndrome. Orthopedics 2006; 29:347-353.
5. Asamoto S, Boker DK, Jodicke A. Surgical treatment for ulnar nerve entrapment at the elbow. Neurol Med Chir (Tokyo) 2005; 45:240-244; discussion 244-245.
6. Nabhan A, Ahlhelm F, Kelm J, et al. Simple decompression or subcutaneous anterior transposition of the ulnar nerve for cubital tunnel syndrome. J Hand Surg [Br] 2005; 30:521-524.
7. Muermans S, De Smet L. Partial medial epicondylectomy for cubital tunnel syndrome: outcome and complications. J Shoulder Elbow Surg 2002; 11:248-252.
8. Ogata K, Manske PR, Lesker PA. The effect of surgical dissection on regional blood flow to the ulnar nerve in the cubital tunnel. Clin Orthop Relat Res 1985; (193):195-198.
9. Ogata K, Shimon S, Owen J, Manske PR. Effects of compression and devascularisation on ulnar nerve function: a quantitative study of regional blood flow and nerve conduction in monkeys. J Hand Surg [Br] 1991; 16:104-108.
10. Messina A, Messina JC. Transposition of the ulnar nerve and its vascular bundle for the entrapment syndrome at the elbow. J Hand Surg [Br] 1995; 20:638-648.
11. Adelaar RS, Foster WC, McDowell C. The treatment of the cubital tunnel syndrome. J Hand Surg [Am] 1984; 9A:90-95.
12. Bartels RH, Verhagen WI, van der Wilt GJ, et al. Prospective randomized controlled study comparing simple decompression versus anterior subcutaneous transposition for idiopathic neuropathy of the ulnar nerve at the elbow: I. Neurosurgery 2005; 56:522-530; discussion 522-530.
13. Biggs M, Curtis JA. Randomized, prospective study comparing ulnar neurolysis in situ with submuscular transposition. Neurosurgery 2006; 58:296-304; discussion 296-304.
14. Gervasio O, Gambardella G, Zaccone C, Branca D. Simple decompression versus anterior submuscular transposition of the ulnar nerve in severe cubital tunnel syndrome: a prospective randomized study. Neurosurgery 2005; 56:108-117; discussion 117.
15. Froimson AI, Anouchi YS, Seitz WH Jr, Winsberg DD. Ulnar nerve decompression with medial epicondylectomy for neuropathy at the elbow. Clin Orthop Relat Res 1991; (265):200-206.
16. Froimson AI, Zahrawi F. Treatment of compression neuropathy of the ulnar nerve at the elbow by epicondylectomy and neurolysis. J Hand Surg [Am] 1980; 5:391-395.
17. Artico M, Pastore FS, Nucci F, Giuffre R. 290 surgical procedures for ulnar nerve entrapment at the elbow: physiopathology, clinical experience and results. Acta Neurochir (Wien) 2000; 142:303-308.
18. Bartels RH. History of the surgical treatment of ulnar nerve compression at the elbow. Neurosurgery 2001; 49:391-399; discussion 399-400.
19. Amako M, Nemoto K, Kawaguchi M, et al. Comparison between partial and minimal medial epicondylectomy combined with decompression for the treatment of cubital tunnel syndrome. J Hand Surg [Am] 2000; 25:1043-1050.
20. Grewal R, Varitimidis SE, Vardakas DG, et al. Ulnar nerve elongation and excursion in the cubital tunnel after decompression and anterior transposition. J Hand Surg [Br] 2000; 25:457-460.
21. Black BT, Barron OA, Townsend PF, et al. Stabilized subcutaneous ulnar nerve transposition with immediate range of motion: long-term follow-up. J Bone Joint Surg Am 2000; 82:1544-1551.
22. Osterman AL, Davis CA. Subcutaneous transposition of the ulnar nerve for treatment of cubital tunnel syndrome. Hand Clin 1996; 12:421-433.
23. Amadio PC, Beckenbaugh RD. Entrapment of the ulnar nerve by the deep flexor-pronator aponeurosis. J Hand Surg [Am] 1986; 11:83-87.
24. Broudy AS, Leffert RD, Smith RJ. Technical problems with ulnar nerve transposition at the elbow: findings and results of reoperation. J Hand Surg [Am] 1978; 3:85-89.
25. Davis GA, Bulluss KJ. Submuscular transposition of the ulnar nerve: review of safety, efficacy and correlation with neurophysiological outcome. J Clin Neurosci 2005; 12:524-528.
26. Lundborg G. Surgical treatment for ulnar nerve entrapment at the elbow. J Hand Surg [Br] 1992; 17:245-247.
27. Nathan PA. Surgical treatment of ulnar nerve entrapment at the elbow. J Hand Surg [Br] 1993; 18:133.
28. Posner MA. Compressive ulnar neuropathies at the elbow: II. Treatment. J Am Acad Orthop Surg 1998; 6:289-297.
29. Posner MA. Compressive ulnar neuropathies at the elbow: I. Etiology and diagnosis. J Am Acad Orthop Surg 1998; 6:282-288.
30. Posner MA. Compressive neuropathies of the ulnar nerve at the elbow and wrist. Instr Course Lect 2000; 49:305-317.
31. Hollerhage HG, Stolke D. [Results of volar transposition of the ulnar nerve in cubital tunnel syndrome]. Neurochirurgia 1985; 28:64-67.

Epicondylitis

DESCRIPTION, INDICATIONS, CONTRAINDICATIONS, PURPOSE, UNDERLYING MECHANICS

Lateral and medial pain and localized tenderness that occurs at the distal humeral epicondyles with repetitive eccentric or concentric loading of the flexor or extensor muscles is termed *epicondylitis*. This word is a misnomer because the pain is related to microtraumatic events that lead to tendinosis and tears of the tendons and muscles rather than inflammation.

Epicondylitis is more common laterally than medially by a ratio ranging from 4-7:1,[1,2] affecting the dominant elbow twice as often as the nondominant one. Men and women have epicondylitis with equal incidence with an average peak age of 42 years. Young patients tend to have acute pain after tennis or throwing activities. Lateral epicondylitis, also called "tennis elbow," is almost exclusively related to tennis and is felt with the backhand stroke when extensor tendons are tensed up to absorb the impact from the tennis ball. Medial epicondylitis, also referred to as golfer's elbow, can affect golfers or throwing athletes. Baseball pitchers and javelin throwers are especially affected due to valgus overload of the elbow. The chronic pain that presents in the older individual is usually related to occupational exposure or activity overload.

The most common sites for pathology are the tendons of the extensor carpi radialis brevis laterally and the flexor carpi radialis and pronator teres medially. An ulnar neuropathy can coexist with medial epicondylitis in up to 50% of cases.[3]

Except for acute injuries that are commonly seen in elite or upper-level athletes, most cases of epicondylitis are treated nonoperatively with a 90% success rate. Conservative therapy includes physical therapy, anti-inflammatory medication, icing, bracing, and splinting with reduction in activities that provoke the problem. If pain remains after 3 months, corticosteroid is usually injected into the area of pain. If pain persists and limits activity and function after 6 months, operative treatment is considered.

Surgical options for epicondylitis include débridement or excision of tendinosis or partial tears, production of neovascularization, repair, or release. This can be done by open or arthroscopic procedures. Percutaneous extensor tenotomy has been recently described.[4] Laterally, a synovial fringe or a radiohumeral bursa can be resected.

Excellent results are seen after resection and repair for lateral epicondylitis with a success rate of more than 90%.[5] The outcomes are not as good for medial epicondylitis with a 50% success rate. This depends on the presence of concomitant ulnar nerve abnormalities. Release of the tendon may lead to weakness of the muscle.

Contraindications to surgery include a noncompliant patient or one who has not completed the nonoperative regimen stated earlier. If a patient with medial epicondylitis has symptoms associated with the ulnar nerve, the nerve is released at surgery.

EXPECTED APPEARANCE ON IMAGING

Stress radiographs can be obtained to evaluate for valgus or varus instability. If damage is suspected to the tendons, MRI or ultrasonography may be obtained before surgery. These tests will quantitate the degree or tendon damage, allowing for accurate preoperative assessment, determination of the best procedure for therapy, as well as postoperative recovery time course. Little has been written about the MRI appearance of the postoperative tendon. In our experience, it may take some time for the signal intensity to return to normal after surgery. The tendon should demonstrate continuity and will become low

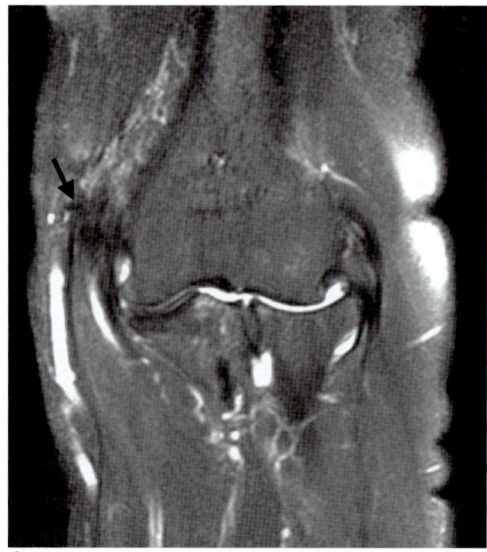 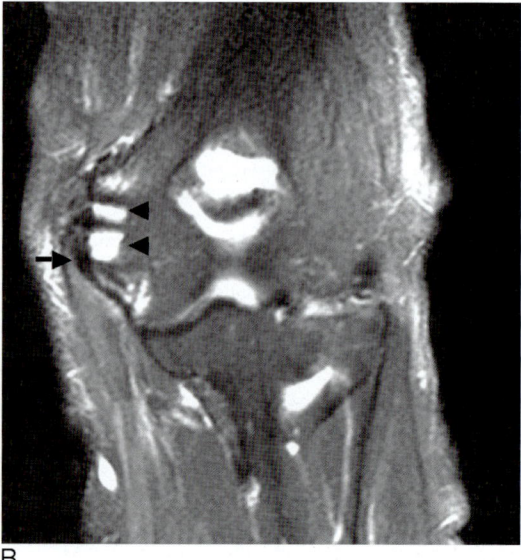

A B

■ **FIGURE 107-10** This patient had a repair of the flexor tendons with medial epicondylar suture anchors and ulnar nerve transposition. **A** and **B,** The tendon repair appears intact with normal continuity, signal intensity, and thickening on these coronal, fat-suppressed, T2-weighted MR images of the elbow (*arrows*). Suture anchors are attached to bone in proper position in **B** (*arrowheads*). (*Courtesy of William Morrison, MD, Philadelphia, PA.*)

in signal intensity, often with thickening (Fig. 107-10). Metallic artifact may lie in the area, obscuring evaluation by MRI, especially on gradient-echo images (Fig. 107-11). Re-tear manifests as architectural disruption of the tendon (Fig. 107-12). It has been shown that epicondylitis can be accompanied by underlying ligament pathology,[6] and such abnormalities should be included in the search pattern on a postoperative MRI. This is particularly important in patients who have continuing pain, and it may further destabilize the elbow in those who have had surgical tendon release.

POTENTIAL COMPLICATIONS AND RADIOLOGIC APPEARANCE

Incomplete resection of abnormal tissue can be a problem, presenting with an appearance similar to tendinosis or tendon tear. Ligament abnormalities and adventitial bursa

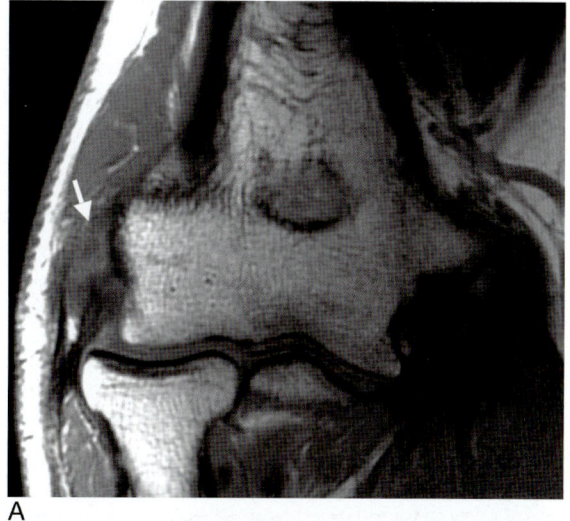

A

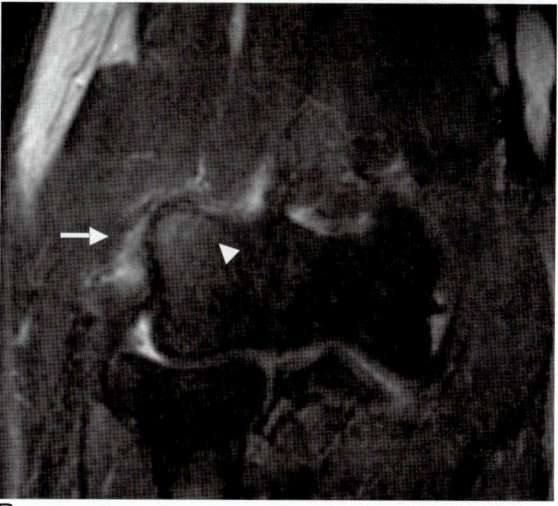

B

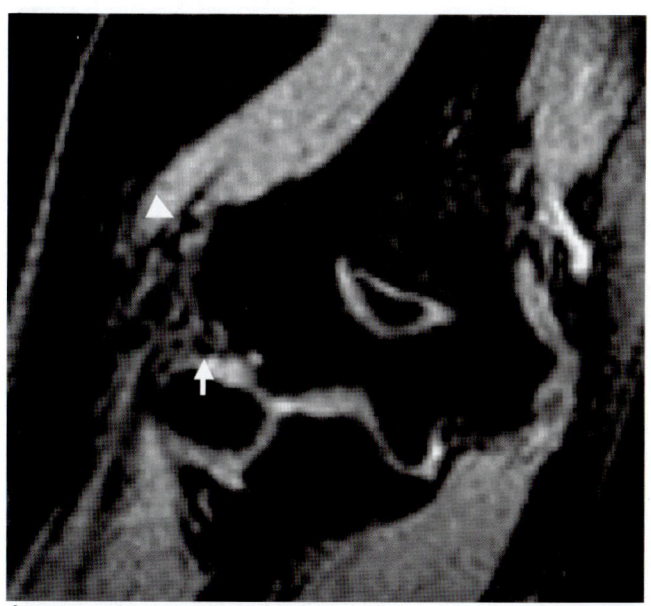

A

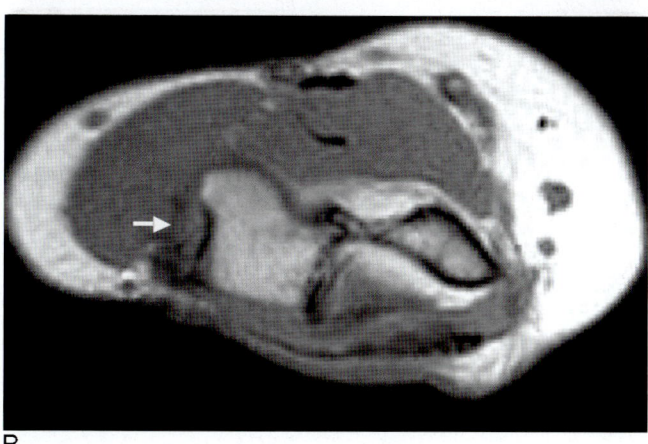

B

■ **FIGURE 107-11**   Normal postoperative lateral epicondylitis repair. Coronal, gradient-echo (**A**) and axial T1-weighted (**B**) MR images show an intact extensor tendon repair after lateral epicondylitis (*arrows*). The micrometallic artifact is obscuring the tendon on the gradient-echo image (*arrowhead*). (*Courtesy of William Morrison, MD, Philadelphia, PA.*)

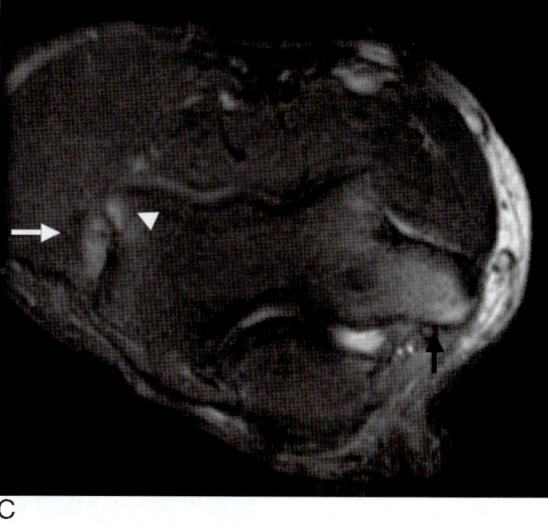

C

■ **FIGURE 107-12**   Lateral epicondylar débridement with re-tear. Coronal, T1-weighted (**A**) and coronal (**B**) and axial (**C**) fat-suppressed, T2-weighted MR images demonstrate fiber disruption consistent with a partial tear (*white arrows*). Note the adjacent bone marrow edema in the lateral epicondyle on the fluid-sensitive sequences (*arrowheads*). There is poor fat suppression on the other side, mimicking edema in the axial plane (*black arrow*). The underlying radial collateral ligament is intact. (*Courtesy of William Morrison, MD, Philadelphia, PA.*)

formation may be seen postoperatively. Percutaneous techniques occasionally result in synovial fistula formation. Excessive scar tissue may be a problem in the surgical bed. Medial procedures could affect the ulnar nerve as stated earlier. Care should be taken when interpreting an MRI when a failed surgical tendon has been injected with corticosteroid or anesthetic. The injectate will elevate signal intensity on T2-weighted sequences. A failed postoperative tendon can undergo another excision and repair.[7]

SUGGESTED READINGS

Cain EL, Dugas JR, Wolf RS, et al. Elbow injuries in throwing athletes: A current concepts review. Am J Sports Med 2003; 621–635.
Kraushaar B, Nirschl RP. Tendinosis of the elbow (tennis elbow). J Bone Joint Surg Am 1999; 81:259–278.

REFERENCES

1. Gabel GT, Morrey BF. Tennis elbow. Instr Course Lect 1998; 47:165–172.
2. Leach RE, Miller JK. Lateral and medial epicondylitis of the elbow. Clin Sports Med 1987; 6:259–272.
3. Gabel GT, Morrey BF. Operative treatment of medical epicondylitis: influence of concomitant ulnar neuropathy at the elbow. J Bone Joint Surg Am 1995; 77:1065–1069.
4. Yerger B, Turner T. Percutaneous extensor tenotomy for chronic tennis elbow: an office procedure. Orthopedics 1985; 8:1261–1263.
5. Nirschl RP, Pettrone FA. Tennis elbow: the surgical treatment of lateral epicondylitis. J Bone Joint Surg Am 1979; 61:832–839.
6. Bredella MA, Tirman PF, Fritz RC, et al. MR imaging findings of lateral ulnar collateral ligament abnormalities in patients with lateral epicondylitis. AJR Am J Roentgenol 1999; 173:1379–1382.
7. Organ SW, Nirschl RP, Kraushaar BS, Guidi EJ. Salvage surgery for lateral tennis elbow. Am J Sports Med 1997; 25:746–750.

Biceps Tendon

DESCRIPTION, INDICATIONS, CONTRAINDICATIONS, PURPOSE, UNDERLYING MECHANICS

Biceps tendon tears usually result from eccentric loading of the muscle. They may result from athletic activities such as weightlifting but are also seen after routine activities such as carrying a heavy unbalanced load. In these cases in which there is minimal trauma, weakening of a tendon that has undergone degeneration is suspect.[1] Mechanical impingement during pronation and a radial tuberosity enthesophyte can also cause tears of the tendon.[2] Most tears occur 1 to 2 cm above the radial tuberosity where the tendon is less vascular and there is a histologic transition.[3] Disruption of the biceps tendon is more common in men between 40 and 60 years of age.

Surgery is preferred over nonoperative treatment in cases of ruptured biceps tendon. Surgery restores supination and improves cosmetic appearance when there is biceps tendon retraction. When possible, the torn tendon is reattached to the radial tuberosity with suture anchors via an anterior approach.[4] In instances of delayed diagnosis, scarring of the muscle makes reattachment of the tendon more difficult.[2] An Achilles tendon allograft may be required or the biceps tendon can be attached to the brachialis tendon.[5]

EXPECTED APPEARANCE ON IMAGING

On MRI and ultrasonography, the biceps tendon may appear thickened postoperatively. It should be continuous from the muscle to the radial tuberosity if it has been reattached or if a graft has been placed (Fig. 107-13). It may be reattached to the brachialis muscle in some cases (Fig. 107-14).

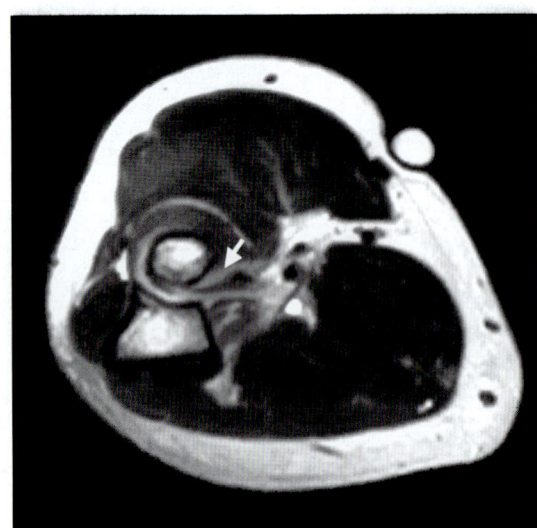
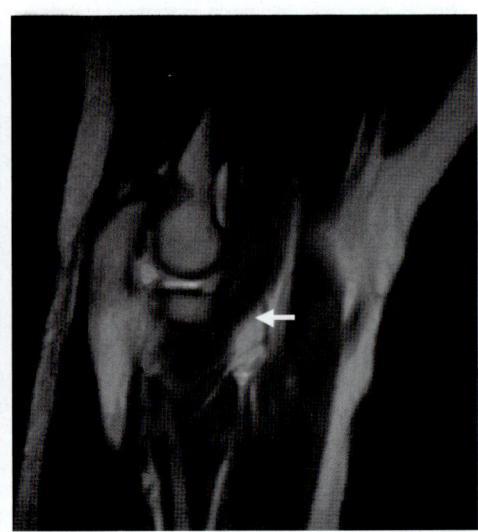

■ **FIGURE 107-13** Normal postoperative biceps tendon. Axial T1-weighted (**A**) and sagittal T2-weighted (**B**) MR images of the elbow show an intact biceps tendon repair (*arrows*). The tendon is of normal caliber and in continuity to its distal attachment on the bicipital tuberosity. (*Courtesy of William Morrison, MD, Philadelphia, PA.*)

A

B

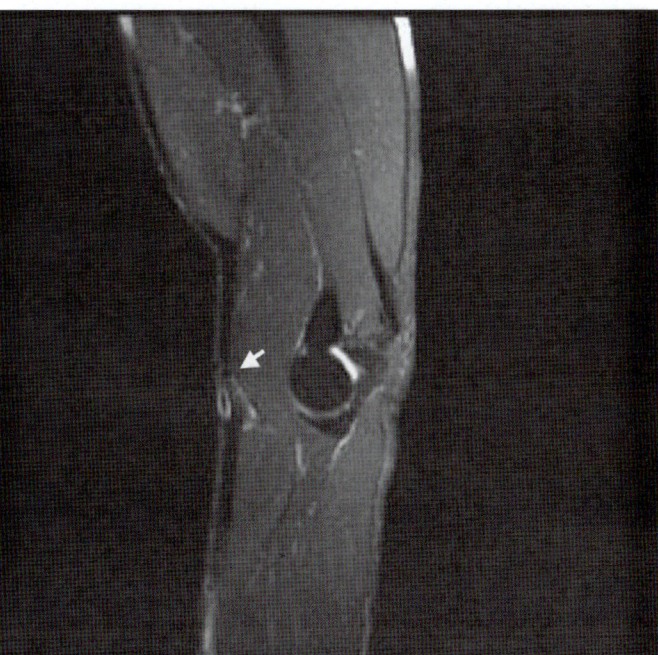

■ **FIGURE 107-14** Normal biceps tendon repair inserted on brachialis (*arrow*) on this sagittal, fat-suppressed T2-weighted MR image. *(Courtesy of Tim Sanders, MD, Charlottesville, VA.)*

The normal tendon occasionally displays intermediate signal intensity on MRI.[6] Suture anchors or an osseous defect may be present at the radial tuberosity. The tendon can be imaged with the elbow in flexion, abduction, and supination that places slight tension on the tendon and allows

for visualization of the tendon from the musculotendinous junction to the insertion on a single image.[6]

POTENTIAL COMPLICATIONS AND RADIOLOGIC APPEARANCE

Complications of distal biceps tendon repair are uncommon. They include re-rupture (Figs. 107-15 to 107-17) and nerve injuries involving the median and radial nerves and the branch of the radial nerve, the posterior interosseous nerve. Proximal radioulnar synostosis[7] and heterotopic ossification around the elbow are also complications that can best be seen on radiographs or CT.[6,8] The latter may be related to the degree of soft tissue dissection during surgery as well as exposure of the periosteal surface of the ulna.

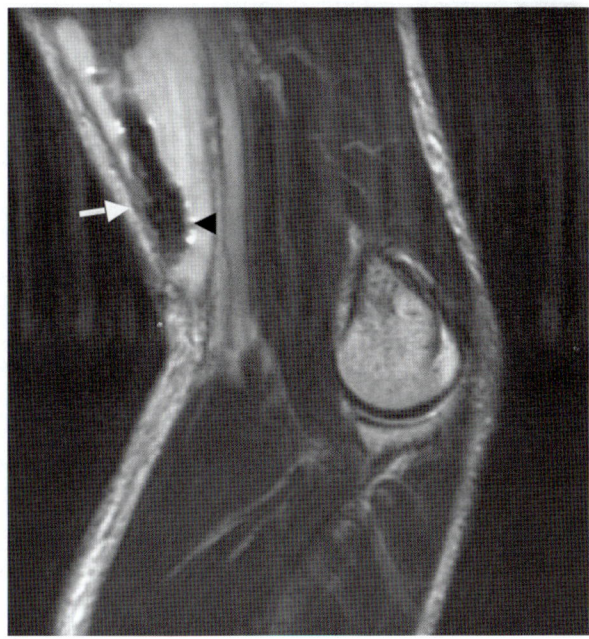

A

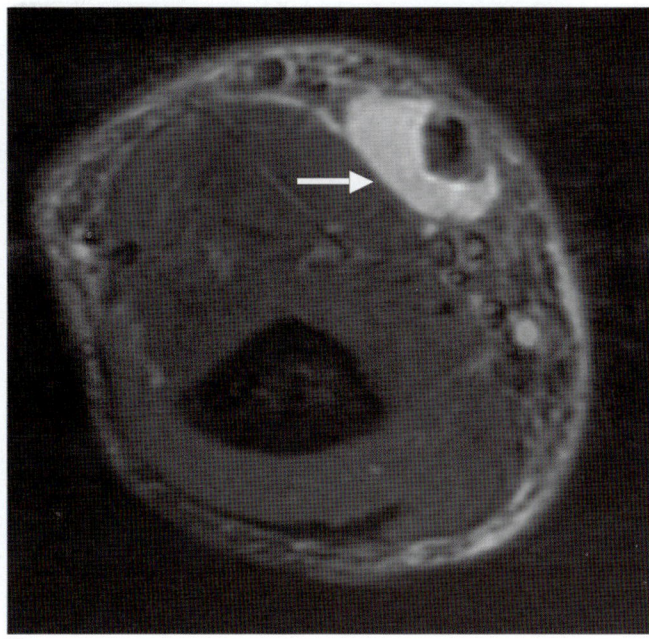

B

■ **FIGURE 107-15** Re-rupture of biceps tendon after surgery. The biceps tendon is proximally retracted on sagittal, proton density–weighted (**A**) and axial, fat-suppressed (**B**) T2-weighted MR images (*arrows*). Metallic artifact is seen in the elbow proximal biceps (*arrowhead*). *(Courtesy of William Morrison, MD, Philadelphia, PA.)*

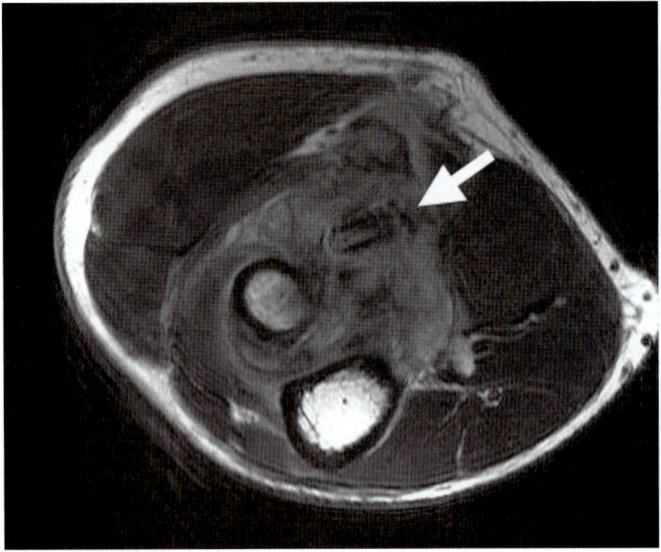

A

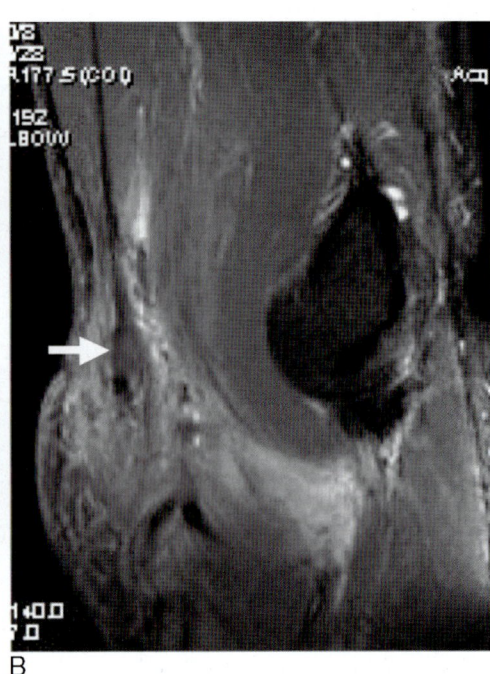

B

■ FIGURE 107-16   Re-rupture of a biceps repair as shown on axial T2-weighted (**A**) and sagittal (**B**) MR images (*arrows*). (*Courtesy of Tim Sanders, MD, Charlottesville, VA.*)

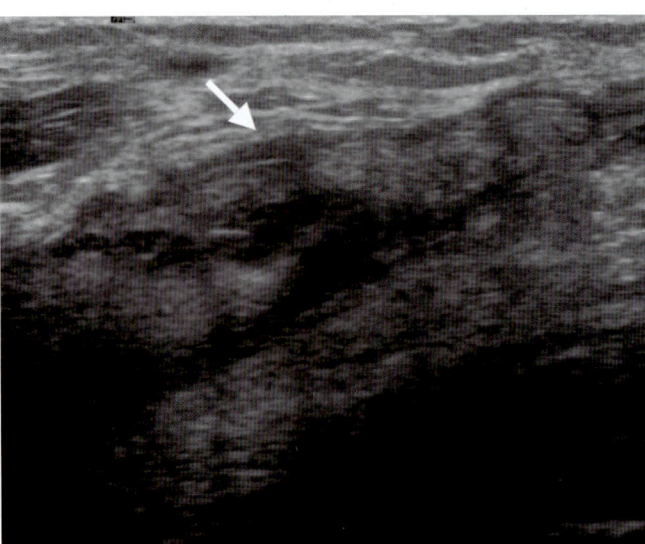

■ FIGURE 107-17   Re-ruptured distal biceps repair on a sagittal ultrasound image (*arrow*). (*Courtesy of Gina Allen, MD, Birmingham, England.*)

SUGGESTED READINGS

Chung CB, Chew FS, Steinbach L. MR imaging of tendon abnormalities of the elbow. Magn Reson Imaging Clin North Am 2004; 12:233-245.

Falchook FS, Zlatkin MB, Erbacher GE, et al. Rupture of the distal biceps tendon: evaluation with MR imaging. Radiology 1994; 190:659-663.

Morrey BF. The Elbow. Philadelphia, Lippincott Williams & Wilkins, 2002.

Safran MR, Graham SM. Distal biceps tendon ruptures. Clin Orthop 2002; 404:275-283.

REFERENCES

1. Morrey BF, Askew IJ, An KN, Dobyns JH. Rupture of the distal tendon of the biceps brachii: a biomechanical study. J Bone Joint Surg Am 1985; 67:418-421.

2. Seiler JG 3rd, Parker LM, Chamberland PD, et al. The distal biceps tendon: two potential mechanisms involved in its rupture: arterial supply and mechanical impingement. J Shoulder Elbow Surg 1995; 4:149-156.

3. Koch S, Tillmann B. The distal tendon of the biceps brachii: structure and clinical correlations. Ann Anat 1995; 177:467-474.

4. Lintner S, Fischer T. Repair of the distal biceps tendon using suture anchors and an anterior approach. Clin Orthop Relat Res 1996; (322):116-119.

5. Hovelius L, Josefsson G. Rupture of the distal biceps tendon: report of five cases. Acta Orthop Scand 1977; 48:280-282.

6. Giuffre BM, Moss MJ. Optimal positioning for MRI of the distal biceps brachii tendon: flexed abducted supinated view. AJR Am J Roentgenol 2004; 182:944-946.

7. Failla JM, Amadio PC, Morrey BF, Beckenbaugh RD. Proximal radio-ulnar synostosis after repair of distal biceps brachii rupture by the two-incision technique: report of four cases. Clin Orthop Relat Res 1990; (253):133-136.

8. Davison BL, Engber WD, Tigert LJ. Long term evaluation of repaired distal biceps brachii tendon ruptures. Clin Orthop Relat Res 1996; (333):186-191.

Triceps Tendon

DESCRIPTION, INDICATIONS, CONTRAINDICATIONS, PURPOSE, UNDERLYING MECHANICS

The triceps tendon is composed of three components: the long, lateral, and medial muscles. It inserts as a common tendon on the posterosuperior surface of the olecranon process. Triceps tendon ruptures are rare.[1] They usually occur as a result of eccentric contraction against resistance, deceleration stress on a contracted muscle, or direct insult to the posterior arm. Radial head fractures may also be seen with triceps tendon tears.

Involvement at the musculotendinous junction or avulsion of the tendon from the olecranon with a small osseous fragment are more common presentations of injury to this muscle, but the insult can occur anywhere.[2,3] Underlying systemic diseases such as chronic renal failure and hyperparathyroidism are also causes for this problem. Chronic olecranon bursitis or bursectomy can also lead to triceps tears. Rupture is usually accompanied by ecchymosis. Elbow extension is either weak or absent.

Partial ruptures of the triceps are treated nonoperatively. Because nonoperative treatment of a full-thickness tear results in weakness and incomplete extension, those tears are repaired surgically with a good prognosis and almost full range of motion. The tendon is reattached to the ulna with drill holes. Periosteum may be closed over the tendon or a proximal flap of forearm fascia or distal triceps can be used to reinforce the repair. Tendon grafts can also be used. If a large avulsion fragment is present, then it is fixed with a screw and washer.

KEY POINTS

■ Triceps tendon tears are rare.
■ Surgery is reserved for full-thickness triceps tendon tears.
■ The triceps tendon is reattached to the olecranon.
■ Excluding re-tear, there are few complications of repair.

EXPECTED APPEARANCE ON IMAGING

On radiographs, one may see soft tissue swelling and hardware after surgery. Drill holes are sometimes present in the olecranon. An avulsion fragment should be attached to the olecranon. On MRI and ultrasonography, the tendon should be continuous without architectural disruption to suggest a partial- or full-thickness tear. It can be slightly elevated in signal intensity on MRI in the early repair stage but should decrease to a normal tendinous signal intensity within a year. A re-tear of a surgical repair could demonstrate an avulsion fragment of the olecranon.

POTENTIAL COMPLICATIONS AND RADIOLOGIC APPEARANCE

The triceps tendon can re-rupture after surgical repair. This is manifest as discontinuity of the tendon with high signal intensity on fluid-sensitive sequences (Fig. 107-18). Except for re-tear, there are few complications of triceps tendon repair. One should look for excessive scar tissue, olecranon bursitis, heterotopic bone formation, evidence of infection, or nerve damage including ulnar neuropathy (Fig. 107-19), which may result in anconeus denervation.

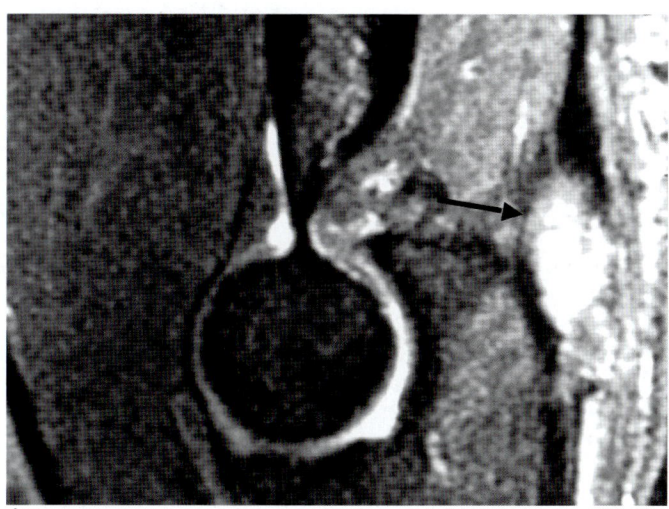
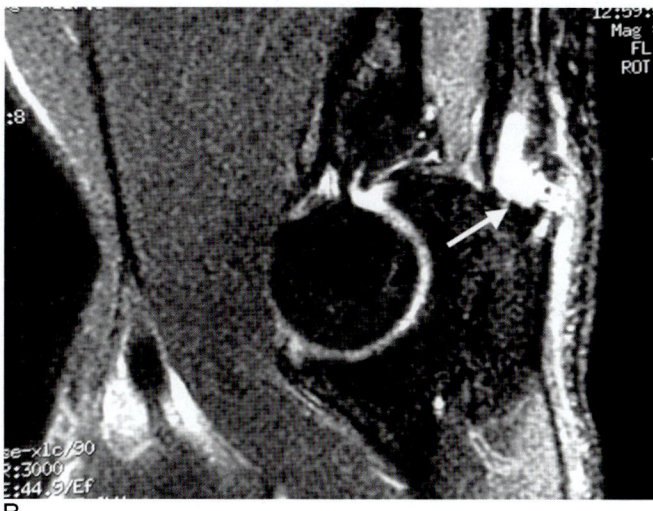

A   B

■ FIGURE 107-18 Disrupted triceps tendon repair. **A,** Sagittal, fat-suppressed, T2-weighted image of the elbow preoperatively shows a full-thickness tear of the distal triceps at the olecranon attachment. **B,** The follow-up sagittal, fat-suppressed, T2-weighted image shows a partial re-tear of the triceps (*arrow*).

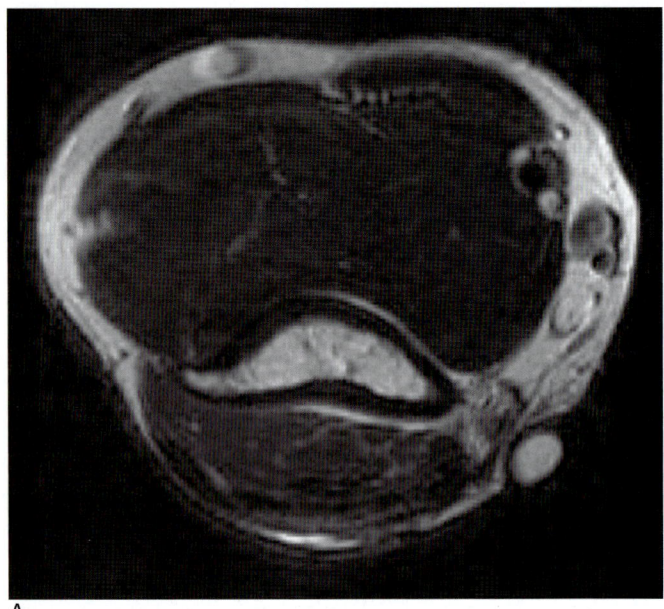 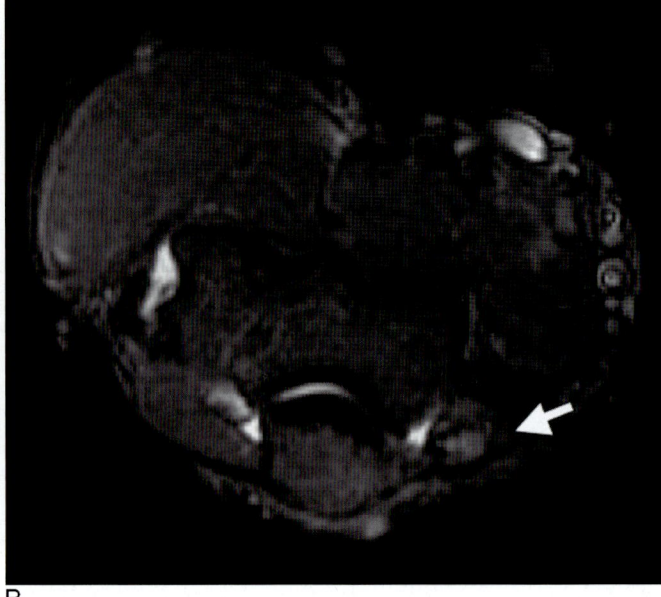

■ **FIGURE 107-19** Ulnar neuritis after triceps repair seen on axial, T1-weighted (**A**) and fat-suppressed T2-weighted (**B**) MR images (under marker). *(Courtesy of Tim Sanders, MD, Charlottesville, VA.)*

SUGGESTED READINGS

Chung CB, Chew FS, Steinbach L. MR imaging of tendon abnormalities of the elbow. Magn Reson Imaging Clin North Am 2004; 12:233–245.
Morrey BF. The Elbow. Philadelphia, Lippincott Williams & Wilkins, 2002.
Tarnsey FF. Rupture and avulsion of the triceps. Clin Orthop 1972; 83:177–183.

REFERENCES

1. Anzel SH, Covey KW, Weiner AD, Lipscomb PR. Disruption of muscles and tendons; an analysis of 1,014 cases. Surgery 1959; 45:406–414.
2. Farrar EL 3rd, Lippert FG 3rd. Avulsion of the triceps tendon. Clin Orthop Relat Res 1981; (161):242–246.
3. Pina A, Garcia I, Sabater M. Traumatic avulsion of the triceps brachii. J Orthop Trauma 2002; 16:273–276.

KEY POINTS

■ Olecranon bursitis is usually treated conservatively.
■ Operative treatment of olecranon bursitis is reserved for chronic pain and discomfort.
■ The surgery can be performed open or arthroscopically.
■ Complications include poor wound healing, scar tissue that envelops the adjacent tendon and bone, and fistula formation.

Olecranon Bursitis

DESCRIPTION, INDICATIONS, CONTRAINDICATIONS, PURPOSE, UNDERLYING MECHANICS

The olecranon bursa is located in the subcutaneous tissues posterior to the olecranon process. It serves to reduce friction in the region. Distention of the bursa can occur after trauma, infection, or arthropathy, such as gout or rheumatoid arthritis. In addition, infection is a cause of olecranon bursitis.[1] Calcium pyrophosphate dihydrate deposition has also been implicated.[2]

Most patients with noninfectious olecranon bursitis are treated with aspiration and corticosteroid injections. If this fails and pain and discomfort persist, surgical excision of the olecranon bursa is performed.[3] This can be performed along with open surgical drainage or endoscopically using an arthroscope. The latter procedure is thought to have fewer complications such as poor wound healing, infection, and loss of joint mobility, although it does not fare well in rheumatoid patients who have bursae that communicate with the elbow joint.[4] A prominent adjacent olecranon process or spur can be resected.

EXPECTED APPEARANCE ON IMAGING

A postoperative MRI or ultrasonography should show lack of fluid in the region of the olecranon bursa. A small amount of scar tissue may be present (Fig. 107-20).

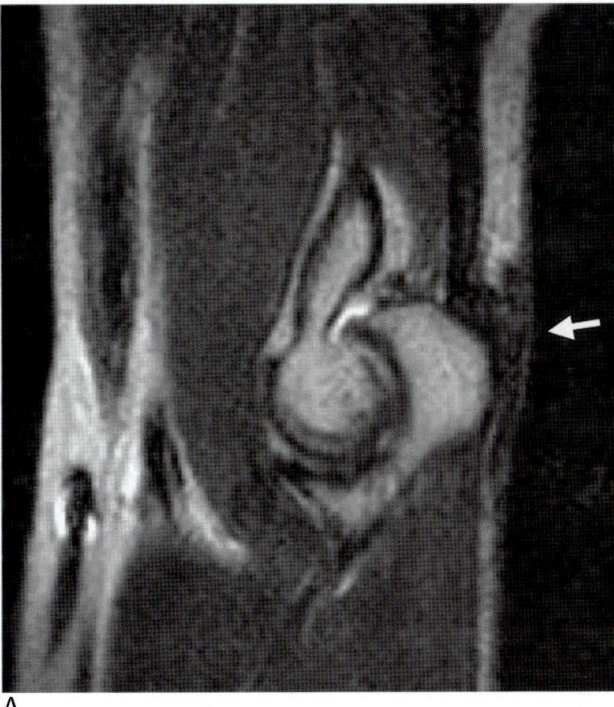

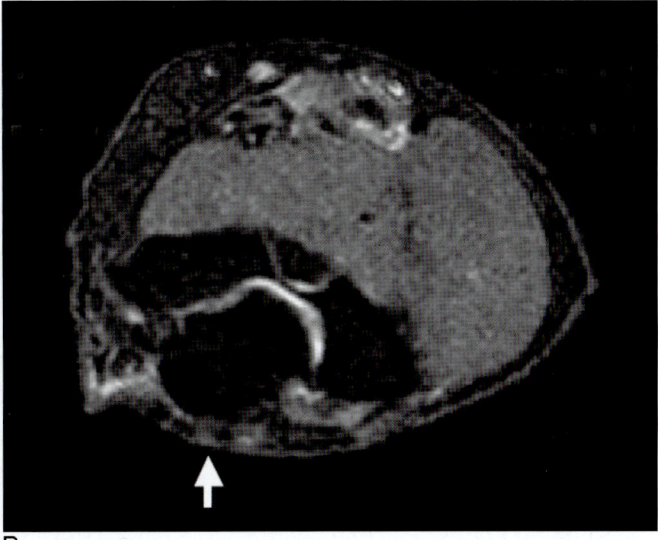

■ **FIGURE 107-20** Olecranon bursectomy. Sagittal fast spin-echo, T2-weighted (**A**) and axial, gradient-echo (**B**) MR images show low signal scarring in the location of prior olecranon bursectomy (*arrows*). (*Courtesy of Javier Beltran, MD, Brooklyn, NY.*)

POTENTIAL COMPLICATIONS AND RADIOLOGIC APPEARANCE

The most common complication of open olecranon bursectomy is poor wound healing.[4] Scar can adhere to tendon or bone.[3] A synovial-cutaneous fistula may form.[5] Fluid should not be present within the olecranon bursa. A triceps tendon tear may result after olecranon bursectomy.

SUGGESTED READINGS

Degreef I, De Smet L. Complications following resection of the olecranon bursa. Acta Orthop Belg 2006; 72:400–403.
Ogilvie-Harris DJ, Gilbart M. Endoscopic bursal resection: the olecranon bursa and prepatellar bursa. Arthroscopy 2000; 16:249–253.

REFERENCES

1. Ho G Jr, Tice AD, Kaplan SR. Septic bursitis in the prepatellar and olecranon bursae: an analysis of 25 cases. Ann Intern Med 1978; 89:21–27.
2. Gerster JC, Lagier R, Boivin G. Olecranon bursitis related to calcium pyrophosphate dihydrate crystal deposition disease. Arthritis Rheum 1982; 25:989–996.
3. Kerr DR. Prepatellar and olecranon arthroscopic bursectomy. Clin Sports Med 1993; 12:137–142.
4. Quayle JB, Robinson MP. A useful procedure in the treatment of chronic olecranon bursitis. Injury 1978; 9:299–302.
5. Thompson GR, Manshady BM, Weiss JJ. Septic bursitis. JAMA 1978; 240:2280–2281.

Common Elbow Fractures

DESCRIPTION, INDICATIONS, CONTRAINDICATIONS, PURPOSE, UNDERLYING MECHANICS

Fractures commonly affect the elbow in the supracondylar region of the distal humerus, radial head, coronoid process, and ulna. Insults to the capitellum result in osteochondral lesions.

Supracondylar fractures are the second most common type of fracture in children.[1] In 95% of cases these are caused by a fall on an outstretched hand with an extended elbow. The distal fragment is posteriorly displaced. Five percent of supracondylar fractures occur with the elbow flexed and result in anterior displacement of the distal fragment. These types of fractures are associated with ulnar nerve injury.[2,3] A severely displaced fracture can buttonhole the triceps muscle.[3] Supracondylar fractures may be treated conservatively with closed reduction and splinting or casting. Percutaneous pinning is often an option that provides superior results to closed reduction.[4] The elbow is less flexed, decreasing the chance of Volkmann's ischemic contracture. Displaced, comminuted, or open fractures or any that are associated with nerve entrapment or vascular injury are treated with open reduction and internal fixation.

Radial head fractures are seen mainly in adults between the ages of 30 and 60 years. They result from a fall on the outstretched arm or less commonly from a direct impact from the lateral side of the elbow. They can be nondisplaced, displaced with marginal fractures, or comminuted. The elbow may be dislocated in between 10% to 30% of injuries.[5] Most radial head fractures are treated conservatively. Comminuted or cleavage fractures of the radial head often require open reduction and internal fixation, especially if they block motion of the elbow.[6,7] Complete or partial excision of the radial head is also performed as an open or arthroscopic procedure.[8] Radial head prostheses are used for complex injuries about the elbow.

Coronoid process fractures are usually associated with posterior elbow dislocation.[9,10] Type I fracture is an avulsion of the tip of the coronoid process. A type II fracture is called when the fragment that is less than 50% of the coronoid process. Type II fractures are those where the fragment is more than 50% of the coronoid process. Nondisplaced type I and II fractures are treated conservatively whereas type III fractures

and displaced fractures are highly unstable and are treated with open reduction and internal fixation using a compression screw or similar hardware.

Olecranon fractures usually result from a sudden contraction of the triceps hyperextension injury with high force trauma or a direct force from a fall on the flexed elbow. Displaced olecranon fractures are treated with internal fixation with tension-band wiring using parallel Kirschner wires or an intramedullary cancellous screw.[11] Small avulsion fractures at the triceps are excised with reattachment of the triceps.

Osteochondral injury to the capitellum is often the result of valgus stress. This produces compression on the capitellum. It is more common in adolescents who perform throwing sports in the dominant elbow. Nondisplaced, stable fragments are treated conservatively or with arthroscopic drilling. Loose fragments can be arthroscopically removed or reattached to the parent bone. Newer techniques to reduce complications such as arthritis such as osteochondral plug transfer (mosaicplasty), chondrocyte transplant, or allograft reconstruction have not been thoroughly evaluated.[12,13]

EXPECTED APPEARANCE ON IMAGING

In general, normal postoperative radiographs show fractures reduced to near anatomic alignment. Nonunion and malunion is commented on. Hardware remains in the same position as shown on the postoperative radiograph, and there is no evidence of lucency or periosteal reaction around the hardware to suggest loosening or infection. The elbow is not subluxed or dislocated on a normal postoperative radiograph. A line drawn through the radius should intersect with the capitellum on anteroposterior and lateral radiographs. Intra-articular bodies may be present and are noted in the report.

The supracondylar fracture should be reduced to near anatomic alignment (Fig. 107-21). Occasionally the line drawn down the front of the humerus does not intersect

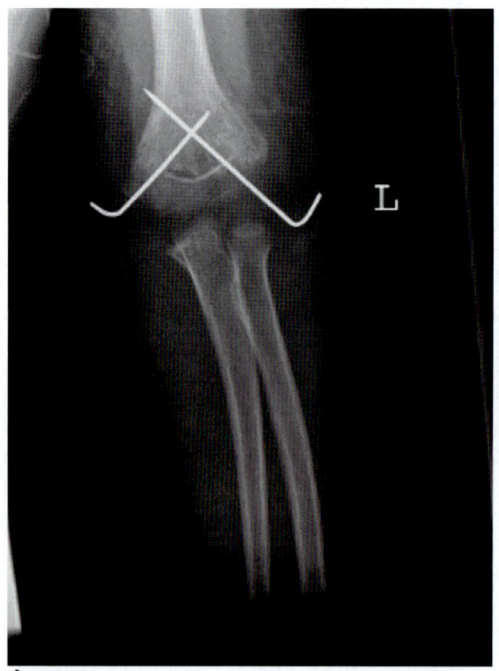
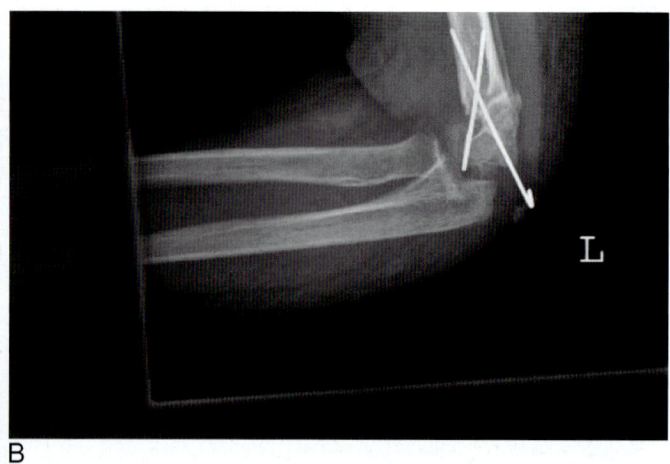

■ **FIGURE 107-21** Supracondylar fracture fixation. Anteroposterior (**A**) and lateral (**B**) radiographs of the left elbow demonstrate two crossed Kirschner wires traversing a supracondylar fracture of the distal humerus near the elbow. The fracture is in anatomic alignment.

the capitellum at the junction of the anterior and middle third even with satisfactory reduction. The elbow should be in mild valgus. Pins may have four configurations, including medial and lateral crossed pins, three lateral pins, two lateral parallel pins, or two lateral crossed pins. Pins are removed at 3 weeks if the fracture appears healed.

The radial head should line up with the capitellum on anteroposterior and lateral views. It can be evaluated on a radial head view obtained with the elbow in lateral position, flexed to 90 degrees with the beam projected over the capitellum, and angled at 45 degrees to the forearm. Fracture fragments are noted. The radial head may be absent or replaced with a metallic or plastic prosthesis on the postoperative radiograph (Fig. 107-22).

Olecranon fractures are usually seen with tension-band wiring using parallel Kirschner wires or an intramedullary cancellous screw (Fig. 107-23). Radiographs should show anatomic alignment of the fragments with progressive fracture healing.

It may be difficult to see coronoid process fractures well on radiographs due to the overlap of the radius. Reformatted CT images are useful in such cases. Small fractures are usually treated conservatively, whereas large fractures are pinned back to the parent bone.

Osteochondral lesions are treated in a variety of ways. If the fragment is pinned back to the parent bone, it should be in anatomic alignment. Bone plugs and chondrocyte transplant can be assessed with MRI. Radiographically, the graft is incorporated with a normal contour of the subchondral cortex. MRI shows normalization of the signal intensity of cartilage overlying the lesion.[13]

POTENTIAL COMPLICATIONS AND RADIOLOGIC APPEARANCE

Complications of elbow fractures include malunion and nonunion. Alignment, callus formation, and healing of the fracture line should be assessed on radiographs taken at 90 degrees to each other. If there is any question of malunion or nonunion, multiplanar reformatted CT images can be performed. Plates and screws should not pull out of the fracture. New periosteal reaction or increasing lucency around hardware can suggest loosening or infection (Fig. 107-24). The elbow may be subluxed or dislocated. Heterotopic bone frequently forms around the elbow and restricts motion.

Specific complications are seen for the various fractures. These are discussed in the following paragraphs.

Treatment of supracondylar fracture may cause the elbow to go into varus. This is related to poor reduction or loss of reduction and can be seen in up to 58% of supracondylar fractures.[14,15] Cubitus varus can interfere with throwing sports, swimming, and push-ups and may lead to lateral condylar fracture.[15] Cubitus varus can be treated with osteotomy.[16] Pin tract infections and nerve injuries, particularly of the ulnar nerve, related to the pins or reduction may occur.[17,18] Posterolateral displacement is associated with median nerve and brachial artery injury.[2] Posteromedial displacement is more often associated with radial nerve injury.[2,19] The brachial artery may also be compromised. Volkmann's ischemic contracture can result. This may be evaluated with arteriography, MR angiography or Doppler ultrasonography before exploration.[20]

Radial head fracture reductions may displace postoperatively. The hardware can loosen. Radial head excision can result in injury to the radial nerve or its branches as well as the ulnar nerve. These nerves can be studied with MRI or ultrasonography as well as electromyography. Radial head excision also results in occasional proximal radial migration and asymptomatic subluxation at the distal radioulnar joint that can lead to degenerative arthropathy in that region.[4] Radial head prostheses may loosen, sublux (Fig. 107-25), dislocate, or break.[21] Silicone synovitis is another complication that results in a destructive arthropathy that requires removal of the prosthesis.[22]

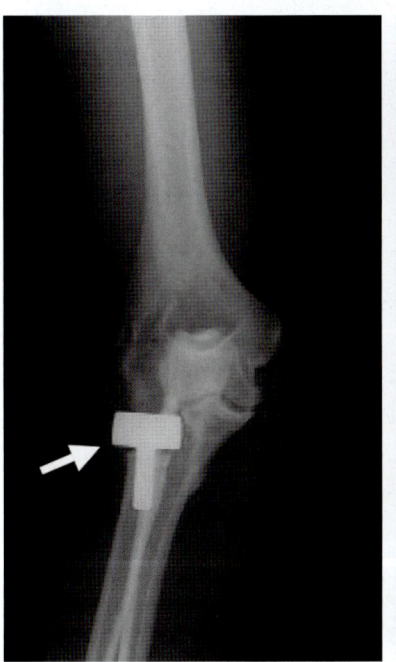 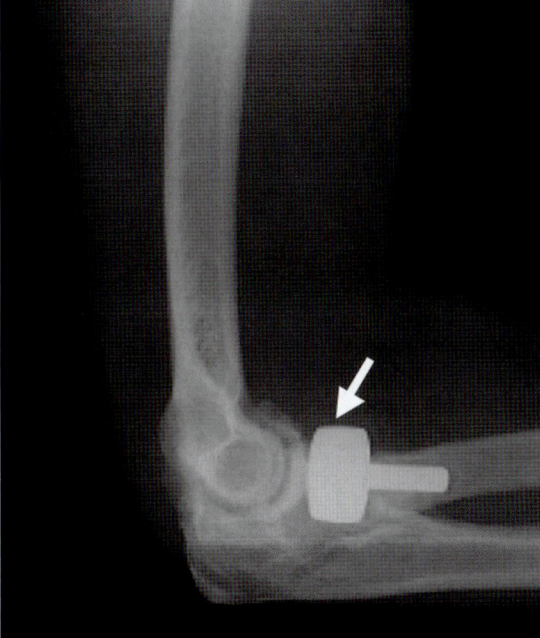

■ **FIGURE 107-22** Radial head replacement in anatomic alignment. Anteroposterior (**A**) and lateral (**B**) views show the radial head replacement in anatomic alignment (*arrows*).

A   B

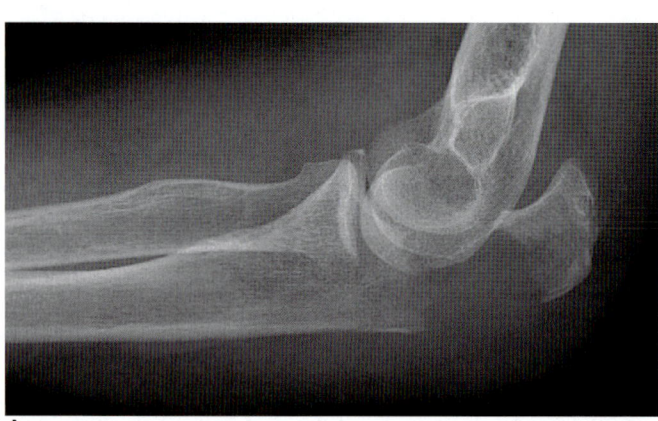

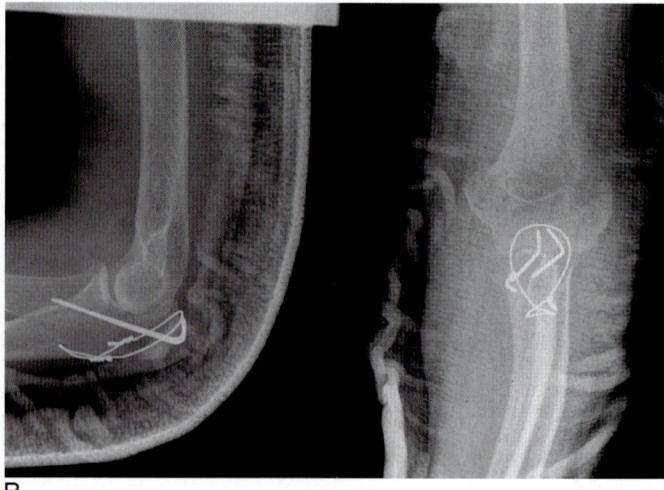

A   B

■ **FIGURE 107-23**   Olecranon fracture with distraction of the fragments. **A** and **B,** Postoperative radiographs demonstrate figure-of-eight tension band and two Kirschner wires with the elbow in a plaster splint. The fracture is reduced to anatomic alignment.

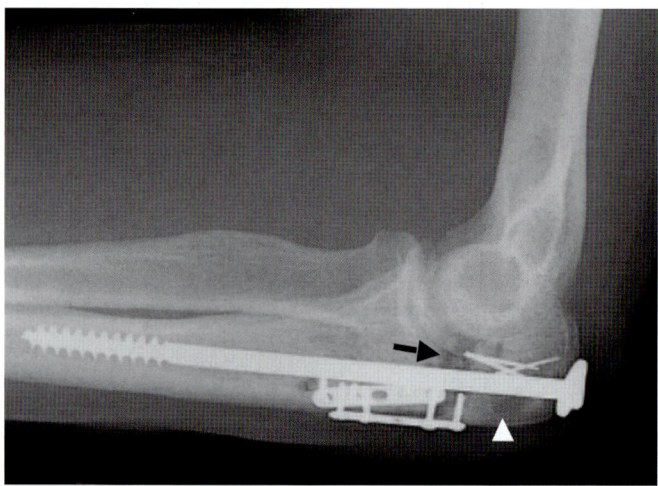

■ **FIGURE 107-24**   Infected postsurgical reduction of an olecranon fracture. There is a Brodie abscess in the proximal fragment (*arrowhead*) with a nonunion of the fracture (*arrow*).

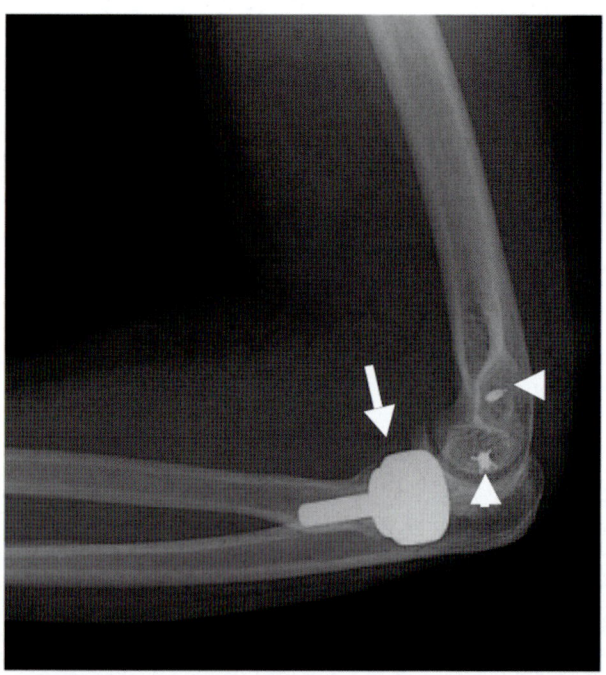

■ **FIGURE 107-25**   Posteriorly subluxed radial head replacement (*arrow*) on lateral radiograph. Note the suture anchors for extensor and flexor tendon repairs (*arrowheads*).

Olecranon fractures may displace. Olecranon bursitis is a complication of open reduction and internal fixation of the olecranon fracture. It will be seen as a soft tissue swelling on radiographs and a fluid-filled mass on CT, MRI, and ultrasonography.

Fragments associated with osteochondral lesions should be removed from the joint and not visible on imaging. Arthrography can be useful to look for these bodies and to determine if they are intra-articular. CT arthrography and MR arthrography also demonstrate cartilaginous bodies not seen on radiographs. Loosening of osteochondral fragments are recognized by the development of increasing lucency at the interface of the fragment with the parent bone. This can be evaluated with MRI or MR arthrography. Radiographic degenerative changes are frequently seen in the radiocapitellar joint and may be associated with radial head enlargement.[23]

SUGGESTED READINGS

Anderson SE, Otsuka NY, Steinbach LS. MR imaging of pediatric elbow trauma. Semin Musculoskelet Radiol 1998; 2:185–198.
Green NE. Fractures and dislocations about the elbow. In Green NE (ed). Skeletal Trauma in Children. Philadelphia, WB Saunders, 1994, pp 213–256.

REFERENCES

1. Farnsworth CL, Silva PD, Mubarak SJ. Etiology of supracondylar humerus fractures. J Pediatr Orthop 1998; 18:38–42.
2. Campbell CC, Waters PM, Emans JB, et al. Neurovascular injury and displacement in type III supracondylar humerus fractures. J Pediatr Orthop 1995; 15:47–52.
3. Williamson DM, Cole WG. Flexion supracondylar fractures of the humerus in children: treatment by manipulation and extension cast. Injury 1991; 22:451–455.
4. Pirone AM, Graham HK, Krajbich JI. Management of displaced extension-type supracondylar fractures of the humerus in children. J Bone Joint Surg Am 1988; 70:641–650.
5. Gaston SR, Smith FM, Baab OD. Adult injuries of the radial head and neck; importance of time element in treatment. Am J Surg 1949; 78:631–635; discussion, 647–651.
6. Sanders RA, French HG. Open reduction and internal fixation of comminuted radial head fractures. Am J Sports Med 1986; 14:130–135.
7. Esser RD, Davis S, Taavao T. Fractures of the radial head treated by internal fixation: late results in 26 cases. J Orthop Trauma 1995; 9:318–323.
8. Coleman DA, Blair WF, Shurr D. Resection of the radial head for fracture of the radial head: long-term follow-up of seventeen cases. J Bone Joint Surg Am 1987; 69:385–392.
9. Regan W, Morrey B. Fractures of the coronoid process of the ulna. J Bone Joint Surg Am 1989; 71:1348–1354.
10. Regan W, Morrey BF. Classification and treatment of coronoid process fractures. Orthopedics 1992; 15:845–848.
11. Gartsman GM, Sculco TP, Otis JC. Operative treatment of olecranon fractures: excision or open reduction with internal fixation. J Bone Joint Surg Am 1981; 63:718–721.
12. Oka Y, Ohta K, Fukuda H. Bone-peg grafting for osteochondritis dissecans of the elbow. Int Orthop 1999; 23:53–57.
13. Iwasaki N, Kato H, Ishikawa J, et al. Autologous osteochondral mosaicplasty for capitellar osteochondritis dissecans in teenaged patients. Am J Sports Med 2006; 34:1233–1239.
14. Levine MJ, Horn BD, Pizzutillo PD. Treatment of posttraumatic cubitus varus in the pediatric population with humeral osteotomy and external fixation. J Pediatr Orthop 1996; 16:597–601.
15. Davids JR, Maguire MF, Mubarak SJ, Wenger DR. Lateral condylar fracture of the humerus following posttraumatic cubitus varus. J Pediatr Orthop 1994; 14:466–470.
16. Barrett IR, Bellemore MC, Kwon YM. Cosmetic results of supracondylar osteotomy for correction of cubitus varus. J Pediatr Orthop 1998; 18:445–447.
17. Brown IC, Zinar DM. Traumatic and iatrogenic neurological complications after supracondylar humerus fractures in children. J Pediatr Orthop 1995; 15:440–443.
18. Rasool MN. Ulnar nerve injury after K-wire fixation of supracondylar humerus fractures in children. J Pediatr Orthop 1998; 18:686–690.
19. Sairyo K, Henmi T, Kanematsu Y, et al. Radial nerve palsy associated with slightly angulated pediatric supracondylar humerus fracture. J Orthop Trauma 1997; 11:227–229.
20. Copley LA, Dormans JP, Davidson RS. Vascular injuries and their sequelae in pediatric supracondylar humeral fractures: toward a goal of prevention. J Pediatr Orthop 1996; 16:99–103.
21. Knight DJ, Rymaszewski LA, Amis AA, Miller JH. Primary replacement of the fractured radial head with a metal prosthesis. J Bone Joint Surg Br 1993; 75:572–576.
22. Vanderwilde RS, Morrey BF, Melberg MW, Vinh TN. Inflammatory arthritis after failure of silicone rubber replacement of the radial head. J Bone Joint Surg Br 1994; 76:78–81.
23. Jackson DW, Silvino N, Reiman P. Osteochondritis in the female gymnast's elbow. Arthroscopy 1989; 5:129–136.

Distal Forearm Fractures at the Wrist

DESCRIPTION, INDICATIONS, CONTRAINDICATIONS, PURPOSE, UNDERLYING MECHANICS

Fractures of the distal forearm at the wrist are common after a fall on an outstretched hand. Distal radial fractures may be accompanied by a fracture of the ulnar styloid. Isolated distal ulnar fractures are much less common. There are many types of distal radial fractures. The distal radius may have a fracture that extends to the articular surface or the fracture may be extra-articular. Colles' fracture typically occurs 2 to 3 cm from the articular surface in the distal radial metaphysis and may extend to the articular surface. It is characterized by a dorsal tilt of the radius. The Barton's fracture also has a dorsal tilt and occurs on the dorsal or volar (reverse Barton's) lip of the radius with associated subluxation of the carpus. Smith's fractures are characterized by an extra- or intra-articular fracture with a volar tilt of the radial articular surface. The chauffer's fracture (also called Hutchinson's or bumper fracture) occurs in the radial styloid. A die-punch fracture refers to fractures that involve the lunate fossa of the distal radius. The Galeazzi fracture-dislocation consists of a fracture of the distal third of the radius that may extend to the articular surface, is often dorsally displaced, and is associated with dorsal ulnar dislocation of the distal radioulnar joint.

A fracture can be treated conservatively with closed reduction in a cast if it appears stable, being minimally displaced or impacted. Distal fractures that have significant displacement or comminution require surgery. Articular fractures that unite with more than 2 mm of surface incongruity result in arthrosis and are treated surgically. The unstable lesions can be semi-constrained with closed reduction and external fixation, percutaneous pins, or pins and plaster. Those fractures that cannot be reduced with this method or are severely comminuted with soft tissue

---

KEY POINTS

- Distal forearm fractures at the wrist may require closed reduction with or without fixation.
- Unstable fractures are treated with open reduction and internal fixation.
- Distal radial articular surface should be in neutral or volar tilt after treatment.
- The ulnar inclination of the distal radius should be more than 15 degrees.
- The radius and ulna should be at approximately the same length at the distal radioulnar joint.
- Arthrography, CT, ultrasonography, and MRI can be helpful in assessing for complications such as malunion, nonunion, and soft tissue injury after treatment.

injury require fixation of the distal radius. The fractures that require open reduction and internal fixation include Barton's, reverse Barton's, and radial styloid fractures. Buttress plate fixation is often performed on these types of fractures.[1,2] Compression fractures of the radial articular surface or fractures with displaced and rotated fragments also require open reduction and internal fixation.

EXPECTED APPEARANCE ON IMAGING

After treatment, the fracture fragments should be reduced to anatomic alignment without significant displacement. The distal radius is expected to have a neutral or volar tilt on lateral radiographs (Fig. 107-26). On the posteroanterior view, the radius may have an ulnar inclination of greater than 15 degrees. The radial articular surface may be compromised if it contains more than a 2-mm stepoff. The ulna should be equal to the length of the radius at the distal radioulnar joint on a neutral wrist view obtained with the wrist on the radiographic table, in neutral forearm rotation, and with 90 degrees of elbow flexion and shoulder abduction. Bone graft may be used to fill in the fracture site[3] and should not be misinterpreted for fracture fragments. An ulnar styloid fracture is usually left alone and variably unites with the shaft.

POTENTIAL COMPLICATIONS AND RADIOLOGIC APPEARANCE

Malunion of the distal radius is more common in the wrist than in any other site in the body, occurring in 5% of patients.[4] Complications of radial fractures include malunion, nonunion, neurologic complications due to nerve retraction, unstable internal fixation, extension of fixation screws into the articulation (Fig. 107-27), loss of reduction or fixation, infection, and peritendinous adhesions. If the radius has not been adequately reduced from impaction, continued radial shortening is associated with positive ulnar variance, which can lead to ulnocarpal impaction syndrome. The distal radial cartilage can be damaged, leading to radiocarpal arthropathy. The triangular fibrocartilage, proximal row intrinsic carpal ligaments, and extrinsic carpal ligaments may also be torn in the presence of a fracture of the distal forearm. Osseous displacement, malunion, and nonunion can be identified on CT. The soft tissue abnormalities are best seen on MRI if there is not too much hardware in place to obscure them. Arthrography can be used to evaluate for ligament or triangular fibrocartilage damage in those situations in which the hardware would produce significant artifact on MRI.

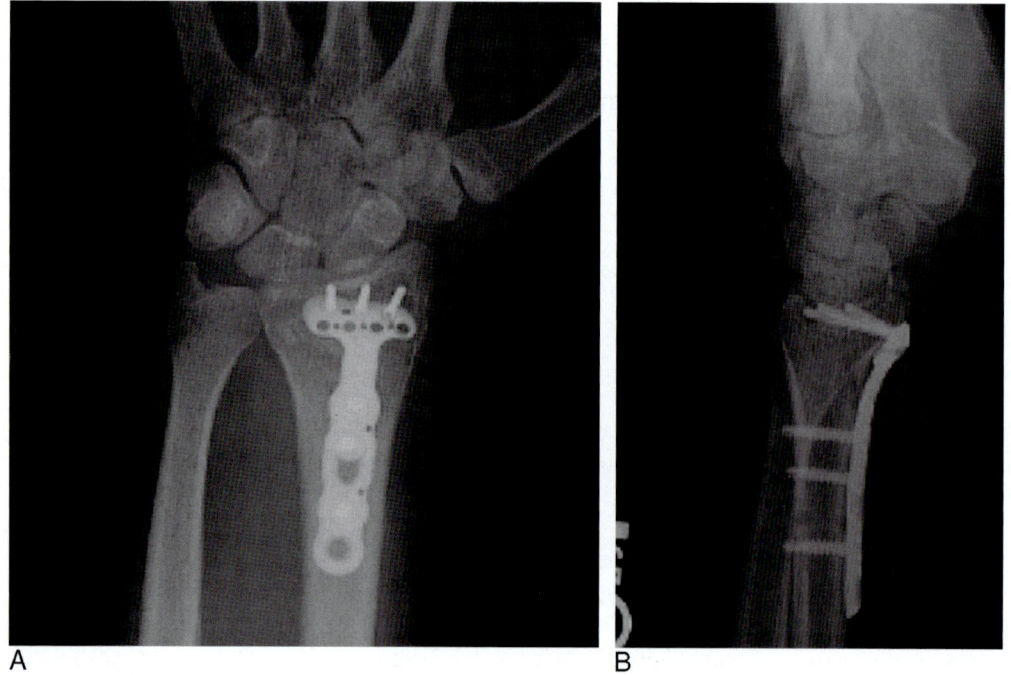

A **B**

■ **FIGURE 107-26** Colles' fracture reduced to anatomic alignment and treated with plate and screws. Posteroanterior (**A**) and lateral (**B**) radiographs.

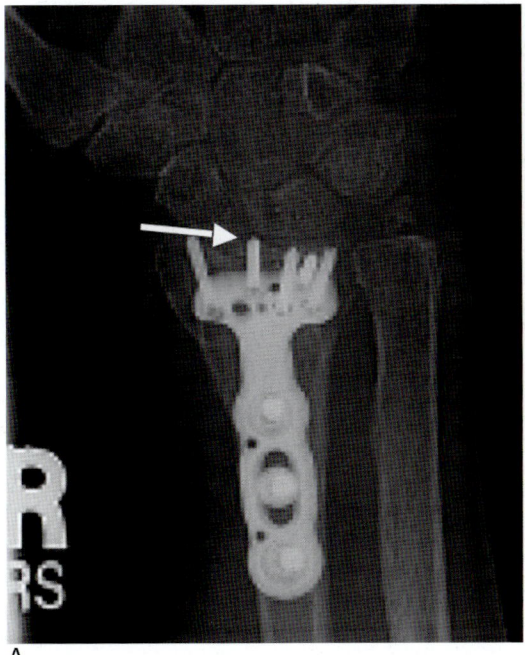
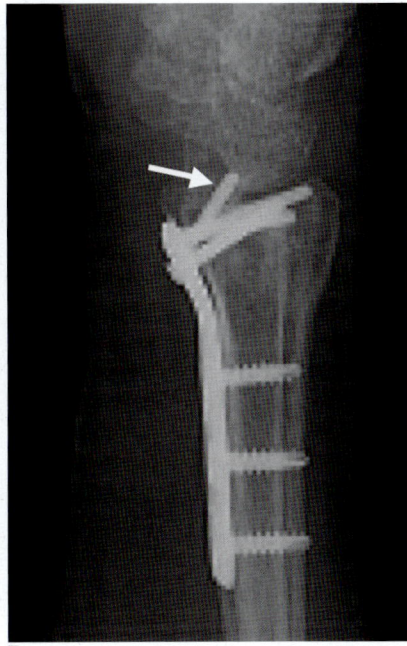

■ **FIGURE 107-27** Colles' fracture with internal fixation plate. The distal screws extend into the radiocarpal joint (*arrows*). Posteroanterior (**A**) and lateral (**B**) radiographs.

A

B

SUGGESTED READINGS

Fernandez DL. Correction of post-traumatic wrist deformity in adults by osteotomy, bone-grafting, and internal fixation. J Bone Joint Surg Am 1982; 64:1164–1178.

Goldfarb CA, Yin Y, Gilula LA, et al. Wrist fractures: what the clinician wants to know. Radiology 2001; 219:11–28.

REFERENCES

1. Axelrod TS, McMurtry RY. Open reduction and internal fixation of comminuted, intraarticular fractures of the distal radius. J Hand Surg [Am] 1990; 15:1–11.
2. Bradway JK, Amadio PC, Cooney WP. Open reduction and internal fixation of displaced, comminuted intra-articular fractures of the distal end of the radius. J Bone Joint Surg Am 1989; 71:839–847.
3. Herrera M, Chapman CB, Roh M, et al. Treatment of unstable distal radius fractures with cancellous allograft and external fixation. J Hand Surg [Am] 1999; 24:1269–1278.
4. Cooney WP 3rd, Dobyns JH, Linscheid RL. Complications of Colles' fractures. J Bone Joint Surg Am 1980; 62:613–619.

Carpal Tunnel Syndrome

DESCRIPTION, INDICATIONS, CONTRAINDICATIONS, PURPOSE, UNDERLYING MECHANICS

Carpal tunnel syndrome is the most common nerve entrapment syndrome in the upper extremity. It can be caused by repetitive motion, acute trauma, infection, mass lesions, variant anatomy, infiltrative disorders, and intrinsic nerve abnormalities or a combination of these factors. The syndrome may disappear with splinting, medication, injections, and a decrease in or avoidance of certain activities. In patients with excisable masses such as ganglia or neurogenic tumors, excision of the mass is performed. Most other patients require surgical decompression of the transverse carpal ligament. The flexor retinaculum is usually divided at its ulnar aspect with complete release. Additional epineurotomy for thickened and scarred epineurium is also occasionally performed. This may be done with an open procedure or with endoscopic release.

EXPECTED APPEARANCE ON IMAGING

The postoperative appearance of the carpal tunnel presents several challenges to the radiologist. Normal postoperative findings must be differentiated from persistent pathologic changes. The carpal tunnel volume is usually increased in the anteroposterior dimension with volar displacement of the contents. The transverse carpal ligament

KEY POINTS

- The content of the carpal tunnel displaces volarly after transverse carpal ligament release.
- The median nerve may decrease in size and signal intensity on T2 weighting after surgery.
- The transverse carpal ligament should be discontinuous from the level of the pisiform to the hook of the hamate.
- The median nerve and ulnar nerve may be lacerated, and a neuroma could result.
- A mass in or around the carpal tunnel may be responsible for symptoms if not diagnosed preoperatively.

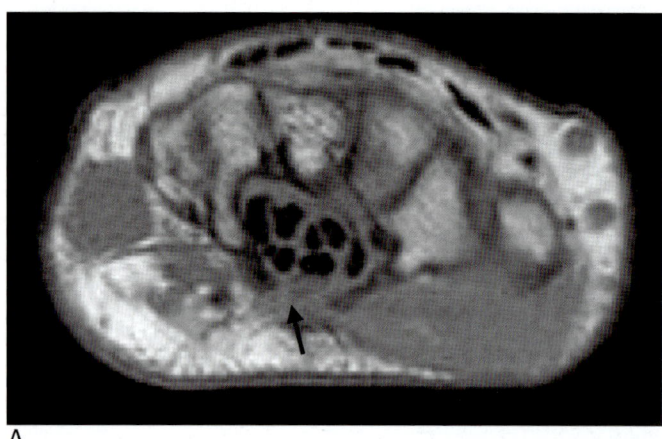 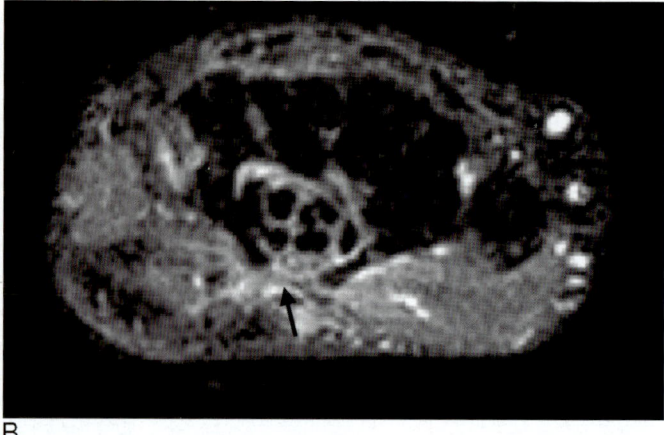

■ **FIGURE 107-28** Normal postoperative carpal tunnel release. There is discontinuity of the central flexor retinaculum where it has been surgically released on axial T1-weighted and gradient-echo sequences (*arrows*). The contents of the carpal tunnel are shifted volarly. *(Courtesy of Javier Beltran, MD, Brooklyn, NY.)*

is discontinuous at the site of surgical release (Fig. 107-28). Widening of the fat stripe in Perona's space at the floor of the carpal tunnel dorsal to the flexor digitorum profundus tendons is another common finding. If preoperative imaging is available, comparison will generally demonstrate some improvement in the signal intensity and size of the median nerve without complete resolution. Both MRI and ultrasound imaging have been advocated for the assessment of the asymptomatic, postoperative patient.

Several normal postoperative changes are routinely demonstrated with ultrasonography. In a study comparing the appearance of the median nerve before and after successful carpal tunnel release in 20 hands, significant increase in median nerve volume was documented at the level of the pisiform and hamate.[1] Also, the carpal volume increased in volume at the level of the hamate, largely owing to increased volar displacement of the transverse carpal ligament.

After successful carpal tunnel surgery, the MR appearance of the median nerve normalizes. The nerve decreases in size at the level of the pisiform, flattening at the level of the hook of the hamate, and signal intensity usually returns to normal.[2,3] Wu and colleagues[4] found that the best MR predictor of recurrent carpal tunnel syndrome was enlargement of

the median nerve at the level of the pisiform. Enlargement was seen in 40% of patients with recurrent carpal tunnel syndrome and only 8% with clinically successful surgery ($P = .007$). Another good predictor of persistent carpal tunnel syndrome in this study was persistent tenosynovitis seen in 60% compared with 35% of controls ($P = .02$).

POTENTIAL COMPLICATIONS AND RADIOLOGIC APPEARANCE

A small number of patients continue to experience symptoms after surgical release of the retinaculum. This clinical scenario is a difficult clinical problem. Nerve conduction studies are generally positive for weeks to months after successful carpal tunnel release and are not helpful in this clinical setting. Several complications should be sought on MRI and ultrasonography. Incomplete release of the transverse carpal ligament results in continued symptoms. This occurs more frequently with the endoscopic procedure. The imaging characteristics include a continuous transverse carpal ligament spanning the carpal tunnel anywhere between the pisiform and hook of the hamate levels (Fig. 107-29).[5] It is hard to differentiate an incom-

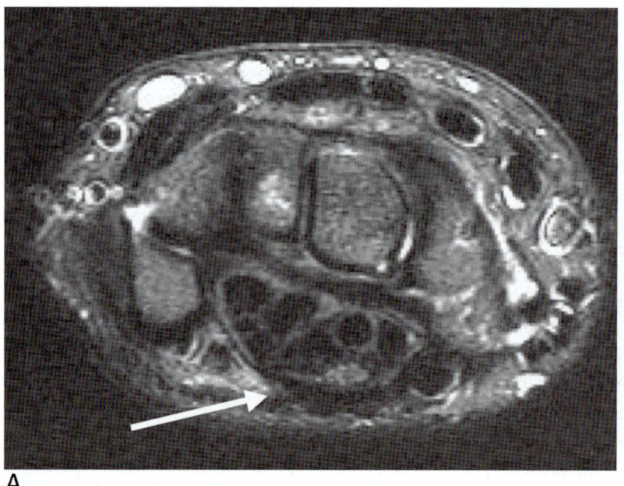 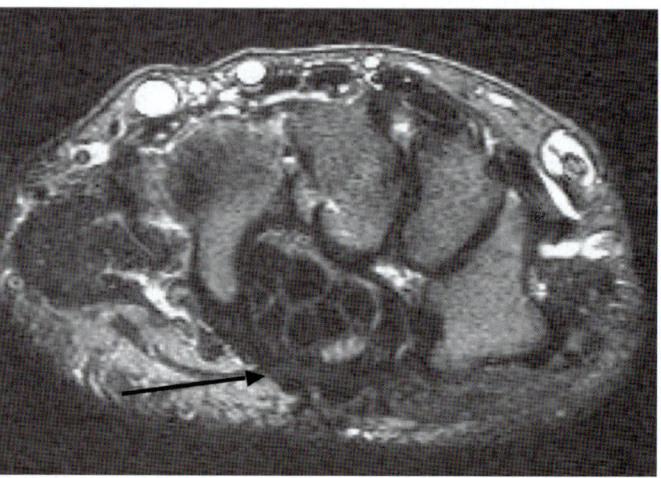

■ **FIGURE 107-29** Recurrent carpal tunnel syndrome after retinacular release presents with continuity of the flexor retinaculum at the level of the pisiform (**A**) and hook of the hamate (**B**) (*arrows*). *(Courtesy of Javier Beltran, MD, Brooklyn, NY.)*

plete release from a transverse carpal ligament that has reconstituted due to inflammation and scarring. In some of those cases, the carpal tunnel pressure decreases after surgery but increases the second month due to the filling in of the defect.[6] Occasionally, this reconstitution of the transverse carpal ligament is associated with increased volume in the carpal tunnel and there are no symptoms of carpal tunnel.[4] Other complications include laceration of the median nerve, which can result in nerve deficits and a neuroma, ulnar artery laceration, and fracture of the hook of the hamate.[7] When imaging is not performed preoperatively, failure to diagnose a mass in or around the carpal tunnel will result in the mass being visualized on postoperative studies.

KEY POINTS

- Scaphoid fractures are treated operatively when there is displacement, comminution, malunion, or nonunion.
- Kirschner wires and compression screws are used.
- Complications of surgically treated scaphoid fractures include nonunion, avascular necrosis, SNAC wrist, and neuroma.
- Sagittal cross sectional imaging is useful to detect the humpback deformity.
- Avascular necrosis is difficult to diagnose and can be overlooked if the proximal fragment is sclerotic. MRI with intravenous contrast is more sensitive than routine MRI for diagnosis.

SUGGESTED READINGS

Berquist TH. Nerve compression syndromes. In Berquist TH (ed). MRI of the Hand and Wrist. Philadelphia, Lippincott Williams & Wilkins, 2003.

Bordalo-Rodrigues M, Amin P, Rosenberg AS. MR imaging of common entrapment neuropathies at the wrist. Magn Reson Imaging Clin North Am 2004; 12:265-279.

REFERENCES

1. Lee CH, Kim TK, Yoon ES, Dhong ES. Postoperative morphologic analysis of carpal tunnel syndrome using high resolution ultrasonography. Ann Plast Surg 2005; 54:143-146.
2. Cudlip SA, Howe FA, Clifton A, et al. Magnetic resonance neurography studies of the median nerve before and after carpal tunnel decompression. J Neurosurg 2002; 96:1046-1051.
3. Allmann KH, Horch R, Gabelmann A, et al. Morphology of the carpal tunnel. Movement studies in patients with constriction symptoms and healthy probands using MR tomography. Unhallchinurgie 1996; 22:5-11.
4. Wu HT, Schweitzer ME, Culp RW. Potential MR signs of recurrent carpal tunnel syndrome: initial experience. J Comput Assist Tomogr 2004; 28:860-864.
5. Bonel HM, Heuck A, Frei KA, et al. Carpal tunnel syndrome: assessment by turbo spin echo, spin echo and magnetization transfer imaging applied in a low-field MR system. J Comput Assist Tomogr 2001; 25:137-145.
6. Sanz J, Lizaur A, Sanchez Del Campo F. Post-operative changes of carpal canal pressure in carpal tunnel syndrome: a prospective study with follow-up of 1 year. J Hand Surg [Br] 2005; 30:611-614.
7. Rowland EB, Kleinert JM. Endoscopic carpal tunnel release in cadavera: an investigation of the results of 12 surgeons with this training model. J Bone Joint Surg Am 1994; 76:266-268.

Scaphoid Fractures

DESCRIPTION, INDICATIONS, CONTRAINDICATIONS, PURPOSE, UNDERLYING MECHANICS

Scaphoid fractures are the most common carpal bone fractures and usually result from a fall on an outstretched hand. The waist of the scaphoid is the most frequent site of fracture, followed by the proximal and the distal pole. The more proximal the fracture, the higher the risk of osteonecrosis in the proximal fragment, because the vascular supply to the scaphoid runs from distal to proximal. Instability of the fracture is characterized by greater than 1 mm of fragment displacement, a scapholunate angle of more than 60 degrees (normal, 30–60 degrees), and/or a radiolunate or capitolunate angle greater than 15 degrees (normal, 0 ± 15 degrees). Displaced fractures can lead to malunion or nonunion, which results in carpal collapse and degenerative arthritis. After casting, the scaphoid fracture should show healing within 20 weeks. If no healing occurs, surgical fixation is indicated. Fractures of the waist displaying more than 1 mm of displacement, comminution, angulation, or malrotation are treated with open reduction and internal fixation. Surgery can be performed via open procedure or arthroscopy. Options include closed reduction with percutaneous pinning or compression screw insertion,[1] and open reduction with Kirschner wires or a compression screw. Comminuted fractures may require bone grafting. Most scaphoid fractures detected more than 4 weeks after injury are best treated surgically.

EXPECTED APPEARANCE ON IMAGING

Posteroanterior and lateral radiographs (Fig. 107-30) along with an ulnarly deviated posteroanterior (scaphoid) view (Fig. 107-31) allow for assessment of alignment, nonunion, and avascular necrosis. The fracture may be located in the proximal, middle, or distal third. Hardware such as a pin or compression screw normally traverses the fracture site (see Figs. 107-30 and 107-31). The fragments should be reduced, and the fracture should heal over a few months. CT can be used to evaluate the fracture for nonunion and malunion when deciding if surgery is needed (Fig. 107-32) and after surgical intervention (Fig. 107-33). Use of metal reduction techniques such as higher kVp and mAs as well as narrower x-ray beam collimation and lower pitch setting improves evaluation of the postoperative scaphoid by CT.[2] MRI is helpful for identifying avascular necrosis in the postoperative setting, although hardware artifact may make it difficult to evaluate (Fig. 107-34). Special techniques to reduce artifact on MRI have been described.[3]

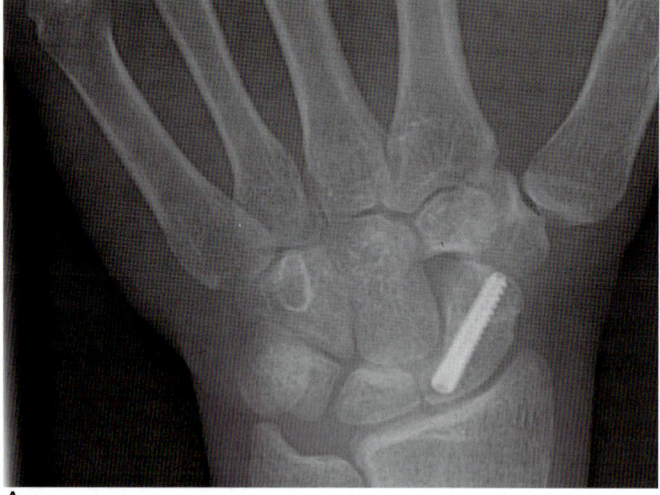

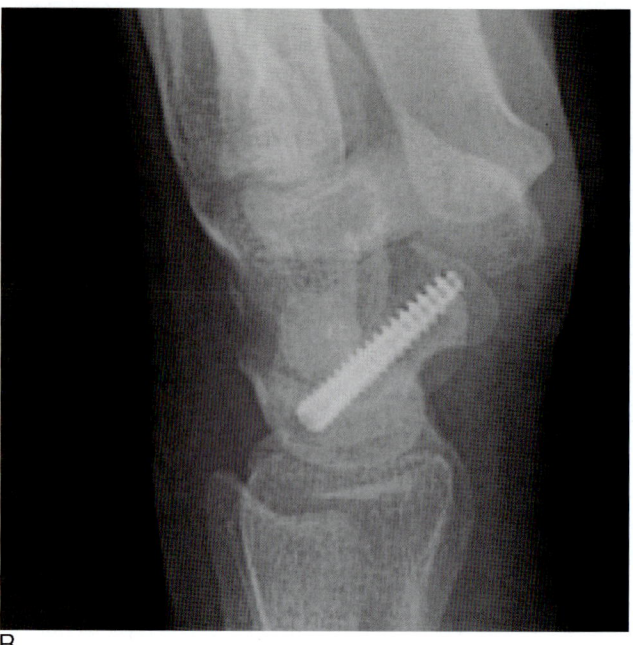

■ **FIGURE 107-30** Scaphoid fracture after surgery with good result. A screw traverses the healed fracture on posteroanterior (**A**) and lateral (**B**) views without evidence of nonunion or avascular necrosis.

POTENTIAL COMPLICATIONS AND RADIOLOGIC APPEARANCE

Scaphoid nonunion, characterized by a lack of fusion at the surgical site, can be a complication of conservative treatment or surgical repair (see Fig. 107-32). There is often sclerosis and/or cyst formation at the margins of the fracture. Fractures of the waist of the scaphoid may collapse and dorsally angulate, resulting in a flexion (humpback) deformity (see Fig. 107-32). This is best

seen on sagittal CT and MRI studies. Osteotomies are performed when a humpback deformity is discovered. Dorsal intercalated segment instability (DISI) may also be seen. This should be diagnosed on a neutral lateral wrist radiograph. Nonunion leads to a pattern of instability and articular degeneration known as SNAC (scaphoid nonunion advanced collapse) wrist. Four progressive stages of SNAC wrist have been identified, including arthritis of the radial styloid, extension of the arthritic

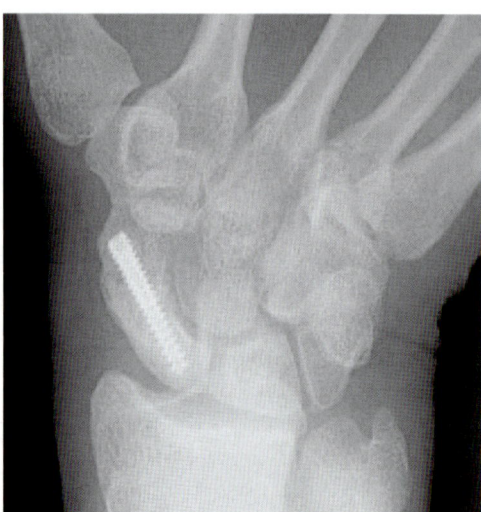

■ **FIGURE 107-31** This scaphoid view shows postoperative pinning for the scaphoid fracture shown in Figure 107-34. The patient did well postoperatively with fracture healing and no avascular necrosis.

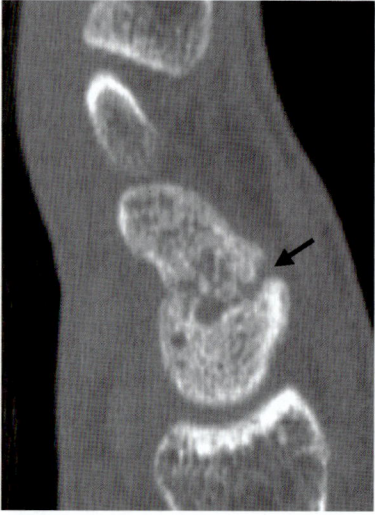

■ **FIGURE 107-32** There is a scaphoid fracture nonunion (*arrow*) with possible avascular necrosis in the proximal pole presenting as sclerosis on this sagittal CT reformatted image. There is also excessive dorsal angulation at the apex of the fracture consistent with a humpback deformity. These three criteria are indications for surgery.

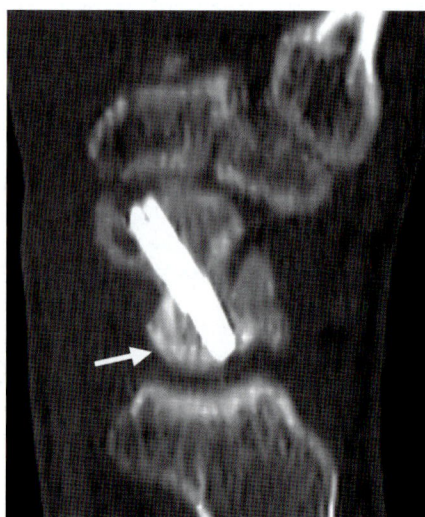

■ **FIGURE 107-33** Treated scaphoid fracture with traversing screw shows healed fracture with proximal scaphoid sclerosis that may represent avascular necrosis (*arrow*). The bone posteriorly is the adjacent displaced carpal bone.

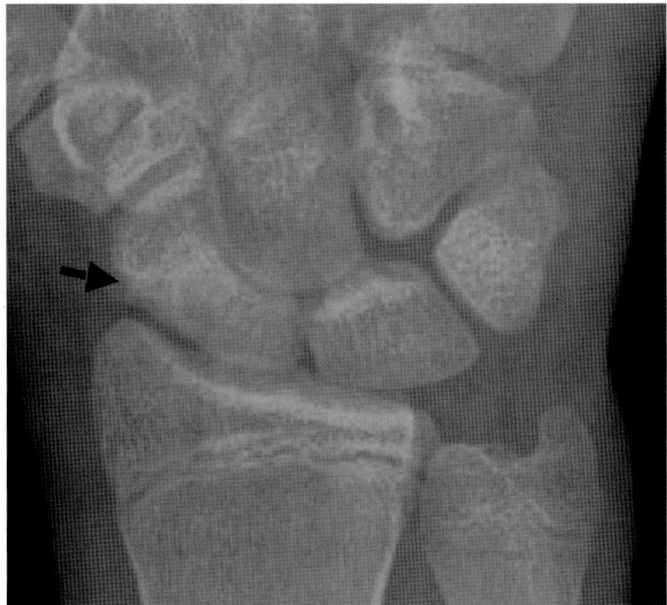

A

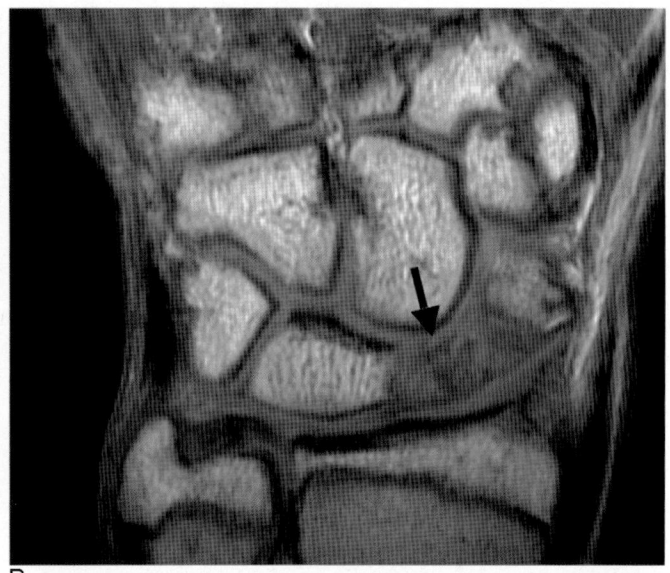

B

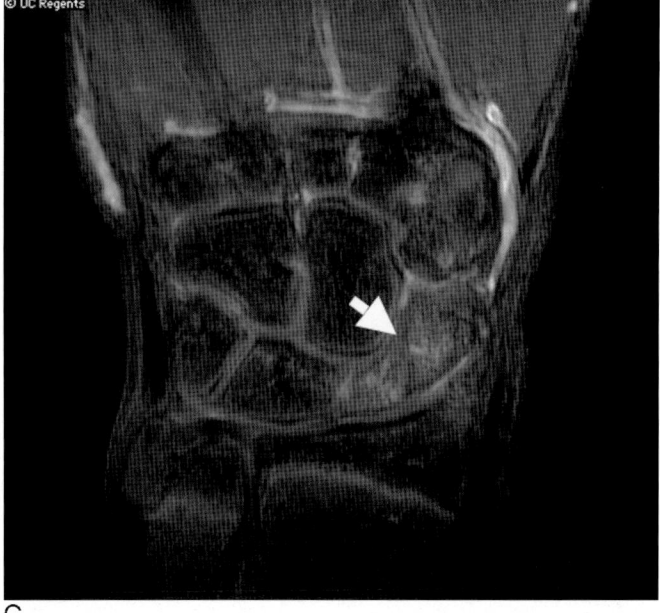

C

■ **FIGURE 107-34** Scaphoid fracture. **A,** There is a subtle fracture of the scaphoid on this posteroanterior radiograph manifest as sclerosis and stepoff in the waist portion (*arrow*). **B,** Coronal, T1-weighted MR image shows the fracture with low signal intensity in the proximal pole (*arrow*). **C,** The entire scaphoid enhances after intravenous administration of gadolinium (*arrow*) on this T1-weighted, fat-suppressed image. The patient had a scaphoid pinning and did well postoperatively with fracture healing and no avascular necrosis as shown in Figure 107-31.

change to the scaphoid fossa of the radius, capitolunate arthritis, and diffuse carpal arthritis. Avascular necrosis can result with or without nonunion. It is usually seen in the proximal portion of the scaphoid. Sclerosis of the proximal fragment on radiographs or CT suggests the presence of avascular necrosis, but this is not always a specific finding.[4] MRI with intravenous contrast can be useful in this setting.[5] If the proximal fragment shows low signal intensity on T1 and T2 weighting without contrast medium enhancement, it is likely affected by avascular necrosis. However, contrast enhancement and high signal intensity on T2 weighting are not always specific

for viability (see Fig. 107-34). Avascular necrosis is more accurately diagnosed by intraoperative assessment, and, when diagnosed, it is treated with bone grafting. MRI can also be used to detect avascular necrosis in cases of nonunion treated with a vascular pedicle graft.[6] Nonviable or fragmented proximal poles are treated with salvage procedures that include fragment excision, intercarpal arthrodesis, and proximal row carpectomy. Adhesions cause stiffness, nerve damage, and development of a neuroma at the surgical site. Silastic implants are no longer used because they cause synovitis that produces bone and cartilage destruction (Fig. 107-35).

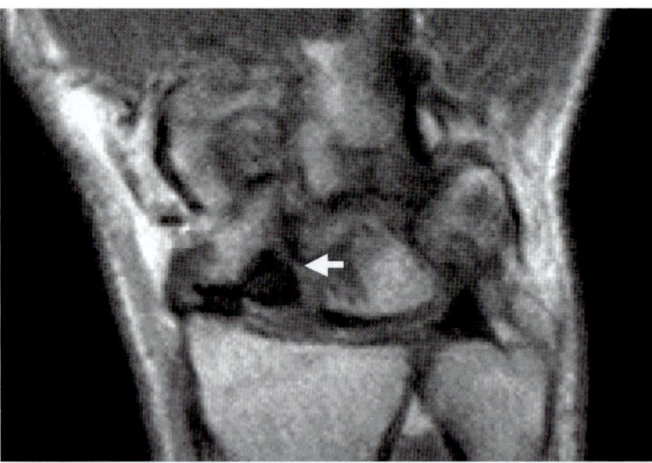

A

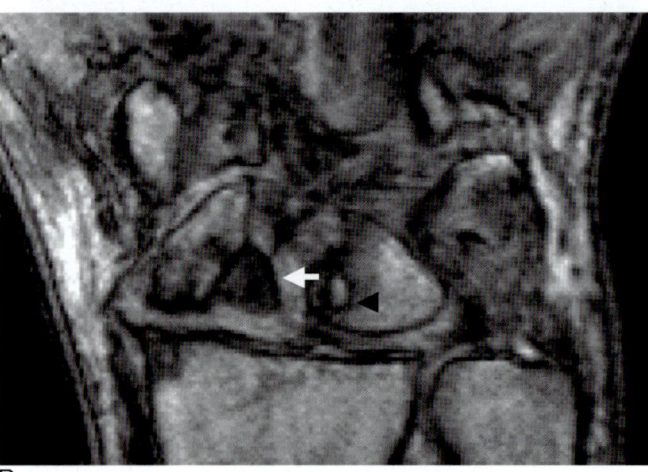

B

■ FIGURE 107-35 Silastic implant for scaphoid fracture caused Silastic synovitis. Coronal T1-weighted (**A**) and gradient-echo (**B**) MR images demonstrate the low signal intensity Silastic implant (*arrows*). There was a reaction to the Silastic material that produced bone destruction, including the cyst in the lunate (*arrowhead*). (*Courtesy of Javier Beltran, MD, Brooklyn, NY.*)

SUGGESTED READINGS

Amadio PC, Taleisnik J. Fractures of the carpal bones. In Green DP, Hotchkiss RN, Pederson WC (eds). Green's Operative Hand Surgery, 4th ed. New York, Churchill Livingstone, 1999.

Gelberman RH, Wollock BS, Siegel DB. Current concepts review: fractures and nonunions of the carpal scaphoid. J Bone Joint Surg Am 1989; 71:1560-1565.

REFERENCES

1. Herbert TJ, Fisher WE. Management of the fractured scaphoid using a new bone screw. J Bone Joint Surg Br 1984; 66:114-123.
2. Buckwalter KA, Parr JA, Choplin RH, Capello WN. Multichannel CT imaging of orthopedic hardware and implants. Semin Musculoskelet Radiol 2006; 10:86-97.
3. Olsen RV, Munk PL, Lee MJ, et al. Metal artifact reduction sequence: early clinical applications. RadioGraphics 2000; 20:699-712.
4. Cheung YY, Naspinsky SR, Goodwin DW, et al. Increased radiodensity of the proximal pole of the scaphoid: a common finding in computed tomography imaging of the wrist. J Comput Assist Tomogr 2006; 30:850-857.
5. Cerezal L, Abascal F, Canga A, et al. Usefulness of gadolinium-enhanced MR imaging in the evaluation of the vascularity of scaphoid nonunions. AJR Am J Roentgenol 2000; 174:141-149.
6. Anderson SE, Steinbach LS, Tschering-Vogel D, et al. MR imaging of avascular scaphoid nonunion before and after vascularized bone grafting. Skeletal Radiol 2005; 34:314-320.

Postoperative Evaluation of Carpometacarpal, Metacarpal, and Phalangeal Trauma including the Surrounding Soft Tissue Structures

DESCRIPTION, INDICATIONS, CONTRAINDICATIONS, PURPOSE, UNDERLYING MECHANICS

Nondisplaced fractures of metacarpals and phalanges that do not extend to the articular surface are often treated conservatively with immobilization. Surgery is usually indicated for unstable fractures of the metacarpals and phalanges. Fractures with articular stepoff, open fractures, displaced or angulated fractures, those with bone loss or shortening, as well as multiple fractures or joint displacement usually require open reduction and internal fixation. Most fractures can be treated with initial traction and then percutaneous fixation techniques. Hardware used include Kirschner wires, plates, and screws that are placed so that they avoid the tendons, blood vessels and nerves. Kirschner wires are eventually removed and therefore are either cut off under the skin or protrude above the skin surface. Some intra-articular fractures may also be stabilized with hardware placed arthroscopically.

Arthritis of the thumb carpometacarpal joint can be treated with resection arthroplasty, ligament reconstruction, and tendon interposition with the entire flexor carpi radialis tendon (Fig. 107-36). The flexor carpi radialis

---

KEY POINTS

- Surgery is indicated for unstable fractures of the metacarpals and phalanges.
- Kirschner wires, plates, screws, and external fixators are used for fractures of the hand.
- Three views of the affected bone are recommended for evaluation.
- There should not be a stepoff at the joint surface.
- MRI and ultrasonography are useful for evaluation of ligament and tendon repairs in the hand.

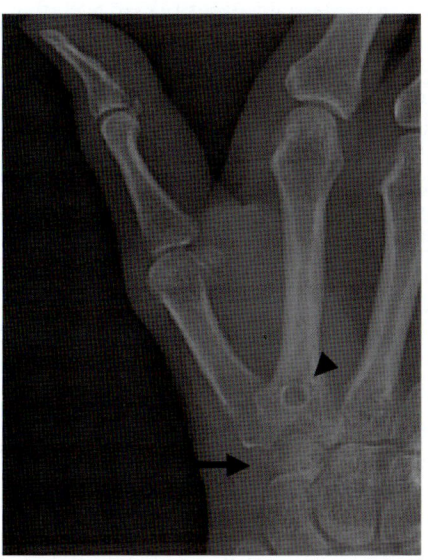

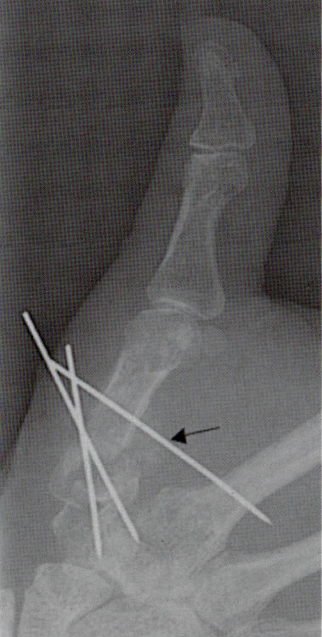

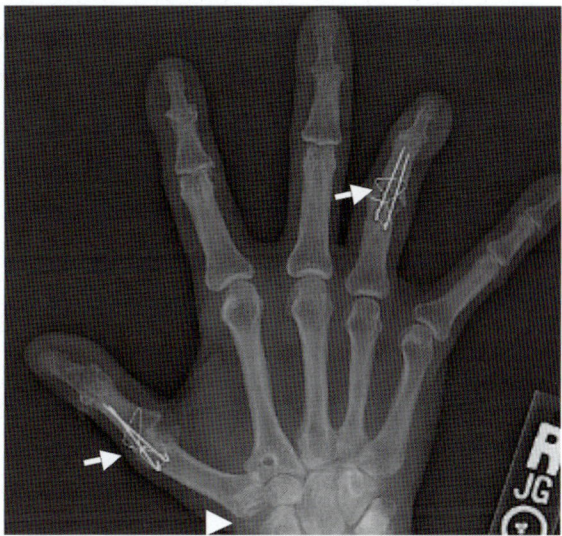

■ **FIGURE 107-36** Postoperative appearance of trapeziometacarpal arthroplasty using the flexor carpi radialis tendon. The trapezoid has been resected (*arrow*). There is a hole drilled at the base of the second metacarpal through which the reinforcing tendon traverses (*arrowhead*).

■ **FIGURE 107-37** Rolando fracture at the base of the first metacarpal treated with Kirschner wires. The fracture line is still visualized, and there is some callus formation around the site (*arrow*).

■ **FIGURE 107-38** Postoperative appearance in psoriatic involvement of the hand. Trapeziometacarpal arthroplasty (*arrowhead*) with first metacarpophalangeal and fourth proximal interphalangeal joint fusions with Kirschner and cerclage wires for arthritis (*arrows*). Note the distal interphalangeal joint erosions characteristic of psoriatic arthropathy.

tendon is used for reconstruction and interposition. A partial trapezoidectomy is provides excellent pain relief and restoration of function. No morbidity is usually observed with use of the entire flexor carpi radialis tendon.[1]

Fractures at the carpometacarpal joints are often unstable and require surgery. Frank or subtle dislocations may be present in this region. Fractures at the base of the first metacarpal include the Bennett's fracture, which is a small intra-articular avulsion fracture at the attachment of the first metacarpocarpal ligament that produces a single fragment with volar lip fracture. Bennett's fractures are often treated with closed reduction, but if the volar lip fragment involves more than 25% to 30% of the articular surface, it is considered unstable and screw fixation can be performed. The comminuted fracture at the base of the first metacarpal that extends to the carpometacarpal joint is called the Rolando fracture. Rolando's fractures are considered unstable and are treated with open reduction and internal fixation (Fig. 107-37).

Unstable fractures of the metacarpal shafts usually angulate with the apex dorsal. This is due to pull by wrist extensors proximally and interosseous muscles and long finger flexors distally. Many of these fractures are treated with immobilization. Open reduction and internal fixation is indicated if there is severe dorsal angulation. Fractures of the metacarpal head are intra-articular, and precise reduction is indicated. Large fragments are treated with open reduction and internal fixation using Kirschner wires. Metacarpophalangeal joints that have comminuted fractures or arthritis can be treated with fusion using pins, wires, and bone graft (Fig. 107-38).

Fractures that involve the base of a proximal phalanx that extend to the articular surface are unstable and treated surgically. Phalangeal shaft fractures may be treated surgically if they are comminuted or displaced (Fig. 107-39). Fractures of the mid proximal phalanges often angulate with the apex volar owing to forces from the extensor tendons and intrinsic muscles. Proximal interphalangeal joint injuries are usually treated conservatively unless they are severely comminuted with large fracture fragments.[2]

The gamekeeper's thumb represents a tear of the ulnar collateral ligament. This is caused by a valgus stress. The ligament may avulse off of the base of the first metacarpal or may be disrupted distally without bony avulsion (Fig. 107-40).

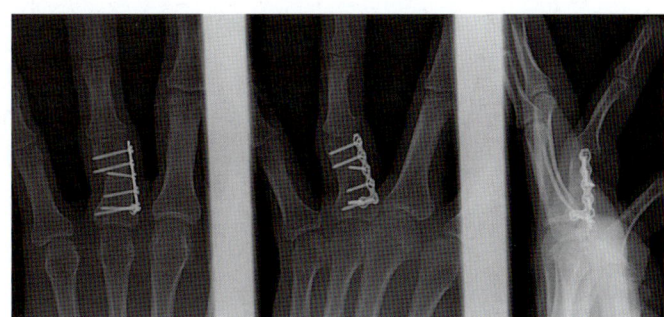

■ **FIGURE 107-39** Posteroanterior, oblique, and lateral radiographic views of a healed comminuted fracture of the diaphysis of the fourth proximal phalanx after open reduction and internal fixation with side plate and screws.

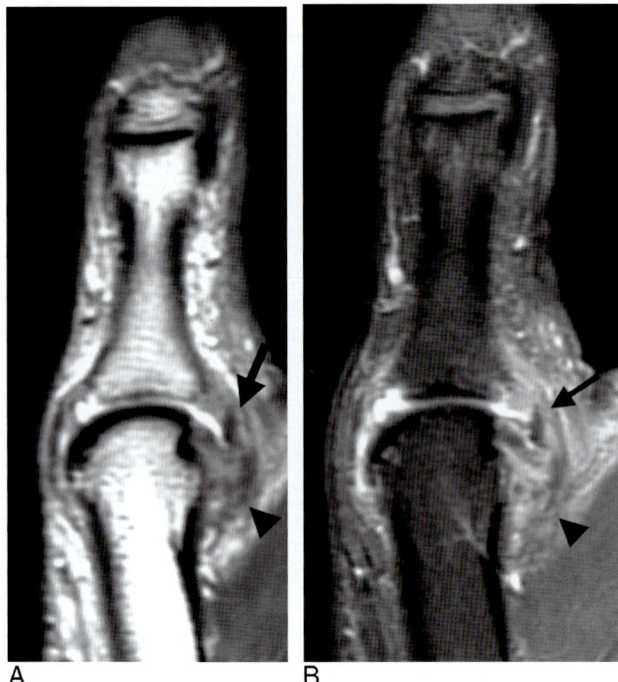

■ FIGURE 107-40 Stener lesion that was surgically repaired. Coronal, T1-weighted (**A**) and T2-weighted (**B**) MR images of the thumb demonstrated a disrupted retracted ulnar collateral ligament of the thumb consistent with a Stener lesion. The ligament lies over the adductor hood, indicating a surgical lesion (*arrows*).

Nondisplaced bony avulsions are immobilized in a cast or splint while displaced fragments are pinned back to the parent bone.[3,4] Partial ligament tears are treated with immobilization for 2 to 3 weeks. A complete ligament tear may remain near the proximal phalanx under the adductor aponeurosis or can displace superficial to the adductor aponeurosis. The latter arrangement is called a Stener lesion.[5] Ligament healing is prevented when there is interposition of the adductor aponeurosis between the ligament and the bone (see Fig. 107-40). This type of lesion requires reattachment of the ligament to the proximal phalanx under the adductor aponeurosis with surgical reduction and internal fixation. It is ideal to perform this surgery within 10 days of injury.

Fractures that are treated surgically in the distal phalanx include a type II hyperflexion fracture of the base of the distal phalanx that involves more than a third of the articular surface or the type III fracture called a mallet finger, which is a hyperextension injury of the articular surface that usually involves more than half of the articular surface.

EXPECTED APPEARANCE ON IMAGING

After surgery, the metacarpals and phalanges as well as the neighboring articulations should be restored to near anatomic alignment without articular subluxation or dislocation. It is best to do posteroanterior, lateral, and oblique radiographic views of the region (see Fig. 107-39). Joint surfaces should be reduced without stepoff. Radiographic

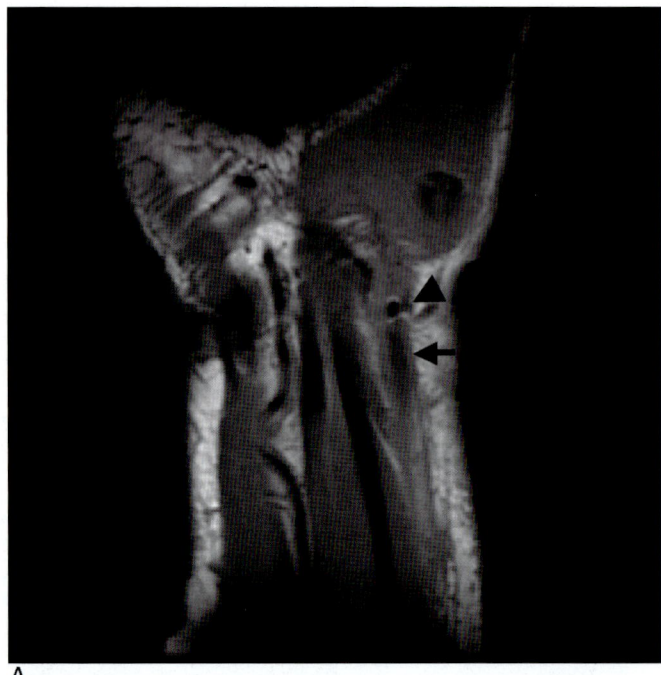

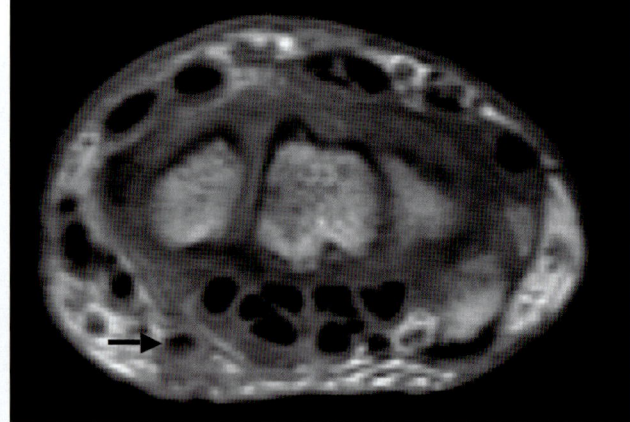

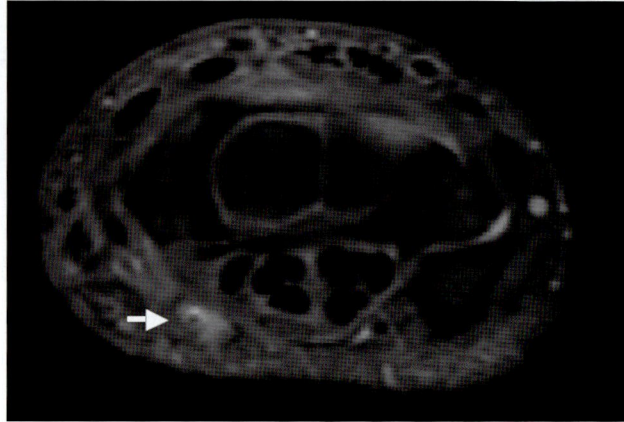

■ FIGURE 107-41 Flexor carpi radialis tendon repair re-tear. Coronal T1-weighted (**A**), axial T1-weighted (**B**), and axial T2-weighted (**C**) MR images demonstrate the retracted flexor carpi radialis tendon after repair (*arrows*). Note the micrometallic artifact at the tendon end (*arrowhead*). (*Courtesy of Mark Skirgaudas, MD, Hartford, CT.*)

evaluation requires serial comparison of fracture alignment and hardware location. MRI or ultrasonography are useful for evaluation of ligament and tendon healing after surgical repair. These structures may thicken but should appear continuous. On MRI, the signal intensity will decrease with time. Surrounding hardware and micrometallic artifacts related to surgical instrument placement during repair may make MRI less reliable for evaluation.

POTENTIAL COMPLICATIONS AND RADIOLOGIC APPEARANCE

Each follow-up examination should be scrutinized for hardware fractures, displacement, or pullout. Fracture alignment changes should be noted. Ligament and tendon re-tears present as partial- or full-thickness loss in continuity of the structure after breakdown of a suture repair on MRI and ultrasonography (Fig. 107-41). The tendon or ligament may retract from its attachment site. Scarring around ligament and tendon tears along with involvement of adjacent structures by scar, seen with MRI or ultrasonography, should be noted (Figs. 107-42 and 107-43). In one study of flexor tendon repair of the hand by MRI,[6] MRI showed isolated low signal intensity peritendinous adhesions as a frequent finding around intact tendons. Tendon ruptures were of two types: frank rupture or elongated scar tissue that the authors called callus. Tendon gaps were significantly larger in frank rupture. With elongated fibrous scarring, there was a thin fibrous continuity to the tendon. Tenolysis was used for short and mature callus. MRI is useful for evaluating partial or complete tears of the collateral ligaments around the metacarpophalangeal joints of the fingers and their surgical

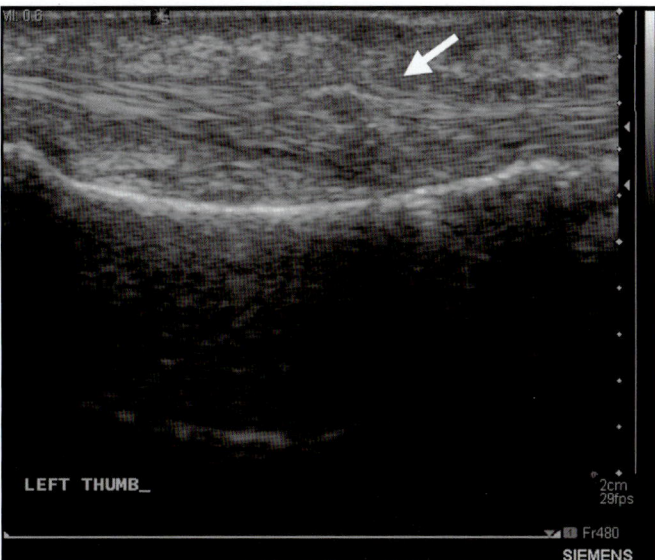

■ **FIGURE 107-42** Previously repaired scarred flexor tendon of the left thumb. The flexor tendon is dynamically not working smoothly because of the repair. Postoperative ultrasound image shows scarring/sutures and loss of clarity between the superficialis and profundus tendons (*arrow*). *(Courtesy of Gina Allen, MD, Birmingham, England.)*

complications.[7] Infection is rare but should be considered when there is bone destruction, cortical loss or periosteal reaction, lucency surrounding pins, or soft tissue swelling. Abscesses present with fluid collections that can be identified by ultrasonography, CT, or MRI.

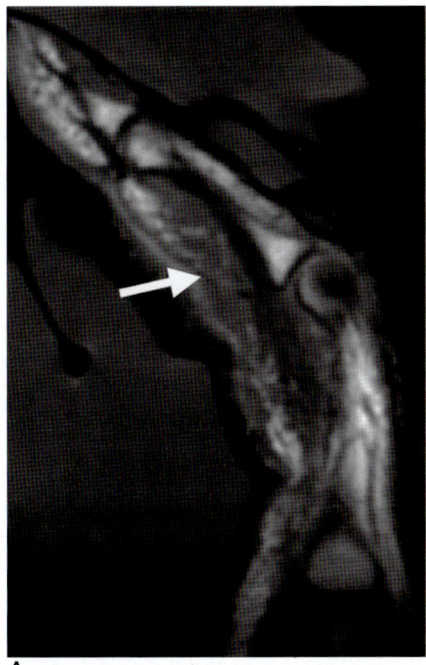

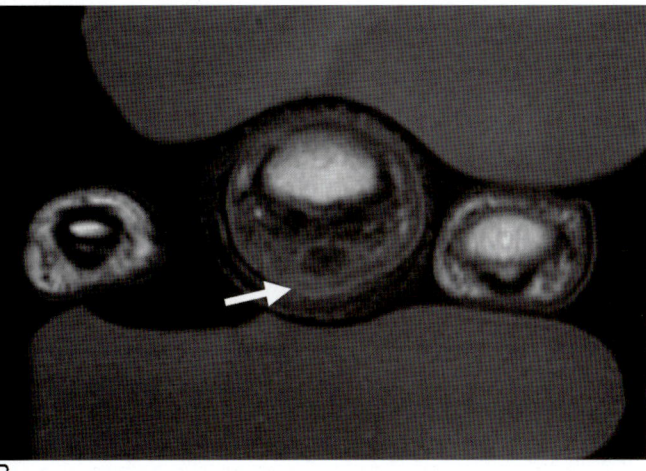

■ **FIGURE 107-43** Excess scar tissue after flexor digitorum profundus tendon repair with contracture of the finger. Sagittal T1-weighted (**A**) and axial T2-weighted (**B**) MR images of the finger demonstrate intermediate signal intensity scar tissue in the surgical region (*arrows*).

SUGGESTED READINGS

Ebrahim FS, De Maeseneer M, Jager T, et al. US diagnosis of UCL tears of the thumb and Stener lesions: Technique, pattern-based approach, and differential diagnosis. RadioGraphics 2006; 26:1007–1020.

Gutow AP, Slade JF, Mahoney JD. Phalangeal injuries. In Trumble T (ed). Hand Surgery Update 3: Hand, Elbow and Shoulder. Rosemont, IL, American Society for Surgery of the Hand, 2003, pp 1–27.

Markiewitz AD. Metacarpal fractures. In Trumble T (ed). Hand Surgery Update 3: Hand, Elbow and Shoulder. Rosemont, IL, American Society for Surgery of the Hand, 2003, pp 29–35.

REFERENCES

1. Varitimidis SE, Fox RJ, King JA, et al. Trapeziometacarpal arthroplasty using the entire flexor carpi radialis tendon. Clin Orthop Relat Res 2000; 370:164–170.
2. Blazar PE, Steinberg DR. Fractures of the proximal interphalangeal joint. J Am Acad Orthop Surg 2000; 8:383–390.
3. Kozin SH, Bishop AT. Gamekeeper's thumb: Early diagnosis and treatment. Orthop Rev 1994; 23:797–804.
4. Weiland AJ, Berner SH, Hotchkiss RN, et al. Repair of acute ulnar collateral ligament injuries of the thumb metacarpophalangeal joint with an intraosseous suture anchor. J Hand Surg [Am] 1997; 22:585–591.
5. Stener B. Skeletal injuries associated with rupture of the ulnar collateral ligament of the metacarpophalangeal joint of the thumb: a clinical and anatomical study. Acta Chir Scand 1963; 125: 583–586.
6. Drape JL, Silbermann-Hoffman O, Houvet P, et al. Complications of flexor tendon repair in the hand: MR imaging assessment. Radiology 1996; 198:219–224.
7. Theumann NH, Pessis E, Lecompte M, et al. MR imaging of the metacarpophalangeal joints of the fingers: evaluation of 38 patients with chronic joint disability. Skeletal Radiol 2005; 34:210–216.

108

The Postoperative Hip

Derek R. Armfield, Jon K. Sekiya, Marc J. Philippon, Eoin C. Kavanagh, and George Koulouris

Postoperative Imaging in Arthroscopic Hip Surgery

Derek R. Armfield, Jon K. Sekiya, and Marc J. Phillipon

Although first described in 1931, hip arthroscopy has only recently gained acceptance as a major tool for diagnosing and treating hip disorders, especially for the athlete. Consequently, the diagnosis of intra-articular pathology, particularly labral tears, has increased. MR arthrography is the accepted modality for the definitive evaluation of labral injury.[1-3] Patients with labral injuries often undergo labral débridement for symptomatic treatment.[4]

It is known that injury to fibrocartilaginous structures in other joints can cause increased contact forces across the joint (i.e., glenoid labrum, knee meniscus) and can predispose to arthritis.[5,6] The exact etiology of acetabular labral tears and the relation to the development of osteoarthritis is unclear and unique for each patient, but several theories have been postulated, including trauma, degeneration, femoroacetabular impingement, and rotational capsular laxity.

Therefore, the concept of labral repair is increasing in an effort to preserve joint mechanics and avoid the long-term possibility of the development of osteoarthritis.[7] Currently, treatment is primarily directed toward pain relief and long-term studies of the efficacy of labral repairs and prevention of osteoarthritis do not exist. One of the authors (M.J.P.) has significant experience with repair of labral tears with initial good results.[7-9] A recent 2-year study compared patients who underwent labral debridement with those who underwent labral repair and found that the repair group had better outcome at 2 years (80% vs. 28% excellent results and less radiographic findings of osteoarthritis), prompting the authors to recommend labral repair over resection.[10]

Repair techniques of the labrum are based on experience and analogous arthroscopic techniques in the shoulder and knee. For example, suture banding of intrasubstance labral tears is similar to meniscal repairs and using suture anchors to reattach detached labral tears is similar to a glenoid labral repair in the shoulder (Fig. 108-1).

The labrum, however, is not the only intra-articular structure that can be injured or cause pain. Chondral injuries are another obvious source of pain and injury. Recently, tears of the ligamentum teres have been found to be a significant source of intra-articular hip pain.[11] Capsular injuries of the hip have been associated with hip injury and subject to repair as well. Techniques to treat these nonlabral injuries include microfracture and cartilage transfer techniques, bony arthroscopic osteochondroplasty for femoroacetabular impingement (i.e., similar to subacromial decompression), and capsular shrinkage or plication of the hip for rotational instability (i.e., similar to shoulder capsule surgery).

KEY POINTS

- Arthroscopic treatment of hip pathology is increasing and addresses the labrum and other structures, including ligamentum teres, joint capsule, cartilage, and femoroacetabular impingement.
- MRI evaluation of the hip should include description of tears as either intrasubstance or detached, along with the length and extent of intact tissue to guide preoperative planning.
- Femoroacetabular impingement is a more recently recognized structural abnormality associated with labral tears and chondral injury that can be treated arthroscopically and with open procedures.
- Each hip should be carefully assessed for femoroacetabular impingement because radiographic findings may be subtle.
- Ligamentum teres pathology can be a significant source of hip pain and should be evaluated.
- Capsular laxity is often a clinical diagnosis, although some MR findings may exist.
- Cartilage injuries can be difficult to detect with MRI.

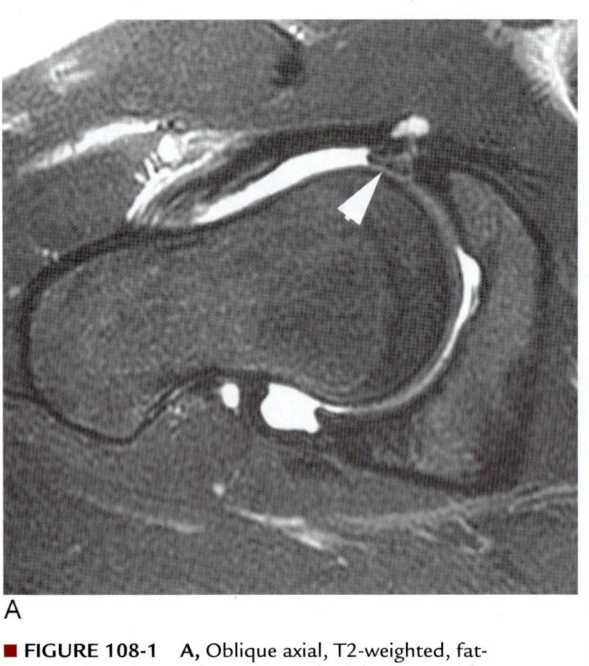

A

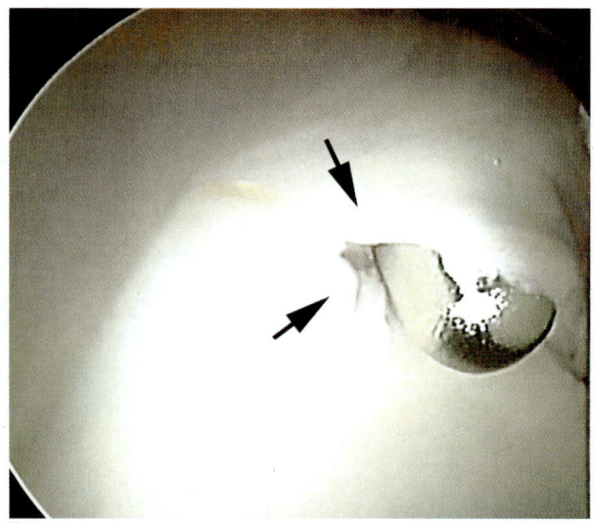

B

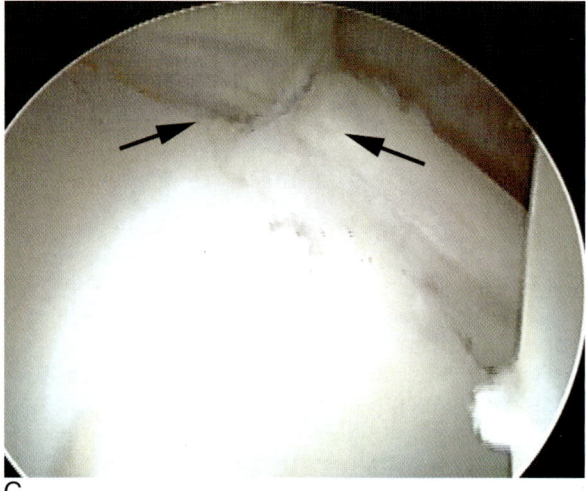

C

■ **FIGURE 108-1 A,** Oblique axial, T2-weighted, fat-saturated MR image shows a complex labral tear with intrasubstance tearing (*white arrow*) and detachment that underwent intrasubstance suture banding and reattachment. **B,** Arthroscopic image shows a probe in a labral tear (*black arrows*) that was surgically treated with intrasubstance suture banding (**C,** *black arrows*).

Although the common end point and manifestation of clinical symptoms may be related to labral injury, one should evaluate all structures of the hip, including surrounding soft tissues, because treatment may involve several anatomic problems. This chapter reviews the current leading edge arthroscopic techniques and imaging findings associated with intra-articular hip pathology to form a basis for understanding this new and rapidly changing field.

LABRAL INJURY

Labral injuries are a common source of hip pain and intra-articular pathology, often presenting with mechanical symptoms. The diagnosis is largely clinical and similar to patients with meniscal injury. Patients may have distinct mechanical symptoms or subtle positional symptoms or dull pain. MR arthrography is currently the preferred imaging modality for preoperative assessment with improved sensitivity and specificity over nonarthrogram MRI.

Indications, Contraindications, Purpose, and Underlying Mechanics

Patients with intra-articular pathology are often treated for several months before the diagnosis of labral abnormalities is made. One study of athletes showed that nearly 60% required 7 months before the source of pain was recognized.[12] Patients commonly experience deep hip pain that can emanate toward the groin. The log-rolling test for labral pathology is the most specific maneuver because it prevents confounding stressing of surrounding structures. Arthroscopy is typically performed under general anesthesia with the patient in supine or lateral position. Multiple ports are available, with the two most common being the anterior and the anterolateral portals. Mild distraction is used to access the intra-articular portion of the joint.[13] Contraindications to arthroscopy include, are but not limited to, advanced arthritis, superficial infection, obesity, and joint ankylosis.

Biomechanical studies suggest that the labrum has an important role in hip mechanics.[14] It provides negative intra-articular pressure by maintaining seal, enhancing joint stability and containment of the femoral head. Removal of labral tissue can have deleterious biomechanical effects on cartilage. Based on techniques from the shoulder and knee, labral repair techniques have been applied to the hip.

New techniques comprise primarily intrasubstance suture banding for intrasubstance tears and suture anchor reattachment for detached labral tears. Some tears are complex and may undergo several repair techniques, including débridement (Figs. 108-2 to 108-4). Our preoperative MRI evaluation includes evaluation of the type of tear (intrasubstance vs. detached), length, location, and assessment of amount of residual tissue, which helps the surgeon determine which type of procedures may be used.

Expected Appearance on Relevant Modalities

Postoperative imaging of the labrum requires understanding of the techniques utilized. Postoperative MR arthrography in patients who have undergone traditional labral débridement portray the normal triangular labrum as a blunted structure with volume loss proportional to the degree of surgical resection. It is not uncommon for two thirds of the preoperative volume of the labrum to be resected. The residual tissue should still have decreased signal intensity on T1- and T2-weighted images, but the normal triangular morphology no longer exists. It is important to ensure that the residual labral tissue remains firmly adhered to the acetabular margin.

The postoperative appearance of the labrum that has undergone surgical intervention with suture banding or acetabular reattachment can have a different appearance. In these cases the volume of labral tissue should be similar to that shown on preoperative imaging. The labral morphology, however, may be altered with loss of the normal triangular structure. The residual labral tissue should be closely approximated to the acetabular rim. Intrasubstance suture material may have mildly increased signal on long and short echo time sequences compatible with suture and granulation tissue, which can last months or longer; but unless fluid and contrast equivalent signal intensity is present, caution should be exercised before diagnosing a recurrent tear (Fig. 108-5).

Potential Complications and Radiologic Appearances

Complications from prior surgery include primarily recurrent tears. Interposition of contrast/fluid between the labrum and the acetabular margin or within the labral tissue itself suggests recurrent detachment or tearing (Fig. 108-6). Suture material and granulation tissue may have increased signal on long and short echo time images but generally not that of fluid or intensity on long echo time sequences, as in the case of recurrent tears. Postoperative adhesions may also occur between the labrum and capsule, which appear as thin, fibrous strands and may be symptomatic (Fig. 108-7).

Complications associated with hip arthroscopy include postoperative bleeding, infection, soft tissue injury, and nerve injury (traction or direct) as well as traumatic injury to the joint from scope placement. Postprocedural imaging is rarely performed except for refractory cases and persistent pain. Sometimes in cases of nerve injury, MRI may be obtained to exclude a macroscopic abnormality. Postoperative myositis ossificans has been seen owing to localized trauma and bleeding. In these rare instances, matured ossification can be resected (Fig. 108-8).

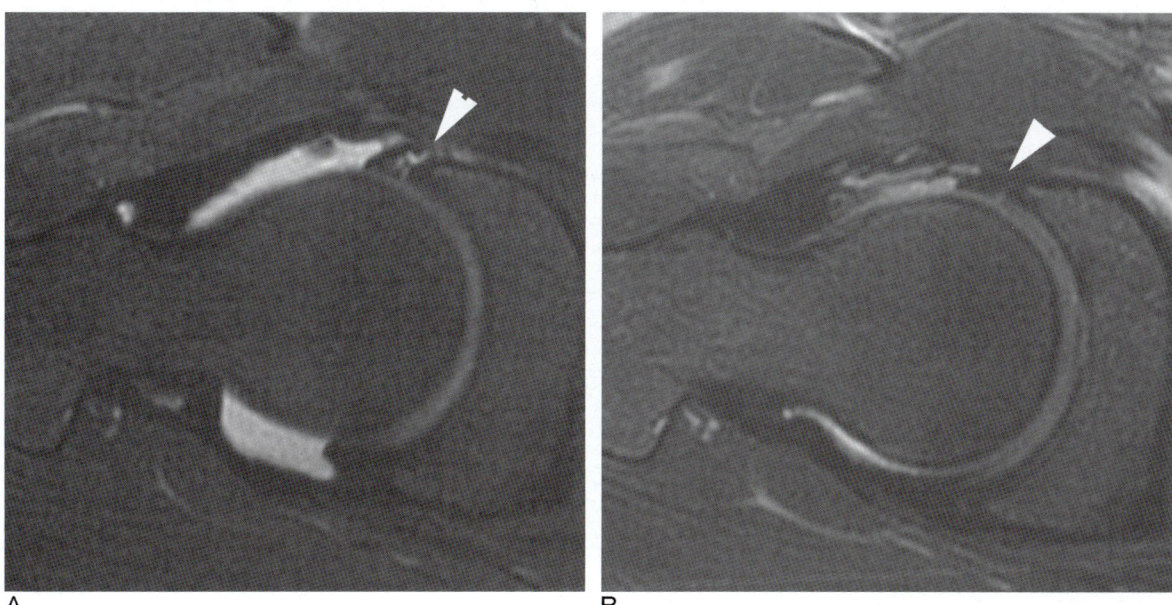

A   B

■ **FIGURE 108-2** **A,** Oblique axial, T2-weighted, fat-saturated MR image depicts capsular-side-only tear of the labrum treated with débridement (*arrowhead*). **B,** Postoperative images in same patient show healing of previous tear (*arrowhead*).

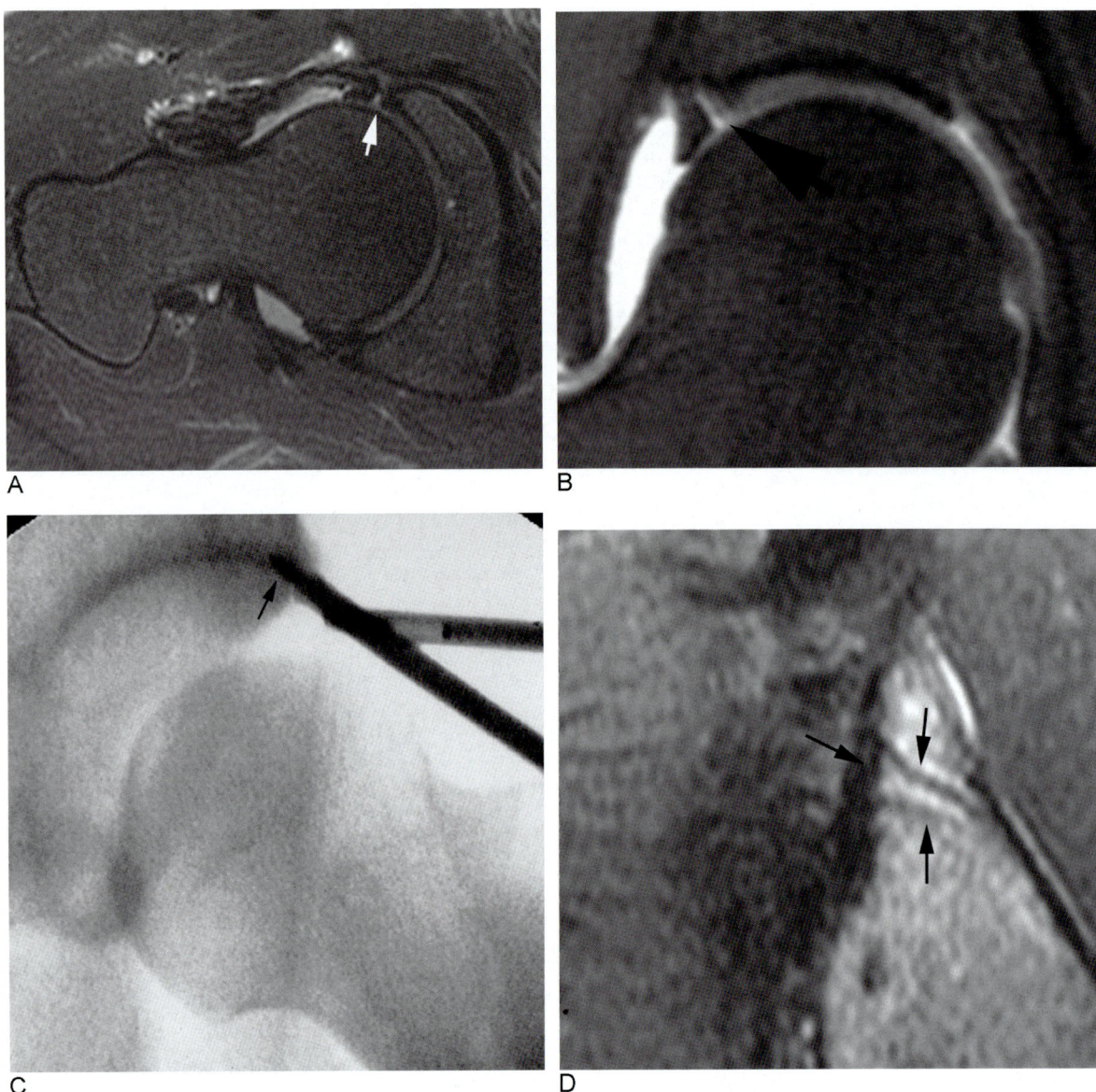

■ **FIGURE 108-3** Detached anterosuperior labral tear seen in oblique axial (*white arrow*) (**A**) and coronal (*black arrow*) (**B**) planes before surgery that was treated with suture anchor reattachment. **C,** Fluoroscopic spot film demonstrates placement of suture anchor in the acetabular rim (*black arrow*). **D,** Oblique axial, T2-weighted, fat-saturated MR image shows minimal artifact from suture anchor within the acetabulum (*black arrows*).

CARTILAGE INJURY

Chondral injuries of the hip may be difficult to see owing to the relative thinness and curvilinear articular surfaces of the hip with cross-sectional imaging. Chondral injuries are often associated with labral tears and involve the anterosuperior aspect of the hip. This area is not evaluated with weight-bearing anteroposterior views of the hip; therefore, cross-sectional imaging and/or arthroscopic visualization is needed when a chondral injury is clinically suspected and radiographs are negative. MR arthrography can help identify chondral injury, and the sensitivity is decreased as compared with the gold standard of arthroscopy.[16,17] Delamination cartilage injuries have also been described using MR arthrography. Multidetector or multichannel CT allows for higher spatial resolution to evalu-

ate cartilage with initial promising results when applied to dysplastic hips with CT arthrography.[18]

Indications, Contraindications, Purpose, and Underlying Mechanics

Arthroscopic techniques for repair are limited and consist primarily of chondroplasty for low-grade, partial-thickness defects and microfracture for full-thickness defects or an unstable flap lesion on a weight-bearing surface.[19] Occasional arthritis may be an indication for intervention.

Chondroplasty is performed with either a bur or a radiofrequency device to stabilize cartilage defects. The technique of microfracture has been used successfully in the knee and other joints. This technique utilizes a surgical

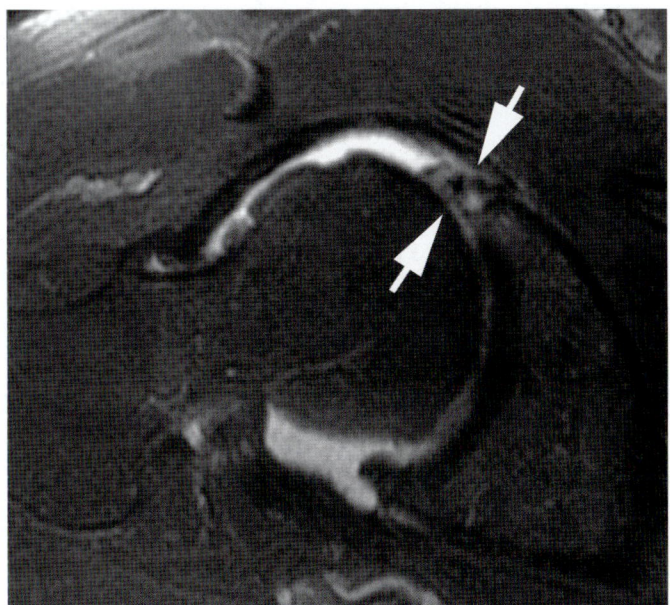

■ **FIGURE 108-4** Macerated tear (*white arrows*) of anterosuperior labrum treated with combination of débridement, intrasubstance sutures, and suture anchor reattachment.

awl to puncture the subchondral bone, which allows marrow blood (and associated undifferentiated stem cells) to form a clot and ultimately develop into fibrocartilage (not articular cartilage). Anecdotally, defects have been repaired using chondral plugs. Contraindications include inabililty to follow the extensive postprocedural rehabilitation, partial-thickness lesion, and lesion with an underlying bone defect.

Expected Appearance on Relevant Modalities

Again due to the nature of spherocity and thinning, cartilage defects can be difficult to image. In our experience, MR arthrography often underestimates the degree of chondrosis when compared with arthroscopy. Rarely is postprocedural imaging performed and only in refractory cases. Cartilage injuries are often associated with labral problems. Postoperative appearance of microfracture technique in the first few months includes subchondral marrow edema (Fig. 108-9).

Potential Complications and Radiologic Appearances

Postoperative imaging is usually limited. Radiographs can be used to assess for osteoarthritis progression.

CAPSULAR INJURY

Although considered a stable joint due to large bony contact areas and coverage, the hip can be subject to soft tissue instability. The diagnosis of instability is often clinical and difficult to diagnose.[8] Instability may be due to chronic overuse from microinstability in athletes or culminate in hip pain from generalized ligamentous laxity in the average patient (advanced cases related to connective tissue disorders would be included in this category). Soft tissue restraints of the hip include the iliofemoral ligament, labrum, and ligamentum teres as well as surrounding musculature. The iliofemoral ligament form the joint capsule anteriorly and are usually the injured structures that undergo repair.

Indications, Contraindications, Purpose, and Underlying Mechanics

The role of arthroscopic treatment is unclear at this time but consists of either thermal capsulorrhaphy or suture plication. Thermal treatment uses a radiofrequency probe that heats the collagen of capsule causing collagen damage, which the body subsequently heals over time with decreased laxity. This technique has been used in the shoulder with marginal success, but in the hip (potentially due to the much thicker capsule than seen in the shoulder) the technique seems to work well. Suture plication may be used in conjunction or separately from thermal treatment. The medial and lateral limbs of the iliofemoral ligament are sutured together until the appropriate tension of the capsule is achieved as assessed during arthroscopy.[8]

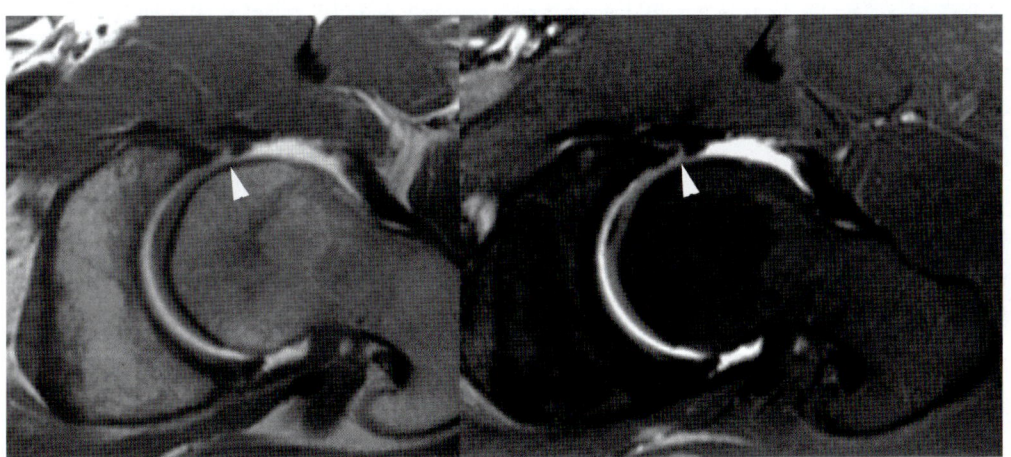

■ **FIGURE 108-5** Oblique axial image from an MR arthrogram in a 30-year-old professional football player shows postoperative granulation tissue seen on T1- (*left*) and T2- (*right*) weighted images within the labral substance (*white arrowheads*) 2 months after intrasubstance banding.

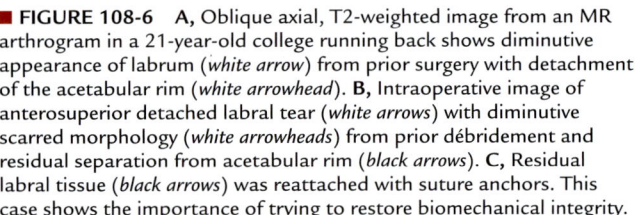

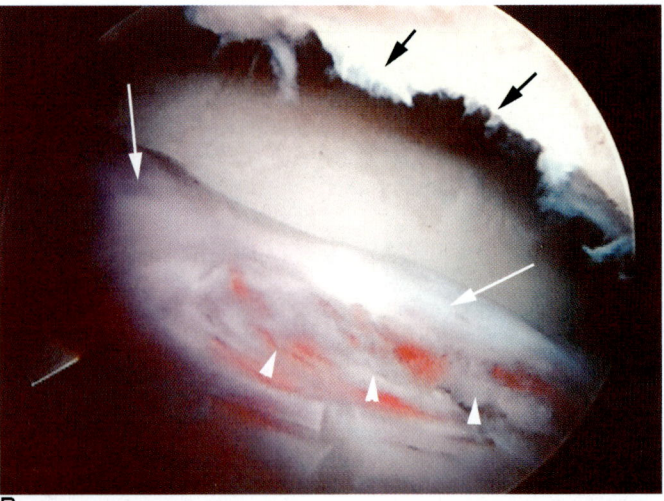

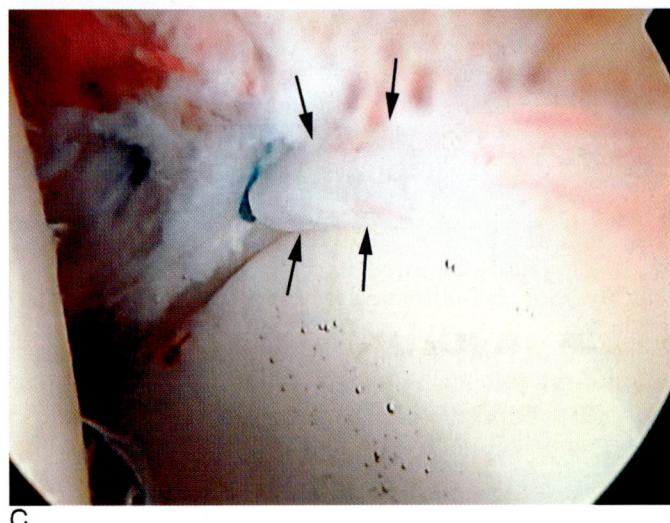

■ **FIGURE 108-6 A,** Oblique axial, T2-weighted image from an MR arthrogram in a 21-year-old college running back shows diminutive appearance of labrum (*white arrow*) from prior surgery with detachment of the acetabular rim (*white arrowhead*). **B,** Intraoperative image of anterosuperior detached labral tear (*white arrows*) with diminutive scarred morphology (*white arrowheads*) from prior débridement and residual separation from acetabular rim (*black arrows*). **C,** Residual labral tissue (*black arrows*) was reattached with suture anchors. This case shows the importance of trying to restore biomechanical integrity.

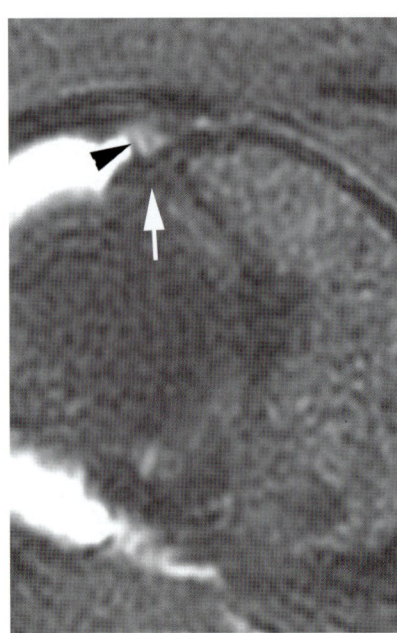

■ **FIGURE 108-7** Oblique axial, T2-weighted image from a postoperative MR arthrogram shows arthroscopically proven adhesions (*black arrowhead*) between the capsule and previously repaired anterosuperior labrum (*white arrow*).

Expected Appearance on Relevant Modalities

Hip instability is usually a clinical diagnosis confirmed with arthroscopy. Some have found that gentle traction of the hip under fluoroscopy may show asymmetric joint space widening, which can be associated with instability. Our preliminary investigations have found that the morphology of the anterior capsule can be altered in cases of capsular laxity. In our experience, the anterior capsule without laxity is of uniform thickness and does not demonstrate undersurface fraying or perforation. In cases of laxity, the lateral aspect of the joint capsule is hypertrophic with an irregular undersurface (Fig. 108-10). Postoperatively, the capsule appears thicker as compared with preoperative imaging using either thermal treatment or plication (Fig. 108-11). Depending on the type of suture there is minimal magnetic field inhomogeneity artifact (Fig. 108-12).

Potential Complications and Radiologic Appearances

Occasionally, patients may experience an inflammatory reaction, possibly to the suture material, and develop synovitis, resulting in hip pain. In our experience this is

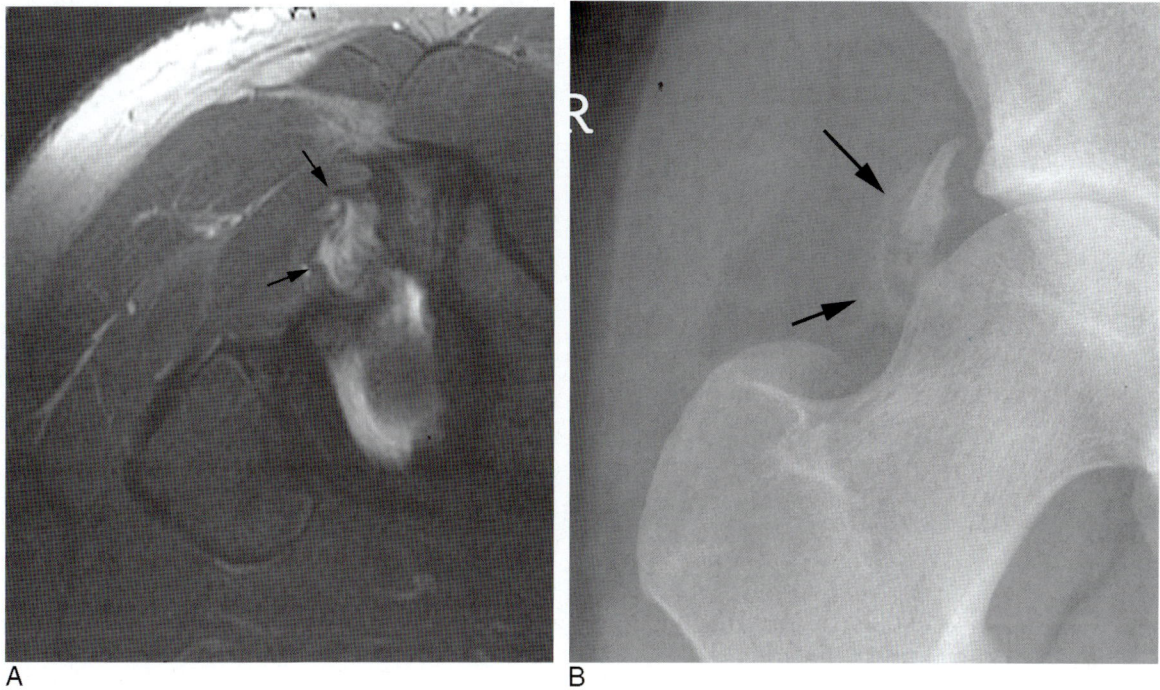

A   B

■ FIGURE 108-8   **A,** Oblique axial, T2-weighted, fat-saturated MR image shows hyperintensity involving the proximal anterior capsule at a portal site consistent with postsurgical hematoma (*black arrows*). **B,** Anteroposterior radiograph shows mature ossification of myositis ossificans (*black arrows*) due to soft tissue hemorrhage at a portal site. Treatment with resection was successful.

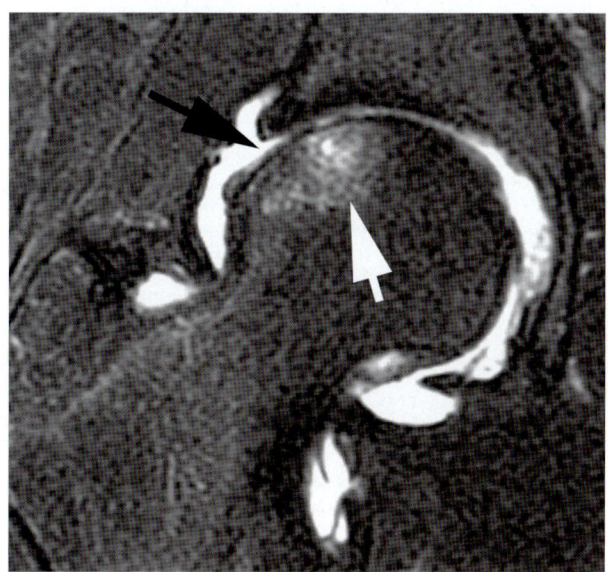

■ FIGURE 108-9   Coronal T2-weighted, fat-saturated image from an MR arthrogram shows advanced chondrosis of the femoral head (*black arrow*) with postoperative marrow edema in the femoral head (*white arrow*) from microfracture technique.

not seen on conventional MR arthrography. Postcontrast imaging with an intravenous contrast agent may have a role. Occasionally, additional surgery may be needed to remove excessive granulation tissue. Unlike the shoulder, thermal capsulorrhaphy of the hip capsule has been used successfully without complications.

FEMOROACETABULAR IMPINGEMENT

Femoroacetabular impingement is a recently recognized source of hip pain that is related to labral tears. The exact etiology is controversial and could be congenital, acquired during trauma in skeletal development, or even secondary to underlying soft tissue injury with subsequent bone remodeling. There are two basic types: type 1 (cam) and type 2 (pincer), with cam impingement being more common.[20,21] The radiographic findings can be very subtle and best seen as aspherocity on anteroposterior radiographs or loss of offset of the normal femoral head-neck junction on a cross-table lateral radiograph.[22] Cross-sectional imaging on CT and MRI can be used to generate an alpha angle to evaluate the degree of offset. Pincer impingement is often associated with acetabular retroversion best seen on a well-centered anteroposterior radiograph of the hip showing a crossover sign where the anterior bone of the acetabular rim projects beyond the margin of the posterior rim.[23] This can be seen with cross-sectional imaging as well but often must be measured at the superior aspect of the acetabular, not the midpoint; otherwise, it looks normal.

Two basic procedures are available for treatment.[20,21,24,25] Open osteoplasty requires an extensive approach including a trochanteric osteotomy and, more recently, an all-arthroscopic version called osteochondroplasty. The second technique essentially removes the bone bump or excessive acetabular coverage. Recent studies have shown the accuracy of bone removal is similar to that in an open procedure. In general, one can remove 30% of the diameter of the femur without risk of postintervention fracture.[26] Postoperative radiographs can assess the degree of residual bony impingement (Fig. 108-13).

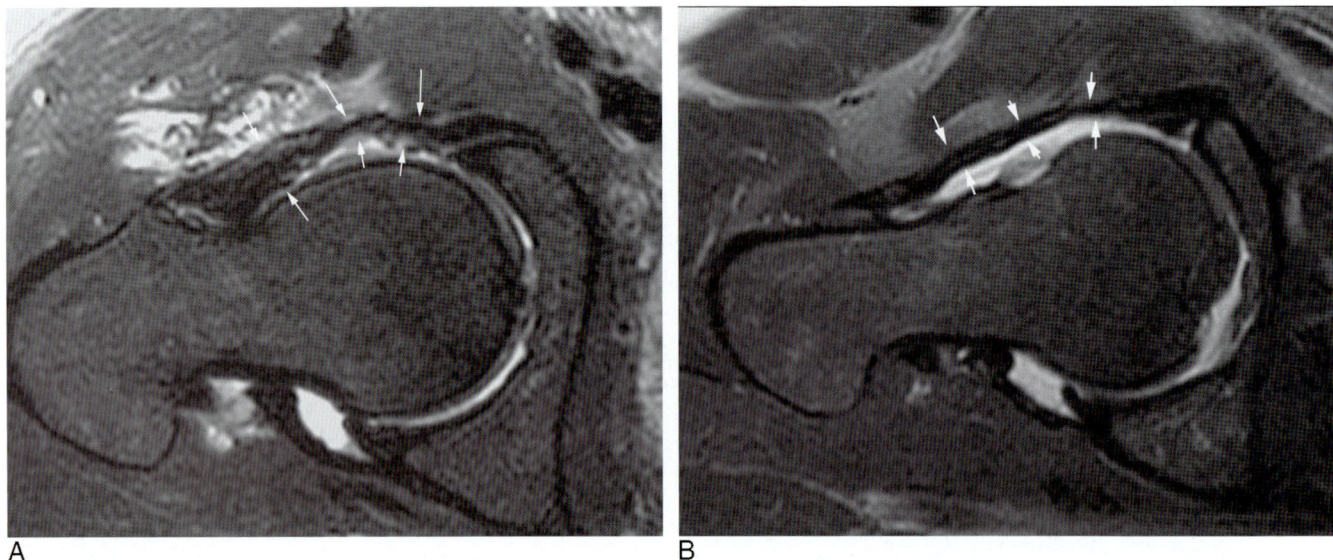

■ **FIGURE 108-10   A,** Oblique axial, T2-weighted, fat-saturated MR image with irregular anterior capsule undersurface (*white arrows*) with nonuniform thickness compatible with anterior capsular laxity on this surgically proven case. **B,** Normal-appearing capsule in a different patient for comparison. Note smooth undersurface and uniform thickness of the anterior capsule (*white arrows*) in this surgically proven case without laxity.

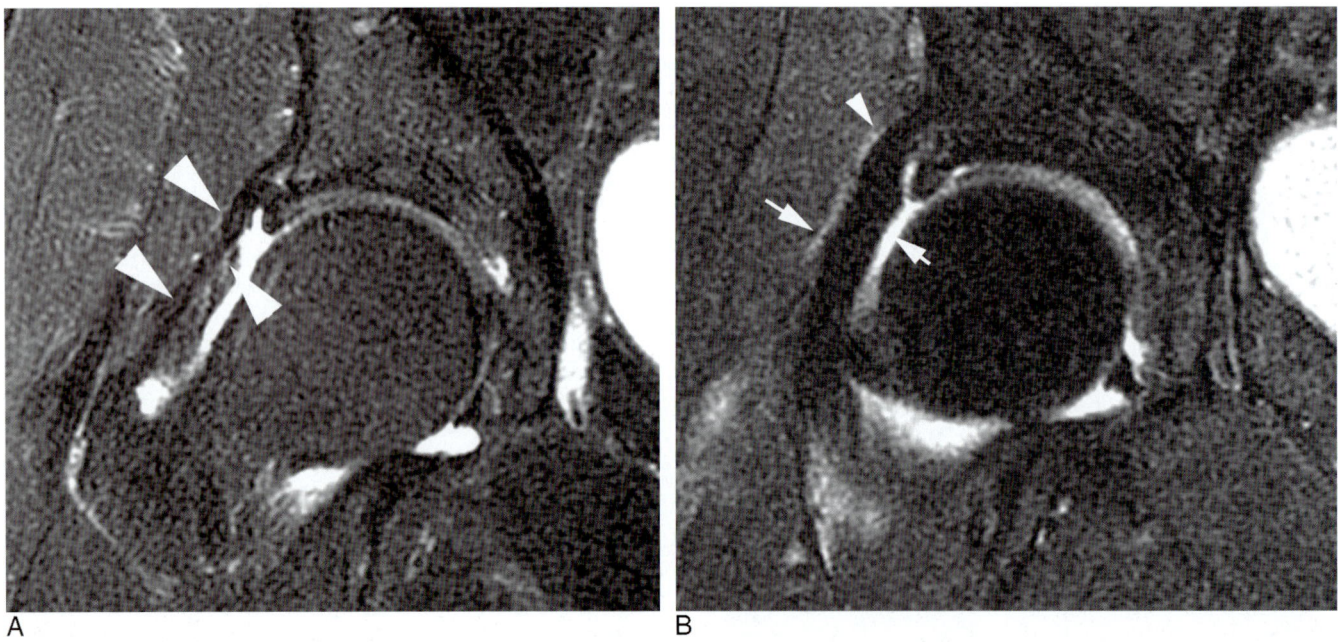

■ **FIGURE 108-11   A,** Coronal T2-weighted, fat-saturated image from MR arthrogram shows markedly attenuated iliofemoral ligament (*white arrows*) and capsule that was treated with thermal capsulorrhaphy. **B,** Note the postoperative hypertrophic change and enlarged morphology of the ligament (*white arrows*) as compared with the preoperative state 6 months earlier.

Indications, Contraindications, Purpose, and Underlying Mechanics

Before surgical intervention patients often have failed conservative management, which is not surprising owing to the underlying mechanical process. The choice between open and arthroscopic treatments is primarily dependent on the surgeon's preference. Similar to situations that occur in many other fields, arthroscopic treatment appears to offer similar treatment with decreased recovery time and iatrogenic trauma. Contraindications are similar to those of hip arthroscopic procedures in general, as described earlier. Whatever method is utilized, it is important that all relevant pathology is addressed, including labral and chondral injuries.

The goal of the surgery is to remove the mechanical source of impingement, which in the case of cam type impingement occurs at the femoral head/neck junction. It is essential to restore the appropriate contour and remove the bony bump. This is performed using an arthroscopic motorized bur. Once the procedure is

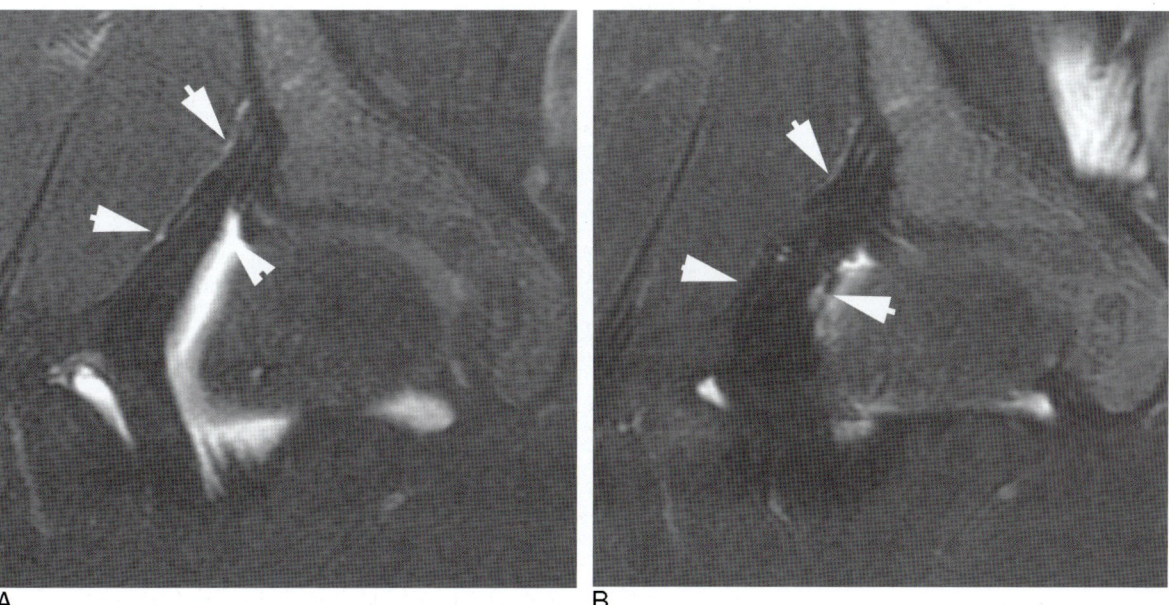

A   B

■ **FIGURE 108-12** **A,** Coronal T2-weighted, fat-saturated MR image shows attenuated iliofemoral ligament (*white arrows*) that was treated with suture plication. **B,** Postoperative image shows minimal artifact from suture material with enlarged appearance of the iliofemoral ligament (*white arrows*), implying improved structural integrity.

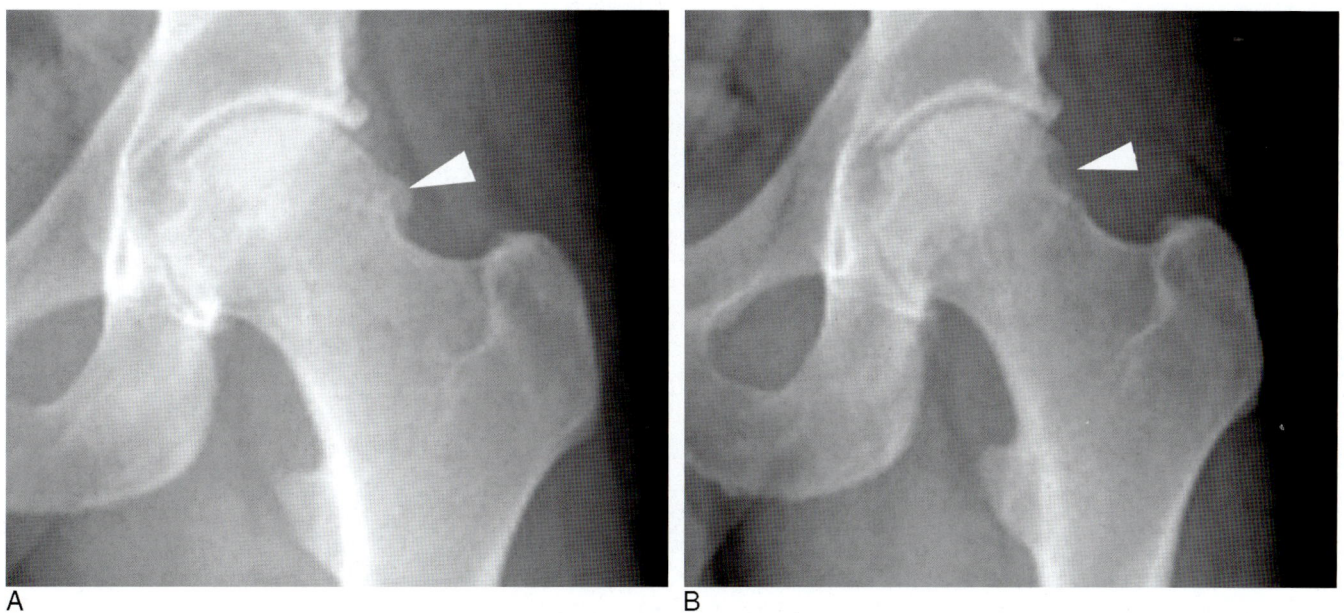

A   B

■ **FIGURE 108-13** **A,** Anteroposterior radiograph of a patient with degenerative change and femoroacetabular impingement (*white arrowhead*) of the hip who underwent arthroscopic osteochondroplasty. **B,** Postoperative appearance demonstrated removal of impinging bony excrescence (*white arrowhead*).

performed, the hip joint is evaluated during arthroscopy with passive range of motion to ensure clearance at the femoral head/neck junction. Open procedures often require transient dislocation of the hip for exposure of the femoral head/neck junction and removal with a chisel to accomplish the same means. Unfortunately, the open procedure requires a greater trochanteric osteotomy, which violates the hip abductor attachments. Although these are rigidly fixed after comple-

tion of the procedure, nonunions have been described. In addition, with either open or arthroscopic surgery, care should be exercised to protect as many perforating vessels as possible so that the blood supply to the femoral head is preserved.

Pincer-type impingement can be treated arthroscopically in a similar fashion using an osteotome and motorized bur (Fig. 108-14).[24] The open surgical approach counterpart is an acetabular osteotomy.

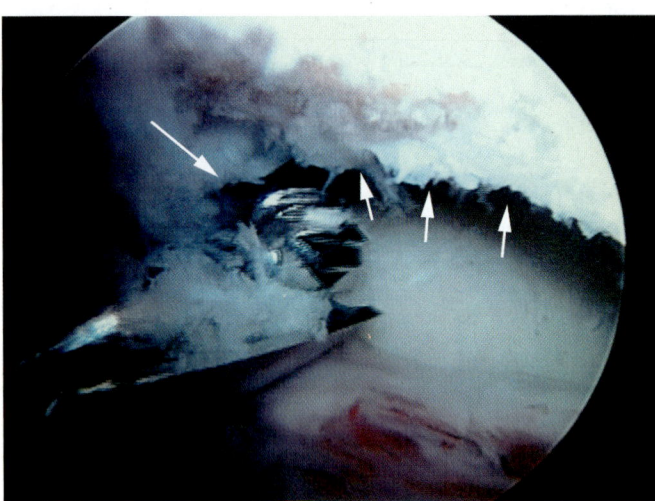

■ **FIGURE 108-14** Intraoperative image shows arthroscopic burring of prominent acetabular rim (*white arrows*) before labral reattachment.

Expected Appearance on Relevant Modalities

A recent study found no increased fracture risk when less than 30% of the femoral head/neck junction is removed. Postoperative appearances for arthroscopic repair demonstrate focal notched defects at the site of surgical intervention. Radiographs are obtained for documentation and assessment of the amount of bone removed.

Potential Complications and Radiologic Appearances

If symptoms persist, recurrent labral injuries can be a source of this pain. Postoperative fractures would be a potential complication but are very uncommon. Excessive bone removal can be detected with radiographs. Postprocedural avascular necrosis during long open procedures is also a theoretical concern that could

be visualized with MRI. Intra-articular bleeding is a possible complication as well but rarely imaged. If the original symptoms persist, an MR arthrogram may demonstrate recurrent labral injuries or progression of chondrosis.

LIGAMENTUM TERES INJURY

Tears of the ligamentum teres are a recently recognized source of hip pain. In one large series, this was the third most common cause of hip pain among athletes.[11] Other studies have shown that tears of the ligamentum teres can affect at least 8% of patients.[27] These tears have been arthroscopically classified previously as complete, partial, and degenerative.

Indications, Contraindications, Purpose, and Underlying Mechanics

The role of the ligamentum teres is unclear. It does contain nerve fibers, and biomechanically it tightens with external rotation and, therefore, may play a role in joint stability, particularly if there is underlying rotational instability. Partial tears of the ligamentum teres are often treated by débridement with an arthroscopic shaver to remove excessive or irregular tissue, which may be a source of impingement or pain.[8] Complete tears of ligamentum teres may also be resected and rarely reconstructed in patients in whom their hips undergo extremes of motion and are exposed to high axial forces, such as enthusiasts of the martial arts.

In the past, partial tears have been difficult to diagnose with MR arthrography because there is little if any published literature. We recently found MR arthrography demonstrated good correlation with arthroscopy for detecting partial tears. Criteria for partial tears included abnormal increased signal on T2-weighted images and/or abnormal irregular morphology, depending on the presence of foveal hypertrophy, which is defined as greater than 2-mm medial extension of ligamentum teres tissue around a best fit circle of the femoral head on oblique axial images parallel to the femoral neck (Fig. 108-15).

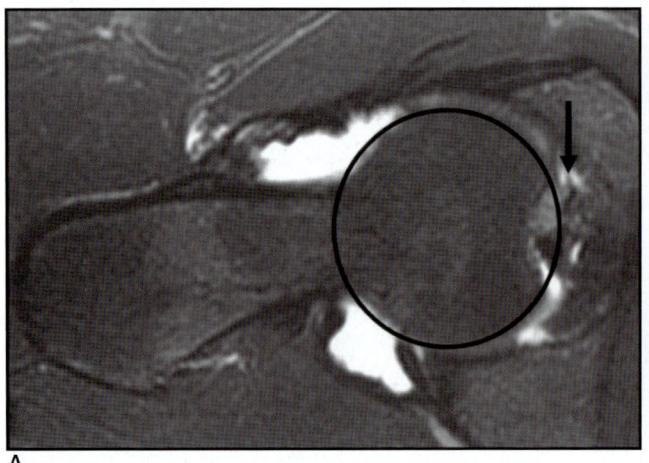
A

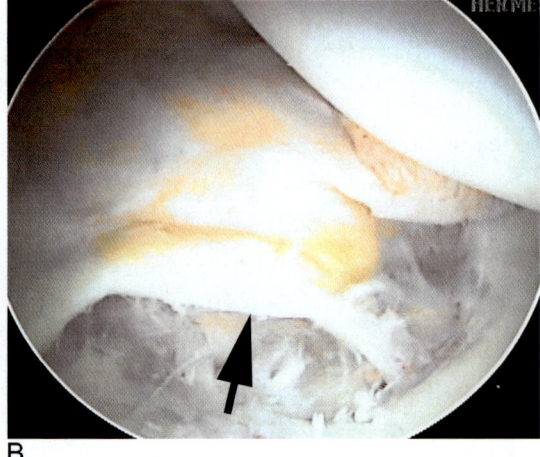
B

■ **FIGURE 108-15** **A,** Hypertrophic appearance of the ligamentum teres (*black arrow*) with abnormal signal and enlarged morphology extending several millimeters beyond a best fit circle of the femoral head, a useful measuring technique in our practice. **B,** Arthroscopic image of partially torn ligamentum teres (*black arrow*) in a different patient.

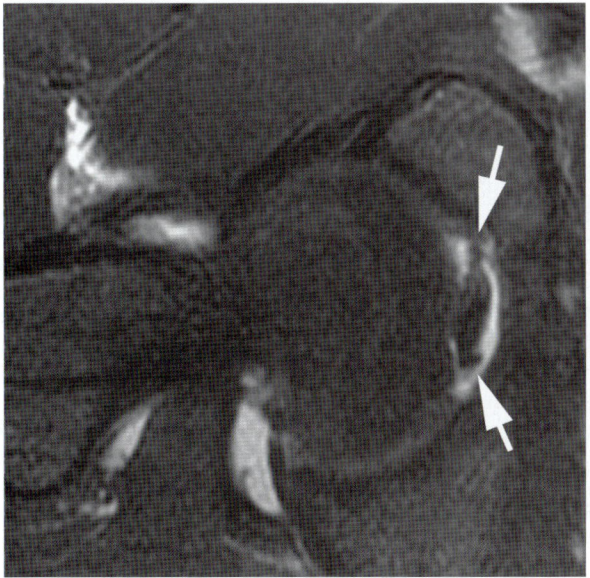 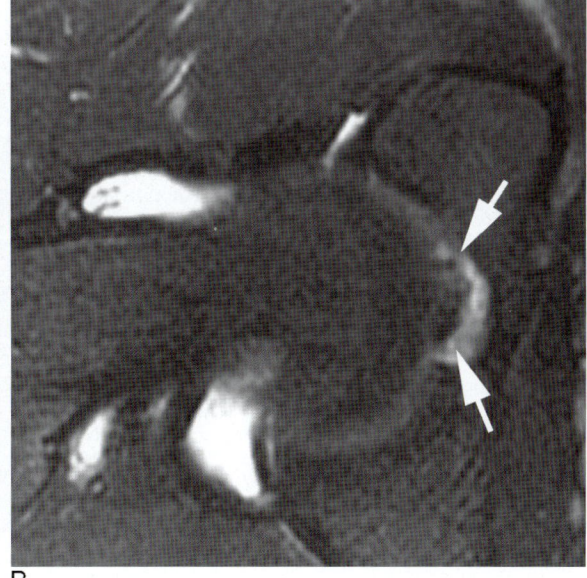

A   B

■ **FIGURE 108-16** **A,** Oblique axial, T2-weighted, fat-saturated MR image from MR arthrogram with hypertrophic and irregular appearance of partial torn ligamentum teres (*white arrows*) that was confirmed arthroscopically and débrided. **B,** Postoperative image 6 months later in same patient demonstrates smooth well-marginated appearance of the ligamentum teres (*white arrows*).

Expected Appearance on Relevant Modalities

Postoperative imaging is often unremarkable using MR arthrography. The ligament often has a smooth surface with decreased volume due to partial resection. Signal characteristics on MR arthrography demonstrate uniform decreased T2 signal intensity (Fig. 108-16). Recurrent tears are a possibility.

Potential Complications and Radiologic Appearances

No known complications of ligamentum teres débridement have been identified as of yet with MRI. Complications associated with arthroscopy in general, however, remain.

SUGGESTED READINGS

Armfield DR, Towers JD, Robertson DD. Radiographic and MR imaging of the athletic hip. Clin Sports Med 2006; 25:211–239, viii.

Kelly BT, et al. Arthroscopic labral repair in the hip: surgical technique and review of the literature. Arthroscopy 2005; 21:1496–1504.

Kelly BT, Williams RJ 3rd, Philippon MJ. Hip arthroscopy: current indications, treatment options, and management issues. Am J Sports Med 2003; 31:1020–1037.

Philippon MJ. New frontiers in hip arthroscopy: the role of arthroscopic hip labral repair and capsulorrhaphy in the treatment of hip disorders. Instr Course Lect 2006; 55:309–316.

REFERENCES

1. Petersilge CA. From the RSNA Refresher Courses. Radiological Society of North America. Chronic adult hip pain: MR arthrography of the hip. RadioGraphics 2000; 20(Spec No):S43–S52.

2. Czerny C, et al. Lesions of the acetabular labrum: accuracy of MR imaging and MR arthrography in detection and staging. Radiology 1996; 200:225–230.

3. Toomayan GA, et al. Sensitivity of MR arthrography in the evaluation of acetabular labral tears. AJR Am J Roentgenol 2006; 186:449–453.

4. McCarthy JC. The diagnosis and treatment of labral and chondral injuries. Instr Course Lect 2004; 53:573–577.

5. Baratz ME, Fu FH, Mengato R. Meniscal tears: the effect of meniscectomy and of repair on intraarticular contact areas and stress in the human knee: a preliminary report. Am J Sports Med 1986; 14:270–275.

6. Greis PE, et al. Glenohumeral articular contact areas and pressures following labral and osseous injury to the anteroinferior quadrant of the glenoid. J Shoulder Elbow Surg 2002; 11:442–451.

7. Kelly BT, et al. Arthroscopic labral repair in the hip: surgical technique and review of the literature. Arthroscopy 2005; 21:1496–1504.

8. Kelly BT, Williams RJ 3rd, Philippon MJ. Hip arthroscopy: current indications, treatment options, and management issues. Am J Sports Med 2003; 31:1020–1037.

9. Philippon MJ. New frontiers in hip arthroscopy: the role of arthroscopic hip labral repair and capsulorrhaphy in the treatment of hip disorders. Instr Course Lect 2006; 55:309–316.

10. Espinosa N, et al. Treatment of femoro-acetabular impingement: preliminary results of labral refixation. J Bone Joint Surg Am 2006; 88:925–935.

11. Byrd JW, Jones KS. Traumatic rupture of the ligamentum teres as a source of hip pain. Arthroscopy 2004; 20:385–391.

12. Byrd JW, Jones KS. Hip arthroscopy in athletes. Clin Sports Med 2001; 20:749–761.

13. Byrd JW. The role of hip arthroscopy in the athletic hip. Clin Sports Med 2006; 25:255–278, viii.

14. Ferguson SJ, et al. The influence of the acetabular labrum on hip joint cartilage consolidation: a poroelastic finite element model. J Biomech 2000; 33:953–960.

15. Lieberman JR, Altchek DW, Salvati EA. Recurrent dislocation of a hip with a labral lesion: treatment with a modified Bankart-type repair. Case report. J Bone Joint Surg Am 1993; 75:1524–1527.

16. Schmid MR, et al. Cartilage lesions in the hip: diagnostic effectiveness of MR arthrography. Radiology 2003; 226:382–306.

17. Beaule PE, Zaragoza E, Copelan N. Magnetic resonance imaging with gadolinium arthrography to assess acetabular cartilage delamination: a report of four cases. J Bone Joint Surg Am 2004; 86:2294–2298.

18. Nishii T, et al. Fat-suppressed 3D spoiled gradient-echo MRI and MDCT arthrography of articular cartilage in patients with hip dysplasia. AJR Am J Roentgenol 2005; 185:379–385.
19. Crawford K, et al. Microfracture of the hip in athletes. Clin Sports Med 2006; 25:327–335, x.
20. Ganz R, et al. Femoroacetabular impingement: a cause for osteoarthritis of the hip. Clin Orthop Relat Res 2003; (417):112–120.
21. Lavigne M, et al. Anterior femoroacetabular impingement: part I. Techniques of joint preserving surgery. Clin Orthop Relat Res 2004; (418):61–66.
22. Meyer DC, et al. Comparison of six radiographic projections to assess femoral head/neck asphericity. Clin Orthop Relat Res 2006; 445:181–185.
23. Li, PL, Ganz R. Morphologic features of congenital acetabular dysplasia: one in six is retroverted. Clin Orthop Relat Res 2003; (416):245–253.
24. Philippon MJ, Schenker ML. A new method for acetabular rim trimming and labral repair. Clin Sports Med 2006; 25:293–297, ix.
25. Philippon MJ, Schenker ML. Arthroscopy for the treatment of femoroacetabular impingement in the athlete. Clin Sports Med 2006; 25:299–308, ix.
26. Mardones RM, et al. Surgical treatment of femoroacetabular impingement: evaluation of the effect of the size of the resection. J Bone Joint Surg Am 2005; 87:273–279.
27. Gray AJ, Villar RN. The ligamentum teres of the hip: an arthroscopic classification of its pathology. Arthroscopy 1997; 13:575–578.

Postoperative Imaging in Arthroplastic Hip Surgery

Eoin C. Kavanagh and George Koulouris

Radiographic evaluation of the hip, both before and after any operative procedure, is the cornerstone of radiologic assessment. Radiographic evaluation serves as the first line of investigation in the postoperative hip, providing an overall view of the hip joint, where the diagnosis is often made, before the introduction of cross-sectional imaging, which may be used for disease confirmation and determination of severity and extent. The relative ease of radiographic comparison allows for accurate monitoring of disease progression. Importantly, in the postarthroplasty patient, subtle changes are often indicators of loosening and thus hardware failure. More sophisticated imaging and image-guided interventions may then be used to determine the cause of hardware failure, primarily to exclude sepsis.

The high prevalence of hip pathology and the general success of hip replacement surgery have resulted in hip arthroplasty becoming a routine procedure, with an estimated 170,000 such procedures performed on an annual basis in the United States as a primary procedure and approximately 35,000 as revision surgery.[1] Although the types of prostheses continuously evolve, hip prostheses may be divided simply into unipolar, bipolar, and total arthroplasty, with the latter further divided into metal on polyethylene, metal on metal, and ceramic on ceramic systems. Hip fractures requiring orthopedic fixation are also very common, with many types of internal fixation devices currently available. Given sufficient time, all prostheses and fixation devices eventually fail. Because component

failure may have a protracted subclinical course, detecting any findings of malfunction relies heavily on routine radiographic assessment. Although these findings may be subtle, a high index of suspicion of hardware failure is critical. Close monitoring is paramount to prevent complications, which may limit the success of possible future revision surgery, such as the loss of adequate bone stock.

Indications, Contraindications, Purpose, and Underlying Biomechanics

There are myriad indications for hip arthroplasty, including osteoarthritis, rheumatoid arthritis, gout, seronegative arthropathies, hemophilia, developmental dysplasia, and femoroacetabular impingement. Most fractures of the femoral neck and head will require operative internal fixation, with either dynamic hip screw placement or arthroplasty. Many operative procedures are also performed for avascular necrosis of the hip, depending on its severity, including core decompression, placement of vascularized fibular grafts, and arthroplasty. There are not many contraindications for arthroplasty and fracture fixation, but they include active sepsis at the operative site, bleeding diathesis, and concomitant medical illness rendering the patient unfit for anesthesia. The goal of these procedures is to restore the affected hip with normal biomechanics, thereby allowing the patient to ambulate more affectively.

Expected Appearance on Relevant Modalities

The radiographic appearance of the postoperative hip should show the entire fixation device or prosthesis in at least two planes. These images should demonstrate the components in their entirety, extending above and beyond the hardware by several centimeters, such that adjacent soft tissues, bones, and cement restrictors may be analyzed. Typically, anteroposterior and lateral radiographs are obtained to evaluate the anatomic alignment of the prosthetic device and to check for any potential complications, such as periprosthetic fracture or malalignment. The strength of the radiograph includes the general overview

---

KEY POINTS

- The imaging assessment of the postoperative hip begins with the presurgical radiologic examination, which is often accompanied by sophisticated cross-sectional imaging studies.
- After hip surgery, the radiograph is the most important imaging modality in routine and symptomatic assessment, with comparison with any prior radiographs with the prosthesis in situ critical.
- Although the differential diagnostic possibilities of postarthroplasty pain are broad, mechanical, or aseptic, loosening is the most common condition confronting the clinician and radiologist. Because loosening is a diagnosis of exclusion, ensuring infection is not the cause of loosening is paramount and, as such, cross-sectional imaging, scintigraphy, and arthrocentesis may be required.

that may be obtained, as well as the ability to directly compare for any changes, often subtle, with the most recent prior examination. Postoperative CT can be performed to evaluate hardware alignment, but usually postoperative radiographs will suffice. MRI with metal reduction techniques can be employed to evaluate the postoperative hip, but this modality is typically reserved for more complicated cases, as discussed later.

Potential Complications and Radiologic Appearance

Detecting complications after hip fracture fixation and hip arthroplasty is the result of thorough clinical history taking and examination and with the judicious use of supportive radiologic and laboratory parameters. Again, as for the preoperative hip, radiologic examination begins with the basic radiographic examination, with an anteroposterior and lateral radiograph as a minimum. Routine radiographic surveillance after arthroplasty and fracture fixation commences in the acute postoperative period. This is repeated at regular intervals, with many prosthetic hips often observed clinically and radiographically on an annual basis for the life of the patient.

Although the specific causes and modes of failure for an individual prosthesis vary, prosthetic failure most commonly manifests as loosening and, as such, radiographic assessment is aimed at the detection of this finding. The diagnosis and detection of sepsis has the critical therapeutic implication of requiring a two-stage revision arthroplasty, which is first performed with hardware removal and insertion of antibiotic-impregnated cement, followed by insertion of the new prosthesis 6 weeks later. This contrasts to the typical single-stage revision for all other causes of component failure. Imaging modalities thus available include arthrography, with the ability to also perform simultaneous arthrocentesis, ultrasonography, CT, MRI, and nuclear scintigraphy. Soft tissue pathologic processes should also be evaluated as possible sources of pain.

LOOSENING

Aseptic, or mechanical, loosening is the most common cause for revision arthroplasty,[2] followed by osteolysis ("particle disease") and infection (septic loosening). Aseptic loosening is often a diagnosis of exclusion, when investigations for the cause of loosening are importantly negative for infection and the radiologic findings are not typical for osteolysis. Unfortunately, with respect to loosening, it is unrealistic to rely on radiographic observation to have the desired precision of detecting submillimeter motion, particularly within the first 2 years after replacement where early motion is equated with a universally poor outcome. This precise measurement is now possible with the use of template matching algorithms,[3] further improved with the use of bone marking and stereometry.[4] Despite these advanced methods, knowledge of the more familiar radiographic manifestations of loosening as assessed on observation is critical.

An alteration in component position as when compared with prior radiographs is unequivocally diagnostic of loosening. In addition to this, motion on stress views is also diagnostic. On stress views obtained with CT, a difference

in femoral component version of greater than 2 degrees is diagnostic when comparing views obtained with maximal external and internal rotation.[5] Irrespective of the cause, loosening of a cemented prosthesis manifests as an increase in periprosthetic lucency at the bone-cement interface of 2 mm or more. Progression of lucency (even if less than 2 mm) or fracture of cement is also consistent with loosening.[6] In the setting of revision arthroplasty, lucency greater than 2 mm is allowed, but reference in this instance should be made with the early postrevision radiographs.

Ideally, the flange of the femoral stem should sit flush with the cut surface of the femoral shaft. Movement occurring inferior to this level, or subsidence, is consistent with femoral prosthesis loosening. Lucency adjacent to the femoral stem should be described with reference made to the standardized Gruen zones (Fig. 108-17).[7] Insertion of a femoral component results in the well-known localized form of disuse osteopenia known as stress shielding, a phenomenon occurring secondary to the bypassing of mechanical forces. In most instances, only proximal loss occurs[8]; however, in a proportion of cases, loss of periprosthetic bone density along the entire femoral stem may result in loosening (Fig. 108-18). In these circumstances, the osteopenia is typically more prominent laterally along the femoral stem (Fig. 108-19) and in the retroacetabular region, with the latter best appreciated with CT.[9] Stress shielding may predispose to periprosthetic fracture, usually at the tip of the femoral component (Fig. 108-20). Note should be made that a distal femoral cement restrictor plug may be utilized, which acts to form a seal, preventing distal cement migration such that adequate contact with the prosthesis may be optimized. Often, a small focus of entrapped gas may be visualized and should not be confused as the consequence of infection.

Although loosening of the femoral component may be simply evaluated on the standard anteroposterior and lateral

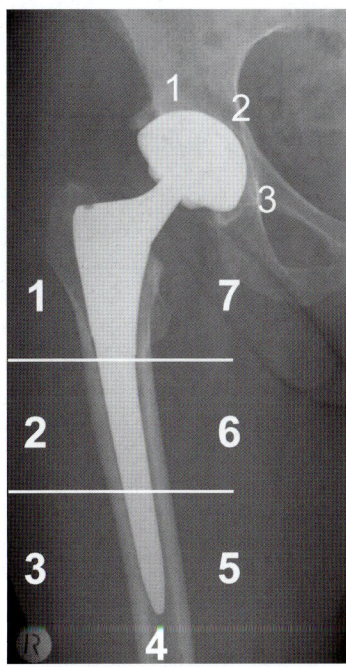

■ **FIGURE 108-17** Anteroposterior radiograph delineating the standard seven Gruen zones for the referencing of abnormality.

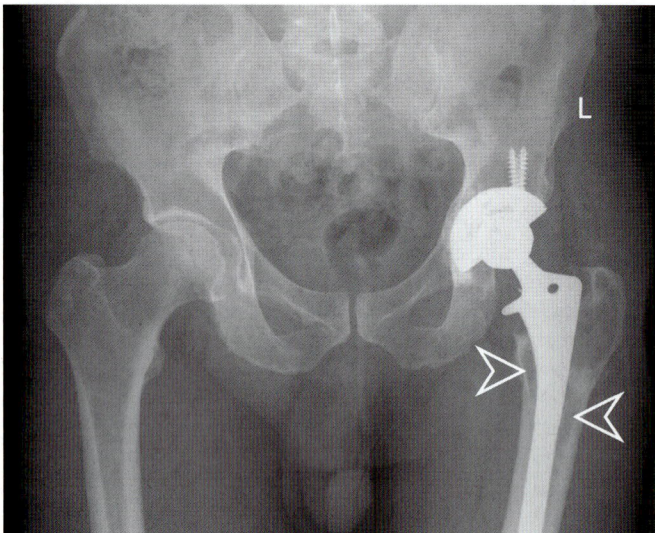

■ **FIGURE 108-18** Anteroposterior radiograph of the left hip demonstrating stress shielding at both trochanters, with periprosthetic lucency extending distally, ultimately resulting in loosening of the femoral stem (*arrowheads*).

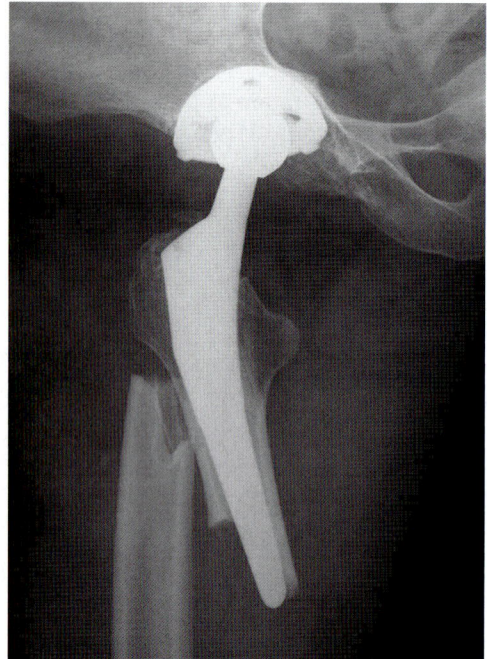

■ **FIGURE 108-20** Oblique anteroposterior radiograph of the right hip demonstrating a displaced periprosthetic fracture as a consequence of loosening.

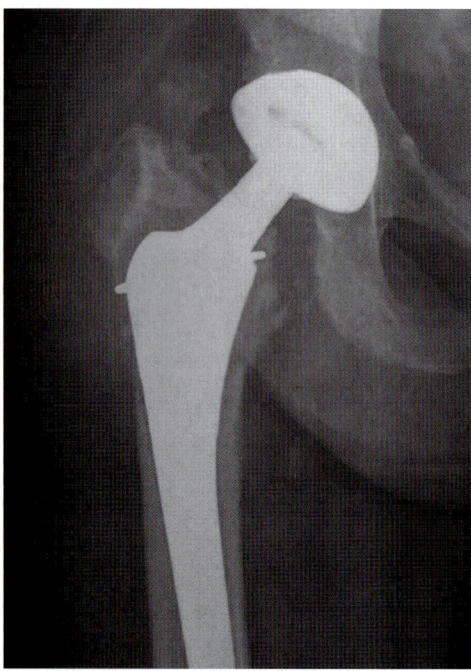

■ **FIGURE 108-19** Anteroposterior radiograph of the right hip demonstrating breach of the cortex of the proximal femur at the flange of the femoral stem, diagnostic of loosening.

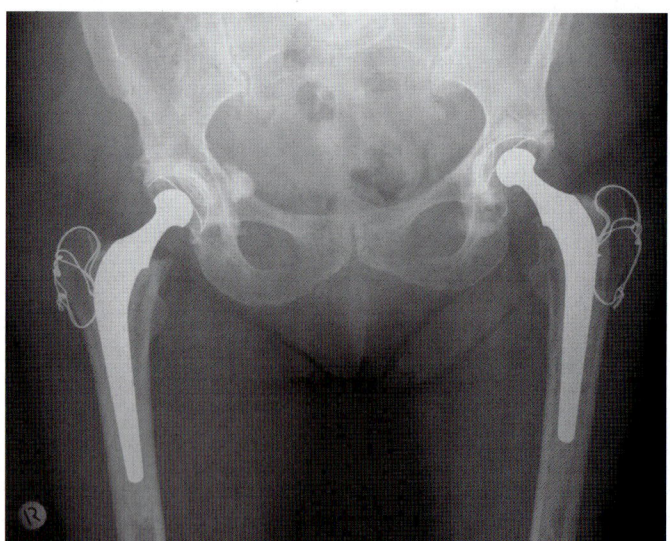

■ **FIGURE 108-21** Anteroposterior radiograph of the pelvis after bilateral arthroplasty demonstrates lucency at bone-cement interface of all three Gruen zones of the acetabulum involving the left hip.

views of a hip radiographic series, radiographic assessment of the acetabulum is relatively more difficult owing to its shape. Apart from measuring the lucent interval at the bone-cement interface, additional criteria for loosening of the acetabular component have been described and include lucent zones developing or progressing after 2 years in uncemented systems, radiolucent lines in all three zones (Figs. 108-21 and 108-22), radiolucent lines greater than 2 mm in any area, and migration.[10] The sensitivity and specificity of these findings is 94% and 100%, respectively. Often, the

subtle findings of lucency are not detected early, such that the diagnosis of loosening may only be made radiographically finally when component malalignment or migration has occurred, typically medially and/or superiorly.[11,12] The inclination of the acetabulum is an important and simple measurement, which is the angle of tilt that the acetabular component makes with the horizontal. Despite patient positioning, a horizontal line forms a standard reference and is drawn either connecting the inferiormost aspect of both ischial tuberosities (the bi-ischial line) or both teardrops

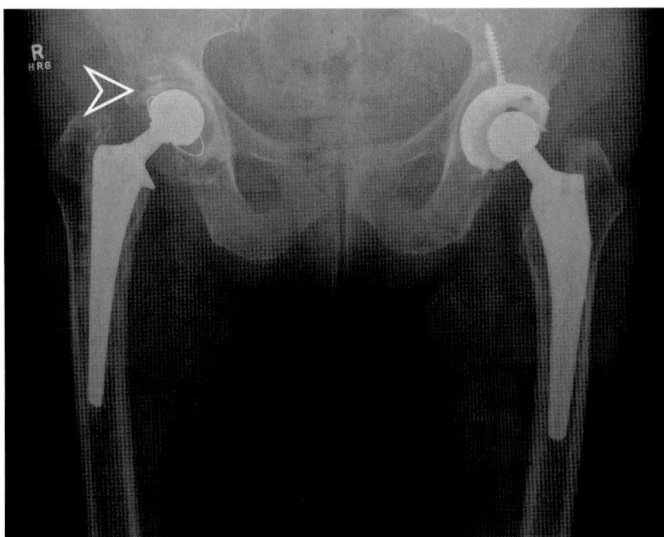

■ **FIGURE 108-22** Anteroposterior radiograph of the pelvis after bilateral arthroplasty demonstrates lucency at bone-cement interface (*arrowhead*) of all three Gruen zones of the acetabulum involving the right hip.

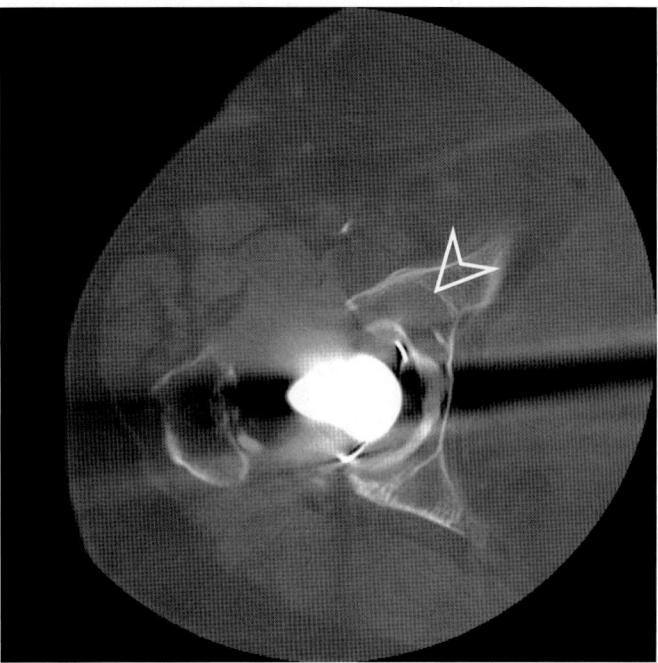

■ **FIGURE 108-23** CT scan of the right hip clearly delineates a region of extensive periacetabular lucency compatible with loosening, as well as the general poor quality of the bone stock.

(the bi-teardrop line). Ideally, this angle should approximate 45 degrees (range: 35-55 degrees), with an alteration of angle of greater than 4 degrees or movement greater than 4 mm compatible with loosening.[13] A line drawn from Kohler's line to either the acetabular margin or femoral head is utilized to exclude medial migration on subsequent evaluation. Any form of protrusion or intrapelvic migration is also consistent with acetabular component loosening.[14]

Multidetector CT (MDCT), with its ability to reduce beam-hardening artifact, has a higher sensitivity for the detection of periacetabular lucency (Fig. 108-23) and thus a higher pick-up rate for diagnosing early component loosening.[15] This modality may be utilized in the setting in which radiographic assessment is equivocal or clinical suspicion for loosening is high but radiographic findings are negative.[15] CT allows for highly accurate measurement of cup orientation despite the degree of patient pelvic tilt and rotation.[16,17] Although acetabular anteversion may be roughly estimated on a lateral radiograph, this technique suffers from poor reliability and lacks the high degree of precision required in accurately assessing component migration. Lateral radiographs in particular suffers from variation in patient positioning and are too imprecise when an exact measurement is required.[18] Anteversion, however, may be measured with great accuracy on CT, first by drawing a line tangential to the opening of the acetabulum, which is then measured in comparison to the anteroposterior plane. Anatomic derivation of the antero-posterior plane is made by first accurately drawing a true horizontal line, which may vary depending on patient positioning. As such, a line drawn along the posterior aspect of the posterior columns serves as the basis from which a line in the anteroposterior plane is drawn perpendicular to it. The intersection made with the line drawn tangential to the acetabulum therefore defines the degree of acetabular version.[19]

CT has the additional advantage of accurately assessing further parameters of acetabular geometry, specifically, the acetabular depth and degree of anterior and posterior wall cover.[20,21] These measurements are of particular use in preoperative planning for revision arthroplasty.[22] The quality of screw fixation[23] and the assessment of the degree and quality of osseointegration of bone substitutes[24] can also be made. Furthermore, the quality and degree of bone stock[25] may be assessed on CT, with dual-energy x-ray absorptiometry (DEXA) scanning[26] being an alternative imaging modality. Finally, CT-guided obturator nerve block may also be used for control of chronic, recalcitrant hip pain, including that in patients for whom surgery is not suitable.[27,28]

Several arthrographic techniques have been described in the diagnosis of prosthetic loosening. After successful needle placement into the prosthetic hip, these techniques rely on the principle of demonstrating the presence of contrast material below the level of the intertrochanteric line interposed between the bone-cement interface. In its simplest form, standard fluoroscopic demonstration of contrast agent may be utilized, but digital subtraction techniques are superior.[29,30] Contrast medium insinuating between the bone-cement interface is diagnostic of loosening and may be more apparent after ambulation.[31] High-pressure techniques have decreased the false-positive rate of this technique, but a false-negative result may occur in the setting of adhesions and fibrous tissue formation, limiting the spread of contrast. In addition, a negative result may still be obtained despite the presence of loosening owing to the inability to achieve adequate high pressures and distention in the patient with a lax pseudocapsule or communicating bursae. The sensitivity and specificity of the test may reach up to 100%, with the addition of the less viscous radiotracer technetium-99 m (^{99m}Tc) sulfur colloid.[32-34] Overall, arthrography tends to have a lower accuracy for acetabular component loosening.[35]

Bone scintigraphy with ^{99m}Tc-labeled methylene diphosphonate (^{99m}Tc-MDP) is a sensitive, although nonspecific, modality for determining aseptic loosening of the prosthetic hip. Increased tracer uptake, consistent with increased marginal osteoblastic activity, is considered physiologic for up to 12 months after surgery. After this time, uptake is reflective of microinstability and thus diagnostic of loosening, typically occurring medial to the inferior aspect of the femoral stem and at the greater trochanter (Figs. 108-24 and 108-25). This appearance, however, also

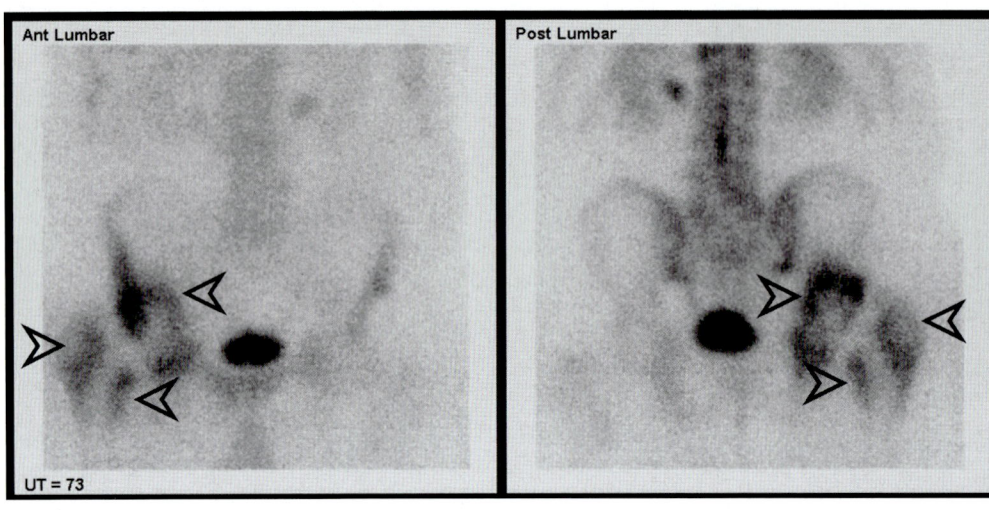

■ FIGURE 108-24 Anterior and posterior images of a ^{99m}Tc MDP bone scan in two separate patients demonstrating abnormal scintigraphic periprosthetic uptake (*arrowheads*) compatible with loosening.

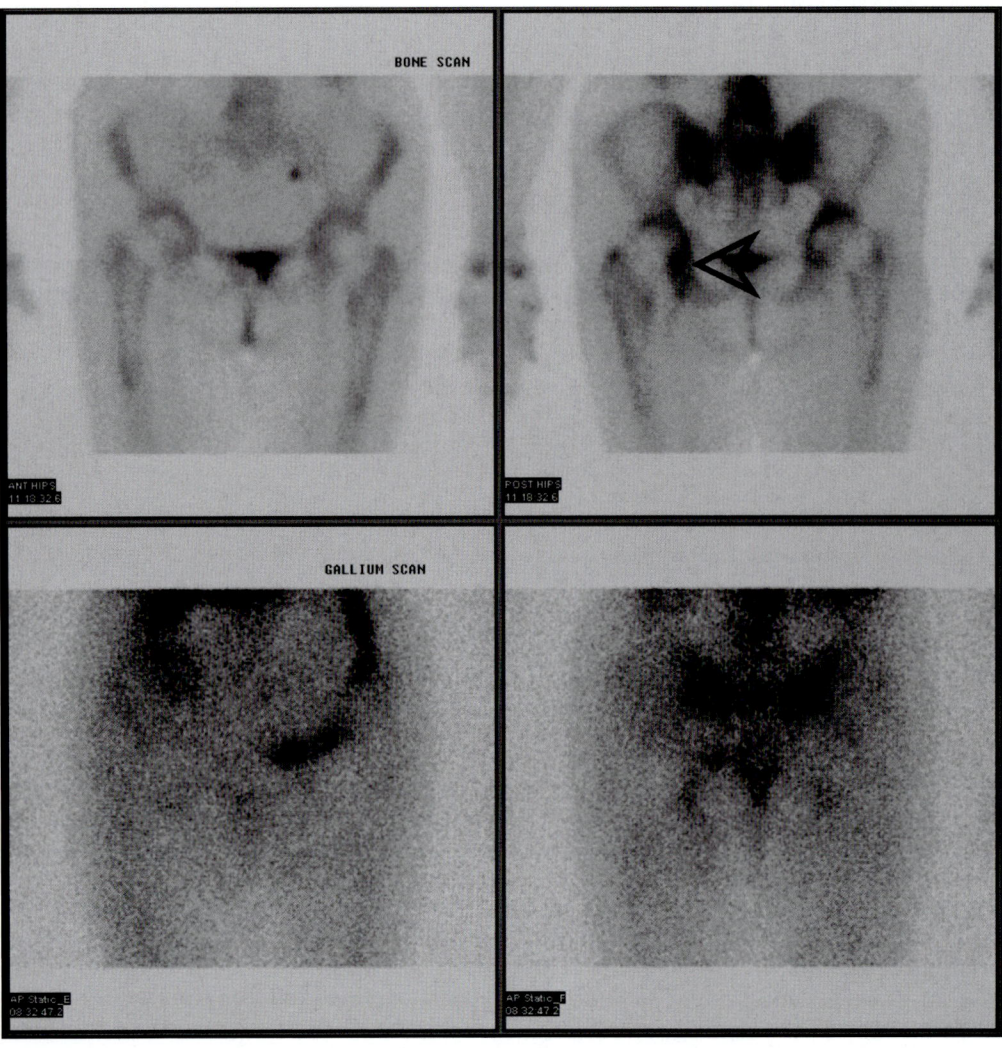

■ FIGURE 108-25 Anterior and posterior images (*upper images*) of a ^{99m}Tc MDP bone scan in two separate patients demonstrating abnormal scintigraphic periprosthetic uptake compatible with loosening. Gallium scintigraphy in both cases was negative (*lower images*), thereby excluding infection as a cause of loosening.

may be seen in infection, which may be excluded in the setting when other tests are negative for infection, including a negative ^{99m}Tc sulfur colloid or labeled white blood cell scan. In the setting in which a standard ^{99m}Tc-MDP study is negative, any cause of hardware loosening, including infection, may be confidently excluded.

With the aim of improving stability, uncemented prostheses have recently gained popularity. These systems are also indicated in the young patient in whom preserving bone stock is critical, given that future revisions are likely. Simplistically, uncemented systems achieve fixation by using components causing either bone ingrowth or chemical bonding between the metal-bone interface. Bone ingrowth systems achieve fixation via fibrous and osseous ingrowth between metallic beads coating the prosthesis. On the other hand, chemical bonding occurs as the result of coating a prosthesis with hydroxyapatite. Stability is further enhanced by limited reaming of the femoral medullary canal so that a very close fit between the prosthesis and the femoral canal and endosteum occurs. Unfortunately, the lack of a cement-bone interface makes the diagnosis of prosthetic loosening difficult radiographically. A lucent line may be produced at the bone-prosthesis interface consistent with a fibrous union but should not be confused with loosening. After 2 years, progression of lucency and an increase in the number of free metal beads, or "bead shedding," is consistent with loosening. Loosening due to stress shielding is more common in uncemented prostheses. Serial nuclear medicine bone scans are required to determine loosening, and, unfortunately, arthrography may lead to false-positive results.

DISLOCATION

Dislocation is the second most common reason for revision surgery.[36] It was previously more common utilizing the traditional posterior approach but has been minimized with the standard lateral (Hardinger) approach. Dislocation occurring soon after surgery is usually due to a lax pseudocapsule (Fig. 108-26). This has been correlated arthrographically, where leakage of contrast agent may be seen in the patient with early dislocation, consistent with the lack of adequate pseudocapsule formation.[37] After the first 3 months, dislocation is usually due to acetabular malposition, such as excessive anteversion (>20 degrees) or inclination (>60 degrees). After 5 years, dislocation is usually due to progressive pseudocapsule laxity, the latter more common in elderly females. In this subgroup of patients, no leakage is seen, consistent with progressive, chronic stretching.[37] Postoperative abductor muscle avulsion results in the loss of the vital dynamic hip stability that these muscles provide and, thus, is also a risk factor for dislocation. MRI, ultrasonography,[38] and CT[39] may be utilized to visualize the integrity of the abductor muscles, as well as the sequelae of avulsion, particularly muscle denervation and atrophy, with success.

INFECTION

Improved sterility, operative technique, and patient care has resulted in a decrease in the frequency of infection, such that it is now the third most common reason for revision

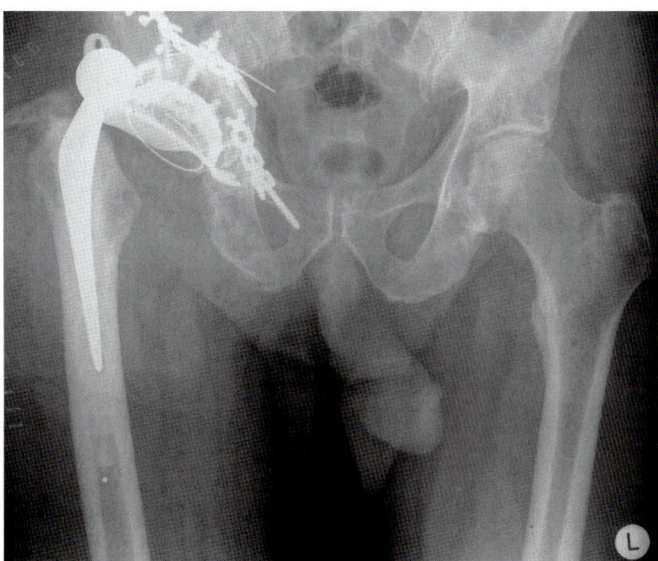

■ **FIGURE 108-26** Anteroposterior radiograph of the pelvis demonstrating acute postoperative dislocation of a revised right hip prosthesis, initially indicated after complex traumatic pelvic fractures.

arthroplasty, occurring in 1% to 5% of hip replacements.[36] The radiographic signs of infection may be identical to that of mechanical aseptic loosening, particularly in low-grade chronic sepsis. With increasing severity, however, several additional signs may be present that may alert the clinician to the diagnosis of infection. Radiographic abnormality developing rapidly and with an aggressive appearance favors the diagnosis of infection, whereas aseptic loosening typically has a gradual and progressive course of clinical symptoms, similarly matched radiographically. Overt, well-established radiographic findings of septic arthritis and osteomyelitis, such as rapidly developing osseous erosions and periosteal reaction, are diagnostic. The diagnosis may be also be suggested by the presence of irregular joint capsules, loculation, complex effusions, pseudobursae, sinus tracts, fistulas, and abscesses on arthrography, ultrasonography, CT, and contrast-enhanced MRI.

The imaging modality of choice in the diagnosis of infection, however, has been with the use of scintigraphy. Identifying the presence of loosening, as evidenced by increased scintigraphic uptake using standard ^{99m}Tc scintigraphy is nonspecific, because this does not reliably distinguish septic loosening from mechanical loosening or particle disease. In addition to this, standard bone scintigraphy may remain positive for years after arthroplasty when using an uncemented prosthesis in which bone ingrowth is designed to occur. As such, additional radioisotopes must be employed to increase specificity. Gallium-67 (^{67}Ga)-labeled white blood cells are highly sensitive for infection, given the recruitment of neutrophils in the inflammatory cascade. When negative, ^{67}Ga-labeled white blood cell scintigraphy effectively excludes infection. Infection may also be excluded when the degree of uptake is less than that demonstrated on technetium scanning or when radiotracer uptake is concordant. Gallium uptake specifically within the joint is consistent with septic arthritis.

Diagnostic accuracy of greater than 90% is now possible combining a marrow sensitive study (typically

^{99m}Tc-labeled sulfur colloid) with a white blood cell–labeled study (^{99m}Tc or indium-110). ^{110}In-labeled white blood cell scintigraphy is the test of choice, but it is time consuming, labor intensive, and expensive.[40] Because the labeled white blood cells accumulate in areas of infection, however, not as avidly in areas of normal marrow, the characteristic finding of radiotracer discordance is diagnostic of infection (Fig. 108-27). Conversely, ^{99m}Tc sulfur colloid accumulation may occur in normal marrow but not to the same extent as in areas of infection. Other criteria for infection using scintigraphy include areas of indium uptake exceeding that of technetium.[41] As seen in standard ^{99m}Tc scintigraphy, uptake on white blood cell–labeled imaging may be part of the normal postoperative response for up to 2 years, although the degree of uptake is less than that seen with technetium. More recently, positron emission tomography is finding wider applications in musculoskeletal imaging and may be combined with CT to diagnose infection. Although the presence of increased glucose metabolism adjacent to a prosthesis is consistent with an inflammatory reaction,[42,43] the site of infection is critical for specificity as opposed to the degree of intensity of fluorodeoxyglucose uptake.[44] Abnormal increased glucose metabolism consistent with infection occurs in the prosthesis-bone interface along the

femoral component. Increased glucose metabolism around the head and neck of the prosthesis is nonspecific, because it may be normal or even seen in aseptic loosening.

Preoperative joint aspiration and culture may be the most useful single test in the workup of the patient with painful joint arthroplasty.[45,46] The sensitivity of arthrocentesis, however, varies from 50% to greater than 90%,[47,48] with a negative predictive value approaching 100%. In some series, arthrocentesis may have a low sensitivity in detecting chronic, low-grade, occult sepsis,[47] when operative culture is used as a gold standard. Furthermore, false-positive findings may be due to skin contaminants. Careful attention to technique is vital, with avoidance of a dry tap by passing the needle past the lateral aspect so that the needle goes into the most dependent portion of the pseudojoint.[49]

More recently, using techniques designed to reduce magnetic susceptibility artifact, MRI may also be used to evaluate the postoperative hip and has particular use in defining surrounding soft tissue complications of infection, such as abscess, sinuses tracts, and fistulas. By replacing standard fat-saturation techniques with short tau inversion recovery (STIR) sequences, "blooming" secondary to metallic artifact is minimized, although STIR sequences are of slightly poorer resolution when com-

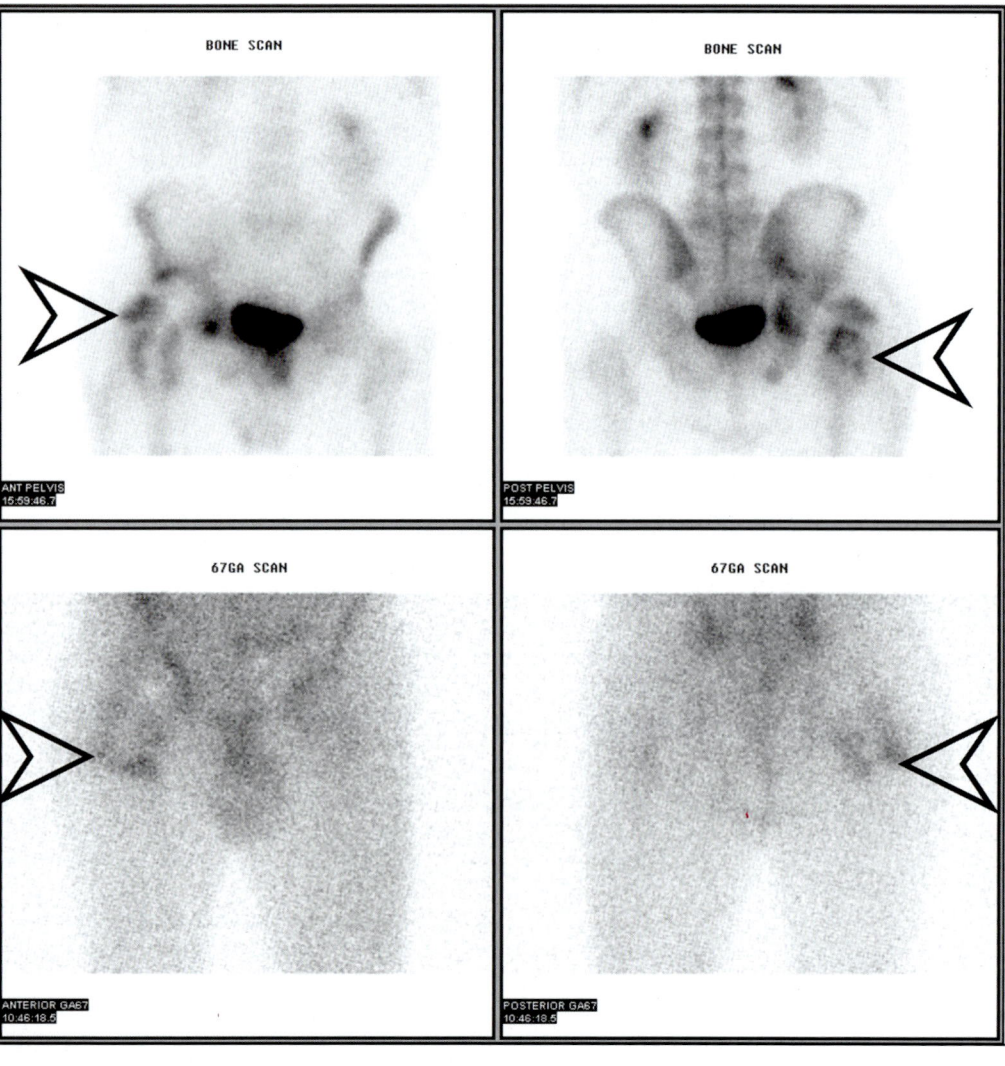

■ **FIGURE 108-27** Combined ^{99m}Tc MDP (*top: anterior and posterior*) and gallium-67–labeled white blood cell (*bottom: anterior and posterior*) scintigraphy status after right total hip arthroplasty demonstrating discordant areas of uptake, compatible with infection.

pared with routine T2-weighted fat-saturation imaging. One advantage, however, of STIR imaging is the robustness of this sequence because T2-weighted fat saturation suffers from inhomogeneous suppression of fat signal, which may potentially be confused with hyperintense signal and thus incorrectly attributed to a pathologic process. Other options also include using thin sections, increasing the receiver and slice select bandwidth (with the subsequent decrease in resolution partially offset by increasing the number of excitations), minimizing echo time (by using fast spin-echo imaging), using increased frequency encoding gradient strengths, and orienting the frequency encoding direction along the longitudinal axis of the prosthesis.[50] Also, lower magnetic field strength (less than 1.0 T) systems may decrease metallic susceptibility artifact. As such, MRI may reliably diagnose cellulitis, abscesses, sinus tracts, fistulas, periprosthetic collections, osteomyelitis, and septic arthritis. It may also be utilized for anatomic delineation and further characterization of equivocal scintigraphic findings. CT is also sensitive for similar pathology involving the soft tissues,[51] including intrapelvic extension and psoas muscle involvement.[52]

Ultrasonography also is particularly sensitive for evaluating soft tissue collections and joint effusions. Again, it may be utilized for guidance in performing arthrocentesis, as well as evaluating postoperative collections, reliably distinguishing a hematoma or abscess from a seroma. Power and color flow Doppler imaging is an added feature, enabling the detection of hyperemia indicative of inflammation, which would favor an effusion or collection being infected. Ultrasonographic demonstration of an effusion resulting in less than 3.2 mm in distention of the anterior pseudocapsule from the anterior femoral cortex indicates that infection is unlikely. Conversely, an infected prosthesis typically demonstrates an effusion with an average anterior displacement of the pseudocapsule of 10.2 mm.[53]

PERIPROSTHETIC FRACTURE

Periprosthetic fracture is an uncommon, although increasingly noted complication after arthroplasty,[54] attributed to in part by the increasing frequency of revision arthroplasty (poorer bone stock) as well as the popularity of uncemented prostheses (tight press fit required for ingrowth). Periprosthetic fractures typically occur at the tip of the femoral stem, often preceded by an area of increased cortical thickening or "stress riser" (Fig. 108-28). Cerclage wires may be utilized for reinforcement. Should a fracture occur, a long-stem femoral prosthesis is usually indicated, bypassing the fracture. Periprosthetic fracture involvement of the acetabulum is extremely uncommon.[55]

ACETABULAR LINER WEAR

The polyethylene cup lining the acetabulum commonly progressively wears in a steady manner over the years after arthroplasty, preferentially involving its superior, weight-bearing aspect. Ideally, the femoral head should be demonstrated radiographically to be equidistant between the superior and inferior margins of the acetabular cup on the anteroposterior radiograph. Wear therefore manifests as eccentric positioning of the femoral head, resulting in a

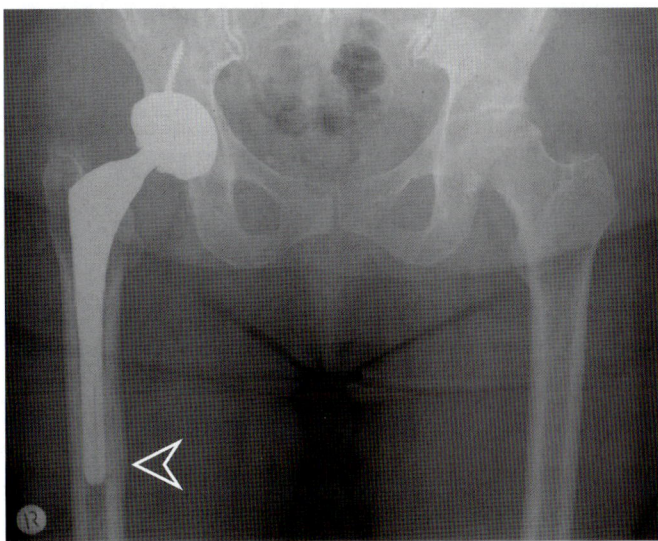

■ **FIGURE 108-28** Anteroposterior pelvic radiograph demonstrating an area of cortical thickening of the medial aspect of the right femoral stem tip in keeping with a "stress riser."

decrease in distance between the femoral head and superior margin of the acetabulum, with a concomitant increase in distance between the femoral head and inferior acetabular margin. Serial comparison with radiographs is paramount, with wear up to 1.5 mm per year within the normal range. Rarely the acetabular liner may fracture or completely dislocate, in which case the femoral head typically articulates directly with the acetabular cup superiorly and the liner may be visualized as a distinct radiolucent focus (Fig. 108-29). Positron emission tomography may show polyethylene wear, owing to the inflammatory reaction elicited, which is a potential pitfall for infection.[56]

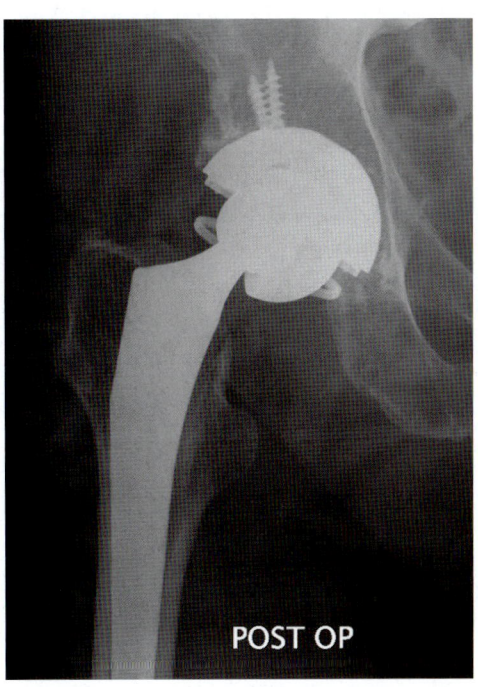

POST OP

■ **FIGURE 108-29** Anteroposterior radiograph of the right hip demonstrating dislocation of the polyethylene liner, as indicated by the metallic marker and adjacent lucency encircling the femoral head.

PARTICLE DISEASE

Particle disease, also known as particle inclusion disease or giant cell granulomatous response, is most commonly secondary to microabrasive wear and shedding of any portion of the prosthesis, with the polyethylene used in the acetabular liner and/or polymethyl methacrylate (PMMA) cement having a higher inflammatory profile than metal and ceramic particles. The foreign materials are engulfed by macrophages, resulting in the release of cytokines and therefore attracting inflammatory cells. With time, chronic inflammation ensues, with a granulomatous response and giant cells (histiocytes). This cascade causes an increase in osteoclastic activity, ultimately radiographically manifesting as osteolysis. Early detection of osteolysis is critical, because the condition is asymptomatic until substantial bone loss has occurred, which may limit or complicate future surgical options. Particle diseases typically occur 1 to 5 years after arthroplasty, with the presence of lucency during this time interval at the prosthesis/bone (or bone/cement) interface, in the setting of acetabular liner wear, consistent with the diagnosis. Such lesions are lytic, are characteristically expansile, and demonstrate smooth endosteal scalloping (Fig. 108-30).[57] This scalloped morphology is in contrast to the linear areas of osseous resorption characteristic of aseptic mechanical loosening. CT and MRI are sensitive modalities in detecting and estimating the size of osteolytic foci due to particle disease, as well as the often associated soft tissue fluid collections. Although these collections have an underlying inflammatory cause, extension to the pelvis or skin implies the diagnosis of infection and thus is an important differentiating feature. In an effort to reduce the incidence of particle disease, the polyethylene liner has been eliminated from the design of modern systems, resulting in either ceramic-on-ceramic or metal-on-metal designs. These designs. however, are not without their disadvantages, with ceramic-on-ceramic systems having been associated with catastrophic breakage in 2% of patients. The concern of a carcinogenic effect of metal-on-metal systems has limited its universal application until further long-term data become available.

HETEROTOPIC BONE FORMATION

Heterotopic ossification is a common, although rarely clinically significant, finding after arthroplasty. Risk factors for extensive heterotopic ossification limiting joint range of motion include ankylosing spondylitis, diffuse idiopathic skeletal hyperostosis, and a past history of heterotopic ossification. If extensive enough, heterotopic ossification may result in complete ankylosis (Fig. 108-31). In such instances, confirmation of stability or maturation of the ossification is vital, because early surgery may worsen the extent of ossification. This may be evaluated radiographically, where lesion stability of 3 months is consistent with quiescence. [99m]Tc scintigraphic uptake of similar intensity to the native bone, or less, also implies that osteoblastic activity is minimal, as is the absence of edema within the heterotopic foci on MRI. MDCT is useful in staging the extent of bone formation and helping guide therapeutic radiotherapy and surgery.[58] CT is also useful in guiding needle placement in cases in which ossification makes aspiration with routine fluoroscopy difficult.[59]

PSEUDOBURSAE

After arthroplasty, pseudobursae commonly form typically adjacent to both trochanters[60] and may limit the maximal achievable joint pressure and thus provide a false-negative result on arthrography. Pseudobursae may be assessed with MRI, CT, and ultrasonography, with the

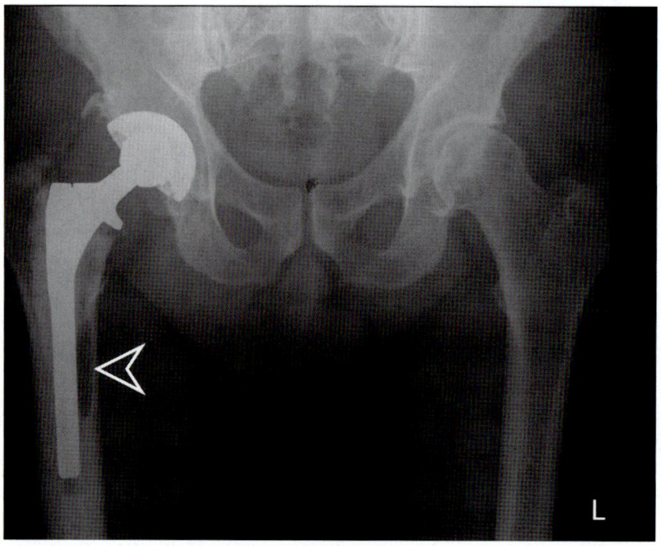

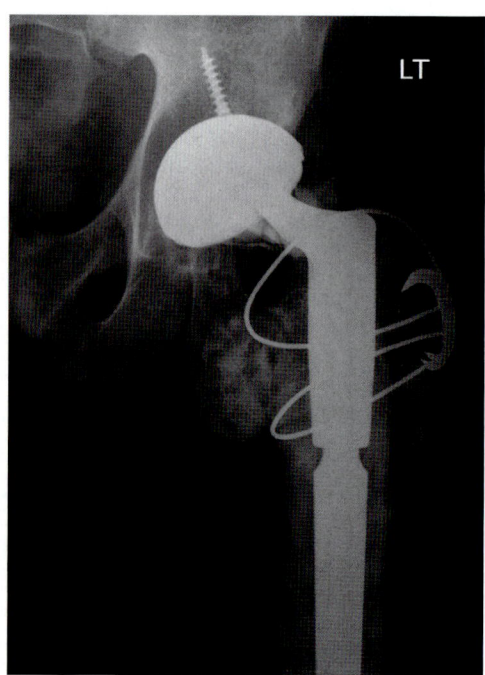

■ **FIGURE 108-31** Anteroposterior radiograph of the left hip status after revision arthroplasty demonstrating complete ankylosis secondary to postoperative heterotopic ossification.

■ **FIGURE 108-30** Anteroposterior radiograph of a prosthetic right hip demonstrating a scalloped lucency at Gruen zone 6 typical of particle disease.

latter modality providing the capability for simultaneous treatment with image-guided corticosteroid administration, as well as the ability to aspirate where infection within these structures is considered a possibility.

ILIOPSOAS IMPINGEMENT

Impingement of the iliopsoas tendon occurs secondary to an oversized acetabular cup. In conjunction with positive clinical findings, overhang of greater than 12 mm,[61] as assessed on CT, is consistent with the diagnosis. An effusion of the hip joint, as may occur in loosening,[62] may result in iliopsoas bursitis[63] and thus result in the clinical findings of iliopsoas impingement. Rarely, this may be mimicked by iliopectineal bursitis.[64] Iliopsoas impingement may also be diagnosed sonographically,[65] as evidenced by the loss of normal tendon fibrillar echogenicity (compatible with tendinosis), as well as the normal smooth movement and glide that the tendon makes during dynamic assessment. Ultrasonography may again be utilized to percutaneously administer corticosteroid into the iliopsoas bursa for symptomatic relief. Depending on the exact cause of iliopsoas impingement, surgical release[66] may be occasionally required.

REFERENCES

1. American Academy of Orthopaedic Surgeons. Osteoarthritis of the Hip: A Compendium of Evidence-based Information and Resources; Joint Replacement. http://www.aaos.org/Research/documents/oainfo_hip.asp. Accessed November 13, 2006.
2. Clohisy JC, Calvert G, Tull F, et al. Reasons for revision hip surgery: a retrospective review. Clin Orthop Relat Res 2004; 429:188-192.
3. Burkhardt K, Szekely G, Notzli H, et al. Submillimeter measurement of cup migration in clinical standard radiographs. IEEE Trans Med Imaging 2005; 24:676-688.
4. Karrholm J, Hultmark P, Carlsson L, et al. Subsidence of a non-polished stem in revisions of the hip using impaction allograft: evaluation with radiostereometry and dual-energy X-ray absorptiometry. J Bone Joint Surg Br 1999; 81:135-142.
5. Berger R, Fletcher F, Donaldson T, et al. Dynamic test to diagnose loose uncemented femoral total hip components. Clin Orthop Relat Res 1996; 330:115-123.
6. Weissman BN. Current topics in the radiology of joint replacement surgery. Radiol Clin North Am 1990; 28:1111-1134.
7. Gruen TA, McNiece GM, Amstutz HC. "Modes of failure" of cemented stem-type femoral components: a radiographic analysis of loosening. Clin Orthop Relat Res 1979; 141:17-27.
8. Boden H, Adolphson P, Oberg M. Unstable versus stable uncemented femoral stems: a radiological study of periprosthetic bone changes in two types of uncemented stems with different concepts of fixation. Arch Orthop Trauma Surg 2004; 124:382-392.
9. Schmidt R, Muller L, Kress A, et al. A computed tomography assessment of femoral and acetabular bone changes after total hip arthroplasty. Int Orthop 2002; 26:299-302.
10. Udomkiat P, Wan Z, Dorr LD. Comparison of preoperative radiographs and intra operative findings of fixation of hemispheric porous-coated sockets. J Bone Joint Surg Am 2001; 83:1865-1871.
11. Bassett LW, Gold RH, Hedley AK. Radiology of failed surface-replacement total-hip arthroplasty. AJR Am J Roentgenol 1982; 139:1083-1088.
12. Puri L, Wixson RL, Stern SH, et al. Use of helical computed tomography for the assessment of acetabular osteolysis after total hip arthroplasty. J Bone Joint Surg Am 2002; 84:609-614.
13. Yoder SA, Brand RA, Pederson DR, et al. Total hip acetabular component position affects component loosening rates. Clin Orthop 1988; 220:79-87.
14. Sudanese A, Giardina F, Garagnani L. Intrapelvic migration of prosthetic acetabular component. Chir Organi Mov 2004; 89:223-232.
15. Claus AM, Engh CA Jr, Sychterz CJ, et al. Computed tomography to assess pelvis lysis after total hip replacement. Clin Orthop Relat Res 2004; 422:167-174.
16. Tannast M, Langlotz U, Siebenrock KA, et al. Anatomic referencing of cup orientation in total hip arthroplasty. Clin Orthop Relat Res 2005; 436:144-150.
17. Olivecrona H, Weidenheim L, Olivecrona L, et al. A new CT method for measuring cup orientation after total hip arthroplasty: a study of 10 patients. Acta Orthop Scand 2004; 75:252-260.
18. Marx A, von Knoch M, Pfortner J, et al. Misinterpretation of cup anteversion in total hip arthroplasty using planar radiography. Arch Orthop Trauma Surg 2006; 126:487-492.
19. Goodman SB, Adler SJ, Fyhrie DP, et al. The acetabular teardrop and its relevance to acetabular migration. Clin Orthop 1988; 236:199-204.
20. Dias JJ, Johnson GV, Finlay DB, et al. Pre-operative evaluation for uncemented hip arthroplasty: the role of computerized tomography. J Bone Joint Surg Br 1989; 71:43-46.
21. Chiang PP, Burke DW, Freiberg AA, et al. Osteolysis of the pelvis: evaluation and treatment. Clin Orthop Relat Res 2003; 417:164-174.
22. Berman AT, McGovern KM, Paret RS, et al. The use of preoperative computed tomography scanning in total hip arthroplasty. Clin Orthop Relat Res 1987; 222:190-196.
23. Seel MJ, Hafez MA, Eckman K, et al. Three-dimensional planning and virtual radiographs in revision total arthroplasty for instability. Clin Orthop Relat Res 2006; 442:35-38.
24. Nishii T, Sugano N, Miki H, et al. Multidetector-CT evaluation of bone substitutes remodeling after revision hip surgery. Clin Orthop Relat Res 2006; 442:158-164.
25. Howard JL, Hui AJ, Bourne RB, et al. Computed tomographic analysis of bone support for three acetabular cup designs. Clin Orthop Relat Res 2005; 434:163-169.
26. Laursen MB, Nielsen PT, Sobaile K. J Clin Densitom 2005; 8:476-483.
27. Heywang-Kobrunner SH, Amaya B, Okoniewski M, et al. CT-guided obturator nerve block for diagnosis and treatment of painful conditions of the hip. Eur Radiol 2001; 11:1047-1053.
28. House CV, Ali KE, Bradshaw C, et al. CT-guided obturator nerve block via the posterior approach. Skeletal Radiol 2006; 35:227-232.
29. Walker CW, FitzRandolph RL, Collins DN, et al. Arthrography of painful hips following arthroplasty: digital versus plain film subtraction. Skeletal Radiol 1991; 20:403-407.
30. Ginai AZ, van Biezen FC, Kint PA. Digital subtraction arthrography in preoperative evaluation of painful total hip arthroplasty. Skeletal Radiol 1996; 25:357-363.
31. Hardy DC, Reinus WR, Totty WG, et al. Arthrography after total hip arthroplasty: utility of postambulation radiographs. Skeletal Radiol 1988; 17:20-23.
32. Resnik CS, Fratkin MJ, Cardea A. Arthroscintigraphic evaluation of the painful total hip prosthesis. Clin Nucl Med 1986; 11:242-244.
33. Swan JS, Braunstein EM, Wellman HN, et al. Contrast and nuclear arthrography in loosening of the uncemented hip prosthesis. Skeletal Radiol 1991; 20:15-19.
34. Koster G, Munz DL, Kohler HP. Clinical value of combined contrast and radionuclide arthrography in suspected loosening of hip prostheses. Arch Orthop Trauma Surg 1993; 112:247-254.
35. Tehranzadeh J, Gubernick I, Blaha D. Prospective study of sequential technetium-99 m phosphate and gallium scanning in painful hip prostheses (comparison of diagnostic modalities). Clin Nucl Med 1988; 13:229-236.
36. Bauer TW, Schils J. The pathology of total joint arthroplasty: II: Mechanisms of implant failure. Skeletal Radiol 1999; 28:483-497.
37. Miki H, Masuhara K. Arthrographic examination of the pseudocapsule of the hip after posterior dislocation of total hip arthroplasty. Int Orthop 2000; 24:256-259.
38. Connell DA, Bass C, Sykes CA, et al. Sonographic evaluation of gluteus medius and minimus tendinopathy. Eur Radiol 2003; 13:1339-1347.

39. Roy BR, Binns MS, Horsfall H. Radiological diagnosis of abductor denervation after hip surgery. Skeletal Radiol 2001; 30:117-118.
40. Palestro CJ, Roumanas P, Swyer AJ, et al. Diagnosis of musculoskeletal infection using combined In-111 labeled leukocyte and Tc-99 m SC marrow imaging. Clin Nucl Med 1992; 17:269-273.
41. Love C, Tomas MB, Marwin SE, et al. Role of nuclear medicine in diagnosis of the infected joint replacement. RadioGraphics 2001; 21:1229-1238.
42. Zhuang H, Duarte DS, Pourdehnad M, et al. Exclusion of chronic osteomyelitis with F-18 fluorodeoxyglucose positron emission tomographic imaging. Clin Nucl Med 2000; 25:281-284.
43. Zhuang H, Chacko TK, Hickeson M, et al. Persistent non-specific FDG uptake on PET imaging following hip arthroplasty. Eur J Nucl Med 2002; 29:1328-1333.
44. Chacko TK, Zhuang H, Stevenson K, et al. The importance of the location of fluorodeoxyglucose uptake in periprosthetic infection in painful hip prostheses. Nucl Med Commun 2002; 23:851-855.
45. Levitsky KA, Hozack WJ, Balderston RA, et al. Evaluation of the painful prosthetic joint. Relative value of bone scan, sedimentation rate and joint aspiration. J Arthroplasty 1991; 6:237-244.
46. Ali FD, Wilkinson JM, Copper JR, et al. Accuracy of joint aspiration for the preoperative diagnosis of infection in total hip arthroplasty. J Arthroplasty 2006; 21:221-2226.
47. Fehring Tk, Cohen B. Aspiration as a guide to sepsis in revision total hip arthroplasty. J Arthroplasty 1996; 11:543-547.
48. Tigges S, Stiles RG, Meli RJ, et al. Hip aspiration: a cost effective and accurate method of evaluating the potentially infected hip prosthesis. Radiology 1993; 189:485-488.
49. Brandser EA, El-Khoury GY, FitzRandolph RL. Modified technique for fluid aspiration from the hip in patients with prosthetic hips. Radiology 1997; 204:580-582.
50. White LM, Kim JK, Mehta M, et al. Complication of total hip arthroplasty: MR imaging—initial experience. Radiology 2000; 215:254-262.
51. Jacquier A, Champsaur P, Vidal V, et al. CT evaluation of total hip infection. J Radiol 2004; 85:2005-2012.
52. Buttaro M, Della Valle AG, Piccaluga F. Psoas abscess associated with infected total hip arthroplasty. J Arthroplasty 2002; 17:230-234.
53. Van Holsbeeck MT, Eyler WR, Sherman LS, et al. Detection of infection in loosened hip prostheses: efficacy of sonography. AJR Am J Roentgenol 1992; 163:318-384.
54. Younger ASE, Dunwoody J, Duncan CP. Periprosthetic hip and knee fractures: the scope of the problem. Instr Course Lect 1998; 47:251-256.
55. Peterson CA, Lewallen DG. Periprosthetic fracture of the acetabulum after total hip arthroplasty. J Bone Joint Surg Am 1996; 78:426-431.
56. Kisielinski K, Cremerius U, Reinartz P, et al. Fluorodeoxyglucose positron emission tomography detection of reactions due to polyethylene wear in total hip arthroplasty. J Arthroplasty 2003; 18:528-532.
57. Reinus WR, Gilula LA, Kyriakos M, et al. Histiocytic reaction to hip arthroplasty. Radiology 1985; 155:315-318.
58. Magid D. Preoperative interactive 2D-3D computed tomography assessment of heterotopic bone. Semin Arthroplast 1992; 3:191-199.
59. Chew FS, Bwon JH, Palner WE, et al. CT-guided aspiration in potentially infected total hip replacements complicated by heterotopic bone. Eur J Radiol 1995; 20:72-74.
60. Berquist TH, Bender CE, Maus TP, et al. Pseudobursae: a useful finding in patients with painful hip arthroplasty. AJR Am J Roentgenol 1987; 148:103-106.
61. Cyteval C, Sarrabere MP, Cottin A, et al. Iliopsoas impingement on the acetabular component: radiologic and computed tomography findings of a rare hip prosthesis complication in eight cases. J Comput Assist Tomogr 2003; 27:183-188.
62. Morrison KM, Apelgren KN, Mahany BD. Back pain, femoral vein thrombosis, and an iliopsoas cyst: unusual presentation of a loose total hip arthroplasty. Orthopedics 1997; 20:347-348.
63. Matsumoto K, Hukuda S, Nishioka J, et al. Iliopsoas bursal distension caused by acetabular loosening after total hip arthroplasty: a rare complication of total hip arthroplasty. Clin Orthop Relat Res 1992; 279:144-148.
64. Lin YM, Ho TF, Lee TS. Iliopectineal bursitis complicating hemiarthroplasty: a case report. Clin Orthop Relat Res 2001; 392:366-371.
65. Cheung YM, Gupte CM, Beverly MJ. Iliopsoas bursitis following total hip replacement. Arch Orthop Trauma Surg 2004; 124:720-723.
66. Della Valle CJ, Rafii M, Jaffe WL. Iliopsoas tendonitis after total hip arthroplasty. J Arthroplasty 2001; 16:923-926.

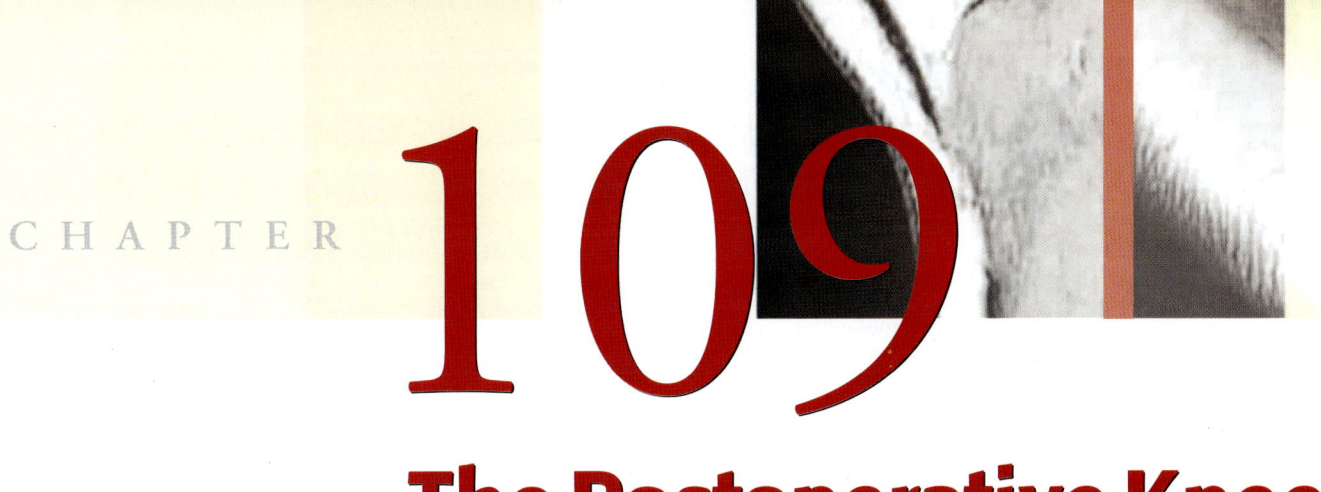

109

The Postoperative Knee

Douglas Mintz

Imaging the postoperative knee can be challenging. The postoperative knee can have all of the pathologic processes of the preoperative knee in addition to specific issues related to the surgery performed, general problems with surgery, and specific postoperative complications. The imaging is often confounded by artifact produced from instrumentation or surgical scar, so that often special imaging technique is required, especially for CT and MRI. Because imaging is used to answer clinical questions, knowledge of the procedures performed and the reason for the postoperative imaging can be very helpful and important in interpreting studies. If not provided on the ordering physician's request, this information usually can be obtained with a telephone call. Because surgical procedures have evolved and continue to evolve, it helps to have a working knowledge of these procedures and interaction with the referring physicians fosters that knowledge.

The discussion in this chapter is on some of the postoperative findings one may encounter. The emphasis is on MRI because that is the modality most commonly used. Radiography, fluoroscopy, CT, ultrasonography, and nuclear imaging also have roles for some postoperative issues.

ARTHROSCOPY

Description

Arthroscopy is the technique of percutaneous visualization of a joint. By adapting a cystoscope, Takagi, a Japanese surgeon, first used arthroscopy in the early 1900s to diagnose tuberculosis of the knee. His student, Wantanabe, worked on the technique, producing the first modern arthroscope in the late 1950s. With the advent of fiberoptics and improvement of cameras, arthroscopy became much better in the 1970s and widely used in the 1980s.[1]

Indications, Contraindications, Purpose, and Underlying Mechanics

Before good noninvasive diagnostic procedures became available, arthroscopy was used as a diagnostic tool. Now it is commonly used to perform therapeutic interventions and has largely replaced arthrotomy for many operative procedures in the knee. It has the advantages of reduced morbidity and shorter recovery times.

Some of the procedures that are commonly performed through an arthroscope include cruciate ligament reconstructions, meniscectomies and meniscal repairs, chondroplasty, removal of intra-articular bodies, and removal of other masses.

The importance of knowing if arthroscopy has been performed lies in the need to know if a finding on the study is postsurgical. For example, if a meniscus is small, and no surgery was performed, a more thorough search for a displaced flap will ensue.

Expected Appearance on Relevant Modalities

On radiography, it is impossible to tell that arthroscopy has been performed unless there has been some kind of instrumentation. On MRI, arthroscopic portals cause scar that appears as low signal on all pulse sequences (Fig. 109-1). They are characteristic in location in the medial and lateral aspects of the infrapatellar fat. Evidence of whatever procedure was performed through the arthroscope may also be seen.

Potential Complications and Radiologic Appearance

Whenever a foreign body is placed in a joint the potential for infection exists. The appearance of septic arthritis is described elsewhere and has the same appearance in the postoperative as well as the native state—effusion with rapidly progressive joint space narrowing on the radiograph with eventual resorption/destruction of subchondral bone. The MRI features of infection are effusion with synovitis and reactive abnormal signal in the surrounding tissues. Noninfectious inflammatory arthropathy does not generally cause the degree of soft tissue signal abnormality on MRI.

Occasionally, an arthroscopic portal is placed through a portion of the patellar tendon. This often causes an extensive reaction in the tendon, with focal thickening on MRI (Fig. 109-2).

It used to be thought that patients who undergo arthroscopy can develop avascular necrosis. The theory was that the increase in pressure from the joint distention during arthroscopy could decrease blood flow and cause necrosis. More likely, the sudden new pain that patients get after arthroscopy has to do with subtle subchondral insufficiency fractures (Fig. 109-3).[2] Rarely, the arthroscope can directly hit and injure the articular surface.

Another complication is complex regional pain syndrome, formerly known as reflex sympathetic dystrophy. Although it can occur after trauma without surgery, it may also be related to surgery (Fig. 109-4).

ARTHROTOMY

Description

Before arthroscopy was common, orthopedic surgeons performed knee surgeries through long incisions made lateral or medial to the patella. These incisions give excellent exposure to the joint.

Indications, Contraindications, Purpose, and Underlying Mechanics

An arthrotomy is currently used when a procedure cannot be performed arthroscopically. Before arthroscopy became available and popular, arthrotomies were more common. Meniscectomies and reconstructions of the anterior cruciate ligament (ACL), now done arthroscopically, used to require arthrotomy.

The most common indication for arthrotomy is joint arthroplasty. Tumor resections and chondral repair and replacement procedures require arthrotomy, as does meniscal transplantation. Pigmented villonodular synovitis may require arthrotomy for complete resection, depending on the extent of disease and ability of the arthroscopist.

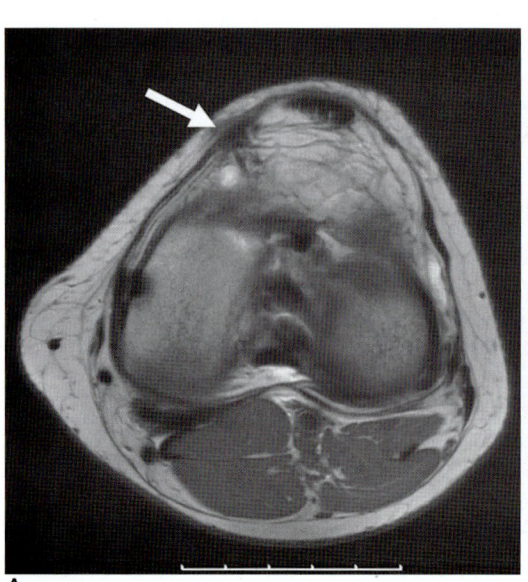
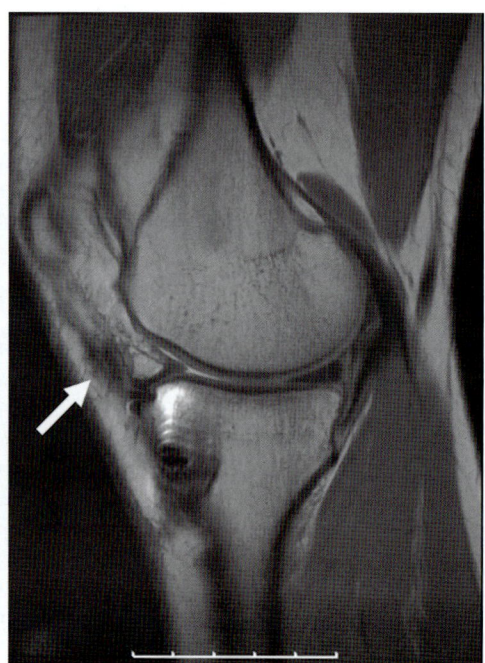

■ FIGURE 109-1 Arthroscopy scars. Axial (**A**) and sagittal (**B**) intermediate echo time MR images show the typical scars (*arrows*) from arthroscopic portal placement. There are usually medial and lateral scars. (©Hospital for Special Surgery, New York, New York.)

A   B

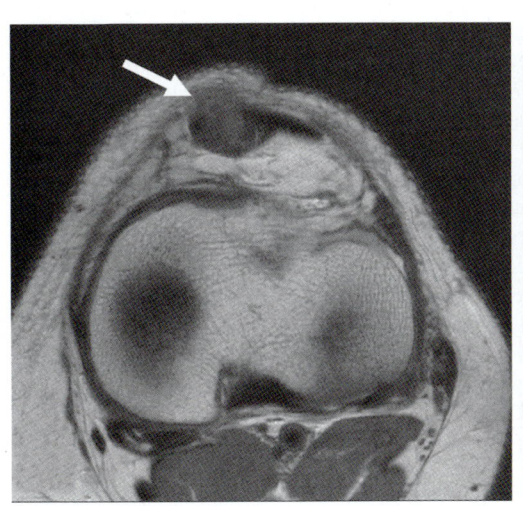
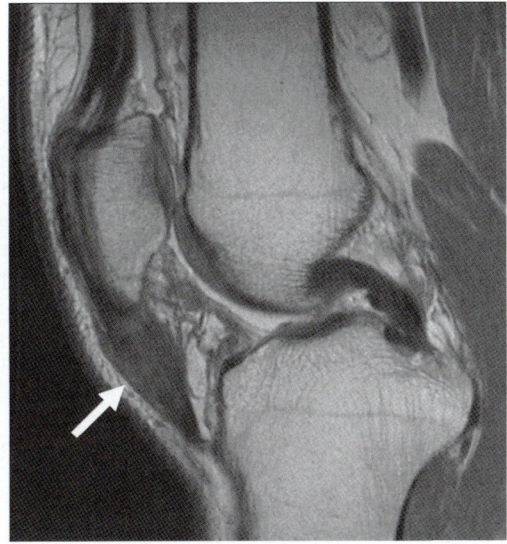

A

B

■ **FIGURE 109-2** Patellar tendon scar. Axial (**A**) and sagittal (**B**) MR images show patellar tendon abnormality (*arrows*) from an arthroscopic portal being placed through it. (©Hospital for Special Surgery, New York, New York.)

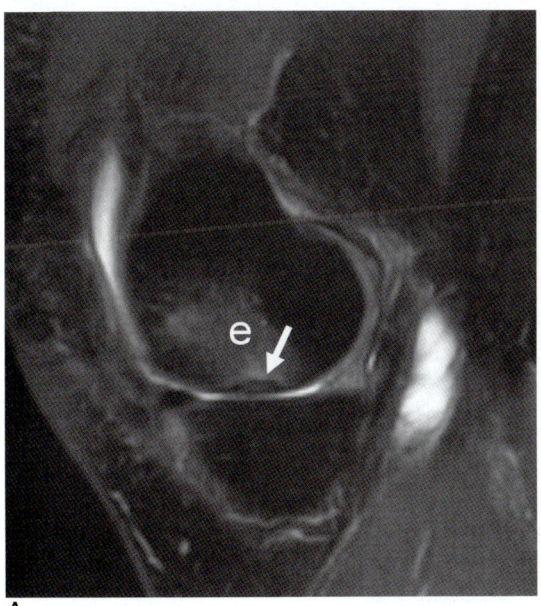
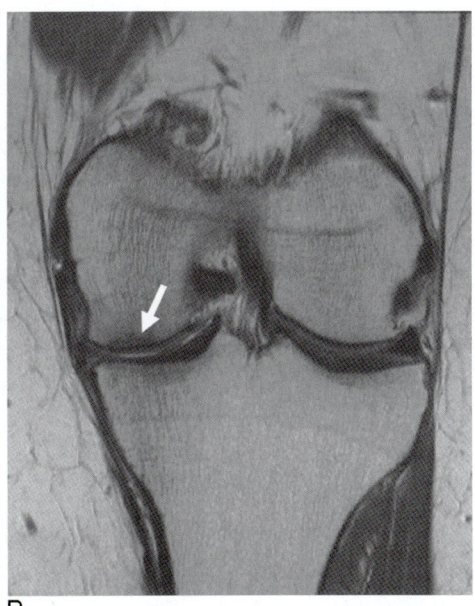

A

B

■ **FIGURE 109-3** Subchondral fracture. Some weeks after partial medial meniscectomy, this patient's sudden onset of pain was due to a subchondral fracture. Sagittal, fat-suppressed MR image (**A**) better shows the high signal intensity of the bone marrow edema (e) associated with the fracture, which is shown by the low signal intensity line (*arrow*, **A, B**). (©Hospital for Special Surgery, New York, New York.)

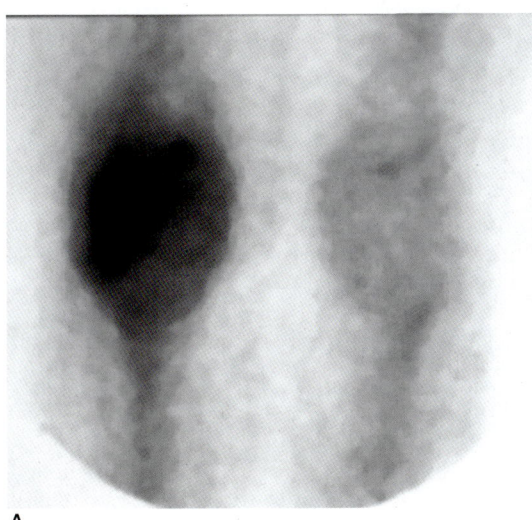
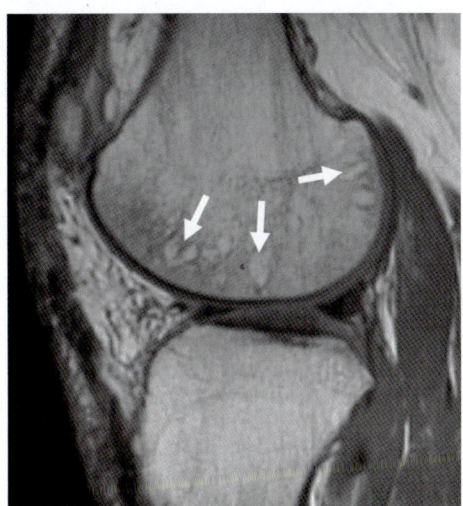

A

B

■ **FIGURE 109-4** Complex regional pain syndrome (reflex sympathetic dystrophy). Blood pool images from a bone scintiscan (**A**) show diffuse uptake around the knee. Sagittal, intermediate echo time MR image (**B**) shows patchy, rounded periarticular foci of relative increased signal (*arrows*) that appear to be associated with complex regional pain syndrome. (©Hospital for Special Surgery, New York, New York.)

Expected Appearance on Relevant Modalities

As with arthroscopy, an arthrotomy itself leaves no radiographic findings. It is other findings on a radiograph that indicate that arthrotomy was performed, such as the implant placed for knee replacement.

On MRI, a long vertical low signal line represents the scar left from arthrotomy (Fig. 109-5). It lies either lateral or medial to the patella, depending on the approach used. The incision is long enough to be able to peel back the patella to expose the joint. With time, these scars become less conspicuous so that after many years it may be difficult to tell if an arthrotomy was performed.

Potential Complications and Radiologic Appearance

The arthrotomy itself has few associated complications. As in arthroscopy, the potential for infection exists and has the same appearance, regardless of etiology.

ANTERIOR CRUCIATE LIGAMENT RECONSTRUCTION

Description

Tears of the ACL of the knee can lead to joint instability and subsequent arthrosis. First repaired in 1895 and reconstructed in 1903, many materials and techniques have been used to fix ACL tears. The first patellar autograft was used in 1935. A hamstring graft followed shortly thereafter in 1939. Despite these early descriptions, people tried to primarily repair the ACL for many years afterward. Most of the primary repairs failed: only the proximal tears repaired early had success. Other than in proximal tears and bony avulsions (a minority of ACL injuries) we see reconstructions. During the 1970s extra-articular stabilizations were used (Fig. 109-6). During the 1980s different graft materials such as carbon fiber and Dacron were used. Reconstructions as they are currently performed became popular in the late 1980s because of the introduction of interference screws and advances in arthroscopic surgery.[1,3]

Because the ACL is the most commonly reconstructed knee ligament, we are most often called upon to evaluate it. There are about 100,000 ACL reconstructions performed in the United States annually. There is an about 10% failure rate (often due to reinjury). Radiologists in a busy MRI practice will see many knees with ACL reconstruction for problems with the graft or a different problem in the same knee. Because they are so common, one should know how they look and what can go wrong with them.

Indications, Contraindications, Purpose, and Underlying Mechanics

Tears of the ACL are reconstructed in active patients whose tears cause instability that impedes normal activities for that individual. An ACL-deficient, unstable knee will, over time, progress to premature arthrosis. In patients whose knees are not unstable (because of arthritis, for example) or who are not very active, the ligament may remain torn.

The purpose of the reconstruction is to restore the stabilizer of the tibia to anterior translation.

Expected Appearance on Relevant Modalities

Over the years, different techniques and materials have been used for reconstructions. Artificial grafts have been used but failed because the grafts would fall apart or the

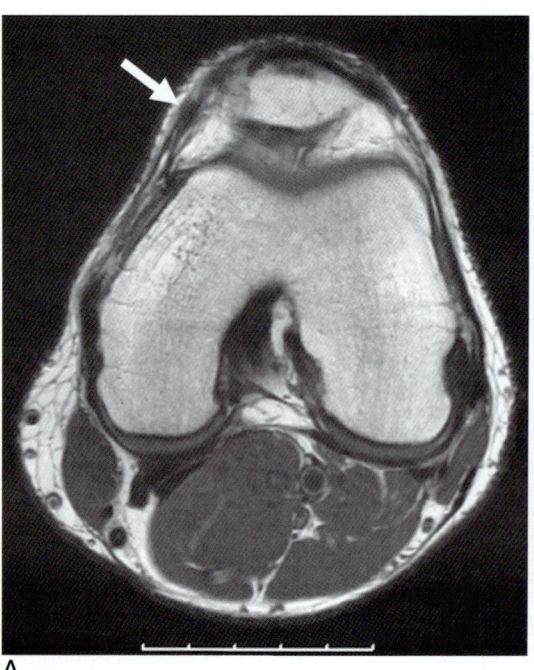
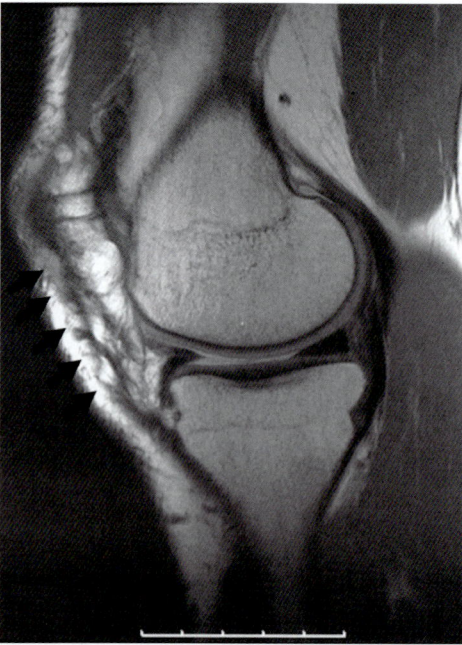

■ **FIGURE 109-5** Arthrotomy scar. Axial (**A**) and sagittal (**B**) MR images show scar from medial arthrotomy (*white arrow* and *black arrows*) for cartilage repair. The scar is similar to that for arthroscopy but more extensive. (©Hospital for Special Surgery, New York, New York.)

A

B

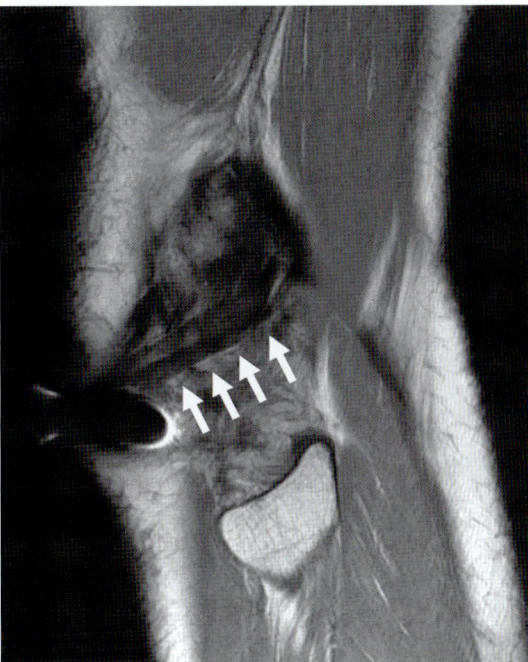

■ **FIGURE 109-6** Extra-articular stabilization. Sagittal MR image through the lateral side of the knee showing an extra-articular graft (*arrows*) that was used to stabilize the knee after ACL tear, before constructions were commonly performed. (©Hospital for Special Surgery, New York, New York.)

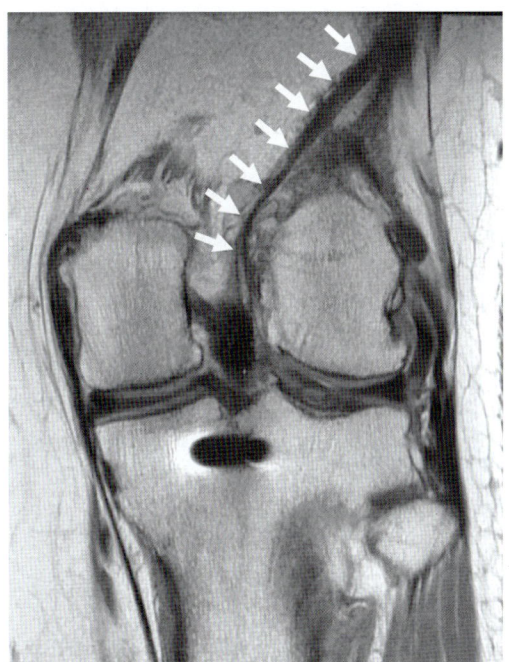

■ **FIGURE 109-7** Iliotibial band autograft for ACL reconstruction. Coronal, intermediate echo time MR image shows ACL autograft with iliotibial band (*arrows*). This technique was popular in the 1970s. The only way to know that the reconstruction was done with an iliotibial band is to follow the structure over sequential images. (©Hospital for Special Surgery, New York, New York.)

body would react to them. A variety of autograft reconstructions have been used from the extra-articular ACL reconstruction (essentially a stabilization procedure that was not with an in-situ graft) to the autologous patellar tendon remaining fixated on the tibial tubercle (Marshall Mackintosh) to a variety of other autografts—iliotibial band (Fig. 109-7), patellar tendon with bone plugs, or hamstring autograft. Allografts are also used (usually Achilles tendon but also patellar tendon). Rarely, contralateral patellar tendon is used.

The commonly used current material is either bone-patella-bone or hamstring autograft or allograft. A variety of fixation devices are also in use: fixation screws that grab bone plug and native bone (interference screws), endobuttons (plastic buttons that the graft that holds the graft outside the bone preventing it from sliding back), and a few other devices including horizontal femoral fixation devices and staples (Figs. 109-8 to 109-10). The interference screws can be made from metal or bioabsorbable radiolucent materials (polymers such as polylactic acid [PLA] or polyglycolic acid [PGA]). They have a similar appearance on MRI, although the nonmetallic ones have less artifact.

When hamstring is used, it is often folded on itself and one can see up to four strands of tendon used for ligament reconstruction. Any of the grafts can be augmented with suture. This augmentation gives rise to a dephasing artifact that runs along the graft (Fig. 109-11).

The proximal and distal ends of a graft arthroscopically placed through tunnels in the tibia and femur line up in the maximally flexed knee. The outline of the tunnels are discernible on radiography (see Fig. 109-8). More important than knowing what graft was used or what fixation was used is knowing its integrity and appropriateness of placement (position). Recently, some surgeons have reconstructed the two discrete bands of native ligament, yielding two separate proximal points of fixation.

Position

Appropriate placement of the graft is important to prevent some of the complications of inappropriate placement—graft impingement, knee instability, and laxity. Whereas some surgeons are starting to use two bands of graft to better simulate the native ACL, most use only one. To mimic function of the native ligament, the tibial tunnel should be at the back of the native ACL footprint (it used to be placed more anterior than that). The femoral tunnel hugs the posterior cortex of the femur such that the graft parallels Blumensaat's line in the sagittal plane (Fig. 109-12). In the coronal plane, the graft should be angled about 15 degrees to prevent the knee from turning on itself (see Fig. 109-8).[4] Some surgeons place the graft a bit looser than others. This is a matter of technique and preference so that just because a tibia appears a bit more anterior than a native ACL it does not imply inappropriate laxity, re-tear, or misplacement. The position thought to be optimal for the tibial tunnel has moved over the years. It is now believed that the tibial graft should enter the tibia at the posterior portion of the native ligament. This practice will likely be modified with the increasing use of two bundle grafts and with further research into biomechanics.

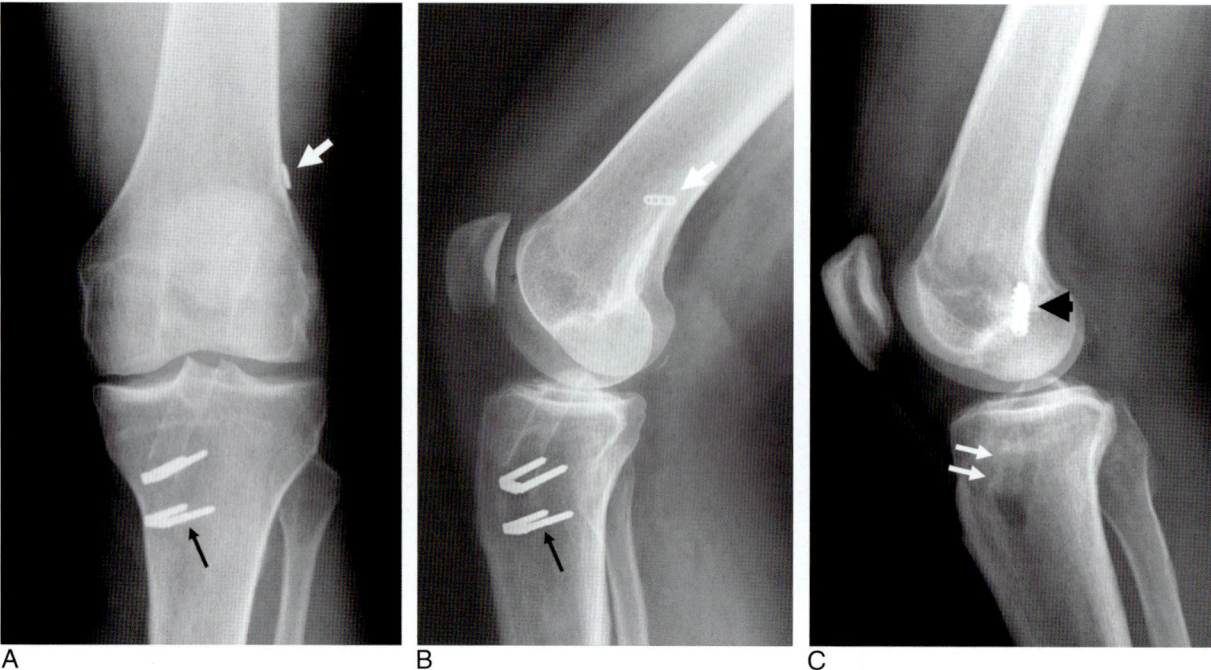

■ FIGURE 109-8 ACL reconstruction. Radiographs show the different types of fixation: staples (*thin black arrows*, **A, B**), buttons (*short white arrow*, **A**), and screws (*black arrowhead*, **C**). Some devices, such as bioabsorbable screws (*small white arrows*, **C**) are not easily visible on radiography. Sometimes the bone plug of a bone-patella-bone construct can be seen. On the frontal view the graft should be angulated about 15 degrees. On the lateral view the tibial tunnel should be at the posterior aspect of the anterior tibial spine. (©Hospital for Special Surgery, New York, New York.)

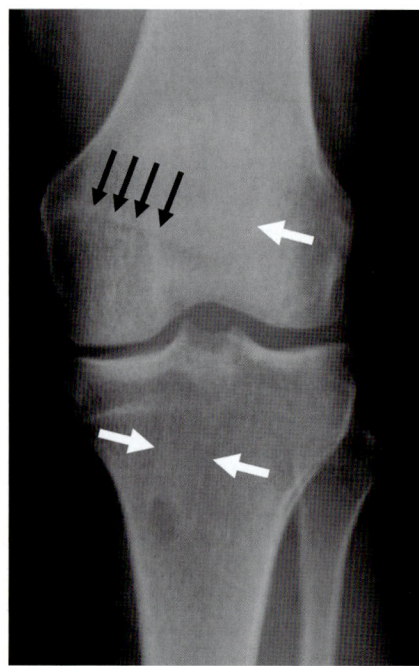

■ FIGURE 109-9 Transverse fixation. Some surgeons prefer a transverse fixation. Frontal radiograph in a patient with ACL reconstruction shows tibial tunnel and lateral wall of the femoral tunnel. A transverse lucency represents a bioabsorbable fixation device of the proximal graft (*small black arrows*). (©Hospital for Special Surgery, New York, New York.)

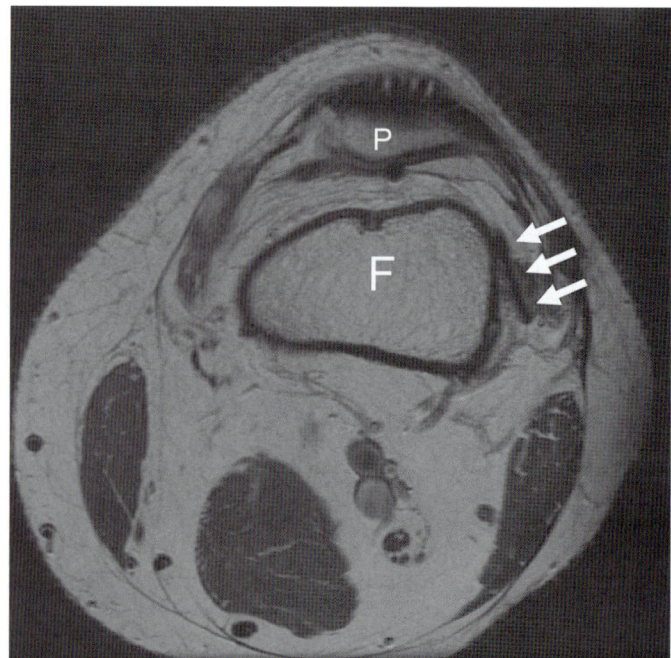

■ FIGURE 109-10 Endobutton. Axial MR image at the level of the distal femur (F) shows the radiolucent endobutton (*arrows*), which can be used for fixation of cruciate ligament reconstructions. The graft is tied through the button with a suture, but the button is too large to pull back through the graft's tunnel. The top of the patella is visible (P). (©Hospital for Special Surgery, New York, New York.)

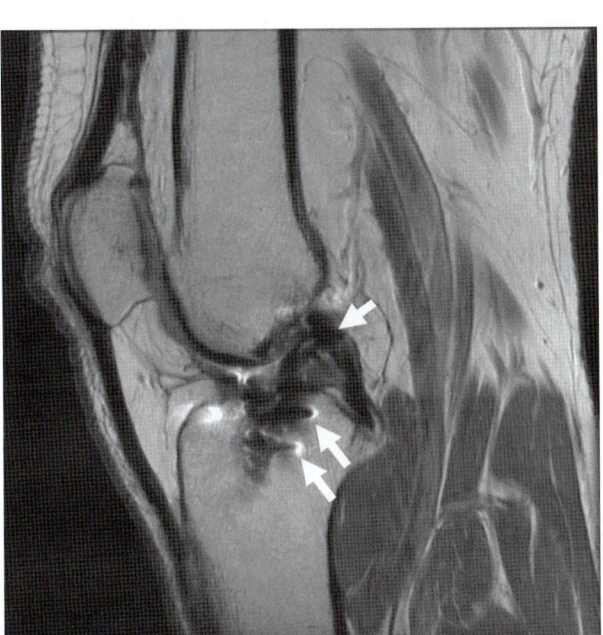

■ **FIGURE 109-11** Hamstring reconstruction augmentation. Sagittal, intermediate echo time MR image shows ACL reconstruction. Multiple low signal foci with dephasing artifact are related to graft augmentation, often done with suture (*arrows*). (©Hospital for Special Surgery, New York, New York.)

Signal

Ligament reconstructions go through a well-documented pattern of incorporation in which the graft initially serves as a stabilizer and then as a scaffold for a new fibrous support to form. For this to happen, the graft must become vascularized, resorbed to some extent, and then replaced. The MRI appearance reflects those changes.

Initially a graft is of homogeneously low signal intensity. Over a couple of months the graft becomes higher in signal intensity during the vascularization phase. Over 6 months to 2 years it again becomes of homogeneously high signal intensity. During the revascularization stage the graft is weak and susceptible to re-injury. Normally, a graft should be a continuous low signal structure (Fig. 109-12).

Harvest Site

The site of allograft harvest shows postoperative abnormalities. For patellar harvest, the defect in the central third may or may not be apposed by suture and the patellar bone plug harvest side may or may not have bone graft placed into it. Both bone plug harvest sites are usually visible on the axial images forever. The patellar tendon is initially thick and high signal on MR and, with time, becomes more normal.

There are more subtle findings in hamstring harvest: there is loss of the semitendinosus and often the gracilis tendon with a thin, and eventually thicker, fibrous sheath over the length of the harvest (Fig. 109-13). Regeneration of the tendon that results in a fibrous scar in the region from where the tendon was harvested has been described.

Potential Complications and Radiologic Appearance

Complications of ACL grafts include problems related to placement (e.g., persistent instability or graft impingement); reactions to the graft (scar, inflammation, infection); and trauma (re-tears, degeneration, ganglion formation).

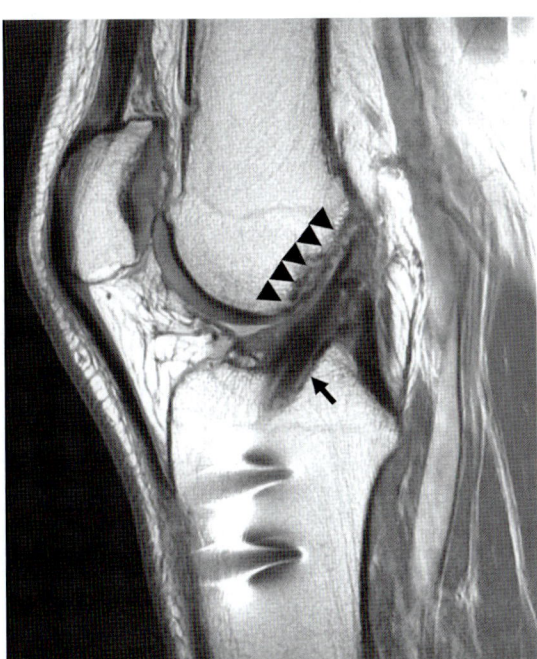

■ **FIGURE 109-12** Normal ACL reconstruction. Sagittal, fast spin-echo, intermediate echo time MR image shows a low signal graft parallel to Blumensaat's line (*arrowheads*). The tibial tunnel (*black arrow*) enters the tibia at the posterior portion of the native ligament, and the femoral attachment is posterior, at the posterior cortex of the distal femur. (©Hospital for Special Surgery, New York, New York.)

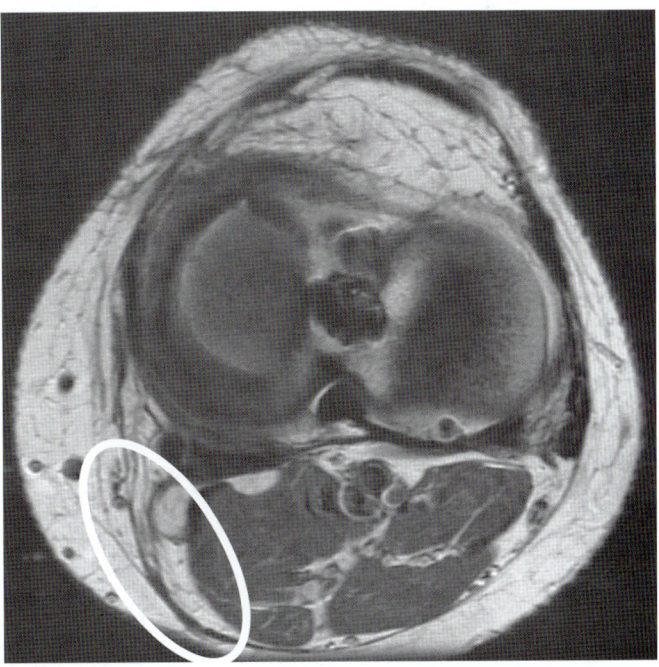

■ FIGURE 109-13 Hamstring harvest. Axial, intermediate echo time MR image at the level of the femorotibial joint demonstrates poor definition of the hamstring tendons, indicating that they have been harvested for the patient's ACL reconstruction. (©Hospital for Special Surgery, New York, New York.)

When a graft is malpositioned, impingement can occur either against the bone of the tibia or at the intercondylar notch. The graft curves around or rubs against bone. This can wear down the graft or impede its function (Fig. 109-14). During the graft placement some surgeons will remove some of the bone around the intercondylar notch (notchplasty) to prevent this from happening (Fig. 109-15).

If the graft is too vertical, the knee will be unstable to rotation and the femur and tibial can twist on each other (Figs. 109-16 and 109-17).

Focal scar formation in the intercondylar notch can block terminal extension and cause pain. This phenomenon is the so-called Cyclops lesion because of its similar appearance to the single eye of the Cyclops. This lesion may be related to inadequate removal of the native ACL or simply exuberant inflammatory response (Fig. 109-18). More extensive inflammatory response can lead to arthrofibrosis, which is characterized on MRI as low signal intensity tissue replacing the infrapatellar fat and extending from the femoral trochlea to the patella and patellar tendon (Fig. 109-19). Clinically, these involved knees will be painful and have limited flexibility.

Some patients develop an inflammatory reaction to the graft. This traditionally was a greater problem with synthetic grafts because there would be bone resorption and the tunnels would widen. This same phenomenon occasionally happens with allografts. In this circumstance, it can be difficult to differentiate this inflammatory

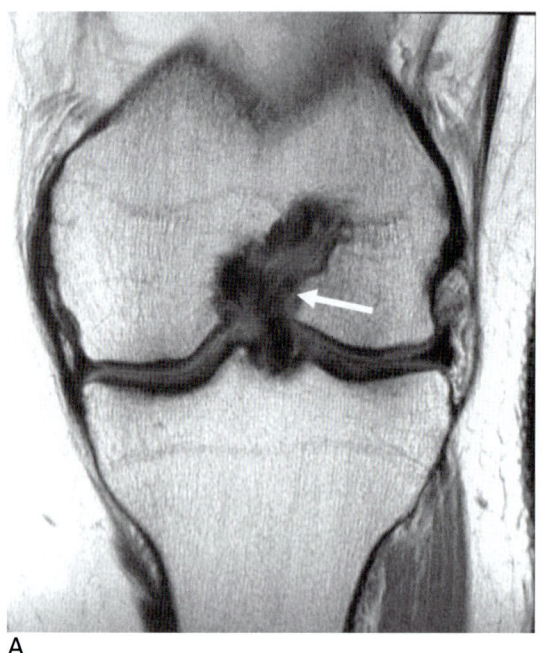

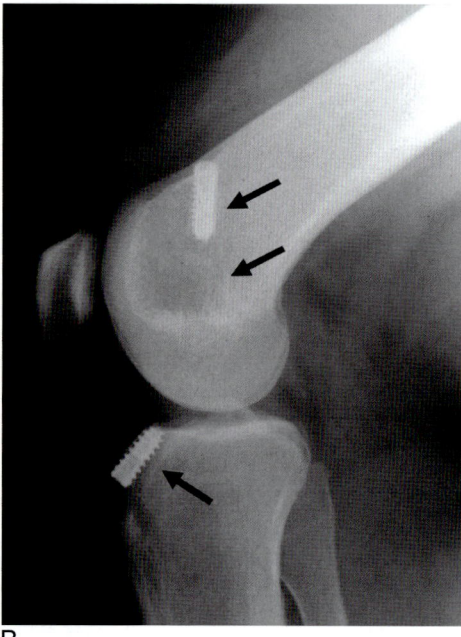

■ **FIGURE 109-14** Graft impingement. **A,** Coronal MR image of the knee shows that the ACL graft is displaced by the lateral femoral condyle in the intercondylar notch (*white arrow*). This is related to poor placement of the graft. **B,** Lateral radiograph shows by the position of the interference screws that the femoral tunnel is too far anterior and the tibial tunnel is too anterior and shallow (*black arrows*). (©Hospital for Special Surgery, New York, New York.)

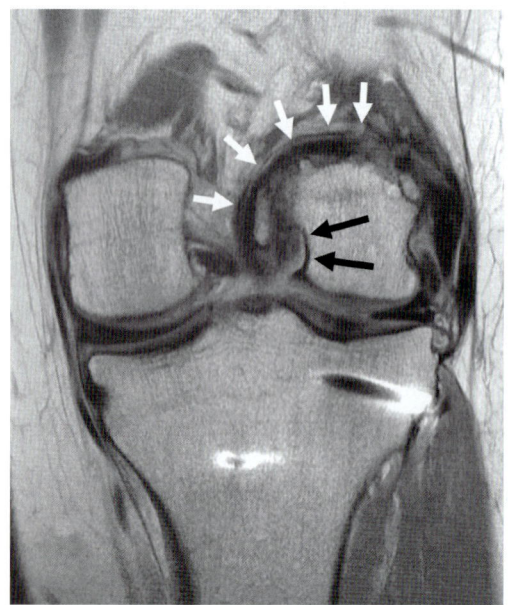

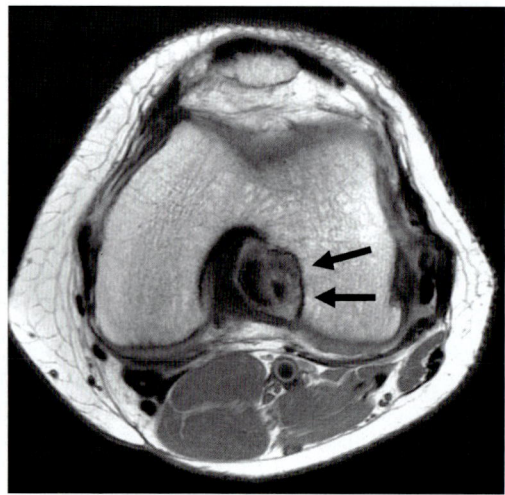

■ **FIGURE 109-15** Over-the-top ACL reconstruction. Notchplasty. **A,** Coronal intermediate echo time MR image shows an ACL reconstruction (*white arrows*) that courses over the lateral femoral condyle, rather than going through an osseous femoral tunnel. **B,** Both the coronal and the axial (**B**) MR image show notchplasty (*black arrows*) in which bone is removed from the condyle to prevent graft impingement. (©Hospital for Special Surgery, New York, New York.)

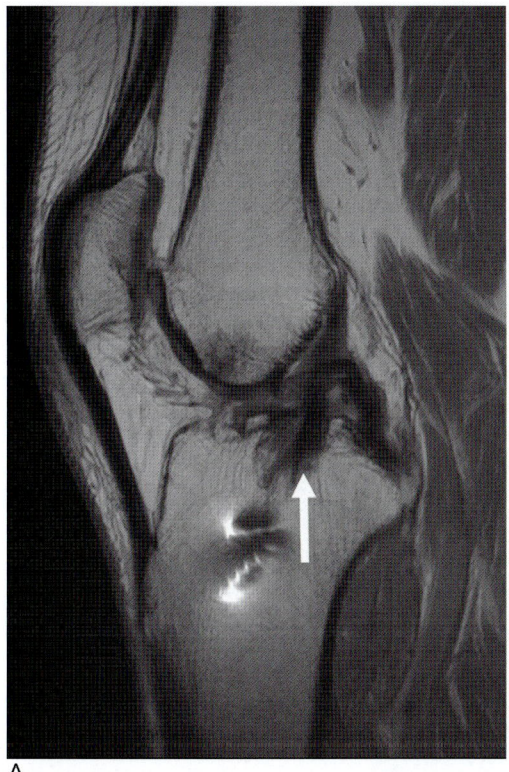
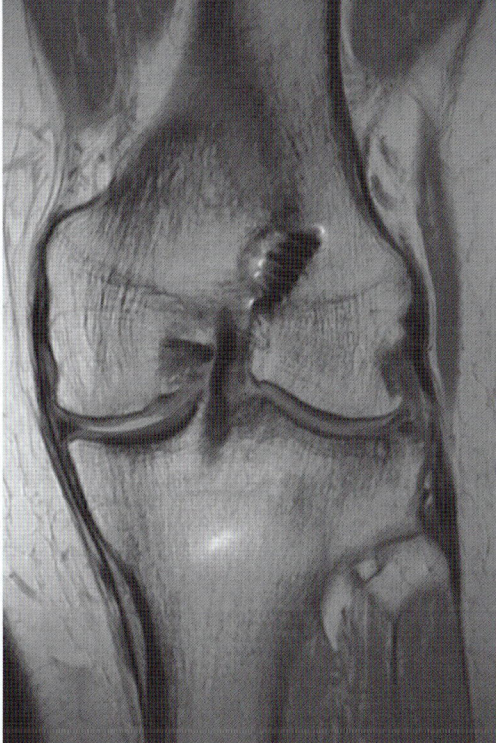

A   B

■ **FIGURE 109-16**   Poor ACL graft placement. Proper graft placement is important to the proper function of the graft. Sagittal (**A**), and coronal (**B**), intermediate echo time MR images show posterior placement of the ACL graft (**A**, *arrow*), causing a relative vertical orientation in the sagittal plane. The graft is also vertical in the coronal plane. Early arthrosis is evident, with chondral loss in all compartments, a lateral tibial plateau small subchondral cyst, prior partial medial meniscectomy, and lateral meniscal surgery with persistent signal. (©Hospital for Special Surgery, New York, New York.)

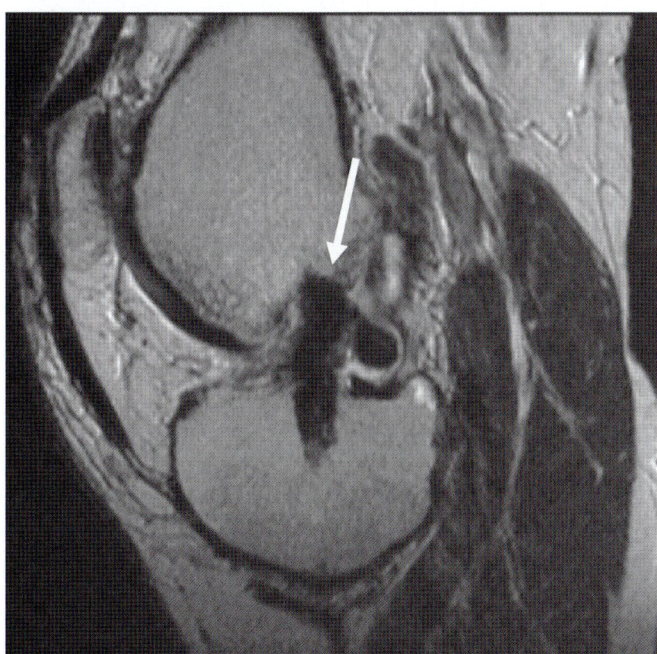

■ **FIGURE 109-17**   Poor ACL graft placement. Oblique sagittal T2-weighted MR sequence shows anterior placement on the femoral side (*arrow*), causing vertical orientation of the graft. This contributes to rotational instability. (©Hospital for Special Surgery, New York, New York.)

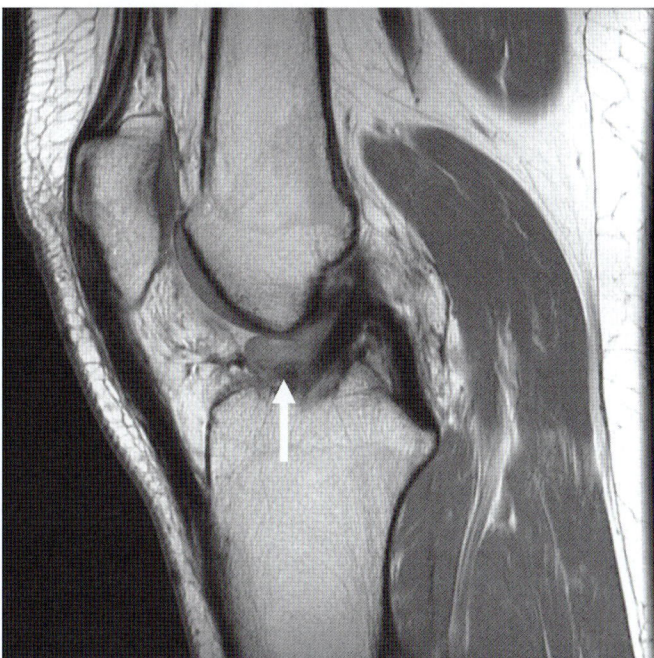

■ **FIGURE 109-18**   Cyclops lesion. Sagittal, midline, intermediate echo time MR image shows intermediate signal scar in the intercondylar notch anterior to the ACL, called a Cyclops lesion (*arrow*). (©Hospital for Special Surgery, New York, New York.)

reaction from infection. The graft and tunnels show high signal intensity, and the knee has a generalized inflammatory response, with joint effusion and synovitis being the most prominent features. The diagnosis of infection can best be confirmed with joint aspiration (Figs. 109-20 and 109-21).

Like the native ligament, one can perceive tears—both partial and complete. They are evaluated in the same way as for the native ligament, looking for contiguous low signal fibers (Fig. 109-22). As with the native ligament, ganglia can form in the reconstructed ligament. These ganglia (fluid

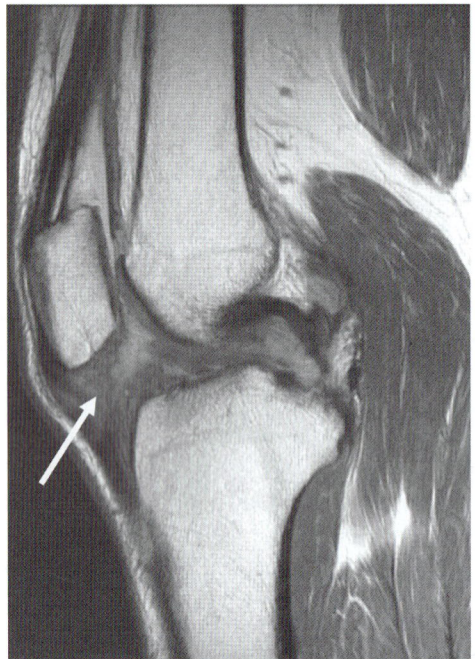

■ FIGURE 109-19 Arthrofibrosis. Some patients have an inflammatory reaction that results in dense scar of the joint and limited motion. This sagittal MR image shows complete filling of the infrapatellar fat with abnormal low signal (*arrow*)—the hallmark of arthrofibrosis. (©Hospital for Special Surgery, New York, New York.)

signal regions) can extend into the bone tunnels and cause widening of the tunnel (Fig. 109-23). Other pathologic processes that occur in the unoperated knee, such as stress fractures, are also "fair game" for the postoperative knee (Fig. 109-24).

POSTERIOR CRUCIATE LIGAMENT RECONSTRUCTION

Description

Posterior cruciate ligament (PCL) tears are less common than ACL tears. The PCL stops posterior translation of the tibia, and tears most commonly occur from direct impaction of the tibia with the knee flexed (the so-called dashboard injury). Hyperextension and knee dislocation are the other major mechanisms of injury to the PCL.

PCL reconstruction can be performed using a one- or two-bundle technique (Fig. 109-25). Two bundles are more commonly used for the PCL than for the ACL reconstruction.

Indications, Contraindications, Purpose, and Underlying Mechanics

As with ACL tears, instability can lead to arthrosis. To prevent this, reconstruction of the ligament is performed. Isolated PCL tears may not be fixed, especially in an older or inactive individual.

Expected Appearance on Relevant Modalities

Posterior cruciate ligament reconstruction is less common but has a similar appearance to ACL reconstruction. More often with the PCL reconstruction two bands are used with slightly different insertion points on the femur. The ligaments themselves should maintain the same signal as the ACL and be of homogeneously low signal intensity and continuous.[5]

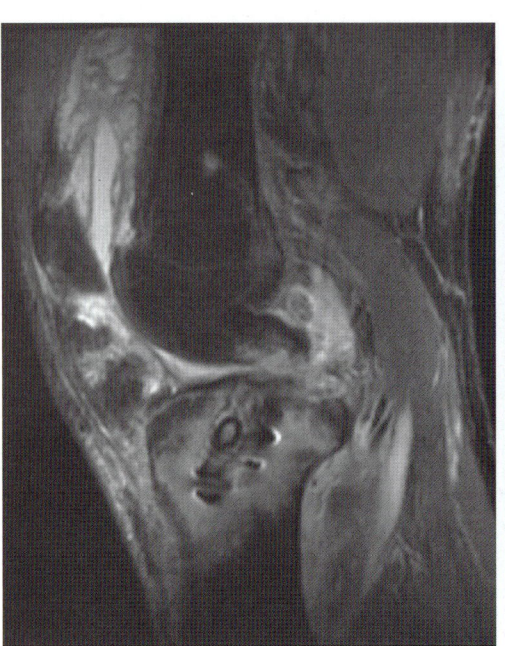
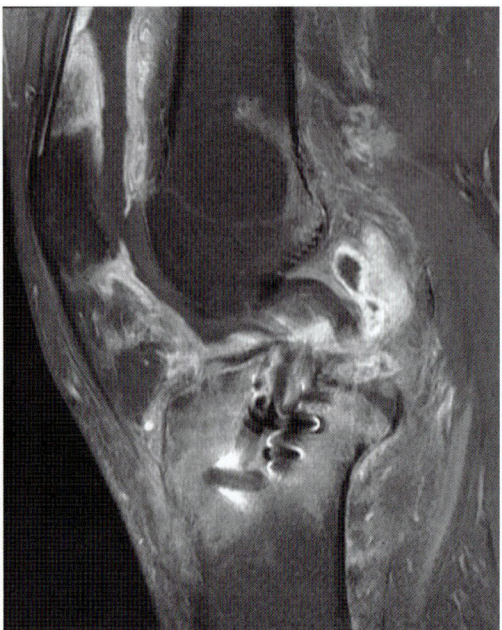

A   B

■ FIGURE 109-20 Infected ACL reconstruction. Sagittal short tau inversion recovery (**A**) and fat-suppressed, contrast-enhanced, T1-weighted (**B**) MR images show high signal with enhancement in the tibia, around the graft, in the joint, and in the surrounding soft tissues anterior and posterior to the tibia, indicating graft infection with associated septic arthritis. (©Hospital for Special Surgery, New York, New York.)

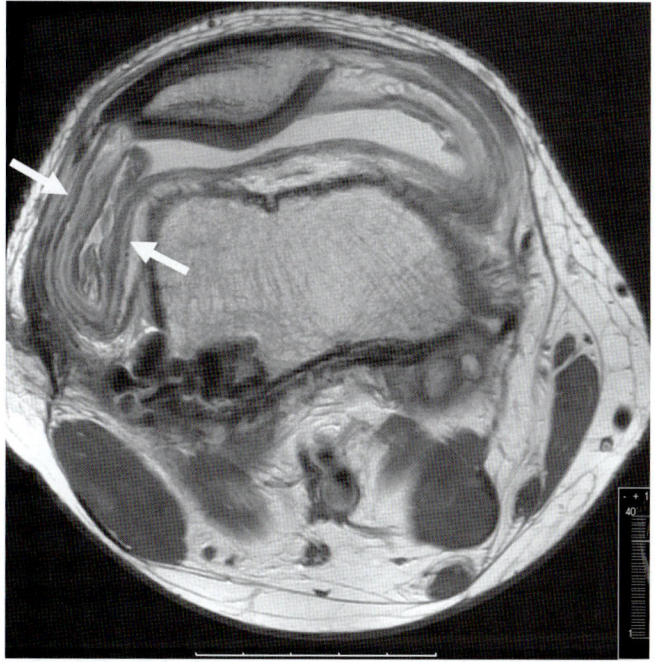

■ FIGURE 109-21 Infected ACL reconstruction. Same patient as in Figure 109-20. On this axial, intermediate echo time MR image, the layered synovial thickening suggests the presence of infection (*arrows*). (©Hospital for Special Surgery, New York, New York.)

Potential Complications and Radiologic Appearance

The complications of PCL reconstruction are the same as those associated with ACL reconstruction: infection, graft re-tear, and malposition. Arthrofibrosis and intercondylar notch scarring are not as common.

MEDIAL COLLATERAL LIGAMENT RECONSTRUCTION

Description

Tears of the medial collateral ligament (MCL) are common sports injuries. The ligament usually heals without help, but repair/reconstruction is sometimes necessary. Autograft reconstruction of the MCL was first reported in 1914. The common technique currently used was published by Bosworth in 1952 and is referred to as a Bosworth procedure.[1]

Indications, Contraindications, Purpose, and Underlying Mechanics

Because most tears heal on their own, we see relatively few repairs and reconstructions. As with the ACL, primary

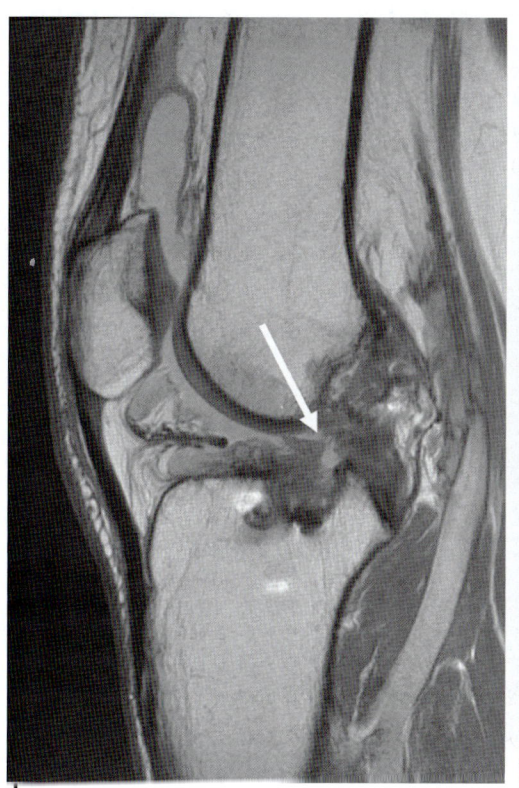

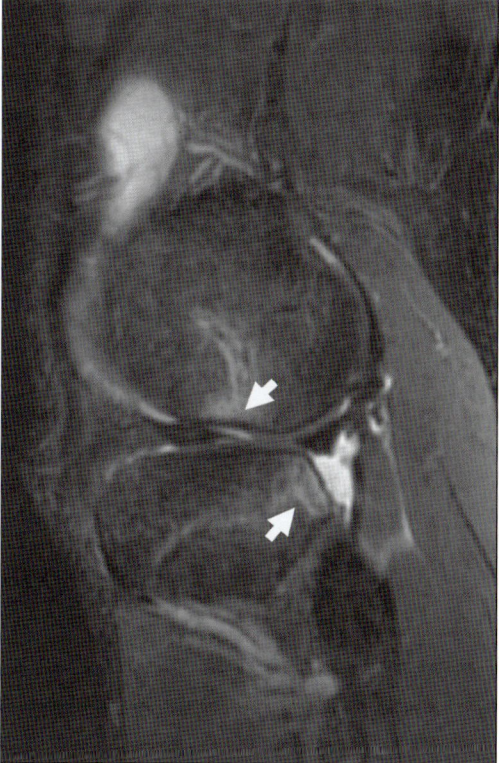

A B

■ FIGURE 109-22 Re-tear of ACL reconstruction. **A,** Sagittal MR image shows a defect (*long arrow*) in the middle third of this ACL reconstruction, reflecting acute complete tear. Anterior tibial translation is a secondary sign. **B,** Sagittal fat-suppressed image of a different patient with acute ACL reconstruction re-tear shows the characteristic translational impaction injuries (*short arrows*). (©Hospital for Special Surgery, New York, New York.)

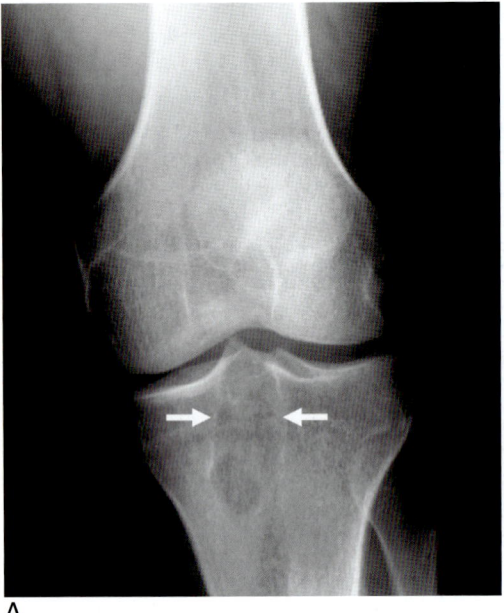
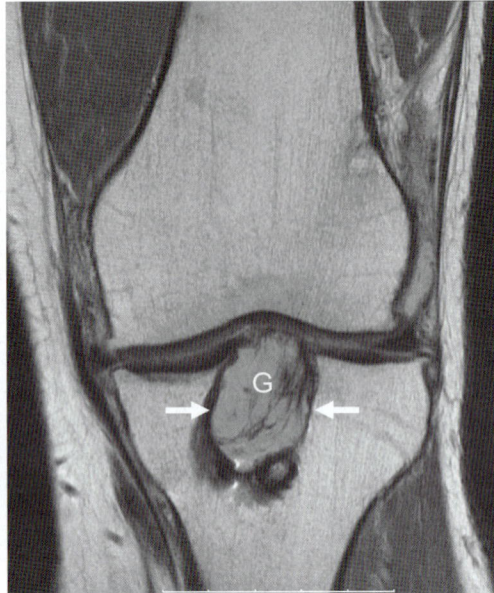

A   B

■ FIGURE 109-23 Postoperative tibial tunnel widening/ACL ganglion. Frontal radiograph (**A**) and coronal MR image using an intermediate echo time sequence (**B**) show evidence of ACL reconstruction with widening of the tibial tunnel (*between the arrows*) related to ganglion (G) within the reconstructed ligament. Normally the tunnel width is less than 1.5 cm. (©Hospital for Special Surgery, New York, New York.)

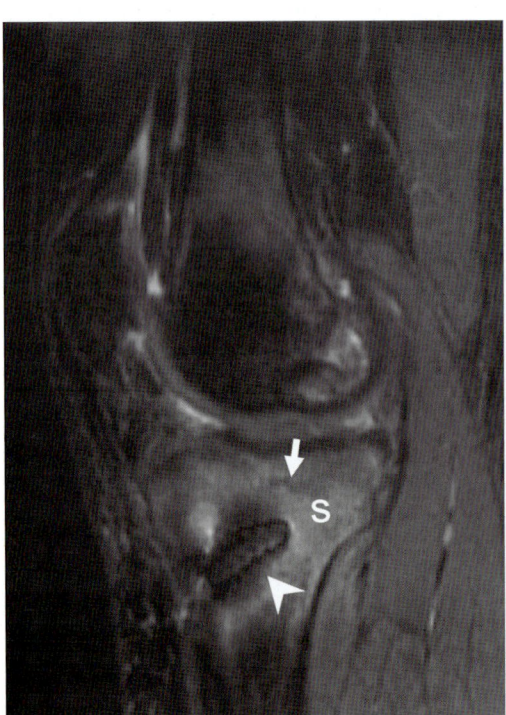
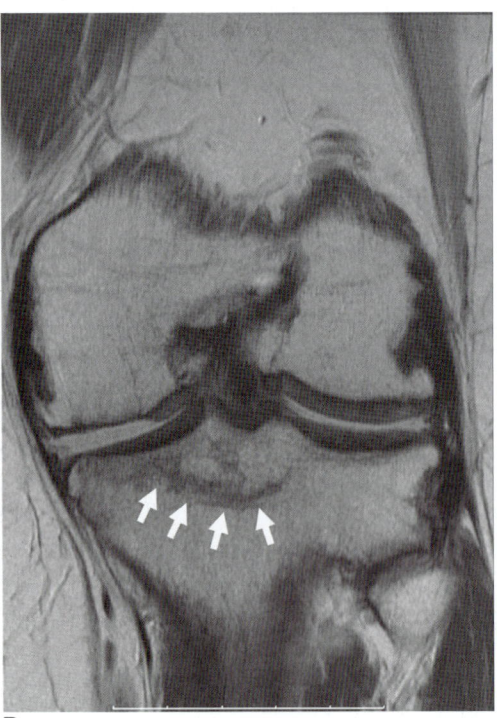

A   B

■ FIGURE 109-24 Stress fracture. Sagittal short tau inversion recovery (**A**) and coronal intermediate echo time (**B**) MR images in a patient who has undergone ACL reconstruction and has a stress fracture of the proximal tibia. On **A** there is extensive reactive high signal (s) and the hint of the fracture line (*arrow*). The higher-resolution, fast spin-echo sequence in **B** shows the medullary fracture (*small arrows*). The interference screw is visible (*arrowhead*). The appearance is the same as it would be if there had been no surgery. (©Hospital for Special Surgery, New York, New York.)

repairs are less common than reconstructions. The setting for reconstruction is usually that of an unstable knee, such as in multiple ligament injuries. Occasionally, patients who have ACL and MCL tears will have the MCL reconstructed if the surgeon thinks the knee is too unstable to valgus load after the ACL reconstruction. Sometimes high-performance athletes with repeated MCL injury will undergo ACL reconstruction.

Expected Appearance on Relevant Modalities

The healing MCL can be quite thick and exhibit high signal intensity on MRI. A reconstructed ligament will have either interference screws or staples in the medial femoral condyle related to the surgery. The fixation devices (or holes associated with them), but not the ligament, are visible

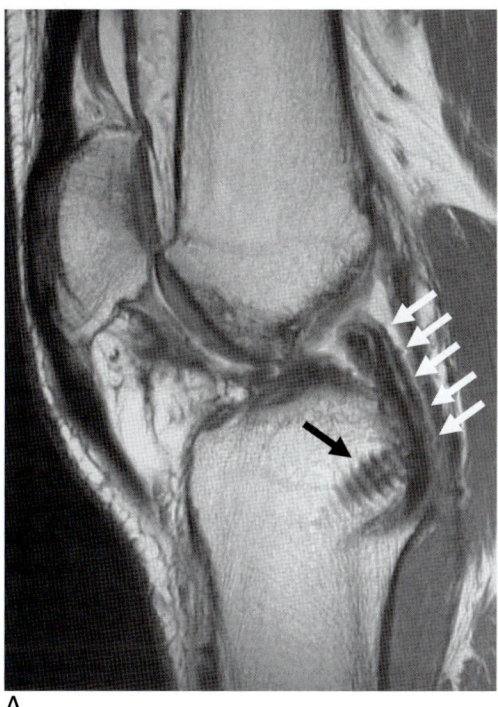
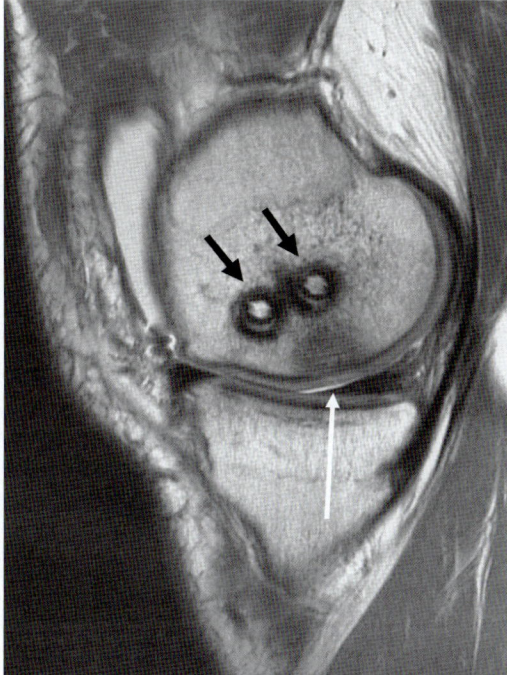

■ FIGURE 109-25 Posterior cruciate ligament reconstruction. Sagittal midline (**A**) and medial (**B**) MR sections through the knee demonstrate an intact reconstruction (*white arrows*) (the proximal aspect is just not visible on these slices). There is one distal and two proximal interference screws (*black arrows*) to better approximate the native ligament. Previous chondroplasty was performed (**B**, *long arrow*), and the overlying reparative cartilage is minimally thin and mildly of high signal. (©Hospital for Special Surgery, New York, New York.)

on radiography. On MRI the reconstructed ligament can be thick but should be low in signal and continuous. On ultrasonography, it should also be continuous and show homogeneous echogenicity.

Potential Complications and Radiologic Appearance

As with other ligaments, re-tear and failure of fixation are the most common complications. Failure is rare, and the MRI findings of a re-tear or a discontinuous or thick ligament are the same as in a torn native MCL.

POSTEROLATERAL CORNER RECONSTRUCTION

Description

The important implication of posterolateral corner injuries of the knee is relatively recent, as is their repair or reconstruction. The anatomy is complex, and it is only with improvements in MRI technique and therapeutic arthroscopy that the details of these injuries have been elucidated.

Indications, Contraindications, Purpose, and Underlying Mechanics

The need for repair or reconstruction of the posterolateral corner of the knee (posterior capsule, popliteofibular ligament, popliteus tendon, lateral collateral ligament, biceps femoris, and lateral meniscus) derives from preventing instability and preserving other ligament repairs.

Posterolateral corner injury and instability can result in ACL reconstruction failure. To prevent this, for high-grade injuries, the posterolateral corner is augmented, repaired, or reconstructed. The need for repair or reconstruction can be made after the ACL is treated. The surgeon examines the knee for stability in the operating room to determine whether the posterolateral corner needs attention. Isolated posterolateral injuries are rarely severe enough to require ligament or tendon repair or reconstruction.

Expected Appearance on Relevant Modalities

There are various techniques for providing more stability to the posterolateral corner. An anatomic reconstruction requires an allograft tendon to be placed and fixed along the lines of the native structures. As many as three grafts can be placed for reconstruction (Fig. 109-26). As with the grafts described previously, they should be of low signal intensity and continuous. Because they do not always perfectly follow the native structures, simple description of the course and assessment of integrity suffices because there is often significant associated scar tissue.

Reconstruction of the lateral structures is often combined with reconstruction of the ACL (Fig. 109-27).

Potential Complications and Radiologic Appearance

Whereas hardware failure and re-injury would be the most common complications, other typical problems such as infection may also occur. As with all surgeries, there may be an inflammatory or granulomatous reaction to the graft or suture.

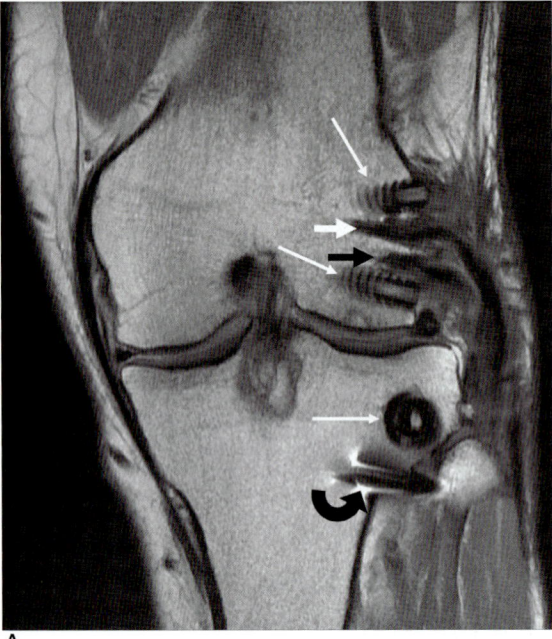

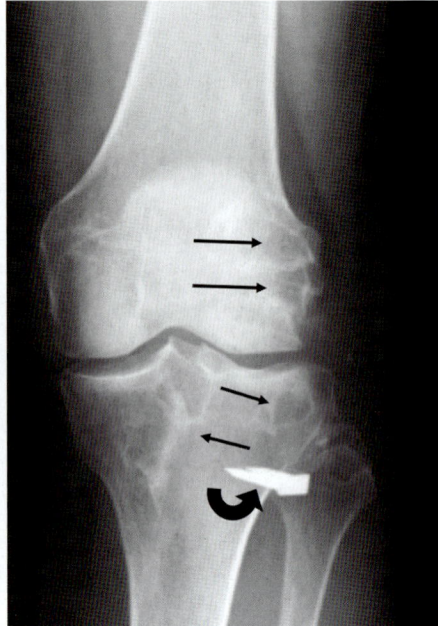

A   B

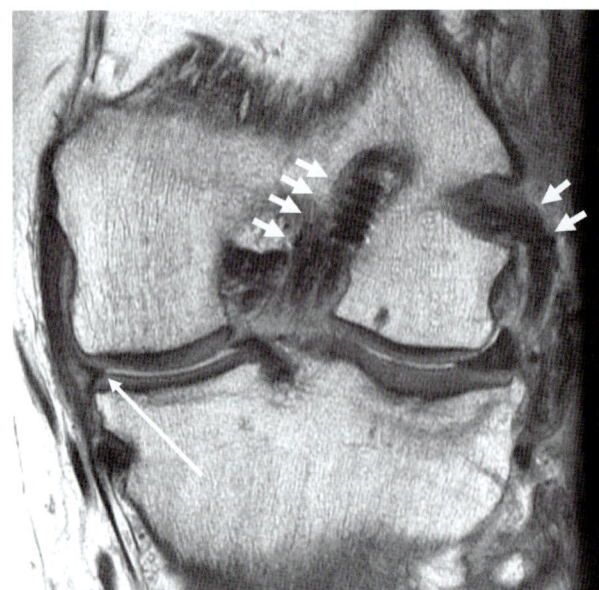

■ **FIGURE 109-27** Posterolateral corner and ACL reconstruction. Coronal, intermediate echo time MR image shows ACL and fibular collateral ligament reconstructions (*short white arrows*). After meniscectomy, change is noted in the medial meniscus (*long white arrow*). (©Hospital for Special Surgery, New York, New York.)

MULTIPLE LIGAMENT RECONSTRUCTION

Description

Severe trauma, such as knee dislocations, can injure many structures and render the knee unstable. For any hinged joint, if both collateral ligaments are torn the cause is likely to be dislocation.

Indications, Contraindications, Purpose, and Underlying Mechanics

To restore stability in a joint where many structures have been injured, many structures need to be repaired. Multiple ligament reconstructions can be difficult. From an imaging standpoint, one need merely to evaluate each structure and its integrity, as described earlier.

Expected Appearance on Relevant Modalities

The expected appearance of a multiligament reconstruction is a composite of the individual ligaments. They should all be anatomic in position and continuous. On MRI, they are of low signal intensity. On radiography, the fixation devices should not extend into the joint or excessively into the soft tissues.

Potential Complications and Radiologic Appearance

Complications have also been discussed previously and include poor graft placement, re-injury, infection, and reactive scar formation, none of which is specific to multiligament reconstruction.

MENISCECTOMY

Description

Meniscectomy is the process of removing a portion or all of a meniscus. Partial removal, the process of shaving an irregular edge, may simply be referred to as débridement. Meniscal resections are commonly performed arthroscopically, but in the past they required an open procedure through an arthrotomy.

Indications, Contraindications, Purpose, and Underlying Mechanics

Meniscal tears are common and can be caused by both degenerative and traumatic processes. The tears can cause pain, catching, and clicking. Displacement of potions of the torn meniscus can cause locking of the knee or the inability to flex or extend the knee.

Because the meniscus is important for the normal function of the joint—to dissipated load and add stability—surgeons try to preserve meniscal tissue. This can be done by repairing or sometimes replacing or transplanting meniscal tissue. If the meniscal tissue is abnormal, is thought to be the source of the patient's symptoms, and cannot be salvaged, it is resected. Formerly, before the importance of preserving meniscal tissue was realized, surgeons resected the entire meniscus. Now they resect only as much as they have to for relief of symptoms and restoration of function.

Expected Appearance on Relevant Modalities

The appearance of the postoperative meniscus depends on the surgery performed. In partial meniscectomy, in which a portion of the meniscus is shaved to restore a smooth edge, the meniscus may simply appear smaller on MRI (Fig. 109-27). If there was a large tear, such as a long oblique tear, the appearance may be that of a smaller meniscus with persistent oblique increased signal intensity in the meniscal remnant that can persist for years after surgery.[6]

If the meniscus is severely degenerated or so extensively torn that it cannot be salvaged, all or most of the meniscus will be removed (resected).

Potential Complications and Radiologic Appearance

The primary complication of partial meniscectomy for meniscal tear is re-tear or degeneration of that meniscus. If the meniscus is re-torn, it can appear very similar to a torn native meniscus: on arthrography or MR arthrography, contrast medium would get into the tear. Without contrast medium enhancement we have to rely on signal intensity, and it can be difficult to distinguish on MRI between the residual healing or healed scar after partial meniscectomy from a re-tear. The re-tear is supposed to have higher abnormal signal intensity than fluid, whereas the repaired, healed, or healing meniscus is supposed to have slightly lower signal intensity. Often we do not have the preoperative study to see where a meniscus was torn originally. Of course if the new signal abnormality is in a different place from the original tear, the abnormality is evaluated as if there was no surgery and careful examination for tears and flaps should be undertaken as usual.

An almost expected result of meniscal resection is joint arthrosis. It is not so much a complication as a consequence. Evaluation of articular cartilage is at least as important in the postoperative knee as in an unoperated knee.

MENISCAL REPAIR

Description

Because the meniscus is important for the normal function of the joint—to dissipate load and add stability—surgeons try to preserve meniscal tissue. This can be done by repairing or sometimes replacing/transplanting meniscal tissue. Different methods of meniscal repair (tack fixation and inside-out and outside-in techniques) are at the discretion of the surgeon.

Indications, Contraindications, Purpose, and Underlying Mechanics

The peripheral aspect of the meniscus (toward the capsule) is more vascular than the central aspect. This vascularity may allow healing and repair so that peripheral tears may be repaired, whereas central tears cannot be repaired, because they will not heal. The peripheral part of the meniscus is called the red zone, the midportion is called the red-white zone, and the central portion is the white zone. The red zone corresponds to zones 0 and 1; the red-white zone is zone 2; and the white zone is zone 3.

Meniscocapsular separations fall into zone 0 tears and can be repaired. Complete radial tears are difficult because they extend to the nonvascular zone and, if approximated, have a lot of stress put on a repair during weight bearing. In young people, attempts may be made to repair these with suture and blot clot to promote healing, because the resection would remove a large portion of meniscus and accelerate arthrosis. In oblique tears the central portion may be resected, with the peripheral portion being repaired.

Expected Appearance on Relevant Modalities

On conventional MR or CT arthrography, a meniscal repair would look like a normal meniscus, unless partially resected, in which case it would look like a partial meniscectomy. There may be some irregularity at the repair site, but there will be no contrast imbibition.[6]

On MRI, we usually see scar from the repair, with small foci of dephasing near the capsule that indicate that there has been surgery. Often scar extends to the subcutaneous fat in the region of the repair. Artifact may also be present in the meniscus, depending on the method of repair used, with tack fixation having slightly more artifact.

The site of a normal meniscal repair can have abnormal signal in the orientation of the original tear that represents fibrous tissue (Fig. 109-28). There may also be high signal that is more extensive than in the original tear, related to the repair (Fig. 109-29). Persistent increased signal intensity is part of the normal healing process and can remain for up to 2 years after surgery. This intermediate signal, however, will not be as high as the signal intensity of joint fluid.

Unless the signal intensity is as high as that as fluid, or fluid is definitely in the prior defect, one cannot say

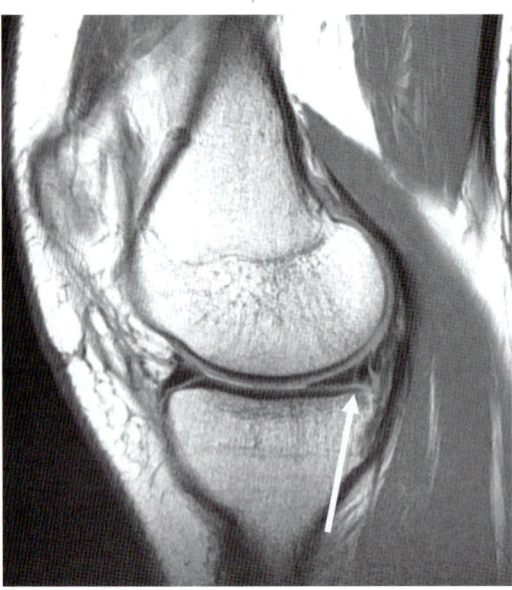

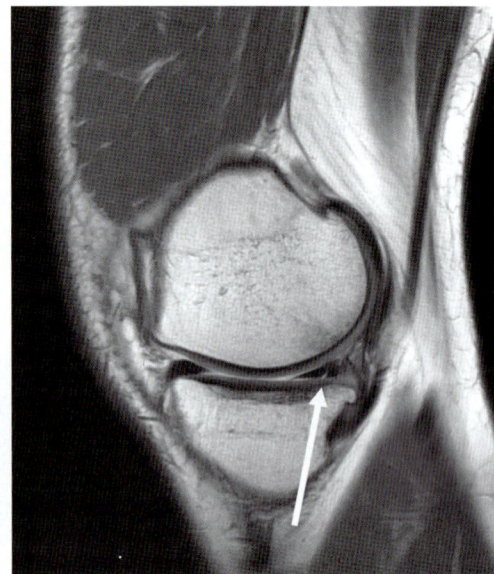

■ **FIGURE 109-28** Meniscal healing versus re-tear. Sagittal intermediate echo time MR images of the medial compartment. Abnormal signal in these postoperative medial menisci meets the tibial articular surface. The higher (fluid) signal in **B** reflects re-tear, whereas the intermediate signal in **A** represents healing (fibrous tissue). These subtle criteria apply whether evaluating the meniscus after débridement in that location or repair. (©Hospital for Special Surgery, New York, New York.)

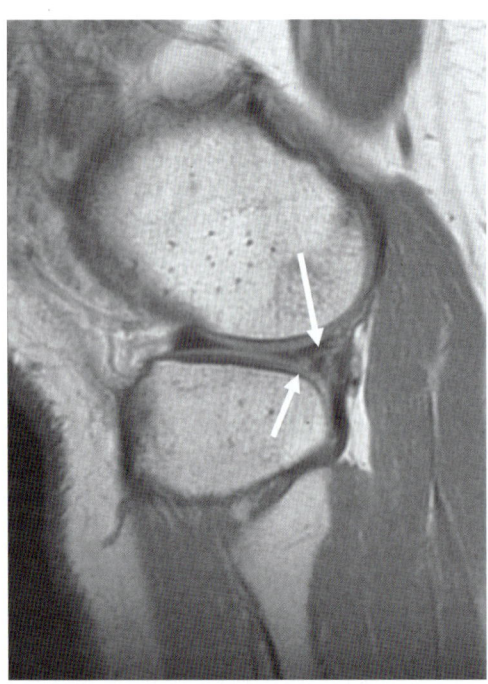

■ **FIGURE 109-29** Meniscal repair. Sagittal, short echo time MR image shows the multiple areas of high signal (*arrows*) that can be present after meniscal repair, without re-tear. (©Hospital for Special Surgery, New York, New York.)

that the meniscus has re-torn. This is also true on MR arthrography where it would be easier to see re-tears. Parameniscal cysts are usually, but not always, drained at the time of meniscal surgery, so their presence does not indicate there is a re-tear. Fluid can also dissect into the meniscus from the capsular side. Whereas this suggests that the meniscal repair is not healing well and that there is breakdown of the repair, this fluid, if it does not extend to an articular surface, is not considered a re-tear (Fig. 109-30).

A promising technique to evaluate healing, forwarded by Dr. Lawrence White of Mt. Sinai Hospital in Toronto, is to perform an MR meniscal perfusion study to look for contrast medium flowing across the meniscus in the region of prior tear/repair. If the contrast medium passes, then blood is crossing the gap and the meniscus is healed.

It is also true that menisci can tear in places different from where the repair was performed. In that case they are treated as an unoperated meniscus.

Potential Complications and Radiologic Appearance

The most common complication of meniscal repair is lack of healing and re-tear. As described earlier, re-tear is characterized by fluid imbibition into the repair site (Fig. 109-31). Fluid at the capsule extending into the meniscus suggests that the meniscus is not healing well (see Fig. 109-30).

In repairing menisci, sutures are fed percutaneously into the joint. Although an attempt is made to avoid important structures while doing this, occasionally a suture will tether the peroneal nerve, causing early postoperative neuralgia and requiring surgery to remove the offending suture (Fig. 109-32). Subcutaneous scar is less likely to do this postoperatively.

MENISCAL TRANSPLANT

Description

Because the meniscus is important for the normal function of the joint—to dissipate load and add stability—surgeons try to preserve meniscal tissue. This can be done by repairing or sometimes replacing or transplanting meniscal tissue. It would be ideal for patients to be able to regenerate meniscal tissue, and scaffolds are being developed to help promote this.[7] Until those or other techniques for tissue regeneration or replacement are available and successful,

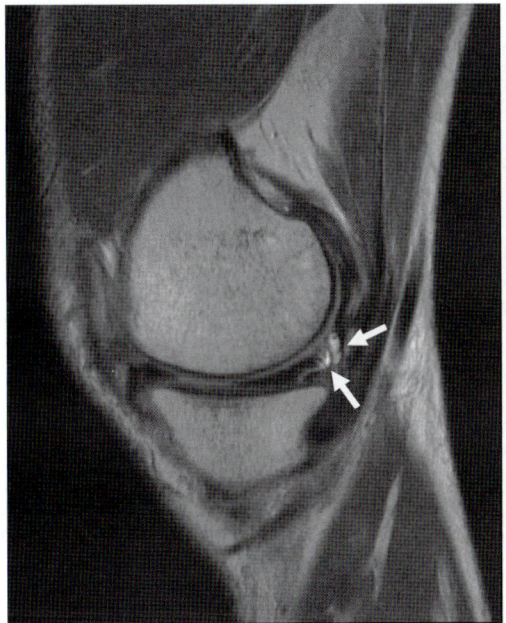
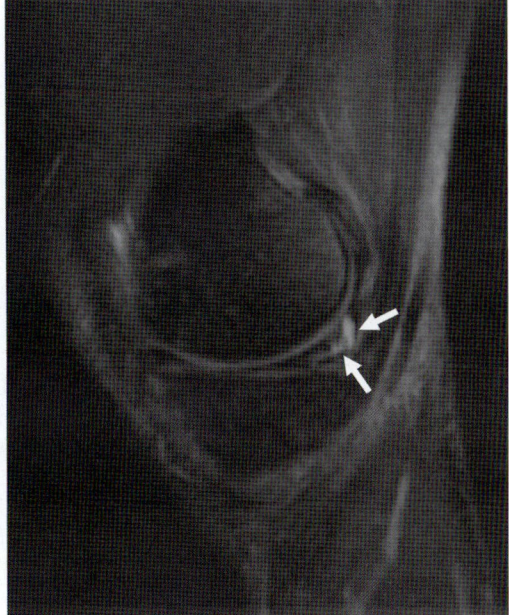

A   B

■ **FIGURE 109-30** Postoperative meniscal repair. Sagittal, intermediate echo time MR images through the medial compartment without (**A**) and with (**B**) fat suppression demonstrate high signal with fluid intensity at the capsule and extending into the meniscus (*arrows*), indicating capsular-sided breakdown of the repair. When the fluid clearly extends to the articular surface, it defines a re-tear. (©Hospital for Special Surgery, New York, New York.)

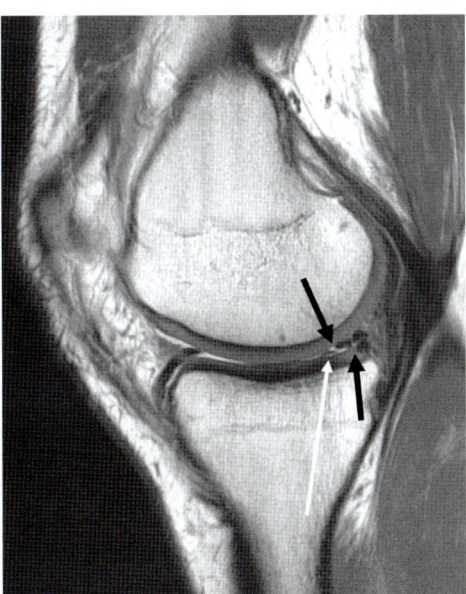

■ **FIGURE 109-31** Re-tear meniscal repair. This sagittal intermediate echo time MR image of an orthopedic surgery resident shows fluid signal coursing through the posterior horn of the medial meniscus (*black arrows*), indicating complex (more than one plane) tear. There is a small apical flap (*long white arrow*). (©Hospital for Special Surgery, New York, New York.)

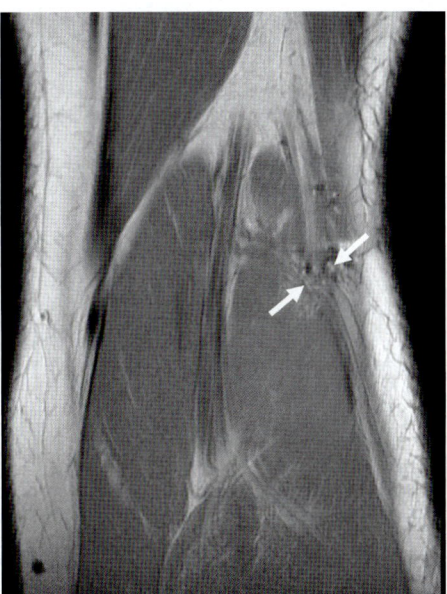

■ **FIGURE 109-32** Peroneal nerve injury. Coronal, intermediate echo time MR image shows a deviation in the course of the peroneal nerve (*arrows*) after lateral meniscus repair. There are specks of dark signal with dephasing in this area. The finding is related to suture tethering of the peroneal nerve, requiring surgery to release the nerve. It is important to extend the coronal images far enough posterior to include the peroneal nerve if that is a clinical concern. (©Hospital for Special Surgery, New York, New York.)

the only option that patients have is to have their menisci replaced with cadaveric meniscal transplants.[8]

Meniscal allografts were first performed almost 100 years ago as partial knee transplantation to avoid amputation. The first isolated meniscal allografts were placed in the mid 1980s.[9]

Artificial menisci that would allow native fibrocartilage to grow into an artificial scaffold are being developed but are not yet available in the United States.

Indications, Contraindications, Purpose, and Underlying Mechanics

Because meniscal transplantation is a potential way to prevent arthrosis in patients who have required meniscectomy, the indication is just that—for patients without menisci who have not yet developed arthrosis. Once the knee is arthritic, the transplant has a high likelihood of failure. Therefore, arthrosis is a relative contraindication to meniscal transplantation.[10]

For the allograft to work, alignment and, therefore, mechanics of the joint have to be normal. For this reason, in some individuals, standing hip to ankle radiographs are performed to see if a concomitant osteotomy is necessary to correct any abnormal mechanical axis of the knee before transplantation.

The clinical and radiographic outcome measures for meniscal allografts do not always agree. Patients can be asymptomatic but still have a torn, extruded, or degenerated graft. Likewise, a patient can have a normal graft from an imaging standpoint but have continued symptoms. Imaging becomes an important way to objectively judge success and evaluate new techniques, such as meniscal allografts.

Expected Appearance on Relevant Modalities

Recognizing that a patient has had a meniscal allograft placed is half the battle. Once that is realized, there are five things to evaluate on postoperative meniscal transplants: the meniscus integrity itself, attachment to the joint capsule, attachment to bone, degree of extrusion, and underlying joint (Fig. 109-33).[10]

Whereas there are different ways to treat the allograft, the radiographic appearances of these methods are the same. The meniscus should maintain normal signal and morphology: it should be of low signal intensity without tear (using the criteria for a native meniscus) (Fig. 109-34).

The allograft is sutured to the native capsule circumferentially. This attachment can have high signal, but there should be no separation or fluid interposition. They usually heal to the capsule very well (see Figs. 109-33 and 109-34).

Two methods of meniscal attachment to bone are commonly used: the plug method and the slot method. In the plug method the tibial attachments of the anterior and posterior horns are harvested with a small plug of bone that is inserted into holes made in the native knee (much like the mosaicplasty technique described for osteochondral autograft discussed later). These plugs are incorporated into the native bone. In the slot method, a cylindrical slot of bone is harvested. This slot incorporates the bony attachments of the anterior and posterior horns of the allograft. A similar cylinder of bone removed from the native tibia allows the allograft cylinder to be slotted in to fill the gap. The slotted bone becomes incorporated into the native bone. Initially, the allograft bone is of high signal intensity on fat-suppressed sequences and the interface between it and native bone is clearly visible. Over time, the allograft develops normal bony signal intensity and this interface disappears.

Because the lateral tibial plateau is smaller and there is less room to place separate plugs, slots are almost always used on the lateral side.

The degree of meniscal extrusion (the amount that the meniscus extends beyond the tibial margin on the coronal view) is one of the measurements associated with graft failure. The more it is extruded (and this can be measured in millimeters or percent), the more likely the meniscus is to have lost its integrity and the worse it will function to

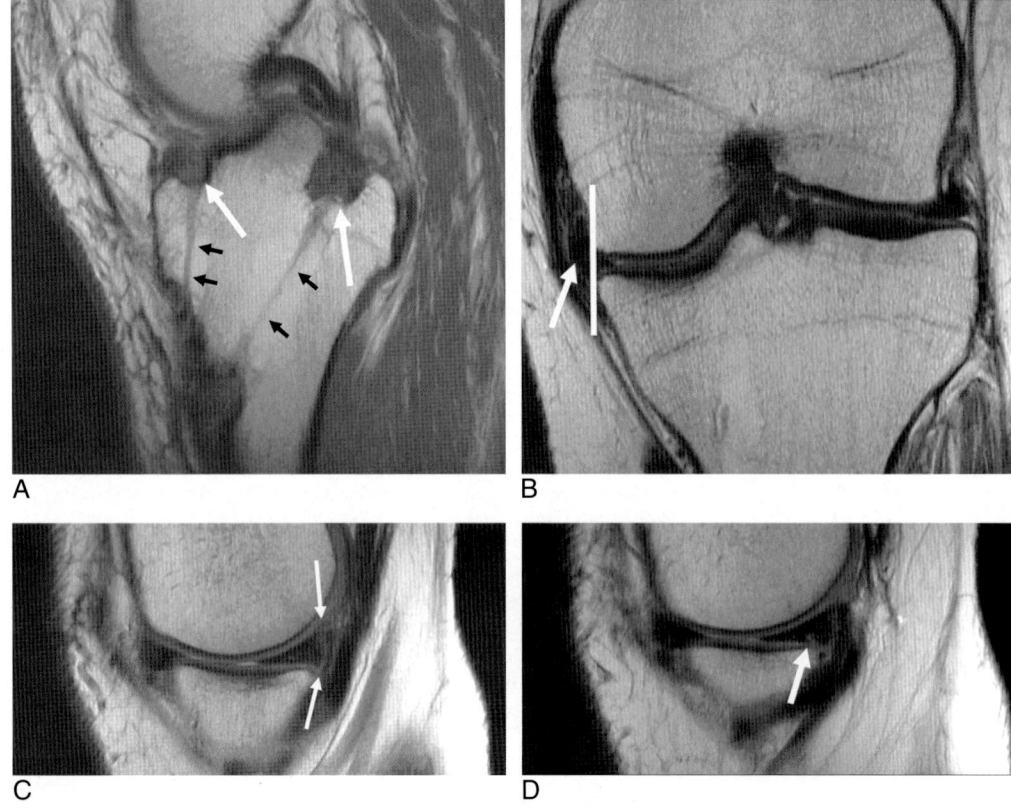

A B C D

■ **FIGURE 109-33** Medial meniscal allograft. One of the hardest parts about evaluating meniscal allografts is knowing that one has been placed. Evaluation for bone plug incorporation, capsular healing, meniscal integrity, and meniscal extrusion follow. **A,** Midline sagittal MR image shows the two plugs with suture lines (*small black arrows*) extending from them in this patient with a medial meniscal allograft. The plugs are not normal bony signal and may have necrosed (*white arrows*). **B,** Coronal MR image shows meniscal extrusion (*arrow*) beyond the medial joint line (*line*). **C,** Sagittal MR image shows persistent high signal at the capsule, indicating that it has not entirely incorporated (*small arrows*). **D,** Sagittal MR image shows peripheral high signal extending to the tibial articular surface reflecting subtle tear of the allograft meniscus (*arrow*). (©Hospital for Special Surgery, New York, New York.)

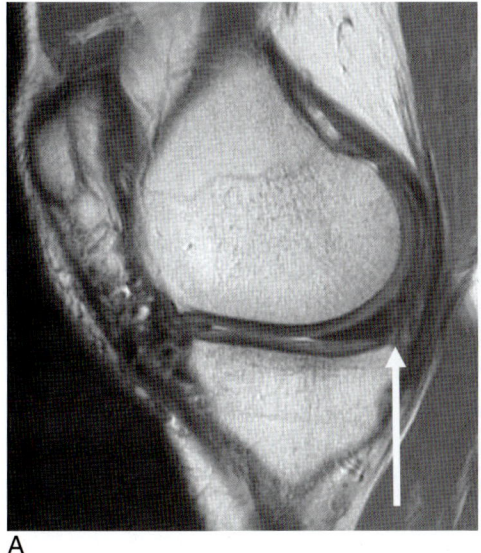 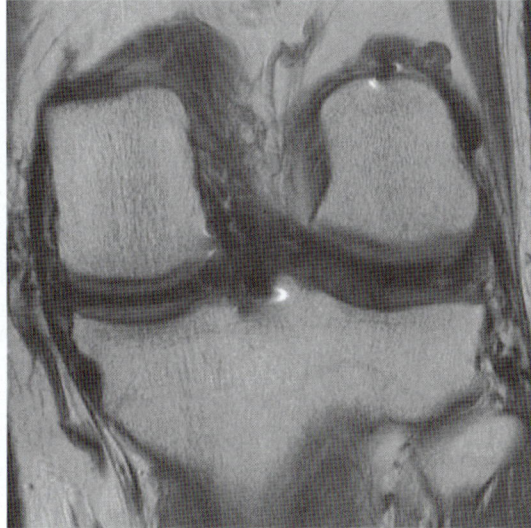

■ **FIGURE 109-34** Meniscal transplant. Sagittal (**A**) and coronal (**B**), intermediate echo time MR images 6 years after successful medial meniscal transplant using plugs. The meniscus is not torn or extruded. The anterior capsule and infrapatellar fat are scarred. The posterior capsule is healed (**A**, *arrow*). (©Hospital for Special Surgery, New York, New York.)

A   B

dissipate force. Some surgeons like to evaluate the knee with weight-bearing views to get an idea of extrusion in a more functional situation.[8]

Lastly, as with all joints, whether or not surgery has been performed, the rest of the joint must be evaluated for chondral loss, status of the other meniscus, and any other pathologic process.

Potential Complications and Radiologic Appearance

The specific complications of meniscal allograft involve each of the things that are listed as needing to be evaluated and have to do with failure of the allograft, either by poorly incorporating or intrinsically failing, such as

from tearing or losing its characteristics. There is also the possibility that the meniscus was poorly sized or poorly placed. The size that is requested for the meniscal allograft is determined by measurements made from preoperative radiographs.

Re-tears of the meniscal allograft have the same appearance as that of the native meniscus and are evaluated and described similarly (Figs. 109-35 and 109-36).

The capsular attachment may show dephasing related to suture. Otherwise the signal of the capsule varies from high to low on intermediate echo time, T2-weighted sequences. Fluid signal indicates capsular detachment.

Bone plugs or slots can fail to incorporate, yielding a persistent line of demarcation. This may occur when the bone becomes ischemic (persistent increased intermediate

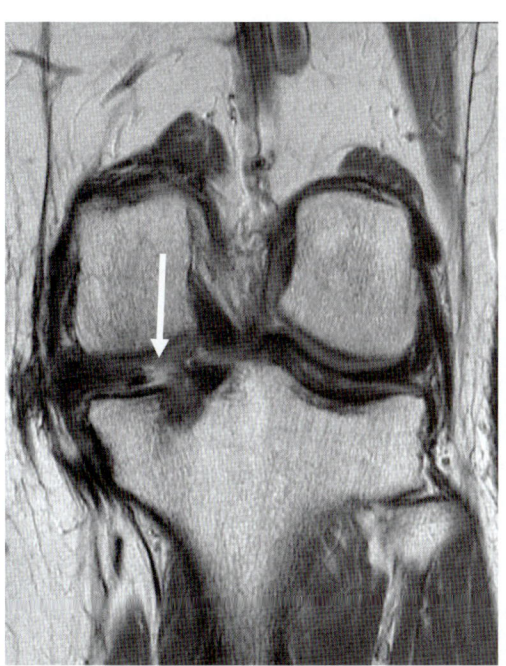 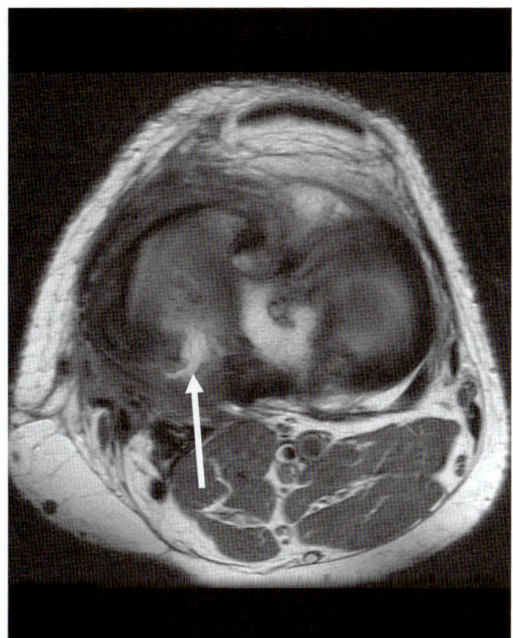

■ **FIGURE 109-35** Medial meniscal transplant, plug technique. Posterior coronal (**A**) and axial (**B**) MR images in a patient with meniscal transplant show a radial tear of the posterior horn (*arrows*). (©Hospital for Special Surgery, New York, New York.)

A   B

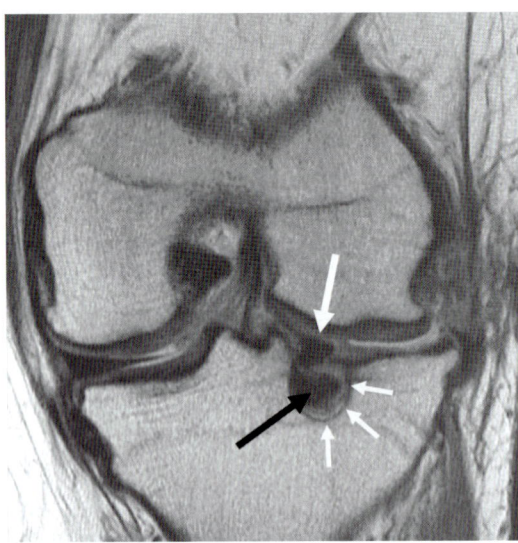

A

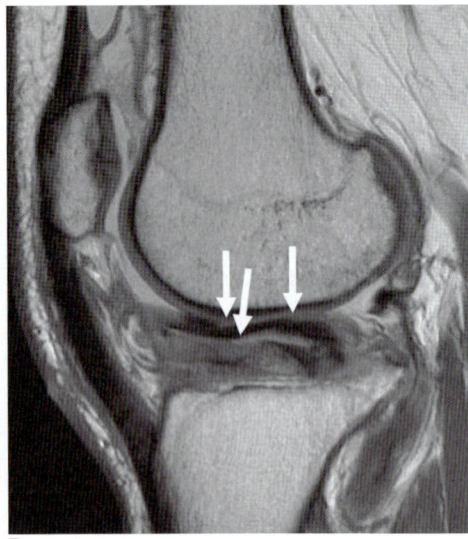

B

■ **FIGURE 109-36** Lateral meniscal transplant, slot technique. Bucket handle tear. Coronal (**A**) and axial (**B**) MR images in a patient with meniscal transplant show displacement of the entire meniscus into the intercondylar notch (*arrows*). The slot appears low in signal, indicating fibrosis (*black arrow*). An interface surrounding it indicates that it has not incorporated (*small arrows*). (©Hospital for Special Surgery, New York, New York.)

echo time T2-weighted signal) or necrotic (low signal on all sequences) (see Figs. 109-33 and 109-36).

The plugs should be placed near to the native tibial attachments so the meniscus can perform the same job with the same orientation. Sometimes it is hard to place the plugs exactly: many meniscal transplants have concomitant ACL grafts, and the room for plugs is limited. Occasionally, the allograft was badly sized and the allograft is too big or too small for the knee. It would appear that way if the meniscus is not getting to the edge of the joint (too small) or looks redundant.

CHONDRAL STIMULATION

Description

With the ability to see inside the knee joint, first with arthrotomy and arthrography and now with arthroscopy and MRI, we are identifying subtle abnormalities that might have previously gone undetected or tolerated. One of these abnormalities is articular chondral injuries that can cause pain, catching, clicking, or locking.

The simplest treatment for a chondral injury, and one that can be performed at the time of arthroscopy without preparation, is to make holes in the subchondral bone, promoting bleeding. The blood fills the chondral defect and promotes the creation of reparative cartilage (usually fibrocartilage rather than articular cartilage).

Chondroplasty involves smoothing the chondral edges and base of a chondral lesion. When the chondral abnormality extends to bone, stimulating bleeding is done by techniques called picking, abrasion arthroplasty, drilling, and microfracture, which are the same from an imaging standpoint.[11]

Indications, Contraindications, Purpose, and Underlying Mechanics

Chondral stimulation by making the subchondral bone bleed is performed for small (<2 cm²) full-thickness chondral defects. Reparative cartilage fills some or all of the defect, re-creating a smooth chondral surface to prevent further damage (Fig. 109-37).

Expected Appearance on Relevant Modalities

It is sometimes hard to tell on MRI that an area has undergone a chondral stimulation technique. Often the only clue is the characteristic reactive bone marrow signal under the chondral lesion (Fig. 109-38). This bone marrow signal lasts for many months after the procedure but is fairly localized to the chondral repair site. Often the stimulated bleeding causes small osteophytes, which appear as raised areas of bone under the healing chondral surface. The new cartilage is fibrocartilage and is usually initially higher in signal intensity than the native cartilage, but it may be lower or the same (Figs. 109-37 and 109-38).

The chondral surface itself tends to look like normal cartilage when the procedure is successful. There can be persistent defects of a portion or all of the original defect, and the new chondral surface may be irregular/fibrillated. It may have any of the characteristics of the native chondral defect: full-thickness loss, partial-thickness loss, and fibrillation.

Potential Complications and Radiologic Appearance

This procedure is generally safe and has very few complications. It also does not prevent additional, more involved, techniques to be performed in the patient's future. The only problem with the procedure is that it may not work in all instances.

MOSAICPLASTY/OATS

Description

Moasicplasty and OATS (osteoarticular transfer system) are essentially the same. They involve taking

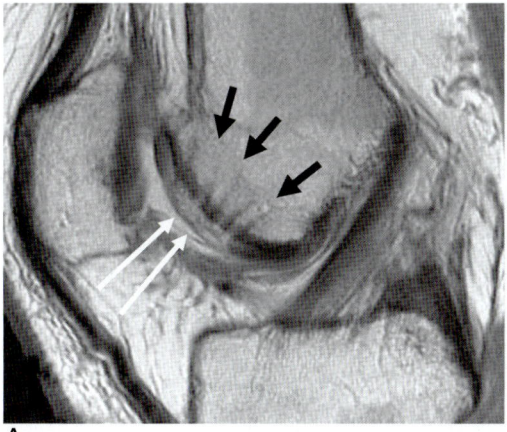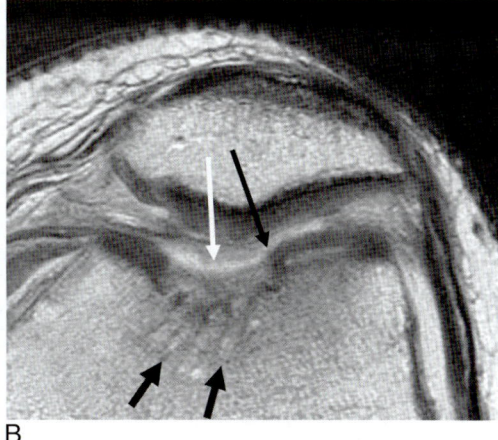

A B

■ **FIGURE 109-37** Chondral stimulation. Sagittal, intermediate echo time MR images of the medial compartment without (**A**) and with (**B**) fat suppression of the same patient as in Figure 109-25. Before the PCL reconstruction. Picking has stimulated reparative fibrocartilage that is fibrillated and of high signal intensity (*long arrow*). Note the reactive bone marrow signal that can last for many months (*short arrow*). Subchondral bone irregularity and overgrowth is not uncommon. (©Hospital for Special Surgery, New York, New York.)

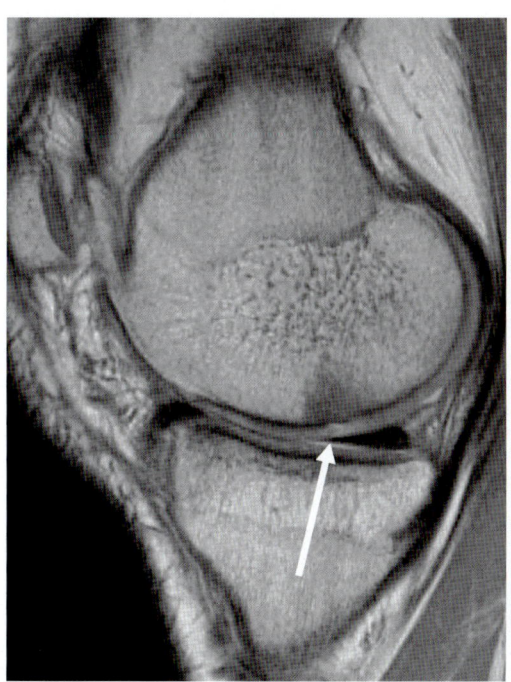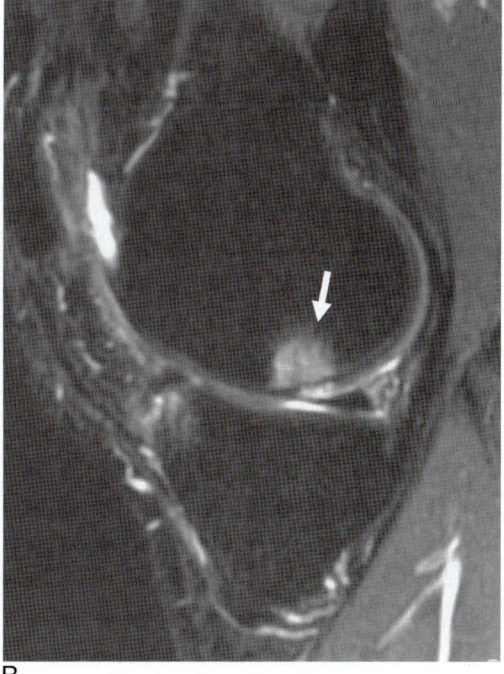

A B

■ **FIGURE 109-38** Lateral collateral ligament and ACL reconstruction. Medial meniscectomy. **A** and **B**, Coronal, intermediate echo time images show a portion of the LCL and ACL reconstructions (*small arrows*). The medial meniscal body (*long arrow*) is small, smaller than the lateral, indicating meniscal resection (unless a displaced meniscal fragment is evident). (©Hospital for Special Surgery, New York, New York.)

osteochondral plugs from one aspect of the joint to another part, usually of the same joint. In the knee, a round plug up to 1 cm wide and about 1 cm deep is removed from a region of the trochlea and placed into the region of chondral defect that has been prepared by having a hole drilled of the same size. The donor site fills in with bone and reparative fibrocartilage. The hope is that the cartilage at the receiver site blends with the adjacent cartilage and a new smooth surface is created.[12]

Recently, scaffolds have been created to use in the donor sites to promote healing, or even as a treatment for a chondral injury. These scaffolds are resorbable and designed to promote healing.

Indications, Contraindications, Purpose, and Underlying Mechanics

Mosaicplasty is usually used for lesions larger than microfracture or when microfracture has failed. The hope is to produce a normal hyaline cartilage surface. As with other techniques, the lesions should be focal. Multiple plugs may be needed to fill a defect (Fig. 109-39).

Expected Appearance on Relevant Modalities

There are two sites to be evaluated: the donor site and the recipient site. The donor site, if not filled with a scaffolding

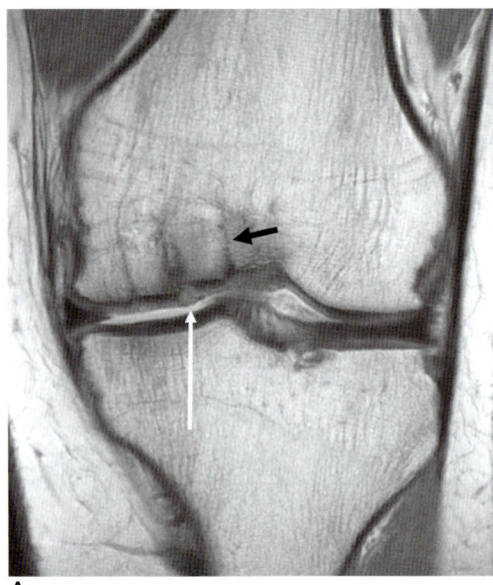

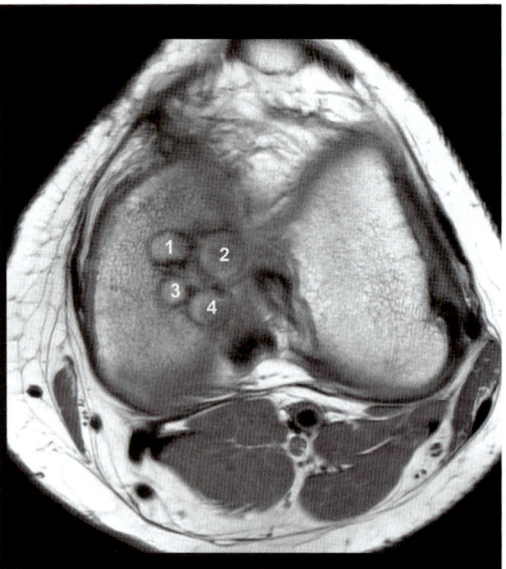

■ **FIGURE 109-39** Mosaicplasty for osteochondritis dissecans. Coronal (**A**) and axial (**B**) MR images show at least four osteochondral autograft plugs placed to treat an osteochondral lesion in the medial femoral condyle. The space between the plugs has filled in with fibrocartilage (**A**, *long white arrow*), and the articular surface is smooth. The interface between the plugs and native bone (**A**, *black arrow*) is still visible, but not wide, and the signal from the plugs is of normal bone. (©Hospital for Special Surgery, New York, New York.)

plug, looks initially like a hole and gradually, over a few months, fills in. The site is of high signal intensity on fat-suppressed images, with grafted sites being lower in signal intensity.

At the receiver site, the bone and cartilage are both important. The plug is initially of high signal intensity and becomes of lower signal intensity over time. An interface between native and transferred bone (or adjacent plugs) is, at first, sharp. Over time, the interface disappears as the bone becomes incorporated, similar to the bone plugs of bone-tendon-bone cruciate ligament reconstructions or meniscal allografts. The cartilage should have the appearance of normal hyaline cartilage with a smooth interface with the surface of surrounding cartilage. Whereas the surface should be flush with the adjacent cartilage, the thickness of the cartilage may be different. This is normal

because the thickness of cartilage in different parts of the knee does vary (Fig. 109-40). Sometimes, because of the geometry of the defect the plugs do not fill the entire defect and there are some gaps. The hope is that cartilage spreads between the native and transferred cartilage to fill these gaps (see Fig. 109-39).

In the cases in which scaffold plugs are used to fill the primary defect, they have a similar appearance to those used to fill donor sites (Fig. 109-41). Some of the composite plugs (those with different substances on the surface and deep layer) look remarkably like autograft plugs on MRI.

The donor sites should fill in with time, with reparative fibrocartilage at the site of the original defect (Fig. 109-42). These tend to be at the peripheral trochlear where there is less stress on the cartilage.

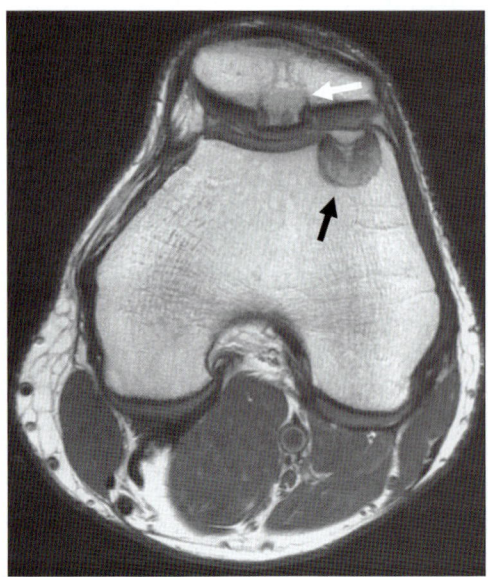

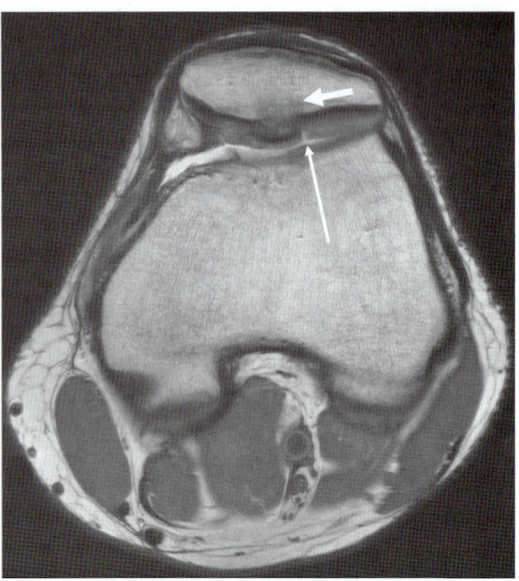

■ **FIGURE 109-40** Mosaicplasty. Axial, intermediate echo time images show patellar osteochondral autograft (*white arrow*) and trochlear harvest site (*black arrow*). Because the donor site (trochlear) cartilage is thinner than the recipient site (patella), the autograft plug is proud so that the cartilage surface can be flush. Note the small persistent defect at the interface of the autograft with the native patellar cartilage. The autograft is mostly incorporated, without an obvious demarcation between the autograft plug and recipient bone (*long thin arrow*). The cartilage over the autograft plug looks normal. (©Hospital for Special Surgery, New York, New York.)

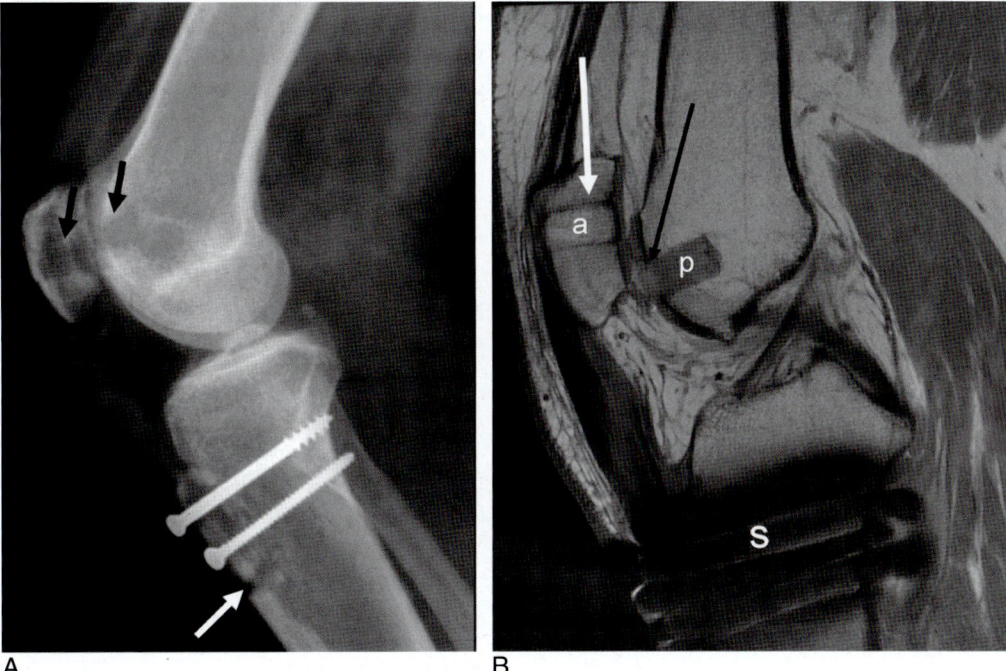

A   B

■ **FIGURE 109-41** Patellar realignment and cartilage repair. Lateral radiograph (**A**) shows screws fixating the tibial tubercle osteotomy performed for distal realignment. This has not yet entirely healed, because there is a demarcation between the native bone and the osteotomized portion (*white arrow*). The defects from cartilage repair are also evident, especially the trochlear harvest site and a patellar site. On the corresponding sagittal, midline, intermediate echo time MR image (**B**), artifact from the two screws is present (s). The patellar tendon is thick and has high signal intensity. It has not entirely remodeled since surgery. There is a patellar osteochondral autograft and a trochlear biphasic artificial composite graft. On the autograft (a), the cartilage surface is smooth and the cartilage itself appears normal. The bone signal is normal. The interface with native bone is visible, indicating that the graft has not yet entirely incorporated (*long white arrow*). At the artificial plug (p), barely discernible on this image, is the interface between the two substances that make up the graft (*long black arrow*). (©Hospital for Special Surgery, New York, New York.)

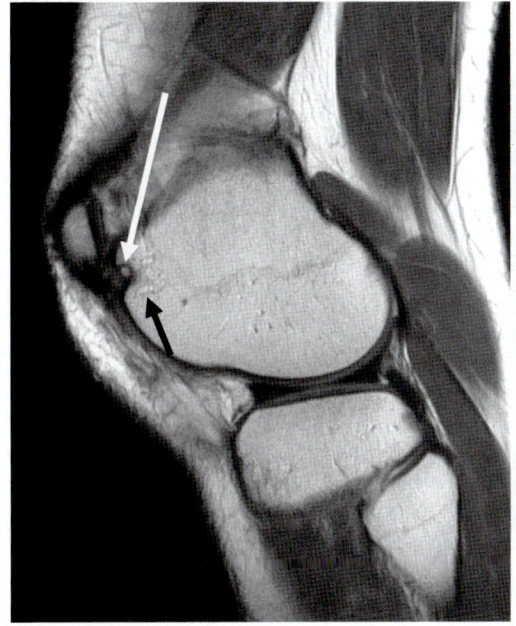

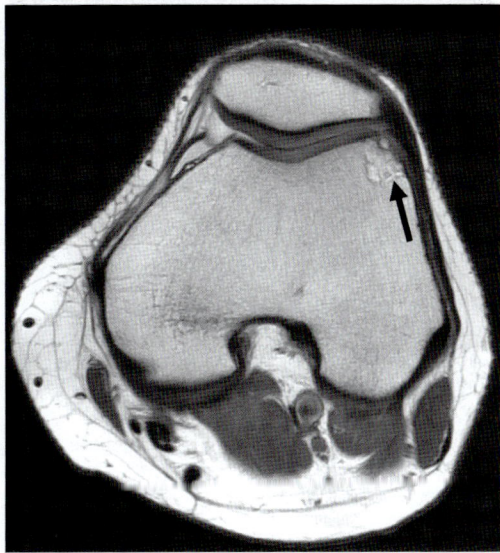

A   B

■ **FIGURE 109-42** Healed graft harvest. Sagittal (**A**) and axial (**B**) intermediate echo time MR images show healed harvest site (*black arrows*) for osteochondral autograft taken for ankle mosaicplasty. A small cortical defect at the articular surface (*long white arrow*) shows mild irregularity of the overlying reparative fibrocartilage. (©Hospital for Special Surgery, New York, New York.)

Potential Complications and Radiologic Appearance

The problems with osteochondral autografts are mostly those of geometry. Sometimes the curvature of the donor site may be different from that of the receiver site, causing an irregular surface. The graft may also be placed slightly proud or, less importantly, slightly deep.

The cartilage over the donor plug usually looks normal. It can, however, become softened or fibrillated or come off. The bone plug may, rarely, slowly or poorly incorporate or become necrotic and appear as low signal intensity on all pulse sequences.

AUTOLOGOUS CHONDROCYTE IMPLANTATION

Description

Autologous chondrocyte implantation (ACI) is an alternative to mosaicplasty for lesions that are too big for microfracture or in whom microfracture has failed. The procedure involves harvesting normal chondrocytes, growing them in cell culture in vitro, and placing them onto a chondral defect. They are usually injected underneath a piece of periosteum that is sewn on to keep them in place over the defect.

Indications, Contraindications, Purpose, and Underlying Mechanics

Some surgeons and institutions prefer ACI to mosaicplasty and vice versa. They have similar indications, and neither is clearly better than the other. A mosaicplasty can be performed if ACI fails.

Expected Appearance on Relevant Modalities

With high-resolution scanning, one sometimes see the periosteal flap, especially if it is thickened. Underneath the flap, the cartilage should be similar in signal to normal hyaline cartilage but may vary. The morphology, although often a bit proud, should be smooth as should the interface with adjacent cartilage (Fig. 109-43).[13]

Potential Complications and Radiologic Appearance

One potential problem with ACI is that chondrocytes may not take well to the underlying bone and not grow. The other potential problem has to do with the periosteal graft. It can tear and displace. It may also hypertrophy, sometimes to the thickness of normal cartilage, and interfere with chondrocyte adherence or growth.

OSTEOCHONDRAL ALLOGRAFT

Description

When an osteochondral defect is too large for other chondral repair techniques, the only option is to replace the osteochondral surface with an allograft. The allograft, which includes bone and overlying cartilage, is placed into an appropriately sized defect, in the area where the chondral defect is, usually on the femoral condyle of the recipient. The allograft should heal to the native bone and restore the articular surface, ideally blending the articular surfaces of the allograft and host cartilage.

Osteochondral allograft may be used after other techniques have failed. Eventually, a good artificial scaffold will replace the need for allograft.

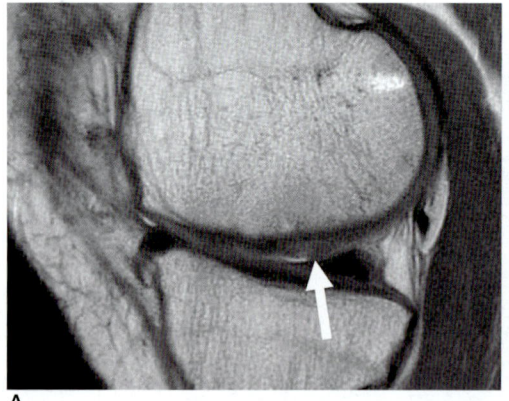
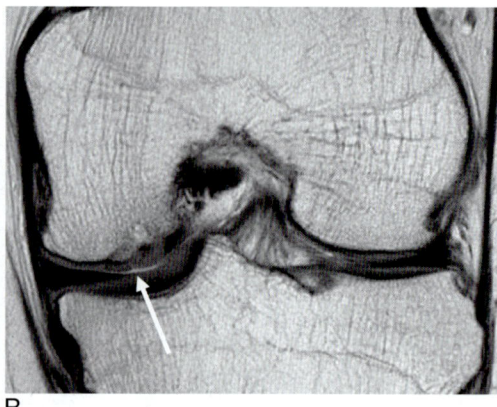

A   B

■ **FIGURE 109-43**   Autologous chondrocyte implantation. Sagittal (**A**) and coronal (**B**), intermediate echo time MR images after the procedure. Often the chondral repair site is slightly proud and bulging initially (**A**, *fat arrow*). The periosteal flap is not well seen here. There is a small area of focal thinning (**B**, *thin arrow*), but the surface appears well covered. The patient, however, subsequently had a mosaicplasty because of the failure of this procedure. (©Hospital for Special Surgery, New York, New York.)

Indications, Contraindications, Purpose, and Underlying Mechanics

Osteochondral allografts are used on large but isolated chondral defects on one articular surface. Ideally, they restore the articular surface and heal over time.

Expected Appearance on Relevant Modalities

Like autograft graft and meniscal plugs, initially the allograft bone shows high signal with a sharp interface of native bone. Over time, the interface becomes less sharp and gradually the allograft and native bone are indistinguishable (Fig. 109-44). Ideally, the articular surfaces are smooth and the geometry of the allograft is similar to the geometry of the native bone it is replacing.[14]

Potential Complications and Radiologic Appearance

The three main problems with allografts are incongruity, necrosis, and loss of overlying cartilage.

It can be difficult to appropriately size an allograft, given differences in geometry of the knees of different patients as well as the varied configuration of the bone of different parts of the knee and thickness of articular cartilage. It is difficult to create exactly the same size allograft as the recipient site, and the contour of the allograft may be different from that of the native bone. This incongruity will not prevent healing but may cause small stepoffs at the articular surface and variable pressures on weight-bearing and lead to chondral loss.

The allografts may not incorporate well and may undergo ischemia and eventually necrose. The articular surface of the allograft may also fracture and collapse.

Lastly, the cartilage over the allograft may become damaged or lost. Although some of the chondrocytes die during processing, the rest regenerate and multiply.

Rejection is not a common problem, but mainly it is caused by ischemia or necrosis.

OSTEOCHONDRITIS DISSECANS REPAIR

Description

Osteochondritis dissecans, described elsewhere, is an osteochondral defect that occurs in characteristic locations and is probably post-traumatic. The fragment may loosen and displace, creating an osteochondral defect.

If the fragment appears loose but has not displaced or if it has displaced but appears viable, it can be reattached with thin absorbable nails whose head is sunken below the chondral surface. If the articular surface is intact, the lesion can be drilled from the nonarticular side to try to promote healing.

Indications, Contraindications, Purpose, and Underlying Mechanics

Because osteochondritis dissecans can leave a large defect, repairing or replacing native bone is beneficial. In younger patients especially, if a thin piece of bone, even if invisible on imaging, is on a chondral surface, it can heal if reattached. If the bone has not displaced, drilling may be attempted to stimulate adherence of the fragment.

When the defect and viable bone are not present on the fragment or the fragment is not available to be replaced, symptomatic patients may undergo the chondral repair techniques described previously.

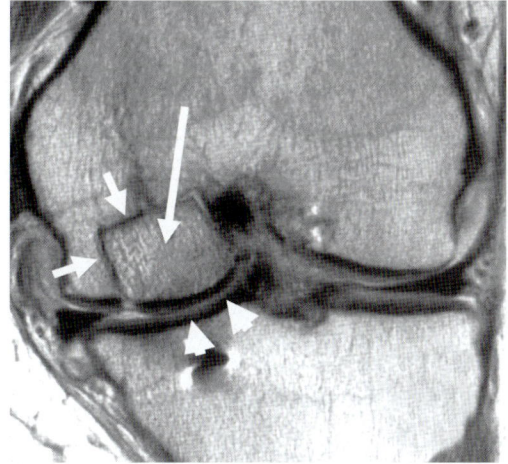 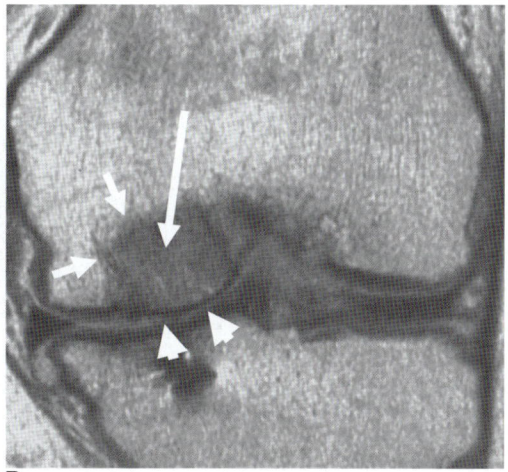

A   B

■ **FIGURE 109-44**   Osteochondral allograft. Medial femoral condylar fresh frozen allograft (*long arrow*) at 10 days (**A**) and 6 months (**B**) after placement. Initially, the graft has normal signal intensity. There is a sharp interface between the allograft and native bone (*small arrows*). The articular cartilage is intact (*arrowheads*). At 6 months, the interface is less sharp (partial incorporation) (*small arrows*) but the graft has lost its normal signal—not low enough signal to be fibrotic and not normal enough to be fully incorporated. The articular cartilage is partly lost (*arrowheads*). (©Hospital for Special Surgery, New York, New York.)

Expected Appearance on Relevant Modalities

The nails used for fixation have a typical appearance on MRI as thin, straight, low signal intensity lines. They are radiolucent, so they are not seen on radiographs. Drilling can also have the appearance of thin, low signal intensity lines. The repaired fragment initially has high signal intensity and irregularity at the interface with underlying bone, but eventually it should heal and blend in with the underlying bone (Fig. 109-45).

If the overlying chondral surface deteriorates, or if the defect is left untreated, the subchondral bone, with time, becomes of normal signal intensity but a defect remains in overlying cartilage.

Potential Complications and Radiologic Appearance

The potential complication of treated osteochondritis dissecans is that the treatment may fail: the piece may displace or collapse to have the same appearance as untreated osteochondritis dissecans. The osteochondral fragment may not become incorporated; it may displace and become a loose intra-articular body, or it may collapse. This may necessitate the use of mosaicplasty to try to fill the defect (see Fig. 109-39).

ARTHROPLASTY

Description

Total arthroplasty is one of the most successful operations conceived. Arthroplasty, or joint replacement, uses various materials to replace a patient's normal joints. In the knee, a portion of the patient's normal distal femur, proximal tibia, and patella is shaved away to create a flat surface on which metal pieces are fitted and glued. A piece of polyethylene between the metal surfaces helps them glide against each other and distributes the load. The design of artificial joints continues to evolve. Current arthroplasty can be performed through a relatively small incision.

The two major types of arthroplasty are constrained (Fig. 109-46), in which the patient's normal ligaments are not used to support the knee structure, and unconstrained, in which the patient's normal ligaments are used to stabilize the joint (Fig. 109-47).[15] Some unconstrained prostheses are able to spare the patient's native posterior cruciate ligament.

Recently, replacements of one compartment have made a resurgence. The unicondylar arthroplasty, or partial replacement, is a less invasive procedure and can delay the need for total replacement in patients with one compartment disease.

Indications, Contraindications, Purpose, and Underlying Mechanics

The primary indication for arthroplasty is arthrosis, whether degenerative or inflammatory. The arthroplasty replaces articular surfaces and restores alignment. Generally, it works quiet well and has been lasting longer because of advances in the materials used.

Another indication for arthroplasty is the surgical removal of a lesion, usually an osseous neoplasm, that results in joint resection. Extensive reconstructions may require both soft tissue and bony reconstructions, and the use of a custom prostheses, especially in growing children, may be necessary.

A unicondylar arthroplasty (partial knee replacement) is used in patients with only medial or lateral compartment arthrosis as an alternative to osteotomy to relieve pain, improve alignment, and delay the need for a total arthroplasty. The implant should not be used if there is arthrosis of the other compartment.

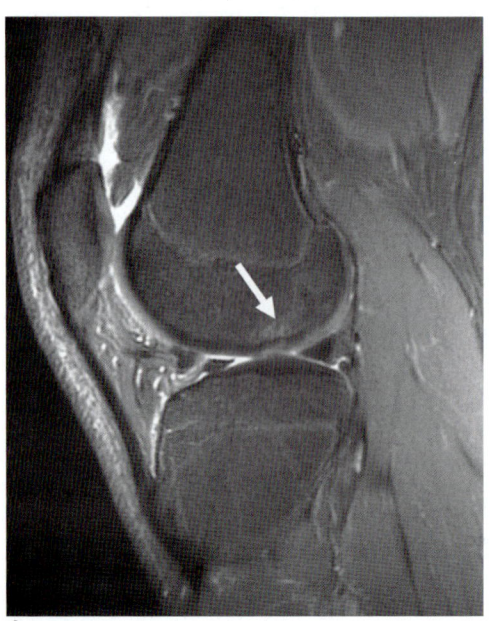

A

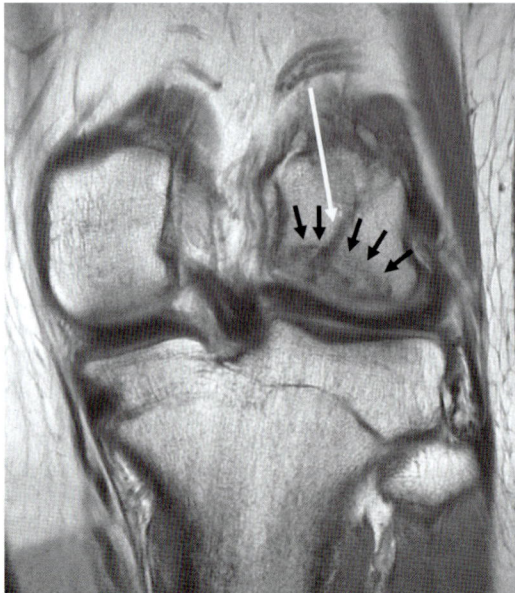

B

■ **FIGURE 109-45** Healed osteochondritis dissecans. **A,** Sagittal, fat-suppressed MR image shows only minimal reactive signal around lesion of osteochondritis dissecans that has been pinned. **B,** On the coronal MR image, black arrows outline the lesion, which exhibits no clear interface with the native bone. One of the pins used for fixation the lesion is visible (*long arrow*). The articular surface is smooth. (©Hospital for Special Surgery, New York, New York.)

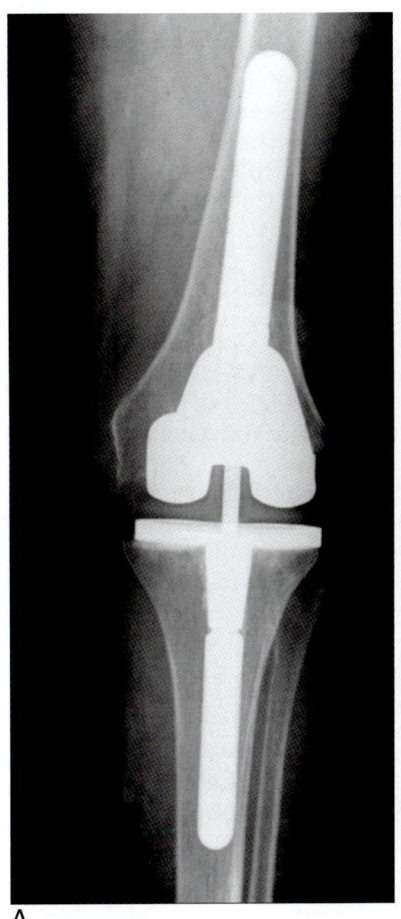

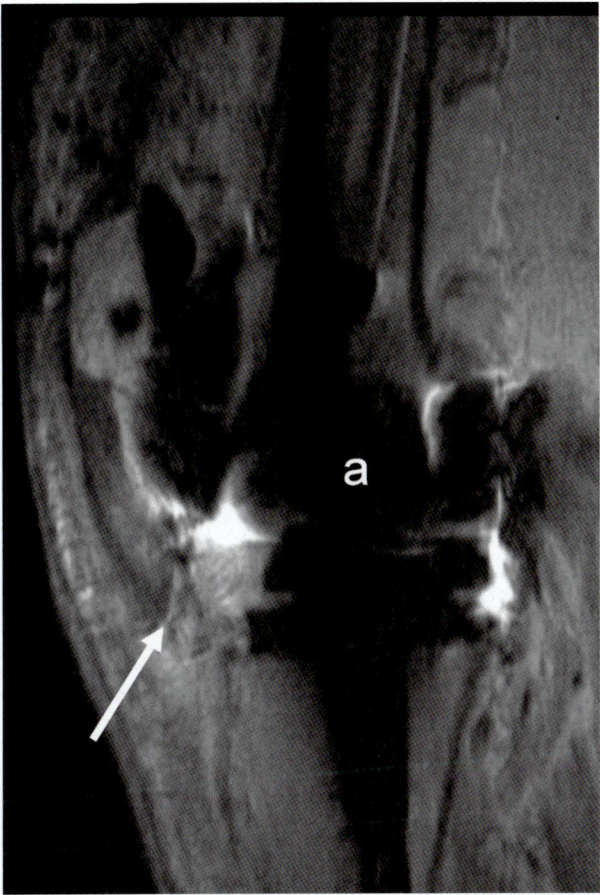

A

B

■ **FIGURE 109-46** Patellar tendon tear. Frontal radiograph (**A**) shows a constrained long-stem knee arthroplasty. Note that the radiograph should include the ends of the stems, no matter how long, to exclude a periprosthetic fracture. Motion-degraded sagittal MR image (**B**) of the same patient shows artifact (a) from the prosthesis and a distal patellar tendon tear (*arrow*). Ultrasound imaging may have been a better choice for evaluating this lesion. (©Hospital for Special Surgery, New York, New York.)

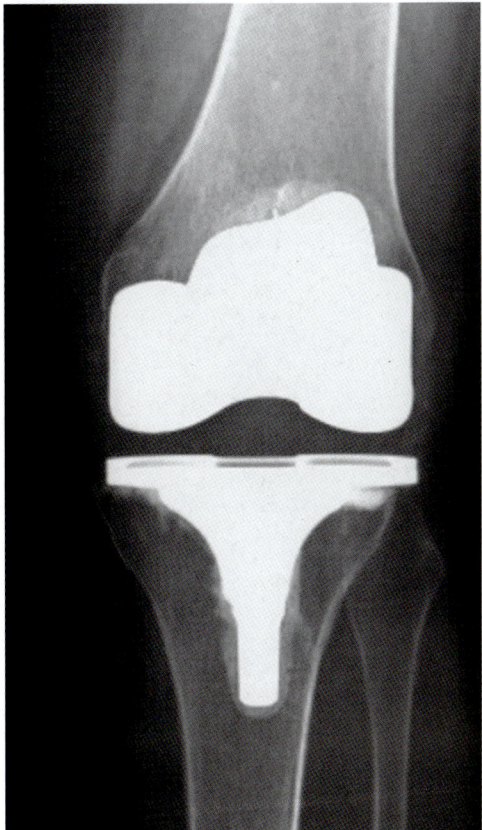

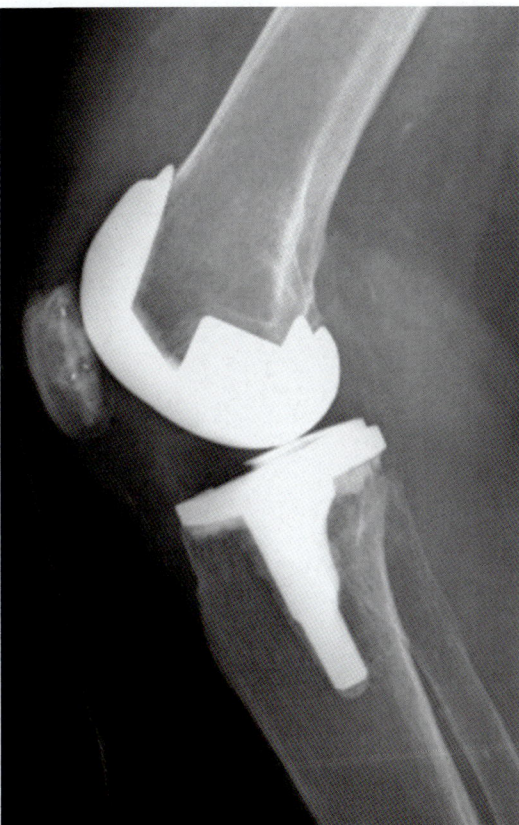

A

B

■ **FIGURE 109-47** Normal knee arthroplasty. Standing frontal (**A**) and lateral (**B**) radiographs of the knee show knee arthroplasty in good position, without bone resorption around the femoral, tibial, or patellar components, all of which are cemented. (©Hospital for Special Surgery, New York, New York.)

Expected Appearance on Relevant Modalities

In a normal arthroplasty, the joint alignment is normal. The arthroplasty is radiopaque, because it is metal, with the space in between the femoral and tibial components being radiolucent (see Fig. 109-47). The constrained arthroplasty has an additional metal piece between the femoral and tibial components (see Fig. 109-46).

When an arthroplasty fails or needs to be replaced, a larger component with more extension into the tibia and femur is used (see Fig. 109-46). Often a layer of cement is used around the arthroplasty that is radiopaque (because of the addition of barium to the methylmethacrylate that is usually used).

Initial radiographs are taken as a baseline for comparison of future radiographs of the joint. Generally no more than 2 mm of lucency between the cement and bone or between the cement and component is present. If the immediate postoperative radiographs show more than 2 mm of lucency, then subsequent radiographs can as well. An increase in the amount of lucency suggests that there is bone absorption (osteolysis), which often occurs from component wear and the body's reaction to the particles produced by that wear (particle disease). The patella should be aligned on the femoral component.

On CT, extensive artifact comes from the instrumentation but the components can be discerned, as can the underlying bone.[16,17] On MRI, there are extensive artifacts but the interface is visible between the tibial and patellar components and the underlying bone. Patience, however, will be rewarded. As one continues to look at the images (after the initial hesitation and disbelief that they are at all useful), the ligaments and the quadriceps tendon become discernible and should be intact. The bone/cement interfaces will become clear and sharp (though sometimes they are irregular, depending on the shape the cement takes) (Fig. 109-48). There will be anterior and infrapatellar scar related to the arthrotomy.[12]

Ultrasound examination can be used to accurately measure the width of the polyethylene piece to look for wear (thinning).[18] Ultrasonography can also be used for evaluation of the quadriceps tendon and the ligaments around the knee, which should be echogenic.

On bone scintigraphy, moderate uptake around a knee prosthesis can continue for up to a year. Thereafter, mild uptake can continue for the life of the prosthesis.

Unicondylar replacements radiographically have smaller tibial and femoral components that should be aligned and, as in total arthroplasty, should be without lucency around the cement.

Potential Complications and Radiologic Appearance

Complications include loosening/osteolysis, infection, fracture, and recurrence of other pathologic processes such as tumor and synovitis. Tendon and ligament injuries may also occur.

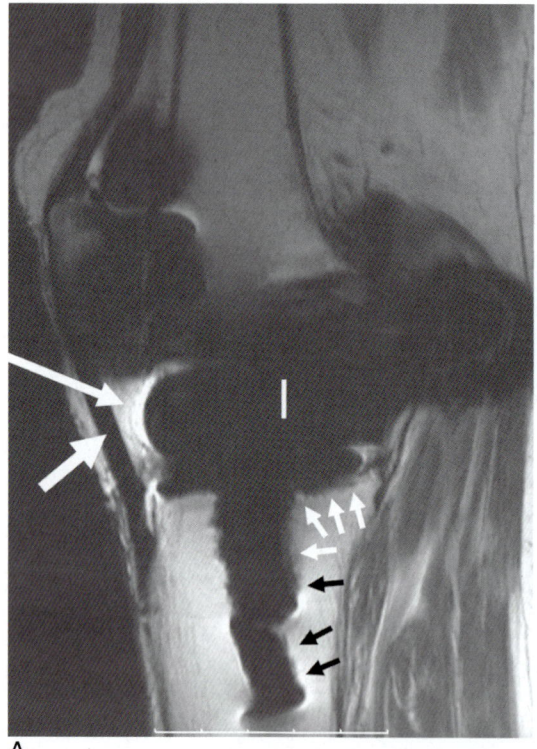 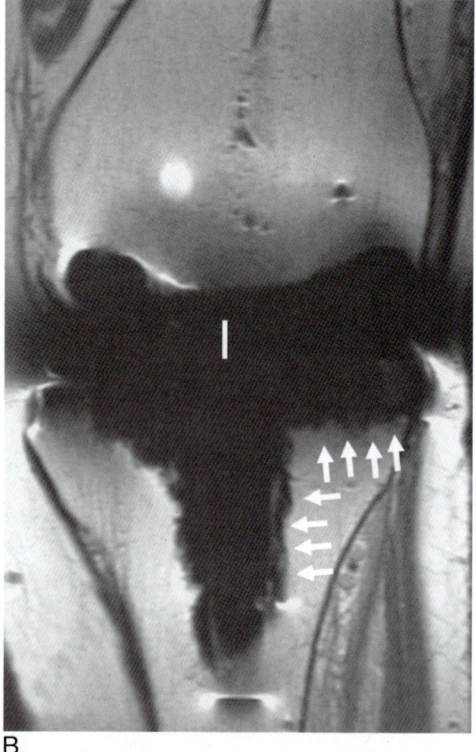

A   B

■ **FIGURE 109-48** Normal knee arthroplasty. Sagittal (**A**) and coronal (**B**), intermediate echo time MR images of knee arthroplasty. The metallic implant causes artifact (I). In addition to evaluating the collateral ligaments, the patellar tendon (*arrow*), and the infrapatellar fat (*long arrow*), careful evaluation of the cement bone interface (*small arrows*) can detect small areas of osteolysis. High signal (especially on fat-suppressed images, not shown) normally extends well up into the femoral diaphysis for months after surgery. (©Hospital for Special Surgery, New York, New York.)

On radiography, fractures are apparent in the distal femur or proximal tibia with or without displacement as it would be without the instrumentation (Fig. 109-49). Patellar fracture around the component is not uncommon and may or may not be visible on radiographs. Cross-sectional imaging such as CT, MRI, or ultrasonography may be necessary (see Fig. 109-49).

Osteolysis is evidenced as increased lucency between the bone and cement or bone and metal. Large defects are visible on radiography (Fig. 109-50). Smaller lucencies can be detected on CT and MRI where well-defined regions of bone loss indicate osteolysis (see Fig. 109-50). With extensive osteolysis, the components may become loose and need to be replaced (Figs. 109-51 and 109-52). The

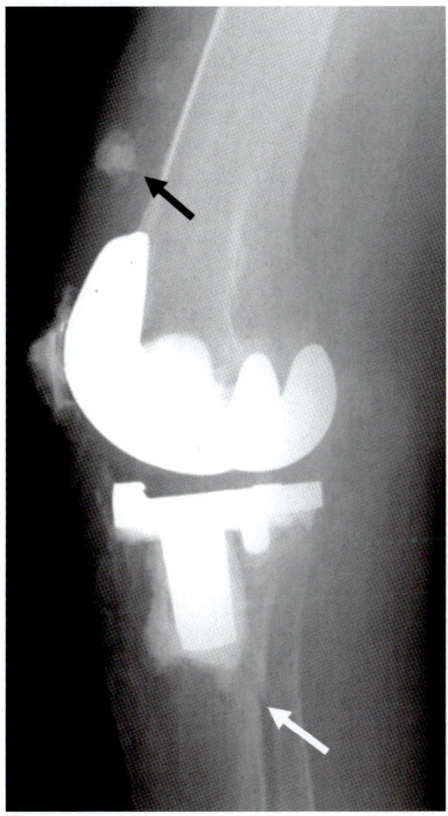
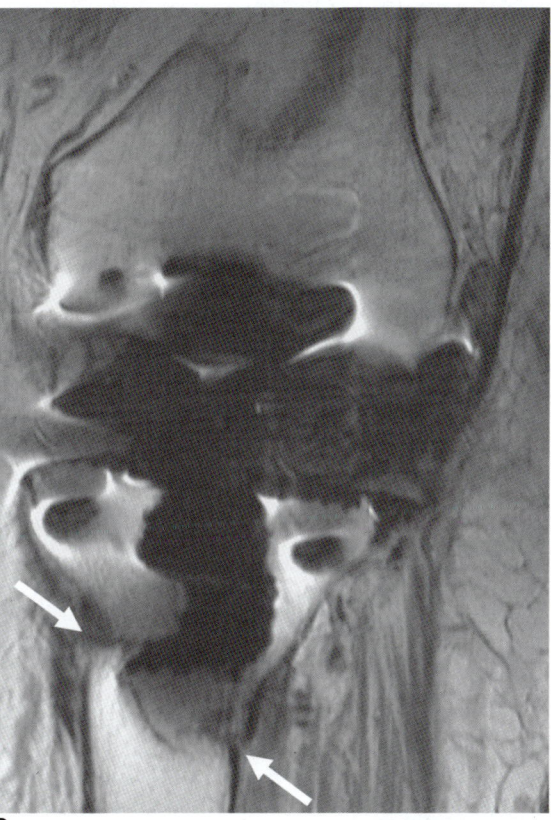

A B

■ **FIGURE 109-49** Fracture. Oblique lateral (**A**) radiograph and coronal intermediate echo time MR image (**B**) show periprosthetic fracture of the tibia (*white arrows*). Patellar fracture (*black arrow*) is also evident. (©Hospital for Special Surgery, New York, New York.)

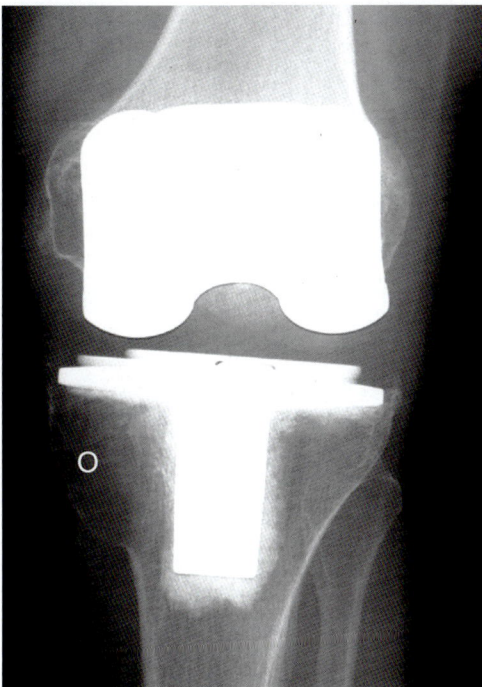
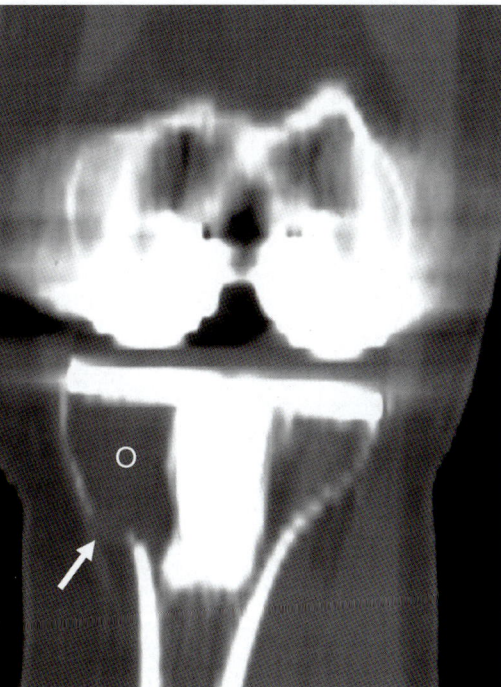

A B

■ **FIGURE 109-50** Osteolysis around knee arthroplasty. Frontal radiograph (**A**) shows relative lucency and mild cortical expansion under the medial aspect of the tibial tray, representing osteolysis (O). This is better defined on CT, in which coronal reformatted imaging defines the area of osteolysis and demonstrates an area of cortical breech (*arrow*). (*Courtesy of Dr. Kevin Math, Beth Israel Hospital, New York, NY.*)

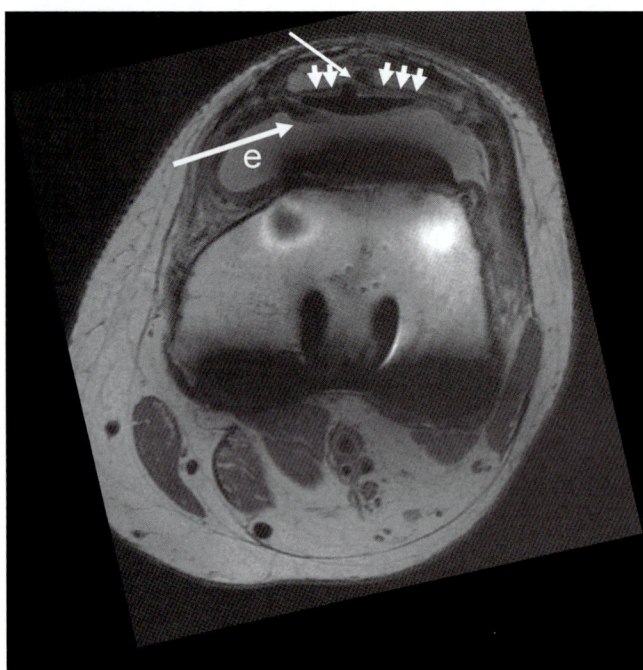

■ **FIGURE 109-51** Loose patellar component. Axial, intermediate echo time MR image shows high signal between the native bone ant the low signal patellar component/cement, indicating osteolysis. Fracture through the cement confirms loosening (*thin arrow*). There is effusion (e). Synovial tissue (*long arrow*) extends around the patellar component and can be the source of pain and clunking. (©Hospital for Special Surgery, New York, New York.)

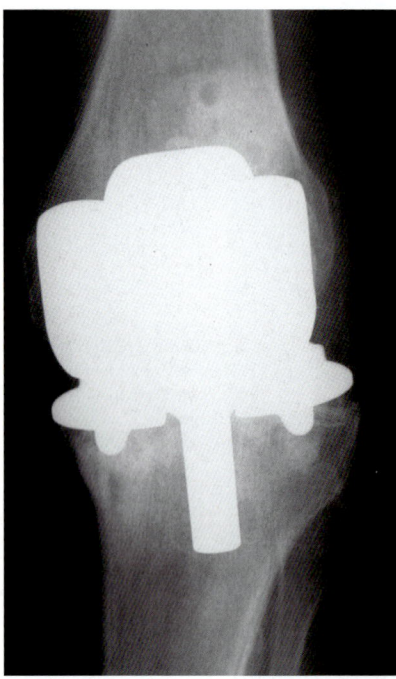

■ **FIGURE 109-52** Loosening of knee arthroplasty. Frontal radiograph of the knee shows malalignment of the tibial component with the tibia, indicating loosening of the tibial component. Fracture of the medial tibial plateau with collapse may have a similar appearance in the acute setting with underlying osteoporosis. (*Courtesy of Dr. Kevin Math, Beth Israel Hospital, New York, NY.*)

osteolysis can lead to a dense synovitis-particle disease. If a component is loose, bone scan should show increased uptake. Positron emission tomography, reportedly a technique that can be used to identify loosening, is not widely employed.[19]

Infection is suggested on MRI when there is abnormal increased signal extending into the soft tissues (Fig. 109-53). Infection can also cause osteolysis, and aspiration is required to confirm this diagnosis. However, rapid osteolysis on radiographs or CT suggests infection. Bone scan with be diffusely and intensely positive, and an indium-labeled white blood cell study will also be positive (and incongruent with a bone marrow uptake from sulfur colloid).[20]

Quadriceps and patellar tendon rupture has similar appearance on ultrasonography, MRI, and radiographs as if it were the native knee (see Fig. 109-46).

Recurrent synovitis may be apparent on MRI and is best seen on the axial images anteriorly around the patella. MRI may also show subtle abnormalities, such as synovial hypertrophy within the patellofemoral joint that can cause a click or clunk (see Fig. 109-51). Dense scar tissue within the infrapatellar fat, easily identified by MRI, can cause pain and stiffness (Fig. 109-54).

QUADRICEPS REPAIR

Description

The quadriceps mechanism, including the quadriceps muscle tendon junction, the quadriceps tendon, the patella, and the patellar tendon (the infrapatellar portion of the quadriceps tendon), can fail. Injuries of the muscle tendon junction and nondisplaced patellar fractures are usually treated nonoperatively.[21]

Tendon tears tend to occur in abnormal tendon, and both complete quadriceps and patellar tendon tears are usually (and have been for over 100 years) treated surgically. Usually, the repair is primary and often includes holes made through the patella for reinforcement. Rarely, tendon augmentation is necessary. The repair can be made with absorbable, nonabsorbable, or wire suture.

The quadriceps often requires augmentation rather than a simple primary repair. Occasionally the patellar tendon is reconstructed rather than repaired.

Indications, Contraindications, Purpose, and Underlying Mechanics

The quadriceps mechanism is the primary knee extender. With lack of use, the muscle rapidly atrophies. Complete tears of the quadriceps and patellar tendons, and partial tears if causing weakness, require repair to restore function and prevent atrophy. Patellar fractures are discussed later in the chapter.

Expected Appearance on Relevant Modalities

The patellar and quadriceps tendons are unusual in that shortly after repair they may still appear markedly abnormal on imaging: on MRI they are thick and have high signal intensity and have the appearance of severe tendonitis.

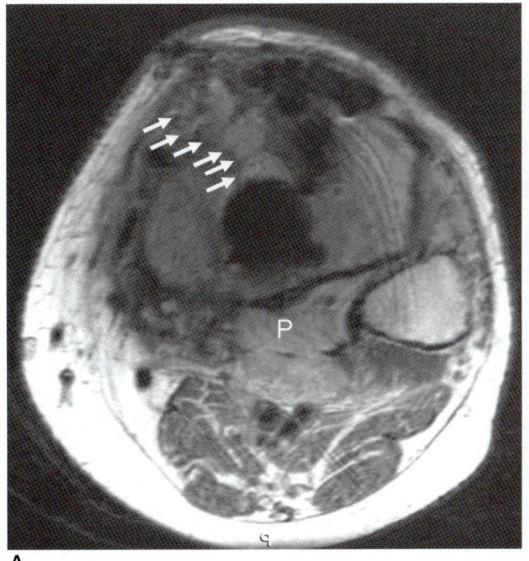

A

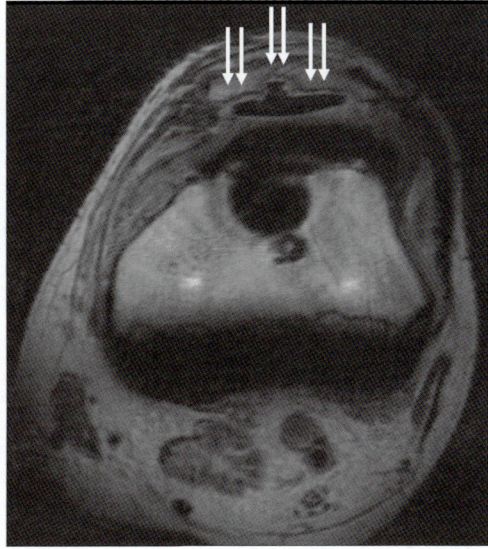

B

■ **FIGURE 109-53**   Infected total knee replacement. Axial intermediate echo time MR images. **A,** High signal representing abscess anterior to the tibial stem extends through bone toward skin (*small arrows*). Posteriorly, reactive signal permeates the popliteus muscle (P). **B,** The patellar component is loose with high signal between the bone and the cement (*long arrows*). (©Hospital for Special Surgery, New York, New York.)

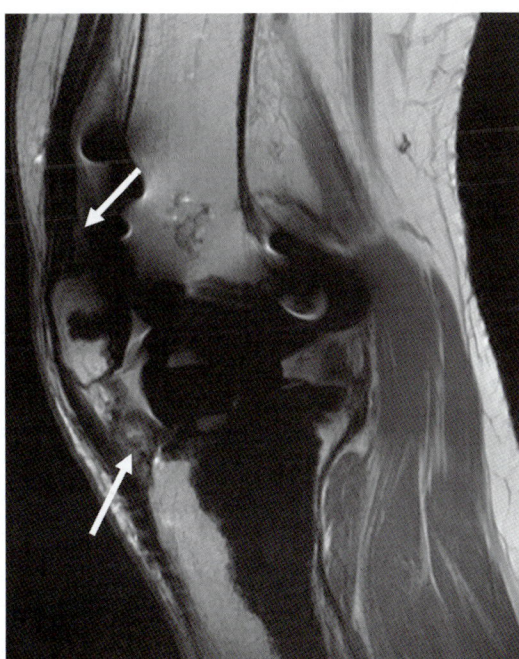

■ **FIGURE 109-54**   Fat pad scar. Sagittal, intermediate echo time image through a knee replacement shows artifact related to the arthroplasty. In the infrapatellar fat, focal scar (*upward arrow*) is abnormal and can be symptomatic. Suprapatellar fat scar (*downward arrow*) is less apparent on this image. (©Hospital for Special Surgery, New York, New York.)

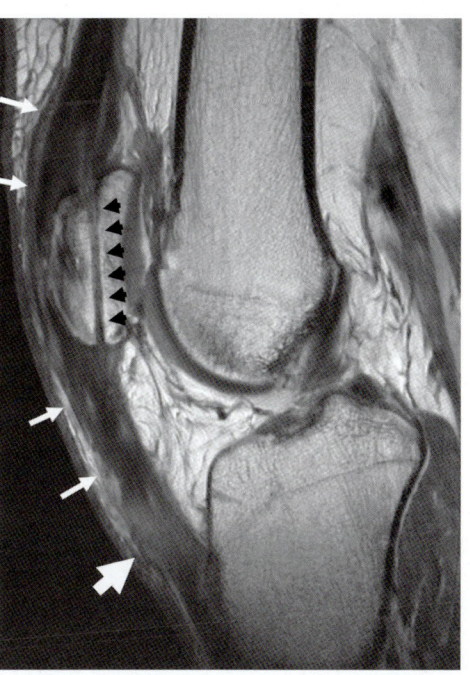

■ **FIGURE 109-55**   Patellar tendon repair. Sagittal, midline intermediate echo time MR image of the knee demonstrates thickening (*white arrows*) and distal high signal (*large white arrow*) in the patellar tendon and thickening of the quadriceps tendon after patellar tendon repair. Linear signal in the patella (*black arrow heads*) is related to fixation that is passed through the patella. Thickening and high signal can remain for many months after tendon repair. (©Hospital for Special Surgery, New York, New York.)

Avoiding early postoperative imaging will prevent moderate worry on the part of the orthopedic surgeon or radiologist. The tendon should be continuous, and (in the case of the quadriceps) all portions of the tendon should be approximated (Fig. 109-55).

After some months, the tendon becomes thinner again and more normal in appearance—thin and of low signal intensity. The holes made in the patella for reinforcement are evident, and sometimes the suture appears as areas of dephasing on MRI. On radiography, the patella should regain its normal position. The tendon thickening is apparent. On ultrasonography, the morphology of the tendon is thick and initially heterogeneous and hyperemic. With time, it acquires a more normal echogenic appearance.

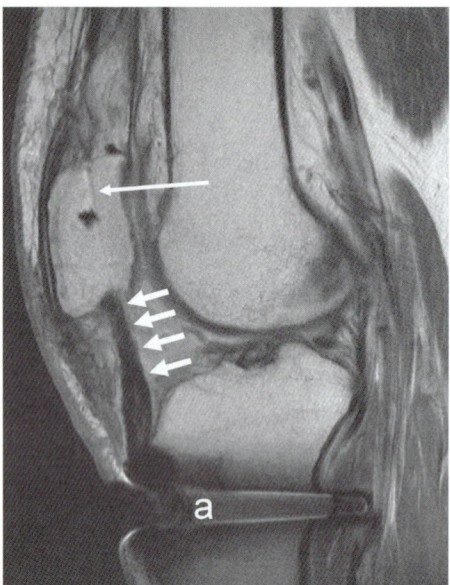

■ **FIGURE 109-56** Patellar tendon reconstruction. Sagittal, intermediate echo time MR image shows prior patellar tendon reconstruction. The origin of the graft is posterior to the native tendon. Thin fixation is present in the patella (*long arrow*). The patient subsequently had a quadriceps tendon tear. Tibial fixation causes artifact (a) on the study. (©Hospital for Special Surgery, New York, New York.)

The reconstructed tendon will have a more normal appearance from the beginning—low signal intensity on MRI and echogenic on ultrasonography (Fig. 109-56).

Potential Complications and Radiologic Appearance

The primary complication of quadriceps repair is re-tear (Fig. 109-57). A re-torn tendon is discontinuous on cross-sectional imaging, and the patellar location is either high

or low on radiography in complete tears. A less common complication is that of patellar fracture, in part related to abnormal forces and stress risers from the fixation through the patella.

PROXIMAL PATELLAR REALIGNMENT

Description

Anterior knee pain is a common orthopedic problem. Although most patients with anterior knee pain respond to strengthening exercises, there are surgical treatments. If deemed necessary because of abnormal patellofemoral tracking in the presence of anterior knee pain, the patella can be realigned to create more normal tracking and patellofemoral mechanics.[1]

The patella can be realigned proximally, usually by releasing the lateral retinaculum and patellofemoral ligament, to allow the patella to shift more medially and decrease the chance for lateral dislocation (the overwhelmingly common direction). Along with this, the medial retinaculum (especially if torn from patellar dislocation) can be repaired or tightened. Distal realignment is discussed later.

Indications, Contraindications, Purpose, and Underlying Mechanics

Proximal realignment is the first surgical line of defense in patients with patellofemoral tracking problems. The procedure should decrease the Q angle and, it is hoped, prevent further dislocations. The lateral release can be performed arthroscopically.

Expected Appearance on Relevant Modalities

The findings can be appreciated at MRI as a fascial defect just anterior to the iliotibial band on axial and coronal images at the level of the patella (Fig. 109-58). It has a

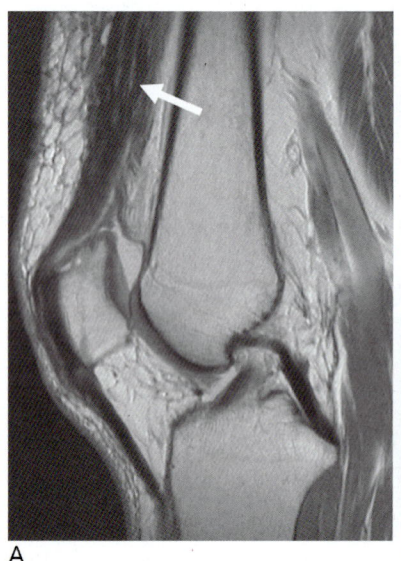
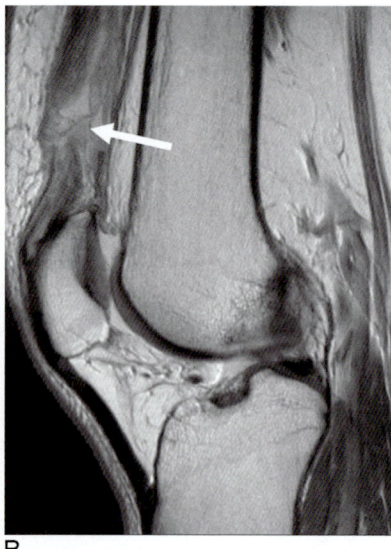
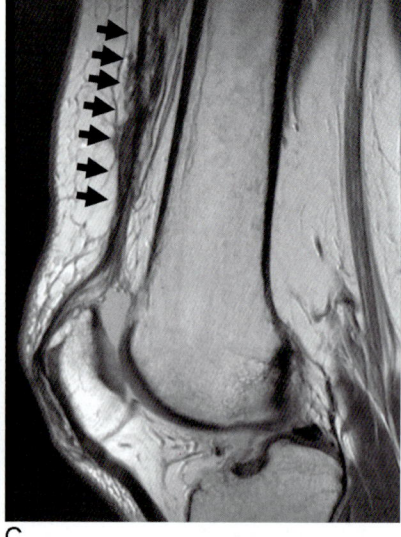

A B C

■ **FIGURE 109-57** Quadriceps tendon re-tear. Sagittal, intermediate echo time MR images show quadriceps thickening after repair (**A**) (*white arrow*), acute re-tear (**B**) (*white arrow*), and chronic tear after a second repair (**C**) (*black arrows*). (©Hospital for Special Surgery, New York, New York.)

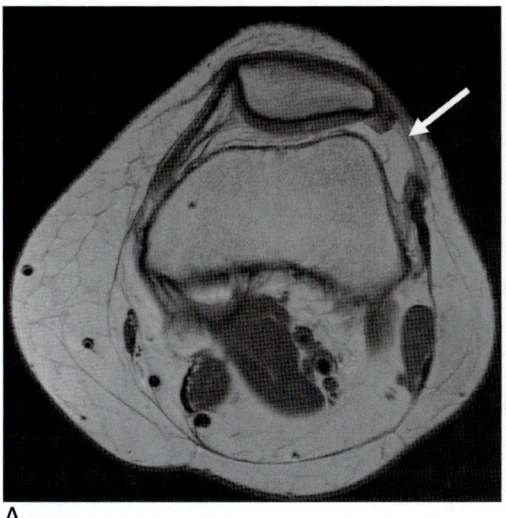
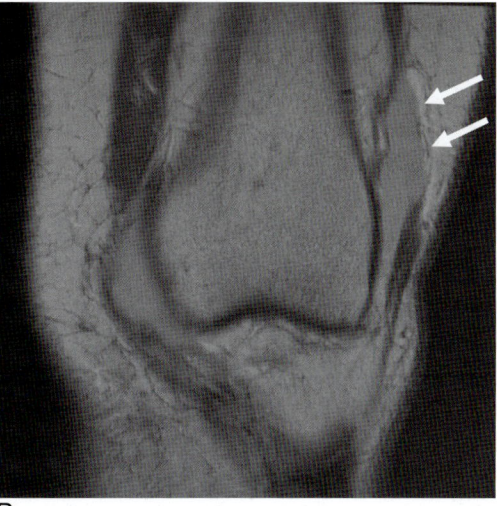

A   B

■ FIGURE 109-58   Lateral release. Axial (**A**) and coronal (**B**) intermediate echo time images demonstrate lateral release for proximal patellar realignment (*arrows*). Coronal images through the anterior knee are sometimes useful to detect this surgical defect. Over time, the retinaculum can re-form. (©Hospital for Special Surgery, New York, New York.)

similar appearance to arthrotomy scar. Medial retinacular plication is more subtle and may not be apparent or simply appear as a scarred medial retinaculum.

Potential Complications and Radiologic Appearance

Proximal realignments are simple procedures. As with some similar procedures, the divided fibrous retinacular tissue can re-form, negating any beneficial effect of the procedure.

DISTAL PATELLAR REALIGNMENT

Description

Distal realignment has been performed for about 100 years (initially it was referred to as medial displacement of the tendon insertion by Roux and described in 1888). The idea of changing the dynamics of the patellofemoral joint is of long standing and has taken various turns. The procedure should fulfill a few goals, including decreasing patellofemoral pain, decreasing the incidence of patellar dislocations, and preventing premature patellofemoral arthrosis. A procedure by Hauser that includes a transfer of the tibial tubercle medially and distally does decrease the dislocation rate but, at the same time, increases patellofemoral contact pressures and may result in increased pain and the development of arthrosis. Medialization of the tibial tubercle through osteotomy (Elmslie-Trillat procedure) decreases patellar dislocations by decreasing the Q angle but do not improve contact pressures. The Maquet procedure (putting a block of bone under a tibial tubercle osteotomy) causes a decrease in contact pressure and decreases pain but does not change tracking. Other procedures that include transfer of a portion of the patellar tendon are uncommon. Finally, the Fulkerson procedure successfully combines approaches by anteriorizing

and medializing the tibial tubercle with osteotomy and placement of bone graft to improve tracking, reduce pain, and retard arthrosis.[1]

Indications, Contraindications, Purpose, and Underlying Mechanics

Distal realignments are used when there is chondral loss to prevent further loss, when there is clear dysplasia that would not respond to noninvolved or less involved surgical methods, and when proximal realignments fail to solve the problem. Distal realignments are contraindicated in children because they would affect the anterior growth plate and potentially lead to genu recurvatum.

Expected Appearance on Relevant Modalities

Radiographically, one sees the fixation screws (usually two) (see Fig. 109-41). The osteotomy site and bone block are also visible until they become incorporated, after which there is simply a prominent anterior tubercle. On patellar views there should be a more normal Q angle. Patella alta, however, will persist.

On MRI, once the osteotomy has healed, only the remaining instrumentation and artifact persist. The remainder of the examination should look similar to the preoperative examination, but careful attention should be paid to patellar cartilage.

Potential Complications and Radiologic Appearance

The major radiographically visible complications to the procedure include failure of fixation, with the appearance of an ununited osteotomy. A problem, especially with the Maquet procedure, is healing anteriorly. Another is pain at the site of the anterior fixation that may be relieved by removal of the screws used for fixation.

TIBIAL PLATEAU FRACTURE FIXATION

Description

The severity of fractures of the tibial plateau governs the need for and the technique of fixation. Tibial plateau fractures are discussed elsewhere but range from the subtle subchondral insufficiency fracture that requires no local treatment to the comminuted Schatzker VI fracture (meta-diaphyseal dissociation), which will require surgical intervention. Other fractures, such as tibial spine avulsion, although fractures of the tibial plateau, may require fixation to secure the ACL and are not considered here.

Indications, Contraindications, Purpose, and Underlying Mechanics

The goal of fracture fixation is to aid fracture healing and to re-create the articular surfaces to prevent early the development of arthrosis (Fig. 109-59). Fixation is usually considered for any splits and depression of the articular surface by more than 3 mm (some will accept up to 1 cm) or angulation by more than 5 degrees.

The two major types of fixation are internal and external. The internal fixation is usually by a plate and screws but may involve percutaneous screw placement and Kirschner wires to augment fixation.

External fixators may be used to unload the joint by spanning the joint with one or more solid bars connecting intraosseous fixation points in the femoral and tibial diaphyses.

Tibial nails (rods) are usually used for more distal fractures.

Expected Appearance on Relevant Modalities

Radiographic spaces and stepoffs should be resolved no matter what fixation method is used (see Figs. 109-59 and 109-60). The imaging appearance of the fixation immediately after surgery should be identical on follow-up evaluations. The screws should not be broken, and normal anatomy should be restored.

As with other fractures, the fracture lines disappear over time. However, as long as a portion of the fracture is healing and creating a stable fixation, fracture lines may still be visible. This finding may be more apparent at fluoroscopy or at CT because of its tomographic abilities. Instrumentation causes artifact on CT (Fig. 109-60).

On MRI, acute or active healing fractures show high signal on fat-suppressed T2 or inversion recovery sequences. With healing, the high signal intensity resolves and the fractures become less apparent. Fracture healing is underappreciated on MRI where signal persists for months, as do the remnants of the fracture. The articular surface should have cartilage, and the ligaments and menisci of the knee should have healed (Fig. 109-59).

Occasionally a screw is placed during or before surgery; it is used for manipulation or stability and is removed before surgery is completed. Thus, screw holes can be seen that eventually fill in.

Rarely, a cortical window is made in the metaphysis to obtain bone graft to aid in the fixation at the articular surface. This may be visible until it heals. Artificial substances (bone graft or bone scaffolds, such as coral, and cement) may be used. They have characteristic radiographic appearances, with cement being dense and homogeneous, coral being dense and particulate, and bone graft being less dense and eventually disappearing.[22]

Potential Complications and Radiologic Appearance

Fracture nonunion is clinically apparent by persistent pain. Radiographically, loss of fixation heralds nonunion, although proximal are rare. If fixation was adequate, infection may lead to a nonunion.

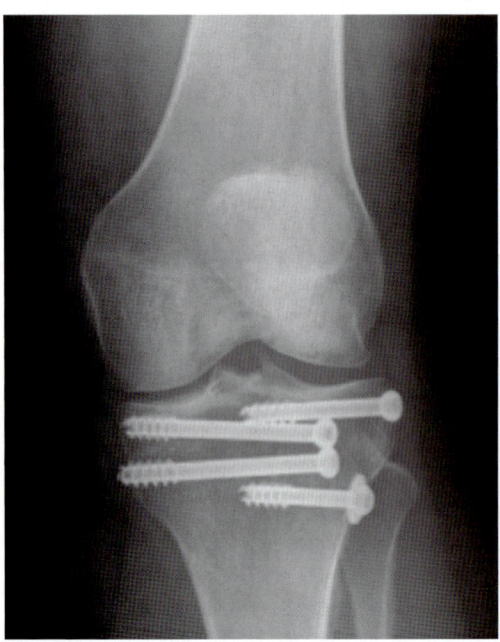

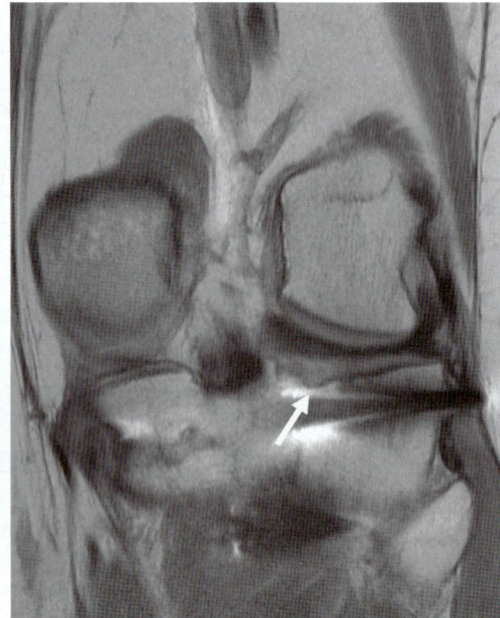

■ FIGURE 109-59 Fixation of lateral tibial plateau fracture. **A,** Frontal radiograph shows the articular surface of the lateral tibial plateau is smooth and defined by a sharp cortical line. **B,** MRI is able better to define the articular surface and demonstrate the articular cartilage, despite instrumentation. There is a small area of cortical depression related to the fracture (*arrow*), but the overlying articular cartilage is intact. (©Hospital for Special Surgery, New York, New York.)

A

B

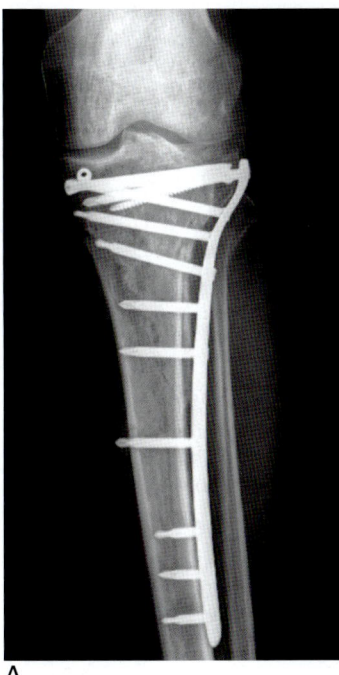
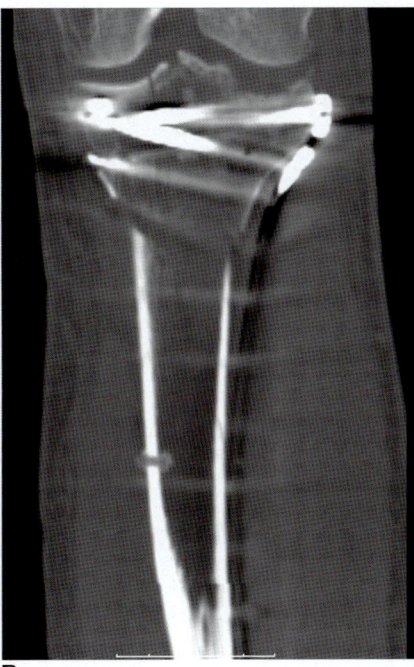

A   B

■ FIGURE 109-60 Tibial plateau fracture fixation. **A,** Frontal radiographs show that this patient has undergone fixation of a tibial plateau fracture using a LISS (Less Invasive Stabilization System) plate. Because this plate is placed subcutaneously, it is often not contoured as well as the older style plates, leaving a larger gap between the bone and the plate. At the articular surface, the lateral tibial plateau cortex is irregular and the articular surface is not smooth. A fibular fracture is also present. **B,** Coronal reformatted CT image shows that, despite instrumentation, the tibial plateau is visible. The CT image better demonstrates a poor reduction of the articular surface. (©Hospital for Special Surgery, New York, New York.)

Malunion can occur if fixation is lost before healing has occurred.

Infection after open fracture may cause a fracture not to heal. Soft tissue damage, as might occur in high-energy and open trauma, disposes an injury to become infected. The infection has the appearance of osteomyelitis elsewhere. Unfortunately, high MR signal intensity and enhancement are common after trauma, both in the bone marrow and in the soft tissues. Infected fractures are often characterized by a sinus tract that can be identified as a high signal tract extending to skin. If the central area does not enhance, the tract likely contains an abscess. Indium-labeled white blood cell studies are specific for infection and can identify osteomyelitis in the presence of trauma, especially if adjacent cellulitis has been treated.

Peroneal nerve palsy can occur. Tibial plateau fractures can extend to involve the fibula. Proximal fibular fractures, because of the close proximity of the peroneal nerve to the fibula, can displace, injure, or otherwise affect the peroneal nerve.

PATELLAR FRACTURE TREATMENT

Description

There are many different procedures for repairing a patellar fracture. The major ones include circumferential (cerclage) fixation with suture or suture wire, figure-of-eight (tension band) suture or suture wire, screw fixation (usually vertical because most fractures are horizontal), Kirschner wire fixation (usually combined with suture or suture wire), and combinations of these (Figs. 109-61 and 109-62).[1]

Severely comminuted fractures may require surgical removal of the patella, which is also a treatment for painful advanced patellofemoral arthrosis.

Indications, Contraindications, Purpose, and Underlying Mechanics

A displaced fracture or more than 2 mm of articular stepoff requires fixation to prevent premature arthrosis. Patients who cannot or prefer not to undergo extension splinting would also undergo fixation. Often fixation includes tension banding so that the tension of the fracture from quadriceps contraction further apposes the fixated fracture.

Concomitant injuries to the quadriceps or patellar tendons may also require surgery.

Expected Appearance on Relevant Modalities

No matter what type of fixation is undertaken, the principles of imaging and fracture healing are the same. On radiographs or at CT, the fragments should be anatomically aligned. The fracture lines, which may first widen (from early bone resorption during healing) should then narrow and disappear.

At MRI, instrumentation may cause artifact and fracture lines and abnormal bone marrow signal will be present even in the late stages of healing. MRI is also useful for evaluation of the cartilage surface. Ideally, the fracture was only of bone and the cartilage surface remained intact. Otherwise, there will be at least a fissure at the level of the fracture.

Potential Complications and Radiologic Appearance

The potential complications for patellar fracture and fixation are the same as with almost any other and include loss of fixation, misplaced hardware, nonunion, malunion, and

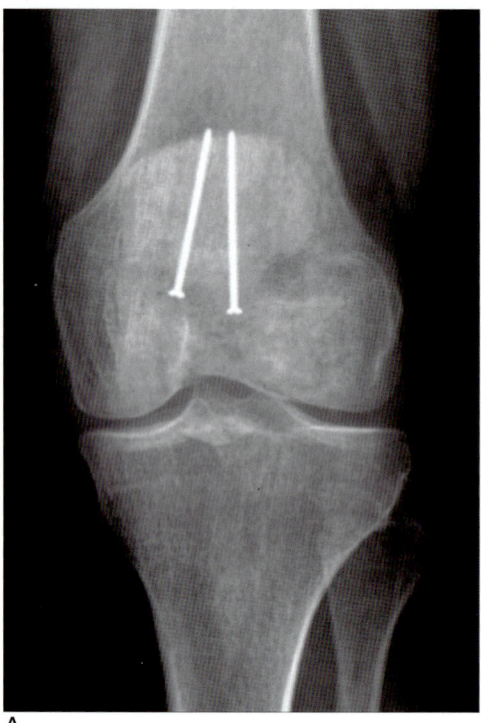

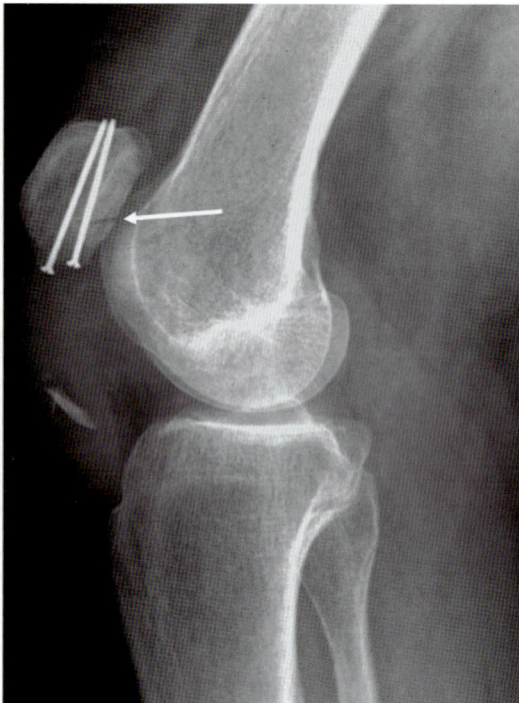

A   B

■ **FIGURE 109-61** Patellar fracture fixation. Frontal (**A**) and lateral (**B**) views show patellar fracture fixation with two screws. There is a small gap in the bone at the articular surface (**B**, *arrow*). Patellar tendon thickening and focal ossification are present. (©Hospital for Special Surgery, New York, New York.)

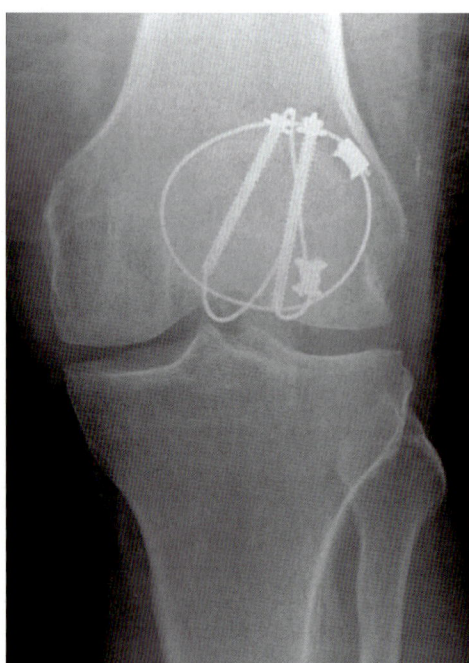

■ **FIGURE 109-62** Patellar fracture fixation. Frontal radiograph shows fixation of a patellar fracture with screws, a figure-of-eight wire, and a cerclage wire. Note that the figure-of-eight wire passes through the cannulated screws. (©Hospital for Special Surgery, New York, New York.)

infection. These have a similar appearance as one would expect with other bones.

Additionally, as with some other fractures, because the patella is superficial, the hardware can become painful and needs to be removed (Fig. 109-63). Lastly, chondral loss over the patella can occur at the time of initial injury or subsequently, but chondromalacia patellae and eventual patellofemoral arthrosis is the outcome that we are trying to avoid.

The major complication of patellectomy is functional, with loss of quadriceps muscle strength.

TUMOR RESECTION WITHOUT INSTRUMENTATION

Description

A variety of soft tissue and bony tumors occur in and around the knee. Imaging the postoperative knee after tumoral resection is primarily performed to look for tumoral recurrence but may also be used to look for complications from the surgery. If there is no instrumentation, the imaging is fairly routine. Immediate postoperative studies are useful for comparison, as are preoperative studies, to know the tumor location and appearance.

The radiographic follow-up after tumor resection is, in part, based on the tumor histology and the postoperative course of the patient. Evaluation for the surgical complications of fracture, infection, or nerve injury in this setting is similar to the search for these in a native knee and is discussed elsewhere.

The evaluation of potential tumor recurrence depends on what surgery has been performed and may simply require imaging of the operative site.

Indications, Contraindications, Purpose, and Underlying Mechanics

The indications for tumor surgery are threefold: to obtain a diagnosis (incisional or excisional biopsy), to treat the

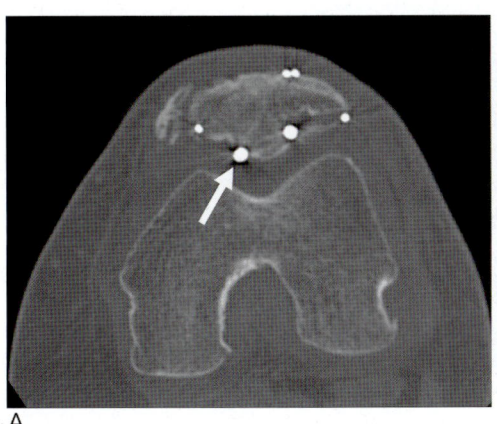

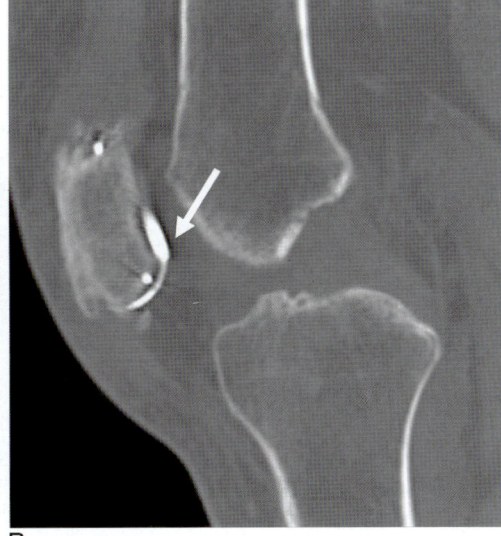

A   B

tumor to relieve pain or discomfort (osteochondroma, nonaggressive lipomatous tumor removal), and to treat the tumor to prevent spread of tumor or complications from its presence or evolution (osteosarcoma, large nonossifying fibroma that may fracture).

After a soft tissue tumor is removed, a new mass will require imaging whose approach will be the same as for the original lesion. After resection of pigmented villonodular synovitis, recurrent pain may warrant examination for recurrence (Fig. 109-64).

In the case of bone tumors, especially aggressive ones or ones with close margins, regular postoperative follow-up is performed at least with radiography, if not additional cross-sectional imaging such as MRI.

Expected Appearance on Relevant Modalities

The wide range of techniques of tumor resection lead to different postoperative radiographic appearances. For most

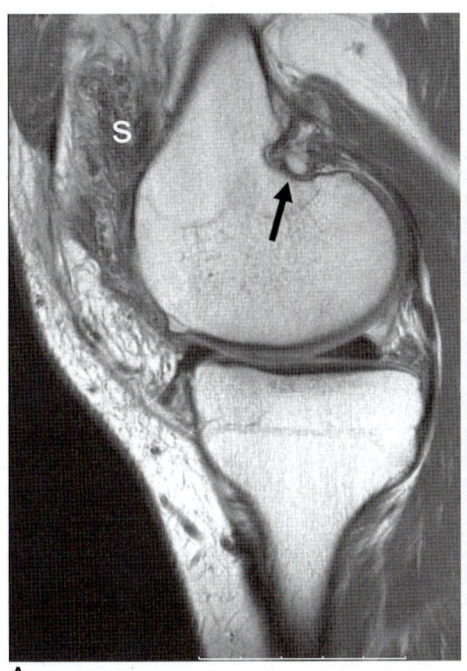

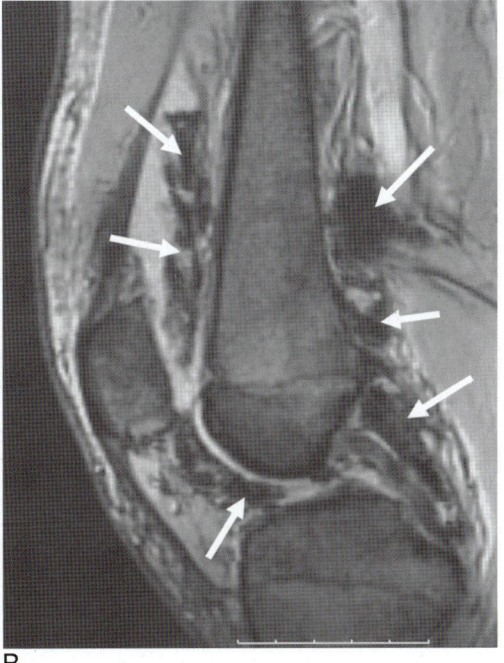

A   B

■ **FIGURE 109-64** Recurrent pigmented villonodular synovitis. **A,** Sagittal intermediate echo time MR sequence shows heterogeneous synovitis (s) with foci of low signal. There is an erosion at the medial gastrocnemius origin from the medial femoral condyle (*black arrow*). **B,** Midline sagittal gradient echo image shows that much of the synovitis has very low signal, related to hemosiderin deposition (*white arrows*). The appearance is the same as it would be for diffuse pigmented villonodular synovitis in the native knee, but this patient had prior surgery. For small areas of disease, it can be difficult to distinguish between recurrent pigmented villonodular synovitis and dephasing related to a surgical procedure performed. (©Hospital for Special Surgery, New York, New York.)

imaging modalities, postoperative bone and soft tissue lesions will have different appearances and are discussed separately. For positron emission tomography, if the original lesion had increased metabolic activity, so will the recurrence, if it is large enough.

Soft Tissue Tumors

Often radiographs will be normal or show only contour abnormalities from resected tissue or added tissue (as from soft tissue flaps). CT will add visualization of the resection scar and the soft tissue deformity. Identification of recurrent tumor may be aided by the use of intravenous contrast, but small recurrences will be difficult to see. Ultrasonography will show the postoperative scar and be able to demonstrate and, to some degree, characterize any new mass that is present. For those comfortable with ultrasonography, it is an excellent way to image soft tissue masses.[23]

MRI will show the postoperative scar as of low signal intensity and within the subcutaneous fat but, depending on the length of time from surgery and the degree of scar, there will be higher signal intensity within the deep soft tissues. The normal anatomy will almost always be distorted, depending on what has been removed or transferred. It can be difficult to distinguish between this scar and recurrent tumor. Some believe that enhancement with intravenous administration of a contrast agent is helpful. Others believe that characterizing the lesion with high-resolution intermediate imaging can help to define abnormal signal as tumor or scar, especially if one is able to compare the appearance with that of the preoperative tumor. Patients who have undergone external-beam irradiation have reaction in the soft tissues for years afterward, with diffuse high signal intensity and fat infiltration. Muscle flaps appear as soft tissue masses but can be distinguished from neoplasm by the persistent muscle fibers. These muscle flaps undergo a process of denervation and atrophy (with a similar appearance to muscle elsewhere going through the same processes) that gives it an abnormal but characteristic appearance.

Intra-articular surgery will cause capsular scar, characterized by low signal intensity along the synovial surfaces of the joint with thickening of the joint capsule.

Bone scintigraphy will be positive in the initial postoperative period but becomes negative (except for the hyperemia after radiation treatment). Most soft tissue tumors are not positive on bone scintigraphy, and it is not a good way to look for local recurrence.

Bone Tumors

Small defects, such as those from osteoid osteoma resection, may appear simply as a cortical defect in all imaging or as hole after radiofrequency ablation. However, the defect from most bone tumor resections needs to be filled, even if the bone does not require stabilization. They can be filled with cement, bone graft, coral, or other scaffolds. All of these have a slightly different imaging appearance. They should fill the defect, and normal anatomy should, if possible, be restored.

On MRI, reactive signal to the surgery is present for months and the bone defect shows abnormal increased

signal for as long as it continues to remodel, sometimes years (as with bone scan). Once returning to normal, the signal should remain normal so that interval postoperative imaging can be useful to compare with later imaging if a patient has new symptoms.

Potential Complications and Radiologic Appearance

The most worrisome complication of tumor resection is tumor recurrence. Often the recurrent tumor has signal characteristics that are the same as the original tumor. Sometimes a transformation will occur or a secondary lesion (e.g., aneurysmal bone cyst) will appear (Figs. 109-65 and 109-66). It is always a good idea to compare radiographs with ones that were taken soon after surgery: this may make subtle, progressive abnormalities stand out and allow one to tell whether a bone defect was simply the resection margin. Sequential studies are very useful in the follow-up of patients with tumors.

Less serious complications such as postoperative seromas appear, as they would for any other surgery.

Soft Tissue

One of the frustrating lesions around the knee is pigmented villonodular synovitis. In the diffuse form, this lesion often recurs and appears as multiple intra-articular masses, often with dephasing on T2*-weighted images (gradient-echo) because of the hemosiderin that comes from the lesion's bleeding (see Fig. 109-64). It has the appearance of the original lesion.

Other soft tissue masses have the MRI and ultrasound appearance of the primary lesion, as do other complications, such as postoperative infection.

Bone

Recurrence of bone tumors is characterized by reappearance of the lesion. On radiography this is seen as new lucency in the bone either by itself or around graft or cement that has been placed. The same is true for CT, in which bone defects have the same appearance whether due to tumor, recurrent tumor, or osteolysis from another cause. On MRI, despite some artifact from cement, one can see soft tissue tumor around graft or cement.

There are also complications related to radiation that may be used as an adjuvant for soft tissue or bone tumors, before, after, or in lieu of surgery. Radiation causes tremendous tissue damage (that is why it can work). The reactive edema from radiation lasts more than a year. Radiation, in addition to inducing secondary tumors, can also weaken bone and result in pathologic fractures (Fig. 109-67).

TUMOR RESECTION WITH INSTRUMENTATION/ALLOGRAFT

Description

The orthopedic oncologic surgeon treating a bone tumor must often reconstruct the bone if it is not entirely amputated. In the diaphysis or metaphysis, this can be done with a combination of filler and stabilization that can

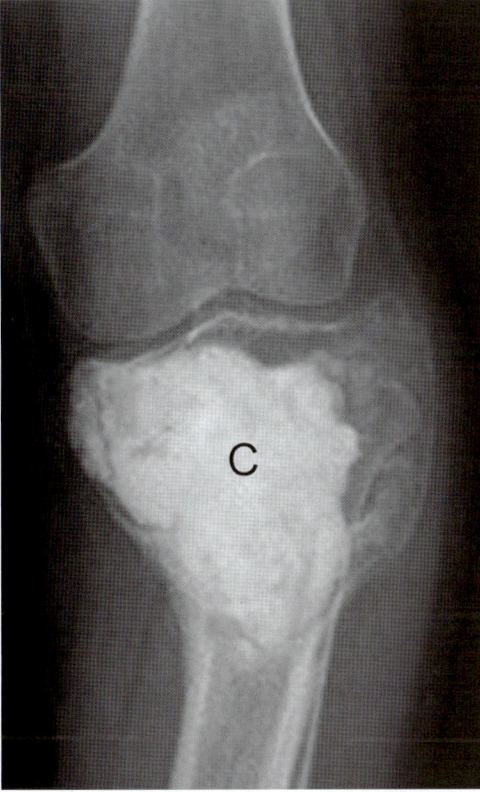

A

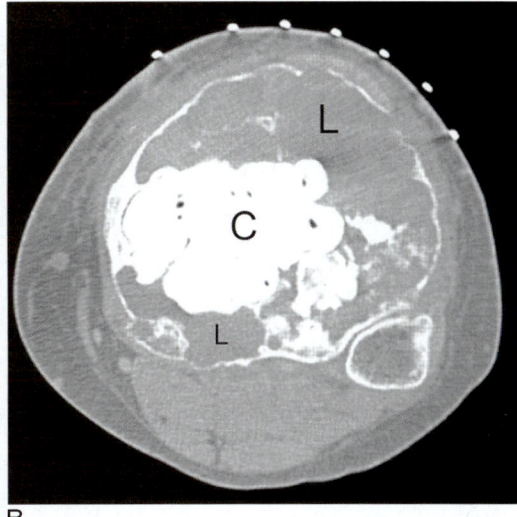

B

■ **FIGURE 109-65** Tumor recurrence. Frontal view of the tibia (**A**) shows cement (C) from prior curettage and packing for giant cell tumor of bone. The lateral bone irregularity and expansion heralds the recurrence, better seen on CT (**B**) at the time of needle biopsy, where there is expansion and lucency (L) around the cement (C). (©Hospital for Special Surgery, New York, New York.)

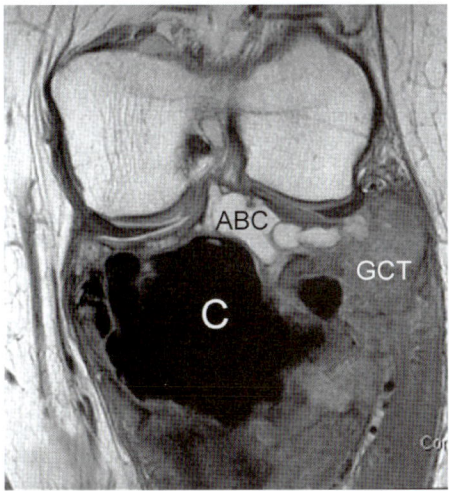

A

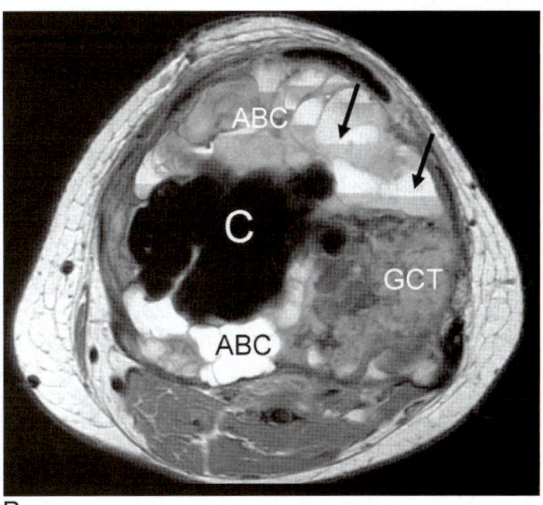

B

■ **FIGURE 109-66** Tumoral recurrence. The same patient as in Figure 109-65. Coronal (**A**) and axial (**B**), intermediate echo time MR images show low signal cement (C), with intermediate signal recurrence of giant cell tumor of bone, with superimposed higher signal aneurysmal bone cyst containing multiple fluid-fluid levels. (©Hospital for Special Surgery, New York, New York.)

be performed with allograft, autograft, internal fixation, external fixation, cement, and bone scaffold. At the joint, some kind of artificial joint may be required. As technology and adjuvant treatments have improved, so have limb-sparing operations. Instrumentation can cause artifact on CT and MRI, but techniques to limit this artifact make them valuable tools to look for complications and recurrence.

Indications, Contraindications, Purpose, and Underlying Mechanics

The reason for the surgery is to remove the tumor. The most common reasons for postoperative imaging include routine follow-up and new pain, which requires a search for recurrence or a complication of the surgery. Instrumentation is used to prevent fractures from weakened bone or to

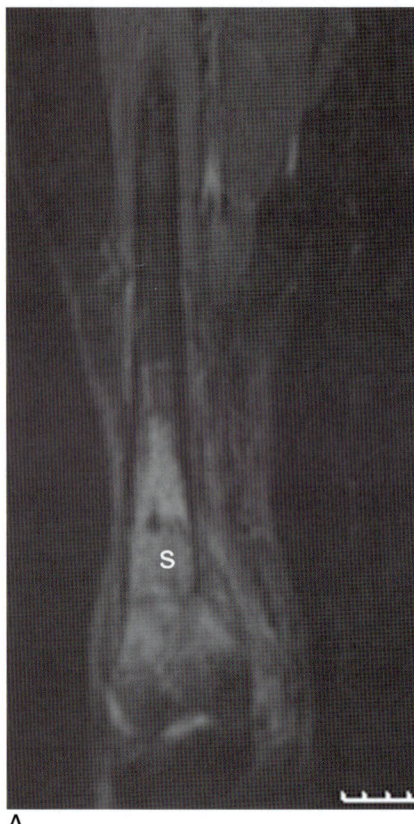
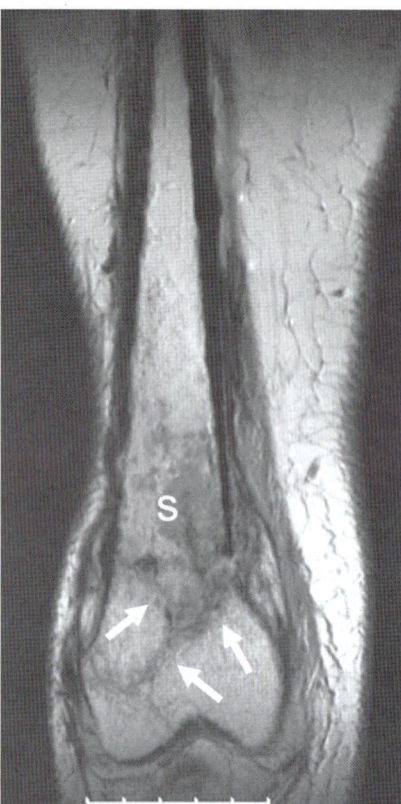

A   B

■ **FIGURE 109-67**   Postirradiation fracture. Coronal, short tau inversion recovery (**A**) and intermediate echo time, fast spin-echo (**B**) MR images demonstrate distal femoral bone marrow signal heterogeneity (s) related to radiation with superimposed fracture (*arrows*). No tumoral recurrence is evident. The pathologic fracture was related to the radiation. Radiation can cause abnormal bone marrow and soft tissue reactive signal on MR for more than a year after the treatment has stopped. (©Hospital for Special Surgery, New York, New York.)

reconstruct a limb that has had a large area of bone or a joint removed. In growing children, prostheses with growth potential have been designed to prevent the need for repeated replacements.

Expected Appearance on Relevant Modalities

The postoperative appearance will depend on the type of reconstruction performed. Joint prostheses for tumor will often be custom made and have long stems compared with a normal knee replacement. Its appearance abides by the same principles as other prostheses: normal alignment should be restored, and the bone around the prosthesis should appose the metal (or cement if used) with no more than a 2-mm gap. Cross-sectional imaging will also be similar, although the soft tissues may be more distorted by surgery and the artifact greater because of a larger prosthesis.

For other fixation the appearance will be similar to the postoperative trauma patient with normal alignment, hardware next to bone, and screws intact. The difference between the appearance of tumor and trauma is the more liberal use of cement (or other agents) in tumor surgery and the absence of the comminuted bone fragments common in high-energy trauma. This difference creates better definition of the defects in tumor resections. Those defects are sometimes filled with allograft or autograft that contains cortex for stability. The appearance will depend on the bone used for the allograft (often fibula). On radiographs the fibular margins will be quite clear initially. It may take years for the bone to be fully incorporated, and

sequential radiographs should show no difference in the graft position.

Allografts, sometimes in conjunction with hardware or joint replacements (composite grafts), are sometimes used to reconstruct large resections. The allograft (just as in the osteochondral allografts of the knee) ultimately becomes incorporated. The interface with native bone is at first sharp but becomes less defined at the graft heals to native bone. The graft itself can become dense from reversible ischemia that is high signal on fat-suppressed (non–T1-weighted) MRI but eventually should have the appearance of normal bone.

Potential Complications and Radiologic Appearance

The most worrisome complication of tumor resection is tumor recurrence. On radiography this will have the appearance of the original lesion, causing a focal bone defect along the prosthesis. Associated soft tissue masses will be easier to see on MRI or identifiable on positron emission tomography.

Hardware failure or prosthesis loosening has a similar appearance as when hardware is placed for other reasons, with screw fracture, loss of fixation, or lucencies around the prosthesis.

Allografts may not incorporate and fail by developing necrosis and/or fracture (Fig. 109-68). Allograft stress fractures can be subtle and barely visible, except on MRI or CT (Fig. 109-69). Infection can also occur, as after any surgery, with a similar radiographic appearance to infection from other sources.

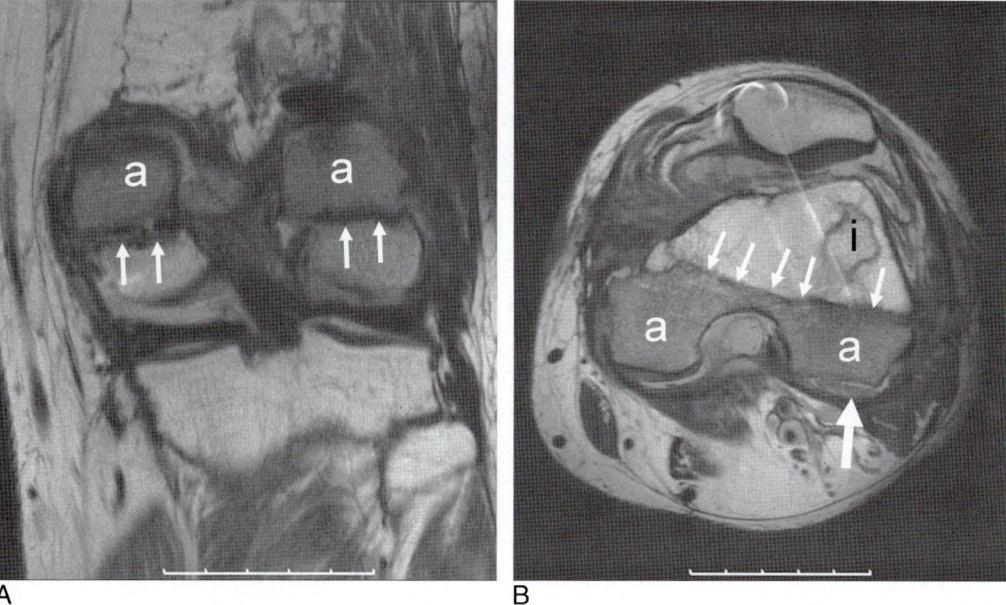

A   B

■ **FIGURE 109-68**   Osteochondral allograft. Coronal (**A**) and axial (**B**), intermediate echo time MR images show that an osteochondral allograft replaced the cranial portions of the femoral condyles (a). The allograft is of low signal, indicating it has not incorporated. This is supported by the well-defined line of demarcation between the graft and the native bone (*small arrows*). The graft is starting to collapse (**B**, *large arrow*) at the articular surface. A bone infarct is incidentally demonstrated (i) as high signal intensity with a serpentine surrounding area of low signal intensity. (©Hospital for Special Surgery, New York, New York.)

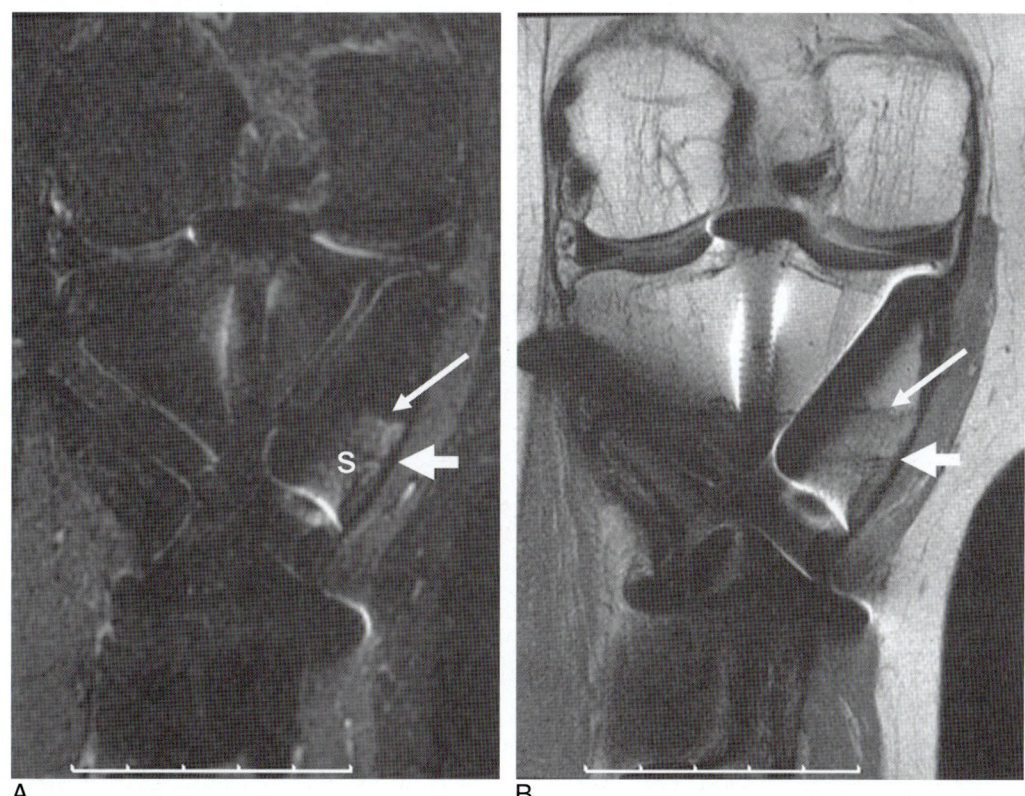

A   B

■ **FIGURE 109-69**   Stress fracture of allograft. Coronal, short tau inversion recovery (**A**) and intermediate echo time (**B**) MR images. The patient has undergone tibial allograft placement with screw fixation that causes artifact. Below the line of demarcation between the native bone and the allograft (*small arrow*) there is a line (*larger arrow*) with surrounding high signal (s) on the fat-suppressed images. This line represents a fracture that was not visible on a radiograph. The entire allograft is lower in signal intensity than the native bone because it has not yet completely incorporated. (©Hospital for Special Surgery, New York, New York.)

TIBIAL OSTEOTOMY

Description

An osteotomy is a purposeful, controlled surgically created fracture that is often done to realign bone. In the proximal tibia or distal femur, after the cut is made, a bone wedge is usually removed (closing wedge) or placed (opening wedge) to rotate the articular surface so that it lies at the correct angle.

Indications, Contraindications, Purpose, and Underlying Mechanics

Osteotomies are still performed around the knee predominantly to correct deformities, whether traumatic, degenerative (arthrosis), or developmental (e.g., Blount's). This procedure is an acceptable alternative to joint arthroplasty in younger patients or patients with unicompartmental disease with deformity. Underlying inflammatory arthropathy is a contraindication. The mechanics involved are that the knee bears at least twice a patient's body weight, mostly through the medial compartment. With varus deformity, the burden to the medial compartment is much greater. This will accelerate arthrosis and cause pain. Restoring the normal valgus of the knee reverses these problems.

The same indication applies in Blount's disease (tibia vara), in which osteotomy with correction of the deformity should be performed early.

Expected Appearance on Relevant Modalities

The osteotomy is usually fixated by a staple or plate with screws (Fig. 109-70). For proximal tibial osteotomies, the fibula may need to be cut also or the fibula may be allowed to ride up alongside the tibia. At first the osteotomy site is visible as a sclerotic line. This eventually disappears as the bone heals.

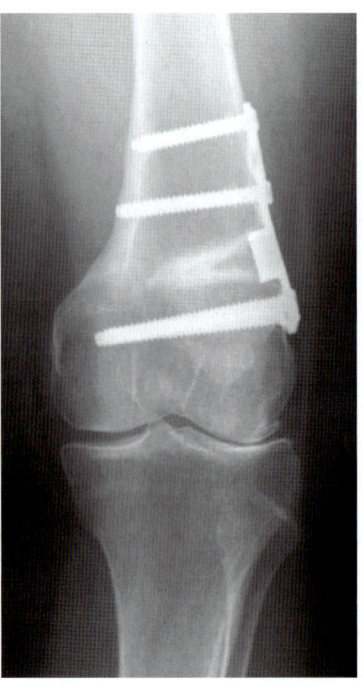

■ **FIGURE 109-70** Femoral osteotomy. Although high tibial osteotomy is more commonly used to correct deformity, this distal femoral osteotomy corrects the exaggerated valgus that was present because of the lateral compartment cartilage loss. There is persistent lateral joint space narrow. Malalignment should be corrected before or concurrently in patients who will undergo meniscal transplant. It is an effective alternative to arthroplasty in patients with knee arthritis. (©Hospital for Special Surgery, New York, New York.)

Potential Complications and Radiologic Appearance

The procedure is relatively safe and effective, although as with any surgery with instrumentation there can be a loss of fixation from nonunion (rare) or infection. In the case of arthritis, the arthritis may still progress, necessitating a joint arthroplasty. With Blount's disease, the deformity can also continue, especially if not fixed early, necessitating further surgery.

SUGGESTED READINGS

Buckwalter KA, Parr JA, Choplin RH, Capello WN. Multichannel CT imaging of orthopedic hardware and implants. Semin Musculoskelet Radiol 2006; 10:86–97.

Frick MA, Collins MS, Adkins MC. Postoperative imaging of the knee. Radiol Clin North Am 2006; 44:367–389.

Gold GE, McCauley TR, Gray ML, Disler DG. What's new in cartilage? RadioGraphics 2003; 23:1227–1242.

Gopez AG, Kavanagh EC. MR imaging of the postoperative meniscus: repair, resection, and replacement. Semin Musculoskelet Radiol 2006; 10:229–240.

Ilaslan H, Sundaram M, Miniaci A. Imaging evaluation of the postoperative knee ligaments. Eur J Radiol 2005; 54:178–188.

Jacobson JA, Lax MJ. Musculoskeletal sonography of the postoperative orthopedic patient. Semin Musculoskelet Radiol 2002; 6:67–77.

Math KR, Zaidi SF, Petchprapa C, Harwin SF. Imaging of total knee arthroplasty. Semin Musculoskelet Radiol 2006; 10:47–63.

Miller TT. Imaging of knee arthroplasty. Eur J Radiol 2005; 54:164–177.

Miller TT. Sonography of joint replacements. Semin Musculoskelet Radiol 2006; 10:79–85.

Polster J, Recht M. Postoperative MR evaluation of chondral repair in the knee. Eur J Radiol 2005; 54:206–213.

Recht MP, Kramer J. MR imaging of the postoperative knee: a pictorial essay. RadioGraphics 2002; 22:765–774.

White LM, Buckwalter KA. Technical considerations: CT and MR imaging in the postoperative orthopedic patient. Semin Musculoskelet Radiol 2002; 6:5–17.

White LM, Kramer J, Recht MP. MR imaging evaluation of the postoperative knee: ligaments, menisci, and articular cartilage. Skeletal Radiol 2005; 34:431–452.

REFERENCES

1. Andrews J, Timmerman LA. Diagnostic and Operative Arthroscopy. Philadelphia, WB Saunders, 1997.
2. Hall FM. Osteonecrosis in the postoperative knee. Radiology 2005; 236:370-371; author reply 371.
3. Colombet P, Allard M, Bousquet V, et al. The history of ACL surgery. Le Journal Francais de l'Orthopedie. Maitrise Orthopedique, France, 5: 2002.
4. Sekiya JK, Wojtys E. Sports medicine: implants of knee ligament repair and reconstructive surgery. In Freiberg AA (ed). The Radiology of Orthopaedic Implants: An Atlas of Techniques and Assessment. St. Louis, Mosby, 2001.
5. Mariani PP, Margheritini F, Camillieri G, Bellelli A. Serial magnetic resonance imaging evaluation of the patellar tendon after posterior cruciate ligament reconstruction. Arthroscopy 2002; 18:38-45.
6. van Trommel MF, Potter HG, Ernberg LA, et al. The use of noncontrast magnetic resonance imaging in evaluating meniscal repair: comparison with conventional arthrography. Arthroscopy 1998; 14:2-8.
7. Kelly BT, Robertson W, Potter HG, et al. Hydrogel meniscal replacement in the sheep knee: preliminary evaluation of chondroprotective effects. Am J Sports Med 2007; 35:43-52.
8. Noyes FR, Barber-Westin SD, Rankin M. Meniscal transplantation in symptomatic patients less than fifty years old. J Bone Joint Surg Am 2005; 87(Suppl 1; pt 2):149-165.
9. Cole BJ, Carter TR, Rodeo SA. Allograft meniscal transplantation: background, techniques, and results. Instr Course Lect 2003; 52:383-396.
10. Potter HG, Rodeo SA, Wickiewicz TL, Warren RF. MR imaging of meniscal allografts: correlation with clinical and arthroscopic outcomes. Radiology 1996; 198:509-514.
11. Polster J, Recht M. Postoperative MR evaluation of chondral repair in the knee. Eur J Radiol 2005; 54:206-213.
12. Potter HG, Foo LF. Magnetic resonance imaging of joint arthroplasty. Orthop Clin North Am 2006; 37:361-373, vi-vii.
13. James SL, Connell DA, Saifuddin A, et al. MR imaging of autologous chondrocyte implantation of the knee. Eur Radiol 2006; 16:1022-1030.
14. Potter HG, Foo L. MR imaging of articular cartilage and of cartilage degeneration. In Stoller D (ed). Magnetic Resonance Imaging in Orthopaedics and Sports Medicine, 3rd ed. Philadelphia, Lipinncott Williams & Wilkins, 2006.
15. Math KR, Zaidi SF, Petchprapa C, Harwin SF. Imaging of total knee arthroplasty. Semin Musculoskelet Radiol 2006; 10:47-63.
16. Buckwalter KA, Parr JA, Choplin RH, Capello WN. Multichannel CT imaging of orthopedic hardware and implants. Semin Musculoskelet Radiol 2006; 10:86-97.
17. Vande Berg B, Malghem J, Maldague B, Lecouvet F. Multi-detector CT imaging in the postoperative orthopedic patient with metal hardware. Eur J Radiol 2006; 60:470-479.
18. Adler RS. Ultrasound of joint replacements. In Freiberg AA (ed). The Radiology of Orthopaedic Implants. St. Louis, Mosby, 2001.
19. Delank KS, Schmidt M, Michael JW, et al. The implications of ^{18}F-FDG PET for the diagnosis of endoprosthetic loosening and infection in hip and knee arthroplasty: results from a prospective, blinded study. BMC Musculoskelet Disord 2006; 7:20.
20. Kantor SG, Schneider R, Insall JN, Becker MW. Radionuclide imaging of asymptomatic versus symptomatic total knee arthroplasties. Clin Orthop Relat Res 1990; (260):118-123.
21. Ilan DI, Tejwani N, Keschner M, Leibman M. Quadriceps tendon rupture. J Am Acad Orthop Surg 2003; 11:192-200.
22. Beaman FD, Bancroft LW, Peterson JJ, Kransdorf MJ. Bone graft materials and synthetic substitutes. Radiol Clin North Am 2006; 44:451-461.
23. Arya S, Nagarkatti DG, Dudhat SB, et al. Soft tissue sarcomas: ultrasonographic evaluation of local recurrences. Clin Radiol 2000; 55:193-197.

110

The Postoperative Ankle and Foot

David Rubin

More than 200 distinct operations are performed in the ankle and foot. Indications for operative intervention include traumatic, overuse, degenerative, arthritic, congenital, neoplastic, and inflammatory conditions. The same general principles of orthopedic care and postoperative imaging that apply to the rest of the appendicular skeleton also apply to the foot and ankle. For example, methods to evaluate fracture fixation in the ankle or tumor excision in the foot parallel those for other skeletal regions. The procedures unique to the foot and ankle are reviewed here, with emphasis on the imaging techniques used to evaluate successful and complicated operations.

OSTEOSYNTHESIS

Description

The most commonly performed operations in the foot and ankle—fracture treatment, osteotomies, and arthrodeses—are designed to fuse bones. After proper positioning of the bones or bone fragments (and preparation of the bone surfaces, in the case of nonunion repair or arthrodesis), the surgeon will employ some form of fixation to maintain alignment while healing occurs. Internal, metallic implants are most commonly used for this purpose, and their presence affects the selection and interpretation of postoperative imaging studies.

Indications, Contraindications, Purpose, and Underlying Mechanics

The indications and principles of fracture fixation in the foot and ankle are the same as those in the rest of the appendicular skeleton (see Chapter 105). The operative principle is to restore the normal anatomic position of the fragments by either closed or open reduction and then to maintain the fragment position until healing can occur. Simple casting or splinting combined with non–weight bearing will suffice for most stable fractures, whereas internal fixation is desirable for inherently unstable or intra-articular fractures. Established nonunions also require freshening of the fractured bone ends and bone grafting.[1] Internal fixation is contraindicated in the presence of ongoing infection, severe comminution, and deficient soft tissue coverage and during the acute phase of neuropathic disease.[2] In these instances, an external fixator can provide fragment stability while healing progresses.

Osteotomies are performed to correct malalignments. The surgeon cuts the bone with an osteotome and then reassembles the pieces to correct any length, angulation, position, or rotational abnormality. Internal fixation with or without bone grafting then allows the bone to heal in its new orientation (Fig. 110-1A). Common indications for hindfoot and midfoot osteotomies include cavus, planus, equinus, varus, valgus, adductus, and abductus deformities due to neuromuscular, traumatic, degenerative, and arthritic causes, as well as complex malalignments due to congenital conditions.[3,4] Forefoot osteotomies may be combined with fusions or soft tissue procedures for malalignments of the great toe (e.g., hallux valgus, metatarsus primum varus)[5] and lesser toes (e.g., bunionette, cock-up, hammer, and crossover deformities.[6]

Arthrodesis is surgical fusion of a joint. Ankle and foot joint replacements succeed only for a few, isolated indications.[7] Thus, severe arthritis that causes pain unresponsive to nonsurgical treatment usually requires fusion.[8,9] The most common causes in the foot and ankle are post-traumatic osteoarthritis and rheumatoid arthritis. Arthrodesis alone, or in addition to a soft tissue operation, is often indicated to restore and maintain plantigrade alignment in a variety of congenital and acquired conditions. A common example is hindfoot triple arthrodesis (surgical fusion of the subtalar, talonavicular, and calcaneocuboid joints) when severe planovalgus results from end-stage posterior tibial tendon dysfunction.[10,11]

To fuse a joint, the surgeon must first decorticate the apposing bone surfaces, exposing the subchondral bone. Bone graft serves as scaffolding for new bone growth and as a source of growth factors and osteoprogenitor material. Finally, compressive fixation is applied with internal, or less commonly, external fixation.[9,12] Newer surgical techniques now allow the surgeon to perform selected fusions arthroscopically.[13] The contraindications to attempting an arthrodesis are the same as those for internal fixation of fractures and osteotomies.[2]

Expected Appearance on Relevant Modalities

Radiographs usually suffice after surgical treatment of ankle and foot fracture fixation, osteotomies, and/or arthrodeses (see Fig. 110-1B). Progressive blurring and narrowing of the interface between opposing bone surfaces indicates healing by callus formation or by incorporation of bone graft. Successful fusion establishes continuity of mature trabeculae and/or cortex between the bones or bone fragments. Obliteration of the space between the bones by itself does not indicate fusion, because with rigid internal fixation, the bone surfaces will often be in full contact immediately after the procedure. Sequential examination is often required to fully document full osseous incorporation and healing. How much mature bony bridging is necessary for surgical success is not known, but often as little as 20% will translate into clinical success, which is defined by (1) lack of pain and tenderness at the operative site, (2) absence of motion between the bones under stress, and (3) ability to function (bear weight). When evaluating postoperative alignment in addition to the completeness of fusion, standing radiographs are needed.

When extensive callus formation, bone graft, or metal implants obscure the plane between the bones multidetector CT examination is the study of choice to evaluate healing.[14] To minimize streak artifact from internal fixation, relatively high kilovolts peak (typically 140 kVp), thin-section collimation (1 mm or less), and a soft reconstruction kernel are useful.[15] Direct scanning perpendicular to the joint or osteotomy is ideal, but multiplanar reformatted images in the required planes will usually be diagnostic. Lastly, including the contralateral foot and ankle in the CT images often provides a baseline reference for the normal anatomy and alignment. On CT images, complete fusion appears as mature bridging trabeculae and/or cortex across the operative bed; in earlier stages of healing indistinct callus and bone graft between the bones will progressively increase in amount and attenuation before bridging the gap.[14]

MRI is not a primary modality for the routine assessment of osteosynthesis operations, but because these procedures are common, an arthrodesis or osteotomy site will often be present on MR examinations performed for other foot and ankle soft tissue conditions. During the healing phase, marrow edema will be present in the bones adjacent to the operation site, representing a combination of mechanical trauma from the procedure and granulation tissue. Similar to the case for radiographs and CT, continuity of mature bone (represented by normal-appearing marrow) indicates fusion (Fig. 110-2), although mild surrounding marrow edema may persist even after fusion occurs, owing to ongoing bone remodeling.

For osteotomies and arthrodesis procedures, healing of the bone graft harvest site should also be evaluated. The distal tibia or calcaneus may be used as a source of bone graft for foot and ankle procedures.[16] Periosteal callus around cortical windows and gradual filling-in of the lytic defect radiographically indicate healing of the donor site. The harvest site often fills with primarily fatty marrow, which is recognized by its paucity of trabeculae and lipid content on CT and MRI. Before complete healing, these are areas of relative weakness, which may be exacerbated because of disuse. During this stage, insufficiency fractures through the donor site are important sources of morbidity.

Potential Complications and Radiologic Appearance

After incisional morbidity (e.g., wound infection, dehiscence, traumatic neuroma) nonunion is the most common complication of attempted osteosynthesis.[10,17] Nonunion means that healing stops before solid bone fusion occurs. The risk of nonunion relates to the integrity of the surgical bed (surrounding infection, tissue ischemia, and a deficient soft tissue envelope all tend to inhibit bone production), the quality of the bone (osteoporotic bone and bone compromised by prior nonunion, osteonecrosis, osteomyelitis, radiation, tumor, or Paget's disease take longer to heal), the adequacy of the surgical reduction and fixation, and host factors such as cigarette smoking, diabetes, and obesity.[9,18] Radiographically, motion between the bone fragments from one examination to the next, often accompanied by loose or fractured implants, is diagnostic of nonunion (see Fig. 110-1C).[18] When signs of motion are lacking, progressive resorption of bone graft, a persistent gap between the bone surfaces, and lack of

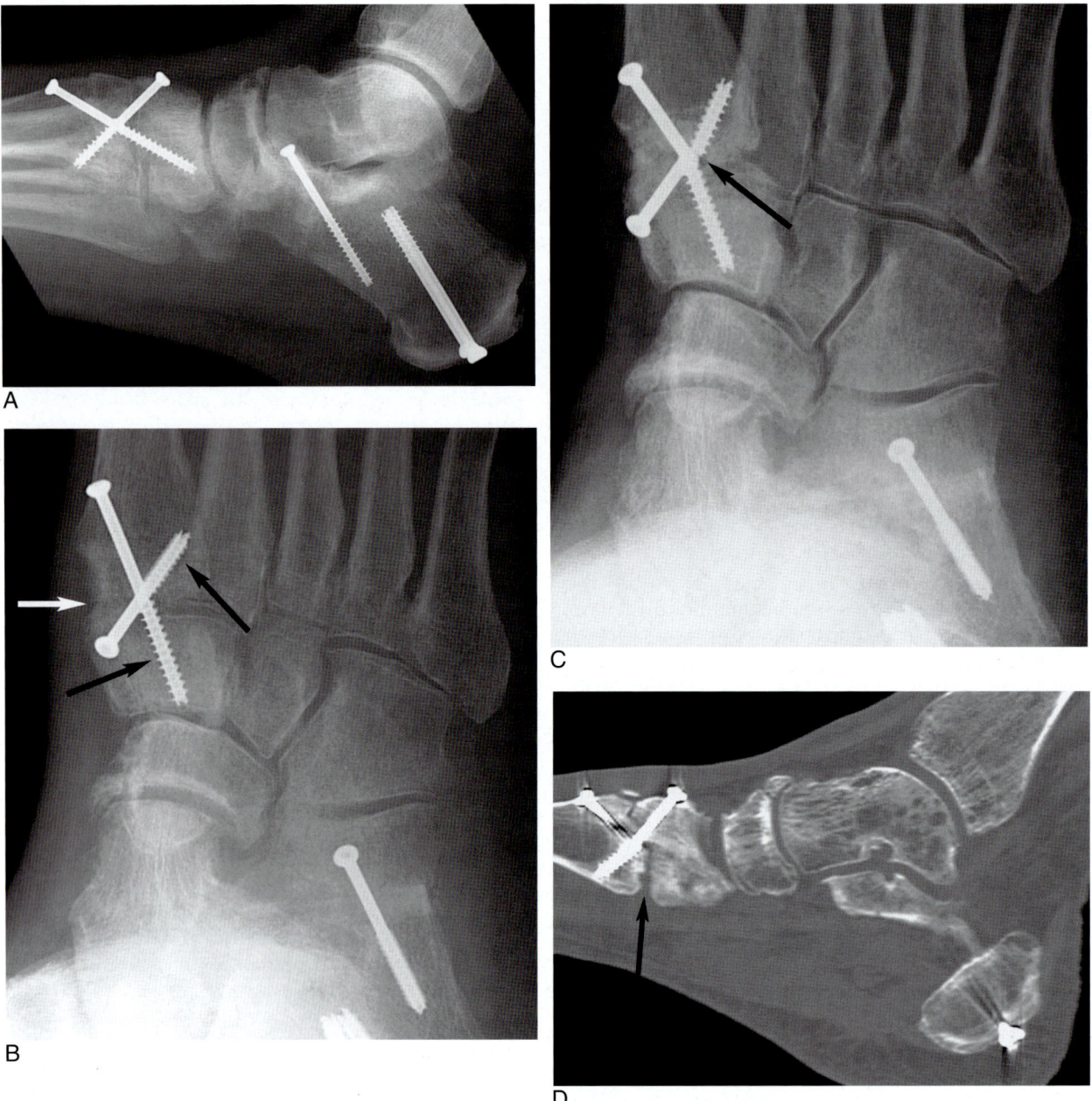

■ **FIGURE 110-1** Failed midfoot arthrodesis. **A,** Lateral projection immediately after surgery. Two screws transfix an attempted first tarsometatarsal joint arthrodesis. Note also the internally fixated calcaneal slide and lateral column-lengthening osteotomies. **B,** Oblique projection 1 month later. A persistent gap is present at the first tarsometatarsal joint space (*white arrow*), and there is bone resorption around the screws (*black arrows*), indicating micromotion. **C,** Three months later, the screws transfixing the fusion site have fatigued and fractured (*arrow*) owing to chronic motion. **D,** Sagittal CT reformatted image shows nonunion, with a persistent gap between the bones, lack of bridging trabeculae, and formation of neocortex along the bone ends (*arrow*). Disuse osteoporosis is present in the hindfoot.

osseous bridging each suggests nonunion but neocortex formation along the bone ends is diagnostic. On CT examination the findings of nonunion are often easier to recognize without obscuration by overlying structures (see Fig. 110-1D).[15] When there is lack of bridging bone, but new cortex has not formed, it may be unclear whether delayed union or nonunion is present. In those circumstances, simply noting that the site is ununited and obtaining a short-term follow-up examination may be necessary.

On MRI, distinguishing nonunion from delayed union is difficult; however, identification of a synovial pseudarticulation containing fluid and lined by a capsule indicates nonunion.

Whereas delayed union may be managed nonoperatively (by casting, decreased weight bearing, or electrical stimulation), symptomatic nonunion typically requires repeat operation. For small, noncritical locations, excision of the nonunited fragment may be curative. In most cases,

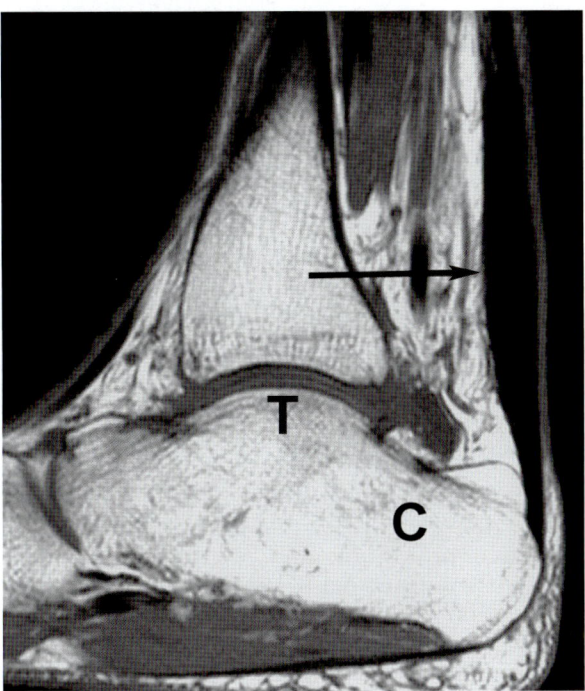

■ **FIGURE 110-2** Solid subtalar arthrodesis. A sagittal T1-weighted MR image shows continuity of the marrow between the talus (T) and calcaneus (C). Focal thickening of the Achilles tendon (*arrow*) represents tendinopathy. *(Courtesy of W. B. Morrison, Philadelphia, PA.)*

however, a revision of the operation, including removal of prior implants, decortication of the bone surfaces, application of fresh bone graft with or without bone-stimulating factors, and reapplication of new internal fixation, is needed. Extending the surgery to include fusion of surrounding joints may be necessary if postoperative instability contributed to the original nonunion. The risk of recurrent nonunion increases with each operation.[17]

Other complications manifest on imaging studies just as they would in the absence of a prior procedure. These include osteomyelitis, residual or recurrent deformity, accelerated osteoarthritis at adjacent joints, osteonecrosis, and stress fractures.[8,10] Arthrodesis may accelerate the development of osteoarthritis in adjacent joints; however, radiographic demonstration of osteoarthritis in these cases does not necessarily equate with a poor outcome or patient satisfaction.[11] Implants may become symptomatic because of impingement on adjacent structures or intra-articular extension. If the location of an orthopedic implant is not clear radiographically, CT examination can easily depict its course. Symptomatic devices can be removed after osseous fusion has occurred.

INSTABILITY OPERATIONS

Description

A lateral ankle sprain is one of the most common musculoskeletal injuries. The typical sprain results in partial or complete tear of the anterior talofibular ligament. In more severe injuries the calcaneofibular ligament will also be affected. A "high" ankle sprain involves the tibiofibular ligament(s) and syndesmotic membrane. Acute sprains of

either type generally heal with conservative therapy, with high sprains taking longer.[19,20] A minority of patients who suffer one or repeated sprains develop chronic instability that interferes with their daily activities.

Chronic instability of the distal tibiofibular syndesmosis is treated by internal fixation, typically with screws (Fig. 110-3).[21] Injuries of the deltoid and sinus tarsi ligaments rarely require surgery.[22] Acute midfoot instability involving the Lisfranc ligament and tarsometatarsal joints is usually managed by open reduction and internal fixation of the subluxated joints or by limited arthrodesis.[23] Chronic midfoot instability requires arthrodesis. Similarly, instability of the toes due to collateral ligament or plantar plate dysfunction is treated by a combination of osteotomies, fusions, and tendon transfers when conservative treatment fails.[24,25]

Indications, Contraindications, Purpose, and Underlying Mechanics

The primary indication for operative management of chronic lateral ankle instability is failure of conservative treatment.[26,27] Imaging findings, including those from stress examinations, MRI, or MR arthrography do not necessarily predict clinical instability. At least a dozen operations have been described to restore the lost function of the anterior talofibular and calcaneofibular ligaments.

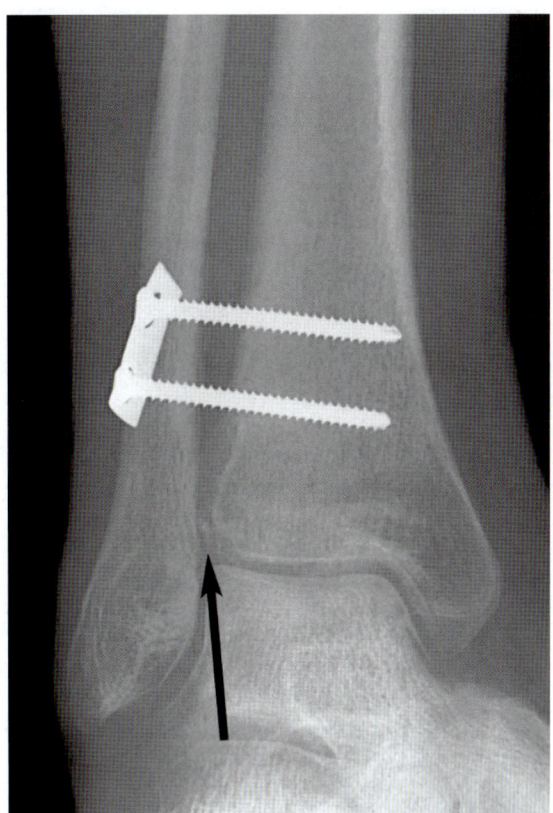

■ **FIGURE 110-3** Syndesmotic injury. A mortise projection of the ankle shows a short semitubular plate and two tricortical screws transfixing the distal tibiofibular syndesmosis in a patient with an unstable high ankle sprain. The alignment is normal, but there is post-traumatic heterotopic ossification in the anteroinferior syndesmotic ligament (*arrow*).

When adequate tissue is present, a primary (Broström) repair is done. The surgeon sews the torn ligament ends and uses suture anchors to reattach the torn ligament(s) to bone. Often surrounding structures (e.g., the inferior extensor retinaculum or a regional periosteal flap) are used to reinforce the repair (the modified Broström technique).[28]

Poor quality ligament tissue necessitates reconstruction rather than repair.[29,30] Most lateral ankle reconstruction procedures use the peroneus brevis tendon to substitute for the nonfunctional ankle ligaments.[31] The tendon (or a split portion of it) is passed through an anterior-to-posterior tunnel drilled in the distal fibula. The transposed peroneal tendon is then either resutured to itself or to the peroneus longus or is anchored to the talus. The tendon may also be tunneled under the periosteum of the talus or calcaneus. The rerouted peroneus brevis tendon replaces the biomechanical function of the ruptured ligaments, maintaining lateral ankle stability. Other reconstructions have been described using a transferred extensor digitorum brevis or plantaris tendon.[32,33]

Expected Appearance on Relevant Modalities

The appearance of the ankle after lateral instability surgery depends on the particular operation performed. After primary ligament repair, radiography may be normal or there may be suture anchors visible in the talus, fibular tip, or calcaneus (Fig. 110-4). The presence of one or more surgical tunnels in the lateral malleolus is the key radiographic finding, indicating a peroneus brevis tendon transfer procedure (Fig. 110-5).

On MR images, low signal intensity scar tissue in the incision and operative bed are typically visible, as well as a fibular tunnel if one was created. Ligament or tendon thickening and ferromagnetic artifact from sutures or anchors indicate the location of reanastomoses. Most importantly, the entire course of the peroneus brevis tendon (which may be in two slips if a tendon-splitting operation was done) should be traced and correlated with the clinical details of the reconstruction (Fig. 110-6). Tendon should be seen both entering and exiting any drilled fibular tunnels, although metal artifact from drilling often precludes visualization of the tendon within the bone.

Potential Complications and Radiologic Appearance

Ankle ligament repair or reconstruction is more likely to fail when there is coexistent osteoarthritis or hindfoot varus. Failed procedures and recurrent ankle instability are best evaluated with MRI or MR arthrography.[34] Reconstructions typically fail because the substituted structure was not properly tightened or stretched out over time. This condition must be recognized clinically because abnormal imaging findings are often absent.[35] Discontinuity of the repaired tissue or of the rerouted peroneus brevis is relatively unusual (Fig. 110-7). Before diagnosing a ruptured reconstruction, close consultation with the operating surgeon helps establish a thorough understanding of the exact procedure performed. Depending on the type of surgery, normal structures may no longer be expected in their anatomic positions.

Peroneal tendon tears or subluxation can accompany lateral ankle instability.[36] Whereas peroneal tendon

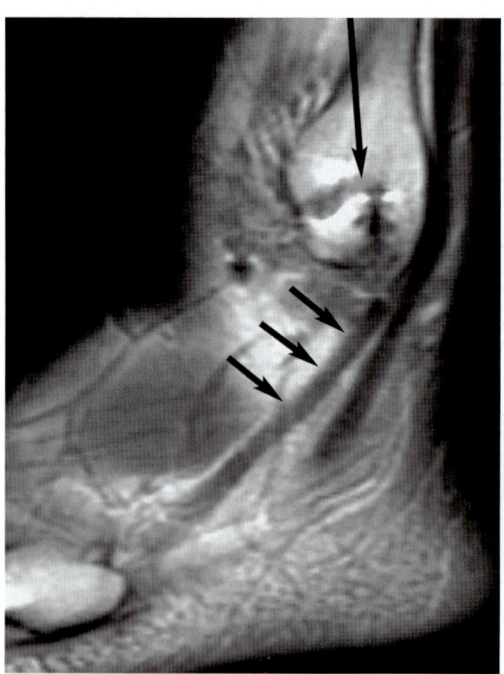
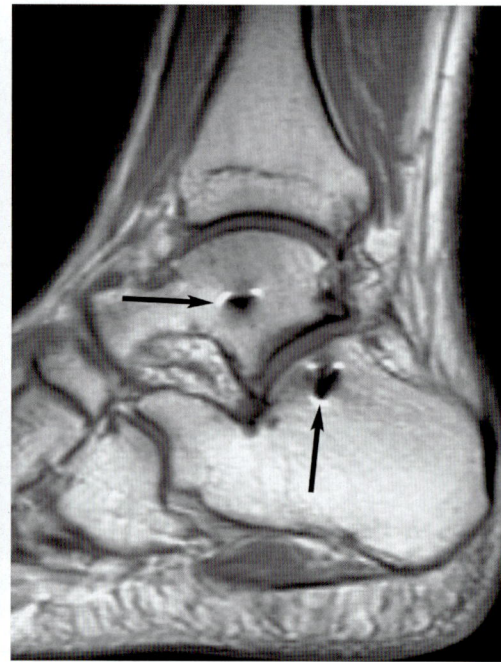

A   B

■ **FIGURE 110-4** Lateral ankle ligament repair. **A,** Sagittal T1-weighted MR image demonstrates ferromagnetic artifact (*long arrow*) in the distal fibula from suture anchors. Note the normal course of the peroneus brevis tendon (*short arrows*). **B,** A sagittal image located more medially shows artifact from anchors at the distal attachments of the repaired anterior talofibular and calcaneofibular ligaments (*arrows*). *(Courtesy of W. B. Morrison, Philadelphia, PA.)*

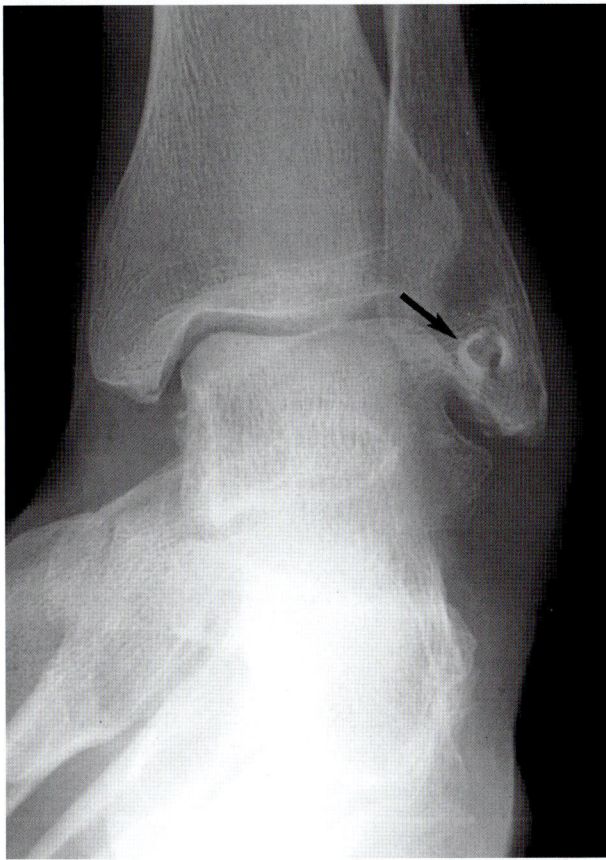

A

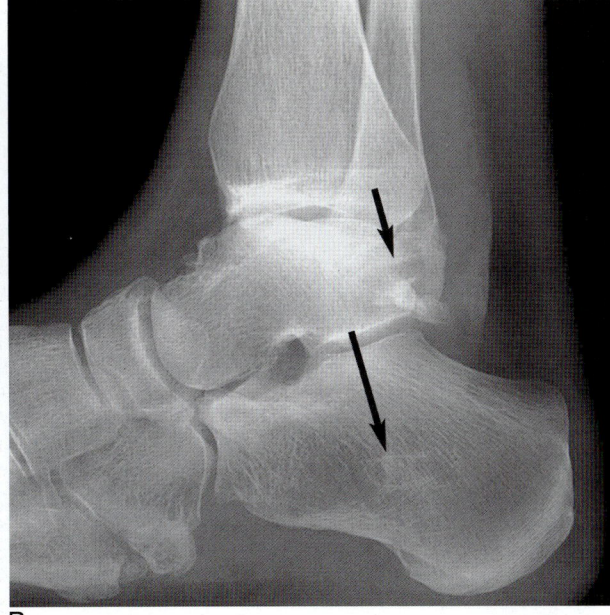

B

■ **FIGURE 110-5** Lateral ankle ligament reconstruction.
A, Anteroposterior radiograph shows a tunnel (*arrow*) drilled
through the distal fibula for passage of a portion of the split
peroneus brevis tendon. The tunnel is an integral part of almost
all reconstruction procedures. **B,** On the lateral radiograph, in
addition to the fibular tunnel (*short arrow*), there is an elevated
periosteal flap of the lateral calcaneus (*long arrow*) corresponding
to the course of the rerouted peroneus brevis tendon slip in a
patient who underwent a Chrisman-Snook procedure.

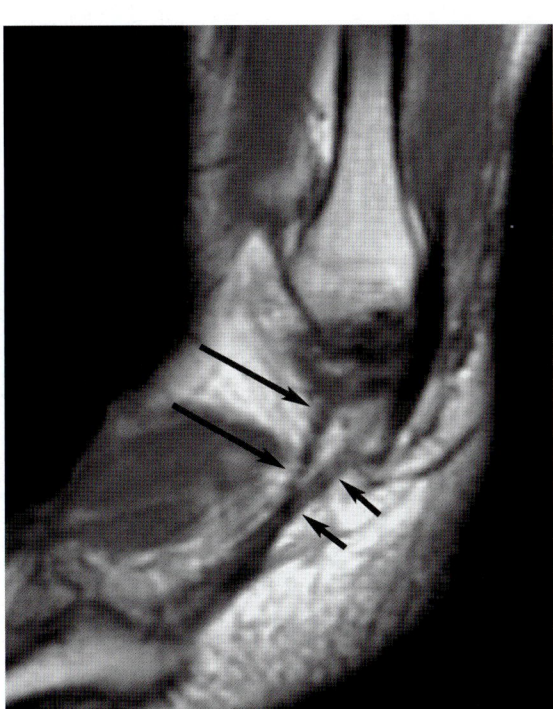

■ **FIGURE 110-6** Normal lateral ligament reconstruction. Sagittal
T1-weighted MR image shows a surgically split peroneus brevis tendon,
one half of which lies anterior to its native position (*long arrows*) after
emerging from a fibular tunnel, merging with the other tendon half
(*short arrows*) proximal to the tendon insertion on the fifth metatarsal
base. A portion of the peroneus longus is visible posterior to the lateral
malleolus. Contrast to Figure 110-4A. (*Courtesy of W. B. Morrison,
Philadelphia, PA.*)

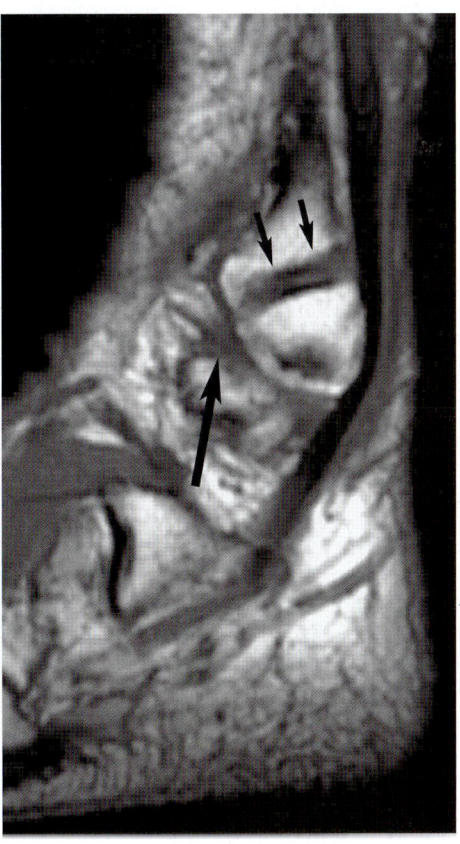

■ **FIGURE 110-7** Failed lateral ankle ligament reconstruction. Sagittal
T1-weighted MR image demonstrates a small focus of low signal-
intensity scar tissue (*long arrow*) but no peroneal tendon exiting from the
fibular tunnel (*short arrows*). Contrast to Figure 110-6. (*Courtesy of M. E.
Schweitzer, New York, NY.*)

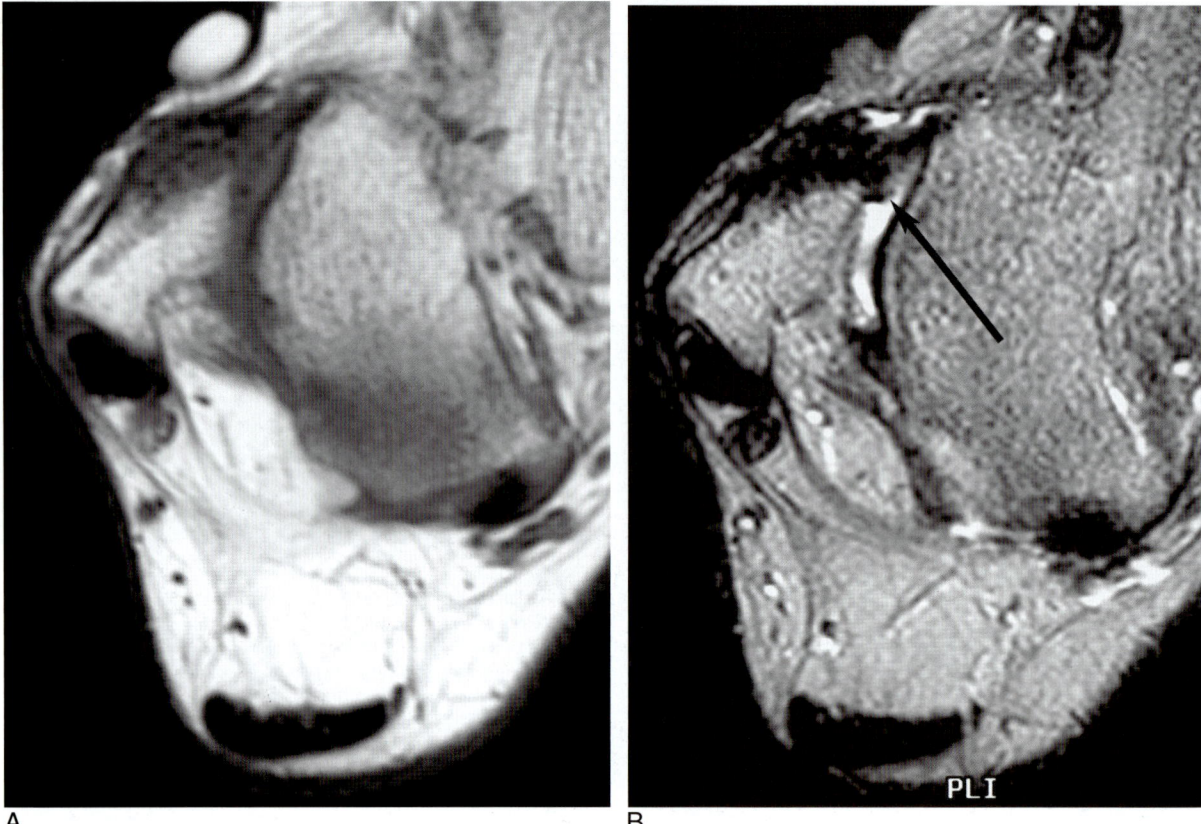

A

B

■ **FIGURE 110-8** Anterolateral soft tissue impingement after lateral ankle ligament repair. **A,** Transverse T1-weighted MR image shows intermediate signal intensity scarring and ferromagnetic artifact at the site of anterior talofibular ligament (Broström) repair. The marker indicates the location of the patient's recurrent pain. **B,** The T2-weighted MR image shows very low signal intensity scar tissue (*arrow*) within the anterolateral gutter adherent to the deep surface of the repaired ligament. Symptoms resolved after arthroscopic débridement.

abnormalities are readily diagnosed on MR images, in postoperative cases extra caution is needed to ensure that the MRI appearance is due to true pathology and not surgical reconstruction. Intra-articular conditions that may coexist with or follow lateral ligament injuries include anterolateral soft tissue impingement, talar dome osteochondral injuries, and loose bodies.[36,37] Postoperative MR images can be used to identify each of these conditions (Fig. 110-8).[38,39]

TENDON PROCEDURES

Description

Tendon disorders are a major source of morbidity in the hindfoot and ankle. The Achilles, posterior tibial, anterior tibial, flexor hallucis longus, and peroneal tendons are most frequently affected. True inflammatory tendonitis in the foot is managed nonoperatively. Lacerations follow penetrating injury can be repaired primarily (Fig. 110-9). However, most tendon disorders result from of chronic degeneration, overuse, and incomplete healing. A spectrum of pathology from tendinopathy through partial tears through complete tears and surgery has a role at any stage when symptoms are refractory to conservative treatment or in specific clinical scenarios when outcome studies show a clear advantage to surgical over conservative management.[40,41]

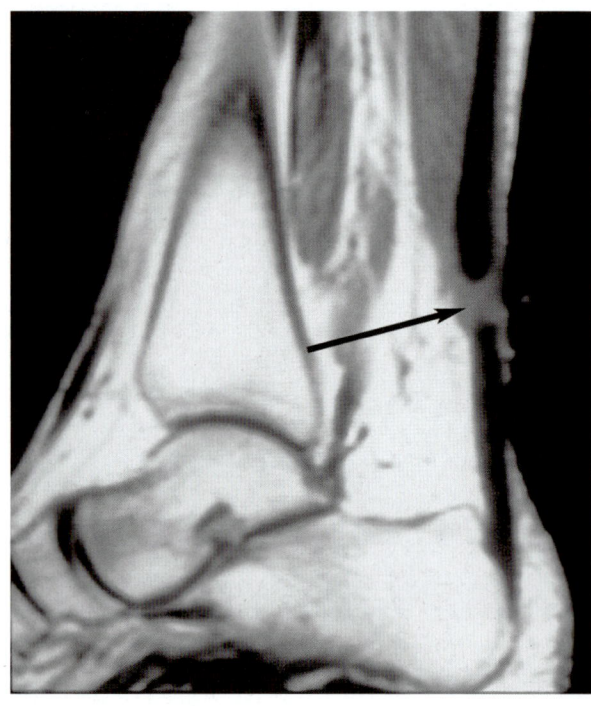

■ **FIGURE 110-9** Achilles tendon laceration. Sagittal T1-weighted MR image shows a severed tendon (*arrow*) from a broken glass injury. The absence of tendinopathy in the underlying tendon makes it an ideal candidate for primary repair.

Indications, Contraindications, Purpose, and Underlying Mechanics

For symptomatic tendinopathy that has not progressed to tendon rupture but is nevertheless refractory to conservative treatment, tenosynovectomy, brisement (distention arthrography of the tendon sheath), and/or tendon débridement can be effective.[42,43] Primary repair may be considered for tendon ruptures with relatively normal tendon quality. The torn tendons ends are reapposed and sutured, using a technique that minimizes scarring and allows smooth gliding but that is strong enough so that passive motion can be instituted quickly. Longitudinal split tears, which most often involve the peroneus brevis and posterior tibial tendons, can also be sutured.[44] When tendinopathy is present, the diseased tendon tissue is first débrided and the repair may be augmented with adjacent healthier tissue, including parts of neighboring tendons.

A tendon transfer or graft becomes necessary when tendon repair is not possible, for example when there is a large gap between the ends of a completely torn tendon, when muscle contracture prevents tendon end reapposition, or when a tendon has been stretched beyond its viscoelastic limits. Autologous sources of tendon grafts include the plantaris, palmaris, peroneus tertius, extensor digitorum, tibialis anterior, flexor digitorum longus, and flexor hallucis longus tendons.[45,46] Cadaveric and synthetic grafts are also available.[47] In cases where advanced tendon dysfunction results in a fixed hindfoot malalignment or osteoarthritis, a salvage procedure such as triple arthrodesis is indicated.[48] Corrective osteotomies combined with tendon transfer procedures can avoid the need for joint fusion when a flexible malalignment is present.[3,46,49]

Malalignments or anatomic features that predispose tendons to injury may be addressed at the time of tendon repair or transfer, or earlier in the course of disease when only tendinopathy is present. Examples include release of the posterior talar fibro-osseous tunnel or os trigonum resection in patients with posterior impingement of the flexor hallucis longus tendon[50] (Fig. 110-10); excision of the posterosuperior calcaneus for Achilles tendon disorders[51]; deepening of the fibular groove for peroneal tendon subluxation[52,53]; and removal of an accessory navicular bone when insertional posterior tibial tendon disease is present.[54] In each case, tendon débridement and/or re-anchoring may accompany the osseous operation (Fig. 110-11).

Tendon lengthening, especially for the Achilles tendon, is often required as an adjunct procedure to redistribute forces on the foot in patients with conditions ranging from midfoot neuropathy to calcaneal equinus to plantar fasciitis.[55] Controlled open or percutaneous tenotomy incisions relax the tendon and allow it to heal elongated. More extensive lengthening may be accomplished by a ZY-plasty, whereby a zigzag incision in the tendon is resewn after the tendon is stretched longitudinally.

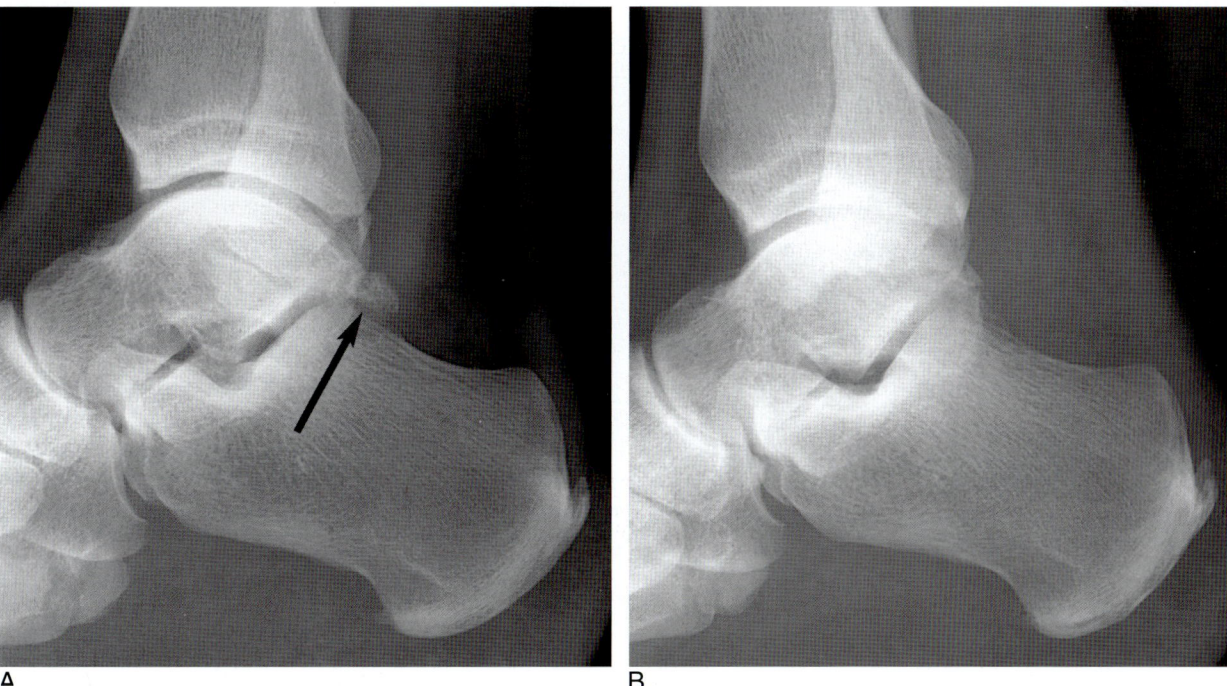

A   B

■ **FIGURE 110-10**   Excision of os trigonum for flexor hallucis longus tendinopathy and tenosynovitis. **A,** Lateral preoperative radiograph shows an os trigonum (*arrow*) in this dancer with posterior ankle pain. **B,** The postoperative radiograph shows that the os has been excised. The diseased tendon was débrided during the operation. Note that a nonunited fragment at the inferior fibular tip was also removed.

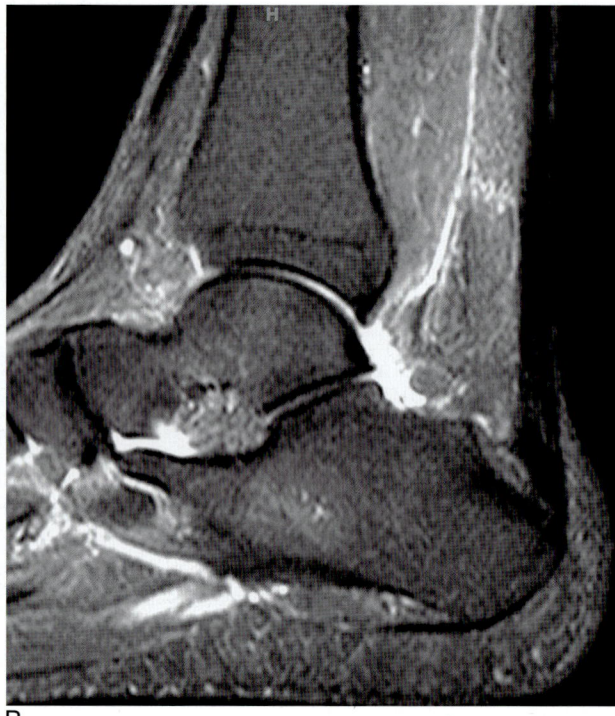

A   B

■ **FIGURE 110-11**   Removal of Haglund process for insertional Achilles tendinopathy. **A,** Postoperative lateral radiograph shows resection of the posterosuperior calcaneus (*arrow*). Note the small amount of heterotopic ossification in the distal Achilles tendon. **B,** Sagittal STIR MR image demonstrating the reattachment of the distal Achilles tendon to the posterior calcaneus.

Expected Appearance on Relevant Modalities

Magnetic resonance imaging and ultrasonography are most commonly used for assessment of tendon procedures. Successfully repaired tendons are initially markedly thickened, with maximum girth peaking approximately 3 months after surgery, but often remain thicker than the native tendon for years.[56,57] Regions of heterogeneous fiber orientation and mixed signal intensity on both T1-weighted and T2-weighted MR images within the tendon are common and do not correlate with clinical parameters (Fig. 110-12A).[57] Tracing the course of the other tendons may be an important clue that a tendon transfer or augmentation has been performed (see Fig. 110-12B). Careful correlation with the details of the operation is crucial to avoid misdiagnosing alterations in other structures as pathologic when they have been incorporated into the repair (Fig. 110-13). Tendons that have undergone a lengthening procedure will be focally thickened where the tendon has been re-sewn to itself (Fig. 110-14).

Potential Complications and Radiologic Appearance

The imaging diagnosis of an incompletely healed or retorn tendon should be made with caution because not infrequently, even a normally healed tendon will not return to its normal preinjury baseline appearance. MR signal and morphologic changes alone are often insufficient; tendon fiber discontinuity is the most reliable sign of a failed repair (Fig. 110-15).[56,57] Intravenous administration of a contrast agent is useful when there is clinical suspicion of postoperative infection involving bone or tendon.[58,59] Rim-enhancing tissue, especially associated with a sinus tract, is highly suggestive of infection (Fig. 110-16).

PLANTAR FASCIA SURGERY

Description

Plantar fasciitis is a common painful heel condition due to overuse. The disorder is usually self limited, but symptoms may last many months. Most cases are successfully managed nonoperatively, with treatment emphasizing rest, stretching, orthotics, and nonsteroidal anti-inflammatory medicines.[60] Surgical resection is generally successful when these measures fail.[61]

Plantar fibromatosis is benign but locally aggressive tumor that occurs within the plantar fascia.[62] Treatment is surgical excision, but local recurrences are common.

Indications, Contraindications, Purpose, and Underlying Mechanics

Refractory heel pain is the main indication for plantar fasciotomy, which may be performed open, percutaneously,

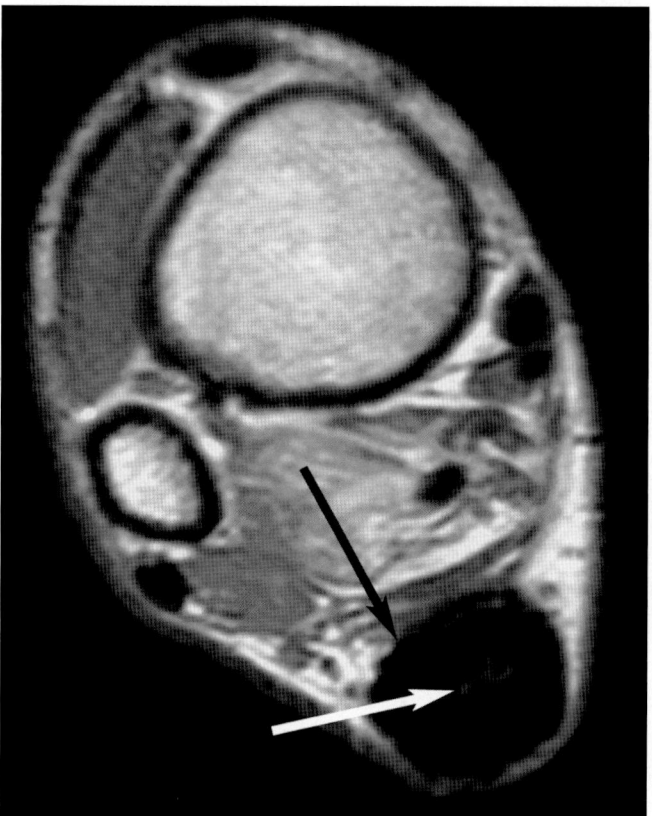

A

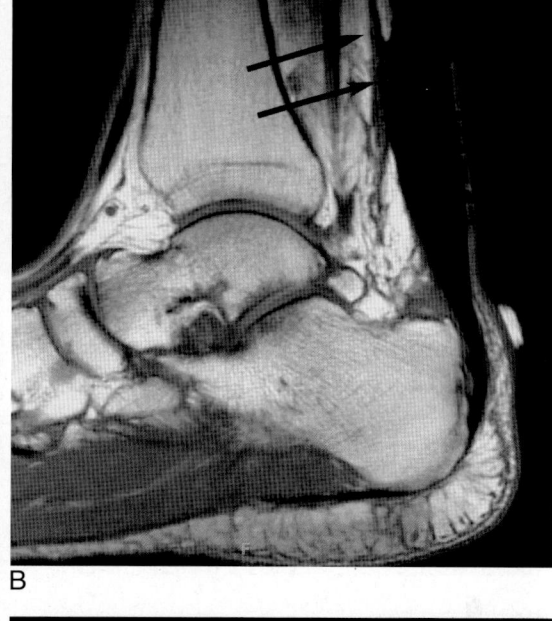

B

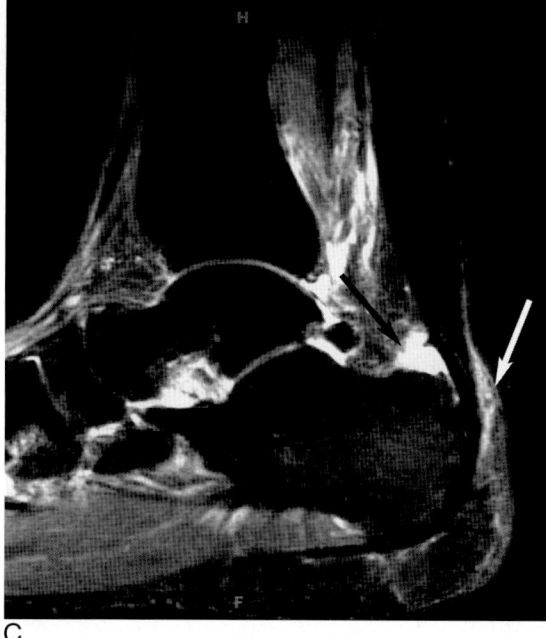

C

■ **FIGURE 110-12** Augmented Achilles tendon repair. **A,** Transverse T1-weighted MR image shows that the repaired tendon is severely thickened (*black arrow*). Note the focus of intermediate signal intensity within the tendon (*white arrow*). Clinically, the repair was intact and asymptomatic. **B,** Sagittal T1-weighted MR image shows the altered course of the flexor hallucis longus tendon (*arrows*), which has been used to augment the repair. **C,** Sagittal STIR MR image shows new insertional Achilles tendon disease including retrocalcaneal bursitis (*black arrow*) and distal Achilles paratenonitis (*white arrow*).

or endoscopically.[63,64] Typically, resection of the fascia is subtotal, sparing the most lateral fibers, in an effort to preserve the longitudinal arch of the foot and avoid injury to adjacent nerves. The goal of surgery is to remove the diseased tissue and promote normal healing. Radiofrequency ablation of the fascia and shock-wave lithotripsy have also been advocated as methods to incite a healing response in the plantar fascia.[65,66]

Initial treatment of plantar fibromatosis depends on the extent of the lesion and may be local excision, wide excision, or plantar fasciectomy. Whereas complete removal reduces the chance of recurrence, large resections are associated with higher morbidity.[67,68] In very aggressive cases, adjuvant radiotherapy is an option to help reduce the incidence of local recurrence.[69]

Expected Appearance on Relevant Modalities

After plantar fasciotomy, the fascia will typically appear thickened with indistinct margins on cross-sectional imaging studies, although in successfully treated cases, edema should not be seen in the adjacent heel fat.[70,71] A gap in the fascia at the site of resection may or may not be present (Fig. 110-17).[71]

Potential Complications and Radiologic Appearance

Recalcitrant or recurrent plantar fasciitis typically demonstrates perifascial edema on T2-weighted or STIR

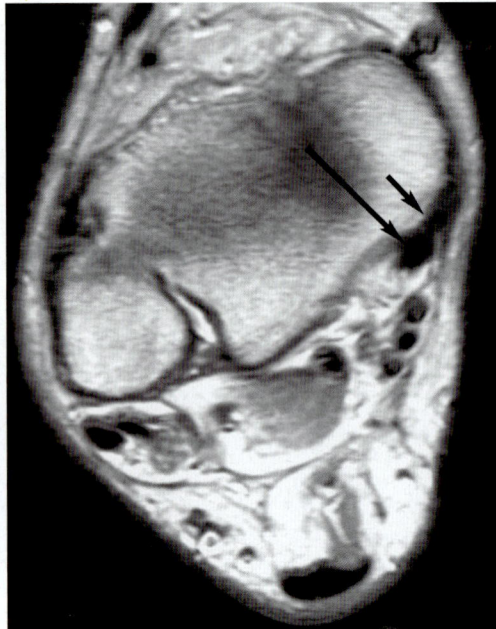

■ **FIGURE 110-13** Posterior tibial tendon rupture managed with a flexor digitorum longus tendon transfer. **A** and **B,** Sequential transverse T1-weighted MR images show the flexor digitorum longus tendon (*long arrow*) displaced medially and anastomosed side-to-side with an atrophic portion of the posterior tibial tendon (*short arrow*). *(Courtesy of W. B. Morrison, Philadelphia, PA.)*

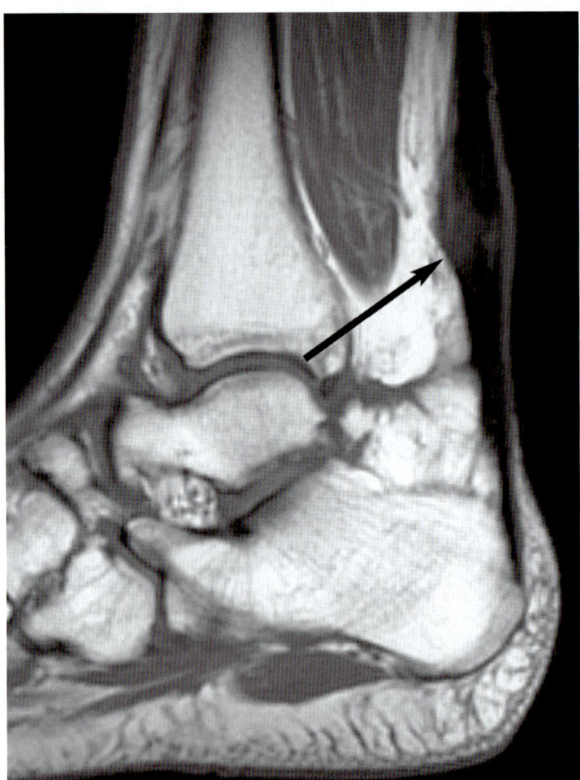

■ **FIGURE 110-14** Achilles lengthening procedure as part of clubfoot surgery. Sagittal T1-weighted image demonstrates focal thickening of the tendon (*arrow*) at the site of a Z-plasty. *(Courtesy of W. B. Morrison, Philadelphia, PA.)*

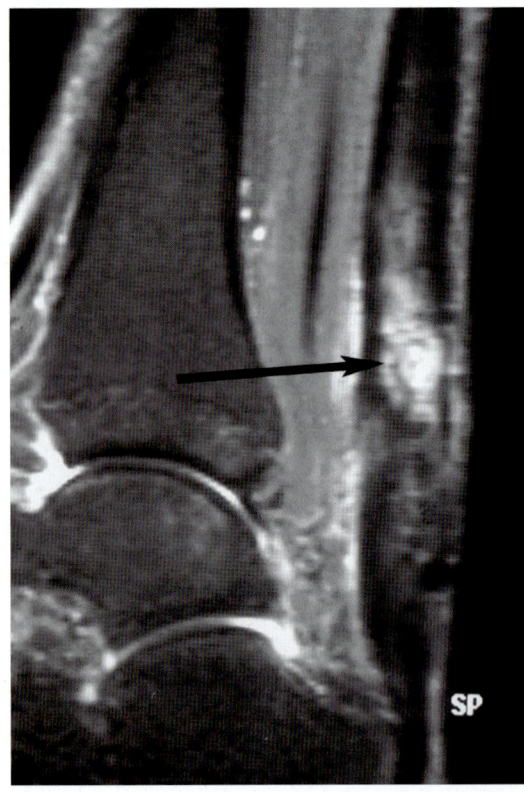

■ **FIGURE 110-15** Achilles tendon re-rupture. Sagittal STIR MR image showing disrupted tendon fibers centrally (*arrow*) within the thickened, repaired Achilles tendon. *(Courtesy of Z. S. Rosenberg, New York, NY.)*

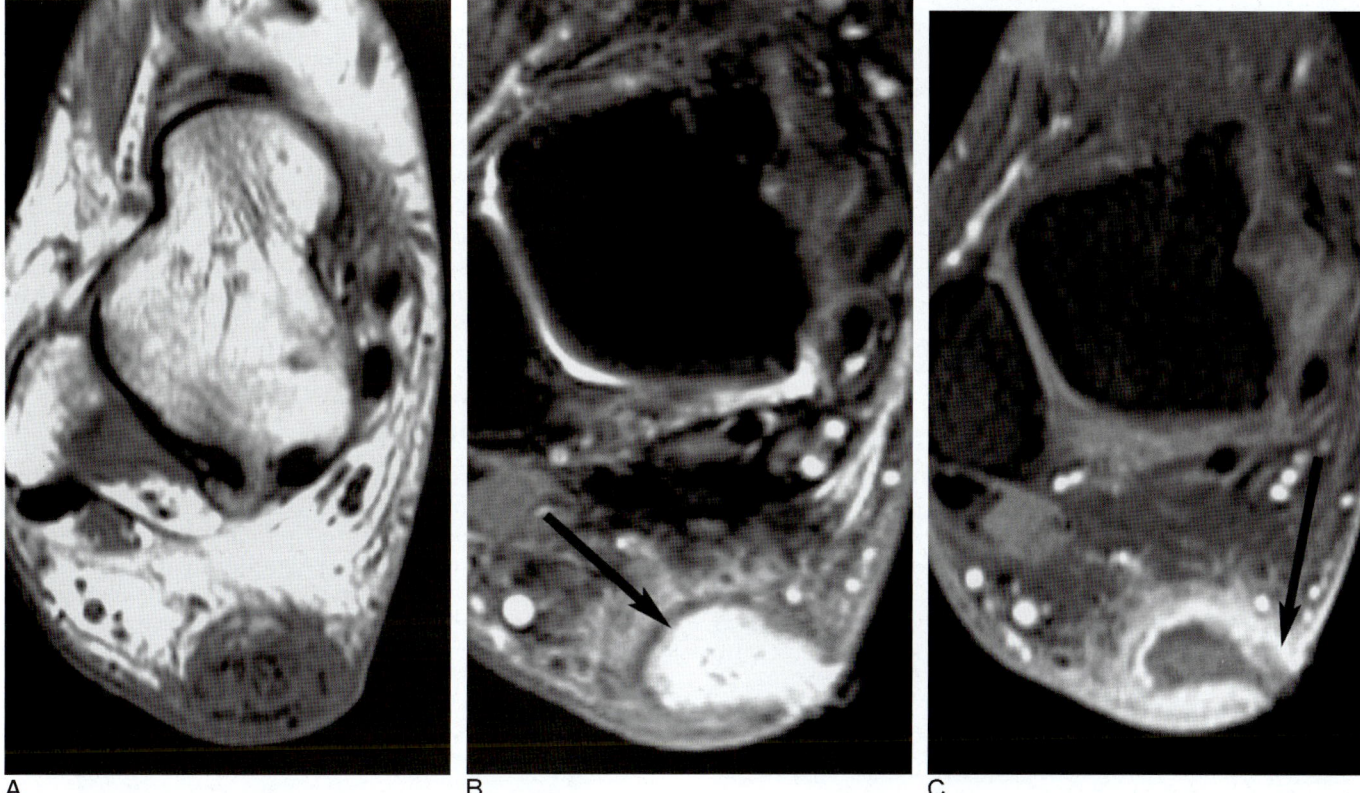

A   B   C

■ **FIGURE 110-16** Infected Achilles tendon repair. **A,** Transverse T1-weighted MR image shows little identifiable low-signal intensity tendon tissue in the operative bed. **B,** T2-weighted MR image shows fluid-intensity signal replacing the repaired tendon (*arrow*). **C,** Fat-suppressed T1-weighted MR image after intravenous contrast medium administration demonstrates that the center of the fluid collection does not enhance but is surrounded by a thick, enhancing rim. Note the sinus tract extending to the skin (*arrow*). *(Courtesy of M. E. Schweitzer, New York, NY.)*

MR pulse sequences.[72] Other potential complications of plantar fasciotomy include development of a flatfoot deformity, which in turn may lead to failure of the posterior tibial and peroneus brevis tendons and accelerated

midfoot osteoarthritis; numbness of the lateral foot from iatrogenic injury to the lateral plantar branch of the posterior tibial nerve; and acute fascial rupture. These conditions are rare but are best evaluated with MRI.[70,72]

Recurrent plantar fibromatosis after resection may be difficult to distinguish from postoperative scarring on cross-sectional imaging studies. Enhancement in the operative bed with associated mass effect favors tumor recurrence (Fig. 110-18).

NERVE DECOMPRESSION

Description

Compression neuropathy of the foot most frequently involves the branches of the posterior tibial nerve. Within the tarsal tunnel, masses such as ganglia, nerve sheath tumors, or muscle anomalies can compress the nerves, or, analogous to carpal tunnel syndrome in the wrist, the increased pressure within the tunnel may be idiopathic.[73,74] Surgical treatment consists of tarsal tunnel decompression and excision of any offending masses.[75]

Indications, Contraindications, Purpose, and Underlying Mechanics

Surgery for tarsal tunnel syndrome is indicated when a space-occupying lesion is identified or in idiopathic cases

■ **FIGURE 110-17** Plantar fasciotomy for refractory plantar fasciitis. Sagittal STIR MR image shows a surgical defect (*arrow*) in the plantar fascia, with minimal edema in the adjacent subcutaneous fat. *(Courtesy of W. B. Morrison, Philadelphia, PA.)*

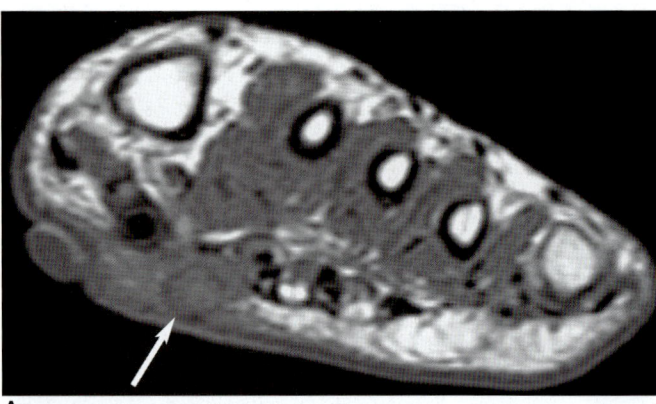

A

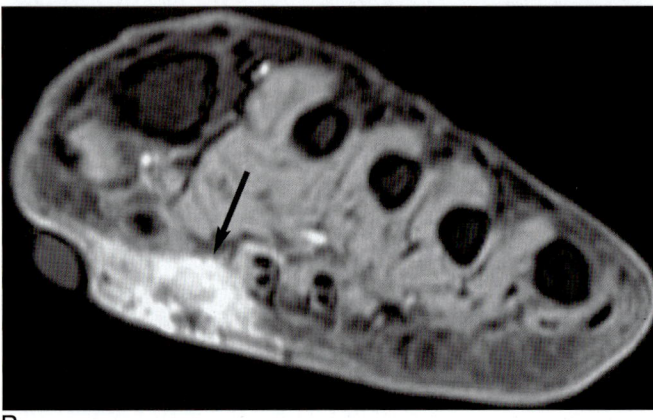

B

■ **FIGURE 110-18** Recurrent plantar fibromatosis. **A,** Short-axis T1-weighted MR image of the forefoot after plantar fibroma resection shows a focal mass (*arrow*) in the operative bed, isointense to muscle. **B,** Fat-suppressed T1-weighted image made after intravenous contrast administration shows intense enhancement of the mass (*arrow*). (*Courtesy of W. B. Morrison, Philadelphia, PA.*)

after a trial of nonoperative care has failed.[73] Neurologic symptoms (pain, paresthesias, numbness) should correspond to a nerve distribution, and a Tinel sign should be elicited over the tarsal tunnel. Ideally, electrodiagnostic studies will confirm the diagnosis, but abnormal nerve conduction tests are not present in all cases.[75] Successful relief of symptoms is more predictable when surgery is performed for a defined mass.[76,77] Tarsal tunnel release is contraindicated when signs and symptoms, imaging, or electrophysiologic data indicate that nerve compression is occurring elsewhere in the neuraxis, such as in the spine. Surgery should also not be performed when the nerve deficit is part of a generalized polyneuropathy due to a metabolic, endocrine, or toxic cause.

The goal of surgery is to relive the pressure on the posterior tibial nerve branches, primarily by decompressing the space surrounding the nerves. This is accomplished by sectioning of the flexor retinaculum, dividing the deep fascia of the abductor hallucis, and neurolysis.[75,78]

Expected Appearance on Relevant Modalities

After tarsal tunnel release, varying amounts of low-signal intensity scar tissue will be present in the surrounding

subcutaneous fat on MR images. Typically, the sectioned retinaculum will be visible (Fig. 110-19). Denervation changes in the muscles supplied by the posterior tibial nerve (abductor hallucis and flexor digitorum brevis for the medial branch; quadratus plantae and abductor digiti minimi for the lateral branch) that predated treatment will usually persist, especially if fatty atrophy representing chronic denervation is present. Because tarsal tunnel syndrome may coexist with other hindfoot conditions such as plantar fasciitis or posterior tibial tendon dysfunction, postoperative images may show evidence of procedures in addition to nerve decompression.[79]

Potential Complications and Radiologic Appearance

Unresolved or recurrent symptoms after tarsal tunnel release are relatively common, involving more than a third of the surgically treated patients in one review,[76] and may be due to incomplete sectioning of the retinaculum or abductor hallucis fascia,[75] scar tissue entrapping the nerve roots or re-establishing the flexor retinaculum, or a persistent or recurrent mass (Fig. 110-20). MRI can

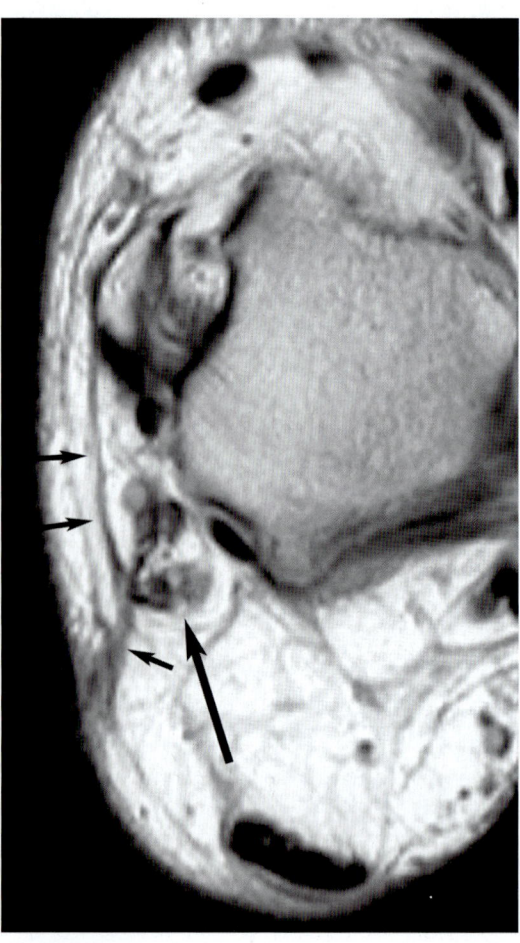

■ **FIGURE 110-19** Tarsal tunnel decompression. Transverse T1-weighted MR image shows the sectioned tarsal tunnel retinaculum (*short arrows*), which has allowed decompression of the posterior tibial nerve branches (*long arrow*). Note the fat surrounding the nerves. (*Courtesy of W. B. Morrison, Philadelphia, PA.*)

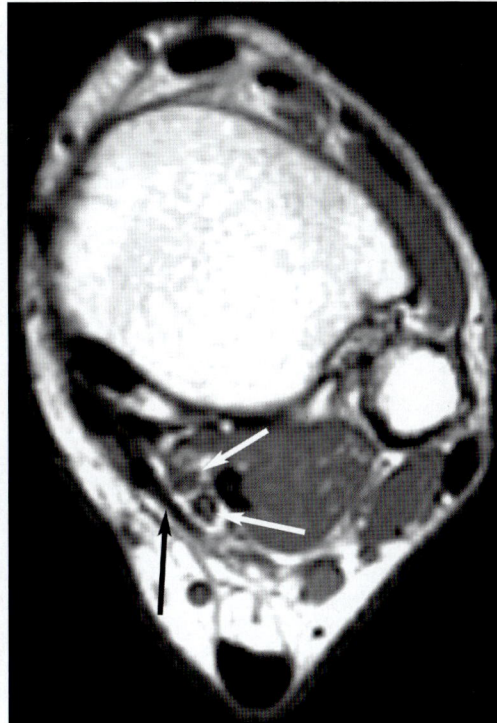

A

B

■ **FIGURE 110-20** Recurrent tarsal tunnel syndrome due to persistent retinaculum. **A,** Transverse T1-weighted MR image at the entrance of the tarsal tunnel shows scarring in the skin incision (*arrow*) extending to the flexor retinaculum. **B,** A transverse image distal to the view in A demonstrates an intact retinaculum (*black arrow*) forming a roof over the branches of the posterior tibial nerve (*white arrows*). Either the retinaculum was incompletely sectioned, or it reconstituted after the release. The patient's symptoms resolved after a repeat tarsal tunnel decompression. Contrast this figure to Figure 110-19.

typically distinguish among these possibilities. The course of the nerves should be traced through the tarsal tunnel on sequential images to identify potential compressing lesions. Low-signal intensity scar completely encircling a nerve branch suggests entrapment (Fig. 110-21) and may be easier to identify after intravenous administration of a contrast agent. Although repeat decompression and neurolysis can be attempted in these cases, surgical outcomes for recurrent tarsal tunnel syndrome are disappointing overall.[80,81]

Other than symptom recurrence, complications from tarsal tunnel syndrome are uncommon and include wound infection, iatrogenic injury to the posterior tibial artery, and inadvertent sectioning of the posterior tibial nerve.[76,80,82] These potentially devastating complications are typically obvious from physical examination findings but can be confirmed with cross-sectional imaging if necessary.

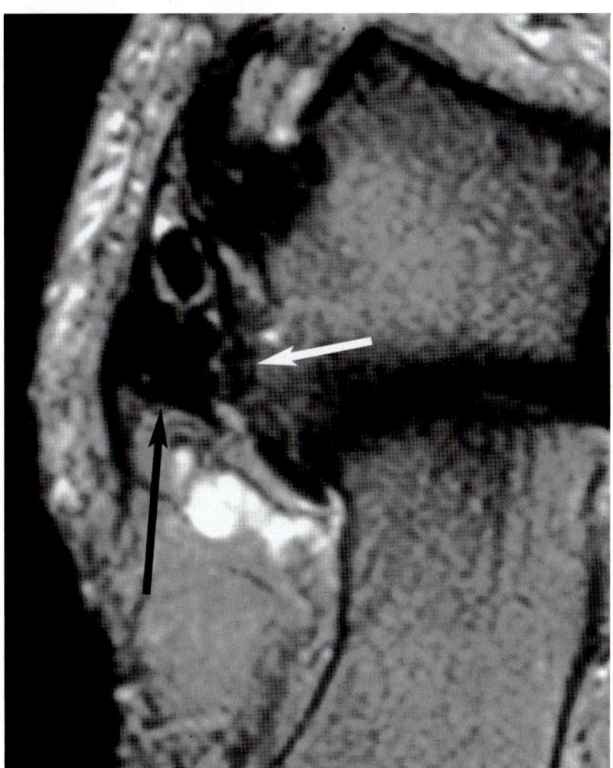

■ **FIGURE 110-21** Recurrent tarsal tunnel syndrome due to scar tissue. Coronal T2-weighted image shows thick, low signal intensity scar tissue (*black arrow*) in the operative bed, obliterating the fat surrounding the nerves (*white arrow*). Extensive neurolysis was necessary at the time of repeat tarsal tunnel decompression. Contrast this figure to Figure 110-19.

SUGGESTED READINGS

Ashman CJ, Klecker RJ, Yu JS. Forefoot pain involving the metatarsal region: differential diagnosis with MR imaging. RadioGraphics 2001; 21:1425–1440.

Bergin D, Morrison WB. Postoperative imaging of the ankle and foot. Radiol Clin North Am 2006; 44:391–406.

Chien AJ, Jacobson JA, Jamadar DA, et al. Imaging appearances of lateral ankle ligament reconstruction. RadioGraphics 2004; 24:999–1008.

Mizel MS, Hecht PJ, Marymont JV, Temple HT. Evaluation and treatment of chronic ankle pain. Instr Course Lect 2004; 53:311–321.

Recht MP, Donley BG. Magnetic resonance imaging of the foot and ankle. J Am Acad Orthop Surg 2001; 9:187–199.

Rosenberg ZS, Beltran J, Bencardino JT. From the RSNA Refresher Courses. Radiological Society of North America. MR imaging of the ankle and foot. RadioGraphics 2000; 20(Spec No):S153–S179.

Tasto JP. Arthroscopy of the subtalar joint and arthroscopic subtalar arthrodesis. Instr Course Lect 2006; 55:555–564.

REFERENCES

1. Rodriguez-Merchan EC, Forriol F. Nonunion: general principles and experimental data. Clin Orthop 2004; 419:4–12.
2. Johnson JE. Surgical treatment for neuropathic arthropathy of the foot and ankle. Instr Course Lect 1999; 48:269–277.
3. Vora AM, Tien TR, Parks BG, Schon LC. Correction of moderate and severe acquired flexible flatfoot with medializing calcaneal osteotomy and flexor digitorum longus transfer. J Bone Joint Surg Am 2006; 88:1726–1734.
4. Joseph TN, Myerson MS. Correction of multiplanar hindfoot deformity with osteotomy, arthrodesis, and internal fixation. Instr Course Lect 2005; 54:269–276.
5. Trnka HJ. Osteotomies for hallux valgus correction. Foot Ankle Clin 2005; 10:15–33.
6. Feibel JB, Tisdel CL, Donley BG. Lesser metatarsal osteotomies: a biomechanical approach to metatarsalgia. Foot Ankle Clin 2001; 6:473–489.
7. Neufeld SK, Lee TH. Total ankle arthroplasty: indications, results, and biomechanical rationale. Am J Orthop 2000; 29:593–602.
8. Wapner KL. Triple arthrodesis in adults. J Am Acad Orthop Surg 1998; 6:188–196.
9. Abidi NA, Gruen GS, Conti SF. Ankle arthrodesis: indications and techniques. J Am Acad Orthop Surg 2000; 8:200–209.
10. Graves SC, Mann RA, Graves KO. Triple arthrodesis in older adults: results after long-term follow-up. J Bone Joint Surg Am 1993; 75:355–362.
11. Pell RF 4th, Myerson MS, Schon LC. Clinical outcome after primary triple arthrodesis. J Bone Joint Surg Am 2000; 82:47–57.
12. Paley D, Lamm BM, Katsenis D, et al. Treatment of malunion and nonunion at the site of an ankle fusion with the Ilizarov apparatus: surgical technique. J Bone Joint Surg Am 2006; 88(Suppl 1 pt 1):119–134.
13. Stroud CC. Arthroscopic arthrodesis of the ankle, subtalar, and first metatarsophalangeal joint. Foot Ankle Clin 2002; 7:135–146.
14. Coughlin MJ, Grimes JS, Traughber PD, Jones CP. Comparison of radiographs and CT scans in the prospective evaluation of the fusion of hindfoot arthrodesis. Foot Ankle Int 2006; 27:780–787.
15. Buckwalter KA, Parr JA, Choplin RH, Capello WN. Multichannel CT imaging of orthopedic hardware and implants. Semin Musculoskelet Radiol 2006; 10:86–97.
16. Raikin SM, Brislin K. Local bone graft harvested from the distal tibia or calcaneus for surgery of the foot and ankle. Foot Ankle Int 2005; 26:449–453.
17. Cooper PS. Complications of ankle and tibiotalocalcaneal arthrodesis. Clin Orthop 2001; 391:33–44.
18. Saxena A, DiDomenico LA, Widtfeldt A, et al. Implantable electrical bone stimulation for arthrodeses of the foot and ankle in high-risk patients: a multicenter study. J Foot Ankle Surg 2005; 44:450–454.
19. Boytim MJ, Fischer DA, Neumann L. Syndesmotic ankle sprains. Am J Sports Med 1991; 19:294–298.
20. Gerber JP, Williams GN, Scoville CR, et al. Persistent disability associated with ankle sprains: a prospective examination. Foot Ankle Int 1998; 19:653–660.
21. Thompson MC, Gesink DS. Biomechanical comparison of syndesmosis fixation with 3.5- and 4.5-millimeter stainless steel screws. Foot Ankle Int 2000; 21:736–741.
22. Harper MC. The deltoid ligament: an evaluation of need for surgical repair. Clin Orthop 1988; 226:156–168.
23. Ly TV, Coetzee JC. Treatment of primarily ligamentous Lisfranc joint injuries: primary arthrodesis compared with open reduction and internal fixation: a prospective, randomized study. J Bone Joint Surg Am 2006; 88:514–520.
24. Myerson MS, Jung HG. The role of toe flexor-to-extensor transfer in correcting metatarsophalangeal joint instability of the second toe. Foot Ankle Int 2005; 26:675–679.
25. Ford LA, Collins KB, Christensen JC. Stabilization of the subluxed second metatarsophalangeal joint: flexor tendon transfer versus primary repair of the plantar plate. J Foot Ankle Surg 1998; 37:217–222.
26. Lynch SA, Renstrom PA. Treatment of acute lateral ankle ligament rupture in the athlete: conservative versus surgical treatment. Sports Med 1999; 27:61–71.
27. Pijnenburg AC, Van Dijk CN, Bossuyt PM, Marti RK. Treatment of ruptures of the lateral ankle ligaments: a meta-analysis. J Bone Joint Surg Am 2000; 82:761–773.
28. Messer TM, Cummins CA, Ahn J, Kelikian AS. Outcome of the modified Brostrom procedure for chronic lateral ankle instability. Foot Ankle Int 2000; 21:996–1003.
29. Liu SH, Baker CL. Comparison of lateral ankle ligamentous reconstruction procedures. Am J Sports Med 1994; 22:313–317.
30. St Pierre R, Allman F Jr, Bassett FH 3rd, et al. A review of lateral ankle ligamentous reconstructions. Foot Ankle 1982; 3:114–123.
31. Larsen E. Static or dynamic repair of chronic lateral ankle instability: a prospective randomized study. Clin Orthop 1990; 257:184–192.
32. Westlin NE, Vogler HW, Albertsson MP, et al. Treatment of lateral ankle instability with transfer of the extensor digitorum. J Foot Ankle Surg 2003; 42:183–192.
33. Anderson ME. Reconstruction of the lateral ligaments of the ankle using the plantaris tendon. J Bone Joint Surg Am 1985; 67:930–934.
34. Chandnani VP, Harper MT, Ficke JR, et al. Chronic ankle instability: evaluation with MR arthrography, MR imaging, and stress radiography. Radiology 1994; 192:189–194.
35. Leach RE, Namiki O, Paul GR, Stockel J. Secondary reconstruction of the lateral ligaments of the ankle. Clin Orthop 1981; 160:201–211.
36. DiGiovanni BF, Fraga CJ, Cohen BE, Shereff MJ. Associated injuries found in chronic lateral ankle instability. Foot Ankle Int 2000; 21:809–815.
37. Renstrom PA. Persistently painful sprained ankle. J Am Acad Orthop Surg 1994; 2:270–280.
38. Rubin DA, Tishkoff NW, Britton CA, et al. Anterolateral soft-tissue impingement in the ankle: diagnosis using MR imaging. AJR Am J Roentgenol 1997; 169:829–835.
39. Magee TH, Hinson GW. Usefulness of MR imaging in the detection of talar dome injuries. AJR Am J Roentgenol 1998; 170:1227–1230.
40. Cetti R, Christensen SE, Ejsted R, et al. Operative versus nonoperative treatment of Achilles tendon rupture: a prospective randomized study and review of the literature. Am J Sports Med 1993; 21:791–799.
41. Khan RJ, Fick D, Keogh A, et al. Treatment of acute Achilles tendon ruptures: a meta-analysis of randomized, controlled trials. J Bone Joint Surg Am 2005; 87:2202–2210.

42. Teasdall RD, Johnson KA. Surgical treatment of stage I posterior tibial tendon dysfunction. Foot Ankle Int 1994; 15:646-648.

43. Johnston E, Scranton P Jr, Pfeffer GB. Chronic disorders of the Achilles tendon: results of conservative and surgical treatments. Foot Ankle Int 1997; 18:570-574.

44. Krause JO, Brodsky JW. Peroneus brevis tendon tears: pathophysiology, surgical reconstruction, and clinical results. Foot Ankle Int 1998; 19:271-279.

45. Wilcox DK, Bohay DR, Anderson JG. Treatment of chronic Achilles tendon disorders with flexor hallucis longus tendon transfer/augmentation. Foot Ankle Int 2000; 21:1004-1010.

46. Sammarco GJ, Hockenbury RT. Treatment of stage II posterior tibial tendon dysfunction with flexor hallucis longus transfer and medial displacement calcaneal osteotomy. Foot Ankle Int 2001; 22:305-312.

47. Lieberman JR, Lozman J, Czajka J, Dougherty J. Repair of Achilles tendon ruptures with Dacron vascular graft. Clin Orthop 1988; 234:204-208.

48. Johnson JE, Yu JR. Arthrodesis techniques in the management of stage II and III acquired adult flatfoot deformity. Instr Course Lect 2006; 55:531-542.

49. Moseir-LaClair S, Pomeroy G, Manoli A 2nd. Intermediate follow-up on the double osteotomy and tendon transfer procedure for stage II posterior tibial tendon insufficiency. Foot Ankle Int 2001; 22:283-291.

50. Hedrick MR, McBryde AM. Posterior ankle impingement. Foot Ankle Int 1994; 15:2-8.

51. Sammarco GJ, Taylor AL. Operative management of Haglund's deformity in the nonathlete: a retrospective study. Foot Ankle Int 1998; 19:724-729.

52. Kollias SL, Ferkel RD. Fibular grooving for recurrent peroneal tendon subluxation Am J Sports Med 1997; 25:329-335.

53. Porter D, McCarroll J, Knapp E, Torma J. Peroneal tendon subluxation in athletes: fibular groove deepening and retinacular reconstruction. Foot Ankle Int 2005; 26:436-441.

54. Sella EJ, Lawson JP, Ogden JA. The accessory navicular synchondrosis. Clin Orthop 1986; 209:280-285.

55. Myerson MS, Henderson MR, Saxby T, Short KW. Management of midfoot diabetic neuroarthropathy. Foot Ankle Int 1994; 15:233-241.

56. Karjalainen PT, Aronen HJ, Pihlajamaki HK, et al. Magnetic resonance imaging during healing of surgically repaired Achilles tendon ruptures. Am J Sports Med 1997; 25:164-171.

57. Moller M, Kalebo P, Tidebrant G, et al. The ultrasonographic appearance of the ruptured Achilles tendon during healing: a longitudinal evaluation of surgical and nonsurgical treatment, with comparisons to MRI appearance. Knee Surg Sports Traumatol Arthrosc 2002; 10:49-56.

58. Morrison WB, Schweitzer ME, Bock GW, et al. Diagnosis of osteomyelitis: utility of fat-suppressed contrast-enhanced MR imaging. Radiology 1993; 189:251-257.

59. Ledermann HP, Morrison WB, Schweitzer ME, Raikin SM. Tendon involvement in pedal infection: MR analysis of frequency, distribution, and spread of infection. AJR Am J Roentgenol 2002; 179:939-947.

60. Wolgin M, Cook C, Graham C, Mauldin D. Conservative treatment of plantar heel pain: long-term follow-up. Foot Ankle Int 1994; 15:97-102.

61. Leach RE, Seavey MS, Salter DK. Results of surgery in athletes with plantar fasciitis. Foot Ankle 1986; 7:156-161.

62. Zgonis T, Jolly GP, Polyzois V, et al. Plantar fibromatosis. Clin Podiatr Med Surg 2005; 22:11-18.

63. Daly PJ, Kitaoka HB, Chao EY. Plantar fasciotomy for intractable plantar fasciitis: clinical results and biomechanical evaluation. Foot Ankle 1992; 13:188-195.

64. Benton-Weil W, Borrelli AH, Weil LS Jr, Weil LS Sr. Percutaneous plantar fasciotomy: a minimally invasive procedure for recalcitrant plantar fasciitis. J Foot Ankle Surg 1988; 37:269-272.

65. Sollitto RJ, Plotkin EL, Klein PG, Mullin P. Early clinical results of the use of radiofrequency lesioning in the treatment of plantar fasciitis. vJ Foot Ankle Surg 1997; 36:215-219.

66. Rompe JD, Decking J, Schoellner C, Nafe B. Shock wave application for chronic plantar fasciitis in running athletes: a prospective, randomized, placebo-controlled trial. Am J Sports Med 2003; 31:268-275.

67. Durr HR, Krodel A, Trouillier H, et al. Fibromatosis of the plantar fascia: diagnosis and indications for surgical treatment. Foot Ankle Int 1999; 20:13-17.

68. Sammarco GJ, Mangone PG. Classification and treatment of plantar fibromatosis. Foot Ankle Int 2000; 21:563-569.

69. de Bree E, Zoetmulder FA, Keus RB, et al. Incidence and treatment of recurrent plantar fibromatosis by surgery and postoperative radiotherapy. Am J Surg 2004; 187:33-38.

70. Woelffer KE, Figura MA, Sandberg NS, Snyder NS. Five-year follow-up results of instep plantar fasciotomy for chronic heel pain. J Foot Ankle Surg 2000; 39:218-223.

71. Yu JS, Smith G, Ashman C, Kaeding C. The plantar fasciotomy: MR imaging findings in asymptomatic volunteers. Skeletal Radiol 1999; 28:447-452.

72. Yu JS, Spigos D, Tomczak R. Foot pain after a plantar fasciotomy: an MR analysis to determine potential causes. J Comput Assist Tomogr 1999; 23:707-712.

73. Sammarco GJ, Chang L. Outcome of surgical treatment of tarsal tunnel syndrome. Foot Ankle Int 2003; 24:125-131.

74. Hirose CB, McGarvey WC. Peripheral nerve entrapments. Foot Ankle Clin 2004; 9:255-269.

75. Bailie DS, Kelikian AS. Tarsal tunnel syndrome: diagnosis, surgical technique, and functional outcome. Foot Ankle Int 1998; 19:65-72.

76. Pfeiffer WH, Cracchiolo A 3rd. Clinical results after tarsal tunnel decompression. J Bone Joint Surg Am 1994; 76:1222-1230.

77. Urguden M, Bilbasar H, Ozdemir H, et al. Tarsal tunnel syndrome—the effect of the associated features on outcome of surgery. Int Orthop 2002; 26:253-256.

78. Gondring WH, Shields B, Wenger S. An outcomes analysis of surgical treatment of tarsal tunnel syndrome. Foot Ankle Int 2003; 24:545-550.

79. Labib SA, Gould JS, Rodriguez-del-Rio FA, Lyman S. Heel pain triad (HPT): the combination of plantar fasciitis, posterior tibial tendon dysfunction and tarsal tunnel syndrome. Foot Ankle Int 2002; 23:212-220.

80. Skalley TC, Schon LC, Hinton RY, Myerson MS. Clinical results following revision tibial nerve release. Foot Ankle Int 1994; 15:360-367.

81. Raikin SM, Minnich JM. Failed tarsal tunnel syndrome surgery. Foot Ankle Clin 2003; 8:159-174.

82. Rosson GD, Spinner RJ, Dellon AL. Tarsal tunnel surgery for treatment of tarsal ganglion: a rewarding operation with devastating potential complications. J Am Podiatr Med Assoc 2005; 95:459-463.

83. Karlsson J, Eriksson BI, Renstrom P. Subtalar instability of the foot: a review and results after surgical treatment. Scand J Med Sci Sports 1998; 8:191-197.

111

Imaging of the Residual Limb after Amputation

Laura M. Fayad

Amputation surgery is an ancient procedure dating back to prehistoric times. Although there have been numerous advances in limb salvage techniques, amputation is still performed today and may be the treatment of choice in cases of severe vascular disease, severe trauma, and malignant neoplasms. In the United States, most amputations are performed in patients with diabetes mellitus and peripheral vascular disease, with amputations in this population accounting for up to 82% of all amputations[1] and lower-extremity amputations accounting for approximately 85% of all amputations.[2,3]

AMPUTATION SURGERY

Description

Amputation is considered a reconstructive procedure and, as such, the approaches and techniques of the surgery are designed to maximize the postoperative functionality of the residual limb and to receive a prosthesis when possible for restoration of locomotion. Although there are several important factors that influence the outcome of amputation surgery, of greatest consequence is the level of amputation (Table 111-1). The length of the residual limb has strong implications for postoperative rehabilitation[4-8] and is decided by the need to eradicate pathology in the limb, the adequacy of the vascular supply, and length requirements for fitting of a prosthesis.[6]

A successful amputation surgery involves the appropriate management of all the amputated tissue layers, including the skin, muscles, nerves, vessels, and bones. First, because the skin is the most important organ for wound healing, the greatest skin length possible is maintained and the cutaneous scar is localized away from the weight-bearing area. Second, muscle is placed over the cut end of the bone with a myodesis to the bone or a myoplasty to give sufficient volume to pad the bone and ensure a good residual limb-prosthetic fit. Third, the nerves are transected under tension and placed in an environment

proximal to the musculocutaneous scar of the amputation site, thereby reducing the possibility that a neuroma will form. Fourth, the larger arteries and veins are dissected and ligated to prevent the occurrence of arteriovenous fistulas and aneurysms. Fifth, bony prominences around the amputated bone are removed. Because ectopic bone formation can occur when the periosteum covering the bone that is retained is stripped, some surgeons prefer to resect the periosteum longer than the residual bone to adequately cover the bone end and deter ectopic ossification.[9]

INDICATIONS, CONTRAINDICATIONS, PURPOSE, AND UNDERLYING MECHANICS

Indications

The general indication for amputation surgery is the case in which a diseased limb cannot be reconstructed or when an attempted reconstruction will lead to a functionally unsatisfactory limb. Specific indications are as follows:

- Peripheral vascular disease: most commonly, for elderly patients with diabetes mellitus.
- Trauma: in some patients with severe open fractures with neurovascular injuries.
- Thermal and electric injury: for severe cases that result in a nonvascular extremity.
- Tumors: reserved for tumors not amenable to limb-salvage techniques, such as tumors with neurovascular invasion or pathologic fractures.
- Infection: for severe cases leading to extremity necrosis. Also, eradication of an infection sometimes necessitates amputation of the infected limb or portion of it.
- Congenital limb deficiency: for failure of formation of a complete limb in children.
- Cosmetic indications: for example, amputation of the fifth toe when it overrides the fourth toe.

KEY POINTS

- Pain is commonly encountered in the residual limb of an amputee. The role of imaging is to distinguish intrinsic from extrinsic causes of pain.
- Adventitial bursae are common and form in response to friction at the residual limb/prosthesis interface. They may be physiologic but can be complicated by inflammation and infection.
- Osseous overgrowth is a common complication of amputation in the pediatric patient, but in an adult the incidence is unclear, although evidence of an aggressive bone edge or heterotopic ossification should be sought, because these lead to overlying soft tissue irritation.
- Osteomyelitis is a common cause of bone marrow signal alterations by MRI, but other bone marrow abnormalities such as a stress fracture, contusion, or postsurgical alterations should be entertained.
- In the differential diagnosis of a soft tissue mass at the residual limb in the first year after amputation, a postoperative neuroma should be considered.

TABLE 111-1 Levels of Surgical Amputation

Upper Extremity	Lower Extremity
Phalangeal	Toe
Ray	Ray
Transcarpal	Transmetatarsal
Wrist disarticulation	Lisfranc's (through the Lisfranc joint)
Transradial/below elbow	Chopart's (through calcaneocuboid or talonavicular joint)
Krukenberg's (separation of ulna and radius to provide pincer-like grasp)	Syme's (just above ankle)
Elbow disarticulation	Transtibial
Transhumeral	Knee disarticulation
Shoulder disarticulation	Transfemoral
Forequarter (upper extremity amputation, scapula, and clavicle)	Hip disarticulation
	Hindquarter (hemipelvectomy through sacroiliac joint

Contraindications

The main contraindication to amputation surgery is poor health impairing the patient's ability to tolerate anesthesia and surgery. The only other contraindication to amputation is a spared limb or part of a limb that would be functionally superior to its amputation.

Expected Appearance on Relevant Modalities

By radiography, the appearance of the bone end should be blunt and the covering soft tissues free of osseous overgrowth. For an understanding of the residual limb/ prosthetic socket interface, weight-bearing static views or videofluoroscopy may be performed to demonstrate any signs of impingement on the covering soft tissues.[10]

Skeletal scintigraphy produces nonspecific areas of increased uptake in the residual limb due to tissue remodeling and is limited by its lack of anatomic resolution. Hence, it is usually reserved for amputees with a high clinical suspicion for osteomyelitis.[11]

With positron emission tomography (PET), there is diffuse postoperative fluorodeoxyglucose (FDG) uptake in the residual limb for up to 18 months. Focal areas of FDG uptake are most commonly due to pressure points and areas of skin breakdown rather than tumor. When focal uptake does not correspond to a clinical area of skin disturbance, locally recurrent tumor is suspected.[12,13] Recently, FDG PET was used to determine basic metabolic changes in the skeletal muscle of amputees, for the purpose of refining rehabilitation techniques.[14]

In the normal postoperative examination, CT will show blunted bony margins at the amputation site without extreme edges. The overlying soft tissues may show areas of ill-defined edema in the early postoperative period with later possible formation of uncomplicated bursae at sites of contact between the residual limb and a prosthesis.[15] With 3D CT, volume modeling of the residual limb may be performed for the purpose of modifying the prosthesis fit and advancing rehabilitation efforts.[16,17]

MRI is a high contrast-resolution technique that affords a superior evaluation of the soft tissues and bone marrow of the amputated extremity. In the noncomplicated amputee there is preservation of normal fatty and hematopoietic marrow signal intensity in the residual bone on T1-weighted imaging, confirming the absence of osteomyelitis or recurrent tumor. The surrounding soft tissues may contain areas of increased fluid signal in the early postoperative period with later development of uncomplicated adventitial bursae. MRI can be used to assist rehabilitation efforts by providing a precise assessment of the soft tissue changes at the residual limb that can lead to corrections at the prosthesis/residual limb interface.[18] Postcontrast imaging is often obtained to increase specificity for the presence of infection and recurrent tumor, assist with characterization of abnormalities, and determine areas of devitalized tissue.

Ultrasonography is more commonly used as a guidance device for therapy in the residual limb rather than a primary diagnostic tool,[19] although it is the study of choice for the evaluation of potential deep venous thrombosis.

Potential Complications and Radiologic Appearance

In its early history, the main complications of amputation surgery included hemorrhage, shock, and sepsis, but with the advent of modern-day anesthesia and refinements in surgical technique, such severe complications have been ameliorated and the life expectancy of an amputee has increased. Nevertheless, difficulties with wound healing and pain at the residual limb are common and imaging plays a vital role in elucidating their causes.

Pain in the residual limb occurs in a high percentage of patients after amputation, with a recent report stating that 95% of patients experience some type of amputation-related pain and 67.7% experience severe pain.[20] In fact, the primary role of imaging in these patients is to differentiate intrinsic causes of pain (those involving the residual limb itself) from extrinsic causes of pain (those that are the result of conflict between the residual limb and the prosthesis due to improper fit or alignment), because extrinsic causes may be abolished by revising the prosthesis rather than treating the residual limb. Table 111-2 provides a listing of potential complications that can be detected and characterized through imaging. Some specific complications are discussed here.

Osseous overgrowth occurs in three varieties: (1) ectopic bone at the site of periosteal avulsion, (2) endosteal bone overgrowth, and (3) heterotopic bone that occurs within the adjacent soft tissues. Osseous overgrowth is a well-known complication of amputation in the pediatric patient, most commonly encountered in a patient younger than the age of 12, with a 20% to 43% incidence of severe overgrowth necessitating surgical revision.[21,22] The anatomic location of the amputation plays a role in formation of the osseous overgrowth, with metaphyseal amputations showing a greater tendency toward heterotopic bone formation compared with diaphyseal amputations and joint disarticulations showing no evidence of bone overgrowth.[23,24] However, in the adult population, bone overgrowth incidence is unclear[25] and can include the development of irregular bone growth with an aggressive bone edge that is continuous with the residual limb as well as heterotopic bone formation in the soft tissues. (An aggressive bone edge occurs when the bone end of a residual limb is not blunted and may develop when extremity alignment is not maintained.)

All forms of osseous overgrowth may result in soft tissue stress and ulceration (Fig. 111-1), leading to pain. Conventional radiography can well demonstrate ossification without the aid of cross-sectional imaging, and radiography with weight-bearing views is adequate for demonstrating soft tissue compression by an area of bone overgrowth. However, CT can map the location of ossification accurately and demonstrate associated inflammatory fluid collections (Fig. 111-2). MRI is most useful for documenting areas of soft tissue inflammation in this setting.[11]

Infection at the site of amputation may manifest as cellulitis, abscess, or osteomyelitis (Fig. 111-3; also see Fig. 111-1). Osteomyelitis is almost always caused by pyogenic bacteria, with fungal, parasitic, and viral infections being uncommon in amputees. Osteomyelitis may occur

TABLE 111-2	**Complications after Amputation**
Imaging Complication	**Potential Etiology**
Skin thickening	Cellulitis
	Scar/keloid
Persistent postoperative edema in skin and subcutaneous tissues	Deficient prosthesis/residual limb interface causing inflammation
	Cellulitis
	Lymphedema
	Deep venous thrombosis
	Underlying medical diseases
Fluid collections	Physiologic adventitial bursa
	Inflamed or infected adventitious bursa
	Hematoma
	Abscess
Soft tissue mass	Neuroma
	Recurrent tumor
Osseous overgrowth	Ectopic bone at site of periosteal avulsion
	Endosteal bone overgrowth
	Aggressive bone edge due to malalignment of extremity
	Heterotopic bone formation in adjacent soft tissues
Bone marrow abnormality	Postoperative reactive bone marrow edema
	Osteomyelitis
	Stress fracture or bone contusion
	Recurrent tumor
Joint abnormality	Joint contracture
	Other joint deformity

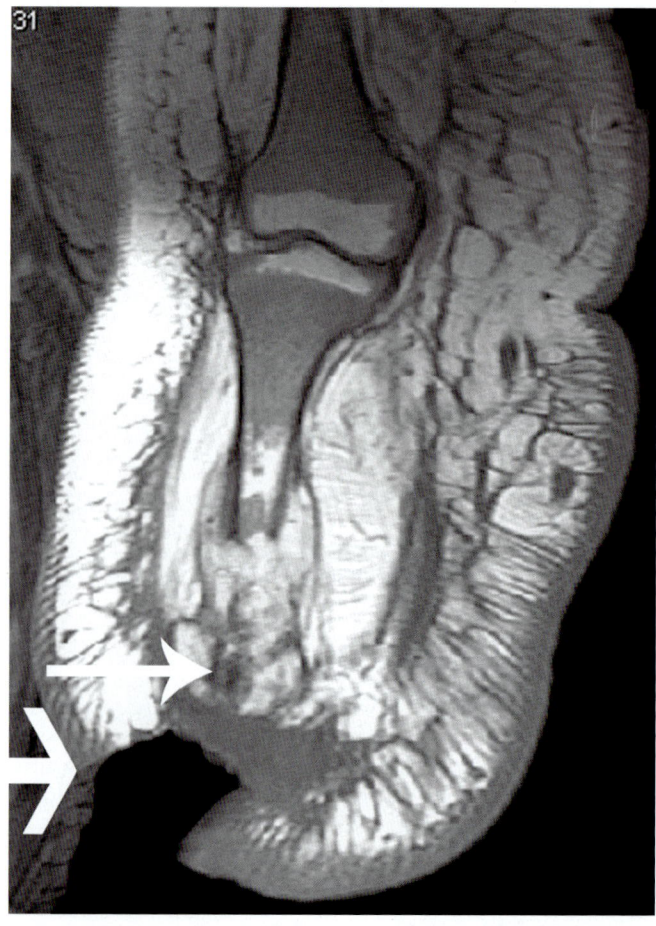

■ **FIGURE 111-1** Coronal T1-weighted spin-echo MR image (TR/TE 520/12) in a patient who underwent transtibial amputation for peripheral vascular disease complicated by heterotopic bone formation (*long arrow*) and adjacent ulceration (*thick arrow*). Note marked skin thickening and subcutaneous signal changes due to cellulitis.

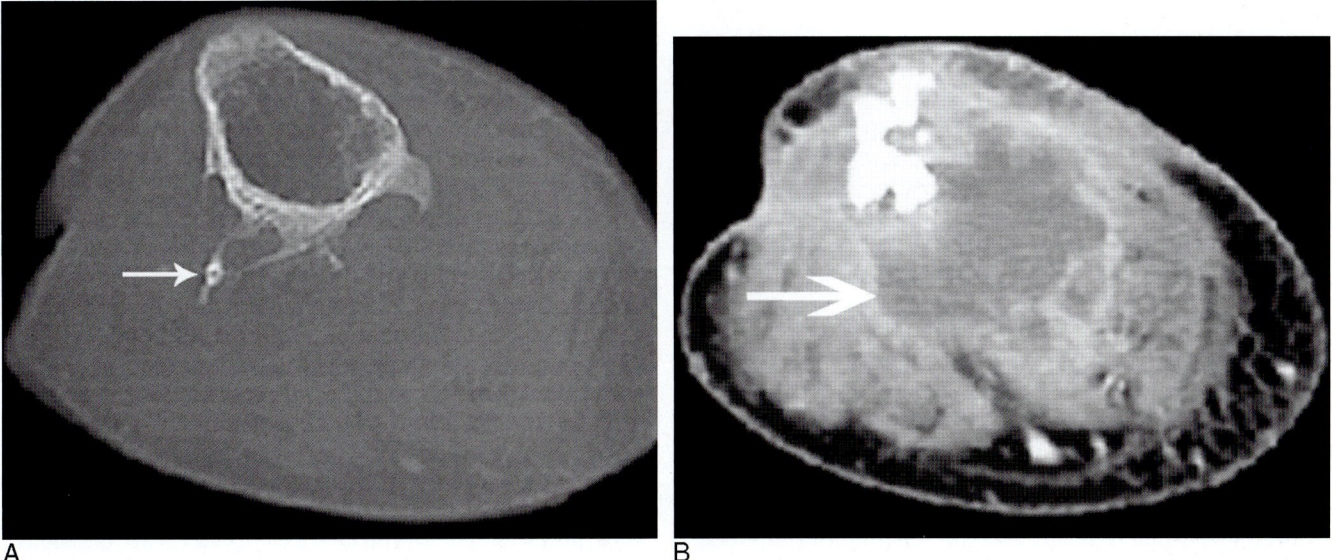

■ **FIGURE 111-2** Axial contrast-enhanced CT images in bone (**A**) and soft tissue (**B**) display obtained from a patient with a transtibial amputation for peripheral vascular disease showing aggressive bone edges (*small arrows* in **A**) associated with a rim-enhancing fluid collection (*arrow* in **B**) that was complicated by infection.

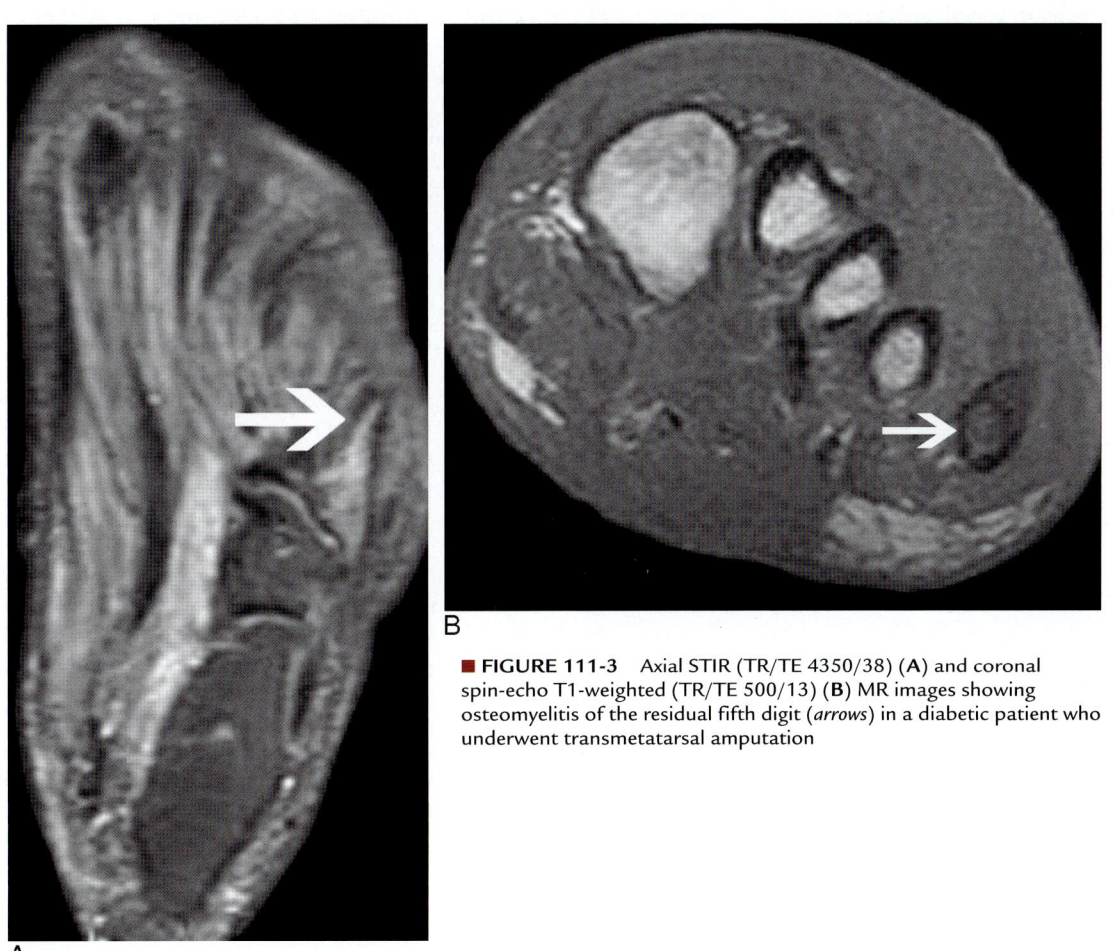

■ **FIGURE 111-3** Axial STIR (TR/TE 4350/38) (**A**) and coronal spin-echo T1-weighted (TR/TE 500/13) (**B**) MR images showing osteomyelitis of the residual fifth digit (*arrows*) in a diabetic patient who underwent transmetatarsal amputation many years after amputation, related to late recurrence of a quiescent septic focus, spread from a contiguous soft tissue infection, or secondary to hematogenous spread from another site. Both MRI and bone scintigraphy may be used for detecting and localizing osteomyelitis, but MRI is at least as sensitive and more specific than many scintigraphic techniques for diagnosing osteomyelitis[26] and is exceedingly useful for its high negative predictive value in the setting of potential infection.[27] MRI is also more advantageous because it provides the ability to demonstrate soft tissue inflammation and fluid collections requiring drainage, as well as sinus tracts.

Osteomyelitis is seen as of low to intermediate signal intensity in the bone marrow on T1-weighted imaging and of high signal intensity on T2-weighted imaging; the latter signal changes are highly sensitive but not specific for infection because other causes such as postsurgical alterations can have a similar appearance (Fig. 111-4). Additional findings that are specific for infection include intraosseous abscess formation, a sinus tract, and development of a sequestrum, which can be detected by CT. Ultrasonography is helpful for identifying fluid collections but is more commonly used for therapy than diagnosis.

Adventitial bursae and areas of localized soft tissue inflammation can develop in the subcutaneous tissues of the amputee in response to friction between the residual limb and its prosthesis. Adventitial bursae are fairly common in clinical practice[15] and are made of mucoid and myxomatous degeneration of connective tissue that, in fact, allows smooth movement of the prosthesis against the residual limb.[18] Bursae are located at typical points of pressure that include the head of the fibula, patella, anterior tibial tuberosity, and the end of the residual bone. Hence, these bursae may be physiologic but can become dysfunctional and painful when inflamed. They are well demonstrated by cross-sectional imaging methods as fluid collections that demonstrate enhancement of their walls after contrast medium administration (see Fig. 111-4). Adventitial bursitis can be distinguished from diffuse inflammation without a localized fluid collection by MRI or CT.

Postoperative neuromas usually arise between 1 and 12 months after transection and are benign. They may be asymptomatic or symptomatic.[19,28] They can be focal or generalized, although they are typically oval and exhibit isointense signal to muscle on T1-weighted imaging, have slightly heterogeneous or increased signal intensity on T2-weighted imaging, and enhance after contrast medium administration (Fig. 111-5).[27-29]

Postamputation recurrence of tumor may be observed months to years after amputation with a variable incidence depending on the original histology of the tumor. A recent report shows that there is a 4% local recurrence rate after amputation for a localized soft tissue sarcoma of the extremity,[30] although up to a 50% recurrence rate for soft tissue sarcomas has been reported.[31] In addition, there are rare instances of development of malignancy at an amputation site that include malignant degeneration of chronically infected tissues and the rare occurrence of Steward-Treves syndrome (the development of angiosarcoma with chronic lymphedema).[32] MRI is the modality of choice for detecting and characterizing local recurrent tumor (Fig. 111-6).[27]

Stress fractures and bone bruises may occur with uneven loading on the prosthesis socket or improper alignment of the prosthesis. Radiographic diagnosis is delayed, but early diagnosis may be performed with MRI or bone scintigraphy (although scintigraphy shows nonspecific uptake). The treatment primarily involves remodeling of the prosthesis and optimization of the residual limb-prosthesis fit.[15]

Joint contractures occur from inactivity and prolonged wheelchair ambulation. These are diagnosed clinically and resolve with physical therapy. Imaging plays a role in identifying atrophy of specific muscle groups and its affect on the development of joint contracture.[33] Joint deformities are specific to certain sites of amputation and may be severe following certain amputation levels: for example, after amputation of the second toe, a severe hallux valgus deformity can develop. For Lisfranc's and Chopart's amputations there is a tendency toward an equinus deformity from loss of the dorsiflexor attachments.

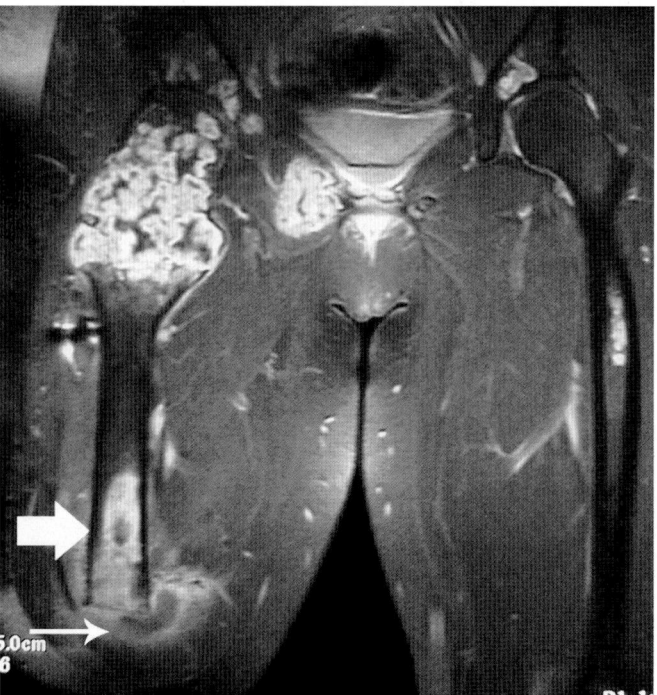

■ **FIGURE 111-4** Coronal postcontrast spin-echo T1-weighted MR image (TR/TE 540/10) in a patient with Ollier's disease who underwent a right transfemoral amputation for chondrosarcoma. The image shows increased signal in the residual femur (*thick arrow*), due to surgical manipulation rather than osteomyelitis or tumor. Note also overlying adventitial bursitis (*thin arrow*). Multiple enchondromas are present in the remaining skeleton.

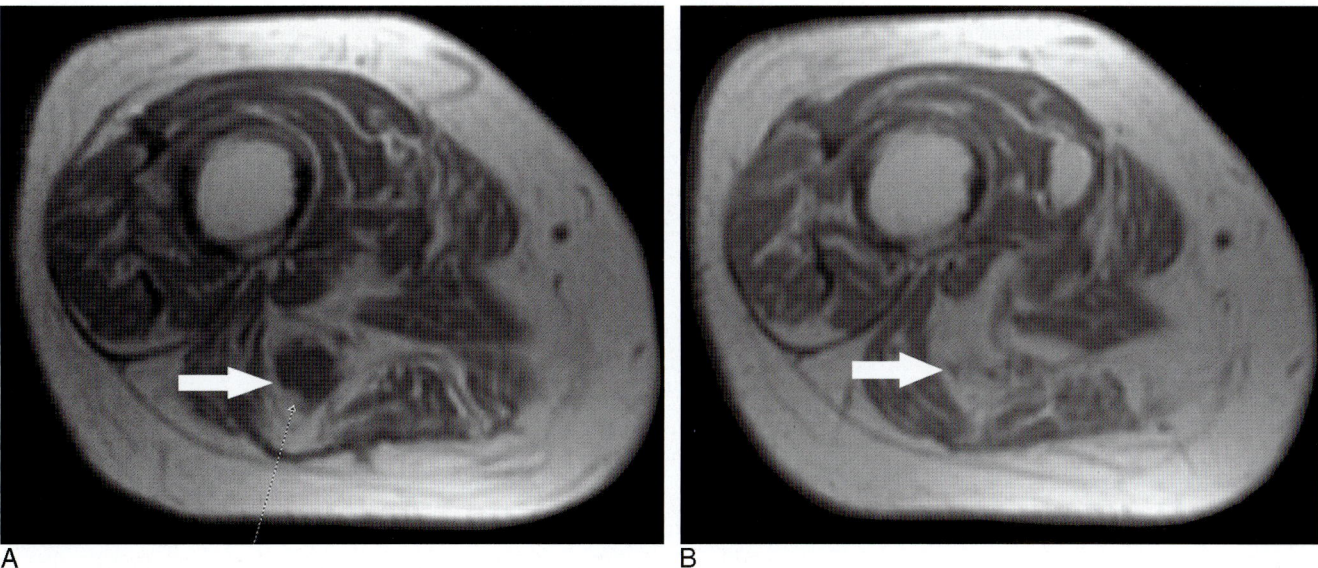

■ **FIGURE 111-5** Axial fast spin-echo T1-weighted MR images obtained before (**A**) and after (**B**) contrast medium administration (TR/TE 550/9) of a 56-year-old man who underwent a transfemoral amputation for chondrosarcoma complicated by a postoperative neuroma. *(Courtesy of Dr. Tamara Haygood, Department of Radiology, M.D. Anderson Cancer Center, Houston, TX.)*

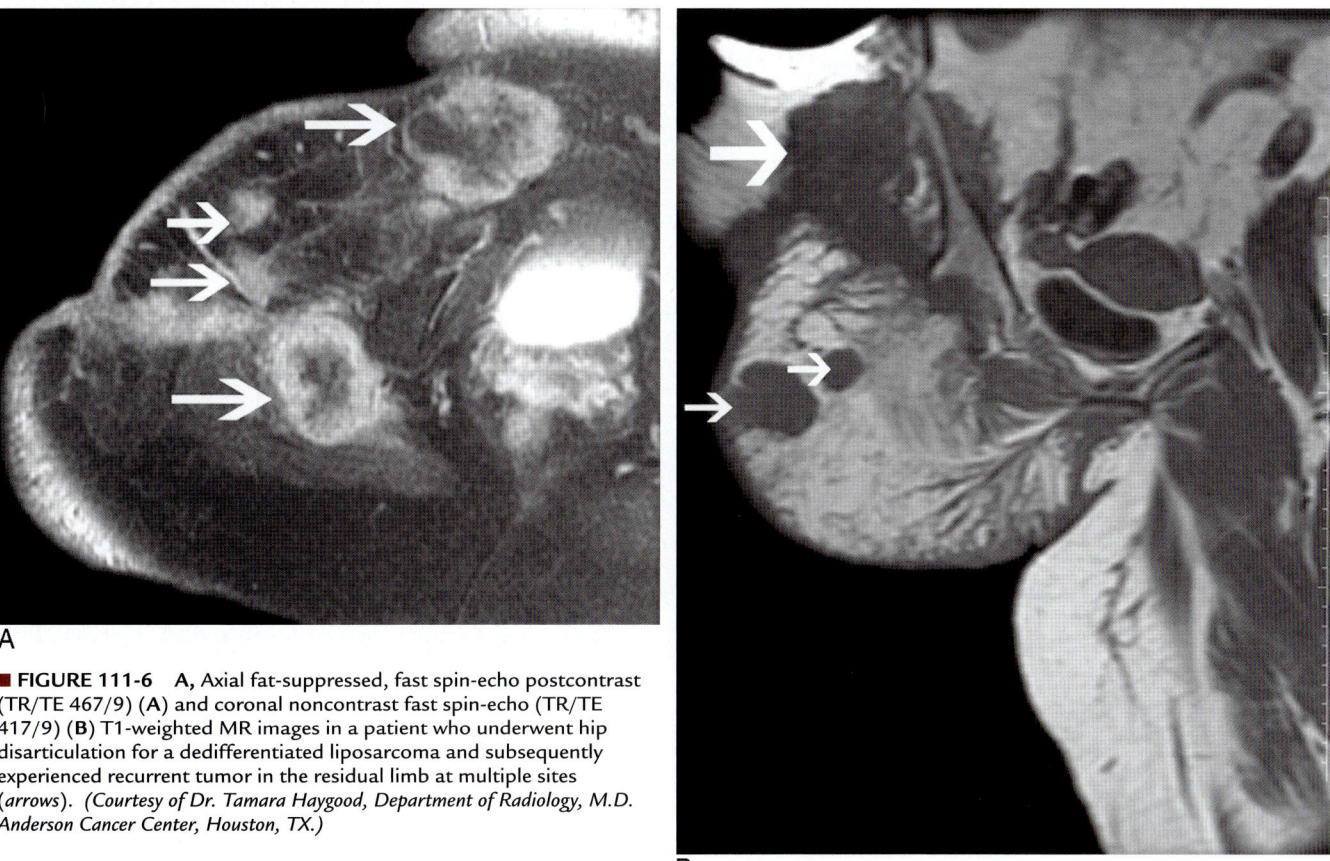

■ **FIGURE 111-6** **A,** Axial fat-suppressed, fast spin-echo postcontrast (TR/TE 467/9) (**A**) and coronal noncontrast fast spin-echo (TR/TE 417/9) (**B**) T1-weighted MR images in a patient who underwent hip disarticulation for a dedifferentiated liposarcoma and subsequently experienced recurrent tumor in the residual limb at multiple sites (*arrows*). *(Courtesy of Dr. Tamara Haygood, Department of Radiology, M.D. Anderson Cancer Center, Houston, TX.)*

SUGGESTED READINGS

Boutin RD, Pathria MN, Resnick D. Disorders in the stumps of amputee patients: MR imaging. AJR Am J Roentgenol 1998; 171:497–501.

Henrot P, Stines J, Walter F, et al. Imaging of the painful lower limb stump. RadioGraphics 2000; 20:S219–S235.

Hurvitz EA, Ellenberg M, Lerner AM, et al. Ultrasound imaging of residual limbs: new use for an old technique. Arch Phys Med Rehabil 1989; 70:556–558.

Knetsche RP, Leopold SS, Brage ME. Inpatient management of lower extremity amputations. Foot Ankle Clin 2001; 6:229–241.

Pasquina PF, Bryant PR, Huang ME, et al. Advances in amputee care. Arch Phys Med Rehabil 2006; 87:34–43.

Provost N, Bonaldi VM, Sarazin L, et al. Amputation stump neuroma: Ultrasound features. J Clin Ultrasound 1997; 25:85–89.

Sammak B, Abd El Bagi M, Al Shahed M, et al. Osteomyelitis: A review of currently used imaging techniques. Eur Radiol 1999; 9:894–900.

Wafa H, Grimer RJ. Surgical options and outcomes in bone sarcoma. Expert Rev Anticancer Ther 2006; 6:239–248.

Weisstein JS, Goldsby RE, O'Donnell RJ. Oncologic approaches to pediatric limb preservation. J Am Acad Orthop Surg 2005; 13:544–554.

Williams HB. The painful stump neuroma and its treatment. Clin Plast Surg 1984; 11:79–84.

REFERENCES

1. Dillingham TR. Pezzin LE, Mackenzie EJ. Limb amputation and limb deficiency: epidemiology and recent trends in the United States. South Med J 2002; 95:875–883.

2. Group TG. Epidemiology of lower extremity amputation in centres in Europe, North America and East Asia. The global lower extremity amputation study group. Br J Surg 2000; 87:328–337.

3. Taylor SM, Kalbaugh CA, Blackhurst DW, et al. Preoperative clinical factors predict postoperative functional outcomes after major lower limb amputation: an analysis of 553 consecutive patients. J Vasc Surg 2005; 42:227–235.

4. Water RL, Perry J, Antonelli D, Hislop H. Energy cost of walking of amputees: the influence of level of amputation. J Bone Joint Surg Am 1976; 58:42–46.

5. Jaegers SM, Arendzen JH, de Jongh HJ. Prosthetic gait of unilateral transfemoral amputees: a kinematic study. Arch Phys Med Rehabil 1995; 76:736–743.

6. Chiodo CP, Stroud CC. Optimal surgical preparation of the residual limb for prosthetic fitting in below-knee amputations. Foot Ankle Clin 2001; 6:253–264.

7. Geertzen JH, Bosmans JC, van der Schans CP, Dijkstra PU. Claimed walking distance of lower limb amputees. Disabil Rehabil 2005; 27:101–104.

8. Fleckenstein JL, Chason DP, Bonte FJ, et al. High-voltage electric injury: assessment of muscle viability with MR imaging and Tc-99 m pyrophosphate scintigraphy. Radiology 1995; 195:205–210.

9. Bowker JH, Keagy RD, Poonekar PD. Musculoskeletal complications in amputees: their prevention and management. In Bowker JH, Michael JW. Atlas of Limb Prosthetics: Surgical, Prosthetic and Rehabilitation Principles, 2nd ed. St. Louis, Mosby–Year Book, 1992, p 678.

10. Bocobo CR, Castellote JM, MacKinnon D, Gabrielle-Bergman A. Videofluoroscopic evaluation of prosthetic fit and residual limbs following transtibial amputation. J Rehabil Res Dev 1998; 35:6–13.

11. Henrot P, Stines J, Walter F, et al. Imaging of the painful lower limb stump. RadioGraphics 2000; 20:S219–S235.

12. Hain SF, O'Doherty MJ, Lucas JD, Smith MA. Fluorodeoxyglucose PET in the evaluation of amputation for soft tissue sarcoma. Nucl Med Commun 1999; 20:845–848.

13. Johnson GR, Zhuang H, Khan J, et al. Roles of positron emission tomography with fluorine-18-deoxyglucose in the detection of local recurrent and distant metastatic sarcoma. Clin Nucl Med 2003; 28:815–820.

14. Shinozaki T, Suzuki K, Yamaji T, et al. Evaluation of muscle metabolic activity in the lower limb of a transfemoral amputee using a prosthesis by using ^{18}F-FDG PET imaging—an application of PET imaging to rehabilitation. J Orthop Res 2004; 22:878–883.

15. Ahmed A, Bayol MG, Ha SB. Adventitious bursae in below knee amputees: case reports and a review of the literature. Am J Phys Med Rehabil 1994; 73:124–129.

16. Commean PK, Burnsden BS, Smith KE, Vannier MW. Below-knee residual limb shape change measurement and visualization. Arch Phys Med Rehabil 1998; 779:772–782.

17. Smith KE, Commean PK, Vannier MW. Residual-limb shape change: three-dimensional CT scan measurement and depiction in vivo. Radiology 1996; 200:843–850.

18. Foisneau-Lottin A, Martinet N, Henrot P, et al. Bursitis, adventitious bursa, localized soft-tissue inflammation, and bone marrow edema in tibial stumps: the contribution of magnetic resonance imaging to the diagnosis and management of mechanical stress complications. Arch Phys Med Rehabil 2003; 84:770–777.

19. Ernberg LA, Adler RS, Lane J. Ultrasound in the detection and treatment of a painful stump neuroma. Skelet Radiol 2003; 32:306–309.

20. Ephraim PL, Wegener ST, MacKenzie EJ, et al. Phantom pain, residual limb pain, and back pain in amputees: results of a national survey. Arch Phys Med Rehabil 2005; 86:1910–1919.

21. Pellicore RS, Sciora J, Lambert CN, et al. Incidence of bone overgrowth in the juvenile amputee population. Int Clin Inform Bull 1974; 13:1–8.

22. O'Neal ML, Bahner R, Ganey TM, Ogden JA. Osseous overgrowth after amputation in adolescents and children. J Pediatr Orthop 1996; 16:78–84.

23. Vocke Ak, Schmid A. Osseous overgrowth after post-traumatic amputation of the lower extremity in childhood. Arch Orthop Trauma Surg 2000; 120:452–454.

24. Speer DP. The pathogenesis of amputation stump overgrowth. Clin Orthop 1981; 159:294–307.

25. Dudek NL, DeHaan MN, Marks MB. Bone overgrowth in the adult traumatic amputee. Am J Phys Med Rehabil 2003; 82:897–900.

26. Beltran J, Noto AM, McGhee RB, et al. Infections of the musculoskeletal system: high-field strength MR imaging. Radiology 1987; 164:449–454.

27. Boutin RD, Pathria MN, Resnick D. Disorders in the stumps of amputee patients: MR imaging. AJR 1998; 171:497–501.

28. Singson RD, Feldman F, Slipma CW, et al. Post-amputation neuromas and other symptomatic stump abnormalities: detection with CT. Radiology 1987; 162:743–745.

29. Singson RD, Feldman F, Staron R, et al. MRI of postamputation neuromas. Skelet Radiol 1990; 19:259–262.

30. Ghert MA, Abudu A, Driver N, et al. The indications for and the prognostic significance of amputation as the primary surgical procedure for localized soft tissue sarcoma of the extremity. Ann Surg Oncol 2004; 12:10–17.

31. Kransdorf MJ, Murphey MD. Imaging of Soft Tissue Tumors. Philadelphia, WB Saunders, 1997, pp 42–56.

32. Kazerooni E, Hessler C. CT appearance of angiosarcoma associated with chronic lymphedema. AJR Am J Roentgenol 1991; 156:543–544.

33. Jaegers SM, Arendzen JH, de Jongh HJ. Changes in hip muscles after above-knee amputations. Clin Orthop Relat Res 1995; 319:276–284.

Abstracts from CD

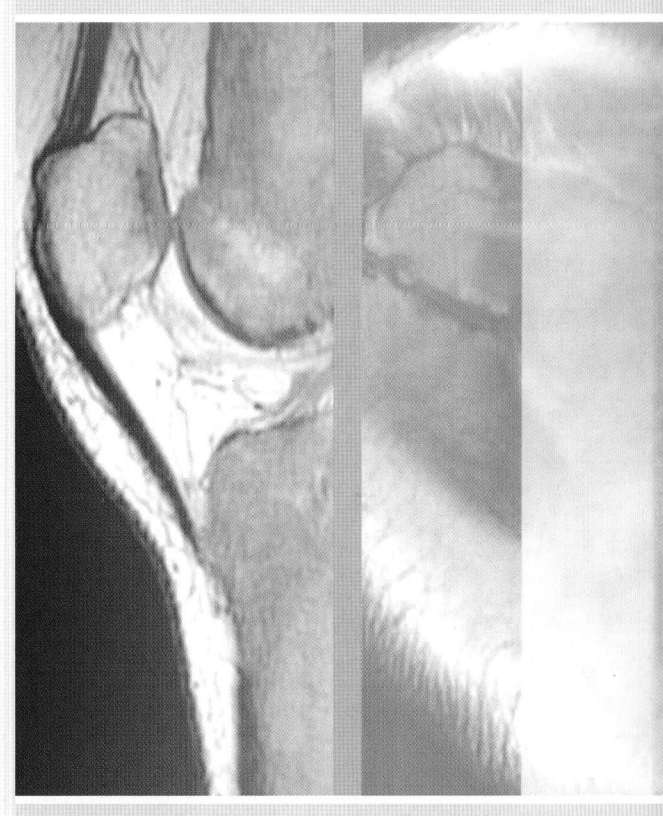

Dental Imaging

See the full chapter by Michael Pharoah on CD.

The interpretation of diagnostic images of abnormalities of the jaws is complex, due to the fact that, in addition to bone pathology common to other bones, the jaws contain diseases of odontogenic origin. Instead of simply listing diseases with their imaging characteristics, this chapter presents an approach to the interpretation of diseases of the jaws. This approach is based on the importance of location (epicenter or point of origin), periphery, internal structure, and effects on surrounding structures. For instance, all odontogenic lesions have an epicenter above the inferior alveolar nerve canal and those derived from odontogenic epithelium such as ameloblastoma or dentigerous cyst originate coronal to the tooth.

Common inflammatory diseases, such as periapical inflammatory disease, have an epicenter at the root apex of teeth, but periodontal disease has an epicenter at the crest of the alveolar process of the maxilla or mandible. Due to the presence of teeth, the occurrence of osteomyelitis is relatively high compared to other osseous structures. The presence of sequestra and the inflammatory periosteal reaction needed for the diagnosis are best seen on CT imaging. The high number of false negative gallium nuclear studies, likely reflecting both the chronic nature and poor vascularity of chronic osteomyelitis of the jaws, leaves CT imaging as the modality of choice. Care must be taken to differentiate osteomyelitis from fibrous dysplasia and osteosarcoma. With the exception of thickening of the lamina dura seen in bisphosphonate treatment, bone necrosis resulting from therapeutic radiation or bisphosphonate treatment is similar to osteomyelitis except for the absence of periosteal reaction.

Odontogenic cysts have specific epicenters related to the tooth structure, with dentigerous cysts in a pericoronal location, radicular cysts in a periapical position, and buccal bifurcation cysts located at the bifurcation of molars. The internal aspect of the cysts usually has a high signal on T2-weighted images, but keratocysts may be more heterogeneous and chronic cysts may have low signal regions from dystrophic calcification. Most cysts grow and expand in a concentric fashion, but keratocysts and simple bone cysts have a predilection for growing along the bone with less expansion.

Odontogenic benign tumors often have a common location relative to the teeth, with ameloblastomas and ameloblastic fibromas typically occurring coronal to teeth, whereas benign cementoblastomas have an apical location. The internal structure of some tumors is described as multilocular, but a careful analysis of the morphology of internal septa can be used to differentiate ameloblastomas, central giant cell granulomas, and odontogenic myxomas. In addition there is commonly a high signal in odontogenic myxomas in T2-weighted images. Giant cell granulomas commonly have a granular, less defined periphery where they have caused expansion of the outer cortical plate.

Of the bone dysplasias, cemental dysplasia is the most common and can express itself as one single lesion or

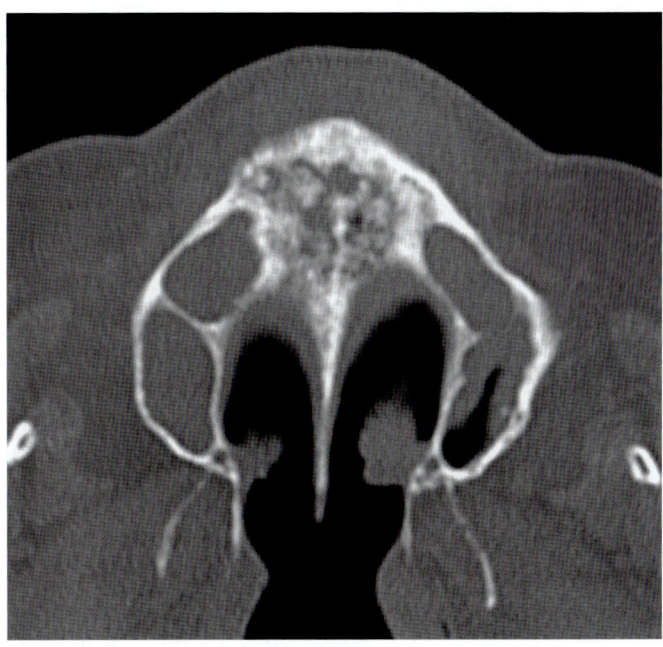

■ **FIGURE 1** Axial CT image (bone algorithm) through the hard palate of the maxilla showing several sequestra from osteonecrosis due to bisphosphonate therapy in a case of multiple myeloma.

2124 ABSTRACT ● *Dental Imaging*

multiple lesions. The epicenter is always periapical and above the inferior alveolar canal even after the teeth have been extracted. When these lesions become secondarily infected, it is important to differentiate this disease from conventional osteomyelitis. Fibrous dysplasia especially involving the maxilla may be differentiated from ossifying fibroma by the shape of the expanded bone.

Other lesions such as those resulting from cherubism, which has no relationship to fibrous dysplasia, always have an epicenter in the posterior of the jaws and a tendency to displace teeth in an anterior direction. Langerhans cell histiocytosis has a characteristic pattern of bone destruction involving the alveolar process of the jaws and produces a periosteal reaction very similar to inflammatory disease.

Normal Variants

See the full chapter by Thomas Pope, Theodore E. Keats, and Mark W. Anderson on CD.

Normal variants in the skeleton are commonly encountered in the practice of radiology. Variation is inseparably related to the study of normal anatomy. An educated familiarity with normal variation is a requirement for any radiologist who interprets images.

Any imaging finding suspected of being a normal variant should be investigated by consulting the *Atlas of Normal Roentgen Variants That May Simulate Disease*. The entities in this book are based on the personal experiences of Drs. Keats and Anderson and on the published work of others. Many of the entities are unproven. However, proof of the normal character of these lesions/abnormalities is that we have seen the entities many times and follow-up shows no change radiographically or no adverse effects to the patients/individuals. Another indication of normality is that follow-up studies prove the lesion to be a consequence of growth. For example, on a lateral projection the fusion of an anterior fontanelle may be confused with a depressed fracture (Fig. 1). Still other findings prove to be normal variants because they occur on the contralateral side with great frequency, and, finally, many of the patients are asymptomatic at the site of the "normal variant."

The error of overdiagnosis of a normal variation as evidence of a pathologic process may be more serious than omission and may lead to needless and harmful therapy. On the other hand, the radiologist should be aware that some normal variants may be associated with symptoms.

Variations of the accepted norm are expected and predicted from the study of science and development. Causes of normal variants include aberrations at the genetic level, aberrations of growth, and unusual activity. No proven single etiology of normal variants has been discovered, and we must assume that skeletal "variants" are part of the daily imaging experience without having a satisfying explanation of exactly how or why they occur.

Normal variations are extremely common occurrences in the daily practice of radiology, and there is no way to estimate their prevalence and epidemiology.

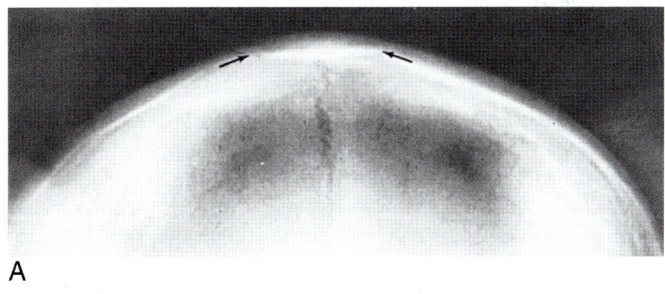

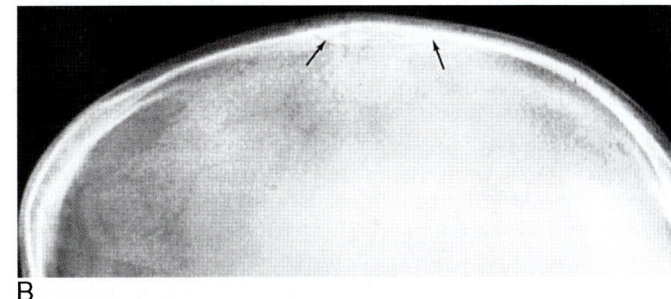

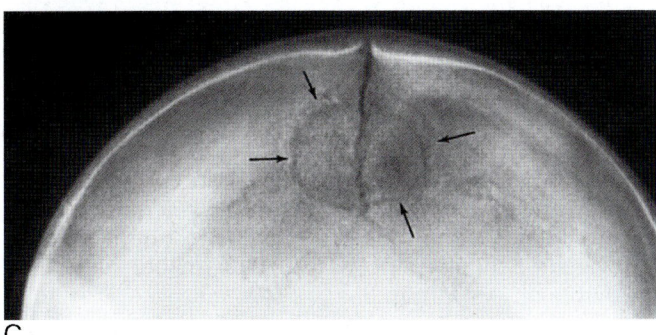

■ **FIGURE 1** (A-C), Fusing anterior fontanelle bone (*arrows*) in a 3-year-old boy. This appearance may be confused with that of a depressed fracture in the lateral projection. *Reference:* Girdany BR, Blank E. Anterior fontanel bones. Am J Roentgenol Radium Ther Nucl Med 1965; 95:148. (*From Keats TE, Anderson MW. Atlas of Normal Roentgen Variants That May Simulate Disease, 8th ed. Philadelphia, Mosby, 2007.*)

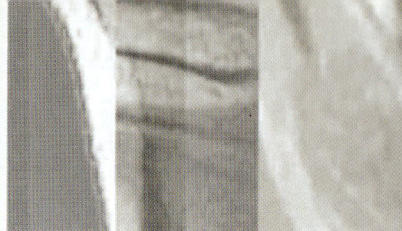

Biopsy: Soft Tissue

See the full chapter by Patrick T. Liu and Catherine C. Roberts on CD.

Soft tissue sarcomas occur most often in the extremities. If an extremity soft tissue mass is not obviously benign, then it should be considered a potential sarcoma until proven otherwise. Because orthopedic oncologic principles call for different avenues of therapy for each lesion type, achieving accurate presurgical diagnosis is a critical step for treatment planning. Biopsies should be performed only by experienced personnel.

Open technique can obtain larger sample sizes, but well-planned percutaneous needle biopsy is a safer and highly accurate procedure for diagnosis of soft tissue masses.

Abnormal patient blood coagulation is a relative contraindication to needle biopsy.

Image guidance for biopsy has the ability to visualize and avoid surrounding neurovascular structures and confirm needle placement within a solid and viable portion of the mass. The choice of guidance modality includes the location of the target mass, ability of the modality to depict the mass, equipment availability, radiation exposure, cost, and the radiologist's familiarity with the modality. Ultrasonography is an excellent means of biopsy guidance. Color Doppler ultrasonography is useful for delineating vessels adjacent to and within the target mass. Avascular regions should not be sampled because of the possibility of necrosis and a nondiagnostic yield (Fig. 1). For lesions not compatible with ultrasonography, CT should be used. MRI best defines soft tissue masses but is usually not necessary for biopsy.

Core needle biopsy is a more accurate biopsy method than fine-needle aspiration. It can rapidly acquire a small core of tissue, permitting more accurate tumor grading. Fine-needle aspiration biopsy provides smaller specimens for cytologic evaluation.

The radiologist should consult with the orthopedic oncologic surgeon to determine the preferred surgical approach. Biopsy needle tracts should be aligned with surgical incisions that would be used if the biopsy reveals a diagnosis of resectable sarcoma. If the surgeon is unavailable for consultation, be sure to place the biopsy tract within the same compartment that contains the mass, placing the skin site directly over that compartment. Joint capsules should also be avoided during biopsies of an extremity.

In CT, the field of view of the guiding images should be kept as small as possible to maximize spatial resolution. CT fluoroscopy can be used to closely follow the trajectory of the biopsy needle.

The ultrasound transducer should be chosen according to the depth and location of the lesion. Higher-frequency transducers can be used for superficial lesions whereas deep lesions require lower-frequency transducers.

Use 1% lidocaine for local anesthesia. With larger sarcomas, the pseudocapsule and immediate surrounding tissues may be hyperesthetic and require anesthetic infiltration.

Any incision used for biopsies should be oriented parallel to the long axis of the limb. Multiple passes with the biopsy needle directed at various angles through the target lesion should be performed to sample multiple regions.

Achieve strict hemostasis after biopsy, to avoid hematoma formation and potential local tumor seeding. Most complications have resulted from bleeding. Patients should be given verbal and written instructions for wound care, analgesic use, and infection precautions.

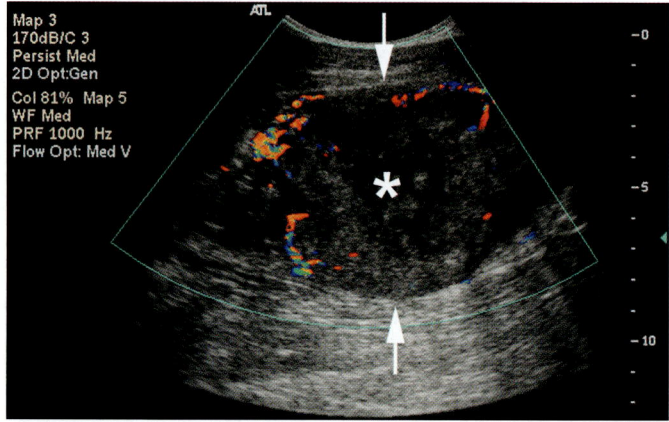

■ **FIGURE 1** Doppler ultrasound study of a soft tissue mass (*arrows*) in the thigh shows peripheral tumor vessels demarcating areas of viable tissue. The central hypovascular region (*) would not be a good target for biopsy because of the possibility of necrosis. Biopsy of peripheral tissue in the vicinity of the vessels was diagnostic for malignant fibrous histiocytoma.

Percutaneous Biopsy of the Appendicular Skeleton

See the full chapter by Raphaëlle Souillard, Patrick Chastanet, and Anne Cotten on CD.

Percutaneous biopsy of appendicular skeletal lesions is a minimally invasive, safe, and inexpensive procedure compared with open biopsy. Therefore, this procedure is indicated in many cases when bone metastasis is suggested. In the region of the pelvis, a focal osteolytic lesion in a patient older than 50 years of age may represent a chondrosarcoma and a careful analysis of CT or MR images is necessary before biopsy to evaluate for signs of a primary lesion (e.g., cartilaginous calcifications, hyperintense cartilaginous lobules on T2-weighted images). In primary bone tumors, percutaneous biopsy may be prone to sampling bias, yielding lower diagnostic accuracy because portions of tumors can have different appearances and histologic aggressiveness. This procedure may be indicated when the benign nature of the lesion cannot be confirmed by clinical, biologic, or imaging features.

Radiologic guidance guarantees the exact site of biopsy and correct needle biopsy position. Radiologic control of needle position during percutaneous biopsy can be accomplished by fluoroscopic, CT, MRI, or ultrasonographic guidance, with the modality selected depending on the biopsy site, imaging appearance, size of lesion, and radiologist's preference. CT-guided biopsy is generally the method of choice for biopsy of small deep lesions close to vital or neurovascular structures or when anatomy is complex.

Radiographs and CT or MR images of the lesion are required before biopsy. Biopsy of an osteolytic lesion provides a better diagnostic accuracy than biopsy of an osteosclerotic lesion. Areas of the lesion that most enhance represent the most active areas of the lesion. On the other hand, cystic areas usually correspond to necrotic areas and should be avoided. In case of suspicion of a primary bone tumor, lesion site and puncture approach have to be selected with the orthopedic surgeon to choose a route that may be removed at the time of definitive surgery.

In lesions involving long bones, the needle has to be introduced perpendicular to the shaft of the bone because the needle tip may skid along the surface to an undesirable position. With peripheral and flat bones, CT rather than fluoroscopic guidance should be used, such as in the case of biopsy of an osteolytic lesion of the rib or a lesion close to vital structures or nerves. Regarding flat bones, such as the scapula, ribs, sternum, and iliac bone, a tangential approach is preferred to avoid damage to vital organs in case of excessive needle advancement (Fig. 1). In case of a sclerotic lesion, a preoperative CT is used to localize less mineralized areas, which are useful to select as the target for biopsy. Joint biopsy is particularly performed when joint infection is suggested. Multiple samplings should be performed from different sites of the lesion.

Complications related to percutaneous skeletal biopsy are rare. The overall accuracy of percutaneous skeletal biopsy reported in the literature varies from 66% to 96%. Diagnostic accuracy is found to be better for osteolytic lesions than for osteosclerotic lesions. Cystic lesions, predominantly filled with necrotic material, blood, or cystic formation, show much lower diagnostic accuracy.

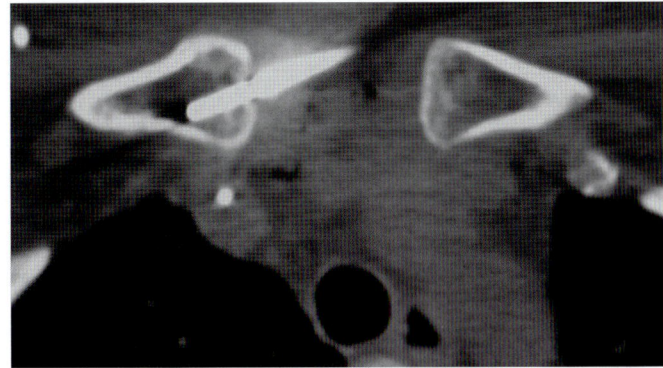

■ **FIGURE 1** Tangential approach to a metastasis of the right clavicle under CT guidance.

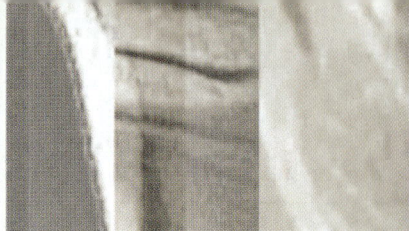

Percutaneous Biopsy of the Spine

See the full chapter by Patrick Chastanet, Anne Cotten,
and Raphaëlle Souillard on CD.

Percutaneous biopsy of spinal lesions is an effective, reliable, safe, and rapid procedure, offering high diagnostic accuracy, especially in metastases or infection. A suspicion of bone metastasis represents the main indication for percutaneous biopsy of the spine (Fig. 1). It may also be indicated in suspicion of other malignant lesions (e.g., osseous lymphoma, plasmocytoma) or when the benign nature of the lesions cannot be confirmed by the clinical, biologic, or imaging features (e.g., osteoporotic vertebral collapse, eosinophilic granuloma).

This procedure can be performed using either fluoroscopic or CT guidance depending on the biopsy site, the habit of the radiologist, the radiographic appearance, and the size of the lesion. The choice of specific needles, on the other hand, depends on the lytic or sclerotic appearance of the lesion and on the integrity and thickness of the overlying bone.

Percutaneous biopsy of the lumbar spine is usually performed under fluoroscopic guidance, which is the method of choice in most cases because of the benefits of less time and less expense. Depending on the location of the lesion, a posterolateral or a transpedicular approach can be used.

On the other hand, CT is essential for thoracic spine biopsies because of the complex anatomy and adjacent vital structures. Cervical spine biopsy can be performed with either CT or fluoroscopic guidance. Sacral spine biopsies are carried out safely with CT guidance.

Preoperative assessment requires review of radiographs and CT or MRI images before biopsy. Procedures are done under strict aseptic conditions. Premedication is recommended.

Pain and infection are generic complications but are relatively low in occurrence. Potential complications mainly

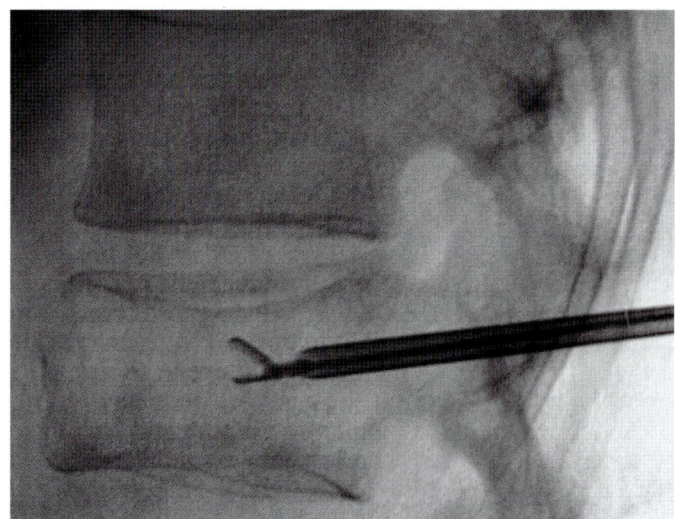

■ **FIGURE 1** Lateral fluoroscopic view of a biopsy forceps used through an external cannula for a biopsy of an osteolytic metastasis.

depend on the anatomic location of the lesion and the route that is used.

A multidisciplinary approach is essential to obtain optimal results. Diagnostic accuracy depends on the nature of the lesion, its radiologic appearance, and its location.

High diagnostic accuracy is generally achieved in metastases and infections. Diagnostic accuracy is similar between lesions in the thoracic and lumbar spine and slightly higher for lesions in the cervical spine and sacrum.

Tumor Ablation

See the full chapter by Willem Obermann on CD.

Radiofrequency (RF) ablation involves positioning an RF-emitting needle within a lesion with radiologic guidance with special care taken in the spine to not injure nerve roots, the spinal cord, the vertebral artery, and vital structures (Fig. 1). RF energy provokes a locally concentrated alternating electrical current in the surrounding soft tissues, causing quick ion movements resulting in local heating. Knowledge of principles of ablation (e.g., temperature, duration, size of destruction), different generator systems and their operation, and different needle choices is critical for success.

Tumors that can be cured with this modality include osteoid osteoma, residual giant cell tumor, and chondroid tumor. Tumor palliation can be successful for large recurrent chordoma, large recurrent chondroid tumors, and metastatic bone lesions with or without cementoplasty. The presence of an electronic implant, such as a pacemaker, serves as a contraindication, owing to electronic interference.

Knowledge of biopsy systems best used with RF ablation needles is essential. There are different types of generators with different sized needles (with or without water cooling), each of which has a specific tissue "kill zone" or radius of tissue death from the needle at the recommended temperature/current.

Umbrella-shaped needles are suitable in soft tissues or for soft tissue components of bone lesions. In calcified bone only straight, rigid needles can be used. For penetrating needles in calcified bone the Bonopty coaxial bone biopsy system is very practical. It can do tissue biopsy and at the same time precisely introduce an RF ablation needle into the lesion.

General or spinal anesthesia is performed for potential intraprocedural pain.

The anatomic safest route should be taken, which means sometimes a longer route through more bone or soft tissue. A preliminary scan should be performed with skin markers on the region where entry is anticipated. A precise approach is needed, optimally under CT guidance and preferably with CT fluoroscopy. The puncture route(s) should be drawn on the monitor. Needle angulations in the scan plane should be noted. It is wise to stay as much in the scan plane as possible to ensure correct needle positioning.

An important concept is that within bone due to variable ion/water content and resultant electrical impedance the heating may not be uniform; the "kill zone" cannot be predicted precisely, so it is better to underestimate than to overestimate the region of destruction.

RF ablation of musculoskeletal tumors being equal or even better than open surgery is controversial. Based on location (e.g., the spine and around the hip joint), surgery may be technically difficult, resulting in a higher frequency of postprocedural morbidity.

Procedural outcomes in osteoid osteoma and other benign tumors were reportedly good. Tumor control of other tumors, particularly malignant tumors, is still experimental.

Aside from puncture complications, other potential risks include burns in the adjacent tissues and skin. Skin burns increase the risk of secondary infection of soft tissues and bone.

Postprocedural pain care is needed. If the tumor is malignant, regular MRI follow-up should be done; if it is benign, only regular clinical follow-up is necessary.

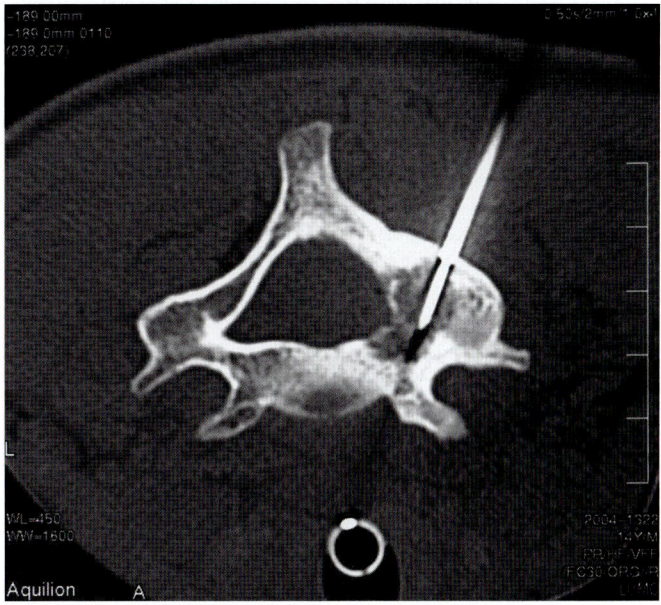

■ FIGURE 1 Big osteoid osteoma C6. Patient positioned prone. One of the six coagulation positions, somewhat lateral (10 mm of ablation, treated at each position for 4 minutes at 90° C).

Spinal Injections

See the full chapter by Michelle S. Barr on CD.

There are various injection types performed in the lumbar spine to provide either short- or long-term relief of back pain from different causes. Most injections should be performed using image guidance, with fluoroscopy currently the most popular but CT, ultrasonography, and MRI also employed.

Epidural corticosteroid injections using interlaminar technique (Fig. 1) require a C-arm fluoroscopy unit. Initial fluoroscopic images are employed to detect segmentation anomalies and rotation of spine. Rotation is determined by identifying spinous process of the vertebrae at the level to be injected and rotating the fluoroscopic unit so that the spinous process lies midway between the pedicles. The C-arm is then positioned approximately 11 degrees away from midline toward the side of maximal pain for the patient, opening up the view of the junction of the spinous process and lamina on that side. A metallic clamp or other radiodense device localizes site of skin entry.

A 22-gauge, 3.5-inch spinal needle is advanced to the spinolaminar junction under posteroanterior oblique fluoroscopy. During this advancement, occasional depth checks may be required by moving the image intensifier into the lateral position. Once the needle tip approximates the posterior aspect of facet joints, the C-arm unit is placed into a lateral position. The spinal needle is slowly advanced into the epidural space under continuous lateral fluoroscopy.

Transforaminal injection is performed with the spinal needle directed into the neural foramen, attempting to parallel the exit plane of the nerve root instead of striking it at a 90-degree angle. The needle should not pass medial to the outer third of the neural foramen on posteroanterior imaging, especially at L4-L5 and L5-S1. At the lower levels the dorsal root ganglia lie within the neural foramen. Confirmation of appropriate needle placement is done with contrast agent, which should travel up the nerve root sheath into the spinal canal, curving immediately beneath the pedicle. Verification of accurate placement of the needle must be performed with lateral fluoroscopy.

Caudal injections are performed with fluoroscopic guidance. A curved needle tip is advanced through the skin to the sacral hiatus, using the curve to maneuver through the kyphosis of the sacrum and to straighten any lateral deviations occurring as the needle is advanced. Confirmation of accurate needle placement is performed with posteroanterior and lateral images.

Articulating facet injections can be performed with an inferior recess approach or oblique approach. The inferior approach takes advantage of a small dish-shaped concavity that lies at the inferior and medial aspect of each facet joint in the lumbar spine. With the use of fluoroscopy, spinous processes are aligned midline between the pedicles. The inferior portions of the facet joints can be found by identifying the spinous process and following the lamina laterally and inferiorly to where it terminates at the lower aspect of inferior articulating facet. The x-ray tube is rotated toward the side of targeted facet until the facet joint line is well visualized. The second commonly used approach is the oblique approach. The x-ray tube is turned oblique toward the side for injection.

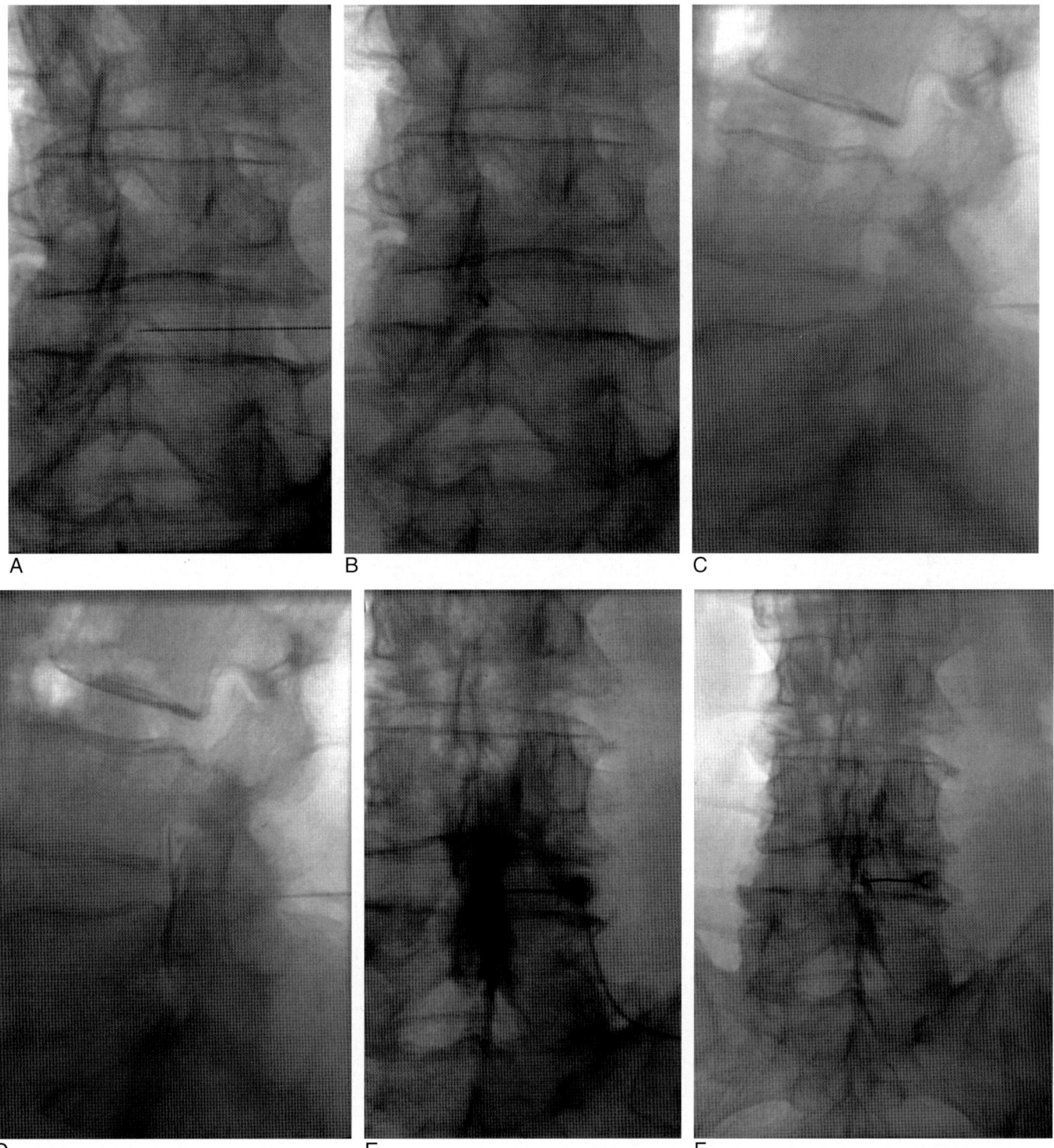

■ **FIGURE 1** Interlaminar epidural corticosteroid injection. **A,** Posteroanterior oblique view reveals the tip of the spinal needle marking the dome-shaped space beneath the junction of the spinous process and lamina. This region is used to gain access into the epidural space. **B,** Once the skin is anesthetized, the needle is advanced into the epidural space, paralleling the needle with the x-ray beam. **C,** Depth confirmation is performed with a lateral view. When the needle tip reaches the level of the facet joints, the syringe with contrast medium and extension tubing can be connected to the needle. **D,** Steady pressure is applied to the syringe as the needle is advanced toward the epidural space. The epidural space has been reached when syringe resistance abruptly decreases and a flash of contrast medium is seen within the epidural space under continuous lateral fluoroscopy. **E,** The injection is evaluated in the posteroanterior plane and shows extension of contrast below the level of injection. **F,** Posteroanterior view after injection of the medications reveals dilution of the contrast agent, providing assurance that the needle position was accurately maintained during the injection.

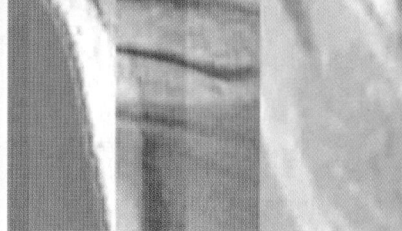

Discography

See the full chapter by Peyman Borghei, Arash Anavim, and Jamshid Tehranzadeh on CD.

Discography is an invasive diagnostic procedure for evaluation of specific cervical, thoracic, or lumbar disc disease in patients who are candidates for surgery when other test results are equivocal or negative. It is not used for initial examination and should not be performed in patients with infection, bleeding diathesis, or spinal instability. The goal of discography is to inject the contrast agent into the nucleus of the disc to assess pain provocation and disc morphology and to identify abnormalities.

The procedure is performed with the patient under enough sedation to provide analgesia without eliminating pain sensation. With the use of fluoroscopic C-arm guidance with digital subtraction, the needle tip is positioned precisely in the center of the disc to access the nucleus pulposus and prevent faulty injection into the annulus fibrosus. Slow injection of contrast agent is performed until the pain response is equal to the patient's "usual" response. Avoid rapid injection, which may elicit a false-positive pain response. The volume of injected contrast agent and the quality of resistance to injection are recorded. Radiographs in anteroposterior and lateral projections are obtained within 20 minutes. CT or MRI may additionally be used for better evaluation of morphologic abnormalities.

Six specific terminologies are used to describe discographic findings: normal disc, in which contrast agent is contained within the nucleus pulposus (Fig. 1); disc degeneration, with complex or multiple annular fissures with or without leakage of contrast agent; bulging disc, showing annular fissures with diffuse, circumferentially bulging but intact peripheral annulus; focal disc protrusion with single annular fissure, with or without leakage of the contrast agent; disc extrusion, in which the annular fissure shows contrast agent extravasation into the epidural space;

and sequestered disc, with demonstration of extruded nuclear material separate from the disc. Annular tears are morphologically described using the modified Dallas classification.

Results of discography have been found to be highly concordant with severity of MRI findings and quite reliable in identification of the exact source of the patient's pain.

Patients may be discharged 2 hours after the procedure after monitoring. They are instructed to report any fever or unusual pain or symptoms in the next few days. The most common complication after discography is discitis. The use of prophylactic antibiotics decreases the prevalence of this complication. Residual diminishing back pain over a few days is a normal sequela.

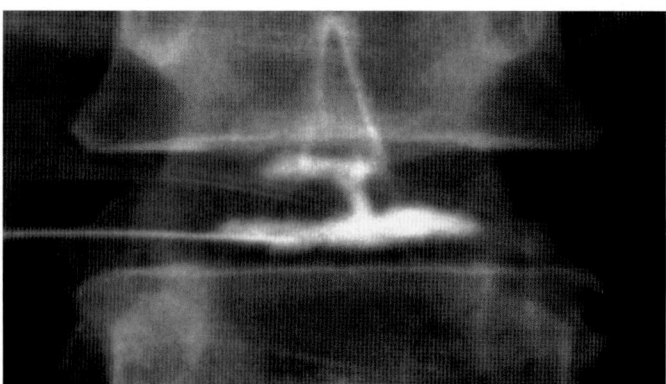

■ **FIGURE 1** Normal discogram at L3-4 level. Note normal bilocular or "hamburger" appearance of contrast agent in the disc. *(From Tehranzadeh J. Discography 2000. Radiol Clin North Am 1998; 36:463-495.)*

Vertebroplasty and Kyphoplasty

See the full chapter by David Wilson on CD.

Vertebroplasty and other percutaneous vertebral treatments are designed to treat pain by stabilizing the fracture using an intravertebral injection of cement. This is indicated in patients who failed to respond to at least 4 weeks of conservative treatment and in patients suffering from a painful vertebral fracture that was identified on cross-sectional imaging and concordant with findings on clinical examination. The underlying conditions of vertebral fractures are osteoporosis, metastasis, hemangioma, myeloma, congenital bony weakness (e.g., osteogenesis imperfecta), acute trauma, and burnt out infection. A maximum of three vertebral fractures may be treated in a single procedure.

Use of this procedure in vertebra plana, osteomyelitis, acute trauma, kyphosis, disseminated myeloma, sacral insufficiency, and other bony fractures is controversial. In myeloma causing vertebral fracture a debate is ongoing regarding the prophylactic use of vertebroplasty in this group of patients in whom the life expectancy is short and the need to treat multiple levels is high (Fig. 1). Compressed vertebral bodies may be expanded before cement injection using either a balloon (kyphoplasty) or a Skybone inflation device.

Needle placement is via a transpedicular, parapedicular, or oblique approach with the patient under continuous monitoring and conscious sedation. Strict aseptic technique, possibly with antibiotic cover, should be employed. Vertebroplasty kits and vertebroplasty specific cement (methylmethacrylate or Cortoss) should be used. Cement injections should be under direct continuous fluoroscopy in the lateral plane and should be discontinued at the slightest suggestion of extravasation. The needle is removed once the cement has set and postprocedural images are taken. Postprocedural management includes rehabilitation and the potential for further injections.

Contraindications include infection and coagulopathies. The integrity of the posterior part of the vertebral body must be documented to decrease the risk of cement extravasation.

Complications include allergy, infection, transient nerve root irritation, nerve root damage, paralysis, pulmonary embolus, and death. Complications may be minimized by the use of premedication antibiotics; careful avoidance of cement extrusion, extravasation, and inadvertent vascular cement injection; and precise placement of the needle before injection. There is a slight increased risk of fracture of adjacent vertebrae after successful vertebroplasty.

Overall, 85% improvement to symptoms might be expected in properly selected patients. Favorable outcome does not correlate with amount of cement injected; therefore, the least amount of cement required to fill cleavage fractures is used.

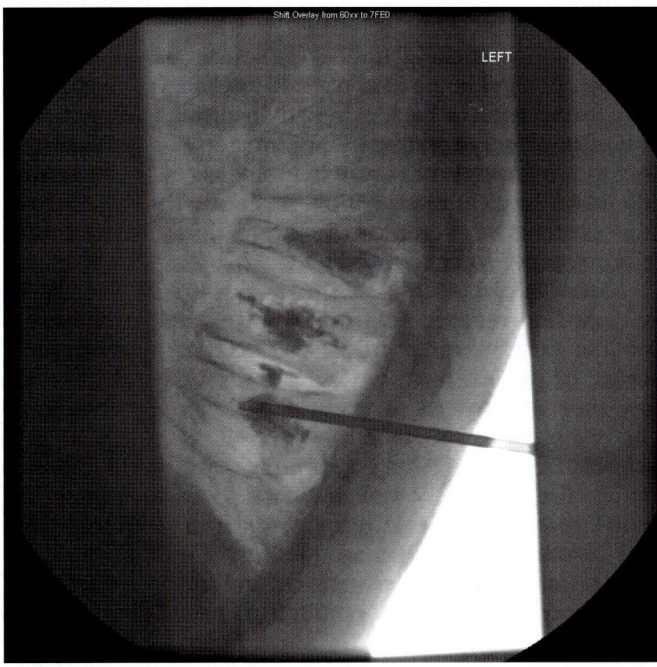

■ **FIGURE 1** Injection of cement was performed at T9 to T11. It was believed that injection to T9 and T11 only would place T10 at risk of fracture. There was some extrusion into the T10/11 disc.

Percutaneous Intradiscal Therapies

See the full chapter by Patrick A. Brouwer and Barry Schenk on CD.

Percutaneous intradiscal therapies are used in the treatment of chronic low back pain and sciatica. Knowledge of disc anatomy and pathophysiology is essential because both conditions result from intervertebral disc disease. Degenerative disease with annular tears causes back pain due to mechanical and chemical stimulation of annular nerve fibers, whereas sciatica is caused by compression of exiting nerve roots by herniated nucleus pulposus. These minimally invasive alternatives to open surgery reduce nucleus pulposus volume by removing intradiscal water or changing nuclear protein structure, resulting in decreased intradiscal hydraulic pressure and pain relief. The procedures discussed are chemonucleolysis, automated percutaneous lumbar discectomy, percutaneous laser disc decompression, nucleoplasty, and intradiscal electrothermal therapy.

Indications include lumbar radicular syndrome, with discography evidence of contained lumbar disc herniation, and discogenic low back pain with insufficient response to 6 weeks of conservative management. Contraindications include sequestration, severe neurologic symptoms requiring acute surgical intervention, severe disc space narrowing, obstructive vertebral abnormalities, previous disc surgery, active infection, and coagulopathy.

Posterolateral access to the nucleus pulposus under biplane fluoroscopic guidance is required. Alternatively, a midline extrathecal approach may be used. Careful monitoring of patient reaction and appropriate use of visual guidance are crucial to prevent damage to nerve roots and surrounding tissues during needle placement or subsequent treatment. Taking appropriate antiseptic measures during the procedure can minimize the risk of infection. Preprocedural antibiotic prophylaxis is not supported by the literature. Procedures are performed on an outpatient basis requiring minimal postprocedural and follow-up care.

Chemonucleolysis uses intradiscal proteolytic enzyme (chymopapain) injection to induce hydrolysis of nuclear proteoglycan molecules. Major complications are enzyme leakage with extradiscal tissue damage and anaphylactic reactions. Studies have shown long-term success rates of up to 80% in properly selected patients

Automated percutaneous lumbar discectomy or nucleotomy involves mechanical removal of nuclear material using an automated nucleotome. When a straight approach

of the disc is difficult, a curved cannula may be helpful. Results of preliminary studies are ambiguous.

Percutaneous laser disc decompression uses laser energy delivered via laser fiber (980 nm diode laser) through a hollow needle to evaporate water in the nucleus pulposus and to reduce intradiscal pressure (Fig. 1). Approach is contralaterally from the unaffected side. Complications are primarily referable to thermal tissue damage. Preliminary studies show promising results.

Nucleoplasty uses "controlled ablation (coblation)" with radiofrequency energy generation of a highly focused plasma field capable of cleaving molecular bonds. This procedure may also be used for cervical vertebrae. Efficacy of this procedure is still unproven.

Intradiscal electrothermal annuloplasty uses a catheter containing a radiofrequency heating element to heat the posterior annulus fibrosus to ablate annular nociceptors, presumably the cause of discogenic pain. This proposed mechanism is controversial, and further studies are required for further evaluation.

There is no evidence from randomized controlled trials warranting the use of therapies listed earlier. Until the results of ongoing trials are published these treatments can be regarded controversial at the least, no matter how many positive case reports and cohorts have been published.

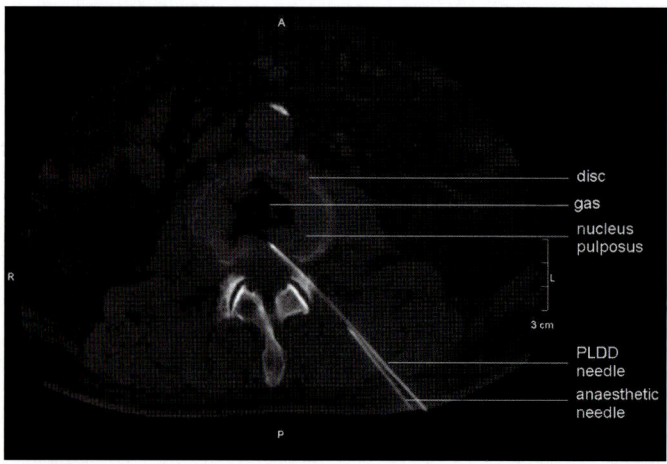

■ **FIGURE 1** CT image taken during percutaneous laser disc decompression.

Ultrasound Procedures

See the full chapter by David Wilson on CD.

Ultrasound guidance may be used in local anesthetic and corticosteroid injections, needle placement for MR or CT arthrography, aspiration biopsy and drainage of fluid for diagnostic and therapeutic reasons, localization of foreign bodies, and cannula placement before thermal and radio-frequency ablation.

It is imperative that the structures to be punctured and those that must be avoided should be visible. A more precise placement of the active agents into the affected area is likely to achieve better results, and a more precise injection into a potential cavity rather than muscle or tendon (Fig. 1) may be less painful. This, therefore, guides the choice of ultrasound machine and the preference for the more effective linear array probe. The location of the target is practically limited to the first 5 to 10 cm of soft tissue and is deemed inaccessible if there is intervening bone or gas.

Approach to the lesion are planned using a diagnostic ultrasound examination. The needle track should take into consideration the possibility of contamination and the option of future surgery. Informed consent should be obtained and documented. Sterility and aseptic techniques with probe covers are essential. In the case of biopsies, close collaboration with the pathologist is mandatory.

Freehand technique is generally preferred, with the operator holding the probe in one hand and the needle in the other. Needles should be placed at 90 degrees to the transducer beam, with visualization of the needle tip during the entire procedure. Verification and image documentation of position must be made before aspiration or sampling. Outcomes must be recorded and audited to improve practice and accuracy.

Ultrasound-guided needle procedures are contraindicated when important structures that might be damaged cannot be visualized by the technique. If gas or gas-containing structures intervene or the structure in question lies behind bone or metal, then ultrasound would not be an appropriate technique. The deeper the mass, the more difficult it is to visualize using ultrasound; and, therefore, injection or biopsy of deeper structures is a relative contraindication, Other potential contraindications are those related to the drugs or penetration of skin, which includes potential allergies, infection at the site of injection, and concurrent administration of drugs that might interact with those being injected.

Risks include allergy, infection, and nerve and vascular damage. Proper technique should minimize these complications. Most procedures are performed on an outpatient basis, without the need for postprocedural medication.

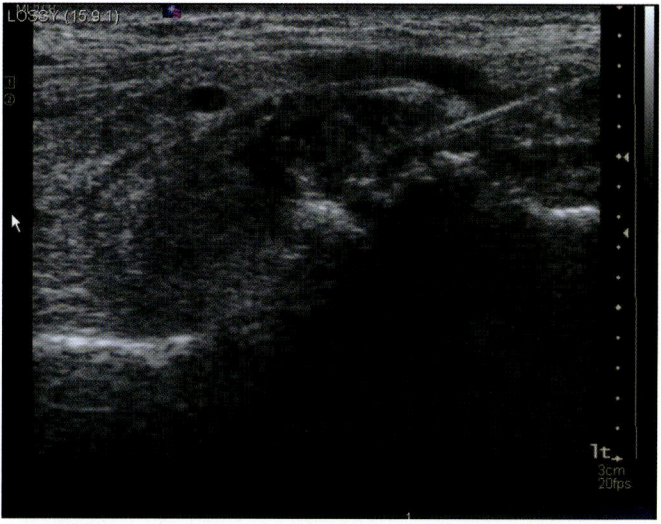

■ **FIGURE 1** Ultrasound-guided injection of a tarsometatarsal joint. The needle tip is placed close to the joint space where the capsule bulges outward. Injection shows that the needle must be in the joint as the images show the capsule enlarging and the new fluid confined to the joint. This is much easier to appreciate on a moving image.

APPENDIX 1

Measurements Most Frequently Used in Orthopedic Imaging

See the full chapter by José Luis del Cura on CD.

Orthopedic radiologic measurements can be used in diagnosis, evaluation, and treatment planning for specific conditions. Normal measurements show significant variations, and measurements only acquire full relevance in the proper clinical context. Impeccable technique is necessary to reduce false-positive results.

Spine measurements are made on radiographs. The Cobb angle (Fig. 1) is the standard system for scoliosis, kyphosis, and lordosis. Vertebral rotation for prognostication is assessed using the Nash and Moe technique. Mehta's rib-vertebral angle difference diagnoses resolving or progressive infantile scoliosis.

In congenital, traumatic, and deficiency diseases, the axial angle of the shoulder is abnormal. Acromioclavicular distance widening is associated with joint trauma or clavicular osteolysis whereas glenohumeral joint space widening suggests shoulder dislocation. Abnormal elbow-carrying angle implies supracondylar humeral, ulnar, or radial fractures. Ulnar variance, measured using the method of perpendiculars, is useful in wrist disorders. Carpal collapse severity and progression are assessed by carpal height ratio. Abnormal radial inclination is seen in distal radial metaphyseal and Madelung deformity. Palmar tilt is used in assessment and surgical planning of distal radial fractures. Radial length is used to quantify distal deformity whereas radial shift is used to measure fracture fragment shift. Ulnar translocation of the carpus is a ratio used to assess radiocarpal ligament disruption. Widened scapholunate distance (Terry-Thomas sign) implies dissociation. Scapholunate and capitolunate angles are used to assess carpal instabilities. The carpal angle is altered in many congenital deformities.

Hip dysplasia evaluation on radiographs can be made using Wiberg's center-edge angle or C-E angle, horizontal toit externe angle, acetabular index, and femoral head coverage. Diagnosis of infantile developmental hip dysplasia is made using the acetabular angle. Ultrasound measurements include acetabular coverage and Graf angles (α and β). Widened hip joint is seen in Legg-Calvé-Perthes disease, hip dysplasia, and synovial effusion. Distance from acetabulum to ilioischiatic line identifies acetabular protrusion in rheumatoid arthritis and trauma. The femoral or neck-shaft angle may show coxa vara or coxa valga deformity. Acetabular sector angles enable assessment and quantification of adult acetabular dysplasia on CT. The angle of anteversion of the femoral head on radiograph, CT, or MRI is used to predict the need for corrective surgery.

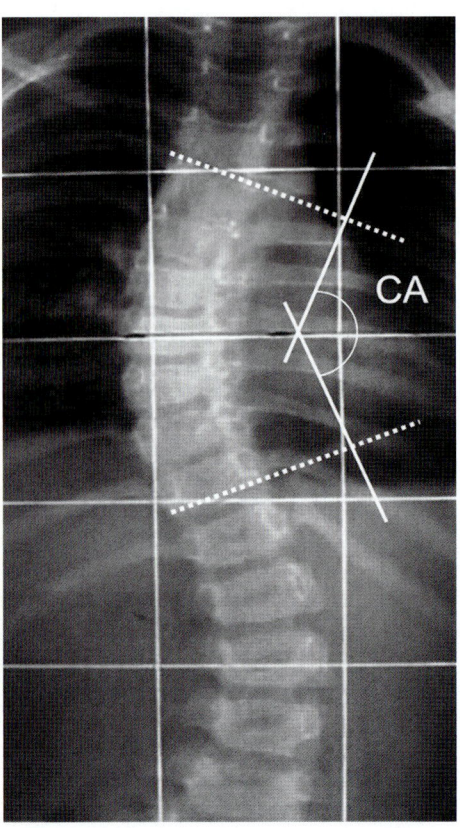

■ **FIGURE 1** Measurement of Cobb angle (CA) in scoliosis.

Lower-leg radiographic measurements include axial (femoral, tibial, and tibiofemoral) angles of the knee for assessing varus and valgus deformities, tibial metaphyseal-diaphyseal angle to identify varus deformity, tibial plateau angle to measure depression in fractures, and patellar relative height determination using the Insall-Salvati and De Carvalho methods in patella alta. Tibial torsion is measured on CT or MRI, whereas patellar alignment is assessed on radiographs, CT, or MRI with congruence, sulcus, and patellar tilt angles and tibial tubercle-femoral sulcus distance. Ankle radiographs use the Boehler angle to identify and prognosticate calcaneal deformity and use axial (talotibial and talofibular) angles for ligamentous ruptures. The dorsoplantar talocalcaneal, or Kite angle, talus/first metatarsal angle, lateral talocalcaneal angle, and calcaneal pitch are used to assess foot deformities. Localization and severity of hallux valgus anomalies are evaluated using first intermetatarsal, metatarsus primus varus, hallux valgus, and hallux interphalangeal angles.

APPENDIX 2
Orthopedic Devices

See the full chapter by Angela Gopez and Aaron Cho on CD.

Blade plate and screws are used with subtrochanteric and supracondylar femoral fractures. Reconstruction plate is used for stabilization of fractures with complex bony surfaces. Buttress plate and screws are commonly used for stabilization of periarticular fractures.

Cortical screws are utilized for stabilization of cortical bone. Cancellous screws are used in metaphyses of long bones. Cannulated screws are used for metaphyseal fractures. The Acutrak screw system is used for scaphoid fractures. The Herbert screw allows compression of fracture margins during insertion and fracture healing and is used for scaphoid fracture. Interference screws are most commonly seen in anterior cruciate ligament reconstruction. Bioabsorbable screws can produce inflammatory synovitis, as seen on follow-up MRI examinations but do not cause metallic susceptibility artifact on postoperative imaging. The Maxwell-Brancheau screw is utilized in arthroereisis. A dynamic hip screw is used in intertrochanteric, subtrochanteric, basilar neck, and femoral condylar fractures causing dynamic compression at fracture margins with weight bearing.

An intramedullary nail is used in the treatment of long-bone diaphyseal femur and tibial fractures. An elastic stable intramedullary nail is indicated in diaphyseal and metaphyseal long-bone fractures in pediatric patients. A cephalomedullary nail is used in unstable peritrochanteric, intratrochanteric, and subtrochanteric femoral fractures. Kirschner wires are generally placed percutaneously, remain contiguous with skin surface, and thus are prone to infection.

Shoulder arthroplasty is indicated in degenerative and inflammatory arthropathy, fracture, and avascular necrosis. Complications include loosening of the glenoid prosthetic component, glenohumeral instability, periprosthetic fracture, rotator cuff tear, and infection. Reverse total-shoulder arthroplasty is utilized for a torn rotator cuff, for rotator cuff arthropathy, or for previous failed arthroplasty. Complications include scapular notching, hematoma, glenohumeral dislocation, and acromial and scapular fractures. Arthrosurface HemiCAP is indicated in treatment of cartilage lesions in major joints. Radial head hemiarthroplasty is indicated in comminuted radial head fracture with concomitant ligamentous injury, dislocation, or radioulnar joint disruption but may cause decreased range of motion, heterotopic ossification, loosening, and infection. Bipolar hip hemiarthroplasty results in increased range of motion. In total-hip arthroplasty, multidetector CT (MDCT) may be helpful in assessing prosthetic positioning (Fig. 1), specifically acetabular version as well as complications such as osteolysis. Hip resurfacing arthroplasty is associated with lower rates of dislocation but has a risk for femoral neck fracture. Unicompartmental (partial)

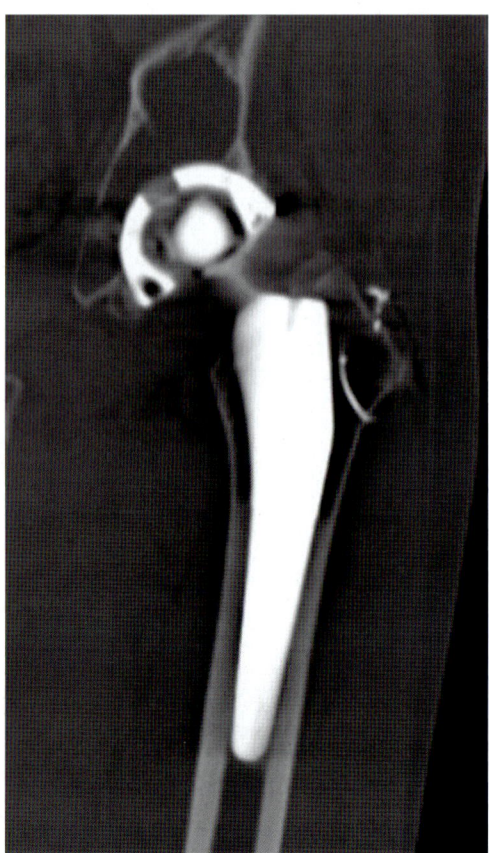

■ **FIGURE 1** MDCT shows periacetabular osteolysis. MDCT capabilities allow for prosthetic imaging with minimal image degradation by metal artifact.

knee arthroplasty is generally indicated for arthropathy confined to a single compartment. Total-knee arthroplasty is done in degenerative and inflammatory arthropathies but causes complications such as patellofemoral malalignment, loosening, osteolysis, infection, periprosthetic fracture, and dislocation. Total ankle arthroplasty is associated with heterotopic ossification, axial malalignment, loosening, and infection. Metatarsophalangeal joint arthroplasty is mainly performed in rheumatoid arthritis. Antibiotic-impregnated cement spacer is inserted after removal of infected arthroplasty.

Corpectomy and fusion removes vertebral body and disc spaces for decompression of spinal canal due to stenosis, spinal deformity (kyphosis), trauma, neoplasm, and infection. Discectomy and fusion is removal of herniated or degenerative disc causing neurologic symptomatology. Disc replacement is utilized in cervical and lumbar degenerative disc disease. X-STOP refers to a titanium metal spacer placed between spinous processes to alleviate symptoms of lumbar spinal stenosis by increasing spinal canal diameter. Lateral mass plate and screws are the preferred surgical technique for posterior cervical stabilization.

APPENDIX 3
Fractures with Names

See the full chapter by José Martel and Ángel Bueno on CD.

Fractures with the most commonly used eponyms include the following.

Bankart fracture refers to glenoid labrum fracture at its anteroinferior portion detected using CT or MRI. Bennett fracture is fracture-dislocation at the first metacarpal base. A Chance/seat belt fracture is a horizontal fracture line in vertebral body or posterior elements commonly affecting L1 or L2. A Colles fracture/Pouteau affects the distal radius with dorsal displacement of the distal fragment and volar angulation (dinner fork deformity) and sometimes is associated with an ulnar styloid process fracture. De Quervain's fracture refers to a scaphoid fracture associated with semilunar bone dislocation. Dupuytren's fracture affects the tibia above the lateral malleolus with an associated medial malleolar fracture and laterally displaced talus. The Galeazzi fracture involves usually the radial diaphysis with dislocation of the distal radioulnar joint (Fig. 1). A Hutchinson/chauffeur fracture is an oblique radial styloid process fracture. The Jefferson fracture is a complex atlas fracture, usually affecting both anterior and posterior arches and lateral masses. The Jones fracture affects the fifth metatarsal base distal to the tuberosity.

Le Fort fracture type I is a bilateral horizontal upper maxillary fracture. Le Fort type II has vertical fracture line and can reach the floor of the orbit, nasal cavity, or hard palate. Le Fort type III has complete maxillary detachment and one or more facial bones from the remaining craniofacial skeleton. A Le Fort ankle fracture is a vertical fracture of the fibula with avulsion of the tibiofibular ligament. Lisfranc's fracture is associated with tarsometatarsal joint dislocation, second metatarsal base fracture, and posterolateral dislocation of four or all five metatarsals. A Maisonneuve fracture is a spiral proximal third fibular fracture with disruption of the distal tibiofibular syndesmosis and interosseous membrane. A Malgaigne fracture involves both pubic rami with sacroiliac dislocation or fracture of the sacrum. A Monteggia fracture is a proximal ulnar fracture with anteriorly dislocated radial head. Rolando's fracture is a comminuted fracture affecting the first metacarpal base. A Segond fracture is fracture-detachment of proximal tibial epiphysis. Shepherd's fracture is a talar fracture at its posterolateral process. A Tillaux fracture is fracture-avulsion of the anterior tibial tubercle.

Some fractures are identified by the mechanism by which they are produced, by profession in which they most frequently occur, or by morphology. A hangman's fracture consists of fracture of the C2 posterior elements and anterior displacement of the C2 vertebral body relative to the C3 body. Boxer's fracture is produced at the fifth metacarpal neck with volar angulation of distal fragment. Clay shoveler's fracture refers to fracture of a lower cervical spinous process. Gamekeeper's thumb/skier's thumb involves fracture-dislocation of the ulnar aspect of

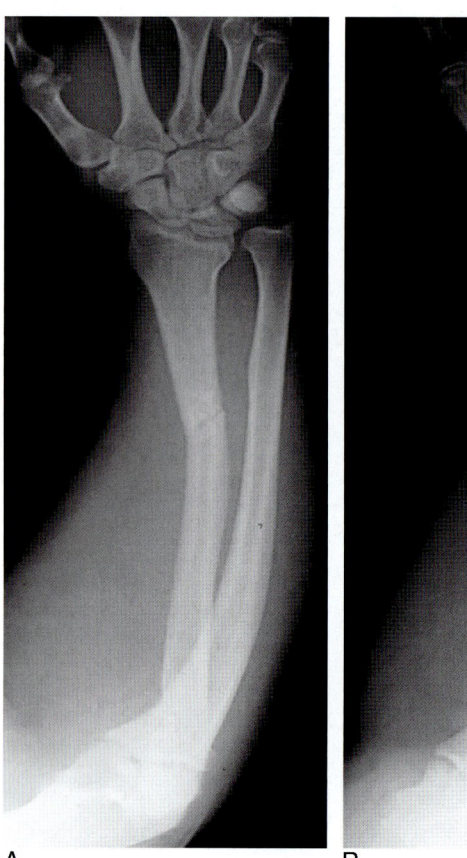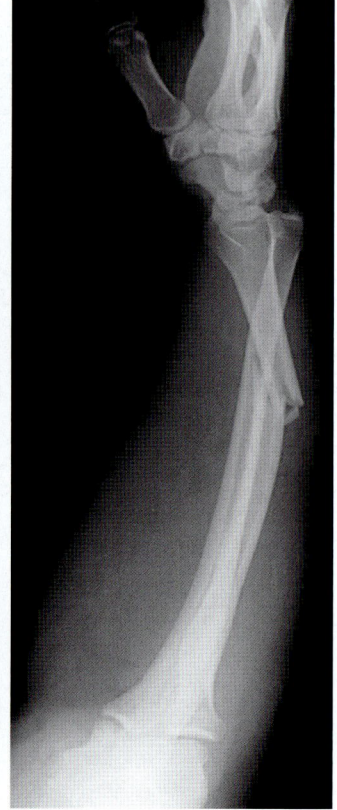

A   B

■ FIGURE 1   Galeazzi fracture.

the first phalangeal base. Greenstick fracture is characterized by fracture at one side of the bone while the opposite side remains intact. Dancer's fracture is fracture-avulsion of the fifth metatarsal base.

Salter-Harris type 1 fracture involves separation of the epiphysis from the diaphysis. Type 2 involves detach-ment of a triangular metaphyseal fragment of bone. Type 3 produces an epiphyseal fragment with a vertical line separating it from remaining epiphysis. Type 4 fractures affect the metaphysis, physis, and epiphysis. Type 5 has crushing of the growth plate with consequent union of epiphysis and diaphysis.

Diseases with Names

See the full chapter by Oleg Opsha and Steven Shankman on CD.

The following is a list of eponyms related to musculo-skeletal disorders, excluding trauma:

Achondrogenesis type I (Parenti-Fraccaro) has deficient ossification in the lumbar vertebrae and absent ossification in the sacral, pubic, and ischial bones. Type II (Langer-Saldino) is characterized by short trunk, large head, and micromelia.

Albright's hereditary osteodystrophy is characterized by shortening of metacarpal and metatarsal bones.

Cartilaginous node formation, enthesopathy, and fracture in **Andersson lesion** are associated with discovertebral destructive lesions.

Baastrup's disease is characterized by apposition of adjacent spinous processes with reactive sclerosis.

Enthesophytes at the posteroinferior glenoid rim at insertion of the posterior band of the inferior glenohumeral ligament complex are termed **Bennett's lesion**.

Bouchard's node is a bony enlargement or osteophytosis at the proximal interphalangeal joints of fingers in osteoarthritis.

Burnett's syndrome is characterized by unilateral or bilateral periarticular calcium deposits.

Diaphyseal dysplasia has cortical thickening at the midshaft area of long bones progressing toward epiphyses.

Charcot-Marie-Tooth disease is characterized by bilateral muscle atrophy in the lower extremities.

Dyggve-Melchior-Clausen syndrome is characterized by short trunk, exaggerated lordosis, protrusion of sternum, flattened vertebral bodies, small hands and feet, and clawed fingers.

Erdheim-Chester disease shows patchy/diffuse increase in density, coarsened trabecular pattern, medullary sclerosis, and cortical thickening.

Ewing's sarcoma is characterized by saucerization of the cortex, by patchy, permeative destruction, and by a large soft tissue mass.

Fabry's disease causes enlargement of joint capsules, osteoporosis, and osteonecrosis.

Fairbank-Ribbing disease shows delayed appearing centers of ossification, fragmented appearance, and premature arthrosis of weight-bearing joints.

Gaucher's disease is characterized by modeling deformities such as Erlenmeyer's flask deformity, osteonecrosis, and fracture.

Goltz's syndrome includes syndactyly, microcephaly, vertebral segmentation defects, and scoliosis.

Gorlin's cyst (calcifying odontogenic cyst) is seen as a mixed radiolucent-radiopaque lesion of jaws with features of both cyst and solid neoplasm.

Hardcastle's syndrome includes pathologic fractures, diaphyseal sclerosis, and marrow infarction with sclerosis.

Bony enlargement or osteophytosis at the distal interphalangeal joints of fingers characterizes **Heberden's nodes**.

Jansen-type metaphyseal dysplasia has marked metaphyseal irregularity, widened growth plates, diffuse osteopenia, and mild bowing of tubular bones.

Köhler's disease shows flattening and sclerosis of tarsal navicular in children.

Lenz-Majewski dysplasia is characterized by a large head, delayed closure of anterior fontanelle, and thickening and sclerosis of skull, orbital rims, and facial bones.

Menkes' syndrome consists of osteopenia, flaring of ends of tubular bones, metaphyseal cupping and irregularity, and osseous spurs.

Pyle's syndrome is characterized by hyperostosis of the cranial vault, an obtuse mandibular angle and mandibular prognathism, an expansion of ribs, clavicles, and pubic and ischial bones, a metaphyseal flare of tubular bones, and an Erlenmeyer flask–like appearance of diaphyses in femur and tibia.

Stickler's syndrome comprises mild epiphyseal dysplasia and overtubulation of long bones.

Van Buchem's syndrome consists of periosteal excrescences in tubular bones, osteosclerotic and enlarged ribs and clavicles, and increased radiodensity of spine.

Voorhoeve's disease (osteopathia striata) is characterized by linear sclerotic striations in metaphyses of long bones and flat bones.

Worth's syndrome consists of cortical thickening in tubular bones, which are not expanded and show normal modeling. In the skull, osteosclerosis begins in the base and later involves facial bones. Sclerosis in the spine is most evident in the spinous processes.

Classic Signs and Findings in Musculoskeletal Radiology

See the full chapter by Imran Omar on CD.

Over time, radiologic signs have become reliable in predicting conditions and have become part of a standard radiologic lexicon. In this section, the most common radiologic signs are described along with the imaging modalities where the sign is observed.

The medial humeral head normally overlapping the posterior glenoid rim on a standard anteroposterior shoulder view in external rotation (half-moon sign) is absent in posterior dislocation of shoulder.

In achondroplasia, the iliac wings are flat with increased acetabular angles and small sacrosciatic notches. The pelvic appearance is similar to that of a champagne glass. Trident hand is also seen in achondroplasia as divergence of fingers when placed on flat surface.

Signs associated with anterior cruciate ligament tears mostly seen in MR images include empty notch sign where nonvisualization of the ligament at the level of the distal femoral intercondylar notch is seen on an axial view.

Fluid-fluid levels are most common in aneurysmal bone cysts and occasionally in telangiectatic osteosarcoma, giant cell tumor, or chondroblastoma.

Teardrop-shaped density anterior to the tibiotalar joint along the talar neck on lateral ankle radiograph indicates a tibiotalar joint effusion. This sign may also refer to blowout fracture of the orbits.

Different signs are seen associated with ankylosing spondylitis such as bamboo spine seen on anteroposterior and lateral views referring to vertebral body squaring and continuous syndesmophytes.

A vascular necrosis is represented by a crescent sign, which refers to thin curvilinear lucency parallel to the cortical surface.

Bucket-handle tear of menisci can be represented by anterior bow-tie sign seen on sagittal MR image, where body of menisci is not seen.

Chronic renal failure is associated with signs such as rugger jersey spine in which horizontal bands of sclerosis in the vertebral bodies resemble an English rugby jersey.

Celery stalk metaphysis is commonly seen in congenital rubella, where vertical striations in bone resemble celery stalk.

Floating teeth sign is seen in eosinophilic granuloma, where there is alveolar osteolysis with sparing of tooth, giving the appearance of tooth unsupported by jaw.

Patients with fibrous dysplasia of the femur often have an exaggerated outward bowing of the femoral head, neck, and shaft producing varus deformity resembling curvature of a shepherd's staff, hence the name shepherd's crook deformity.

In hemangioma, axial CT and MR images show paucity of horizontal trabeculae and thickening of regularly interspersed vertical trabeculae within a vertebral body hemangioma that appear like polka dots.

On lateral radiographs of the skull there is thinning of the outer table with thickened linear, intradiploic trabeculae perpendicular to the inner table called hair-on-end sign in hemolytic anemia.

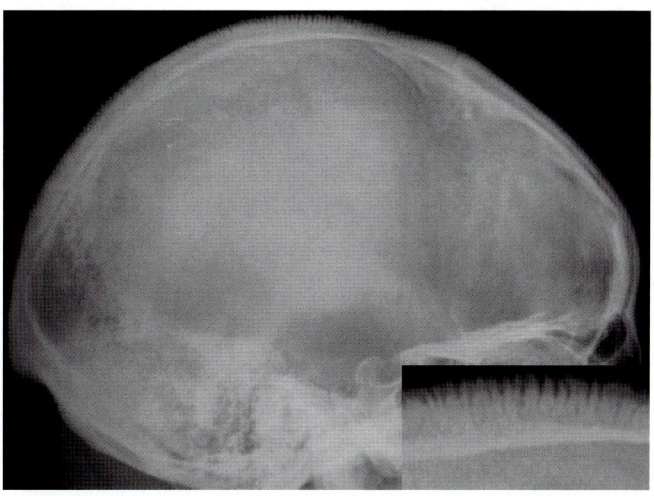

Salt and pepper calvaria is seen in hyperparathyroidism when there is uniform calvarial military mottling.

Blade of grass sign is seen as a flame-shaped diaphysis of long bone associated with Paget's disease.

In psoriasis, signs such as pencil-in-cup deformity showing the eroded head of one phalanx abutting the base of a more distal phalanx may be seen.

APPENDIX 6

Compressive and Entrapment Neuropathies of the Upper and Lower Extremities

See the full chapter by Luis Beltran, Calvin Ma, and Javier Beltran on CD.

Conditions involving compression/entrapment neuropathies can be appreciated on MRI.

In the shoulder region, suprascapular nerve syndrome causes denervation edema/fatty atrophy of the supraspinatus and infraspinatus muscles. Quadrilateral space syndrome causes denervation edema/fatty atrophy of the teres minor and deltoid muscles (Fig. 1).

In the region of the elbow, median nerve compression results in pronator syndrome seen as signal abnormalities/atrophy of flexor pronator muscles. Anterior interosseous nerve syndrome causes denervation edema/fatty atrophy

of deep ventral muscles of forearm. Cubital tunnel syndrome results in denervation edema/fatty atrophy of the flexor carpi ulnaris, flexor digitorum profundus, and ulnar intrinsic muscles of hand. Posterior interosseous nerve syndrome is seen as denervation edema/atrophy of supinator and extensor muscles of forearm.

In the wrist region, carpal tunnel syndrome results in thenar muscle edema/fatty atrophy. Volar bowing of the flexor retinaculum at the distal carpal tunnel (level of hook of hamate) is also seen. Ulnar tunnel syndrome results in denervation edema/atrophy of the hypothenar muscles,

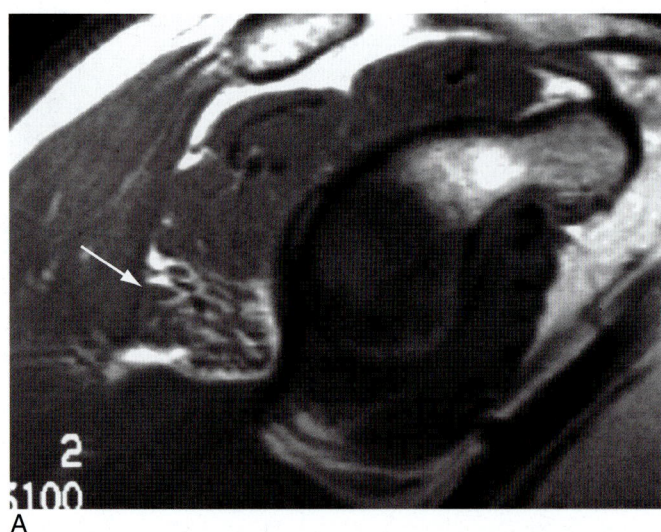

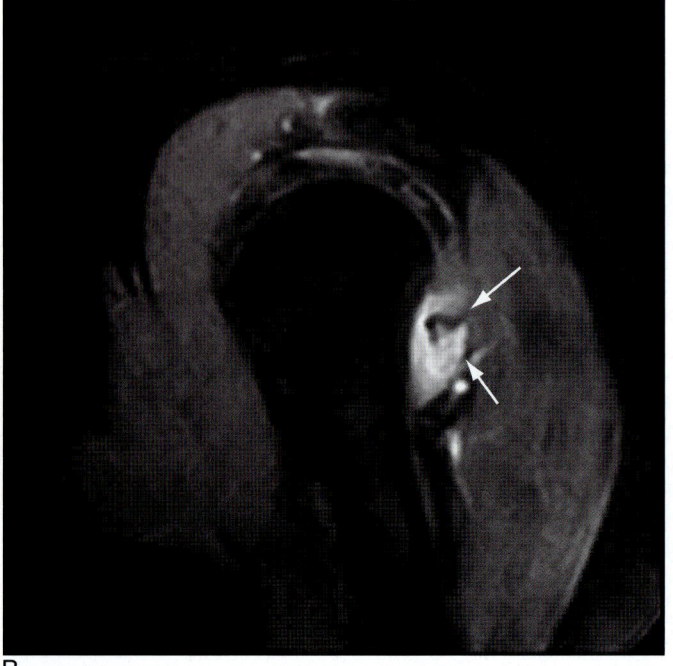

■ **FIGURE 1** Teres minor denervation. **A,** T1-weighted sagittal MR image demonstrates atrophy of the teres minor muscle (*arrow*), indicating late stage. **B,** Sagittal STIR MR image demonstrates early denervation with edema of the teres minor muscle (*arrows*).

adductor pollicis, third and fourth lumbricals, and interosseous muscles. Superficial radial nerve syndrome results in increased signal intensity of the radial nerve on T2-weighted/STIR sequences and increased girth of nerve.

In the pelvis/thigh region, piriformis syndrome causes hypertrophy or atrophy of piriformis muscle and increased signal in piriformis muscle and sciatic nerve. Iliacus syndrome is seen as a mass effect from tears of the iliacus/iliopsoas muscle, hematomas, post-traumatic pseudoaneurysm of iliac vessels, and denervation edema of quadriceps muscle. There are no muscle denervation changes seen in saphenous neuropathy, but there is nerve displacement by space-occupying lesions. In obturator neuropathy, alterations in size/signal of nerve are noted. Mass effect from space-occupying lesions such as soft tissue or osseous pelvic tumors is noted. There is also denervation edema/atrophy of medial thigh muscles. Lateral femoral cutaneous neuropathy causes alteration of signal/size of lateral cutaneous nerve at the site of entrapment, without muscle denervation signal changes.

In the knee region, proximal tibial neuropathy results in denervation changes in gastrocnemius and popliteus muscles. Increased signal intensity of the common peroneal nerve evident on fluid sensitive sequences is seen in common peroneal neuropathy. There is associated denervation edema/atrophy of the anterior and lateral compartment muscles.

In the ankle/foot region, sparing of the lateral compartment muscles is seen in deep peroneal neuropathy. Superficial peroneal neuropathy caused by thickening of fascia and tenting of nerve associated with fascial defect with muscle herniation is best seen on the axial plane. Tarsal tunnel syndrome results in increased size/signal of tibial nerve, which is difficult to detect owing to small-sized nerves. Soft tissue enhancement of the tarsal tunnel in post-gadolinium images is seen. Baxter's neuritis causes absence of inflammation around the proximal fascia and normal fascial thickness with denervation edema/atrophy of the abductor digiti quinti muscle. Suggestive findings include abductor hallucis muscle hypertrophy, plantar fasciitis with medial calcaneal spur, and surrounding soft tissue edema. Jogger's foot results in muscle denervation edema/atrophy of abductor hallucis, flexor digitorum brevis, flexor hallucis brevis, and first lumbrical. Morton's neuroma is seen as plantar interdigital nerve branches embedded in perineural fibrosis. Signal intensity is low on T1- and T2-weighted images and variable on STIR/contrast-enhanced, T1-weighted, fat-suppressed images.

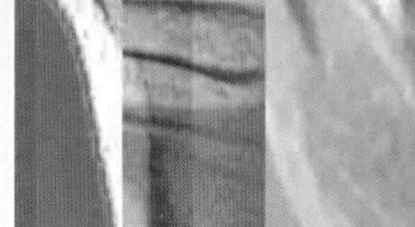

Case Studies

See full text on CD

Index

Note: Page numbers followed by *f* and *t* indicate figures and tables, respectively.